Biochemical, Physiological, *and* Molecular Aspects *of* Human Nutrition

Biochemical, Physiological, *and* Molecular Aspects *of* Human Nutrition

Martha H. Stipanuk, PhD
Professor
Division of Nutritional Sciences
Colleges of Human Ecology and
Agriculture and Life Sciences
Cornell University
Ithaca, New York

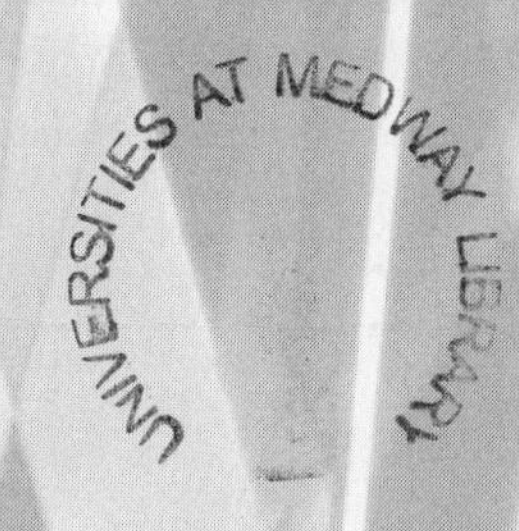

Marie A. Caudill, PhD, RD
Associate Professor
Division of Nutritional Sciences
Colleges of Human Ecology and
Agriculture and Life Sciences
Cornell University
Ithaca, New York

ELSEVIER

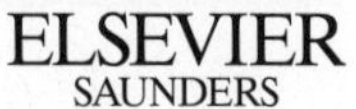

ELSEVIER
SAUNDERS

3251 Riverport Lane
St. Louis, Missouri 63043

BIOCHEMICAL, PHYSIOLOGICAL, AND MOLECULAR
ASPECTS OF HUMAN NUTRITION ISBN: 978-1-4377-0959-9

Notices

Knowledge and best practice in this field are constantly changing. As new research and experience broaden our understanding, changes in research methods, professional practices, or medical treatment may become necessary.

Practitioners and researchers must always rely on their own experience and knowledge in evaluating and using any information, methods, compounds, or experiments described herein. In using such information or methods they should be mindful of their own safety and the safety of others, including parties for whom they have a professional responsibility.

With respect to any drug or pharmaceutical products identified, readers are advised to check the most current information provided (i) on procedures featured or (ii) by the manufacturer of each product to be administered, to verify the recommended dose or formula, the method and duration of administration, and contraindications. It is the responsibility of practitioners, relying on their own experience and knowledge of their patients, to make diagnoses, to determine dosages and the best treatment for each individual patient, and to take all appropriate safety precautions.

To the fullest extent of the law, neither the Publisher nor the authors, contributors, or editors, assume any liability for any injury and/or damage to persons or property as a matter of products liability, negligence or otherwise, or from any use or operation of any methods, products, instructions, or ideas contained in the material herein.

Library of Congress Cataloging-in-Publication Data

Biochemical, physiological, and molecular aspects of human nutrition/[edited by] Martha H. Stipanuk, Marie A. Caudill. – 3rd ed.
p. ; cm.
Includes bibliographical references and index.
ISBN 978-1-4377-0959-9 (pbk.)
I. Stipanuk, Martha H. II. Caudill, Marie A.
[DNLM: 1. Nutritional Physiological Phenomena. 2. Metabolism--physiology. QU 145]
LC classification not assigned
612.3′9–dc23

2011031519

Senior Editor: Yvonne Alexopoulos
Senior Developmental Editors: Lisa P. Newton and Karen C. Turner
Editorial Assistant: Kit Blanke
Publishing Services Manager: Jeff Patterson
Project Manager: Megan Isenberg
Designer: Jessica Williams

Front cover image copyright Dennis Kunkel Microscopy, Inc.

Printed in the United States of America

Last digit is the print number: 9 8 7 6 5 4 3 2

Chapter Contributors

TRACY G. ANTHONY, PhD
Associate Professor
Department of Biochemistry and Molecular Biology
School of Medicine
Indiana University
Evansville, Indiana

RONALD O. BALL, PhD
Professor Emeritus
Department of Agricultural, Food and Nutritional Science
University of Alberta
Edmonton, Alberta, Canada

RICHARD P. BAZINET, PhD
Assistant Professor
Department of Nutritional Sciences
Faculty of Medicine
University of Toronto
Toronto, Ontario, Canada

DARLENE E. BERRYMAN, PhD, RD
Associate Professor, Nutrition
School of Applied Health Sciences and Wellness
Edison Biotechnology Institute
Ohio University
Athens, Ohio

PATSY M. BRANNON, PhD, RD
Professor
Division of Nutritional Sciences
Cornell University
Ithaca, New York

J. THOMAS BRENNA, PhD
Professor
Division of Nutritional Sciences
Cornell University
Ithaca, New York

JOHN T. BROSNAN, DPhil, DSc
University Research Professor
Department of Biochemistry
Memorial University of Newfoundland
St. John's, Newfoundland, Canada

MARGARET E. BROSNAN, PhD
Professor
Department of Biochemistry
Memorial University of Newfoundland
St John's, Newfoundland, Canada

EDITH BROT-LAROCHE, PhD
Research Scientist
Cordeliers Research Center
Department of Physiology, Metabolism, Differentiation
INSERM/Université Pierre et Marie Curie/CNRS
Paris, France

CHUCK T. CHEN, BSc
PhD Candidate
Department of Nutritional Sciences
University of Toronto
Toronto, Ontario, Canada

STEVEN K. CLINTON, MD, PhD
Professor
Division of Medical Oncology
Department of Internal Medicine
The Ohio State University
Columbus, Ohio

GERALD F. COMBS, Jr., PhD
Professor Emeritus
Cornell University
Ithaca, New York
Center Director
Grand Forks Human Nutrition Research Center
USDA-ARS
Grand Forks, North Dakota

ROBERT R. CRICHTON, PhD, FRSC
Professor Emeritus
IMCN, Bâtiment Lavoisier
Université Catholique de Louvain
Louvain-la-Neuve, Belgium

BRENDA M. DAVY, PhD, RD
Associate Professor
Department of Human Nutrition, Foods and Exercise
College of Agriculture and Life Sciences
Virginia Polytechnic Institute and State University
Blacksburg, Virginia

HEDLEY C. FREAKE, PhD
Professor
Department of Nutritional Sciences
College of Agriculture and Natural Resources
University of Connecticut
Storrs, Connecticut

BALZ FREI, PhD
Director and Endowed Chair
Distinguished Professor of Biochemistry and Biophysics
Linus Pauling Institute
Oregon State University
Corvallis, Oregon

JESSE F. GREGORY III, PhD
Professor
Department of Food Science and Human Nutrition
University of Florida
Gainesville, Florida

ARTHUR GRIDER, PhD
Associate Professor
Department of Foods and Nutrition
College of Family and Consumer Sciences
University of Georgia
Athens, Georgia

MATTHEW W. HULVER, PhD
Associate Professor
Department of Human Nutrition, Foods and Exercise
College of Agriculture and Life Sciences
Virginia Polytechnic Institute and State University
Blacksburg, Virginia

RONALD J. JANDACEK, PhD
Adjunct Professor
Department of Pathology and Laboratory Medicine
University of Cincinnati
Cincinnati, Ohio

ELIZABETH H. JEFFERY, PhD
Professor
Department of Food Science and Human Nutrition
College of Agricultural, Consumer and Environmental Sciences
Department of Pharmacology
College of Medicine
University of Illinois
Urbana, Illinois

ANNA-SIGRID KECK, PhD, CIP
Executive Director of the Research Institute
Carle Foundation Hospital
Adjunct Assistant Professor
Department of Food Science and Human Nutrition
University of Illinois
Urbana, Illinois

ARMELLE LETURQUE, PhD
Research Scientist
Cordeliers Research Center
Department of Physiology, Metabolism, Differentiation
INSERM/Université Pierre et Marie Curie/CNRS
Paris, France

CRYSTAL L. LEVESQUE, PhD
Postdoctoral Fellow
Department of Animal & Poultry Science
University of Guelph
Guelph, Ontario, Canada

EDWARD O. LIST, PhD
Senior Scientist
Edison Biotechnology Institute
Ohio University
Athens, Ohio

NELL I. MATTHEWS, BA
Research Associate
Department of Biochemistry
College of Medicine
University of Arkansas for Medical Sciences
Little Rock, Arkansas

MARY M. McGRANE, PhD
Professor—Retired
Departments of Nutritional Sciences and Molecular and Cell Biology
The University of Connecticut
Storrs, Connecticut

MARGARET McNURLAN, PhD
Professor of Surgery
Stony Brook University Medical Center
Stony Brook, New York

ALEXANDER MICHELS, PhD
Research Associate
Linus Pauling Institute
Oregon State University
Corvallis, Oregon

JOSHUA W. MILLER, PhD
Professor
Department of Medical Pathology and Laboratory Medicine
School of Medicine
University of California, Davis
Sacramento, California

DONALD M. MOCK, MD, PhD
Professor
Department of Biochemistry and Molecular Biology
Department of Pediatrics
College of Medicine
University of Arkansas for Medical Sciences
Little Rock, Arkansas

PAUL J. MOUGHAN, PhD, DSc, FRSC, FRSNZ
Distinguished Professor and Director
Riddet Institute
Massey University
Palmerston North, New Zealand

FORREST H. NIELSEN, PhD
Research Nutritionist
U.S. Department Agriculture, Agricultural Research Service
Grand Forks Human Nutrition Research Center
Grand Forks, North Dakota

NOA NOY, PhD
Professor
Departments of Pharmacology and Nutrition
Case Western Reserve University
School of Medicine
Cleveland, Ohio

SARAH K. ORR, BSc
PhD Candidate
Department of Nutritional Sciences
University of Toronto
Toronto, Ontario, Canada

ROBERT S. PARKER, PhD
Associate Professor
Division of Nutritional Sciences
Cornell University
Ithaca, New York

ELIZABETH N. PEARCE, MD, MSc
Associate Professor of Medicine
Section of Endocrinology, Diabetes, and Nutrition
Boston University School of Medicine
Boston, Massachusetts

W. TODD PENBERTHY, PhD
Professor
Department of Molecular Biology and Microbiology
College of Medicine
University of Central Florida
Orlando, Florida

GAVIN L. SACKS, PhD
Assistant Professor
Department of Food Science
Cornell University, New York State Agricultural Experiment Station
Geneva, New York

BARRY SHANE, PhD
Professor
Department of Nutritional Science and Toxicology
University of California
Berkeley, California

SUE A. SHAPSES, PhD
Professor
Department of Nutritional Sciences
Rutgers University
New Brunswick, New Jersey

HWAI-PING SHENG, PhD
Honorary Associate Professor
Departments of Physiology, Pharmacology, and Pharmacy
Li Ka Shing Faculty of Medicine
The University of Hong Kong
Hong Kong, China

JOANNE L. SLAVIN, PhD, RD
Professor
Department of Food Science and Nutrition
College of Food, Agricultural and Natural Resource Sciences
University of Minnesota
Minneapolis, Minnesota

ARTHUR A. SPECTOR, MD
Professor Emeritus
Department of Biochemistry
Carver College of Medicine
University of Iowa
Iowa City, Iowa

CHRISTINA STARK, MS, RD, CDN
Nutrition Specialist
Division of Nutritional Sciences
Cornell University
Ithaca, New York

BRUCE R. STEVENS, PhD
Professor
Department of Physiology & Functional Genomics
College of Medicine
University of Florida
Gainesville, Florida

JUDITH STORCH, PhD
Professor
Department of Nutritional Sciences
School of Environmental and Biological Sciences
Rutgers University
New Brunswick, New Jersey

HEI SOOK SUL, PhD
Professor, Calloway Chair in Human Nutrition
Department of Nutritional Science and Toxicology
University of California
Berkeley, California

KELLY A. TAPPENDEN, PhD, RD
Professor
Department of Food Science and Human Nutrition
University of Illinois at Urbana-Champaign
Champaign, Illinois

CHRISTOPHER A. TAYLOR, PhD, RD, LD
Associate Professor
Medical Dietetics Division and Department of Family Medicine
School of Allied Medical Professions
College of Medicine
The Ohio State University
Columbus, Ohio

ALAN B. R. THOMSON, MD, PhD
Distinguished University Professor
University of Alberta
Adjunct Professor
University of Western Ontario
Canada

PATRICK TSO, PhD
Professor
Department of Pathology and Laboratory Medicine
College of Medicine
University of Cincinnati
Cincinnati, Ohio

JÜRGEN VORMANN, Dr. rer. nat.
Director and Professor
Institute for Prevention and Nutrition
Ismaning/Munich, Germany

REIDAR WALLIN, PhD
Professor Emeritus
Department of Internal Medicine
Section on Molecular Medicine
Wake Forest University School of Medicine
Winston-Salem, North Carolina

GARY M. WHITFORD, PhD, DMD
Regents' Professor
Department of Oral Biology
College of Dental Medicine
Georgia Health Sciences University
Augusta, Georgia

CONTRIBUTORS OF NUTRITION INSIGHTS AND CLINICAL CORRELATIONS

SABRINA BARDOWELL, RD
PhD Candidate
Division of Nutritional Sciences
Cornell University
Ithaca, New York

PATSY M. BRANNON, PhD, RD
Professor
Division of Nutritional Sciences
Cornell University
Ithaca, New York

ELANGO KATHIRVEL, PhD
Research Scientist
Southern California Institute for Research and Education
Long Beach, California

JOEL B. MASON, MD
Professor of Medicine and Nutrition, Tufts University
Scientist I and Director, Vitamins & Carcinogenesis Laboratory, Jean Mayer USDA Human Nutrition Research Center on Aging at Tufts University
Boston, Massachusetts

KENGATHEVY MORGAN, PhD
Research Scientist
Southern California Institute for Research and Education
Long Beach, California

TIMOTHY R. MORGAN, MD
Chief of Hepatology
VA Long Beach Healthcare System
Long Beach, California
Professor of Medicine
University of California, Irvine
Irvine, California

MARGARET P. RAYMAN, DPhil
Professor
Division of Nutritional Sciences
Faculty of Health and Medical Sciences
University of Surrey
Guildford, United Kingdom

KELSEY SHIELDS, BS
Nutritional Sciences Major
Division of Nutritional Sciences
Cornell University
Ithaca, New York

PATRICK J. STOVER, PhD
Professor and Director
Division of Nutritional Sciences
Cornell University
Ithaca, New York

BARBARA J. STRUPP, PhD
Professor
Division of Nutritional Sciences and Department of Psychology
Cornell University
Ithaca, New York

Reviewers

JOSHUA A. BOMSER, PhD
Associate Professor
Department of Human Nutrition
The Ohio State University
Columbus, Ohio

SARAH L. BOOTH, PhD
Professor, Friedman School of Nutrition Science and Policy, Tufts University
Senior Scientist and Associate Director, Jean Mayer USDA Human Nutrition Research Center on Aging at Tufts University
Boston, Massachusetts

PHYLLIS E. BOWEN, PhD, RD
Professor
Department of Kinesiology and Nutrition
University of Illinois at Chicago
Chicago, Illinois

KIMBERLY K. BUHMAN, PhD
Assistant Professor
Department of Foods and Nutrition
Purdue University
West Lafayette, Indiana

JOHN E. DOMINY, PhD
Postdoctoral Fellow
Dana-Farber Cancer Institute
Harvard Medical School
Boston, Massachusetts

CARRIE EARTHMAN, PhD, RD
Assistant Professor
Department of Food Science and Nutrition
University of Minnesota
St. Paul, Minnesota

ALISON B. KOHAN, PhD
Postdoctoral Fellow
College of Medicine
University of Cincinnati
Cincinnati, Ohio

STEFANIA LAMON-FAVA, MD, PhD
Associate Professor
Friedman School of Nutrition Science
Tufts University
Boston, Massachusetts

KIMBERLY O'BRIEN, PhD
Professor
Division of Nutritional Sciences
Cornell University
Ithaca, New York

MICHAEL E. SPURLOCK, PhD
Professor
Department of Food Science and Human Nutrition
Iowa State University
Ames, Iowa

JANE ZIEGLER, DCN, RD, LDN, CNSD
Department of Nutritional Sciences
School of Health Related Professions
University of Medicine and Dentistry of New Jersey
Newark, New Jersey

Preface

We are pleased to present the third edition of *Biochemical, Physiological, and Molecular Aspects of Human Nutrition.* Our understanding of nutrition and its role in health and disease has grown immensely over the past two decades, and much of this progress has been made at the biochemical, physiological, and molecular levels. Recognizing that it is difficult for students, instructors, clinicians, and practitioners to obtain and sustain a deep understanding of the biology of human nutrition, we have worked to develop a textbook that provides a comprehensive, accessible, scientifically accurate, and up-to-date overview of the current understanding of the biological bases of human nutrition. Individuals specializing in nutrition and its effects on health will want to have the third edition of *Biochemical, Physiological, and Molecular Aspects of Human Nutrition* on their shelves as a convenient resource.

The third edition of *Biochemical, Physiological, and Molecular Aspects of Human Nutrition* reflects the contributions of over 60 researchers and academicians who represent a diverse range of expertise. These individuals have written, revised, and reviewed chapters, helping us distill complex scientific information into readable chapters and helpful illustrations. Input from experts was deemed essential to ensure up-to-date and accurate information. As editors, we have done our best to ensure consistency of style and approach so that the individual chapters and units work together as a whole, especially for those who will use this text to teach the biology of nutrition or to acquire a solid understanding of this topic for themselves.

AUDIENCE FOR THE BOOK

Students in nutrition, metabolism, and other life sciences— This book is intended largely for upper-level undergraduate students and graduate students who have completed studies in organic chemistry, biochemistry, molecular biology, and physiology. Hence topics are covered at a more advanced level than in introductory and intermediate textbooks that assume less background in these supporting disciplines. Nevertheless, an effort has been made to present material in a manner that allows a reader who is unfamiliar with a particular topic to obtain a clear, concise, and thorough understanding of the essential concepts. Particular attention has been given to the design of figures and choice of tabular material to ensure that illustrations and tables clarify, extend, and enrich the text.

Instructors in nutrition, metabolism, and other life sciences— Although the topics are logically arranged for reading from first to last, each chapter is also written to be a self-contained unit to facilitate use of a subset of chapters or a different sequence of presentation of chapters according to instructional needs. The depth and breadth of coverage make this text somewhat unique among nutrition texts. It is an especially good choice for courses on macronutrient metabolism and for courses on micronutrient (vitamin and mineral) metabolism. Teaching resources for instructors, including an image collection (which includes all images and selected tables from the text) and three supplementary tables for chapter 24, are available on CD. *To obtain a copy, please contact your local Elsevier rep or call Faculty Support at 1-800-222-9570.*

Dietitians, clinicians, and other health professionals— Given the broad availability of scientific and pseudoscientific information to the general public, it is important that dietitians and other health practitioners have a solid understanding of the biology of human nutrition and health. *Biochemical, Physiological, and Molecular Aspects of Human Nutrition* provides insights into recommended nutritional practices as well as the science behind the advice.

ORGANIZATION OF THE BOOK

The text consists of six units that encompass a traditional coverage of nutrients by classification (macronutrients, vitamins, and minerals) as well as the integrated metabolism and use of these nutrients. In recognition of new paradigms in thinking about nutrition, Unit I considers the historical foundations of nutrition, changes in how nutrients are being defined and in how dietary recommendations are being made, as well as the potentially beneficial nonnutrient components of food. The macronutrients or energy-yielding nutrients (carbohydrates, proteins, and lipids) are discussed in Units II through V. Unit II provides an overview of the structure and properties of the macronutrients. The digestion and absorption of the macronutrients are discussed in Unit III, and the metabolism of the macronutrients is the topic of Unit IV. The last two chapters in Unit IV provide an integrated overview of the regulation of metabolism of macronutrients. Finally, the relation of these macronutrients to energy balance is discussed in Unit V. The vitamins are discussed in Unit VI. The B vitamins have been grouped and discussed in three chapters in a manner that facilitates an understanding of their functions in macronutrient metabolism. The unique functions of vitamins C, K, E, A, and D are described in individual chapters. The minerals and water are the subjects of Unit VII; those with well-characterized nutritional or health-related roles are discussed in detail. Included within each chapter are feature boxes with Nutrition Insights, Clinical Correlations, Life Cycle Considerations, and Historical Tidbits. Significant disease-related aspects of nutrition are incorporated into the individual chapters and also are highlighted in many of the feature boxes scattered throughout the book.

The third edition includes many new figures drawn specifically for this book. Illustrations have been carefully prepared to enhance the text, providing further insights and facilitating understanding. References to the research literature and recommended readings, as well as related websites, are provided for each chapter as appropriate.

Acknowledgments

Working on the third edition of *Biochemical, Physiological, and Molecular Aspects of Human Nutrition* has been a very positive experience for us. All of those who helped us as we worked on this project contributed to our enjoyment of this work, and we extend our deep gratitude to each of you.

In particular, our deep appreciation goes to the chapter contributors. The text is much enriched by the contributions of so many talented researchers and teachers. Their commitment to making scientific advances available and accessible to our audiences is clear from the willingness of these busy individuals to accept the challenge and devote the time and effort required to see their chapters through the entire process. Their willingness to respond to queries, to discuss and resolve apparent differences of opinion among authors, and to allow the editorial flexibility needed to turn individual chapters into a coherent and integrated text was superb.

It has been a delight to work with the amazing staff at Elsevier who handled the publication process. Senior Editor Yvonne Alexopoulos and Developmental Editor Lisa Newton kept the process running smoothly and efficiently and made our job so much easier in many ways. The support and efforts of Developmental Editor Karen Turner on the art and of Project Manager Megan Isenberg on the production process are also greatly appreciated. We would also like to acknowledge Dennis Kunkel Microscopy, Inc. for supplying the front cover image.

During the time we worked on this book, our colleagues in the Division of Nutritional Sciences in the College of Human Ecology and the College of Agriculture and Life Sciences at Cornell University supported our efforts in many ways, especially by serving as sources of expertise and by contributing several of the chapters. We also acknowledge our own graduate students and research staff, who kept our research programs moving forward with full force during our work on this book, and our families and friends who supported and encouraged us in this work. A special thank you is extended to Kelsey Shields for her assistance with chapter formatting.

THE EDITORS
Martha H. Stipanuk
Marie A. Caudill

Contents

UNIT I

Nutrients: Essential and Nonessential

Nutrition may be defined simply as the utilization of foods by living organisms for normal growth, reproduction, and maintenance of health. Nutrients can be divided into two broad groups: (1) organic and (2) inorganic.

Inorganic nutrients include minerals and water. Those nutrients that can be used in inorganic form do not need to come from living sources such as plants or animals. Minerals are present in the earth's crust and are taken up from soil or water by plants and microorganisms, thereby making their way into the food chain. In some cases, the mineral elements are incorporated into organic compounds; for example, selenium and phosphate are present in food proteins. The amount of some minerals in foods can vary substantially depending on the concentration of that mineral in the soil or water in which the food was grown. Humans require more than a dozen different minerals in their diets. These include calcium and phosphorus that we need to make bones and teeth, iodine that we need to make thyroid hormone, and iron that we need as part of certain proteins including the hemoglobin in red blood cells. Much of our mineral intake comes from the foods we eat, but we also obtain minerals from water sources, salts, and food additives.

Nutrients in the organic or carbon-containing group make up the bulk of our diets and provide us with energy as well as many essential organic compounds. Organic nutrients include proteins, carbohydrates (sugars and starches), fats, and vitamins. These organic compounds are synthesized by living cells from simpler compounds. Green plants and photoplankton (such as algae and a special group of photosynthetic bacteria) form the base of the organic nutrient chain. These chlorophyll-containing forms of life use energy from sunlight to combine carbon dioxide from the atmosphere and water to make carbohydrates by a process we call photosynthesis. Therefore plants and photoplankton are able to make organic compounds (such as sugars and carbohydrates) from inorganic compounds (CO_2 and H_2O) in the environment. Animals and most microorganisms, however, cannot carry out photosynthesis and must have preformed organic material in their diets. These species obtain organic nutrients by eating other organisms. Bacteria generally have simple nutrient needs. Most bacteria need a simple organic carbon source, usually decaying plant or animal life. Conversely, animals and humans have complex nutritional needs and require a number of different organic compounds in their diets. We obtain organic nutrients—protein, carbohydrates, fats including some essential fatty acids, and 13 essential vitamins—by consuming a variety of plant and animal foods.

This first unit contains three chapters. Chapter 1 explores the scientific efforts that resulted in the identification and definition of essential nutrients. Much of this work took place during the first half of the twentieth century, with the goals of preventing nutrient deficiency disease and determining the actual amount of each nutrient that is required to prevent deficiency symptoms. Much more attention was given during the latter decades of the twentieth century to the role of nutrition in the maintenance or enhancement of health and in the reduction of risk of certain chronic diseases, such as heart disease and cancer. This latter focus is continuing in the twenty-first century as much remains to be understood about the relationships of nutrition, diet, and health, and about beneficial or harmful "nonnutrient" components of foods. In Chapter 2, various groups of compounds that are actively being studied for their health effects and the current state of knowledge of how these compounds impact health are presented. How we put the knowledge of the science of nutrition into practice is of only academic interest unless it is applied to improvement of the health and well-being of individuals and populations. Chapter 3 presents various means by which the understanding of biological needs and functions of nutrients is translated into information that allows consumers to make healthy dietary choices.

CHAPTER 1

Nutrients: History and Definitions

Martha H. Stipanuk, PhD

Nutrients are defined as chemical substances found in foods that are necessary for human life and growth, maintenance, and repair of body tissues. It is now commonly accepted that proteins, fats, carbohydrates, vitamins, minerals, and water are the major nutritional constituents of foods.

DISCOVERY OF THE NUTRIENTS

Before the chemical nature of food was understood, food was believed to be made up of nutriment, medicines, and poisons. In ancient Greece (~500-300 BC), differences in the physical properties of foods and in their content of medicinal and toxic substances were recognized. The role of diet in the causation and treatment of disease was recognized, as evidenced by the use of liver to treat night blindness. However, the physicians of this era had no understanding of the chemical nature of foods and believed that foods contained only a single nutritional principle that was called aliment. In some ways this ancient understanding is still appropriate in that foods do contain nutrients, substances beneficial to health, and substances that have adverse effects on health, although we now know that each of the three principles in fact includes many different chemical compounds.

EARLY OBSERVATIONS

The belief that foods contained a single nutritional principle persisted for more than two millennia up until the nineteenth century and impeded progress in understanding nutrition. Some recorded observations made during the seventeenth and eighteenth centuries hinted at scientific progress to come. For example, during the 1670s Thomas Sydenham, a British physician, observed that a tonic of iron filings in wine produced a clinical response in patients with chlorosis, a condition now recognized as hypochromic or iron-deficiency anemia (McCollum, 1957). In 1747 James Lind of Scotland, while serving as a naval surgeon, conducted a clinical trial of various proposed treatments of sailors who were ill with scurvy. He observed that consumption of citrus fruits (oranges and lemons), but not other typical foods and medicines, cured the disease (Carpenter, 1986). Nevertheless, chlorosis and scurvy were not viewed as nutritional diseases, and the concept that a disease might be caused by a deficit of a substance that was nutritionally essential did not exist. Before 1900, toxins, heredity, and infections, but not yet nutrition, were recognized as causes of disease.

RECOGNITION THAT FOOD IS A SOURCE OF SPECIFIC NUTRIENTS

By the early 1800s the elements carbon, nitrogen, hydrogen, and oxygen were recognized as the primary components of food, and the need for the carbon-containing components of food as a substrate for combustion (heat production) was recognized (Carpenter, 2003a). Protein was identified as a specific essential dietary component by the observations of François Magendie in Paris in 1816. Magendie showed that dogs fed only carbohydrate or fat lost considerable body protein and weight within a few weeks, whereas dogs fed foods that contained nitrogen (protein) remained healthy. In 1827 William Prout, a physician and scientist in London, proposed that the nutrition of higher animals could be explained by their need for proteins, carbohydrates, and fats, and this explanation was widely accepted. During the next two decades, the need of animals for several mineral elements was demonstrated, and at least six mineral elements (Ca, P, Na, K, Cl, and Fe) had been established as essential for higher animals by 1850 (Harper, 1999; Carpenter et al., 1997).

The nineteenth century German chemist Justus von Liebig postulated that energy-yielding substances (carbohydrates and fats) and proteins, together with a few minerals, represented the essentials of a nutritionally adequate diet, and he proposed that the nutritive value of foods and feeds could be predicted from knowledge of their gross chemical composition. Liebig prepared tables of food values based on this concept—work that was facilitated by the work of Wilhelm Henneberg, who devised the Weende system, known as proximate analysis, for analyzing foods and feeds for protein, fat, fiber, nitrogen-free extract (carbohydrate), and ash (McCollum, 1957). Throughout the remainder of the nineteenth century, nutritional thinking continued to be dominated by the belief that sources of energy, protein, and a few minerals were the sole principles of a nutritionally adequate diet.

Despite the dominance of Liebig's views during the mid to late nineteenth century, it should be noted that the

HISTORICAL TIDBIT 1-1

The Connection between Combustion and Respiration

The Experiments of Antoine Lavoisier

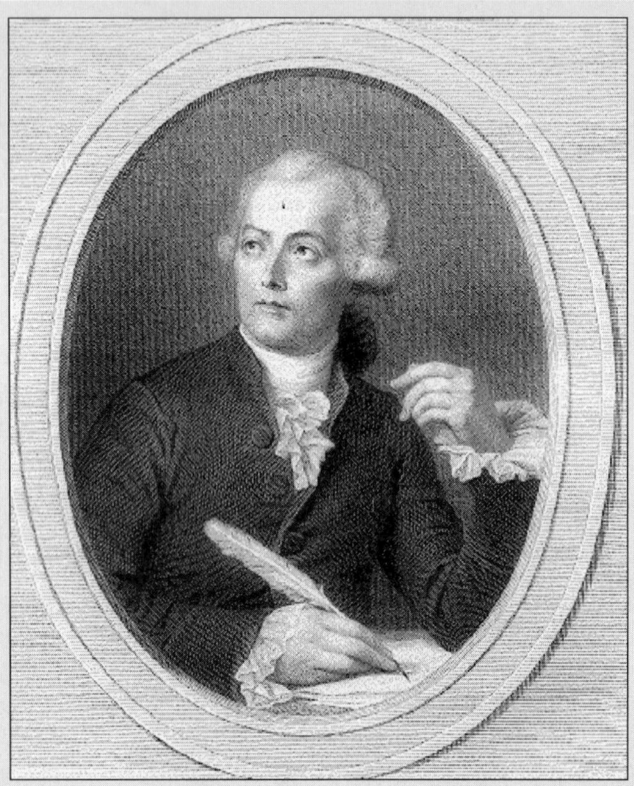

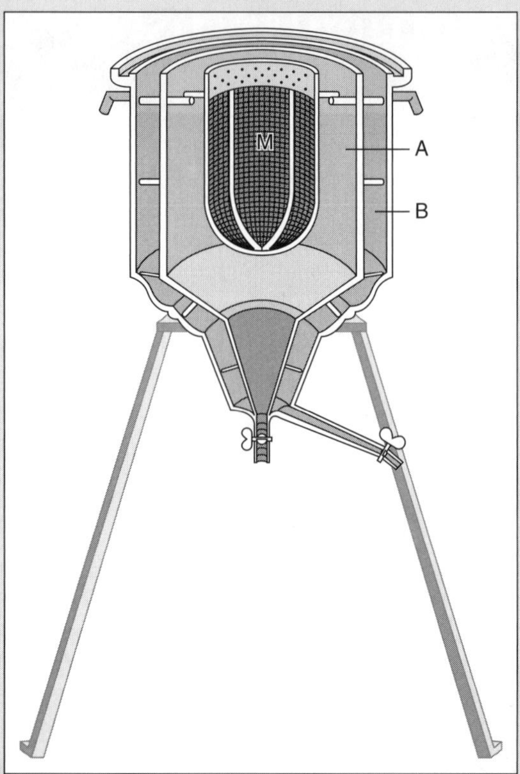

The world's first ice-calorimeter, used in the winter of 1782-83 by Antoine Lavoisier and Pierre-Simon Laplace. The guinea pig was placed in a mesh chamber (M) surrounded by two shells (A and B) filled with ice. Heat produced by the animal melted the ice and the water that flowed out of the calorimeter was collected and weighed.

Nearly 300 years before Lavoisier, during the sixteenth century, the artist and scientist Leonardo da Vinci noted the part played by air in combustion. The ancients realized that air was necessary for burning but did not understand the nature of the combustion process. Leonardo arranged deliberate experiments on enclosed combustion and arrived at the correct answer to a problem that continued to worry experimenters for years afterward. In manuscripts deposited as the *Codex Leicester,* Leonardo noted that "air is consumed by the introduction of the fire." He also noted, in the *Codice Atlantico,* that "where flame cannot live, no animal that draws breath can live," clearly correlating the phenomenon of combustion with the one of animal respiration. Like Leonardo, Robert Fludd and John Mayow came to their own correct interpretations of the phenomenon of combustion in the seventeenth century. However, despite the work of these early insightful scientists, the phlogiston theory dominated the view of combustion from the late seventeenth century through much of the eighteenth century. The phlogiston theory posited the existence of the substance called phlogiston in combustible materials; the process of combustion was thought to involve the release of phlogiston into the air. Because substances in a sealed container were observed to burn for only a limited period of time, air was thought to have a limited capacity to accept phlogiston.

This phlogiston theory of combustion was widely accepted until it was refuted by Antoine Lavoisier's experiments showing that respiration was essentially a slow combustion of organic material using inhaled oxygen and producing carbon dioxide and water (Wilkinson, 2004). Lavoisier and mathematician Pierre-Simon Laplace performed experiments in 1780 with guinea pigs in which they quantified the oxygen consumed and carbon dioxide produced by metabolism. They also developed an ice-calorimeter apparatus to measure the amount of heat given off during combustion or respiration (see drawing). They measured the quantity of carbon dioxide and heat produced by a live guinea pig that was confined in this apparatus and then determined the amount of heat produced when sufficient carbon was burned in the ice-calorimeter to produce the same amount of carbon dioxide as had been exhaled by the guinea pig. They found the same ratio of heat to carbon dioxide for both processes, leading to the conclusion that animals produced energy by a type of combustion reaction. Lavoisier further showed that combustion involved the reaction of the combustible substance with oxygen and that heat or light were released as weightless by-products. Lavoisier and his colleagues viewed respiration as a very slow combustion phenomenon that is conducted inside the lungs. About 50 years later in 1837, German physiologist Heinrich Gustav Magnus performed his famous experiments showing that

HISTORICAL TIDBIT 1-1—cont'd

The Connection between Combustion and Respiration
The Experiments of Antoine Lavoisier

both carbon dioxide and oxygen existed in both arterial and venous blood, with oxygen higher and carbon dioxide lower in arterial blood compared to venous blood. Magnus correctly concluded that combustion (oxygen uptake; carbon dioxide, water, and heat production) must occur throughout the body (not just in the lungs), and other scientists subsequently showed that oxidation occurs in the tissues, not in the blood plasma.

With Armand Sequin, Lavoisier pushed his studies further to investigate the influence of work, food, and environmental temperature on metabolism. By measuring the amount of carbon dioxide exhaled, they showed that respiration (oxygen consumption or carbon dioxide production) increased by about 10% in a cold environment, by 50% due solely to food intake, and by 200% with exercise. They also showed a direct correlation between the heart rate (pulse) and the amount of work performed (sum of weights lifted to a predetermined height) and between the heart rate and the quantity of oxygen consumed. These studies, along with some knowledge of the chemical composition of plant and animal foods, allowed Lavoisier to make the fundamental conclusion that the oxidation of carbon compounds was the source of energy for activity and other bodily functions of animals.

Although Lavoisier's experiments were cut short by the French Revolution and his execution by the French revolutionists during the Reign of Terror (because of Lavoisier's service as a tax collector), Lavoisier's seminal contributions to modern chemistry, metabolism, nutrition, and exercise physiology were enormous. He is often called the "Father of Modern Chemistry."

validity of his assumptions was challenged during the nineteenth century (McCollum, 1957). In 1843 Jonathan Pereira in England stated that diets containing a wide variety of foods were essential for human well-being, whereas diets containing only a few foods were associated with the acquisition of diseases such as scurvy. Jean Baptist Dumas, based on his observation that an artificial milk formula that contained all of the known dietary constituents failed to prevent deterioration of health of children during the siege of Paris (1870-1871), also questioned the validity of Liebig's assumptions. In addition, Nikolai Lunin (~1881), who worked in Gustav von Bunge's laboratory in Dorpat, Estonia, conducting studies with mice in an effort to identify inadequacies in the mineral component of purified diets, demonstrated that mice fed a diet composed of purified proteins, fats, carbohydrates, and a mineral mixture survived less than 5 weeks, whereas mice that received milk or egg yolk in addition to the purified components remained healthy throughout the experiment. Lunin concluded that milk must contain small quantities of other unknown substances essential to life, but von Bunge apparently did not encourage him or subsequent students in his laboratory who made similar observations to investigate what the active factor in milk might be. The Liebig–von Bunge view that nutritional requirements consisted only of protein, energy-yielding substances, and a few minerals still had such hold on scientific thought that, rather than consider that these observations might point to the presence of other essential nutrients in foods, the inadequacies of the purified diets were attributed to mineral imbalances, failure to supply minerals as organic complexes, or lack of palatability (Wolf and Carpenter, 1997).

Also of significance were the studies of beriberi that were conducted during the nineteenth century. Kanchiro Takaki was concerned during the 1880s with the devastating effects of beriberi on sailors in the Japanese navy. Because of the superior health of British sailors, he compared the food supplies of the two navies and was struck by the higher protein content of the British rations. He, therefore, included evaporated milk and meat in the diet and substituted barley for part of the polished rice in the Japanese rations. These changes eradicated beriberi. He attributed this to the additional protein. In retrospect, we know that this was incorrect (i.e., beriberi is caused by thiamin deficiency), but his conclusion does imply that he correctly considered beriberi to be a disease caused by a nutritional inadequacy (Takaki, 1906). Christiaan Eijkman, an army physician in the Dutch East Indies, began his investigations of beriberi in the 1890s (Jansen, 1956). He had observed a high incidence of beriberi in the prisons in Java in which polished rice was a staple. He assumed it was caused by chronic consumption of a diet consisting largely of polished rice. He noted during his experimental studies that chickens fed on a military hospital diet composed mainly of polished rice developed a neurological disease resembling beriberi, whereas birds fed rice with the pericarp intact remained healthy. He concluded that ingestion of the high starch diet resulted in formation in the intestine of a substance that acted as a nerve poison and that rice hulls contained an antidote. Eijkman's conclusion illustrates the fact that a connection between nutrient deficiency and disease was still a foreign concept at the end of the nineteenth century.

RECOGNITION OF THE CONNECTION OF DIET AND DISEASE

Resistance to the notion of nutritional deficiency diseases continued into the early twentieth century. With the accumulating number of diet-associated diseases, however, the concept that a disease might be caused by a deficit of an essential nutrient slowly gained acceptance (Carpenter, 2003b).

In 1901 Gerrit Grijns, who took over Eijkman's research in the Dutch East Indies in 1896, showed through feeding trials that Eijkman's active substance was present in other foods

(Jansen, 1956; Carpenter, 1995). After demonstrating that beriberi could be prevented by including rice polishings, beans, or water extracts of these foods in the diet, he proposed that beriberi was a dietary deficiency disease caused by the absence of an essential nutrient present in rice hulls. Grijns thus interpreted Eijkman's results correctly and provided for the first time a clear concept of a dietary deficiency disease. The broad implications of Grijns' interpretation of his investigation of beriberi were not appreciated for some years, however.

In 1907 Alex Holst and Theodore Fröhlich in Norway reported that guinea pigs fed dry diets with no fresh vegetables developed a disease resembling scurvy; supplying them with fresh vegetables cured the disease—giving rise to a second example of a dietary deficiency disease (Carpenter, 1986). Interestingly, Holst and Fröhlich had been looking for a mammal to test a diet that had earlier produced beriberi in pigeons; they were surprised that scurvy resulted instead because, up until that time, scurvy had not been considered to occur in any species other than humans. This was a fortuitous occurrence because the guinea pig allowed assessment of the antiscorbutic value of different foodstuffs, leading to the isolation and identification of vitamin C.

In 1914 Joseph Goldberger was appointed by the Surgeon General of the United States to study the disease pellagra, which was prevalent in the southern United States. At the time, pellagra was thought to be an infectious disease, but Goldberger correctly theorized that the disease was caused by malnutrition (Carpenter, 2003c). He observed that those who treated the sick never developed the disease and noticed that people with restricted diets (mainly corn bread, molasses, and a little pork fat) were more likely to develop pellagra. Goldberger, however, had difficulty convincing others of this theory. Eventually, Goldberger's group found that dogs developed a condition called "blacktongue" when fed mixtures with mostly cornmeal and no meat or milk powder, allowing dogs to be used to "assay"' fractions from various foods for anti-blacktongue potency. The dogs responded rapidly to yeast, and yeast was also found to cure pellagra in humans. After Goldberger's death, Conrad Elvehjem at the University of Wisconsin went on to show in 1937 that nicotinic acid, which had been discovered to be a bacterial growth factor, was extremely potent in curing blacktongue and also prevented and healed pellagra.

The iodination of salt in the 1920s, the fortification of milk with vitamin D in the 1930s (even before vitamin D had been purified and synthesized), and the addition of niacin, thiamin, and iron to cereal flours and products in the 1930s were successful efforts to reduce the incidence of goiter, rickets, and pellagra (Bishai and Nalubola, 2002), respectively. The concept of nutritional deficiency disease was firmly established.

DISCOVERY OF THE FIRST SMALL ORGANIC MOLECULE ESSENTIAL FOR GROWTH

The first evidence of essentiality of a specific small organic molecule was the discovery by Edith Willcock and Fredrick G. Hopkins (1906) that a supplement of the amino acid tryptophan, which had been discovered in 1900, prolonged survival of mice fed a zein-based diet. Zein is the major storage protein in corn endosperm and it contains only a small proportion of tryptophan. It was also recognized at this time that enzyme hydrolysates of protein supported adequate growth rates, whereas acid hydrolysates of protein failed to support growth (Carpenter, 2003b). This difference was also attributed to a deficiency of tryptophan due to the destruction of tryptophan by acid digestion (Henriques and Hansen, 1905). But the growth rate of rats fed on semipurified diets was not satisfactory, so further work on amino acid requirements was delayed until this problem was solved.

DISPROVING LIEBIG'S HYPOTHESIS

The validity of Liebig's hypothesis—that the nutritive value of foods and feeds could be predicted from measurements of their gross composition—was directly tested at the University of Wisconsin from 1907 to 1911 in what has become known as the Wisconsin single-grain experiment (Carpenter et al., 1997; Hart et al., 1911). This study was suggested to E. B. Hart by his predecessor at the University of Wisconsin, Stephen M. Babcock, who had observed that milk production by cows consuming rations composed of different feedstuffs differed considerably, even when the rations were formulated to have the same gross composition and energy content. Hart and colleagues compared the performance of four groups of heifers fed rations composed entirely of corn (cornmeal, corn gluten, and corn stover), wheat (ground wheat, wheat gluten, and wheat straw), or oats (oat meal and oat straw), all formulated to be closely similar in gross composition and energy content; or a mixed ration consisting of equal parts of the three plants. Six-month-old heifers were fed the assigned rations to maturity and through two reproductive periods. Differences between performance of the corn and wheat groups were marked, with other groups being intermediate. Calves born to cows consuming the corn ration were strong and vigorous and all lived, but cows consuming the wheat ration all delivered 3 to 4 weeks prematurely and none of the calves lived beyond 12 days. Cows fed the corn ration produced almost double the amount of milk produced by those fed the wheat ration. Thus Hart and colleagues demonstrated that the nutritive value of a ration could not be predicted solely from measurements of its content of protein, energy, and a few minerals. In hindsight, the signs of inadequacy in the wheat and oat groups resembled those of vitamin A deficiency, which was probably prevented by the carotene in the ration that contained corn.

THE ANIMAL GROWTH MODEL AND THE DISCOVERIES OF ESSENTIAL VITAMINS AND AMINO ACIDS

Although investigators were beginning to conduct nutritional studies with rodents fed purified diets in the early 1900s, it was difficult to maintain growth in rats using diets composed of starch, lard, isolated protein, and mineral mixes, even with casein as the protein source. This problem was overcome by addition of a protein-free extract of milk to these diets (Willcock and Hopkins, 1906; Block and Mitchell, 1946). In 1912 Hopkins suggested that an organic complex that animals cannot synthesize was absent from the purified diets. Also in 1912, Casimir Funk, a young Polish chemist who had been trying to purify the antiberiberi principle from rice polishings, expressed the opinion that beriberi, as well as scurvy and pellagra, were dietary deficiency diseases (Rosenfeld, 1997). Funk believed these diseases were caused by a dietary lack of "special substances which are in the nature of organic bases, which we will call vitamines" (from the Latin *vita,* meaning "life," and amine, because he thought all of these compounds contained an amine functional group). Soon after these ideas were proposed, the concept that foods contained small quantities of organic substances that were essential nutrients was generally accepted. The name *vitamine* soon became synonymous with Hopkins' "accessory factor." By the time it was shown that not all vitamines were amines, the word was already ubiquitous. In 1920 Jack Cecil Drummond proposed that the final "e" be dropped to deemphasize the "amine" implication.

Between 1909 and 1913 Elmer V. McCollum and Margaret Davis noted that growth of rats was satisfactory if the fat was supplied as butterfat, but not if butterfat was replaced by lard or olive oil. Meanwhile, Thomas Osborne and Lafayette Mendel in Connecticut observed that if they further purified the protein-free milk included in their diets by a process that included removal of ether-soluble compounds, growth failure of rats again occurred; if they substituted butterfat for the lard in this diet, growth was restored (Osborne and Mendel, 1911, 1914). Both groups concluded that butterfat contained an unidentified substance essential for growth. McCollum and Davis proceeded to extract an active substance from butterfat and transferred it to olive oil, which then promoted growth. They called this substance *fat-soluble A.* When they further tested this substance in a polished rice diet of the type used by Eijkman and Grijns in their studies of beriberi, they found that even though the diet contained the fat-soluble A, it still failed to support growth. An aqueous extract of either wheat germ or boiled eggs provided the missing factor needed to cure beriberi; this factor was designated *water-soluble B.* The then-unknown substance preventing scurvy was named *water-soluble C.* Following Drummond's recommendations in 1920, these substances were subsequently referred to as vitamins A, B, and C.

The work of McCollum and colleagues in Wisconsin and of Osborne and Mendel in Connecticut in developing rodent models and the use of long-term growth of rats as a measure of nutritional adequacy opened up a new approach to the search for essential amino acids as well as vitamins. Using semipurified diets supplemented with a protein-free milk extract, Osborne and Mendel (~1915) demonstrated that proteins from different sources differed in nutritive value; and they discovered that lysine, sulfur-containing amino acids, and histidine were required by rats for growth (Block and Mitchell, 1946).

RAPID DISCOVERY OF OTHER ESSENTIAL NUTRIENTS

The emergence of the use of the animal growth model and semipurified diets was extremely important to the identification of essential nutrients. By 1915 six minerals (Ca, P, Na, K, Cl, and Fe), four amino acids (tryptophan, lysine, sulfur-containing amino acids, and histidine), and three vitamins (A, B, and C) had been identified as essential nutrients. By 1918 the concept of the presence of "accessory factors or vitamins" or "minor constituents of foods" that are essential for health was established. Also, the importance of consuming a wide variety of foods to ensure that diets provided adequate quantities of these substances was being emphasized in health programs for the public in the United States and Great Britain and by the League of Nations; this was followed by a decline in the incidence of dietary deficiency diseases during the next three decades. Acceptance of the new paradigm was followed by a period of unparalleled discovery in nutritional science from about 1915 to the 1950s (Carpenter, 2003c).

In 1919 Sir Edward Mellanby incorrectly identified rickets as a vitamin A deficiency based on the ability of cod liver oil to cure rickets in dogs. In 1922 McCollum destroyed the vitamin A in cod liver oil but found that it still cured rickets, indicating that fat-soluble A was really two substances. The factor capable of curing xerophthalmia was then named vitamin A, and the substance that prevented rickets was named vitamin D. Also in 1922 Herbert McLean Evans and Katharine Scott Bishop discovered vitamin E as a factor essential for rat pregnancy; this new vitamin was called "food factor X" until 1925. In 1929 Henrik Dam found that a factor present in green leaves and in liver, vitamin K, was necessary for blood clotting. Vitamin B was found to have components in addition to the heat-labile thiamin (vitamin B_1). In 1933 Richard Kuhn, Paul György, and Theodor Wagner-Jauregg found that thiamin-free extracts of yeast, liver, or rice bran prevented the growth failure of rats fed a thiamin-supplemented diet, and this vitamin B_2 was found to be a fluorescent substance subsequently called riboflavin. The remaining components of the vitamin B complex were discovered between 1920 and 1941.

The essentiality of the long-chain polyunsaturated fatty acids (linoleic and α-linolenic acids) was shown by George and Mildred Burr in 1929 (Burr and Burr, 1929, 1930; Holman, 1988) at the University of Minnesota Medical School. To show the essentiality of fatty acids, they prepared diets that were completely fat-free by using sucrose instead of cornstarch (which contained 0.7% lipid unextractable with ether); they supplied vitamins A and D by adding the nonsaponifiable fraction of cod liver oil to the diet.

The animal growth model also facilitated the further identification of the essential components provided by dietary protein. William C. Rose and colleagues at the University of Illinois purified 13 of the known amino acids and synthesized 6 others. They then tested the ability of a mixture of these 19 amino acids to substitute for dietary protein. Rats lost weight when fed diets containing these 19 amino acids, suggesting a missing essential component of protein (Rose, 1931). They then went on to identify the yet undiscovered amino acid, threonine, and to show that a mixture of all 20 amino acids could substitute for dietary protein (McCoy et al., 1935). With the identification of all of the amino acid components of protein, Rose and colleagues later identified which of these amino acids were indispensable in the diet of humans.

With the discovery of the presence of minute organic factors (vitamins) essential to the diet came also the recognition and research into minute amounts of certain minerals that are essential in the diet (Mertz, 1981). Discovery of the role of trace minerals in the diet was facilitated by the development of analytical procedures using emission spectroscopy in 1929. The importance of iodine, copper, manganese, and magnesium in animal nutrition had been established by 1940 (Carpenter, 2003d). The essentiality of zinc was firmly established during the 1950s and 1960s, and the roles of selenium and molybdenum as essential elements were first recognized and explored during the same decades. Recognition of the essentiality of some of the ultratrace elements has been facilitated by the discovery of unique roles of these elements in normal metabolism (e.g., selenium for formation of selenocysteine moieties of proteins, iodine for formation of thyroid hormones, and molybdenum for enzyme cofactor formation). Clear essentiality of some other elements present in minute amounts in the diet (e.g., chromium and boron) have been much more difficult to demonstrate and will likely remain so unless they also are shown to be critical components of normal physiological compounds in the animal.

Thus, by 1960, most of the essential nutrients had been identified and characterized and their functions explored. These essential nutrients included essential polyunsaturated fatty acids, 9 amino acids, 12 vitamins, and 11 minerals (Box 1-1).

SETTING CRITERIA FOR ESSENTIALITY

In the late 1950s, after rats had been maintained successfully through four generations fed diets composed of constituents with known chemical structures (Schultze, 1957), it was generally accepted that all (or, at least, most) of the essential nutrients for rats had been discovered. Later, when human subjects were maintained for long periods on intravenous fluids containing only highly purified constituents, it was accepted that the conclusion also applied to humans. Nevertheless, an avid search for additional essential nutrients continued for some years. Over the course of studies to identify nutrients, specific criteria were established for declaring a food constituent to be an essential nutrient. Alfred E. Harper (1999) summarized the following criteria of essentiality that had evolved by about 1950:

- The substance is required in the diet for growth, health, and survival.
- The absence of the substance from the diet or inadequate intake results in characteristic signs of a deficiency disease and, ultimately, death.

BOX 1-1 List of Essential Nutrients for Humans

WATER

AMINO ACIDS

- Histidine
- Isoleucine
- Leucine
- Lysine
- Methionine
- Phenylalanine
- Threonine
- Tryptophan
- Valine
- Other amino acids to supply sufficient amino groups/nitrogen

ENERGY SOURCES (CARBOHYDRATE, FAT, OR PROTEIN)

POLYUNSATURATED FATTY ACIDS

- Linoleic (n-6)
- α-Linolenic (n-3)

VITAMINS

- Ascorbic acid
- Vitamin A
- Vitamin D
- Vitamin E
- Vitamin K
- Thiamin
- Riboflavin
- Niacin
- Vitamin B_6
- Pantothenic acid
- Folate
- Biotin
- Vitamin B_{12}

MINERALS

- Calcium
- Phosphorus
- Magnesium
- Iron
- Sodium
- Potassium
- Chloride
- Zinc
- Copper
- Manganese
- Iodine
- Selenium
- Molybdenum
- Chromium (probably)
- Boron (probably)

- Growth failure and characteristic signs of deficiency are prevented only by the nutrient or a specific precursor of it, not by other substances.
- Below some critical level of intake of the nutrient, growth response and severity of signs of deficiency are proportional to the amount consumed.
- The substance is not synthesized in the body and is therefore required for some critical function throughout life.

Harper also emphasized that nutritional essentiality is characteristic of the species, not the nutrient. For example, ascorbic acid is required by humans and guinea pigs but not by most other species that can synthesize the nutrient from glucose.

During the 1960s and 1970s, the concept of essentiality was modified for the mineral elements that could not be fed at dietary concentrations sufficiently low to interfere with growth, development, maturation, or reproduction—some of the ultratrace elements. The most commonly used criterion was that a dietary deficiency must consistently and adversely change a biological function from optimal, and this change must be preventable or reversible by physiological amounts of the element (Nielsen, 2000). However, this latter basis for establishing essentiality of minerals ultimately was not very satisfactory for the ultratrace elements, because it was impossible to determine whether some of the changes were really the result of low intakes causing suboptimal functions or whether the mineral supplements had pharmacological actions in the body. Today, most scientists do not consider an element essential unless it has a defined biochemical function. Nevertheless, there is no universally accepted list of ultratrace elements that are considered essential.

Forest Nielsen suggests that a nutritionally beneficial element be defined as "one with health restorative effects in response to an apparent deficient intake of that element, at intakes that are found with normal diets; these

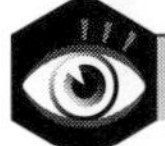

NUTRITION INSIGHT

The History of American Food Composition Tables

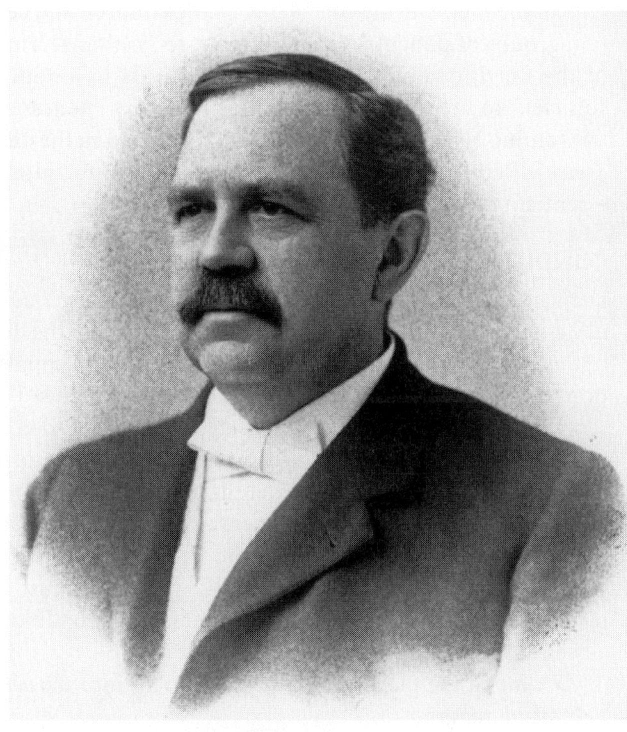

The U.S. Department of Agriculture (USDA) has been compiling food composition data for well over a century. The food composition data it maintains is widely used by nutritionists, researchers, and individuals. Tabulation of food composition data began with the work of Wilbur Olin Atwater scarcely 50 years after the classical studies of Justus von Liebig in Germany. Atwater received his PhD from Yale in 1869 and then studied in Germany, where he became familiar with the works of Carl von Voit, Max Rubner, and Nathan Zuntz.

In 1896 Atwater and A. P. Bryant published the proximate composition of 2,600 American foodstuffs in a bulletin called *The Chemical Composition of American Food Materials.* Within 4 years, an additional 4,000 new foods had been analyzed and a revised edition of the bulletin was published; about a quarter of these new analyses were performed by Atwater and his associates in the chemical laboratory at Wesleyan College (Middletown, CT). A 1906 reprinting of the bulletin stood until 1940 when the USDA Circular No. 549, *Proximate Composition of American Food Materials,* was published. In addition to determining the proximate composition of foodstuffs (protein, fat, carbohydrate, and ash), Atwater and his associates devised a method for calculating the physiological energy value of foodstuffs. By correcting the heat of combustion of food components (i.e., the heat released by the complete combustion of the food in a calorimeter) by factors for incomplete digestion and incomplete oxidation of the food in the body, they calculated the physiological fuel values of protein, fat, and carbohydrate isolated from various foods. They then applied these factors to the proximate composition of individual foods to calculate their available energy, or caloric, values. The caloric values in current food composition tables and on food product labels are still calculated this way today.

The first extensive revision of Atwater's work was in 1950 with the publication of the USDA Agriculture Handbook No. 8, *Composition of Foods—Raw, Processed, Prepared,* which contained values for 11 nutrients. Agriculture Handbook No. 8 was subsequently revised in 1963 and then expanded into a series of publications from 1976 to 1992. The *USDA Nutrient Database for Standard Reference* is the current form of the food composition tables. It has been maintained electronically since 1980, with frequent updates, and can be downloaded from the USDA's Nutrient Data Laboratory Home Page: *www.ars.usda.gov/ba/bhnrc/ndl.*

health restorative effects can be amplified or inhibited by nutritional, physiologic, hormonal, or metabolic stressors" (Nielsen, 2000, p. 116). Nielsen (2000) gives the following examples of nutritionally beneficial elements:

- Boron, the effects of which can be amplified by a marginal vitamin D deficiency,
- Vanadium, the effects of which can be amplified by deficient or luxuriant dietary iodine, and
- Nickel, the beneficial effects of which are inhibited by vitamin B_{12}, pyridoxine, or folic acid deficiency.

Nielsen (2000, pp. 116-117) suggested use of the following four categories of evidence to support the contention that a trace element is nutritionally essential:

1. A dietary deprivation in some animal models consistently results in a changed biological function, body structure, or tissue composition that is preventable or reversible by an intake of an apparent physiological amount of the element in question.
2. The element fills the need at physiological concentrations for a known in vivo biochemical action to proceed in vitro.
3. The element is a component of known biologically important molecules in some life form.
4. The element has an essential function in lower forms of life.

Using Nielsen's criteria, there is strong circumstantial evidence for the essentiality of arsenic, boron, chromium, nickel, silicon, and vanadium, and limited circumstantial evidence for essentiality of aluminum, bromine, cadmium, fluorine, germanium, lead, lithium, rubidium, and tin. The strongest evidence for essentiality exists for boron and chromium, and these two elements likely belong in the category of established essential nutrients for higher animals including humans.

CONCERNS ABOUT EXCESSIVE INTAKES

With the successive discoveries of essential nutrients between 1915 and 1950 and the virtual disappearance of dietary deficiency diseases in developed countries, emphasis in nutrition changed to ensuring that diets would provide adequate quantities of all essential nutrients to prevent impairment of growth and development. In 1940 the Food and Nutrition Board of the National Research Council was organized in the United States with the function of advising on problems of nutrition in connection with national defense. This committee recognized the need for standards or allowances for intake of nutrients needed for maintenance of good health. The Food and Nutrition Board formulated the first set of Recommended Dietary Allowances (RDAs) for Americans in 1941. This committee has subsequently published nine revisions of the RDAs up through the 10th edition in 1989 and now has established the more extensive Dietary Reference Intakes.

During the first half of the twentieth century, relatively little attention was given to total food intake and its effects on health. An exception during this time was the work of Clive McCay at Cornell in the 1930s (McCay et al., 1939). McCay argued that short-term trials with an emphasis on rapid growth did not provide an adequate test of the most desirable nutritional state throughout life. His studies showed that rats fed restricted amounts of a nutritionally adequate diet grew slower and survived longer than those allowed to eat freely. Concern about total food intake and health, however, increased during the second half of the twentieth century, as evidenced by the introduction of dietary guidelines for Americans in 1977 and by the growing concerns about obesity, metabolic syndrome, and chronic disease. Various editions of dietary guidelines for Americans have addressed concerns about excessive intakes of fat, saturated fat, cholesterol, salt and sodium, sugar, alcohol, and total energy.

NUTRIENTS THAT DO NOT MEET THE STRICT CRITERIA FOR ESSENTIALITY

As knowledge of nutritional needs grew, it became clear that there were conditions under which individuals required the presence of dispensable (nonessential) nutrients in the diet. During the 1970s, young children and certain groups of patients were found not to synthesize some of the nutritionally dispensable amino acids in amounts sufficient to meet their needs. These normally "nonessential" amino acids, therefore, had to be provided in the diet. These discoveries expanded the concept of "nutritional essentiality."

CONDITIONALLY ESSENTIAL NUTRIENTS

Daniel Rudman and associates proposed the term *conditionally essential* for nutrients not ordinarily required in the diet but which must be supplied exogenously to specific populations that do not synthesize them in adequate amounts. The term was initially applied to dispensable nutrients needed by seriously ill patients maintained on total parenteral nutrition, but the term has been expanded to apply to similar needs that result from developmental immaturity, pathological states, or genetic defects. Rudman and A. G. Feller (1986) proposed the following three criteria that must be met to establish unequivocally that a nutrient is conditionally essential:

1. Decline in the plasma level of the nutrient into the subnormal range
2. Appearance of chemical, structural, or functional abnormalities
3. Correction of both of these by a dietary supplement of the nutrient

Harper (1999) stressed that conditional essentiality represents a qualitative change in requirements, that is, the need for a nutrient that is ordinarily dispensable. He further stressed that this term should not be used for alterations in the need for an essential nutrient, for health benefits from consumption of nonnutrients, or for health benefits from consumption of dispensable nutrients or essential nutrients in excess of amounts needed for normal physiological function. Examples of conditionally essential nutrients include the requirement of premature infants for cysteine and tyrosine, which cannot yet be synthesized in adequate amounts from their precursor amino acids; a possible requirement of long-chain n-3 fatty acids in preterm infants, because preterm infants are not able to synthesize these from α-linolenic acid at a rate that meets the infant's need; a requirement of some patients with cirrhosis of the liver for cysteine, tyrosine, and taurine, owing to decreased hepatic capacity for synthesis of these amino acids from their precursors; and requirements for carnitine or tetrahydrobiopterin by individuals with genetic defects preventing their synthesis. Although choline can be synthesized in the body, a dietary source is required to prevent choline inadequacy in men, postmenopausal women, and populations with an increased demand (i.e., pregnant and lactating women and individuals with certain genetic variants affecting choline metabolism).

MODIFICATION OF REQUIREMENTS FOR AN ESSENTIAL NUTRIENT

Requirements for essential nutrients may be influenced by the presence in the diet of substances that are precursors or metabolic products of the nutrient or substances that interfere with the absorption or use of the nutrient imbalances and disproportions of other related nutrients; malabsorptive conditions; some genetic defects; and use of drugs that impair use of nutrients. These conditions do not alter basic requirements but rather increase or decrease the amounts that must be consumed to meet requirements. For example, tryptophan serves as a precursor in niacin synthesis; vitamin A is derived from β-carotene; phytic acid impairs absorption of zinc and other cations; thiomolybdate forms complexes with copper and prevents its absorption; anticonvulsant medications interfere with folate use; atrophic gastritis decreases absorption of vitamin B_{12}; and genetic defects in the enzyme responsible for reuse of biotin increase the dietary need for this vitamin. Many more examples will be discussed throughout the other chapters of this book.

HEALTH EFFECTS OF NUTRIENTS AND NONNUTRIENT COMPONENTS OF FOOD

In recent years diet–disease relationships have become major areas of investigation in nutrition, and a new paradigm is emerging. Previously, the concept of deficiency was the primary factor in determining nutritional requirements, but new research suggests that total health effects of a nutrient should also be considered (Mertz, 1993). Individual food constituents that may confer health benefits different from those of physiologically required quantities of essential nutrients, whether they are nonnutrients, dispensable nutrients, or essential nutrients in quantities exceeding those obtainable from diet, are appropriately included in guidelines for health. This new paradigm includes the determination of upper safe levels of intake for nutrients as well as nonnutrients that may have harmful effects on health.

This leads us to a new class of substances to consider in terms of nutrition: nonnutritional components of foods that are beneficial to health. The contribution of both fluoride and fiber to health has resulted in their inclusion in the list of nutrients for which the Institute of Medicine has now established Dietary Reference Intakes. Fluoride is prophylactic in low doses, protecting teeth against the action of bacteria, but whether fluoride is essential for tooth and bone development is controversial. Fiber, in moderate amounts, is recognized to be beneficial for gastrointestinal function, and some forms of fiber may be fermented into products that can be absorbed and oxidized to yield energy. But there is no basis for classifying fiber as an essential nutrient. Numerous food constituents, including certain fatty acids, fiber, carotenoids, and various nonnutrient substances in plants, have been associated with lower incidences of chronic or degenerative diseases such as heart disease and cancer.

Health benefits of essential nutrients have also been given greater weight in making nutritional recommendations. Higher intakes of some essential nutrients (especially vitamins E and C, which may function as antioxidants) have also been shown to be associated with lower risk of chronic disease or with enhanced immune system function. Recommendations for folic acid intake for women of childbearing age have taken into account the ability of folic acid to reduce the incidence of neural tube defects.

Obviously, any health benefits of nonnutritive food constituents or higher intakes of essential nutrients may depend upon genetic differences among individuals, differences in lifestyle, and diet–genetic interactions that influence expression of genetic traits. With increasing knowledge of differences in genetic makeup of persons and population groups, more attention will likely be given to making nutritional recommendations relative to genetically determined metabolic differences.

USE OF NUTRIENTS AS PHARMACOLOGICAL AGENTS

Some nutrients or food components, in large doses, may function as drugs. The use of nutrients as pharmacological agents should not be considered under the category of nutrients. Nicotinic acid in large doses (up to 9 g daily) is used to lower serum cholesterol. Tryptophan has been used to induce sleep. The continuous intravenous infusion of magnesium is used in the treatment of preeclampsia and myocardial infarction. Many herbal and natural remedies are based on the use of food components as pharmacological agents.

THINKING CRITICALLY

Concepts of nutrition have clearly changed over the course of history. In the search for essential and beneficial dietary components, it has been necessary to establish definitions and criteria, and these will likely continue to be modified as our understanding and aims related to nutrition and health undergo change.

1. Would use of growth of young mammals or prevention of deficiency diseases as the criterion for establishing requirements or recommended intake levels of essential nutrients necessarily provide a measure of optimal intake? What other types of criteria related to normal physiological processes might be used?
2. What would be the implications of defining all food components that have beneficial effects on health or disease prevention as essential nutrients? What effect would this have on the list of nutrients shown in Box 1-1? Which nutrients for which we currently have recommended intakes fall into the category of beneficial but not essential food components?
3. What is the definition of a conditionally essential nutrient? How would the process of establishing requirements for conditionally essential nutrients differ from the approaches used thus far in establishing nutrient requirements of healthy populations?
4. We are in the early stages of understanding how genetic diversity affects nutritional requirements of the population. For example, it is known that individuals who are homozygous for specific mutations in the gene encoding methyltetrahydrofolate reductase have higher requirements for dietary folate. How do you think the issue of individual variability should be addressed in setting recommended dietary intakes for the population in the future?

REFERENCES

Bishai, D., & Nalubola, R. (2002). The history of food fortification in the United States: Its relevance for current fortification efforts in developing countries. *Economic Development and Cultural Change*, *51*, 37–63.

Block, R. J., & Mitchell, H. H. (1946). The correlation of the amino-acid composition of proteins with their nutritive value. *Nutrition Abstracts and Reviews*, *16*, 249–278.

Burr, G. O., & Burr, M. M. (1929). A new deficiency disease produced by the rigid exclusion of fat from the diet. *The Journal of Biological Chemistry*, *82*, 345–367.

Burr, G. O., & Burr, M. M. (1930). The nature and role of the fatty acids essential in nutrition. *The Journal of Biological Chemistry*, *86*, 587–621.

Carpenter, K. J. (1986). *The history of scurvy and vitamin C*. New York: Cambridge University Press.

Carpenter, K. J. (2003a). A short history of nutritional science: Part 1 (1785-1885). *The Journal of Nutrition*, *133*, 638–645.

Carpenter, K. J. (2003b). A short history of nutritional science: Part 2 (1885-1912). *The Journal of Nutrition*, *133*, 975–984.

Carpenter, K. J. (2003c). A short history of nutritional science: Part 3 (1912-1944). *The Journal of Nutrition*, *133*, 3023–3032.

Carpenter, K. J. (2003d). A short history of nutritional science: Part 4 (1945-1985). *The Journal of Nutrition*, *133*, 3331–3342.

Carpenter, K. J., & Sutherland, B. (1995). Eijkman's contribution to the discovery of vitamins. *The Journal of Nutrition*, *125*, 155–163.

Carpenter, K. J., Harper, A. E., & Olson, R. E. (1997). Experiments that changed nutritional thinking. *The Journal of Nutrition*, *127*, S1017–S1053.

Harper, A. E. (1999). Defining the essentiality of nutrients. In M. E. Shils, J. A. Olson, M. Shike, & A. C. Ross (Eds.), *Modern nutrition in health and disease* (9th ed, pp. 3–10). Baltimore: Williams & Wilkins.

Hart, E. B., McCollum, E. V., Steenbock, H., & Humphrey, G. C. (1911). Physiological effect on growth and reproduction of rations balanced from restricted sources. *University of Wisconsin Agricultural Experiment Station Research Bulletin*, *17*, 131–205.

Henriques, V., & Hansen, C. (1905). Über Eiweis-synthese im Tierkörper. *Hoppe-Seyler's Zeitschrift für Physiologische Chemie*, *43*, 417–446.

Holman, R. T. (1988). George O. Burr and the discovery of essential fatty acids. *The Journal of Nutrition*, *118*, 535–540.

Jansen, B. C. P. (1956). Early nutrition researches on beriberi leading to the discovery of vitamin B1. *Nutrition Abstracts and Reviews*, *26*, 1–14.

McCay, C. M., Maynard, L. A., Sperling, G., & Barnes, L. L. (1939). Retarded growth, life span, ultimate body size and age changes in the albino rat after feeding diets restricted in calories. *The Journal of Nutrition*, *18*, 1–13.

McCollum, E. V. (1957). *A history of nutrition: The sequence of ideas in nutrition investigations*. Boston: Houghton-Mifflin.

McCoy, R. H., Meyer, C. E., & Rose, W. C. (1935). Feeding experiments with mixtures of highly purified amino acids: VIII. Isolation and identification of a new essential amino acid. *The Journal of Biological Chemistry*, *112*, 283–302.

Mertz, W. (1981). The essential trace elements. *Science*, *213*, 1332–1338.

Mertz, W. (1993). Essential trace metals: New definitions based on new paradigms. *Nutrition Reviews*, *51*, 287–295.

Nielsen, F. H. (2000). Importance of making dietary recommendations for elements designated as nutritionally beneficial, pharmacologically beneficial, or conditionally essential. *The Journal of Trace Elements in Experimental Medicine*, *13*, 113–129.

Osborne, T., & Mendel, L. B. (1911). *Feeding experiments with isolated food substances*. Washington, DC: Carnegie Institution of Washington, Publication no. 156.

Osborne, T., & Mendel, L. B. (1914). Amino-acids in nutrition and growth. *The Journal of Biological Chemistry*, *17*, 325–349.

Rose, W. C. (1931). Feeding experiments with mixtures of highly purified amino acids: I. The inadequacy of diets containing nineteen amino acids. *The Journal of Biological Chemistry*, *94*, 155–165.

Rosenfeld, L. (1997). Vitamine-vitamin. The early years of discovery. *Clinical Chemistry*, *43*, 680–685.

Rudman, D., & Feller, A. (1986). Evidence for deficiencies of conditionally essential nutrients during total parenteral nutrition. *Journal of the American College of Nutrition*, *5*, 101–106.

Schultze, M. O. (1957). Nutrition of rats with compounds of known chemical structure. *The Journal of Nutrition*, *61*, 585–595.

Takaki, K. (1906). Three lectures on the preservation of health amongst the personnel of the Japanese navy and army. *Lancet*, *1*(1369), 1451–1520.

Wilkinson, D. J. (2004). The contributions of Lavoisier, Scheele and Priestley to the early understanding of respiratory physiology in the eighteenth century. *Resuscitation*, *61*, 249–255.

Willcock, E. G., & Hopkins, F. G. (1906). The importance of individual amino acids in metabolism. *The Journal of Physiology*, *35*, 88–102.

Wolf, G., & Carpenter, K. J. (1997). Early research into the vitamins: The work of Wilhelm Stepp. *The Journal of Nutrition*, 127, 1255–1259.

RECOMMENDED READING

Carpenter, K. J., Harper, A. E., & Olson, R. E. (1997). Experiments that changed nutritional thinking. *The Journal of Nutrition*, *127*, S1017–S1053.

CHAPTER 2

Food Components with Health Benefits

Elizabeth H. Jeffery, PhD; Kelly A. Tappenden, RD, PhD; and Anna-Sigrid Keck, PhD, CIP

COMMON ABBREVIATIONS

ALA	α-linolenic acid
CLA	conjugated linoleic acid
CVD	cardiovascular disease
DHA	docosahexaenoic acid
EPA	eicosapentaenoic acid
FDA	U.S. Food and Drug Administration
GRAS	generally recognized as safe
ROS	reactive oxygen species
SCFA	short-chain fatty acid
USDA	U.S. Department of Agriculture

One of the most rapidly moving, exciting areas in nutrition research today is the study of foods and food components that decrease risk for chronic diseases, including cardiovascular disease (CVD), chronic inflammatory diseases, and cancer. Food components for which there is emerging or strong scientific evidence suggesting health benefits beyond basic nutrition are discussed in this chapter. In general, these food components are not essential for growth and development as are the essential nutrients, but it should be noted that some essential nutrients can also have beneficial effects on chronic diseases, albeit often at exposure levels greater than what is provided in normal diets. Discovery of bioactive food components that provide health benefits may prove to be as important to good nutrition as the discovery of vitamins and minerals in the last century. Epidemiological studies comparing diet and disease incidence have identified foods—including certain fruits, vegetables, whole grains, and fatty fish—that provide these health benefits. Food choices can greatly influence our risk for chronic disease.

FUNCTIONAL FOODS AND DIETARY SUPPLEMENTS

Many bioactive food components have been purified and characterized chemically (Figure 2-1). When studied in purified form, most of these compounds exhibit specific biochemical actions, giving rise to the term *nutraceutical,* which derives from the idea of a "druglike" nutrient or food component. However, although the study of purified components is frequently used to study mechanism, studies with purified components do not always reflect the full physiological effect of a whole food within the diet (Canene-Adams et al., 2007). This may be due to the presence of multiple compounds in a single food, or the bioavailability of the compound when it is provided as a purified component may be very different than when it is provided within its original food matrix.

DEFINITIONS OF FUNCTIONAL FOODS AND DIETARY SUPPLEMENTS

Foods rich in bioactive food components have been termed functional foods. Although there is no universally accepted definition of a functional food, the International Food Information Council Foundation defines functional foods as those foods that provide health benefits beyond basic nutrition (*www.foodinsight.org/Resources/Detail.aspx?topic=Background_on_Functional_Foods*). The content of bioactive components in a given food varies with genotype of the plant or animal and the growing, storage, and processing conditions. Extracts or concentrates sold as dietary supplements may be labeled with analytical information, but such labeling is not currently required. Supplements are typically advertised to "maintain health," such as normalizing blood pressure, whereas researchers more typically use the term *disease prevention* to describe the same action.

Use of the term *dietary disease prevention* is not limited to maintenance of health but may also refer to the prevention of disease recurrence following successful therapy or the prevention of chronic disease progression, such as bone loss or growth of slow-growing tumors (Mehta et al., 2010). For example, research suggests a possible role for green tea components in slowing increases in white blood cell count in chronic lymphocytic leukemia (Zhang et al., 2008) and a role for tomatoes in slowing increases in prostate-specific antibody, a biomarker for slow-growing prostate cancer (Bowen et al., 2002). Of course for diseases that are aggravated by poor food choices, other aspects of the diet should also be addressed.

Dietary disease prevention does not include active treatment of disease. Once a drug therapy or treatment is initiated, the patient should consult closely with the physician about any supplement use, because bioactive food components can alter drug efficacy. For example, bioactive food components may enhance glutathione synthesis and

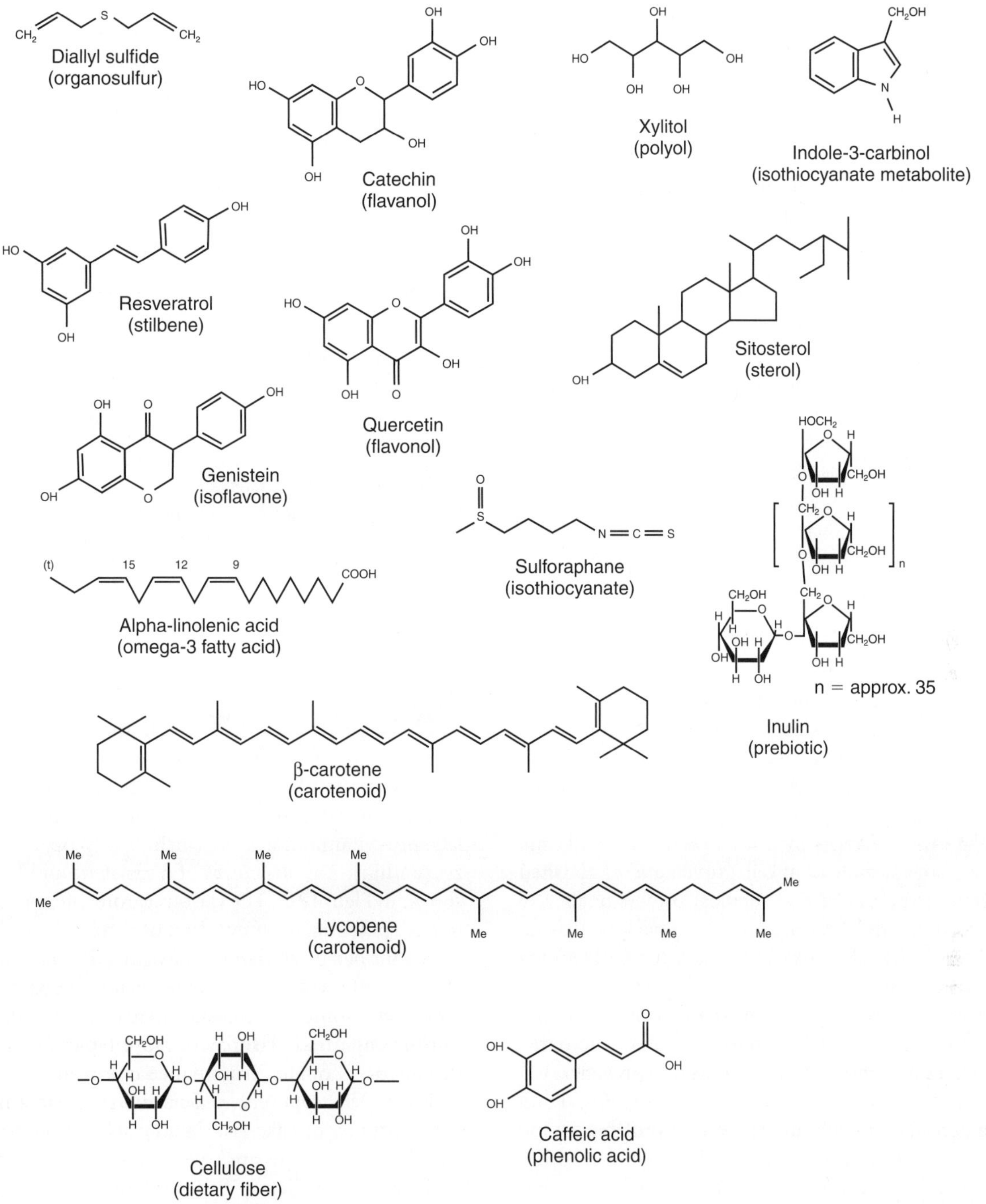

Diallyl sulfide (organosulfur)
Catechin (flavanol)
Xylitol (polyol)
Indole-3-carbinol (isothiocyanate metabolite)
Resveratrol (stilbene)
Quercetin (flavonol)
Sitosterol (sterol)
Genistein (isoflavone)
Sulforaphane (isothiocyanate)
Inulin (prebiotic)
n = approx. 35
Alpha-linolenic acid (omega-3 fatty acid)
β-carotene (carotenoid)
Lycopene (carotenoid)
Cellulose (dietary fiber)
Caffeic acid (phenolic acid)

FIGURE 2-1 Examples of nonessential bioactive food components.

upregulate detoxification enzymes, resulting in rapid clearance of drugs and limiting their intended action.

REGULATIONS AFFECTING DIETARY SUPPLEMENTS

The Dietary Supplement Health and Education Act (DSHEA), passed by the U.S. Congress in 1994, defined dietary supplements as "products that are intended to supplement the diet, and that contain one or more of the following: vitamins, minerals, herbs or other botanicals, amino acids, or other dietary substance for use by man to supplement the diet by increasing the total dietary intake, or concentrates, metabolites, constituents, extracts, or combinations of these ingredients." The DSHEA regulates dietary supplements as foods, thereby distinguishing between dietary supplements aimed to "supplement one's diet" and drugs that are to "treat, mitigate or prevent a disease." Despite these definitions, there is a fine legal line between the physiological activity of a bioactive food component within a dietary supplement and the pharmacological effects of a drug. A key practical difference between drugs and dietary supplements is that drugs must pass through safety and efficacy evaluation, tightly regulated by the U.S. Food and Drug Administration (FDA), before appearing on the market, whereas dietary supplements are not required to undergo formal safety or efficacy evaluation. The safety of dietary supplements is regulated by the FDA only after they have entered the market. DSHEA states that a dietary supplement is "adulterated" only if it presents "a significant or unreasonable risk of illness or injury" under normal conditions of use.

The FDA allows manufacturers of dietary supplements to state health claims and qualified health claims for their products based on the same approval process required for health claims on conventional foods (see Chapter 3 for further explanation of these claims). In addition, under provisions of the DSHEA, dietary supplements may also carry "structure/function" claims that have not been preapproved by the FDA. Because conventional foods are now allowed to carry these structure/function claims, some foods are also marketed as dietary supplements. However, foods may be marketed as dietary supplements only if it is not a product designed to substitute for a food in a meal rather than being used to supplement the diet. For example, a spread that is used in place of butter could not be marketed as a dietary supplement.

THE NEED FOR SURROGATE ENDPOINT BIOMARKERS OF EFFICACY

For the disease prevention field to move forward, there is a dire need for accurate surrogate endpoint biomarkers of efficacy of foods or bioactive food components in disease prevention in humans. A useful biomarker should be closely linked to the progressive pathway for the disease and correlate with changes in risk (Bowen, 2005). Plasma cholesterol is an example of a well-proven and established biomarker that the public and medical professionals rely on to understand the health status of a person. Plasma cholesterol is a reversible measure of risk for CVD and is used by science researchers for testing hypotheses, as well as by consumers monitoring the impact of a change in diet on risk factors for CVD. Cholesterol and other biomarkers have aided the identification of foods that prevent CVD (Figure 2-2).

On the other hand, tools are not readily available for the assessment of risk for cancer, inflammation, and many other chronic diseases. One potential biomarker of hormone-dependent cancer risk in women is the pattern of urinary estrogen metabolites, which is altered by indole-3-carbinol from cruciferous vegetables. Although the mechanism is still under study, increased levels of urinary 2-hydroxyestradiol correlate with a lower risk for breast and uterine cancer. Chronic inflammation, often as a result of obesity, increases risk for many chronic diseases, including cancer. Bioactive food components decrease inflammation via multiple mechanisms, including activation of the transcription factor Nrf2 and epigenetic regulation of gene expression (Thimmulappa et al., 2006; Szarc vel Szic et al., 2010; Kim et al., 2009; Figure 2-3). Research, followed by public education, is needed to develop robust biomarkers in humans for use by consumers and medical professionals in evaluating the impact of diet on disease prevention.

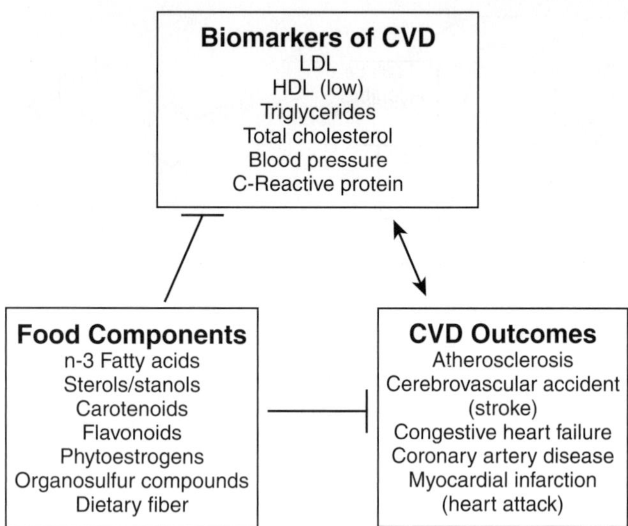

FIGURE 2-2 Cardioprotective food components. Many foods and food components decrease risk for cardiovascular disease (CVD). Impact of diet can be followed by observing the normalization of one or more biomarkers of risk for CVD. For mechanisms, see text for the individual components. *HDL*, High-density lipoprotein; *LDL*, low-density lipoprotein.

CAROTENOIDS

The family of tetraterpenes, or carotenoids, contains both vitamin A precursors (α- and β-carotene and β-cryptoxanthin) and a number of other compounds that lack pro–vitamin A activity (including lycopene, lutein, and zeaxanthin). The structures of β-carotene and lycopene are shown in Figure 2-1. The various carotenoids are considered to have potential for prevention of chronic disease.

A number of epidemiological studies have found correlations of plasma β-carotene with reduced disease risk. However, some β-carotene intervention studies have found enhanced risk with supplementation. Several explanations of the discordance of research findings are possible. The apparent association of plasma β-carotene with reduced disease risk in the epidemiological studies could be simply because the plasma β-carotene level is an indicator of dietary fruit and vegetable intake. Exposure to other common plant food components such as fiber or other phytonutrients could be responsible for the health benefits. On the other hand, the adverse effects of β-carotene supplementation may be related to total dose or exposure. The β-Carotene and Retinol Efficacy Trial (CARET) reported plasma β-carotene levels of about 2 to 6 μmol/L and the Alpha-Tocopherol, Beta-Carotene Cancer Prevention (ATBC) Trial produced levels of about 4 to 8 μmol/L (Erdman et al., 2010; Greenwald, 2002); both of these studies showed adverse effects. In contrast, the Linxian trial and the Physicians' Health Study, which yielded plasma β-carotene levels of about 2 μmol/L or less, did not show adverse effects. Nonsupplemented individuals typically have plasma β-carotene levels of less than 1 μmol/L. Another potential

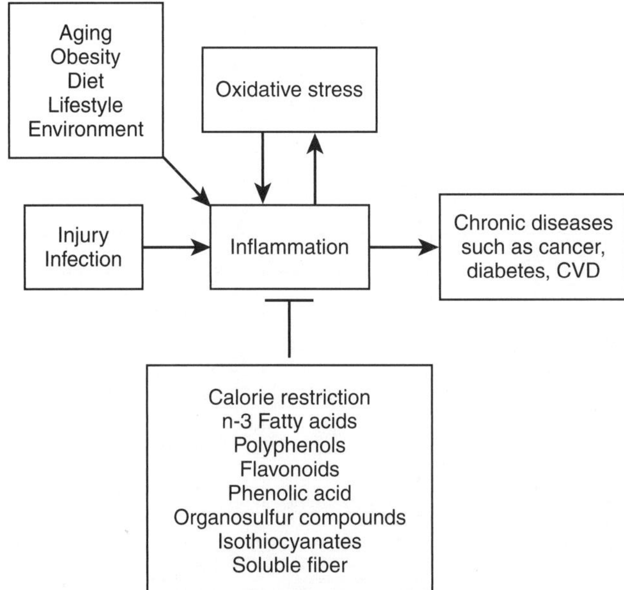

FIGURE 2-3 Antiinflammatory food components. Many foods and food components decrease chronic inflammation, slowing or inhibiting inflammation-enhanced chronic diseases such as cancer and cardiovascular diseases (CVD). For mechanisms, see text for the individual components.

explanation might be that high intakes of β-carotene adversely affect intakes of other lipid-soluble nutrients, but this does not appear to be the case. Plasma lycopene, lutein, zeaxanthin, retinol, and α-tocopherol were unaffected by a tenfold increase in plasma β-carotene (Mayne et al., 1998). The unanticipated outcomes of the β-carotene intervention trials is a reminder that whole foods and food components are not the same thing, that associations do not imply a causal relationship, and that dose or exposure matters.

Lycopene accumulates preferentially in a few tissues, including prostate. Evidence is accumulating that tomatoes and tomato products rich in lycopene may slow or prevent prostate cancer. There is a qualified health claim associated with lycopene and prostate health (Fleshner and Zlotta, 2007). It remains to be determined if lycopene is effective alone, or possibly requires other components from tomatoes (Canene-Adams et al., 2007). In plasma, lycopene is mostly associated with low-density lipoproteins (LDLs), whereas lutein and zeaxanthin binding is shifted toward high-density lipoproteins (HDLs) (Carroll et al., 2000). In the U.S. population, lycopene is the predominant plasma carotenoid.

Lutein and zeaxanthin, but not other carotenoids, accumulate in the macula lutea region of the retina, where they may act as photoprotectors, inhibiting ultraviolet (UV)-induced oxidative damage. One study found a greatly reduced incidence of macular degeneration in those individuals with plasma lutein/zeaxanthin levels in the highest quartile (Bone et al., 2001). The Carotenoids in Age-Related Eye Disease Study (CAREDS) found that lutein and zeaxanthin may protect against macular degeneration in women less than 75 years of age (Seddon et al., 1994; Bone et al., 2001).

Until further studies on safety are conducted, foods rich in carotenoids, such as spinach and corn, may provide a safer alternative to taking purified dietary supplements. Five servings of fruits and vegetables a day contain about 6 mg of carotenoids (Ghiselli et al., 1997), which is considered sufficient to provide any possible carotenoid-related health benefits in preventing chronic disease. A typical Western diet contains about 6 mg/day of carotenoids, but about 60% of this is derived from animal sources, which are lower in lutein and zeaxanthin than fruits and vegetables. Good dietary sources of all carotenoids are yellow and orange fruits and vegetables and dark green leafy vegetables. Tomatoes and watermelon are good sources of lycopene. Spinach is a good source of lutein and zeaxanthin as are marigold petals, which are used as a source of these carotenoids for dietary supplements. Bioavailability of all carotenoids is enhanced by the presence of fat in the diet because carotenoids are fat soluble.

POLYUNSATURATED FATTY ACIDS

Polyunsaturated fatty acids (PUFAs) are essential components of our diets as both n-3 and n-6 PUFAs are required for growth, reproduction, and prevention of deficiency diseases (see Chapter 18). Certain n-3 PUFAs have been identified as possibly lowering the risk for chronic disease (Ruxton et al., 2007), and conjugated linoleic acids (CLAs) may also provide health benefits beyond basic nutrition (Bhattacharya et al., 2006). (See Chapter 6 for information about fatty acid structure and nomenclature.)

The n-3 fatty acids include α-linolenic acid (C18:3, or ALA), eicosapentaenoic acid (C20:5, or EPA), and docosahexaenoic acid (C22:6, or DHA). ALA is present in plant-based food products such as canola oil, flaxseed, and walnuts (Table 2-1). ALA can serve as a precursor to EPA and DHA, but humans metabolize only about 10% of dietary ALA to EPA and DHA. In the United States, typical intake of ALA is much higher than that of EPA and DHA, unless the diet is supplemented with a good source of the C20 and C22 n-3 fatty acids such as wild-caught (not farmed) oily fish and fish products or fish oil capsules. Cow's milk may also contain EPA and DHA, depending on bovine genotype and diet. In Iceland, where cows are fed diets that include fish oils, cow's milk is an excellent source of EPA (Thorsdottir et al., 2004).

Studies suggest that consumption of fish and fish products rich in n-3 PUFAs may provide protection against CVD, cataracts, depression, immune function diseases, and cancer. The strongest association between disease prevention and dietary n-3 PUFAs is for reduction in risk for CVD. A 30-year study of middle-aged men showed an inverse relationship between fish consumption and death from CVD (Daviglus et al., 1997). In the Lyon Diet Heart Study, adults consuming a "Mediterranean" diet high in

TABLE 2-1 Abundant Dietary Sources of the n-3 Fatty Acids ALA, DHA, and EPA

FOOD	ALA (g/TBSP)	EPA AND DHA (g/3 OZ* OR g/TBSP OIL)	AMOUNT OF FOOD THAT PROVIDES ~1 g OF n-3 FATTY ACIDS
Tuna, light, canned in water, drained		0.23	12 oz
Tuna, white, canned in water, drained		0.73	4 oz
Salmon, pink		0.86	3.5 oz
Salmon, Atlantic, farmed		1.62-1.83	1.5-2 oz
Salmon, Atlantic, wild		1.22-1.56	2-2.5 oz
Herring, Pacific		1.41-1.81	1.5-2 oz
Trout, rainbow, farmed		0.79-0.98	3-4 oz
Cod, Pacific		0.18-0.24	12.5-16.5 oz
Shrimp, mixed species		0.46	6 oz
Fish oil, cod liver		2.43	5.6 oz
Fish oil, salmon		4.25	3.2 oz
Canola oil	1.30		10.6 g
Flaxseeds	2.18		5.5 g
Flaxseed oil	7.25		1.9 g
Olive oil, salad or cooking	0.11		126.3 g
Soybean oil, salad or cooking	0.93		14.7 g
Walnuts, English	0.71		11.0 g

Data from U.S. Department of Agriculture, Agricultural Research Service. (2010). *USDA National Nutrient Database for Standard Reference, Release 23.* Retrieved from www.ars.usda.gov/ba/bhnrc.ndl
ALA, α-Linolenic acid; *DHA*, docosahexaenoic acid; *EPA*, eicosapentaenoic acid.
*1 oz = 28.3 g

canola and olive oils had significantly lower blood cholesterol and triglyceride levels, higher HDL cholesterol level, and a 70% reduction in coronary events and cardiac deaths compared to the control group that consumed a normal American diet low in ALA (de Lorgeril et al., 1999). A recent systematic review of the evidence concludes that there is moderate evidence for a relationship between protection against CVD and intake of fish or n-3 PUFAs (Mente et al., 2009).

The n-3 PUFAs may also protect against a number of other chronic diseases. For example, changes in mental health may correlate with low dietary intake of n-3 PUFAs, including incidence of depression, although more studies are needed to clarify this (Hallahan and Garland, 2005; Sinn et al., 2010). Inflammatory conditions, including asthma and inflammatory bowel disease, may be abated or prevented by consumption of fish, but there are insufficient data to support a recommendation for the use of EPA/DHA for these purposes (Chapkin et al., 2009). Similarly, although cell culture studies support a role for n-3 PUFAs in prevention of prostate cancer, this is not supported by clinical findings (Kristal et al., 2010).

The health benefit of dietary n-3 PUFAs may depend not only on the amount in the diet but also on the ratio of n-6 to n-3 PUFAs. Between a 5:1 and 1.8:1 ratio of n-6 to n-3 PUFAs was associated with a decreased risk for colon cancer (Roynette et al., 2004; Simonsen et al., 1998). A typical American diet provides more n-6 PUFAs than n-3 PUFAs, with a typical ratio of n-6 to n-3 greater than 10:1. This is due to the high seed oil content in the U.S. diet; the ratio of n-6 to n-3 PUFAs in corn oil is 46:1, and it is 7:1 in soy oil. One possible explanation for the importance of this ratio from a health perspective is competition between substrates for enzymes involved in prostaglandin synthesis. For example, dietary linoleic acid is a precursor of arachidonic acid, the n-6 C20 PUFA that serves as substrate for prostaglandin E_2 synthesis. Linoleic acid, the n-6 precursor of arachidonic acid, has been associated with stimulation of tumor growth, whereas the n-3 EPA is metabolized to prostaglandin E_3, a compound shown to lower tumor growth in vitro.

Further research is needed to reach significant scientific agreement about the balance of positive and negative health effects from dietary fish or other sources of n-3 PUFAs. The American Heart Association recommends consuming fish rich in n-3 PUFAs twice a week and choosing oils and foods that are rich in ALA (American Heart Association, 2010). Concerns over heavy metal and toxin contamination of wild fish caution against recommending a higher intake of fish. Some species of wild fish may contain high levels of environmental contaminants, including methyl mercury, dioxins, and polychlorinated biphenyls. Levels of these substances are low in fresh and sea waters, but they accumulate in the food chain; hence bigger and older fish contain the highest levels. In the United States, the Environmental Protection Agency and the FDA are responsible for sport-caught fish and commercial fish, respectively. These federal agencies provide consumer information on mercury levels in fish.

CLAs are isomeric forms of linoleic acid (C18:2n-6) with the double bonds separated by one single bond, which adds unique properties to the molecule. CLAs are produced both in the rumen of ruminant animals and in the mammary gland from unsaturated C18 precursor fatty acids; CLAs constitute about 0.5% of the fatty acid content of foods of ruminant origin, with the most abundant CLA being the *cis* 9, *trans* 11 isomer. Major dietary sources of CLAs are dairy products and beef fat.

There is some evidence suggesting that CLAs protect against CVD and certain cancers. CLAs may lower the risk for atherosclerosis by altering the metabolism of very-low-density lipoprotein cholesterol (McLeod et al., 2004). Protection against cancer by CLAs has been reported in animal models, but clinical studies are not definitive (Bhattacharya et al., 2006; Voorrips et al., 2002).

It should be noted that these naturally occurring CLA with *trans* bonds are very different than the *trans* isomers of fatty acids that are formed as a result of hydrogenation or partial hydrogenation of vegetable oils. Although there are limited data in humans, the intake of *trans* fatty acids in hydrogenated fats has been suggested to increase LDL cholesterol, decrease HDL cholesterol, and promote both CVD and cancer growth (de Roos et al., 2003; Benatar, 2010).

PLANT STEROLS/STANOLS

More than 200 sterols and stanols have been identified in plants. The most abundant sterols are β-sitosterol, stigmasterol, and campesterol, whereas the most abundant stanols are sitostanol and campestanol (Moreau et al., 2002). Sterols are essential components of cell membranes. All sterols contain the sterol ring structure but differ in the side chain (see structure of sitosterol in Figure 2-1). Stanols are the saturated form of sterols, with no double bond in the sterol ring. The extent of phytosterol absorption from the intestine is 10% to 15% for campesterol and campestanol, 4% to 7% for sitosterol, and about 1% for sitostanol, compared to 50% for a bolus of cholesterol (Katan et al., 2003). Cholesterol, the most abundant sterol in animals, is not synthesized in plants.

The cholesterol-lowering effect of plant sterols was first identified in the 1950s. Plant stanol and sterol esters lower plasma cholesterol by reducing intestinal cholesterol absorption. More than 50 trials suggest that 1.5 g/day or more of stanol and sterol esters can decrease LDL cholesterol by 10% (Katan et al., 2003). There appears to be little additional benefit from ingesting larger amounts. The addition of stanol or sterol esters is also effective in patients already on a heart-healthy diet or in those taking cholesterol-lowering medications. In one study, the addition of 2.3 g/day of stanol esters to the diet of patients following the National Cholesterol Education Program (NCEP) Step I diet produced an 8% to 11% greater decrease in total cholesterol and a 9% to 14% greater decrease in LDL cholesterol than was observed in control subjects (Hallikainen and Uusitupa, 1999). Many studies have shown that stanols and sterols can provide a further cholesterol-lowering effect in hypercholesterolemic patients taking statin medications. In one such study, intake of 3 g/day of stanol esters resulted in an additional 10% reduction in LDL cholesterol levels compared to statins alone (Blair et al., 2000); this improvement was substantially better than that obtained by doubling the statin dose, which would be expected to decrease plasma LDL cholesterol by an additional 6%.

The American Heart Association currently recommends that hypercholesteremic patients consume plant sterols or stanols in combination with other dietary strategies (e.g., limited intake of saturated fat, *trans*-fatty acids, and cholesterol; intake of more than 10 g/day of viscous fiber) for lowering LDL cholesterol. In 2000 the FDA authorized the use of health claims for the association between plant sterol and stanol esters and reduced risks for CVD. According to the FDA ruling, foods bearing the health claim must contain at least 0.65 g of plant sterol esters or 1.7 g stanol esters per serving, with the assumption that two servings a day would provide an effective amount. Products usually contain the ester forms of sterols and stanols because the esters have a higher lipid solubility and thus are more easily incorporated into foods than free sterols or stanols. The typical Western diet provides 0.15 to 0.40 g/day of plant sterols (~85%) and plant stanols (~15%), mostly from vegetable oils, cereals, vegetables, and fruits. To obtain 1.5 g/day or more of plant stanol and sterol esters in the diet, use of food products containing supplemental sterol or stanol esters, such as a cholesterol-lowering spread containing 1.7 g stanol ester/serving, is necessary.

Emerging evidence indicates that plant sterols and stanols may have other biological roles, including the reduction of various forms of cancer (Jones and AbuMweis, 2009). Mounting evidence indicates that phytosterols inhibit growth of various forms of lung, stomach, ovarian, and breast cancer. Mechanisms identified include inhibition of carcinogen activation, cancer cell growth, angiogenesis, invasion and metastasis, and apoptosis of cancerous cells. Phytosterol consumption may also increase antioxidant enzyme activities and thereby reduce cellular damage induced by oxidative stress.

Plant stanol and sterol esters are considered to be generally recognized as safe (GRAS) by the FDA, and phytosterol ester margarine has been determined to be safe by the Scientific Committee on Foods of the European Union. A meta-analysis of 41 studies led to the conclusion that consumption of phytosterols by healthy humans at the level of 2 g/day is not associated with any major health risks (Katan et al., 2003).

POLYPHENOLICS

Polyphenolics constitute a broad category of secondary plant compounds including simple phenols as well as highly polymerized compounds with molecular masses greater than 30 kDa; the most common forms in food are the flavonoids and phenolic acids. Typically polyphenolics are present in their free (i.e., aglycone) form or as *O*-glycosides (Bravo, 1998). The biological characteristic that brings this broad group of more than 8,000 different compounds together is the hypothesis that the hydroxyl groups might provide reducing power or "antioxidant potential" that might protect the body from oxidative damage due to reactive oxygen species (ROS). This has led to the chemical evaluation of the radical "quenching power" of purified polyphenolics and plant extracts.

FLAVONOIDS

Flavonoids are the most prominent subclass of dietary polyphenolics (Beecher, 2003). Chemically, the flavonoids are low-molecular-weight diphenylpropanes consisting of two aromatic rings joined by a 3-carbon chain that most frequently incorporates oxygen into a cyclic arrangement to form a third interconnecting ring (see catechin, quercetin, and genistein in Figure 2-1). Common flavonoid subclasses are flavones (e.g., apigenin and luteolin), flavonols (e.g., quercetin and kaempferol), isoflavones (e.g., genistein and daidzein), flavanols (e.g., catechins and epigallocatechin gallate), flavanones (e.g., naringenin), and anthocyanidins (e.g., cyanidin and petunidin). Proanthocyanidins, sometimes called tannins, are oligomers or polymers of flavanol units. Flavonoids are present in most plant-based foods, with the majority of dietary flavonoids being derived from teas, berries, other colorful fruit, red wine, and dark chocolate. In addition, flavonoids may be key bioactive components in several herbs used as dietary supplements, such as ginger, licorice, ginseng, kava kava, ginkgo biloba, and St. John's wort.

Flavonoids have been proposed to exert a wide variety of biological activities in humans, including antiinflammatory, antioxidative, antiallergic, and anticarcinogenic activities (Kostyuk and Potapovich, 1998; Guo et al., 2009; Jagtap et al., 2009). Epidemiological studies support a role for flavonoids in prevention of both CVD and cancer (Hertog et al.,

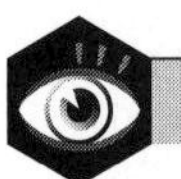

NUTRITION INSIGHT

In Vitro Assessment of Antioxidant Activity

A large number of chronic diseases, including CVD, cancer, diabetes, macular degeneration, Alzheimer disease, arthritis, Parkinson disease, and multiple sclerosis, are considered to be initiated, aggravated, and/or promoted by reactive oxygen species (ROS) and oxidative damage. Epidemiological data show that a diet rich in fruits, vegetables, and whole grains is both rich in polyphenolics and associated with a lower incidence of many of these chronic diseases (Hirvonen et al., 2001; Hollman and Katan, 1999). A possible mechanism for the beneficial effects of polyphenols is their action as antioxidants.

A number of different chemical assays are used to measure radical quenching in vitro. The oxygen radical absorbance capacity (ORAC) assay evaluates the effect of "antioxidant-rich" samples (plant tissue, purified compounds, or even plasma from animals fed antioxidant-rich diets) to inhibit peroxyl radical oxidization of the fluorescent probe, fluorescein (FL) (Prior et al., 2003). Relative activity is compared to that of trolox, a water-soluble analog of α-tocopherol. The major radical quenching compounds in plants are the polyphenolics, shown in the following equations as P-OH.

$$\text{FL-H (reduced; fluorescent)} + \text{ROO}^{\cdot} \rightarrow \text{ROOH} + \text{FL (oxidized; no fluorescence)}$$

$$\text{FL-H} + \text{P-OH} + \text{ROO}^{\cdot} \rightarrow \text{ROOH} + \text{PO} + \text{FL-H (FL-H remains reduced; fluorescent)}$$

A second chemical characteristic of antioxidants is their ability to chelate metals, particularly iron. The Fenton reaction describes how iron reduces peroxide to produce reactive hydroxyl radicals; chelation of iron by an antioxidant inhibits the ROS formation.

$$H_2O_2 + Fe^{2+} \rightarrow OH^{\cdot} + OH^{-} + Fe^{3+}$$

The capacity of a sample or compound to chelate iron and thus prevent oxidation is also often estimated in vitro, through the ferric-reducing antioxidant power (FRAP) assay.

Several other related assays have been developed, notably the trolox equivalent antioxidant capacity (TEAC) assay, commonly used in research at European laboratories. It is very similar to the ORAC assay, except that values are on a very different scale (Aruoma, 2003). Because values for individual bioactive components vary among the assays, only trends can be compared (Proteggente et al., 2002).

What is not clear from the literature is how well the in vitro antioxidant measures (ORAC, TEAC, etc.) reflect health promotion or disease prevention activity. The role of polyphenolics as antioxidants is not well defined, and clinical trial data are inconclusive. Chemical measurements of antioxidant potential do not correlate well with measurement of antioxidant activity within cultured cells (Eberhardt et al., 2005) or plasma (Kris-Etherton et al., 2002). For at least some polyphenolics, other mechanisms such as altered cell signaling or protection from bacterial adhesion may be responsible for the health benefits (Yang and Wang, 2011; Howell, 2002). In other cases, the bioactive substances such as sulforaphane that are not direct-acting antioxidants may upregulate endogenous antioxidant enzymes.

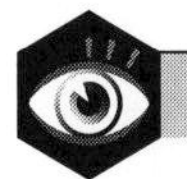

NUTRITION INSIGHT

Synergy

It is common to study a single compound derived from a food to test its bioactivity and mechanism(s) of action. However, a single food contains many nonessential bioactive components that are consumed as a mixture held within the food matrix. To add to this complexity, our diet is made up of many different kinds of foods, which are often ingested simultaneously. These different dietary factors may result in different bioavailabilities and bioactivities compared to those of the individual purified components. Frequently, consumption of the whole food does not have the same effect as the sum of the individual recognized bioactive components within that food. Some components may have additive effects, whereas others may act to enhance, inhibit, mask, or even antagonize the bioactivity of another component.

Synergy occurs when two or more components have a greater effect when given together than can be accounted for by the sum of their individual activities. Synergistic effects may occur between components present in the same food or in different foods or even between a food component and a drug. For example, vitamin C and isoflavones synergistically inhibit LDL-cholesterol oxidation in vitro; green tea and capsicum synergistically exert anticancer effects; curcumin and resveratrol synergistically have an antioxidant effect; and quercetin and catechin synergistically inhibit platelet aggregation (Morre and Morre, 2003; Pignatelli et al., 2000; Aftab and Vieira 2010; Hwang et al., 2000). The overall effect of a combination of whole foods that contain these components, such as orange juice with a soy breakfast bar or green tea with a stir-fry containing peppers, has not been evaluated. One example of synergy of two bioactive components from a single food is the glucosinolate hydrolysis products crambene and indole-3-carbinol from Brussels sprouts. When fed to rodents, crambene and indole-3-carbinol individually and synergistically increased the activity of the anticancer biomarker quinone reductase (Nho and Jeffery, 2001). Not all interactions are synergistic. For example, the probiotic inulin slowed intestinal microbial production of equol from the soy isoflavone daidzein, a negative effect (Zafar et al., 2004). In a recent study broccoli and tomatoes eaten together slowed prostate cancer growth in rats more than the individual foods (52% versus 34% for tomatoes and 42% for broccoli), but the impact was less than additive (Canene-Adams et al., 2007).

The potential benefits of additive or synergistic effects are enormous, and more research needs to focus on the integrated effects of whole foods, or combinations of different foods, and not only on the mechanism of action of single components. The idea of synergy between components in a food provides not only a reason to test the bioactivity of the whole food in addition to that of the individual components but also a rationale to promote the consumption of whole foods as the sources of bioactive components. In addition, foods are less likely to be associated with adverse effects caused by excess intake.

1995). In addition, both clinical and animal studies have suggested an inverse relationship between intake of flavonoids and the incidence of a number of cancers. In a cohort study of 10,000 Finnish men and women, diets that were high in flavonoids (e.g., apples and onions) were associated with a 20% lower incidence of cancer at all sites and a 46% decrease in incidence of lung cancer in particular (Knekt et al., 1997). Animal studies showed a cancer preventive effect of green tea or pure epigallocatechin-3-gallate (Yang et al., 2009). A double blind placebo control study showed that 1 g/day of quercetin for 12 weeks reduced severity of upper respiratory tract infection by 36%, resulting in 31% fewer sick days in a group of middle-aged and older subjects who rated themselves as physically fit (Heinz et al., 2010). Licorice extracts rich in flavonoids may provide protection against peptic ulcer or gastric cancer by inhibiting growth of *Helicobacter pylori* in humans (Fukai et al., 2002).

Whereas free flavonoids can be absorbed across the small intestinal mucosa (Manach et al., 1997), flavonoid glycosides require hydrolysis by digestive enzymes and/or the colonic microbiota to release the flavonoid before it can be absorbed (Hollman and Katan, 1997). After absorption, flavonoids undergo methylation and/or conjugation to glucuronic acid or sulfate before excretion. Conjugates excreted in the bile undergo deconjugation in the gut, catalyzed by gut microbiota, and the flavonoid may be reabsorbed (Manach et al., 1997). Many published studies indicate that flavonoids are only partially absorbed, depending on both the compound and the food matrix. For example, 52% of quercetin in quercetin glycoside from onions was absorbed, whereas only 24% of a pure test sample of free quercetin was absorbed (Hollman and Katan, 1999). Disposition and excretion also depend on both the form of the compound and on other components in the food or meal. For example, tea catechins reached maximum blood levels 2 hours after ingestion of either black or green tea, but green tea catechins were eliminated more rapidly with the half-life for green tea catechins being 4.8 hours compared to 6.9 hours for black tea catechins (van het Hof et al., 1998).

Intake of total flavonoids ranges from about 20 mg/day in the United States, Denmark, and Finland to about 70 mg/day in Holland and Japan (Beecher, 2003). There are two excellent databases of flavonoid content of foods: the USDA Database for the Flavonoid Content of Selected Foods (USDA, 2007) and Phenol-Explorer (Neveu et al., 2010).

Several observations suggest caution in the use of flavonoid supplements. First, as previously seen with β-carotene, flavonoids may act as antioxidants at one dose but as prooxidants at a higher dose (Babich et al., 2008). Second, bioactive food components that are potentially anticarcinogenic in adults may be associated with adverse effects in the developing fetus. For example, pregnant women ingesting unusually large amounts of foods containing topoisomerase II inhibitors, which include flavonoids in soy, coffee, wine, tea, and cocoa, may have a greater risk for giving birth to a child with acute myeloid leukemia (Ross, 1998).

PHENOLIC ACIDS

Phenolic acids, the second largest subclass of polyphenols, are phenols that contain a carboxylic acid group. Phenolic acids can be categorized into one of two groups based on the R group on the carbon ring: hydroxycinnamic acids (cinnamic acid, coumaric acid, ferulic acid, sinapic acid, and caffeic acid) or hydroxybenzoic acids (benzoic acid, salicylic acid, hydroxybenzoic acid, vanillic acid, syringic acid, gallic acid, protocatechuic acid, gentisic acid, and veratric acid). Sometimes the aldehyde analogs (vanillin and syrinaldehyde) are included under hydroxybenzoic acids (Robbins, 2003). The structure of caffeic acid is shown in Figure 2-1.

As for most of the polyphenolics, the primary health benefit of dietary phenolic acids is presently considered to be the provision of "antioxidant capacity" (Morton et al., 2000; Nardini et al., 1997). In addition, hydroxycinnamic acid esters may inhibit 5′-lipoxygenases and thus inhibit the inflammatory process and carcinogenesis (Rao et al., 1993). Both caffeic acid and ellagic acid lowered triglyceride levels, elevated insulin level, and lowered glucose level in the plasma of diabetic mice (Chao et al., 2009); these compounds also lowered the level of ROS, interleukin-6 (IL-6), and tumor necrosis factor-alpha (TNF-α) in cardiac tissue of these animals. Natural caffeic acid derivatives, such as dicaffeoylquinic and dicaffeoyltartaric acids, have been reported to inhibit human immunodeficiency virus type 1 (HIV-1) integrase, the enzyme responsible for integration of viral DNA into the host DNA (Reinke et al., 2004). The phenolic acids found in the serum of rats fed blueberries stimulated osteoblast differentiation, resulting in significantly increased bone mass (Chen et al., 2010). Clinical studies are needed to confirm these effects in humans.

Major dietary sources of phenolic acids include fruits, vegetables, and grains. Coffee is a rich source of caffeic and chlorogenic acids. Human consumption of phenolic acids ranges from 0.025 to 1 g/day, depending on dietary habits (Clifford, 1999), and phenolic acid intake makes up about one third of the total dietary polyphenolic compound intake. Compared to that for flavonoids, little information is available about the bioavailability and metabolism of phenolic acids (Lafay and Gil-Izquierdo, 2008).

There are few reports of adverse effects of phenolic acids in the literature. However, studies of bioactive components are sufficiently incomplete that lack of reported adverse effects cannot be interpreted to mean lack of actual adverse effects. Until sufficient research has been carried out, we cannot know the extent to which these compounds, at various doses, are healthful and/or unsafe.

PHYTOESTROGENS

Dietary phytoestrogens are plant-derived dietary components that structurally and functionally mimic the effects of the hormone estrogen and its metabolites. The major dietary phytoestrogens belong to four subclasses of the polyphenolics: isoflavonoid coumestans (e.g., coumestrol and 4′-methoxycoumestrol), isoflavones (e.g., daidzein and genistein), lignans (e.g., secoisolariciresinol and enterolactone), and stilbenes (e.g., resveratrol) (see structures of genistein and resveratrol in Figure 2-1 and classes of polyphenols in Figure 2-4). Phytoestrogens are present in many common botanicals sold as dietary supplements; they include flavonoids in licorice, isoflavones and lignans in kudzu and soy, isoflavones and coumestans in red clover, and unidentified phytoestrogens in saw palmetto and bloodroot (Ososki and Kennelly, 2003). These polyphenolic compounds, like estrogen, are composed of a planar aromatic ring system (one to three rings) with one or more hydroxyl groups. A chemically, mechanistically, and phylogenetically separate phytoestrogen is indole-3-carbinol (see Figure 2-1), which is an isothiocyanate from cruciferous vegetables. Indole-3-carbinol is not an estrogen mimic, but it alters estrogen metabolism.

The normal roles of estrogens in the body include growth, function of reproductive organs, maintenance of the integrity of the skeleton and central nervous system, and other functions (Ososki and Kennelly, 2003). In part, because phytoestrogens mimic the effect of estrogens (but with lower potency) they are proposed to favorably affect hormone-dependent cancers, menopausal symptoms, glycemic control, and weight maintenance; to decrease thrombus formation and platelet aggregation; and to lower plasma levels of triglycerides, LDL cholesterol, and total cholesterol (Cederroth and Nef, 2009). Many of the current results must be carefully interpreted, and additional studies are needed before general conclusions and recommendations can be finalized.

With particular regard to cancer, whether phytoestrogens diminish or enhance cancer growth is controversial. One possibility is that the effect varies, depending upon a woman's estrogen status. Phytoestrogens are weak agonists, binding to the estrogen receptor (with a greater affinity for the β-receptor than the α-receptor). Therefore they diminish estrogen binding and thus work as antiestrogens in the presence of estrogen, but they bind receptors and promote estrogen receptor signaling in the absence of estrogen. Thus the effect of phytoestrogens would be expected to differ in premenopausal and postmenopausal women. The strongest evidence for breast cancer prevention by soy isoflavones is related to consumption in adolescents, in whom endogenous estrogen production is high (Peeters et al., 2003). Another possibility is that the effect of phytoestrogens varies with the microbial flora. Some studies suggest that cancer prevention is greatest in individuals who support an intestinal microbiota that metabolizes daidzein to the metabolite equol, which binds with greater affinity to estrogen receptors and also has very high antioxidant activity. Protection seems to be reduced in individuals with lower intestinal levels of equol, but more data are needed to confirm this finding (Nagata, 2010).

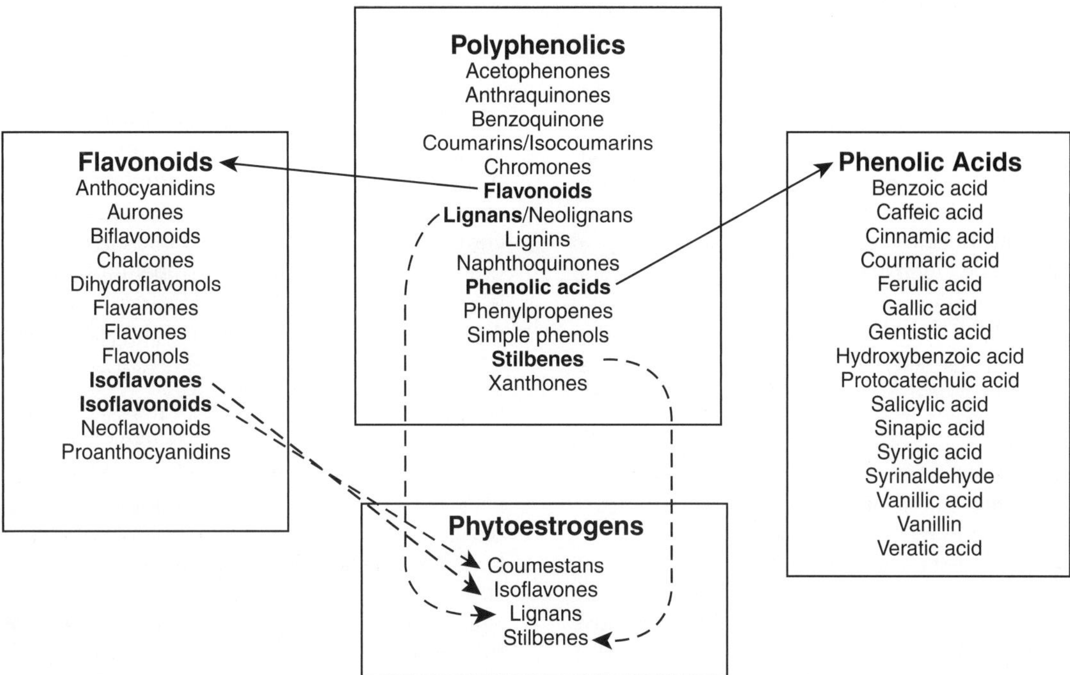

FIGURE 2-4 Polyphenolics and key subclasses. Flavonoids and phenolic acids are the two major subclasses, making up greater than 90% of polyphenolics. Solid lines indicate further classification of these two major subclasses. Bold font for subclass members with dotted lines leading to the Phytoestrogen box indicate that some compounds in these subclasses are also phytoestrogens. The coumestans are derivatives of isoflavonoids.

Extracts, concentrates, and semipurified phytoestrogens from a wide variety of herbs are now on the market, targeted toward postmenopausal women, with no safety information available. Commonly, phytoestrogens are recommended as an alternative to hormone replacement therapy based on the idea that these less potent estrogens may decrease menopausal symptoms, such as hot flashes, while exerting fewer side effects. To date there is little evidence of efficacy or safety. Because bone turnover is under the control of estrogen, phytoestrogens have also been proposed to decrease postmenopausal bone loss, but this remains controversial.

There is concern about the potential for dietary isoflavones to interact with current breast cancer therapies. For example, dietary genistein negated the beneficial effects of tamoxifen on growth of estrogen-dependent breast tumors in vivo (Ju et al., 2002). Concentrates and extracts may contain unnaturally high levels of these bioactive compounds. Because growth of many cancers is enhanced by steroid hormones, it is imperative that more studies be done, using a variety of animal models, to determine the safety of these products. Some animal studies indicate that the effects of purified phytoestrogens in the body may be very different from phytoestrogens within whole food. When ovariectomized mice with estrogen-dependent tumor xenografts were given soy protein isolates enriched in phytoestrogens or purified phytoestrogens, the mice exhibited increased tumor growth, whereas dietary whole soy flour did not support growth of these mammary tumors (Allred et al., 2004).

Legume-containing foods, especially soy products, are high in isoflavones (e.g., up to ~68 mg/100 g wet weight in tofu) and coumestans (e.g., up to ~7 mg/100 g dry weight in soybean sprouts) (Cornwell et al., 2004). In 1999, with more than 30 clinical trials as supporting material, the FDA reviewed and approved a health claim for maintenance of cardiovascular health from foods containing 6.25 g soy flour per serving, with the understanding that four servings per day would reach an effective dose of 25 g soy flour. The benefits of soy could be related to its content of various phytoestrogens such as daidzein and genistein. Wine, grapes, and peanuts are major dietary sources of resveratrol (30 to 1,450 μg/100 mL, 3 to 980 μg/100 g, and 16 to 300 μg/100 g wet weight, respectively). Flax seed, whole grain products, vegetables, and tea are major dietary sources of lignans (up to 370 mg/100 g dry weight).

Indole-3-carbinol, a structurally distinct phytoestrogen, increases estrogenicity via a different mechanism. The acid condensate of indole-3-carbinol, 3,3′-diindolylmethane, potently binds to the aryl hydrocarbon receptor, which then travels to the nucleus to upregulate expression of cytochrome P450 1A1/2, an enzyme intricately involved in endogenous estrogen metabolism (Horn et al., 2002). Upregulation of cytochrome P450 1A1/2 shifts levels of urinary estrogen metabolites to more 2-hydroxyestradiol and less 16α-hydroxyestradiol and estrone, suggesting indole-3-carbinol may act by shifting estrogen metabolism toward formation of the less estrogenic metabolite. The 2-hydroxy metabolites are less estrogenic, and both animal and clinical trials show a decrease in precancerous lesions with intake of 200 or 400 mg per day of indole-3-carbinol (Bradlow et al., 1999). Indole-3-carbinol and its derivatives may also act by interfering with phosphorylation of the estrogen receptor, lowering the estrogenic response (Wang et al., 2006).

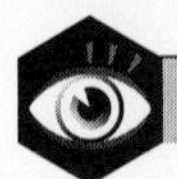

NUTRITION INSIGHT

Safety of Dietary Supplements

Because the concentrations of bioactive components in herbs, spices, and botanical supplements are often much higher than in fruits or vegetables, even small servings of these items may have profound physiological effects. Information on health benefits of herbs, spices, and botanical supplements can be found in various review articles (Craig, 1999; Bent and Ko, 2004; Lampe, 2003; Sparreboom et al., 2004; Wargovich et al., 2001). Interest in herbal supplements has greatly increased in recent years (Sparreboom et al., 2004). The top-selling herbal supplements in the United States according to the market report in 2007 were garlic, echinacea, saw palmetto, ginkgo, cranberry, soy isoflavones, ginseng, black cohosh, St. John's wort, and milk thistle. There is a general lack of data showing efficacy or safety of many dietary supplements.

The FDA may only ban a product that is shown to pose a "significant or unreasonable risk of illness or injury," but proof of risk for harm is difficult to obtain because the manufacturer is not required to disclose any details and the FDA's budget does not support basic research into safety. It took many years and a report contracted by the National Institutes of Health before sufficient data were accumulated for the FDA to successfully ban ephedra-containing products, even though circumstantial evidence had long connected several fatalities to use of these supplements (Shekelle et al., 2003). Almost immediately after the ban was instituted, supplements containing citrus aurantium (bitter orange) came onto the market. The safety of this herbal product is not known in detail, but the active principal, synephrine, is closely related to ephedrine, the active ingredient in ephedra (Fugh-Berman and Myers, 2004).

A second area of safety concern is the interaction between prescription drugs and herbal products, which may enhance or decrease the therapeutic effect of the drug or even cause new side effects (Sparreboom et al., 2004). The most common interactions are related to changed levels of detoxification enzymes, particularly cytochrome P450 3A4, which is responsible for metabolism of most cancer drugs (Sparreboom et al., 2004). Elevated cytochrome P450 activities can lead to more rapid clearance of drugs, hence lowering the therapeutic effects. For example, echinacea taken for 8 days increased clearance of midazolam, a substrate for cytochrome P450 3A4 and 3A5, by 42%. However, echinacea also increased the bioavailability of midazolam from 24% to 36%, demonstrating that interactions between drugs and herbal supplements may be complex.

A third very important issue associated with safety of herbal supplements is that the content and the profile of bioactive components in herbal supplements are not controlled. Regulations for good manufacturing practices now ensure consistency in processing, but this does not regulate the content of the starting material, which can change substantially with genotype of the plant, growing conditions, harvesting procedures, and storage conditions. This results in large variations in the efficacy and toxicity of the supplements and also confounds prediction of interactions of supplements with drugs. A study of ginseng products revealed that different preparations, or "lots," can contain variable amounts of two steroid alcohols, one of which supports and one of which inhibits angiogenesis (Sengupta et al., 2004).

Also of concern is the ease with which high doses of supplements can be consumed. Although dietary supplements are regulated as foods rather than drugs (U.S. Department of Health and Human Services, 1994), many consumers use supplements to treat disease instead of to maintain a healthy lifestyle. Safety of a supplement, or even a traditional food, is based on dose. Even some common foods are associated with toxicity if consumed in excess (e.g., almonds contain cyanoglycosides that release cyanide).

ISOTHIOCYANATES

Cruciferous vegetables (Brassicaceae [syn. Cruciferae]) and related plant species contain glucosinolates, which are the source of isothiocyanates. A glucosinolate consists of a β-D-thioglucose group, a sulfonated aldoxime group, and a side chain made up of one of several different modified amino acids. More than 120 glucosinolates have been identified, and there are commonly three or four major glucosinolates in each plant species. When the plant cell is disrupted, through chopping or chewing, the plant enzyme myrosinase, a thioglucohydrolase, comes into contact with the biologically inactive glucosinolate and hydrolyzes it, releasing an isothiocyanate, a thiocyanate, or a nitrile. The isothiocyanate is usually the most bioactive, and the electrophilic nature of isothiocyanates is thought to be required for their bioactivity. An example of an isothiocyanate is sulforaphane (see Figure 2-1), which is formed from the glucosinolate glucoraphanin found in broccoli.

The source and dietary intake of isothiocyanates and/or their parent glucosinolates vary among cultures and countries. Vegetables of the family Brassicaceae, which are also known as the crucifers or cabbage family, are rich sources of glucosinolates. Cabbage, broccoli, bok choy, and wasabi are examples of glucosinolate-rich crucifers. Per capita consumption of glucosinolates from crucifers in the United States is estimated to range from 10 to 40 mg/day (Kushad et al., 1999; McNaughton and Mark, 2003), whereas per capita consumption of crucifers in Asian diets is generally two to five times as much (Fowke et al., 2003). Little is known about factors that affect isothiocyanate bioavailability, but urinary excretion of isothiocyanates (as *N*-acetylcysteine conjugates) is a substantially greater fraction following ingestion of raw (30% to 60% of intake) rather than cooked (~10% of intake) vegetables, suggesting higher bioavailability of isothiocyanates from raw vegetables (Rouzaud et al., 2004; Getahun and Chung, 1999; Cramer and Jeffery, 2011).

Brassica plants have been used medicinally for millennia. Today, glucosinolates and their hydrolysis products are recognized as important because epidemiological evidence and animal and cell culture studies indicate that isothiocyanates have positive health effects. In particular, they slow the progression of or prevent common cancers (Jeffery and Araya, 2008). Clinical studies show that as little as three to five servings of crucifers each week may significantly lower risk for developing cancer. In a prospective study, three or more servings per week, as compared to one or fewer, decreased risk for prostate cancer by 41% (Cohen et al., 2000). In two other studies, five or more servings per week, compared to one or fewer servings, lowered bladder cancer risk by 51% (Michaud et al., 1999), and compared to two or fewer servings, lowered risk for non-Hodgkin lymphoma by 33% (Zhang et al., 2000). These data suggest that the amount of isothiocyanates needed for crucifers to lower cancer risk by 30% to 50% may be achievable in a normal healthy diet. Whether a mix of isothiocyanates is more effective than a single type, and whether more frequent servings can provide even greater protection remains to be determined. Increased detoxification of carcinogens and prevention of activation of procarcinogens are suggested as major mechanisms by which isothiocyanates protect against cancer. Isothiocyanates have been shown to upregulate phase II detoxification enzymes, such as glutathione sulfurtransferase, that are involved in detoxification of carcinogens (Hayes et al., 2008; Bogaards et al., 1994). Some isothiocyanates have been found to inhibit cytochrome P450 bioactivation of procarcinogens (Maheo et al., 1997; Rose et al., 2000). Isothiocyanates also have the ability to protect against cancer promotion and progression by slowing the growth of tumor cells, arresting the cell cycle, increasing apoptosis, and inhibiting histone deacetylase (Conaway et al., 2002; Myzak et al., 2006).

Few studies have evaluated the effect of crucifers on prevention of chronic diseases other than cancer. In a spontaneously hypertensive strain of rat, feeding dried broccoli sprouts daily for 14 weeks decreased oxidative stress, increased glutathione levels, increased endothelial-dependent relaxation of the aorta, and significantly lowered blood pressure (Wu et al., 2004). There was little or no change in these parameters in healthy rats. More recently, sulforaphane was found to protect against ischemic injury in isolated rat hearts (Piao, 2010) and against inflammation in vitro (Brandenburg et al., 2010). These studies suggest that crucifers may provide the greatest efficacy to individuals at highest disease risk.

Adverse effects of crucifer intake have not been reported in healthy humans with balanced diets, even with high intakes of crucifers. In addition, consumption of extracts of raw or cooked broccoli sprouts up to 50 g wet weight caused no adverse effects (Shapiro et al., 2006). The urinary bladder may be the most sensitive organ to isothiocyanates: in rats, phenethyl isothiocyanate (~75 $mg{\cdot}kg^{-1}{\cdot}day^{-1}$) and benzyl isothiocyanate (~80 $mg{\cdot}kg^{-1}{\cdot}day^{-1}$) both caused preneoplastic changes in the urinary bladder in as little as 2 weeks, inducing bladder cancer when treatment was extended (Akagi et al., 2003; Hirose et al., 1998). Very high dietary levels of glucosinolates and their isothiocyanate and nitrile hydrolysis products irritated the intestine of F344 rats (Lai et al., 2008). Some crucifers also contain compounds other than glucosinolates that are known to have adverse effects in humans. For example, crucifers contain goiter-promoting, thyroid-enlarging compounds such as thiocyanate ion and goitrin (5-vinyloxazolidine-2-thione) (Fenwick et al., 1983). These goitrogens have been a problem in livestock, and goiters were observed in Europeans between World Wars I and II in famine-stricken areas where cabbage was almost the only food available. Erucic acid, a fatty acid that has been associated with cardiac toxicity, is present in a number of crucifer seeds, including rapeseed and broccoli seeds, although it is absent from seedlings and whole plants.

ORGANOSULFURS

Organosulfur or sulfur-rich compounds are present in allium vegetables. The alliums contain a derivative of cysteine called alliin, or *S*-allyl-L-cysteine sulfoxide. When allium vegetables are crushed, alliin comes into contact with the enzyme alliinase to produce a lipid-soluble, unstable intermediate called allicin (diallyl thiosulfinate) that decomposes to produce several lipid-soluble allyl sulfides including diallyl sulfide (DAS), diallyl disulfide (DADS), and diallyl trisulfide (DATS). In addition, ajoene (4,5,9-trithiadodeca-1,6,11-triene-9-oxide) is formed from allicin when garlic is crushed in oil. In addition, *S*-allylcysteine (SAC) and *S*-allylmethylcysteine (SAMC) are found in aged garlic. The structure of DAS is shown in Figure 2-1.

Common dietary sources of organosulfurs are onions, leaks, chives, scallions, and garlic. Garlic is the richest dietary source of organosulfurs. In 2009 garlic sales were the third highest of all botanical supplements, with retail sales estimated at $19.3 million. The strongest clinical support for a health benefit of garlic is a lipid-lowering and an antithrombotic role in patients with CVD (Butt et al., 2009). Garlic appears to exert its antithrombotic effect via inhibition of platelet aggregation and enhanced fibrinolysis (Rahman, 2001). The action of ajoene in inhibiting platelet aggregation has been studied in vitro and may be a result of inhibition of cyclooxygenase/prostaglandin synthesis, inhibition of mobilization of platelet calcium, and/or disruption of fibrinogen binding to the platelet glycoprotein IIb/IIIa receptor, integrin. Not all clinical studies have found a lipid-lowering effect of garlic, possibly because of differences in formulation and/or serving size.

Garlic is proposed to also exert anticancer actions. Epidemiological studies provide a link between intake of allium vegetables and decreased risk for a number of cancers (Sengupta et al., 2004; Milner, 2001). Possible mechanisms have been identified from cell culture studies, and a few have been taken through to whole animal studies, but clinical studies are lacking. SAC and SAMC from aged garlic have been shown to exhibit excellent radical scavenging activity (Thomson and Ali, 2003). DAS increased apoptosis of human bladder cancer cells by a caspase 3–dependent pathway (Lu et al., 2004).

Rats given purified DADS and DATS (0.1 mmol/kg body weight by intraperitoneal injection) exhibited significantly increased hepatic phase II detoxification enzyme activities, supporting results from cell culture (Fukao et al., 2004). Prevention of DNA oxidation and inhibition of DNA binding and mutagenesis have also been seen in both cell culture and in animal models (Song and Milner, 2001). Additional animal and clinical studies are needed before a causal link between dietary organosulfur compounds and cancer risk can be concluded. One additional property of allium vegetables, shared with cruciferous vegetables, is the presence of a selenocysteine methyltransferase enzyme that allows the plant to take up inorganic selenium (Se) and accumulate this as Se-methylselenocysteine, which may have anticancer properties (Powolny and Singh, 2008).

Garlic and its bioactive thiols have been studied extensively for drug interactions via effects on the drug-metabolizing isoforms of cytochrome P450. Acute exposure to DAS and DAT inhibit cytochrome P450 2E1, whereas chronic exposure upregulates cytochrome P450 2E1. However, dietary garlic does not appear to affect drug metabolism via effects on either cytochrome P450 3A4 or cytochrome P450 2D6 (Markowitz et al., 2003). Infrequently, dietary garlic has been associated with gastrointestinal distress and even anaphylactic shock, although a more common concern with excess garlic intake is red blood cell hemolysis (de Roos et al., 2003).

POLYOLS

Polyols, or sugar alcohols, include alcohols of monosaccharides (e.g., sorbitol, mannitol, xylitol, and erythritol), disaccharides (e.g., isomaltitol, lactitol, and maltitol), and polysaccharides (e.g., maltitol syrup and hydrogenated starch hydrolysates) (Van Loveren, 2004). Sugar alcohols are used as sweeteners in foods, gum, candy, and beverages. Commonly used sugar alcohols are xylitol (see structure in Figure 2-1), sorbitol, mannitol, and lactitol. Natural sugar alcohols are present in many fruits and vegetables, but commercial products may contain synthetically produced polyols.

Sugar alcohols provide fewer calories than sugars (1.5 to 3 kcal/g compared to 4 kcal/g). This is partly due to reduced absorption (via passive diffusion) from the intestine, which results in some of the sugar alcohol bypassing absorption and becoming substrate for fermentation by the colonic microflora (American Dietetic Association, 2004; Mäkinen et al., 1985). The lower and slower absorption of sugar alcohols results in a lower glycemic response than from an equivalent molar amount of sugar. Many low-calorie foods contain sugar alcohols. Sugarless chewing gum often contains 1 g sugar alcohol per piece; a ¼ cup serving of low-calorie maple syrup may contain 6 g of sugar alcohols; and a low-carbohydrate cookie (28 g) may contain as much as 8 g of sugar alcohols.

The potential health benefits from consuming sugar alcohols are a reduced glycemic response, a decreased risk for caries, and a prebiotic effect (Van Loveren, 2004; Mäkinen et al., 1985). Evidence strongly suggests that in people who chew gum, use of gums containing sugar alcohols in place of sugar can significantly protect against caries (Van Loveren, 2004). There is an FDA-approved health claim stating that sugar alcohols do not promote tooth decay. Use of gum containing sugar alcohols limits acid production by plaque bacteria, reduces plaque, decreases levels of the caries-producing mutans streptococci in plaque and saliva, and promotes remineralization (Mäkinen, 2010). In a Finnish study, children who used gum containing sugar alcohols during 1982 had significantly fewer caries during 1988 than children not using gum (Isokangas et al., 1991). This effect of low-calorie sweeteners may be due to more than simply elimination of sugar; sugar alcohols may stimulate saliva flow and possibly even have a direct antimicrobial effect (Van Loveren, 2004). The preventative effects depend on frequency of chewing (e.g., three to five pieces of gum per day are considered effective) as well as the type and amount of sugar alcohol present in the gum (e.g., xylitol and sorbitol appear to have the strongest preventive effects) (Soderling et al., 1989). If there is a claim on the product containing sugar alcohols, a declaration of content is required on the nutrition label.

Excessive consumption of sugar alcohols may lead to an osmotic diarrhea owing to their slow absorption from the gut. Amounts greater than 50 g sorbitol or 20 g mannitol per day can cause diarrhea (Van Loveren, 2004). Because of the risk for diarrhea and malabsorption, all products containing either of these polyols must have a label stating, "excess consumption may have a laxative effect."

Stevia or sweetleaf *(Stevia rebaudiana)* is a South American herb with a long history of use as a sweetener (Ulbricht et al., 2010). In 2008 the FDA declared stevia a natural zero calorie sweetener safe for use in foods and beverages, clearing a path for companies to market it in a variety of products. Steviol, which contains two hydroxyl groups, is the aglycone of the glycosides present in stevia. Sugar residues (glucose and to a lesser extent rhamnose) are esterified to one or both of the hydroxyl groups in steviol to form the glycosides; these ester linkages are not hydrolyzed by enzymes of the human digestive system. The main glycosides present in stevia are stevioside and rebaudioside A, which are 200 to 450 times sweeter than sucrose. Products containing sugar alcohols or stevia in place of sweeteners such as sucrose or corn syrup can be labeled as sugar-free. Glycosides in stevia extracts are hydrolyzed by the microflora in the large intestine to release the sugars and the aglycone, steviol. Two long-term studies indicate that stevia may be effective in lowering blood pressure in hypertensive patients, whereas shorter studies did not find this effect (Ulbricht et al., 2010). Stevia may also possibly improve glucose tolerance, but more research is needed in this area.

DIETARY FIBER

The definition of fiber has varied over the years, in large part as our understanding has increased. Recently the Institute of Medicine (IOM, 2002) defined dietary fiber as "nondigestible carbohydrates and lignins that are intrinsic and intact in plants" and defined added fiber as "isolated, nondigestible carbohydrates that have beneficial physiological effects in humans." Total fiber is the sum of dietary and added fiber. Different plant food products contain different mixtures of fiber components. Various components of dietary fiber differ in their solubility, fermentability, and viscosity. Fermentable fibers may be fermented by the microbiota in the human intestine, resulting in production of short-chain fatty acids (SCFAs), which include acetate, propionate, and butyrate.

Forms of dietary fiber that are commonly available in over-the-counter supplements are psyllium husk, methylcellulose, polycarbophil, guar gum, wheat dextrins, β-glucan, and inulin. Fruits, vegetables, and whole grains are all good sources of dietary fiber. In addition, some processed food products containing psyllium and cellulose are sold specifically as good sources of fiber. The USDA nutrient database includes fiber content of common foods. Examples of high fiber foods are apples and broccoli (3 to 5 g fiber/serving). The IOM (2002) recommends a fiber intake of 14 g for each 1,000 kcal of energy consumed, which translates to approximately 25 g/day for women (based on a caloric intake of 1,800 kcal/day) and 38 g/day for men (based on a caloric intake of 2,700 kcal/day). Americans typically consume far less dietary fiber than current recommendations.

A high fiber diet protects against many of the chronic diseases such as cancer, CVD, diabetes, and obesity. It is possible that fiber may adsorb cholesterol and prevent its absorption, aiding cardiovascular health by decreasing cholesterol absorption. Mechanisms that might be involved in the proposed protective effects of fiber against colon and certain other cancers include dilution of and/or binding to toxic and carcinogenic components in the diet, both of which lead to lowered exposure to these substances (Gonzalez and Riboli, 2010; Park et al., 2009). Lignins and other components of fiber may chelate both essential metals such as iron and carcinogenic or toxic metals such as cadmium. Studies using colon cancer cells in culture suggest that butyrate produced by fermentation of dietary fiber may inhibit proliferation and promote differentiation and enhanced apoptosis of colon cancer cells. Animals fed sodium gluconate (50 g/kg) plus azoxymethane (a carcinogen) exhibited higher cecal butyrate and significantly fewer tumors than animals receiving the carcinogen but no fermentable substrate (Kameue et al., 2004). Although there are substantial animal data to support a role for fiber in prevention of colon cancer, epidemiological data have not supported this claim (Alberts et al., 2000; Lawlor and Ness, 2003; Mai et al., 2003).

The proposed protective actions of fiber against obesity and diabetes may occur in part because fiber dilutes the nutrient content or energy density of the diet by adding bulk but relatively little energy, and in part because dietary fiber prolongs chewing time, potentially enhancing satiety and decreasing energy intake. In addition, viscous fiber is thought to add bulk to chyme, slowing stomach emptying and further affecting satiety. Added bulk might also provide for more rapid transfer of chyme through the colon, which is less irritating to the epithelial tissue and musculature, thus preventing diverticulosis.

Fermentable fiber is hydrolyzed to SCFAs by the intestinal microbiota, mostly in the distal ileum and colon. Some bacterial populations, including bifidobacteria, are supported better than others by a high fiber diet, leading to a change in the microbiota community that is present (Gorbach and Goldin, 1990). The SCFAs produced by fiber fermentation provide an energy source for the epithelial cells lining the intestine. Cell culture studies showed that butyrate supports differentiation and apoptosis, consistent with protection against colon cancer (Cai et al., 2004). In contrast, resection studies in neonatal piglets showed that butyrate promoted proliferation and villus growth and inhibited apoptosis in this model of short bowel syndrome (Bartholome et al., 2004). Given the opposing actions of butyrate in different model systems, the mechanisms underlying the benefit of butyrate production need further study.

Health claims approved by the FDA that support a relationship between health and dietary fiber for prevention of both CVD and cancer are based on the content of the soluble fiber β-glucan. Data on cholesterol-lowering effects of soluble dietary fiber provide a strong and consistent basis for the health claims for oats and psyllium. In addition, numerous studies support a beneficial role for whole grain fiber, including a meta-analysis of 12 studies that showed that persons who consume about three servings of whole grain fiber per day had a 26% decrease in risk for CVD (Anderson et al., 2000). Claims for the cholesterol-lowering effects of fruits and vegetables may, at least in part, be due to the presence of fiber in these foods. The claim for lowering of cholesterol by soy protein isolate (25 g/day) may also be in part due to its fiber content (~5%), although it is likely also due to other components, such as estrogenic isoflavones (Erdman, 2000).

PREBIOTICS/PROBIOTICS

Prebiotics are nondigestible dietary substances found within foods that encourage the growth and activity of favorable intestinal bacteria, thereby improving the host health. They may include fructans, resistant starch, and other indigestible fibers and oligosaccharides (Madley, 2001). In contrast, probiotics are living microorganisms that, upon ingestion in sufficient numbers, exert health benefits. Probiotics and prebiotics are sold both as components within conventional foods and as dietary supplements, making consumption difficult to estimate. Good whole food sources of prebiotics include Jerusalem artichokes, bananas, onions, garlic, honey, and leeks. Commercially used probiotics include bacterial species of lactobacilli and bifidobacteria, and the yeast *Saccharomyces boulardii.* Probiotics are often found in yogurt, yogurt drinks, kefir, and dietary supplements. In some countries such as Japan, both probiotics and prebiotics are included in hundreds of products. The recommended amount per day to confer health benefits is estimated at 3 to 10 g/day for prebiotics and 1 to 2 billion colony-forming units (cfu) per day for probiotics (Hasler et al., 2004).

There are more than 400 different types of bacteria and approximately 10^{14} bacterial cells in the human intestine: tenfold the number of eukaryotic cells in the human body. Common types of bacteria include bacteroides, eubacteria, peptostreptococci, bifidobacteria, enterobacteria, streptococci, lactobacilli, clostridia, and staphylococci (Sekirov et al., 2010). Loss of optimal bacterial composition in the intestine may play a role in many disease states. The primary benefits of probiotics and prebiotics are thought to reside in their support of a healthy microbiota community by promoting the population of beneficial bacteria, such as bifidobacteria, and reducing the number of harmful bacteria, such as *Escherichia coli.* A robust, stable commensal microbiota reduces the risk for infectious diarrhea, stimulates turnover and integrity of the intestinal cells, enhances immunity, and increases gut motility. Probiotics and prebiotics are proposed to improve intestinal health, enhance immunity, enhance the bioavailability of nutrients, reduce symptoms of lactose intolerance, decrease the prevalence of allergy in susceptible individuals, and reduce the risk for certain cancers (Tappenden and Deutsch, 2007).

Although the mechanisms by which probiotics and prebiotics exert these beneficial effects are not fully elucidated, several have been proposed. Probiotics may antagonize pathogens through production of antimicrobial and antibacterial compounds; they may compete for pathogen binding at receptor sites and for available nutrients and growth factors; and they may stimulate cells involved in the immune response (Kopp-Hoolihan, 2001; Fedorak and Madsen, 2004, Tappenden and Deutsch, 2007). Probiotics, including *Lactobacillus rhamnosus, Lactobacillus reuteri, Lactobacillus casei,* and *Bifidobacterium lactis,* may shorten the duration of acute retroviral diarrhea in children (Fedorak and Madsen, 2004). In a study of patients with irritable bowel syndrome, patients who received a probiotic preparation containing *Lactobacillus plantarum* LP 01 and *Bifidobacterium breve* BRO for 28 days had less abdominal pain (scores decreased by 52% compared to 11% for the placebo group) and fewer symptoms (a decrease of 44.4% for the treatment group compared to 8.5% for the placebo group) (Saggioro, 2004). Prebiotics provide substrate for the microbiota to ferment to SCFAs, which are preferentially available to the cells lining the colon and which lower the pH of the intestinal environment. The benefit of these nutrients may be particularly important in infants, because the consumption of prebiotics by formula-fed infants during the first 6 months of life is reported to reduce the cumulative incidence of infections during that period (Arslanoglu et al., 2007) and to reduce the incidence of allergic manifestations during the first 2 years of life (Arslanoglu et al., 2008).

Cases of infection caused by probiotics such as lactobacilli and bifidobacteria organisms are rare. It has been estimated that probiotics are responsible for 0.05% to 0.4% of cases of infective endocarditis and bacteremia (Borriello et al., 2003). Occasional reports of bacteremia and endocarditis associated with lactobacilli have been noted to most likely occur in severely immunocompromised individuals (Kopp-Hoolihan, 2001).

OVERALL RECOMMENDATIONS

Although evidence exists to support various health claims for food supplements and functional foods, much additional research is needed to identify food components and determine their bioactivity as well as the effect of the whole food and food matrix on efficacy and potency. More information is needed before specific recommendations can be made about which bioactive compounds and what amounts of bioactive compounds should be consumed for optimal health, whether from food supplements or whole foods. Nevertheless, this is an active area of research and our understanding of the effects of nonnutritional components of foods will continue to increase over the coming decades.

THINKING CRITICALLY

Standard dietary advice from nutritionists has long been to consume a variety of foods, eat a diet rich in plant foods, and choose whole foods rather than highly processed prepared foods or supplements. Whether from the viewpoint of our current understanding of essential nutrient requirements or from the viewpoint of our current understanding of the role of other food components on health or prevention of chronic disease, list as many reasons as you can that support consumption of:

1. a variety of foods in the diet;
2. five or more servings per day of fruits and vegetables; and
3. whole foods such as fruits, vegetables, and whole grains rather than highly processed foods.

REFERENCES

Aftab, N., & Vieira, A. (2010). Antioxidant activities of curcumin and combinations of this curcuminoid with other phytochemicals. *Phytotherapy Research, 24,* 500–502.

Akagi, K., Sano, M., Ogawa, K., Hirose, M., Goshima, H., & Shirai, T. (2003). Involvement of toxicity as an early event in urinary bladder carcinogenesis induced by phenethyl isothiocyanate, benzyl isothiocyanate, and analogues in F344 rats. *Toxicologic Pathology, 31,* 388–396.

Alberts, D. S., Martinez, M. E., Roe, D. J., Guillen-Rodriguez, J. M., Marshall, J. R., van Leeuwen, J. B., … Sampliner, R. E. (2000). Lack of effect of a high-fiber cereal supplement on the recurrence of colorectal adenomas. Phoenix Colon Cancer Prevention Physicians' Network. *New England Journal of Medicine, 342,* 1156–1162.

Allred, C. D., Allred, K. F., Ju, Y. H., Clausen, L. M., Doerge, D. R., Schantz, S. L., … Helferich, W. G. (2004). Dietary genistein results in larger MNU-induced, estrogen-dependent mammary tumors following ovariectomy of Sprague-Dawley rats. *Carcinogenesis, 25*, 211–218.

American Dietetic Association. (2004). Position of the American Dietetic Association: Use of nutritive and nonnutritive sweeteners. *Journal of the American Dietetic Association, 104*, 255–275.

American Heart Association. (2010). *Fish and Omega-3 Fatty Acids*. Retrieved from http://www.heart.org/HEARTORG/GettingHealthy/NutritionCenter/HealthyDietGoals/Fish-and-Omega-3-Fatty-Acids_UCM_303248_Article.jsp

Anderson, J. W., Hanna, T. J., Peng, X., & Kryscio, R. J. (2000). Whole grain foods and heart disease risk. *Journal of the American College of Nutrition, 19*, 291S–299S.

Arslanoglu, S., Moro, G. E., & Boehm, G. (2007). Early supplementation of prebiotic oligosaccharides protects formula-fed infants against infections during the first 6 months of life. *The Journal of Nutrition, 137*, 2420–2424.

Arslanoglu, S., Moro, G. E., Schmitt, J., Tandoi, L., Rizzardi, S., & Boehm, G. (2008). Early dietary intervention with a mixture of prebiotic oligosaccharides reduces the incidence of allergic manifestations and infections during the first two years of life. *The Journal of Nutrition, 138*, 1091–1095.

Aruoma, O. I. (2003). Methodological considerations for characterizing potential antioxidant actions of bioactive components in plant foods. *Mutation Research, 523–524*, 9–20.

Babich, H., Gottesman, R. T., Liebling, E. J., & Schuck, A. G. (2008). Theaflavin-3-gallate and theaflavin-3′-gallate, polyphenols in black tea with prooxidant properties. *Basic & Clinical Pharmacology & Toxicology, 103*, 66–74.

Bartholome, A. L., Albin, D. M., Baker, D. H., Holst, J. J., & Tappenden, K. A. (2004). Supplementation of total parenteral nutrition with butyrate acutely increases structural aspects of intestinal adaptation after an 80% jejunoileal resection in neonatal piglets. *Journal of Parenteral and Enteral Nutrition, 28*, 210–222, discussion 222–223.

Beecher, G. R. (2003). Overview of dietary flavonoids: Nomenclature, occurrence and intake. *The Journal of Nutrition, 133*, 3248S–3254S.

Benatar, J. R. (2010). Trans fatty acids and coronary artery disease. *Open Access Journal of Clinical Trials, 2*, 9–13.

Bent, S., & Ko, R. (2004). Commonly used herbal medicines in the United States: A review. *The American Journal of Medicine, 116*, 478–485.

Bhattacharya, A., Banu, J., Rahman, M., Causey, J., & Fernandes, G. (2006). Biological effects of conjugated linoleic acids in health and disease. *The Journal of Nutritional Biochemistry, 17*, 789–810.

Blair, S. N., Capuzzi, D. M., Gottlieb, S. O., Nguyen, T., Morgan, J. M., & Cater, N. B. (2000). Incremental reduction of serum total cholesterol and low-density lipoprotein cholesterol with the addition of plant stanol ester-containing spread to statin therapy. *The American Journal of Cardiology, 86*, 46–52.

Bogaards, J. J., Verhagen, H., Willems, M. I., van Poppel, G., & van Bladeren, P. J. (1994). Consumption of Brussels sprouts results in elevated alpha-class glutathione S-transferase levels in human blood plasma. *Carcinogenesis, 15*, 1073–1075.

Bone, R. A., Landrum, J. T., Mayne, S. T., Gomez, C. M., Tibor, S. E., & Twaroska, E. E. (2001). Macular pigment in donor eyes with and without AMD: A case-control study. *Investigative Ophthalmology & Visual Science, 42*, 235–240.

Borriello, S. P., Hammes, W. P., Holzapfel, W., Marteau, P., Schrezenmeir, J., Vaara, M., & Valtonen, V. (2003). Safety of probiotics that contain lactobacilli or bifidobacteria. *Clinical Infectious Diseases, 36*, 775–780.

Bowen, P. (2005). Selection of surrogate endpoint biomarkers to evaluate the efficacy of lycopene/tomatoes for the prevention/progression of prostate cancer. *The Journal of Nutrition, 135*, 2068S–2070S.

Bowen, P., Chen, L., Stacewicz-Sapuntzakis, M., Duncan, C., Sharifi, R., Ghosh, L., … Van Breemen, R. (2002). Tomato sauce supplementation and prostate cancer: Lycopene accumulation and modulation of biomarkers of carcinogenesis. *Experimental Biology and Medicine (Maywood, N.J.), 227*, 886–893.

Bradlow, H. L., Sepkovic, D. W., Telang, N. T., & Osborne, M. P. (1999). Multifunctional aspects of the action of indole-3-carbinol as an antitumor agent. *Annals of the New York Academy of Sciences, 889*, 204–213.

Brandenburg, L. O., Kipp, M., Lucius, R., Pufe, T., & Wruck, C. J. (2010). Sulforaphane suppresses LPS-induced inflammation in primary rat microglia. *Inflammation Research, 59*, 443–450.

Bravo, L. (1998). Polyphenols: Chemistry, dietary sources, metabolism, and nutritional significance. *Nutrition Reviews, 56*, 317–333.

Butt, M. S., Sultan, M. T., Butt, M. S., & Iqbal, J. (2009). Garlic: Nature's protection against physiological threats. *Critical Reviews in Food Science and Nutrition, 49*, 538–551.

Cai, J., Chen, Y., Murphy, T. J., Jones, D. P., & Sartorelli, A. C. (2004). Role of caspase activation in butyrate-induced terminal differentiation of HT29 colon carcinoma cells. *Archives of Biochemistry and Biophysics, 424*, 119–127.

Canene-Adams, K., Lindshield, B. L., Wang, S., Jeffery, E. H., Clinton, S. K., & Erdman, J. W., Jr. (2007). Combinations of tomato and broccoli enhance antitumor activity in dunning r3327-h prostate adenocarcinomas. *Cancer Research, 67*, 836–843.

Carroll, Y. L., Corridan, B. M., & Morrissey, P. A. (2000). Lipoprotein carotenoid profiles and the susceptibility of low density lipoprotein to oxidative modification in healthy elderly volunteers. *European Journal of Clinical Nutrition, 54*, 500–507.

Cederroth, C. R., & Nef, S. (2009). Soy, phytoestrogens and metabolism: A review. *Molecular and Cellular Endocrinology, 304*, 30–42.

Chao, P. C., Hsu, C. C., & Yin, M. C. (2009). Anti-inflammatory and anti-coagulatory activities of caffeic acid and ellagic acid in cardiac tissue of diabetic mice. *Nutrition & Metabolism, 14*, 33–40.

Chapkin, R. S., Kim, W., Lupton, J. R., & McMurray, D. N. (2009). Dietary docosahexaenoic and eicosapentaenoic acid: Emerging mediators of inflammation. *Prostaglandins, Leukotrienes, and Essential Fatty Acids, 81*, 187–191.

Chen, J.-R., Lazarenko, O. P., Wu, X., Kang, H., Blackburn, M. L., Shankar, K., … Ronis, M. J. (2010). Dietary induced serum phenolic acids promote bone growth via p38 MAPK/b-catenin canonical Wnt signaling. *Journal of Bone and Mineral Research, 25*, 2399–2411.

Clifford, M. N. (1999). Chlorogenic acids and other cinnamates—Nature, occurrence, and dietary burden. *Journal of the Science of Food and Agriculture, 79*, 362–372.

Cohen, J. H., Kristal, A. R., & Stanford, J. L. (2000). Fruit and vegetable intakes and prostate cancer risk. *Journal of the National Cancer Institute, 92*, 61–68.

Conaway, C. C., Yang, Y. M., & Chung, F. L. (2002). Isothiocyanates as cancer chemopreventive agents: Their biological activities and metabolism in rodents and humans. *Current Drug Metabolism, 3*, 233–255.

Cornwell, T., Cohick, W., & Raskin, I. (2004). Dietary phytoestrogens and health. *Phytochemistry, 65*, 995–1016.

Craig, W. J. (1999). Health-promoting properties of common herbs. *The American Journal of Clinical Nutrition, 70*, 491S–499S.

Cramer, J., & Jeffery, E. H. (2011). Sulforaphane absorption and excretion following ingestion of a semi-purified broccoli powder rich in glucoraphanin and broccoli sprouts in healthy men. *Nutrition and Cancer, 63*, 196–201.

Daviglus, M. L., Stamler, J., Orencia, A. J., Dyer, A. R., Liu, K., Greenland, P., … Shekelle, R. B. (1997). Fish consumption and the 30-year risk of fatal myocardial infarction. *New England Journal of Medicine, 336*, 1046–1053.

de Lorgeril, M., Salen, P., Martin, J. L., Monjaud, I., Delaye, J., & Mamelle, N. (1999). Mediterranean diet, traditional risk factors, and the rate of cardiovascular complications after myocardial infarction: Final report of the Lyon Diet Heart Study. *Circulation, 99*, 779–785.

de Roos, N. M., Schouten, E. G., & Katan, M. B. (2003). Trans fatty acids, HDL-cholesterol, and cardiovascular disease. Effects of dietary changes on vascular reactivity. *European Journal of Medical Research, 8*, 355–357.

Eberhardt, M. V., Kobira, K., Keck, A.-S., Juvik, J. A., & Jeffery, E. H. (2005). Correlation analyses of phytochemical composition, chemical, and cellular measures of antioxidant activity of broccoli (*Brassica oleracea* L. Var. italica). *Journal of Agricultural and Food Chemistry, 53*, 7421–7431.

Erdman, J. W., Jr. (2000). AHA Science Advisory: Soy protein and cardiovascular disease: A statement for healthcare professionals from the Nutrition Committee of the AHA. *Circulation, 102*, 2555–2559.

Erdman, J. W., Liu, A. G., & Zuniga, K. (2010). Lessons learned from β-carotene supplement trials. *Sight and Life Magazine, 2*, 7–10.

Fedorak, R. N., & Madsen, K. L. (2004). Probiotics and prebiotics in gastrointestinal disorders. *Current Opinion in Gastroenterology, 20*, 146–155.

Fenwick, G. R., Heaney, R. K., & Mullin, W. J. (1983). Glucosinolates and their breakdown products in food and food plants. *Critical Reviews in Food Science and Nutrition, 18*, 123–201.

Fleshner, N., & Zlotta, E. R. (2007). Prostate cancer prevention: Past, present and future. *Cancer, 110*, 1889–1899.

Fowke, J. H., Shu, X. O., Dai, Q., Shintani, A., Conaway, C. C., Chung, F. L., … Zheng, W. (2003). Urinary isothiocyanate excretion, brassica consumption, and gene polymorphisms among women living in Shanghai, China. *Cancer Epidemiology, Biomarkers & Prevention, 12*, 1536–1539.

Fugh-Berman, A., & Myers, A. (2004). Citrus aurantium, an ingredient of dietary supplements marketed for weight loss: Current status of clinical and basic research. *Experimental Biology and Medicine (Maywood, N.J.), 229*, 698–704.

Fukai, T., Marumo, A., Kaitou, K., Kanda, T., Terada, S., & Nomura, T. (2002). Anti-*Helicobacter pylori* flavonoids from licorice extract. *Life Sciences, 71*, 1449–1463.

Fukao, T., Hosono, T., Misawa, S., Seki, T., & Ariga, T. (2004). The effects of allyl sulfides on the induction of phase II detoxification enzymes and liver injury by carbon tetrachloride. *Food and Chemical Toxicology, 42*, 743–749.

Getahun, S. M., & Chung, F. L. (1999). Conversion of glucosinolates to isothiocyanates in humans after ingestion of cooked watercress. *Cancer Epidemiology, Biomarkers & Prevention, 8*, 447–451.

Ghiselli, A., D'Amicis, A., & Giacosa, A. (1997). The antioxidant potential of the Mediterranean diet. *European Journal of Cancer Prevention, 6*, S15–S19.

Gonzalez, C. A., & Riboli, E. (2010). Diet and cancer prevention: Contributions from the European Prospective Investigation into Cancer and Nutrition (EPIC) study. *European Journal of Cancer, 46*, 2555–2562.

Gorbach, S. L., & Goldin, B. R. (1990). The intestinal microflora and the colon cancer connection. *Reviews of Infectious Diseases, 12*, S252–S261.

Greenwald, P. (2002). Cancer prevention clinical trials. *Journal of Clinical Oncology, 20*, 14S–22S.

Guo, W., Kong, E., & Meydani, M. (2009). Dietary polyphenols, inflammation, and cancer. *Nutrition and Cancer, 61*, 807–910.

Hallahan, B., & Garland, M. R. (2005). Essential fatty acids and mental health. *British Journal of Psychiatry, 186*, 275–277.

Hallikainen, M. A., & Uusitupa, M. I. (1999). Effects of 2 low-fat stanol ester-containing margarines on serum cholesterol concentrations as part of a low-fat diet in hypercholesterolemic subjects. *The American Journal of Clinical Nutrition, 69*, 403–410.

Hasler, C. M., Bloch, A. S., Thomson, C. A., Enrione, E., & Manning, C. (2004). Position of the American Dietetic Association: Functional foods. *Journal of the American Dietetic Association, 104*, 814–826.

Hayes, J. D., Kelleher, M. O., & Eggleston, I. M. (2008). The cancer chemopreventive actions of phytochemicals derived from glucosinolates. *European Journal of Nutrition, 47*(S2), 73–88.

Heinz, S. A., Henson, D. A., Austin, M. D., Jin, F., & Nieman, D. C. (2010). Quercetin supplementation and upper respiratory tract infection: A randomized community clinical trial. *Pharmacological Research, 62*, 237–242.

Hertog, M. G., Kromhout, D., Aravanis, C., Blackburn, H., Buzina, R., Fidanza, F., … Nedeljkovic, S. (1995). Flavonoid intake and long-term risk of coronary heart disease and cancer in the seven countries study. *Archives of Internal Medicine, 155*, 381–386.

Hirose, M., Yamaguchi, T., Kimoto, N., Ogawa, K., Futakuchi, M., Sano, M., & Shirai, T. (1998). Strong promoting activity of phenylethyl isothiocyanate and benzyl isothiocyanate on urinary bladder carcinogenesis in F344 male rats. *International Journal of Cancer, 77*, 773–777.

Hirvonen, T., Pietinen, P., Virtanen, M., Ovaskainen, M. L., Hakkinen, S., Albanes, D., & Virtamo, J. (2001). Intake of flavonols and flavones and risk of coronary heart disease in male smokers. *Epidemiology, 12*, 62–67.

Hollman, P. C., & Katan, M. B. (1997). Absorption, metabolism and health effects of dietary flavonoids in man. *Biomedicine & Pharmacotherapy, 51*, 305–310.

Hollman, P. C., & Katan, M. B. (1999). Dietary flavonoids: Intake, health effects and bioavailability. *Food and Chemical Toxicology, 37*, 937–942.

Horn, T. L., Reichert, M. A., Bliss, R. L., & Malejka-Giganti, D. (2002). Modulations of P450 mRNA in liver and mammary gland and P450 activities and metabolism of estrogen in liver by treatment of rats with indole-3-carbinol. *Biochemical Pharmacology, 64*, 393–404.

Howell, A. B. (2002). Cranberry proanthocyanidins and the maintenance of urinary tract health. *Critical Reviews in Food Science and Nutrition, 42*, 273–278.

Hwang, J., Sevanian, A., Hodis, H. N., & Ursini, F. (2000). Synergistic inhibition of LDL oxidation by phytoestrogens and ascorbic acid. *Free Radical Biology & Medicine, 29*, 79–89.

Institute of Medicine. (2002). *Dietary reference intakes: Energy, carbohydrate, fiber, fat, fatty acids, cholesterol, protein, and amino acids.* Part 2. Washington, DC: National Academies Press.

Isokangas, P., Tenovuo, J., Soderling, E., Mannisto, H., & Makinen, K. K. (1991). Dental caries and mutans streptococci in the proximal areas of molars affected by the habitual use of xylitol chewing gum. *Caries Research, 25*, 444–448.

Jagtap, S., Meganathan, K., Wagh, V., Winkler, J., Hescheler, J., & Sachinidis, A. (2009). Chemoprotective mechanism of the natural compounds, epigallocatechin-3-O-gallate, quercetin and curcumin against cancer and cardiovascular diseases. *Current Medicinal Chemistry, 16*, 1451–1462.

Jeffery, E. H., & Araya, M. (2008). Physiological effects of broccoli consumption. *Phytochemistry Reviews, 8*, 283–298.

Jones, P. J., & AbuMweis, S. S. (2009). Phytosterols as functional food ingredients: Linkages to cardiovascular disease and cancer. *Current Opinion in Clinical Nutrition and Metabolic Care, 12*, 147–151.

Ju, Y. H., Doerge, D. R., Allred, K. F., Allred, C. D., & Helferich, W. G. (2002). Dietary genistein negates the inhibitory effect of tamoxifen on growth of estrogen-dependent human breast cancer (MCF-7) cells implanted in athymic mice. *Cancer Research, 62*, 2474–2477.

Kameue, C., Tsukahara, T., Yamada, K., Koyama, H., Iwasaki, Y., Nakayama, K., & Ushida, K. (2004). Dietary sodium gluconate protects rats from large bowel cancer by stimulating butyrate production. *The Journal of Nutrition, 134,* 940–944.

Katan, M. B., Grundy, S. M., Jones, P., Law, M., Miettinen, T., & Paoletti, R. (2003). Efficacy and safety of plant stanols and sterols in the management of blood cholesterol levels. *Mayo Clinic Proceedings, 78,* 965–978.

Kim, Y. S., Young, M. R., Bobe, G., Colburn, N. H., & Milner, J. A. (2009). Bioactive food components, inflammatory targets, and cancer prevention. *Cancer Prevention Research, 2,* 200–208.

Knekt, P., Jarvinen, R., Seppanen, R., Hellovaara, M., Teppo, L., Pukkala, E., & Aromaa, A. (1997). Dietary flavonoids and the risk of lung cancer and other malignant neoplasms. *American Journal of Epidemiology, 146,* 223–230.

Kopp-Hoolihan, L. (2001). Prophylactic and therapeutic uses of probiotics: A review. *Journal of the American Dietetic Association, 101,* 229–238.

Kostyuk, V. A., & Potapovich, A. I. (1998). Antiradical and chelating effects in flavonoid protection against silica-induced cell injury. *Archives of Biochemistry and Biophysics, 355,* 43–48.

Kris-Etherton, P. M., Hecker, K. D., Bonanome, A., Coval, S. M., Binkoski, A. E., Hilpert, K. F., … Etherton, T. D. (2002). Bioactive compounds in foods: Their role in the prevention of cardiovascular disease and cancer. *The American Journal of Medicine, 113,* 71S–88S.

Kristal, A. R., Arnold, K. B., Neuhouser, M. L., Goodman, P., Platz, E. A., Albanes, D., & Thompson, I. M. (2010). Diet, supplement use, and prostate cancer risk: Results from the prostate cancer prevention trial. *American Journal of Epidemiology, 172,* 566–577.

Kushad, M., Brown, A. F., Kurilich, A. C., Juvik, J., Klein, B. P., Wallig, M. A., & Jeffery, E. H. (1999). Variation of glucosinolates in vegetable crops of *Brassica oleracea*. *Journal of Agricultural and Food Chemistry, 47,* 1541–1548.

Lafay, S., & Gil-Izquierdo (2008). Bioavailability of phenolic acids. *Phytochemistry Reviews, 7,* 301–311.

Lai, R. H., Keck, A. S., Wallig, M. A., West, L., & Jeffery, E. H. (2008). Evaluation of the safety and bioactivity of purified and semipurified glucoraphanin. *Food and Chemical Toxicology, 46,* 195–202.

Lampe, J. W. (2003). Spicing up a vegetarian diet: Chemopreventive effects of phytochemicals. *The American Journal of Clinical Nutrition, 78,* 579S–583S.

Lawlor, D. A., & Ness, A. R. (2003). Commentary: The rough world of nutritional epidemiology: Does dietary fibre prevent large bowel cancer? *International Journal of Epidemiology, 32,* 239–243.

Lu, H. F., Sue, C. C., Yu, C. S., Chen, S. C., Chen, G. W., & Chung, J. G. (2004). Diallyl disulfide (DADS) induced apoptosis undergo caspase-3 activity in human bladder cancer T24 cells. *Food and Chemical Toxicology, 42,* 1543–1552.

Madley, R. (2001). Probiotics, prebiotics, & synbiotics: Harnessing enormous potential. *Nutraceuticals World, 4,* 50–76.

Maheo, K., Morel, F., Langouet, S., Kramer, H., Le Ferrec, E., Ketterer, B., & Guillouzo, A. (1997). Inhibition of cytochromes P-450 and induction of glutathione S-transferases by sulforaphane in primary human and rat hepatocytes. *Cancer Research, 57,* 3649–3652.

Mai, V., Flood, A., Peters, U., Lacey, J. V., Jr., Schairer, C., & Schatzkin, A. (2003). Dietary fibre and risk of colorectal cancer in the Breast Cancer Detection Demonstration Project (BCDDP) follow-up cohort. *International Journal of Epidemiology, 32,* 234–239.

Mäkinen, K. K. (2010). Sugar alcohols, caries incidence, and remineralization of caries lesions: A literature review. *International Journal of Dentistry, 98,* 1072–1095.

Mäkinen, K. K., Soderling, E., Hurttia, H., Lehtonen, O. P., & Luukkala, E. (1985). Biochemical, microbiologic, and clinical comparisons between two dentifrices that contain different mixtures of sugar alcohols. *Journal of the American Dental Association, 111,* 745–751.

Manach, C., Morand, C., Demigne, C., Texier, O., Regerat, F., & Remesy, C. (1997). Bioavailability of rutin and quercetin in rats. *FEBS Letters, 409,* 12–16.

Markowitz, J. S., Devane, C. L., Chavin, K. D., Taylor, R. M., Ruan, Y., & Donovan, J. L. (2003). Effects of garlic (*Allium sativum* L.) supplementation on cytochrome P450 2D6 and 3A4 activity in healthy volunteers. *Clinical Pharmacology and Therapeutics, 74,* 170–177.

Mayne, S. T., Cartmel, B., Silva, F., Kim, C. S., Fallon, B. G., Briskin, K., … Goodwin, W. J., Jr. (1998). Effect of supplemental beta-carotene on plasma concentrations of carotenoids, retinol, and alpha-tocopherol in humans. *The American Journal of Clinical Nutrition, 68,* 642–647.

McLeod, R. S., LeBlanc, A. M., Langille, M. A., Mitchell, P. L., & Currie, D. L. (2004). Conjugated linoleic acids, atherosclerosis, and hepatic very-low-density lipoprotein metabolism. *The American Journal of Clinical Nutrition, 79,* 1169S–1174S.

McNaughton, S. A., & Marks, G. C. (2003). Development of a food composition database for the estimation of dietary intakes of glucosinolates, the biologically active constituents of cruciferous vegetables. *The British Journal of Nutrition, 90,* 687–697.

Mehta, R. G., Murillo, G., Naithani, R., & Peng, X. (2010). Cancer chemoprevention by natural products: How far have we come? *Pharmaceutical Research, 27,* 950–961.

Mente, A., De Koning, L., Shannon, H. S., & Anand, S. S. (2009). A systematic review of the evidence supporting a causal link between dietary factors and coronary heart disease. *Archives of Internal Medicine, 169,* 659–669.

Michaud, D. S., Spiegelman, D., Clinton, S. K., Rimm, E. B., Willett, W. C., & Giovannucci, E. L. (1999). Fruit and vegetable intake and incidence of bladder cancer in a male prospective cohort. *Journal of the National Cancer Institute, 91,* 605–613.

Milner, J. A. (2001). A historical perspective on garlic and cancer. *The Journal of Nutrition, 131,* 1027S–1031S.

Moreau, R. A., Whitaker, B. D., & Hicks, K. B. (2002). Phytosterols, phytostanols, and their conjugates in foods: Structural diversity, quantitative analysis, and health-promoting uses. *Progress in Lipid Research, 41,* 457–500.

Morre, D. J., & Morre, D. M. (2003). Synergistic Capsicum-tea mixtures with anticancer activity. *The Journal of Pharmacy and Pharmacology, 55,* 987–994.

Morton, L. W., Croft, K. D., Puddey, I. B., & Byrne, L. (2000). Phenolic acids protect low density lipoproteins from peroxynitrite-mediated modification in vitro. *Redox Report, 5,* 124–125.

Myzak, M. C., Hardin, K., Wang, R., Dashwood, R. H., & Ho, E. (2006). Sulforaphane inhibits histone deacetylase activity in BPH-1, LnCaP and PC-3 prostate epithelial cells. *Carcinogenesis, 27,* 811–819.

Nagata, C. (2010). Factors to consider in the association between soy isoflavone intake and breast cancer risk. *Journal of Epidemiology, 20,* 83–89.

Nardini, M., Natella, F., Gentili, V., Di Felice, M., & Scaccini, C. (1997). Effect of caffeic acid dietary supplementation on the antioxidant defense system in rat: An in vivo study. *Archives of Biochemistry and Biophysics, 342,* 157–160.

Neveu, V., Perez-Jiménez, J., Vos, F., Crespy, V., du Chaffaut, L., Mennen, L., … Scalbert, A. (2010). Phenol-Explorer: An online comprehensive database on polyphenol contents in foods. *Database (Oxford), 2010*:bap024.

Nho, C. W., & Jeffery, E. (2001). The synergistic upregulation of phase II detoxification enzymes by glucosinolate breakdown products in cruciferous vegetables. *Toxicology and Applied Pharmacology, 174,* 146–152.

Ososki, A. L., & Kennelly, E. J. (2003). Phytoestrogens: A review of the present state of research. *Phytotherapy Research, 17*, 845–869.

Park, Y., Brinton, L. A., Subar, A. F., Hollenbeck, A., & Schatzkin, A. (2009). Dietary fiber intake and risk of breast cancer in postmenopausal women: The National Institutes of Health-AARP Diet and Health Study. *The American Journal of Clinical Nutrition, 90*, 664–671.

Peeters, P. H., Keinan-Boker, L., van der Schouw, Y. T., & Grobbee, D. E. (2003). Phytoestrogens and breast cancer risk. Review of the epidemiological evidence. *Breast Cancer Research and Treatment, 77*, 171–183.

Piao, C. S., Gao, S., Lee, G. H., Kim, D. S., Park, B. H., Chae, S. W., … Kim, S. H. (2010). Sulforaphane protects ischemic injury of hearts through antioxidant pathway and mitochondrial K(ATP) channels. *Pharmacological Research, 61*, 342–348.

Pignatelli, P., Pulcinelli, F. M., Celestini, A., Lenti, L., Ghiselli, A., Gazzaniga, P. P., & Violi, F. (2000). The flavonoids quercetin and catechin synergistically inhibit platelet function by antagonizing the intracellular production of hydrogen peroxide. *The American Journal of Clinical Nutrition, 72*, 1150–1155.

Powolny, A. A., & Singh, S. V. (2008). Multitargeted prevention and therapy of cancer by diallyl trisulfide and related *Allium* vegetable-derived organosulfur compounds. *Cancer Letters, 269*, 305–314.

Prior, R. L., Hoang, H., Gu, L., Wu, X., Bacchiocca, M., Howard, L., … Jacob, R. (2003). Assays for hydrophilic and lipophilic antioxidant capacity [oxygen radical absorbance capacity (ORAC(FL))] of plasma and other biological and food samples. *Journal of Agricultural and Food Chemistry, 51*, 3273–3279.

Proteggente, A. R., Pannala, A. S., Paganga, G., Van Buren, L., Wagner, E., Wiseman, S., … Rice-Evans, C. A. (2002). The antioxidant activity of regularly consumed fruit and vegetables reflects their phenolic and vitamin C composition. *Free Radical Research, 36*, 217–233.

Rahman, K. (2001). Historical perspective on garlic and cardiovascular disease. *The Journal of Nutrition, 131*, 977S–979S.

Rao, C. V., Desai, D., Simi, B., Kulkarni, N., Amin, S., & Reddy, B. S. (1993). Inhibitory effect of caffeic acid esters on azoxymethane-induced biochemical changes and aberrant crypt foci formation in rat colon. *Cancer Research, 53*, 4182–4188.

Reinke, R. A., Lee, D. J., McDougall, B. R., King, P. J., Victoria, J., Mao, Y., … Robinson, W. E., Jr. (2004). L-Chicoric acid inhibits human immunodeficiency virus type 1 integration in vivo and is a noncompetitive but reversible inhibitor of HIV-1 integrase in vitro. *Virology, 326*, 203–219.

Robbins, R. J. (2003). Phenolic acids in foods: An overview of analytical methodology. *Journal of Agricultural and Food Chemistry, 51*, 2866–2887.

Rose, P., Faulkner, K., Williamson, G., & Mithen, R. (2000). 7-Methylsulfinylheptyl and 8-methylsulfinyloctyl isothiocyanates from watercress are potent inducers of phase II enzymes. *Carcinogenesis, 21*, 1983–1988.

Ross, J. A. (1998). Maternal diet and infant leukemia: A role for DNA topoisomerase II inhibitors? *International Journal of Cancer Supplement, 11*, 26–28.

Rouzaud, G., Young, S. A., & Duncan, A. J. (2004). Hydrolysis of glucosinolates to isothiocyanates after ingestion of raw or microwaved cabbage by human volunteers. *Cancer Epidemiology, Biomarkers & Prevention, 13*, 125–131.

Roynette, C. E., Calder, P. C., Dupertuis, Y. M., & Pichard, C. (2004). n-3 polyunsaturated fatty acids and colon cancer prevention. *Clinical Nutrition, 23*, 139–151.

Ruxton, C. H. S., Reed, S. C., Simpson, J. A., & Millington, K. J. (2007). The health benefits of omega-3 polyunsaturated fatty acids: A review of the evidence. *Journal of Human Nutrition and Dietetics, 20*, 275–285.

Saggioro, A. (2004). Probiotics in the treatment of irritable bowel syndrome. *Journal of Clinical Gastroenterology, 38*, S104–S106.

Seddon, J. M., Ajani, U. A., Sperduto, R. D., Hiller, R., Blair, N., Burton, T. C., … Willett, W. (1994). Dietary carotenoids, vitamins A, C, and E, and advanced age-related macular degeneration. *The Journal of the American Medical Association, 272*, 1413–1420.

Sekirov, I., Russell, S. L., Antunes, L. C., & Finlay, B. B. (2010). Gut microbiota in health and disease. *Physiological Reviews, 90*, 859–904.

Sengupta, A., Ghosh, S., & Das, S. (2004). Modulatory influence of garlic and tomato on cyclooxygenase-2 activity, cell proliferation and apoptosis during azoxymethane induced colon carcinogenesis in rat. *Cancer Letters, 208*, 127–136.

Shapiro, T. A., Fahey, J. W., Dinkova-Kostova, A. T., Holtzclaw, W. D., Stephenson, K. K., Wade, K. L., … Talalay, P. (2006). Safety, tolerance, and metabolism of broccoli sprout glucosinolates and isothiocyanates: A clinical phase I study. *Nutrition and Cancer, 55*, 53–62.

Shekelle, P. G., Hardy, M. L., Morton, S. C., Maglione, M., Mojica, W. A., Suttorp, M. J., … Gagne, J. (2003). Efficacy and safety of ephedra and ephedrine for weight loss and athletic performance: A meta-analysis. *The Journal of the American Medical Association, 289*, 1537–1545.

Simonsen, N., van't Veer, P., Strain, J. J., Martin-Moreno, J. M., Huttunen, J. K., Navajas, J. F., … Kohlmeier, L. (1998). Adipose tissue omega-3 and omega-6 fatty acid content and breast cancer in the EURAMIC study. European Community Multicenter Study on Antioxidants, Myocardial Infarction, and Breast Cancer. *American Journal of Epidemiology, 147*, 342–352.

Sinn, N., Milte, C., & Howe, P. R. C. (2010). Oiling the brain: A review of randomized controlled trials of omega-3 fatty acids in psychopathology across the lifespan. *Nutrients, 2*, 128–170.

Soderling, E., Makinen, K. K., Chen, C. Y., Pape, H. R., Jr., Loesche, W., & Makinen, P. L. (1989). Effect of sorbitol, xylitol, and xylitol/sorbitol chewing gums on dental plaque. *Caries Research, 23*, 378–384.

Song, K., & Milner, J. A. (2001). The influence of heating on the anticancer properties of garlic. *The Journal of Nutrition, 131*, 1054S–1057S.

Sparreboom, A., Cox, M. C., Acharya, M. R., & Figg, W. D. (2004). Herbal remedies in the United States: Potential adverse interactions with anticancer agents. *Journal of Clinical Oncology, 22*, 2489–2503.

Szarc vel Szic, K., Ndlovu, M. N., Haegeman, G., & Vanden Berghe, W. (2010). Nature or nurture: Let food be your epigenetic medicine in chronic inflammatory disorders. *Biochemical Pharmacology, 80*, 1816–1832.

Tappenden, K. A., & Deutsch, A. S. (2007). The physiological relevance of the intestinal microbiota–contributions to human health. *Journal of the American College of Nutrition, 26*, 679S–683S.

Thimmulappa, R. K., Lee, H., Rangasamy, T., Reddy, S. P., Yamamoto, M., Kensler, T. W., & Biswal, S. (2006). Nrf2 is a critical regulator of the innate immune response and survival during experimental sepsis. *The Journal of Clinical Investigation, 116*, 984–995.

Thomson, M., & Ali, M. (2003). Garlic [*Allium sativum*]: A review of its potential use as an anti-cancer agent. *Current Cancer Drug Targets, 3*, 67–81.

Thorsdottir, I., Hill, J., & Ramel, A. (2004). Omega-3 fatty acid supply from milk associates with lower type 2 diabetes in men and coronary heart disease in women. *Preventative Medicine, 39*, 630–634.

Ulbricht, C., Isaac, R., Milkin, T., Poole, E. A., Rusie, E., Serrano, J. M. G., … Woods, J. (2010). An evidence-based systematic review of stevia by the Natural Standard Research Collaboration. *Cardiovascular & Hematological Agents in Medicinal Chemistry, 8*, 113–127.

U. S. Department of Agriculture. Nutrient Analysis Laboratory. (2007). *USDA database for the flavonoid content of selected foods, Release 2.1 (2007).* Retrieved from http://www.ars.usda.gov/services/docs.htm?docid=6231

U. S. Department of Health and Human Services. (1994). Dietary supplements: Establishment of date of application. *Federal Register, 61*, 350–437.

van het Hof, K. H., Wisesman, S. A., Yang, C. S., & Tijburg, L. B. M. (1999). Plasma and lipoprotein levels of tea catechins following repeated tea consumption. *Proceedings of the Society for Experimental Biology and Medicine, 220*, 203–209.

Van Loveren, C. (2004). Sugar alcohols: What is the evidence for caries-preventive and caries-therapeutic effects? *Caries Research, 38*, 286–293.

Voorrips, L. E., Brants, H. A., Kardinaal, A. F., Hiddink, G. J., van den Brandt, P. A., & Goldbohm, R. A. (2002). Intake of conjugated linoleic acid, fat, and other fatty acids in relation to postmenopausal breast cancer: The Netherlands Cohort Study on Diet and Cancer. *The American Journal of Clinical Nutrition, 76*, 873–882.

Wang, T., Milner, M., Milner, J., & Kim, Y. (2006). Estrogen receptor alpha as a target for indole-3-carbinol. *The Journal of Nutritional Biochemistry, 17*, 659–664.

Wargovich, M. J., Woods, C., Hollis, D. M., & Zander, M. E. (2001). Herbals, cancer prevention and health. *The Journal of Nutrition, 131*, 3034S–3036S.

Wu, L., Ashraf, M. H., Facci, M., Wang, R., Paterson, P. G., Ferrie, A., & Juurlink, B. H. (2004). Dietary approach to attenuate oxidative stress, hypertension, and inflammation in the cardiovascular system. *Proceedings of the National Academy of Sciences of the United States of America, 101*, 7094–7099.

Yang, C. S., Wang, X., Lu, G., & Picinich, S. C. (2009). Cancer prevention by tea: Animal studies, molecular mechanisms and human relevance. *Nature Reviews. Cancer, 9*, 429–439.

Yang, C. S., & Wang, H. (2011). Mechanistic issues concerning cancer prevention by tea catechins. *Molecular Nutrition and Food Research, 55*, 819–831.

Zafar, T. A., Weaver, C. M., Jones, K., Moore, D. R., 2nd, & Barnes, S. (2004). Inulin effects on bioavailability of soy isoflavones and their calcium absorption enhancing ability. *Journal of Agricultural and Food Chemistry, 52*, 2827–2831.

Zhang, M., Zhao, X., Zhang, X., & Holman, C. (2008). Possible protective effect of green tea intake on risk of adult leukaemia. *British Journal of Cancer, 98*, 168–170.

Zhang, S. M., Hunter, D. J., Rosner, B. A., Giovannucci, E. L., Colditz, G. A., Speizer, F. E., & Willett, W. C. (2000). Intakes of fruits, vegetables, and related nutrients and the risk of non-Hodgkin's lymphoma among women. *Cancer Epidemiology, Biomarkers & Prevention, 9*, 477–485.

RECOMMENDED READINGS

Hasler, C. M., Bloch, A. S., & Thomson, C. A. (2004). Position of the American Dietetic Association: Functional foods. *Journal of the American Dietetic Association, 104*, 814–826.

Kris-Etherton, P. M., Hecker, K. D., Bonanome, A., Coval, S. M., Binkoski, A. E., Hilpert, K. F., … Etherton, T. D. (2002). Bioactive compounds in foods: Their role in the prevention of cardiovascular disease and cancer. *The American Journal of Medicine, 113*, 71S–88S.

RECOMMENDED WEBSITES

Code of Federal Regulations. National Archives and Records Administration. List of substances generally recognized as safe. http://www.access.gpo.gov/nara/cfr/waisidx_02/21cfr182_02.html

Food and Nutrition Information Center. United States Department of Agriculture. Information about antioxidants, phytochemicals, and functional foods. http://fnic.nal.usda.gov

National Center for Complementary and Alternative Medicine. National Institutes of Health. Research and consumer health information about herbal supplements and alternative medicine. http://nccam.nih.gov

Nutrient Data Laboratory. United States Department of Agriculture. Links to data on bioactive compound (flavonoids) content of American foods. http://www.ars.usda.gov/services

Phenol-Explorer. An online comprehensive database on polyphenol contents in foods. http://www.phenol-explorer.eu

United States Food and Drug Administration. United States Department of Health and Human Services. Information on regulation of dietary supplements and labeling requirements. http://www.cfsan.fda.gov

CHAPTER 3

Guidelines for Food and Nutrient Intake

Christina Stark, MS, RD, CDN

COMMON ABBREVIATIONS

Nutrient Standards

AI	Adequate Intake
AMDR	Acceptable Macronutrient Distribution Range
DRI	Dietary Reference Intake
DRV	Daily Reference Value
DV	Daily Value
EAR	Estimated Average Requirement
EER	Estimated Energy Requirement
RDA	Recommended Dietary Allowance
RDI	Reference Daily Intake
RNI	Recommended Nutrient Intake
UL	Tolerable Upper Intake Level

Agencies/Organizations

FAO	Food and Agriculture Organization
FDA	U.S. Food and Drug Administration
IOM	Institute of Medicine
NRC	National Research Council
USDA	U.S. Department of Agriculture
USDHHS	U.S. Department of Health and Human Services
WHO	World Health Organization

When people sit down to a meal, they eat food, not nutrients. Most people do not think about the individual nutrients they are consuming, but instead focus on the flavor, texture, and aroma of the food. Although consumers do indicate that nutrition is an important factor when making food selections, other factors such as taste, cost, and convenience may outweigh any nutritional considerations. The challenge is to translate the biochemical and physiological requirements for nutrients into practical guidelines so that people can make healthful food choices. Simply knowing nutrient requirements does not ensure that someone will consume an adequate diet.

This chapter explores various types of dietary recommendations, ranging from those focused on specific nutrients to those based on entire food groups. In the United States these include the Dietary Reference Intakes (DRIs), the Dietary Guidelines for Americans, and the United States Department of Agriculture (USDA) Food Patterns. Many other countries around the world have developed their own sets of recommended dietary intakes, dietary guidelines, and/or food guides. In addition, the Food and Agriculture Organization (FAO) and World Health Organization (WHO) of the United Nations system routinely establish recommendations for nutrient intake (FAO, 2009, 2010). Both professionals and consumers can use these recommendations and guidelines in the promotion and selection of healthful diets.

DIETARY REFERENCE INTAKES

In the United States the DRIs are the current reference values for recommended intakes and safe upper levels of intake of nutrients. The term *DRI* was introduced in 1994 and superceded the former term, *Recommended Dietary Allowance* (RDA), which had been the standard since 1941. The DRIs were developed jointly by the Institute of Medicine (IOM), which is the health arm of the National Academies in the United States, and the Canadian government. The DRIs have replaced Canada's previous reference values known as Recommended Nutrient Intakes (RNIs) (IOM, 2006). In contrast to the previous RDAs and RNIs, which provided single values for each nutrient, the DRIs are a set of reference values.

DRIs were developed to address some of the limitations of having only a single set of reference values for applying dietary recommendations to individuals and groups. They were developed using a risk assessment framework that considers not only the relationship between nutrient intakes and indicators of adequacy, but also the potential reduction in the risk of chronic disease. The framework also considers the potential health problems from intakes that are too high. The DRIs were issued as a series of reports, with each report covering a group of related nutrients (IOM, 1997, 1998, 2000a, 2001, 2002, 2004).

The reports, which cover a total of 45 nutrients, energy, and food components, group them as follows:

- Calcium, phosphorus, magnesium, vitamin D, and fluoride
- Thiamin, riboflavin, niacin, vitamin B_6, folate, vitamin B_{12}, pantothenic acid, biotin, and choline
- Vitamin C, vitamin E, selenium, and carotenoids
- Vitamin A, vitamin K, arsenic, boron, chromium, copper, iodine, iron, manganese, molybdenum, nickel, silicon, vanadium, and zinc

- Energy, carbohydrate, fiber, fat, fatty acids, cholesterol, protein, and amino acids
- Water, potassium, sodium, chloride, and sulfate

A selective summary of these reports has also been published, which serves as a more accessible and compact reference for professionals (IOM, 2006). In late 2010 a new DRI report was issued for vitamin D and calcium after it was determined there were sufficient new data to justify reviewing and updating the original DRIs for these two nutrients (IOM, 2011).

DEFINITIONS

The DRIs consist of the following nutrient-based reference values: Estimated Average Requirement (EAR), Recommended Dietary Allowance (RDA), Adequate Intake (AI), and Tolerable Upper Intake Level (UL). For macronutrients, there is also the Acceptable Macronutrient Distribution Range (AMDR) and the Estimated Energy Requirement (EER). The scientific data for developing DRIs consist of clinical trials and observations in humans and other studies including dose–response, balance, depletion–repletion, prospective observation, and case–control approaches. The EARs, RDAs, AIs, and ULs refer to average daily intakes over a number of days. The IOM describes each value in the following way:

- EAR: the average daily nutrient intake level that is estimated to meet the requirements of half of the healthy individuals in a particular life stage and gender group (IOM, 2006, p. 8).

This value is used as the basis for developing the RDA and can be used for assessing the adequacy of estimated nutrient intakes of individuals and groups and for planning intakes for groups.

In the case of energy, an Estimated Energy Requirement (EER) is provided.

- EER: the average dietary energy intake that is predicted to maintain energy balance in a healthy adult of a defined age, gender, weight, height, and level of physical activity consistent with good health (IOM, 2006, p. 8).
- RDA: the average daily dietary nutrient intake level that is sufficient to meet the nutrient requirements of nearly all (97% to 98%) healthy individuals in a particular life stage and gender group (IOM, 2006, p. 8).

The RDA can be used as a guide for daily intake by individuals. Intakes below the RDA, however, cannot be considered inadequate, because the RDA falls above the requirements of most people. It is based on an estimate of the average requirement plus an increase (typically two standard deviations above the EAR) to account for the variation within a particular group.

- AI: the recommended average daily intake level based on observed or experimentally determined approximations or estimates of nutrient intake by a group (or groups) of apparently healthy people that are assumed to be adequate; used when an RDA cannot be determined (IOM, 2006, p. 8).

Individuals should use the AI as a guide for intake of a nutrient for which no RDA exists. The AI is an intake level that is derived through experimental or observational data that appears to sustain a desired indicator of health in a group (or groups) of apparently healthy people.

- UL: the highest average daily nutrient intake level that is likely to pose no risk of adverse health effects to almost all individuals in the general population. As intake increases above the UL, the potential risk of adverse effects may increase (IOM, 2006 p. 8).

This value is not intended to be a recommended level of intake, and there is no established benefit for individuals to consume nutrients at levels above the RDA or AI. For most nutrients, this value refers to total intakes from food, fortified food, and nutrient supplements.

- AMDR: the range of intakes of an energy source that is associated with a reduced risk of chronic disease, yet can provide adequate amounts of essential nutrients (IOM, 2006, p. 11).

These values, which are estimated for fat, fatty acids, carbohydrate, and protein, are expressed as percent of energy since the requirement is not independent of other energy sources or the total energy requirement of an individual.

Figure 3-1 shows how the DRI values relate to the risks of either inadequacy or adverse effects. The DRIs provide a set of reference values for 12 life-stage groups for the United States and Canada. Similar sets of recommendations, typically called recommended dietary intakes, exist for other countries or in some cases for a worldwide audience (FAO/WHO, 2002, 2004).

CRITERIA FOR SETTING DIETARY RECOMMENDATIONS

The first edition of the *Recommended Dietary Allowances,* published by the National Academy of Sciences in 1943, provided recommended intakes for energy and nine essential nutrients. The RDAs were revised periodically based on new scientific knowledge and interpretations. With each revision there were changes in the numbers of nutrients considered and the levels recommended, but the basic philosophy was to define RDAs as levels sufficient to cover individual variations and provide a margin of safety above minimum requirements (IOM, 1994). In contrast, the criteria used to determine the DRIs goes beyond preventing a nutrient deficiency disease and also includes optimizing health, reducing the risk of chronic disease, and avoiding overconsumption of a nutrient (IOM, 2006). For example, the DRI for vitamin C is higher than simply the amount to prevent scurvy. It also considers the amount needed for antioxidant protection and tissue saturation while at the same time minimizing urinary loss. Like the former RDAs, the DRIs apply to the healthy general population and are not intended to apply to people who have an acute or chronic disease or who are already malnourished.

Other countries with recommended dietary intakes have also debated how to define their levels—should they use a minimal amount that prevents deficiency disease in all healthy people, an intermediate amount that allows for a large margin of safety, or a level that supports optimal nutrition? For example, when setting the requirement for

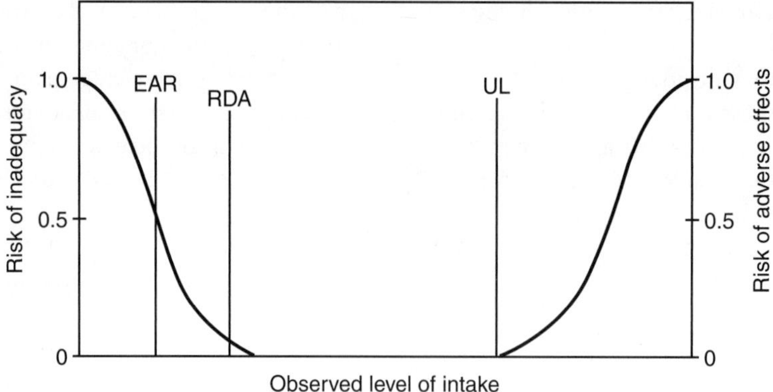

FIGURE 3-1 Relationship between Dietary Reference Intakes. This figure shows that the Estimated Average Requirement (*EAR*) is the intake at which the risk of inadequacy is 0.5 (50%) to an individual. The Recommended Dietary Allowance (*RDA*) is the intake at which the risk of inadequacy is very small—only 0.02 to 0.03 (2% to 3%). The Adequate Intake (*AI*) does not bear a consistent relationship to the EAR or the RDA because it is set without an estimate of the requirement. At intakes between the RDA and the Tolerable Upper Intake Level (*UL*), the risks of inadequacy and of excess are both close to 0. At intakes above the UL, the risk of adverse effects may increase. (From IOM. [2006]. *Dietary Reference Intakes: The essential guide to nutrient requirements.* Washington, DC: National Academies Press, p. 12.)

vitamin C, Australia and New Zealand considered several criteria, including biochemical indices, clinical outcomes, vitamin C turnover, and interactions with other protective phytochemicals in fruits and vegetables. Going on the strength of the evidence, the final recommendation was set based on the prevention of scurvy, vitamin C turnover, and biochemical indices of vitamin C status, such as in plasma, urine, and leukocytes. However, it was not based on the potential interaction with other food components eaten at the same time (National Health and Medical Research Council, 2006).

The use of professional judgment and interpretation to set an RDA, DRI, or other recommended intake is illustrated by the range of values for some nutrients in sets of standards in different countries. For example, a review of nutrient requirements for children in 29 European countries found a twofold to fourfold difference among countries in their established reference values for vitamin and mineral requirements (Prentice et al., 2004; Pavlovic et al., 2007). Although different standards may be due in part to biology, much of the difference can be explained by the varied approaches used in setting the standards. The IOM has examined the conceptual framework used to develop the DRIs and has identified ways the development process could be enhanced (IOM, 2008).

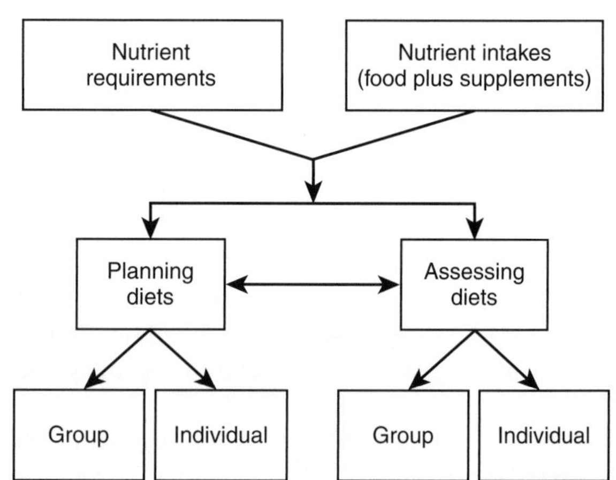

FIGURE 3-2 Conceptual framwork: Uses of Dietary Reference Intakes. (From IOM. [2007]. *Dietary Reference Intakes research synthesis: Workshop summary.* Washington, DC: National Academies Press, p. 135. Adapted from Beaton, G. H. [1994]. Criteria of an adequate diet. In M. E. Shils, J. A. Olson, & M. Shike (Eds.), *Modern nutrition in health and disease* (9th ed., pp. 1491–1505). Philadelphia, PA: Lea & Febiger.

HOW DRIs ARE USED

The various DRI values relate to the distribution of requirements and the distribution of intakes, and they can be used to both assess and plan diets of individuals and groups. Dietary assessment is done to determine if the nutrient intake of an individual or group meets their nutrient requirement. Dietary planning is used to recommend a diet that provides adequate, but not excessive, levels of nutrients for either an individual or a group (IOM, 2006). Figure 3-2 provides the conceptual framework for these uses, although using the DRIs to assess and plan diets of individuals is more challenging because the exact nutritional requirements of an individual cannot be readily determined. Both nutrient requirements and nutrient intakes are only estimates based on available data, so any assessment results or dietary recommendations are at best approximations. Nutrient intake data should be considered in the context of other data, such as clinical, biochemical, or anthropometric information.

Over the years, the former RDAs were often inappropriately interpreted as the amounts of essential nutrients a healthy individual needs over time. They were also used for several other purposes, including establishing nutrient standards for food assistance programs such as the National School Lunch Program and School Breakfast Program, evaluating dietary survey data, designing nutrition education programs, developing and fortifying food products, and setting standards for food labels (IOM, 1994). The DRIs were purposely developed to address some of the limitations and inappropriate applications of the former RDAs in assessing and planning diets. In general, EARs are used to assess intakes of both individuals and groups. If no EAR exists, the AI can be used in a limited way to assess intakes of individuals and groups. EARs can also be used for planning nutrient intakes of groups. RDAs should only be used as a guide for planning nutrient intakes of individuals. If no EAR (hence no RDA) exists, the AI can be used as a guide for planning nutrient intakes of individuals or as a target for the mean or median intake when planning for groups. The IOM has issued two separate reports describing in more detail how the DRIs can be applied to dietary assessment and planning (IOM, 2000b, 2003). Boxes 3-1 and 3-2 summarize how these applications differ between individuals and groups.

BOX 3-1 Uses of DRIs for Assessing Intakes of Individual and Groups

FOR AN INDIVIDUAL

EAR: Use to examine the probability that usual intake is inadequate.
RDA: Usual intake at or above this level has a low probability of inadequacy.
AI: Usual intake at or above this level has a low probability of inadequacy.
UL: Usual intake above this level may place an individual at risk of adverse effects from excessive nutrient intake.

FOR A GROUP

EAR: Use to estimate the prevalence of inadequate intakes within a group.
RDA: Do not use to assess intakes of groups.
AI: Mean usual intake at or above this level implies a low prevalence of inadequate intakes.
UL: Use to estimate the percentage of the population at potential risk of adverse effects from excessive nutrient intake.

From IOM. (2000b). *Dietary Reference Intakes: Applications in dietary assessment.* Washington, DC: National Academy Press, p. 4.
AI, Adequate Intake; *DRI,* Dietary Reference Intake; *EAR,* Estimated Average Requirement; *RDA,* Recommended Dietary Allowance; *UL,* Tolerable Upper Intake Level.

BOX 3-2 Uses of DRIs for Planning Intakes of Apparently Healthy Individuals and Groups

FOR AN INDIVIDUAL

EAR: Should not be used as an intake goal for the individual.
RDA: Plan for this intake; usual intake at or above this level has a low probability of inadequacy.
AI: Plan for this intake; usual intake at or above this level has a low probability of inadequacy.
UL: Plan for usual intake below this level to avoid potential risk of adverse effects from excessive nutrient intake.

FOR A GROUP

EAR: Use to plan for an acceptably low prevalence of inadequate intakes within a group.
RDA: Should not be used to plan intakes of groups.
AI: Plan for mean intake at this level; mean usual intake at or above this level implies a low prevalence of inadequate intakes.
UL: Use in planning to minimize the proportion of the population at potential risk of excessive nutrient intake.

From IOM. (2003). *Dietary Reference Intakes: Applications in dietary planning.* Washington, DC: National Academies Press, p. 4.
AI, Adequate Intake; *DRI,* Dietary Reference Intake; *EAR,* Estimated Average Requirement; *RDA,* Recommended Dietary Allowance; *UL,* Tolerable Upper Intake Level.

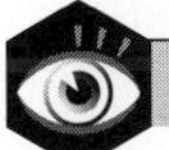

NUTRITION INSIGHT

Translating Evidence into Policy: Using a Risk Assessment Framework for the 2011 Dietary Reference Intakes for Calcium and Vitamin D

Patsy M. Brannon, PhD, RD

The Institute of Medicine released the 2011 Dietary Reference Intakes (DRIs) for calcium and vitamin D in November 2010, following a nearly two-year process by a committee of 14 research scientists and clinicians from a broad array of disciplines, including nutrition, pediatrics, gerontology, endocrinology, cancer biology, dermatology, immunology, biostatistics, and epidemiology (IOM, 2011). The committee was charged to review the evidence for all relevant health outcomes for calcium and vitamin D; to update the DRIs as appropriate, assessing how much is required and how much is too much; and to identify the research gaps and needs. Specifically and for the first time, this committee was also charged to incorporate a risk assessment framework and systematic evidence-based reviews (SEBRs) to enhance the objectivity and the transparency of the decision-making process leading to the committee's conclusions. A risk assessment framework is a structured four-step process that is based on the probability, prevalence, and distribution of risk for an adverse health outcome. This probability emphasis is well-suited to determination of a DRI, which is also a probability-based public health model of assessing the distribution of risk of an adverse health outcome both at low and high intakes.

The first step in the risk assessment framework is the identification of the specific health outcome(s) for both the Estimated Average Requirement (EAR) and the Tolerable Upper Intake Level (UL), based on a critical and comprehensive review of the totality of the evidence available. The IOM committee carefully examined two SEBRs that were conducted by the Tufts and Ottawa Evidence-based Practice Centers, which are funded by the Agency for Healthcare Research Quality, USDHHS (Chung et al., 2009; Cranney et al., 2007). The committee also

Continued

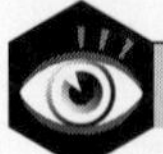

NUTRITION INSIGHT—cont'd

identified and reviewed additional literature. In total, over 1,000 primary research articles, meta-analyses, and other evidence reviews were critiqued in addition to the SEBRs; over 25 specific health outcomes were analyzed. The committee integrated all these data, used expert opinion, and made scientific judgments based on this evidence. Selection of the health outcome indicator(s) required consistency of effect, evidence of causality, and sufficient evidence for determination of the dose–response.

Only one health outcome—skeletal health—met these criteria for the EAR for either vitamin D or calcium. Measurements of skeletal health that were used included bone mineral content/density, rickets/osteomalacia, calcium absorption, and fracture risk. For the UL, kidney stones were selected as the indicator for calcium. Hypercalciuria/hypercalcemia of acute toxicity, adjusted for the emerging evidence of a U-shaped risk with low and high vitamin D levels for all-cause mortality, cardiovascular disease, selected cancers, falls, fractures, and small for gestational age, were selected as the UL indicators for vitamin D.

The second step in the risk assessment framework is the specification of the DRIs based on the dose–response for the selected indicator. In the case of vitamin D, many challenges presented in determining this dose–response, including the issues surrounding sun exposure, the hormonal nature of vitamin D, and the need to combine evidence from observational and randomized clinical trials to link serum 25-hydroxyvitamin D levels (the biomarker of total vitamin D "exposure" from both intake and its endogenous synthesis) with the skeletal health outcomes. Many of the studies assessed this biomarker but not vitamin D intake. Serum 25-hydroxyvitamin D levels of 40 nmol/L and 50 nmol/L were linked to the EAR and RDA, respectively, enabling the specification of daily intakes of 400 IU and 600 IU, respectively, as the EAR and the RDA for individuals ages 1 to 70 years.

The third and fourth steps are the evaluation of the intake data for the U.S. and Canadian populations and the characterization of the public health implications, including the prevalence of inadequate intakes in these populations. The latest National Health and Nutrition Examination Survey data reveal that 19% of the U.S. population has inadequate intakes based on having levels of serum 25-hydroxyvitamin D that are less than 40 nmol/L. The prevalence of inadequate vitamin D status is much higher (53%) in African Americans.

An advantage of the risk assessment framework is that it allows for easier updating of the DRIs if new evidence accumulates that is sufficient to justify a revision of the 2011 DRIs. Evidence on the nonskeletal health outcomes associated with vitamin D presently lack consistency of effect and evidence of causality, and additional evidence for these outcomes would be helpful in considering further revisions.

DIETARY ADVICE: GOALS AND GUIDELINES

Although the DRIs can be used for dietary planning, they are not a practical guide for use by consumers in selecting a healthful diet. The DRIs focus on specific nutrients, whereas people make food selections based on individual foods and food groups. Dietary advice for consumers needs to focus on recommended food selections in the context of the total diet.

DEVELOPMENT OF DIETARY GUIDELINES

Over the years as the relationship between diet and health became clearer, a new type of dietary advice emerged in the form of dietary goals and guidelines. Unlike the former RDAs, which focused on ensuring adequate intakes of essential nutrients, these guidelines emphasize the need to increase or decrease consumption of those food components that have been shown to affect the risk of certain chronic diseases. Another difference is that RDAs and DRIs state the amount (weight) of intake recommended on a daily basis for various nutrients with no indication of whether typical intake is high or low; whereas dietary guidelines often start with the estimated national diet and express recommended changes, generally in terms of increasing or reducing various foods and food components.

In the United States this shift in focus from obtaining adequate intakes to minimizing excessive intakes began in 1977 when a United States Senate Select Committee on Nutrition and Human Needs issued a set of recommendations known as the *Dietary Goals for the United States* (United States Senate, 1977). These goals provided quantitative recommendations on the amounts of complex carbohydrates, sugar, fat, saturated fat, cholesterol, and sodium that should be consumed. The Dietary Goals were controversial, in part because the diet plans developed to meet the goals were so different from the food patterns of typical Americans.

Subsequently, a new publication, *Nutrition and Your Health: Dietary Guidelines for Americans*, was jointly issued in 1980 by the USDA and the U.S. Department of Health, Education, and Welfare (now the U.S. Department of Health and Human Services [USDHHS]). This publication has been revised six times since 1980. The 1995 revision was the first one to be mandated by the government as a result of the National Nutrition Monitoring and Related Research Act (NNMRRA), which requires the Secretaries of Agriculture and Health and Human Services to review and jointly issue the Guidelines every 5 years (NNMRRA, 1990).

The purpose of the Dietary Guidelines is to translate information about individual nutrients and food components into an interrelated set of recommendations to help the public choose a healthy diet. The process used to create the Dietary Guidelines has evolved to include three stages: (1) an evidence-based review of the scientific literature; (2) the development of a policy document for professionals such as policy makers, nutrition educators, nutritionists, and health care providers; and (3) the development of messages and materials that communicate the Guidelines to the public. The seventh edition of the Guidelines—*Dietary Guidelines for Americans 2010*—provides recommendations that encompass two overarching concepts (USDA/USDHHS, 2010):

- Maintain calorie balance over time to achieve and sustain a healthy weight.
- Focus on consuming nutrient-dense foods and beverages.

The policy document identifies 23 key recommendations for the general population and 6 for specific population groups, such as pregnant women and older adults. The key recommendations are intended as an integrated set of advice, grouped into four categories: (1) balancing calories to manage weight, (2) reducing intake of certain foods and food components, (3) increasing intake of certain foods and nutrients, and (4) building healthy eating patterns. Examples of key recommendations are "Prevent and/or reduce overweight and obesity through improved eating and physical activity behaviors" and "Reduce the intake of calories from solid fats and added sugars." To help consumers implement the Guidelines, these recommendations are translated into consumer-friendly messages and materials by the USDA, USDHHS, and others.

The Dietary Guidelines have traditionally been intended for healthy Americans ages 2 years and over. However, the latest recommendations recognize the large percentage of Americans who are overweight or obese and/or at risk for chronic disease. Compared to previous Guidelines, the 2010 Dietary Guidelines place stronger emphasis on reducing calorie consumption and increasing physical activity and are intended for Americans ages 2 years and over, including those at risk for chronic disease. The Guidelines are not intended for younger children and infants, whose dietary needs differ.

SOURCES OF DIETARY GUIDELINES

The Dietary Guidelines form the base of federal nutrition policy in the United States, but it is not the only set of dietary advice. Other agencies, organizations, and countries have also issued dietary goals or guidelines. For example, nutrition-related goals are included in the U.S. government's initiative *Healthy People 2020,* which provides 10-year national objectives for promoting health and preventing disease (USDHHS, 2010a). The Nutrition and Weight Status topic area has 22 specific health objectives that fall into categories such as food and nutrient consumption (for example, increase intake of fruits, vegetables, and whole grains; decrease intake of saturated fat, solid fats, added sugars, and sodium; increase calcium; and decrease iron deficiency); weight status (prevent inappropriate weight gain in youth and adults); food insecurity (eliminate very low food security among children); and healthier food access (increase the percentage of schools that offer nutritious foods and beverages outside the school meals). In 2010 the U.S. Surgeon General released a report, *Vision for a Healthy and Fit Nation,* which provides guidelines related to reducing the risk of becoming overweight or obese (USDHHS, 2010b). Some of these guidelines are directed at individual food choices, but others relate to creating healthy environments—in the home, school, work site, and community—as a way to support healthy choices.

Various health organizations and expert panels have also issued dietary guidelines, often to reduce the risk of a specific disease. For example, guidelines from the American Heart Association and the American Cancer Society are aimed at reducing the risk of heart disease and cancer, respectively (Lichtenstein et al., 2006; Kushi et al., 2006). Dietary recommendations developed by a WHO/FAO Expert Consultation are aimed at reducing the risk of six nutrition-related chronic diseases considered to be the greatest public health burden worldwide: obesity, diabetes, cardiovascular diseases, cancer, osteoporosis, and dental diseases (WHO/FAO, 2003).

FOOD GUIDES

The key recommendations in the Dietary Guidelines provide general goals for how Americans should eat, but there is still a need for more specific food-related advice if the Guidelines are to be implemented. Advising someone to choose a diet that is low in saturated fats and *trans* fats and rich in calcium is not helpful if the person does not know which foods are sources of these fats or calcium. Food guides are designed to translate recommendations on nutrient intake into recommendations on food intake.

DEVELOPMENT OF FOOD GUIDES

Over the years, the U.S. government has published various food guides (Welsh et al., 1993). The first federal food guide, based on five food groups, was issued in 1916. The five groups (namely milk and meat, cereals, vegetables and fruits, fats and fatty foods, and sugars and sugary foods) were chosen based on the knowledge at that time of food composition and nutritional needs. During the Great Depression in the 1930s, there was an increased need for advice on how to select foods economically, so family food plans were developed to serve as buying guides. These food plans still exist today, adjusted for inflation, and serve as the basis for food stamp allotments.

In 1943 a food guide known as the "Basic Seven" was issued; this food guide recommended a certain number of daily servings from each of seven food groups. This guide was simplified and modified in 1956 to what became known as the "Basic Four." The Basic Four guide was meant to represent a foundation diet that would supply a major portion of the RDAs for nutrients but only part of the energy needs. It was expected that people would eat additional foods to fulfill their needs for additional energy and nutrients.

Because the Basic Four and previous food guides were developed in the context of preventing deficiency diseases, the primary focus was on getting enough nutrients from a variety of foods. This advice complemented the USDA's goal of promoting the consumption of various agricultural products.

In 1979 following the publication of the Dietary Goals, the USDA published *The Hassle-Free Guide to a Better Diet.* This food guide included the same foundation diet as recommended in the Basic Four, but identified a fifth group of fats, sweets, and alcohol, for which moderation was advised. This was a significant change from previous food guides, as the government had now identified a food group for which there was no recommended number of daily servings.

Instead, consumers were simply being urged to eat sparingly from this group.

After publication of *The Hassle-Free Guide to a Better Diet*, the first edition of the *Dietary Guidelines for Americans* was issued, and it became clear that a new food guide was needed to help consumers translate the advice in the Guidelines into actual food choices. In developing the new food guide, the USDA first identified several philosophical goals for the guide: it should promote overall health, focus on the total diet, be useful to the target audience, and allow flexibility (Welsh et al., 1993). To improve the visibility and usefulness of the new food guide, *The Food Guide Pyramid*, released in 1992, was developed as a graphic representation of the guide (USDA, 1992). The Food Guide Pyramid was designed to help Americans choose a diet that was nutritionally adequate but also moderate in energy and limited in food components often consumed in excess.

Although the pyramid-shaped graphic was familiar to many consumers, the daily food intake patterns (i.e., the what and how much to eat) are what form the scientific foundation behind the Pyramid. In 2005 the daily food intake patterns were updated to reflect the latest nutritional standards as well as current food consumption choices in determining nutrient sources. The process involved the following five steps (Britten et al., 2006), which were similar to those used to develop the original Pyramid food patterns:

1. Establishing energy levels. Estimates of the energy needs for various age/gender groups within the population were identified.
2. Establishing nutritional goals. Goals were set based on the DRI reports released between 1997 and 2004 for various vitamins, minerals, and macronutrients.
3. Establishing food groupings. Foods and food subgroups were identified based on nutrient content, use in meals, and familiarity.
4. Identifying nutrient contributions from each food group. The nutrient profiles of each food group were calculated based on the consumption-weighted averages of the nutrient content of foods in each food group. Foods in their lowest fat form and with no added sugar were selected for determining the nutrient profile of each food group.
5. Determining recommended amounts from each food group. Starting from the original Pyramid food pattern, the amounts of each food group or subgroup were iteratively increased or decreased until the pattern for each calorie level achieved its nutritional goal or came within

TABLE 3-1 USDA Food Patterns*

FOOD GROUP	1,600 KILOCALORIES	2,000 KILOCALORIES	2,400 KILOCALORIES
Fruits	1.5 cups	2 cups	2 cups
Vegetables	2 cups	2.5 cups	3 cups
Dark-green	1.5 cups/week	1.5 cups/week	2 cups/week
Red and orange	4 cups/week	5.5 cups/week	6 cups/week
Beans and peas (legumes)	1 cup/week	1.5 cups/week	2 cups/week
Starchy	4 cups/week	5 cups/week	6 cups/week
Other	3.5 cups/week	4 cups/week	5 cups/week
Grains	5 oz-eq†	6 oz-eq	8 oz-eq
Whole grains	3 oz-eq	3 oz-eq	4 oz-eq
Enriched grains	2 oz-eq	3 oz-eq	4 oz-eq
Protein foods	5 oz-eq	5.5 oz-eq	6.5 oz-eq
Seafood	8 oz/week	8 oz/week	10 oz/week
Meat, poultry, eggs	24 oz/week	26 oz/week	31 oz/week
Nuts, seeds, soy products	4 oz/week	4 oz/week	5 oz/week
Dairy	3 cups	3 cups	3 cups
Oils	22 g	27 g	31 g
Maximum SoFAS‡ limit, kilocalories (% of total calories)	121 (8%)	258 (13%)	330 (14%)

Condensed from USDA/USDHHS. (2010). *Dietary Guidelines for Americans 2010* (7th ed). Washington, DC: U.S. Government Printing Office, p. 79. Retrieved from http://www.cnpp.usda.gov/Publications/DietaryGuidelines/2010/PolicyDoc/PolicyDoc.pdf

*Recommended average intake amounts for selected calorie levels. Recommended amounts are daily intakes except for the amounts of vegetable and protein foods subgroups, which are recommended intakes per week. All foods are assumed to be in nutrient-dense forms, lean or low-fat and prepared without added fats, sugars, or salt. Solid fats and added sugars may be included up to the daily maximum limit identified in the table.

†*oz-eq,* Ounce-equivalent.

‡*SoFAS,* Solid fats and added sugars.

a reasonable range. After nutrient needs were met using foods in their lowest fat and no-added-sugar forms, the number of remaining calories needed to meet estimated energy needs were determined. These calories could be obtained by increasing the amount of food from each group; by consuming higher fat or added-sugar forms of foods; by adding oil, fat, and sugars to foods; or by consuming alcohol.

As a result of this process, new daily food intake patterns were created that meet the DRIs for almost all nutrients at all calorie-intake levels. The food intake patterns were released as part of *Dietary Guidelines for Americans* in 2005 and updated in 2010 (USDHHS/USDA, 2005; USDA/USDHHS, 2010). Table 3-1 shows the recommended average daily amounts of food from each food group for 3 of the 12 calorie levels: (1) 1,600, (2) 2,000, and (3) 2,400. Table 3-2 identifies what counts as an equivalent amount of food for different food choices within each food group.

The USDA Food Patterns (Table 3-1) list food group recommendations as total amounts in household measures (e.g., cups or ounces), rather than in number of servings. USDA made this change to help address some of the confusion about what constitutes a "serving." In addition, the "portion" of a food someone chooses to eat may not equal what the government previously identified as a serving in the original Food Guide Pyramid. Care must be taken not to use how many portions someone eats as a way to assess how well his or her diet meets the recommendations. In fact, studies have shown the typical portion sizes eaten at home and away from home have increased over the years. It has been suggested that these larger portion sizes are contributing to the obesity epidemic (Dietary Guidelines Advisory Committee, 2010).

TABLE 3-2 Quantity Equivalents for Each Food Group

FOOD GROUP	QUANTITY EQUIVALENT
Fruits	1 cup-equivalent is: • 1 cup raw or cooked fruit • ½ cup dried fruit • 1 cup fruit juice
Vegetables	1 cup-equivalent is: • 1 cup raw or cooked vegetable • ½ cup dried vegetable • 1 cup vegetable juice • 2 cups leafy salad greens
Grains	1 ounce-equivalent is: • 1 1-oz slice bread • 1 oz uncooked pasta or rice • ½ cup cooked rice, pasta, or cereal • 1 tortilla (6″ diameter) • 1 pancake (5″ diameter) • 1 ounce ready-to-eat cereal (about 1 cup cereal flakes)
Protein foods	1 ounce-equivalent is: • 1 ounce lean meat, poultry, seafood • 1 egg • 1 Tbsp peanut butter • ½ oz nuts or seeds • ¼ cup cooked beans or peas
Milk	1 cup-equivalent is: • 1 cup milk, fortified soy beverage, or yogurt • 1½ oz natural cheese (e.g., cheddar) • 2 oz processed cheese (e.g., American)

Condensed from USDA/USDHHS. (2010). *Dietary Guidelines for Americans 2010* (7th ed). Washington, DC: U.S. Government Printing Office, p. 80. Retrieved from http://www.cnpp.usda.gov/Publications/DietaryGuidelines/2010/PolicyDoc/PolicyDoc.pdf

To help consumers put the new food intake patterns into practice in order to improve their food choices, a food guidance system, called MyPyramid, was developed and released shortly after the Dietary Guidelines in 2005 (USDA, 2005). In 2011 USDA released MyPlate (Figure 3-3), a new symbol representing USDA's food guidance system (USDA, 2011). This new food icon is a visual cue to remind consumers to make healthier food choices consistent with the Dietary Guidelines.

Consumers can get more in-depth information and individualized guidance by going to *www.ChooseMyPlate.gov*. The website provides advice and interactive tools for specific audiences, such as preschoolers and pregnant and breastfeeding women. It also provides a variety of resources for professionals.

CHALLENGES OF USING FOOD GUIDES

As is true with all food guides, the adequacy of the diet depends upon the food choices within food groups. Within each food group, foods vary in nutrient density (i.e., nutrients provided per kilocalorie). For example, the 2010 USDA Food Patterns are based on choosing nutrient-dense foods

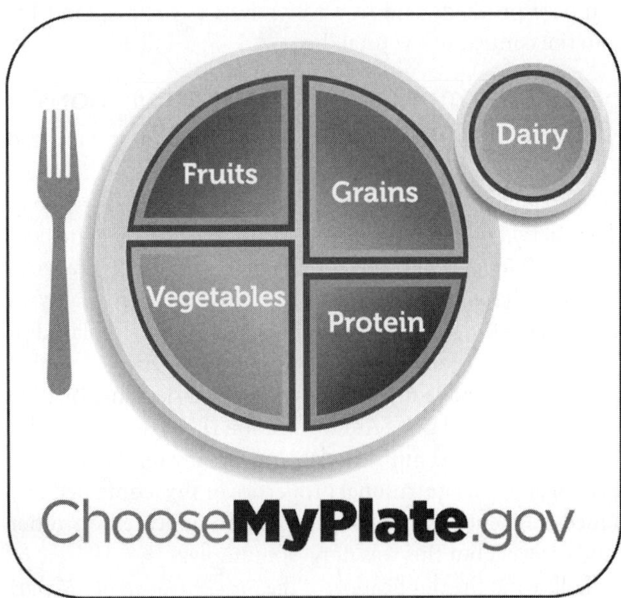

FIGURE 3-3 MyPlate. (From USDA. [2011]. *MyPlate.* Retrieved from http://www.ChooseMyPlate.gov)

and assume that the recommendations are followed in totality (USDA/USDHHS, 2010). A poor diet could be selected consisting primarily of foods with low nutrient density that still satisfies the recommended quantities from each food group. Consumers also need to account for fats contained in milk products and meat, fats and sugars that are added when foods are processed or prepared, and calories from alcohol. The allowance for calories from solid fats and added sugars, or "SoFAS," provides for some additional fats and sugars in the diet, but many consumers do not recognize the "extra" fats and sugars already consumed as part of their food choices. Also, any calories from alcohol need to be considered as part of the total calorie intake, and these calories would reduce the allowance for calories from SoFAS.

Developing a useful food guide for a population group is a challenge. It requires a balance between starting with what people typically eat and recommending achievable changes versus recommending an ideal eating pattern that is unlikely to be followed because it differs so much from customary food choices. In addition, the food intake pattern may not reflect diverse cultures or eating styles within the population. To address this issue, nutrition educators have adapted food guides to be more relevant to culturally diverse audiences, those who eat a vegetarian diet, or different age groups, such as young children and older adults (USDA, 2010).

LABELING OF FOODS AND SUPPLEMENTS

The USDA Food Patterns are only one tool to help Americans implement the Dietary Guidelines; food labels are another tool. Many consumers make food choices at the point of purchase, typically in a grocery store. The food label, which includes the "Nutrition Facts" panel, provides consumers with information about the ingredients and nutrients contained in individual foods. This information can be used to compare products and to assess how a particular food fits into the context of the total diet.

DEVELOPMENT OF FOOD LABELING REGULATIONS

Nutrition information has been required on most packaged foods since 1994, although the government has been involved in the regulation of food labels since 1906 with the passage of the Federal Food and Drugs Act and the Federal Meat Inspection Act (Golan et al., 2001). These laws gave the federal government the authority to regulate the safety and quality of food. The 1906 Federal Food and Drugs Act was replaced in 1938 with the Federal Food, Drug and Cosmetic Act, which prohibited any labeling that was false or misleading. In 1973 the U.S. Food and Drug Administration (FDA) issued regulations that required nutrition labeling on any food that made a claim about its nutritional properties or that contained any added nutrients. Nutrition information appeared on other foods as well, but this was done voluntarily.

Following the publication of the *Surgeon General's Report on Nutrition and Health* (USDHHS, 1988) and *Diet and Health,* a report by the National Research Council (NRC) (NRC, 1989), the FDA and the USDA's Food Safety and Inspection Service (which regulates meat and poultry products) asked the Food and Nutrition Board of the NRC to make recommendations on how to improve food labels so they could be used to select healthful diets. In the following year the Nutrition Labeling and Education Act (1990) was passed, which required several changes in the food label, including mandatory nutrition labeling. The FDA issued the final regulations implementing the Nutrition Labeling and Education Act in 1993 (USDHHS, 1993). Although not required to do so by law, USDA's Food Safety and Inspection Service also issued new regulations at the same time mandating nutrition labeling on processed meat and poultry products and providing for voluntary nutrition information for raw meat and poultry products. Both sets of regulations went into effect in 1994.

The Nutrition Labeling and Education Act (1990) was originally intended to apply to both foods and dietary supplements, including vitamins, minerals, amino acids, herbs, and similar products. Controversy over the proposed rules on health claims affecting supplements led to the Dietary Supplement Act (1992), which exempted dietary supplements from any new labeling requirements for 1 year to allow for further discussion. Eventually the FDA issued regulations on January 4, 1994, stating that dietary supplements have to provide the same basic nutrition information that is found on labels of other foods (USDHHS, 1994).

NUTRITION INFORMATION ON LABELS

Current labeling regulations require labeling of most packaged foods to list the following components on a per serving basis: total calories (kilocalories); calories from fat; and amounts of total fat, saturated fat, *trans* fat, cholesterol, sodium, total carbohydrate, dietary fiber, sugars, protein, vitamin A, vitamin C, calcium, and iron (USDHHS, 2009a). Figure 3-4 shows an example of the required format for a Nutrition Facts panel. The list of required nutrients has evolved over time to reflect new information about diet and health. For example, evidence about the health effects of *trans* fatty acids led to a requirement that *trans* fat content must be listed on the label as of January 2006 (USDHHS, 2003a). In contrast, the listing of thiamin, riboflavin and niacin, which was required on labels before 1994, is now optional because there is less concern about getting adequate amounts of these three vitamins than in the past. Other values that are optional include calories from saturated fat and the amounts of polyunsaturated fat, monounsaturated fat, potassium, soluble fiber, insoluble fiber, sugar alcohol, other carbohydrates, vitamins, and minerals for which RDIs have been established, and the percent of vitamin A that is present as β-carotene (USDHHS, 2009a).

DAILY VALUES ON LABELS

As required by law, the nutrition information on the food label must be presented in a way that enables consumers to put the information into the context of the total daily diet.

Nutrition Facts

Serving Size 1 cup (228g)
Servings Per Container 2

Amount Per Serving

Calories 260 Calories from Fat 120

	% Daily Value*
Total Fat 13g	**20%**
Saturated Fat 5g	**25%**
Trans Fat 2g	
Cholesterol 30mg	**10%**
Sodium 660mg	**28%**
Total Carbohydrate 31g	**10%**
Dietary Fiber 0g	**0%**
Sugars 5g	
Protein 5g	

Vitamin A 4% • Vitamin C 2%
Calcium 15% • Iron 4%

* Percent Daily Values are based on a 2,000 calorie diet. Your Daily Values may be higher or lower depending on your calorie needs:

	Calories:	2,000	2,500
Total Fat	Less than	65g	80g
Sat Fat	Less than	20g	25g
Cholesterol	Less than	300mg	300mg
Sodium	Less than	2,400mg	2,400mg
Total Carbohydrate		300g	375g
Dietary Fiber		25g	30g

Calories per gram:
Fat 9 • Carbohydrate 4 • Protein 4

FIGURE 3-4 Required format for nutrition information on food labels: The Nutrition Facts Panel. (From USDHHS. [2009]. *Examples of revised nutrition facts panel listing* trans *fat.* College Park, MD: FDA. Retrieved from http://www.fda.gov/Food/GuidanceComplianceRegulatoryInformation/GuidanceDocuments/FoodLabelingNutrition/ucm173838.htm)

To meet this objective, nutrients are listed in terms of the percentage of Daily Value (DV) they provide. The DVs are based on two sets of reference values for nutrients: the Daily Reference Values (DRVs) and the Reference Daily Intakes (RDIs) (USDHHS, 2009a).

The DRVs were developed for nutrients such as fat, carbohydrate, cholesterol, and fiber for which no previous standards existed. The DRVs for the energy-providing nutrients are calculated based on the caloric content of the daily diet, which for labeling purposes was chosen as 2,000 kcal. The RDIs provide reference values for vitamins and minerals and are based on previously established standards. The single term DV, which encompasses both DRVs and RDIs, was chosen for food labels to limit consumer confusion. Consumers can use the %DV to determine if a food product is high or low in certain nutrients. The %DV is based on a single serving of that food. A DV of 5% or less of a nutrient is considered low; 20% or more is considered high. The %DV also makes it easy to compare the nutrient content between similar products. Table 3-3 shows the DVs based on a 2,000 calorie intake.

TABLE 3-3 Daily Value (DV) Reference Amounts

FOOD COMPONENT	DV*
Total fat	65 g
Saturated fat	20 g
Cholesterol	300 mg
Sodium	2,400 mg
Potassium	3,500 mg
Total carbohydrate	300 g
Dietary fiber	25 g
Protein	50 g
Vitamin A	5,000 IU
Vitamin C	60 mg
Calcium	1,000 mg
Iron	18 mg
Vitamin D	400 IU
Vitamin E	30 IU
Vitamin K	80 μg
Thiamin	1.5 mg
Riboflavin	1.7 mg
Niacin	20 mg
Vitamin B_6	2 mg
Folate	400 μg
Vitamin B_{12}	6 μg
Biotin	300 μg
Pantothenic acid	10 mg
Phosphorus	1,000 mg
Iodine	150 μg
Magnesium	400 mg
Zinc	15 mg
Selenium	70 μg
Copper	2 mg
Manganese	2 mg
Chromium	120 μg
Molybdenum	75 μg
Chloride	3,400 mg

From USDHHS. (2009a). *Guidance for industry: A food labeling guide.* Appendix F: Calculate the percent daily value for the appropriate nutrients. College Park, MD: FDA. Retrieved from http://www.fda.gov/Food/GuidanceComplianceRegulatoryInformation/GuidanceDocuments/FoodLabelingNutrition/FoodLabelingGuide/ucm064928.htm

*Based on a daily energy intake of 2,000 kcal, for adults and children 4 or more years of age.

SERVING SIZES ON LABELS

The nutrition information on a food label is based on a specified serving size. In the past, food manufacturers determined the serving size; under the current labeling regulations, serving sizes are more uniform within a food category and reflect the amount of that food customarily eaten at one time (USDHHS, 2009a). The uniformity in serving sizes makes it easier for consumers to compare nutritional qualities of similar products than in the past. Consumers must keep in mind that the serving size on the label does not necessarily represent the amount any given individual eats. Someone who eats more or less than the specified serving size of a given food will need to adjust the nutrition information accordingly.

CLAIMS ON LABELS

Claims that can be used on conventional foods and dietary supplements fall into three categories: nutrient content claims, health claims, and structure/function claims (USDHHS, 2003b).

Nutrient Content Claims

Nutrient content claims describe the level of a nutrient or dietary substance in a serving of a product such as ones labeled "low-fat" or "high-fiber." The 1993 food labeling regulations provide standardized definitions for certain terms (USDHHS, 1993). For example, a low-fat food must have 3 g or less of fat per serving, a fat-free food must have less than 0.5 g of fat per serving, and a high-fiber food must have 5 g or more of fiber per serving. Nutrient content claims can also be used to compare the level of a nutrient in one food to another. For example, a "reduced" calorie food must have at least 25% fewer calories per standard serving size than an appropriate reference food.

Health Claims

Health claims are those that link the consumption of a food, food component, or dietary supplement with reduction in risk of a certain disease or health-related condition. For years health claims were explicitly prohibited by federal regulations because any claim that a substance could affect the course of a disease was considered equivalent to a drug claim. That meant a food carrying a health claim on the label could be considered an unapproved new drug and technically could be seized. As the relationship between diet and disease became more established, the FDA modified its policy and now allows three basic types of health claims (USDHHS, 2003b): (1) health claims authorized by the Nutritional Labeling and Education Act (NLEA), (2) health claims based on authoritative statements, and (3) qualified health claims. The main difference between the three types of health claims is the level of scientific evidence that is required to support the claim.

The first type, NLEA-approved health claims, requires the most rigorous standard of "significant scientific agreement (SSA)." The Dietary Supplement Act (1992) and the Dietary Supplement Health and Education Act (1994) also allow for approved health claims that meet SSA on supplements. To date, the FDA has approved 12 specific health claims that foods or supplements can make that meet the SSA criteria. These include claims related to links between calcium and osteoporosis; dietary fat and cancer; sodium and hypertension; and folate and neural tube defects.

The Food and Drug Administration Modernization Act (1997) provided the second way for health claims to be approved. In this case, health claims have to be based on "authoritative statements" from federal scientific bodies or the National Academies. Claims allowed under this category are authorized for foods but not for dietary supplements. To date the FDA has approved four claims under this category: whole grain foods and reduced risk of heart disease and certain cancers; potassium and reduced risk of high blood pressure and stroke; fluoridated water and reduced risk of dental caries; and low intakes of saturated fat, cholesterol, and *trans* fat and reduced risk of heart disease.

In 2002 the FDA allowed for the third type of health claim to be used on food and supplement labels when there is only emerging evidence to suggest a relationship between a substance and a health-related condition. These are known as qualified health claims because a qualifying statement regarding the strength of the evidence is required on the label to prevent the claim from being misleading. For example, a qualified health claim about walnuts and heart disease requires the following statement:

> Supportive but not conclusive research shows that eating 1.5 ounces per day of walnuts, as part of a low saturated fat and low cholesterol diet and not resulting in increased caloric intake, may reduce the risk of coronary heart disease. See nutrition information for fat [and calorie] content (USDHHS, 2009a, Appendix D).

A qualified health claim about selenium and cancer permitted on a dietary supplement label would require the following statement:

> Selenium may reduce the risk of certain cancers. Some scientific evidence suggests that consumption of selenium may reduce the risk of certain forms of cancer. However, FDA has determined that this evidence is limited and not conclusive (USDHHS, 2009a, Appendix D).

To help companies who want to make a health claim on their product, the FDA issued a guidance document to industry in 2009 that clarifies the agency's current thinking on (1) the process for evaluating the scientific evidence, (2) the meaning of the SSA standard, and (3) credible scientific evidence to support a qualified health claim (USDHHS, 2009b). The document describes the evidence-based review system that the FDA intends to use for the scientific evaluation of various types of health claims.

Structure/Function Claims

Structure/function claims describe a product's ability to maintain the normal structure or function of the body or to affect a person's general well-being. On conventional foods, structure/function claims relate to the effects of a nutrient, whereas on dietary supplements these claims can relate to a nutrient or other dietary ingredient. "Calcium builds strong bones" and "fiber maintains bowel regularity" are examples of structure/function claims. Unlike health claims, structure/function claims do not need to be preapproved by the FDA, although they must still be truthful and not misleading. The Dietary Supplement Health and Education Act (1994) established some specific regulatory procedures for structure/function claims on dietary supplements. The dietary supplement label must contain a "disclaimer" that the FDA has not evaluated the claim, and a statement that the product is not intended to "diagnose, treat, cure or prevent any disease." The supplement manufacturer is required to notify the FDA about the text of the claim no later than 30 days after the product is first marketed. In contrast, food manufacturers do not need to include the disclaimer and are not required to notify the FDA about their structure/function claims (USDHHS, 2010c).

OTHER POINT-OF-PURCHASE LABELING

The Nutrition Facts panel is only one place consumers can get nutrition information about a product. Food manufacturers can use other point-of-purchase methods, such as front-of-package labeling, to convey similar information. This information, often in the form of symbols such as checkmarks, stars, or numerical scores, is intended to give consumers information about the nutritional attributes of a food at a glance. These rating systems, which provide either nutrient-specific, summary indicator, or food group information, are based on nutritional criteria that have been developed by food manufacturers, retailers, or trade or health organizations. There is concern that the use of different and sometimes conflicting criteria can lead to consumer confusion (IOM, 2010). The FDA currently provides guidance to industry on the use of this type of point-of-purchase labeling, but is developing regulations to provide more standardized, science-based criteria on which to base front-of-package nutrition labeling (USDHHS, 2009c).

Foods bought from certain restaurants or vending machines are also subject to labeling requirements. Section 4205 of the Patient Protection and Affordable Care Act (2010) requires restaurants with 20 or more locations to list the calorie count for standard items on their menus and menu boards and to make other nutrition information available upon request. They must also provide a prominent statement about suggested daily caloric intake to help consumers put the calorie information into context. Vending machine operators with 20 or more machines are required to provide the calorie count for certain items. This information must be available to the consumer prior to purchase.

THINKING CRITICALLY

A great deal of food and nutrient information and recommendations are available to individuals concerned about nutrition.

1. Keep a record of your food and beverage intake for 1 or more days. Compare your intake to the USDA Food Patterns (Table 3-1) and nutrient standards for recommended intakes of protein, fat, carbohydrate, and one or more vitamins and minerals. Interactive tools to help you do both tasks can be found on USDA's ChooseMyPlate website at *www.ChooseMyPlate.gov.* Based on the results, how might you improve your diet?
2. Compare the results of your food pattern analysis with your nutrient analysis. Do you see any areas where you have high or low intakes of particular foods and also of nutrients particularly abundant in those foods? Would following current dietary guidelines result in dietary changes that would improve your nutrient intake?
3. Compare the Daily Value (DV) reference amounts used for food labeling (Table 3-3) with the current RDA values for the same nutrients. How closely does each current DV match the current adult RDA? A summary table of the DRIs (including RDAs) can be found on the Institute of Medicine's website at *www.iom.edu/Activities/Nutrition/SummaryDRIs/DRI-Tables.aspx.*
4. Look at food or supplement packaging for claims. Identify the category each claim falls under: nutrient content, health, or structure/function. For each health claim, identify which of the three subtypes of health claims it falls under.

REFERENCES

Britten, P., Marcoe, K., Yamini, S., & Davis, C. (2006). Development of food intake patterns for the MyPyramid food guidance system. *Journal of Nutrition Education and Behavior, 38,* S78–S92.

Chung, M., Balk, E. M., Brendel, M., Ip, S., Lau, J., Lee, J.,… Trikalinos, T. A. (2009). Vitamin D and Calcium: A Systematic Review of Health Outcomes. Evidence Report No. 183. (Prepared by the Tufts Evidence-based Practice Center under Contract No. HHSA 290-2007-10055-I.) AHRQ Publication No. 09-E015. Rockville, MD: Agency for Healthcare Research and Quality.

Cranney, A., Horsley, T., O'Donnell, S., Weiler, H. A., Puil, L., Ooi, D. S., … Mamaladze, V. (2007). Effectiveness and Safety of Vitamin D in Relation to Bone Health. Evidence Report/Technology Assessment No. 158. (Prepared by the University of Ottawa Evidence-based Practice Center (UO-EPC) under Contract No. 290-02-0021.) AHRQ Publication No. 07-E013. Rockville, MD: Agency for Healthcare Research and Quality.

Dietary Guidelines Advisory Committee. (2010). *Report of the Dietary Guidelines Advisory Committee on the Dietary Guidelines for Americans, 2010.* Washington, DC: U.S. Department of Agriculture, Agricultural Research Service.

Dietary Supplement Act of 1992, Public Law 102-571. 102nd Congress, 2nd session. October 29, 1992.

Dietary Supplement Health and Education Act of 1994, Public Law 103-417. 103rd Congress, 2nd session. October 25, 1994.

Food and Agriculture Organization. (2009). *Food-based dietary guidelines.* Retrieved from http://www.fao.org/ag/humannutrition/nutritioneducation/fbdg/en

Food and Agriculture Organization. (2010). *Nutritional requirements.* Retrieved from http://www.fao.org/ag/agn/nutrition/requirements_ pubs_en.stm

Food and Agriculture Organization/World Health Organization Expert Consultation. (2002). *Human vitamin and mineral requirements.* Bangkok, Thailand: FAO/WHO. Retrieved from http://www.fao.org/docrep/004/y2809e/y2809e00.htm

Food and Agriculture Organization/World Health Organization Expert Consultation. (2004). *Human energy requirements.* Rome, Italy: FAO/WHO. Retrieved from http://www.fao.org/docrep/007/y5686e/y5686e00.htm

Food and Drug Administration Modernization Act of 1997, Public Law 105-115. 105th Congress, 1st Session. November 21, 1997.

Golan, E., Kuchler, F., Mitchell, L., Green, C., & Jessup, A. (2001). Economics of food labeling. *Journal of Consumer Policy, 24,* 117–184.

Institute of Medicine. (1994). *How should the Recommended Dietary Allowances be revised?* Washington, DC: National Academy Press.

Institute of Medicine. (1997). *Dietary Reference Intakes for calcium, phosphorus, magnesium, vitamin D, and fluoride.* Washington, DC: National Academy Press.

Institute of Medicine. (1998). *Dietary Reference Intakes for thiamin, riboflavin, niacin, vitamin B_6, folate, vitamin B_{12}, pantothenic acid, biotin, and choline.* Washington, DC: National Academy Press.

Institute of Medicine. (2000a). *Dietary Reference Intakes for vitamin C, vitamin E, selenium and carotenoids.* Washington, DC: National Academy Press.

Institute of Medicine. (2000b). *Dietary Reference Intakes: Applications in dietary assessment.* Washington, DC: National Academy Press.

Institute of Medicine. (2001). *Dietary Reference Intakes for vitamin A, vitamin K, arsenic, boron, chromium, copper, iodine, iron, manganese, molybdenum, nickel, silicon, vanadium, and zinc.* Washington, DC: National Academy Press.

Institute of Medicine. (2002). *Dietary Reference Intakes for energy, carbohydrate, fiber, fat, fatty acids, cholesterol, protein, and amino acids.* Washington, DC: The National Academies Press.

Institute of Medicine. (2003). *Dietary Reference Intakes: Applications in dietary planning.* Washington, DC: The National Academies Press.

Institute of Medicine. (2004). *Dietary Reference Intakes for water, potassium, sodium, chloride, and sulfate.* Washington, DC: The National Academies Press.

Institute of Medicine. (2006). *Dietary Reference Intakes: The essential guide to nutrient requirements.* Washington, DC: The National Academies Press.

Institute of Medicine. (2007). *Dietary Reference Intakes research synthesis: Workshop summary.* Washington, DC: The National Academies Press.

Institute of Medicine. (2008). *The development of the DRIs 1994–2004: Lessons learned and new challenges: Workshop summary.* Washington, DC: The National Academies Press.

Institute of Medicine. (2010). *Front-of-package nutrition rating systems and symbols.* Washington, DC: The National Academies Press.

Institute of Medicine. (2011). *Dietary Reference Intakes for calcium and vitamin D.* Washington, DC: The National Academies Press.

Kushi, L. H., Byers, T., Doyle, C., Bandera, E. V., McCullough, M., Gansler, T.,… American Cancer Society 2006 Nutrition and Physical Activity Guidelines Advisory Committee. (2006). American Cancer Society guidelines on nutrition and physical activity for cancer prevention: Reducing the risk of cancer with healthy food choices and physical activity. *CA: A Cancer Journal for Clinicians, 56,* 254–281.

Lichtenstein, A. H., Appel, L. J., Brands, M., Carnethon, M., Daniels, S., Franch, H. A., … Wylie-Rosett, J. (2006). Diet and lifestyle recommendations revision 2006: A scientific statement from the American Heart Association Nutrition Committee. *Circulation, 114,* 82–96.

National Health and Medical Research Council. (2006). *Nutrient reference values for Australia and New Zealand: Including recommended dietary intakes.* Canberra: NHMRC Publications. Retrieved from http://www.nhmrc.gov.au/_files_nhmrc/file/publications/synopses/n35.pdf

National Nutrition Monitoring and Related Research Act of 1990, Public Law 101-445. 101st Congress, 2nd session. October 22, 1990.

National Research Council. (1989). *Diet and health: Implications for reducing chronic disease risk.* Washington, DC: National Academy Press.

Nutrition Labeling and Education Act of 1990, Public Law 101-535. 101st Congress, 2nd session. November 8, 1990.

Patient Protection and Affordable Care Act. (2010). Public Law 111-148. 111th Congress, 2nd session. March 23, 2010.

Pavlovic, M., Prentice, A., Thorsdottir, I., Wolfram, G., & Branca, F. (2007). Challenges in harmonizing energy and nutrient recommendations in Europe. *Annals of Nutrition & Metabolism, 51,* 108–114.

Prentice, A., Branca, F., Desci, T., Michaelsen, K. F., Fletcher, R. J., Guesry, P., … Samartín, S. (2004). Energy and nutrient dietary reference values for children in Europe: Methodological approaches and current nutritional recommendations. *British Journal of Nutrition, 92,* S83–S146.

U.S. Department of Agriculture. (1992). The Food Guide Pyramid. *USDA Home and Garden Bulletin 252.* Washington, DC: U.S. Government Printing Office.

U.S. Department of Agriculture. (2005). *USDA Secretary Mike Johanns reveals USDA's steps to a healthier you.* USDA press release, April 19. Retrieved from http://www.choosemyplate.gov/global_nav/media_press_release.html

U.S. Department of Agriculture. (2010). *Dietary guidance, Food Guide Pyramid.* Beltsville, MD: Food and Nutrition Information Center. Retrieved from http://fnic.nal.usda.gov/nal_display/index.php?info_center=4&tax_level=2&tax_subject=256&topic_id=1348

U.S. Department of Agriculture. (2011). *First Lady, Agriculture Secretary launch MyPlate icon as a new reminder to help consumers to make healthier food choices.* USDA press release, June 2. Retrieved from http://www.cnpp.usda.gov/Publications/MyPlate/PressRelease.pdf

U.S. Department of Agriculture/U.S. Department of Health and Human Services. (2010). *Dietary Guidelines for Americans 2010* (7th ed.). Washington, DC: U.S. Government Printing Office.

U.S. Department of Health and Human Services. (1988). *The Surgeon General's report on nutrition and health.* DHHS Publication No. (PHS) 88-50210. Washington, DC: U.S. Government Printing Office.

U.S. Department of Health and Human Services. (1993). Food labeling; General provisions; Nutrition labeling; Label format; Nutrient content claims; Health claims; Ingredient labeling; State and local requirements and exemptions; Final rules. *Federal Register, 58,* 2066–2941.

U.S. Department of Health and Human Services. (1994). Dietary supplements; Establishment of date of application. *Federal Register, 61,* 350–437.

U.S. Department of Health and Human Services. (2003a). Food labeling; Trans fatty acids in nutrition labeling; Consumer research to consider nutrient content and health claims and possible footnote or disclosure statements; Final rule and proposed rule. *Federal Register, 68,* 41433–41506.

U.S. Department of Health and Human Services. (2003b). *Claims that can be used on conventional foods and dietary supplements.* College Park, MD: Food and Drug Administration. Retrieved from http://www.fda.gov/Food/GuidanceCompliance RegulatoryInformation/GuidanceDocuments/FoodLabelingNutrition/FoodLabelingGuide/ucm111447.htm

U.S. Department of Health and Human Services. (2009a). *Guidance for industry: A food labeling guide.* College Park, MD: Food and Drug Administration. Retrieved from http://www.fda.gov/Food/GuidanceComplianceRegulatoryInformation/Guidance Documents/FoodLabelingNutrition/FoodLabelingGuide

U.S. Department of Health and Human Services. (2009b). *Guidance for industry: Evidence-based review system for the scientific evaluation of health claims.* College Park, MD: Food and Drug Administration. Retrieved from http://www.fda.gov/Food/GuidanceComplianceRegulatoryInformation/GuidanceDocuments/FoodLabelingNutrition/ucm073332.htm

U.S. Department of Health and Human Services. (2009c). *Guidance for industry: Letter regarding point of purchase food labeling.* College Park, MD: Food and Drug Administration. Retrieved from http://www.fda.gov/Food/GuidanceComplianceRegulatoryInformation/GuidanceDocuments/FoodLabelingNutrition/ucm187208.htm

U.S. Department of Health and Human Services. (2010a). *Healthy People 2020: Objective topic areas.* Retrieved from http://www.healthypeople.gov/2020/topicsobjectives2020/pdfs/HP2020objectives.pdf

U.S. Department of Health and Human Services. (2010b). *The Surgeon General's vision for a healthy and fit nation 2010.* Rockville, MD: Office of the Surgeon General. Retrieved from http://www.surgeongeneral.gov/library/obesityvision/obesityvision2010.pdf

U.S. Department of Health and Human Services. (2010c). *Structure/function claims.* College Park, MD: Food and Drug Administration. Retrieved from http://www.fda.gov/Food/LabelingNutrition/LabelClaims/StructureFunctionClaims

U.S. Department of Health and Human Services/U.S. Department of Agriculture. (2005). *Dietary Guidelines for Americans 2005* (6th ed.). Washington, DC: U.S. Government Printing Office. Retrieved from http://www.health.gov/dietaryguidelines/dga2005/document/pdf/DGA2005.pdf

United States Senate Select Committee on Nutrition and Human Needs. (1977). *Dietary goals for the United States* (2nd ed.). Washington, DC: U.S. Government Printing Office.

Welsh, S., Davis, C., & Shaw, A. (1993). *USDA's food guide: Background and development.* U.S. Department of Agriculture, Human Nutrition Information Service, Miscellaneous Publication 1514.

World Health Organization/Food and Agriculture Organization Expert Consultation. (2003). *Diet, nutrition and the prevention of chronic diseases.* WHO Technical Report Series 916. Geneva: WHO. Retrieved from ftp://ftp.fao.org/docrep/fao/005/ac911e/ac911e00.pdf

RECOMMENDED WEBSITES

Institute of Medicine of the National Academies. Information about the Dietary Reference Intakes. http://www.iom.edu/Global/Topics/Food-Nutrition

U.S Department of Agriculture, Center for Nutrition Policy and Promotion. Information about the Dietary Guidelines and the Dietary Guidelines Advisory Committee. http://www.dietaryguidelines.gov

U.S. Department of Agriculture, Center for Nutrition Policy and Promotion. Information for consumers and professionals about MyPlate, the USDA Food Patterns, guidance for healthful eating, and interactive dietary assessment tools. http://www.ChooseMyPlate.gov

U.S. Department of Health and Human Services, Food and Drug Administration, Food Labeling and Nutrition. Information about labeling of foods and dietary supplements. http://www.fda.gov/Food/LabelingNutrition

UNIT II

Structure and Properties of the Macronutrients

The organic macronutrients are carbon compounds synthesized by living organisms. They include carbohydrates, proteins or amino acids, and lipids. In the individual chapters in this unit on the structure and properties of the organic macronutrients, specific compounds in each class are described, from the viewpoint of both dietary macronutrients and organic compounds formed in the human body during metabolism of the macronutrients. Compounds in the fourth group of organic nutrients, the vitamins, are micronutrients and are considered in Unit VI. Organic macronutrients are required in large amounts and are sources of energy for the body.

Like all organic compounds, proteins, carbohydrates, and lipids are made up largely of six elements: (1) hydrogen, (2) oxygen, (3) carbon, and (4) nitrogen along with some (5) phosphorus and (6) sulfur. These six relatively small elements, with atomic weights less than or equal to 32, make up the basic structures of proteins, carbohydrates, lipids, and vitamins, as well as nucleic acids and intermediates of metabolism. If water (H_2O), which makes up approximately 63% of the human body, is not considered, carbon, oxygen, hydrogen, and nitrogen (in organic compounds) make up 92% of the "dry weight" of the human body; these elements are present in about 11 kg of protein, 10 kg of fat, and about 1 kg of carbohydrate (mainly glycogen) in a lean 65-kg man.

The ability of carbon to form carbon-to-carbon bonds, extended carbon chains, and cyclic compounds permits the formation of a myriad of organic compounds; the structures of a number of these compounds are considered in this unit. In organic molecules, the atoms of carbon, hydrogen, oxygen, phosphorus, and sulfur are held together by covalent bonds, which are formed when two atoms share a pair of outer orbital electrons. Each covalent bond of every molecule represents a small amount of stored energy, thereby allowing organic molecules to serve as a source of energy to the body. Units III, IV, and V describe the processes involved in the assimilation of dietary organic macronutrients, how these are used by the body for growth and maintenance via synthesis of the structural and functional components of the human body, and how these macronutrients are used as fuels with conversion of excess substrate to stored fuels for subsequent use.

CHAPTER 4

Structure, Nomenclature, and Properties of Carbohydrates

*Joanne L. Slavin, PhD, RD**

Carbohydrates are the most abundant organic components in most fruits, vegetables, legumes, and cereal grains, and they provide texture and flavor in many processed foods. They are the major energy source for humans by digestion and absorption in the small intestine and, to a lesser extent, by microbial fermentation in the large intestine. Food carbohydrates are often classified as available or unavailable carbohydrates. Available carbohydrates are those that are hydrolyzed by enzymes of the human gastrointestinal tract to monosaccharides that are absorbed in the small intestine and enter the pathways of carbohydrate metabolism. Unavailable carbohydrates are not hydrolyzed by human digestive enzymes, but they may be partially or totally fermented by bacteria in the large intestine, forming short-chain fatty acids that may be absorbed and contribute to the body's energy needs.

Glucose is an essential energy source for human tissues; some types of cells such as red blood cells are not able to use other fuels. Glucose for the body's use may be derived from dietary starches and sugars, from glycogen stores in the body, or by synthesis in vivo from gluconeogenic precursors such as amino acid carbon skeletons. Glucose also serves as a precursor for synthesis of all other carbohydrates including lactose produced by the mammary gland, the ribose needed for nucleic acid synthesis, and the sugar residues that are found as covalently bound constituents of glycoproteins, glycolipids, and proteoglycans in the body.

Carbohydrates are defined as polyhydroxy aldehydes and ketones and derivatives of these sugars. This definition emphasizes the hydrophilic nature of most carbohydrates and allows inclusion of sugar alcohols (alditols), sugar acids (uronic, aldonic, and aldaric acids), glycosides, and polymerized products (oligosaccharides and polysaccharides) among the classes of carbohydrates. The hydroxyl groups of carbohydrates may be modified by substitution with other groups to give esters and ethers or be replaced to give deoxy and amino sugars. Carbohydrates are also covalently bound to many proteins and lipids. These glycoconjugates include the glycoproteins, proteoglycans, and glycolipids.

*This chapter is a revision of the chapter contributed by Betty A. Lewis, PhD, and Martha H. Stipanuk, PhD, for the second edition.

MONOSACCHARIDES OR SUGAR RESIDUES

Aldoses and ketoses are monosaccharides or simple sugars. Monosaccharides are further classified by the number of carbon atoms in their structures (i.e., the trioses, tetroses, pentoses, hexoses, heptoses, octoses, and nonoses) and by their stereochemistry (i.e., D or L). For chains of sugar residues or "monosaccharide" units, the carbohydrates are classified by the degree to which the sugar units are polymerized (e.g., disaccharides, oligosaccharides, and polysaccharides).

STRUCTURES AND NOMENCLATURE OF THE ALDOSES AND KETOSES

Monosaccharides or simple sugars include the aldoses such as glucose and ketoses such as fructose. Aldoses contain one aldehyde group and hence are polyhydroxy aldehydes. Ketoses contain one ketone group and hence are polyhydroxy ketones. Both have the empirical chemical formula $(CH_2O)_n$.

Chirality of Monosaccharides

A chiral carbon atom is one that is bonded to four different groups. A property of chiral molecules that lack a plane of symmetry is optical activity, or their ability to rotate or turn the plane of linearly polarized light as the light travels through a solution of the compound. Several systems are used to designate the chirality or spatial configuration of atoms on a molecule. The D/L system is commonly used for designating the chirality of sugars and amino acids. In the D/L system, each molecule is named by its relation to glyceraldehyde. Glyceraldehyde is the simplest aldose sugar with a chiral atom, the C2 of glyceraldehyde. Thus, the three-carbon glyceraldehyde exists as both D- and L-enantiomers. The two-carbon aldehyde, glycolaldehyde, does not have a chiral carbon atom and hence has no optical activity.

All D-aldoses are related to D-glyceraldehyde, and L-aldoses are similarly related to L-glyceraldehyde. The relation of D-aldoses to D-glyceraldehyde can be seen clearly by looking at a scheme for the chemical synthesis of the series of D-aldoses from D-glyceraldehyde. In the synthetic scheme shown in Figure 4-1, a nucleophilic cyanide ion (:CN) adds to the carbonyl carbon (C1) of glyceraldehyde, giving two cyanohydrin products. Selective reduction and hydrolysis of the CN group to an aldehyde completes the conversion of the triose D-glyceraldehyde to the pair of aldotetroses having

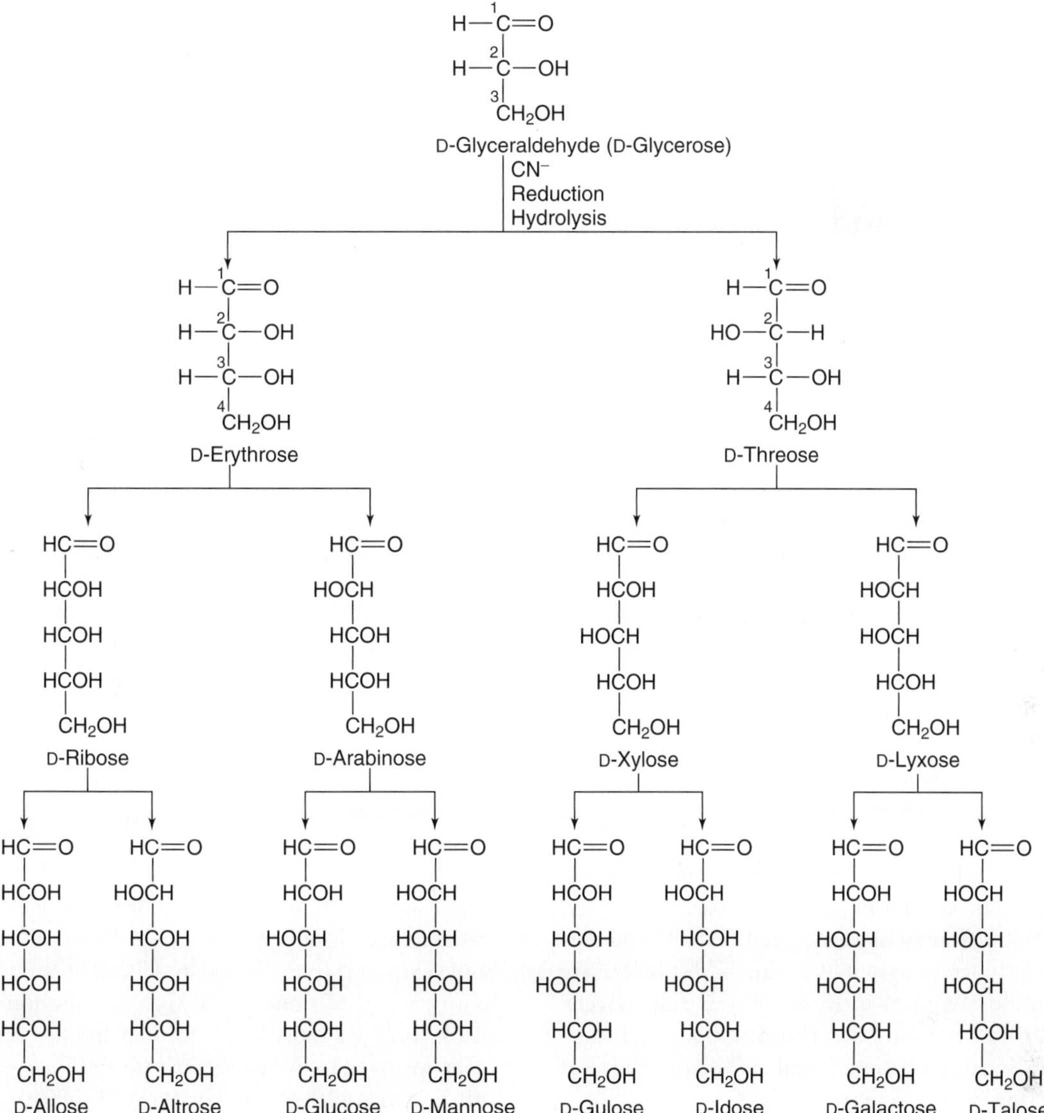

FIGURE 4-1 Structures of the D-aldoses (tetroses, pentoses, and hexoses) showing their derivation from D-glyceraldehyde by chemical synthesis. At each application of this reaction scheme, the :CN anion adds to the carbonyl carbon, lengthening the carbon chain by one carbon and creating a new chiral center at C2 and a new pair of isomers. Reduction and hydrolysis of the cyanide group restore the aldehyde functional group.

a new chiral carbon at C2 (i.e., C1 of the glyceraldehyde precursor). Accordingly, this reaction scheme lengthens the carbon chain from the carbonyl end and gives two new aldoses, the last three carbons of which derive from glyceraldehyde. Therefore the configuration of the hydroxyl on the highest numbered chiral carbon of an aldose or ketose determines its D or L status. For a D-sugar, this hydroxyl is shown drawn to the right of the carbon chain in the Fischer formula.

Each cycle of the synthesis creates a new chiral center (i.e., at C2 of the successive aldoses) and a pair of stereoisomers. Accordingly, there are two tetroses, four pentoses, and eight hexoses in the D- (see Figure 4-1) and also in the L-series; not all of these occur commonly in nature. The nutritionally important glucose is one of the eight possible D-aldohexose monosaccharides. The L-sugars are mirror images (enantiomers) of the D-sugars, with the configuration of all chiral carbons reversed (e.g., D-glucose and L-glucose).

Similarly, D-ketoses are related to D-glyceraldehyde, and L-ketoses are related to L-glyceraldehyde. The simplest ketose sugar is the three-carbon dihydroxyacetone, which does not have a chiral carbon. The simplest ketose sugar with enantiomers is the four-carbon erythrulose.

Epimers

Sugars that vary in their configuration at only one carbon are epimers: for example, D-glucose and D-mannose are C2 epimers, whereas D-glucose and D-galactose are C4 epimers. Enzymes that catalyze epimer formation are called epimerases.

Systematic Naming of Aldoses and Ketoses

The names of each of the two aldotetroses, four aldopentoses and eight aldohexoses are shown in Figure 4-1. The carbonyl group in aldoses is always C1, but carbonyl groups

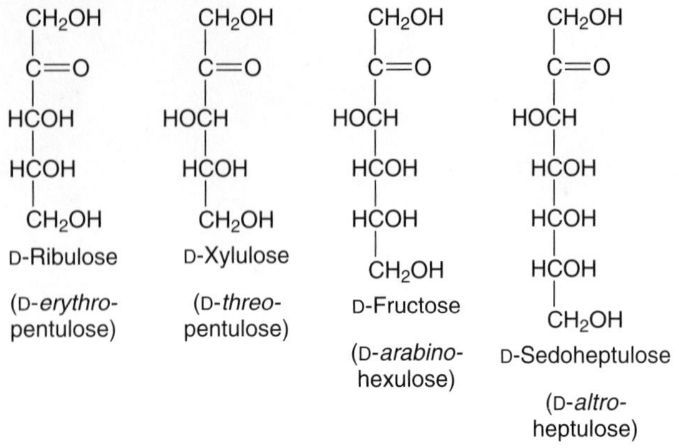

CH$_2$OH	CH$_2$OH	CH$_2$OH	CH$_2$OH
C=O	C=O	C=O	C=O
HCOH	HOCH	HOCH	HOCH
HCOH	HCOH	HCOH	HCOH
CH$_2$OH	CH$_2$OH	HCOH	HCOH
		CH$_2$OH	HCOH
			CH$_2$OH
D-Ribulose (D-*erythro*-pentulose)	D-Xylulose (D-*threo*-pentulose)	D-Fructose (D-*arabino*-hexulose)	D-Sedoheptulose (D-*altro*-heptulose)

FIGURE 4-2 Physiologically important ketoses and their common names. Systematic names are shown in parentheses.

may occur at any internal carbon atom in ketoses. In the common ketoses (Figure 4-2), the carbonyl group is usually at C2. A few ketoses, such as fructose, are known by their trivial names, but ketoses also are named systematically with the suffix "-ulose" denoting a ketose sugar. In this nomenclature, a group of up to four consecutive chiral carbons is named after the corresponding aldose sugar (e.g., triose, tetrose, pentose, or hexose) that possesses the same chiral group, and the number of carbon atoms is designated also. D-Fructose is the most common ketose, and its systematic name is D-*arabino*-hexulose, showing that the three chiral carbons in D-fructose have the same configuration as the three chiral carbons in D-arabinose. Frequently, the names ribulose and xylulose are used for the two ketopentoses. Their correct systematic names, however, are D-*erythro*-pentulose and D-*threo*-pentulose, respectively, showing that they have only two chiral carbons and indicating the relationship of these chiral carbons to those of erythrose and threose (see Figure 4-1).

Although the common monosaccharides are pentoses and hexoses, sugars with more than six carbon atoms also occur naturally. Some have trivial names, but most sugars having more than six carbons and possessing four or more chiral carbons are named systematically, as described in the preceding text for the aldoses and ketoses. Sedoheptulose (D-*altro*-heptulose), a seven-carbon sugar, and the other ketoses shown in Figure 4-2 are involved as phosphorylated intermediates in carbohydrate metabolism. *N*-Acetylneuraminic acid, a nine-carbon acidic ketose, is an important signaling epitope in glycoproteins.

The abbreviations or symbols for the sugars usually consist of the first three letters of their names (Table 4-1). The abbreviations of glucose (Glc) and some ketoses are exceptions to this rule.

CYCLIC AND CONFORMATIONAL STRUCTURES FOR MONOSACCHARIDES AND SUGAR RESIDUES

Hemiacetals and hemiketals are compounds that are formed by addition of an alcohol to a carbonyl group of an aldehyde or ketone, respectively. Reaction of an intramolecular hydroxyl group with the carbonyl group of an aldose or

TABLE 4-1 Abbreviated Names for Some Common Carbohydrates

NAME	ABBREVIATION
Arabinose	Ara
Fructose	Fru
Fucose	Fuc
Galactose	Gal
Galacturonic acid	GalA
N-Acetylgalactosamine	GalNAc
Glucose	Glc
Glucuronic acid	GlcA
N-Acetylglucosamine	GlcNAc
Iduronic acid	IdoA
Mannose	Man
N-Acetylneuraminic acid	Neu5Ac
Rhamnose	Rha
Xylose	Xyl

Abbreviations for di-, oligo-, and polysaccharides often add D- or L- to indicate the enantiomeric form, *p* or *f* to indicate the pyranose or furanose ring form, α- or β- to indicate the stereochemistry of the glycosidic linkage, and carbon numbers to indicate the carbon atoms that are *O*-linked by the glycosidic bond. The designation is often omitted for the more common D-enantiomers and *p*-ring form.

ketose forms a cyclic hemiacetal or cyclic hemiketal, which are also called lactols. When a ring structure forms, the carbonyl carbon is transformed into a chiral carbon, giving rise to a new pair of isomers called α- and β-anomers. Aldoses and ketoses are more stable in their five- or six-membered cyclic forms than in their acyclic forms. Thus glucose, fructose, and many other sugars exist mainly in their cyclic forms.

Cyclization of Aldoses and Ketoses to Pyranose and Furanose Ring Structures

Cyclization of an aldose occurs via an intramolecular reaction of the nucleophilic hydroxyl group on C4 or C5 with the C1 aldehyde, as shown for glucose in Figure 4-3. This spontaneous reaction transforms the carbonyl carbon (i.e., C1 of an aldose) into a chiral carbon (the anomeric carbon), giving the α- and β-anomers of both the furanose and pyranose ring forms. The same type of cyclization reaction occurs with the ketoses in which the C5 or C6 hydroxyl group reacts with the C2 ketose carbonyl. In the Fischer formula, the hemiacetal (anomeric) –OH of the α-anomer is drawn on the same side of the carbon chain as the D designator oxygen (e.g., C5–O– of a hexose). In aqueous solution, the acyclic and cyclic isomers are in equilibrium, with the most energetically stable isomers predominating. For most aldoses, the six-membered pyranose ring is more stable than the five-membered furanose ring. However, some sugars (e.g., arabinose, ribose, and fructose) frequently occur in the furanose ring form in disaccharides, oligosaccharides, and polymers. The equilibrium nature of the hemiacetal reaction dictates that all hydroxyls

β-D-Glucopyranose ⇌ *aldehydo*-D-Glucose ⇌ α-D-Glucopyranose

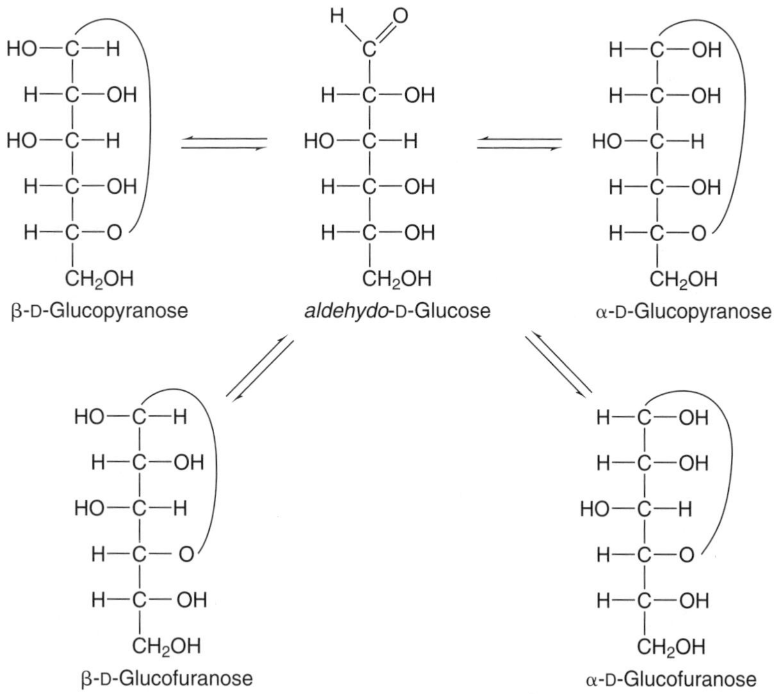

β-D-Glucofuranose α-D-Glucofuranose

FIGURE 4-3 The equilibrium mixture of cyclic anomeric and acyclic forms of D-glucose in aqueous solution.

and the carbonyl group can undergo reactions; that is, the sugar can react in acyclic or in ring form.

Drawing Sugar Ring Structures

Sugar ring structures are depicted in several ways, as shown for glucose and fructose in Figure 4-4. The Fischer projection formula is a convention used to depict a stereoformula in two dimensions. The Haworth formula was introduced as a more realistic depiction of the bond lengths in the cyclic sugars. Hydroxyl groups on the right of the carbon chain in the Fischer projection are below the plane of the ring in the Haworth formula, and those on the left of the carbon chain in the Fischer projection are above the plane of the ring in the Haworth formula. The exocyclic group (e.g., the $-CH_2OH$ group attached to C5 of hexoses such as glucose and fructose shown in Figure 4-4) is placed above or below the plane in the Haworth formula, depending on the stereochemistry of the ring oxygen. If the hydroxyl group that contributes the ring oxygen is on the right of the carbon chain in the Fischer structure, then the exocyclic group is above the plane in the Haworth structure. If the ring connects from a hydroxyl group on the left of the carbon chain in the Fischer structure, then the exocyclic group is drawn below the plane in the Haworth structure.

Because five- and six-membered rings are not planar but have a three-dimensional characteristic, the chair conformational formula is preferred for showing spatial relationships, such as in enzyme-catalyzed reactions where fit of substrate to enzyme binding site is important. In chair conformations, C2, C3, C5, and the ring oxygen are planar, and C1 and C4 are out of the plane and on opposite sides of the plane. The orientations of the hydroxyls are axial (almost perpendicular to the mean plane of the ring) or equatorial (almost parallel to the mean plane). Pyranose sugars assume a chair conformation based in part on maximizing the number of large groups ($-OH$ and $-CH_2OH$) at equatorial positions, which are less sterically hindered than are axial positions. The $^4C_1$ conformation, in which C4 is above and C1 is below the plane, is preferred (lower energy) for α- and β-D-glucopyranose and most of the other aldohexoses.

CHEMICAL REACTIVITY OF THE MONOSACCHARIDES AND SUGAR RESIDUES

Sugars are relatively stable when pure and dry. In solution, their alcohol, aldehyde, and keto groups are involved in various reactions that are both nonenzymatic and enzymatic.

General Reactivity of Sugars

Aldoses are reducing agents, and the carbonyl group of an aldose is simultaneously oxidized to a carboxyl group when aldoses act as reducing agents. Ketoses are not good reducing agents because simultaneous oxidation of the carbonyl would require carbon chain cleavage. However, ketoses can isomerize to aldoses in an alkaline reducing sugar test and therefore result in a positive reducing sugar test even though they are nonreducing sugars. Formerly, glucose in urine was analyzed by an assay for reducing sugars, but more specific methods are now available. In vivo, oxidation of the aldehyde group of glucose is catalyzed enzymatically by a dehydrogenase, and this reaction yields the lactone (an intramolecular ester of the newly formed carboxylic acid) as the product. An example of this type of reaction is the conversion of glucose 6-phosphate to 6-phosphoglucono-δ-lactone in the pentose phosphate pathway of metabolism (see Chapter 12, Figure 12-20).

β-D-Glucopyranose:

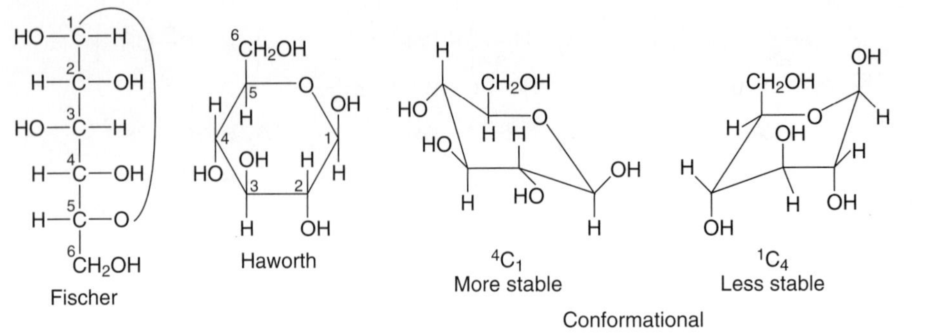

Fischer

Haworth

$^4C_1$ More stable

$^1C_4$ Less stable

Conformational

β-D-Fructofuranose:

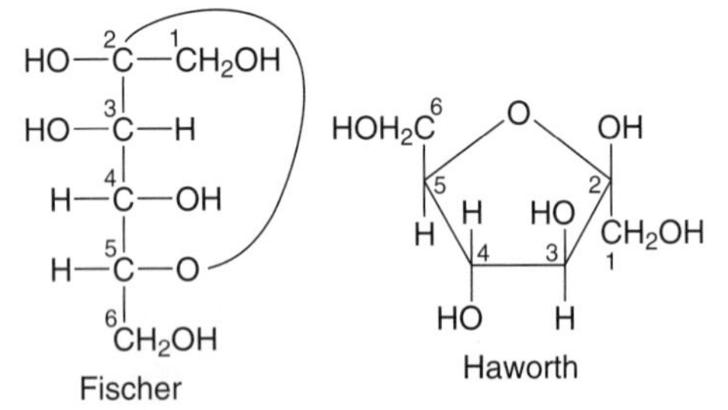

Fischer

Haworth

FIGURE 4-4 Representations of the cyclic structures of β-D-glucopyranose and β-D-fructofuranose. The chair conformations are designated "C" with a superscript number on the left that indicates the number of the sugar carbon that lies above the plane, and with a subscript number on the right that indicates the number of the sugar carbon that lies below the plane. The other three ring carbons and the ring oxygen lie within the plane.

The carbonyl group of an aldose or ketose is readily reduced to an alcohol by chemical catalysis, giving an alditol from an aldose or an epimeric pair of alditols from a ketose. These alditols (sugar alcohols), which lack a carbonyl group, are more stable than the aldoses and ketoses, and they are not reducing agents. Aldehyde reductases catalyze a similar reduction in vivo (e.g., in conversion of glucose to glucitol, which is also known as sorbitol).

The carbon proton adjacent to the carbonyl (i.e., the C2 or α-carbon proton) in aldoses is acidic and easily abstracted in basic solution, leading to epimerization of the aldoses at C2 as well as their isomerization to ketoses. Thus glucose is epimerized to mannose and isomerized to fructose. Similar reactions occur in carbohydrate metabolism, as seen in the phosphoglucose isomerase–catalyzed conversion of glucose 6-phosphate to fructose 6-phosphate and in the phosphomannose isomerase-catalyzed conversion of mannose 6-phosphate to fructose 6-phosphate (see Chapter 12, Figures 12-4 and 12-5). Similar reactions occur with ketoses.

Hydroxyl groups of carbohydrates are readily converted into a variety of esters, but the phosphate esters of the monosaccharides are particularly important as intermediates in metabolism. Sugar phosphates are also components of biological polymers. This is illustrated by the nucleic acids, which have ribose phosphates and 2-deoxyribose phosphates as key constituents. Other derivatives of hydroxyls, including ethers, are also important in modification of monosaccharides in living systems and contribute to the diversity of carbohydrate structure.

Formation of Glycosidic Linkages

The general term *glycoside* is used to describe any molecule in which a sugar group is bonded through its anomeric carbon to another group via a glycosidic bond. As an example, the acid-catalyzed reaction of a sugar (glucose) with an alcohol (methanol) to form methyl D-glucopyranoside, which is an example of an *O*-glycoside, is shown in Figure 4-5. Although only the α-glycoside is shown, both α- and β-glycosides form in nonenzymatic reactions. When properly activated, sugars react with each other to form specific oligosaccharides and polysaccharides in which a sugar residue is linked by a new bond between its anomeric carbon and one of the hydroxyl groups of the second sugar residue. Thus the sugar residues in oligosaccharides and polysaccharides are linked by *O*-glycosidic bonds.

The terms *glycone* and *aglycone* are commonly used to refer to the two molecules linked by a glycosidic bond, particularly when the compound being described is not a chain of sugar residues (i.e., not an oligosaccharide or polysaccharide). The sugar group is the glycone and the nonsugar group is the aglycone part of the glycoside; for example, in Figure 4-5 glucose is the glycone and methanol is the aglycone portion of methyl D-glucopyranoside. The glycone can consist of a single sugar group (monosaccharide) or several sugar groups (oligosaccharide). Glycosides may be classified by the sugar group. If the sugar group is glucose, the molecule is a glucoside; if it is glucuronic acid (glucuronate), the molecule is a glucuronide. Various hydroxylated compounds are glycosylated in the liver by linkage to glucuronic

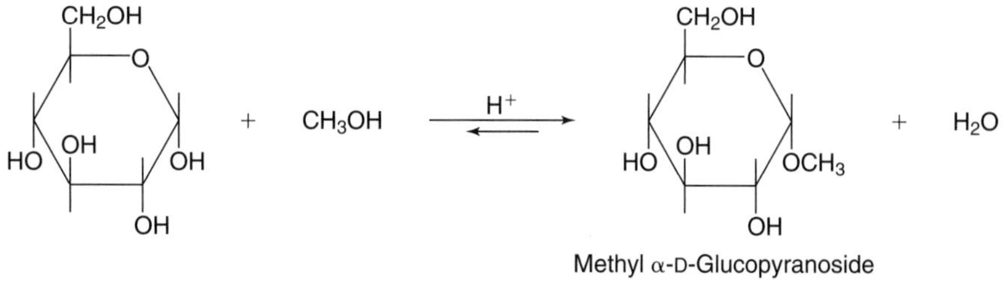

FIGURE 4-5 Reactions of sugars with alcohols. Acid-catalyzed synthesis of the glycoside methyl α-D-glucopyranoside. This reaction is reversible. The glycosidic bond is hydrolyzed by cleavage between the anomeric carbon of the glucosyl group and the oxygen of the bond.

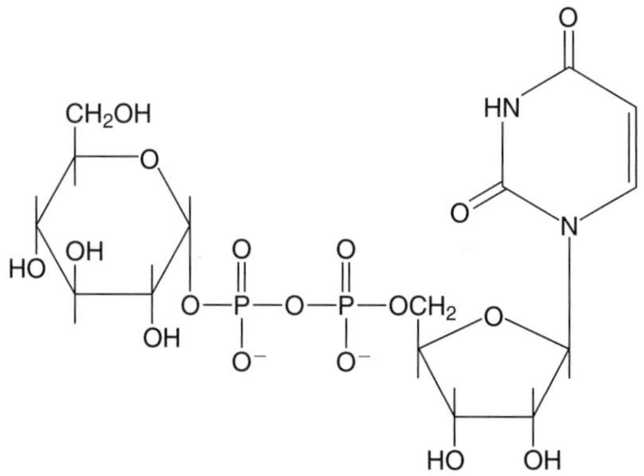

FIGURE 4-6 The structure of uridine diphosphate (UDP)–glucose (UDPG), an activated form of glucose and an intermediate in glycogen synthesis in vivo. In this structure, β-D-ribose is linked to the amine uracil by an *N*-glycosidic bond, and the α-D-glucose unit is esterified to phosphate by an *O*-glycosidic bond.

acid, which increases their water solubility; formation of β-D-glucuronides is a major means of detoxification and excretion of both endogenous (e.g., bilirubin) and exogenous (e.g., acetaminophen) compounds.

Sugars also react with amines or thiols to give *N*- or *S*-glycosides, respectively. For example, β-D-ribose and 2-deoxy-β-D-ribose in nucleic acids are bonded to purines and pyrimidines by *N*-glycosidic bonds. In uridine diphosphate (UDP)–glucose, the β-D-ribose is linked to uracil by an *N*-glycosidic bond, and the α-D-glucose and β-D-ribose units are each ester-linked to phosphate, as shown in Figure 4-6. The sugar nucleotides are used extensively in vivo for enzymatic synthesis of carbohydrates, including lactose and glycogen. In glycoproteins, oligosaccharide chains are linked to the β-carboxamide nitrogen of asparagine (an *N*-glycosidic bond) or to the hydroxyl of serine/threonine (an *O*-glycosidic bond). Plants use the glycosidic bond extensively in synthesizing different glycosides, many of which are physiologically active.

Glycosides are more stable than aldoses and ketoses in several respects. The carbonyl/hemiacetal carbon in the glycoside is protected from base-catalyzed reactions and from reduction and oxidation. The pyranose and furanose ring structures and the anomeric configuration are also stabilized and do not undergo the interconversions shown in Figure 4-3. However, the glycosidic bonds can be hydrolyzed by acid or enzyme catalysis releasing the free sugar and the alcohol (with the alcohol often being another sugar molecule). Glycosidases, which catalyze hydrolysis of glycosides, typically have high specificity for the sugar or glycone portion and the stereochemistry of the anomeric linkage (α or β) but lower specificity for the aglycone or sugar that donates the hydroxyl group for the glycosidic bond. Such specificity has important implications for the enzymatic digestion of carbohydrates, as is discussed in Chapter 8.

Maillard Reaction of Reducing Sugars with Amines

Aldoses and ketoses react with aliphatic primary and secondary amines, including amino acids and proteins, to form *N*-glycosides, which readily dehydrate to the respective Schiff base by the Maillard reaction, as shown in Figure 4-7 (reactions i and ii). The aldose Schiff base spontaneously undergoes an Amadori rearrangement at C1 and C2, giving a substituted 1-amino-1-deoxyketose (reaction iii). A ketose Schiff base will rearrange to a substituted 2-amino-2-deoxyaldose (not shown). These sugar amines undergo additional very complex reactions, leading to formation of highly reactive dicarbonyls (such as 3-deoxy-D-glucosone), cross-linking of proteins (as in reaction iv), formation of fluorescent compounds and brown pigments, and formation of low-molecular-weight compounds, some of which are useful flavoring agents. Although the Maillard complex of reactions has been studied extensively, the reactions are understood only in part. Lysine residues in proteins often react with sugars by the Maillard reaction. The reaction of glucose with hemoglobin was discovered first. Blood glucose reacts with hemoglobins via the Maillard reaction, and the modified protein, detected by gel electrophoresis, is an indicator of plasma glucose levels in diabetics over the lifespan of the erythrocytes. The term *glycated* protein is used to distinguish these Maillard-derived, carbohydrate-modified proteins from true glycosylated proteins (glycoproteins). The Maillard and subsequent reactions also occur in food products exposed to heat, such as in powdered or evaporated milk during processing or storage, giving an off-white color to the product and decreasing the nutritive value of food proteins. Lysine residues in proteins are irreversibly modified by the Maillard reaction, and modification of lysine residues is partially responsible for the nonenzymatic browning and decrease in nutritive value.

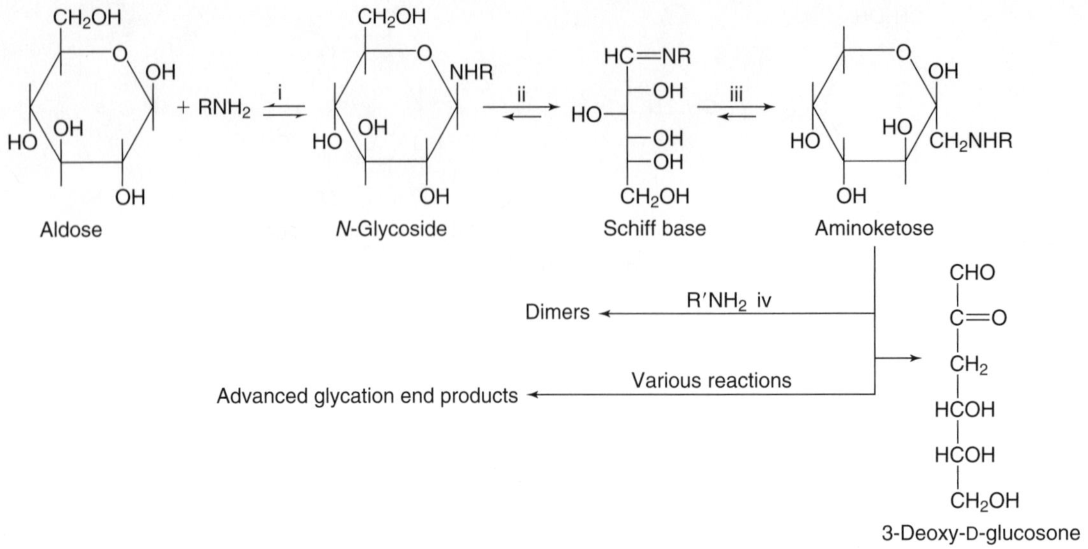

FIGURE 4-7 Initiation of the Maillard reaction of amines with aldoses. The aminoketose intermediate formed by reaction iii undergoes various reactions, including conversion to a highly reactive dicarbonyl compound (3-deoxy-D-glucosone). When the amino group ($R'NH_2$) for reaction iv is from a protein, the reaction may result in cross-linked proteins.

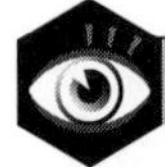

NUTRITION INSIGHT

Sugar-Protein Reactions in Diabetes and Aging

The Maillard/Amadori reactions of sugars with amino acids and proteins lead to a cascade of reactions. Products of these reactions are referred to as *advanced glycation end products.* These reaction end products have been observed in collagen-rich tissues in vivo and in vitro, and they are associated with stiffening of artery walls, lung tissue, and joints and with other aging symptoms. Considerable evidence links hyperglycemia with increased formation of these end products; these products accumulate in the blood vessel wall proteins and may contribute to vascular complications of diabetes. Glycation of lens proteins increases somewhat with aging, but acceleration is associated with diabetes. Incubation of lens proteins with glucose or glucose 6-phosphate in vitro results in changes in the lens proteins that mimic most of those observed with age- and cataract-related changes in the lens. Drug-induced inhibition of the reactions leading to these end products in diabetic animals prevents various disease-associated pathologies of the arteries, kidneys, nerves, and retina.

OTHER CLASSES OF CARBOHYDRATE UNITS

Monosaccharides or monosaccharide residues may be modified or derived in several ways. Carbonyl groups can be reduced or oxidized, and terminal $-CH_2OH$ groups can be oxidized. Hydroxyl groups on any of the carbons are subject to various modifications.

ALDITOLS

The alditols, or polyols, which occur naturally in plants and other organisms, are reduction products of aldoses and ketoses in which the carbonyl has been reduced to an alcohol. Two common alditols are shown in Figure 4-8, xylitol and sorbitol (glucitol). Reduction of ketoses gives an epimeric pair of alditols unless the reaction is enzyme-catalyzed and therefore stereospecific. The alditols, like the sugars, are soluble in water and vary in degree of sweetness. Xylitol, the sweetest, approaches the sweetness of sucrose. Because the alditols do not have a carbonyl group, they are considerably less reactive than their corresponding sugars. They do not undergo base-catalyzed reactions of epimerization and isomerization, the Maillard reaction, or the formation of glycosides (unless they are participating as the "alcohol" or aglycone component). Alditols share the same hydrophilic character as the sugars and are used in products as humectants to prevent excessive drying. Sorbitol and xylitol are not readily metabolized by oral bacteria and are used in chewing gums and candies for this noncariogenic characteristic. Both sorbitol and xylitol are

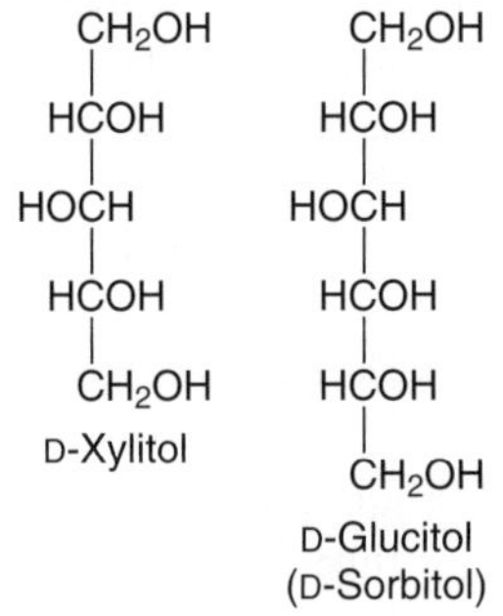

FIGURE 4-8 Structures of the common sugar alcohols (alditols), D-xylitol and D-glucitol.

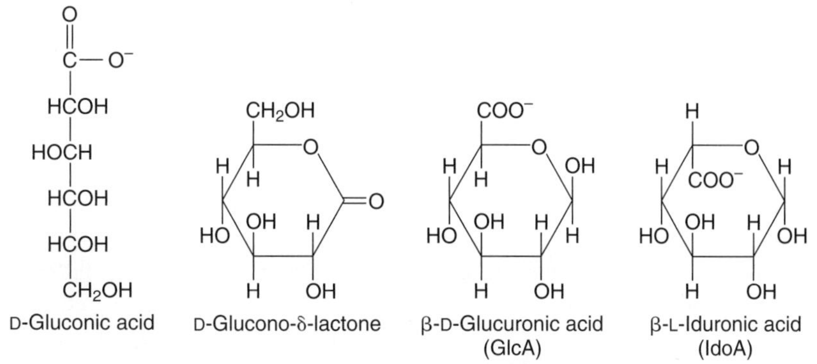

D-Gluconic acid D-Glucono-δ-lactone β-D-Glucuronic acid (GlcA) β-L-Iduronic acid (IdoA)

FIGURE 4-9 Carboxylic acid derivatives of D-glucose and L-idose. D-Gluconic acid is shown along with its 1,5-lactone, an intramolecular ester. D-Glucuronic and L-iduronic acids are shown as their β anomers; uronic acids are important constituents of glycosaminoglycans. The acids are shown in their anionic forms (gluconate, glucuronate, and iduronate), which are the major species at physiological pH.

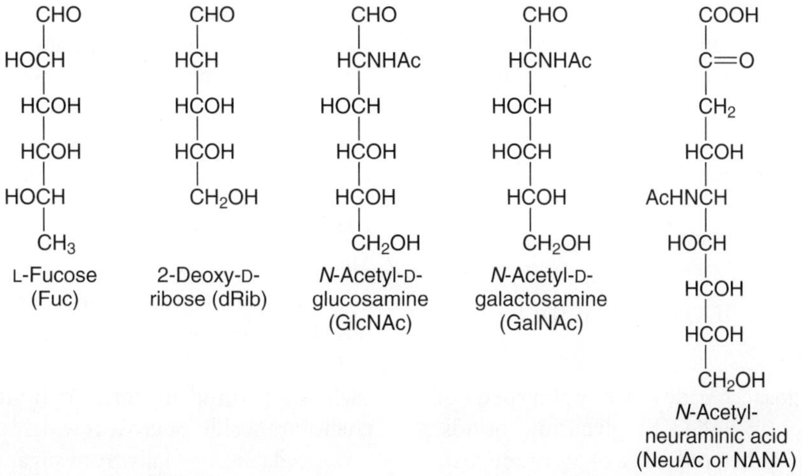

L-Fucose (Fuc) 2-Deoxy-D-ribose (dRib) *N*-Acetyl-D-glucosamine (GlcNAc) *N*-Acetyl-D-galactosamine (GalNAc) *N*-Acetyl-neuraminic acid (NeuAc or NANA)

FIGURE 4-10 Examples of deoxy and amino sugars that are constituents of important biological compounds such as DNA, glycoproteins, and glycoconjugates.

passively absorbed in the small intestine and metabolized in the liver. Excessive amounts of alditols passing into the colon may induce diarrhea owing to their fermentation leading to increased luminal osmolarity (Grabitske and Slavin, 2009).

GLYCURONIC, GLYCONIC, AND GLYCARIC ACIDS

Sugar acids are sugars in which the carbonyl group and/or the terminal $-CH_2OH$ group has been oxidized to a carboxyl group ($-COOH$). Uronic acids are formed when the terminal $-CH_2OH$ group of an aldose or ketose is oxidized to a terminal carboxyl group ($-COOH$). Two examples of uronic acids are shown in Figure 4-9. D-Glucuronic acid is an important constituent of glycosaminoglycans in mammalian systems, and its C5 epimer, L-iduronic acid, is present to a lesser extent. Glucuronic acid (and its 4-*O*-methyl ether), D-galacturonic acid, D-mannuronic acid, and the less common L-guluronic acid are constituents of the nondigestible polysaccharides of plants and algae, which contribute to dietary fiber.

Aldonic acids are oxidation products of the aldoses in which the C1 aldehyde functional group ($-CHO$) has been oxidized to a carboxyl group ($-COOH$). Aldonic acids such as gluconic acid readily undergo internal ester bond formation (between the carboxylic acid and an alcohol substituent) to yield the respective neutral cyclic lactone. D-Gluconic acid and its lactone are shown in Figure 4-10. Aldaric acids are dicarboxylic acids in which both terminal groups of the aldose have been oxidized to carboxyl groups. Ulosonic acids are formed when the C1 ($-CH_2OH$) group of a 2-ketose sugar is oxidized to a carboxyl group, creating an α-ketoacid. These sugar acids are much less common than the uronic acids.

DEOXY AND AMINO SUGARS

Several common sugars lack the complete complement of hydroxyl groups; examples of these are shown in Figure 4-10. Deoxy sugars, in which a hydroxyl group is replaced by a hydrogen, include 2-deoxy-D-ribose, L-fucose (6-deoxy-L-galactose), and L-rhamnose (6-deoxy-L-mannose). L-Fucose is a constituent of many glycoproteins and serves as a signaling epitope for physiological events (e.g., in the inflammatory response). The presence of fucose in crucial oligosaccharides of cell-surface glycoproteins is required for recruitment of leukocytes to sites of inflammation and injury. L-Rhamnose (6-deoxy-L-mannose) occurs in plant polysaccharides, and

2-deoxy-D-ribose is the sugar constituent of deoxyribonucleotides that make up DNA.

In the common amino sugars, the C2 hydroxyl group is replaced by an amino group. These common amino sugars are D-glucosamine (2-amino-2-deoxy-D-glucose) and D-galactosamine (2-amino-2-deoxy-D-galactose), which usually occur as the *N*-acetyl derivatives (*N*-acetyl-D-glucosamine and *N*-acetyl-D-galactosamine) as shown in Figure 4-10. They are constituents of glycosaminoglycans and of many glycoproteins.

Glycoproteins and a class of glycolipids known as gangliosides may also contain derivatives of neuraminic acid. Neuraminic acid is a unique nine-carbon amino deoxy keto sugar acid. The *N*- or *O*-substituted derivatives of neuraminic acid are collectively known as sialic acids, the predominant form in mammalian cells being *N*-acetylneuraminic acid, which is shown in Figure 4-10. Although the amino group of neuraminic acid is most frequently acetylated in sialic acids, it may be glycosylated instead. Hydroxyl substituents of gangliosides are much more varied and may include acetyl, lactyl, methyl, sulfate, and phosphate groups. Sialic acids play a number of important biological roles. They are present in mucins and cell-surface glycoproteins and are a critical part of the innate immune system. Chemically, neuraminic acid is very sensitive to acid degradation, and its glycosidic linkages in glycoproteins and gangliosides are very easily hydrolyzed.

DISACCHARIDES AND OLIGOSACCHARIDES AND THEIR PROPERTIES

Disaccharides and oligosaccharides are composed of monosaccharides covalently linked by glycosidic bonds. They can be classified as either reducing or nonreducing. A disaccharide or oligosaccharide terminating with a residue that has an unsubstituted anomeric –OH group is reducing. An oligosaccharide that has the final sugar unit joined by linkage of its anomeric carbon to the anomeric carbon of the preceding sugar so that the oligosaccharide does not have a free anomeric –OH is nonreducing. If the disaccharide or oligosaccharide has a free anomeric carbon (i.e., not involved in a glycosidic bond), the hemiacetal or hemiketal is in equilibrium with the free aldehyde or ketone form. Because reducing oligosaccharides have an unsubstituted anomeric –OH group at their reducing end, this sugar residue can essentially undergo any of the reactions that the simple sugars undergo, including reduction, oxidation, and base-catalyzed epimerization and isomerization.

Disaccharides and oligosaccharides are readily hydrolyzed to their constituent monosaccharides by acid or enzymatic hydrolysis of their glycosidic linkages, with enzymes showing strong specificity for the specific sugar units and anomeric forms involved in the glycosidic bonds. As a result of this specificity, humans digest only a subset of the carbohydrates present in foods. The structures of the three major dietary disaccharides (sucrose, lactose, and maltose) are shown in Figure 4-11.

DISACCHARIDES

Sucrose

Sucrose (table sugar), a nonreducing disaccharide, is composed of α-D-glucopyranosyl and β-D-fructofuranosyl units covalently linked through the anomeric carbon of each sugar unit to form α-D-glucopyranosyl-(1,2)-β-D-fructofuranoside. Sucrose is widely distributed in plants. It is produced commercially from sugar cane and sugar beets but

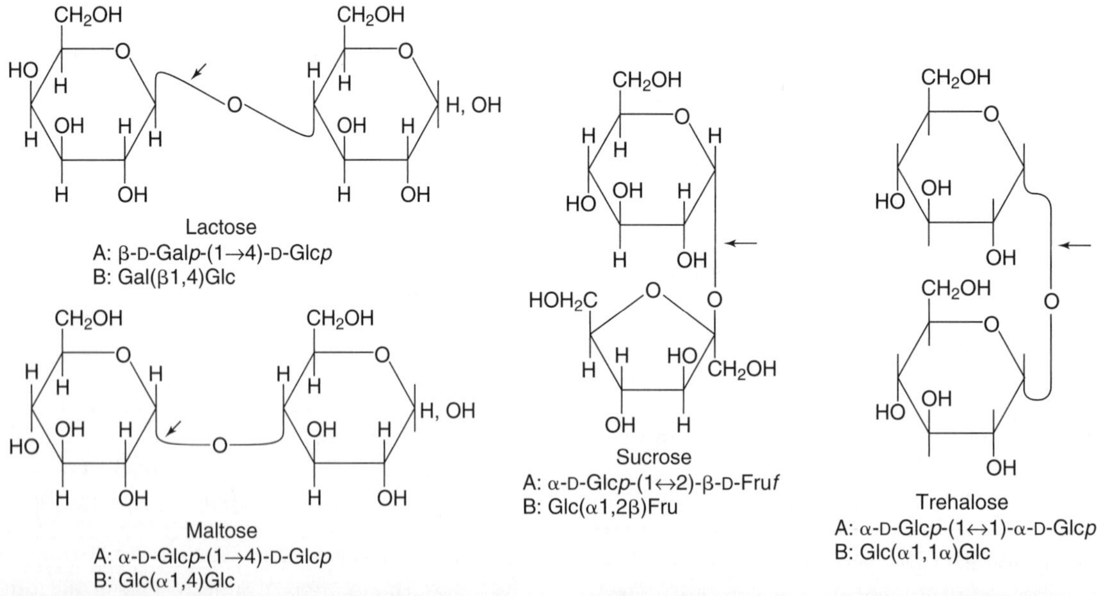

FIGURE 4-11 Reducing (lactose and maltose) and nonreducing (sucrose and trehalose) disaccharides. The free anomeric –OH of the glucosyl unit of lactose and of maltose indicates the reducing nature of these disaccharides. In sucrose and trehalose, both anomeric carbons are involved in the glycosidic bond, and these disaccharides are nonreducing. The arrows point to the glycosidic bonds. Two abbreviated structural notations are shown for these disaccharides. Notation *A* defines the complete structure, whereas *B* assumes the more common ring form and D-configuration for each sugar unit.

is typically called cane sugar regardless of its source. It is easily hydrolyzed to glucose and fructose in acid solution and rapidly digested by sucrase, an α-glucosidase of the intestinal villi. Sucrose is a major caloric sweetener for commercial or home use, and the term *sugar* on food labels refers specifically to sucrose.

Lactose

Lactose [β-D-galactopyranosyl-(1,4)-D-glucopyranose, milk sugar] is synthesized in the mammary glands of mammals. The concentration in milk varies with species and constitutes about 4 g/100 mL of bovine milk compared with 7 g/100 mL of human milk. Lactose is present in dairy products and also in processed foods that contain whey products formed from the watery part of milk that remains after the manufacture of cheese. Lactose has about one third the sweetness of sucrose. It is readily digested to glucose and galactose by a β-galactosidase (lactase) of the small intestine. Lactose is a reducing disaccharide and therefore susceptible to reactions of the glucose carbonyl group, including the Maillard reaction. Alkaline isomerization of lactose gives lactulose [β-D-galactopyranosyl-(1,4)-D-fructofuranose], in which the

NUTRITION INSIGHT

Derivatives of Sucrose Used by the Food Industry: Noncaloric Fat and Sugar Substitutes

The low cost and purity of sucrose and the eight hydroxyl groups in its structure make sucrose an appealing starting material for chemical modification. In 1968 Procter & Gamble, while searching for a way to increase the fat intake of premature babies, created a fat substitute, sucrose polyester. Sucrose polyester, which is known as olestra or Olean, is a sucrose molecule to which as many as eight fatty acid residues (usually six to eight long-chain fatty acids) derived from vegetable oil have been esterified. Olestra has so many fatty acid "spokes" around the central sucrose core that digestive enzymes and bacteria in the intestinal tract cannot find an entry point to break down the molecule. Thus it passes through the body largely unhydrolyzed. Olestra was approved by the U.S. Food and Drug Administration (FDA) in 1996 as a replacement for regular cooking oil in production of savory snack foods such as crackers, potato chips, and corn chips (U.S. Department of Health and Human Services, 1996).

In 1976 Tate & Lyle, in conjunction with researchers at Queen Elizabeth College, University of London, discovered that chlorination of three hydroxyl groups on sucrose produced a modified sucrose that is about 600 times as sweet as sucrose. They subsequently developed the product in partnership with McNeil Nutritionals. Use of this chlorinated sucrose derivative, which is known as sucralose or Splenda, was approved by Canada in 1991. In 1998 the FDA granted approval for use of sucralose as a tabletop sweetener in the United States, and in 1999 the FDA granted approval for use of sucralose as a general purpose sweetener in food products (U.S. Department of Health and Human Services, 1998, 1999). Sucralose is currently used as a sugar substitute in numerous food products, including beverages, baked goods, dairy products, canned fruits, syrups, and condiments, and it is also sold to consumers, under its trade name Splenda, for use as a table and baking sugar substitute.

CLINICAL CORRELATION

Sugars and Dental Caries

Sugars are readily metabolized by oral bacteria, leading to production of organic acids in sufficient concentration to lower the pH of dental plaque. Most studies have focused on the contribution of sucrose, but monosaccharides are also readily fermented by the bacteria in the dental plaque. The acids demineralize (dissolve) the nearby tooth enamel. If the degree of demineralization exceeds remineralization over repeated cycles of changing acid concentrations, dissolution of the tooth enamel leads to tooth decay.

Although many studies done in the past clearly demonstrated the relationship between sucrose consumption and dental caries at the population level (e.g., association between sugar consumption and dental caries among countries) and at the individual level (e.g., persons with hereditary fructose intolerance who strictly limit sugar consumption), the apparent relationship between sugar consumption and dental caries has weakened in industrialized countries in recent decades. The weakening of the observed relationship is due, at least partially, to the decreased prevalence of caries in children owing to widespread use of fluoride, which raises the threshold of sugar intake at which caries will progress to cavitation. Furthermore, studies have shown that the amount of carbohydrate consumed is not as significant in the formation of dental caries as is the frequency of consumption. The form of the carbohydrate is also important because sticky carbohydrates are retained on the teeth and allow acid production to be prolonged. The American Dental Association recommends that the number of between-meal snacks eaten each day be minimized, that sweet consumption be limited to meal time, and that infants not be allowed to sleep with bottles containing sweetened liquids, fruit juices, milk, or formula *(www.ada.org)*.

glucose unit has been isomerized to fructose. This isomerization also occurs to some extent during heating of milk. Lactulose is not digested or absorbed from the small intestine and it therefore acts as substrate for fermentation and, hence, as a colonic acidifier and an osmotic laxative.

Trehalose

α,α-Trehalose [α-D-glucopyranosyl-(1,1)-α-D-glucopyranoside] is a nonreducing disaccharide found in fungi, such as young mushrooms and yeasts, and in invertebrates, such as insect hemolymph. It is digested by an intestinal α-glucosidase called trehalase. Trehalose is a rather insignificant dietary disaccharide in most modern diets.

Maltose

Only small amounts of maltose [α-D-glucopyranosyl-(1,4)-D-glucopyranose] are consumed as such in the diet. Maltose occurs naturally in the seeds of starch-producing plants, and small amounts are used in processed foods. Isomaltose [α-D-glucopyranosyl-(1,6)-D-glucopyranose] probably does not occur naturally, but both maltose and isomaltose are formed by acidic hydrolysis of starch; the isomaltose results from the structural branch points of amylopectin. Digestion of starch by α-amylases in the lumen of the gastrointestinal tract yields maltose, maltotriose, and α-dextrins containing the isomaltose moiety. Digestion of these glucose disaccharides and oligosaccharides is accomplished by intestinal α-glucosidases (maltase–glucoamylase and sucrase–isomaltase). Digestion of carbohydrates is discussed in detail in Chapter 8.

OLIGOSACCHARIDES

Although disaccharides are common components of the diet, oligosaccharides containing 3 to 10 sugar residues are not abundant.

α-Galactosides

A series of α-galactosides, known as raffinose, stachyose, verbascose, and ajucose, occur in relatively large amounts in soybeans, lentils, and other legume seeds. As shown in Figure 4-12, these oligosaccharides contain a sucrose moiety to which one or more residues of α-galactose are attached by a 1,6 linkage to the glucose moiety of sucrose. Raffinose, stachyose, verbascose, and ajucose contain one, two, three, or four residues of α-D-galactose, respectively. Multiple residues of α-D-galactose are attached to each other by 1,6 linkages; for example, stachyose contains an α-D-galactopyranosyl-(1,6)-D-galactopyranosyl unit attached to C6 of the glucose unit of sucrose. During plant seed development, a galactosyl derivative of inositol [i.e., α-D-galactosyl-(1,3)-D-*myo*-inositol] serves as the donor of the galactose residues in the galactosyltransferase reactions that catalyze the synthesis of raffinose family oligosaccharides. Because humans do not have a digestive α-D-galactosidase, the α-galactosides consumed in legumes pass into the lower gut to be metabolized by gut microorganisms. Excessive flatulence may result from fermentation of these oligosaccharides.

β-Fructans

Fructose oligosaccharides are produced by hydrolysis of inulin, which is a β-fructan obtained from chicory roots. Inulin is a polymer of fructose residues with the fructose residues present as furanose rings joined by β(2,1)-glycosidic linkages. The partial hydrolysate of inulin (oligofructose) is used as a food ingredient. Although pyranose rings are more stable thermodynamically and occur more frequently in polymers than do furanose rings, furanose rings are found in inulin and in sucrose because the biosynthesis of these molecules in plants involves the 6-phosphate ester of fructose as the fructose donor. In fructose 6-phosphate, the −OH on C6 is tied up and not free to cyclize with the carbonyl carbon to form a pyranose ring, so fructose 6-phosphate forms only furanose rings. The food industry also produces synthetic fructose oligosaccharides that are sucrose molecules to which fructose units have been added by β(2,1)-linkages. Fructose oligosaccharides are about 30% as sweet as sucrose and are used as bulking agents, emulsifiers, sugar substitutes, fat replacers, and prebiotics in a variety of food products. Fructose oligosaccharides are not hydrolyzed by enzymes of the digestive tract but can be fermented by bacteria in the large intestine.

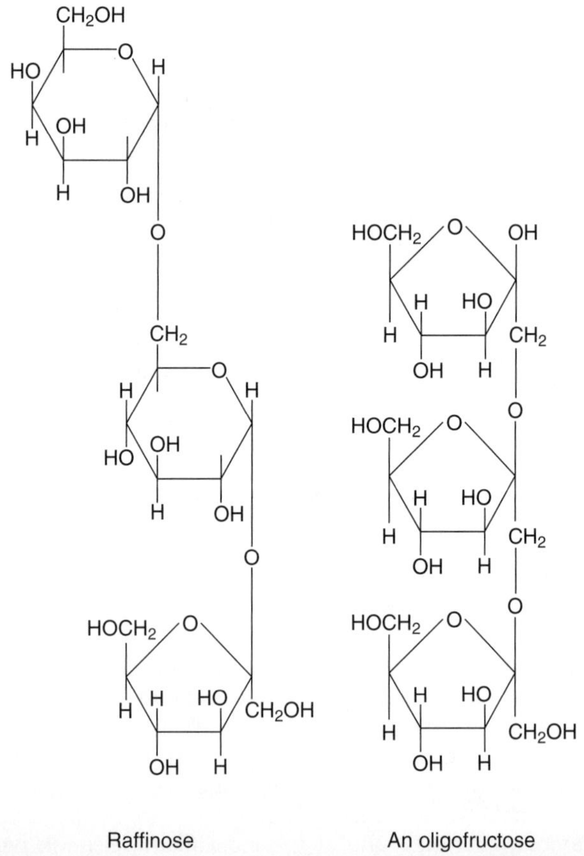

Raffinose

An oligofructose

FIGURE 4-12 Structures of two oligosaccharides: raffinose [α-D-galactopyranosyl-(1,6)-α-D-glucopyranosyl-(1,2)-β-D-fructofuranose] and an oligofructose product of inulin hydrolysis [β-D-fructofuranosyl-(2,1)-β-D-fructofuranosyl-(2,1)-β-D-fructofuranose].

Products of Starch Digestion

Although α-glucan oligosaccharides are not common in natural foods, they are added to many processed foods and they form to a limited extent during baking. Maltodextrins are produced by the hydrolysis of starch and consist of a mixture of variable length chains of D-glucose residues (e.g., 3 to 19 glucose units long) linked by α(1,4)- or α(1,6)-glycosidic bonds. Maltodextrins are classified by the degree of hydrolysis, and those with shorter glucose chains have a higher degree of sweetness and solubility. Those with shorter glucose chains are called glucose syrups, or commonly corn syrup, because glucose syrup is usually made from cornstarch. Corn, wheat, rice, and potatoes are the main sources of starch for production of maltodextrins, and the dextrins are produced by enzymatic digestion or by acid hydrolysis. Maltodextrins are used in many commercially prepared foods as thickeners, sweeteners, and humectants, and corn syrup is widely used in home preparation of candy and other desserts.

POLYSACCHARIDES OF NUTRITIONAL IMPORTANCE

Polysaccharides are polymers composed of sugars linked by glycosidic bonds. They vary in size from approximately 20 to more than 10^7 sugar units. The structural diversity includes molecular size, kinds and proportions of sugars, ring size (furanose or pyranose), anomeric configuration (α or β), and linkage site of the glycosidic bonds, as well as the sequence of these sugars and linkages in the polysaccharide and the presence of noncarbohydrate components.

GENERAL CHARACTERISTICS OF POLYSACCHARIDES

Polysaccharides may be linear or branched, and the latter exhibit various branching modes that range from a single sugar unit to longer extensions carrying additional branches, as illustrated in Figure 4-13. Polysaccharides may be classified by whether they are polymers of only one type of sugar residue (homopolysaccharides) or of two or more different sugar residues (heteropolysaccharides). Homopolysaccharides are designated either by a trivial name, such as starch and cellulose, or by a systematic name constructed from the constituent sugar names and the suffix "an." Thus α(1,4)-D-glucan is the systematic name for amylose, and β(1,4)-D-glucan is the systematic name for cellulose. Both are made up of glucose units linked C1→C4 but contain different C1 stereoisomers (anomers) of glucose.

In heteropolysaccharides composed of more than one kind of sugar, the sugar units may be linked in many different arrangements. Repeating units of a two- or three-sugar sequence is common. The physical properties of polysaccharides depend highly on their chemical and conformational structures. In general, polysaccharides that are highly branched are water soluble, whereas linear polysaccharides tend to be insoluble. However, linear polysaccharides possessing structural irregularities that hinder intermolecular hydrogen bonding may be soluble and give viscous solutions. Hyaluronic acid, a linear polysaccharide with two different sugars in alternating sequence, shows this mucilaginous characteristic. In contrast, glycogen, which is highly branched and very soluble, gives relatively nonviscous solutions. Many different polysaccharide structures are represented in the plant kingdom, whereas only a few have been identified in vertebrates. Bacteria synthesize many unusual sugars, thereby greatly increasing the diversity of their polysaccharide antigens.

DIGESTIBLE POLYSACCHARIDES

Starch and glycogen are digestible polysaccharides of glucose. Both linear and branched forms of starch are found in plant cells. Glycogen has a highly branched structure and is found in animal tissues, particularly muscle and liver.

Starch: Amylose and Amylopectin

Starch is one of the most abundant polysaccharides in plants, where it is stored in the seeds, tubers, roots, and some fruits. It is composed of two families of polymers, a mostly linear amylose [α(1,4)-D-glucan] and the branched amylopectin [α(1,4)-D-glucan with branches linked to C6]. Starches from different sources vary in structure, but typically amylopectin has an average chain length between branch points of 20 to 25 glucose units. Typical starches contain 20% to 30% amylose and 70% to 80% amylopectin; however, high amylopectin (e.g., waxy corn, 98% amylopectin) and high amylose (e.g., high amylose corn, 55% to 85% amylose) starches are also available. Starches for food processing are produced

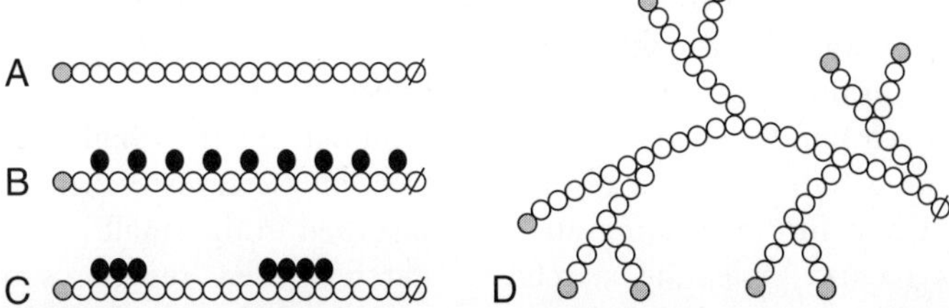

FIGURE 4-13 Branching structures of polysaccharides. **A,** Linear polysaccharide. Circles represent sugar units linked by glycosidic bonds. **B,** Alternating branches consisting of a single sugar unit, ●. **C,** Blocks of consecutive single sugar unit branches, ●. **D,** Ramified structure (branches on branches). Ø, Reducing end; ◯, Nonreducing end; ●, one sugar residue linked as a branch to the main chain.

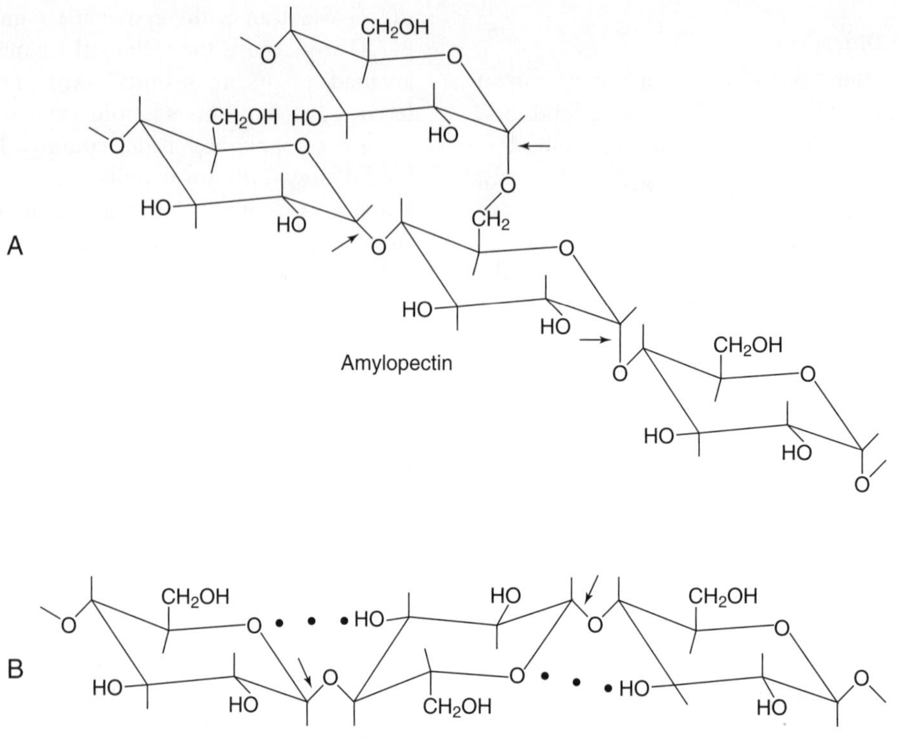

A

Amylopectin

B

Cellulose

FIGURE 4-14 **A,** A segment of starch amylopectin structure showing the α-D-glycosidic bonds and the branch points. Glycogen has a similar structure. **B,** The conformational structure of cellulose shows that alternate β-D-glucosyl units are flipped 180 degrees, giving a flat, ribbonlike structure stabilized by hydrogen bonds (• • •). The glycosidic bonds are indicated by the arrows.

from many sources. The most important sources are corn (regular, waxy, and high amylose), potato, rice, tapioca, and wheat. The physical properties and, to some extent, the digestibility of the starches vary with their fine structure and reflect their source.

Amylose and amylopectin molecules are laid down in plants during biosynthesis in highly organized particles called granules. The highly organized or crystalline structure of starch granules makes amylose and amylopectin less susceptible to digestion by α-amylase. The linear molecular structure of amylose results in more tightly packed granules, which are more insoluble and more resistant to digestion than those containing more of the branched and less tightly packed amylopectin. Therefore certain raw starch granules with high amylose content, particularly those in raw potatoes and green bananas, resist digestion.

Although hydrogen bonding of the starch components renders the granules insoluble in water below approximately 55° C, cooking or heating in the presence of water breaks the intermolecular hydrogen bonds and the starch takes up water or swells, causing a transition to a disorganized amorphous structure. Upon further heating and further swelling, the granules rupture, releasing starch into the liquid. This process is called starch gelatinization. The hydration and disruption of starch granule structure that normally occurs during cooking and food processing makes the starch more accessible. Thus in contrast to the raw starches, cooked potato and green banana starch are readily digested.

Gelatinized starch is hydrolyzed to glucose in the gastrointestinal tract by the combined action of salivary and pancreatic α-amylases and the intestinal mucosal α-glucosidases (maltase–glucoamylase, sucrase–isomaltase). The α-amylases, which cleave the α(1,4)-linkages only, catalyze hydrolysis of starch to maltose, maltotriose, maltotetrose, and oligosaccharides called α-limit dextrins that contain at least four glucose units and include an α(1,6)-linked branch point. These disaccharides and oligosaccharides are then converted to glucose by the α-glucosidases. Figure 4-14 shows a fragment of the amylopectin structure and the α(1,4)- and α(1,6)-glycosidic linkages that can be hydrolyzed by human digestive enzymes. The human upper digestive tract does not possess an endogenous (1,4)-β-D-glucanase, and therefore cellulose, with its β-linkages, is not digestible.

Resistant Starch

Although starch is highly digestible, it appears that about 15% of dietary starches may not be well digested and absorbed in the small intestine (Sajilata et al., 2006). This starch is called "resistant starch." Several factors may cause starch to be resistant to digestion and absorption in the small intestine. One of these factors is the physical structure or food matrix. Starch granules in whole or partly ground cereal grains and legumes may be resistant to

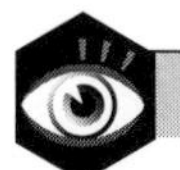

NUTRITION INSIGHT

Corn Syrups: A Major Source of Dietary Sugars

The development of various types of corn syrups and maltodextrins from cornstarch sources has brought about major changes in the food industry. Starch is separated from other parts of the corn kernels and is then hydrolyzed by acid- or enzyme-catalyzed processes to produce a mixture of glucose and glucose oligosaccharides. Corn syrups or maltodextrins with various degrees of hydrolysis are produced and classified according to reducing sugar content; the higher the reducing sugar value, the greater the degree of hydrolysis and the smaller the oligosaccharides.

More recently, a glucose isomerase has been used to convert some of the glucose in corn syrup to fructose to produce high-fructose corn syrups. If a higher percentage of fructose is desired, fructose is chromatographically separated and then backmixed to produce a syrup with the desired fructose concentration. High-fructose corn syrup is classified according to its fructose content (e.g., 42%, 55%). High-fructose corn syrup is listed as Generally Recognized as Safe (GRAS) for use by the food industry in the United States on the basis that its saccharide composition (glucose to fructose ratio) is approximately the same as that of honey, invert sugar, and the disaccharide sucrose. Several features of high-fructose corn syrup have led to its widespread use as a sweetening agent in processed foods. On a weight basis, glucose is less sweet than sucrose, whereas fructose is sweeter. Fructose is also twice as soluble as glucose at low temperatures. Thus conversion of half of the glucose to fructose produces a syrup that is more stable and sweeter than a glucose solution of the same sugar concentration. In addition, high-fructose corn syrup is less expensive than sucrose.

Because fructose is processed differently in the body than glucose, which is the more common sugar unit in dietary carbohydrates, fructose bypasses many of the regulatory points that control glucose uptake and metabolism. There is concern that high intakes of either sucrose or high-fructose corn syrup may have adverse effects in terms of obesity and diabetes beyond those associated with the intake of calories from refined products. The basis of these concerns is addressed more fully in Chapters 8 and 12.

digestion due to trapping of starch inside intact plant cells. Digestive enzymes may be unable to penetrate or break down the plant cell walls. Furthermore, the starch trapped inside these plant cell walls may not be easily gelatinized during cooking. Milling, grinding, and other types of food processing that disrupt the food matrix may make starch more accessible to the digestive enzymes in the gastrointestinal tract.

Another factor that affects starch digestion by the gastrointestinal tract is the tight packing of starch in crystalline structures in starch granules. As discussed earlier, certain raw starch granules with high amylose content, particularly those in raw potatoes and green bananas, are very resistant to digestion. High-amylose corn starches have high gelatinization temperatures and typically resist digestion, even after cooking. Legumes are also a rich source of resistant starch.

A third physical process that affects starch availability is retrogradation. When a starch is cooked and then cooled, a gel is formed from the starch and trapped water. Because of the limited solubility of amylose and amylopectin in water, however, there is a tendency for the solubilized amylose chains, and to a lesser extent the branched amylopectin chains, to realign or reaggregate through hydrogen bonding over time in the process known as retrogradation. Starches that have a high amylose to amylopectin ratio tend to have an earlier onset of retrogradation and to form firmer gels that are more resistant to dispersion in water and digestion by α-amylase. Retrogradation occurs in foods that have been cooked and then cooled (e.g., potatoes, bread, or pasta) and in food products that undergo repeated moist heat treatments during food processing (e.g., canned beans and peas). Retrogradation in starch-based products is frequently undesirable, as in the staling or undesirable hardening of bread or in the syneresis (expulsion of liquid from the gel) of starch-thickened puddings.

Finally, certain chemically modified and cross-linked starches that are used in processed foods such as cakes and breads are resistant to digestion by human digestive enzymes.

Glycogen

Glycogen, like amylopectin, is an α(1,4)-D-glucan with branches on branches that are α(1,6)-linked. Glycogen has a high molecular mass, in the range of 10^6 to 10^9 Da. The average length of the α(1,4)-linked chain between branch points is 10 to 14 glucose units. Because of its greater degree of branching compared with amylopectin, glycogen is readily soluble in cold water and gives solutions of relatively low viscosity, which facilitate its use as a readily available endogenous energy source. The branching pattern interferes with intramolecular and intermolecular hydrogen bonding of the glycogen chains, thereby permitting rapid solvation and easy access to enzymes. A low viscosity of the solution facilitates diffusion of the substrate to the enzymes and diffusion of products away from the enzymes that hydrolyze glycosidic bonds in glycogen.

Glycogen is present in most animal tissues, with the highest content in liver and skeletal muscle. It may constitute up to 10% (wet weight) of the human liver. Mammalian tissue levels of glycogen are highly variable and affected by factors such as nutritional status and time of day. Electron microscopy of native glycogen in mammalian cells has revealed glycogen particles (β-particles) with diameters of about 10 to 30 nm. In liver, but not in muscle, supramolecular complexes called α-particles with diameters as large as 300 nm are also observed. These α-particles consist of several covalently linked β-particles (Sullivan et al., 2010).

TABLE 4-2 Nondigestible Food Polysaccharides of Plant, Algal, and Bacterial Origin

POLYSACCHARIDE	MAIN CHAIN OR REPEAT UNIT*	BRANCHES, OTHER SUBSTITUENTS†
PLANTS		
Cellulose	-Glc(β1,4)Glc-	None
Arabinoxylan	-Xyl(β1,4)Xyl-	L-Araf(α1,2 or α1,3)- or Acetate at C2 or C3 of Xyl
Xyloglucan	Glc(β1,4)Glc-	Xyl(α1,6)-; Gal (β1,2) or Araf(α1,3) linked to Xyl(α1,6)-; Fuc(α1,2)Gal (β1,2)Xyl(α1,6)-; or Araf(α1,3)Araf(α1,3)Xyl(α1,6)-
Galactomannan	-Man(β1,4)Man-	Gal(α1,6)-
Cereal β-glucan	-[Glc(β1,4)]$_n$Glc(β1,3)-	None
Rhamnogalacturonan-1	-[GalA(α1,4)L-Rha(α1,2)]-	Oligosaccharide side chains (rich in Gal and L-Araf) attached to L-Rha at C4; main chain contains some methyl esters of GalA
ALGAE		
Alginic acid	-[ManA(β1,4)]$_n$[L-GulA(α1,4)]$_n$-	None
Carrageenan	-[Gal(β1,4)3,6-anhydroGal(α1,3]-	-SO_3^- at C4, C2†
BACTERIA		
Xanthan gum	-Glc(β1,4)Glc‡	4,6-Pyr-Man(β1,4)Glc(β1,2)6-Ac-Man(α1,3)- side chains attached to alternate glucose resides in the main chain. Pyr (pyruvate) is linked by bonds between its C2 and the C4 and C6 of the terminal Man of some of the side chains. Ac (acetate) is linked to the C6 of many internal Man residues of the side chain

*Sugars are D isomers and pyranose ring forms unless otherwise indicated.
†The substituent group replaces the proton of the –OH of a sugar unit in the main chain.
‡Alternating glucose units are substituted at C3 by the trisaccharide branch. The nonreducing terminal Man carries a pyruvate substituent and the other Man is substituted at C6 by an acetyl group.

NONDIGESTIBLE PLANT POLYSACCHARIDES (DIETARY FIBER)

Polysaccharides are the major components of plant cell walls and interstitial spaces. Plants also synthesize storage polysaccharides other than starch, including galactomannans, the β(1,3)(1,4)-D-glucans of cereal grains, and the fructans of grasses and some tubers. All of these nonstarch polysaccharides present in plants, as well as those added during food processing, constitute dietary fiber (Table 4-2).

Cellulose and Hemicelluloses

Cellulose is a linear β(1,4)-D-glucan with a flat, ribbonlike conformation in which alternate glucose units are flipped 180 degrees and hydrogen bonded intramolecularly (see Figure 4-14). These ribbonlike chains are aligned in parallel arrays called microfibrils, in which the chains are strongly hydrogen bonded to each other. The microfibrils are similarly packed together into strong fibers, which are very insoluble and stiffen the plant cell wall. Associated with cellulose in the cell wall are several other insoluble polysaccharides, the hemicelluloses. These include the xyloglucans, which have a cellulose-like backbone with α-D-xylose units linked to C6 of glucosyl units, and arabinoxylans, in which the β(1,4)-D-xylan chain has α-L-arabinofuranose and D-glucuronic acid branches at C2 or C3.

Pectic Polysaccharides

Pectic polysaccharides [α(1,4)-D-galacturonans with occasional α-L-rhamnose units] and other associated polysaccharides (galactans and arabinans) are present in the interstitial spaces and cell walls of immature plant tissues. Native pectic galacturonan in the plant tissue is relatively insoluble, but isolated commercial pectin is soluble in hot water. Calcium ions form complexes with the galacturonic acid units of pectin, cross-linking the chains into a gel network. This is thought to account partially for the insolubility of native pectin in the plant tissue. The calcium–pectin complex is also the basis for dietary low-sugar, low-calorie fruit jams and jellies, whereas jellies prepared without calcium require a high sugar content to form a gel structure.

NATURAL AND MODIFIED POLYSACCHARIDES FOR USE IN PROCESSED FOODS

Several natural polysaccharides are used in processed foods for their functional properties. These natural polysaccharides include guar and locust bean galactomannans, alginic acid and carrageenan from seaweed, xanthan gum, and starches from several sources. Polysaccharides are also modified physically and chemically to enhance their functionality (Tharanathan, 2005). Some examples of modified starch and cellulose are listed in Table 4-3. Starch and cellulose are

TABLE 4-3 Modified Polysaccharides Added to Processed Foods

POLYSACCHARIDE	MODIFYING GROUP OR TREATMENT*	PRODUCT
Starch	$-COCH_3$	Starch acetate (ester)
	$-CH_2CHOHCH_3$	Hydroxypropyl starch (ether)
	$-PO_2^-$–	Phosphate cross-linked starch (diester)
	Acid, heat	Dextrins
	Water, heat	Cold water–soluble starch
Cellulose	$-CH_2COOH$	Carboxymethylcellulose (CMC)
	$-CH_2CHOHCH_3$	Hydroxypropylcellulose
	$-CH_3$	Methylcellulose
	Acid, heat	Microcrystalline cellulose

*The modifying group replaces the proton of one of the three free hydroxyls of the glucose units at a degree of substitution usually less than 1 per 10 glucose units.

alkylated or esterified to convert a very small proportion of the hydroxyls into ethers or esters for increased solubility. Starches are also subjected to partial acid or enzymatic hydrolysis, yielding starch dextrins with greater solubility. Industrial production of starch dextrins by pyrolysis (dry heat under acidic conditions) promotes further alteration of the structure, including new linkages, increased branching, and some decrease in size. Maltodextrins, which are smaller than the dextrins, usually in the oligosaccharide range, are formed by enzymatic hydrolysis of gelatinized starch without structural alterations. Modified starch products designed for enhanced solubility would be expected to favor rapid digestion and absorption, whereas those designed for greater cross-linking may result in starch that is resistant to digestion. In general, the modified starches are digestible by human digestive enzymes, whereas the other polysaccharides added to foods contribute to dietary fiber. The interest in functional foods aimed at obesity and diabetes control may lead to the use of more resistant starches by the food industry (Zhang and Hamaker, 2009; Grabitske and Slavin, 2008).

GLYCOCONJUGATES OF PHYSIOLOGICAL INTEREST

Conjugates of sugars and oligosaccharides play essential physiological roles. These glycoconjugates include the glycosaminoglycans and proteoglycans, the glycoproteins, and the glycolipids.

TABLE 4-4 Structural Repeating Units of the Glycosaminoglycans, Showing Sulfation Patterns and Structural Variation

GLYCOSAMINOGLYCAN	REPEAT UNIT*
Hyaluronan	[-GlcNAc(β1,4)GlcA(β1,3)-]$_n$
Chondroitin 4-sulfate and 6-sulfate	[-GalNAc(β1,4)GlcA(β1,3)-]$_n$ with 4 (or 6) – SO_3^-
Dermatan sulfate	[-GalNAc(β1,4)L-IdoA(α1,3)-]$_n$ with 4 – SO_3^- and 2 – R; R = H or SO_3^- and [-GalNAc(β1,4)GlcA(β1,3)-]$_n$ with 4 (or 6) – SO_3^-
Keratan sulfate	[-Gal(β1,4)GlcNAc(β1,3)-]$_n$ with 6 – R and 6 – R; R = H or SO_3^-
Heparan sulfate and heparin	[-GlcN**R**(α1,4)GlcA(β1,4)-]$_n$ with 6 – R′; **R** = Ac or SO_3^-; R′ = H or SO_3^- and [-GlcNAc(α1,4)L-IdoA(α1,4)-]$_n$ with 2 – R; R = H or SO_3^-

With the exception of hyaluronan and keratan sulfate, the glycosaminoglycans are glycosidically linked to the core protein chain by the sequence -4GlcA(β1,3)Gal(β1,4)Xyl(β1,3)L-serine. Keratan sulfate is glycosidically linked to core proteins by either *N*-linkage to an asparagine residue or *O*-linked to a serine/threonine residue. Hyaluronan is not covalently linked to proteins. Sugars are D unless noted as L.

*R in the abbreviated structure format refers to the proton of an –OH or $-NH_2$ group or a substitution for the proton (e.g., esterification of the sugar residue with sulfate or acetate).

GLYCOSAMINOGLYCANS

Glycosaminoglycans (Table 4-4) are linear polysaccharides that have a disaccharide repeat unit composed of a hexosamine and a uronic acid. They are constituents of the extracellular spaces of mammalian tissues and vary in molecular mass and in fine structure. Many are sulfated and thus more highly charged. Most glycosaminoglycans are covalently bound to proteins, and the resulting proteoglycans vary considerably in the number and types of bound glycan chains.

Hyaluronic Acid

Hyaluronic acid (hyaluronan) is a negatively charged, soluble, high-molecular-weight, linear glycan composed of D-glucuronic acid and *N*-acetyl-D-glucosamine. It is found in the extracellular matrix, especially in soft connective tissue. Unlike most glycosaminoglycans, it is not covalently linked to protein but binds physically to receptor proteins on many different cells. Hyaluronic acid is noted for its ability to form highly viscous solutions, and some of its clinical applications depend on this rheology. The viscosity stems from the extended helical conformation, high molecular weight, and network of aggregated chains. Thus hyaluronic acid may have a role in water and protein homeostasis in the extracellular matrix. Interaction between hyaluronic acid and its cell receptors is involved in cell locomotion and migration, as shown for lymphocytes. Hyaluronic acid is synthesized by transfer of sugar units from their nucleotide diphosphate derivatives to the reducing end of the growing hyaluronic acid chain. This is in contrast to the usual mode of chain lengthening of oligosaccharides and polysaccharides, which involves addition of sugar units to the nonreducing end of the growing chain.

Chondroitin Sulfate

Chondroitin sulfate has a disaccharide repeat unit of D-glucuronic acid and *N*-acetyl-D-galactosamine, with sulfate ester groups added at C2 of glucuronic acid units and C4 or C6 of the galactosamine units. This sulfation adds sequence heterogeneity, defined by the amount and position of the sulfate esters along the chain. The large number of ionized sulfate groups and the weaker uronic acid carboxylate groups ensure that this large polysaccharide will attract counter cations and water for osmotic balance and hydration of the polysaccharide.

Dermatan Sulfate

Dermatan sulfate is synthesized from chondroitin sulfate by intracellular C5 epimerization of some of the D-glucuronic acid units to L-iduronic acid. This both produces a new uronic acid and increases structural diversity relative to the proportion and sequence of each acid. The other major differences between dermatan sulfate and chondroitin sulfate reside in the number of sulfate groups and their positions.

Keratan Sulfate

Keratan sulfate, composed of alternating D-galactose and *N*-acetyl-D-glucosamine units, lacks a uronic acid constituent, but it is heavily sulfated. The *N*-acetyl-D-glucosamine units carry sulfate groups at C6, and some of the galactose units are sulfated also at C6.

Heparin and Heparan Sulfate

Heparin and heparan sulfate have disaccharide repeat units of D-glucuronic acid and D-glucosamine with some L-iduronic acid. The glucosamine units may be *N*-acetylated or *N*-sulfated, and all sugar residues may be *O*-sulfated. Heparin is extensively epimerized and thus has many iduronic acid residues. Heparin also has a high proportion of *N*-sulfates and total sulfate. Heparin is found predominantly in the secretory granules of mast cells. Heparan sulfate chains vary widely in extent of epimerization and sulfation, with some chains having little iduronic acid or sulfate. Despite its name, heparan sulfate has less sulfate than heparin. Heparan sulfate is found linked to many cell-surface proteins and as a component of matrix proteoglycans. Lipoprotein lipase in the capillaries of muscle and adipose tissue is closely associated with a heparan sulfate proteoglycan.

PROTEOGLYCANS

Proteoglycans are large, complex macromolecules that consist of a protein core to which glycosaminoglycans are covalently linked. These proteoglycans are found in the plasma membrane and extracellular matrices of most eukaryotic cells, where they have many functions. They may play a role in cell–cell and cell–matrix interactions and bind to a variety of ligands. The size and complexity of proteoglycans varies. A proteoglycan may carry more than one covalently linked glycosaminoglycan as well as additional oligosaccharides that are *N*- and *O*-linked to the core protein. Heparan sulfate/heparin proteoglycans contain at least one heparan sulfate chain and usually *O*- and *N*-linked oligosaccharides in addition. The proteoglycans containing chondroitin sulfate, dermatan sulfate, and heparan sulfate frequently share a common tetrasaccharide-linkage region (GlcA-Gal-Gal-Xyl-) by which the glycosaminoglycan is covalently *O*-linked to a serine residue of the protein. Keratan sulfate is an exception and is found both *O*-linked and *N*-linked to serine/threonine or asparagine residues, respectively, of core proteins. The biosynthesis of the glycosaminoglycan portion of proteoglycans occurs posttranslationally and takes place in the lumen of the endoplasmic reticulum and Golgi apparatus.

GLYCOPROTEINS

Many proteins carry covalently linked oligosaccharides as minor components. The number and size of the oligosaccharide chains vary. The *N*-linked oligosaccharides tend to have a common core and are β-glycosidically linked from the *N*-acetyl-D-glucosamine unit to the nitrogen of the β-carboxamide of asparagine. Mucin-type glycoproteins have an α-D-galactosyl unit *O*-linked to the hydroxyl group of serine or threonine. Collagen is unique in that the carbohydrate chains are *O*-linked to the C5 of 5-hydroxylysine. The carbohydrate moieties of glycoproteins may help stabilize proteins, thus inhibiting denaturation, and may be involved in protein folding in addition to other specific biological roles (Figure 4-15).

GLYCOLIPIDS

Glycolipids are widespread in nature but only as minor components of the lipid fraction and usually in association with proteins. The common glycolipids of mammalian systems include cerebrosides and gangliosides, which are glycosyl (glucosyl or galactosyl) derivatives of sphingolipids. Glycolipids are sometimes classified as neutral or acidic based on the absence or presence of ionizable sulfate or sialic acid constituents. These glycosphingolipids contain a base

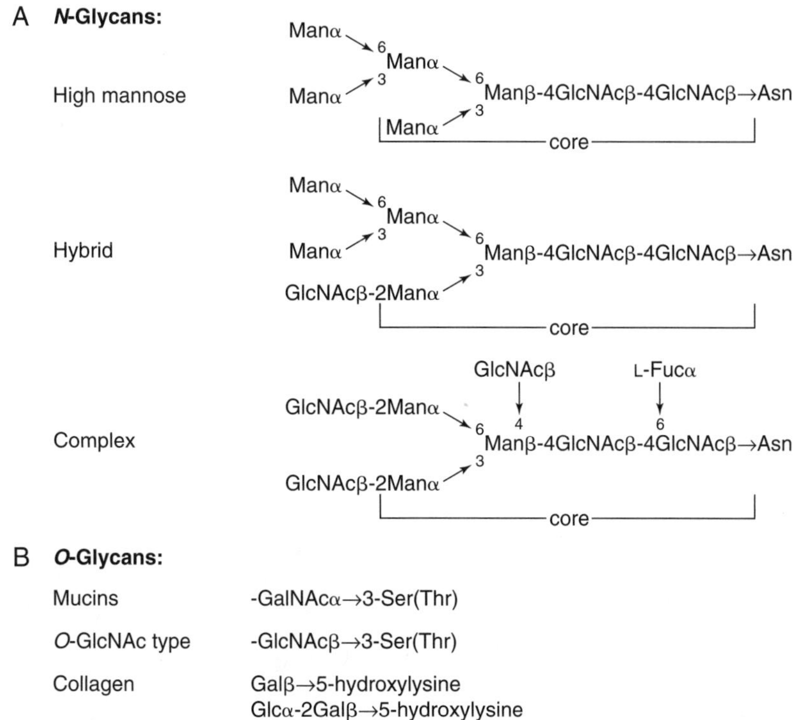

FIGURE 4-15 Structural variations in oligosaccharide chains of glycoproteins and their attachment site in the protein. **A,** Examples of *N*-linked oligosaccharides. A core of five sugar units, common to all three types of *N*-linked glycans, is linked to an asparagine (Asn) residue in the protein. High-mannose *N*-glycans contain an additional two to six mannose (Man) units. *N*-Glycans of the hybrid and complex types have N-acetylglucosamine (GlcNAc)-bearing branches. The two core Man branches of complex *N*-glycans include one containing only Man residues and one containing GlcNAc. In the complex *N*-glycans, both Man branches contain GlcNAc. Additional GlcNAc branches (antennae) may occur on hybrid and complex *N*-glycans. Other sugars, including galactose and sialic acid, also may be linked to the nonreducing ends of the GlcNAc-containing chains in the hybrid and complex *N*-glycans. **B,** Examples of *O*-linked oligosaccharides, linked to serine (Ser) or threonine (Thr) residues of various proteins or to 5-hydroxylysine residues in posttranslationally modified collagen. *O*-Linked oligosaccharides in the mucins and *O*-GlcNAc-type oligosaccharides in glycoproteins may be extended at the nonreducing end by addition of *N*-acetylglucosamine, galactose, L-fucose, and sialic acid. Sugars are D-enantiomers unless noted otherwise.

such as sphingosine, which has an 18-carbon monounsaturated chain substituted with two hydroxyl groups and an amine group. The amine nitrogen of the sphingosine unit is acylated with a long-chain (14- to 26-carbon) fatty acid. A carbohydrate unit (usually glucose or galactose) is glycosidically attached to the *N*-acylsphingosine (ceramide) at its C1 hydroxyl group to form a cerebroside (monoglycosylceramide). The sugar unit of a cerebroside may also be sulfated to form a sulfatide. Cerebrosides are neutral glycosphingolipids, whereas sulfatides are acidic glycosphingolipids. Large amounts of galactocerebroside and galactocerebroside 3-sulfate are found in the brain. The major glycolipids in milk are shown in Table 4-5.

TABLE 4-5 The Major Neutral and Acidic Glycolipids of Bovine and Human Milk

NEUTRAL GLYCOLIPIDS	ACIDIC GLYCOLIPIDS
Gal(β1,1)Cer	Neu5Ac(α2,3)Gal(β1,4) Glc(β1-1)Cer
Glc(β1,1)Cer	Neu5Ac(α2,8)Neu5Ac(α2,3) Gal(β1,4)Glc(β1,1)Cer
Gal(β1,4)Glc(β1,1)Cer	

Cer, Ceramide. $HOCH_2$-C(H)(NHR)-C(H)(OH)-CH=CH-$C_{13}H_{27}$, with *R* representing a long-chain acyl group.

Additional sugar residues (usually glucose, galactose, L-fucose, or *N*-acetylgalactosamine) are attached to cerebrosides (usually to glucosylceramide) to form globosides and gangliosides, which are also sphingolipids. Globosides are ceramides with two or more neutral sugar residues. The neutral diglycosylceramide, called lactosylceramide [Gal(β1,4) Glc(β1,1)Cer], is the precursor of other globosides and of gangliosides; lactosylceramide is also found in the membrane of red blood cells. Tetraglycosylceramides ("aminoglycolipids") are globosides that contain an additional sugar (i.e., galactose) and an *N*-acetylhexosamine unit (i.e., *N*-acetylgalactosamine); certain globosides are antigenic determinants of blood group types. Gangliosides are formed by the addition of sialic acid (*N*-acetylneuraminic acid) to diglycosylceramide; additional sugar residues such as galactose, *N*-acetylgalactosamine, and *N*-acetylglucosamine may also be added to form a variety of gangliosides, many containing branches formed by the addition of one or two sialic acid units to the linear portion of the oligosaccharide chain. Gangliosides are found on the surface membranes of most cells, and they make up about 6% by weight of total brain lipids. Gangliosides are most highly concentrated in the ganglion cells of the central nervous system.

Aberrant glycosylation of glycosphingolipids in tumor cells is strongly implicated as an essential mechanism in tumor progression. Abnormal accumulation of specific glycosphingolipids in specific cancers has been correlated with altered cell–cell or cell–substratum interactions, and reagents that block glycosylation have been shown to inhibit tumor cell metastasis.

Plants and microorganisms synthesize several simple glycolipids, which include fatty acid esters of the sugars and glycosides of diglycerides, hydroxy fatty acids, and *myo*-inositol-containing phospholipids. Highly complex lipopolysaccharides of cell walls of pathogenic gram-negative bacteria act as endotoxins, inducing a strong response from the animal immune system, and as pyrogens, inducing fever. The lipopolysaccharides, or endotoxins, are composed of three domains: the terminal carbohydrate chain, which defines the antigenicity; the lipid A, which is embedded in the outer membrane and is the source of the endotoxin activity (probably after it is released from the cell in soluble form); and an oligosaccharide core, which is sandwiched between. Endotoxins are responsible for many of the clinical manifestations of infections with pathogenic gram-negative bacteria such as *Neisseria meningitidis, Escherichia coli,* and *Salmonella* spp.

THINKING CRITICALLY

Most of the substrates for bacterial fermentation in the colon, leading to production of short-chain fatty acids and gases (hydrogen, carbon dioxide, and methane), are carbohydrates rather than proteins or fats. Some dietary carbohydrates that promote gas production include raffinose and related oligosaccharides found in legume seeds, sorbitol and other sugar alcohols, lactose (particularly in lactose-intolerant individuals), resistant starches, and dietary fiber.

1. What is the chemical or structural basis for the lack of digestion and/or absorption of each of these carbohydrates in the human small intestine?
2. Dietary supplements or digestive aids contain α-galactosidase (e.g., Beano) or β-galactosidase (e.g., Lactaid). What are the substrates for each of these enzymes? How do these supplements reduce gas production in the lower gastrointestinal tract?
3. What are common sources of dietary resistant starch? How can food processing and/or food preparation techniques alter the amount of total starch that is resistant to digestion in the human small intestine?

REFERENCES

Grabitske, H. A., & Slavin, J. L. (2008). Low-digestible carbohydrates in practice. *Journal of the American Dietetic Association, 108*, 1677–1681.

Grabitske, H. A., & Slavin, J. L. (2009). Gastrointestinal effects of low-digestible carbohydrates. *Critical Reviews in Food Science and Nutrition, 49*, 327–360.

Sajilata, M. G., Singhal, R. S., & Kulkarni, P. R. (2006). Resistant starch—A review. *Comprehensive Reviews in Food Science and Food Safety, 5*, 1–17.

Sullivan, M. A., Vilaplana, F., Cave, R. A., Stapleton, D., Gray-Weale, A. A., & Gilbert, R. G. (2010). Nature of alpha and beta particles in glycogen using molecular size distributions. *Biomacromolecules, 11*, 1094–1100.

Tharanathan, R. N. (2005). Starch—Value addition by modification. *Critical Reviews in Food Science and Nutrition, 45*, 371–384.

U.S. Department of Health and Human Services. (1996). Food additives permitted for direct addition to food for human consumption: olestra; final rule. *Federal Register, 61*, 3118–3173.

U.S. Department of Health and Human Services. (1998). Food Additives Permitted for Direct Addition to Food for Human Consumption: Sucralose; final rule. *Federal Register, 63*, 16417–16433.

U.S. Department of Health and Human Services. (1999). Food Additives Permitted for Direct Addition to Food for Human Consumption: Sucralose; final rule. *Federal Register, 64*, 43908–43909.

Zhang, G., & Hamaker, B. R. (2009). Slowly digestible starch: Concept, mechanism, and proposed extended glycemic index. *Critical Reviews in Food Science and Nutrition, 49*, 852–867.

RECOMMENDED READINGS

Bode, L. (2009). Human milk oligosaccharides: Prebiotics and beyond. *Nutrition Reviews, 67*(Suppl. 2), S183–S191.

Cummings, J. H., & Stephen, A. M. (2007). Carbohydrate terminology and classification. *European Journal of Clinical Nutrition, 61*(Suppl. 1), S5–S18.

Elbein, A. D., Pan, Y. T., Pastuszak, I., & Carroll, D. (2003). New insights on trehalose: A multifunctional molecule. *Glycobiology, 13*, 17R–27R.

Englyst, K. N., Liu, S., & Englyst, H. N. (2007). Nutritional characterization and measurement of dietary carbohydrates. *European Journal of Clinical Nutrition, 61*(Suppl. 1), S19–S39.

Kaur, N., & Gupta, A. K. (2002). Applications of inulin and oligofructose in health and nutrition. *Journal of Biosciences, 27*, 703–714.

Slavin, J. (2003). Why whole grains are protective: Biological mechanisms. *The Proceedings of the Nutrition Society, 62*, 129–134.

RECOMMENDED WEBSITE

Recommendations of the International Union of Pure and Applied Chemistry (IUPAC) and the International Union of Biochemistry and Molecular Biology (IUBMB). IUPAC-IUBMB Joint Commission on Biochemical Nomenclature (JCBN). Nomenclature of Carbohydrates. http://www.chem.qmw.ac.uk/iupac/2carb/

CHAPTER 5

Structure, Nomenclature, and Properties of Proteins and Amino Acids

*Martha H. Stipanuk, PhD**

Proteins were first recognized as a distinct class of biological molecules in the eighteenth century by Antoine Fourcroy and others, evidenced by the ability of egg whites, wheat gluten, plasma albumin, and fibrin (from clotted blood) to coagulate when treated with heat or acid. The Dutch chemist Gerhadus Johannes Mulder carried out elemental analysis of common proteins and found that nearly all proteins had a similar empirical formula, $C_{400}H_{620}N_{100}O_{120}P_1S_1$, leading him to conclude that all "albuminous" compounds might be composed mainly of a single type of compound. The name "protein" (from the Greek word *proteios,* meaning "primary") was first given to this class of molecules in 1838 by Mulder's associate, Jöns Jakob Berzelius.

We now know that proteins, often called polypeptides, are made up of amino acid residues linked by peptide bonds. Proteins are involved in essentially every process that takes place in cells, and these proteins have a remarkable diversity of functions. Proteins function as enzymes, transcription factors, binding proteins, transmembrane transporters and channels, hormones, immunoglobulins, motor proteins, receptors, structural proteins, and signaling proteins.

The human genome contains about 23,000 protein-coding genes, and proteins make up 20% to 50% of the dry mass of the adult human body, with fat being the other major component. These proteins and peptides are synthesized using amino acids as the building blocks, much as complex carbohydrates are synthesized using sugar residues as the building blocks. In addition to the important role of amino acids as precursors for protein synthesis, amino acids have important roles as intermediates in metabolism; as precursors of nonpeptide compounds, such as the neurotransmitter γ-aminobutyric acid and the coenzyme nicotinamide adenine dinucleotide; and as precursors for synthesis of several unique small peptides, such as glutathione.

In terms of diet, humans and other animals must consume protein to meet needs for amino acids including specific amino acids that cannot be synthesized by the organism. Protein in human diets includes both animal sources, such as meat, milk, fish, and eggs; and plant sources, such as cereal seeds (wheat, rice, maize) and legume seeds (soybeans, peanuts). The major proteins in meat and fish include myofibrillar, sarcoplasmic, and connective tissue proteins. The major protein in egg is ovalbumin in the egg white, which is present as a source of protein for growth of the embryo, whereas the major protein in milk is casein, which is present as a source of protein for the mammalian newborn. The majority of protein in plant seeds consists of globulins or storage proteins that are synthesized during seed development and stored in protein bodies. These proteins are hydrolyzed during seed germination to provide nutrients for the developing seedling.

THE PROTEINOGENIC AMINO ACIDS

All peptides and proteins, regardless of their origin, are constructed from amino acids that are covalently linked together, usually in a linear sequence. Twenty-one amino acids are naturally incorporated into polypeptides in mammals. Twenty of these are directly encoded by the universal genetic code. The twenty-first of the amino acid precursors for protein synthesis, selenocysteine, is incorporated into a small number of proteins by a unique cotranslational mechanism requiring special secondary structure in the messenger RNA (mRNA) (i.e., a selenocysteine insertion sequence, SECIS) that causes the UGA stop codon to encode selenocysteine (see Chapter 39). Another unusual amino acid called pyrrolysine is considered the twenty-second proteinogenic amino acid, but it is found only in some methane-producing enzymes in methanogenic archaea. The structures of the 20 common amino acids and selenocysteine are shown in Figure 5-1.

Amino acids have distinctive "side chains" or "R" groups that give each amino acid size, shape, and characteristics that dictate solubility and electrochemical properties. A given R group confers novel, sometimes unique, chemical properties to an amino acid, and amino acids are often classified based on the chemical properties of their respective R groups. With such diverse building blocks, it is easy to understand how peptides and proteins can be designed for complex activities.

CHIRALITY AND OPTICAL ROTATION

As shown in Figure 5-2, each amino acid contains an amino group and a carboxylic acid group. Both of these functional moieties are bonded directly to a central carbon atom designated as the α-carbon. Except for glycine, the α-carbon for

*This chapter is a revision of the chapter written by Robert B. Rucker, PhD, and Taru Kosonen, PhD, for the second edition.

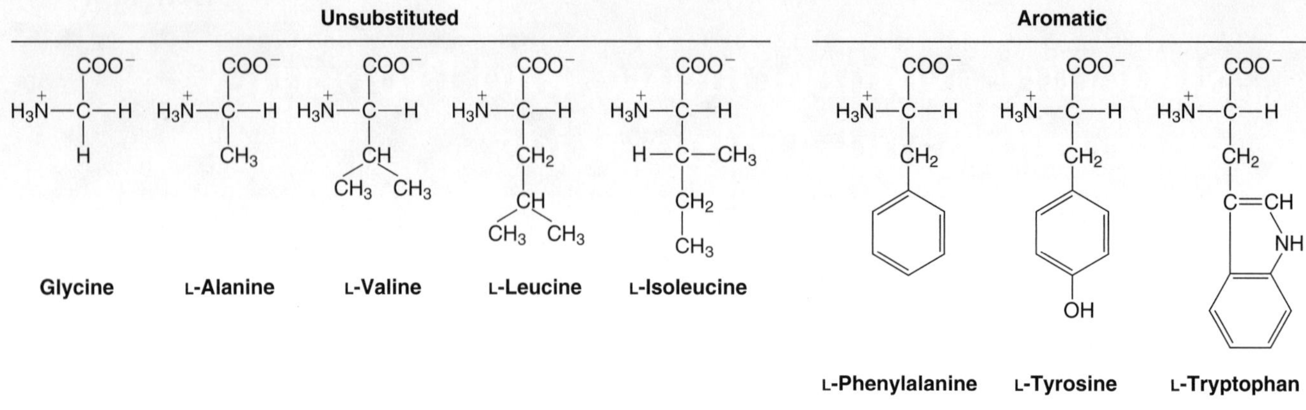

FIGURE 5-1 Structures of the common proteinogenic amino acids. The ionic species shown for each amino acid is the dominant species at pH 7.4.

each of the amino acids has four different functional groups bonded to it: an amino group, a carboxylic acid group, hydrogen, and its R group. The α-carbon of glycine does not have an R group or side chain, so two hydrogen atoms are attached to the α-carbon.

The presence of four different functional groups creates a chiral center. A chiral center exists when an arrangement around a given molecule cannot be superimposed. For all amino acids (with the exception of glycine), there are two non-superimposable, mirror-image forms. These two forms are referred to as stereoisomers, designated as L- and D-isomers. This terminology comes from the Latin terms *laevus* and *dexter* or *levo* and *dextro,* meaning left and right, respectively. The D- and L-isomers of a given amino acid will rotate plane polarized

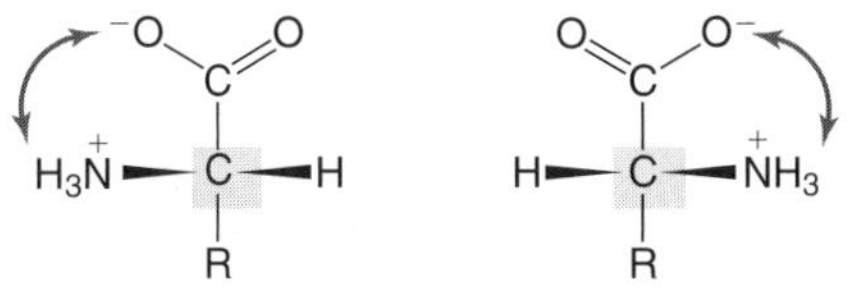

L-Isomer D-Isomer

FIGURE 5-2 General structure for the α-amino acids. Stereoisomers are shown in their L and D forms. Note the position of the α-carbon. Because carbon can form four valence bonds, the α-carbon of an amino acid can be viewed as being at the center with its four substituents located at the corners of a tetrahedron. When a carbon atom has four different substituents, two distinct spatial arrangements are possible. Fisher projections are used to depict the L and D isomers. In a Fisher projection, bonds pointing horizontally are viewed as coming out of the plane on which they are depicted, whereas those pointing vertically go below the plane. A zwitterion is also depicted, wherein the arrows designate the potential balance and interaction between the positive (+) charge of the amino group and the negative (–) charge of the carboxylate group.

light in opposite directions, but amino acids are designated D or L not by the direction in which they themselves rotate light. Instead, the L and D convention for amino acid stereochemistry refers to the optical activity of the isomer of glyceraldehyde from which the amino acid can theoretically be synthesized. D-Glyceraldehyde is dextrorotary, whereas L-glyceraldehyde is levorotary. Thus the designation L or D in combination with the given name of an amino acid implies a specific spatial configuration around the amino acid's α-carbon.

Proline also deserves special comment, because its R group is joined both at the α-carbon and amino group to form a 5-membered ring. Thus, the α-amino nitrogen of proline has two alkyl substituents but only one hydrogen in its unprotonated state. For this reason, proline is referred to as a secondary amino acid or *imino* acid. The α-carbon of proline remains a chiral center.

Although the L and D designations remain in common usage for most amino acids, another system for assigning stereochemistry, the RS system, is used most often in organic chemistry. The symbol *R* comes from the Latin *rectus* for "right," and *S* comes from the Latin *sinister* for "left." The RS system denotes the absolute stereochemistry of the molecule, with each stereogenic center in a molecule being assigned a prefix (R or S) according to whether its configuration is right- or left-handed. In order to make the R or S assignment, relative priority values are assigned to each of the four substituents on the chiral carbon based on the mass of the groups (heaviest to lightest) according to basic rules. Almost all of the amino acids in proteins are S at the α-carbon, but cysteine and selenocysteine are R and glycine is nonchiral at their α-carbons.

In proteins and peptides, amino acids are found almost exclusively in the L form, although D-amino acids are found in some bacterial proteins and peptides (Petsko and Ringe, 2004). The almost exclusive presence of L-amino acids in proteins indicates that reactions that involve amino acid and protein synthesis must be highly stereospecific. The metabolic pathways for amino acid synthesis create predominantly amino acids in their L forms. Moreover, the biological machinery required for protein assembly recognizes L-amino acids almost exclusively. It should be noted that D-aspartate and D-serine are produced by the mammalian brain by enzymes that catalyze the racemization of L-aspartate and L-serine, respectively, and these D-amino acids are involved in activation of the *N*-methyl-D-aspartate type of excitatory amino acid receptors (Wolosker et al., 2008).

THE ACID AND BASE CHARACTERISTICS OF AMINO ACIDS

In aqueous solutions, amino acids are easily ionized. The most abundant ionic species present when amino acids are dissolved in an aqueous medium at neutral pH are shown in Figure 5-1, and the pK_as for all dissociable groups are shown in Table 5-1. The acid dissociation constant K_a is used to define characteristics of titratable groups in organic acids and amines. The negative log of the dissociation constant K_a is called the pK_a of the titratable group. In a practical sense, this means that when the pH is equal to the pK_a, the associated (AH, protonated) and dissociated (A^-, unprotonated) species will be present in equal molar concentrations.

$$K_a = [H^+]([A^-]/[AH])$$

$$\log K_a = \log [H^+] + \log([A^-]/[AH])$$

$$-\log K_a = -\log [H^+] - \log([A^-]/[AH])$$

$$pK_a = pH - \log([A^-]/[AH])$$

The pK_as of carboxylic acid groups are relatively low, usually 2 to 4, so these groups are almost always negatively charged at physiological pH. Amino groups have pK_as that are relatively high, usually 9 to 11, so these groups are almost always positively charged at physiological pH. Most amino acids have neutral side chains at physiological pH and have an overall net charge of 0. However, these amino acids still have a positively charged amino group and a negatively charged carboxyl group. Thus they are not uncharged molecules, nor are they cations or anions. The name "zwitterion" or "dipolar ion" is given to such molecules that have both positive and negative charges but a net charge of zero.

In a nonhydrated state, most amino acids exist as nonvolatile crystalline solids. In this case, an internal transfer of a hydrogen ion from the –COOH group to the $-NH_2$ group of the amino acid leaves an ion with both a negative charge and a positive charge. The zwitterionic character of amino acids causes them to be held together by electrostatic forces, or ionic bonds, in a crystalline lattice (i.e., analogous to the crystalline lattice of sodium chloride and other salt crystals). These ionic attractions between oppositely charged ions are strong, and consequently thermal decomposition of amino acids usually requires high temperatures (e.g., above 200° C).

Ionizable groups of amino acids can be characterized by titrating a solution of the amino acid with acid or base to obtain a titration curve. The types and number of the functional

TABLE 5-1 Properties of the Amino Acids That Serve as Common Building Blocks of Proteins

	AMINO ACID	MOLECULAR MASS (g/mol)	pK_a α-COOH	pK_a α-NH_3^+	pK_a R GROUP	HYDROPATHY INDEX (KYTE-DOOLITTLE SCALE)
Hydrophilic amino acids (charged and very polar)	Arginine	155	2.17	9.04	12.48	−4.5
	Lysine	146	2.18	8.95	10.53	−3.9
	Asparagine	132	2.04	9.82		−3.5
	Aspartate	133	2.09	9.82	3.86	−3.5
	Glutamine	146	2.17	9.13		−3.5
	Glutamate	147	2.19	9.67	4.25	−3.5
	Histidine	174	1.82	9.17	6.0	−3.2
Amino acids with intermediate hydrophobicity (Tyr and moderately/weakly polar amino acids)	Tyrosine	181	2.20	10.07	9.11	−1.3
	Tryptophan	204	2.38	9.39		−0.9
	Serine	105	2.21	9.15		−0.8
	Threonine	119	2.63	10.43		−0.7
	Glycine	75	2.34	9.60		−0.4
	Proline	115	1.99	10.6 (NH_2^+)		1.6
	Alanine	89	2.34	9.69		1.8
	Methionine	149	2.28	9.31		1.9
	Cysteine	121	1.71	10.78	8.33	2.5
Hydrophobic amino acids (uncharged and nonpolar)	Phenylalanine	165	1.83	9.13		2.8
	Leucine	131	2.36	9.68		3.8
	Valine	117	2.32	9.62		4.2
	Isoleucine	131	2.36	9.68		4.5

groups capable of reacting with or exchanging a hydrogen ion (proton) influence the shape of this curve. Addition of base (or acid) will result in a rapid change in the pH of the solution when no group is being titrated, whereas a much slower rate of change in the pH of the solution will be observed when an ionizable group is being titrated. For example, alanine contains two titratable groups: one carboxylic acid group and one amino group. In aqueous solution at a very low or acidic pH (i.e., a high hydrogen ion concentration), both the amino group and the carboxylic acid group of alanine will be protonated, and as a result alanine will be positively charged. If base is gradually added (to decrease the concentration of hydrogen ions), the carboxylic acid group will lose its proton and alanine will become a zwitterion with one negative charge and one positive charge. If more base is added to increase the pH, eventually the positively charged amino group will lose its proton and alanine will become negatively charged.

The presence of a titratable group can be easily observed on a titration curve as a marked decrease in the change in pH per unit of base added; this will appear as a flattening of the curve when pH is plotted on the vertical axis and units of base are plotted on the horizontal axis. In essence, the titratable group acts as a buffer to resist changes in pH by donating protons to neutralize the base that is added. A curve obtained by the titration of histidine, which contains three titratable functional groups, is shown in Figure 5-3. On a titration curve, the pK_a can be observed as the point of inflection near the center of the "plateau." The inflection point is where the curvature changes from concave up to concave down. For histidine in Figure 5-3, three pK_as can be detected: the carboxyl group has a pK_a = 1.82 the imidazole group has a pK_a = 6.0, and the α-amino group has a pK_a = 9.17.

Because pK_a is a $\log_{10}$ scale, a 1.0 unit change in pH on either side of the pK_a will be associated with a tenfold change in the ratio of the associated and dissociated species, and a 2.0 unit change in pH on either side of the pK_a will be associated with a 100-fold change in the ratio.

$$pH - pK_a = \log([A^-]/[AH])$$

$$[A^-]/[AH] = 10^{(pH - pK_a)}$$

Thus if the pK_a for an ionizable group is 6.0, the ratio of the unprotonated to the protonated species will be 0.01 (mainly protonated) at pH 4.0 and 100 (mainly unprotonated) at pH 8.0. On the titration curve, the rate of change in pH per unit of base (or acid) added increases as one moves away from the pK_a of a titratable group.

When amino acids are incorporated into peptides, they lose their ability to form zwitterions because the α-carboxyl and α-amino groups are in peptide linkage with other amino acid residues. Other than the charges due to ionization of the

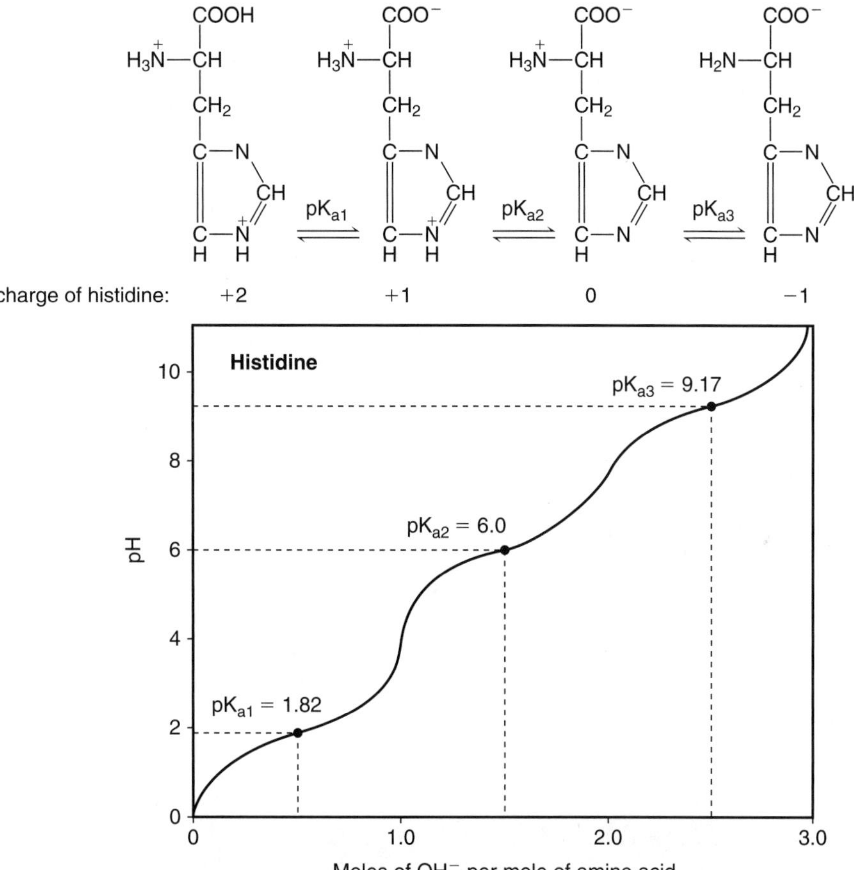

FIGURE 5-3 Titration curve for histidine.

C-terminal carboxyl group and N-terminal amino group, it is ionization of the R groups of the amino acids in the polypeptide that comprises the electrical charge of the macromolecule. Aspartate and glutamate have carboxylate groups on their side chains, whereas lysine has an ε-amino group and arginine has a basic guanidinium group; these groups are normally charged at physiological pH. In contrast, the imidazole ring of histidine ($pK_a = 6.0$) and the thiol group (−SH) of cysteine ($pK_a = 8.3$) have pK_as that are closer to neutral and undergo partial ionization within the range of physiological pH, meaning that relatively small shifts in cellular pH can change the charge of these residues. The seleno group of selenocysteine has a pK_a of about 5.2, such that selenocysteine residues are mostly ionized at physiological pH.

The ionization state of these side chains affects the physical and chemical properties of proteins and is important for their interactions with other proteins, substrates or ligands, and other macromolecules as well as for their physiological functions. Within chromatin, the basic amino acid residues in histones form ionic bonds with the acidic sugar–phosphate backbone of DNA. Acidic amino acid residues are involved in chelation of calcium ions by calcium-binding proteins. The histidine side chain and the carboxylate of acidic amino acids often serve as coordinating ligands for metals in metalloproteins. Within the native protein structure, pK_a values for ionizable groups can be substantially altered because of interactions with nearby residues or the hydrophobicity of the interior of the protein. Such alterations can be critical for the catalytic function of proteins such as enzymes (Harris and Turner, 2002).

HYDROPHOBICITY OR HYDROPHILICITY OF AMINO ACID RESIDUES

In addition to differences in size and charge, amino acids also differ in hydrophobicity or hydrophilicity (i.e., the tendency to interact with a polar or nonpolar solvent or environment). This property of amino acid R groups can vary widely, ranging from totally nonpolar or hydrophobic (water insoluble) to polar or hydrophilic (water soluble). The hydrophobic character of amino acid residues is believed to be the major driving force in protein folding. The amino acid residues with high positive hydropathy scores (e.g., isoleucine and valine) tend to repel the aqueous environment and consequently tend to pack together in the interior of the protein to avoid contact with water. On the other hand, amino acid residues with high negative hydropathy scores (e.g., arginine and lysine) will most likely be found on the surface of the protein in contact with the aqueous environment.

Jack Kyte and Russell Doolittle (1982) proposed a hydropathy index that is now widely used to predict aspects of protein structure; this scale assigns negative numbers to the most hydrophilic side chains and positive numbers to the

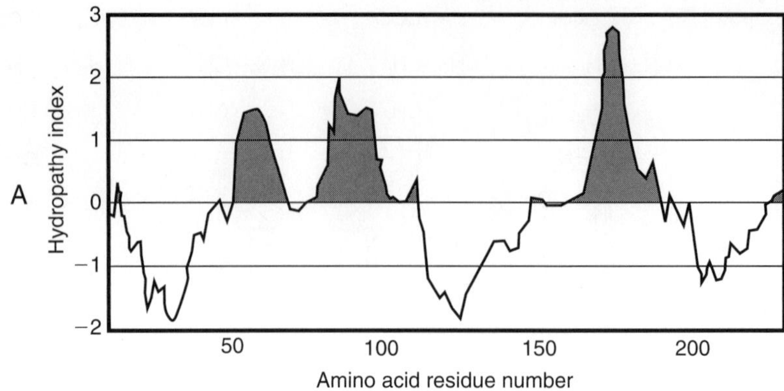

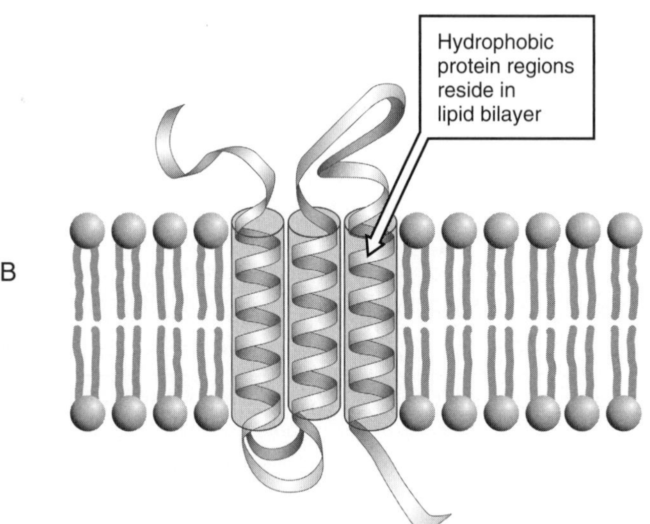

FIGURE 5-4 A hydropathy plot. Hydrophobic regions are usually found in the interior of proteins, whereas hydrophilic regions are likely to interact with aqueous or ionic environments. See Table 5-1 for hydropathic index values for given amino acids. A hydropathy plot (**A**) identifies regions of a polypeptide chain that contain amino acids that are predominantly hydrophobic (*shaded*) or, in contrast, hydrophilic in nature. The example shown could apply to a transmembrane protein (**B**). Transmembrane proteins often cross the lipid bilayers of cell membranes. The hydrophobic regions (positive hydropathic values) are associated with the interior of the membrane, whereas the hydrophilic regions may extend into the cytoplasmic compartment or toward the exterior of the cell.

most hydrophobic side chains (see Table 5-1). Other scales have been developed, some of which assign quite different values to some of the amino acids. Efforts to develop better methods of predicting protein structure continue. An example of the use of a hydropathy index to predict the transmembrane segments of a protein sequence is shown in Figure 5-4. Transmembrane segments of transmembrane proteins can be predicted from the average hydrophobicity scores for small regions of the polypeptide chain (e.g., segments of 9 to 19 amino acids). Transmembrane regions of proteins, which must pass through the lipid bilayers of cell membranes, tend to have high hydropathy scores (greater than 1.6 units).

MODIFICATIONS OF AMINO ACID SIDE CHAINS

As was noted in the previous section, the properties of the common amino acids can vary markedly depending upon their innate characteristics (e.g., size, charge, polarity, and hydropathy). The characteristics of some amino acids can also be altered by additional enzymatic and nonenzymatic modifications of the R group. Such modifications can occur as cotranslational or posttranslational events following incorporation of the amino acid into proteins (see Chapter 13). These specific amino acid modifications are introduced to modulate or modify a given chemical property. Posttranslational modifications extend the structures and properties of amino acids in proteins well beyond those of the 20 (or 21, if selenocysteine is included) amino acids used for protein translation in mammals.

Specific chemical properties can be altered subtly or dynamically by posttranslational modification. Some examples of posttranslational modifications of amino acid R groups in proteins include the methylation of lysine and histidine residues, the acetylation of lysine residues, the hydroxylation of proline and lysine residues, and the carboxylation of glutamate residues (Figure 5-5). These types of modifications of R groups are essential in defining the structural and functional

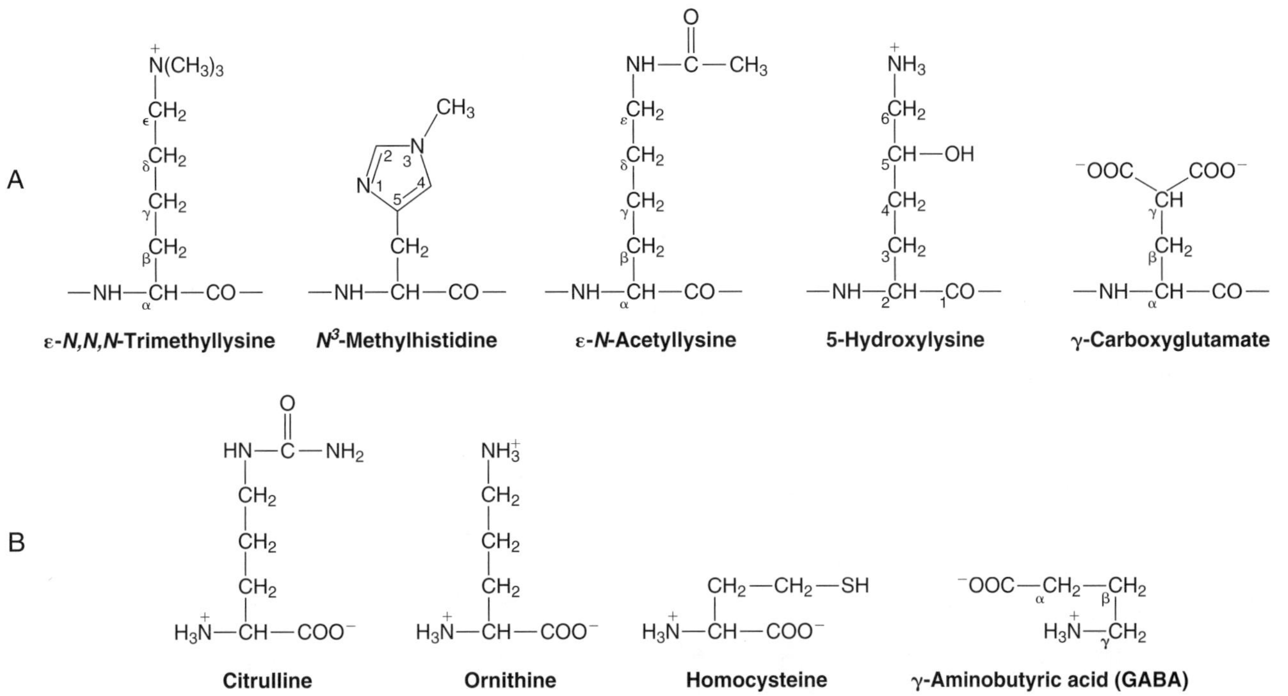

FIGURE 5-5 Examples of posttranslationally modified and less conventional amino acids. **A,** Examples of posttranslationally modified amino acids. An amino acid is first incorporated into a given peptide or protein and then altered by an enzyme catalyzed reaction. The modified amino acid may be released when the protein is degraded. Examples of the products of methylation (ε-*N,N,N*-trimethyllysine residue and N^3 methylhistidine residue formation), N-acetylation (ε-N-acetyllysine), hydroxylation (5-hydroxylysine residue formation), and γ-carboxylation (γ-carboxyglutamate residue formation) are shown. **B,** Examples of nonproteinogenic amino acids formed from free amino acids. The structures for citrulline, ornithine, homocysteine, and γ-aminobutyric acid are shown. Arginine and glutamate are precursors of citrulline and ornithine. Homocysteine is the demethylation product of methionine. GABA is formed by decarboxylation of glutamate.

properties of proteins. For example, the γ-carboxylation of glutamate residues in prothrombin and other blood clotting factors is critical for calcium binding and the proper function of these clotting factors in the blood clotting cascade.

A number of other amino acids are derived from metabolism of the free (nonpeptide) forms of the common amino acids. For example, ornithine can be formed from glutamate, proline, or arginine; citrulline is formed from ornithine; homocysteine is formed from methionine; γ-aminobutyrate is formed from glutamate; and 5-hydroxytryptophan is formed from tryptophan. Many of these amino acids and the distinct metabolic pathways by which they are synthesized are discussed in Chapter 14.

SYNTHESIS OF PEPTIDES AND PROTEINS

The synthesis of peptides or polypeptides involves the covalent linkage of amino acids by peptide bonds, as shown in Figure 5-6. Once linked in a peptide chain, an individual amino acid is called a residue.

PEPTIDE BOND FORMATION

Peptide bond formation is endergonic (i.e., it requires energy) with a positive free energy change of about 20 kJ/mol (~4.8 kcal/mol) at physiological pH. A positive free energy change of this magnitude means that combining an amino group of one amino acid with the carboxyl group of another does not occur spontaneously to any appreciable extent. Consequently, peptide synthesis requires both energy and specialized mechanisms (see Chapter 13).

The linked series of peptide bonds (carbon, nitrogen, and oxygen atoms) forms the main chain or protein backbone, and the R groups of amino acids extend from the chain. *Protein, polypeptide,* and *peptide* are used somewhat ambiguously and often overlap in meaning and usage. *Protein* is generally used to refer to the complete biological molecule in a stable conformation. *Peptide* is typically used for short oligomers of less than 30 amino acid residues, which often lack a stable three-dimensional structure. *Polypeptide* is used to refer to any linear chain of amino acid residues, regardless of length, and sometimes is used to imply an absence of defined conformation.

The amino acid sequence of peptides or proteins is conventionally written from the N-terminus (amino acid with a free α-amino group) to the C-terminus (amino acid with a free α-carboxyl group), which is the same order as that in which amino acid residues are added to the growing peptide chain during protein synthesis. Residues are also numbered, beginning with the N-terminal residue and moving toward the C-terminus. Because of the large number of amino acid residues in protein, both three-letter and one-letter abbreviations have been assigned to amino acids and are often used for writing out primary sequences (Table 5-2).

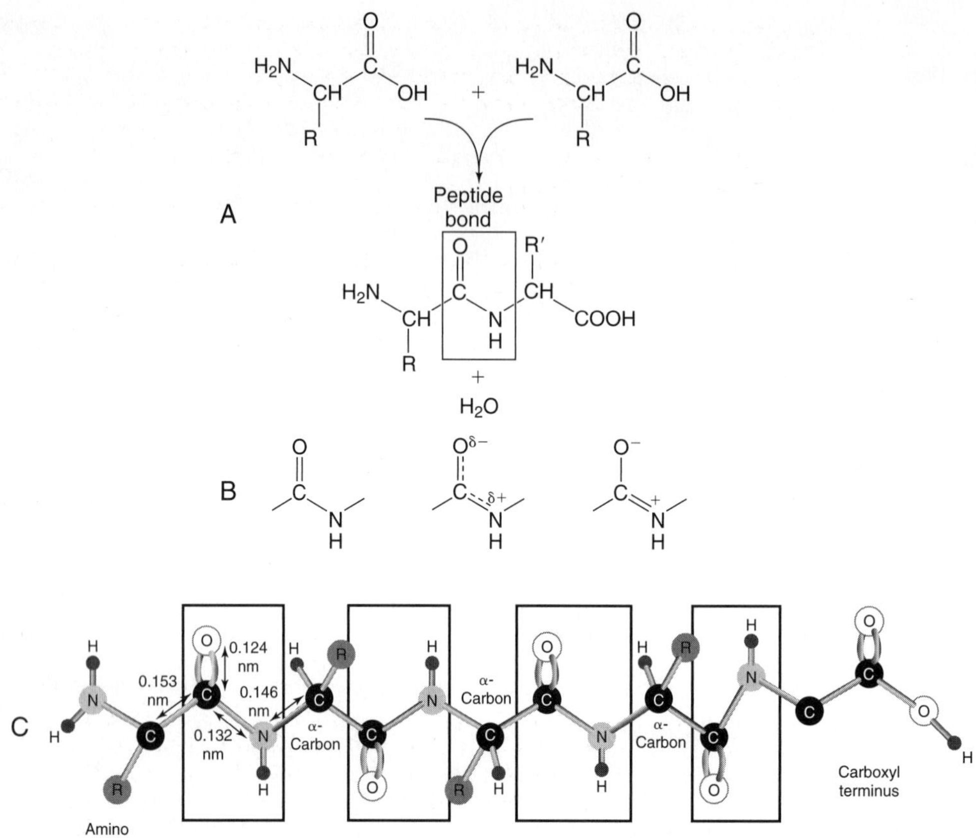

FIGURE 5-6 Formation of a peptide bond. As shown in **A**, the α-amino group of one amino acid displaces the hydroxyl of the carboxyl group in another. Although amino acids are good nucleophiles, the hydroxyl group is a poor leaving group. Therefore the reaction is endergonic with a free energy of change of about 20 kJ, or about 4.8 kcal per mole. As shown in **B**, the peptide bond is capable of resonance and charge separation. As indicated in **C**, the oxygen and nitrogen of the amide bond lie in a plane, which contributes to peptide bond stabilization. The hydrogen of the amino group is usually *trans* to the oxygen in the peptide backbone. Note that the bond length between the oxygen and carbon originating from the carboxyl group is 0.124 nm, which is typical of a C=O double bond. The nitrogen that is attached to the C=O forming the peptide bond also has a relatively short bond length (0.132 nm), indicating some double bond character. This causes an electric dipole. Because each bond has some double bond character, there is also restricted rotation. However, the nitrogen to α-carbon bond is 0.146 nm, which is typical of a single bond. Rotation can occur around this bond, unless it is hindered by the presence of an amino acid with a bulky R group (e.g., valine or isoleucine) or the presence of a proline residue.

As mentioned previously, residues within polypeptide chains can be modified after the amino acid precursors have been incorporated into the polypeptide chain, and this can occur either as the polypeptide is coming off the ribosome before the mRNA has been completely translated or after the complete polypeptide is released. In addition, the polypeptide can be cleaved during the process of synthesis and translocation.

The amino acid sequence for methionine enkephalin is shown in Figure 5-7. Methionine enkephalin is a pentapeptide. It is derived from an enkephalin precursor protein containing 267 amino acid residues, which is cleaved by a processing protease to yield several molecules of methionine enkephalin and one of leucine enkephalin (Comb et al., 1982). Peptides that play important functions in the body include a number of hormones, such as glucagon, antidiuretic hormone (vasopressin), and adrenocorticotrophic hormone (ACTH), and neuropeptides, which include the enkephalins, endorphins, and substance P. Most of these physiologically active peptides are produced by cleavage of large protein precursors.

Polypeptides or proteins have linear sequences that range from about 30 amino acid residues to those that contain thousands of residues. The largest known protein is titan, a component of the muscle sarcomere, with a molecular mass of almost 3,000 kDa and a total length of almost 27,000 amino acid residues. Bovine insulin, whose sequence is shown in Figure 5-8, was the first protein to be sequenced. This was accomplished by Frederick Sanger at Cambridge between 1950 and 1958 (Stretton, 2002). One of the reasons Sanger chose insulin for his work is that it was one of a few proteins readily available in pure form at the time. It was purified from bovine pancreas to treat patients with diabetes mellitus. Sanger used a variety of methods, many of which he developed, to first determine that there were two different chains in insulin (based on N-terminal residue analysis), that these two chains were linked by disulfide bonds between cysteine residues (by splitting these bonds with performic acid oxidation), and that the two chains had different amino acid compositions. Then, using partial hydrolysis followed by

TABLE 5-2 Abbreviations and Codons for Proteinogenic Amino Acids

AMINO ACID	THREE-LETTER CODE	ONE-LETTER CODE	POSSIBLE CODONS (CODON-BEARING STRAND OF DNA)
Alanine	Ala	A	GCA, GCC, GCG, GCT
Cysteine	Cys	C	TGC, TGT
Aspartate	Asp	D	GAC, GAT
Glutamate	Glu	E	GAA, GAG
Phenylalanine	Phe	F	TTC, TTT
Glycine	Gly	G	GGA, GGC, GGG, GGT
Histidine	His	H	CAC, CAT
Isoleucine	Ile	I	ATA, ATC, ATT
Lysine	Lys	K	AAA, AAG
Leucine	Leu	L	CTA, CTC, CTG, CTT, TTA, TTG
Methionine	Met	M	ATG
Asparagine	Asn	N	AAC, AAT
Proline	Pro	P	CCA, CCC, CCG, CCT
Glutamine	Gln	Q	CAA, CAG
Arginine	Arg	R	AGA, AGG, CGA, CGC, CGG, CGT
Serine	Ser	S	AGC, AGT, TCA, TCC, TCG, TCT
Threonine	Thr	T	ACA, ACC, ACG, ACT
Selenocysteine	Sec	U	TGA + SECIS element in mRNA
Valine	Val	V	GTA, GTC, GTG, GTT
Tryptophan	Trp	W	TGG
Tyrosine	Tyr	Y	TAC, TAT
Stop codon			TAA, TAG, TGA

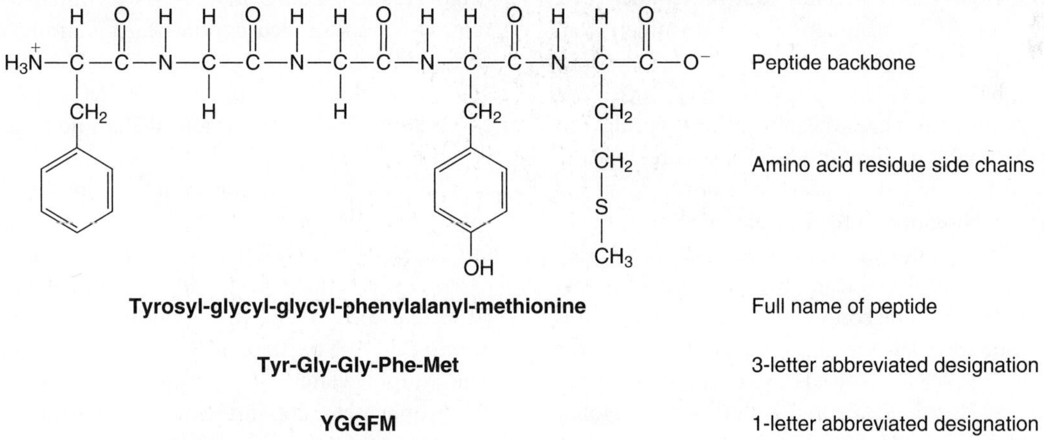

FIGURE 5-7 Amino acid sequence of the pentapeptide, methionine enkephalin.

fractionation of the products and end-group analysis, further partial hydrolysis and analysis of the longer products, addition of reagents to block formation of new disulfide bonds, and the mapping of sequences of overlapping fragments, he and his coworkers determined the amino acid sequence of both chains, A and B. They also identified the locations of the disulfide bonds. Sanger's work clearly showed, for the first time, that polypeptides consisted of linear polymers of amino acids rather than branched polymers or colloids. This was a seminal discovery, and Sanger was awarded a Nobel Prize for this work in 1958.

THE GENETIC CODE

The fact that there was a well-defined sequence in polypeptides led to the thought that information about the specific sequence of amino acids for each protein had to be encoded

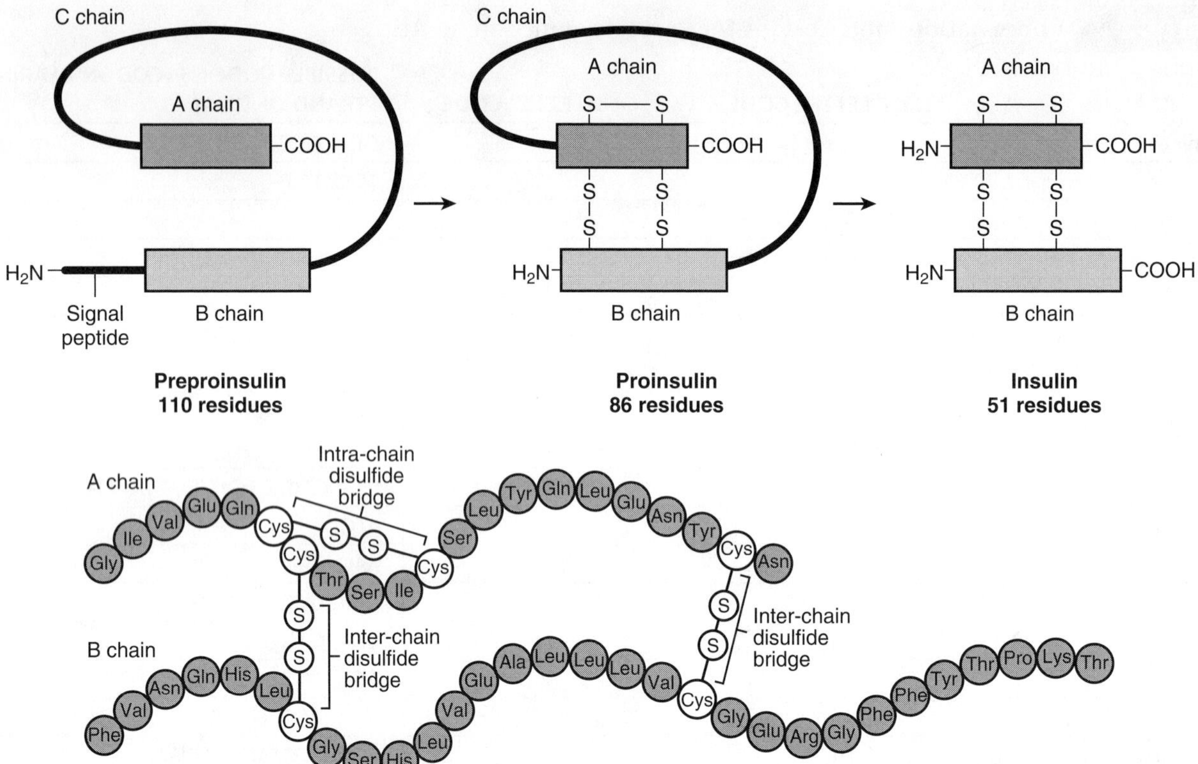

FIGURE 5-8 The primary sequence of insulin. Insulin is synthesized as a preproinsulin precursor polypeptide. A signal peptide of 24 amino acid residues is cleaved from the amino terminus of the polypeptide. Subsequently, the so-called C peptide of 31 amino acid residues is cleaved from the center of the polypeptide, leaving the insulin A chain (30 amino acid residues) and B chain (21 amino acid residues) held together by two interchain disulfide bridges. An additional intrachain disulfide bond is part of the tertiary structure.

in the genomic DNA. In both deoxynucleic acid (DNA) and ribonucleic acid (RNA) there are only four nucleotide bases: adenine (A), cytosine (C), guanine (G), and thymine (T) in DNA or uracil (U) in RNA. Guanine base-pairs with cytosine, whereas adenine base-pairs with thymine or uracil. Once it was known that only four bases are available for base pairing, scientists concluded that a minimum sequence of three nucleotide bases would be required to specify one of the 20 amino acids. Marshall W. Nirenberg at the U.S. National Institutes of Health was the first to crack the genetic code by discovering that UUU encoded phenylalanine in 1961, demonstrating that indeed a unit of genetic code consists of three bases, which is now called a codon. By 1966 Nirenberg had deciphered all the RNA codons, and in 1968 he received the Nobel Prize in Physiology or Medicine. He shared the prize with Robert W. Holley and Har Gobind Khorana. Holley discovered and determined the sequence of the first transfer RNA (tRNA), which was key to explaining how proteins are synthesized from mRNA. Khorana developed methods for synthesis of nucleotide polymers (i.e., synthetic RNA), which were used to crack the genetic code.

Information about the specific sequence of amino acids for each protein is encoded in the DNA. Certain portions of a gene encode sequences that are transcribed and processed into mature mRNAs, which in turn serve as the templates for protein synthesis. The DNA and mRNA contain nucleotide base sequences that in turn determine amino acid sequences (Figure 5-9). Codons in the DNA (which by convention refers to the so-called codon-bearing strand of the DNA) and codons in the mRNA are identical, except that mRNA contains uridine (U) in place of the thymidine (T) present in DNA. A list of the codons and the amino acids they specify is given in Table 5-2.

The link between the genetic code and amino acid sequence is the specificity provided by a set of tRNAs and aminoacyl-tRNA synthetases. Transfer RNA molecules each carry a specific nucleotide sequence called an anticodon. A particular aminoacyl-tRNA synthetase esterifies a specific amino acid to a particular tRNA with its unique anticodon. The aminoacylated tRNA thus carries the amino acid to the proper place for insertion in the growing polypeptide chain, a process that depends on the ability of the anticodon to base pair with the proper codon on the mRNA. Today, amino acid sequences of proteins are frequently inferred from the nucleotide sequence of the protein's gene or the nucleotide sequence of its corresponding mRNA.

Genetic diseases are caused by inheritable changes in the DNA sequence. Phenylketonuria (PKU) is an example of a genetic metabolic disease caused by the inheritance of a "disease" allele for phenylalanine hydroxylase from both parents. Phenylalanine hydroxylase is the enzyme that converts phenylalanine to tyrosine. In the absence of a

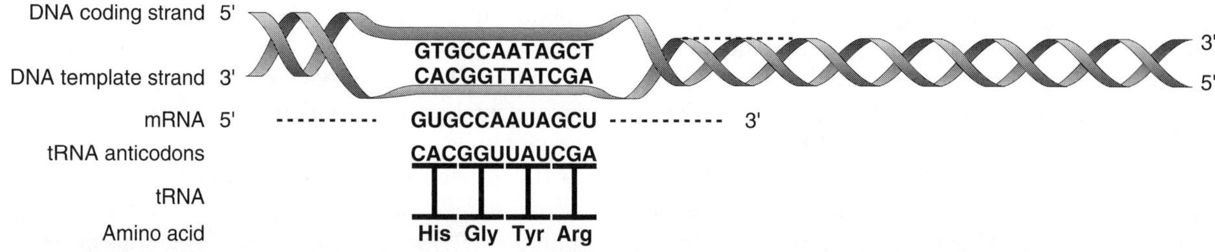

FIGURE 5-9 Illustration of use of nucleotide sequences to encode the amino acid sequence of polypeptides. The nucleotide codons and anticodons for an unwound section of DNA double helix are shown. Messenger RNA (mRNA) is transcribed from the so-called template strand of DNA, not from the so-called coding or sense strand. Which strand of DNA is the template depends on the particular gene being transcribed. The coding region of the mRNA is translated into protein by base-pairing of the anticodons of the transfer RNA (tRNA) molecules with the mRNA. The tRNA molecules are aminoacylated with the appropriate amino acid by aminoacyl-tRNA synthetases that uniquely recognize their specific tRNA and their specific amino acid substrates.

functional enzyme, phenylalanine accumulates in the blood, and abnormal phenylalanine metabolites are excreted in the urine. A disease allele is one in which a nucleotide substitution or a deletion or insertion of one or more nucleotides has either changed the coding for a critical amino acid residue, introduced a premature termination codon, or disrupted the correct three-nucleotide reading frame. Many mutations have little or no consequence because they do not change the amino acid that is inserted (especially a substitution of the third nucleotide in a codon) or because the amino acid change may still yield a functional protein. At least 67 allelic variants of the phenylalanine hydroxylase gene have been identified in individuals with PKU. Most of these variants are single point mutations (i.e., a single nucleotide substitution causing a change in the encoded amino acid) that map to the catalytic domain of the enzyme. The incidence of PKU is about 1 in 15,000 births.

An example of a single nucleotide substitution that does not cause disease but alters nutrient requirements is the C677T mutation in the gene for 5,10-methylenetetrahydrofolate reductase. Individuals who are homozygous for this polymorphism have a higher requirement for folate. About 5% to 10% of the general white population is homozygous for this point mutation.

PROTEIN STRUCTURE

Proteins do not naturally exist as long linear polymers, but rather the polypeptide chain folds in three dimensions. Protein structure forms in a hierarchical manner from so-called primary structure to quaternary structure. The first atomic resolution structures of proteins were solved by X-ray crystallography in the 1960s (Strandberg et al., 2009) and by nuclear magnetic resonance (NMR) spectroscopy in the 1980s (Wüthrich, 2001). Much has been learned about the three-dimensional structure of proteins by application of these two methodologies.

PRIMARY STRUCTURE

The linear sequence of amino acids in the polypeptide chain is called the *primary structure* of the protein. Once the polypeptide is synthesized, the amino acids in the polypeptide interact with each other to produce a well-defined three-dimensional structure, which is known as the folded or native state of the protein. The primary structure determines most of the higher level structure of the protein. In fact, considerable information about the three-dimensional structure of the protein can be inferred from the primary structure. The wide variety of primary sequences in proteins underlies the many different three-dimensional conformations of proteins.

In addition, many small sequences or motifs within the primary structure act as specific signals for certain protein modifications that impact biological regulation. Examples include (1) the sequences Asn-X-Ser and Asn-X-Thr, which are common sites for *N*-linked glycosylation in proteins (i.e., the addition of sugars to asparagine side chains at specified sites along the polypeptide chain); (2) the sequence Arg-Gly-Asp-Ser, which corresponds to a cell surface–binding domain in certain proteins (e.g., fibronectin) and allows a protein to bind to a cell's surface; and (3) the sequence Lys-Asp-Glu-Leu, which is one of the signals important for the vectoral movement of soluble proteins within the endoplasmic reticulum (ER). The use of X in the first example indicates that a number of given amino acids can be substituted for X without affecting the functional significance of the sequence when it appears in a protein. When an amino acid sequence is associated with a definable and consistent function, it is often designated as a consensus sequence, particularly if the sequence is found in a diversity of animal, plant, or bacterial cells.

SECONDARY STRUCTURE

The backbone of the polypeptide chain is highly polar and prefers contact with water, but the hydrophobic amino acids have side chains that are nonpolar and prefer to be on the inside of the protein. A major way this problem is solved is the formation of regular secondary structures that allow the −NH and −C=O groups along the backbone to form hydrogen bonds with each other. Thus the term *secondary structure* refers to local regularly occurring structure in proteins that is mainly formed through hydrogen bonds between backbone atoms. A single polypeptide may contain multiple sections of secondary structure, and these regions may be connected to each other by loop regions of various lengths and irregular shapes. These loop regions or regions of random coil do not have secondary structure and are found mainly at the surface of the folded protein molecule.

Protein secondary structure consists largely of α-helices and β-pleated sheets, which are illustrated in Figure 5-10. Sequences within polypeptide chains that form α-helices are enriched in amino acids with free rotation around the polypeptide chain. The backbone chain in the α-helix adopts a right-handed spiral conformation such that the carbonyl group of amino acid n forms a hydrogen bond with the amino group of amino acid $n + 4$ (see Figure 5-10, *B*). Occasionally, the different spacing between hydrogen bonds gives rise to a more tightly or loosely coiled helix. In the α-helix, all of the R groups point outward.

In the polypeptides that form β-sheets, a common feature is segmental repeats of amino acids whose side chains restrict free rotation around the polypeptide backbone. In contrast to the α-helix, the polypeptide backbone of these regions is almost fully extended. Beta-sheets are formed when the amino (−NH) and carbonyl (−C=O) groups of one part of the polypeptide backbone form hydrogen bonds with the carbonyl and amino groups of another strand of the polypeptide backbone that is adjacent to the first strand in the folded protein (see Figure 5-10, *C* and *D*). The adjacent stretches

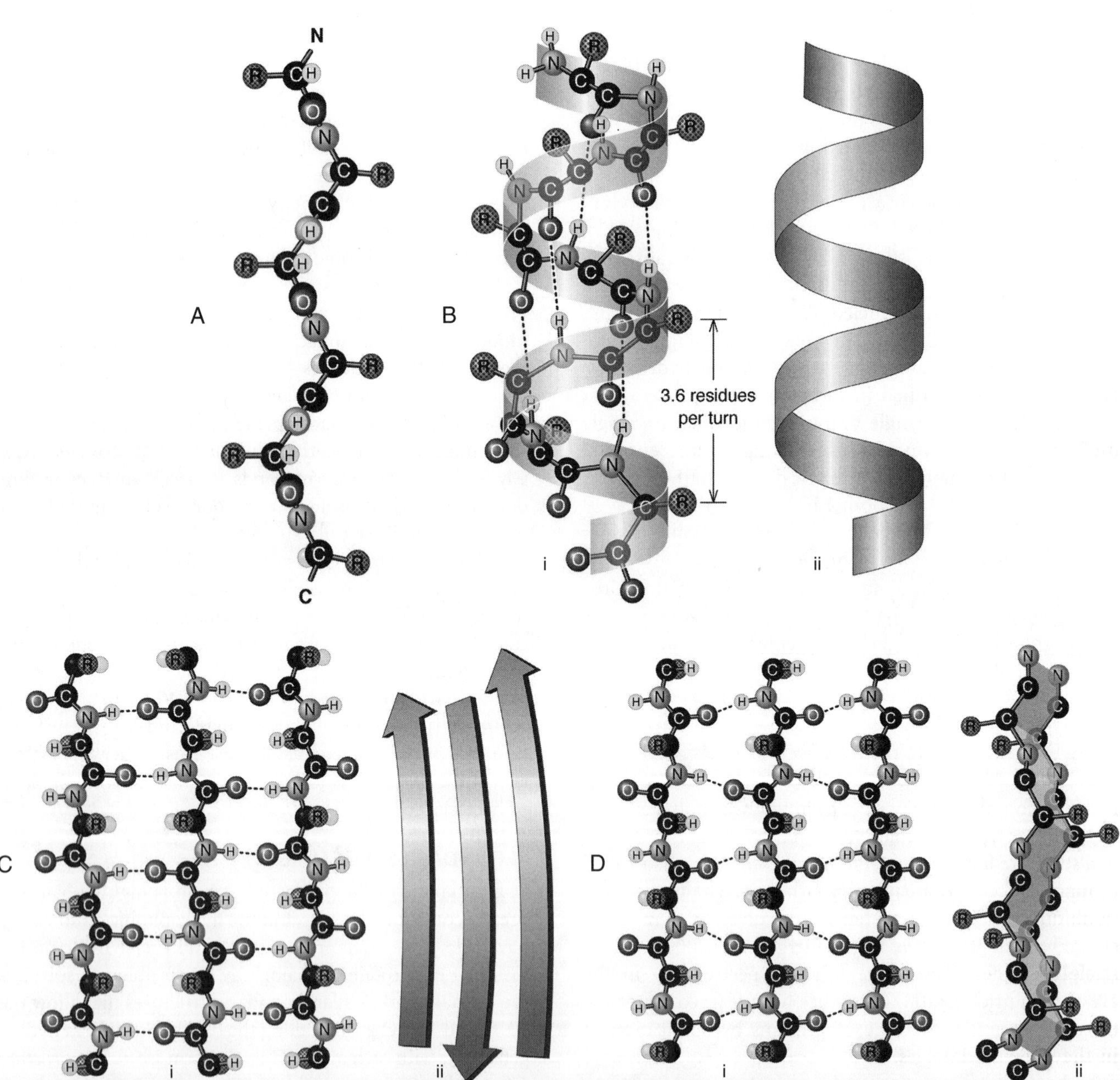

FIGURE 5-10 Types of secondary structure. **A,** A polypeptide strand with no secondary structure. **B,** Representations of α-helices: i. Peptide backbone showing hydrogen bonds and R groups sticking outward from the α-helix. ii. Ribbon representation. **C,** Representations of antiparallel β-sheets. i. Model of antiparallel beta sheet showing hydrogen bonds. ii. Ribbon model of antiparallel β-strands. **D,** Representations of parallel β-sheets. i. Model of parallel β-sheets showing hydrogen bonds. ii. Side view showing pleated shape of β-sheets. See text for more details.

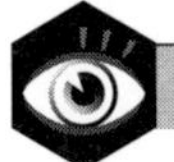

NUTRITION INSIGHT

Wheat Proteins: The Good and the Bad

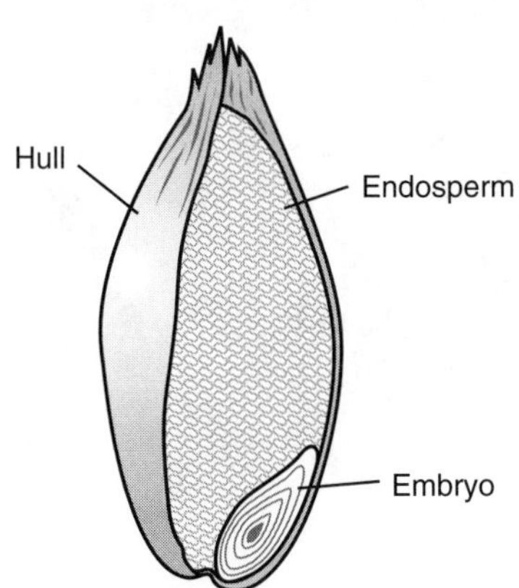

The good: Gluten is an important nutritional and functional protein in foods. Many food proteins have functional properties that are used in cooking and food processing. An important example is gluten, which is the major protein in the seed portion of wheat. Gluten comes from the Latin *gluten,* meaning "glue." Interestingly, the amino acid glutamate was so named because it was first isolated from gluten. Gluten refers collectively to two proteins called gliadin and glutenin that exist in the endosperm of wheat. When dough made with wheat flour is kneaded, gluten forms as glutenin molecules cross-link to make a submicroscopic network. These glutenin molecules associate with gliadin, and this contributes viscosity and extensibility to the mix. Bread flours are high in gluten, whereas cake flours are lower in gluten. Kneading and increased wetness promotes the formation of gluten strands and cross-links, which result in a chewier product. Shortening inhibits formation of cross-links, so it is used along with diminished water and minimal working when a tender and flaky product such as a pie crust is desired.

The bad: Celiac disease is an autoimmune response triggered by consumption of wheat protein. Wheat is a major source of protein in human diets. Celiac disease is an autoimmune disorder of the small intestine that is caused by a reaction to gliadin from wheat and to similar proteins such as the prolamins found in barley and rye. One region of α-gliadin stimulates disruption of tight junctions between the intestinal epithelial cells so that protease-resistant peptides of α-gliadin can enter the circulation to stimulate an immune response.

In addition, the enzyme tissue transglutaminase modifies gliadin peptides by cross-linking the gliadin peptide to a lysine residue of the transglutaminase via a γ-glutamyl-lysine isopeptide bond; this results in formation of new epitopes that are believed to trigger the primary immune response by which autoantibodies to transglutaminase develop. Thus when susceptible individuals eat gliadin or other similar proteins, their immune system reacts to the cross-linked gliadin–transglutaminase and, in effect, attacks the normal tissue of the small intestine.

The cause of celiac disease is polyfactorial, but genetic susceptibility is an important factor. Most susceptible individuals have either the DQ2 or DQ8 isoform of the HLA-DQ gene, which encodes a component of the MHC class II antigen-presenting receptor. The reason that presence of these genes increases the risk of celiac disease is that receptors with these isoforms bind to gliadin peptides more tightly than other forms of the antigen-presenting receptor. Therefore these forms are more likely to activate T lymphocytes and initiate the autoimmune process.

The inflammatory process leads to disruption of the structure and function of the small intestine's mucosal lining (villous atrophy), which impairs the body's ability to absorb nutrients. The villous atrophy may also cause secondary lactose intolerance due to the decreased absorptive surface area and reduced production of lactase. There is no effective treatment for celiac disease other than avoidance of gluten in the diet. It should be noted that celiac disease is different from a wheat allergy. Although wheat allergy is also due to ingestion of and treated by avoidance of wheat, allergies to wheat (or other food proteins) do not cause the severe intestinal damage associated with celiac disease.

of polypeptide chain do not need to be near each other in the linear sequence of the polypeptide but only near each other in the folded three-dimensional structure. The hydrogen bonds between β-strands lie roughly in the plane of the β-sheet, with the peptide carbonyl groups pointing in alternating directions for each successive residue. The R groups of successive α-carbons within an individual strand point outward, roughly perpendicularly to the plane of the sheet, with these successive residues alternately pointing straight up or straight down. Adjacent strands in a β-sheet are aligned so that their α-carbons are adjacent and so that the R groups attached to these adjacent α-carbons point in the same direction. Beta-sheets have a pleated appearance because of the tetrahedral chemical bonding at the α-carbons.

Because peptide chains have a directionality conferred by their N-terminus and C-terminus, adjacent stands (regions of the polypeptide) may have the same (parallel) or opposite (antiparallel) directionality. All strands within a β-sheet do not need to be consistently parallel or antiparallel. In fact, an individual strand may exhibit a mixed bonding pattern, with a parallel strand on one side and an antiparallel strand on the other. However, antiparallel arrangements of β-strands are the most stable and the most common. The hydrogen bonds between carbonyls and amines are stronger for antiparallel strands than for parallel strands. In models of protein structures, the directionality of β-strands are often represented by an arrow pointing toward the C-terminus (see Figure 5-10, *C, ii*).

Fibrous proteins are distinguished by their extensive regions of regular secondary structure. Most fibrous proteins are filamentous and elongated and play structural roles in tissues. A good example of a fibrous protein in the human body is the α-keratins, which are the major proteins of hair, fingernails, and skin calluses. The secondary structure of α-keratins is composed predominantly of α-helices.

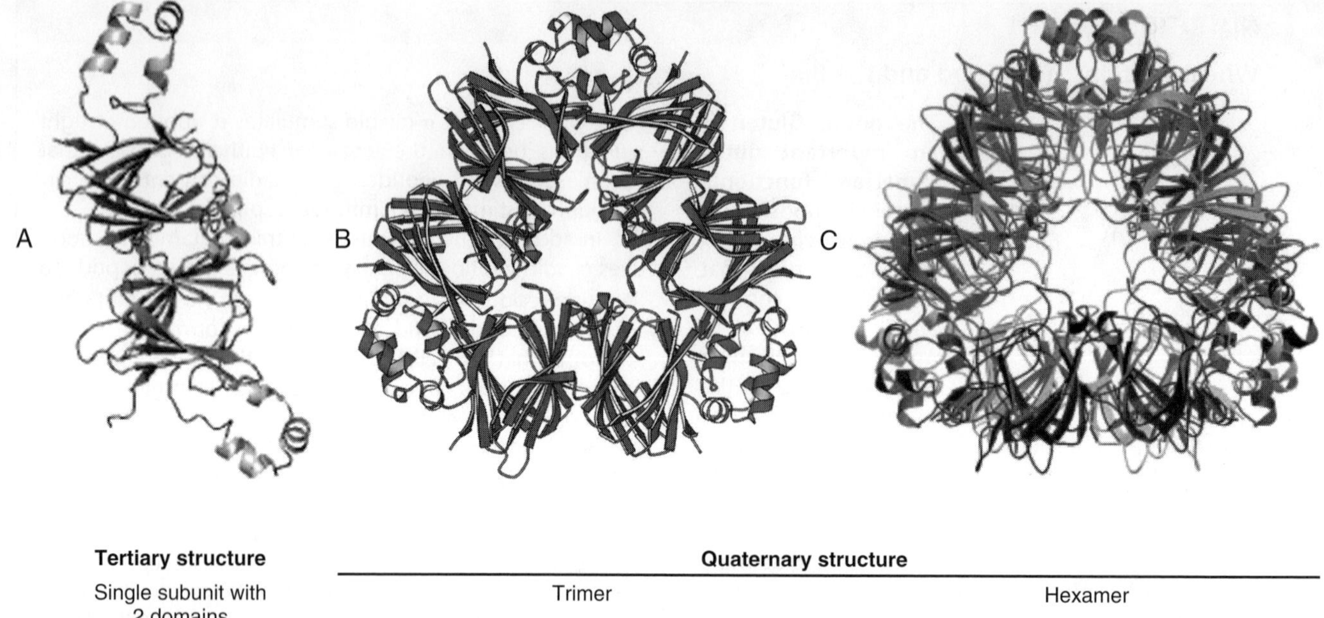

FIGURE 5-11 Ribbon representations of the structure of seed storage proteins. **A,** The canavalin subunit. Canavalin is a vicilin from jack bean. Each domain of the symmetrical subunit can be divided into a β-barrel subdomain and a helix–loop–helix subdomain. **B,** The trimeric structure of canavalin. **C,** The hexameric structure of glycinin, a leguminin found in soybeans. The hexameric structure is made up of two leguminin trimers. (Based on work of Ko, T. P., Day, J., & McPherson, A. [2000]. The refined structure of canavalin from jack bean in two crystal forms at 2.1 and 2.0 A resolution. *Acta Crystallographica. Section D, Biological Crystallography, 56,* 411–420; Adachi, M., Kanamori, J., Masuda, T., Yagasaki, K., Kitamura, K., Mikami, B., & Utsumi, S. [2003]. Crystal structure of soybean 11S globulin: Glycinin A3B4 homohexamer. *Proceedings of the National Academy of Sciences of the United States of America, 100,* 7395–7400. Copyright 2003 National Academy of Sciences, U.S.A.)

Collagen, which provides much of the extracellular matrix of bone and other tissues, has a more unusual secondary structure. It contains chains of left-handed helical structure that are wound together with two other chains to form a right-handed helical structure. Other fibrous proteins such as the β-keratins found in feathers and scales and the fibroin made by silkworms and spiders contain mainly β-sheet structures.

TERTIARY STRUCTURE

The secondary structural elements of the polypeptide fold together to give a closely packed, three-dimensional structure. The term *tertiary structure* is used to describe this overall three-dimensional arrangement of amino acids within a protein. In addition to regions of secondary structure that lock the positions of some atoms relative to each other, the overall three-dimensional shape of a protein molecule is a compromise structure that has the best balance of attractive and repulsive forces between different regions of the molecule. Frequently the tertiary structure of proteins involves the formation of two or more structurally independent parts of the protein, known as domains, that are held together by a relatively thin stretch of polypeptide backbone. Tertiary structure may also include the formation of covalent, disulfide bonds between cysteine residues within the polypeptide chain. Complex protein structures can be determined to an atomic level by X-ray diffraction of crystallized proteins or by NMR spectroscopy of small (less than 30 kDa) proteins in solution. An example of the tertiary structure of a protein is shown in Figure 5-11, *A*.

Tertiary structures may also accommodate specific functional groups called prosthetic groups or cofactors. The term *prosthetic group* is used to describe a unique moiety or defined chemical structure that confers a specific function or additional property to a given protein. Prosthetic groups may be covalently or noncovalently linked to the proteins they serve. Examples of prosthetic groups include the heme group in hemoglobin and myoglobin, enzyme cofactors such as lipoic acid or pyridoxal 5′-phosphate, and metal ligands such as iron and copper.

QUATERNARY STRUCTURE

For proteins made up of more than one polypeptide chain, an additional term, *quaternary structure,* is used to describe the three-dimensional arrangement of multiple polypeptide chains in the complex. The protein may be made up of identical or different polypeptide chains, usually called subunits or monomers, that interact with each other to form an oligomer. The subunits are held together by hydrophobic interactions and other attractive forces such as ionic and hydrogen bonds; covalent disulfide bonds between chains are rarely involved. Many proteins form homodimers or heterodimers. Some examples of proteins with more than two subunits include (1) hemoglobin, a heterotetramer made up of two identical α subunits and two identical β subunits, (2) antibodies of the IgG form, which have two light chains and two heavy chains, with disulfide bonds within each chain as well as between the two heavy chains, (3) the insulin receptor, which is a transmembrane receptor tyrosine kinase that is a disulfide-linked dimer composed of two heterodimers, each of which contains an α-chain and a β-chain, and (4) myosin, which is a hexamer made up of two trimers, with each trimer composed of a heavy chain, an essential light chain, and a regulatory light chain. Examples of important food proteins that have quaternary structure are the globulin family proteins called vicilins and legumins, which are shown in Figure 5-11. These oligomeric proteins are the major storage proteins in legume seeds, such as soybeans and peas, and are important sources of dietary protein. Legumins exist as hexamers, which are synthesized from six molecules of a precursor protein that has an N-terminal acidic and a C-terminal basic domain. Vicilins are trimeric molecules formed from three molecules of a precursor that has structurally similar N- and C-terminal domains.

HIGHER LEVELS OF PROTEIN ASSEMBLY

Many supramolecular protein assemblies are made of multiple subunits or proteins that are held together by noncovalent interactions. For example, the pyruvate dehydrogenase complex, which converts pyruvate to acetyl-CoA, contains multiple copies of three different enzymes (E1, E2, E3), a binding protein, and five different coenzymes. The estimated mass of the human pyruvate dehydrogenase complex is 950,000 kDa, with 40 molecules of E2, 20 molecules of E3 binding protein, 40 E1 heterotetramers, and 20 E3 dimers (Brautigam et al., 2009). Two other examples of supramolecular protein assembles are shown in Figure 5-12. The 26S proteasome, which carries out much of intracellular protein degradation in mammalian cells, contains about 66 subunits and has a molecular mass of about 2,000 kDa. The contractile units of muscle are made up of actin, myosin, and accessory proteins that are organized into the myofilaments that ultimately form the contractile units of muscle. The basic unit of the myofibrils is the sarcomere, which is a multiprotein complex composed of the thick filament (myosin, myosin-binding protein C) system, the thin filament (actin, tropomyosin, troponin) system (Figure 5-12), and nebulin and titan, which give stability.

For stabilization of protein structures, it is often essential to cross-link specific polypeptide chains. For structural proteins, such as collagen and elastin, the formation of interchain cross-links facilitates the formation of fibers and protein complexes, whose molecular masses can range into the millions of daltons. For example, collagen fibrils are made of many molecules of collagen, each of which is a cross-linked triple helix formed from three procollagen α-chains. The process of collagen fibril assembly, which is dependent upon a number of cotranslational and posttranslational modifications, is illustrated in Figure 5-13

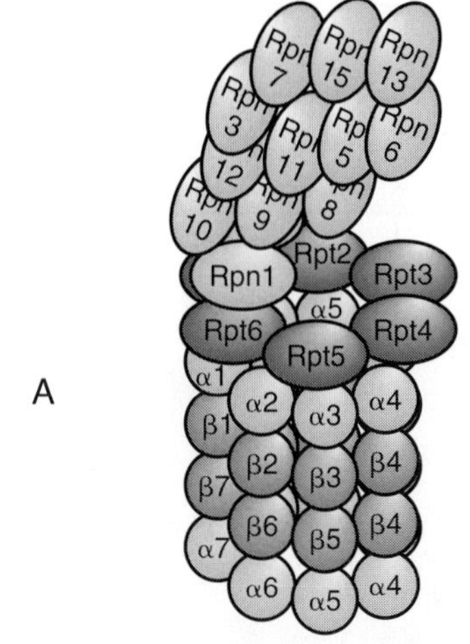

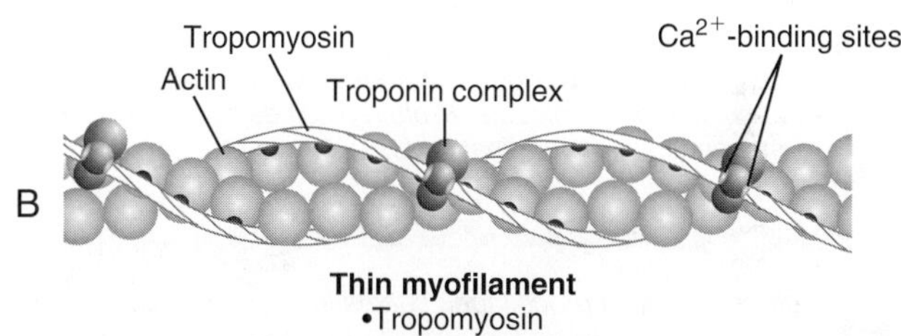

FIGURE 5-12 Examples of supramolecular protein complexes. **A,** 26S Proteasome. **B,** Thin myofilament.

(Kagan, 2000). The formation of interchain cross-links also renders collagen and elastin resistant to the action of many proteinases so that these proteins can exist in a proteinase-enriched environment without significant damage or alteration.

STABILIZATION OF PROTEIN CONFORMATIONS

The final shape of a protein determines how it functions. Protein conformations are stabilized by weak noncovalent forces or interactions. A large number of these weak interactions can substantially stabilize the native protein structure. Important noncovalent interactions in folded proteins include hydrophobic interactions with free energy change of association in the range of 8 to 13 kJ/mol (2 to 3 kcal/mol); hydrogen bonds with typical strengths of 5 to 30 kJ/mol (1 to 7 kcal/mol); electrostatic interactions (attractive or repulsive) with bond strengths of 4 to 25 kJ/mol (1 to 7 kcal/mol); and the very weak van der Waals forces with strengths of less than 4 kJ/mol (less than 1 kcal/mol). For comparison, the amount of energy needed to break a covalent C–C bond is about 350 kJ/mol, or 83 kcal/mol. Disulfide bridges

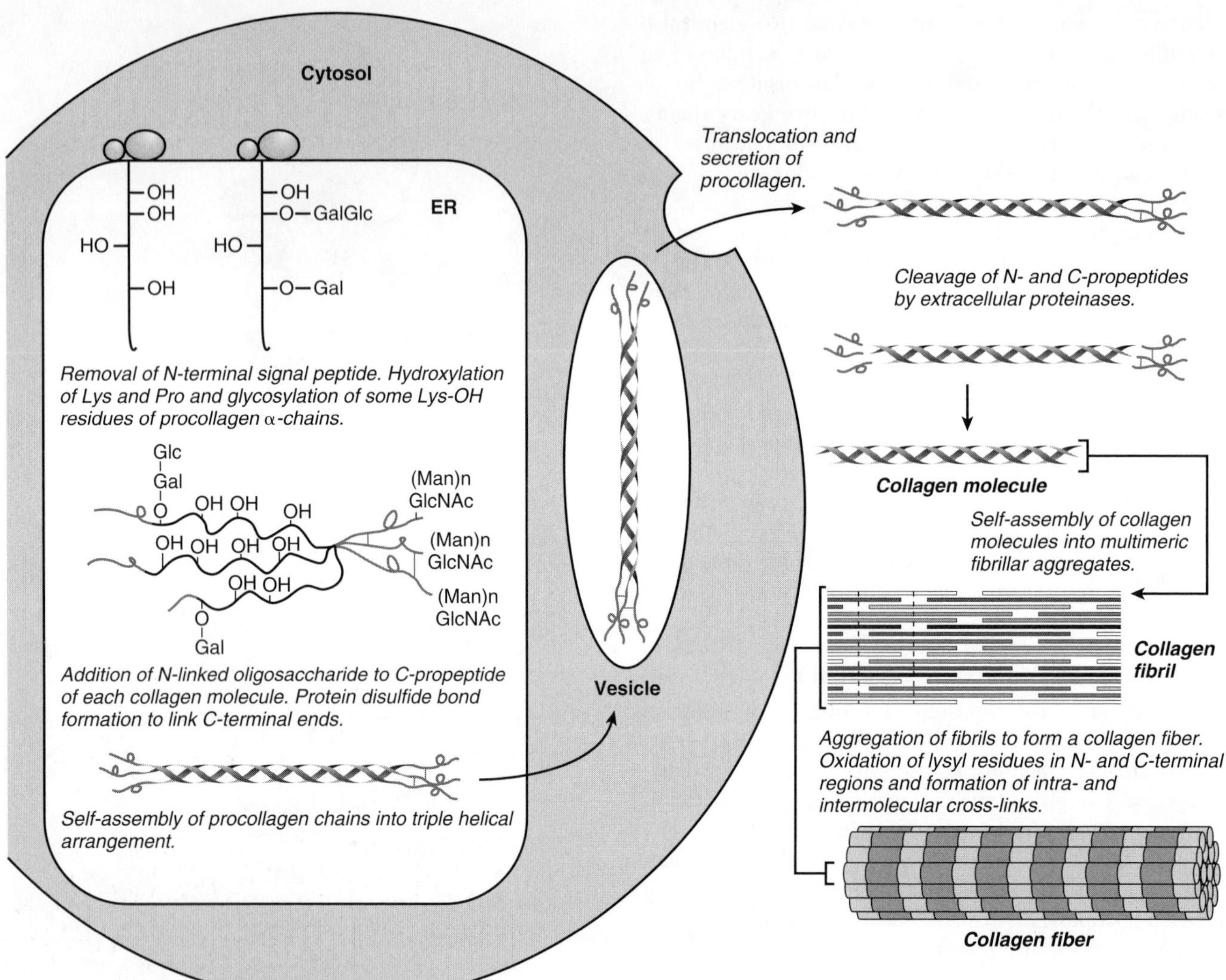

FIGURE 5-13 Collagen synthesis involves a number of cotranslational and posttranslational modifications. The fibril-forming collagens are synthesized as procollagens on the ribosomes of the rough ER. Modifications that occur in the ER include the removal of signal peptides; hydroxylation of proline and lysine residues to 4-hydroxyproline, 3-hydroxyproline, and hydroxylysine residues; glycosylation of certain hydroxylysine residues to galactosylhydroxylysine and glucosylgalactosylhydroxylysine residues; glycosylation of a mannose-rich oligosaccharide on the C-terminal propeptide of each chain; chain association; disulfide bonding between chains; and formation of a triple helix. The procollagen triple helix moves through the Golgi complex and is secreted to the extracellular space. Extracellular modifications consist of removal of large peptides from both N- and C-termini of the procollagen, which converts the procollagen to collagen. The collagen forms ordered aggregates, and the collagen units are cross-linked to form stable collagen fibrils. Cross-linking of collagen is based upon aldehyde formation from lysine or hydroxylysine residues, which involves the deamination of these residues by lysyl oxidase (protein-lysine 6-oxidase) to form allysine or hydroxyallysine residues, respectively. These aldehyde residues then react spontaneously with each other or with lysine residues to form cross-links.

between cysteine residues at different locations can stabilize parts of a three-dimensional structure by introducing a covalent cross-link; the covalent S–S bond strength is about 228 kJ/mol, or 54 kcal/mol.

The amino acid sequence of each protein contains the information that specifies both the native structure and the pathway to attain that state. In general, proteins fold so that hydrophobic elements of the protein are buried deep inside the structure and hydrophilic side chains end up on the outside. Minimizing the number of hydrophobic side chains exposed to water is an important driving force behind the folding process. Most globular proteins are able to assume their native state unassisted. Some proteins require chaperone proteins for assistance in folding or in remaining folded under certain environmental conditions such as exposure to heat. Chaperones also assist in the refolding of misfolded proteins.

The process of folding and unfolding of proteins is dynamic. For most proteins, this process results from a programmed sequence of events. When a protein is folded so that it is functional, the process is referred to as naturation. Denaturation of a protein involves disruption of the weak, noncovalent interactions responsible for quaternary, tertiary, and secondary structure. Thus a

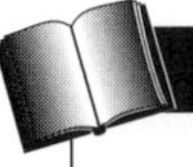

HISTORICAL TIDBIT

What Is a Dalton? Why Are Daltons Used to Express the Molecular Mass of Proteins?

Although scientists in the 1800s discovered that chemical elements are composed of atoms and that each chemical compound was composed of molecules in which atoms were combined in a fixed way, they did not have a way to define the mass of atoms or molecules. However, chemists realized they could use relative masses to describe and predict the outcome of chemical reactions. The general idea was that atoms of hydrogen, known to be the lightest element, should have a relative mass of 1, and other atoms should have masses that are multiples of this (then unknown) mass of the hydrogen atom. Although we now have good estimates of atomic masses, the concept of relative atomic mass is still widely used. In 1960 chemists and physicists agreed on the definition of the unified atomic mass unit as 1⁄12 the mass of the most common isotope of carbon, known as carbon-12 atoms. Thus the mass of an atom or molecule is calculated based on the ratio of its mass to that of carbon-12, which has six protons and six neutrons in its nucleus. Roughly, relative mass = number of protons + neutrons. An alternate name for the unified atomic mass unit is the dalton (Da), which was named after the English chemist John Dalton, who proposed the atomic theory of matter in 1803. The latter unit is often used to state the masses of large organic molecules such as proteins, with the masses typically stated in kilodaltons (kDa).

The use of relative units does not provide a measure of actual mass of a molecule. To get around this problem, the "mole" was defined as the number of elementary entities (atoms or molecules) in exactly 12 g of carbon-12. Thus the mass of one mole of any atom or molecule is its relative atomic or molecular mass in grams. The then unknown number of "entities" in one mole was called Avogadro's number, named for the Italian chemist and physicist Amedeo Avogadro. Hence, Avogadro's number was defined as the number of atoms in exactly 12 g of carbon-12. This allowed mass to be defined as g/mol, a unit widely used in chemistry today. The mass of one mole of an atom or molecule is its atomic or molecular mass in grams. Thus hydrogen atoms have a mass of 1 g/mol. The relative atomic mass of alanine is 89, so 89 g of alanine contains 1 mol of alanine molecules, giving alanine a molecular mass of 89 g/mol. The same approach is used to describe the mass of macromolecules such as proteins. For example, apolipoprotein B-100, which is involved in lipid transport, is a very large protein composed of a single polypeptide chain of 4,536 amino acid residues (Law et al., 1986). Apolipoprotein B-100 has a relative molecular mass of 513 kDa, and one mole of apolipoprotein B-100 molecules has a mass of 513 kg, so the molecular mass of apolipoprotein B-100 is said to be 513 kg/mol.

Many scientists in the nineteenth and twentieth centuries used various approaches to try to determine Avogadro's number, resulting in progressively more accurate determinations. The current value is $6.02214179 \times 10^{23}$, with an uncertainty of $0.00000047 \times 10^{23}$. Thus the atomic mass unit (or dalton) can be calculated as equal to 1 g divided by Avogadro's number. Using the current estimate of Avogadro's number, the size of the mass represented by a single relative atomic mass unit is $1.660538782 \times 10^{-27}$ kg.

fully denatured protein will lack both tertiary and secondary structure and exist as a so-called random coil. Loss of three-dimensional structure usually produces a loss of biological function.

In vitro, denaturation can be brought about by heating, by treatment with alkali or acid to change pH, by chemical denaturants such as urea, by detergents, and by mechanical forces such as vigorous shaking. Depending on the protein, the degree of the denaturation, and the environment, a denatured protein may be able to refold. In many cases, however, denaturation is irreversible. Heating and/or addition of acid are used to irreversibly denature proteins in cooking or food processing, as evidenced by the "cooking" of fish by either heat or acid. Disulfide bonds can be broken by treatment of proteins with mercaptoethanol or other reducing agents.

STABLE POSTTRANSLATIONAL MODIFICATIONS OF PROTEINS

As mentioned earlier with the discussion of amino acids, posttranslational modifications extend the range of chemical properties of the common amino acids within proteins. These modified amino acid residues are important to the processing, localization, and function of the protein. Such modifications of the polypeptide chain residues may occur as the polypeptide is being translated or after the polypeptide has been released from the ribosome. Posttranslational modifications of proteins often occur during their movement through the cell to their final destinations. A defect in posttranslational modification can produce a dysfunctional product, just as can defects in the primary sequence or in protein folding.

Most posttranslational modifications can be placed in one of three broad categories: (1) those that involve peptide bond cleavage, (2) those that involve modification of the amino- or carboxy-terminal amino acid, and (3) those that involve modification of specific amino acid side chains. Examples of posttranslational peptide bond cleavage include activation of many peptide hormones and conversion of zymogens to active enzymes. For example, trypsinogen and other protease zymogens are converted to active proteases by hydrolysis of an internal peptide bond to release an N-terminal segment. Formation of the hormone insulin from its precursor polypeptide, proinsulin, occurs by proteolytic excision (cleavage) of an internal segment, leaving two polypeptide chains attached by disulfide bonds (see Figure 5-8). Proopiomelanocortin produced by the pituitary gland can be cleaved to yield seven different polypeptide hormones, including ACTH and α-melanocyte–stimulating hormone (α-MSH). Similarly, as mentioned before, the enkephalins are formed by cleavage of a precursor protein. In other cases, the N-terminal sequence is used to direct polypeptide trafficking but is cleaved after it has served its purpose; for example, the N-terminal signal peptide targets nascent proteins to the ER. In addition, the removal of the initial N-terminal methionine from many polypeptides permits proteins to have amino acids other than methionine at the N-terminus.

The second category of cotranslational or posttranslational modifications, modifications of the N- or C-terminus of the protein, are important in the selective activation of enzymes and hormones and in allowing proteins to be inserted into membranes without the protein having a transmembrane region. These N- and C-terminal modifications usually occur in conjunction with cleavage of an N-terminal amino acid or C-terminal peptide from the precursor polypeptide. For example, amidation of the C-terminal amino acid is a common posttranslational modification that is essential for activation of many hormones and neuropeptides (e.g., calcitonin, vasopressin, and α-MSH). The amide group for C-terminal amidation is contributed by a glycine residue that is oxidized and then cleaved, producing the C-terminally amidated peptide and a small *N*-glyoxylated peptide. Some proteins undergo N-terminal *N*-acetylation or *N*-myristoylation in conjunction with removal of the N-terminal methionine. Other proteins are modified by addition of lipid membrane anchors to their C-terminal amino acid to facilitate the association of these proteins with membranes. Examples include the addition of a farnesyl or geranylgeranyl group to the sulfur atom of a C-terminal cysteine residue and the addition of glycosylphosphatidylinositol to the carboxyl group of a C-terminal amino acid. Both of these lipidation processes are coupled with cleavage of several amino acids from the C-terminus to expose the new modified C-terminal amino acid. Following attachment of an isoprenyl group, the carboxylate of the cysteine is methylated in a reaction utilizing S-adenosylmethionine as the methyl donor.

The third category of posttranslational modifications, in which R groups or side chains are modified, provides chemical features important for cellular compartmentalization and trafficking, receptor binding, regulatory signaling, prosthetic group addition or formation, protein cross-linking, and the creation of novel chemical sites such as those important to metal binding. Table 5-3 lists some examples of chemical modifications of side chains of amino acid residues in proteins and the amino acid residues that are common targets

TABLE 5-3 Examples of Posttranslational Modifications Involving Amino Acid Side Chains

SELECTED FUNCTIONS	PROCESS OR EXAMPLE	COMMONLY TARGETED AMINO ACIDS IN PROTEINS
Compartmentalization, trafficking, receptor binding	Acylation	Asn, Cys, Gln, Lys, Ser
	Acetylation	Ala, Arg, Gly, His, Lys
	Glycosylation	Asn, Cys, Gln, Hyp, Lys, Ser, Thr, Tyr
	Ubiquitin-like protein addition	Lys
Regulatory signaling	Acetylation	Lys
	Adenylylation	Tyr
	ADP-ribosylation	Cys, Glu, Arg, Lys, Ser
	Methylation	Arg, Asp, Glu, His, Lys, Ser, The
	Phosphorylation	Ser, Thr, Tyr, His, Lys
	Ubiquitin addition	Lys
	Sulfation	Tyr
Prosthetic group addition or formation	Biotinylation	Lys
	Flavin addition	Cys, His
	Phosphopantetheine addition	Ser
	Pyridoxal phosphate addition	Lys
	Retinal addition	Lys
Other	Disulfide bond formation	Cys-Cys
	Carboxylation	Asp, Glu
	Halogen addition (iodine)	Tyr
	Hydroxylation	Asp, Lys, Pro, Asn
	Nonenzymatic glycosylation	Arg, Lys
	Sulfoxide formation	Met
	Glutamylation	Glu
	Glutathionylation	Cys
	Palmitoylation	Cys

for the modifications, and the structures of a few of these are shown in Figure 5-5. Glycosylation, the attachment of oligosaccharide chains, occurs in many proteins synthesized in the ER. Glycosylation plays important roles in protein folding, trafficking, and function. The formation or incorporation of various prosthetic groups in proteins usually occurs as a posttranslational protein modification, such as the covalent addition of biotin to carboxylases or the association of pyridoxal phosphate with aminotransferases. The addition of a given prosthetic group may be essential to the creation of an enzymatic or functional active site. Hydroxylation of lysine and proline side chains in collagen is an essential step in their association to form the tropocollagen triple helix; and the γ-carboxylation of glutamate residues in prothrombin is essential for its activity as a clotting factor.

REGULATION OF THE AMOUNT OF PROTEIN AND ITS FUNCTIONAL STATE

The amount of protein in a cell is a function of the balance between its rate of synthesis and its rate of degradation. In addition, the ability of the protein to correctly function depends upon many additional factors, including localization of the protein within the cell or its secretion from the cell, reversible or irreversible posttranslational modifications that affect its function or activity, and cofactor synthesis. Either an increase in the amount of a protein or an increase in the function of the protein will increase the cell's capacity for the process carried out by that protein. Steps at which protein concentration or function are regulated are summarized in Figure 5-14.

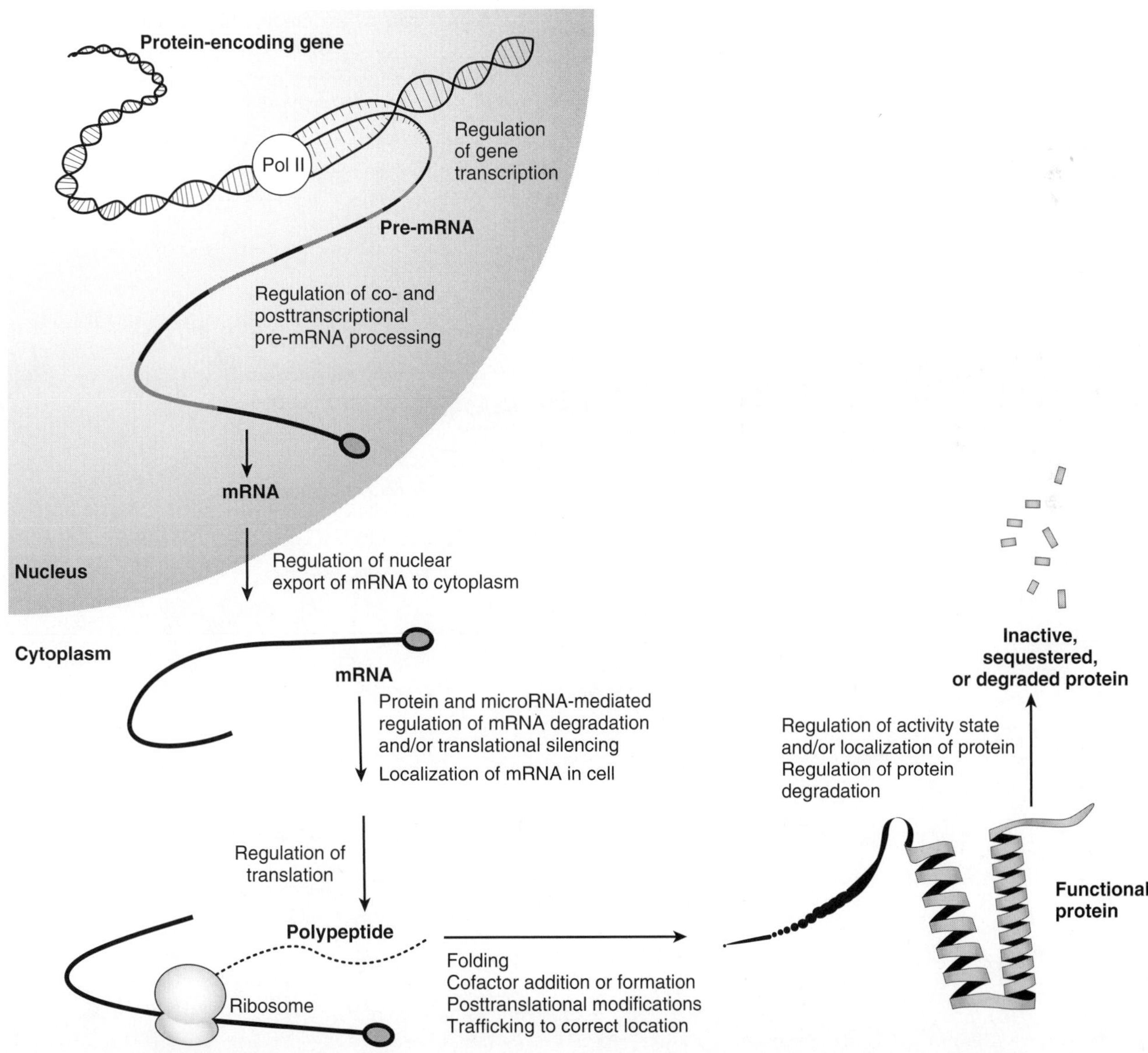

FIGURE 5-14 Illustration of multiple points at which protein concentration and function can be regulated.

NUTRITION INSIGHT

Nutrition Insight: Vitamin C and Connective Tissue Protein Synthesis

The nutritional deficiency disease scurvy has a dynamic and important impact on connective tissue and extracellular matrix integrity. With respect to extracellular matrix stability, ascorbic acid is a cofactor for lysyl and prolyl hydroxylases (i.e., procollagen-lysine α-ketoglutarate 5-dioxygenase and prolyl 4-hydroxylase), which form 5-hydroxylysine, 3-hydroxyproline, and 4-hydroxyproline residues in proteins. A decrease in prolyl and lysyl hydroxylase activities causes a net decrease in the production of hydroxyproline and hydroxylysine residues in collagen and related proteins. Collagen constitutes one third of the total protein in the body and is the major protein in the extracellular matrix of the connective tissue. Underhydroxylated collagen polypeptide chains do not associate properly and are more susceptible to degradation than normal forms of collagen; this is an underlying factor in many of the lesions associated with scurvy.

The hydroxylation of lysine and proline residues in collagen α-chains serves several specific functions. The formation of hydroxyproline residues is very important for the stabilization of the triple helical conformation of collagen by hydrogen bonds and water bridges. About 25% of the total amino acids in type I collagen (the major type) are proline, and 40% to 45% of the proline is hydroxylated. The hydroxylation of lysine residues is important for two additional subsequent modifications of collagen. First, the hydroxylation of lysine residues is necessary for glycosylation. In type I collagen α-chains, glycosylation occurs only at the hydroxyl group of certain hydrolysine residues in the helical domain to form galactosylhydroxylysine or glucosylgalactosylhydroxylysine residues. Second, the hydroxylation of lysine residues in collagen is necessary for formation of the covalent intramolecular and intermolecular cross-links between modified lysine side chains that are critical for the stability of collagen fibrils. Lysine and hydroxylysine are deaminated by lysyl oxidase (protein-lysine 6-oxidase), which creates highly reactive aldehyde groups. These groups then spontaneously react to form covalent bonds and complex cross-linked structures such as pyridinoline and deoxypyridinoline.

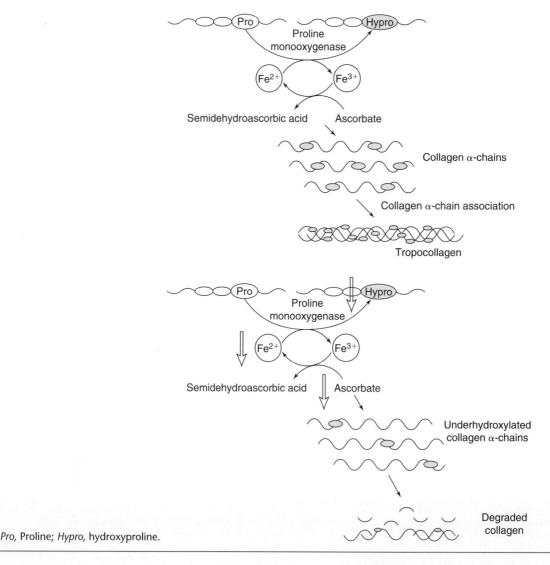

Pro, Proline; *Hypro,* hydroxyproline.

Protein synthesis involves the transcription of the protein-encoding gene to form mRNA, followed by translation of the mRNA to produce the encoded polypeptide. Transcription occurs in the nucleus, with RNA polymerase II transcribing the protein-encoding genes. Transcription of a gene depends on the direct interaction of specific nucleotide sequences or secondary structural elements in the DNA, particularly in the promoter region, with proteins known as transcription factors. Transcription factors act as enhancers or repressors to change transcription levels of individual genes. In addition to proteins that interact directly with the DNA, many other proteins influence transcription by protein–protein interactions. The production, localization, and activity of these transcription factors is regulated in the cell in response to various stimuli, and this in turn regulates gene transcription. In addition, because chromosomes are packaged with histones and other proteins to form a compacted chromatin structure that must be unwound to allow access of the transcriptional apparatus and regulatory proteins, changes to chromatin structure further regulate protein synthesis. Modifications of chromatin include the methylation of DNA and the acetylation of histones.

Once gene transcription has started, the nascent transcript is extensively processed and modified, which includes capping of the 5′ end, splicing of intron–exon junctions, and cleavage and polyadenylation at the 3′ end. Steps in pre-mRNA processing can be regulated to affect the amount of mature mRNA produced, and in genes with alternative splice sites, the identity of the protein product can be changed. Before the mature mRNA can be translated into protein, it must be exported through a nuclear pore into the cytoplasm where it associates with the ER and nuclear envelope and spreads throughout the cytosol. The export of mRNA is regulated by a number of binding proteins that ensure only mature mRNAs are exported.

The stability of mRNAs varies greatly and this affects their cellular concentrations. Certain sequences in the untranslated portion, usually the 3′ end of the mRNA, are specific binding sites for small regulatory RNAs (e.g., microRNA) or binding proteins (e.g., AU-rich element binding proteins). Binding of a small regulatory RNA (as part of a ribonucleoprotein complex) to its element in the mRNA induces cleavage (leading to mRNA degradation) or translational silencing (which sometimes leads to increased degradation). Binding of regulatory proteins can result in either increased stability or increased degradation of the mRNA. Under certain conditions, mRNA is sequestered in stress granules or processing bodies but not degraded, although it is not being actively translated.

In addition to its dependence on mRNA concentration and localization, the process of translation itself is regulated. The major mechanisms affect translation initiation. Several mechanisms for regulation of translation are discussed in Chapter 13.

Once a polypeptide is synthesized, it must be correctly folded and in many cases trafficked to its site of action. Many proteins require stable posttranslational modifications (e.g., glycosylation, acetylation, disulfide bond formation) or cofactor addition before they are functional or can be correctly trafficked. All of these factors determine the amount of functional protein that is synthesized.

The steady state concentration of any protein is also influenced by its rate of turnover or degradation. If the rate of synthesis remains constant, an increase in the degradation rate will decrease the steady state concentration of the protein, and a decrease in the degradation rate will increase the concentration. All proteins, like mRNAs, have a constitutive turnover rate, but for many proteins the rate of degradation can be regulated to alter the pool of functional protein. In addition, quality control mechanisms target improperly folded or damaged proteins for degradation. The function or activity state of a protein may also be regulated by reversible covalent modification (e.g., phosphorylation), by interactions with other proteins (e.g., binding proteins), by sequestration in a cellular compartment or protein aggregate where the protein is nonfunctional, and through activation or inhibition by small molecules.

THINKING CRITICALLY

Denaturation of food proteins has many desirable, and some undesirable, effects. A variety of mechanisms are involved in this denaturation. Once the food protein is denatured, it can form new bonds and associations and often forms aggregates or "gels."

1. Identify examples of how protein denaturation by heat (e.g., cooking), mechanical force (e.g., beating), changes in acid or base (e.g., addition of lemon juice), or enzymes (e.g., rennin or chymosin) is used in food processing and preparation.
2. Describe the processes involved in denaturation of the protein.

REFERENCES

Brautigam, C. A., Wynn, R. M., Chuang, J. L., & Chuang, D. T. (2009). Subunit and catalytic component stoichiometries of an in vitro reconstituted human pyruvate dehydrogenase complex. *The Journal of Biological Chemistry, 284*, 13086–13098.

Comb, M., Seeburg, P. H., Adelman, J., Eiden, L., & Herbert, E. (1982). Primary structure of the human Met- and Leu-enkephalin precursor and its mRNA. *Nature, 295*, 663–666.

Harris, T. K., & Turner, G. J. (2002). Structural basis of perturbed pKa values of catalytic groups in enzyme active sites. *International Union of Biochemistry and Molecular Biology Life, 53*, 85–98.

Kagan, H. M. (2000). Intra- and extracellular enzymes of collagen biosynthesis as biological and chemical targets in the control of fibrosis. *Acta Tropica, 77*, 147–152.

Kyte, J., & Doolittle, R. F. (1982). A simple method for displaying the hydropathic character of a protein. *Journal of Molecular Biology, 157*, 105–132.

Law, S. W., Grant, S. M., Higuchi, K., Hospattankar, A., Lackner, K., Lee, N., & Brewer, H. B., Jr. (1986). Human liver apolipoprotein B-100 cDNA: complete nucleic acid and derived amino acid sequence. *Proceedings of the National Academy of Sciences U.S.A., 83*, 8142–8146.

Petsko, G. A., & Ringe, D. (2004). *Protein structure and function.* Sunderland, MA: New Science Press.

Strandberg, B., Dickerson, R. E., & Rossmann, M. G. (2009). 50 years of protein structure analysis. *Journal of Molecular Biology, 392*, 2–32.

Stretton, A. O. W. (2002). The first sequence: Fred Sanger and insulin. *Genetics, 162*, 527–532.

Wolosker, H., Dumin, E., Balan, L., & Foltyn, V. N. (2008). D-Amino acids in the brain: D-Serine in neurotransmission and neurodegeneration. *The FEBS Journal, 275*, 3514–3526.

Wüthrich, K. (2001). The way to NMR structures of proteins. *Nature Structural Biology, 8*, 923–925.

RECOMMENDED WEBSITES

International Union of Pure and Applied Chemistry (IUPAC) and International Union of Biochemistry and Molecular Biology (IUBMB) Joint Commission on Biochemical Nomenclature. IUPAC-IUBMB Joint Commission on Biochemical Nomenclature (JCBN). Nomenclature and symbolism for amino acids and peptides. http://www.chem.qmul.ac.uk/iupac/AminoAcid

The National Center for Biotechnology Information. U.S. National Library of Medicine. This site provides many tools and data bases useful in the study of the genome and gene products. http://www.ncbi.nlm.nih.gov/guide

CHAPTER 6

Structure, Nomenclature, and Properties of Lipids

J. Thomas Brenna, PhD, and Gavin L. Sacks, PhD

COMMON ABBREVIATIONS

CMC	critical micellar concentration
FFA	free fatty acids
LT	leukotrienes
LX	lipoxins
MP	melting point
NEFA	nonesterified fatty acids
PG	prostaglandins
PtdCho	phosphatidylcholine
PtdEtn	phosphatidylethanolamine
PtdIns	phosphatidylinositol
PtdSer	phosphatidylserine
PUFA	polyunsaturated fatty acids
TAG	triacylglycerol
TX	thromboxanes

Lipids are a diverse set of small molecules that are unified by their solubility in nonpolar solvents. They have many biological functions, and the amounts of lipids present in humans range from many kilograms for fatty acids to nanograms for docosanoids. The major biological functions of lipids include serving as structural components of cell membranes, serving as a form of energy storage, providing lubrication and conditioning for body surfaces, and functioning as signaling molecules of various types, including activators of nuclear receptors and G protein–coupled receptors and second messengers from phosphatidylinositol and sphingolipids. Lipids also function as receptors, antigens, sensors, electrical insulators, biological detergents, and membrane anchors for proteins.

Fats represent a major source of dietary and cellular energy. Although *fat* is sometimes used as a synonym for *lipid,* the subgroup of lipids called triacylglycerols (TAGs) is the dominant component of dietary fats and oils. In addition to TAGs, sterols (such as cholesterol and plant sterols) and membrane phospholipids (glycerophospholipids) are present in dietary lipids. TAGs and phospholipids all contain fatty acids esterified to glycerol and are important sources of fatty acids for oxidation to supply energy, essential fatty acids, and the gluconeogenic substrate glycerol. Most of the dietary lipid by far is TAG from fat droplets in plant and animal cells, and fat intake in the United States accounts, on average, for 32% to 37% of total caloric intake in adults.

Fat in animals is stored in specialized cells called adipocytes that contain very large fat droplets that push most of the cytoplasm toward the plasma membrane; fat is also found in smaller lipid droplets in other cell types. Fat in plants is found primarily as storage lipid droplets in the embryo or endosperm of seeds, where its purpose is to provide nutrition during germination. Important exceptions are olive and palm, where the lipids are mostly in the pulp. The fats and oils used in cooking are ones that have been separated from their animal and plant sources. Important animal fats are lard, tallow, and butterfat, and widely used plant oils include those extracted from soybeans, rapeseed/canola, cottonseed, peanuts, sunflower, corn, and olives.

THE CHEMICAL CLASSES OF LIPIDS—THEIR STRUCTURE AND NOMENCLATURE

Lipids do not share any overall characteristic chemical structural similarity, but they can nevertheless be categorized into subclasses according to structural similarities. One system for categorizing major classes of lipids is listed in Box 6-1, emphasizing those that are directly and indirectly of nutritional importance. A comprehensive system oriented toward detailed molecular studies is available at Lipidomics Gateway *(www.lipidmaps.org/)*. The nomenclature of lipids is dominated by trivial names that are either historical or driven by systematics of metabolism. As with all organic compounds, systematic organic chemical naming rules have been established for lipids, but traditional lipid nomenclature persists for good reason. Most traditional lipid naming conventions are convenient when viewed in the context of mammalian lipid metabolism and, to a lesser extent, are logical extensions of the traditional methods used to analyze lipids. Thus study of lipid nomenclature also reveals structural and metabolic relationships among lipids, and familiarity with nomenclature makes the study of lipid metabolism much clearer.

FATTY ACIDS

Fatty acyl chains are the basic units of glycerolipids that render these compounds nonpolar. They are referred to as fatty acids in part because many traditional analytical methods

BOX 6-1 A Chemical Classification of Biologically Important Lipids*

I. Nonesterified fatty acids
  A. Saturated fatty acids
  B. Unsaturated fatty acids
  C. *Trans* fatty acids
  D. Conjugated fatty acids
II. Glycerolipids
  A. Monoacylglycerols, diacylglycerols, triacylglycerols (esters of fatty acids with glycerol)
III. Glycerophospholipids
  A. Common phospholipids (PtdCho, PtdEtn, PtdIns, PtdSer, phosphatidylglycerol)
  B. Lysophospholipids
  C. Diphosphatidylglycerols (cardiolipins)
  D. Ether phospholipids (platelet-activating factors, plasmalogens)
IV. Glycoglycerolipids (including sulfates)
V. Sphingolipids
  A. Sphingosine
  B. Ceramide
  C. Sphingomyelin
  D. Neutral glycosphingolipids (e.g., cerebrosides)
  E. Acidic glycosphingolipids (e.g., gangliosides)
VI. Isoprenoids (carotenoids, retinoids, prenols)
VII. Steroids
  A. Sterols
  B. Steroid hormones (sex hormones, corticosteroids)
  C. Bile acids
VIII. Biological waxes (long-chain ester waxes and related compounds)
IX. Eicosanoids
  A. Cyclooxygenase products (prostaglandins, thromboxanes)
  B. Lipoxygenase products (leukotrienes, lipoxins)
  C. Cytochrome P450 products
X. Other lipids (acyl CoA, acylcarnitine, anandamide, lipopolysaccharides)

Adapted from Small, D. M., & Zoeller, R. A. (1991). Lipids. In *Encyclopedia of human biology* (Vol. 4, pp. 725–748). Orlando, FL: Academic Press, Inc.

*The chemical classification of lipids given in this table is necessarily incomplete and arbitrary. It progresses from hydrocarbons to more complex chemical structures. Simple esters and glycerol esters yield, on hydrolysis, alcohol and/or glycerol and fatty acid. The major membrane lipids, glycerophospholipids, yield fatty acid (or alcohol), glycerol, phosphate, and the appropriate base (choline, ethanolamine, etc.). Sphingolipids yield the base sphingosine and a fatty acid on hydrolysis. A comprehensive classification scheme can be found at *www.lipidmaps.org/* and in abbreviated form at *en.wikipedia.org/wiki/Lipid.*

first hydrolyze all fatty esters into fatty acids. However, the level of free fatty acids (FFA), which are also called nonesterified fatty acids (NEFA), is very low compared to the amount of fatty acids present in esterifed forms, primarily as glycerolipids. The plasma concentration of FFA is about 0.3 to 0.6 mmol/L with about 99% of these FFA noncovalently bound to albumin. Higher concentrations of plasma FFA may occur locally at sites of high lipolytic activity (e.g., the capillary beds in adipose tissue, muscle, and heart) where FFA are liberated during lipolysis of TAG present in chylomicrons or very-low-density lipoproteins by lipoprotein lipase.

Fatty acids are characterized by their carboxylic acid head group and their hydrocarbon chain tail. Fatty acyl chains in glycerolipids are the result of condensation of the carboxylic acid head group with a hydroxyl (alcohol) group in the glycerol backbone via an ester bond. In mammals, fatty acids or fatty acyl chains may range from 2 carbons (C_2) to as many as 40 carbons (C_{40}) in length but primarily exist as C_{12} to C_{22} chains. Fatty acids are sometimes most conveniently classified according to chain length, although these categories are not rigidly defined. We can define *short-chain* fatty acids as those that have 6 or fewer carbon atoms. The chemistry of short-chain fatty acids is sufficiently dominated by the carboxyl group that they are soluble at least to some extent in water. *Medium-chain* fatty acids have 8 to 14 carbon atoms, and *long-chain* fatty acids have more than 14 carbons. Fatty acids are also classified according to their degree of unsaturation, which is the number of double bonds in their hydrocarbon chains.

Saturated Fatty Acids

The term *saturated* in the context of fatty acids refers specifically to fatty acyl chains that are exclusively made up of sp^3 hybridized (tetrahedral geometry) carbon atoms arranged as linear $-CH_2-$ chains as shown in Figure 6-1. Such chains are said to be saturated with hydrogen because the chain has no double (or triple) bonds across which hydrogen may be added.

Fatty acids are synthesized predominantly through the successive addition of two-carbon units to a growing acyl chain by the fatty acid synthase enzyme. Chain-elongation ceases at 16 carbons to create palmitic acid in mammals, although small amounts of fatty acids with 14- (myristic acid) and 18- (stearic acid) carbons are also produced. Additional two-carbon units may be added to these fatty acids by elongation enzyme systems to yield longer saturated fatty acids. Table 6-1 presents the chain lengths, systematic

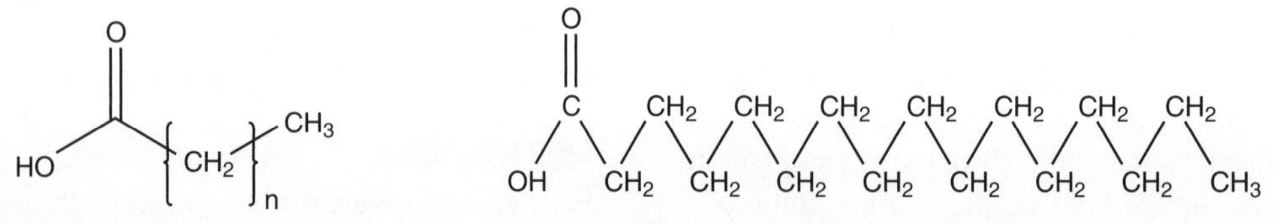

FIGURE 6-1 Structure of saturated fatty acids. On the left is a general structure for a saturated nonesterified (or free) fatty acid. The right shows the structure of a specific saturated fatty acid, *n*-hexadecanoic acid (palmitic acid).

names, trivial names, and melting points of the most abundant saturated fatty acids in mammalian tissues.

In mammals, the majority of saturated fatty acids are configured as straight chains, but in rare cases methyl groups extend from the main chain, usually near its terminal methyl.

TABLE 6-1 Naturally Occurring Straight-Chain Saturated Carboxylic Acids and Their Melting Points

# OF CARBONS	SYSTEMATIC NAME	TRIVIAL NAME	MP (° C)
2	Ethanoic	Acetic	17
3	Propanoic	Propionic	−21
4	*n*-Butanoic	Butyric	−8
6	*n*-Hexanoic	Caproic	−3
8	*n*-Octanoic	Caprylic	17
10	*n*-Decanoic	Capric	32
12	*n*-Dodecanoic	Lauric	44
14	*n*-Tetradecanoic Acid	Myristic	54
16	*n*-Hexadecanoic Acid	Palmitic	63
18	*n*-Octadecanoic Acid	Stearic	70
20	*n*-Eicosanoic Acid	Arachidic	75
22	*n*-Docosanoic Acid	Behenic	80
24	*n*-Tetracosanoic Acid	Lignoceric	84

MP, Melting point; *n,* normal, straight-chain structural isomer.

A fatty acid that terminates with two methyl groups (i.e., an isopropyl configuration) at the end of a hydrocarbon chain is referred to as *iso.* If the chain terminates with a methyl and an ethyl group (i.e., an isobutyl configuration), the fatty acid is said to be *anteiso,* as shown in Figure 6-2. In humans, branched-chain fatty acids appear in vernix, the protective waxy white substance that coats and protects the fetus during late gestation. They have also been detected as minor components of skin, blood, and hair, as well as in cancer cells. Iso and anteiso C_{15} and C_{17} saturated fatty acids are major components of some microorganisms such as gram-positive bacteria.

Unsaturated Fatty Acids

Unsaturated is used to describe fatty acids with at least one double bond, consisting of two adjacent sp^2 hybridized carbon atoms, with a trigonal, approximately planar geometry. They are unsaturated with respect to hydrogen, because hydrogen can be covalently added across the double bond to yield sp^3 carbon atoms. The overwhelming majority of unsaturated sites in mammalian fatty acids are double bonds configured in the *cis* geometry. When two or more double bonds are present in a molecule, the fatty acid is said to be polyunsaturated. Generally, double bonds in mammalian polyunsaturated fatty acids (PUFAs) are separated by a methylene ($-CH_2-$) group ("methylene-interrupted"). This structural property of PUFAs confers special chemical properties. One important chemical property is that the double bonds are not conjugated, and thus there is free rotation about the $-CH_2-$ group. As with saturated fatty acids, use of trivial names is very common for unsaturated fatty acids. Table 6-2 is a compilation of the systematic and trivial names for the most common unsaturated fatty acids.

PUFA biosynthesis is discussed in depth in Chapter 18; however, a brief overview is necessary to rationalize PUFA

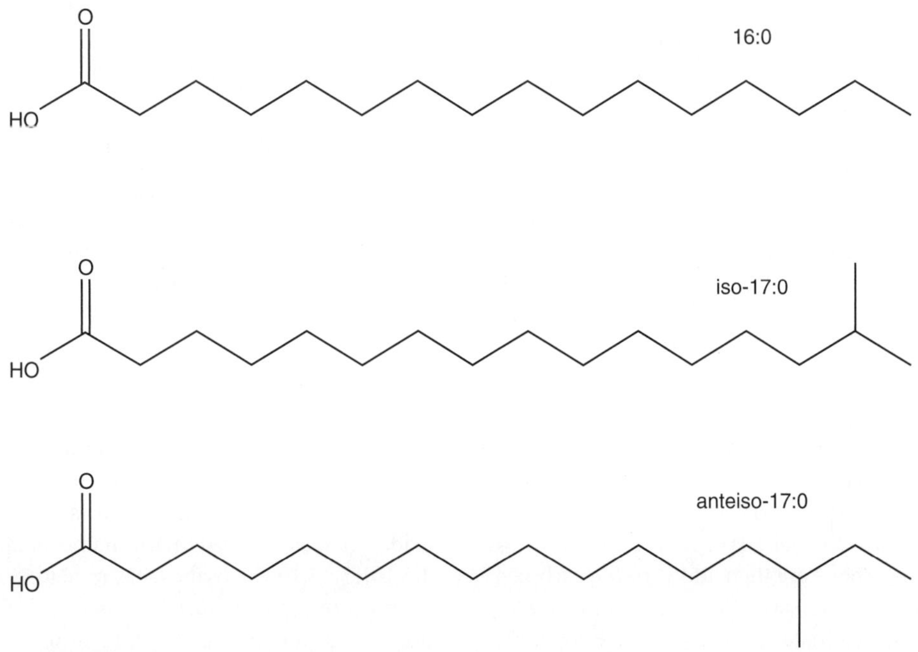

FIGURE 6-2 Structures of straight-chain versus branched-chain (iso and anteiso) fatty acids.

TABLE 6-2 Naturally Occurring Straight-Chain Unsaturated Fatty Acids and Their Melting Points

ABBREVIATED NOTATION	SYSTEMATIC NAME	TRIVIAL NAME	MP (° C)
14:1n–5	*cis*-9-tetradecenoic	Myristoleic	–4
16:1n–7	*cis*-9-hexadecenoic	Palmitoleic	0.5
18:1n–7	*cis*-11-octadecenoic	*cis*-Vaccenic	15
t-18:1n–7	*trans*-11-octadecenoic	trans-Vaccenic	44
18:1n–9	*cis*-9-octadecenoic	Oleic	16
t-18:1n–9	*trans*-9-octadecenoic	Elaidic	47
20:3n–9	All *cis*-5,8,11-eicosatrienoic	Mead	
22:1n–9	All *cis*-13-docosenoic	Erucic	35
18:2n–6	All *cis*-9,12-octadecadienoic	Linoleic (LA)	–5
18:3n–6	All *cis*-6,9,12-octadecatrienoic	γ-Linolenic (GLA)	–11
20:4n–6	All *cis*-5,8,11,14-eicosatetraenoic	Arachidonic (AA)	–50
22:5n–6	All *cis*-4,7,10,13,16-docosapentaenoic	DPA	
18:3n–3	All *cis*-9,12,15-octadecatrienoic	α-Linolenic (ALA)	–10
20:5n–3	All *cis*-5,8,11,14-eicosapentaenoic	EPA	–54
22:6n–3	All *cis*-4,7,10,13,16,19-docosahexaenoic	DHA	–44

MP, Melting point.

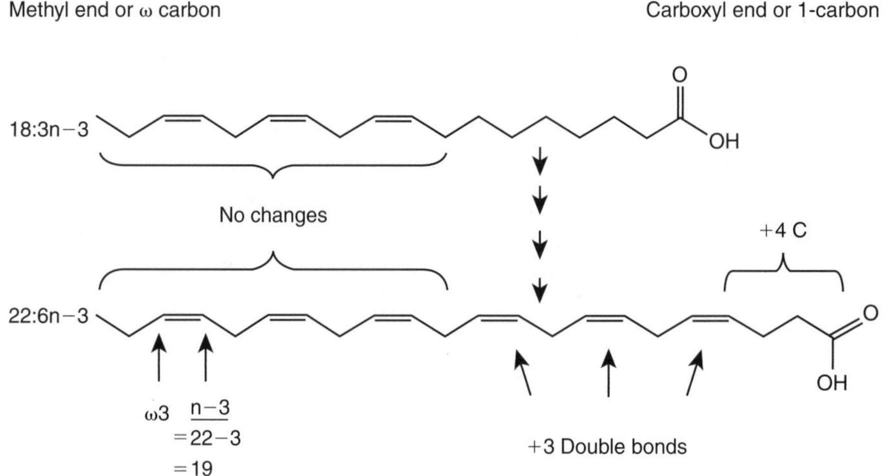

FIGURE 6-3 Synthesis of long-chain PUFA. The conversion of one PUFA into another proceeds from the carboxyl end of the molecule in mammals, and there are no changes to the methyl end. Shown here is the conversion of α-linolenic acid (systematic name: 9,12,15-octatrienoic acid) to 4,7,10,13,16,19-docosahexaenoic acid. Several steps of elongation and desaturation are required (indicated by arrows). Numbering the first double bond from the methyl end of the molecule (using the ω numbering system) or the IUPAC system ("n–", where "n" is the number of C atoms in the molecule) locates the double bond closest to the methyl end of the molecule. Thus PUFA names also reveal metabolic relationships, for example, 18:3n–3 and 22:6n–3. Because double bonds are methylene-interrupted and all-*cis*, this designation fully defines the molecular structure.

nomenclature. Consider the pathway for synthesis of docosahexaenoic acid (C_{22}, 6 double bonds) from α-linolenic acid (C_{18}, 3 double bonds). This pathway begins with the insertion of a double bond between carbons 6 and 7 of α-linoleic acid by a Δ6-desaturase to make stearidonic acid (C_{18}, 4 double bonds). Two carbons are then added to the carboxyl end of the molecule by an elongase, followed by insertion of a double bond to make eicosatetraenoic acid (C_{20}, 5 double bonds). Additional desaturation, elongation, and oxidation steps finally result in docosahexaenoic acid. Figure 6-3 shows the systematic organic chemistry names and numbering for the first and last structures in this pathway. The systematic name of α-linoleic acid is 9,12,15-octadecadienoic acid, whereas the systematic name of the final product is 4,7,10,13,16,19-docosahexaenoic acid. Counting from the C1 position, as is required in systematic naming, the double bonds that were numbered 9, 12, and 15 in the precursor are now numbered 13, 16, and 19 in the product (9 → 13; 12 →

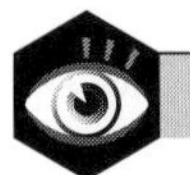

NUTRITION INSIGHT

Fat Matters: Quality as well as Quantity

The rise of obesity in America in the last decade of the twentieth century has led to an explosion of research on metabolic consequences of excess adipose tissue. Diet fads that focus on either low-fat foods or low-carbohydrate (and thus high-fat) foods have prompted many studies of the metabolic consequences of dietary fat levels. Remarkably, much of this research has completely ignored the composition of fat and focused only on dietary amount, implying that the composition is unimportant. Many papers, including ones published in highly ranked research journals, report animal studies in which one group is fed a high-fat diet of unspecified composition that induces overeating and obesity and a control group is fed a standard rodent diet that contains a lower amount of fat, again of unspecified and almost certainly different composition.

That so little attention would be given to the composition of the dietary fat is remarkable in light of the large number of human and animal studies showing that dietary fatty acid composition has a profound influence on many aspects of metabolism. Detailed studies in humans and experimental animals, conducted in the 1950s and since, have shown that each fatty acid has unique but overlapping sets of metabolic properties (Warden and Fisler, 2008).

Could changes in dietary fatty acid composition have a role in the obesity epidemic? Do some fats adversely affect human health more than others? Alternatively, does obesity so overwhelm metabolism that the role of fat composition becomes much less significant? Whatever the answer, the issue cannot be overlooked.

The fatty acids consumed by Americans changed dramatically in the twentieth century. Seed oils such as soy, corn, and canola oils were rare before the industrial revolution of the 1800s because they require mechanical crushing or solvent extraction for efficient production. Fruit oils such as olive and palm oils, along with rendered animal fat (lard and tallow), were more widely used. The high-quality taste and low cost of seed oils drove a rise in seed oil production throughout the twentieth century. Today, soybean oil accounts for a staggering 20% of calories consumed by Americans, in the form of mayonnaise, deep frying fat, salad dressings, margarine, nondairy coffee creamers, snack foods, and sandwich spreads. It may be found in any food with an ingredient list that refers generically to "vegetable oil."

The application of conventional and modern molecular methods (genetically modified) to engineer fatty acid composition of various food oils is resulting in the introduction of oils with modified fatty acid content into the food supply. A notable example is the genetic modification of soybeans to produce oils high in oleic acid. High oleic soy oil was developed to replace the use of *trans* fatty acid–rich hydrogenated fats for deep frying and other purposes for which an oil with high oxidative stability is needed. The high oleic soybean oil was generated by downregulating expression of the fatty acid desaturase gene that encodes the enzyme that converts monounsaturated oleic acid to the polyunsaturated linoleic acid. The oil from these soybeans contains about 80% oleic acid, compared to 25% for conventional soybean oil. At the same time, it contains less than 9% linoleic acid compared to 54% in conventional soybean oil, and less α-linolenic acid, 3% compared to 7% in conventional soybean oil. Commercial production of these high oleic soybeans was approved in North American countries in 2009–2010. Further modification of the fatty acid composition (e.g., increasing the α-linolenic acid content) is under development. Similarly, high oleic acid peanuts, with only 3% linoleic acid, are already on the consumer market in Australia as peanut butter and peanut-containing snacks. These current and upcoming changes to the fatty acid composition of the food supply will result in a major change, once again, in the fatty acid composition of fats in our diets and, with this change, we will likely see physiological consequences related to fatty acid composition rather than amount of fat.

16; 15 → 19). Repeated many times for PUFAs, these changes in bond position number when counted from the carboxyl carbon make it difficult to track double bonds and, more importantly, fatty acids that are derived from one another.

A solution is to number double bonds from the other end of the molecule, taking advantage of the fact that mammals cannot insert double bonds into the methyl end portion of the PUFA chain. Two conventions that are routinely used, which are effectively identical, are the *IUPAC* (International Union of Pure and Applied Chemistry) "n minus" convention and the *omega* convention. Examples of these notations are shown in Figure 6-3 for α-linolenic acid (18:3n−3) and docosahexaenoic acid (22:6n−3).

The IUPAC notation retains a close connection to the systematic organic chemistry notation. The "n" represents the number of carbons in the whole molecule, 18 in the case of α-linolenic acid and 22 in the case of docosahexaenoic acid. The number of double bonds follows the number of carbons, with the two separated by a colon (e.g., C18:3, or simply 18:3 for α-linolenic acid with three double bonds and 22:6 for docosahexaenoic acid with six double bonds). The location of the double bond closest to the methyl end of the fatty acid is indicated by the "n minus" nomenclature; for α-linolenic acid (18:3n−3), the double bond closest to the methyl end is carbon 18−3 or C15 (i.e., between C15 and C16). For docosahexaenoic acid (22:6n−3), the double bond closest to the methyl end is carbon 22−3 or C19 (i.e., between C19 and C20).

An alternative system called the *omega* notation, proposed by Holman, recognizes that the systematic organic chemistry numbering designates the carbon next to the carboxyl as "α," and labels the last carbon in the acyl chain "ω." The first double bond counting from the methyl end of α-linolenic or of docosahexaenoic acid appears at the third carbon and hence is designated ω3 (i.e., "omega three"). Although the IUPAC and omega numbering systems technically refer to different carbon atoms (e.g., C15 in 18:3n−3 versus C16 in 18:3ω3; or C19 in 22:6n−3 versus C20 in 22:6ω3), the n− and omega nomenclature effectively designate the equivalent fatty acids when the numeral following the n− or omega is the same. For example, 18:3n−3 and 18:3ω3 designate the same fatty acid (α-linolenic acid) and 20:4n−6 and 20:4ω6 both designate arachidonic acid.

Because all common PUFAs have *cis* double bonds arranged in methylene-interrupted positions, both notations are taken to imply *cis* geometry and methylene interruption of the double bonds. Thus a designation of n−6 (ω6) or n−3 (ω3), along with the number of carbons and number of double bonds, fully defines the structure of the PUFAs. For instance, "18:3n−6" or "18:3ω6" completely defines the structure of γ-linolenic acid as the fatty acid with the systematic name all-*cis*-6,9,12-octadecatrienoic acid.

Fatty acids with *trans* or conjugated double bonds do not ordinarily appear at other than trace levels in mammalian tissues (other than in the skin surface lipids), although they may be consumed as part of the diet. Example structures of *trans* and conjugated unsaturated fatty acids are shown in Figure 6-4. These fatty acids should **not** be designated with the n− or ω notation, unless further specification is provided. Unlike the situation with common fatty acids, there is no universal specialized notation for these more unusual fatty acids. Either systematic notation or some convenient adaptation of systematic numbering may be used. An example of acceptable notation would be "*trans*-18:1n−9" to specify the monounsaturated C_{18} fatty acid with a *trans* double bond between C9 and C10. For fatty acids with more than one double bond, a "Δ" notation system is frequently used. The superscript Δ precedes the designation of the sites of unsaturation counting from the carboxyl carbon. For instance, $18{:}3^{\Delta 6,9,12}$ designates γ-linolenic acid.

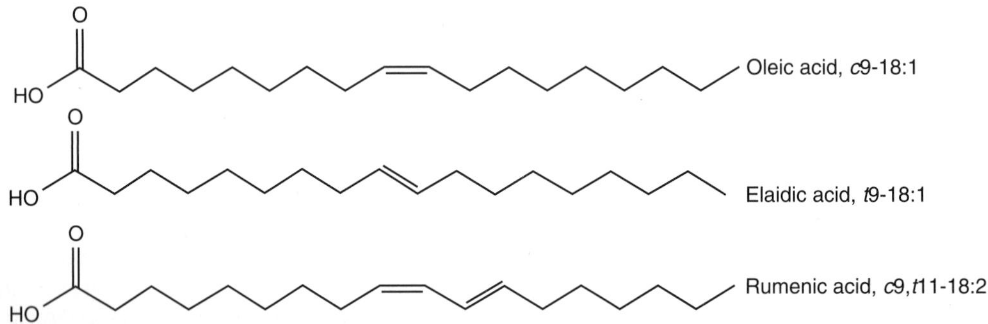

FIGURE 6-4 Structures of oleic acid (*c*9-18:1), elaidic acid (*t*9-18:1), and rumenic acid (*c*9,*t*11-18:2).

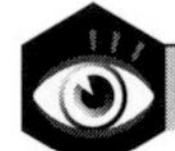

NUTRITION INSIGHT

Vitamin F

The odd list of designations we now have for vitamins—A, D, E, and K for the fat-soluble vitamins, several Bs (with a few numbers missing) and C for the water-soluble vitamins, and some with no letters or numbers—is a remnant of the uneven but eventual progress in scientific understanding of the group of essential nutrients we call vitamins. What of other letters between E and K?

Vitamin F was proposed as the name of a factor associated with fat, and this proposal appeared in several papers in the 1920s. The discovery that fat-containing diets are essential for health is usually assigned to a 1929 paper of George and Mildred Burr (Burr and Burr, 1929), then working in the attic of the University of Minnesota medical school (Holman, 1992). They showed that rats fed fat-free diets developed scaly and sore skin, especially on the face and tail; had hair loss; grew at about two thirds of the normal rate; had a shortened life span; and were unable to reproduce. Animals that were emaciated and covered with very scaly skin were placed on 10 "drops" of lard per day. The animals immediately showed signs of recovery and within 10 weeks were fully "cured." No recovery was seen when the non–fatty acid (nonsaponifiable) fraction of lard was used, thus indicating that the essential fat consisted of fatty acid(s). Subsequent studies established that the fat of greater unsaturation improved the ability of the fat to cure eczema (Brown et al., 1938). However, the inability of scientists to reproduce these effects in humans reduced their interest in vitamin F. We now know that periods greater than 6 months on fat-free diets are required to cause overt deficiency symptoms in humans. Today, the essentiality of the n–6 and n–3 fatty acids, linoleic (18:2n–6) and α-linolenic (18:3n–3) acid, is clearly established, and we would consider these to be components of the so-called vitamin F. There is still controversy about whether humans can synthesize sufficient long-chain PUFAs from 18:2n–6 and 18:3n–3 for optimum health. If, in fact, long-chain fatty acids are essential at some or all stages of the life cycle, PUFAs such as 20:4n–6, 20:5n–3, and 22:6n–3 might also be considered separate components of vitamin F. As progress continues toward defining the details of human requirements for PUFAs, as well as the role of specific PUFAs in human metabolism, the concept of a series of vitamin Fs may yet prove useful.

γ-Linolenic acid is also similarly designated as 9,12,15-18:3. Notations in which the individual double bonds are denoted, by counting from the carboxyl end, lend themselves to designation of isomers of γ-linolenic acid, often by adding leading "*c*" or "*t*" to specify double bond *cis* or *trans* geometry (e.g., *c*9,*t*11-octadecadienoic acid, or $18{:}2^{\Delta\, c9,t11}$, for rumenic acid.

ACYLGLYCEROLS

Acylglycerols are esters of glycerol and fatty acids. Acylglycerols are synthesized by esterification of fatty acids to the hydroxyl groups of the three-carbon sugar, glycerol. Thus acylglycerols may have up to three fatty acid moieties esterified to the glycerol "backbone." Dietary fats and oils are mainly mixtures of triacylglycerols. Before we can discuss the nomenclature of acylglycerols (and glycerophospholipids in the next section), it is important to understand the stereochemistry of glycerol.

Prochiral Glycerol

Stereochemistry is an important property of glycerolipids. The glycerol molecule possesses a plane of symmetry such that the central carbon atom can be considered *prochiral,* a chemical term referring to a carbon atom with four substituents, three of which are different. A prochiral carbon is not chiral, but substitution of one of the equivalent substituent groups with a fourth, nonequivalent group renders the central carbon chiral. This is the case for the central carbon of glycerol: when non–chemically equivalent moieties are added to the $-CH_2OH$ groups, the central carbon becomes chiral. Chirality is very important to biochemical properties and thus must be described unambiguously. Here, the systematic notation of organic chemistry, with rules for designating chiral centers as R or S, leads to even more confusing designations than in the case of fatty acid double bond position. However, a single notation that closely parallels metabolism was introduced in the 1960s and is widely used. As shown in Figure 6-5, glycerol can be positioned so that the top and bottom $-CH_2OH$ are oriented with their $-OH$ groups extending to the right and the middle $-OH$ extending to the left. By convention, the positions are referred to as *sn*-1, *sn*-2, and *sn*-3 (top to bottom), with *sn* being an abbreviation for "stereospecific numbering." In some contexts, the *sn*-1 and *sn*-3 positions are metabolically equivalent and are designated the α positions, with the center *sn*-2 position then being designated the β position. When non–chemically equivalent groups are added to the *sn*-1 and *sn*-3 positions, glycerol becomes chiral.

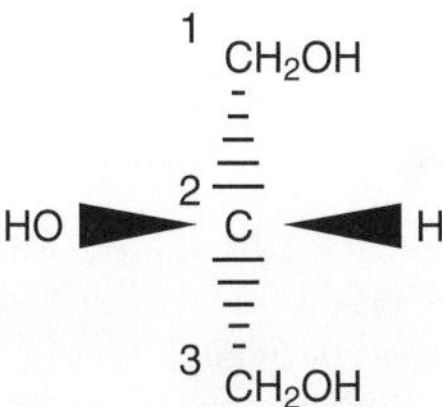

FIGURE 6-5 Glycerol. The carbon positions are numbered according to the *sn* convention.

Monoacylglycerols, Diacylglycerols, and Triacylglycerols

Acylglycerols are formed by the esterification of one or more of the glycerol –OH groups with a fatty acid carboxyl group by means of an ester linkage. A single acyl substitution to form an ester bond forms a monoacylglycerol, which may be designated as a 1-, 2-, or 3-monoacyl-*sn*-glycerol, depending on location of the fatty acid on the glycerol moiety. For example, esterification of hexadecanoic acid (palmitic acid) to the 1-position of glycerol produces 1-hexadecanoyl-*sn*-glycerol (1-palmitoyl-*sn*-glycerol). When two fatty acids are reacted with glycerol to form ester bonds, a diacylglycerol is formed (e.g., 1,3-diacyl-*sn*-glycerol or 1,2-diacyl-*sn*-glycerol). Both monoacylglycerols and diacylglycerols occur in relatively low proportion in mammals but are important as biochemical intermediates in many lipolytic reactions and are critical building blocks in the synthesis of more complex phospholipids and triacylglycerols. Diacylglycerols also act as second messengers for some membrane-triggered reactions.

A triacylglycerol (TAG) is formed when all three hydroxyls of glycerol form ester bonds with fatty acids. TAGs are the most common form of lipids in food and in mammalian tissues. The older abbreviated term *triglyceride* and its abbreviation TG are also used as synonyms for TAG, primarily in the medical literature. The properties of acylglycerols (e.g., melting point) depend greatly on the fatty acid chains involved. The fatty acids in a TAG may be all the same, all different, or two of a kind with one different one. If all three fatty acids are the same, the TAG is called a simple TAG (e.g., triolein). If one of the fatty acids is different, it becomes a complex TAG. If the fatty acids at the *sn*-1 and *sn*-3 positions are different, the TAG is chiral. Chirality in TAG is of less physiological importance than in other glycerolipids because many enzymes catalyzing reactions involving TAGs do not distinguish between the *sn*-1 and *sn*-3 (i.e., α) positions. Saturated fatty acyl chains tend to be found in the *sn*-1 and *sn*-3 positions, whereas unsaturated fatty acyl chains tend to be found in the *sn*-2 position of acylglycerols. There are notable exceptions, however, as in lard (pork fat) and human milk, for which 16:0 is predominantly in the *sn*-2 position and unsaturated fatty acyl chains are in the *sn*-1 and *sn*-3 positions.

The three unique positions of the glycerol backbone permit a tremendous number of positional isomers—that is, TAG with the same three fatty acids arranged in many different ways on the three positions of glycerol. For instance, consider the number of isomeric TAGs with the three fatty acids: palmitic (P), oleic (O), and stearic (S) acids. They could be arranged in six different ways listed in *sn*-1,2,3 order: POS and SOP, PSO and OSP, OPS and SPO, where the pairs are stereoisomers. Moreover, a fat containing these three fatty acids may not contain all fatty acids on all distinct TAG molecules; it may also contain PPP, PPS, OSO, and other combinations. In general, the number of unique TAG isomers is F^3, where F is the number of fatty acids present in a sample. Even simple fats have more than 10 different fatty acids, which could be present as 10^3, or 1,000, chemically distinct TAG molecules.

TAGs are the major storage lipids of plants and higher animals. Both plant oils (olive, corn, safflower) and animal fats (lard, suet, tallow) are predominantly mixtures of complex TAGs. A few percent of sterols, vitamins, free fatty acids, carotenoids, and other fat-soluble molecules are usually present in oils and fats. In animals, adipose tissue is the main source of fat, but skeletal muscle, heart, liver, skin, and bone marrow often contain appreciable amounts of TAGs in intracellular oil droplets.

Examples of structures and nomenclature for monoacylglycerols, diacylglycerols, and triacylglycerols are shown in Figure 6-6. Use of the IUPAC-IUB *sn* nomenclature is generally preferred over the use of the trivial names in most cases, although trivial names are commonly used for simple acylglycerols (e.g., the use of triolein for 1,2,3-tri-*cis*-9-octadecenoyl-*sn*-glycerol). A benefit of the *sn* nomenclature is that it clearly reveals the relationship between the precursor TAG and its DAG and MAG hydrolysis products. For example, the hydrolysis of 1-palmitoyl-2-stearoyl-3-myristoyl-*sn*-glycerol at the 1 position yields 2-stearoyl-3-myristoyl-*sn*-glycerol (Figure 6-7).

GLYCEROPHOSPHOLIPIDS

Glycerophospholipids are commonly described as phospholipids or phosphoglycerides. These lipids are derived from the parent compound phosphatidic acid, which is also known as diacylglycerol 3-phosphate. Other members of the glycerophospholipids include lysophospholipids and diphosphatidylglycerols. All glycerophospholipids contain at least one fatty acid esterified to the glycerol backbone.

Diacylphospholipids, the Common Phospholipids

The general structure of the diacylphospholipids is presented in Figure 6-8, and the several classes of common phospholipids and their structures are shown in Figure 6-9. In all cases, a phosphate group is esterified to the *sn*-3 position of glycerol,

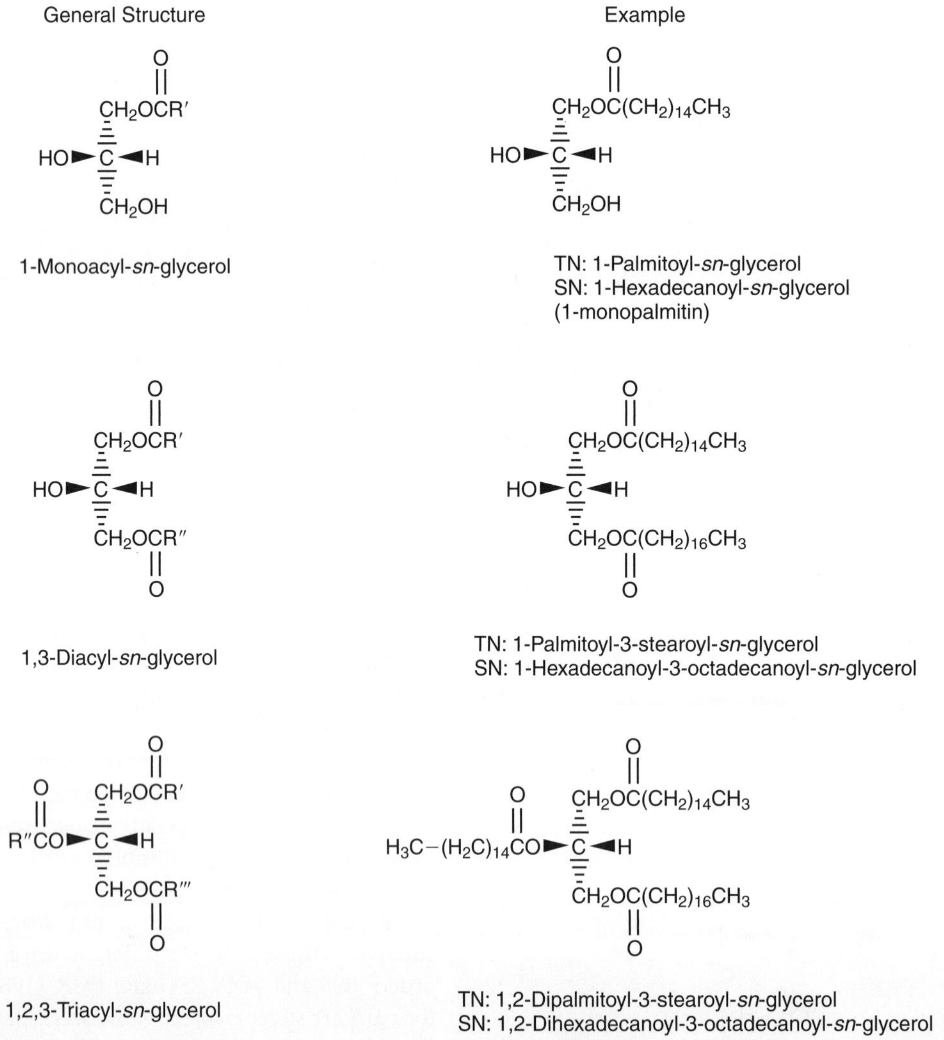

FIGURE 6-6 Examples of structures and nomenclatures for monoacylglycerols, diacylglycerols, and triacylglycerols. *SN,* Systematic name; *TN,* trivial name.

and fatty acids are esterified to the *sn*-1 and *sn*-2 positions. Most commonly, the *sn*-2 position is occupied by an unsaturated acyl chain, whereas the *sn*-1 position is occupied by a saturated chain. However, there are notable exceptions to this generality. For instance, the major surfactant lipid of the lung has 16:0 in both positions, and some of the phospholipids of the retinal photoreceptors have very high concentrations of unsaturated fatty acyl chains in both positions.

The simplest phospholipid is phosphatidic acid (diacylglycerol 3-phosphate), in which phosphoric acid is esterified to

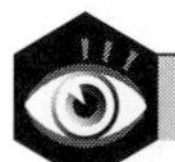

NUTRITION INSIGHT

Trans Fatty Acids: The Good, the Bad, and the Ugly

Trans fats refers to the presence of *trans* double bonds in an unsaturated fatty acyl group in the fat. *Trans* double bonds arise from two sources: chemical catalytic hydrogenation of unsaturated oils and as normal products of rumen bacterial and bovine physiology in dairy products. Those arising from hydrogenation of oils have a generally bad reputation as unnatural promoters of heart disease. Food labeling rules implemented by the U.S. Food and Drug Administration in 2006 specified that the content of *trans* fats be shown on all food labels, and this resulted in many food producers removing *trans* fats from their prepared foods. In contrast to the *trans* fats in hydrogenated fats, the *trans* fats in dairy products are associated with beneficial physiological effects, at least in animal studies.

Chemical hydrogenation adjusts the melting point of oils, turning them into solid fats, by saturating many double bonds with hydrogen and isomerizing others from *cis* to *trans*. Saturated and *trans* fatty acids in oils have higher melting points than corresponding fatty acids with *cis* double bonds, and thus any oil can have its melting point finely adjusted by adding just the right amount of hydrogen. Hydrogenation lowers the cost of shortening for baked goods because any inexpensive, high-quality, deodorized/flavor-neutral oil available at a particular time can be hydrogenated to make shortening. Furthermore, hydrogenation destroys PUFAs, particularly α-linolenic acid, which is considered to be a major cause of rancidity that limits the life of frying oil and other high temperature–treated foods.

The *trans* fatty acids resulting from hydrogenation mainly constitute a series of monoenes with *trans* double bonds distributed at various positions along the hydrocarbon chain, centered at the site of the original *cis* double bond. Conjugated double bonds of various positions and geometries are also created. These distributions of *trans* monoene and diene fatty acids are thought to be atherogenic due to their increasing plasma cholesterol in a manner similar to some saturated fats (Hu and Willett, 2002), especially myristic and lauric acids.

In contrast to hydrogenated fats, dairy products have a very specific distribution of *trans* fatty acids. The most prominent dairy *trans* fat is a monoene, *trans*-11-18:1 (vaccenic acid), with smaller amounts of other monoenes with double bonds located at the C4 to C16 positions. Also present at lower concentrations are dienes known as conjugated linoleic acids (CLAs). The most prominent of these is the *cis*-9, *trans*-11-18:2 fatty acid, named rumenic acid (Kramer et al., 1998), constituting around 90% of all CLA in dairy products. This fatty acid is a product of the rumen production of vaccenic acid, which is acted upon by a Δ9-desaturase in the cow's mammary gland (Kay et al., 2004). The conversion of vaccenic acid to rumenic acid also occurs in humans (Turpeinen et al., 2002). The *trans*-7, *cis*-9 isomer of 18:2 is made in a similar way but accounts for much less of the total. Rumenic acid has potent anticarcinogenic properties in rats, and a close structural isomer, *trans*-10, *cis*-12-18:2, has antiobesity effects in rats (Pariza, 2004). Neither effect has been confirmed in humans, but research is continuing on the possible health benefits of these *trans* double bond–containing isomers of monoene and diene fatty acids found in dairy products.

Most regulatory definitions of *trans* fat, such as those of the U.S. Food and Drug Administration and the Codex Alimentarius for international trade, define *trans* fat as the geometrical isomers of monounsaturated and polyunsaturated fatty acids having nonconjugated carbon–carbon double bonds in the *trans* configuration. These definitions thus specifically exclude the *trans* fats (CLA and vaccenic acid) that are found in dairy products and beef.

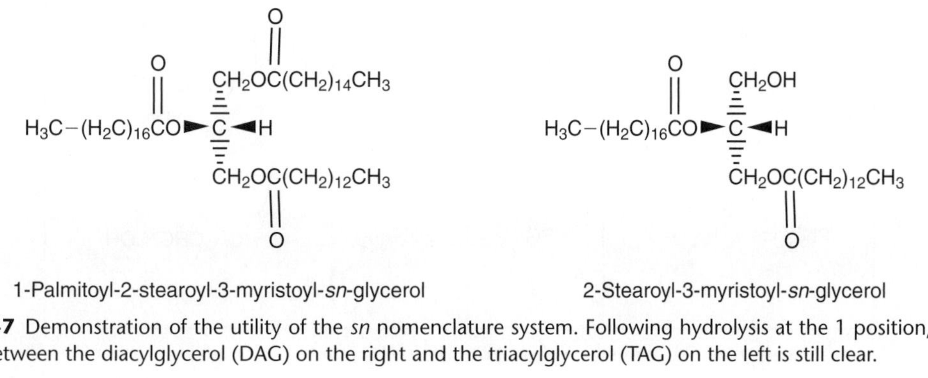

1-Palmitoyl-2-stearoyl-3-myristoyl-*sn*-glycerol

2-Stearoyl-3-myristoyl-*sn*-glycerol

FIGURE 6-7 Demonstration of the utility of the *sn* nomenclature system. Following hydrolysis at the 1 position, the relationship between the diacylglycerol (DAG) on the right and the triacylglycerol (TAG) on the left is still clear.

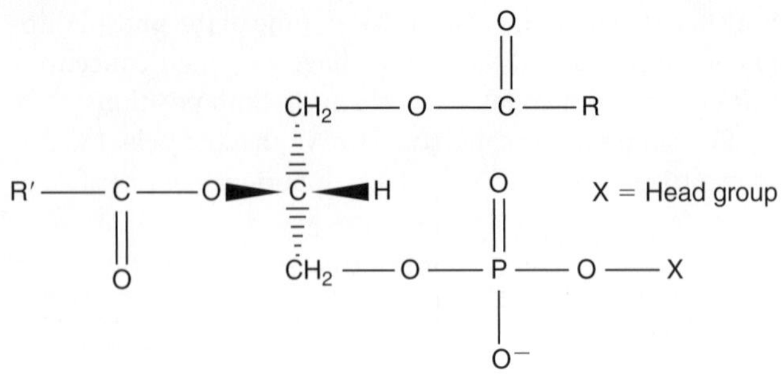

FIGURE 6-8 General structure of the common diacylphospholipids. *X*, Choline, ethanolamine, serine, inositol, glycerol, others.

the *sn*-3 position of glycerol but no polar head group is esterified to the phosphate. Although phosphatidic acid is an important intermediate in lipid metabolism, it is a very minor constituent of the phospholipid fraction of tissues. For all of the other common phospholipids, one of five polar head groups (choline, ethanolamine, serine, inositol, or glycerol) is esterified to the phosphate group. Phospholipids are classified on the basis of their head group. The five major classes of phospholipids thus are phosphatidylcholine (PtdCho, also called lecithin), phosphatidylethanolamine (PtdEtn), phosphatidylserine (PtdSer), phosphatidylinositol (PtdIns), and phosphatidylglycerol. The structures of these phospholipids are shown in Figure 6-9.

Addition of these polar head groups imparts amphiphilic character to phospholipids so that, effectively, the head group of the molecule dissolves in aqueous solution while the fatty acyl chains congregate together. This property allows phospholipids to form membranes and the outer layers of lipid droplets. The various structures of polar head groups lead to different metabolic and structural roles. Although most phospholipids are part of the main structure of membranes, some, such as PS and PI, also have very specific functions.

In many of the phospholipid bilayer membranes in cells, the inner and outer leaflets have different lipid compositions. For example, in human erythrocytes, the inner or cytoplasmic leaflet is rich in PtdEtn, PtdSer, and PtdIns and their phosphorylated derivatives, whereas the outer leaflet is made up of mainly PtdCho, sphingomyelin, and a variety of glycolipids. The asymmetrical distribution of PtdSer has important biological implications because it imparts specific biophysical properties and also enables specific signaling. For example, PtdSer enables certain proteins with PtdSer-specific binding domains to dock with the membrane. Movement of PtdSer to the outer leaflet of the cell during apoptosis is a signal for macrophages to scavenge the cell. Redistribution of platelet PtdSer triggers the conversion of prothrombin to thrombin in blood clotting.

Phosphatidylinositol is a substrate for phosphorylation at the 3-, 4-, and/or 5-positions of the inositol group, and thus up to eight different phosphoinositides are possible. These are often abbreviated as PtdInsP (or PIP) along with numbers that indicate the number and positions of the phosphate groups. For example, phosphatidylinositol 4,5-bisphosphate is abbreviated PtdIns(4,5)P_2 (or PIP_2) Glycosylphosphatidylinositols (GPIs) are lipid moieties that are attached to certain proteins posttranslationally via an oligosaccharide linker. GPI acts as a

Common Phospholipid	Trivial Abbreviation	IUPAC Abbreviation	Structure of Head Group ("X")
Phosphatidylcholine	PC	PtdCho	$-CH_2CH_2\overset{+}{N}(CH_3)_3$
Phosphatidylethanolamine	PE	PtdEtn	$-CH_2CH_2\overset{+}{N}H_3$
Phosphatidylserine	PS	PtdSer	$-CH_2CH(COO^-)\overset{+}{N}H_3$
Phosphatidylinositol	PI	PtdIns	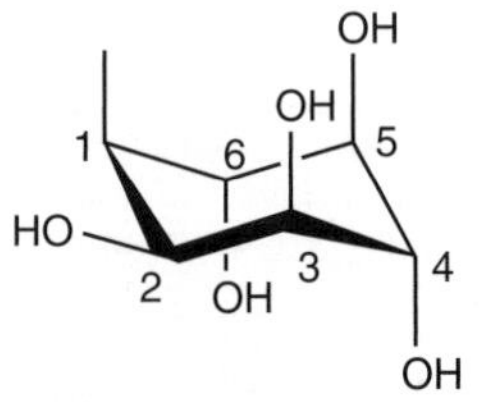
Phosphatidylglycerol	PG	PtdGro	$-CH_2CH(OH)CH_2OH$

FIGURE 6-9 Common head groups in mammalian phospholipids. *IUPAC*, International Union of Pure and Applied Chemistry.

membrane anchor for a number of cell surface proteins. The two fatty acids within the GPI moiety interact loosely with the cell membrane to bind the protein to the membrane.

Lysophospholipids and Diphosphatidylglycerols

Lysophospholipids and diphosphatidylglycerols are two additional subclasses of glycerophospholipids. The structures of these compounds are shown in Figure 6-10.

When one of the acyl groups of a phospholipid is removed by hydrolysis, the resulting phospholipid is called a lysophospholipid. Lysophospholipids, with a single fatty acyl chain, are formed by the action of phospholipases, which hydrolyze the fatty acyl group in the *sn*-2 or *sn*-1 position. Lysophospholipids are good detergents or emulsifiers because of their strong water-soluble head group and their lipid-soluble hydrocarbon chain.

Diphosphatidylglycerols contain two phosphatidic acids linked via a shared glycerol head group. They are more commonly referred to as cardiolipins, because they were first isolated from heart tissue, but they are present in all tissues. In eukaryotes, cardiolipins are synthesized in mitochondria and are particularly enriched in the inner mitochondrial membrane. Cardiolipins interact with various proteins and are essential for mitochondrial function. In mammalian tissues, cardiolipins contain mostly C_{18} fatty acids with most of this being linoleic acid (18:2n−6), although notable exceptions occur in certain tissues, such as testes and brain.

Ether Phospholipids: Platelet-Activating Factors and Plasmalogens

Although glycerolphospholipids typically exist as 1,2-*sn*-diacylphospholipids, in some cases glycerolphospholipids have an alkyl or alkenyl chain joined to the glycerol moiety by an ether linkage (–C–O–C–) instead of a fatty acyl chain joined by an ester linkage. Platelet-activating factors, which have the general formula 1-alkyl-2-acetyl-*sn*-glycerol-3-phosphocholine, are the best-characterized ether-linked glycerophospholipids. They were first discovered because of their ability to induce the aggregation of blood platelets but are now known to have various biological activities, including the mediation of cell–cell interactions and the receptor-mediated activation of phospholipases. In response to cell-specific stimuli, appreciable amounts of platelet-activating factors are produced by inflammatory cells. Plasmalogens are ether lipids in which the *sn*-1 position of glycerol is bound to an alkenyl moiety with the double bond of the alkenyl chain next to the ether bond (i.e., a vinyl ether –C–O–C=C– linkage). A typical ester-linked fatty acid is at the *sn*-1 position, and the *sn*-3 position has a phospholipid head group such as choline or ethanolamine.

PL Class	Glycerol Linkages	General Name	General Structure
Common phospholipids	*sn*-1: Ester *sn*-2: Ester	1,2-Diacyl-*sn*-phospholipids	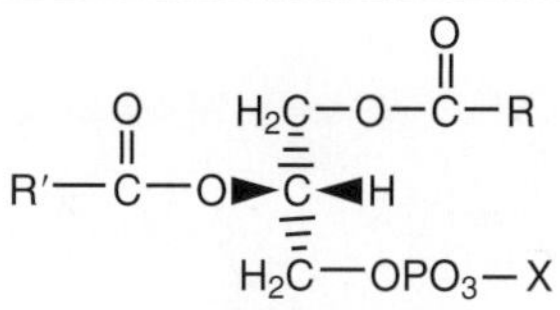 H_2C—O—C(=O)—R R′—C(=O)—O►C◄H H_2C—OPO_3—X
Lysophospholipids	*sn*-1: Ester *sn*-2: none (or vice versa)	1-Acyl-*sn*-phospholipids (or 2-Acyl-*sn*-phospholipids)	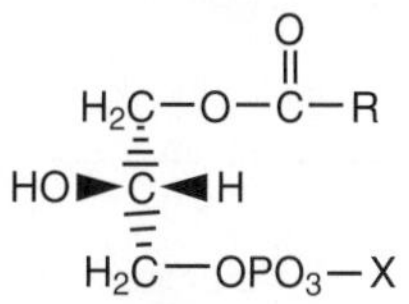 H_2C—O—C(=O)—R HO►C◄H H_2C—OPO_3—X
Platelet-activating factors	*sn*-1: Alkyl ether *sn*-2: Ester (Acetyl)	1-Alkyl-2-acetyl-*sn*-glycero-3-phosphocholine	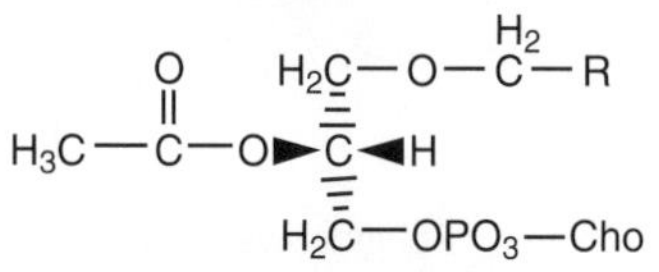 H_2C—O—CH_2—R H_3C—C(=O)—O►C◄H H_2C—OPO_3—Cho
Plasmalogens	*sn*-1: Vinyl ether *sn*-2: Ester	1-Alkenyl-2-acyl-phospholipids (PtdCho, PtdEt, PtdSer)	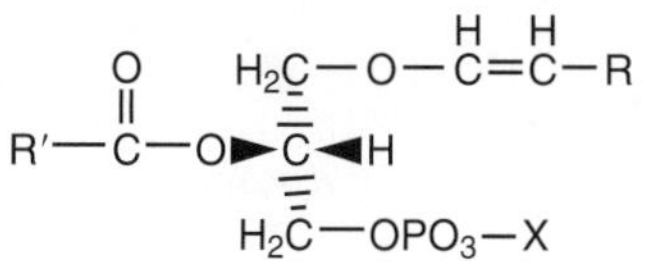 H_2C—O—CH=CH—R R′—C(=O)—O►C◄H H_2C—OPO_3—X
Cardiolipin	Phosphoester and Acyl ester	1,3-Bis(*sn*-3′-phosphatidyl)-*sn*-glycerol	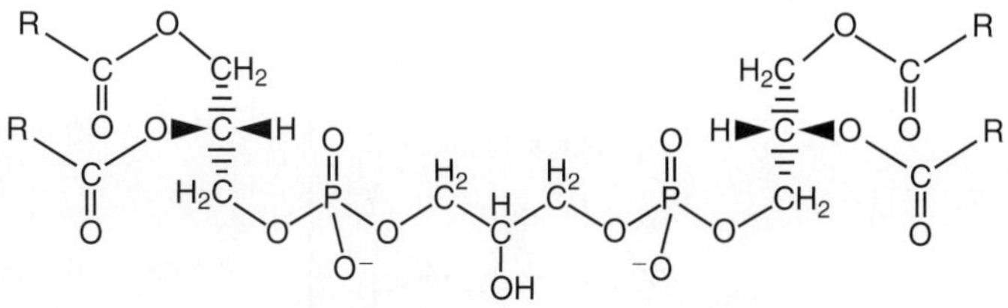 [R—C(=O)—O—CH_2; R—C(=O)—O►C◄H; H_2C]—O—P(=O)(O⁻)—O—CH_2—CH(OH)—CH_2—O—P(=O)(O⁻)—O—[CH_2; H►C◄O—C(=O)—R; H_2C—O—C(=O)—R]

FIGURE 6-10 Major classes of phospholipids. *PL*, Phospholipid; *X*, choline, ethanolamine, serine, inositol, glycerol, others.

Plasmalogens constitute 50% of choline glycerophospholipids in the heart, and they are also present at a significant concentration in several other tissues, particularly as membrane constituents.

Glycerophospholipid Molecular Complexity

The variety of fatty acids and polar head groups that are used in the synthesis of glycerophospholipids, as well as variations in the number of acyl groups that are attached and the type of linkage involved, gives rise to a diverse group of compounds. The term *radyl* is used to refer to hydrocarbon chains linked to a glycerol without specifying the chemical linkage and thus refers collectively to the acyl, alkyl, and alkenyl substituents of glycerophospholipids. With the large number of radyl groups, polar groups, and related substituents that can be linked to the three positions of glycerol, the number of possible, distinct glycerophospholipids is vast. We saw earlier that random distribution of three different substituent groups in TAGs gives rise to F^3 isomers. The number of possibilities is more restricted for phospholipids because the polar head group is always found in the *sn*-3 position.

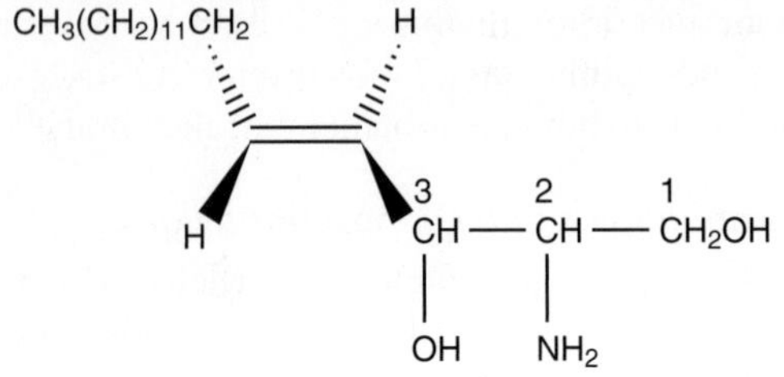

FIGURE 6-11 Sphingosine (2-amino-*trans*-4-octadecene-1,3-diol).

SPHINGOLIPIDS

Not all mammalian lipids contain a glycerol backbone; the class of lipids called sphingolipids is formed by the addition of fatty acids or sugars to sphingosine, a long-chain amino alcohol (Figure 6-11). Sphingosine is a C18 amino alcohol with an unsaturated hydrocarbon chain (2-amino-*trans*-4-octadecene-1,3-diol). Sphingolipids are found in membranes and have various signaling functions. A table of the most common sphingolipids is shown in Figure 6-12, and the metabolism of sphingolipids is discussed in Chapter 16.

Ceramide is formed when a fatty acid is linked to sphingosine through an amide bond to the C2 amine substituent

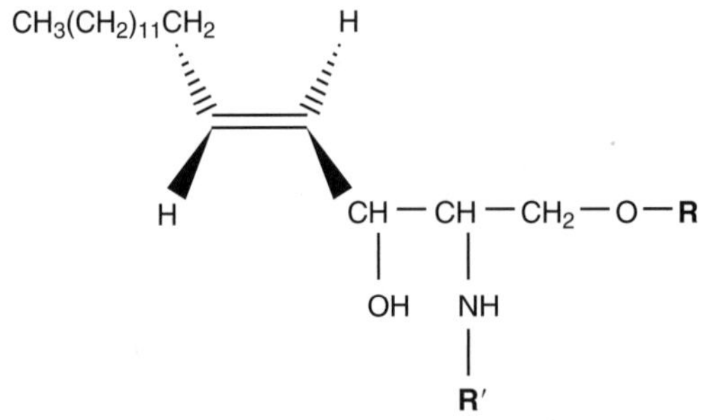

Neutral Sphingolipids	R	R′
Ceramide	H	–C(=O)–$(CH_2)_nCH_3$
Sphingomyelin	–PO_3– Cho	–C(=O)–$(CH_2)_nCH_3$
Psychosine	– Sugar	H
<u>Glycosylceramides</u>		
Cerebroside (mono-)	– Sugar	–C(=O)–$(CH_2)_nCH_3$
Oligoglycosylceramides	– $(Sugar)_n$	

FIGURE 6-12 Structures of neutral sphingolipid classes. *Cho,* Choline.

(see Figure 6-11). Substituted ceramides are important constituents of skin lipids. When phosphocholine is esterified to the C1 alcohol group of the sphingosine moiety of ceramide, sphingomyelin is formed. Sphingomyelin is an abundant sphingolipid in animal cell membranes and is particularly abundant in the plasma membrane. It is also an important constituent of the myelin sheaths surrounding neuronal axons.

Glycosphingolipid is a general term for any compound containing one or more glycosyl residues and a sphingoid base such as sphingosine. The simplest neutral glycosphingolipids, the psychosines, have a monosaccharide (usually galactose) linked to the C1 alcohol of sphingosine via a glycosidic bond. The psychosines are important as biochemical intermediates but may have some other functions not yet well understood. Monoglycosylceramides, or cerebrosides, are similarly formed by the linking of a monosaccharide to ceramide. In animals, galactosylcerebroside is a major component of the myelin sheath insulating the nerves, whereas glucosylcerebroside is an important constituent of the skin lipids that are necessary to maintain the water permeability barrier of the skin. Successive addition of monosaccharides to cerebrosides generates di-, tri-, and tetra-glycosylceramides. Typically, the names of the oligoglycosylceramides are written in shorthand, with abbreviations for the sugars and the linkages. For example, the triglucosylcerebroside globotriaose has the structure Gal(α1,4)Gal(β1,4)GlcCer.

Glycosphingolipids are often divided into two categories, neutral and acidic, a reflection of the extraction procedure typically used for their isolation. Neutral glycosphingolipids possess unsubstituted glycosyl groups. Acidic glycosphingolipids have glycosyl groups with negatively charged substituents, either sulfate groups or sialic acid residues. In higher animals, the most important class of acidic glycosphingolipids is the gangliosides, which are formed when negatively charged sialic acid (*N*-acetylneuraminic acid, Figure 6-13) is added to the oligosaccharide or sugar side chain of the sphingolipid. The C2 of sialic acid links to the sphingolipid either through an ether bond to the C3 of one (or more) of the sugars or through an ether linkage to the C8 position of another sialic acid moiety. Gangliosides are firmly anchored to the outer surfaces of many plasma membranes and appear to be involved in various functions, including cell-to-cell contact, ion conductance, and acting as receptors. High concentrations of gangliosides are found on neuronal membranes in the brain.

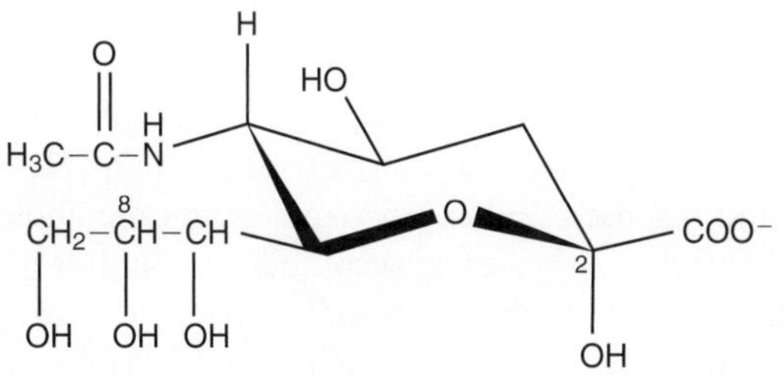

FIGURE 6-13 Sialic acid (*N*-acetylneuraminic acid, NANA).

ISOPRENOIDS

Many of the compounds responsible for color, aroma, and chemical signaling in plants are derived from the five-carbon monomeric unit, isoprene (Figure 6-14). The isoprenoids are occasionally further classified as terpenes if they are hydrocarbons or as terpenoids if they contain oxygen substituents, although some texts use terpenoid and isoprenoid interchangeably. Some examples of isoprenoid structures are shown in Figure 6-15. Typically, the smaller isoprenoids (C_{25} or smaller) are assembled head-to-tail, whereas the larger isoprenoids are assembled head-to-head from smaller units. Generally, these lipophilic molecules are associated with lipid membranes or bound to specific carrier proteins.

In animals, a pathway from mevalonic acid leads to the formation of the 15-carbon chain, farnesyl pyrophosphate, which is made up of three isoprene units (see Chapter 17). Addition of a fourth isoprene unit converts farnesyl diphosphate to geranylgeranyl diphosphate. Farnesyl diphosphate and geranylgeranyl diphosphate pyrophosphate are donors of isoprenyl groups for the posttranslational prenylation of a variety of proteins including heterotrimeric G-proteins and small GTP binding proteins. These isoprenyl groups are transferred to a cysteine residue near the C-terminus of the protein via a thioether linkage. Farnesyl pyrophosphate also is a precursor of various isoprenoid compounds. Important isoprenoid compounds with specific functions in mammals include ubiquinone (coenzyme Q), which is a component of the mitochondrial electron transport chain; dolichol, which serves as a membrane anchor for the formation of oligosaccharide chains for *N*-glycosylation of proteins in the ER and Golgi; and the 30-carbon polyisoprenoid, squalene, which is a precursor for sterol synthesis. Squalene undergoes cyclization and oxidation to form cholesterol and steroids. The isoprene building blocks are difficult to discern in steroids, however, because three carbons are lost between squalene and cholesterol. The structures of squalene and β-carotene are shown in Figure 6-16.

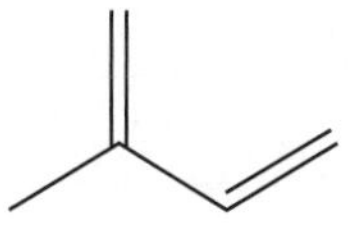

Isoprene

FIGURE 6-14 Structure of isoprene, the building block of isoprenoids.

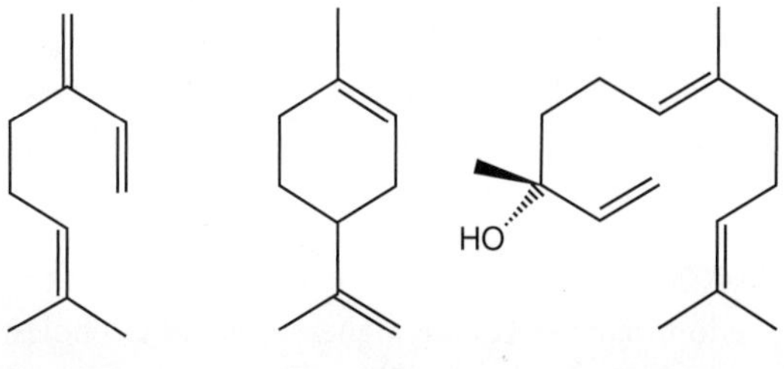

Myrcene Limonene Nerolidol

FIGURE 6-15 Structures of a monoterpene (myrcene), a cyclic monoterpene (limonene), and a sesquiterpene (nerolidol).

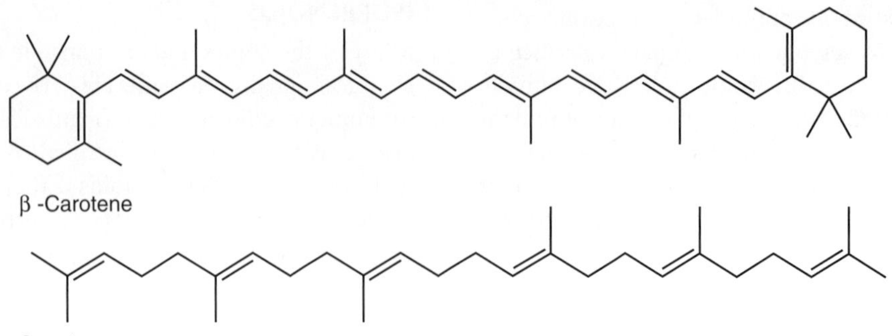

FIGURE 6-16 Structures of β-carotene (*top*) and squalene (*bottom*).

Head-to-tail isoprenoid alcohols, shown in Figure 6-17, are called polyprenols. Polyprenols are produced by plants and are common constituents of essential oils. "Essential" in this context refers to sensory characteristics of oils such as aromas and should be distinguished from the use of "essential" to describe the nutritional properties of PUFAs. Indeed, many of these compounds provide part of the aroma we associate with flowers (e.g., geraniol with geraniums and farsenol with lily-of-the-valley). Dolichols, also shown in Figure 6-17, are similar to polyprenols, except that the isoprene at the hydroxyl (α) end is saturated. Dolichols consist of 15 to 19 isoprene units (75 to 90 carbon atoms) and are typically esterified to a phosphate at the terminal alcohol group.

In esterified form, polyprenols are precursors to the fat-soluble vitamins A, E, and K. The carotenoids are a class of C_{40} isoprenoids (eight isoprene units) that includes lycopene, carotene, and xanthophylls. Carotenoids are synthesized from mevalonic acid in plant cells. These complex hydrocarbons are ingested by animals, and some proportion is taken up into the gut cells. One of these, β-carotene, is oxidatively cleaved in the center to produce vitamin A, a 20-carbon polyisoprenoid alcohol, as discussed in Chapter 26.

STEROIDS

Steroids are structurally related molecules that possess the characteristic perhydro-1,2-cyclopentano-phenanthrene ring system. The core of steroids is composed of twenty carbons bonded together to form four fused rings, three cyclohexane rings (A, B, and C), and one cyclopentane ring (D), as shown in Figure 6-18. Steroids vary by the functional groups attached to the four-ring core and by the oxidation state of the rings. Most steroids fall under the category of sterols, which have a double bond between C5 and C6 (3β unsaturation), a hydroxyl group at C3, methyl groups at C10 and C13, and an alkyl chain at C17, which is also shown in Figure 6-18.

Cholesterol

The predominant sterol in higher animals is cholesterol, which is present mainly in cell membranes where it may play roles in modulating compressibility, permeability, fusibility, thickness, and organization of the membranes. More than 200 plant sterols (phytosterols) are known to exist, including sitosterol, stigmasterol, and campesterol. These plant sterols are similar to cholesterol but contain different alkyl side chains. The side chains associated with cholesterol and some phytosterols are shown in Figure 6-18. More complex molecules with a steroid nucleus, such as digitalis, are also found in plants. Digitalis is a strong stimulant for heart contractions and has been used for centuries to combat heart failure.

Human intestinal absorption of phytosterols is normally negligible and much less than that of cholesterol. Dietary plant sterols are taken up by intestinal cells and then excreted into the intestinal lumen by specific transporters in the ATP-binding cassette (ABC) transporter family. In individuals with a rare genetic condition called β-sitosterolemia, which is due to mutations in the genes encoding the ABCG5 and ABCG8 transporters, large amounts of plant sterols are absorbed and deposited in the body tissues. Phytosterols that are normal constituents of soy oil are also in the intravenous soy emulsions widely used in parenteral nutrition. High amounts of phytosterols infused into the bloodstream appear to be a contributing factor to liver injury induced in infants by intravenous feeding. Plasma plant sterols are normally eliminated by secretion into bile and subsequent fecal excretion, whereas plant sterols taken up from the lumen of the intestine by absorptive cells are secreted back into the lumen of the intestine via the ABCG5 and ABCG8 transporters. Organ damage can occur when clearance cannot keep up with deposition.

Free cholesterol is at relatively low concentration outside of cell membranes. Cholesterol is transported and stored as cholesteryl esters, which are very nonpolar. Cholesteryl esters are formed by addition of a fatty acyl group, often arachidonate, to the hydroxyl group at C3 of cholesterol via an ester linkage. Cholesteryl esters are stored in organs, such as the adrenal gland and the corpus luteum of the ovary, where they serve as precursors for synthesis of steroid hormones. Cholesteryl esters also accumulate in certain disorders (e.g., cholesteryl ester storage disease, familial hypercholesterolemia, and Tangier disease). In atherosclerosis, macrophages in cardiac vessel walls take up low-density lipoprotein (LDL) particles and dispose of all components except the cholesteryl esters. The cholesteryl esters accumulate as lipid droplets in dramatic fashion so that these cells expand to many times their normal size. Regions in which these cells collect appear as fatty streaks in the vessel wall, and under a microscope

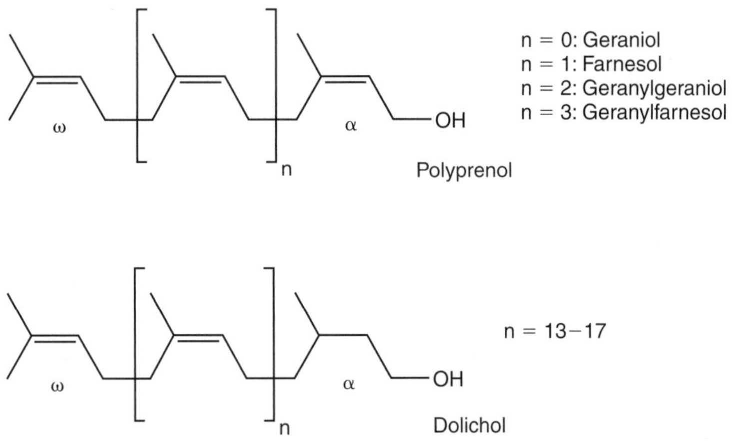

FIGURE 6-17 General structures for polyprenols and dolichols. The isoprene unit is shown in brackets and is the basic repeating unit for synthesis of many lipids, including carotenoids and steroids. The double bonds are converted to single bonds in many specific lipids.

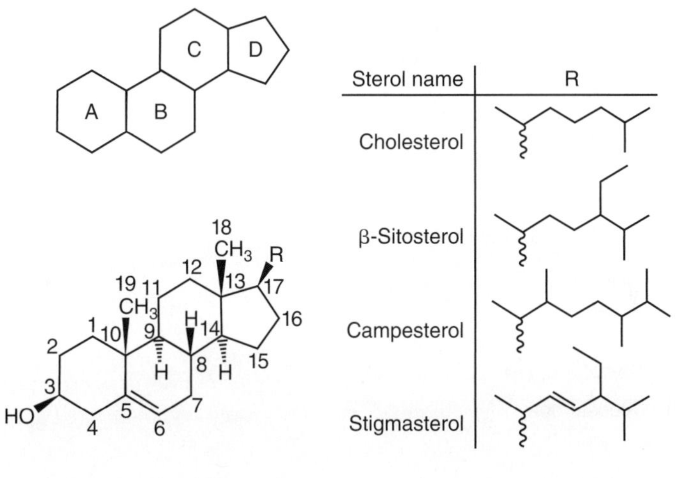

FIGURE 6-18 Steroid structure. *Top left,* Sterane, the base structure for all steroids, showing designation of rings A, B, C, and D. *Bottom left,* General structure for cholesterol and phytosterols, demonstrating the unique sterol numbering system. Alkyl side chains for several naturally occurring sterols are depicted on the right.

they have a bubblelike appearance that gave them the name foam cells. Foam cell formation is an initiating macroscopic anatomical event that can then develop into full atherosclerosis in which large unstable plaques develop and rupture, resulting in vessel occlusion and a myocardial infarction.

Steroid Hormones

Cholesterol is the parent compound for biosynthesis of the steroid hormones that serve as long-range messengers transported in the blood. There are five major classes of steroids in vertebrates: androgens, estrogens, progestagens, glucocorticoids, and mineralocorticoids; examples of these structures are shown in Figure 6-19. Classification of steroid hormones is based on their physiological roles rather than on structural characteristics, although structural characteristics of each group can be defined.

Androgens, estrogens, and progestagens are sex hormones and are produced mainly by the gonads (testes and ovaries). Androgens (e.g., testosterone) promote muscle development and other male secondary sex characteristics. Estrogens (e.g., estradiol) are responsible for regulation of the menstrual cycle and female secondary sex characteristics. The progestagens (e.g., progesterone) suppress ovulation and have antiestrogenic effects. Estrogens, such as estradiol, are characterized by a phenolic ring A and lack of a C19 methyl group, resulting in a C_{18} structure. Androgens, such as testosterone, possess a C_{19} structure and a hydroxyl or keto group at the C17 and C3 positions. Progesterone, the only natural progestatin, has a C_{21} structure and an acetyl moiety at C17. However, synthetic progestagens (progestins) used in oral contraceptives may lack both the acetyl group and the C19 methyl group.

Glucocorticoids and mineralocorticoids are corticosteroids, produced in the cortex of the adrenal gland. Glucocorticoids (e.g., cortisol) have antiinflammatory actions and regulate macronutrient metabolism, whereas the mineralocorticoids (e.g., aldosterone) regulate electrolyte and water balance, mainly by promoting sodium retention in the kidney. Corticosteroids are distinguished by Δ4 desaturation and keto groups at C3 and C20. The glucocorticoids, such as cortisone, also have a C21 hydroxyl group and either a hydroxyl or a keto group at C11. The primary mineralocorticoid, aldosterone, has a keto group at C18.

Vitamin D derivatives, including vitamin D hormone or vitamin D_3, are a closely related group of sterols, although they are not technically steroids.

Bile Acids

Bile acids are formed by degrading the terminal side chain of cholesterol to remove carbons 25 through 27, oxidizing C24 to a carboxylic acid group, and by adding hydroxyl groups to various positions in the ring. The bile acids, cholic and chenodeoxycholic acids, are synthesized from cholesterol in the liver (Figure 6-20). These bile acids are then conjugated with taurine or glycine via a peptide linkage between the terminal carboxyl group on their side chain and the amino group of taurine or glycine; this leaves the sulfonic acid group of taurine or the carboxylic acid group of glycine free and ionizable, making these conjugated bile acids natural emulsifying agents. The addition of a polar, hydrophilic amino acid increases the amphiphilic nature of the bile acid. These conjugated bile acids are secreted in the bile; they are also responsible for emulsifying cholesterol in the bile, and the excretion of both cholesterol and bile acids is the major way cholesterol is removed from the body. Conjugated bile acids are also

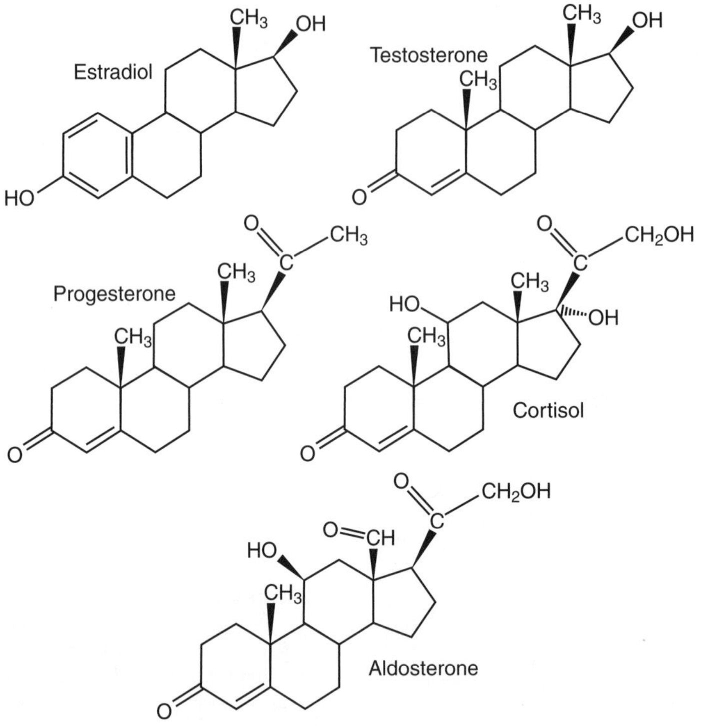

FIGURE 6-19 Representative structures of the five classes of steroid hormones. Examples are estradiol (an estrogen), testosterone (an androgen), progesterone (a progestogen), cortisol (a glucocorticoid), and aldosterone (a mineralocorticoid).

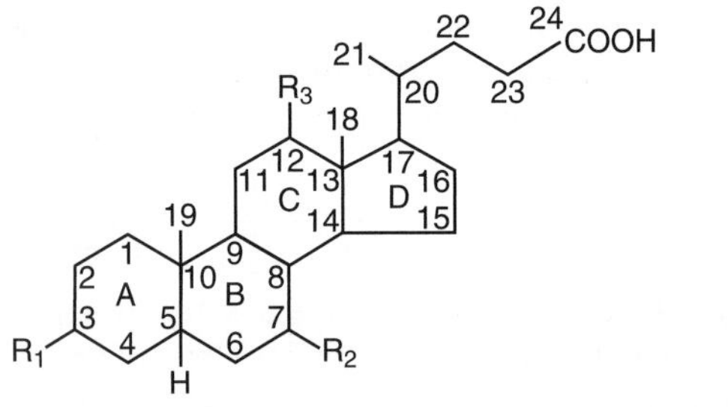

Bile acid	R_1	R_2	R_3
Lithodeoxycholic	αOH	H	H
Deoxycholic	αOH	H	αOH
Chenodeoxycholic	αOH	αOH	H
Ursodeoxycholic	αOH	βOH	H
Cholic	αOH	αOH	αOH
Ursocholic	αOH	βOH	αOH

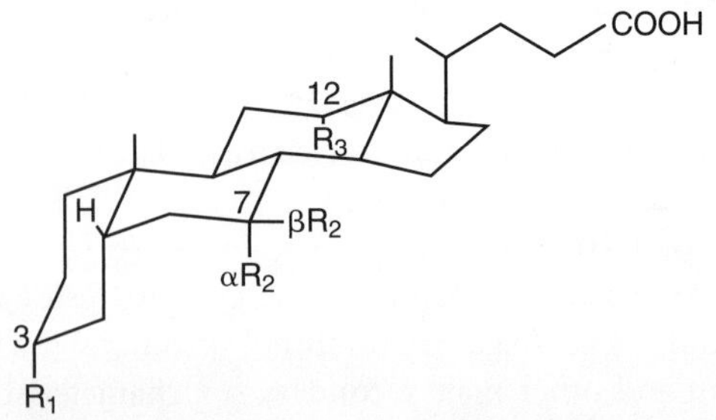

FIGURE 6-20 Molecular structure of common bile acids, showing the common steroid ring and side-chain structure. The location and orientation of hydroxyl group(s) are given for each bile acid. NOTE: Lithodeoxycholic acid is commonly called lithocholic acid.

efficient at emulsifying fats and forming mixed micelles and thus aid in the digestion and absorption of fat and fat-soluble vitamins in the intestine. The terms *bile acid* and *bile salt* are often used interchangeably, but bile acid technically refers to the protonated form, whereas bile salt refers to the deprotonated or ionized form, which needs a cation to neutralize it.

WAXES

Biological waxes are heterogeneous mixtures of long-chain (C_{20} to C_{40}), primarily saturated compounds. The formal definition of a wax is an ester of a long-chain acid and a long-chain alcohol, with the general structure $R{-}COOCH_2{-}R'$. The acyl and alkyl groups are typically unbranched and saturated, although branched or unsaturated chains occur in some waxes. Beeswax contains the ester triacontyl hexadecanoate as a primary component, and the primary component of spermaceti (derived from whale head oil) is hexadecyl hexadecanoate (Figure 6-21).

Waxes are found on the surfaces of plants and animals to provide a hydrophobic barrier. Waxes tend to be solids at ambient temperature, accumulate in intracellular droplets or on surfaces of leaves or skin, and have almost no solubility in cellular membranes. Plankton and higher members of the aquatic food chain, including coral, mollusks, fish, sharks, and even whales, store large quantities of waxes, for a variety of functions, including buoyancy, insulation, and energy stores. Waxes are prominent components of vernix, a unique fatty coating that collects on the skin of human infants in the last weeks of gestation. Vernix is thought to lubricate the fetus during parturition and to serve as a protective barrier against water loss and possibly bacterial infection. Normal human skin lipid (sebum) contains about 25% waxy esters (~C_{40}) along with squalene and TAGs.

EICOSANOIDS AND DOCOSANOIDS

Eicosanoids are oxygenated nonesterified fatty acids principally derived from arachidonic acid (20:4n−6). Smaller amounts are generated from the other C_{20} PUFAs, dihomo-γ-linolenic acid (20:3n−6) and eicosapentaenoic acid (20:5n−3). These derivatives are present in low concentration, are chemically unstable, and have a very short lifetime. They act as autocrine/paracrine hormones to influence contractility, membrane permeability, and many other cellular functions. In contrast to endocrine hormones like steroids, eicosanoids act on cells and tissues local to their site of production, with the eicosanoids binding to receptors on the same cell that secreted the eicosanoid or to receptors on nearby cells.

Eicosanoids are produced by three enzyme classes: cyclooxygenases, lipoxygenases, and cytochrome P450s. The functions and nomenclature of eicosanoids are dependent on their biosynthetic route. In addition to the enzymatically synthesized eicosanoids, some eicosanoids called isoprostanes that are formed nonenzymatically have been described.

Cyclooxygenase Products: Prostaglandins and Thromboxanes

The cyclooxygenase products (prostaglandins and thromboxanes) have a prominent role in reproduction and in the inflammatory response and have prostanoic acid as a general structure (Figure 6-22). They are classified according to the nature of their ring structure. Prostaglandins (PG) have a five-member ring and thromboxanes (TX) have a six-member ring, as shown in Figure 6-23. In nearly all cases, PG and TX have a hydroxyl group on C15. The alphabetical nomenclature of PG (PGA, PGB, etc.) is a vestige of their original classification based on solubility properties: PGA is soluble in acid, PGB is soluble in base, PGE is soluble in ether, and PGF is soluble in phosphate (Marks and Fürstenberger, 1999). The subscript at the end of the name corresponds to the number of double bonds in the molecule and also gives insight into the C_{20} fatty acid precursor. Two double bonds are lost during the cyclization reaction. Thus PGE_1, PGE_2, and PGE_3, which are shown in Figure 6-24, derive from 20:3n−6, 20:4n−6, and 20:5n−3, respectively. Isoprostanes are diastereomers of PG, typically at the C8 or C12 chiral sites. Because they are racemic, they are known to be formed

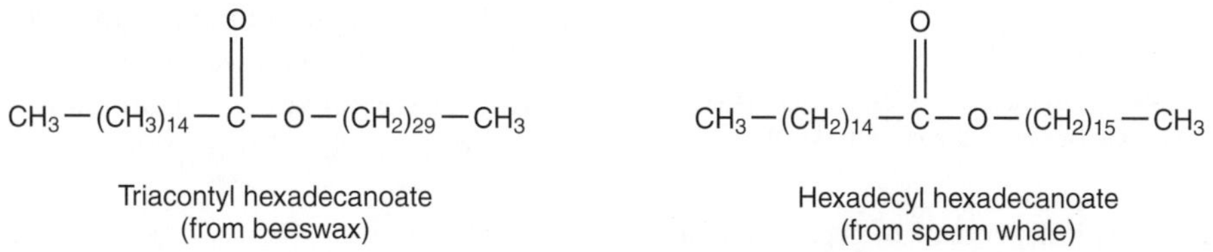

$CH_3{-}(CH_3)_{14}{-}C(=O){-}O{-}(CH_2)_{29}{-}CH_3$

Triacontyl hexadecanoate (from beeswax)

$CH_3{-}(CH_2)_{14}{-}C(=O){-}O{-}(CH_2)_{15}{-}CH_3$

Hexadecyl hexadecanoate (from sperm whale)

FIGURE 6-21 Examples of structures of ester waxes, formed from long-chain fatty alcohols and long-chain fatty acids.

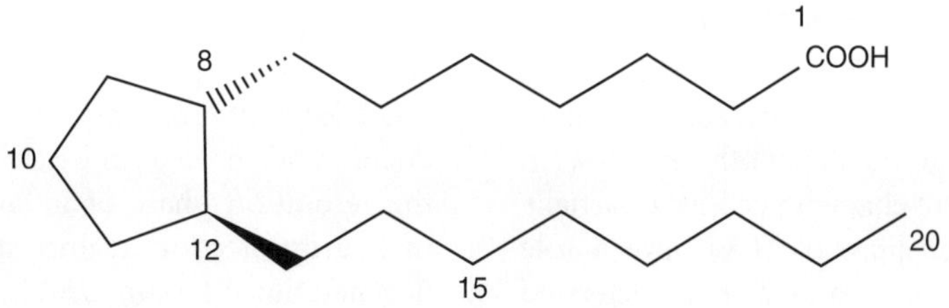

FIGURE 6-22 Prostanoic acid, base structure for all cyclooxygenase products.

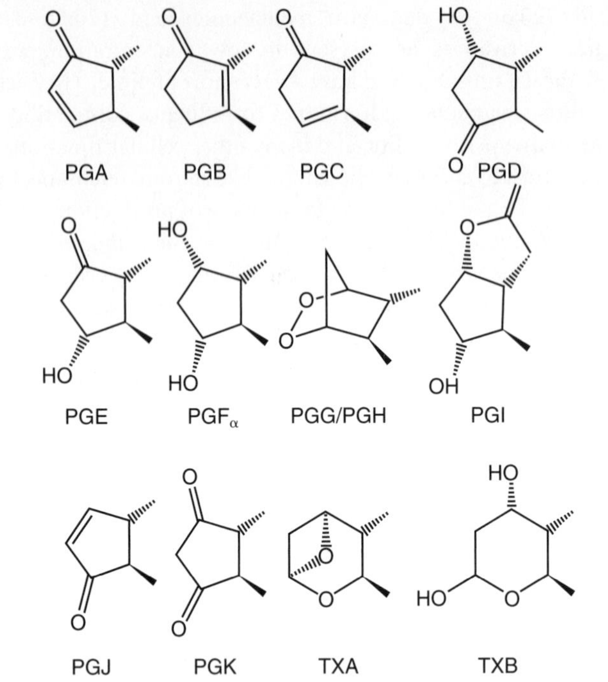

FIGURE 6-23 Nomenclature for ring structures of the prostaglandins (PGs) and thromboxanes (TXs).

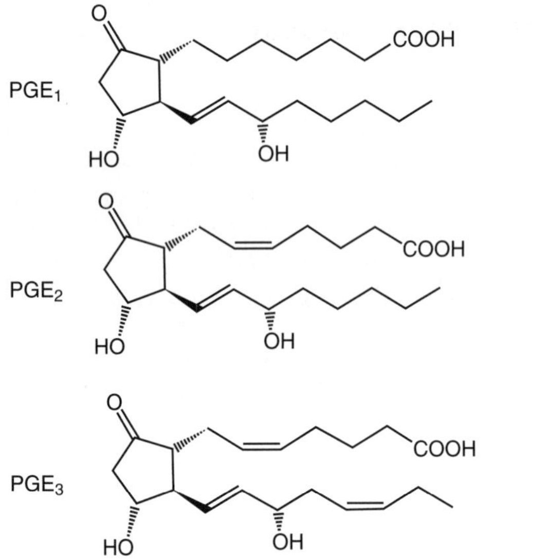

FIGURE 6-24 The E series of prostaglandins. The subscripts correspond to the number of double bonds in the carbon skeleton.

by free radical mechanisms independent of cyclooxygenase and hence are frequently used as biomarkers for oxidative damage.

Lipoxygenase Products: Leukotrienes and Lipoxins

The major lipoxygenase products are the leukotrienes and the lipoxins. The leukotrienes (LTs) cause contraction in respiratory, vascular, and intestinal smooth muscles, in addition to other roles, and are characterized by a partially conjugated C_{20} structure. The lipoxins (LX) have a role in mediating cell-cell interactions and are characterized by a fully conjugated C_{20} structure. There are five major endogenous classes of LT (LTA, LTB, LTC, LTD, LTE) and two classes of LX (LXA, LXB). Analogous to PG nomenclature, the number of double bonds in LT and LX is written as a subscript. Lipoxygenases do not remove double bonds, so LTE_3 derives from 20:3n−6, LTE_4 from 20:4n−6, and LTE_5 from 20:5n−3. Example structures of LT and LX are shown in Figure 6-25. LTC is conjugated with glutathione to form a cysteinyl-leukotriene, and the other cysteinyl-leukotrienes, LTD and LTE, are formed by metabolism of LTC.

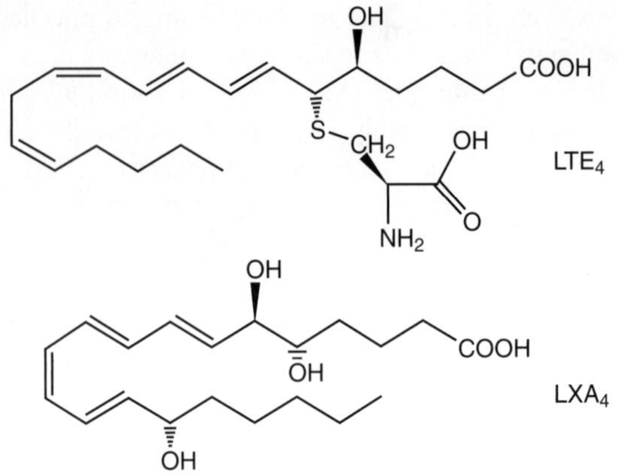

FIGURE 6-25 Structures of a leukotriene (LT) and a lipoxin (LX). The LT (*LTE_4*) possesses a partially conjugated C_{20} skeleton, whereas the LX (*LXA_4*) is fully conjugated. The subscripts correspond to the number of double bonds. A cysteinyl moiety is conjugated in LXA_4.

Other Oxidized Unsaturated Fatty Acid Derivatives

A general nomenclature also exists for oxidized (hydroxy, hydroperoxy, epoxy, and oxo) unsaturated fatty acids that do not qualify as leukotrienes or lipoxins, and this nomenclature is most commonly used when reporting intermediates in the lipoxygenase pathway. Table 6-3 lists the abbreviations for substituents, carbon number, and double bond number, and examples of this nomenclature can be found in Figure 6-26. It is common practice to use shorthand and drop the double bond positions and stereochemistry; for example, 15S-hydroperoxy-5Z,8Z,11Z,13E-eicosatetraenoic acid may be written as 15-HpETE, although the full name will usually be defined at the beginning of the text. Products from the cytochrome P450 pathway, which are primarily epoxy and dihydroxy derivatives of arachidonic acid, such as 5(6)-EpETrE, are also reported using this general nomenclature.

Docosanoids

Docosanoids are C_{22} analogs of eicosanoids that often show agonistic behavior to receptors intended for their C_{20} counterparts. For example, latanoprost and related docosanoids have been shown to lower intraocular pressure by agonistic action on the F-prostanoid (FP) receptor and are thus effective treatments for glaucoma. In recent years, endogenous docosanoids have been described that have potent action in the resolution phase of inflammation (Serhan, 2008) and in neuroprotection against stroke and retinal and neural degeneration (Bazan, 2009). Structural details are under active study.

TABLE 6-3 Nomenclature for Oxidized Derivatives of Unsaturated Fatty Acids

NUMBER OF SUBSTITUENTS	SUBSTITUENT NAME	NUMBER OF CARBONS	NUMBER OF DOUBLE BONDS
1: **no name**	Hydroxy: **H**	12: **D** (dodeca)	1: **ME** (monoenoic)
2: **Di**	Hydroperoxy: **Hp**	14: **T** (tetradeca)	2: **DE** (dienoic)
3: **Tri**	Epoxy: **Ep**	15: **P** (pentadeca)	3: **TrE** (trienoic)
4: **Tetra**	Keto: **Oxo**	16: **Hx** (hexadeca)	4: **TE** (tetraenoic)
5: **Penta**		17: **H** (heptadeca)	5: **PE** (pentaenoic)
6: **Hexa**		18: **O** (octadeca)	6: **HE** (hexaenoic)
		19: **N** (nonadeca)	
		20: **E** (eicosa)	
		22: **Do** (docosa)	

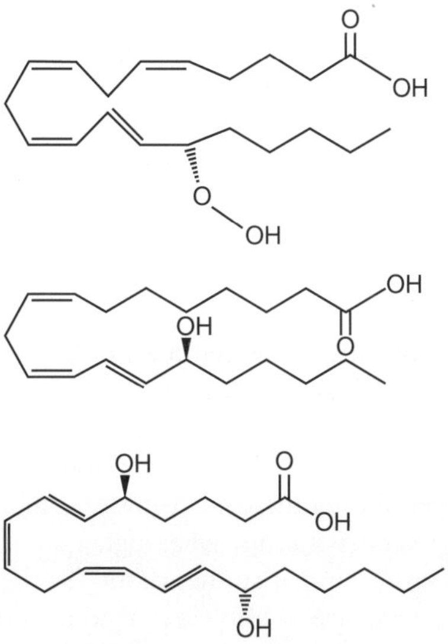

15S-HpETE

15S-Hydroperoxy-5Z,8Z,11Z,13E-eicosatetraenoic acid

15(S)-HETrE

15S-Hydroxy-8Z,11Z,13E-eicosatrienoic acid

5S,15S-DiHETE

5S,15S-Dihydroxy-6E,8Z,11Z,13E-eicosatetraenoic acid

FIGURE 6-26 Examples of general nomenclature for oxidized unsaturated fatty acids.

OTHER LIPIDS

Acyl coenzyme A and acylcarnitine are key intermediates in fatty acid metabolism; they are usually present in low concentrations, but under certain conditions they may accumulate and disrupt cellular functions. Cytidine diphosphate diacylglycerol is an intermediate in phospholipid synthesis and probably partitions into membranes.

N-Acylethanolamines have ethanolamine in place of glycerol as a backbone and are present in low concentration in human plasma. *N*-Arachidonoylethanolamine, also called anandamide, has attracted special attention for its role as the neurotransmitter associated with the cannabinoid receptors. The monoglyceride 2-arachidonylglycerol is also an endogenous (natural) ligand for cannabinoid receptors. Ligand binding to cannabinoid receptors is associated with analgesia, muscle relaxation, improvement of mood, and appetite stimulation (Grotenhermen, 2004). Cannabinoid receptors are also activated by plant cannabinoids such as Δ9-tetrahydrocannabinol, commonly abbreviated as THC. It is produced by the cannabis plant, from which the cannabinoid receptors got their name.

Lipopolysaccharides (endotoxin) are a large, complex class of bacterial glycolipids, present in the outer leaflet of the outer membrane of gram-negative organisms. They are made up of a lipid moiety known as lipid A and an oligosaccharide chain that varies among different bacteria. In higher animals, endotoxins promote inflammation and are responsible for many of the clinical manifestations of infections with pathogenic gram-negative bacteria. The lipid portion of lipopolysaccharides is thought to be responsible for most of these effects.

α-Lipoic acid, also known as thioctic acid, has received attention for its pharmacological function in improving the antioxidant state of the cell. Lipoic acid contains a five-member ring with a disulfide linkage. It is formed from octanoic acid that has been attached to a lysine residue of the apoenzyme before enzymatic insertion of the sulfur atoms. Thus lipoic acid is normally bound to its apoprotein by an amide linkage, and its bound form is called lipoamide. Lipoamide is a required cofactor for certain mitochondrial enzymes such as pyruvate dehydrogenase complex.

SOAPS AND DETERGENTS

Soaps are alkali-metal salts of long-chain fatty acids (e.g., potassium stearate). They are readily produced by treatment of TAGs (such as in tallow or lard) with a strong base. These soaps are amphiphilic compounds with surfactant behavior and have long been used as cleaning agents. Modern synthetic detergents generally have a much stronger acid for the polar head group, which yields amphiphiles that are less sensitive to pH changes. Sodium dodecyl sulfate is a widely used anionic surfactant or detergent that has a tail of 12 carbon atoms attached to a sulfate group.

FATTY ACIDS AND FOOD FATS

From a dietary standpoint, the macronutrient we call fat is more than 90% TAG, with the remaining 10% comprising sterols, phospholipids, and other lipids. TAGs in food products or extracted fats from foods can exist in either solid or liquid form at room temperature, depending on their fatty acyl chain composition. Mixtures of TAGs that are solids at room temperature are called fats, whereas those that are liquid at room temperature are called oils. Table 6-4 shows the fatty acid (or fatty acyl) composition of popular fats and oils (mixtures of TAGs) in the U.S. food supply. In Table 6-4, the units are percent fatty acid by weight, abbreviated %, w/w, which equals the grams of fatty acid per 100 grams total fat. In Table 6-4, the various fats and oils are grouped based on the relative abundance of saturated fatty acids, polyunsaturated linoleic acid, polyunsaturated α-linolenic acid, or monounsaturated oleic acid in the TAGs. Overall, for the fats classified as saturated fats in Table 6-4, a mean of 60% of the total fat is made up of saturated fatty acids, whereas only 5% is made up of PUFAs. Within this group, coconut and palm kernel are rich in the shorter-chain saturated fatty acids 10:0, 12:0, and 14:0. Substantial evidence indicates that saturated fatty acids are atherogenic, resulting in an elevation of LDL cholesterol levels. Palm kernel oil is extracted from the seed of the palm and should not be confused with oil from the fruit of the palm (also shown in Table 6-4), which has a very different distribution of saturated fatty acids and much higher levels of 18:1. Cocoa fat, usually referred to as cocoa butter, is rich in 18:0 and is generally regarded as not atherogenic. Fats of ruminant animals, represented by butterfat and tallow, tend to be very saturated because the ruminal bacteria secrete enzymes that saturate feed PUFAs consumed by the cow. Bacterial enzymes in the rumen also contribute to the formation of the natural *trans* fatty acids found in cow's milk. Lard tends to have more PUFA because the pig is not a ruminant, but production feeding practices tend to produce pork with relatively low PUFA levels.

The PUFA-rich oils are split into those that provide very small amounts of α-linolenic acid (18:3n−3) but high levels of linoleic acid (18:2n−6) and those that are good sources of α-linolenic acid (18:3n−3). Notably, the average total PUFA level in the two groups is very similar, comprising more than half of the total fat. However, the high-linoleic oils contain very low amounts of 18:3n−3 and are insufficient as the sole source of n-3 fatty acids, although they do contain a high level of essential fatty acid 18:2n−6. Conversely, the α-linolenic oils, led by flaxseed and canola, are rich in 18:3n−3, whereas soy and the much rarer walnut oil provide sufficient 18:3n−3 as well as high levels of 18:2n−6. The specific PUFA composition of oils is of nutritional importance, particularly for pregnant and lactating women and for children whose growing central nervous system has an absolute requirement for longer chain n−3 PUFAs, for which α-linolenic acid (18:3n−3) is an important dietary precursor.

Finally, in Table 6-4, oils rich in monounsaturated fatty acids are represented by olive and avocado oils, in which oleic acid (18:1n−9) makes up about 71% of the total fatty acids. These fruit oils are generally considered to be neutral with respect to atherogenesis, neither promoting nor reducing lipid biomarkers related to the coronary artery disease. High oleic soy oil is also shown in the list. This oil is among the newest generation of oils that are from oil seed crops that have been genetically modified specifically for their nutritional properties. The amount of linoleic acid in the high oleic soy oil is typically less than 10% of fatty acids, a fraction of the level of linoleic acid found in normal (conventional or commodity) soy oil, which is about 54% of total fatty acids. In oils under development in 2010, the linoleic-to-linolenic ratio is closer to 1:1 (Pioneer Hi-Bred International, Inc., 2010), more in line with recommendations that have been made by many nutritional scientists. The overall composition of these oils is more similar to that of olive or avocado oil, with somewhat higher levels of α-linolenic acid. Numerous animal studies dating to the 1960s show that a dietary balance of linoleic acid to α-linolenic acids close to 1:1 enhances the biosynthesis and accumulation of long-chain PUFAs and is an effective means to increase 22:6n−3 status. In contrast, recent studies show that 22:6n−3 cannot be enhanced by dietary provision of α-linolenic acid or any other precursor (Brenna et al., 2009).

As in Table 6-4, the TAG composition of oils, fats, and lipoproteins is usually reported as the total overall fatty acid composition of the TAG mixture. This information is widely available from various sources (Firestone, 1999; Shahidi, 2005; Gunstone et al., 1994; Kuksis, 1978; Sonntag, 1979) and is valuable because it tells us which major fatty acids are esterified to the glycerol. However, knowledge of the overall fatty acid composition of TAG mixtures does not provide information about the position of the various fatty acids on the glycerol backbone or about the number of specific TAG species that are present in a given sample. Although various methods are available to determine the position of fatty acids on the TAG molecule and even to fully characterize the molecular forms present in oil, these methods tend to be more expensive or elaborate than analysis of overall fatty acid compositions. For this reason and because for nutritional purposes absorption is very high, fatty acid compositions of TAG mixtures are typically reported without stereochemical information.

TABLE 6-4 Fatty Acid Composition of Edible Fats and Oils*

	Saturated				MUFAs	PUFAs			Sums for		
	10:0 + 12:0	14:0	16:0	18:0	18:1n–9	18:2n–6	18:3n–3		SFAs	MUFAs	PUFAs
SATURATED FATS											
Coconut	54	19	9	3	6	2	<1		85	6	2
Palm kernel	52	16	8	3	15	2	<1		79	15	2
Palm	—	1	44	5	40	9	<1		50	40	9
Cocoa	—	—	26	34	33	3	<1		60	33	3
Butterfat (cow)	6	11	27	12	29	2	<1		56	29	3
Beef tallow	—	3	24	19	43	3	1		46	43	4
Lard (pork fat)	—	2	26	14	44	10	<1		42	44	10
								Mean ± SD	60 ± 16	30 ± 15	5 ± 4
PUFAs (LINOLEIC)											
Peanut	—	—	11	3	52	28	<1		14	52	28
Sesame	—	—	9	5	39	45	<1		14	39	45
Safflower	—	—	7	2	19	75	<1		9	19	75
Cottonseed	—	1	24	3	18	52	<1		28	18	52
Sunflower	—	—	7	5	26	61	<1		13	26	59
Corn	—	—	13	2	31	53	1		14	31	54
								Mean ± SD	15 ± 5	29 ± 14	56 ± 16
PUFAs (α-LINOLENIC)											
Flaxseed (linseed)	—	—	6	3	20	17	53		9	20	70
Canola (rapeseed)	—	—	3	2	60	20	10		5	60	30
Soy (commodity)	—	—	11	4	23	54	7		15	23	61
Walnut	—	—	7	2	18	58	14		9	18	72
								Mean ± SD	11 ± 5	30 ± 19	57 ± 16
MUFAs											
Olive	—	—	13	3	71	10	1		16	71	11
Avocado	—	—	14	—	65 (16:1, n–7)	13	1		14	71	14
Soy (high oleic)†	—	—	11	4	75	<9	3		15	75	5–12
								Mean ± SD	15 ± 1	72 ± 2	<12

*Expressed as percent fatty acid, weight-for-weight (%, w/w); equal to grams fatty acid per 100 grams fat, as a percent. *MUFAs,* Monounsaturated fatty acids; *PUFAs,* polyunsaturated fatty acids; *SD,* standard deviation; *SFAs,* saturated fatty acids.
†Genetically modified, expected availability in the USA, 2012. Data from Firestone (1999) and Pioneer Hi-Bred International (2010).

PHYSICAL AND STRUCTURAL PROPERTIES OF LIPIDS

Lipid structures generally fall into two categories: those that demonstrate a high degree of long-range order, or periodicity, in one or more directions; and those that possess minimal or no long-range order. Most biologically relevant lipid structures (membrane bilayers, vesicles, micelles) fall into the second category. Well-ordered lipid structures with crystalline or crystalline-like properties are relevant to food science and processing but are rarely if ever observed in vivo.

The properties of complex biological lipid structures are often extrapolated from the properties of lipids as isolated compounds. As was mentioned in the previous section, most biological fats are a mixture of many distinct compounds that are impossible to fully characterize. Glycerophospholipids with identical fatty acids at all positions (other than the *sn*-3 position for phospholipids) are easy to synthesize from glycerol and fatty acids, and consequentially their properties have been carefully assessed. Synthesis of glycerophospholipids with fatty acids at stereospecifically defined positions is a much more complex process and such compounds are expensive and rare. As a result, there is rich literature on the biochemical properties of some lipids but not of most lipids.

More importantly, there are no situations where lipids appear in tissues in pure form or where they do not interact with other lipids and with proteins. Chemically, mixtures have drastically different properties than pure compounds. For instance, mixtures have complex phase change behavior that may not even have an analogy in pure systems; for example, as the segregation of like molecules as mixtures cool can lead to fractional crystallization. Within these constraints, a study of the properties of lipids is a useful exercise for understanding the role and function of lipids in biological systems.

EXTRACTION TECHNIQUES

Lipids in real samples, such as cell membranes or food matrices, are usually not studied in situ, because of limitations of analytical techniques. Instead they are typically extracted into solvent before any analysis takes place. These extraction procedures change the lipid composition and properties significantly, sometimes in obvious ways, as for instance in destruction of the bilayer, and sometimes in less obvious ways, such as the loss of water and proteins, which can influence lipid properties. Thus it is important to consider the most commonly employed extraction techniques.

Lipids can be extracted from almost any tissue with several standard methods. A classic method used since the 1950s is called the Folch method (Folch et al., 1957). Tissue is homogenized by a rotating blade device in a mixture of chloroform ($CHCl_3$) and methanol (CH_3OH) at a ratio of 20 parts solvent to 1 part tissue by volume. The mixture is then extracted against a highly polar salt solution, so that polar components dissolve into the aqueous phase, and the lipids stay behind in the nonpolar phase. Much of the methanol also dissolves into the aqueous phase, but enough stays in the lipid phase to dissolve amphiphilic lipids, specifically phospholipids, which are not very soluble in pure chloroform.

An elegant alternative technique known as the Bligh and Dyer method (Bligh and Dyer, 1959) has been more popular in recent decades, because it requires less solvent than the Folch method. The Bligh and Dyer technique uses a ratio of chloroform to methanol to water of approximately 2:1:0.8 to dissolve all components of the tissue homogenate into a single phase. The water component must be adjusted for the water content of every tissue to ensure that there is a single phase or the extraction is very inefficient. Salt water is then added, and polar compounds are removed while lipids remain in the organic phase. Other methods based on methylene chloride, hexane, and other solvents are in common use as well.

These extracted lipids are dissociated from all other noncovalently bound components of their cellular environment. Importantly, phospholipids are removed from membranes where they existed in some complex mixture with other lipids, sugars, and proteins. Properties of these crude lipid extracts, particularly bulk properties such as melting points and dielectric constants, bear little resemblance to those of functional, structurally intact lipids in the cell. As would be expected, these extracted lipids are mixtures with many distinct molecules numbering in the thousands and are never fully characterized.

SURFACE BEHAVIOR OF LIPIDS AT THE WATER INTERFACE

Lipids take on important properties at air–water or oil–water interfaces. The interaction of a specific lipid with an aqueous interface depends on the balance of the hydrophilicity and lipophilicity of the lipid (i.e., the relative strengths of the hydrocarbon and water-seeking parts). Thus when a lipid droplet contacts a water surface of limited area, one of three events will occur: (1) very hydrophobic lipids, such as mineral oils (mixtures of hydrocarbon compounds), will simply sit on the water as an intact droplet or lens; (2) slightly hydrophilic lipids, such as vegetable oils (mixtures of TAGs), will spread to form a continuous insoluble monolayer of molecules in equilibrium with the remainder of the droplet; or (3) highly hydrophilic lipids, such as soap detergents (sodium or potassium salts of fatty acids) or bile salts (e.g., sodium cholate), will spread to form an unstable film from which molecules desorb into the water. Lipids are found at almost all interfaces between cellular compartments. Between two aqueous compartments within a cell, a membrane phospholipid bilayer is present. Between fat and aqueous compartments in the cytoplasm (e.g., a fat droplet in a fat cell) or plasma (e.g., a lipoprotein particle), a phospholipid monolayer forms the interface.

DETERMINANTS OF LIPID MELTING

Lipid melting is the solid to liquid phase change, as is illustrated by the melting of butter or animal fat by heat. Lipid melting is governed by the strength of the molecular interactions of hydrocarbons, primarily of aliphatic chains and sterols. It is affected by chain length, polar substitution, and the presence of double bonds. The effect of increasing chain length on chain-melting transition (solid to liquid) is shown in Figure 6-27 for a variety of lipids. Note that as the chain length increases, the melting temperature rises. Double bonds, triple bonds, methylene branches, and halide substitutions at the end of the chain decrease the melting temperature, but polar substituents, particularly those that can form hydrogen bonds or ionic bonds, increase the melting transition temperature. The order of increasing melting temperatures for a given chain length is as follows: 1-olefins < alkanes < ethyl esters < normal alcohols < carboxylic or fatty acids < TAGs < 1,2 diacylglycerols = 3 monoacylglycerols < anhydrous PtdCho.

LIPID SOLUBILITY AND MICELLES AND EMULSIONS

Solubility of lipids in aqueous phases is a more chemically complex process than for simple dissolution of ionic or polar compounds. True solutions are molecular dispersions in which solutes are surrounded and dynamically interact with many solvent molecules. At very low concentrations, lipids form molecular dispersions in aqueous solution. At higher concentrations, lipids tend to form aggregates of various sizes defined by the composition of the lipid mixture.

The true solubility (i.e., formation of molecular dispersions) of different types of lipids in aqueous systems is quite variable, extending from the virtual insolubility of

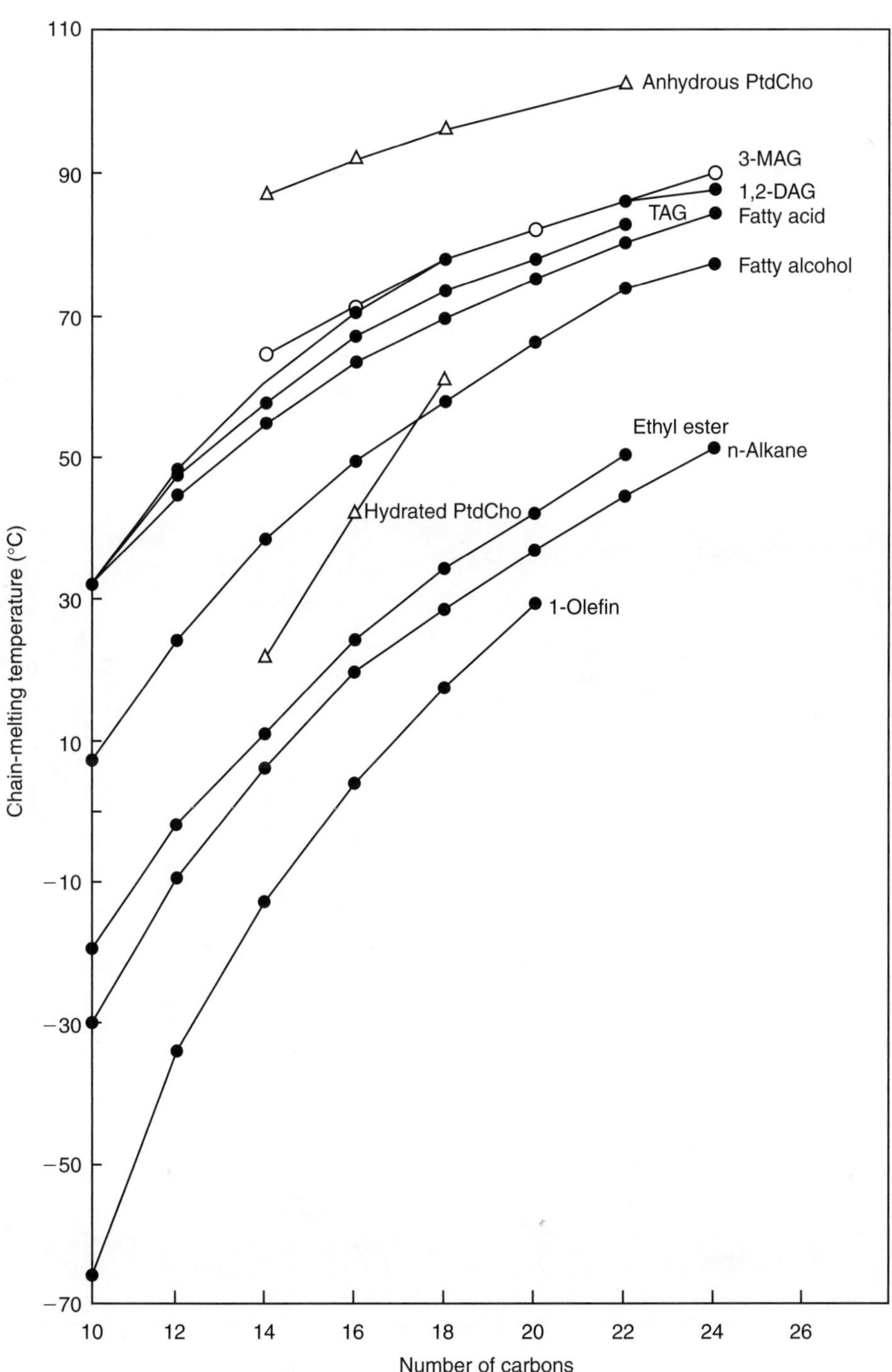

FIGURE 6-27 Effects of polar substituents on melting of the hydrocarbon chain for a variety of lipids. The chain-melting transition (i.e., to liquid chain) temperatures for a variety of lipids are plotted against the number of carbons in the aliphatic chain. The stronger the interaction of the polar groups with each other, the higher the melting point (MP). This is illustrated by the difference between fatty acids, which can form hydrogen bonds between the carboxyl groups, and ethyl esters of fatty acids, which cannot. The MP of the hydrogen-bonded fatty acids is 30° C to 40° C higher. Note that the melting transition temperatures increase with increasing hydrocarbon chain length, even in water. The presence of water, however, lowers the chain transition when compared with the dry lipid, as shown by the difference in chain-melting temperature for hydrated versus anhydrous phosphatidylcholine (PtdCho). *DAG,* Diacylglycerol; *MAG,* monoacylglycerol; *TAG,* triacylglycerol.

high-molecular-weight hydrocarbons and TAGs to the very high solubility of soaps and detergents. The solubility of fatty acids is very low, and it decreases with increasing chain length and thus decreasing polarity. Fatty acid solubility also increases as the temperature increases.

Apparent solubility of lipids may be much higher than the true solubility, because of the formation of aggregates that are smaller than the wavelength of visible light (400 to 700 nm diameter) and thus appear clear even though not all of the lipid molecules are molecularly dispersed. Some of the more polar lipids, such as potassium and sodium soaps and bile salts, form optically clear aqueous solutions in which the apparent solubility may be as high as 60 g of lipid per 100 g of solution. These higher solubilities occur because these more polar lipids can spontaneously form small, spherical aggregates of molecules called *micelles,* and such dispersions are called micellar solutions. Micellar solutions are not a true molecular dispersion but can be considered a dispersion of a lipid-rich phase in a much more abundant aqueous phase. Micelles are spherical structures, about two molecular lengths in diameter in pure water; but when salt is added they often enlarge and assume cylindrical or discoidal shapes.

Micellar solutions are thermodynamically stable and form spontaneously in water when a polar lipid is present above a critical concentration and temperature (Figure 6-28). The molecules within the micelles are in rapid equilibrium with a low concentration of molecularly dispersed solute molecules. This low concentration of molecularly dispersed solute molecules would be considered a saturated true solution of the solute in the solvent, and this concentration is called the critical micellar concentration (CMC) for that particular lipid. Above the CMC, the excess lipid forms micelles. Micellar solutions can solubilize other less soluble lipids to form mixed micelles.

In the intestinal lumen, monoacylglycerols, diacylglycerols, FFA, and bile salts form micelles, which can then incorporate very nonpolar compounds such as cholesterol and fat-soluble vitamins in their hydrophobic interiors. Bile salts enhance formation of mixed micellar solutions in bile and in the intestinal lumen during fat absorption. Such solutions are necessary for the proper absorption of fat and fat-soluble vitamins.

Lipids may also be suspended in aqueous systems as *emulsions,* similar to an oil–water based salad dressing stabilized by amphiphilic protein. Margarine and mayonnaise are two other commonly encountered emulsions that are dominated by the lipid phase. Typically, emulsions have particle sizes between 10 to 100 μm and therefore appear opaque. Insoluble lipids such as TAGs or cholesteryl esters can be made to form relatively stable aqueous–lipid emulsions by adding an emulsifier such as a phospholipid. For instance, emulsions containing particles with a core of TAG and a surface layer of an emulsifier such as PtdCho can be formed in vitro by agitation. Very stable emulsions of soy oil stabilized with phospholipids are used in hospitals for intravenous (parenteral)

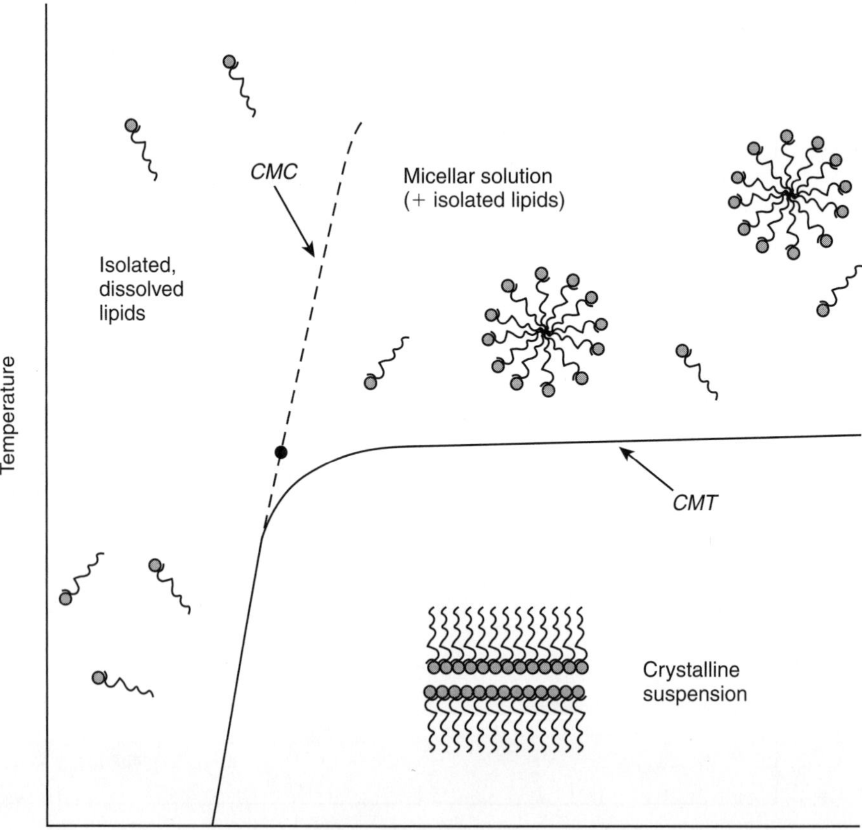

FIGURE 6-28 Behavior of soluble, amphiphilic lipids as a function of temperature and concentration. Micelles occur only at temperatures above the critical micelle temperature (*CMT*) and lipid concentrations above the critical micelle concentration (*CMC*). At concentrations below the CMC, the lipid detergent exists as a molecularly dispersed solute. At high lipid concentration but at temperatures below the CMT, the lipid forms a crystalline suspension.

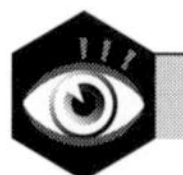

NUTRITION INSIGHT

Lipids and Cell Membranes

The cell membrane, often called the plasma membrane, surrounds all cells and provides a physical barrier between the intracellular and extracellular environments. In addition, various molecules in the cell membrane play roles in selective transport, cell adhesion, ion channel conductance, cell signaling, and attachment of the intracellular cytoskeleton.

The fundamental structural element of membranes is the arrangement of amphiphilic phospholipids in a bilayer, with their more hydrophilic head groups oriented to the cytosolic and extracellular faces and their hydrophobic fatty acyl tails on the interior of the bilayer. This arrangement prevents polar solutes from diffusing across the membrane but allows for passive diffusion of more hydrophobic molecules dissolved at low concentration in the aqueous phase or transported to the membrane in association with carrier proteins. Of course, biological membranes are much more complex than a simple phospholipid bilayer. In addition to phospholipids, membranes contain cholesterol and many proteins as well as glycolipids and glycoproteins that are oriented so their oligosaccharide moieties are on the extracellular surface. Plasma membranes are typically about half lipid and half protein by weight, with the carbohydrate moieties of glycolipids and glycoproteins contributing about 5% to 10% of the total membrane mass. Because proteins have much greater molecular masses than lipids, there is about 1 protein molecule for every 50 to 100 lipid molecules in plasma membranes. The favored concept of the last four decades for the membrane has been the fluid mosaic model proposed by S.J. Singer and G.L. Nicolson (1972). In this model, the membrane is viewed as a fluid, or two-dimensional liquid, wherein molecules are able to laterally diffuse within the layer they are present in and thus are randomly distributed throughout that half of the lipid bilayer.

Although the fluid mosaic model is a useful basic model of the organization of biological membranes, plasma membranes contain several structures or apparent domains that suggest further organization of membrane structure. Membranes contain protein–protein complexes, structures formed by the cytoskeleton, and large stable structures such as synapses or desmosomes, and these structures may act as immobile obstacles that restrict the long-range movement of membrane molecules while playing specific metabolic roles, such as transmitters of signaling molecules.

Another type of specialized membrane region is the lipid raft (Simons and Vaz, 2004). Lipid rafts are lipid-rich microdomains that are more ordered and move as a multimolecular complex in the membrane bilayer. Lipid rafts contain more cholesterol and sphingolipids and tend to contain more saturated phospholipids than the surrounding bilayer. They tend to be transient structures that assemble when a cell is stimulated (activated) in some way, presumably for some specific function. The formation of plasma membrane invaginations containing caveolin proteins, called caveolae, occurs in the lipid raft domains of the plasma membrane, and these are also enriched in cholesterol and sphingolipids. The physical presence of lipid rafts in vivo remains controversial, because if they exist, they are both small (less than 200 nm, below the limit of a light microscope) and evanescent and thus are particularly difficult to study in vivo. New single-particle detection techniques are being explored for this purpose (Cottingham, 2004) and may well clarify the subtle biophysical events within membranes.

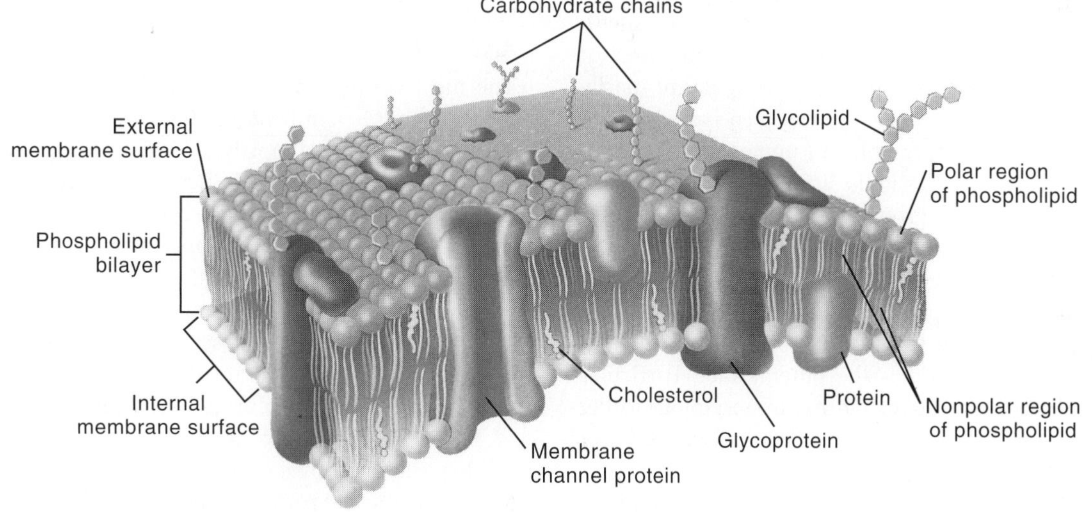

From Thibodeau G.A., & Patton K.T. (2007). *Anatomy & Physiology* (6th ed.). St. Louis, MO: Elsevier.

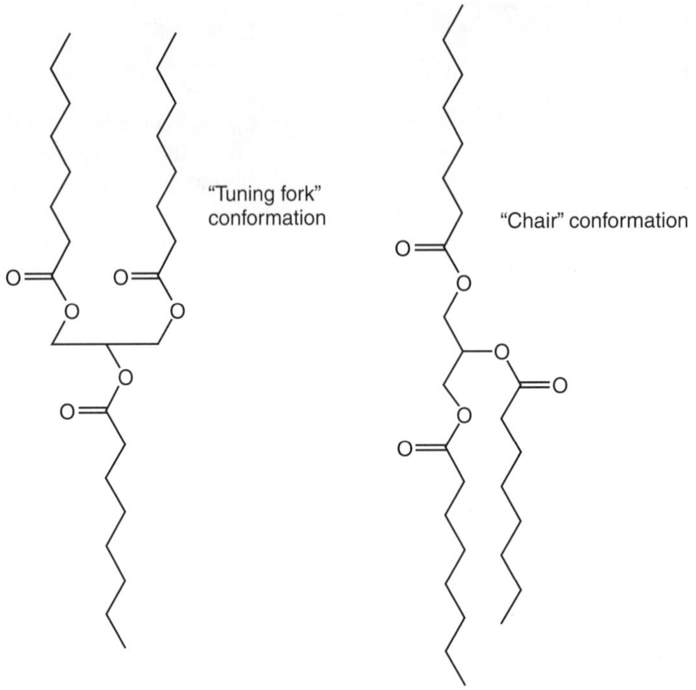

"Tuning fork" conformation

"Chair" conformation

FIGURE 6-29 Tuning fork (*left*) and chair (*right*) conformations of crystalline TAGs.

feeding to provide fat for individuals who are incapable of oral (enteral) feeding. Emulsification of fat is also critical for efficient digestion of fat by pancreatic lipase in the small intestine. Bile salts play an important role in the emulsification of fat in the intestine, breaking large fat droplets into smaller droplets coated with bile acid, which increases the surface area of lipid that is accessible to the digestive enzymes.

THE LIPID BILAYER

In all cells, lipids appear to form barriers between compartments within the cell, such as for specific organelles, and between the cell and the outside chemical environment. These barriers are called membranes and are mixtures of approximately ⅔ lipid and ⅓ protein. The lipid is primarily phospholipid arranged in a bilayer that also includes proteins, cholesterol, and other lipids to impart structure and function. The phospholipids in the lipid bilayer are arranged so that the polar or ionic groups are at the inner and outer surfaces of the bilayer, whereas the hydrocarbon chains are directed inward to form a hydrophobic barrier. For the plasma membrane, the phospholipids in contact with the inside of the cell form the inner leaflet, whereas the side that contacts the outside world is the outer leaflet. Particular phospholipid classes tend to be more common to one leaflet than another; for instance, PtdSer is enriched in the inner leaflet.

Artificial bilayers can be easily made from purified phospholipids. When a pure, very saturated phospholipid, such as dipalmitoyl phosphatidylcholine, is agitated vigorously, a spherical bilayered "cell" called a liposome can be the result. The interior of this bilayer consists of tightly packed, closely interacting hydrocarbon chains, and the bilayer tends to be rigid. As the unsaturation of the phospholipid increases, the bilayer becomes more flexible. When liposomes are made from a mixture of phospholipids and cholesterol, the cholesterol segregates to the interior of the membrane where it interacts with the hydrocarbon chains and in general makes the bilayer less rigid. The strength of molecular interactions in bulk phases is associated with their melting (and boiling) points. By analogy, highly interacting, rigid membranes can be thought of as having more molecular order than membranes that are more unsaturated and include cholesterol and other compounds.

HIGHLY ORDERED LIPIDS: TRIGLYCERIDES AND POLYMORPHIC FORMS

The most commonly encountered ordered lipids, and the most relevant to a nutrition setting, are those found in solid, edible fats composed mostly of TAGs, such as butter, shortening, and cocoa butter. Polymorphism refers to the fact that TAG, and other lipids, can crystallize in different crystal types. TAGs typically align along their long axes with their hydrocarbon chains elongated, which maximizes the van der Waals interactions between their hydrophobic regions. The two most commonly observed orientations for TAGs in crystalline environments are the "tuning-fork" conformation and the "chair" conformation, depicted in Figure 6-29.

These conformations are capable of forming multiple solid crystalline forms, depending on the nature of the conformation and the packing orientation. Thus different crystalline forms have different lattice structures and stabilities, and consequently different melting points, but form the same liquid upon melting. The most common polymorphic forms are the α-, β-, and β′-states, which are depicted in Figure 6-30. The α- and β′-states are based on the tuning fork conformation, whereas the β-state is based on the chair

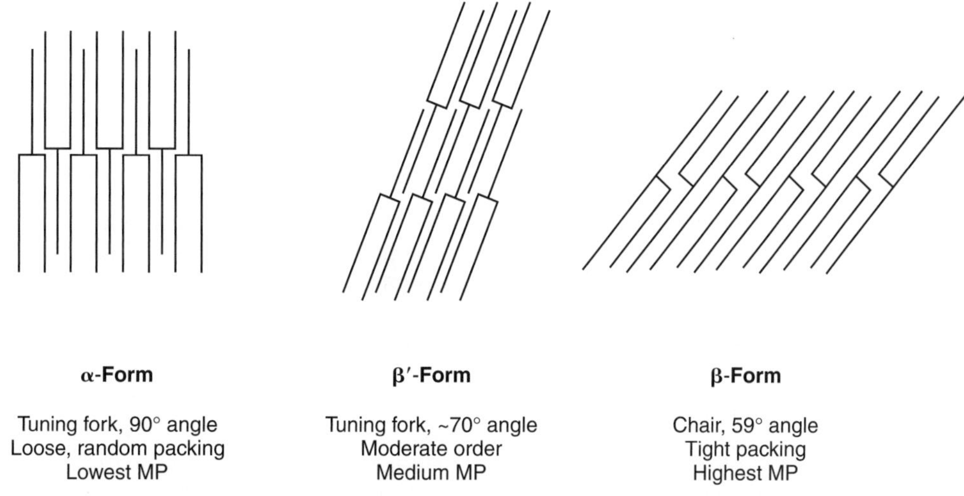

FIGURE 6-30 Common polymorphs of solid triacylglycerols. *MP,* Melting point.

conformation. Packing efficiency and melting point increase in the order $\alpha < \beta' < \beta$. The β-state crystals are more ordered and larger, whereas the α and β′ states form less ordered, smaller crystals. In general, the more disordered, lower melting point polymorphs, such as the α form, are formed by fast cooling of liquid fat, whereas the more organized polymorphs are formed by slower cooling.

Some TAGs have more complicated polymorphic forms, and natural mixtures of TAGs may exist as a combination of polymorphic forms and stoichiometric ratios of molecules in the same crystal. Forming the correct polymorphic form is important in producing palatable and attractive foods. For example, shortening manufacturers prefer to form the β′ rather than β polymorph, because it results in smaller crystals that, in turn, result in a smoother mouthfeel. Conversely, chocolate manufacturers prefer to form the β polymorph of cocoa butter, which has a melting point of 35.5° C, compared to 27° C for the β′ form. Polymorphic transitions from β to β′ forms are responsible for the white, dusty layer (bloom) sometimes seen on old chocolate. While not toxic, bloom is unacceptable to most consumers.

DIGESTION AND ABSORPTION OF DIETARY FATS AND OILS

A single meal often contains dietary fat from a variety of sources (dairy, meat, vegetable). These mix with digestive secretions in the stomach and small intestine and undergo digestion and absorption. Absorption from the lumen is generally quite efficient, with more than 95% of the TAG consumed in the diet typically being absorbed (Carey et al., 1983). About 50% of dietary cholesterol is absorbed.

Although absorption of the mixture of TAGs present in dietary fat is very efficient, the digestion and absorption of specific, highly saturated fats may be much less efficient. The solid–liquid phase change is important for digestion, as evidenced by the poor efficiency of digestion and absorption of saturated TAGs such as tristearin (MP 73° C) and tripalmitin (MP 66° C). These pure TAGs with high melting points (MPs) above body temperature are not hydrolyzed by pancreatic lipase and pass through the gut largely unabsorbed, still in solid form. Dietary fat is nevertheless well absorbed because it is a mixture of TAGs and other lipids. Unlike pure compounds, the MPs of these lipids have a broad range in which they soften and can be emulsified sufficiently to be acted upon by enzymes and other proteins in the aqueous phase. The melting and crystallization temperatures for a variety of TAGs, diacylglycerols, and monoacylglycerols that are present during fat metabolism have been reported (Small, 1991).

TAG structure can also influence digestion and absorption characteristics of some TAGs, particularly those with melting points lower than body temperature. For example, some studies indicate that if the saturated fatty acid is esterified in the *sn*-2 position of glycerol, it is more likely to be absorbed than if it is in the *sn*-1 or *sn*-3 position, at least in studies using pure fats. This relationship between stereospecific position and absorption is due to the specificity of pancreatic lipase, which cleaves TAG at the 1- and 3- positions. For example, consider two positional isomers of dioleoyl stearoyl glycerol, OSO (MP 25° C) and OOS (MP 24° C). Both OSO and OOS are liquids at body temperature. In studies in rats, about 94% of the stearate in OSO was absorbed, whereas only about 62% of the stearate in OOS was absorbed (Redgrave et al., 1988). When intestinal enzymes hydrolyze 1 mol of OSO, they produce 1 mol of 2-monostearin (and 2 mol of oleic acid). The MP of 2-monostearin is close to the body temperature of rats (39° C), and it can be incorporated into micelles by bile salts and thus be absorbed. However, hydrolysis of OOS gives 1 mol of stearic acid. The MPs of stearic acid and its soap are above 50° C, so these digestion products solidify and are poorly absorbed. Although effects of TAG structure can be demonstrated for pure TAGs, it has little effect on dietary fat absorption. On the other hand, these effects are of importance for engineered foods applications, such as the development of low-calorie foods based on low absorption of the engineered food fat.

THINKING CRITICALLY

1. Draw the structure of a triacylglycerol with palmitic acid esterified in the *sn*-1 position, arachidonic acid esterified in the *sn*-2 position, and palmitoleic acid esterified in the *sn*-3 position of glycerol.
2. For the three fatty acids in this triacylglycerol, give an acceptable numerical shorthand description using both the "n minus" and the Δ systems of nomenclature.
3. Consider a mixture of fat produced by esterification of three fatty acids (A, B, C) to the glycerol. There will be triacylglycerol molecules containing various combinations of A, B, and C such as ABC and BBB. There will be isomeric forms of those with a chiral center. How many unique triacylglycerol isomers could be in this mixture? Using a simple shorthand notation (e.g., variations of 3 letter combinations to indicate fatty acid and its position on the glycerol backbone), show all of these isomers.

REFERENCES

Bazan, N. G. (2009). Neuroprotectin D1-mediated anti-inflammatory and survival signaling in stroke, retinal degenerations, and Alzheimer's disease. *Journal of Lipid Research* (Suppl. 50), S400–S405.

Bligh, E. G., & Dyer, W. J. (1959). A rapid method of total lipid extraction and purification. *Canadian Journal of Biochemistry and Physiology, 37*, 911–917.

Brenna, J. T., Salem, N., Jr., Sinclair, A. J., & Cunnane, S. C. (2009). α-Linolenic acid supplementation and conversion to n−3 long-chain polyunsaturated fatty acids in humans. *Prostaglandins, Leukotrienes, and Essential Fatty Acids, 80*, 85–91.

Brown, W. R., Hansen, A. E., Burr, B. O., & McQuarrie, I. (1938). Effects of prolonged use of extremely low-fat diet in an adult human subject. *The Journal of Nutrition, 16*, 511–524.

Burr, G. O., & Burr, M. M. (1929). A new deficiency disease produced by the rigid exclusion of fat from the diet. *The Journal of Biological Chemistry, 82*, 345–367.

Carey, M. C., Small, D. M., & Bliss, C. M. (1983). Lipid digestion and absorption. *Annual Review of Physiology, 45*, 651–677.

Cottingham, K. (2004). Do you believe in lipid rafts? Biologists are turning to several analytical techniques to find out whether lipid rafts really exist. *Analytical Chemistry, 76*, 403A–406A.

Firestone, D. (Ed.). (1999). *Physical and chemical characteristics of oils, fats, and waxes*. Champaign, IL: AOCS Press.

Folch, J., Lees, M., & Sloane-Stanley, G. H. (1957). A simple method for the isolation and purificaiton of total lipides from animal tissues. *The Journal of Biological Chemistry, 226*, 497–509.

Grotenhermen, F. (2004). Pharmacology of cannabinoids. *Neuro Endocrinology Letters, 25*, 14–23.

Gunstone, F. D., Harwood, J. L., & Padley, F. B. (1994). *The lipid handbook* (2nd ed.). London: Chapman and Hall.

Holman, R. T. (1992). *A long scaly tale—The study of essential fatty acid deficiency at the University of Minnesota. Third International Congress on Essential Fatty Acids and Eicosanoids, Adelaide, Australia*. Champaign, IL: AOCS Press.

Hu, F. B., & Willett, W. C. (2002). Optimal diets for prevention of coronary heart disease. *The Journal of the American Medical Association, 288*, 2569–2578.

Kay, J. K., Mackle, T. R., Auldist, M. J., Thomson, N. A., & Bauman, D. E. (2004). Endogenous synthesis of *cis*-9, *trans*-11 conjugated linoleic acid in dairy cows fed fresh pasture. *Journal of Dairy Science, 87*, 369–378.

Kramer, J. K., Parodi, P. W., Jensen, R. G., Mossoba, M. M., Yurawecz, M. P., & Adolf, R. O. (1998). Rumenic acid: A proposed common name for the major conjugated linoleic acid isomer found in natural products. *Lipids, 33*, 835.

Kuksis, A. (Ed.). (1978). *Handbook of lipid research* (Vol. 1). New York: Plenum Press.

Lipidomics Gateway. *Lipid classification system*. Retrieved from http://www.lipidmaps.org/data/classification/LM_classification_exp.php

Marks, F., & Fürstenberger, G. (Eds.). (1999). *Prostaglandins, leukotrienes, and other eicosanoids: From biogenesis to clinical application*. New York: Wiley-VCH.

Pariza, M. W. (2004). Perspective on the safety and effectiveness of conjugated linoleic acid. *The American Journal of Clinical Nutrition, 79*, 1132S–1136S.

Pioneer Hi-Bred International, Inc. (2010). *Plenish High Oleic Soybean Oil*. Retrieved from http://www.plenish.com

Redgrave, T. G., Kodali, D. R., & Small, D. M. (1988). The effect of triacyl-*sn*-glycerol structure on the metabolism of chylomicrons and triacylglycerol-rich emulsions in the rat. *The Journal of Biological Chemistry, 263*, 5118–5123.

Serhan, C. N. (2008). Systems approach with inflammatory exudates uncovers novel anti-inflammatory and pro-resolving mediators. *Prostaglandins, Leukotrienes, and Essential Fatty Acids, 79*, 157–163.

Shahidi, F. (Ed.). (2005). *Bailey's industrial oil and fat products* (6th ed), 5 Volumes. New York: John Wiley & Sons.

Singer, S. J., & Nicolson, G. L. (1972). The fluid mosaic model of the structure of cell membranes. *Science, 175*, 720–731.

Simons, K., & Vaz, W. L. (2004). Model systems, lipid rafts, and cell membranes. *Annual Review of Biophysics and Biomolecular Structure, 33*, 269–295.

Small, D. M. (1991). The effects of glyceride structure on absorption and metabolism. *Annual Review of Nutrition, 11*, 413–434.

Sonntag, N. O. V. (1979). Composition and characteristics of individual fats and oils. In D. Swern (Ed.), *Bailey's industrial oil and fat products* (Vol. 1, pp. 289–478). New York: John Wiley & Sons.

Turpeinen, A. M., Mutanen, M., Aro, A., Salminen, I., Basu, S., Palmquist, D. L., & Griinari, J. M. (2002). Bioconversion of vaccenic acid to conjugated linoleic acid in humans. *The American Journal of Clinical Nutrition, 76*, 504–510.

Warden, C. H., & Fisler, J. S. (2008). Comparisons of diets used in animal models of high-fat feeding. *Cell Metabolism, 7*, 277.

RECOMMENDED READING

Gurr, M., Harwood, J., & Frayn, K. (2002). *Lipid biochemistry*. New York: Blackwell Publishing.

RECOMMENDED WEBSITES

Cyberlipid Center. A student-oriented website describing many aspects of lipidology. http://www.cyberlipid.org/cyberlip/home0001.htm

LipidBank. Database of chemical properties of lipids, by the Japanese Conference on the Biochemistry of Lipids (JCBL). http://lipidbank.jp/index.html

Lipid Library. An elementary to intermediate treatment of lipid structures and analysis. http://lipidlibrary.aocs.org

Lipidomics Gateway. A comprehensive source of information on lipid molecular biology by the LIPID MAPS consortium and Nature Publishing Group. http://www.lipidmaps.org

Moss, G. P. (1976). *Nomenclature of lipids*. Compendium of International Union of Pure and Applied Chemsitry (IUPAC) and International Union of Biochemistry and Molecular Biology (IUBMB) recommendations for naming organic and biological compounds. http://www.chem.qmul.ac.uk/iupac/lipid

UNIT III

Digestion and Absorption of the Macronutrients

Digestion largely involves the processes that result in the enzymatic breakdown of complex macronutrients to their smaller units (e.g., digestion of starch to glucose). Absorption of these smaller molecules across the epithelial cell layer of the intestinal mucosa into the lamina propria (the vascular layer of connective tissue beneath the epithelium) allows them to enter either the blood or the lymph for circulation to the rest of the body. Release and absorption of vitamins and minerals are also essential, and these processes are described in Units VI and VII.

The gastrointestinal (GI) tract can be considered as a tubular structure extending from the mouth to the anus, and the contents in the lumen of the GI tract can be considered as being "outside" of the body. Uptake of nutrients into the circulatory systems (the blood and lymph), which supply cells with nutrients, depends upon several factors, including (1) the efficient enzymatic breakdown of complex nutrients into molecules small enough to be taken up by the intestinal absorptive cells; (2) uptake of nutrients by transporter proteins located at the luminal membrane of the absorptive cells; (3) further hydrolysis (e.g., peptide hydrolysis to amino acids) or processing (e.g., triacylglycerol synthesis and the formation of chylomicrons) within the absorptive cells; and (4) transport out of the absorptive cell across the contraluminal or basolateral membrane into the underlying extracellular connective tissue layer (called the lamina propria) that also contains small blood and lymphatic vessels. Here, the products of digestion and absorption enter either the capillaries (and hence the portal blood) or the lacteals (and hence the lymph and ultimately the blood). These processes involved in the entrance of nutrients into the body's circulation are discussed in this unit, and the subsequent utilization of these absorbed nutrients by body tissues is discussed in Unit IV.

Certain dietary components, especially complex carbohydrates and lignins from plant cell walls, are not hydrolyzed by enzymes of the human digestive system and pass into the large intestine undigested. The undigestible components of plant cells are called dietary fiber. Although fiber is not an essential nutrient, it is considered to be an additional source of energy, to have physiological and health benefits, and to be an important component of healthy diets. Some of the undigestible residues are fermented by colonic bacteria to form short-chain fatty acids and gases, whereas others add directly to the mass of the stool or are used by the colonic bacteria for their own growth. The short-chain fatty acids may cross the colonic epithelium by diffusion, enter the portal blood, and be used as a fuel by tissues.

CHAPTER 7

Overview of Digestion and Absorption

Alan B. R. Thomson, MD, PhD, and Patrick Tso, PhD

COMMON ABBREVIATIONS

CCK	cholecystokinin	GIP	gastric inhibitory peptide
GI	gastrointestinal	GLP	glucagon-like peptide

Most foodstuffs are ingested in forms that are unavailable to the body and must be broken down into smaller molecules before they can be absorbed into the circulation. The gastrointestinal (GI) tract is the system that carries out the functions of ingestion, digestion, and absorption. The major functions of the GI tract are to digest complex molecules in foods (making them absorbable) and to absorb simple nutrients, including monosaccharides, monoacylglycerols, fatty acids, amino acids, vitamins, minerals, and water. In addition, the GI tract serves excretory, secretory, endocrine, and protective functions.

GENERAL STRUCTURE AND FUNCTION OF THE GI TRACT

The GI tract extends from the mouth to the anus and consists of a long muscular tube with a continuous lumen that opens to the exterior at both ends (Figure 7-1). It has openings for the entry of secretions from the salivary glands, the liver, and the pancreas. The GI system includes the oral cavity, pharynx, esophagus, stomach, small intestine, large intestine, and rectum, as well as accessory organs (salivary glands, pancreas, liver, and gallbladder) that provide essential secretions.

BASIC ANATOMICAL STRUCTURE OF THE GI TRACT

Once past the oral cavity, most of the digestive tract has a distinct anatomical structure that is typical of tubular organs (Figure 7-2). Although there are variations along the GI tract, its wall generally comprises four basic tissue layers surrounding the lumen.

Mucosa

The first layer of the GI tract, or the layer facing the lumen, is the mucosa. The mucosa actually has three parts: a lining of epithelium that directly contacts food particles; the underlying lamina propria or connective tissue layer that also contains small blood and lymphatic vessels, nerve fibers, and in some cases exocrine and endocrine glands; and a thin layer of smooth muscle that separates the mucosa from the submucosa.

Submucosa

The second basic layer is the submucosa, which is a compact fibrous connective tissue layer that contains blood vessels, nerve fibers, and in some cases lymphatic structures or exocrine glands. This layer provides support, the blood supply, and nerve input controlling secretion (i.e., the Meissner plexus).

Muscularis Externa

The third basic layer is the muscularis externa, which actually consists of two, sometimes three, layers of muscle. The layer closest to the lumen is composed of circular muscle fibers, which narrow or constrict the lumen when contracted. An outer layer of longitudinal muscle fibers provides longitudinal contraction, which shorten and widen the lumen of the GI tract. Some parts of the GI tract, such as the stomach, have an additional muscle layer. The major nerve supply of the GI tract is contained between the circular and longitudinal muscle layers and is known as the myenteric or Auerbach plexus. This nerve supply controls GI tract motility.

Serosa or Adventitia

The fourth basic layer is either the serosa or the adventitia. The intraperitoneal organs of the digestive tract (i.e., upper 5 cm of duodenum, jejunum, ileum, cecum, appendix, transverse colon, sigmoid colon, and upper part of the rectum) are freely suspended in the peritoneal cavity and have a serosa, which is a thin layer of loose connective tissue covered by simple squamous epithelium. The serosa is basically an extension of the peritoneum that lines the wall of the peritoneal cavity and holds the abdominal organs in place. The serosa secretes a watery lubricant that allows parts of the gut to move smoothly over each other. Other parts of the

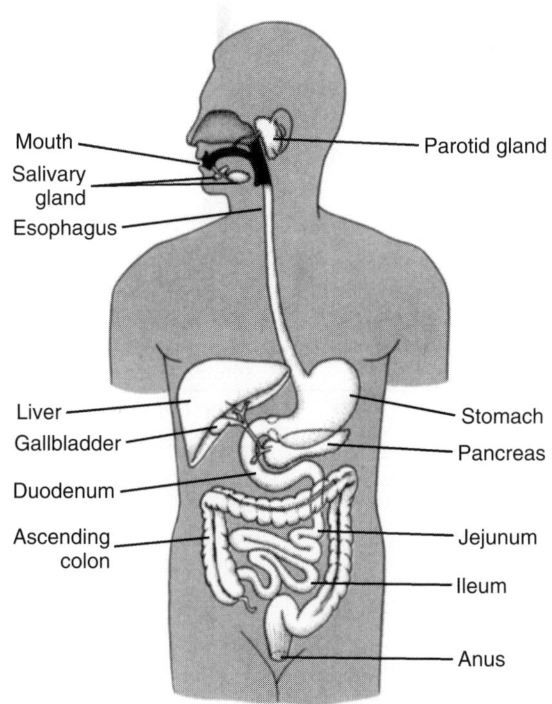

FIGURE 7-1 Gross anatomy of the gastrointestinal system.

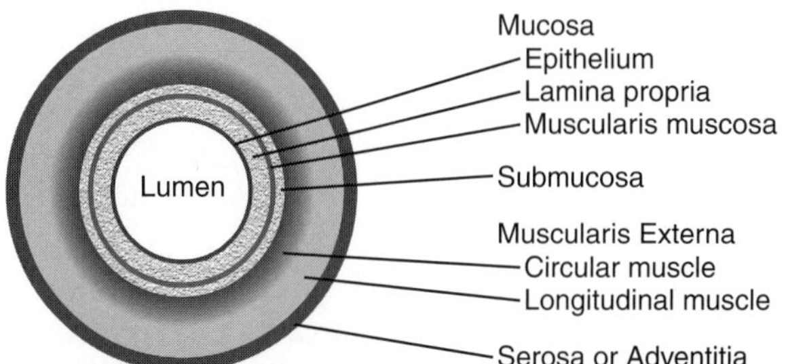

FIGURE 7-2 General organization of the intestinal wall.

GI tract that are outside of the peritoneal cavity, such as the esophagus and lower part of the rectum, have an outermost connective tissue layer known as adventitia. The retroperitoneal organs (i.e., lower part of the duodenum, ascending and descending colon, and middle part of the rectum) are bound to the posterior abdominal wall by adventitia and covered on their free anterior surfaces by serosa.

GENERAL MECHANISMS FOR REGULATION OF GI TRACT FUNCTION

The digestion and absorption of nutrients are both neurally and hormonally regulated.

Intrinsic and Extrinsic Nervous Systems

The GI tract is innervated by both a local intrinsic nervous system and the extrinsic autonomic nervous system. The intrinsic enteric nervous system is responsible for much of the neural regulation of GI motility and function. The enteric nervous system comprises the myenteric plexus, which lies between the muscular layers of the gut and is involved in coordinating the movement of food through the GI tract, and the Meissner plexus, which lies in the submucosa that is under the inner mucosal layer of the gut and is involved in the control of GI secretions and blood flow in the gut wall. The enteric nervous system has both sensory and motor neurons that detect changes in the gut (e.g., as a result of ingesting food or drink) and regulate secretion and motility.

The parasympathetic and sympathetic arms of the autonomic nervous system function along with the enteric nervous system to regulate gut function. In general, parasympathetic stimulation promotes digestion and absorption by increasing GI secretion, increasing muscle tone and peristalsis, and relaxing GI sphincters and blood vessels. On the other hand, sympathetic stimulation has the opposite effects, leading to decreased secretion, decreased muscle tone and movement, and constriction of sphincters and blood vessels. The major parasympathetic supply to the GI tract is via the vagus and pelvic nerves, whose nerve endings in the GI tract release acetylcholine, whereas the major sympathetic nerve endings secrete mainly norepinephrine.

The arrangement of the enteric nervous system and its connections with the sympathetic and parasympathetic systems support several types of GI reflexes that are important in GI control. These reflexes may be integrated entirely within the gut wall enteric nervous system or may involve afferent signals from the receptors in the GI tract that travel back to the central nervous system to trigger efferent output to the same or different parts of the GI tract.

Pacemaker Cells

The GI tract contacts a special type of interstitial cell that seems to serve a pacemaker function. The interstitial cells of Cajal (ICC) create a basal electrical rhythm that generates spontaneous electrical slow waves that spread to smooth muscle cells. These slow waves organize gut smooth muscle contractions into the phasic patterns underlying peristalsis and segmentation. The frequency of ICC activity is about 3 cycles per minute in the stomach and colon, 12 cycles per minute in the duodenum, and 9 cycles per minute in the ileum.

GI Hormones

GI hormones are secreted by enteroendocrine cells located throughout the GI tract (Table 7-1). These enteroendocrine cells do not form endocrine glands but rather secrete GI hormones that exert local effects on the GI tract via paracrine and autocrine actions. They also affect other tissues via endocrine actions after entering the circulation. GI hormones play important roles in regulating GI functions, such as gut motility and the secretion of hydrochloric acid (HCl). The actions of these hormones on other tissues, such as brain, pancreas, liver, and gallbladder, also affect the regulation of the GI tract by these tissues.

BASIC FUNCTIONS OF THE GI TRACT

The major functions of the GI tract are digestion and absorption.

TABLE 7-1 The Endocrine Cells of the GI Tract

CELL NAME	HORMONE	LOCATION	STIMULUS FOR SECRETION	MAIN FUNCTION
G cells	Gastrin	Stomach, mainly pyloric region	Protein in gastric lumen	Stimulates gastric HCl secretion; stimulates pepsinogen secretion; increases gastric motility
X/A-like cells	Ghrelin	Stomach	Fasting	Stimulates gastric emptying; acts via the central nervous system to stimulate appetite
Enterochromaffin-like cells (ECL cells)	Histamine	Stomach	Gastrin	Acts on G cells to stimulate gastrin secretion
D cells in stomach and intestinal mucosa, as well as in pancreatic islets and enteric neurons	Somatostatin	Stomach, intestines, and pancreas	Intake of fat, protein, or glucose; presence of HCl in stomach lumen	Inhibits hormone release from GI tract and pancreas; acts as an enterogastrone to inhibit gastric acid secretion
Enterochromaffin cells (EC cells)	Serotonin	Stomach and intestines	Small intestinal release: intraluminal fluids, nutrients, acid, amino acids, hypertonic and hypotonic solutions; Colonic release: short-chain fatty acids	Stimulates both intrinsic and extrinsic nerves
I cells	Cholecystokinin (CCK)	Duodenum and jejunum	Partially hydrolyzed fat or protein in the duodenum/jejunum; acidic pH of chyme from the stomach entering duodenum	Stimulates contraction of gallbladder; stimulates release of enzymes by exocrine pancreas; inhibits gastric emptying
S cells	Secretin	Duodenum and jejunum	Acidic pH of chyme from the stomach entering duodenum	Stimulates release of bicarbonate-rich secretion by pancreas; inhibits HCl secretion by stomach; decreases gastric motility
K cells	Gastric inhibitory polypeptide (GIP)	Duodenum and proximal jejunum	Food in the small intestine	Stimulates pancreas to secrete insulin
L cells	Glucagon-like peptide-1 (GLP1) Glucagon-like peptide-2 (GLP2)	Small intestine	Food in the small intestine	GLP-1 stimulates pancreas to secrete insulin GLP-2 stimulates nutrient absorption and has trophic effects on the gut mucosa
M cells	Motilin	Duodenum and jejunum	Periodic and recurrent secretion pattern synchronized with phasic contractions during fasting	Stimulates GI motility, regulates phasic contractions

GI, Gastrointestinal; *HCl*, hydrochloric acid.

Digestion

Both mechanical (physical) and enzymatic (chemical) processes are involved in digestion. Mechanical digestion includes the chewing of food and the muscular movements of the stomach and intestines that break food particles into smaller pieces, thus exposing a greater surface area of the food to digestive enzymes. Mechanical digestion also mixes food with various secretions from the GI tract and accessory organs, which facilitates the action of digestive enzymes on the food particles. Chemical digestion is defined as the breakdown of food by enzymes. These enzymes either are secreted into the lumen of the GI tract by glandular cells in the mouth, chief cells in the stomach, or exocrine cells of the pancreas; or they are resident enzymes of the brush border (luminal) membrane or the cytoplasm of mucosal cells of the small intestine. Digestion also involves the effect of gastric acid to denature proteins. Digestion occurs before nutrients can cross the absorptive cells to enter the interstitial fluid/circulatory system.

Absorption

Absorption is the movement of nutrients, including water and electrolytes, across the mucosal epithelial lining facing the lumen of the GI tract into the lamina propria (interstitium), where they enter either the blood or the lymph. Nutrient absorption includes both transcellular (through the epithelial absorptive cells) and paracellular (between the epithelial cells) mechanisms. Most nutrient absorption occurs in the small intestine, which has specialized absorptive cells that effect transcellular uptake. Substances pass from the intestinal lumen into the absorptive cells and then out of the absorptive cells to the extracellular compartment. The processes responsible for movement across the luminal membrane of the absorptive cells are often quite different from those responsible for movement across the basolateral or contraluminal cell membranes to the lamina propria. Paracellular uptake by movement through pores between cells may accomplish absorption of water, ions, and some other small molecules. Once nutrients have entered the lamina propria, they enter either the capillaries (into the blood) or the lacteals (into the lymph).

Other Functions of the GI Tract

In the context of digestion, the GI tract has many secretory functions that help to moisten and lubricate the food, adjust the pH of the GI tract contents, and supply some of the enzymes needed for the luminal digestion process. The GI tract also has important endocrine functions because it contains many enteroendocrine cells that release hormones into the bloodstream. Many of these regulate GI tract function, and some regulate food intake. Excretion is another important function of the GI tract. Undigested food material, bacterial mass, and metabolic wastes excreted by the liver in the bile are all excreted by the GI tract in the feces. In addition, the GI tract is an important part of the immune system. Immunoreactive cells in the lamina propria and submucosa of the GI tract, the layer of mucus covering the epithelium, the tight junctions between the epithelial cells of the mucosa, and lysozyme secretion by Paneth cells in the small intestine all serve to protect the body from pathogens that can enter the body through the GI tract.

THE UPPER GI SYSTEM

Sometimes the GI tract is divided into upper and lower parts. The upper GI regions include the oral cavity, the esophagus, and the stomach. The lower GI tract includes the small intestine, the large intestine, and the rectum. Sometimes the first part of the small intestine, the duodenum, is divided into two parts based upon arterial supply or embryology, with the upper region of the duodenum considered part of the upper GI tract.

THE ORAL CAVITY

The process of digestion and absorption begins with the ingestion of food. A number of factors are involved in regulation of food intake, and the complex process of this regulation is discussed in Chapter 22. In the oral cavity, chewing involves the cutting and grinding of food by the teeth and the crushing of the food bolus into smaller particles. The process of chewing also mixes food with saliva. Secretion of saliva by the salivary glands is stimulated by the parasympathetic nervous system in response to the sight, smell, and taste of food and mechanical stimulation of the oral cavity.

Saliva has many functions, including partial digestion of starch by salivary amylase; antibacterial activity (due to the presence of thiocyanate, lactoferrin, and lysozyme); moistening of the mouth to facilitate speech, chewing, and swallowing; neutralization of acids (due mainly to presence of bicarbonate and carbonic anhydrase in the saliva); moistening and lubricating the bolus of food to facilitate swallowing; and maintaining oroesophageal tissue integrity (due to secretion of epidermal growth factor, which may help to repair the esophagus if it has been damaged, for example by gastric acid). Although salivary amylase is mixed with food in the mouth, most of the digestion by this enzyme is accomplished in the stomach rather than in the oral cavity. The salivary amylase mixed in the food bolus continues to be active in the interior of the bolus for a period of time after the food has been swallowed. Once the food bolus is broken up and the amylase is inactivated by the acidic secretions of the stomach, its action ends. In some species, lingual lipase is secreted by glands in the tongue, and this enzyme is most active in the acidic environment of the gastric lumen. Secretion of lingual lipase is insignificant in humans, but the stomach of humans does secrete a lipase that has similar acid lipase activity.

SWALLOWING

Swallowing is the process by which the food bolus passes from the mouth to the pharynx and on through the esophagus into the stomach. Swallowing begins with the oral phase that is under voluntary neuromuscular control. This initial voluntary action, however, triggers the pharyngeal and esophageal phases, which are under involuntary control by the autonomic nervous system. The swallowing reflex is initiated by touch receptors in the pharynx as the food bolus is pushed to the back of the mouth by the tongue. This swallowing reflex consists of a series of highly coordinated responses that include interruption of breathing, movement of the soft palate to close the entrance to the nasal cavities, movement of the tongue to close the exit from the pharynx back into the mouth, closure of the larynx by the epiglottis so that food does not enter the trachea, contraction of the pharynx to force the bolus into the esophagus, and peristaltic movements in the esophagus that carry the food to the stomach.

THE ESOPHAGUS

The esophagus has a typical tubular organ structure with a sphincter at each end (i.e., at the junctions of the esophagus with the pharynx and the stomach). The mucosa of the esophagus is distensible to accommodate the swallowing of a fairly large bolus of food and hence has a somewhat puckered appearance when the underlying muscle has not been stretched. The mucosal epithelium is a stratified squamous epithelium that is resistant to abrasion. Submucosal glands secrete mucus. In humans, the inner circular and outer longitudinal muscle layers are primarily composed of skeletal muscle fibers in the upper portion of the esophagus and of smooth muscle in the lower part of the esophagus near the junction with the stomach. The food bolus can move through the approximately 25-cm-long esophagus and enter the stomach in less than 10 seconds.

Reflexes initiated during swallowing relax the upper esophageal sphincter to let food pass, after which various muscles of the pharynx as well as peristalsis by the muscles of the esophagus sequentially push the bolus of food through the esophagus. Coordinated contractions of the esophageal muscles produce the waves of peristalsis that propel the bolus through the esophagus. The lower esophageal sphincter relaxes before the contraction wave, allowing food to enter the stomach. The lower esophageal sphincter then closes to prevent the reflux of stomach acid into the esophagus.

When the lower esophageal sphincter does not close properly, the acidic stomach contents rise up into the esophagus. This is known as acid reflux or acid regurgitation. During pregnancy, the lower esophageal sphincter may be more relaxed than usual, and there may be increased pressure on the stomach as a result of the growing baby. This may allow the reflux of acid into the esophagus, giving the feeling of heartburn and regurgitation. Smoking and obesity are also factors that contribute to frequent acid reflux. Certain foods, such as alcohol, chocolate, and peppermints, may worsen symptoms because they relax the lower esophageal sphincter and slow gastric emptying. Occasional gastroesophageal reflux is common, but persistent reflux that occurs more than twice per week is considered more serious because the stomach acid can damage and inflame the esophageal mucosa. Gastroesophageal reflux disease may occur because of weak contraction or abnormal relaxation of the lower esophageal sphincter, a hiatal hernia in which a small portion of the stomach pushes up through the diaphragm, or weak muscle contractions in the esophagus.

THE STOMACH

The food bolus exits the lower esophageal sphincter through the cardiac orifice, the opening that connects the cardia region of the stomach to the esophagus. Vagal reflexes initiated by the cephalic phase of eating (i.e., by the sight, smell, thought, or taste of food) inhibit contractile activity in the proximal stomach even when the stomach is empty, and the entry of food into the stomach promotes relaxation of the cardia of the stomach. Thus the stomach muscles relax in preparation for the entrance of food and in response to the entrance of food. When relaxed and empty, the adult human stomach has a volume of about 0.05 L, but it normally expands to hold about 1 L of food and liquid and can hold up to 2 L or more with associated discomfort.

Functions of the Stomach

The stomach serves several functions in digestion and absorption. First, it temporarily stores the swallowed food and liquid until it is passed to the intestines. Second, the stomach secretes HCl, enzymes or zymogens needed for initiating digestion, endocrine hormones that regulate the process of food assimilation, and intrinsic factor that is essential for vitamin B_{12} absorption in the small intestine. Third, the stomach mixes up the food, liquid, and digestive juice produced by the stomach and then macerates this mixture into a semiliquid state. This semiliquid mass of partly digested food is called chyme. Fourth, the stomach regulates the rate of entry of chyme into the small intestine. Although food undergoes substantial physical and chemical modifications in the stomach, little absorption occurs. Some water, salts, and lipid-soluble substances such as ethanol and short-chain fatty acids are absorbed, however.

Basic Anatomy of the Stomach

The stomach has four gross anatomical regions: cardia, fundus, body (or corpus), and pyloric antrum (Figure 7-3). The body, which is the largest part of the stomach, extends from the cardia to the pylorus, the sections that connect with the esophagus and the small intestine, respectively. The fundus is the upper end of the stomach that lies above the cardia and superior to the opening of the esophagus. The pylorus is sometimes described as having two sections: a pyloric antrum that narrows into the pyloric canal. The pyloric canal is surrounded by thickened, circular smooth muscle fibers to form a pyloric sphincter at the opening of the pyloric canal into the duodenum; this sphincter helps control the evacuation of food from the stomach. The lining of the stomach has folds or plaits called rugae, which are most pronounced toward the pyloric end of the stomach. They flatten and disappear as the stomach is filled and distends.

The tubular structure of the stomach wall follows the basic four-layer structure: mucosa, submucosa, muscle layers, and serosa. The mucosa comprises a simple columnar epithelium, which lines the luminal surface of the stomach and the gastric pits; the lamina propria, which contains various glands, depending on the region of the stomach; and a thin smooth muscle layer. The submucosa of the stomach contains no glands. The muscle layers of the stomach include the circular (middle) and longitudinal (outer) layers of muscle found in other parts of the GI system as well as an inner oblique layer that is responsible for creating the motion that churns and physically grinds the food. The serosa consists of connective tissue that is continuous with the peritoneum. The simple columnar epithelial cells that form the luminal surface layer of the stomach are usually

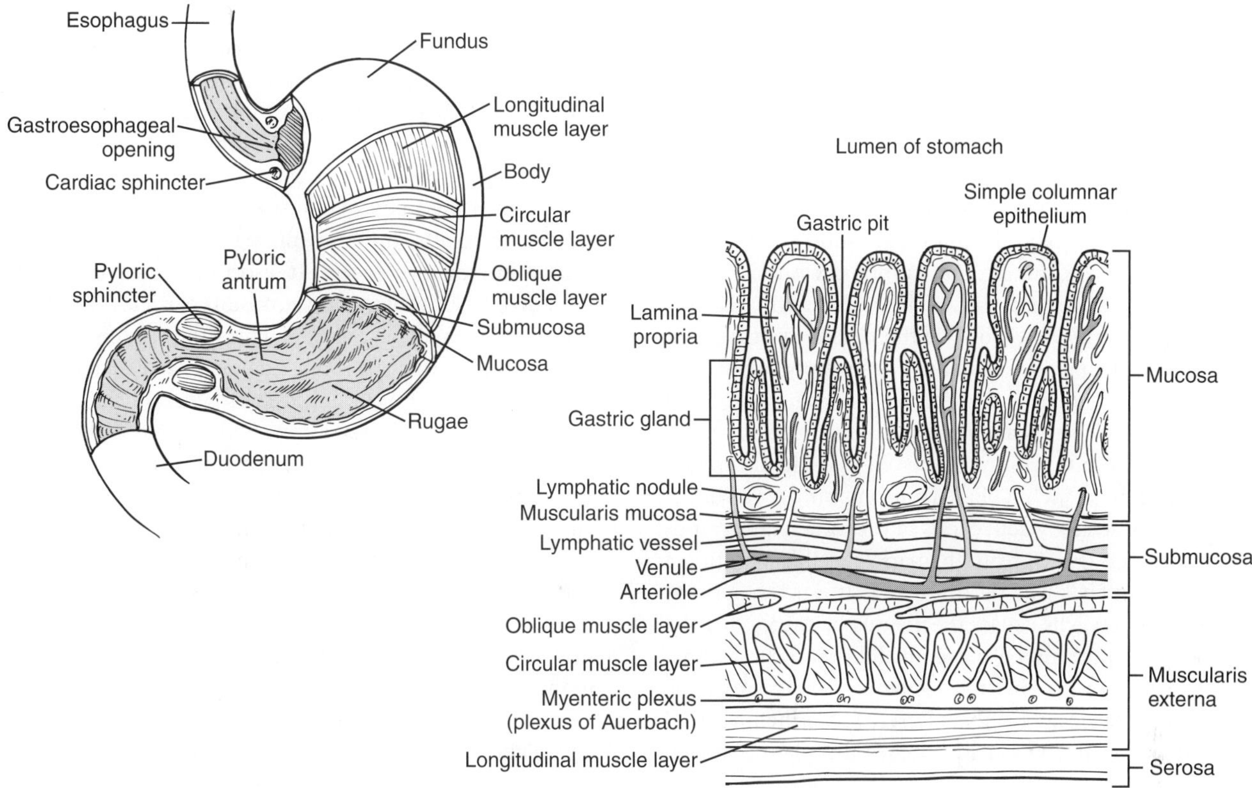

FIGURE 7-3 Diagrams showing the gross anatomy *(left)* and fine anatomy *(right)* of the stomach.

referred to as surface mucous cells because they secrete mucus. The layer of mucus on the surface of the mucosal epithelium is important in protecting the stomach lining from damage by acid and proteolytic enzymes secreted by the gastric glands. In fact, the pH of the mucus layer remains nearly neutral because of secretion of bicarbonate by the underlying mucosa, whereas the pH becomes very acidic (pH ~1 to 3) in the stomach lumen due to HCl secretion from the gastric pits when the gastric glands are stimulated.

Gastric Pits and Gastric Glands

The gastric mucosa contains many minute depressions called gastric pits that extend into the mucosal layer. Glands that contain a mixed population of cell types are associated with these gastric pits. The cell types and secretions of the gastric glands vary somewhat by the region of the stomach in which they are located. The glands extend deep into the mucosa layer, surrounded by the connective tissue of the lamina propria, and they open into the base of the gastric pits. Although connective tissue separates the individual glands, most of the volume of the gastric mucosa is occupied by secretory cells, primarily the parietal and chief cells.

Gastric glands contain a mixture of several cell types, including mucoid cells, parietal cells, chief cells, and enteroendocrine cells. The mixed secretions of the exocrine gastric glands are referred to as the gastric juice. The main components of human gastric juice are mucus, secreted by mucoid cells; HCl and intrinsic factor, secreted by parietal cells; and pepsinogens and gastric lipase, secreted by chief cells, along with water, electrolytes, and bicarbonate. Gastric juice is secreted in response to the vagal stimulation associated with eating (e.g., in response to taste and smell) and in response to gastrin released by enteroendocrine cells in the stomach.

The products of the enteroendocrine cells are not secreted into the lumen of the gastric pit and are not a part of the gastric juice. The enteroendocrine secretions may act locally via paracrine mechanisms or be taken up from the extracellular fluid into the bloodstream to circulate to various tissues as endocrine hormones. Vagal reflexes initiated during the initial phase of eating, as well as the lower luminal acidity and distention caused by the entrance of food into the stomach, stimulate release of hormones, including gastrin, by the enteroendocrine cells of the stomach. Protein in food is also a potent stimulator of gastrin release. Gastrin (from G cells) stimulates HCl production by parietal cells in the gastric glands. The main mechanism of gastrin's action is thought to involve enterochromaffin-like (ECL) cells. ECL cells are stimulated by gastrin to release histamine, and it is thought that the stimulation of parietal cells is mainly due to histamine binding secondary to gastrin's effects on histamine release. Gastrin secretion is inhibited by feedback from acid within the lumen of the stomach. This feedback mechanism regulates the amount of gastrin released and therefore the amount of acid secreted in response to a meal.

Ghrelin is another hormone released by the stomach. The release of ghrelin is stimulated by fasting and is suppressed by the ingestion of food. Ghrelin stimulates gastric emptying and acts via the central nervous system to stimulate appetite.

Hydrochloric Acid Secretion and Function

The parietal cells are the source of gastric HCl. Parietal cells contain secretory channels called canaliculi, from which the gastric acid is secreted into the lumen of the stomach. Gastric acid secretion happens in several steps. First, chloride and hydrogen ions are secreted separately from the cytoplasm of parietal cells and mixed in the canaliculi. H^+ ions are generated within the parietal cell from dissociation of H_2O. The OH^- ions formed in this process combine with CO_2, in a reaction catalyzed by carbonic anhydrase, to form HCO_3^-. The HCO_3^- is transported out of the cell in exchange for Cl^- ions. Thus the parietal cell now has a supply of both H^+ and Cl^- ions for secretion. Cl^- and K^+ ions are transported into the lumen of the canaliculus by conductance channels. H^+ ions are then pumped out of the cell in exchange for K^+ by the membrane H^+,K^+-ATPase (proton pump). The accumulation of osmotically active ions in the canaliculus causes water to diffuse outward from the parietal cell, generating a secretion rich in HCl. The bicarbonate that was transported out of the parietal cells causes the venous blood leaving the stomach to temporarily be more alkaline than the arterial blood delivered to it. This phenomenon is known as the alkaline tide. Gastric acid is then secreted into the lumen of the gastric gland and gradually reaches the main stomach lumen.

The resulting acidic environment (pH ~1 to 3) in the stomach lumen favors the denaturation (unfolding) of proteins, which makes the peptide bonds in the proteins more accessible to proteolytic enzymes. The acidic environment is also necessary to activate the pepsinogens secreted by the chief cells (i.e., to convert pepsinogens to pepsins via autocatalytic cleavage) and to promote the enzymatic activity of the pepsins, which exhibit optimal activity and stability at an acidic pH of approximately 2. Additionally, the gastric acidity destroys many microorganisms that enter the GI tract via the oral cavity. Some organisms such as *Helicobacter pylori* can survive the acidic pH of the lumen long enough to burrow through the mucoid lining of the stomach to find a niche close to the epithelial cell layer. *H. pylori* infection is a common and easily treatable cause of peptic ulcers.

Digestion in the Stomach

Once activated by the acidic environment of the stomach, pepsins begin the process of protein digestion in the stomach by hydrolyzing the protein into large peptide fragments and some free amino acids. Gastric lipase hydrolyzes triacylglycerol in the acidic medium to yield predominantly diacylglycerol and free fatty acids. These products of fat hydrolysis may play a role in beginning the emulsification of lipids in the stomach contents.

Gastric Emptying

Contraction of the stomach muscle layers grinds and mixes the food and gastric secretions to produce the chyme. Gastric motility is stimulated by gastrin and stomach distention. To move from the stomach to the small intestine, chyme must pass through the pyloric sphincter, which is composed of a thickened band of circular muscle that contracts in opposition to an approaching peristalsis. Peristaltic waves squeeze chyme toward the pyloric sphincter and, when there is sufficient pressure, a small amount of the acidic chyme moves through the pyloric sphincter and into the duodenum (the first section of the small intestine). Most, however, squirts back toward the body of the stomach. The retropulsion of the chyme results in better mixing of chyme and breaking of food into smaller pieces. It also facilitates the dispersion of oil droplets into very fine emulsion particles. The dispersion of oil droplets greatly facilitates the subsequent digestion of lipids in the small intestine, because pancreatic lipase acts at the water–lipid interface, and emulsification significantly increases this surface area. Only liquids and small particles in chyme pass through the pyloric sphincter into the small intestine because of the small opening that results from contraction of the pyloric sphincter.

The stomach regulates the amount of food presented to the duodenum so that it does not exceed the absorptive capacity of the small intestine. The rate at which chyme moves from the stomach to the duodenum depends mainly on the tonal contraction of the pyloric sphincter and also on the strength of the peristaltic contractions. The nature of the chyme and the receptivity of the small intestine play important roles in regulating the relaxation of the pyloric sphincter. Gastrin and ghrelin promote gastric emptying, whereas cholecystokinin (CCK), secretin, and gastric inhibitory polypeptide (GIP), which are released by the small intestine in response to the entrance of chyme from the stomach, inhibit gastric motility, gastric secretion, and gastric emptying. It typically takes 3 to 4 hours for the contents of the stomach to empty following a meal, although this depends on the size and composition of the meal as well as other factors such as emotional state.

THE SMALL INTESTINE

Most of the digestion and uptake of nutrients takes place in the small intestine, which is uniquely adapted to accommodate these processes. The small intestine of an adult is about 5 to 7 m in length and 2.5 to 4 cm in diameter. It is divided anatomically into three sections: the duodenum, jejunum, and ileum. The wall of the small intestine has the typical four layers: mucosa, submucosa, smooth muscle with inner circular and outer longitudinal layers, and serosa. The most distinct feature of the small intestine is its highly modified mucosa, which has several features that increase its surface area in support of its important absorptive functions. The lamina propria of the small intestinal mucosa also contains numerous lymphocytes, plasma cells, macrophages, and eosinophils, as well as localized collections of lymphoid tissue called lymphatic nodules.

DUODENUM

The first section of the small intestine is the duodenum, which is approximately 25 cm in length and ends at the point where the ligament of Treitz attaches the intestine

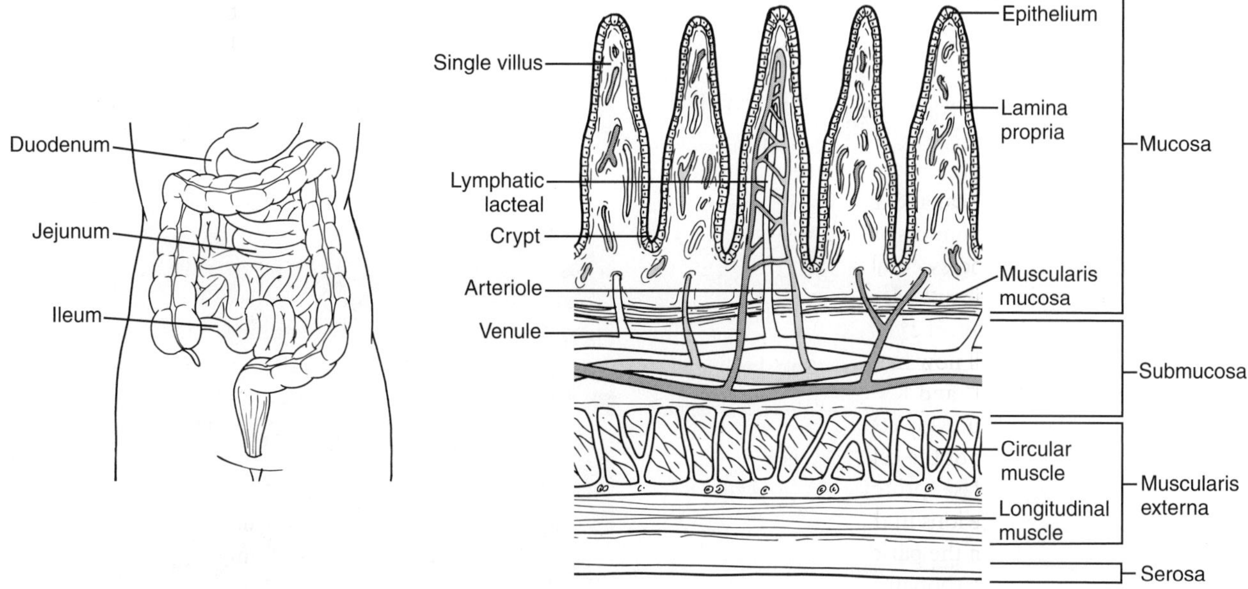

FIGURE 7-4 Diagrams showing the gross anatomy *(left)* and fine anatomy *(right)* of the small intestine.

to the diaphragm. The duodenum receives the acid chyme from the stomach. It also receives secretions from the liver or gallbladder and the pancreas, which enter via the common bile duct. The duodenum has Brunner glands, which in some areas penetrate the muscularis mucosae to enter the submucosa. Brunner glands produce a clear, viscous, alkaline (pH ~8.1 to 9.3) fluid that contains glycoproteins and bicarbonate ions. The secretion of Brunner glands and the bicarbonate-rich secretion from the pancreas protect the proximal small intestine by neutralizing the acidic chyme from the stomach. These alkaline secretions also serve to bring the pH of the intestinal contents close to the optimum for activity of the pancreatic digestive enzymes.

JEJUNUM AND ILEUM

The remainder of the small intestine from the end of the duodenum is arbitrarily divided into jejunum (the upper 40%) and ileum (the lower 60%) (Figure 7-4). There is no clear morphological separation between the two sections, but the character of the intestine does gradually change from the beginning of the jejunum to the end of the ileum. The jejunum has numerous large folds, called plicae circulares. These plicae consist of a core of submucosa and the overlying mucosa. Although they may be present in the duodenum and ileum, they are not as large and are not a significant feature in those regions. Most nutrients are absorbed in the jejunum, with the exceptions of iron and calcium, which are absorbed mostly in the duodenum, and vitamin B_{12} and bile acids, which are absorbed mostly in the ileum. The ileum also serves a reserve function, digesting and absorbing any nutrients that escape these processes in the jejunum.

THE SMALL INTESTINAL MUCOSA

The luminal surface of the small intestine is covered by fingerlike projections called *villi,* which are about 0.5 to 1.5 mm in length. The core of each villus is an extension of the lamina propria, and each villus is covered by a simple columnar epithelium. The core of each villus contains a lymphatic capillary called a lacteal and numerous capillaries. The lacteal is accompanied by smooth muscle fibers arising from the underlying muscularis mucosae, which allow the villus to intermittently contract and expel the contents of the lacteal into the lymphatic network.

Simple tubular structures called *crypts,* which are also covered with simple columnar epithelium, open onto the luminal surface at the bases of the villi and extend downward toward the submucosa. Near the base of the crypts are stem cells that give rise to all epithelial cell types, with the exception of the white blood cells associated with the mucosa. Cells in the crypts secrete a fluid called succus entericus that contains water and electrolytes. These crypt stem cells produce new epithelial cells, allowing the small intestine to continuously renew the cells lining its surface. As the epithelial cells proliferate and migrate up from the crypts to the tips of the villi, the activity of mucosal digestive enzymes and the capacity of the cell to absorb nutrients increases, whereas the cell's capacity to secrete succus entericus decreases. Epithelial cells of the villi have an average life span of approximately 3 to 5 days after they enter the villi from the crypts. Cells are sloughed off from the tips of the villi into the intestinal lumen where they may undergo digestion.

The dominant cell type of the small intestinal columnar epithelium is the *enterocyte* or *absorptive cell,* a tall columnar cell with microvilli that is specialized for the transport of substances (Figure 7-5). Absorbed substances are transported

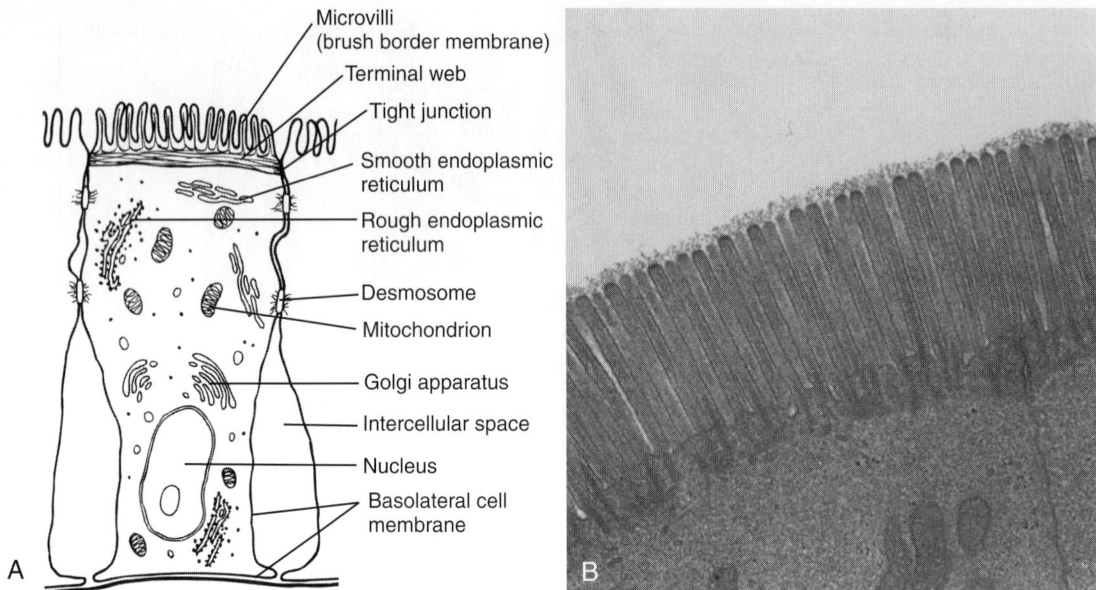

FIGURE 7-5 **A,** Drawing showing the structure of an enterocyte (a small intestinal absorptive cell). **B,** Electron micrograph showing the microvilli, or brush border, membrane of an enterocyte. (From Poley, J. R. [1988]. Loss of the glycocalyx of enterocytes in small intestine. *Journal of Pediatric Gastroenterology and Nutrition 7,* 386–394.)

across these absorptive cells and enter the capillaries or the lymphatic lacteal in the underlying lamina propria. *Microvilli* are minute hairlike projections (approximately 5 μm tall) from the plasma membrane on the apical (lumen-facing) surface of the enterocyte. The microvilli are formed by actin filaments that are attached to the plasma membrane at the tip of the microvillus and that end in a terminal web of actin microfilaments and myosin near the base of the microvillus. Under the microscope, the microvilli resemble the hairs of a paintbrush, giving rise to the term *brush border membrane* to describe the apical membrane of absorptive cells with microvilli. The apical, or brush border, membrane of a single cell has about 3,000 microvilli. The villi and microvilli, along with folds in the submucosa, increase the surface area of the small intestine to about 600 times that of a simple cylinder of the same length and diameter. The final surface area of the small intestine is approximately 200 m^2. The epithelial cells are connected to each other by tight junctions near their apical ends to form a semipermeable seal.

The apical membranes of enterocytes contain numerous glycoproteins. These glycoproteins are inserted into the plasma membrane with their functional domains extending outward toward the lumen. Many of these glycoproteins are digestive enzymes, which are discussed in more detail in Chapters 8 and 9. The matrix formed at the surface of the intestinal epithelium by the carbohydrate side chains of these glycoproteins is known as the *glycocalyx.* This glycocalyx "traps water," giving rise to an *unstirred water layer* near the absorptive surface. Because the fluid layer next to the epithelial cell surface is poorly mixed, the major mechanism for solute movement across the unstirred water layer is diffusion down the concentration gradient.

In addition to enterocytes, the small intestinal mucosal epithelium contains several other kinds of cells. Under the microscope, these nonabsorptive cells can easily be distinguished from the absorptive enterocytes, because the nonabsorptive cells do not have a brush border apical membrane. Mucus-secreting cells, called *goblet cells,* are interspersed among the enterocytes, and their abundance increases from the duodenum to the terminal ileum. *M* or *microfold cells* are associated with underlying aggregates of lymphoid nodules that are called Peyer's patches. M cells sample luminal contents and present antigens to the underlying lymphoid cells where immune responses can be initiated. *Paneth cells* are located at the base of the crypts and secrete antimicrobial substances such as lysozyme and antimicrobial peptides.

Enteroendocrine Cells of the Small Intestine

Enteroendocrine cells are most often found in the lower part of the crypts but can be found anywhere in the epithelium. The most abundant products of these enteroendocrine cells are CCK, secretin, and GIP, all of which are GI hormones that play important roles in regulating GI tract function.

CCK is released by enteroendocrine I cells in the upper small intestine. I cells secrete CCK when they are stimulated by the presence of partially hydrolyzed fat (fatty acids and monoacylglycerol) and protein (amino acids and peptides) in the chyme that enters the duodenum as well as by the initially acidic pH of the chyme. CCK stimulates the release of bile from the gallbladder and secretion of enzyme-rich pancreatic juice by the acinar cells of the exocrine pancreas. CCK also acts on the stomach to inhibit gastric emptying.

Secretin is released by enteroendocrine S cells, which are found in highest densities in the duodenum and jejunum. The S cells are stimulated by the acidic pH of chyme from the stomach to release secretin. In turn, secretin stimulates the secretion of bicarbonate-rich pancreatic juice.

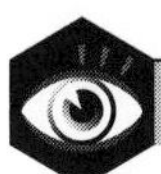

NUTRITION INSIGHT

Oral Tolerance and Food Allergies

The intestinal epithelium has a very large surface area and is exposed to numerous dietary and microbial antigens. The development of oral tolerance is essential for preventing inflammatory responses to these antigens. Oral tolerance refers to the suppression of local and systemic immune responses to an antigen by prior administration of the antigen by the oral route. This can occur because, in addition to forming a barrier that limits penetration of luminal bacteria and dietary allergens, the intestinal epithelium allows antigen sampling by endocytosis and phagocytosis.

Antigens are sampled via their uptake and translocation by epithelial M cells associated with underlying lymphoid tissue, which contains dendritic cells. Dendritic cells are the major intestinal antigen-presenting cells (APCs) in the gut-associated lymphatic tissue. Antigens in the luminal contents are also directly sampled by dentritic cells of the lamina propria that extend their dendrites between the epithelial cells. Subepithelial APCs with captured antigen migrate via the lymph to mesenteric lymph nodes where these cells either mature to become active APCs that stimulate T-effector cells (i.e., T helper cells) for productive immunity or become conditioned for tolerance via the generation and/or expansion of T-regulatory cells. When the intestinal epithelium is exposed to high doses of antigen, oral tolerance can also develop by the clonal deletion, or anergy, of specific T cell clones.

T-regulatory cells are a specialized subpopulation of T cells that suppress activation of the immune system and thereby maintain immune system homeostasis and tolerance to self-antigens. These T-regulatory cells, upon subsequent recognition of antigen, migrate to lymphoid organs, where they suppress immune responses by inhibiting the generation of T-effector cells, and to the target organ, where they suppress disease by releasing cytokines. The T-regulatory cells secrete the suppressive cytokines TGFβ (transforming growth factor beta) and IL10 (interleukin 10), for example.

Interaction of the gut-associated lymphatic tissue with food antigens usually leads to tolerance. However, disruption in the mucosal immune system may lead to food intolerance (also called food hypersensitivity). Food intolerance generally represents either a failure in the development of tolerance or a breakdown of existing tolerance. It may result from defects in immune or nonimmune barriers in the GI tract. A sustained T helper type 2 cell response is one of the major features of food allergy. Risk factors for the development of food allergy include a genetic predisposition to atopy, an immature mucosal immune system, inadequate normal gut flora, an increase in mucosal permeability, immunoglobulin A (IgA) deficiency or other immunological defect, GI infection, formula feeding, and introduction of solid foods before 4 months of age.

Food allergies occur in about 6% to 8% of children and 2% to 4% of adults. The most common food allergens include cow's milk, eggs, peanuts, and seafood. Many studies have indicated that formula feeding of infants and early introduction of solid foods are associated with skewing the immune system toward T helper type 2 cell activity and higher incidence of food allergy (Chahine and Bahna, 2010; Brandtzaeg, 2010). Fortunately, many food allergies of early infancy have a high spontaneous remission rate at around 3 years of age, most likely due to a progressive shift from induction of T helper type 2 cells to induction of T-regulatory cells.

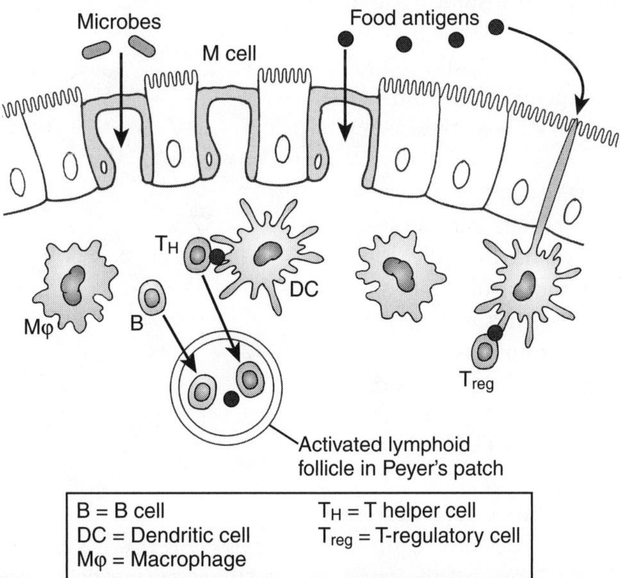

Based on drawing from Brandtzaeg, P. (2010). Food allergy: Separating the science from the mythology. *Nature Reviews Gastroenterology and Hepatology, 7*, 380–400.

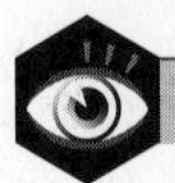

NUTRITION INSIGHT

GI Tract Function in Term and Preterm Infants

The full-term newborn infant exhibits the necessary GI structural and functional characteristics for the assimilation of the nutrients in breast milk. Within the first few days after birth, the mucosal mass and structural features of the mucosa of the intestines undergo dramatic change, with large increases in cellular mass and surface area. The first feedings of colostrum stimulate the growth and development of the GI tract to accommodate the change to oral feeding. Colostrum is the milk produced by the mother during the first few days after delivery; colostrum is enriched in growth factors (e.g., epidermal growth factor, insulin-like growth factors, and transforming growth factors) and immunogenic compounds (e.g., immunoglobulins, immunomodulators, and antimicrobial peptides). Thus term infants are able to consume and assimilate nutrients in adequate quantities to promote the rapid growth that occurs shortly after birth.

Although the unborn infant has a sterile GI tract, a newborn rapidly acquires intestinal microbiota during and after birth from the mother and surrounding environment. The acquired microbiota are a major stimulus for development of the infant's immune system. Initially, the infant is protected by immunoglobulin G (IgG) antibodies that were transferred to the fetus across the placenta, especially during the last few weeks of gestation, and also by the large amounts of secretory IgA obtained after birth from the colostrum and breast milk of the mother. IgA acts in the lumen of the GI tract, where it adheres to mucosal surfaces and prevents pathogens from sticking to or penetrating the barrier provided by the GI epithelium.

Preterm infants, on the other hand, may be unable to consume enteral nutrients because of an underdeveloped swallowing reflex, lack of the enzyme lactase needed to hydrolyze milk sugar, and an immature motility pattern for digestion. The diminished transfer of IgG before birth and the lack of acquisition of IgA by intake of colostrum and milk after birth contribute to the higher risk of infection observed in premature babies. The goals of nutrition therapy for premature infants are to support the overall growth of the infant as well as the development of the digestive, absorptive, and immune functions of the GI tract. Enteral feeding of the preterm infant contributes to body growth and intestinal development as well as to immunological protection. To the extent possible, the preterm neonate will benefit from enteral feeding of colostrum and breast milk (Commare and Tappenden, 2007; Neu, 2007). Infants who require intravenous (parenteral) feeding are likely to benefit from small-volume enteral feedings to supplement the parenteral nutrition, because this will provide additional nutrients for growth, immunoglobulins for protection, and growth factors that promote maturation of the infant's GI tract. Very premature infants (less than 32 weeks gestational age) are not able to coordinate sucking activities during the swallowing process and are usually fed by nasogastric tube.

GIP is synthesized by K cells in the mucosa of the duodenum and jejunum. It is an incretin, which is a name given to GI hormones that increase the amount of insulin released by the pancreas, even before plasma glucose levels become elevated. GIP is also known as glucose-dependent insulinotropic peptide in recognition of this function. Glucagon-like peptide-1 (GLP1) is another incretin. GLP1 is synthesized by L cells in the small intestine.

Hormone secretions of the small intestine serve to (1) stimulate pancreatic and biliary secretions into the small intestine to facilitate the processing of chyme from the stomach; (2) inhibit gastric acid secretion and motility and thus slow the emptying of stomach contents into the small intestine; and (3) prepare the body for the influx of nutrients. When the intestine is full, the stomach acts mainly as storage for food.

ROLES OF THE PANCREAS AND LIVER IN FUNCTION OF THE SMALL INTESTINE

The exocrine cells of the pancreas synthesize and secrete enzymes or the zymogen precursors of enzymes required for digestion of macromolecules in the lumen of the small intestine (Figure 7-6). The pancreatic juice also provides a rich source of bicarbonate to neutralize the HCl in the chyme entering the duodenum from the stomach. Enzymes and zymogens in the pancreatic juice include pancreatic

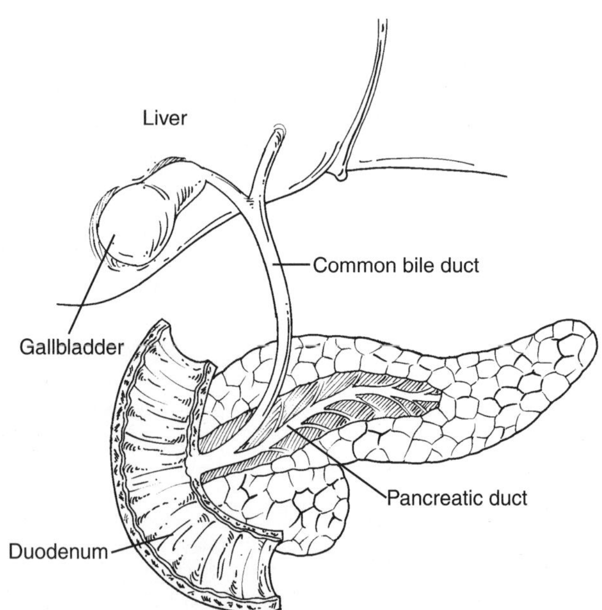

FIGURE 7-6 Diagram showing the bile duct and pancreatic duct and the entrance of both bile and pancreatic secretions into the duodenum via the common bile duct.

α-amylase, lipases (pancreatic lipase and carboxylester lipase), prophospholipase A_2, nucleolytic enzymes (ribonuclease and deoxyribonuclease), several proenzymes for proteolytic enzymes (trypsinogen, chymotrypsinogen, proelastase, and procarboxypeptidases), and a nonenzyme protein called procolipase. Pancreatic enzymes are most active in the neutral pH range, and the rapid neutralization of the gastric acid in the upper duodenum facilitates digestion of nutrients by pancreatic enzymes. CCK and secretin stimulate the secretion of pancreatic juice in response to chyme entering the small intestine.

The liver secretes bile into the bile duct that empties into the duodenum. Between meals, the duodenal opening of this duct is closed and bile flows into the gallbladder, a saccular organ that is attached to the common hepatic bile duct and serves to store and concentrate bile. Secretin stimulates bile secretion by the liver, and CCK stimulates gallbladder contraction to release stored bile. Bile is an alkaline solution containing electrolytes, pigments, bile salts, and other substances. Bile salts play an important role in the normal digestion and absorption of lipids, as is discussed in more detail in Chapter 10.

The pancreatic duct joins with the hepatic bile duct to form the common bile duct just before entering the duodenum, so the bile mixes with pancreatic secretions before they enter the duodenum. Pancreatic and biliary secretions enter the upper duodenum through the sphincter of Oddi, and luminal digestion begins in the duodenum and jejunum. The jejunum is the major site for the uptake of nutrients, and the absorption of most nutrients is complete before the chyme reaches the ileum. If nutrients are still present in chyme that reaches the ileum, the "ileal brake" slows the emptying of chyme from the stomach and also slows intestinal motility. When unabsorbed nutrients, particularly fatty acids, enter the ileum, they stimulate the release of regulatory peptides such as GIP that activate the so-called ileal brake response. It should be noted, however, that products of macronutrient digestion are typically completely absorbed long before the digesta enter the ileum.

DIGESTIVE ENZYMES OF THE SMALL INTESTINE

Although the digestion of most nutrients in the small intestine is extensively carried out by enzymes secreted by the pancreas, enzymes located at the apical surface of the plasma membrane of enterocytes are responsible for the completion of this digestive process to release molecules that can be transported across the membrane. Several α-glucosidases, a β-galactosidase, and several peptidases are present in the membrane. These enzymes are necessary for further digestion of oligosaccharide and peptide products of luminal hydrolysis, as well as hydrolysis of dietary disaccharides and other compounds. These apical or brush border membrane enzymes are called ectoenzymes because they are located outside the cell (i.e., on the luminal rather than the cytoplasmic side of the membrane). As for other membrane glycoproteins, the hydrophobic domain of the protein is generally anchored to the lipid bilayer of the apical membrane, and the bulk of the protein, including the active enzymatic domain(s), is exposed to the extracellular environment of the intestinal lumen.

Some final processes important for completing the process of preparing nutrients to enter the circulation occur inside the enterocytes. In addition to oligopeptide digestion by apical enzymes before absorption of the amino acid, dipeptide, and tripeptide products, enzymes in the cytosol of enterocytes are involved in completing the process of peptide hydrolysis. Peptidases in the cytosol of enterocytes catalyze the hydrolysis of small peptides to free amino acids. Also present in the cytosol of the enterocytes are enzymes that are involved in the assimilation of lipid digestion products to reform triacylglycerols, cholesteryl esters, and phospholipids from the simpler lipids that have been absorbed. This resynthesis process is necessary for the incorporation of lipids into chylomicrons, the lipoprotein complexes in which most products of lipid digestion and absorption ultimately exit across the basolateral membrane and then enter the lymphatic vessels and ultimately the blood.

Digestion of carbohydrates, proteins, and lipids is discussed more extensively in Chapters 8 to 10.

ABSORPTION OF NUTRIENTS IN THE SMALL INTESTINE

Absorption involves the movement of simple nutrients from the lumen of the GI tract across the epithelium into the extracellular matrix of the lamina propria, where they can enter either the capillaries or the small lymphatic vessels. The movement of nutrients and electrolytes across the small intestinal epithelium occurs by both transcellular and paracellular transport mechanisms.

Transcellular Uptake of Nutrients

Absorption of nutrients usually involves their movement through the apical or brush border membrane into the enterocyte and then across the basolateral membrane of the enterocyte into the interstitial fluid. Transcellular uptake is usually mediated by one of several general mechanisms, as illustrated in Figure 7-7, but different transporters may be involved at the apical membrane than at the basolateral membrane.

The uptake of nutrients and electrolytes by the small intestinal epithelial cells may be by passive diffusion down a concentration gradient, with movement occurring through the lipid bilayer of the apical membrane or through water-filled pores that are present either in the membrane or between the cells. Uptake of substances across the apical membrane may also occur by carrier-mediated transport systems, which may be either passive or active. *Passive carrier-mediated transport* is often called facilitated diffusion because, as for simple diffusion, movement is also down an electrochemical gradient from an area of high concentration to one of low concentration. Many compounds require a specific carrier for absorption because they cannot pass through the lipid bilayer of the membrane or through pores or channels. These specific transporters may function as uniports (moving only one compound), symports (moving two compounds together in the same direction), or antiports (or exchangers, which move

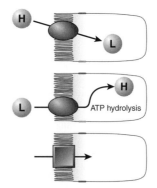

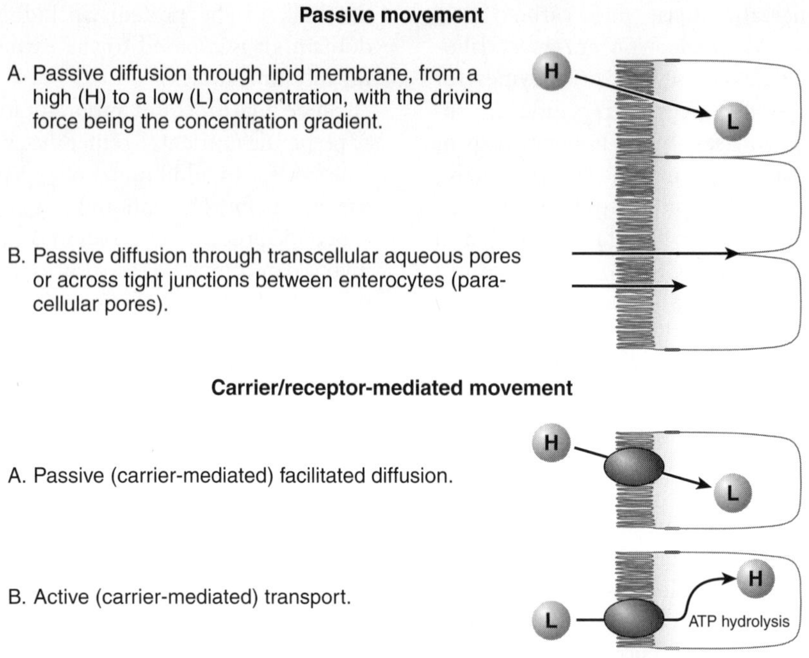

Passive movement
A. Passive diffusion through lipid membrane, from a high (H) to a low (L) concentration, with the driving force being the concentration gradient.
H
L
B. Passive diffusion through transcellular aqueous pores or across tight junctions between enterocytes (paracellular pores).
Carrier/receptor-mediated movement
A. Passive (carrier-mediated) facilitated diffusion.
H
L
B. Active (carrier-mediated) transport.
H
L
ATP hydrolysis
C. Receptor-mediated (exo-/endocytosis, pinocytosis).

FIGURE 7-7 Mechanisms of movement of nutrients across the membranes of intestinal absorptive cells.

one substance in and a different substance out of the cell). Facilitated diffusion can be bidirectional, allowing for an equalization of the concentration of a substance on both sides of the membrane. An example of passive mediated transport systems is the Na^+-independent hexose transporters.

Active carrier-mediated transport involves energy expenditure, and these systems are usually unidirectional and concentrative. Energy is supplied via ATP hydrolysis, but the energy requirement may be *primary* or *secondary.* For example, sodium (Na^+) and potassium (K^+) concentrations in cells are maintained by the Na^+,K^+-ATPase, which pumps Na^+ out of cells and K^+ into cells (against their concentration gradients) at the expense of ATP hydrolysis; this is primary active transport of Na^+ and K^+ by an antiport. The stoichiometry of the Na^+,K^+-ATPase reaction is 1 mol of ATP hydrolysis coupled to the outward pumping of 3 mol of Na^+ and the simultaneous inward pumping of 2 mol of K^+. This generates a low intracellular Na^+ concentration and an electrical potential of about −60 mV in the cytosol relative to the extracellular fluid. Electrochemical gradients such as this one for Na^+ are used to drive what is called secondary active transport. In secondary active transport, the energy is directly derived from a concentration gradient or an electrical potential, or both, across the membrane rather than from the chemical energy of a covalent bond change, such as occurs with ATP hydrolysis. However, energy is still required to establish the gradients, such as that established by the Na^+,K^+-ATPase, that provide the electrochemical "force" for solute uptake. The sodium/glucose cotransporter 1 (SGLT1) is an example of a secondary active transporter that relies on the gradients maintained by the Na^+,K^+-ATPase for transport of glucose across the apical membrane of enterocytes. SGLT1 is a symport, and it is able to transport glucose against its concentration gradient because of the cotransport of Na^+ down its electrochemical gradient. Similarly, there are symports in the gut for H^+ and dipeptides or tripeptides that are coupled to active transport processes.

Mediated transport allows uptake of nutrients and other compounds to be site-specific, because only the segment of the small intestine that expresses the carrier protein is capable of taking up the substrate. The advantage of expressing transporters in a subsegment of the small intestine is illustrated by the concentrative reuptake of bile salts by a Na^+/bile acid cotransport system in the apical membrane of only those enterocytes in the lower portion of the ileum. By delaying the uptake of bile salts until they reach the lower ileum, the presence of adequate bile salts in the lumen of the small intestine for efficient lipid digestion is ensured.

In addition to diffusion and carrier-mediated transport, a third mechanism for uptake of some large molecules is *pinocytosis* (either endocytosis or exocytosis). Receptor-mediated endocytosis may be responsible for uptake of some larger peptides from the lumen of the small intestine. Similarly, molecules may be transported out of cells by exocytosis. An example of exocytosis is the transport of triacylglycerol-rich chylomicrons from the cytosol of enterocytes across the basolateral membrane so that they can enter the lymphatic vessels. Pinocytosis also accomplishes the nonspecific transport of any smaller molecules that are trapped within the endocytic or exocytic vesicles.

CLINICAL CORRELATION

Roux-en-Y Gastric Bypass Surgery

In persons with very severe obesity, surgery may be the only effective means of weight loss when treatment by diet and exercise fails. The most effective surgery is the Roux-en-Y gastric bypass, which is done to both restrict food intake and cause malabsorption. The surgeon first creates a gastric pouch from a small part of the upper stomach. Next, the smaller stomach is connected directly to the middle portion of the small intestine, bypassing the lower stomach, the duodenum, and the first portion of the jejunum. Finally, the bypassed digestive section is attached to the lower section of the small intestine, allowing upper GI tract, pancreatic, and biliary secretions to eventually mix with food. The name of the procedure is derived from the name of the French surgeon (César Roux) who first devised it and the Y-shaped representation of the anastomosis of the bypassed portion of the upper small intestine with the distal small intestine.

The dramatically reduced size of the stomach effectively limits the amount of food that can be consumed. The bypass of the upper small intestine and the delayed mixing of food with pancreatic and biliary secretions reduce the extent of digestion and absorption. Because food does not pass through the duodenum, GI peptides such as CCK and secretin are not released in adequate amounts to trigger normal release of pancreatic exocrine secretions and bile, further impairing macronutrient digestion. It is the combination of reduced food intake and the mild malabsorption caused by the Roux-en-Y bypass that makes this surgery such an effective weight loss treatment.

Patients who undergo Roux-en-Y bypass surgery typically lose 50% to 75% of their initial excess weight, and this weight reduction is sustained with long-term follow-up. Most importantly, the weight loss is sufficient to resolve or significantly reduce most of the life-threatening medical conditions associated with severe clinical obesity. Bariatric surgery frequently improves glucose intolerance and eliminates diabetes. On the other hand, the same principles that induce weight loss (i.e., reduced food intake and malabsorption) can also result in deficiencies of macronutrients, vitamins, and minerals. Deficiencies of iron and calcium, which are normally absorbed in the duodenum, and of vitamin B_{12}, which requires binding to intrinsic factor produced by gastric glands in stomach, are common. Deficiencies of vitamin D and folic acid are also frequently observed (Gasteyger et al., 2008).

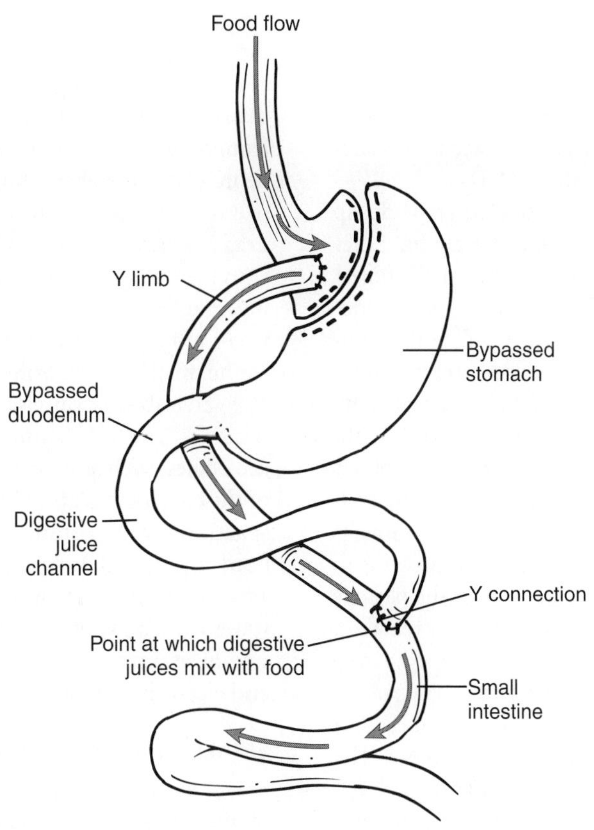

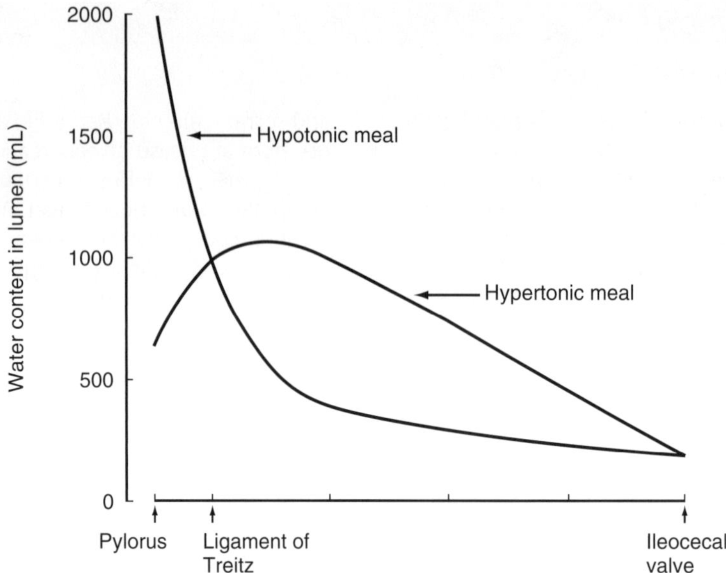

FIGURE 7-8 Water content in the lumen of the small intestine after a hypotonic (steak) meal and a hypertonic (doughnut and milk) meal.

Paracellular Uptake of Nutrients

Paracellular uptake of nutrients occurs through the tight junctions, adherens junctions, and desmosomes between adjacent epithelial cells. This uptake can be described as unmediated passive diffusion, driven by electrochemical or osmotic gradients or by solvent drag, because no specific carrier is involved. Paracellular diffusion of small molecules is mainly restricted by pore size in the tight junction, with most pores being 8 to 9 Å in diameter; in general, the paracellular pathway accommodates molecules with a molecular mass less than 600 Da.

Tight junctions are macromolecular structures made up of several transmembrane proteins (claudins, occludin, junctional adhesion molecules, and tricellulin) that form the pores. These transmembrane proteins interact with membrane-associated zonula occludens proteins that regulate the perijunctional actinomyosin ring. Claudins, a large family consisting of 24 members, determine the size and charge selectivity as well as the permeability of the paracellular pores. Tight junctions regulate paracellular movement of ions and solutes in many physiological and pathological states. Cytokine production in response to allergic and inflammatory reactions is known to lead to reorganization of tight junction proteins to increase intestinal permeability. This can increase the passage of allergens that tend to perpetuate the inflammatory reaction.

Absorption of Water in the Small Intestine

Water is transported both ways across the intestinal epithelium, and this is largely driven by osmotic gradients. The small intestine absorbs a large volume of water, perhaps 7 L, each day, with much of this water coming from salivary, gastric, intestinal, pancreatic, and biliary secretions as well as water taken in as food and beverage. This water is absorbed through both transcellular pores and paracellular pores. Transcellular transport of water across the plasma membranes of enterocytes and other cells is mediated by aquaporins that form selective pores for movement of water along the osmotic gradient. Paracellular uptake occurs across the tight junctions via size- and charge-selective pores.

The osmolality of the plasma is about 300 mOsm. When a hypotonic meal is ingested, water is rapidly absorbed by the duodenum and the jejunum paracellularly (between the cells) through the tight junctions. The tight junctions (pores between intestinal epithelial cells) of the duodenum and the jejunum have a larger diameter (8 Å) than those existing in the ileum (4 Å). The absorption of water facilitates the absorption of electrolytes by the small intestine via a process called solvent drag in which dissolved solutes are carried ("dragged") along with the water. On the other hand, when a hypertonic meal is ingested, water is drawn into the lumen. The accumulation of water in the lumen and the absorption of ions and nutrients by the small intestine bring the luminal contents to isotonicity.

Water absorption also follows the osmotic changes that occur as a result of nutrient absorption. Uptake of small molecules, such as glucose or amino acids, makes the cytosol of the enterocytes and the interstitial fluid in the basolateral spaces more hypertonic, and this may pull water through both transcellular and paracellular pores. The proximal small intestine plays an important role in the absorption of water from a hypotonic meal, whereas the distal small intestine plays a more important role in the absorption of water and electrolytes following a hypertonic meal (Figure 7-8).

SMALL INTESTINAL MOTILITY

Small intestinal motility facilitates both digestion and uptake of nutrients by the small intestine. The rate of digestion depends on the duration of exposure of nutrients to the enzymes in the lumen of the small intestine and on the thorough mixing of intestinal contents. Mixing is achieved by the presence of slow waves of contraction, followed by relaxation of different segments of the small intestine. The frequency of contraction gradually decreases from the duodenum to the ileum, ensuring that the digesta is slowly moved along the length of the small intestine.

CHEMISTRY AND THE ENTEROHEPATIC CIRCULATION OF BILE ACIDS

Because of its role in bile acid synthesis and secretion, the liver plays an important role in the digestion and uptake of lipids by the GI tract. The primary bile acids, cholic acid and chenodeoxycholic acid, are synthesized from cholesterol in the liver. The liver conjugates bile acids with either glycine or taurine to form more polar compounds. The ionizable sulfonate group of taurine or the ionizable carboxyl group of glycine is a stronger acid than the carboxyl group of the unconjugated bile acid. Thus conjugated bile acids exist as negatively charged sulfonate or carboxylate ions. The ratio of glycine to taurine conjugates in adult human bile is about 3:1. Because bile contains significant amounts of Na^+ and K^+ and has an alkaline pH, the bile acids and their conjugates exist in bile in a salt form (i.e., as bile salts). The terms *bile acid* and *bile salt* may be used interchangeably. The bile acids also solubilize cholesterol in the bile, permitting some cholesterol to be transported from the liver to the intestine for excretion in the feces (if it is not reabsorbed).

Conjugated bile acids exhibit detergent properties. At neutral pH values above their pK_as (i.e., above pH 1.5 to 3.7) and at concentrations above 2 to 5 mmol/L, they reversibly form aggregates called micelles. Bile acids facilitate emulsification of dietary fat, increasing the surface area between the lipid and aqueous phases; promote digestion of dietary lipids; and promote the subsequent incorporation of the products of lipid digestion into micelles, favoring their absorption.

Bile acids are absorbed into the portal circulation via passive diffusion along the entire small intestine, and more importantly by receptor-mediated transport in the lower ileum. The recirculation of bile acids (or other compounds) between the small intestine and the liver is called the enterohepatic circulation. The enterohepatic recirculation of bile acids is 99% efficient, with a loss of only about 1% into the colon. The body pool of bile acids (~4 g) is recycled through the intestine about 12 times per day (depending on the frequency of meal intake); a loss of 1% (0.04 g) per pass results in a loss of about 500 mg of bile salts per day via the feces. This loss is compensated by daily synthesis in the liver of an equivalent amount of bile acids from cholesterol. Although only a small percentage of the bile acids is lost in the feces with each pass through the intestinal tract, this loss along with the demand for cholesterol metabolism to replete the bile acid pool represents the major route for excretion of cholesterol from the body.

Some of the primary bile acids in the intestine are metabolized by intestinal bacteria, leading to their deconjugation and 7α-dehydroxylation to produce secondary bile acids; deoxycholate is produced from cholate, and lithocholate is produced from chenodeoxycholate. These secondary bile acids, especially deoxycholate, may be reabsorbed and participate in the enterohepatic circulation along with the primary bile acids.

The enterohepatic circulation of bile acids can be considered as two basic processes: secretion from the liver and absorption from the intestine. Specific transporters of bile acids are required for both processes, as shown in Figure 7-9 (Dawson et al., 2009; Pellicoro and Faber, 2007). The hepatocytes of the liver are polarized with sinusoidal (basolateral) and canalicular (apical) plasma membrane. Bile acids are secreted across the canalicular membrane into the bile by the ATP-dependent bile salt export pump (BSEP) and by the multidrug resistance protein MRP2. Bile acids are then delivered to the intestinal lumen where they emulsify dietary lipids and cholesterol to facilitate their absorption. Intestinal epithelial cells in the distal ileum reabsorb the majority of the secreted bile acids through the apical Na^+-dependent bile acid transporter (ASBT), as well as by Na^+-independent organic anion transporting peptides (OATPs). Cytosolic ileal bile acid binding protein (IBABP) mediates the transcellular movement of bile acids to the basolateral membrane, across which they exit the enterocyte via the heteromeric organic solute transporter (OSTα/OSTβ) to then enter the portal circulation. Upon reaching the liver sinusoids, the majority of conjugated bile acids are taken up across the sinusoidal membranes of hepatocytes via Na^+-dependent and independent mechanisms, mediated by Na^+-taurocholate cotransporting polypeptide (NTCP) and OATPs, respectively. Intracellular transport within hepatocytes back to the canalicular membrane is mediated by several possible transport proteins. An essential role of bile acid transporters is evident from the pathologies associated with their genetic disruption or dysregulation of their functions.

METABOLISM OF NUTRIENTS IN THE ENTEROCYTES

Following the uptake of digestion products into the enterocytes, nutrients are transported across the absorptive cell and exit the basolateral membrane to the interstitium, where they enter the portal blood or the lymphatic vessels for passage to other parts of the body. However, some of the nutrients taken up from the gut are used by the enterocytes themselves and thus do not leave the cell. Because the small intestinal epithelial cells are metabolically very active and are continuously renewed, nutrients taken up from the intestinal lumen, as well as nutrients supplied by the arterial circulation, are necessary for maintenance of the structural and functional integrity of the small intestinal mucosa. The small intestine particularly uses glutamine as a fuel, as is discussed further in Chapters 9 and 14, and glutamine also stimulates the proliferation of enterocytes. Fasting causes atrophy of the small intestinal mucosa, and this atrophy can be reversed by feeding certain amino acids such as glutamine.

Within the enterocytes, most of the products of fat digestion, particularly the monoacylglycerols and long-chain fatty acids, are reesterified to form triacylglcyerols, which are incorporated into chylomicrons and exported across the basolateral membrane. Chylomicrons also contain cholesteryl esters, phospholipids, fat-soluble vitamins, and other lipids.

TRANSPORT OF NUTRIENTS INTO THE CIRCULATION

Nutrients that are absorbed from the GI tract are subsequently transported via either the portal circulation or the lymphatic system. Most of the water-soluble nutrients (amino acids, monosaccharides, glycerol, short-chain fatty acids, electrolytes, and water-soluble vitamins) are transported predominantly by the portal route. These nutrients enter the capillaries that feed into the portal vein, which carries the venous blood draining the splanchnic bed. The liver is unusual in that 75% of its blood supply is the portal venous blood, with the hepatic artery supplying only about 25% of the liver's blood flow. The passage of venous blood from the splanchnic bed through the liver before it is returned to the heart allows the liver to take up nutrients or release metabolites into the venous blood before the blood is returned to the arterial circulation supplying other body tissues.

The lymphatic system in the GI tract plays a pivotal role in the transport of lipophilic substances. Chylomicrons are too large to enter the pores of the capillaries but can pass through the large fenestrations of the lacteals. The lymphatic vessels ultimately empty into the venous circulation by way of the thoracic duct before the circulation enters the heart. A substance transported by the lymphatic system will thus enter the blood just before it goes to the heart and will then circulate throughout the body in the arterial blood with no first pass through the liver.

The lymphatic system is important in maintaining fluid balance in the body because it acts as a drainage system to return excess fluid and proteins in the extracellular fluids back into the circulatory system. Although many of the molecules carried by the portal circulation can also be carried by the lymphatic circulation, the portal blood flow is many times greater than lymphatic flow, so transport by the lymphatic circulation is only of relatively minor significance, compared with the portal circulation, for transport of most water-soluble compounds.

MOVEMENT OF THE REMAINS OF CHYME INTO THE LARGE INTESTINE

At the end of the ileum, the remains of the chyme pass through the ileocecal value into the large intestine. The relaxation of the ileocecal sphincter and contractile activity of the ileum is promoted by gastrin released during the gastric phase. The passage of chyme through the small intestine takes about 3 to 4 hours. It takes about 2 hours for the first part of a meal to reach the large intestine, and all of the undigested portion from a meal leaves the small intestine and enters the colon within about 8 hours of eating. By the time the chyme has reached the colon, most nutrients and about 90% of the water have been absorbed, but some electrolytes, water, and undigested material (which is normally mostly from the indigestible polysaccharides and resistant proteins) remain. Ileostomy

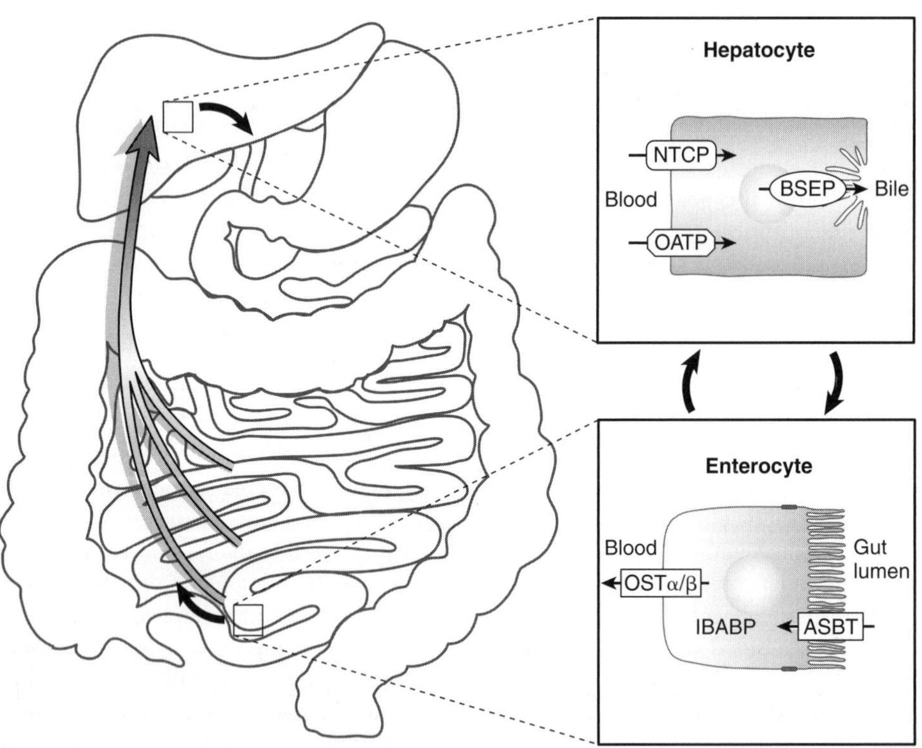

FIGURE 7-9 The enterohepatic recirculation of bile acids. The main hepatocyte and ileal enterocyte transporters responsible for the enterohepatic circulation of bile salts are shown as white boxes. Bile acids synthesized in hepatocytes are secreted through the canalicular membrane into the bile, which eventually is secreted into the duodenum. These bile acids can be reabsorbed by enterocytes and subsequently carried back to the liver by the portal blood. *ASBT (SLCIOA2)*, apical Na^+-dependent bile salt transporter; *BSEP (ABCB11)*, Bile salt export pump; *IBABP*, ileal bile acid binding protein; *NTCP (SLCIOA1)*, sodium-taurocholate cotransporting polypeptide; *OATP (SLCO1)*, organic anion transporting peptide; *OSTα/β*, heteromeric organic solute transporter.

effluent, which was collected from ileostomy patients who consumed a typical British diet, contained about 40 g of dry matter per day, comprising 16 g of carbohydrate, 16 g of protein, 1 g of fat, and 7 g of minerals (ash). The amount of dry matter entering the colon would be higher in individuals consuming high-fiber diets. Some of the protein entering the colon, such as mucins and enzymes secreted into the GI tract, is of endogenous rather than dietary origin.

THE LARGE INTESTINE

The large intestine extends from the ileocecal junction to the anus and consists of the cecum, the colon, and the rectum (Figure 7-10). The large intestine is about 1.5 m long and has a diameter of about 9 cm. Thus the large intestine is so named because it has a much larger diameter than the small intestine; the large intestine is only about 20% to 30% as long as the small intestine. The colon constitutes the majority of the length of the large intestine. The cecum lays just below the opening of the ileum into the colon and is a small pouch that is about 6 cm long. The vermiform appendix hangs off the cecum and opens into it. The colon is continuous with the rectum, the short terminal segment of the digestive tube that includes the anal canal.

The large intestine differs from the small intestine most obviously in its larger diameter and bulged or sacular appearance. The luminal wall of the large intestine is lined with simple columnar epithelium, but it does not have the folds and villi of the small intestine and thus has a flatter surface. The colonic mucosa has numerous deep crypts, and the stem cells that support renewal of the colonic epithelium are near the bottom of these crypts. The colonic epithelium is made up primarily of colonocytes and abundant mucus-secreting goblet cells. Colonocytes (i.e., the absorptive cells of the colon) have much shorter microvilli than do the enterocytes of the small intestine. The inner circular layer of smooth muscle is similar to that in the small intestine, but the outer longitudinal layer in the colon includes the taeniae coli, which are three narrow bands of muscle (~0.5 to 1 cm in width), that run the entire length of the colon and are approximately equally spaced around its circumference. Because the taeniae are shorter than the length of the colon itself, the taeniae force the colon to form its characteristic sacculations or outpocketings arranged into three distinct rows.

FUNCTIONS OF THE LARGE INTESTINE

The primary functions of the colon are (1) absorption of water and electrolytes from the ingesta, (2) microbial fermentation, and (3) formation and storage of feces. As the material that enters the colon from the ileum moves through the large intestine, it is mixed with mucus and bacteria. Some of the undigested organic materials (which are mostly from dietary fiber) undergo fermentation. Much of the remaining water is absorbed by the colonocytes, using mechanisms that are similar to those for the small intestine.

Water and Electrolyte Absorption

In general, the colonic epithelium is more efficient at water absorption than the small intestine, and this is facilitated by uptake of Na^+ ions in the colon, a process that is increased by the hormone aldosterone. As water is absorbed, the stools become semisolid. Cl^- is absorbed in the colon, and bicarbonate is released into the lumen.

Gut Microflora and Fermentation

The large intestine is the natural habitat of a large and diverse bacterial community. The major functions of the gut microbiotica include metabolic activities that salvage energy and absorbable nutrients, trophic effects on intestinal

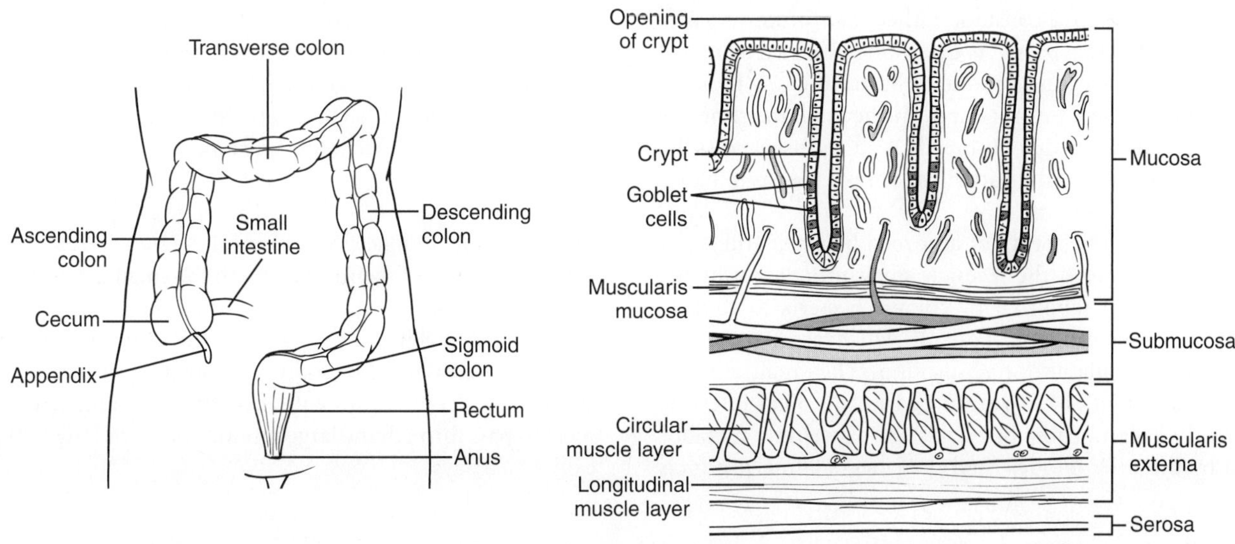

FIGURE 7-10 Diagrams showing the gross anatomy *(left)* and fine anatomy *(right)* of the large intestine.

epithelial cells, and protection of the colonized host against invasion by pathogenic organisms. The genetic diversity of the microorganisms in the gut provides various enzymes and biochemical pathways distinct from those of the host. Bacterial numbers may exceed 10^{11} per gram of dry matter in the colonic contents.

The gut bacteria break down some of the components of the chyme that were not digested in the small intestine (e.g., some components of dietary fiber) as well as the carbohydrate components of mucus (see Chapter 11 for more details as well as a discussion of prebiotics and probiotics). The bacteria use these nutrients for their own needs and for proliferation; they produce some short-chain fatty acids (i.e., acetate, propionate, and butyrate) and gases (e.g., hydrogen [H_2] and carbon dioxide [CO_2]). Short-chain fatty acid production occurs mainly in the cecum and ascending colon and less so in subsequent portions of the colon, mainly because most of the fermentable carbohydrate is consumed before it reaches the distal or descending colon. The short-chain fatty acids produced by fermentation account for more than half of the total anion content of human feces. Bicarbonate secretion into the lumen neutralizes part of the acid load generated by these anions. Protein fermentation occurs mainly after fermentable carbohydrate has been depleted and results in production of ammonia (NH_3), amines, phenols, methane (CH_4), and branched- and short-chain fatty acids.

The human large intestine absorbs significant quantities of the short-chain fatty acids produced by fermentation, primarily by diffusion. Once absorbed, the fatty acids either are metabolized by the cells of the colonic epithelium or enter the portal venous blood. Short-chain fatty acids can be used as an energy source for the body. The nutritional importance of short-chain fatty acid production in the colon remains uncertain for humans, but it is estimated that these short-chain fatty acids may account for more than 5% of total caloric intake.

The gases formed by bacterial fermentation in the colon include H_2, CO_2, and CH_4, which are passed periodically as flatus. Some bacteria consume rather than produce gases. The degree of flatus passed is determined by the balance of production versus consumption of bacterial gases. In addition, some of the gases produced in the large intestine are absorbed and excreted in the breath. A gas diffuses across the mucosa according to the partial pressure of the gas in blood versus luminal contents.

Almost all cholesterol not absorbed before it enters the colon is excreted in the feces. A small proportion of the cholesterol is metabolized by colonic bacteria to coprostanol and coprostanone, both of which are poorly soluble and unavailable for absorption. The small amount of bile acids that is not reabsorbed in the small intestine enters the colon. These bile acids are extensively metabolized by the microbiotica, and their degradation products are lipid-soluble and may be passively absorbed. Both fat (if malabsorbed) and fiber sequester bile acids and their metabolites in the lumen of the intestine and thereby interfere with their absorption. In total, about 50 mg/day of bile acids are passively absorbed in the human colon, primarily as their microbial degradation products.

Approximately 25% of the urea synthesized in the liver reaches the GI tract by diffusion from the blood. Bacterial urease in the colon converts the urea to NH_3. The NH_3 diffuses across the colonic mucosa, enters the portal venous blood, and returns to the liver where it may be used for resynthesis of urea.

Feces Formation and Excretion

Stool formation is occurring throughout the large intestine as the residue from the small intestine is mixed with mucus and bacteria and undergoes fermentation, and as water and electrolytes are absorbed. The muscular action of the colon also compacts the fecal material into a stool. Mass movements of the colon push the stools into the rectum. These are a unique type of movement that strips an area of large intestine clear of its luminal contents. Following a meal, the presence of fat in the proximal small intestine and the distention of the colon are signals for a mass movement of the colon. Distention of the rectum stimulates the defecation reflex, which results in reflex relaxation of the internal anal sphincter followed by voluntary relaxation of the external anal sphincter and defection. Defecation can be prevented by voluntary constriction of the external sphincter, and this is followed by relaxation of the rectum and contraction of the internal sphincter, a state that can be maintained until another bolus of feces is forced into the rectum.

Normal feces are roughly 70% to 75% water and 20% to 25% solids. The bulk of fecal solids are bacteria and undigested organic matter and fiber. Stephen and Cummings (1980) reported that fecal dry matter in subjects who consumed a typical British diet averaged about 27 g per day. Of the 27 g of fecal dry matter, the majority (~18 g) was biomass (bacteria) and the remainder was nonfermented fiber and various water-soluble organic and inorganic compounds. Thus most of the organic material that enters the colon is fermented and used for bacterial growth, unless large amounts of a nonfermentable fiber are consumed.

Transit Time

From the time of ingestion of a meal, it takes about 2 hours for the first part of the meal to reach the small intestine and then another 4 to 6 hours for all of the meal to reach the colon. Thus by 8 hours after a meal, the stomach and small intestine are essentially empty if another meal is not consumed. The length of time it takes for the residue from the meal to pass through the large intestine is much longer, typically 1 to 3 days.

THINKING CRITICALLY

1. Sections of the small intestine may be surgically removed to treat intestinal inflammation, injuries, blockage, or tumors. The effect of such surgeries on GI tract function and nutrition depends on the length and region of the small intestine that is removed. Extensive resection of the ileum is typically associated with vitamin B_{12} deficiency, low luminal concentration of bile acids, fatty diarrhea (steatorrhea), and fat-soluble vitamin deficiencies.
   a. Explain why removal of the ileum would cause a deficiency of vitamin B_{12} but not necessarily of other B vitamins.
   b. Explain why removal of the ileum might lead to a low concentration of bile acids in the lumen of the remaining small intestine.
   c. Explain why removal of the ileum could lead to fat malabsorption and to fat-soluble vitamin deficiencies.
2. Cystic fibrosis is the most common of the lethal inherited diseases in northern Europe and North America. The disease is caused by mutations in the gene encoding a chloride channel protein found in membranes of cells that line passageways of the lungs, liver, pancreas, intestines, reproductive tract, and skin. Cystic fibrosis affects the cells that produce mucus and digestive secretions, and these secretions become thick and sticky. The thick mucus can block tubes that carry digestive enzymes from the pancreas to the small intestine and cause severe nutritional deficiencies. Bile secretion by the liver may also be affected.
   a. Explain how the pancreatic damage that results from cystic fibrosis leads to the malabsorption of fat and protein. How might this problem be treated in patients with cystic fibrosis?
   b. Explain how cystic fibrosis affects the ability of patients to absorb fat-soluble vitamins and to absorb essential fatty acids. How might these particular deficiencies be treated?

REFERENCES

Brandtzaeg, P. (2010). Food allergy: Separating the science from the mythology. *Nature Reviews Gastroenterology and Hepatology, 7*, 380–400.

Chahine, B. G., & Bahna, S. L. (2010). The role of the gut mucosal immunity in the development of tolerance versus development of allergy to food. *Current Opinion in Allergy and Clinical Immunology, 10*, 394–399.

Commare, C. E., & Tappenden, K. A. (2007). Development of the infant intestine: Implications for nutrition support. *Nutrition in Clinical Practice, 22*, 159–173.

Dawson, P. A., Lan, T., & Rao, A. (2009). Bile acid transporters. *Journal of Lipid Research, 50*, 2340–2357.

Gasteyger, C., Suter, M., Gaillard, R. C., & Giusti, V. (2008). Nutritional deficiencies after Roux-en-Y gastric bypass for morbid obesity often cannot be prevented by standard multivitamin supplementation. *The American Journal of Clinical Nutrition, 87*, 1128–1133.

Neu, J. (2007). Gastrointestinal maturation and implications for infant feeding. *Early Human Development, 83*, 767–775.

Pellicoro, A., & Faber, K. N. (2007). Review article: The function and regulation of proteins involved in bile salt biosynthesis and transport. *Alimentary Pharmacology & Therapeutics, 26*(Suppl. 2), 149–160.

Stephen, A. M., & Cummings, J. H. (1980). Mechanism of action of dietary fibre in the human colon. *Nature, 284*, 283–284.

RECOMMENDED READINGS

Anderson, G. J., Fraser, D. M., & McLaren, G. D. (2009). Iron absorption and metabolism. *Current Opinion in Gastroenterology, 25*, 129–135.

Commare, C. E., & Tappenden, K. A. (2007). Development of the infant intestine: Implications for nutrition support. *Nutrition in Clinical Practice, 22*, 159–173.

Drozdowski, L., Iordache, C., Clandinin, M. T., Wild, G., Todd, Z., & Thomson, A. B. (2009). Dexamethasone and GLP-2 given to lactating rat dams influence glucose uptake in suckling and postweanling offspring. *Journal of Parenteral and Enteral Nutrition, 33*, 433–439.

Hofmann, A. F., & Hagey, L. R. (2008). Bile acids: Chemistry, pathochemistry, biology, pathobiology, and therapeutics. *Cellular and Molecular Life Sciences, 65*, 2461–2483.

Hui, D. Y., Labonté, E. D., & Howles, P. N. (2008). Development and physiological regulation of intestinal lipid absorption. III. Intestinal transporters and cholesterol absorption. *American Journal of Physiology Gastrointestinal and Liver Physiology, 294*, G839–G843.

Newberry, E. P., & Davidson, N. O. (2009). Intestinal lipid absorption, GLP-2 and CD36: Still more mysteries to moving fat. *Gastroenterology, 137*, 775–778.

Panlowski, S. W., Warren, C. A., & Guerrant, R. (2009). Diagnosis and treatment of acute or persistent diarrhea. *Gastroenterology, 136*, 1874–1886.

CHAPTER 8

Digestion and Absorption of Carbohydrate

*Armelle Leturque, PhD, and Edith Brot-Laroche, PhD**

COMMON ABBREVIATIONS

GLUT glucose transporter
SGLT sodium/glucose cotransporter

Carbohydrates typically provide 45% to 65% of energy in human diets. Dietary carbohydrates include a variety of simple and complex carbohydrates, some of which are digestible by human gastrointestinal enzymes and some of which are not hydrolyzed by these enzymes. The digestible carbohydrates give rise to monosaccharide units that are absorbed by sugar transport systems. The processes involved in the digestion and absorption of digestible carbohydrates are the focus of this chapter. Dietary fiber is not a source of glucose or other monosaccharides in the small intestine. Dietary fiber is made up mainly of complex nondigestible carbohydrates and resistant starches from plant foods. The fate of the nondigestible carbohydrates is discussed in detail in Chapter 11.

CARBOHYDRATE COMPONENTS OF THE HUMAN DIET

Carbohydrates are the major macronutrient in most human diets. Digestible carbohydrates are considered to include monosaccharides (glucose, fructose, and galactose), disaccharides (sucrose, lactose, maltose, and trehalose), oligosaccharides (often breakdown products of polysaccharides as found in corn syrup), polysaccharides (starches and small amounts of glycogen from meat products), and sugar alcohols (sorbitol and mannitol). In the United States, the median intake of total carbohydrate by adults is approximately 250 g (1,000 kcal) per day (~50% of total calories). Most of this is derived from the starch present in grains and certain vegetables (e.g., corn, tapioca, flour, cereals, popcorn, pasta, rice, and potatoes). Approximately 50 g (200 kcal) per day of the total carbohydrate intake in the United States is from added sugars (monosaccharides and disaccharides), which are defined as sugars and syrups (including honey and maple syrup) that are added to foods during processing or preparation. Added sugars therefore include those added to soft drinks, cakes, cookies, fruit-flavored drinks, ice cream, and candy, but do not include naturally occurring sugars, such as lactose in milk or fructose and sucrose in fruits. Lactose is the major carbohydrate in the diets of breast- or formula-fed infants (~47 g per day).

Carbohydrate intake also includes nondigestible carbohydrates present in foods. Most of these are plant polysaccharides classified as dietary fiber. The median intake of dietary fiber by adults living in the United States is approximately 15 g per day. Nondigestible oligosaccharides, such as raffinose and stachyose, are found in small amounts in legumes. Differences in the proportions of fiber and digestible carbohydrates in foods are responsible for the differences in nutritional and energetic values of food carbohydrates from various sources.

DIGESTION OF STARCHES

Polymers and oligomers of glucose along with dimers of glucose and either galactose, fructose, or glucose are digested efficiently as they travel through the small intestine. Digestion involves the enzymatic cleavage of the oxygen bridges, called glycosidic bonds, that link the hexose units. The released free hexoses, but not the larger sugars or oligosaccharides, are transported across the intestine into the circulation. The processes of enzymatic digestion occur within the lumen of the small intestine under the influence of secreted pancreatic amylase and the abundant constituent oligosaccharidases of the apical membrane of the columnar epithelial enterocytes lining the villi of the small intestine. The fates of the major dietary carbohydrates within the small intestine are summarized in Table 8-1.

LUMINAL DIGESTION OF STARCHES

After infancy, starches are the major food source of glucose for humans. Starches exist as semicrystalline storage granules in all plants, but the structural and chemical composition

*This is a revision of the chapter previously contributed by Roberto Quezada-Calvillo, MD; Claudia C. Robayo, MD; and Buford L. Nichols, MD.

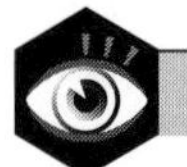

NUTRITION INSIGHT

Effects of Dietary Carbohydrate on Blood Glucose: Glycemic Index and Glycemic Load

The rise in blood glucose level promoted by carbohydrate-rich food is not directly linked to simple or complex carbohydrate content. Indeed many factors influence sugar absorption rates. These include physical entrapment, association with fiber, other components of the diet, processing of food, and physiological state of the subject. David Jenkins and colleagues proposed the concept of glycemic index (GI) to help diabetic patients identify foods that have the smallest effect on blood glucose (Jenkins et al., 1981). GI uses a scale from 0 to 100. A GI of 100 is given to the area under a 2-hour blood glucose curve in response to oral intake of 50 g of glucose. Consumption of 50 g of carbohydrates within desserts, candies, bread, breakfast cereals, rice, and potato products yields a high GI (higher than 70), whereas intake of 50 g of carbohydrates as part of fruits, nonstarchy vegetables, dairy, and nuts generally yields a low GI (less than 55).

The rise in blood glucose is also influenced by the size of the portion consumed; Walter Willett and colleagues defined the glycemic load (GL) in 1997 as the mathematical product of GI and carbohydrate amount (Salmeron et al., 1997). Using this approach, 34 g (one slice) of white bread, 247 g of apple, 68 g of reduced-fat ice cream, and 138 g of lentil were calculated to have equal GL values, although their GI values and carbohydrate amounts varied by as much as threefold (Brand-Miller et al., 2003). When fed to subjects, all but one (lentils) of these foods gave identical areas under the 2-hour glucose response curve. To determine the effects of increasing GL, another group of subjects was given food portions to provide GL doses equivalent to 1, 2, 3, 4, or 6 slices of bread. The incremental increases in GL produced stepwise increases in both glycemia and insulinemia, supporting the concept of GL as a measure of overall glycemic response and insulin demand. The usefulness of the GL concept has also been supported by studies in which mixed meals were fed (Wolever and Bolognesi, 1996) and by studies in which subjects were assigned to diets with different GLs due either to changes in carbohydrate amount or to differences in the GI of foods in the diet (Wolever and Mehling, 2003; Galgani et al., 2006). Limitation of the GL of a meal may limit the extent of postprandial hyperglycemia, which may be related to risk of type 2 diabetes, coronary heart disease, and weight gain.

TABLE 8-1 Summary of Digestion of Dietary Carbohydrate

FOOD SOURCE	% OF DIETARY CARBOHYDRATE	PRODUCTS OF LUMINAL HYDROLYSIS	PRODUCTS OF BRUSH BORDER MEMBRANE HYDROLYSIS
Starches (amylose, amylopectin)	60 to 70	Maltose, maltotriose, and α-dextrins	Glucose
Lactose	0 to 10	None	Glucose and galactose
Sucrose	30	None	Glucose and fructose

of starch granules varies with each plant species and within different parts of the plant. Starch digestion begins by the action of secreted α-amylase in the lumen of the gastrointestinal tract and is completed by the action of α-glucosidases that are associated with the apical membrane of the intestinal mucosal cells.

Digestion of Starches by Soluble α-Amylase

Amylase has the distinction of being the first enzyme to be discovered. In 1833, Anselme Payen and Jean-François Persoz, chemists at a French sugar factory, extracted a substance from malt that converted starch to sugars. Payen and Persoz called this substance diastase (meaning a separation), because the enzyme converts the starch in barley seed to soluble sugars when the beer mash is heated, and this causes the husk to separate from the rest of the seed. The name diastase was subsequently changed to amylase, based on the Latin name for starch *(amylum)* and retaining the -ase suffix (now commonly used for naming enzymes) from the enzyme's original name. Discovery of salivary and pancreatic amylases followed thereafter.

Production and secretion of amylase is restricted to the salivary and pancreatic exocrine glands. The amylases are α(1,4) endoglucosidases that cleave internal α(1,4) glycosidic bonds in linear starch chains to produce a variety of glucose oligomers. The salivary and pancreatic α-amylases are secreted as soluble proteins into the mouth or small intestine via the salivary ducts and pancreatic/common bile duct, respectively.

Thus digestion of starch begins in the mouth by action of salivary α-amylase as food is chewed and mixed with saliva. The action of amylase, however, ceases abruptly after the chewed food mixes with the acidic secretions of the stomach, because amylase activity requires neutral pH. Although the amylase protein is acid labile, the presence of starch in association with the amylase and the protection of amylase within the bolus of food provides some delay in amylase inactivation by the gastric acid (Rosenblum et al., 1988).

Pancreatic amylase is secreted in large quantities into the duodenal lumen. Most of the starch component of grains or legumes establishes contact with the pancreatic α-amylases within the polar bulk phase of the intestinal luminal milieu. The concentration of amylase achieved within the duodenal lumen greatly exceeds that required for cleavage of the bonds joining the glucose components of the starches. Indeed, the cleavage of starches to the final oligosaccharide products normally occurs in the uppermost part of the small intestine and is virtually complete by the time the meal reaches the duodenal–jejunal junction (Fogel and Gray, 1973). Furthermore, refined starches are hydrolyzed efficiently to glucose oligomers, even in patients with exocrine pancreatic insufficiency who have amylase levels that are only about 10% of normal (Fogel and Gray, 1973).

Differences in Structure and Digestion of Amylose and Amylopectin

It is important to consider the structure of the principal dietary starches, because amylase has specificity for only the α(1,4)-linked straight-chain regions of the glucosyl polysaccharide, whereas the most abundant food starches also have α(1,6)-branching links. The simplest starch is the linear and unbranched amylose, which is a polymer of α(1,4)-linked glucosyl units (~600 glucose residues per molecule). Amylase has maximal specificity for the interior links, and its active site binds five consecutive glucose residues at specific subsites and cleaves between the second and third subsites, as shown in Figure 8-1, to form two smaller polymers. Sequential cleavage eventually leads to the production of pentasaccharides that bind with high affinity at all five of the amylase subsites. The pentasaccharide will be hydrolyzed at the penultimate linkage from the reducing end of the pentasaccharide to release the trisaccharide maltotriose and the disaccharide maltose. Products smaller than the pentasaccharide are not able to bind at all subsites and thus have very low affinity for the amylase active site; hence these smaller oligosaccharides are not readily cleaved by amylase. Overall, the sequential actions of amylase promote the release of maltotriose and maltose as the main final products of luminal amylose digestion.

Amylopectin is a more complex form of starch, representing about 80% of dietary polysaccharide. Figure 8-2 depicts the action of amylase on amylopectin to yield the final oligosaccharide products within the distal duodenal lumen. Although its linear segments are similar to those for amylose, amylopectin is branched by virtue of α(1,6) links positioned approximately every 25 residues along the chain. Glycogen, though a minor dietary carbohydrate, has a structure analogous to that of amylopectin and is also digested by amylase. Amylase is unable to cleave the α(1,6) branching link, and the structural angulation created by this linkage inhibits the enzyme from attacking some of the adjacent α(1,4) links. As a consequence, branched oligosaccharides called α-limit dextrins (or α-dextrins), along with maltose and maltotriose, are the final products of amylopectin hydrolysis by α-amylase. Dextrins of average mass of five to six glucose units represent nearly one third the mass of the final breakdown products of amylopectin.

Overall, the hydrolytic activities of salivary and pancreatic amylases on amylose and amylopectin result in production of glucose oligosaccharides and disaccharides containing α(1,4) linkages and glucose oligosaccharides containing both α(1,4) and α(1,6) linkages, with only about 4% of the glucose residues being released as free glucose monomers (Yook and Robyt, 2002). The subsequent steps of starch digestion are ensured by activities of the α-glucosidases associated with the apical membrane of the intestinal mucosal cells, as discussed later.

Regulation of Amylase Secretion

Both salivary and pancreatic amylase levels are low at birth but typically reach adult levels before 1 year of age. Expression of pancreatic amylase activity appears to lag behind the expression of other enzymes synthesized in the acinar cells of the pancreas. This has prompted some pediatricians and nutritionists to recommend withholding starch from the diet until about 6 months of age. Nevertheless, clinical symptoms resulting from cereal feeding before 6 months of age are rare (Lebenthal et al., 1983).

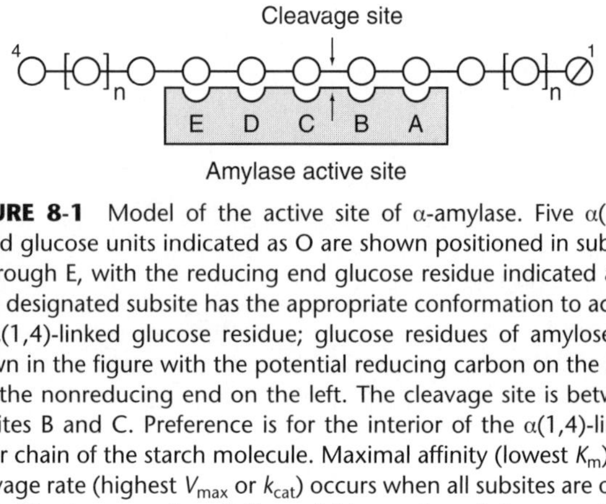

Cleavage site
4
n
n
1
E D C B A
Amylase active site

FIGURE 8-1 Model of the active site of α-amylase. Five α(1,4)-linked glucose units indicated as O are shown positioned in subsites A through E, with the reducing end glucose residue indicated as ⊘. Each designated subsite has the appropriate conformation to accept an α(1,4)-linked glucose residue; glucose residues of amylose are shown in the figure with the potential reducing carbon on the right and the nonreducing end on the left. The cleavage site is between subsites B and C. Preference is for the interior of the α(1,4)-linked linear chain of the starch molecule. Maximal affinity (lowest K_m) and cleavage rate (highest V_{max} or k_{cat}) occurs when all subsites are occupied with glucose units; *n* is the variable number of glucose residues in amylose. When amylopectin is the substrate, the portions of the starch in brackets also contain branches created by α(1,6) links of glucose residues as shown in Figure 8-2.

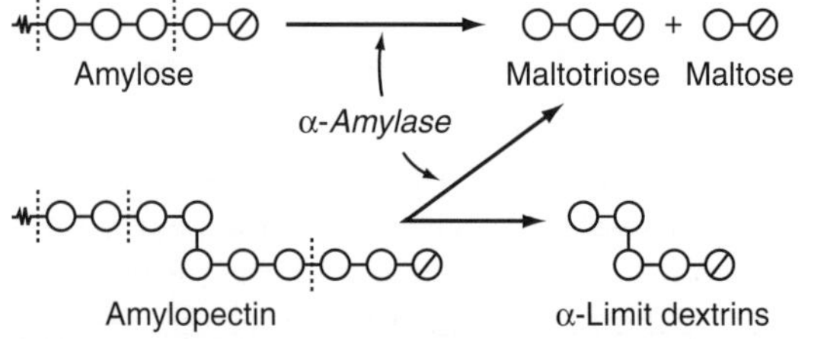

Amylose
Maltotriose Maltose
α-Amylase
Amylopectin
α-Limit dextrins

FIGURE 8-2 Action of salivary and pancreatic α-amylases on linear (amylose) and branched (amylopectin) forms of starch. Horizontal links denote α(1,4) linkages; vertical links indicate α(1,6) linkages. *O,* Glucose units; *Ø,* reducing end glucose unit. (From Gray, G. M. [1981]. Carbohydrate absorption and malabsorption. In L. R. Johnson [Ed.], *Physiology of the gastrointestinal tract* [pp. 1063-1072]. New York: Raven Press.)

Secretion rate patterns for total protein and salivary amylase mirror those of salivary flow rate, suggesting there is little regulation of amylase synthesis or secretion by the salivary gland. Salivary secretion is mainly regulated by neural signals and responds to the sight, smell, and taste of food, which can increase salivary flow by up to eightfold.

In pancreatic acinar cells, amylase along with other digestive enzymes is packaged in large (<1 μm diameter) secretory vesicles known as zymogen granules that are stored in the acinar cells. In the acidic zymogen granule, amylase is inactive. In response to various secretagogues, such as cholecystokinin, or to neural signals, the contents of the zymogen granule undergo exocytosis into the lumen of the acinus, which feeds into the pancreatic duct. Upon release from the acidic zymogen granule into the pancreatic duct, amylase becomes active due to the higher pH of the pancreatic secretions. The higher pH of the pancreatic juice is largely due to the bicarbonate secreted by the pancreas. This bicarbonate secretion is important for neutralizing the acidic contents of the stomach as they enter the duodenum.

COMPLETION OF STARCH DIGESTION BY INTEGRAL MEMBRANE OLIGOSACCHARIDASES

The apical (brush border) membrane surface of the small intestinal enterocytes is replete with oligosaccharidases. Two of these oligosaccharidases are α-glucosidases that carry out the final steps in starch digestion (Semenza and Auricchio, 1991). Each one of these α-glucosidases, as synthesized, possesses two domains, with each domain containing an independent active site. The enzyme molecules are named for the main activities of the two domains: maltase–glucoamylase and sucrase–isomaltase. Both are attached to the apical membrane by an N-terminal hydrophobic sequence that spans the membrane.

Roles of Maltase–Glucoamylase and Sucrase–Isomaltase in Starch Digestion

These α-glucosidase activities are all classified as exoglucosidases because they can cleave one glucose residue at a time from the nonreducing end of starch oligosaccharides. All of these α-glucosidases cleave α(1,4) linkages of glucose residues. The functional differences among maltase–glucoamylase, sucrase, and isomaltase are the degree of their specificity for a particular substrate or glycosidic linkage at the nonreducing terminus of the glucose oligosaccharides. Glucoamylase has high specificity for the α(1,4) link at the nonreducing terminus of straight-chain glucosyl oligosaccharides containing from two to nine glucose units. Maltase hydrolyzes α(1,4) bonds in both starch oligosaccharides and in the disaccharide maltose. Sucrase displays high efficiency for the α(1,4) links of the smallest glucosyl oligosaccharides, maltose and maltotriose, and hence is an efficient maltase. It reinforces maltase–glucoamylase in the release of α(1,4)-linked glucose units, but its name comes from its unique capacity to cleave the link between the glucose and fructose units of sucrose [α-D-glucopyranosyl(1,2′)β′-D-fructofuranoside]. Similarly, isomaltase (α-dextrinase) has appreciable specificity for the α(1,4) links in the oligosaccharide products of starch digestion, but its maximal and unique specificity is for the α(1,6) branching link of the α-dextrins. Because of its α(1,6) specificity and the use of the α(1,6) disaccharide isomaltose as a substrate in the in vitro assay of its activity, it is commonly called isomaltase. Isomaltose, however, is not a natural substrate produced by α-amylase action on amylopectin. The term α-dextrinase is also used for isomaltase to more appropriately describe the enzyme's capacity to cleave both α(1,4) and α(1,6) links in the oligosaccharide products (limit dextrins) of starch digestion.

Maltase–glucoamylase, isomaltase (α-dextrinase), and sucrase work in a complementary manner to cleave the bonds in the α-dextrins in sequence from the nonreducing end to release free glucose units. As shown in Figure 8-3, at each step in the process, one or more of these enzymes has high specificity for the α-glucosyl link closest to the nonreducing end of specific oligosaccharide products. These glucosidases produce free glucose for transport into the enterocyte.

Contributions of Maltase–Glucoamylase and Sucrase–Isomaltase to Oligosaccharide Hydrolysis

The relative contribution of maltase–glucoamylase versus sucrase–isomaltase in the hydrolysis of the α(1,4) linkages in the oligosaccharides released by action of amylase on dietary

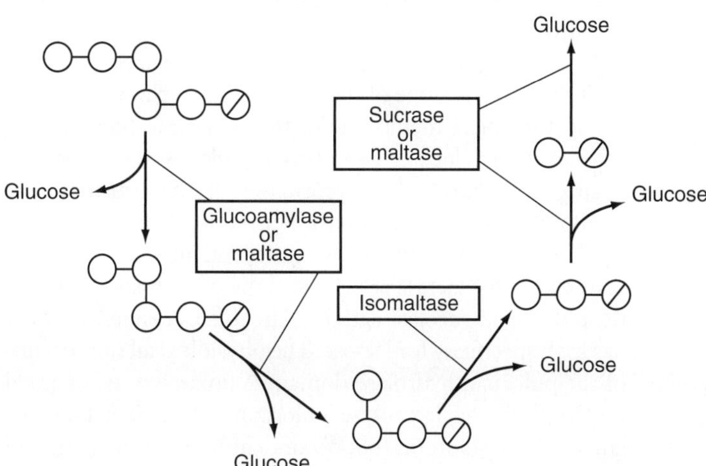

FIGURE 8-3 Concerted action of intestinal surface membrane oligosaccharidases on a typical α-dextrin final product of amylopectin digestion. The major active hydrolases for each removal of a glucose residue from the nonreducing terminus is shown in the boxed area. Note that only the isomaltase is capable of removing the α(1,6)-linked glucose "stub" from the intermediate tetrasaccharide substrate (bottom of figure). ○, Glucose units; ⊘, reducing end glucose unit. (From Gray, G. M. [1981]. Carbohydrate absorption and malabsorption. In L. R. Johnson [Ed.], *Physiology of the gastrointestinal tract* [pp. 1063-1072]. New York: Raven Press.)

TABLE 8-2 Kinetic Constants for α-Glucosidases for Oligosaccharide Hydrolysis

Glucose Residues	Maltase–Glucoamylase		Sucrase–Isomaltase	
N	K_m* (mmol/L)	k_{cat}† (sec^{-1})	K_m (mmol/L)	k_{cat} (sec^{-1})
2	2.1	56	14	3.2
3	1.1	149	21	3.1
4	0.4	78	24	3.5
5	0.4	63	61	3.4
6	0.7	70	57	2.1
7	1.0	80	120	2.2

*K_m, Michaelis constant; the substrate concentration at which an enzyme or transporter is half-saturated with substrate.
†k_{cat}, First-order rate constant corresponding to the slowest step or steps in the overall catalytic reaction; the number of catalytic cycles the active site undergoes per unit time.

starch has historically been difficult to assess. The enzymatic activities of the two proteins overlap, and there is a lack of assays to completely distinguish the contributions of the two intestinal mucosal enzymes to starch digestion in humans as well as the inhibitory effect of starch digestion products on some of the catalytic domains.

Maltase–glucoamylase has a higher affinity (lower K_m) and faster rate of substrate turnover (higher k_{cat}) for hydrolysis of glucose oligomers than does sucrase–isomaltase, and thus it will catalyze a more rapid rate of hydrolysis at low concentrations of glucose oligomers (Table 8-2). However, it appears that maltase–glucoamylase contributes a relatively small fraction of the total glucose oligomer-hydrolyzing activity in humans in vivo. Indeed, sucrase–isomaltase activity in humans is about 20 times that of maltase–glucoamylase activity. Moreover, sucrase–isomaltase is not inhibited by lumenal starch-derived oligosaccharides as is the activity of maltase–glucoamylase in assays performed in vitro (Quezada-Calvillo et al., 2007). Thus sucrase–isomaltase probably contributes most of the α-glucosidase activity when high-starch diets are consumed.

DIGESTION OF DIETARY DISACCHARIDES

In addition to digestion of maltose, as described for the end products of starch breakdown, humans have the capacity to hydrolyze unique linkages present in sucrose, lactose, and trehalose. Kinetic properties of these disaccharidase activities are shown in Table 8-3. These disaccharidases are all associated with the luminal surface of the enterocytes, as illustrated in Figure 8-4.

SUCROSE DIGESTION BY SUCRASE

Sucrose [α-D-glucopyranosyl(1,2′)β′-D-fructofuranoside], which is also known as table sugar, is the most abundantly consumed natural sweetener. Table sugar is refined from sugar cane or sugar beets, and various refined forms of sucrose are used in production of processed foods. Sucrose is also present in relatively large amounts in fruits, such as oranges and apples.

TABLE 8-3 Kinetic Properties of Intestinal Brush Border Membrane Disaccharidases for Hydrolysis of Disaccharides

ENZYME	PRINCIPAL SUBSTRATE	K_m* (mmol/L)	k_{cat}† (sec^{-1})
α-GLUCOSIDASES			
Sucrase	Sucrose	18	120
Trehalase	Trehalose	3	20
β-GALACTOSIDASE			
Lactase	Lactose	2	4

*K_m, Michaelis constant; the substrate concentration at which an enzyme or transporter is half-saturated with substrate.
†k_{cat}, First-order rate constant corresponding to the slowest step or steps in the overall catalytic reaction; the number of catalytic cycles the active site undergoes per unit time.

Intestinal digestion of sucrose requires hydrolysis of the α(1,2′)β′ linkage, which involves the anomeric carbon of both hexoses, to yield glucose and fructose. In mammalian species, the hydrolysis of sucrose is performed by the sucrase activity of the sucrase–isomaltase complex. The resulting monosaccharides are then absorbed by the intestinal epithelial cells.

LACTOSE DIGESTION BY LACTASE

Lactose [β-D-galactopyranosyl(1,4′)D-glucopyranoside] is a disaccharide abundant in the mammalian milk from which it takes its name (from the Latin *lac*, for "milk"). Milk ingestion by breast- or formula-fed infants provides approximately 70 g/L (or 55 g/day) of carbohydrates, of which approximately 60 g/L (or 47 g/day) is lactose. (The remainder of the milk carbohydrates are oligosaccharides that are not digestible by the human gastrointestinal enzymes.) The nutritional relevance of lactose is more limited after infancy because of the introduction of alternative dietary carbohydrates.

Lactose digestion in mammals requires lactase–phlorizin hydrolase activity, one of the intestinal disaccharidases present in the apical membrane of the small intestinal enterocytes. Although lactase–phlorizin hydrolase shows structural analogies with other α-glycosidases of the brush border membrane, it has a distinctive neutral β-galactosidic activity. The molecule contains two independent active sites, one responsible for lactase activity and the other associated with the phlorizin hydrolase activity. The β-galactosidase domain has high specificity for lactose. The physiological significance of the phlorizin hydrolase domain is unknown. It is named for its ability to hydrolyze phlorizin, which is a toxic 2′-glucoside of phloretin that occurs naturally in the bark and seeds of some fruit trees

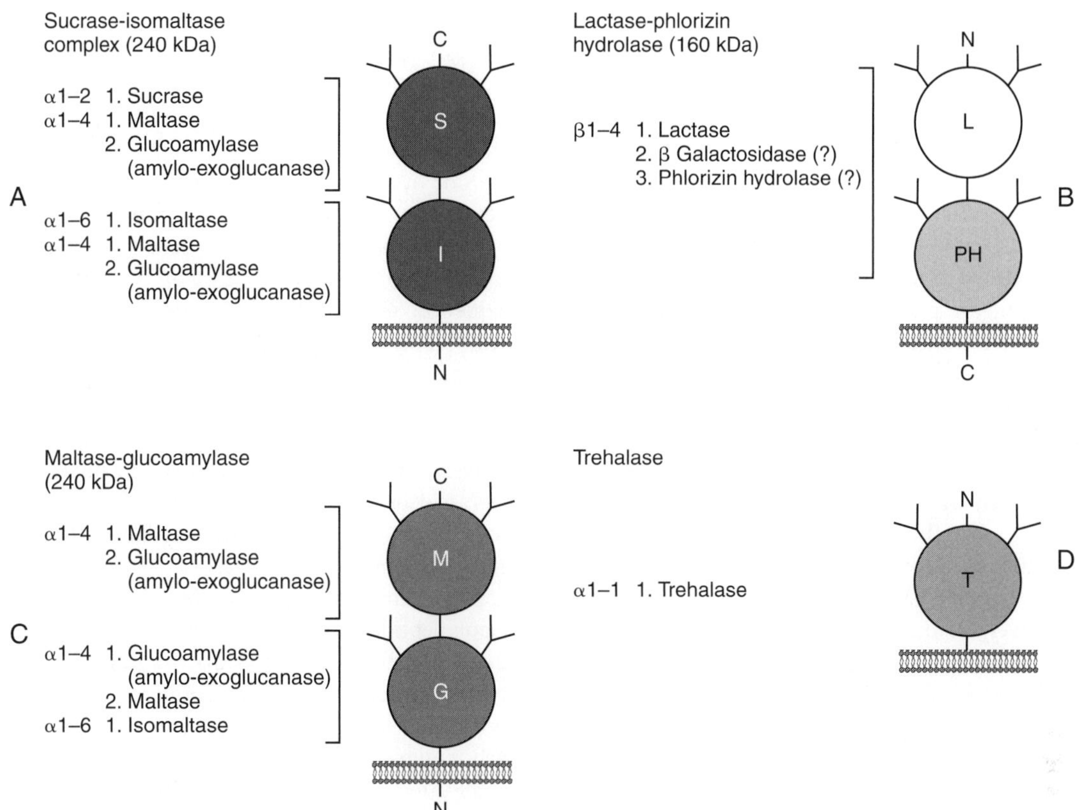

FIGURE 8-4 Schematic structures of human intestinal disaccharidases and their enzyme activities. The activities are ranked (*1, 2, 3*) by importance to carbohydrate nutrition. **A,** Sucrase–isomaltase is a bifunctional enzyme that hydrolyzes α(1,4) glycosidic bonds with low affinity (high K_m) and α(1,6) glycosidic bonds with high affinity (low K_m). Sucrase also hydrolyzes the α(1,2′)β′ linkage in sucrose. Isomaltase is anchored to the apical membrane of enterocytes by its N-terminus; the sucrase domain is cleaved off by action of pancreatic proteases but sucrase remains associated with isomaltase via noncovalent interactions. **B,** Lactase–phlorizin hydrolase hydrolyzes β(1,4) glycosidic bonds, such as that found in lactose. Lactase–phlorizin hydrolase is attached to the apical membrane by the C-terminus of the phlorizin hydrolase domain. **C,** Maltase–glucoamylase has a high affinity (very low K_m) for the α(1,4) glucosidic bonds of glucose oligomers. Maltase–glucoamylase is attached to the apical membrane by the N-terminus of the glucoamylase domain. **D,** Trehalase acts on the α(1,1′)α′ glycosidic bond of trehalose. Trehalase is anchored to the plasma membrane through a glycosylphosphatidylinositol (GPI) anchor.

TREHALOSE DIGESTION BY TREHALASE

Trehalose [α-D-glucopyranosyl-(1,1′)α′-D-glucopyranoside] is a disaccharide present in small amounts in bacteria, fungi, plants, and invertebrates (Elbein et al., 2003; Richards et al., 2002). Significant food sources of trehalose in modern Western diets include baker's yeast, brewer's yeast, cultivated and wild mushrooms, honey, sunflower seeds, sea algae, lobster, shrimp, and processed foods to which trehalose has been added. Trehalose may have constituted a larger source of sugar in the diet of ancient man, and some populations eat a much higher proportion of invertebrates (e.g., insects in which trehalose is the major hemolymph sugar) and fungi (e.g., yeasts, molds, mushrooms, and truffles) as part of their diets and therefore ingest more trehalose than is provided by typical Western diets. Reported concentrations of trehalose from natural sources vary because of experimental conditions, analytical methods, and the life stage of the organism assayed. In organisms, trehalose performs diverse functions that include energy storage and transport as well as protection against extreme temperatures or desiccation (Schiraldi et al., 2002).

The α(1,1′)α′ glucosidic linkage of the glucose residues in trehalose is hydrolyzed by trehalase, which is present in the brush border membrane of the intestinal epithelial cells of humans and most mammals. Hydrolysis of each molecule of trehalose by trehalase renders two molecules of free glucose. The presence of trehalase activity in the human intestine may reflect a widespread dependence of ancient humans on insects and fungi as primary sources of nutrients.

EXPRESSION AND PROCESSING OF THE OLIGOSACCHARIDASES AND DISACCHARIDASES

Oligosaccharidase and disaccharidase activities that can hydrolyze linkages between sugar residues present in the human diet are regulated at the level of gene expression at various developmental stages and during absorptive cell differentiation. Expression of functional enzyme is dependent on posttranslational modifications and appropriate protein trafficking to the apical membrane of enterocytes.

EFFECT OF DEVELOPMENTAL STAGE AND DIET ON SACCHARIDASE EXPRESSION

In humans the oligosaccharidases and disaccharidases are present in the gut before birth and are expressed throughout life. In general, levels of these enzymes are reduced in subjects who have fasted or are receiving parenteral nutrition, and levels are increased in subjects fed a carbohydrate-rich diet or in patients with uncontrolled diabetes. In most other mammals the lactase–phlorizin hydrolase is expressed from birth to weaning, and the other oligosaccharidases appear during the transition from maternal milk to starch-based diets. Lactase–phlorizin hydrolase in the intestinal mucosa of humans reaches maximal activity at an early postnatal age and then declines before adulthood in most people (Simon-Assmann et al., 1986). NF-LPH1 is a transcription factor that is present exclusively in intestinal epithelium and is thought to regulate expression of the lactase–phlorizin hydrolase gene. NF-LPH1 declines simultaneously with lactase–phlorizin hydrolase activity during the postweaning period. Thus a reduction in the expression of NF-LPH1 might be the cause of the decline in lactase activity that occurs before adulthood in most humans (Kuokkanen et al., 2003; Troelsen et al., 2003).

CRYPT–VILLUS EXPRESSION OF SACCHARIDASES

Expression of oligosaccharidase and disaccharidase activities at the cellular level is tightly linked to enterocyte differentiation (Boudreau et al., 2002; Troelsen et al., 1997). For example, immature enterocytes developing from stem cells in crypts of the intestinal mucosa do not have sucrase–isomaltase activity. As enterocytes traverse to the crypt–villus junction, sucrase–isomaltase messenger RNA (mRNA) and sucrose–isomaltase activity are observed to increase. The level of sucrase–isomaltase mRNA reaches its peak when enterocytes are located in the lower and mid villus region and then progressively decreases as these cells move toward the tip (Traber et al., 1992). Expression of other disaccharidase and oligosaccharidase activities follows a similar pattern.

POSTTRANSLATIONAL PROCESSING OF SACCHARIDASES

The posttranslational processing of newly synthesized oligosaccharidases and disaccharidases has been the subject of a number of studies. The general pathways, summarized in Figure 8-5, are similar for lactase–phlorizin hydrolase, sucrase–isomaltase, and maltase–glucoamylase, although each has some specific and unique characteristics (Weisz and Rodriguez-Boulan, 2009). Trehalase expression and processing has little similarity to that of the other disaccharidases. All of these oligosaccharidases and disaccharidases are synthesized in the enterocyte where they are processed in the endoplasmic reticulum (ER) and Golgi apparatus with final vectorial transport to the apical membrane. Lactase–phlorizin hydrolase, sucrase–isomaltase, and maltase–glucoamylase all undergo extensive *N*- and *O*-glycosylation in the ER and Golgi apparatus, but trehalase has only *N*-glycosylation sites. The orientation of these enzymes in the membrane is such that the oligosaccharidase domains, including the active catalytic sites, are on the luminal side of the apical membrane and thus available for efficient cleavage of the luminal substrates.

Maltase–isomaltase and sucrase–isomaltase are both anchored in the membrane by an N-terminal hydrophobic sequence, whereas lactase–phlorizin hydrolase is inserted into the plasma membrane by its C-terminus, as illustrated in Figure 8-4. In contrast to the other disaccharidases, the C-terminus of trehalase is anchored to the plasma membrane via a glycosylphosphatidylinositol (GPI) anchor. Proteolysis is involved in production of the final mature forms of sucrase–isomaltase and lactase–phlorizin hydrolase, whereas no proteolytic processing has been documented to occur for human maltase–glucoamylase.

The human lactase–phlorizin hydrolase gene encodes a polypeptide of four domains, but two of these domains are eliminated during the maturation process to render a mature protein that has two domains containing one potential active site each. Proteolytic processing occurs intracellularly, and proteolytic trimming by pancreatic proteases in the small intestine occurs at a second site after the enzyme has been transferred to the plasma membrane. The N-terminal domains of lactase–phlorizin hydrolase, which are intracellularly cleaved to yield the active brush border enzyme, are required as a chaperone for exit of the mature polypeptide from the ER. The phlorizin hydrolase domain appears to serve an additional chaperone role and is also required for correct folding and trafficking of the lactase domain out of the ER (Behrendt et al., 2010). The *O*-glycosylation that

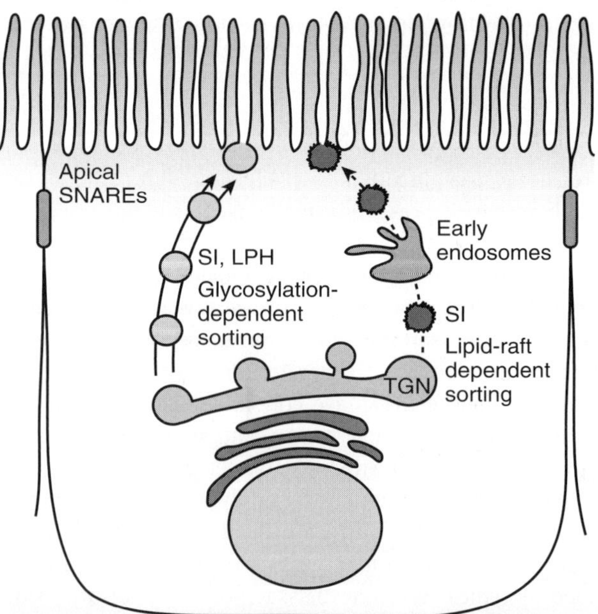

FIGURE 8-5 The apical sorting of sucrase–isomaltase (SI) and lactose–phlorizin hydrolase (LPH) follows glycosylation-dependent pathways (*solid arrows*). In addition, SI can be sorted apically via a lipid-raft (*dark vesicles*) associated pathway (*dotted arrow*).

is added in the Golgi apparatus is required for sorting of lactase–phlorizin hydrolase to the luminal membrane.

Sucrase–isomaltase is transported via the vesicular system to the brush border membrane of enterocytes where it is then subjected to extracellular processing by pancreatic proteolytic enzymes present in the intestinal lumen. The molecule is cleaved to generate a membrane-bound N-terminal isomaltase subunit and a free C-terminal sucrase subunit, which remains associated with the N-terminal isomaltase domain through noncovalent interactions. The C-terminal domain of sucrase–isomaltase appears to act as an intramolecular chaperone for the isomaltase domain and is required for the protein to exit the ER and for subsequent proteolytic processing of the enzyme. In the absence of the sucrase domain, isomaltase remains associated with the ER through its association with the folding chaperone calnexin and is not processed properly (Jacob et al., 2002).

GLYCOSIDIC BONDS NOT HYDROLYZED BY HUMAN DIGESTIVE ENZYMES

Mammals have no digestive capacity for certain oligosaccharides with α-galactosidic linkages (i.e., raffinose, stachyose, verbascose, and ajucose), which are constituents of some legumes, particularly the kidney-shaped beans. Dietary fiber includes polysaccharide components that are homopolymers of glucose or fructose units connected by β-glycosidic linkages (e.g., β-glucans such as cellulose and β-fructans such as inulin) as well as various heteropolysaccharides (e.g., hemicelluloses, pectic substances, gums and mucilages, and algal polysaccharides) that contain a variety of sugar residues and linkage types. Because mammalian pancreatic secretions and integral intestinal oligosaccharidases are incapable of cleaving β-linked glucosyl or fructosyl residues and α-linked galactosyl bonds, these polysaccharides and oligosaccharidases cannot be digested. Instead, they remain intact and may have local probiotic effects on intestinal transport as they travel to lower levels of the ileum and to the colon where the resident bacteria then cleave and modify them extensively to short-chain fatty acids, carbon dioxide, and hydrogen gas. (See Chapter 11 for more discussion of dietary fiber.) (Note that whereas the β(2,1) linkages of fructose polymers found in nature are not hydrolyzed by human digestive enzymes, the α(1,2′)β′ linkage between glucose and fructose in the disaccharide sucrose is readily hydrolyzed, as mentioned earlier.)

ABSORPTION OF MONOSACCHARIDES BY THE ENTEROCYTE

The products of the efficient digestion of starch and disaccharides are essentially the monosaccharides: glucose, galactose, and fructose. Transporters are necessary to promote their entry into and exit from the epithelial absorptive cells (i.e., the enterocytes) of the small intestine. As illustrated in Figure 8-6, a repertoire of transporters in the apical and basolateral membranes of enterocytes regulates the movement of the hexoses across the muscosal epithelium for subsequent delivery to the

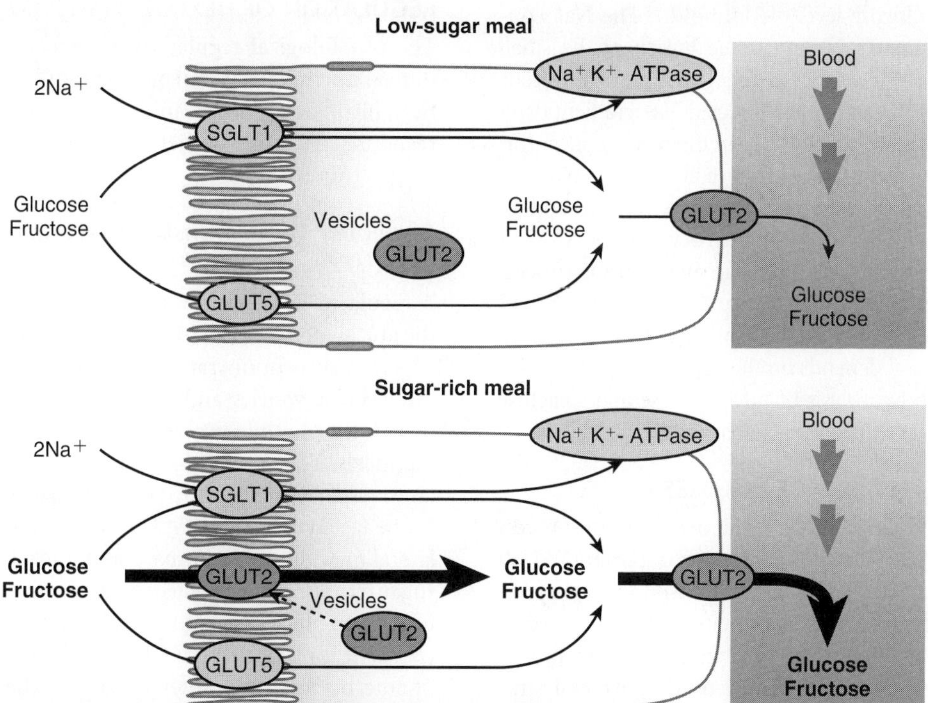

FIGURE 8-6 Physiological regulation of sugar absorption. When hexose concentrations in the lumen are low, hexoses enter enterocytes via SGLT1 and GLUT5, and then they can exit the cells via GLUT2 to enter the bloodstream. The consumption of a sugar-rich meal that saturates SGLT1 and GLUT5 can result in recruitment of GLUT2 into the apical membrane from its intracellular pool. This can triple the sugar uptake by enterocytes. GLUT2 apical translocation is maximal within 10 minutes after consumption of the sugar-rich meal, beyond which GLUT2 is internalized back to intracellular stores, similar to a low-sugar meal condition.

capillaries within the core of each villus. At low luminal concentrations, glucose and galactose are transported across the apical membrane into the enterocyte by the sodium/glucose cotransporter 1 (SGLT1), and fructose is taken up by the facilitated fructose transporter 5 (GLUT5). All three hexoses exit the enterocyte via GLUT2 in the basolateral membrane, a process that delivers these sugars to the capillaries and portal blood.

Pentoses are naturally present in fruits and as part of nucleotides, nucleosides, and nucleic acids in foods. Pentoses are released upon digestion and are taken up into the body. There is little information, however, about the absorption of pentoses, and its nutritional importance has not been investigated. Xylose appears to be absorbed by a passive mechanism that is increased when the integrity of the mucosal epithelium is compromised, and measures of xylose uptake have been used to assess the integrity of the gut epithelia.

SODIUM-DEPENDENT UPTAKE OF HEXOSES

SGLT1 is a transmembrane protein located in the apical membrane of enterocytes. It is a member of family 5 of the solute carrier proteins and is encoded by the *SLC5A1* gene. It cotransports two Na^+ ions and one aldohexose (stoichiometry of 2:1). Glucose and galactose, which differ only by the position of the hydroxyl and hydrogen attached to C4 in the ring structure, are both transported into enterocytes by SGLT1, which has a high affinity for these substrates. The K_m of SGLT1 for glucose and galactose is about 0.5 mmol/L, and its K_m for Na^+ is about 5 mmol/L. Therefore a half-maximal glucose transport rate may be observed even at low luminal glucose concentrations (0.5 mmol/L) that are one tenth of the fasting plasma glucose level (~5 mmol/L). The Na^+ concentration is permanently higher in the lumen of the small intestine than in the enterocyte (e.g., 70 mmol/L versus 12 mmol/L), providing an inward directed Na^+ gradient driving glucose and galactose uptake against their own concentration gradients. After glucose or galactose and its two Na^+ ion partners have entered the enterocyte, they are released and go their separate ways. The Na^+ exits the enterocyte via the Na^+,K^+-ATPase in the basolateral membrane, an energy using process responsible for maintaining the Na^+ and K^+ electrochemical gradients across membranes. Because maintenance of the Na^+ concentration gradient depends on the active pumping of Na^+ out of the cell, with hydrolysis of ATP, glucose and galactose uptake by SGLT1 is classified as secondary active transport.

FACILITATIVE TRANSPORT OF HEXOSES

Hexoses can be transported by a facilitative diffusion process that is mediated by isoforms of the glucose transporter (GLUT) family. These facilitative glucose/hexose transporters are members of family 2 of the solute carrier proteins and are encoded by *SLC2* genes. Facilitative transport involves the movement of a sugar down its concentration gradient across the cell membrane.

GLUT2

GLUT2 is a low-affinity, high-capacity transporter. In contrast to SGLT1, which is half-saturated at approximately 0.5 mmol/L of glucose, GLUT2 does not reach its half-saturation concentration until the glucose concentration is approximately 20 mmol/L. GLUT2 is always found in the basolateral membrane of enterocytes where it transports all three major hexoses (glucose, galactose, and fructose) out of the enterocyte down their concentration gradients (Bell et al., 1990). In mice, GLUT2 is also found in the apical membrane of enterocytes, where it can be transiently involved in the uptake of sugars from the intestinal lumen into the cell following the sugar gradient created by a sugar-rich meal (Gouyon et al., 2003).

GLUT5

GLUT5 is an apical membrane transporter that transports fructose, a ketohexose, into the enterocyte. Unlike GLUT2, GLUT5 is a low-affinity, high-capacity transporter with a K_m for fructose measured in *Xenopus* oocytes to be 5 to 6 mmol/L and estimated in vivo to be about 10 to 15 mmol/L (Douard and Ferraris, 2008). Some GLUT5 transporters are also localized in the basolateral membrane, where they may complement the GLUT2-mediated exit of fructose from the enterocyte.

GLUT7

An additional facilitative hexose transporter, GLUT7, is present in the apical membrane of enterocytes, but the possible role of GLUT7 in dietary sugar absorption is uncertain (Cheeseman, 2008). Its K_m of about 0.5 mmol/L for glucose and fructose indicates saturation at low hexose concentrations compared to GLUT2, but it could be important in the uptake of residual glucose and fructose in the distal small intestine. (See Chapter 12 for more about the GLUT family of transporters.)

REGULATION OF HEXOSE TRANSPORT

The physiological regulation of hexose transport is carried out via different mechanisms to modulate protein translocation, intrinsic activities, and synthesis of new transporters in response to sensing of dietary sugars during meals and after long-term diets.

Regulated Apical Translocation and Internalization of GLUT2

A regulated trafficking of GLUT2 transporters in and out of the apical membrane of the enterocyte provides a fine control of sugar absorption rates. Transporters are cycled between intracellular vesicles and the plasma membranes. Figure 8-6 depicts the physiological regulation of hexose absorption during meals. The regulation of GLUT2 trafficking is conserved among species from insects to mammals (Kellett et al., 2008). In the fasted condition, GLUT2 location is restricted to basolateral membranes in humans and mice. In mice fed a simple sugar meal or a sugar-rich diet, the capacity of the enterocytes to take up glucose, fructose, and galactose was tripled by the transient translocation of GLUT2 into the apical membranes of enterocytes (Gouyon et al., 2003). The presence of apical GLUT2 has been reported when high concentrations of sugars are present in the intestinal lumen (i.e., during refeeding after starvation and during the weaning transition from a high-fat milk to a high-carbohydrate rodent diet) (Kellett et al., 2008). A high concentration of monosaccharides in the lumen

CLINICAL CORRELATION

Glucose and Galactose Malabsorption

Carbohydrate intolerance is a rare but very serious hereditary disorder. Cases due to lack of digestive enzyme (e.g., primary sucrase–isomaltase deficiency) and to impaired hexose transport (i.e., primary glucose–galactose malabsorption) have been reported. On the basis of experience in a Boston hospital, it was estimated that glucose–galactose malabsorption accounted for about 2% of the patients with protracted diarrhea of infancy (Lloyd-Still et al., 1988). In two reported cases of carbohydrate intolerance, the infants developed diarrhea soon after birth. Their stools contained reducing sugars and had an acidic pH. Analysis of tissue obtained by biopsy of the small intestine showed normal villi with normal disaccharidase values. Monosaccharide load tests showed a normal rise in blood glucose following a fructose load dose, which was tolerated well. This result was in contrast to a flat glucose curve in response to a glucose load, which was accompanied by marked abdominal distention, profuse diarrhea, and the presence of reducing sugars in the stools.

Despite feeding a sugar-free formula plus fructose to these two infants with glucose–galactose malabsorption, diarrhea and the excretion of reducing sugars in the stool continued. This was due to a small amount of tapioca starch (25 g/L formula, which supplied more than 12.5 g starch per day for these patients) in the so-called sugar-free formula that was being used. Rigid exclusion of all carbohydrates and sugars except for fructose resulted in cessation of diarrhea and elimination of sugars from the stools.

Thinking Critically

1. These patients were diagnosed before the hexose transporters had been identified. Which hexose transport protein was probably lacking in these patients?
2. If the plasma glucose concentration had been monitored in these two patients following a load dose of sucrose, would a rise in plasma glucose have been observed? What would have been observed following a loading dose of lactose?
3. How would you expect the findings (carbohydrate tolerance, the glucose load test results, and the intestinal biopsy results) to differ in a case of secondary disaccharidase deficiency due to infective gastroenteritis (i.e., rotavirus infection) compared to those reported for these infants with hereditary carbohydrate intolerance?

appears to be instrumental in the process of apical GLUT2 translocation. GLUT2 was not found in the apical membrane of enterocytes of piglets fed high-carbohydrate diets (Moran et al., 2010) or of mice fed diets with complex carbohydrates (Gouyon et al., 2003). This physiological translocation of GLUT2 has not been investigated in humans because invasive jejunal biopsies from fed subjects would be required.

The mechanism triggering apical GLUT2 translocation involves SGLT1. Indeed, a high intraluminal glucose level that saturates SGLT1 capacity can activate a rapid and transient recruitment of GLUT2 into the apical membrane. The GLUT2 trafficking to the apical membrane is reduced by phlorizin, a strong inhibitor of SGLT1, suggesting that a priming of glucose entry via SGLT1 is required to trigger the apical translocation of GLUT2. A fructose load can also activate the translocation of GLUT2 to apical membranes, suggesting that SGLT1 might not be the unique priming system triggering GLUT2 translocation. A possible alternative pathway may be activation of enteroendocrine "sweet taste" G protein–coupled receptors (Tas1R3/Tas1R2). Activation of the dimeric Tas1R receptor by natural and artificial sugars promotes the recruitment of GLUT2 into the apical membrane of murine intestine by a yet unknown mechanism that appears to be mediated through activation of glucagon-like peptide 2 (GLP2) secretion. Indeed, the enterohormone GLP2 induces apical GLUT2 translocation in ex vivo experiments in rodent intestine (Au et al., 2002).

In the intestine the apical location of GLUT2 mediated by dietary sugars is transient. After a glucose load, blood glucose levels increase for 30 minutes and then return to basal levels. A role of the hypoglycemic hormone insulin in GLUT2 internalization back to its intracellular storage compartment in enterocytes has been reported. Internalization of GLUT2 reduces the rate of glucose absorption (Tobin et al., 2008). The intestine is therefore an insulin sensitive tissue contributing to glucose homeostasis. A maximal glucose action on apical GLUT2 translocation is observed within 10 minutes after a glucose load, whereas insulin action occurs later on to internalize GLUT2. The balance between glucose and insulin signaling likely determines the level of apical GLUT2.

In pathological conditions associated with insulin resistance, insulin-induced internalization can be lost, keeping GLUT2 in an apical location. With changes in eating habits and modern Westernized diets, fructose consumption has increased dramatically, as has insulin resistance. Insulin resistance is associated with a higher prevalence of metabolic diseases, obesity, and type 2 diabetes (Basciano et al., 2005). In mice fed high-fructose or high-fat diets and suffering from insulin resistance, a permanent location of GLUT2 in the apical membrane was observed even in fasting conditions, indicating a loss of insulin action on GLUT2 internalization (Tobin et al., 2008). This feature further exacerbates the situation by increasing the capacity for sugar absorption in conditions of already poor glycemic control. In rodents, experimental diabetes mimicking human type 1 diabetes also results in the permanent localization of GLUT2 in the apical membrane. Diabetes and insulin resistance in humans may thus be exacerbated by an increased capacity for sugar absorption via permanent apical GLUT2 location (Ait-Omar et al., 2011).

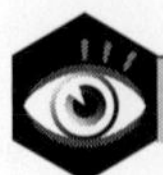

NUTRITION INSIGHT

Glucose Transport Enhances Water Absorption

The absorption of NaCl and solutes is known to be accompanied by the movement of water, presumably because an osmotic gradient is produced by absorption of the electrolytes and solutes such as amino acids and monosaccharides. Glucose uptake also creates an osmotic gradient and promotes water absorption. Expression of SGLT in *Xenopus* oocytes induced a movement of 260 water molecules along with the transport of 2 Na^+ and 1 glucose molecule (Loo et al., 1996). Expression of GLUT2 in *Xenopus* oocytes resulted in the uptake of 35 water molecules for each sugar molecule transported (Zeuthen et al., 2007). According to calculations using these numbers, the transport of the usual quantity of glucose- or hexose-containing nutrients consumed daily (~250 g/day) would support water absorption of several liters by the human intestine. Although this might seem rather amazing, we know that approximately 9 to 11 L of fluid are reabsorbed daily by the human gastrointestinal tract. The osmotic effects of glucose and amino acids are used in oral rehydration therapy; oral rehydration solutions contain these solutes to promote the absorption of water. Although the exact mechanisms for water uptake are still being worked out, we know that water is able to move through both transcellular and paracellular pores in the gut epithelium.

Regulation of SGLT1

SGLT1 activity in the apical membrane of enterocytes is also regulated by mechanisms in addition to SGLT1 expression levels. SGLT1 appears to be regulated by changes in trafficking and activation state (Kellett et al., 2008; Walker et al., 2005; Filatova et al., 2009; Osswald et al., 2005). The involved mechanisms are still being elucidated.

Regulation of Transporter Expression

In addition to the regulation of transporter trafficking, there is regulation of hexose transporter gene expression. The mRNA abundance of all three major hexose transporters displays diurnal variation with an increase just before feeding and a marked increase in response to sugar consumption. In rats, glucose or fructose (released from digestion of polysaccharides and oligosaccharides or perfused directly into the intestinal lumen) increased the expression of the *SGLT1*, *GLUT5*, and *GLUT2* genes (Miyamoto et al., 1993). This effect was not due to a metabolic product of glucose such as phosphorylated glucose, because nonmetabolizable 3-*O*-methylglucose also augmented the mRNA levels. Artificial sugars were shown to increase the expression of *GLUT5* and *SGLT1* in Caco-2 cells (Le Gall et al., 2007). The expression of *SGLT1* was rapidly upregulated in the small intestine of rats exposed to glucose, fructose, or sugar substitutes, with the topology of response matching the expression profile of sweet taste receptor *Tas1R3/Tas1R2* (Stearns et al., 2010). A similar increase in *SGLT1* expression was observed in small intestine of piglets fed diets with more than 50% of energy from carbohydrate (Moran et al., 2010). High concentrations of natural sugars (over 100 mmol/L of glucose or fructose) and low amounts of artificial sugars (in the mmol/L range) can activate sweet taste receptors in the enteroendocrine cells, and it appears that this leads to increased expression of the hexose transporter genes.

Regulation of transporter expression is also tightly linked to enterocyte differentiation. Hexose transporters are absent or present at low levels in immature enterocytes in the crypts of the intestinal mucosa, but their expression increases as the cells mature and move up along the villus toward the tip. Hexose transporter expression also tends to be higher in the duodenum/jejunum and lower in the ileum.

FACTORS AFFECTING CARBOHYDRATE ASSIMILATION

The processes of starch and oligosaccharide digestion as well as final monosaccharide transport are usually very efficient, enabling total assimilation of ingested starch, disaccharides, and monosaccharides. Nevertheless, digestion and absorption of dietary carbohydrate in healthy individuals may be affected by several factors.

EFFECT OF TRANSIT TIME

The initial factors involved in carbohydrate processing are the rate of chewing and residence time in the mouth, which affect the interaction of the starch component with salivary amylase. The oral phase is usually a relatively short period, and the meal is then exposed to the low pH of the stomach, which stops the action of the salivary amylase. Once filled, the stomach reservoir will empty at a rate that is dependent upon the nutrient composition of the meal. The presence of dietary fat, nondigestible carbohydrate (dietary fiber), and high osmolality (such as that present in concentrated desserts sweetened with sucrose) all will retard gastric emptying, thereby slowing the rate of overall carbohydrate assimilation. Gastric emptying and gut motility are under the control of gut signals released in the course of a meal. Gut motility is driven by contractions that occur in wave patterns likely originating in smooth muscle. Both amplitude and duration of the waves depend upon hormones, paracrine signals, and the autonomic nervous system for proper regulation.

Once the stomach does empty, the intraluminal digestion of carbohydrates is a highly efficient process. Indeed, most starch is digested within the lumen of the duodenum, the uppermost part of the small intestine. Complete hydrolysis of the resulting starch oligosaccharides, as well as any dietary disaccharides, and the absorption of the released hexose sugars generally occur within the jejunum of the small intestine before the digesta reaches the ileum. Transit time through the small intestine may have some effect on the rate of carbohydrate assimilation. Meal composition affects intestinal motility and hence transit time through the small intestine. However, in the absence of intestinal or pancreatic disease, the effect of intestinal motility on the overall assimilation of hexoses is small, with sugars being absorbed before the digesta reaches the colon.

EFFECT OF PHYSICAL STATE OF STARCH

Despite the capacity for complete digestion of starch, some properties of foods or starches can inhibit the process in the gastrointestinal tract. Physicochemical properties of particular food carbohydrates, such as the degree of crystallization or moisture or the presence of physical barriers, can limit the extent of starch digestion. For instance, processed retrograde starch, which contains a more crystalline arrangement of molecules than natural starch, is refractory to hydrolysis by amylase and maltase–glucoamylase. Food starches are naturally present in grains and legumes in association with proteins, many of which are hydrophobic and hence hinder the luminal interaction of the secreted polar amylases with the polysaccharide within the interior of the starch granules. Physical processing of grains, such as cracking, milling, or heating at 100° C for several minutes, changes the physical relationship of starch to the accompanying protein, making it more available to the water-soluble amylase. In addition, the presence of nondigestible polysaccharides (cellulose, hemicellulose, and pectin) may interfere with the efficiency of the amylase–starch interaction by blocking the physical association of amylase with its substrate. Therefore, depending upon the physical availability of starch in the prepared food, a small proportion (1% to 10%) of the ingested starch may escape amylase action, and this residual starch passes into the colon where it is fermented by colonic bacteria.

DEFICIENCIES OF CARBOHYDRATE ASSIMILATION

Other than the physical condition of the ingested carbohydrate, particularly if it is starch, the most important factors determining the rate of carbohydrate assimilation are the enzymatic hydrolysis by the apical membrane oligosaccharidases and the transport of the released monosaccharides. Several deficiencies or disorders of carbohydrate assimilation are related to the genetic or functional deficiency of particular membrane oligosaccharidases, disaccharidases, or sugar transporters. The main approach to therapy, once a defect in carbohydrate digestion or absorption has been identified, is the elimination of the unassimilated carbohydrate from the diet.

CARBOHYDRATE MALABSORPTION PHENOTYPE

The carbohydrate malabsorption phenotype is identical regardless of whether it is caused by oligosaccharidase, disaccharidase, or monosaccharide transporter deficiency and whether it is due to gene defects, mucosal atrophy, or inflammatory bowel diseases. The consequences when an oligosaccharidase, disaccharidase, or transporter is appreciably reduced or absent from the enterocyte apical membrane are summarized in Figure 8-7. The proximal malabsorption of lactose (or sucrose or glucose/galactose) results in an increase in intraluminal osmolar load that delivers undigested disaccharides and trapped fluid into the colon. In children and adults, the colon activates a salvage pathway of carbohydrate fermentation to

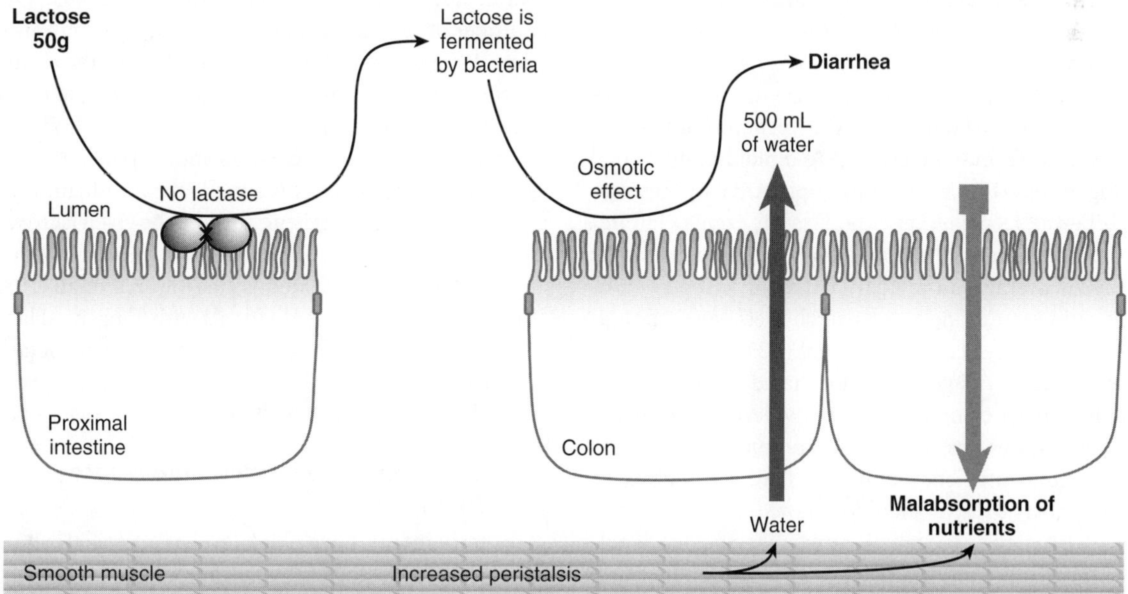

FIGURE 8-7 Pathogenesis of a carbohydrate malabsorption syndrome. Maldigestion of lactose allows bacteria to use it as substrate for fermentation, thereby producing short-chain fatty acids and gases. These products of fermentation increase the lumen osmolarity, in turn inducing an increase in ileal and colonic water and augmentation of peristalsis of the gut, which can lead to secondary malabsorption of other nutrients. Deficiencies in any oligosaccharidase or hexose transporter can result in the same pathological events.

short-chain fatty acids by the bacterial flora (Topping and Clifton, 2001). Some of the short-chain fatty acids (acetate, propionate, and butyrate) are absorbed from the colon. The colonic fermentation of carbohydrates by bacteria also produces carbon dioxide (CO_2) and hydrogen (H_2) gases. An increase in H_2 in the breath is used experimentally as evidence of increased fermentation. The fermentation products increase osmolarity and the quantity of fluid and gas in the lower small intestine and colon; this is manifested by symptoms of abdominal cramping, discomfort, and diarrhea. In infants, the colonic fermentation pathway is often inadequate, and a diet-sensitive acidic osmotic diarrhea may occur with unmetabolized carbohydrate being passed in the stools. More severe symptoms, including vomiting, may develop. Untreated, sugar malabsorption represents a loss of calories and micronutrients, minerals, and vitamins, which may lead to weight loss or failure to thrive.

AMYLASE DEFICIENCY AND ITS TREATMENT

Defects of amylase digestion of starch are rarely found. Although a small percentage of starch escapes amylase action, this is related to the polysaccharide's physical state rather than to a limiting quantity of the amylase. The pancreatic and salivary amylase genes are 97% identical, but the protein products show some slight differences in starch cleavage patterns. The amount of pancreatic amylase secreted in response to a meal is in great excess of the amount that is required for optimal intraluminal digestion of starch to the final oligosaccharide products. Therefore a decrease in amylase amount or activity may not have a physiological consequence. In addition, a genetic redundancy may contribute to the rarity with which defects of amylase are found. In humans, amylase is encoded by two different loci, AMY1 (salivary amylase) and AMY2 (pancreatic amylase),which show strong tissue-specific expression. The human genome contains two identical genes coding for pancreatic amylase (AMY2A and AMY2B), giving each diploid cell four genes encoding pancreatic amylase. The number of copies of the salivary amylase gene in humans is highly variable, with individuals having diploid copy numbers ranging from 2 to 15. These multiple AMY1 genes are believed to be the result of gene duplication events (Iafrate et al., 2004). Individuals from populations eating high-starch diets display, on average, more *AMY1* copies in their genomes than those eating traditionally low-starch diets, suggesting a diet-related pressure selection (Perry et al., 2007).

Amylase deficiency is generally associated with exocrine pancreatic insufficiency that results in low levels of all pancreatic digestive secretions. The most common causes of exocrine pancreatic insufficiency in humans are cystic fibrosis and chronic pancreatitis. It should be noted, however, that an isolated deficiency of pancreatic amylase in the duodenal fluid of a 3-year-old child has been reported (Mehta et al., 2000). The child presented with poor weight gain, abdominal distention, flatulence, and loose stools on an intermittent basis, and supplementation with pancreatic enzymes was associated with a sustained catch-up weight gain and resolution of the gastrointestinal symptoms.

GENETIC OLIGOSACCHARIDASE AND DISACCHARIDASE DEFICIENCIES AND THEIR TREATMENT

The genetically determined decline of lactase–phlorizin hydrolase activities between infancy and adulthood, as well as mutations in an enhancer region of the gene which lead to lactase persistence in some populations, are well recognized. In addition, rare genetic mutations of the lactase–phlorizin hydrolase, sucrase–isomaltase, or trehalase gene, leading to decreased or absent activities of lactase, sucrase, or trehalase, respectively, occur in human populations. Although some cases of isolated maltase–glucoamylase deficiency have been diagnosed based on biochemical assays, no causal genetic mutations in the gene for maltase–glucoamylase or genes encoding proteins involved in its processing have yet been reported (Nichols et al., 2002; Lebenthal et al., 1994). Most reported cases of maltase–glucoamylase deficiencies have been associated with other disaccharidase deficiencies, suggesting that they may be caused by nongenetic factors or by defects in regulatory factors common to all intestinal glycohydrolases (Karnsakul et al., 2002).

Congenital Lactase Deficiency and Its Treatment

Congenital lactase deficiency in which lactase activity is very low or absent from the intestinal epithelium from birth is a severe, but rare, condition. Because lactose is the sugar present in breast milk and in most infant formulas, symptoms occur soon after birth and can lead to severe dehydration, acidosis, and weight loss if left untreated. A variety of mutations of the lactase–phlorizin hydrolase gene have been identified in the past decade that result in a lack of lactase expression or in the expression of a mutant protein with low activity or impaired folding or trafficking (Torniainen et al., 2009; Kuokkanen et al., 2006; Behrendt et al., 2009). The highest number of cases so far has been found in the Finnish population. In these Finnish cases, a mutation in the coding region of the gene results in the substitution of deoxythymidine for deoxyadenosine at nucleotide 4170. This T4170A mutation creates a premature stop codon and expression of a truncated protein that does not contain a lactase domain. Infants with congenital lactase deficiency need to be given lactose-free formula during infancy. Treatment of breast milk with lactase to hydrolyze lactose is also possible (Simila et al., 1982). After infancy, treatment of individuals with congenital lactase deficiency is similar to those of adults with hypolactasia, which involves avoidance or limitation of crude dairy products and use of milk substitutes such as soy milk or rice milk.

Lactase Deficiency or Lactose Intolerance and Its Treatment

Full-term infants have a high level of intestinal lactase activity and are able to efficiently hydrolyze lactose in breast milk or formula. Lactase activity increases between 8 and 34 weeks of gestation and then increases more rapidly until term. Premature infants are born with less lactase activity than full-term infants. In both premature and term infants, lactase activity appears to increase with milk feeding (Tan-Dy and Ohlsson,

2005). The lactose load that premature infants are able to completely digest is less than that of full-term infants, but preterm infants generally are able to handle the amounts of lactose in breast milk or formula.

Lactase deficiency or lactose intolerance occurs in most mammals after weaning because of a genetically determined decline in lactase expression. The transient expression of lactase–phlorizin hydrolase is regulated by the transcription factor NF-LPH1, as described earlier in the chapter. In humans who do not consume dairy products, intestinal lactase–phlorizin hydrolase activity usually drops about 90% during the first 4 years of life (Simoons, 1970). Thus lactose intolerance in adults is considered a common condition.

Individuals with hypolactasia generally avoid or limit their intake of dairy products and use milk substitutes, such as soy milk or rice milk. Most people with low lactase levels can still tolerate small amounts of milk products, especially when consumed as part of a meal. Because milk products are an excellent source of nutrients and a common part of the diet, enzyme replacement approaches are also widely used. For example, a lactose hydrolyzing enzyme, such as purified β-galactosidase, can be added to dairy products to break down lactose. Dairy products treated with lactase are commercially available, as are lactase preparations that can be taken as a digestive aid just before eating lactose-containing foods or added to milk before its consumption. Fermented milk products may be acceptable because of their lower lactose content; lactase-positive strains of bacteria can both provide the lactase activity to hydrolyze and remove the lactose in the product and provide a probiotic with lactase activity to the gastrointestinal tract.

Lactase Persistence

Certain human populations have lactase persistence. The frequency of lactase persistence is high in northern European populations and some pastoralist populations in Africa (e.g., greater than 90% in Swedes, Danes, and Tutsi), moderate across southern Europe and the Middle East and in some pastoralist African populations (e.g., about 50% in Spanish, French, and pastoralist Arab populations), and low in nonpastoralist Asian and African populations (e.g., about 1% in Chinese, 5% to 20% in West African agriculturalists) (Swallow, 2003). Lactase persistence, allowing lactose digestion to continue into adulthood, is due to inheritance of a dominant allele carrying a mutation that promotes lactose persistence. Several different single nucleotide polymorphisms (SNPs) located in an "enhancer" sequence in an intron of a neighboring gene *(MCM6)* are associated with lactase persistence. The particular *cis*-acting polymorphism varies with the population group, suggesting that several independent mutations led to lactase persistence in human populations. For example, different SNPs that originated on different haplotype backgrounds have been identified in European, sub-Saharan African, and Middle Eastern

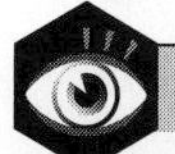

NUTRITION INSIGHT

Is There Too Much Self-Diagnosis of Lactose Intolerance?

Many individuals attribute symptoms of various gastrointestinal tract disorders to lactose intolerance and treat themselves or their children with lactose-restricted diets. Lactose restriction often involves avoiding milk and milk-containing products. This could be a public health concern, because restriction of dairy consumption may predispose individuals to decreased bone accrual, osteoporosis, and other adverse health outcomes. Dairy products are a major source of calcium and an excellent source of many nutrients, including protein, riboflavin, and the fat-soluble vitamins A, D, E, and K. In Western diets, milk consumption is usually critical for taking in the calcium necessary for optimal accumulation of bone mineral. Calcium intake is especially important in young individuals, with calcium needs for bone mineral accrual being greatest at the time of puberty. Pregnant and lactating women need to transfer calcium to the fetus and breast milk; and in elderly persons, higher calcium intake may slow bone mineral loss.

Correct diagnosis of the underlying condition is important, both to resolve the discomfort and prevent the need for unnecessary food restriction. Some people who are clinically lactase deficient do not experience symptomatic lactose intolerance. Most lactose-intolerant persons do not need to completely eliminate the consumption of dairy products; they simply need to reduce the amount consumed. Even adults and adolescents with diagnosed lactose malabsorption should be able to ingest at least 12 g of lactose (equivalent to that in 1 cup of milk) when consumed in a single dose, and larger amounts of lactose can be tolerated if ingested with meals and spread throughout the day. Strategies to reduce lactose intake while maintaining a nutritionally adequate diet might involve inclusion of small amounts of dairy foods and lactase-treated products as well as inclusion of alternative sources for the calcium and other nutrients provided by milk. A table of nondairy sources of calcium is included in the 2005 Dietary Guidelines for Americans, which are available at *www.health.gov*. Nondairy sources of absorbable calcium include dried beans, leafy green vegetables, and any calcium-fortified products.

The National Institutes of Health (NIH) convened a Consensus Development Conference in 2010 to address several questions related to lactose intolerance and health, and its report is available *(http://consensus.nih.gov/2010/lactosestatement.htm)*. For the 2010 conference, the NIH commissioned a systematic review of effective management strategies for lactose intolerance that was conducted by the Minnesota Evidence-based Practice Center (Shaukat et al., 2010). Another review related to the diagnosis of lactose malabsorption and intolerance in primary care was conducted by Jellema and colleagues (2010).

populations (Ingram et al., 2009; Enattah et al., 2008). These evolutionary adaptations appear to have a relatively recent origin (approximately 7,000 years ago), and the convergent adaptation of human lactase appears to be due to a strong selective pressure of adult milk consumption that followed animal domestication by several different pastoralist populations (Tishkoff et al., 2007).

Congenital Sucrase–Isomaltase Deficiency and Its Treatment

Congenital sucrase–isomaltase deficiency (asucrasia) is one of the most frequently reported genetic intestinal disaccharidase deficiencies. The prevalence of congenital sucrase–isomaltase deficiency is estimated to be about 1 in 5,000 people of European descent but has been shown to be much higher in the native Inuit population, affecting about 5% of the population of Greenland (Gudmand-Høyer et al., 1987). It is detected at weaning when infants are first exposed to sucrose- and starch-containing foods. The disorder may be present as an isolated sucrase deficiency, with normal levels of isomaltase activity, or as a combined sucrase and isomaltase deficiency (Jacob et al., 2000). Isolated deficiencies of the isomaltase subunit have not been reported, probably because the correct processing of the sucrase–isomaltase polypeptide depends on the structure and function of the isomaltase subunit. The presence of an immunoreactive sucrase–isomaltase molecule has been demonstrated in all congenital sucrase–isomaltase deficiencies that have been studied, indicating that the protein is synthesized. The bifunctional sucrase–isomaltase that is synthesized, however, either is transported to the apical membrane with a structurally altered and inactive sucrase subunit or contains mutations that block its movement to the apical membrane, causing it to accumulate in the cell until it is degraded.

For individuals with sucrase–isomaltase deficiency, it is necessary to avoid table sugar and other products that contain sucrose. It is also important to limit intake of starch, especially amylopectin, if isomaltase activity is affected. Although sucrase–isomaltase deficiency can be effectively treated by total elimination of sucrose-containing foods, this is difficult to do. Effective enzyme replacement is a highly successful adjunct to dietary restriction. Sacrosidase, an enzyme derived from baker's yeast, hydrolyzes sucrose and is used as a digestive aid for individuals with sucrase–isomaltase deficiency (Treem et al., 1993). Sacrosidase supplements are usually taken before and halfway through a meal or added directly to beverages.

Congenital Trehalase Deficiency

Genetic trehalase deficiencies were first described among Inuit natives with a prevalence of trehalose intolerance of about 8% (Gudmand-Høyer et al., 1988). However, the incidence of primary trehalase deficiency in the United States and Europe is extremely rare, and in many countries no cases are known (Murray et al., 2000). The clinical symptoms observed in subjects with this disorder are similar to those of other disaccharidase deficiencies, but they have been identified because of symptoms associated exclusively with the ingestion of mushrooms or a diagnostic trehalose load dose. Because trehalose has limited distribution in common foods, and trehalose activity is seldom absent but simply low, sufficient elimination of trehalose from the diet to relieve symptoms is usually easily accomplished.

HEXOSE TRANSPORTER DEFICIENCIES WITH A GENETIC CAUSE AND THEIR TREATMENTS

Several relatively rare genetic disorders involve structural defects in the glucose transporters SGLT1 and GLUT2.

Glucose–Galactose Malabsorption

The first hexose transporter mutation to be identified was one that prevents processing and insertion of SGLT1 into the apical membrane, such that the SGLT1 protein accumulates in Golgi compartments. Several additional mutations that impair the transport function of SGLT1 have since been identified (Wright et al., 2003; Brown, 2000). These mutations provoke glucose–galactose malabsorption, which is usually diagnosed in infancy. Unless glucose and galactose sources are eliminated from the diet at an early age, these mutations can lead to death (Meeuwisse and Dahlqvist, 1968). Patients with SGLT1 deficiencies are able to digest fructose-based formulas that are glucose-free, but they cannot tolerate sucrose, which yields both fructose and glucose upon hydrolysis. Tolerance to glucose and galactose may improve with age.

Fanconi-Bickel Syndrome

Mutations in GLUT2 appear to lessen glucose and galactose absorption. Because GLUT2 is expressed in kidney, liver, and pancreatic beta cells as well as in the enterocyte, the phenotype of individuals with GLUT2 deficiency is due to mishandling of glucose by both the intestine and other tissues. A truncated GLUT2 protein was discovered in the first identified patient with Fanconi-Bickel syndrome. More than 30 GLUT2 mutations have been subsequently identified that are thought to be the causative factor of the Fanconi-Bickel syndrome (Santer et al., 2002). This rare inherited recessive autosomal disorder is characterized by hepatorenal glycogen accumulation, proximal renal tubular dysfunction, impaired absorption of glucose and galactose, and failure to thrive. Frequent feeding of slowly absorbed carbohydrates is recommended, and continuous tube feeding of oligosaccharide solutions during the night may be needed. Administration of uncooked cornstarch has been used successfully to promote growth in these patients, underlining an intestinal contribution in this syndrome (Weinstein and Wolfsdorf, 2002).

ACQUIRED DEFICIENCIES OF CARBOHYDRATE DIGESTION AND THEIR TREATMENT

Acquired deficiencies of carbohydrate digestion may be due to surgical removal of part of the intestine, use of antiglycemic drugs, pancreatic exocrine insufficiency, or secondary deficiencies of mucosal surface oligosaccharidase, disaccharidase, and transporter activities due to diet, malnutrition, infection, or bowel disease.

Gastric Bypass Surgery

In morbidly obese patients, gastric bypass surgery is a therapy proposed to lessen obesity. This surgery alters the functional gastrointestinal tract by bypassing about 90% of the stomach, the entire duodenum, and the proximal part of the jejunum of the small intestine. This leaves a reduced stomach pouch that empties into the remaining jejunum. The rapid arrival of poorly digested food into the jejunum may provoke a dumping syndrome (due to adrenergic and vasoactive reactions), and this is a frequent complication observed soon after this surgery. A rare complication of this surgery is postprandial hyperinsulinemic hypoglycemia that usually occurs several months after the surgery. This metabolic abnormality appears to be due to the altered nutrient transit through the gastrointestinal tract (McLaughlin et al., 2010), although hypertrophy and hyperfunction of pancreatic beta cells may also be involved (Mathavan et al., 2010). A reduction in the ingestion of simple carbohydrates and administration of an α-glucosidase inhibitor to slow down sugar assimilation, with the goal of lessening insulin release, is a proposed therapy for treatment of hypoglycemic episodes that occur following gastric bypass surgery (Marsk et al., 2010). Bypass surgery induces profound modifications of intestinal absorption, but postsurgical changes have not been thoroughly studied. Although the ileum usually plays only a limited role in carbohydrate digestion and absorption, it can adapt through cellular proliferation (hyperplasia) to assume a more important role in the case of gastric bypass surgery, extensive jejunal disease, or surgical removal of the upper small intestine (Iqbal et al., 2008).

Use of Antidiabetic Drugs

The development of inhibitors of starch digestion for potential use in treating or preventing human conditions such as diabetes and obesity is an active area of pharmacological research. Acarbose, which is isolated from strains of the bacterium *Actinoplanes,* is a pseudotetrasaccharide composed of maltose bound to an acarviosine group. Acarbose is the most widely used α-glucosidase inhibitor currently on the market (Figure 8-8). Acarbose is an efficient inhibitor of α-amylase and of the C-terminal maltase and sucrase domains of maltase–glucoamylase and sucrose–isomaltase, respectively; it also is a weaker inhibitor of the N-terminal glucoamylase and isomaltase activities (Li et al., 2005; Sim et al., 2010a, 2010b). Acarbose delays the digestion of starch in the small intestine so that glucose from the starch of a meal will enter the bloodstream more slowly, thus matching the impaired insulin response or sensitivity. Therefore acarbose is used therapeutically to control blood glucose levels in patients with type 2 diabetes, particularly those in the early stages of impaired glucose tolerance. However, unpleasant side effects can occur from impaired starch digestion and retention of oligosaccharides in the intestine, and this restricts the acceptability of the drug (Chiasson et al., 2003; Van de Laar et al., 2005). Miglitol, a monosaccharide-like product, is also used as an α-glucosidase inhibitor, but it is not an effective inhibitor of α-amylase.

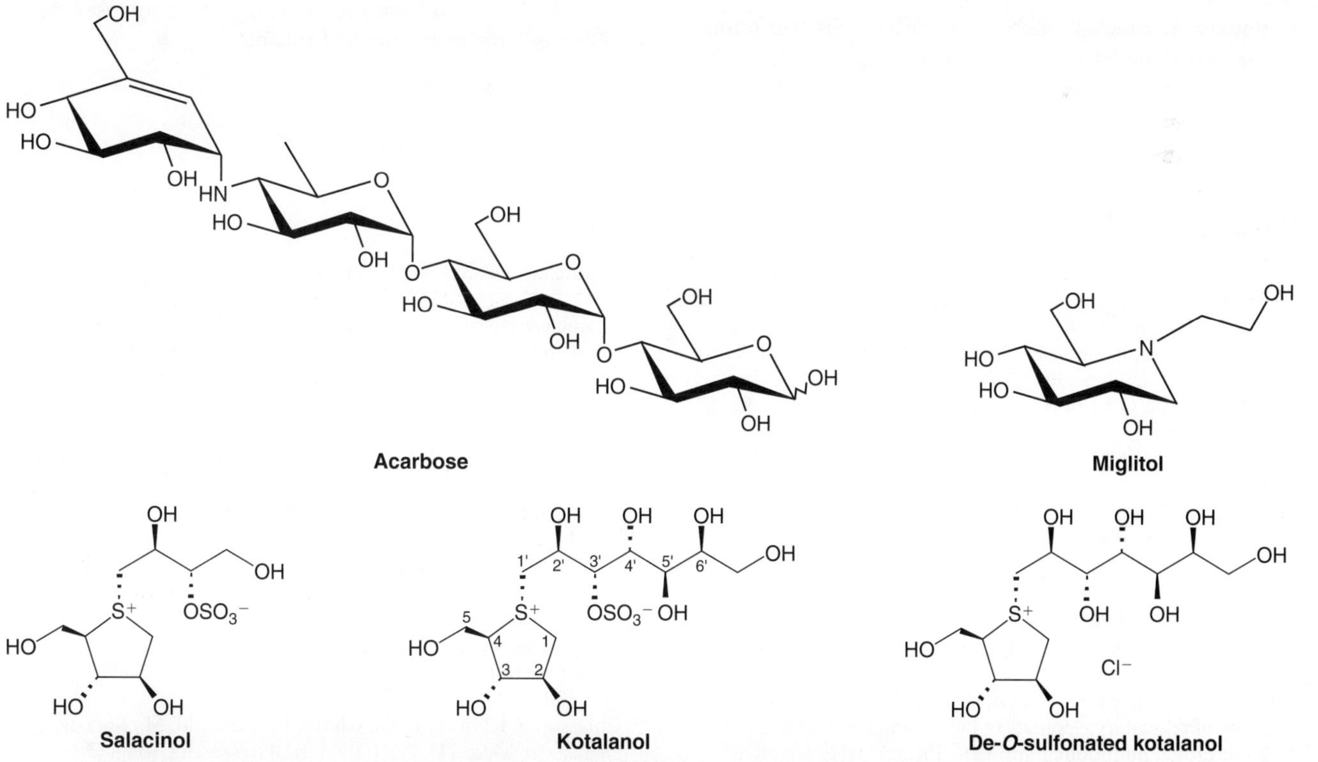

FIGURE 8-8 Structures of α-glucosidase inhibitors. (Modified from Sim, L., Jayakanthan, K., Mohan, S., Nasi, R., Johnston, B. D., Pinto, B. M., & Rose, D. R. [2010]. New glucosidase inhibitors from an ayurvedic herbal treatment for type 2 diabetes: Structures and inhibition of human intestinal maltase-glucoamylase with compounds from *Salacia reticulata. Biochemistry, 49,* 443–451. Copyright 2010 American Chemical Society.)

More recently, studies of a new class of more potent α-glucosidase inhibitors, including the active compounds salacinol, kotalanol, and de-*O*-sulfonated kotalanol, have shown these compounds to be stronger inhibitors than acarbose, particularly of the N-terminal glucoamylase and isomaltase domains of maltase–glucoamylase and sucrose–isomaltase, respectively (Sim et al., 2010a, 2010b). Salacinol, kotalanol, and de-*O*-sulfonated kotalanol are all sulfonium compounds naturally found in *Salacia reticulata*, a shrub native to Sri Lanka and southern India that is used in traditional medicine to prepare natural antidiabetic formulations for diabetic patients (Muraoka et al., 2010). The effectiveness of these compounds in the inhibition of α-glucosidase activities that are not sufficiently decreased by acarbose raises the possibility of combination therapy.

Secondary Oligosaccharidase, Disaccharidase, and Transporter Deficiencies

Diet, malnutrition, pathogen or parasite infections, and inflammatory bowel diseases are associated with intestinal malabsorption that can lead to diarrhea, weight loss, and failure to thrive. Mucosal disaccharidase activity, a marker of the integrity or differentiation of the intestinal epithelium, is perturbed in these pathologies. Indeed, the alteration of the structure and function of the intestinal epithelium impairs not only the absorption of carbohydrates but also the absorption of other nutrients, including minerals and vitamins. Lactose intolerance, in particular, may be observed because of a reduced amount of lactase related to decreased bowel surface, but this resolves once the condition is treated. Secondary lactose or sucrose intolerance is temporary. Dietary restriction for a short period may be helpful, but restricted food intake should not be necessary once the villi have recovered (Di Sabatino and Corazza, 2009).

Fructose intolerance has been reported in some toddlers; a high consumption of fructose in the diet (from refined apple juice or honey) that overwhelms their fructose transport activity was suggested as the main cause of fructose intolerance (Hoekstra et al., 1996). Suppression of offending fructose and sucrose in the diet is sufficient to resolve gut function and may be required until gut maturation is completed.

THINKING CRITICALLY

1. Viral gastroenteritis, parasitic infections, and other conditions that damage the mucosal epithelium can cause secondary lactose intolerance. Why is lactose consumption more of a problem than sucrose or starch consumption for patients with secondary lactose intolerance?
2. Reports of trehalose malabsorption are extremely rare. However, when individuals with suspected trehalose malabsorption have been tested, some have shown a lack of trehalase activity in intestinal biopsies as well as trehalose malabsorption on an oral tolerance test with trehalose. It is possible that trehalase deficiency is more widespread but not frequently diagnosed. What factors might facilitate the lack of detection of a genetic lack of trehalase?
3. A rare inborn error of metabolism is a congenital sucrase–isomaltase deficiency. What reactions in human digestion are catalyzed by this protein? Would you expect patients with sucrase–isomaltase deficiency to have problems digesting sucrose? lactose? maltose? starch? Explain.

REFERENCES

Ait-Omar, A., Monteiro-Sepulveda, M., Poitou, C., Le Gall, M., Cotillard, A., Gilet, J., … Brot-Laroche, E. (2011). GLUT2 accumulation in enterocyte apical and intracellular membranes: A study in morbidly obese human subjects and ob/ob and high fat-fed mice. *Diabetes, 60*, 2598–2607.

Au, A., Gupta, A., Schembri, P., & Cheeseman, C. I. (2002). Rapid insertion of GLUT2 into the rat jejunal brush-border membrane promoted by glucagon-like peptide 2. *The Biochemical Journal, 367*, 247–254.

Basciano, H., Federico, L., & Adeli, K. (2005). Fructose, insulin resistance, and metabolic dyslipidemia. *Nutrition & Metabolism, 2*, 5.

Behrendt, M., Keiser, M., Hoch, M., & Naim, H. Y. (2009). Impaired trafficking and subcellular localization of a mutant lactase associated with congenital lactase deficiency. *Gastroenterology, 136*, 2295–2303.

Behrendt, M., Polaina, J., & Naim, H. Y. (2010). Structural hierarchy of regulatory elements in the folding and transport of an intestinal multidomain protein. *The Journal of Biological Chemistry, 285*, 4143–4152.

Bell, G. I., Kayano, T., Buse, J. B., Burant, C. F., Takeda, J., Lin, D., … Seino, S. (1990). Molecular biology of mammalian glucose transporters. *Diabetes Care, 13*, 198–208.

Boudreau, F., Rings, E. H., van Wering, H. M., Kim, R. K., Swain, G. P., Krasinski, S. D., … Traber, P. G. (2002). Hepatocyte nuclear factor-1 alpha, GATA-4, and caudal related homeodomain protein Cdx2 interact functionally to modulate intestinal gene transcription: Implication for the developmental regulation of the sucrase-isomaltase gene. *The Journal of Biological Chemistry, 277*, 31909–31917.

Brand-Miller, J. C., Thomas, M., Swan, V., Ahmad, Z. I., Petocz, P., & Colagiuri, S. (2003). Physiological validation of the concept of glycemic load in lean young adults. *The Journal of Nutrition, 133*, 2728–2732.

Brown, G. K. (2000). Glucose transporters: Structure, function and consequences of deficiency. *Journal of Inherited Metabolic Disease, 23*, 237–246.

Cheeseman, C. (2008). GLUT7: A new intestinal facilitated hexose transporter. *The American Journal of Physiology, 295*, E238–E241.

Chiasson, J. L., Josse, R. G., Gomis, R., Hanefeld, M., Karasik, A., Laakso, M. & STOP-NIDDM Trial Research Group. (2003). Acarbose treatment and the risk of cardiovascular disease and hypertension in patients with impaired glucose tolerance: The STOP-NIDDM trial. *The Journal of the American Medical Association, 290*, 486–494.

Di Sabatino, A., & Corazza, G. R. (2009). Coeliac disease. *Lancet, 373*, 1480–1493.

Douard, V., & Ferraris, R. P. (2008). Regulation of the fructose transporter GLUT5 in health and disease. *American Journal of Physiology Endocrinology and Metabolism, 295*, E227–E237.

Elbein, A. D., Pan, Y. T., Pastuszak, I., & Carroll, D. (2003). New insights on trehalose: A multifunctional molecule. *Glycobiology, 13*, 17R–27R.

Enattah, N. S., Jensen, T. G., Nielsen, M., Lewinski, R., Kuokkanen, M., Rasinpera, H., … Peltonen, L. (2008). Independent introduction of two lactase-persistence alleles into human populations reflects different history of adaptation to milk culture. *American Journal of Human Genetics, 82*, 57–72.

Filatova, A., Leyerer, M., Gorboulev, V., Chintalapati, C., Reinders, Y., Müller, T. D., … Koepsell, H. (2009). Novel shuttling domain in a regulator (RSC1A1) of transporter SGLT1 steers cell cycle-dependent nuclear location. *Traffic, 10*, 1599–1618.

Fogel, M. R., & Gray, G. M. (1973). Starch hydrolysis in man: An intraluminal process not requiring membrane digestion. *Journal of Applied Physiology, 35*, 263–267.

Galgani, J., Aguirre, C., & Díaz, E. (2006). Acute effect of meal glycemic index and glycemic load on blood glucose and insulin responses in humans. *Nutrition Journal, 5*, 22.

Gouyon, F., Caillaud, L., Carriere, V., Klein, C., Dalet, V., Citadelle, D., … Brot-Laroche, E. (2003). Simple-sugar meals target GLUT2 at enterocyte apical membranes to improve sugar absorption: A study in GLUT2-null mice. *The Journal of Physiology, 552*, 823–832.

Gudmand-Høyer, E., Fenger, H. J., Kern-Hansen, P., & Madsen, P. R. (1987). Sucrase deficiency in Greenland: Incidence and genetic aspects. *Scandinavian Journal of Gastroenterology, 22*, 24–28.

Gudmand-Høyer, E., Fenger, H. J., Skovbjerg, H., Kern-Hansen, P., & Madsen, P. R. (1988). Trehalase deficiency in Greenland. *Scandinavian Journal of Gastroenterology, 23*, 775–778.

Hoekstra, J. H., Van Den Aker, J. H. L., Kneepkens, C. M. F., Stellaard, F., Geypens, B., & Ghoos, Y. F. (1996). Evaluation of $^{13}CO_2$ breath tests for the detection of fructose malabsorption. *The Journal of Laboratory and Clinical Medicine, 127*, 303–309.

Iafrate, A. J., Feuk, L., Rivera, M. N., Listewnik, M. L., Donahoe, P. K., Qi, Y., … Lee, C. (2004). Detection of large-scale variation in the human genome. *Nature Genetics, 36*, 949–951.

Ingram, C. J., Mulcare, C. A., Itan, Y., Thomas, M. G., & Swallow, D. M. (2009). Lactose digestion and the evolutionary genetics of lactase persistence. *Human Genetics, 124*, 579–591.

Iqbal, C. W., Wandeel, H. G., Zheng, Y., Duenes, J. A., & Starr, M. G. (2008). Mechanisms of ileal adaptation for glucose absorption after proximal-based small bowel resection. *Journal of Gastrointestinal Surgery, 12*, 1854–1864.

Jacob, R., Purschel, B., & Naim, H. Y. (2002). Sucrase is an intramolecular chaperone located at the C-terminal end of the sucrase-isomaltase enzyme complex. *The Journal of Biological Chemistry, 277*, 32141–32148.

Jacob, R., Zimmer, K. P., Schmitz, J., & Naim, H. Y. (2000). Congenital sucrase-isomaltase deficiency arising from cleavage and secretion of a mutant form of the enzyme. *The Journal of Clinical Investigation, 106*, 281–287.

Jellema, P., Schellevis, F. G., van der Windt, D. A., Kneepkens, C. M., & van der Horst, H. E. (2010). Lactose malabsorption and intolerance: A systematic review on the diagnostic value of gastrointestinal symptoms and self-reported milk intolerance. *QJM: An International Journal of Medicine, 103*, 555–572.

Jenkins, D. J., Wolever, T. M., Taylor, R. H., Barker, H., Fielden, H., Baldwin, J. M., … Goff, D. V. (1981). Glycemic index of foods: A physiological basis for carbohydrate exchange. *The American Journal of Clinical Nutrition, 34*, 362–366.

Karnsakul, W., Luginbuehl, U., Hahn, D., Sterchi, E., Avery, S., Sen, P., … Nichols, B. (2002). Disaccharidase activities in dyspeptic children: Biochemical and molecular investigations of maltase-glucoamylase activity. *Journal of Pediatric Gastroenterology and Nutrition, 35*, 551–556.

Kellett, G. L., Brot-Laroche, E., Mace, O. J., & Leturque, A. (2008). Sugar absorption in the intestine: The role of GLUT2. *Annual Review of Nutrition, 28*, 35–54.

Kuokkanen, M., Enattah, N. S., Oksanen, A., Savilahti, E., Orpana, A., & Jarvela, I. (2003). Transcriptional regulation of the lactase-phlorizin hydrolase gene by polymorphisms associated with adult-type hypolactasia. *Gut, 52*, 647–652.

Kuokkanen, M., Kokkonen, J., Enattah, N. S., Ylisaukko-Oja, T., Komu, H., Varilo, T., … Jarvela, I. (2006). Mutations in the translated region of the lactase gene (LCT) underlie congenital lactase deficiency. *American Journal of Human Genetics, 78*, 339–344.

Lebenthal, E., Khin, M. U., Zheng, B. Y., Lu, R. B., & Lerner, A. (1994). Small intestinal glucoamylase deficiency and starch malabsorption: A newly recognized alpha-glucosidase deficiency in children. *The Journal of Pediatrics, 124*, 541–546.

Lebenthal, E., Lee, P. C., & Heitlinger, L. A. (1983). Impact of development of the gastrointestinal tract on infant feeding. *The Journal of Pediatrics, 102*, 1–9.

Le Gall, M., Tobin, V., Stolarczyk, E., Dalet, V., Leturque, A., & Brot-Laroche, E. (2007). Sugar sensing by enterocytes combines polarity, membrane bound detectors and sugar metabolism. *Journal of Cellular Physiology 2007, 213*, 834–843.

Li, C., Begum, A., Numao, S., Park, K. H., Withers, S. G., & Brayer, G. D. (2005). Acarbose rearrangement mechanism implied by the kinetic and structural analysis of human pancreatic alpha-amylase in complex with analogues and their elongated counterparts. *Biochemistry, 44*, 3347–3357.

Lloyd-Still, J. D., Listernick, R., & Buentello, G. (1988). Complex carbohydrate intolerance: Diagnostic pitfalls and approach to management. *The Journal of Pediatrics, 112*, 709–713.

Loo, D. D. F., Zeuthen, T., Chandry, G., & Wright, E. M. (1996). Cotransport of water by Na^+/glucose cotransporter. *Proceedings of the National Academy of Sciences of the United States of America, 93*, 13367–13370.

Marsk, R., Jonas, E., Rasmussen, F., & Näslund, E. (2010). Nationwide cohort study of post-gastric bypass hypoglycaemia including 5,040 patients undergoing surgery for obesity in 1986-2006 in Sweden. *Diabetologia, 53*, 2307–2311.

Mathavan, V. K., Arregui, M., Davis, C., Singh, K., Patel, A., & Meacham, J. (2010). Management of postgastric bypass noninsulinoma pancreatogenous hypoglycemia. *Surgical Endoscopy, 24*, 2547–2555.

McLaughlin, T., Peck, M., Holst, J., & Deacon, C. (2010). Reversible hyperinsulinemia hypoglycemia after gastric bypass: A consequence of altered nutrient delivery. *The Journal of Clinical Endocrinology and Metabolism, 95*, 1851–1855.

Meeuwisse, G. W., & Dahlqvist, A. (1968). Glucose-galactose malabsorption. A study with biopsy of the small intestinal mucosa. *Acta Paediatrica Scandinavica, 57*, 273–280.

Mehta, D. I., Wang, H. H., Akins, R. E., Wang, L., & Proujansky, R. (2000). Isolated pancreatic amylase deficiency: Probable error in maturation. *The Journal of Pediatrics, 136*, 844–846.

Miyamoto, K., Hase, K., Takagi, T., Fujii, T., Taketani, Y., Minami, H., … Nakabou, Y. (1993). Differential responses of intestinal glucose transporter mRNA transcripts to levels of dietary sugars. *The Biochemical Journal, 295*, 211–215.

Moran, A. W., Al-Rammahi, M. A., Arora, D. K., Batchelor, D. J., Coulter, E. A., Ionescu, C., … Shirazi-Beechey, S. P. (2010). Expression of Na^+/glucose co-transporter 1 (SGLT1) in the intestine of piglets weaned to different concentrations of dietary carbohydrate. *The British Journal of Nutrition, 104*, 647–655.

Muraoka, O., Morikawa, T., Miyake, S., Akaki, J., Ninomiya, K., & Yoshikawa, M. (2010). Quantitative determination of potent alpha-glucosidase inhibitors, salacinol and kotalanol, in *Salacia* species using liquid chromatography-mass spectrometry. *Journal of Pharmaceutical and Biomedical Analysis, 52*, 770–773.

Murray, I. A., Coupland, K., Smith, J. A., Ansell, I. D., & Long, R. G. (2000). Intestinal trehalase activity in a UK population: Establishing a normal range and the effect of disease. *The British Journal of Nutrition, 83*, 241–245.

Nichols, B. L., Avery, S. E., Karnsakul, W., Jahoor, F., Sen, P., Swallow, D. M., … Sterchi, E. E. (2002). Congenital maltase-glucoamylase deficiency associated with lactase and sucrase deficiencies. *Journal of Pediatric Gastroenterology and Nutrition, 35*, 573–579.

Osswald, C., Baumgarten, K., Stümpel, F., Gorboulev, V., Akimjanova, M., Knobeloch, K. P., … Koepsell, H. (2005). Mice without the regulator gene Rsc1A1 exhibit increased Na+-D-glucose cotransport in small intestine and develop obesity. *Molecular and Cellular Biology, 25*, 78–87.

Perry, G. H., Dominy, N. J., Claw, K. G., Lee, A. S., Fiegler, H., Redon, R., … Stone, A. C. (2007). Diet and the evolution of human amylase gene copy number variation. *Nature Genetics, 39*, 1256–1260.

Quezada-Calvillo, R., Robayo-Torres, C. C., Opekun, A. R., Sen, P., Ao, Z., Hamaker, B. R., … Nichols, B. L. (2007). Contribution of mucosal maltase-glucoamylase activities to mouse small intestinal starch alpha-glucogenesis. *The Journal of Nutrition, 137*, 1725–1733.

Richards, A. B., Krakowka, S., Dexter, L. B., Schmid, H., Wolterbeek, A. P., Waalkens-Berendsen, D. H., … Kurimoto, M. (2002). Trehalose: A review of properties, history of use and human tolerance, and results of multiple safety studies. *Food and Chemical Toxicology, 40*, 871–898.

Rosenblum, J. L., Irwin, C. L., & Alpers, D. H. (1988). Starch and glucose oligosaccharides protect salivary-type amylase activity at acid pH. *The American Journal of Physiology, 254*, G775–G780.

Salmeron, J., Ascherio, A., Rimm, E. B., Colditz, G. A., Spiegelman, D., Jenkins, D. J., … Willett, W. C. (1997). Dietary fiber, glycemic load, and risk of NIDDM in men. *Diabetes Care, 20*, 545–550.

Santer, R., Groth, S., Kinner, M., Dombrowski, A., Berry, G. T., Brodehl, J., … Schaub, J. (2002). The mutation spectrum of the facilitative glucose transporter gene SLC2A2 (GLUT2) in patients with Fanconi-Bickel syndrome. *Human Genetics, 110*, 21–29.

Schiraldi, C., Di Lernia, I., & De Rosa, M. (2002). Trehalose production: Exploiting novel approaches. *Trends in Biotechnology, 20*, 420–425.

Semenza, G., & Auricchio, S. (1991). The lactase history: From physiopathology to biochemistry, molecular and cell biology—and back? In M. Gracey, N. Kretchmer, & E. Rossi (Eds.), *Sugars in nutrition.* (Vol. 25, pp. 93–102) New York: Nestec Ltd., Vevey/Raven Press Ltd.

Shaukat, A., Levitt, M. D., Taylor, B. C., MacDonald, R., Shamliyan, T. A., Kane, R. L., & Wilt, T. J. (2010). Systematic review: Effective management strategies for lactose intolerance. *Annals of Internal Medicine, 152*, 797–803.

Sim, L., Jayakanthan, K., Mohan, S., Nasi, R., Johnston, B. D., Pinto, B. M., & Rose, D. R. (2010a). New glucosidase inhibitors from an ayurvedic herbal treatment for type 2 diabetes: Structures and inhibition of human intestinal maltase-glucoamylase with compounds from *Salacia reticulata*. *Biochemistry, 49*, 443–451.

Sim, L., Willemsma, C., Mohan, S., Naim, H. Y., Pinto, B. M., & Rose, D. R. (2010b). Structural basis for substrate selectivity in human maltase-glucoamylase and sucrase-isomaltase N-terminal domains. *The Journal of Biological Chemistry, 285*, 17763–17770.

Simila, S., Kokkonen, J., & Kouvalainen, K. (1982). Use of lactose-hydrolyzed human milk in congenital lactase deficiency. *The Journal of Pediatrics, 101*, 584–585.

Simon-Assmann, P., Lacroix, B., Kedinger, M., & Haffen, K. (1986). Maturation of brush border hydrolases in human fetal intestine maintained in organ culture. *Early Human Development, 13*, 65–74.

Simoons, F. J. (1970). Primary adult lactose intolerance and the milking habit: A problem in biologic and cultural interrelations. II. A culture historical hypothesis. *The American Journal of Digestive Diseases, 15*, 695–710.

Stearns, A. T., Balakrishnan, A., Rhoads, D. B., & Tavakkolizadeh, A. (2010). Rapid upregulation of sodium-glucose transporter SGLT1 in response to intestinal sweet taste stimulation. *Annals of Surgery, 251*, 865–871.

Swallow, D. M. (2003). Genetics of lactase persistence and lactose intolerance. *Annual Review of Genetics, 37*, 197–210.

Tan-Dy, C. R., & Ohlsson, A. (2005). Lactase treated feeds to promote growth and feeding tolerance in preterm infants. *The Cochrane Database of Systematic Reviews, 18*(2), CD004591.

Tishkoff, S. A., Reed, F. A., Ranciaro, A., Voight, B. F., Babbitt, C. C., Silverman, J. S., … Deloukas, P. (2007). Convergent adaptation of human lactase persistence in Africa and Europe. *Nature Genetics, 39*, 31–40.

Tobin, V., Le Gall, M., Fioramonti, X., Stolarczyk, E., Blazquez, A. G., Klein, C., … Brot-Laroche, E. (2008). Insulin internalizes GLUT2 in the enterocytes of healthy but not insulin-resistant mice. *Diabetes, 57*, 555–562.

Topping, D. L., & Clifton, P. M. (2001). Short-chain fatty acids and human colonic function: Roles of resistant starch and nonstarch polysaccharides. *Physiological Reviews, 81*, 1031–1064.

Torniainen, S., Freddara, R., Routi, T., Gijsbers, C., Catassi, C., Höglund, P., … Järvelä, I. (2009). Four novel mutations in the lactase gene (LCT) underlying congenital lactase deficiency (CLD). *BMC Gastroenterology, 9*, 8.

Traber, P. G., Yu, L., Wu, G. D., & Judge, T. A. (1992). Sucrase-isomaltase gene expression along crypt-villus axis of human small intestine is regulated at level of mRNA abundance. *The American Journal of Physiology, 262*, G123–G130.

Treem, W. R., Ahsan, N., Sullivan, B., Rossi, T., Holmes, R., Fitzgerald, J., … Hyams, J. (1993). Evaluation of liquid yeast-derived sucrase enzyme replacement in patients with sucrase-isomaltase deficiency. *Gastroenterology, 105*, 1061–1068.

Troelsen, J. T., Mitchelmore, C., & Olsen, J. (2003). An enhancer activates the pig lactase phlorizin hydrolase promoter in intestinal cells. *Gene, 305*, 101–111.

Troelsen, J. T., Mitchelmore, C., Spodsberg, N., Jensen, A. M., Noren, O., & Sjostrom, H. (1997). Regulation of lactase-phlorizin hydrolase gene expression by the caudal-related homoeodomain protein Cdx-2. *The Biochemical Journal, 322*, 833–838.

Van de Laar, F. A., Lucassen, P. L., Akkermans, R. P., Van de Lisdonk, E. H., Rutten, G. E., & Van Weel C. (2005). Alpha-glucosidase inhibitors for type 2 diabetes mellitus. *The Cochrane Database of Systematic Reviews, 18*(2), CD003639.

Walker, J., Jijon, H. B., Diaz, H., Salehi, P., Churchill, T., & Madsen, K. L. (2005). 5-Aminoimidazole-4-carboxamide riboside (AICAR) enhances GLUT2-dependent jejunal glucose transport: A possible role for AMPK. *The Biochemical Journal, 385*, 485–491.

Weinstein, D. A., & Wolfsdorf, J. I. (2002). Effect of continuous glucose therapy with uncooked cornstarch on the long-term clinical course of type 1a glycogen storage disease. *European Journal of Pediatrics, 161*(Suppl. 1), S35–S39.

Weisz, O. A., & Rodriguez-Boulan, E. (2009). Apical trafficking in epithelial cells: Signals, clusters, and motors. *Journal of Cell Science, 122*, 4253–4266.

Wolever, T. M., & Bolognesi, C. (1996). Source and amount of carbohydrate affect postprandial glucose and insulin in normal subjects. *The Journal of Nutrition, 126*, 2798–2806.

Wolever, T. M., & Mehling, C. (2003). Long-term effect of varying the source or amount of dietary carbohydrate on postprandial plasma glucose, insulin, triacylglycerol, and free fatty acid concentrations in subjects with impaired glucose tolerance. *The American Journal of Clinical Nutrition, 77*, 612–621.

Wright, E. M., Martin, M. G., & Turk, E. (2003). Intestinal absorption in health and disease—Sugars. *Best Practice & Research Clinical Gastroenterology, 17*, 943–956.

Yook, C., & Robyt, J. F. (2002). Reactions of alpha amylases with starch granules in aqueous suspension giving products in solution and in a minimum amount of water giving products inside the granule. *Carbohydrate Research, 337*, 1113–1117.

Zeuthen, T., Zeuthen, E., & Macaulay, N. (2007). Water transport by GLUT2 expressed in *Xenopus laevis* oocytes. *The Journal of Physiology, 579*, 345–361.

RECOMMENDED READING

Swallow, D. M. (2003). Genetics of lactase persistence and lactose intolerance. *Annual Review of Genetics, 37*, 197–219.

CHAPTER 9

Digestion and Absorption of Protein

Paul J. Moughan, PhD, DSc, FRSC, FRSNZ, and Bruce R. Stevens, PhD

COMMON ABBREVIATIONS

DPPIV dipeptidyl peptidase IV
LPI lysinuric protein intolerance
ORT oral rehydrating therapy
TPN total parenteral nutrition

For the body to assimilate protein, it must be first broken down into small peptides and free amino acids. This occurs to a limited extent in the stomach, with most hydrolysis and absorption occurring in the small intestine. The digestion and absorption processes ultimately supply the circulating blood with primarily free amino acids, in addition to very small amounts of physiologically active small peptide fragments. In the absorptive state, amino acids are transported via the portal blood from the small intestine directly to the liver, with subsequent transport to other organs.

The Food and Agriculture Organization, World Health Organization, and United Nations University (FAO/WHO/UNU, 2007) define a "safe" daily intake of dietary protein as 0.83 g high- quality protein per kg body weight, or 58 g/day for the reference 70-kg man and 47 g/day for the reference 57-kg woman. The approximate median intake of protein for adults aged 31 to 50 years in the United States is 100 g/day for men and 65 g/day for women. In addition to food proteins, the body digests 50 to 100 g per day of endogenous protein that is secreted into or sloughed into the lumen of the gastrointestinal tract. These endogenous proteins include proteins in saliva, gastric juice, and other secretions; pancreatic enzymes; mucoproteins; sloughed intestinal cells; and proteins that leak into the intestinal lumen from the blood. Most of this mixture of exogenous and endogenous proteins (115 to 200 g/day) is efficiently digested and taken up by the absorptive enterocytes as free amino acids and dipeptides and tripeptides. Around 85% of the total protein is absorbed anterior to the end of the small intestine (terminal ileum), with around 10 to 20 g of protein entering the colon each day. Daily fecal nitrogen losses amount to the equivalent of about 10 g of protein. The nitrogen excreted in the feces represents primarily endogenous or dietary nitrogen that was not absorbed from the small intestine; this unabsorbed nitrogen was used in the large intestine by the microflora for growth and is therefore mainly present in the feces as part of the bacterial mass.

DIGESTION OF PROTEIN IN THE GASTROINTESTINAL TRACT

An overall concept diagram of the major aspects of protein digestion and absorption is presented in Figure 9-1, and a typical flow of protein in the adult human is shown in Figure 9-2. The normal events of digestion and absorption are grouped into phases corresponding to physiological events. The six major phases covered in this chapter primarily involve the following:

1. Gastric hydrolysis of peptide linkages in the protein
2. Digestion of protein to smaller peptides by action of pancreatic proteases, which are secreted as zymogens and activated in the lumen of the small intestine where they then carry out digestion
3. Hydrolysis of peptide linkages in oligopeptides by apical (brush border) membrane peptidases and transport of amino acids, dipeptides, and tripeptides across the brush border membrane of the absorptive enterocytes
4. Further digestion of dipeptides and tripeptides by cytoplasmic peptidases in the enterocytes
5. Metabolism of some amino acids within the enterocytes
6. Transport of amino acids across the basolateral membrane of the enterocytes into the interstitial fluid from which the amino acids enter the venous capillaries and hence the portal blood

THE GASTRIC PHASE: DENATURATION AND INITIAL HYDROLYSIS OF PROTEINS

Protein digestion begins with modest processing by the stomach. Here, gastric hydrochloric acid (HCl) and pepsins partially denature and hydrolyze proteins. The stomach plays a minor role in the overall process of protein digestion and serves primarily to prepare polypeptides for the main events of digestion and absorption that take place within the small intestine. Indeed, complete protein assimilation occurs even after surgical removal of the stomach.

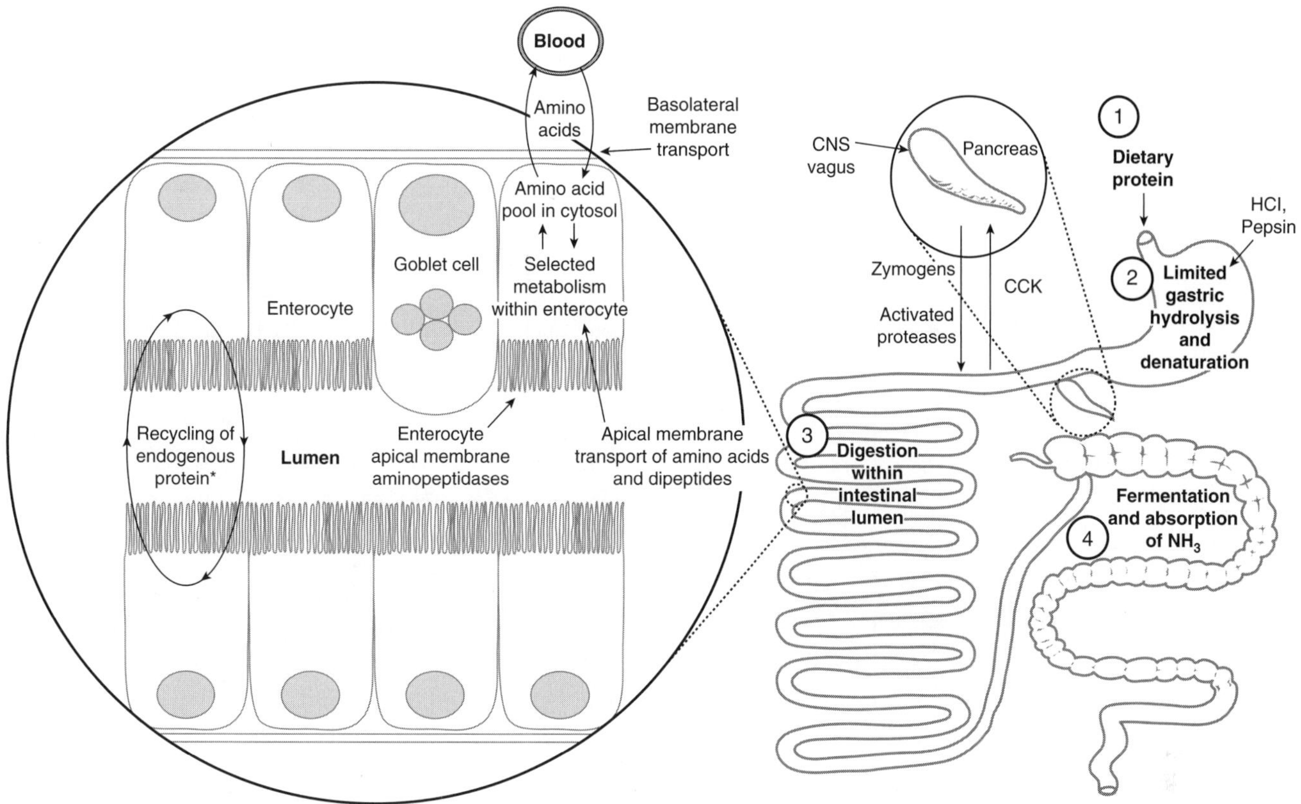

FIGURE 9-1 Overall "concept diagram" of the normal events of protein digestion and absorption. *CCK,* Cholecystokinin; *CNS,* central nervous system; *HCl,* hydrochloric acid.

When food is present in the stomach, or if the appropriate vagal cholinergic efferents are activated, the gastric chief cells secrete inactive pepsinogens. Several isozymes of pepsinogen are released, and each is converted to an active pepsin isozyme by cleavage of a peptide from the amino (N) terminus. Activation occurs spontaneously at a pH of less than 5 by an intramolecular process that involves proteolytic cleavage of a highly basic N-terminal precursor segment. After this autoactivation process forms some pepsin, activation of pepsinogen by active pepsin (autocatalysis) also occurs.

Pepsins are chemically categorized as endopeptidases because they attack peptide bonds within the polypeptide chain. Their catalytic mechanism involves two carboxylic acid groups at the active site of the enzyme, so pepsins are classified as carboxyl proteases. Most digestive enzymes are relatively permissive in the range of substrates they will accept, and the pepsins partially hydrolyze a broad variety of proteins to large peptide fragments and some free amino acids. Pepsins show a preference for hydrolysis of internal peptide bonds that involve the carboxyl groups of tyrosine, phenylalanine, or tryptophan residues and that do not involve a linkage to the imino group of proline.

SMALL INTESTINAL LUMINAL PHASE: ACTIVATION AND ACTION OF PANCREATIC PROTEOLYTIC ENZYMES

Following partial hydrolysis of protein in the stomach, the polypeptides and amino acids enter the lumen of the proximal small intestine where they stimulate the mucosal enterocytes to release the hormone cholecystokinin (CCK) into the circulation. CCK subsequently reaches the pancreas, where it binds to the acinar cells and stimulates the secretion of a variety of enzymes and zymogens by the exocrine pancreas. These exocrine secretions are delivered to the small intestinal lumen by the pancreatic duct, which joins the common bile duct that drains into the duodenum. In addition to the effects of CCK, stomach distention or the sight and smell of food invoke parasympathetic cholinergic vagal nerve efferents that in turn also stimulate the exocrine pancreatic acinar cells to release enzymes and zymogens. *Zymogen* is the general term for the inactive proenzyme form of an enzyme. The structure of the zymogen must be modified for it to be enzymatically active. Like the pepsinogens released by the gastric glands in the stomach, all of the pancreatic proteases are released in zymogen form.

Based on work that originated in the Russian laboratory of Ivan Pavlov in the late 1890s, research has established that protein digestion involves a multistep conversion of inactive zymogens to their active states within the lumen of the small intestine. The current understanding of the activation cascade for these pancreatic zymogens is summarized in Figure 9-3.

PANCREATIC ZYMOGENS AND THEIR ACTIVATION CASCADE

The major pancreatic zymogens are trypsinogen-1, trypsinogen-2, proelastase, chymotrypsinogen, procarboxypeptidase A, and procarboxypeptidase B. The initial step of the activation cascade is catalyzed by enteropeptidase (also called enterokinase). It is bound to the apical membrane of

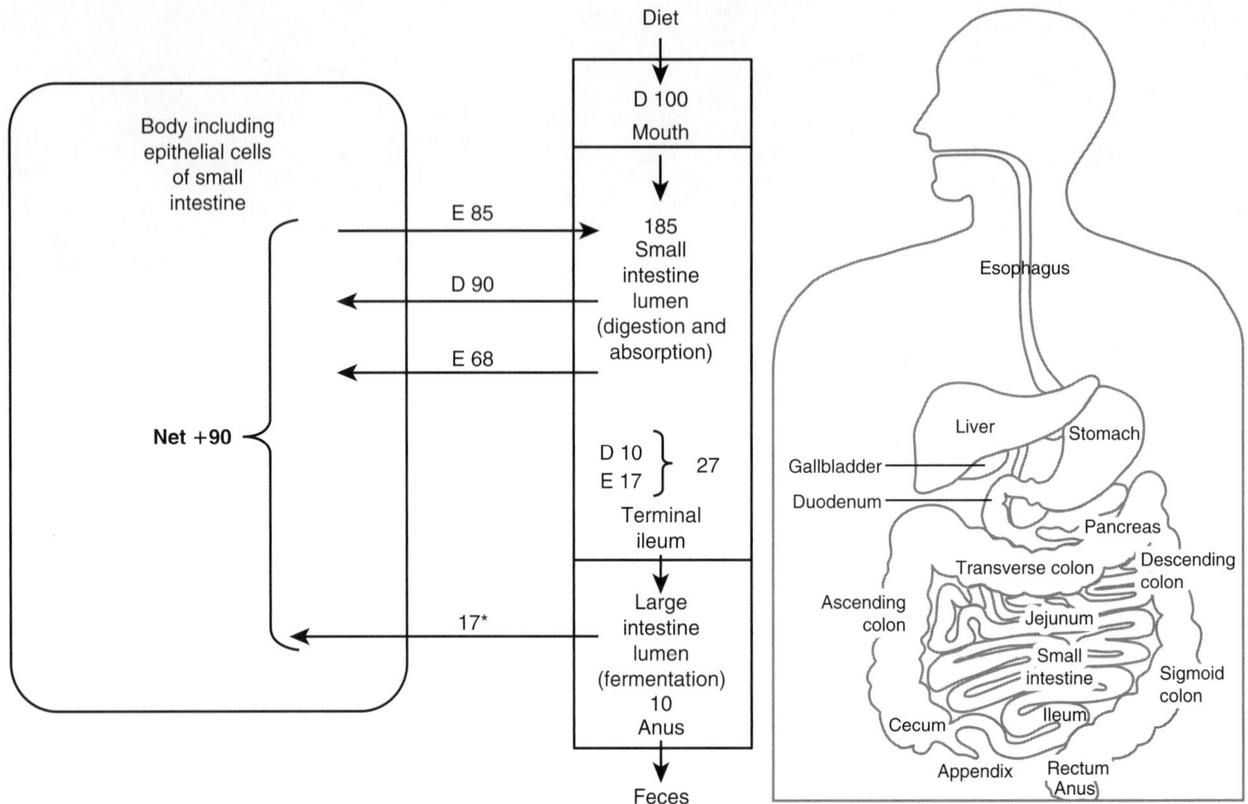

FIGURE 9-2 Typical flow of protein in the adult human. Protein enters the gastrointestinal tract by dietary intake (*D*, ~100 g/day) and endogenous proteins secreted or sloughed off into the lumen of the upper gastrointestinal tract (*E*, ~85 g/day). About 90 g of amino acids from D sources and 68 g of amino acids from E sources are absorbed each day from the small intestine, leaving only about 10 g (D) and 17 g (E) of peptides or related compounds unabsorbed in the terminal ileum, which represents less than 15% of the total protein that entered the upper gastrointestinal tract. *Some of the nitrogen in this undigested/unabsorbed protein is converted to ammonia and other compounds by bacterial fermentation in the large intestine. About 17 g of the products are absorbed, mainly as ammonia. This leaves the equivalent of nitrogen from about 10 g of protein that is excreted in the feces, primarily as part of the microbial mass. *D*, Diet; *E*, endogenous.

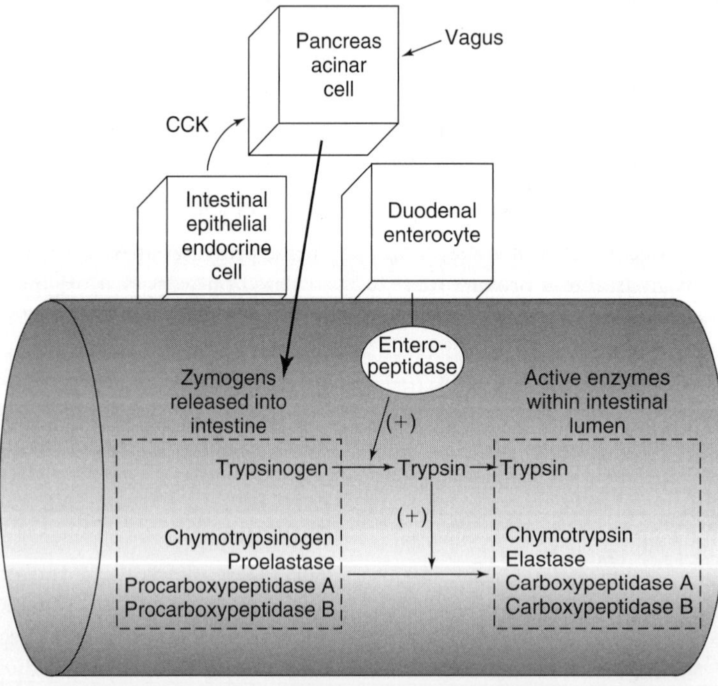

FIGURE 9-3 Cascade activation of pancreatic zymogens within the lumen of the small intestine. *CCK*, Cholecystokinin.

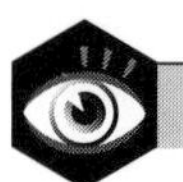

NUTRITION INSIGHT

Trypsin Inhibitors

Low-molecular-weight proteins or polypeptides that act as protease inhibitors are naturally produced by cells in both animals and plants. In particular, legumes (peas, beans, and lentils) and cereals (wheat, buckwheat, and rice bran) contain trypsin inhibitors that can lower the nutritional quality of their proteins. These trypsin inhibitors can be inactivated to a large extent by wet heating or removed by processing techniques used during protein concentration and isolation (e.g., soy protein). Soybean trypsin inhibitors have been widely studied. Although these are inactivated by heating, animals sometimes ingest large amounts of these inhibitors by consuming raw soybeans.

The pancreas, intestinal cells, liver, and other tissues also synthesize a certain amount of trypsin inhibitors. For example, human pancreatic secretory trypsin inhibitor is secreted from pancreatic acinar cells into the pancreatic duct along with the zymogen precursors of the proteolytic digestive enzymes. The possibility that some symptoms observed in diseases such as acute pancreatitis or gastric ulcer result from an absence of normal synthesis/secretion of these inhibitors is under active investigation (Keim, 2008). The therapeutic use of trypsin inhibitors to treat pancreatitis and other inflammatory conditions is also being tested in animal models.

Thinking Critically

1. Why would the presence of trypsin inhibitors in a food decrease the nutritional quality of its protein?
2. Feeding of raw soybean flour or soybean trypsin inhibitor results in an increase in the amounts of secretory products (presumably protein synthesis) within the acinar cells and in enhanced protein secretion by the pancreas. Why might this occur?
3. Why might a lack of trypsin inhibitor result in acute pancreatitis? Why might therapeutic administration of trypsin inhibitor alleviate ulceration or inflammation of tissues?

the enterocytes of the proximal small intestine (duodenum/upper jejunum). Human enteropeptidase is a heavily glycosylated protein with an N-terminal transmembrane domain and a C-terminal extracellular serine protease domain. Enteropeptidase is classified as a serine protease (or serine endopeptidase) because it has a serine residue at its active site as part of a histidine/serine/aspartate catalytic triad.

The importance of enteropeptidase is emphasized by the fact that congenital deficiency of this enzyme leads to life-threatening malabsorption of amino acids. Intestinal enteropeptidase cleaves off an amino terminal octapeptide, Ala-Pro-Phe-Asp-Asp-Asp-Asp-Lys, from trypsinogen-2 and cleaves off the same octapeptide or a pentapeptide, Asp-Asp-Asp-Asp-Lys, from trypsinogen-1. This cleavage yields activated trypsin-1 and trypsin-2 enzymes within the intestinal lumen. The specificity of enteropeptidase for trypsinogen is high; the scissile (to be cleaved) peptide bond in trypsinogen is between the carboxyl group of a lysine residue and the amino group of an isoleucine residue.

Trypsin, which is also a member of the serine protease family but which has a very different specificity than enteropeptidase, then activates the other zymogens required for protein digestion (chymotrypsinogen, proelastase, carboxypeptidases A and B), as well as precursors of proteins required for lipid digestion (procolipase and prophospholipase A_2), by cleaving off selected peptide sequences. The net result of this cascade is a pool of activated proteases within the lumen of the small intestine. Proteolysis is facilitated by the secretion of pancreatic bicarbonate into the intestinal lumen; the bicarbonate neutralizes the gastric acid in the chyme to bring the pH of the intestinal contents to 6 to 7, which is optimal for activity of pancreatic proteases.

It was formerly thought that once some trypsin was formed from trypsinogen by enteropeptidase, the active trypsin could act on trypsinogen as substrate in an autocatalytic process. Although both trypsin and enteropeptidase cleave at scissile bonds that involve a basic residue (lysine or arginine) attached to an isoleucine residue, it is now recognized that the aspartate-rich sequence in the activation peptide segment of trypsinogen suppresses the ability of trypsin to accept trypsinogen as a substrate for autoactivation. Thus enteropeptidase in the small intestine is essential for activation of trypsinogen and the subsequent zymogen activation cascade.

A benefit of synthesis of proteolytic enzymes as zymogens, with activation occurring after the proenzymes have been secreted into the intestinal lumen, is the prevention of proteolytic digestion and tissue damage within the pancreas and pancreatic duct. In addition to this protective mechanism, pancreatic juice normally contains a small peptide that inhibits trypsin to prevent any small amount of trypsin prematurely formed within the pancreatic cells or pancreatic ducts from catalyzing proteolysis. The absence of this protective mechanism leads to pancreatitis. Gain-of-function mutations and copy number variability of the trypsinogen gene, as well as loss-of-function variants for the pancreatic secretory trypsin inhibitor, have firmly established that prematurely activated trypsin causes chronic pancreatitis (Chen and Férec, 2009).

PANCREATIC DIGESTIVE ENZYMES

The pancreatic enzymes can be divided into two general types—serine proteases and carboxypeptidases. Trypsin, chymotrypsin, and elastase are all serine endopeptidases. They are categorized as endopeptidases because they hydrolyze internal peptide bonds within the polypeptide. They are classified as serine proteases because of their catalytic mechanisms, which involve a serine residue in the catalytic site. Serine proteases are normally synthesized in inactive zymogen or proenzyme form. Each of these serine proteases catalyzes the hydrolysis of peptide bonds but with different selectivities or preferences for the side chains flanking the scissile peptide bond. The site of hydrolysis in the polypeptide substrate (i.e., the scissile peptide bond) is flanked by approximately four amino acid residues in both directions that can bind to the enzyme and impact the reactivity of the peptide bond hydrolyzed; the hydrolyzable bond is designated P_1-P'_1 and adjacent amino acids are numbered P_2, P_3, and P_4 toward the N-terminus, and P'_2, P'_3, and P'_4 toward the carboxyl (C) terminus. Trypsin is most likely to cleave peptide bonds with a positively charged residue (arginine or lysine) at the P_1 site (contributing the carboxyl group to the peptide bond); chymotrypsin prefers bonds in which large hydrophobic amino acid residues, such as tryptophan, phenylalanine, tyrosine, methionine, or leucine, are at the P_1 site; and elastase preferentially cleaves peptide bonds that have a small neutral residue, such as alanine, serine, glycine, or valine, at the P_1 site. Proline at the P'_1 site inhibits cleavage by all three serine proteases. The rate at which particular bonds are cleaved also varies with the identities of the amino acid residues in the adjacent positions (P_2-P_4 and P'_2-P'_4).

The second group of proteolytic enzymes secreted by the pancreas, the carboxypeptidases, are exopeptidases that cleave off one amino acid at a time from the C-terminus of the substrate. These exopeptidases can attack the oligopeptides formed by the endopeptidases to sequentially cleave off free amino acids, leaving a mixture of free amino acids and small peptides of two to eight residues. Carboxypeptidases A and B are metalloenzymes that require Zn^{2+} at the active site, where the cation functions as a Lewis acid. (See Chapter 37 for a discussion of zinc metalloenzymes.) Carboxypeptidase B preferentially cleaves C-terminal lysine or arginine residues of peptides, and carboxypeptidase A selectively hydrolyzes most C-terminal amino acids, except proline, lysine, and arginine, with a preference for valine, leucine, isoleucine, and alanine. Neither carboxypeptidase A nor carboxypeptidase B readily cleaves C-terminal amino acids that are linked to a proline residue.

These pancreatic enzymes act as a team within the small intestinal lumen to hydrolyze many of the peptide bonds in proteins and to efficiently digest protein to yield small peptides (two to eight residues) and free amino acids. It is also important to realize that the upper digestive tract of humans contains an active microflora, and bacteria undoubtedly have a role in the digestive breakdown of food and especially of some of the endogenous proteins. Although the size of the microflora in the colon is much greater than that in the upper digestive tract, there is considerable evidence for microbial activity in the upper tract (Moughan, 2003), and it seems likely, though more experimental evidence is needed, that bacterial enzymes complement to some extent the mammalian proteases.

SMALL INTESTINAL MUCOSAL PHASE: BRUSH BORDER AND CYTOSOLIC PEPTIDASES

The products of pancreatic hydrolysis are free amino acids, tripeptides and dipeptides, and larger peptide fragments called oligopeptides. The free amino acids, dipeptides, and tripeptides are transported across the absorptive epithelial cell brush border membrane by specific carriers. Most larger oligopeptides are not transported but must be further hydrolyzed by epithelial brush border membrane–bound enzymes.

These brush border membrane peptidases are dimers that extend into the lumen about 15 nm from the membrane surface. One subunit is anchored to the membrane, and the other subunit participates in the hydrolysis of luminal peptides. These peptidases are all exopeptidases and are further classified as aminopeptidases or carboxypeptidases, depending on whether they hydrolyze the cleavage of amino acids one at a time from the N-terminus or C-terminus of the peptide. A variety of membrane-bound aminopeptidases exist, but the apical membrane of enterocytes possesses only a single known carboxypeptidase, which is peptidyl dipeptidase. As for the pancreatic proteases, these enzymes also show specificities or preferences for the amino acid residues and peptide sequences that they hydrolyze.

For the majority of tripeptides and dipeptides that are transported into the enterocyte, additional cytosolic aminopeptidases act within the absorptive epithelial cells to complete the process of hydrolyzing proteins and peptides to free amino acids. Most protein nitrogen exits the basolateral membrane to the portal blood as free amino acids. As explained later, certain dipeptides, such as carnosine, and a small fraction (~1%) of incompletely digested luminal protein and peptides may enter the portal blood intact.

ABSORPTION OF FREE AMINO ACIDS AND SMALL PEPTIDES

The products of digestion—free amino acids, dipeptides, and tripeptides—are absorbed from the lumen by a variety of transport mechanisms. In this section, free amino acid absorption mechanisms are presented first and are followed by a discussion of dipeptide and tripeptide absorption.

AMINO ACID TRANSPORTERS IN THE APICAL AND BASOLATERAL MEMBRANES

Free amino acids are initially taken up by transporters in the luminal-facing apical membrane of villous absorptive enterocytes and subsequently exit those cells via other basolateral membrane transporters. The amino acids can either pass through the enterocyte unmetabolized, be used for protein synthesis in the enterocyte, be partially (or completely) oxidized for energy, or undergo intermediary metabolic conversion into other amino acids or metabolites that, in turn, are subsequently transported out of the cell across the basolateral membrane. Following basolateral membrane transport to the interstitial fluid, the amino acids move into villus capillaries and on to the liver via the portal circulation, as summarized in Figure 9-1. The intestine is highly efficient in extracting the dietary essential and nonessential amino acids from the lumen as free amino acids. This occurs largely because of the activity of brush border and basolateral membrane transporter systems that handle specific amino acids. Some of the absorbed amino acids are used by the enterocytes themselves, most notably glutamine, which is used as the primary fuel source in enterocytes in place of glucose. Enterocyte basolateral membrane transporters also take up enterocyte-sustaining amino acids from the blood circulation, especially in the postprandial state.

A transport "system" is defined as a physiological functional unit formed from one or more transporter protein subunits. Each transporter subunit type is encoded by a specific gene. A transport system activity may result from the action of a single transporter protein or the multimeric arrangement of transporter proteins within the membrane. Although it is technically correct to use the term *transporter* to mean only a single protein, scientists often informally also refer to multimeric functional units as transporters. Membrane amino acid transporter systems composed of a single protein (monomeric transport systems) are listed in Table 9-1, whereas heterodimeric transporter systems for amino acids are listed in Table 9-2.

Transporters in the apical and basolateral membranes of enterocytes have been identified and characterized, and their messenger RNA (mRNA) and protein expressions have been localized within the intestinal tract (Stevens, 2010). The apical membrane pathways are generally different from those found in the basolateral membrane, as illustrated in Figure 9-4.

Amino acid movement via transport systems occurs by both secondary active transport and facilitated transport mechanisms, depending upon the transport system, as indicated in Tables 9-1 and 9-2. Secondary active transport of amino acids involves the cotransport of a cation with the amino acid and thus is dependent on various ionic and electrical potentials across the enterocyte membranes (Gerencser and Stevens, 1994). These ion gradients provide the electrochemical potential that energizes the secondary active (ion-coupled) transport of amino acids (Stevens, 2010). As indicated in Tables 9-1 and 9-2, Na^+ is the predominate activating ion, but H^+, Cl^-, and K^+ can also play activation roles. Secondary active transporters can move amino acids against steep chemical gradients of roughly 100:1. Although the Iminoacid (PAT1) transporter is H^+-dependent, its amino acid transport activity is also governed by Na^+ ions through energetic coupling to the activity of another apical membrane transporter, the NHE3 Na^+ /H^+ exchanger.

Even in the case of positively charged cationic amino acids moving via the Na^+- or ion-independent (facilitated) transport systems y^+ and $b^{0,+}$, the negative electrical potential across the membrane serves as a driving force along with the chemical gradients for the substrate amino acids. On the other hand, the chemical gradients of neutral amino acids are the sole driving force for absorption via transport system L.

The continual extraction of nutrients from the intestinal lumen results in Na^+ and amino acids moving into the enterocyte cytosol where they are pooled unmetabolized or metabolically converted into other small molecules. In the absorptive state these amino acids subsequently exit from the villous enterocyte into the interstitial fluid via basolateral membrane transporters. In the postabsorptive state, basolateral membrane transporters also serve to supply enterocytes with amino acids from the blood. In both the absorptive and postabsorptive states, the Na^+ electrochemical potential gradient is continually maintained by the Na^+,K^+-ATPase pumps of the basolateral membrane. The Na^+,K^+-ATPase pump maintains a low intracellular Na^+ concentration and a negative electrical potential in the enterocyte.

Intestinal amino acid transport involves cooperation at several levels. First, ion binding to the transporter is required for the activity of all amino acid transporters that depend on ion-coupled cotransport. Second, certain heterodimeric transporter subunits must interact before they are functional in moving their amino acid substrates across the membrane (see Table 9-2). Finally, transepithelial amino acid movement involves the cooperative interaction of transport systems in both the apical and the basolateral membranes (Figures 9-4 and 9-5). As an example of the complexity of multiple levels of cooperation, dibasic amino acid absorption requires uptake by Na^+-independent apical system $b^{0,+}$, which is a heterodimer of $b^{0,+}$AT plus rBAT, into the enterocyte. This is followed by exchange with a neutral amino acid plus Na^+ at the basolateral membrane by system y^+L (heterodimer of y^+LAT1 plus 4F2hc), which releases the amino acid from the enterocyte where it can then enter the portal bloodstream. The exchanged neutral amino acid is ultimately also transported back out of the enterocyte by one of the other basolateral systems selective for that substrate, and the Na^+ ion that was transported in must be transported back out of the cell by the Na^+,K^+-ATPase pump.

REGULATION OF INTESTINAL ABSORPTION OF AMINO ACIDS

One of the major roles of the gastrointestinal tract is to maintain a net positive flow of amino acids in the direction of diet-to-organism. To ensure this, the small intestine is able to adaptively upregulate its capacity for amino acid absorption. As the dietary protein content and the physiological state of the body change over a period of days, the intestine adaptively regulates its capacity to absorb amino acids. The adaptations occur at both tissue and cellular levels. Acting on the intestinal mucosa, various factors can nonspecifically change the absorptive surface area of the intestine. For example, in animal models, mucosal hyperplasia occurs in response to corticosteroids and peptide growth factors; in response to hyperphagia associated with diabetes, hyperthyroidism, neoplasia, and lactation; and in response to accelerated growth. The capacity for amino acid absorption is enhanced in each of these cases.

With the concerted effects of upregulation of transporters in individual cells along with general mucosal hyperplasia, the small intestine can increase its absorptive capacity manyfold compared to its constitutive fasting capacity. On the other hand, when food intake is limited or absent for a period of time, the absorptive capacity of the digestive tract is reduced. Parenteral feeding (i.e., the administration of nutrients by a route other than through the digestive tract, as by intravenous infusion) is widely used in hospitals. In the case of total parenteral nutrition (TPN), the absorptive capacity of the intestine becomes severely reduced as intestinal

TABLE 9-1 Monomeric Amino Acid Transport Systems in Human Small Intestine or Colon

TRANSPORT "SYSTEM" FUNCTIONAL NAME	COMMON ALIAS	GENE (SLC=Solute carrier)	HUMAN GENE LOCUS	TYPICAL SUBSTRATES	ION DEPENDENCY	TISSUE	EPITHELIAL MEMBRANE
SLC1 FAMILY							
X_{AG}^-	EAAT3	*SLC1A1*	9q24	L-Glutamate, D/L-aspartate, cystine (disulfide)	H^+, Na^+, K^+	Small intestine	Apical
ASC	ASCT1	*SLC1A4*	2p13-p15	Alanine, serine, threonine, cysteine, glutamine	Na^+	Small intestine	Apical
ASC	ASCT2 or ATB^0	*SLC1A5*	19q13.3	Alanine, serine, threonine, cysteine, glutamine, branched neutrals	Na^+	Small intestine, colon	Apical
SLC6 FAMILY							
Creatine	CRTR	*SLC6A8*	Xq28	Creatine	Na^+, Cl^-	Small intestine	Apical
GLY	GLYT1	*SLC6A9*	1p33	Glycine	Na^+, Cl^-	Small intestine	Basolateral
$B^{0,+}$	$ATB^{0,+}$	*SLC6A14*	Xq23-q24	Neutrals and dibasics, arginine, D-serine	Na^+, Cl^-	Colon	Apical
B^0 (or B)	B^0AT1	*SLC6A19*	5p15.33	Neutrals, glutamine	Na^+	Small intestine	Apical
IMINO	SIT1	*SLC6A20*	3p21.6	Proline, sarcosine, pipecolate	Na^+	Small intestine, colon	Apical
SLC7 FAMILY							
y^+	CAT-1	*SLC7A1*	13q12-q14	Arginine, ornithine, lysine, histidine, dibasics	None	Small intestine, colon	Basolateral
SLC15 FAMILY							
Pept1	PEPT1	*SLC15A1*	13q33-q34	Dipeptides & tripeptides, carnosine, β-lactam antibiotics, angiotensin-converting enzyme inhibitors	H^+ with NHE3	Small intestine	Apical
SLC16 FAMILY							
T	TAT1	*SLC16A10*	6q21-q22	Aromatics, L-DOPA	None	Small intestine	Basolateral
SLC22 FAMILY							
OCTN2VT	OCTN2	*SLC22A5*	5q23.3	L-Carnitine, acetyl-L-carnitine	Na^+	Small intestine	Apical
SLC36 FAMILY							
Iminoacid	PAT1	*SLC36A1*	5q33.1	Proline, glycine, β-alanine, GABA, taurine, D-serine	H^+ with NHE3	Small intestine, colon	Apical
SLC38 FAMILY							
A	SNAT2	*SLC38A2*	12q	Alanine, asparagine, cysteine, glutamine, glycine, histidine, methionine, proline, serine	Na^+	Small intestine	Basolateral
A	SNAT4	*SLC38A4*	12q13	Alanine, asparagine, cysteine, glycine, threonine	Na^+	Small intestine	Basolateral
N	SNAT5	*SLC38A5*	Xp11.23	Glutamine, histidine, serine, asparagine, alanine	Na^+, H^+	Small intestine (crypt cells)	Apical
SLC43 FAMILY							
LAT4	LAT4	*SLC43A2*	17p13.3	Branched-chain amino acids, phenylalaninine	None	Small intestine	Basolateral

TABLE 9-2 Heterodimer Arrangement of Amino Acid and Peptide Transport Systems in Human Small Intestine

TRANSPORT "SYSTEM" FUNCTIONAL UNIT NAME	HETERODIMER ARRANGEMENT OF SUBUNITS; COMMON ALIASES	SUBUNIT GENES	HUMAN GENE LOCI	REPRESENTATIVE SUBSTRATES	ION DEPENDENCY	TISSUE	EPITHELIAL MEMBRANE
asc	Asc-1 plus 4F2hc*	*SLC7A10* plus *SLC3A2*	19q12-13.1 11q13	Small neutral L- and D-amino acids, alanine, D-serine, cyst(e)ine, glycine	None	Small intestine	Basolateral
$b^{0,+}$	$b^{0,+}$AT plus rBAT	*SLC7A9* plus *SLC3A1*	19q13.1 2p16.3-p21	Dibasics, lysine, arginine, cystine, ornithine, large neutrals (exchange extracellular dibasics with intracellular neutrals)	None	Small intestine	Apical
L	LAT1 plus 4F2hc	*SLC7A5* plus *SLC3A2*	16q24.3 11q13	Branched-chain neutrals, L-DOPA	None	Small intestine	Basolateral
L	LAT2 plus 4F2hc	*SLC7A8* plus *SLC3A2*	14q11.2 11q13	Branched-chain neutrals (small and large)	None	Small intestine	Basolateral
x_c^-	xCT plus 4F2hc	*SLC7A11* plus *SLC3A2*	4q28-q32 11q13	Cystine/glutamate exchange	None	Small intestine	Basolateral (evidence in apical)
y^+L	y^+LAT1 plus 4F2hc	*SLC7A7* plus *SLC3A2*	14q11.2 11q13	Lysine, arginine, dibasics, neutrals	None for dibasics; Na^+ for large neutrals	Small intestine	Basolateral

*The 4F2hc subunit is also commonly called CD98.
SLC, Solute carrier.

atrophy gradually occurs. This phenomenon underlies the importance of enteral feeding in maintaining the integrity of the gut in convalescing patients.

In response to specific peptides, amino acids, and growth factors within the intestinal lumen, individual enterocytes upregulate expression of genes for aminopeptidases and specific membrane transporters, resulting in increased abundance of these enzymes and transport systems in the cell membrane (Pan et al., 2002). Regulation may also occur via posttranslational regulatory mechanisms, as evidenced by the transmembrane stimulation of certain transporters by an increase in the intracellular concentration of one of its amino acid substrates.

Glutamine is a factor critical to many enterocyte functions. The human intestinal transporter ASC that handles glutamine uptake is downregulated in hypoperfused intestine (e.g., with starvation or with TPN) and in ischemic or injured human intestinal epithelial cells, and this is reversed by epidermal growth factor (EGF) exposure (Avissar et al., 2008; Huang et al., 2008). This is important because EGF is found in secretions from intestinal Brunner glands, pancreatic and biliary secretions, swallowed saliva, and breast milk, and is released in response to fasting. Ducroc and colleagues (2010) have shown that leptin downregulates L-glutamine transport via both ASC and B^0 in rat small intestine. B^0 possesses sites that undergo phosphorylation by serum and glucocorticoid inducible kinase isoforms 1 to 3 (SGK1, SGK2, and SGK3), which regulate neutral amino acid transport via this transporter (Böhmer et al., 2010). The expression and enterocyte membrane functional stability of B^0 is further modified by enterocyte apical membrane-bound angiotensin-converting enzyme 2 (ACE2) (Böhmer et al., 2010).

NONPROTEIN AMINO ACIDS AND D-STEREOISOMERS

In addition to serving the amino acids that are used for protein synthesis, gastrointestinal transporters also transport nonproteinogenic amino acids from foods or supplements

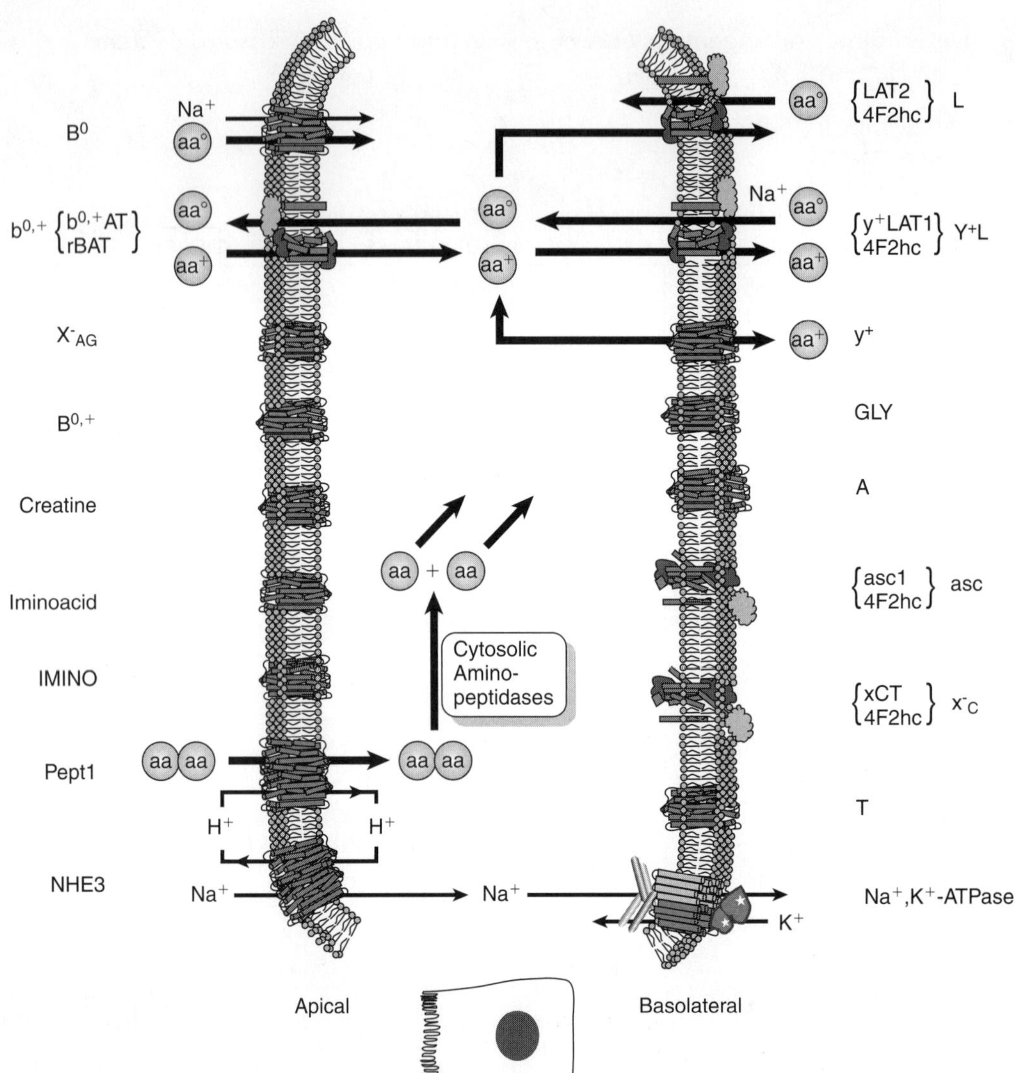

FIGURE 9-4 Amino acid or dipeptide transporter subunits in absorptive enterocyte membranes. Transport systems are functional units that are catalyzed by transporter proteins embedded in the plasma membrane bilayer as either monomers or heterodimers (see details in Tables 9-1 and 9-2). The transport systems and the subunits of the dimeric transporters are denoted by their abbreviated nomenclature. Each transport system serves amino acids or dipeptides with specific structural features. The transporters are localized to either the apical (brush border) or basolateral membrane as shown. Transepithelial movement of amino acids involves interactive, concerted participation among multiple transport systems, multiple subunits, and ion electrochemical gradients. One example is shown for the interplay among neutral/zwitterionic (aa^0) and dibasic/cationic (aa^+) amino acid substrates. Several transport systems actively transport substrates via cotransport with Na^+ or H^+ ions. In the case of H^+ cotransport (e.g., Pept1 and Iminoacid), energetic coupling occurs via the NHE3 Na^+/ H^+ exchanger that is also within the membrane. The Na^+ electrochemical potential is maintained by the basolateral Na^+,K^+-ATPase that transports 3 Na^+ out of the cell in exchange for transport of 2 K^+ ions into the cell.

(see Table 9-2). Creatine is absorbed via the creatine transporter (Verhoeven et al., 2005; Peral et al., 2002). Creatine within the intestinal lumen enhances transepithelial absorption of other nutrients (e.g., other amino acids and glucose) by activating villus actin–myosin motility events. Arginine and leucine influence creatine transport via a putative mechanism involving the mammalian target of rapamycin (mTOR) signaling pathway (Strutz-Seebohm et al., 2007; Stevens, 2010). β-Alanine and taurine are absorbed via system Iminoacid (PAT1). GABA is transported by the Iminoacid (PAT1) system, and L-DOPA is transported by the T (TAT1) system.

The vast majority of absorbed amino acids are L-stereoisomers. However, modern diets contain some D-amino acids due to the racemization of some amino acids during food processing and also due to the presence of a small fraction of naturally occurring D-amino acids derived from plants and bacteria. Neuroactive D-serine is carried by systems $B^{0,+}$, Iminoacid, and asc; D-aspartate is absorbed via X^-_{AG}. Industrial processing of food induces a small fractional racemization of all amino acids. The decreased proteolysis of peptide bonds containing one or two D-amino acids (i.e., D-D, D-L, and L-D peptide bonds) impairs digestibility and bioavailability of these processed proteins (Friedman, 2010).

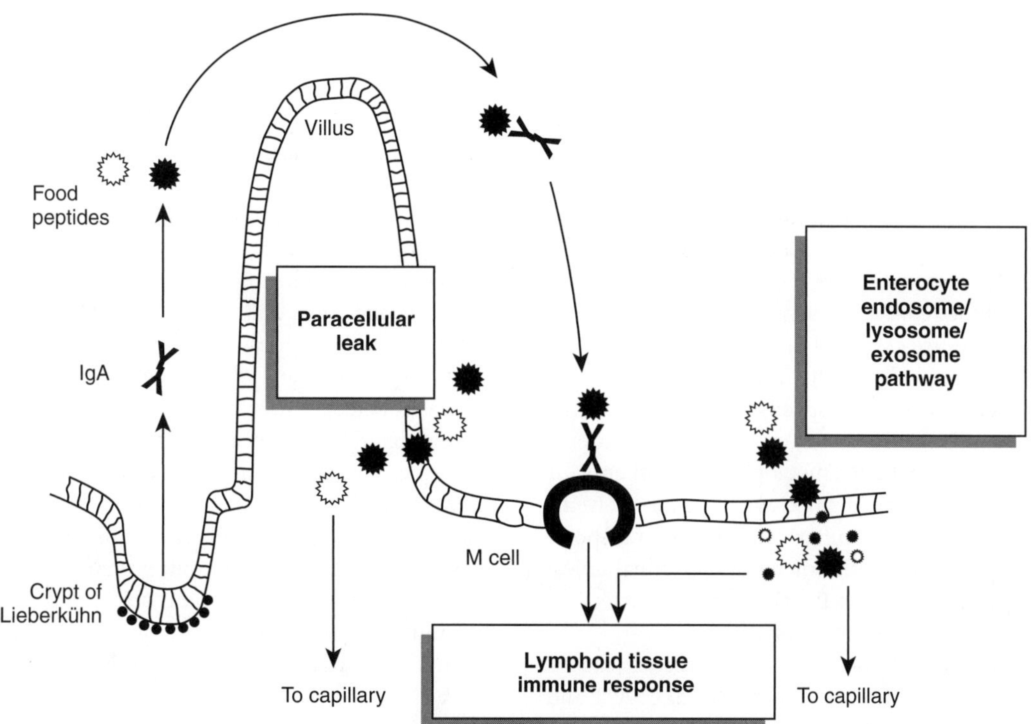

FIGURE 9-5 Intestinal processing of intact large peptides that escape luminal digestion. Intact large, and potentially antigenic, peptide fragments can be taken up across the epithelial barrier of the small intestine by three possible pathways: IgA/M cell presentation to Peyer's patches, paracellular movement across leaky tight junctions, and/or transcellular movement via enterocyte endocytosis/exocytosis processing. Dimeric IgA released from the crypt region can bind to specific epitopes of partially digested food polypeptides within the intestinal lumen. M cells (located within the epithelium adjacent to absorptive enterocytes) are activated by the dimeric IgA/peptide complex. Activated M cells present the food polypeptide as an antigen to lymphoid tissue within the intestinal lining, thereby initiating a local inflammatory immune response that creates leaky tight junctions and thus provides paracellular uptake pathways for additional peptide fragments. Peptide antigens can also bind the enterocyte apical membrane within clathrin-coated pits and be taken up by endocytosis. Further hydrolysis within the enterocyte of the peptides taken up by either method can lead to basolateral exit of digestion products (amino acids or smaller peptides) or intact peptides that escaped complete degradation. MHC II presentation of these peptides to gastrointestinal lymphoid tissues initiates local inflammatory events. The food peptides that escape hydrolysis or processing by the intestinal lymphoid tissue and do enter the bloodstream via the capillaries can cause a systemic immune response.

PEPTIDE TRANSPORT

In addition to free amino acids, dipeptide and tripeptide products of protein hydrolysis are also transported across the apical membrane of absorptive enterocytes. Indeed dipeptides and tripeptides are absorbed more efficiently and to a greater extent across the apical surface than is the equivalent free amino acid mixture. This phenomenon has been exploited in the clinical feeding of partially hydrolyzed proteins in patients with pancreatic insufficiency, rather than feeding purely free amino acids. Once dipeptides are removed from the lumen, they are primarily hydrolyzed to the constituent free amino acids by aminopeptidases within the enterocyte cytoplasm. The free amino acids pooled in the enterocyte cytoplasm are finally transported across the basolateral membrane to the portal blood via appropriate amino acid transporters. The ability to absorb amino nitrogen both as dipeptides and tripeptides and as free amino acids via multiple transporters ensures efficient absorption of amino acids from digested proteins.

Uptake of peptides by enterocytes is primarily due to the high-capacity apical membrane Pept1 transporter, which is expressed throughout the small intestine. Dipeptide and tripeptide secondary active transport via Pept1 is driven by the apical membrane proton (H^+) electrochemical potential, in coordination with the NHE3 Na^+/H^+ exchanger (see Table 9-1 and Figure 9-4). The Pept1 transporters absorb most dipeptides and tripeptides composed of L-amino acids, as well as a variety of peptidomimetic drugs, such as amino β-lactam antibiotics (e.g., pencillins and cephalosporins), angiotensin-converting enzyme inhibitors, angiotensin receptor blockers, and antiviral and anticancer agents (Meredith, 2009).

Pept1 mRNA levels exist in the colon but only at about 1% the level of that in the small intestine. It is of interest that in the condition of chronic inflammatory disorders such as Crohn disease and ulcerative colitis, both colonic and small intestinal Pept1 levels are greatly upregulated (Meier et al., 2007). It is not known whether Pept1 expression in these cases is the cause or the result of chronic inflammation. Another peptide transporter, Pept2, is expressed in kidney and other tissues but is not important for the intestinal transport of peptides.

DISORDERS OF INTESTINAL AMINO ACID TRANSPORT

The absorptive epithelium of the small intestine shares many physiological and functional traits with the reabsorptive epithelium of the kidney proximal tubule. Both tissues possess aminopeptidases on their apical membranes, and both possess many of the same amino acid transport systems. Several inborn disorders of amino acid transport are associated with a defective or absent constitutive transport system in both the intestinal and the renal absorptive epithelial membranes (Bröer, 2008). These are clinically observed as specific aminoacidurias, which display autosomal recessive or dominant inheritance patterns. Although specific amino acid transporters of the intestinal membrane are impaired in patients with aminoacidurias, a patient's metabolic requirements for nutrient amino acids may be met (except in the case of lysinuric protein intolerance) by other amino acid transporters with overlapping specificities or by the intestinal apical dipeptide/tripeptide transporter Pept1. No genetic defects of peptide transporter proteins are known.

Cystinuria is a well-documented inherited disease caused by defects in the genes encoding the rBAT *(SLC3A1)* and $b^{0,+}$AT *(SLC7A9)* transporter subunits that cooperatively comprise the heterodimeric $b^{0,+}$ system (see Table 9-2). This system plays an important transport role in both the kidney and the small intestine, and both are impaired in patients with cystinuria (Chillarón et al., 2010). The signature clinical phenotype of classical cystinuria is simultaneous excretion of lysine, ornithine, arginine, and cystine in the urine due to a lack of reabsorption of these amino acids by the proximal tubular cells of the kidney. The disease can be caused by either recessive transmission of *SLC3A1* mutations or dominant genetics of mutations in *SLC7A9*. Intestinal uptake of cystine does not appear to be affected by *SLC7A9* mutations (although they can affect renal reabsorption). However, SLC3A1 defects impede small intestinal absorption to the extent that cystine appears in the feces; and in babies, cystine stones can even appear in the colon (Benoist et al., 2007). Because the Pept1 transporter gene *(SLC15A1)* is not affected in cystinuria, peptides containing dibasic amino acids are still absorbed sufficiently to prevent protein malnutrition

Human disorders of amino acid uptake are also caused by mutations of genes encoding the y^+LAT1, B^0, T, and IMINO transporters. Patients with lysinuric protein intolerance (LPI; also called hyperdibasic aminoaciduria type 2, or familial protein intolerance) show symptoms of diarrhea and

CLINICAL CORRELATION

Cystinuria

Cystinuria is an inherited disorder of amino acid transport that affects the epithelial cells of the small intestine as well as renal tubules. There are three cystinuria phenotypes, characterized by excretion of cystine and formation of kidney stones in the urinary tract: normal (type I), high stone-forming (type II) range, and moderate (type III) range. A urinary cystine excretion exceeding 1.2 mmol/day (compared with a normal excretion of 0.05 to 0.25 mmol/day) is usually diagnosed as type II. Because cystine, the disulfide of cysteine, is very insoluble in aqueous solution, cystine stones are formed and hexagonal cystine crystals appear in the urine. Stones generally form at cystine excretion rates of greater than 300 mg cystine per gram of creatinine in acidic urine. Treatment is directed at reducing the concentration of cystine in urine by increasing urine volume, increasing cystine solubility by alkalinizing the urine, and reducing cystine excretion by use of D-penicillamine or other sulfhydryl-containing compounds to reduce the disulfide or form more soluble mixed disulfides.

Two distinct genes, *SLC3A1* and *SLC7A9,* are involved in cystinuria. These two genes encode the two subunits of apical membrane transport system $b^{0,+}$, which serves cystine, neutral amino acids, and dibasic amino acids such as lysine, arginine, and ornithine. The *SLC3A1* gene, which is on chromosome 2, encodes the rBAT subunit, which is the heavy chain activator subunit. The *SLC7A9* gene on chromosome 19 encodes the $b^{0,+}$AT light-chain transmembrane channel subunit. Cystine and dibasic amino acid transport occurs in exchange for neutral amino acids, as driven by the enterocyte's interior negative membrane potential.

One form of cystinuria is inherited as an autosomal recessive trait characterized by mutations in *SLC3A1* (rBAT). Other patients with cystinuria display dominant genetics, resulting from mutations in *SLC7A9* ($b^{0,+}$AT). Several allelic variants of the subunit genes have been described as responsible for cystinuria (Nunes et al., 2005a, 2005b; Palacín, 1994). Patients who are homozygous for disease-causing mutations of either gene show type II traits, whereas patients who are heterozygotes for mutations of either or both genes may have a type I, II, or III phenotype. Type I and III patients retain nutritionally significant intestinal absorption of cystine and dibasic amino acids.

Thinking Critically

1. Adequate amino acid nutrition is not a particular problem in individuals with cystinuria. Why? Discuss several factors related to diet, intestinal absorption, or renal reabsorption that could result in this defect having minimal effect on nutrition.
2. The amount of neutral amino acids excreted in the urine is not elevated in individuals with cystinuria. What are some possible reasons for this?
3. At pH values of less than 7.5, approximately 1 mmol (250 mg) of cystine per liter is the aqueous solubility limit of cystine. Cystinuric patients may excrete more than 1 g of cystine per day. What recommendations would you give a cystinuric patient with regard to water intake?

vomiting following a protein meal. LPI is an autosomal recessive disease caused by a defect in the *SLC7A7* gene encoding the y^+LAT1 subunit of the dimeric basolateral transport system y^+L (Bröer, 2008). Hartnup disorder involves Na^+-dependent B^0 transporter serving the neutral amino acids; this is an autosomal recessive phenotype resulting from mutations in the *SLC6A19* gene that is expressed primarily in the intestine and kidney. In Hartnup disorder, the poor absorption of the amino acid tryptophan leads to inadequate synthesis of NAD(P)/nicotinamide; this gives rise to pellagra-like clinical symptoms, such as cerebellar ataxia and diarrhea. (See Chapter 24 for more discussion of tryptophan and the niacin requirement.) In infants, the so-called blue diaper syndrome is the result of excessive, unabsorbed tryptophan reaching the large intestine, where it is converted by bacteria to blue indole derivatives; this defect is attributable to the disruption of the aromatic amino acid transporter T encoded by gene *SLC16A10*. Iminoaciduria can be attributable to defects of the *SLC6A20* gene encoding the IMINO (proline) transporter. Other less understood transport diseases include methionine malabsorptive syndrome, which leads to growth failure due to insufficient delivery and retention of the essential amino acid methionine; and dicarboxylic aminoaciduria, which is due to an impediment in the transport of glutamate and aspartate.

METABOLISM OF AMINO ACIDS IN INTESTINAL EPITHELIAL CELLS

Although most dietary amino acids taken up by enterocytes are subsequently transported across the basolateral membrane and enter the portal blood unchanged, several of the amino acids undergo considerable metabolic conversion to other compounds before exit to the portal circulation. In particular, enterocytes metabolize glutamate, glutamine, aspartate, and arginine taken up from the luminal contents. Glutamine is extensively metabolized by enterocytes as a major energy source, and the two nitrogens of glutamine leave the enterocytes primarily as alanine, proline, citrulline, and ammonia. (See Chapter 14 for further discussion of amino acid metabolism.)

USE OF FREE AMINO ACIDS AND PEPTIDES FOR ORAL REHYDRATION THERAPY

Intestinal absorption normally occurs across the enterocytes of the mucosal epithelium lining the villi of the small intestine, whereas secretion of fluid and electrolytes occurs via mucosal crypt cells. When the intestine becomes infected with microorganisms that release enterotoxin (e.g., *Escherichia coli, Vibrio cholera*), excessive quantities of water and electrolytes are lost by intestinal crypt cells in the form of a secretory diarrhea. The fluid and electrolyte losses can be overcome by the use of oral rehydrating therapy (ORT) solutions. ORT solutions typically contain glucose and electrolytes (salts) and can contain amino acids. ORT exploits the coupled uptake of Na^+ ions, amino acids, glucose, and water that occurs in the absorptive villus cells. ORT solutions are essentially isoosmotic or hypoosmotic fluids containing Na^+, Cl^-, citrate, and K^+ with free amino acids such as glutamine and alanine or sugars such as glucose. The mechanism by which intestinal transporters couple the absorption of Na^+ ions and amino acids was discussed earlier. Water absorption is subsequently osmotically coupled to the uptake of Na^+ and amino acids or glucose (see Chapter 8). Because the enteral administration of amino acids or proteins is also beneficial in promoting the morphological, digestive, and absorptive integrity of the mucosa and preventing the loss of absorptive capacity that occurs with prolonged lack of enteral nutrient intake, the use of peptide/amino acid/Na^+ rehydration is a useful therapeutic aid during infection, surgery, or other trauma of the gut.

PHYSIOLOGICALLY ACTIVE DIETARY PEPTIDES

Although protein digestion is generally an efficient process, very small amounts of certain peptide fragments or intact peptide growth factors resist hydrolysis entirely; they may be absorbed and have bioactive properties in the body after their absorption as intact peptides (Pellegrini, 2003; Zaloga and Siddiqui, 2004; Rutherfurd-Markwick and Moughan, 2005). For example, partial digestion of certain proteins found in cereal grains (gluten and gliadin), soy products, or cow's milk (casein, lactalbumin, β-lactoglobulin) results in incompletely hydrolyzed peptide fragments that can penetrate the mucosal barrier. Small peptides with unusal peptide linkages or unusual amino acids also escape digestion and are absorbed intact; these include L-carnosine (β-alanyl-histidine) and anserine (β-alanyl-1-N-methyl-l-histidine).

EXAMPLES OF BIOACTIVE PEPTIDES

Examples of oligopeptides that are resistant to proteolysis in the gut are peptides that contain proline, which result from the limited ability of proteolytic enzymes to cleave amide bonds involving this imino acid. The apical membrane dipeptidyl peptidase IV (DPPIV), however, is able to cleave N-terminal dipeptides from polypeptides containing proline or alanine in the penultimate position. Enterocyte apical membrane-bound DPPIV is responsible for inactivating many ingested peptides or proteolytic by-products that could impart biological activity. Example substrates for DPPIV are the exorphin type of peptides formed from casomorphin (milk) and gluteomorphin (wheat) fragments. If not inactivated, these food peptides may act as either opioid agonists or antagonists for opioid receptors in the central nervous system. It is widely postulated that individuals lacking sufficient DPPIV activity may be predisposed to certain opioid-related mood, behavior, or thought disturbances, such as those experienced with depression, autism, or psychosis.

The uptake of certain intact peptide growth factors, such as EGF or transforming growth factor alpha (TGFα), are especially important during development and maturation of the gastrointestinal mucosa. A wide spectrum of peptides from plants (e.g., wheat, soybean, spinach) and bovine and human milk are known to enter the general blood circulation intact, whereby they influence neural opioid receptors,

TABLE 9-3 Selected Bioactive Food-Derived Peptides

SOURCE	PEPTIDE NAME	AMINO ACID SEQUENCE	PHYSIOLOGICAL ACTIVITY
Meat	L-Carnosine	β-Alanyl-histidine	Antiinflammatory; antioxidant; prevents glycation
Wheat	Gliadorphin	YPQPQPF	Opioid agonist
Wheat	Gluten exorphin-A5	GYYPT	Peripheral inhibition of stress-induced pain; CNS opioid agonist
Milk	β-Lactorphin	ALPMHIR	ACE inhibitor
Milk	β-Casokinin-7	AVPYPQR	ACE inhibitor
Milk	β-Lactorphin dipeptide	YL	ACE inhibitor
Milk	Casoplatelin	MAIPPKKNQDK	Inhibits platelet aggregation
Milk	Lactotransferrin thrombic inhibitory peptide	KRDS	Inhibits platelet aggregation
Milk	Casoxin D	YVPFPPF	Opioid antagonist
Milk	α-Casein exorphin	RYLGYLE	Opioid agonist
Milk	β-Casomorphin-7	YPFPGPI	Opioid agonist; decreases intestinal motility; enhances NaCl absorption
Milk	Lactoferricin	FKCRRWNRMKKLGA-PSITCVRRAF	Antimicrobial; disrupts bacterial membranes
Milk	Phosphopeptide	SSSEE	Calcium/phosphate-stabilizing to enhance absorption

NOTE: Sequences use standard amino acid symbols (see Chapter 5, Table 5-2).
ACE, Angiotensin-converting enzyme; *CNS,* central nervous system.

the immune system, or the angiotensin-converting enzyme (ACE). Some examples of bioactive food-derived peptides and their physiological activities are listed in Table 9-3.

In addition, some intact proteins as well as polypeptide fragments formed during digestion may modulate intestinal function via local actions before they are fully broken down, with absorption of the amino acid and dipeptide and tripeptide products, or before they are fermented by the microflora of the large intestine. Phosphopeptides from milk casein enhance calcium absorption; soybean peptides inhibit cholesterol and bile acid absorption; and wheat albumin suppresses luminal amylase activity.

MECHANISMS FOR UPTAKE OF BIOACTIVE PEPTIDES

Details describing transepithelial movement of luminal peptide fragments are incompletely understood. However, a general picture has emerged regarding how partially hydrolyzed food peptides interact with the mucosal barrier. One or more of four general mechanisms are involved: (1) specific transport via Pept1, (2) paracellular movement across leaky tight junctions, (3) transcellular movement across the enterocyte via endocytosis and exocytosis, and (4) immunoglobulin A (IgA) or microfold cell (M cell) presentation to Peyer's patches (lymphoid tissue). Pept1 transport has been discussed earlier, and it functions only for small peptides. Peptides of variable size may be transported by the other three mechanisms, as illustrated in Figure 9-5.

Paracellular uptake of peptides occurs by movement of peptides between the mucosal cells instead of through the mucosal cells. This can occur when the tight junctions between the mucosal epithelial cells are damaged and thus leaky. The leaky junctions increase the nonspecific permeability of the intestinal epithelium to all macromolecules. Pathologies associated with chronic or extensive abdominal radiation, malnutrition, or invasive microorganisms (e.g., salmonellae or shigellae) can include damage to the epithelial cells and to the tight junctions of the intestinal mucosal barrier.

Very small amounts of certain intact polypeptides and even some bacteria can escape proteolysis in the lumen of the gastrointestinal tract and be absorbed intact via endocytic uptake across the brush border membrane (Mallegol et al., 2007). This transcellular route starts with receptor-mediated endocytosis across the enterocyte apical membrane into the enterocyte cytoplasm where degradation may occur by the late endosome/lysosome system. Selective peptide fragments can be protected from complete degradation as the result of binding to MHC-II (major histocompatibility complex class II) molecules to form an exosome package. The enterocytes appear to be capable of releasing these exosomes by exocytosis across the basolateral membrane. The epithelial exosome–MHCII–peptide package is presented to dendritic cells residing within the lamina propria. These professional antigen presenting cells complete the peptide digestion process and, in the case of antigenic peptides, are responsible for activating T cells and inducing an immune response.

Finally, proteins and peptide antigens may be nonspecifically absorbed intact from the lumen via an M cell–dependent mechanism. M cells are specialized cells of the small intestinal epithelium that overlay Peyer's patches. These patches are aggregates of lymphoid nodules that are located in the small intestinal mucosa and extend into the submucosa. M cells are considered to be the major pathway for sampling antigens present in the gut. M cells transport peptides into the underlying tissue and present the peptides as antigens to dendritic cells and macrophages in the Peyer's patches, thereby initiating a lymphoid tissue inflammatory immune response that includes IgA secretion. IgA, in dimeric form, is secreted across epithelial cells at the base of the intestinal crypts. Secretory IgA attaches to the mucus overlying the enterocytes, where it can neutralize pathogens or their toxins. This IgA also can bind to specific epitopes of incompletely hydrolyzed food peptides in the lumen and present them as antigens to M cells of the epithelium. This local immune response can create leaky tight junctions in the intestinal epithelium, and thus also promote uptake of large dietary peptides into the portal blood via the paracellular uptake pathway.

DETERMINING DIETARY PROTEIN DIGESTIBILITY

Most dietary proteins and oligopeptides are rapidly degraded in the human digestive tract, but some are quite resistant to hydrolysis. The extent of digestion and the rate of breakdown of a dietary protein is dependent upon its amino acid sequence and on posttranslational modifications such as glycosylation. Further, the total food matrix within which a dietary protein is found may affect digestibility. For example, proteins embedded in plant cell wall material may be poorly accessed by pepsin and pancreatic proteases. Food processing with accompanying Maillard-type reactions and cross-linkages can decrease protein digestibility.

Traditionally, the digestibility of dietary protein was assessed by comparing fecal nitrogen output with dietary nitrogen intake for the test protein. This approach, however, does not provide an accurate assessment of the digestion of the protein by digestive enzymes. This is better assessed by determining nitrogen in the contents of the lower ileum before the remnants from digestion and absorption enter the colon. The large intestine houses a prolific population of microorganisms, which contain or secrete protease enzymes and which take up and use amino acids. Thus the proteins and peptides that enter the colon from the small intestine are rapidly hydrolyzed, and the released amino acids are either used by the bacteria for growth or metabolized with the formation of ammonia, amines (e.g., the foul-smelling diamines, cadaverine and putrescine), and numerous other nitrogenous compounds. Some of the ammonia is used by the bacteria to synthesize amino acids for production of bacterial protein, some is lost via the feces, and some is absorbed and mostly converted to urea in the liver. The urea is either excreted in the urine or may be recycled into the colon, where it can be broken down by the bacteria to again enter the colonic ammonia pool. Although transport systems for both amino acids and peptides have been identified in colonic tissue, it appears that amino acids are not absorbed in nutritionally significant amounts from the adult mammalian large bowel (Wrong et al., 1981; Moughan, 2003; Gilbert et al., 2008), although this matter remains somewhat controversial (Ganapathy et al., 2006).

The important point is that fecal protein is predominantly microbial protoplasmic protein, and its amino acid composition is not directly related to that of the undigested protein in the ileal effluent that enters the colon. For most of the individual amino acids there is a net loss of the amino acid during transit through the colon, although for some amino acids (e.g., methionine) there may be a net gain from ileum to feces due to bacterial synthesis of amino acids. For the determination of protein digestibility as a result of protein digestion, measurement of protein remaining in the luminal contents at the end of the small intestine (terminal ileum) is considered more appropriate than measurement in the feces (Moughan, 2003). Ileal digestibility determination, however, raises practical problems of how representative samples of ileal digesta can be obtained from the terminal ileum. Ileal digesta can be sampled using nasointestinal intubation (Modigliani et al., 1973), or digestibility studies can be done in subjects whose colon has been surgically removed because of ulcerative colitis or other disease conditions (Rowan et al., 1994). Alternatively, animal models of digestibility have been used to assess digestibility of food proteins (Deglaire et al., 2009). The young growing pig is often used for these studies, and digesta may be sampled directly from the intestine of the anesthetized animal or collected from animals with surgically implanted cannulas.

A consideration when determining the ileal digestibility of food protein is the need to correct for the presence of nitrogen of endogenous or bacterial origin, which makes up a significant proportion of the total protein found at the terminal ileum. A number of methods that allow endogenous protein to be distinguished from undigested dietary protein have been developed (Moughan, 2003); these can be applied to measure the nondietary protein component so this can be subtracted from the total ileal protein to estimate dietary protein component. When correction for the endogenous component has been made, the determined digestibility is referred to as "true" digestibility.

Technically, the term *digestibility* refers to the disappearance of a nutrient during the transit of food through the digestive tract. Thus one may refer to protein digestibility or amino acid digestibility, depending upon whether the disappearance of protein or of an individual dietary amino acid has been determined. Amino acid digestibility data are more informative because they provide insight into the extent of absorption of each individual amino acid. Unfortunately, there is not a great deal of published information on ileal amino acid digestibility in humans.

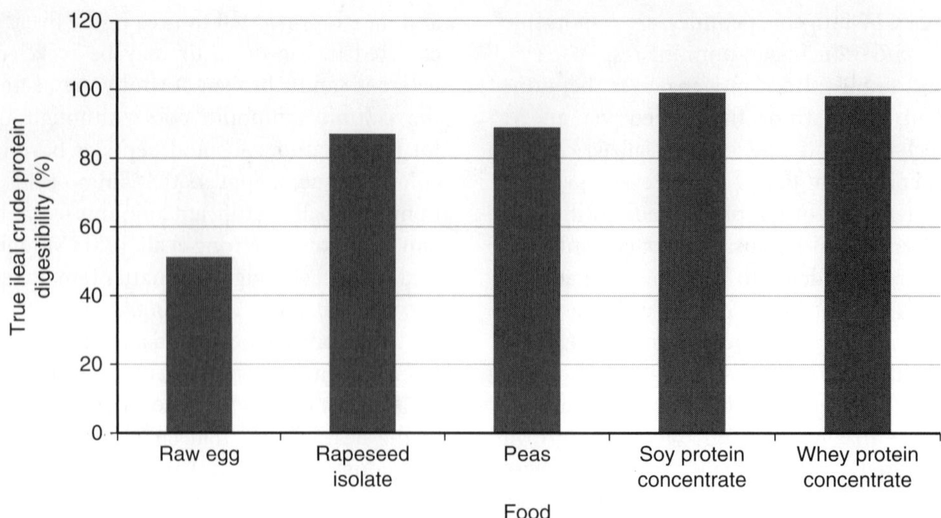

FIGURE 9-6 Measurements in humans of true ileal protein digestibility for a range of foods. Percent digestibility refers to the amount of food nitrogen in the contents of the terminal ileum (corrected for endogenous nitrogen by subtraction of endogenous nitrogen from total ileal nitrogen) expressed as a percentage of the nitrogen content of the food. (Data from Moughan, P. J. [2009]. Digestion and absorption of proteins and peptides. In D. J. McClements & E. A. Decker [Eds.], *Designing functional foods: Measuring and controlling food structure breakdown and nutrient absorption* [pp. 148–170]. Cambridge, UK: Woodhead Publishers.)

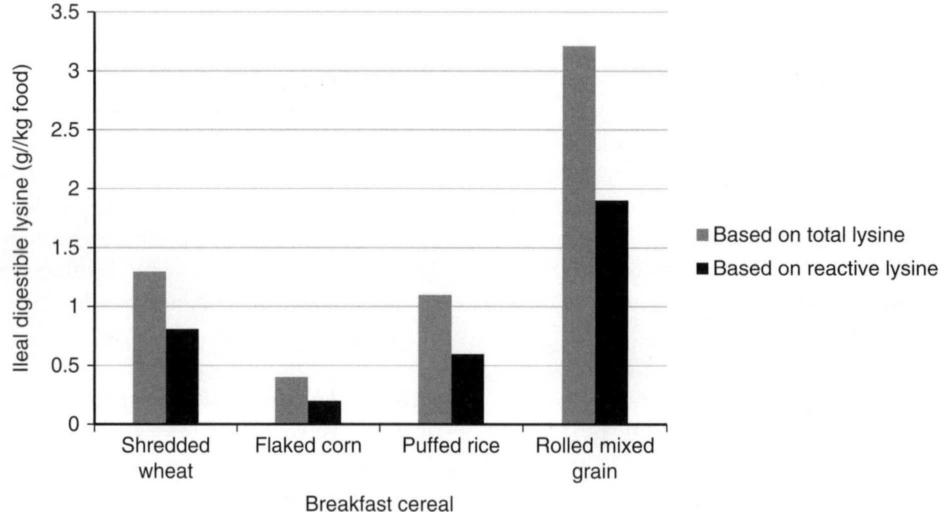

FIGURE 9-7 True ileal digestible lysine content of four cereal products based on determination of either total lysine or bioavailable lysine. The difference in amount of digestible lysine as determined by analysis of total lysine versus reactive or bioavailable lysine represents the extent of damage to lysine during heat processing. Heat processing induces Maillard damage to lysine residues in the food proteins. (Data from Rutherfurd, S. M., Torbatinejad, N. M., & Moughan, P. J. [2006]. Available (ileal digestible reactive) lysine in selected cereal-based food products. *Journal of Agricultural and Food Chemistry, 54,* 9453–9457.)

Figure 9-6 gives information for some highly digestible and for some poorly digestible protein sources. The true ileal digestibility of crude protein ranged from 51% through 87% to 99% for these examples. The variation in actual digestibilities may be greater than that shown here, however, because many of the more poorly digested vegetable proteins (Gilani et al., 2005) have not yet been subjected to ileal digestibility assay.

During the processing of foods and also during the prolonged storage of foods (especially at high ambient temperatures), amino acids and particularly the highly reactive amino acid lysine may undergo structural changes (Moughan, 2003). Generally the structurally altered amino acids are metabolically unavailable even if they are absorbed. When proteins are hydrolyzed by strong acid in preparation for amino acid analysis, these structurally altered amino acids can revert to the parent amino acid. Such reversion does not occur in the milder acidity of the stomach, however, so the reversion that occurs during acid hydrolysis of undigested proteins leads to an unpredictable degree of error in the analysis of available amino acids. This can give rise to misleading values for amino acid digestibility and has implications for the determination of amino acid digestibility based on hydrolysis and analysis of amino acids in ileal contents and for the use of these values. For foods with damaged protein, specific bioassays based on the measurement of the "reactive" (structurally unaltered) as opposed to the "total" amounts of an amino acid in the food and ileal digesta have been developed (Moughan and Rutherfurd, 1996) and are more accurate. Nutritionally significant differences have been reported between true ileal digestible total lysine (traditional method) and true ileal digestible reactive lysine (new assay), indicating a considerable degree of damage to food lysine, as illustrated by the data in Figure 9-7. Such reductions in nutritional value due to food processing or prolonged storage may have serious consequences for nutritional well-being in the developing world, where dietary lysine intakes may be marginal. Considerable scope exists for improving the processing, storage, and cooking of foods to maximize amino acid digestibility.

THINKING CRITICALLY

1. What is an endopeptidase and what is an exopeptidase? Give examples of each.
2. How are amino acids and peptides absorbed? Consider how they cross both the apical and the basolateral membranes of the enterocyte to make their way into the interstitial fluid of the lamina propria.
3. What are the major products of protein digestion that enter the bloodstream? Do absorbed amino acids initially enter the venous or arterial blood? Would this have any implications for their metabolism by tissues?
4. What is the difference between "true" digestibility and "apparent" digestibility of a protein in the gastrointestinal system? Which value more accurately reflects the availability of a specific food protein to the body? Give the rationale for your answer.

REFERENCES

Avissar, N. E., Sax, H. C., & Toia, L. (2008). In human entrocytes, GLN transport and ASCT2 surface expression induced by short-term EGF are MAPK, PI3K, and Rho-dependent. *Digestive Diseases and Sciences, 53*, 2113–2125.

Benoist, J. F., Imbard, A., Dreux, S., Garel, C., Haddad, G., Hoffet, M., … Muller, F. (2007). Antenatal biochemical expression of cystinuria and relation to fetal hyperechogenic colon. *Clinical Chemistry, 53*, 149–150.

Böhmer, C., Sopjani, M., Klaus, F., Lindner, R., Laufer, J., Jeyaraj, S., … Palmada, M. (2010). The serum and glucocorticoid inducible kinases SGK1-3 stimulate the neutral amino acid transporter SLC6A19. *Cellular Physiology and Biochemistry, 25*, 723–732.

Bröer, S. (2008). Amino acid transport across mammalian intestinal and renal epithelia. *Physiological Reviews, 88*, 249–286.

Chen, J. M., & Férec, C. (2009). Chronic pancreatitis: Genetics and pathogenesis. *Annual Review of Genomics and Human Genetics, 10*, 63–87.

Chillarón, J., Font-Llitjós, M., Fort, J., Zorzano, A., Goldfarb, D. S., Nunes, V., & Palacín, M. (2010). Pathophysiology and treatment of cystinuria. *Nature Reviews Nephrology, 6*, 424–434.

Deglaire, A., Bos, C., Tomé, D., & Moughan, P. J. (2009). Ileal digestibility of dietary protein in the growing pig and adult human. *The British Journal of Nutrition, 102*, 1752–1759.

Ducroc, R., Sakar, Y., Fanjul, C., Barber, A., Bado, A., & Lostao, M. P. (2010). Luminal leptin inhibits L-glutamine transport in rat small intestine: Involvement of ASCT2 and B0AT1. *American Journal of Physiology. Gastrointestinal and Liver Physiology, 299*, G179–G185.

Food and Agriculture Organization, World Health Organization, & United Nations University. (2007). *Protein and amino acid requirements in human nutrition.* Report of a joint FAO/WHO/UNU expert consultation. WHO Technical Report Series No 935. Geneva: World Health Organization.

Friedman, M. (2010). Origin, microbiology, nutrition, and pharmacology of d-amino acids. *Chemistry & Biodiversity, 7*, 1491–1530.

Ganapathy, V., Gupta, N., & Martindale, R. G. (2006). Protein digestion and absorption. In L. R. Johnson, K. E. Barrett, F. K. Ghishan, J. L. Merchant, H. M. Said, & J. D. Wood (Eds.). *Physiology of the gastrointestinal tract* (4th ed., pp. 1667–1692). New York: Academic Press.

Gerencser, G. A., & Stevens, B. R. (1994). Thermodynamics of symport and antiport catalyzed by cloned or native transporters. *The Journal of Experimental Biology, 196*, 59–75.

Gilani, G. S., Cockell, K. A., & Sepehr, E. (2005). Effects of antinutritional factors on protein digestibility and amino acid availability in foods. *Journal of AOAC International, 88*, 967–987.

Gilbert, E. R., Wong, E. A., & Webb, K. E., Jr. (2008). Peptide absorption and utilization: Implications for animal nutrition and health. *Journal of Animal Science, 86*, 2135–2155.

Huang, Q., Li, N., Zhang, W., Zhu, W., Li, Q., Wang, B., & Li, J. (2008). Glutamine transporter ASCT2 was down-regulated in ischemic injured human intestinal epithelial cells and reversed by epidermal growth factor. *Journal of Pediatric Gastroenterology and Nutrition, 46*, 71–79.

Keim, V. (2008). Role of genetic disorders in acute recurrent pancreatitis. *World Journal of Gastroenterology, 14*, 1011–1015.

Mallegol, J., van Niel, G., Lebreton, C., Lepelletier, Y., Candalh, C., Dugave, C., … Heyman, M. (2007). T84-intestinal epithelial exosomes bear MHC class II/peptide complexes potentiating antigen presentation by dendritic cells. *Gastroenterology, 132*, 1866–1876.

Meier, Y., Eloranta, J. J., Darimont, J., Ismair, M. G., Hiller, C., Fried, M., … Vavricka, S. R. (2007). Regional distribution of solute carrier mRNA expression along the human intestinal tract. *Drug Metabolism and Disposition: The Biological Fate of Chemicals, 35*, 590–594.

Meredith, D. (2009). The mammalian proton-coupled peptide cotransporter PepT1: Sitting on the transporter-channel fence? *Philosophical Transactions of the Royal Society of London. Series B, Biological Sciences, 364*, 203–207.

Modigliani, R., Rambaud, J. C., & Bernier, J. J. (1973). The method of intraluminal perfusion of the human small intestine. I. Principle and technique. *Digestion, 9*, 176–192.

Moughan, P. J. (2003). Amino acid availability: Aspects of chemical analysis and bioassay methodology. *Nutrition Research Reviews, 16*, 127–141.

Moughan, P. J., & Rutherfurd, S. M. (1996). A new method for determining digestible reactive lysine in foods. *Journal of Agricultural and Food Chemistry, 44*, 2202–2209.

Nunes, V., Font-Llitjos, M., Jimenez-Vidal, M., Bisceglia, L., Di Perna, M., de Sanctis, L., … Nunes, V. (2005a). Gene symbol: SLC3A1. Disease: Cystinuria. *Human Genetics, 116*, 541.

Nunes, V., Font-Llitjos, M., Jimenez-Vidal, M., Bisceglia, L., Di Perna, M., de Sanctis, L., … Palacín, M. (2005b). Gene symbol: SLC7A9. Disease: Cystinuria, type non-I. *Human Genetics, 116*, 244.

Palacín, M. (1994). A new family of proteins (rBAT and 4F2hc) involved in cationic and zwitterionic amino acid transport. A tale of two proteins in search of a transport function. *The Journal of Experimental Biology*, *196*, 123–137.

Pan, M., Souba, W. W., Karinch, A. M., Lin, C. M., & Stevens, B. R. (2002). Epidermal growth factor regulation of system L alanine transport in undifferentiated and differentiated intestinal Caco-2 cells. *Journal of Gastrointestinal Surgery*, *6*, 410–417.

Pellegrini, A. (2003). Bioactive peptides from food proteins. *Current Pharmaceutical Design*, *9*, 16.

Peral, M. J., Garcia-Delgado, M., Calonge, M. L., Duran, J. M., De La Horra, M. C., Wallimann, T., … Ilundain, A. (2002). Human, rat and chicken small intestinal Na-Cl-creatine transporter: Functional, molecular characterization and localization. *The Journal of Physiology*, *545*, 133–144.

Rowan, A. M., Moughan, P. J., Wilson, M. N., Maher, K., & Tasman-Jones, C. (1994). Comparison of the ileal and faecal digestibility of dietary amino acids in adult humans and evaluation of the pig as a model animal for digestion studies in man. *British Journal of Nutrition*, *71*, 29–42.

Rutherfurd-Markwick, K. J., & Moughan, P. J. (2005). Bioactive peptides derived from food. *Journal of AOAC International*, *88*, 955–966.

Stevens, B. R. (2010). Amino acid transport by epithelial membranes. In G. Gerencser (Ed.), *Epithelial transport physiology* (pp. 353–378). New York: Humana Press.

Strutz-Seebohm, N., Shojaiefard, M., Christie, D., Tavare, J., Seebohm, G., & Lang, F. (2007). PIKfyve in the SGK1 mediated regulation of the creatine transporter SLC6A8. *Cellular Physiology and Biochemistry*, *20*, 729–734.

Verhoeven, N. M., Salomons, G. S., & Jakobs, C. (2005). Laboratory diagnosis of defects of creatine biosynthesis and transport. *Clinica Chimica Acta*, *361*, 1–9.

Wrong, O. M., Edmonds, C. J., & Chadwick, V. S. (1981). *The large intestine: Its role in mammalian nutrition and homeostasis*. Lancaster, England: MTP Press Limited.

Zaloga, G. P., & Siddiqui, R. A. (2004). Biologically active dietary peptides. *Mini Reviews in Medicinal Chemistry*, *4*, 815–821.

RECOMMENDED READING

Feldmand, M., Friedman, L. S., & Brandt, L. J. (2010). *Sleisenger and Fordtran's gastrointestinal and liver disease* (9th ed.). Philadelphia: Saunders/Elsevier.

CHAPTER 10

Digestion and Absorption of Lipids

Patsy M. Brannon, PhD, RD; Patrick Tso, PhD; and Ronald J. Jandacek, PhD

COMMON ABBREVIATIONS

ABC	ATP-binding cassette proteins
ACAT	acyl CoA:cholesterol acyltransferase
CE	cholesteryl esters
CoA	coenzyme A
ER	endoplasmic reticulum
FA	fatty acids
FABP	fatty acid–binding protein
MAG	monoacylglycerols
MTP	microsomal triacylglycerol transfer protein
NPC1L1	Niemann-Pick C1 like 1 protein
SCP	sterol carrier protein
SR-B1	scavenger receptor B1
TAG	triacylglycerol

The central challenge for the digestion and absorption of dietary lipids (defined in Chapter 6) is their insolubility in the aqueous environments that characterize the gastrointestinal lumen and enterocyte (small intestinal absorptive cell). To meet this challenge, coordinated and complex processes involving emulsification, digestion, micellar solubilization, uptake, intracellular transport, and packaging into lipoproteins for transport must occur. These processes begin in the stomach, continue in the lumen of the small intestine, and conclude in the enterocyte. Digestion of lipids depends upon actions of amphipathic enzymes, other proteins, and bile acids (bile salts) that act at the lipid–aqueous interface.

Although a variety of lipids are consumed in the diet, nonpolar triacylglycerols represent the largest component (90% or more) and provide the polyunsaturated/essential fatty acids (discussed in Chapter 18). These triacylglycerols contain predominantly long-chain fatty acids (chain lengths of 14 to 20 carbons) esterified to the glycerol backbone. According to the 2000-2006 National Health and Nutrition Examination Survey (NHANES), the average daily consumption of fat (triacylglycerols) by American adults is approximately 65 g for women and 95 g for men (34% of the caloric intake). Other dietary lipids include cholesterol; cholesteryl esters; plant sterols; plant sterol esters; the fat-soluble vitamins A, D, E, and K (discussed in Chapters 28 through 31); carotenoids; and phospholipids. Daily dietary intake of sterols includes 275 mg of cholesterol (NHANES 2000-2006), 100 to 400 mg of plant sterols and other noncholesterol sterols, and 1 to 2 g of phospholipids. Secretion of endogenous biliary lipids into the intestine present far more additional cholesterol (1 g) and phospholipids (10 to 20 g) to the intestine over the course of a day than are consumed in the diet. The fat-soluble vitamins and carotenoids are consumed in vastly smaller amounts, typically in milligram or microgram amounts.

LUMINAL DIGESTION OF LIPIDS

Hydrolysis of triacylglycerols, cholesteryl esters, and phospholipids is absolutely required for their absorption from the intestinal lumen into the enterocyte. Multiple lines of evidence conclusively demonstrate this requirement: (1) the failure to absorb silver-containing oil droplets in electron micrograph studies (Cardell et al., 1967); (2) the nonabsorbability of nonhydrolyzable polyoleate esters (Mattson and Volpenhein, 1972); and (3) the reduction of fat absorption by the partial inhibition of the primary hydrolytic enzymes, gastric and pancreatic lipases; by orlistat (tetrahydrolipstatin, Xenical) in humans (Carrière et al., 2001); or by the combined knockout of pancreatic hydrolytic enzymes (lipase and carboxylester lipases) in mice (Gilham et al., 2007). Thus the first critical process in lipid digestion and absorption is the hydrolysis of the lipid esters.

GASTRIC DIGESTION OF TRIACYLGLYCEROLS

Digestion of triacylglycerols in humans begins in the stomach with the action of the hydrolytic enzyme, gastric lipase, which is secreted by the gastric mucosa. This lipase is most active in an acidic environment. It preferentially hydrolyzes the fatty acid at the *sn*-3 position of the triacylglycerol molecule, regardless of the fatty acid esterified to this position (Aloulou and Carrière, 2008), but it can also hydrolyze fatty acids at the *sn*-1 position (Whitcomb and Lowe, 2007). Although the optimal pH of gastric lipase is around 4, the enzyme is still active at pH 6 to 6.5 and probably continues to hydrolyze triacylglycerol in the upper duodenum where the pH is between 6 and 7. In cases of pancreatic insufficiency, gastric lipase may compensate at least partially for the loss of the pancreatic hydrolytic lipases. Overall, the net digestion of fat in the stomach is limited (less than 10% to 25%), but it contributes to the subsequent digestion of fat in the lumen. Gastric lipase plays an important role in the digestion of fat in human milk and formula by infants, who have low levels of the major hydrolytic enzyme, pancreatic lipase, until weaning (Lindquist and Hernell, 2010; Whitcomb and Lowe, 2007). As discussed later, pancreatic lipase-related protein 2 and carboxylester lipase also contribute to the digestion of fat by the infant.

The 1,2-diacylglycerols and fatty acids produced as a result of the action of gastric lipase may promote some emulsification of dietary fat in the stomach. In addition, grinding and mixing of the gastric contents contribute to dispersion into fine lipid droplets less than 0.5 mm in diameter. These droplets leave the stomach and enter the small intestine where the combined action of bile and pancreatic secretions brings about a marked change in the chemical and physical form of the dietary lipids.

LUMINAL SMALL INTESTINAL DIGESTION OF TRIACYLGLYCEROLS

When the acidic chyme containing the lipid droplets reaches the duodenum, it triggers the secretion of cholecystokinin, which in turn triggers the release of bile from the gallbladder. Bile contains the biological detergents known as bile acids. Some of the bile acids partition onto the surface of the fine lipid droplets and contribute to their emulsification. Mixture of the chyme with the alkaline secretion of the Brunner glands and the bicarbonate-rich secretion from the pancreas occurs in the duodenum, resulting in a neutralization of the gastric acid so that the intestinal contents in humans have a slightly alkaline pH.

Pancreatic lipase, which has a pH optimum around pH 8, digests most of the triacylglycerol that enters the small intestine (Whitcomb and Lowe, 2007), acting along with the contributing activities of carboxylester lipase (Gilham et al., 2007) and possibly pancreatic lipase-related peptide 2 (Figure 10-1). Pancreatic lipase, which is secreted in its active form, works at the lipid–aqueous interface of the emulsified lipid particles and mainly hydrolyzes the *sn*-1 and *sn*-3 positions of triacylglycerol molecules to release 2-monoacylglycerol and free fatty acids. However, the bile acids at the lipid–aqueous interface of the emulsified lipid particles inhibit the action of

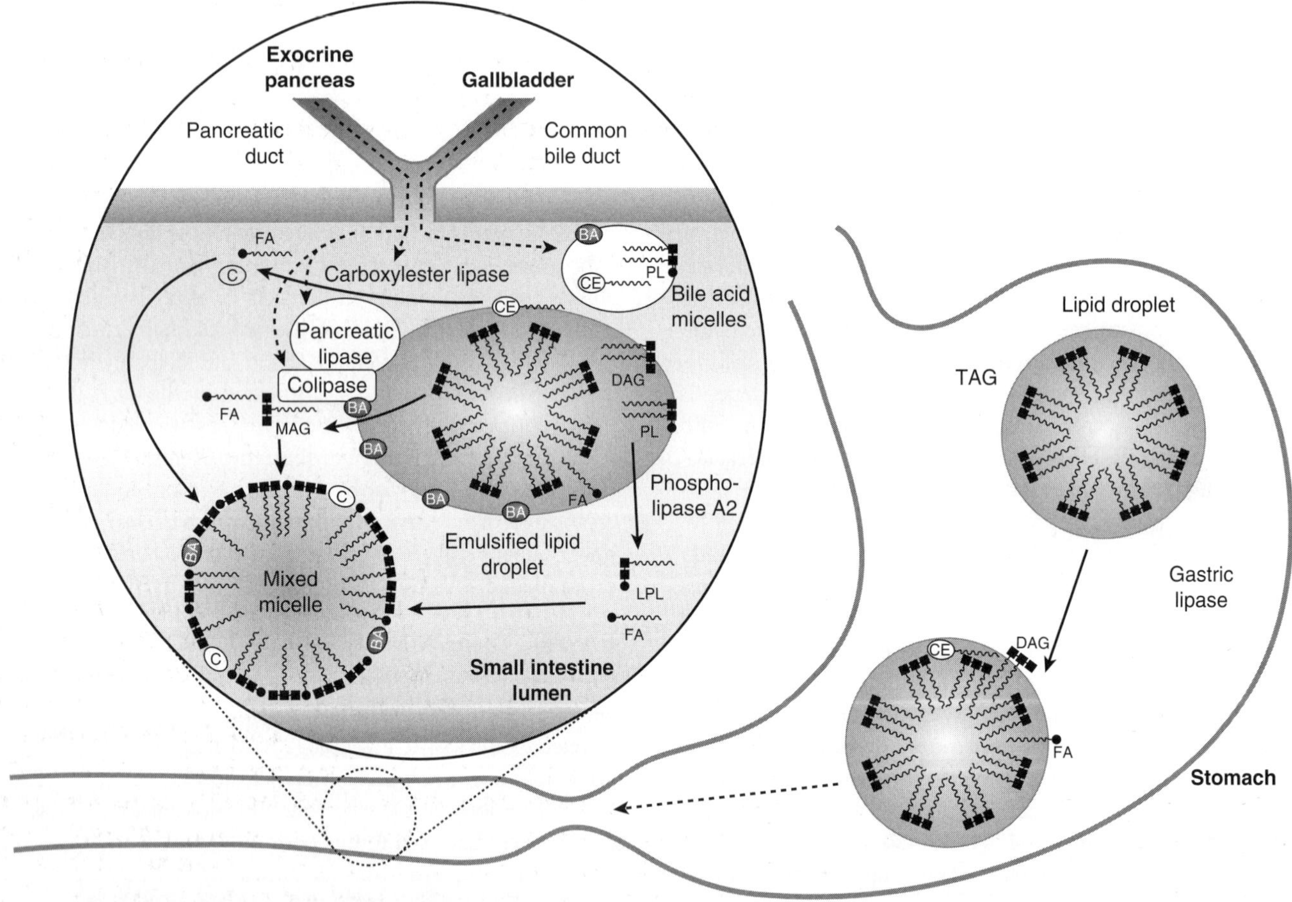

FIGURE 10-1 Lipid digestion in the stomach and small intestine. Gastric lipase hydrolyzes triacylglycerol (*TAG*) in large lipid droplets to diacylglycerol (*DAG*) and fatty acids (*FA*) in the stomach while the mixing and grinding of the stomach emulsifies the lipid. The emulsified lipid droplets enter the small intestine where they stimulate release of cholecystokinin. This in turn causes the gallbladder to release bile acids (*BA*), which are largely in the form of micelles with endogenous cholesteryl ester (*CE*) and phospholipid (*PL*). These bile acids partition into the emulsified lipid droplet. The exocrine pancreas secretes pancreatic lipase and its required cofactor colipase, phospholipase A2, and carboxylester lipase. After activation by the action of trypsin, pancreatic lipase and colipase bind together to the surface of the BA-covered lipid emulsion, inducing a conformational change in phospholipase to enable the hydrolysis of TAG and DAG to monoacylglycerol (*MAG*) and FA. Phospholipase A2 hydrolyzes PL to lysophospholipids (*LPL*) and FA. Carboxylester lipase hydrolyzes CE to cholesterol (*C*) and FA. The lipid digestion products partition into the mixed micelles. Note that lipid droplets and micelles are not drawn to scale. Lipid droplets are about 500 nm in diameter, whereas micelles are about 5 nm in diameter.

pancreatic lipase unless colipase is present. Colipase is also secreted by the pancreas as the inactive procolipase, which is activated by trypsin-mediated proteolytic cleavage in the small intestine. The binding of colipase to the lipid–aqueous interface allows the binding and anchoring of lipase to the interface. This binding in a 1:1 molar ratio also results in important conformational changes in lipase that expose its active site and enable its hydrolytic action. Colipase deficiency in humans and mice results in fat malabsorption.

In contrast, pancreatic lipase-related protein 2 has broad activity and hydrolyzes triacylglycerols, phospholipids, and galactolipids, depending on the species (Whitcomb and Lowe, 2007) and is neither stimulated by colipase nor inhibited by bile acids. Its action appears important for triacylglycerol digestion in the newborn when its secretion is high. In knockout mice lacking pancreatic lipase-related protein 2, fat malabsorption is present in pups until weaning when pancreatic lipase secretion increases (Lindquist and Hernell, 2010).

LUMINAL SMALL INTESTINAL DIGESTION OF PHOSPHOLIPIDS

Digestion of phospholipids occurs in the small intestine through the hydrolytic action of pancreatic phospholipase A2, which acts at the lipid interface of micelles. Pancreatic phospholipase A2 acts on both the dietary and the endogenous phospholipids. The most abundant of these phospholipids is phosphatidylcholine. The pancreas secretes an inactive prophospholipase A2, which is then activated by trypsin-mediated cleavage in the lumen. Phospholipase A2 hydrolyzes the fatty acid from the *sn*-2 position of phosphatidylcholine to yield a fatty acid and lysophosphatidylcholine (Whitcomb and Lowe, 2007). Some minor contribution may also come from the intestinal mucosal intrinsic membrane enzyme known as retinyl ester hydrolase or phospholipase B, which has both phospholipase and retinyl ester hydrolase activities.

LUMINAL SMALL INTESTINAL DIGESTION OF CHOLESTERYL ESTERS

Digestion of cholesteryl esters also occurs in the small intestinal lumen. Although most dietary and biliary cholesterol is present as the free sterol, about 10% to 15% of the total cholesterol is present as cholesteryl esters that require hydrolysis before absorption. Carboxylester lipase (also called cholesteryl ester lipase, bile acid–stimulated lipase, and nonspecific esterase) is secreted by the pancreas as an active enzyme and hydrolyzes cholesteryl ester to free cholesterol and fatty acid. Carboxylester lipase has a broad specificity and can hydrolyze triacylglycerols (at all three positions), phosphoglycerides, sphingolipids, galactolipids, vitamin A esters, and monoacylglycerols, as well as cholesteryl esters. Carboxylester lipase, like phospholipase A2, can act on substrates in bile acid micelles, and it is stimulated by bile acids, particularly trihydroxy bile acids such as cholic acid. This activation occurs through a unique conformational change resulting in the self-aggregation of carboxylester lipase in the presence of trihydroxy bile acids (taurocholate or glycocholate); this change brings about an increase in activity by protecting the enzyme from proteolytic inactivation.

LUMINAL SMALL INTESTINAL DIGESTION OF ESTERS OF FAT-SOLUBLE VITAMINS

Digestion of fat soluble vitamin esters, primarily retinyl ester, occurs in the small intestine by several enzymes including carboxylester lipase, retinyl ester hydrolase (phospholipase B),

NUTRITION INSIGHT

Use of Structured Triacylglycerols to Enhance Absorption of Fatty Acids

Structured triacylglycerols are mixtures of long- and medium-chain fatty acids incorporated on the same glycerol backbone by hydrolysis and random reesterification of the constituent oils. Structured triacylglycerols may have different actions than do mixtures of the starting-point triacylglycerols that have not been reesterified. Currently, structured triacylglycerols having their *sn*-2 acyl group substituted with a long-chain fatty acid are of nutritional interest. Because triacylglycerols are hydrolyzed to 2-monoacylglycerols and fatty acids in the gastrointestinal tract, and because the 2-monoacylglycerols may be taken up and converted to triacylglycerol without further hydrolysis, fatty acids esterified to the 2 position of glycerol may be more likely to be absorbed into the lymphatics. For example, fatty acids with less than 12 carbons are generally transported via the portal route as free fatty acids bound to plasma albumin; but medium-chain fatty acids esterified to the 2 position will be readily absorbed as 2-monoacylglycerols, which are further acylated with long-chain fatty acids in the 1 and 3 positions for lymphatic transport.

Jensen and colleagues (1994) studied the lymphatic absorption of a structured triacylglycerol formed by enzymatic hydrolysis of medium-chain triacylglycerol and fish oils, with random reesterification of the hydrolyzed fatty acids. They compared results to that for an equivalent physical mixture of the constituent medium-chain triacylglycerol and fish oils. Enhanced lymphatic absorption of medium-chain fatty acids in rats was observed when they were delivered as a structured triacylglycerol containing medium-chain fatty acid in the 2 position and long-chain fatty acids in the 1 and 3 positions, compared with the physical mixture. The very-long-chain polyunsaturated fatty acids in fish oil triacylglycerols are generally not well absorbed unless they are in the 2 position. However, because most of the long-chain polyunsaturated fatty acids in fish oils are in the 2 position naturally and because very-long-chain fatty acids cannot be absorbed directly into the portal blood, there was little difference in lymphatic absorption of fish oil fatty acids when structured triacylglycerols and physical mixes were compared.

and also pancreatic lipase (Harrison, 2005). Other fat soluble vitamins (D and E) and carotenoids are present primarily in their free unesterified forms in foods.

RELATIVE CONTRIBUTIONS OF LIPID DIGESTING ENZYMES

The relative contributions of lipid digesting enzymes is not fully understood but is known to depend on the stage of development and the relative availability of the various lipases. As stated earlier, gastric lipase and pancreatic lipase-related peptide 2 appear to be able to digest completely the dietary lipid in breast milk or formula, because pancreatic lipase is very low in the newborn. Carboxylester lipase is present in secreted breast milk and also contributes to fat digestion in the newborn (Whitcomb and Lowe, 2007). Studies in knockout mice lacking one or more lipases also reveal the redundancy and compensation of the lipases in lipid digestion. Deficiency of pancreatic lipase does not affect triacylglycerol absorption in mice fed a low-fat diet but reduces it in those fed a high-fat diet and also reduces cholesterol absorption (Gilham et al., 2007). Loss of carboxylester lipase does not affect retinyl ester absorption, although it does reduce cholesteryl ester absorption. Deficiency of phospholipase A2 does not affect phospholipid absorption. However, deficiency of both pancreatic lipase and carboxylester lipase reduces both triacylglycerol and retinyl palmitate digestion and absorption (Gilham et al., 2007). Similarly during pancreatic insufficiency in humans, gastric lipase contributes to the partial digestion of dietary lipid. Clearly, the overlapping and complementary functions of the lipid digesting enzymes allow for redundancy and compensation in lipid digestion.

UPTAKE OF LIPID DIGESTION PRODUCTS BY THE ENTEROCYTES

To be used by the body, the products of lipid digestion must be taken up by enterocytes and then released into the circulation. Issues related to solubility in the aqueous environment must again be overcome for adequate absorption to occur. Regional differences in intestinal lipid absorption exist; absorption is more efficient in the proximal than in the distal small intestine. As noted later, these variations may reflect differential expression of transport mechanisms or differences in processing and production of chylomicrons due to the higher proximal availability of phospholipids that are needed for prechylomicron formation in the enterocyte.

MICELLAR SOLUBILIZATION OF LIPID DIGESTION PRODUCTS

Micellar solubilization of the digestion products, predominantly monoacylglycerols, fatty acids, lysophosphatidylcholine, and cholesterol, is essential to their uptake by enterocytes. Micellar solubilization enables the lipid digestion products to cross the barrier presented by the unstirred water layer surrounding the epithelial surface of the small intestine. The unstirred water layer varies in thickness depending on how vigorously the intestinal contents are mixed (Figure 10-2). Without micelle formation, the low solubility of lipid digestion products in water would limit their ability to cross this unstirred layer. Micelles form when the bile acid concentration is at or above the critical micellar concentration (~1 to 2 mmol/L, depending on the specific bile acid). In the human small intestinal lumen, the bile acid concentration is almost always above the critical micellar concentration, such that

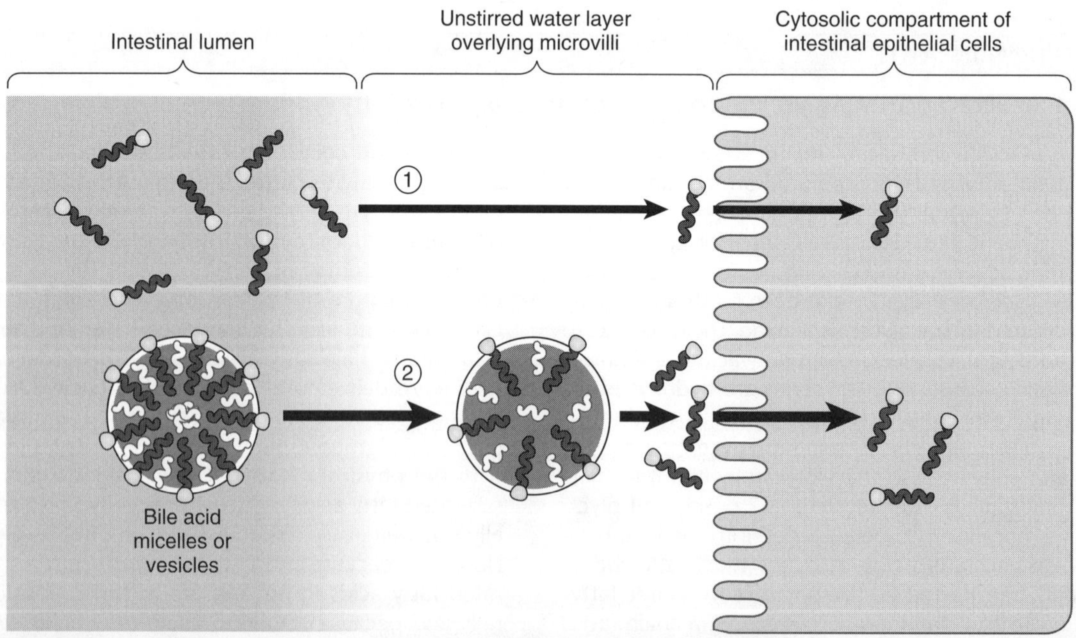

FIGURE 10-2 The role of bile acid micelles in overcoming the diffusion barrier associated with the unstirred water layer. In the absence of bile acids (*1*), only a limited number of lipid molecules diffuse through the unstirred water layer to be taken up across the brush border membrane of the enterocytes. In the presence of bile acids (*2*), more lipid molecules can be delivered to the brush border membrane by bile acid micelles.

bile acid micelles form (Hofmann, 2009). Once incorporated into the mixed micelles (containing bile acids and other lipid moieties), lipid digestion products readily cross the unstirred water layer, resulting in a 100- to 1,000-fold increase in the aqueous concentrations of fatty acids, monoacylglycerols, cholesterol, and lysophosphatidylcholine near the epithelial absorptive surface. Thus micellar solubilization provides an efficient mechanism for diffusion of lipid digestion products across the unstirred water layer, facilitating the subsequent uptake of these lipid molecules by the enterocytes.

The micellar phase, however, is not homogeneous. In addition to the large disc-like mixed bile acid micelles that are more or less saturated with lipids, lipid crystalline or unilamellar vesicles exist and are composed of mixed lipids saturated with bile acids (Carey et al., 1983). These vesicles may play an important role in the uptake of lipid digestion products in patients with low intraluminal bile acid concentrations (Mansbach et al., 1980) or bile fistulae (Porter et al., 1971).

ABSORPTION OF PRODUCTS OF LIPID DIGESTION BY ENTEROCYTES

Absorption of the products of lipid digestion occurs through two mechanisms: passive diffusion and carrier-mediated transport across the apical (brush border) membrane of enterocytes. Observations of saturable uptake supports the involvement of transporters in the uptake of fatty acids and cholesterol, but uptake after proteolytic treatment of the brush border membrane supports a role of passive diffusion as well.

Passive Diffusion

In passive diffusion, the products of lipid digestion in the mixed micelles dissolve in the lipids of the brush border membrane. The concentration gradient between the lipids in the brush border membrane and those in the intracellular compartment of the enterocytes favors initial diffusion of these products into the cell. The rapid intracellular reesterification of the lipid digestion products helps maintain low intracellular concentrations of the digestion products, thus favoring their continued uptake or diffusion. The more water-soluble products of lipid digestion, such as glycerol and short-chain fatty acids, if present, are efficiently taken up by diffusion.

Carrier-Mediated Uptake of Fatty Acids

Identification of specific transporters for fatty acids has been controversial. Although fatty acid transport protein 4 was initially suggested to play a role in the absorption of fatty acids, current evidence suggests that it does not (Shim et al., 2009). Instead, fatty acid transport protein 4 is localized to the endoplasmic reticulum (ER) membrane and plays a role in the intracellular processing of fatty acids (Mansbach and Gorelick, 2007). Emerging instead is the role of the fatty acid translocase, CD36 (Figure 10-3), in the absorption of fatty acids from the proximal, but not distal, intestine (Nassir et al., 2007). CD36, a glycoprotein, is a member of the type B scavenger receptor family that translocates long-chain fatty acids across the apical membrane of the enterocyte, but the precise mechanism of this transfer is not understood. CD36 may act in concert with other membrane and intracellular proteins to effect this transfer, although the nature and identity of these other proteins is not known.

Carrier-Mediated Uptake of Cholesterol

Another transport protein, NPC1L1, plays an essential role in cholesterol and phytosterol uptake (Hui et al., 2008; Betters and Yu, 2010; see Figure 10-3). The highest expression of NPC1L1 in the proximal small intestine colocalizes with the site of maximal cholesterol absorption. Both NPC1L1 and cholesterol absorption are minimal in the distal small intestine. Deficiency of NPC1L1 in knockout mice reduced cholesterol absorption by 70% (Altmann et al., 2004). Further, NPC1L1 is the target of ezetimibe, a potent inhibitor of cholesterol and plant sterol absorption (Betters and Yu, 2010). This transporter protein cycles between the apical surface and intracellular compartments of the enterocyte in a mechanism consistent with cholesterol-regulated, clathrin-mediated

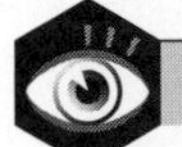

NUTRITION INSIGHT

Absorption of Lipophilic Drugs and Toxins

Many lipophilic compounds, including drugs, fat-soluble vitamins, and other compounds present in food or present on food as contaminants, are incorporated into chylomicrons in the intestinal mucosal cells and transported via the lymph. Hence absorption of these compounds depends upon normal fat digestion and absorption and upon chylomicron formation and secretion. The role of dietary fat in the absorption of fat-soluble vitamins is well-known. Uptake of lipophilic drugs and toxins also may be promoted when ingested along with dietary fat. Factors that limit lipid digestion, such as blockage of biliary flow or chylomicron formation, may interfere with or prevent absorption of these compounds.

Patients are often advised to take lipophilic medications together with their meals to enhance the absorption of the drug by the gastrointestinal tract. Delivery of lipophilic drugs in forms that enhance their absorption and thus require smaller doses is of interest to pharmaceutical manufacturers. Enhancement of absorption of lipophilic compounds by the presence of dietary fat also may affect absorption of environmental contaminants or toxins. For example, absorption of DDT (1,1-*bis*[p-chlorophenyl]-2,2,2-trichloroethane), a toxic chlorinated hydrocarbon pesticide now banned in the United States, is enhanced by concomitant fat feeding. Enhanced absorption of lipophilic compounds by dietary fat also may account for the observation that tetrachloroethylene causes toxic effects when fed with a high-fat meal. Tetrachloroethylene is a drug used for treating hookworm infections, and it is not ordinarily absorbed from the gastrointestinal tract.

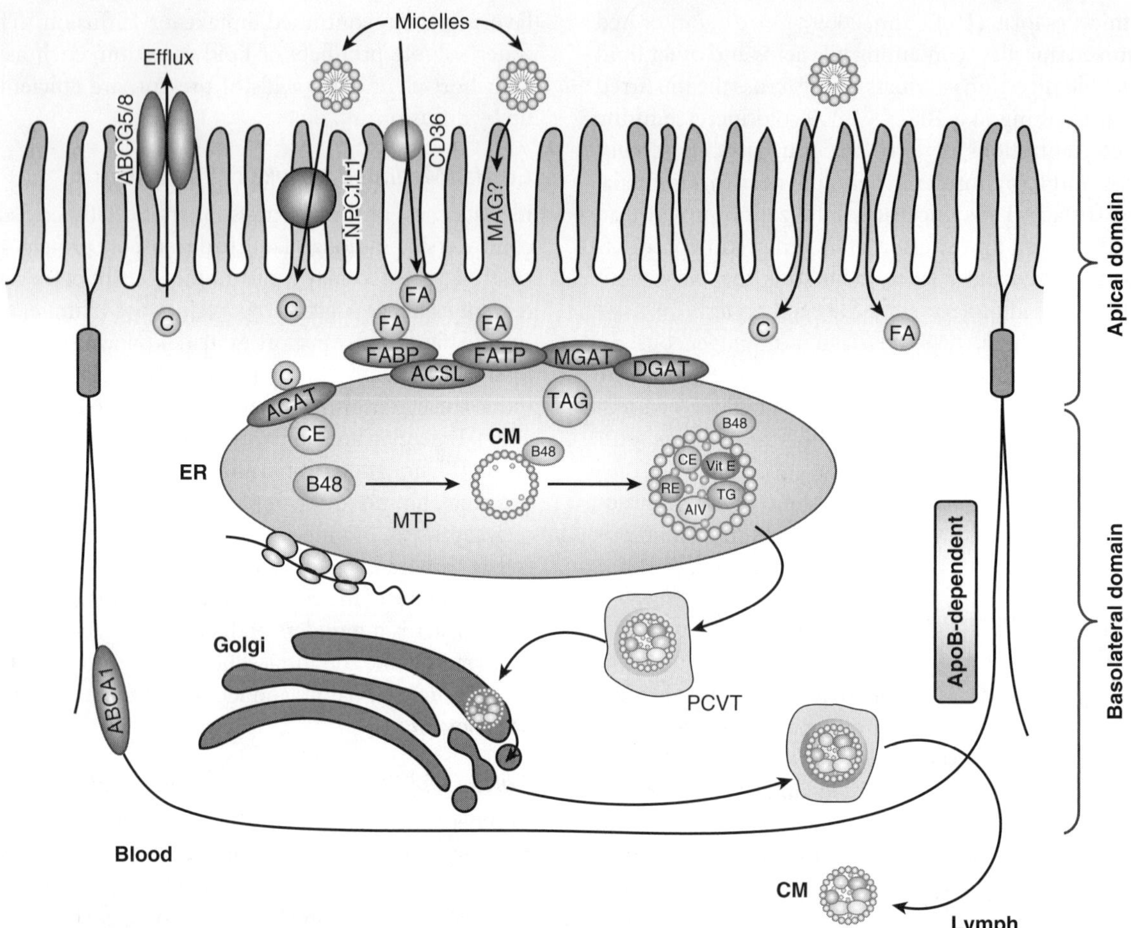

FIGURE 10-3 Intestinal lipid absorption. Products of lipid hydrolysis are solubilized in micelles and presented to the apical membranes of enterocytes. This membrane harbors several transport proteins that participate in the uptake of various types of lipids. Niemann-Pick C1 like 1 (*NPC1L1*) is a protein involved in cholesterol uptake. CD36 participates in fatty acid (*FA*) absorption. In addition, passive diffusion of lipid digestion products also occurs. In the cytosol, FA-binding protein (*FABP*) transports FAs to the ER where fatty acid transport protein-4 (*FATP*) or acyl-CoA synthetase long-chain family members (*ACSL*) activates them to acyl-CoAs for subsequent esterification. Acyl-CoA:cholesterol acyltransferase (*ACAT*), monoacylglycerol transferase (*MGAT*), and diacylglycerol acyltransferase (*DGAT*) are found in the membranes of the endoplasmic reticulum (*ER*), where they facilitate the esterification of cholesterol (*C*), monoacylglycerols (*MAG*), and diacylglycerols (*DAG*), respectively. These esterified products, triacylglycerols (*TAG*) and cholesteryl esters (*CE*), are incorporated into apolipoprotein (apo) B-48–containing chylomicrons (*CM*) in a microsomal triacylglycerol transport protein (*MTP*)-dependent manner. The newly synthesized prechylomicrons are transported in specialized vesicles, the prechylomicron transport vesicles (*PCTV*), to the Golgi apparatus for further processing and for secretion. In addition, enterocytes express ATP-binding cassette (*ABC*) transporter A1 on the basolateral membrane to facilitate the efflux of cholesterol and plant sterols. (Adapted from Iqbal, J., & Hussain, M. M. [2009]. Intestinal lipid absorption. *American Journal of Physiology Endocrinology and Metabolism, 296*, E1183–E1194.)

endocytosis. Details remain to be elucidated, but NPC1L1 may act as an extracellular free cholesterol receptor, recruiting extracellular cholesterol to its N-terminal until the cholesterol content in this microdomain of the apical membrane reaches the threshold necessary for endocytosis and targeting to intracellular compartments (Betters and Yu, 2010). At least two other proteins, scavenger receptor B1 (SR-B1) and CD36 may also play roles in cholesterol absorption, particularly in the proximal intestine (Hui et al., 2008). Like NPC1L1, SR-B1 is inhibited by ezetimibe. The relative contributions of NPC1L1, SR-B1, and CD36 and their potential interactions in cholesterol absorption are not fully understood.

Complicating assessment of the net absorption of cholesterol, however, is the efflux of absorbed cholesterol from the enterocyte through the ATP-binding cassette proteins (ABCG5 and ABCG8) that are located on the enterocyte's apical membranes (Hui et al., 2008; see Figure 10-3). Their expression is highest in the proximal and midsections of the small intestine; they limit net cholesterol absorption by transporting cholesterol back into the lumen of the intestine. Furthermore, these ABC transporters efficiently transport plant sterols, which differ from cholesterol only by a methyl or ethyl group in the side chain, out of the enterocyte. Thus only a small percentage (≈1%) of ingested noncholesterol sterols are absorbed and retained in the body, whereas 50% to 60% of dietary cholesterol is absorbed and retained. This tremendous ability of the small intestine to discriminate against the plant sterols is lost in patients with β-sitosterolemia, a rare autosomal recessive disorder characterized by hyperabsorption of all sterols. Mutations in the *ABCG5* or *ABCG8* genes cause β-sitosterolemia (Lu et al., 2001). Many of these mutations seem to prevent formation of stable heterodimers and to impair trafficking of the sterol transporter to the apical surface of the cells (Graf et al., 2004), thus reducing the efflux of plant sterols back to the lumen of the intestine.

Inhibition of Cholesterol Absorption by Plant Sterols

Plant sterols in the lumen also inhibit cholesterol absorption despite their apparent uptake by the same transport system. Two possible mechanisms for this inhibition are the displacement of cholesterol from the bile acid–lipid mixed micelles by plant sterols (Nissinen et al., 2002) and the inhibition of the rate of cholesterol esterification in the enterocytes (Field and Mathur, 1983).

Margarines and vegetable oil spreads and salad dressings containing fatty acid esters of plant sterols or plant stanols, which are more soluble than unesterified plant sterols or stanols, have been promoted as functional foods for lowering cholesterol levels. Once digested, the free plant sterols or stanols hinder cholesterol solubility in micelles. Intake of 2 to 3 g of phytostanol ester or phytosterol ester per day decreases plasma low-density lipoprotein (LDL)–cholesterol level by approximately 10%, which is, however, less than that predicted based on estimates of decreased cholesterol absorption. This lower than expected decrease in serum LDL-cholesterol might be due to compensatory mechanisms that increase the rate of endogenous cholesterol synthesis when dietary intake is low (Lichtenstein and Deckelbaum, 2001).

Carrier-Mediated Uptake of Fat-Soluble Vitamins

The intestinal absorption of lipid-soluble vitamins is discussed in Chapters 28 through 31. The mechanisms of intestinal uptake of the fat-soluble vitamins are unclear and an area of active investigation. Passive diffusion is suggested for retinol and the carotenoids, but the possibility of carrier-mediated uptake of retinol is also suggested. Particularly for vitamin E, the role of a number of the transporters discussed earlier, including CD36, NPC1L1 and SR-B1, are being explored. Evidence from genetically manipulated mouse models, in vitro studies in cell models, and studies with selective inhibitors suggest a role for SR-B1 and NPC1L1 in intestinal vitamin E absorption (Takada and Suzuki, 2010). Recent evidence demonstrates a potential role of the cholesterol transporters NPC1L1 and SR-B1 in the uptake of vitamin D by the enterocytes in both cell culture and mouse models (Reboul et al., 2011).

INTRACELLULAR METABOLISM OF ABSORBED LIPIDS

Once in the cytosol of the enterocyte, lipid digestion products are again in an aqueous environment and must be transported intracellularly from the apical region, where they are absorbed, to the ER, where the enzymes involved in their metabolism are located. In the ER, these lipids are largely reesterified in preparation for packaging and export in large lipoprotein particles called chylomicrons. These processes are summarized in Figure 10-3.

INTRACELLULAR TRANSPORT OF ABSORBED LIPIDS

Although not yet fully understood, two fatty acid–binding proteins (FABP), I-FABP (intestinal, also called FABP2) and L-FABP (liver, also called FABP1), present in the cytosol of the enterocyte appear to play the key roles in the transport of absorbed fatty acids to the ER (Mansbach and Siddiqi, 2010). Their expression is greater in the proximal small intestine where lipid absorption is higher. Their proportions differ among species, with L-FABP predominant in humans and equal proportions found in rats. Their concentration is also greater in villi than in crypt enterocytes (Ockner and Manning, 1974). These two FABPs differ in their binding specificity (Besnard et al., 1996). I-FABP strongly binds only with fatty acids, but L-FABP binds a number of compounds in addition to long-chain fatty acids (e.g., lysophosphatidylcholine, retinoids, bilirubin, and carcinogens) (Bansal et al., 1989; Bass, 1988; Glatz and Veerkamp, 1985). L-FABP also binds to esters of fatty acids and coenzyme A (fatty acyl-CoAs). They also differ in their delivery of their ligands. I-FABP attaches to the ER membrane and delivers its ligand through a targeted "collision" with the ER membrane that is efficient and rapid, whereas L-FABP delivers fatty acids to the ER randomly, via slower cytosolic diffusion (Mansbach and Siddiqi, 2010). Because of these differences in delivery, I-FABP is proposed to deliver fatty acids from the apical membrane to the ER and L-FABP is proposed as a reservoir for absorbed fatty acids.

The mechanism whereby the absorbed cholesterol that has been internalized via NPC1L1 is released from endocytotic vesicles and transported to the ER is unclear. Before the discovery of the role of NPC1L1 in cholesterol absorption, the sterol carrier protein-2 (SCP-2) was suggested to play a role in the intracellular transport of cholesterol, but its role has not been elucidated.

REESTERIFICATION OF LIPID DIGESTION PRODUCTS

2-Monoacylglycerols and fatty acids are reconstituted to form triacylglycerol, mainly via the monoacylglycerol pathway. First, fatty acids must be activated to fatty acyl-CoAs (Mansbach and Siddiqi, 2010). Fatty acids taken up by the enterocyte are esterified with a fatty acid to form fatty acyl-CoAs, and this esterification may be catalyzed by acyl-CoA synthetase long-chain family members 3 and 5 (ACSL) or by fatty acid transport protein 4 (FATP4), which are localized on the ER membrane of the enterocytes. Formation of fatty acyl-CoA results in the capture of absorbed fatty acids and ensures a concentration gradient favoring further absorption of fatty acids from the lumen.

As shown in Figure 10-4, 2-monoacylglycerol is reacylated into triacylglycerol by the consecutive action of monoacylglycerol acyltransferase (MGAT), which produces *sn*-1,2 diacylglycerol (DAG), and diacylglycerol acyltransferase (DGAT), which produces triacylglycerols. These enzymes are located on the cytosolic surface of the ER. Thus

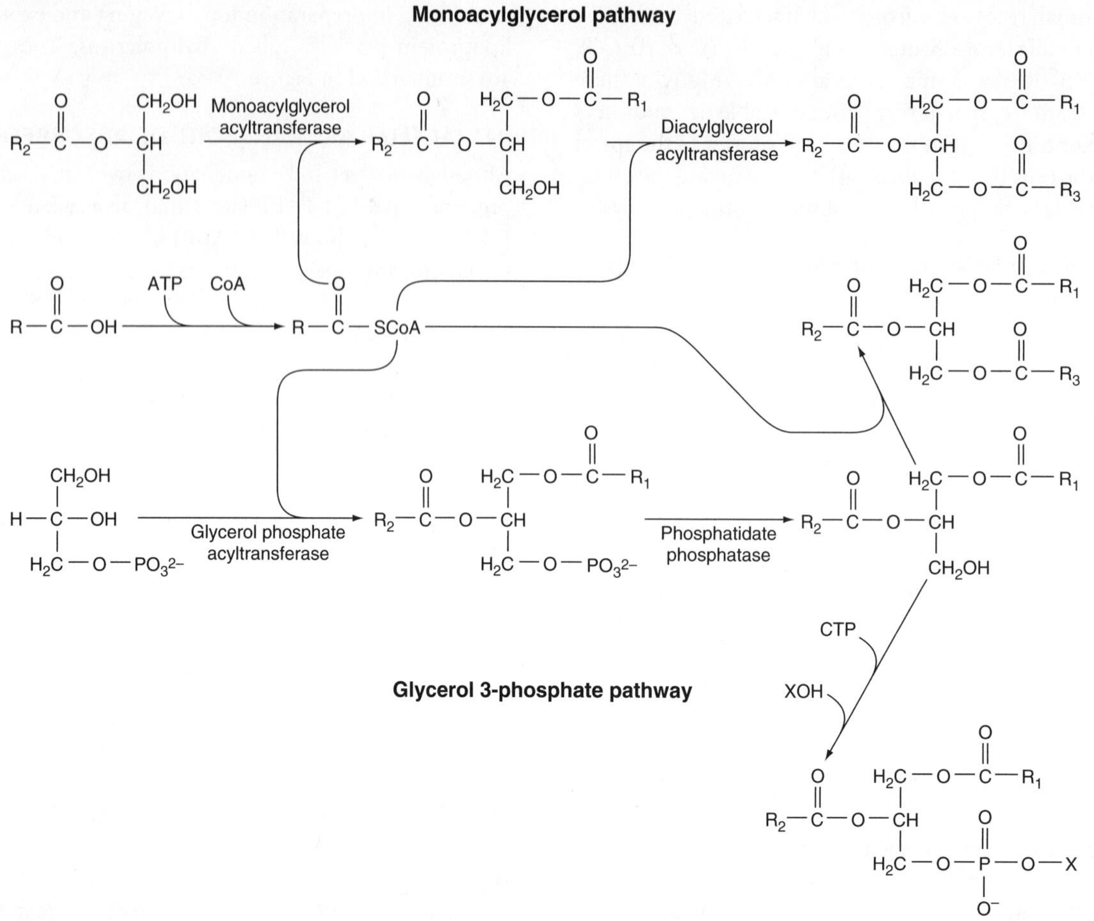

Monoacylglycerol pathway

Glycerol 3-phosphate pathway

FIGURE 10-4 Pathways of triacylglycerol biosynthesis in the intestinal mucosal cells (enterocytes). *R(COOH),* Fatty acid; *X(OH),* alcohol (e.g., choline or serine); both shown in ester linkages.

triacylglycerols are formed at the cytosolic surface of the ER membrane. The triacylglyerols must then cross the ER membrane to enter the lumen or inside of the ER, but the mechanism of transfer is not well understood (Mansbach and Siddiqi, 2010). In one proposed mechanism, triacylglycerols, which have a low solubility in the ER membrane, are assumed to accumulate in the membrane until the saturation point is reached. After this saturation, the triacylglycerols are thought to split the membrane phospholipid bilayer, forming a bulging protrusion into the lumen of the ER that is then internalized (Kindel et al., 2010).

Another pathway present in intestinal mucosa for the formation of triacylglycerol de novo is the glycerol 3-phosphate pathway, which (as shown in Figure 10-4) involves the stepwise acylation of glycerol 3-phosphate to form phosphatidic acid. In the presence of phosphatidate phosphatase, phosphatidic acid is hydrolyzed to release inorganic phosphate and to form diacylglycerol, which is then further esterified to form triacylglycerol. The relative importance of the monoacylglycerol pathway and the glycerol 3-phosphate pathway depends on the supply of 2-monoacylglycerol and fatty acid. During normal lipid absorption, the monoacylglycerol pathway predominates in enterocytes because of the abundant supply of 2-monoacylglycerol and fatty acid and their efficient conversion to triacylglycerol, and also because 2-monoacylglycerol inhibits the glycerol phosphate pathway. However, when the supply of 2-monoacylglycerol is insufficient, the glycerol phosphate pathway becomes the major pathway for the formation of triacylglycerol.

Lysophosphatidylcholine and other lysophospholipids inside the enterocytes can be reacylated to form phosphatidylcholine and other phospholipids, or these lysophospholipids can be hydrolyzed to form glycerol 3-phosphorylcholine. The liberated fatty acids can be used for triacylglycerol synthesis, whereas the glycerol 3-phosphorylcholine can be readily transported via the portal blood for use in the liver. Another reaction that occurs in intestinal mucosal cells is the combination of two molecules of lysophosphatidylcholine to yield one molecule of phosphatidylcholine and one molecule of glycerol 3-phosphorylcholine.

Absorbed cholesterol is transported almost exclusively by the lymphatic system, mainly as esterified cholesterol in chylomicrons. Enterocytes handle cholesterol derived from the intestinal lumen differently than the cholesterol that is synthesized de novo. Cholesterol absorbed from the gut does not mix freely with the free cholesterol pool in the enterocyte and is preferentially esterified for incorporation into chylomicrons and export into the lymph. The rate of esterification of cholesterol probably regulates the rate of its lymphatic transport. Acyl CoA:cholesterol acyltransferase (ACAT) located on the ER membrane esterifies cholesterol (Hui and Howles, 2005). This enzyme is present in both the jejunum and the ileum, but the jejunum, the site most actively involved in cholesterol absorption, has significantly higher levels than the ileum. The activity of this enzyme can be increased by feeding a high-cholesterol diet.

ASSEMBLY OF INTESTINAL LIPOPROTEINS

Lipoproteins are lipid–protein complexes formed by the small intestine and the liver for the export of lipids from these organs. The lipoproteins secreted by the enterocyte include (1) chylomicrons; (2) intestinal very-low-density lipoproteins (VLDLs, also called small chylomicrons); and (3) high-density lipoproteins (HDLs). Both chylomicrons and intestinal VLDLs are triacylglycerol-rich lipoproteins. In this chapter, only chylomicrons and intestinal VLDLs are discussed, because the small intestine secretes only a small amount of HDLs (HDLs are discussed in Chapter 17). During fasting, the major lipoproteins secreted by the small intestine are the intestinal (apo B-48–containing) VLDLs. Chylomicrons are the major lipoproteins secreted by the small intestine following a lipid-rich meal. Chylomicrons are only made and secreted in the small intestine, whereas VLDLs are mainly synthesized by the liver.

Composition of Chylomicrons and VLDLs

The composition of the chylomicron is described in Table 10-1. The major apolipoproteins associated with chylomicrons are apolipoprotein (apo) A-I, apo A-IV, and apo B-48. Traces of apo E and apo C are added to the chylomicrons after their entry into the circulation. Data from both animals and humans indicate that the fatty acid composition of the triacylglycerol of chylomicrons closely resembles that of the dietary lipid consumed. In the example shown in Table 10-2, Kayden and colleagues (1963) studied the changes in human lymph triacylglycerol composition after a subject ingested 100 g of corn oil. The fatty acid composition of chylomicron triacylglycerol collected 8 hours after the lipid dose was virtually identical to that of the corn oil ingested. The fatty acid composition of the phospholipids of chylomicrons is less influenced by dietary fatty acids, however, because phosphatidylcholine from bile is the major source of phospholipids in the intestinal lumen and thus also for chylomicrons. Biliary phosphatidylcholine has a unique fatty acid composition.

As shown in Table 10-1, intestinal VLDLs are smaller and have a different lipid composition than chylomicrons. In contrast, the apolipoprotein composition is not different between lymph chylomicrons and intestinal VLDLs.

Assembly of Chylomicrons in the ER

Formation of chylomicrons in the ER occurs in two steps. First, the ER synthesizes apo B-48, which forms the dense primordial lipid-poor lipoprotein. Then this primordial particle fuses with a lipid-rich, protein-poor particle in a process dependent on microsomal triglyceride transfer proteins (MTPs) to form the lipid-rich prechylomicron containing apo B-48, which will subsequently be transferred to the Golgi apparatus for final processing before secretion into the lymph.

TABLE 10-1 Composition and Characteristics of Nascent Intestinal Chylomicrons and Intestinal VLDLs*

	CHYLOMICRON	INTESTINAL VLDL
Density	<0.95 g/mL	0.95 to 1.006 g/mL
Size	80 to 500 nm	30 to 80 nm
Total lipid	~98% of particle mass	~90% of particle mass
Triacylglycerol	~86%	~60%
Cholesterol (mostly as cholesteryl ester)	~4%	~15%
Phospholipids	~8%	~15%
Total protein	~2% of particle weight	~10% of particle weight
Major apoproteins	B-48, A-1, A-IV, and A-II	Probably similar to chylomicron
Minor apoproteins	C and E (both acquired through interaction with other plasma lipoproteins)	Same as chylomicron

VLDL, Very-low-density lipoprotein.
*Nascent intestinal chylomicrons and VLDLs harvested from intestinal lymph.

TABLE 10-2 Alteration of Fatty Acid Composition (% by Weight) of Human Lymph Chylomicron Triacylglycerol After Feeding Corn Oil (100 g)

		Lymph	
FATTY ACID	CORN OIL (%)	FASTING (%)	8 to 10 hr* (%)
C 12:0		4	0
C 14:0		13	0
C 16:0	11	28	10
C 18:0		10	2
C 18:1	27	32	22
C 18:2	61	10	64

*Time after corn oil feeding.
Data from Kayden, H. J., Karmen, A., & Dumont, A. (1963). Alterations in the fatty acid composition of human lymph and serum lipoproteins by single feeding. *Journal of Clinical Investigation, 42,* 1373–1381.

Synthesis of apo B-48 and the Primordial Lipoprotein

Although two major forms of apolipoprotein B are made by humans (i.e., apo B-100 and apo B-48), the small intestine synthesizes and secretes only apo B-48. Both forms of apo B are encoded by the same gene, but only the N-terminal portion (i.e., 48% translation of the entire gene) is translated in the small intestine. This truncated translation occurs because of a unique mechanism of messenger RNA (mRNA) editing by apo B editing catalytic component 1, which deaminates a cytosine to a uridine, resulting in an earlier stop codon (Mansbach and Siddiqi, 2010). Even though apo B is required for the formation of chylomicrons, the supply of apo B is probably not a rate-limiting step for lipid output in chylomicrons. Nascent apo B-48 is rapidly degraded in the lumen of the ER when lipid is not available to protect it from degradation.

The truncated apo B-48 is clearly not obligatory for chylomicron assembly, because mice without the gene for editing apo B-100 to apo B-48 (*apobec-1* knockout mice) absorb dietary fat even though they only produce apo B-100. Nevertheless, apo B-48 appears superior over apo B-100 in chylomicron assembly and fat absorption (Kendrick et al., 2001), because chylomicron secretion is markedly reduced in mice unable to produce apo B-48.

As apo B-48 is cotranslationally translocated into the lumen of the ER, both luminal lipid and chaperone proteins (MTP and BiP) associate with it. The association of chaperones and lipid with apo B-48 prevents its degradation by the ubiquitin–proteasome degradation pathway. The primordial lipoprotein, containing apo B-48, phospholipids, cholesteryl esters, and small amounts of triacylglycerol, detaches from the ER membrane into the lumen of the ER.

Formation of the Prechylomicron

Formation of the prechylomicron continues in the lumen of the ER, where lipid-rich particles are added in an MTP-dependent process. The lipid-rich particles contain triacylglycerols and cholesteryl esters formed on the cytosolic side of the ER and are then transferred across the ER membrane, as discussed earlier, but these lipid-rich particles do not contain apo B-48 or apo A1, another apolipoprotein made by the enterocyte. The role of MTP in this process is not fully understood, but presumably MTP directs the lipid-rich particle to the primordial particle and ensures the transfer of the lipid to the growing prechylomicron. When dietary fat is high, the rate-limiting step in chylomicron assembly and secretion appears to be the addition of the lipid droplet to the nascent chylomicron particle. The size of these lipid droplets is thought to determine the size of the chylomicrons produced, but apo A-IV, another apolipoprotein made in the enterocyte, also increases the size of the secreted chylomicron (Mansbach and Siddiqi, 2010).

Transfer of the Prechylomicron to the Golgi Apparatus

Transfer of the prechylomicron to the Golgi apparatus from the ER is a complex process that involves a unique and large prechylomicron transport vesicle (PCTV) that is approximately 250 nm in diameter (Mansbach and Siddiqi, 2010). This vesicle encloses the large prechylomicron particle and ferries it from the ER lumen to the Golgi apparatus. The PCTV is far larger than the COPII-coated vesicles formed in the classical pathway of vesicular transfer of proteins from the ER to the Golgi apparatus. Formation of COPII vesicles requires a group of five proteins known as coat protein complex II proteins. These classical vesicles are only 55 to 100 nm in diameter and not large enough to accommodate the prechylomicrons. Formation of PCTVs appears to be a unique process for prechylomicron transport in the enterocyte. Unlike COPII vesicles, PCTVs can form in the absence of COPII proteins, suggesting a unique mechanism for their formation. L-FABP may play a role in the formation of the PCTV, but this is not well understood. Although not needed for their production, the PCTVs do contain the COPII proteins, and the COPII proteins are required for the fusion of PCTVs with the Golgi membranes, suggesting they play a role in target recognition.

The fusion of the PCTV to the *cis*-Golgi complex also depends on the other proteins needed for the targeting, docking, and fusion of the PCTV to the Golgi membrane. Vesicle trafficking in the cell depends on the presence of membrane proteins called SNAREs (soluble *N*-ethylmaleimide-sensitive fusion protein attachment protein receptors). SNAREs are necessary for the fusion of the vesicle and the target membranes. SNAREs exist in matched pairs; one set is in the vesicle (v-SNARE) and the other set is in the target membrane (t-SNARE). A unique set of SNAREs was found to be involved in PCTV targeting to the Golgi complex in rat small intestine (Siddiqi et al., 2006). In this case, VAMP-7 functions as the v-SNARE, and the Golgi membrane recognizes VAMP-7 by a unique set of t-SNAREs comprising syntaxin-5, Rbet 1, and Vtila. The formation of a vesicle and Golgi membrane SNARE complex allows docking of the PCTV to the *cis*-Golgi and its fusion with the Golgi membranes to transfer the prechylomicron to the Golgi apparatus.

Final Processing in the Golgi Apparatus

In the Golgi apparatus of the enterocyte, two final processing steps occur. First is the transfer of apo-AI to the prechylomicron. Second, glycosylation of apo B-48 that began with its *N*-glycosylation in the ER is completed with replacement of mannose residues with other carbohydrate moieties.

Secretion in the Lymph

How prechylomicrons exit the Golgi complex is not well understood, but vesicles transfer the prechylomicrons to the basolateral membrane of the enterocytes, and prechylomicrons are then discharged into the intercellular space through exocytosis. The vesicles fuse with the basolateral membrane and release the chylomicrons through reverse exocytosis into the lamina propria (i.e., the vascular layer of connective tissue beneath the epithelium). The chylomicrons are too large to enter the pores of the capillaries, but they can pass through the large fenestrations of the lacteals into the lymphatic circulation. The lymphatic vessels ultimately empty into the venous circulation by way of the thoracic duct before the point where blood enters the heart.

FACTORS AFFECTING FORMATION AND SECRETION OF CHYLOMICRONS

The formation and the secretion of chylomicrons are tightly regulated by the synthesis of apolipoproteins and lipids in the enterocytes. Although considerable information regarding these factors has been gathered, the mechanisms of how these factors regulate the formation and secretion of chylomicrons remain largely unknown. A major reason for our limited knowledge of this is the lack of good cell models for studying these processes, because it is extremely difficult to maintain intestinal epithelial cells in culture.

ROLE OF APOLIPOPROTEINS A-I AND A-IV

The human small intestine synthesizes both apo A-I and apo A-IV. These apoproteins are secreted in association with chylomicrons. The synthesis and secretion of apo A-IV is markedly stimulated by the ingestion of fat, which is consistent with the marked increase in the amount of lipid secreted in chylomicrons following ingestion of a lipid-rich meal. The synthesis and secretion of apo A-I, however, is not affected by the ingestion of fat. The roles of apo A-I and apo A-IV in the formation and secretion of chylomicrons are not clear. However, following metabolism of chylomicrons in the circulation, apo A-IV detaches and circulates in the plasma either bound to HDLs or as a free protein. A number of recent reports indicate that apo A-IV has a unique physiological role as a circulating signal released in response to fat feeding that may partially mediate the anorectic (inhibition of food intake) effect of lipids.

ROLE OF LUMINAL PHOSPHATIDYLCHOLINE

An adequate supply of intestinal luminal phosphatidylcholine is important for the formation and secretion of intestinal chylomicrons and intestinal VLDLs. It is a major component of the surface coat of chylomicrons. Bile phosphatidylcholine has a unique fatty acid composition that closely resembles that of the phosphatidylcholine in the surface coat of chylomicrons, suggesting that biliary or luminal phosphatidylcholine is preferentially used for the coating of chylomicrons. In a model system, the lipolysis of triacylglycerol emulsions and the rates of clearance of particles from the plasma by hepatocytes versus reticuloendothelial cells depended on the cholesterol content and the phosphatidylcholine species of the lipid emulsion particles (Clark et al., 1991). Consequently, the specific fatty acid composition of the phosphatidylcholine in the chylomicron surface coat may play an important role in the metabolism of chylomicrons by the body.

PORTAL TRANSPORT OF LONG-CHAIN FATTY ACIDS

Most of the absorbed fatty acids are incorporated into triacylglycerols and transported by intestinal lymph in the chylomicrons and intestinal VLDLs, as described earlier. However, fatty acids, perhaps as much as 30%, also can be transported via the portal vein (Mansbach et al., 1991). Medium-chain fatty acids are preferentially transported by the portal vein. Double bonds in long-chain fatty acids also increase portal transport (McDonald et al., 1980). This portal transport increases when rates of lipid absorption are low (McDonald et al., 1980), when there is a defect in the intracellular esterification of fatty acids to form triacylglycerols, or when there is an impairment in chylomicron formation, such as in patients with abetalipoproteinemia (Ways et al., 1967). Portal transport of fatty acids may provide an alternative pathway for triacylglycerol synthesis when the lipid digestion product 2-monoacylglycerol that is needed for reesterification of fatty acids inside the enterocyte is absent; fatty acids transported to the liver by the portal circulation can be esterified to glycerol to form triacylglycerol and hence VLDL in the liver.

HORMONAL REGULATION OF LIPID ABSORPTION

Relatively little is known of how intestinal lipid absorption is regulated by hormones. The intestinal peptide called neurotensin has been reported to enhance lymphatic lipid transport in the rat by enhancing the processing of absorbed dietary fat, but it also induces hemodynamic changes in the gastrointestinal tract (e.g., increased lymph flow). Further experiments are needed to ascertain whether this effect of neurotensin on intestinal lipid transport is an intracellular effect or simply a hemodynamic effect.

More recently, the gastrointestinal hormone, glucagon-like peptide 2 (GLP2), has been reported to increase lipid absorption and chylomicron secretion. GLP2 is released, along with GLP1, from enteroendocrine L cells in response to fat or carbohydrate feeding in humans (Meier et al., 2006), Syrian hamsters, and mice (Hsieh et al., 2009). Administration of GLP2 with a standardized mixed meal of 250 kcal including fat to humans resulted in a small but significantly greater postprandial increase in serum triacylglycerols. If an oral dose of olive oil was given to hamsters and mice with functional CD36, GLP2 administration increased the secretion of apo B-48–containing lipoproteins (i.e., chylomicrons) threefold; the secretion of triacylglycerols in these chylomicrons increased to four times the levels observed in animals that did not receive GLP2. In mice lacking CD36, GLP2 did not affect lipid absorption. Additional studies are needed to understand the signal transduction and mechanism whereby GLP2 regulates lipid absorption and/or chylomicron synthesis, as well as the roles of CD36 and fatty acid absorption in this regulation.

DISORDERS OF INTESTINAL LIPID ABSORPTION

The determination of the amount of fat in the stool is a common test for assessment of intestinal malabsorption. Efficiency of fat digestion is normally high, with 95% of dietary fat absorbed and less than 5% of daily fat intake present in a 24-hour fecal sample. Moreover, the capacities of the enzymatic and transport processes involved in dietary fat absorption greatly exceed those required during normal fat absorption. Complete absorption of dietary fat at intakes of more than 300 g/day and toleration of intakes of more than 600 g/day for a period of 20 days have been reported (Kasper, 1970). Nonetheless, intestinal lipid malabsorption can be caused by a number of clinical conditions.

GENERAL MALABSORPTIVE DISORDERS

A common disorder of the small intestine that results in malabsorption of nutrients, including lipids, is celiac disease, which is a cell-mediated allergy to gluten (a protein rich in proline and glutamine found in wheat, barley, and rye). Celiac disease frequently though not always results in villus atrophy and other intestinal lesions. The resulting malabsorptive state is corrected by a strict gluten-free diet.

PANCREATIC INSUFFICIENCY

A major feature of pancreatic insufficiency, which can occur in individuals with cystic fibrosis (a genetic disorder in the chloride transporter) or chronic pancreatitis, is severe abdominal pain and steatorrhea (the presence of excess fat in feces and the passage of large, pale, frothy stools). These symptoms are caused by the presence of a large amount of undigested fat in the gastrointestinal tract. The lack of adequate pancreatic secretion results in a lack of enzymes for fat digestion in the intestinal lumen. Pancreatic insufficiency is treated by prescribing a low-fat diet or oral supplements of pancreatic enzymes with meals. Oral supplements of pancreatic enzymes are prepared with an enteric coating to prevent release of the enzymes before they reach the small intestine. Severe deficiency of pancreatic secretions may require diets rich in medium-chain triacylglycerols (MCT), which are more readily hydrolyzed by gastric lipase. MCT oils are commercially available and comprise principally triacylglycerols containing esterified octanoic and decanoic acids. However, MCT oil does not provide the essential polyunsaturated fatty acids, linoleic and α-linolenic acid.

DEFICIENCY OF BILE ACIDS

Bile acid deficiency due to gallstones or liver disease results in poor micellar solubilization of lipid digestion products. A deficiency of bile acids does not affect the digestion of triacylglycerol by pancreatic lipase, because bile acids when present actually inhibit pancreatic lipase in the absence of colipase. Thus, the fats present in the stool are mainly lipid digestion products in the form of fatty acid salts (soaps). The small unilamellar vesicles formed by bile acids may also play a role in the delivery of lipid digestion products across the unstirred water layer, resulting in significant amounts of lipid being absorbed, even without bile acid micelle formation, in patients with bile acid deficiencies.

Abetalipoproteinemia

Abetalipoproteinemia, a genetic disorder, results in a near-complete lack of apo B–containing lipoproteins in the circulation. The apo B gene is normal in patients with abetalipoproteinemia (Talmud et al., 1988) and their enterocytes synthesize apo B. However, the large subunit of MTP is mutated (Berriot-Varoqueaux et al., 2000; Wetterau et al., 1992). MTP is the protein that transfers lipids to the apo-B protein as it is translated, allowing it to attain the proper conformation for lipoprotein assembly. In abetalipoproteinemia, transfer of triacylglycerol is blocked and premature degradation of the nascent apo-B protein occurs. Consequently, triacylglycerol droplets accumulate in the intestinal mucosa of these subjects as lipid absorption progresses (Dobbins, 1970). This disorder ultimately results in neurological disorders and acanthocytosis (i.e., the presence of abnormal erythrocytes with spurlike projections in the blood, perhaps due to abnormal composition of membrane lipids).

Chylomicron Retention Disorder

Chylomicron retention disorder is a genetic defect in the transfer of prechylomicrons from the ER to the Golgi apparatus. This results in an absence of chylomicrons in the postprandial plasma due to retention of prechylomicrons in the enterocyte (Roy et al., 1987). The genetic defects causing chylomicron retention disorder are mutations in Sar1b, a small GTPase that is one of the COPII proteins involved in the targeting and fusion of PCTVs to the Golgi apparatus as discussed earlier. The lack of functional Sar1b results in PCTVs that cannot fuse with the Golgi apparatus, and they accumulate in the enterocyte (Peretti et al., 2010). This disorder is associated with chronic diarrhea and steatorrhea, abdominal distention, and failure to thrive in infants, and it should be recognized and treated early. Identification of the genetic mutations underlying this disorder in humans has facilitated the diagnosis of this disorder and thus its earlier treatment.

INTESTINAL FATTY ACIDS AND MUCOSAL INJURY

Long-chain fatty acids in the lumen can be injurious to the intestine, especially to the developing intestine (Velasquez et al., 1994). The magnitude of injury caused by the luminal presence of fatty acids is higher in piglets less than 2 weeks of age than in 1-month-old animals. The change in susceptibility with age suggests that postnatal development of the intestine renders the intestinal mucosa more resistant to lipid-induced injury. Clinically, immaturity or disruption of the intestinal mucosal barrier by fatty acids may result in disease states to which the newborn infant is susceptible, such as necrotizing enterocolitis or toxigenic diarrhea. Esterification of the injurious long-chain fatty acids with ethanol abolished their cytotoxic effects on the intestinal mucosa but still enabled absorption and utilization by the developing intestine.

SATIETY EFFECTS OF FAT FEEDING

There is compelling evidence that the ingestion of fat results in satiation and the inhibition of food intake. A number of characteristics of this lipid-induced satiety suggest that gastrointestinal signals stimulated by lipid digestion and absorption may be mediators. First, long-chain fatty acids are significantly more potent in inducing satiety than are short- or medium-chain fatty acids. Long-chain fatty acids are transported by the small intestine mainly as chylomicrons, whereas medium-chain fatty acids are transported mainly in the portal blood. This observation raises the possibility that chylomicrons are somehow involved in this lipid-induced satiety. Alternatively, long-chain fatty acids may stimulate the release of gastrointestinal hormones such as cholecystokinin from the intestine or ghrelin from the stomach. Second, fatty acids introduced into the small intestinal lumen are more potent in inducing satiety than are fatty acids delivered by direct peripheral venous, portal, or caval routes. Again, this would imply that the gastrointestinal tract, and probably presence of luminal fatty acids or the production of chylomicrons, is somehow involved in this lipid-induced satiety. Third, the lipid-induced satiety is abolished by the presence of orlistat (an inhibitor of pancreatic lipase) in the intestinal lumen, indicating that it is the digestion products and not triacylglycerols per se that elicit the satiety response (Ellrichmann et al., 2008). Therefore most of the observations concerning lipid-induced satiety imply that intestinal lipid digestion and absorption are integral to this regulation.

Evidence exists for involvement of three gastrointestinal peptides or hormones in fat-induced satiety: apo A-IV, cholecystokinin, and ghrelin. First, apo A-IV, which is synthesized in the intestine and incorporated into secreted chylomicrons, may be involved in this lipid-induced satiety (Fujimoto et al., 1992). The synthesis and secretion of apo A-IV is markedly stimulated by the ingestion of fat. Apo A-IV apparently acts on the central nervous system to elicit the satiety response, but the mechanism by which apo A-IV inhibits food intake is not understood. Intravenous (Fujimoto et al., 1992) or central administration (Liu et al., 2003) of apo A-IV inhibits food intake. Therefore apo A-IV appears to be important for the integrated control of digestive function and ingestive behavior. Cholecystokinin, a gastrointestinal hormone produced by the enteroendocrine L cells in the proximal small intestine in response to fat or protein feeding, also inhibits food intake via activating vagal afferent fibers (Delzenne et al., 2010). In contrast to apo A-IV and cholecystokinin, the orexigenic hormone ghrelin produced by gastric endocrine cells in response to hunger and negative energy balance, stimulates appetite directly in the central nervous system (Delzenne et al., 2010). Macronutrients in the small intestine suppress the release of ghrelin. Thus lipid suppression of ghrelin secretion could play a role in its satiety effect. Consistent with a role of digestion products, inhibition of fat digestion blocked the reduction of ghrelin after consumption of a test fat "meal" (Tai et al., 2010). Further research is needed to understand the relative contributions and potential interactions among these three mediators for fat satiety. Gut peptides/hormones are more fully discussed in Chapter 7, and regulation of satiety and food intake is discussed further in Chapter 22.

THINKING CRITICALLY

1. What components of the pancreatic juice are needed for efficient lipid digestion? What is the specific function of each of these in lipid digestion?
2. Lipid digestion and absorption are facilitated by bile acids. If bile secretion and/or gallbladder function are impaired, which specific steps of lipid digestion and lipid absorption would be affected and how would these steps be affected?
3. What are some genetic defects that impair chylomicron synthesis and/or secretion? How might these disorders affect plasma levels of LDL? Total cholesterol? Fat-soluble vitamins? Essential polyunsaturated fatty acid levels?

REFERENCES

Aloulou, A., & Carrière, F. (2008). Gastric lipase: An extremophilic interfacial enzyme with medical applications. *Cellular and Molecular Life Sciences, 65*, 851–854.

Altmann, S. W., Davis, H. R., Jr., Zhu, L. J., Yao, X., Hoos, L., Tetzloff, G., … Graziano, M. P. (2004). Niemann-Pick C1 like 1 protein is critical for intestinal cholesterol absorption. *Science, 303*, 1201–1204.

Bansal, M. P., Cook, R. G., Danielson, K. G., & Medina, D. (1989). A 14-kilodalton selenium-binding protein in mouse liver is fatty acid–binding protein. *The Journal of Biological Chemistry, 264*, 13780–13784.

Bass, N. M. (1988). The cellular fatty acid–binding proteins: Aspects of structure, regulation, and function. *International Review of Cytology, 111*, 143–184.

Berriot-Varoqueaux, N., Aggerbeck, L. P., Samson-Bouma, M., & Wetterau, J. R. (2000). The role of the microsomal triglyceride transfer protein in abetalipoproteinemia. *Annual Review of Nutrition, 20*, 663–697.

Besnard, P., Niot, I., Bernard, A., & Carlier, H. (1996). Cellular and molecular aspects of fat metabolism in the small intestine. *Proceedings of the Nutrition Society, 55*, 19–37.

Betters, J. L., & Yu, L. (2010). NPC1L1 and cholesterol transport. *FEBS Letters, 584*, 2740–2747.

Cardell, R. R., Badenhausen, S., & Porter, K. R. (1967). Intestinal triglyceride absorption in the rat: An electron microscopical study. *The Journal of Cell Biology, 54*, 123–155.

Carey, M. C., Small, D. M., & Bliss, C. M. (1983). Lipid digestion and absorption. *Annual Review of Physiology, 45*, 651–677.

Carrière, F., Renou, C., Ransac, S., Lopez, V., De Caro, J., Ferrato, F., … Laugier, R. (2001). Inhibition of gastrointestinal lipolysis by Orlistat during digestion of test meals in healthy volunteers. *American Journal of Physiology Gastrointestinal and Liver Physiology, 281*, G16–G28.

Clark, S. B., Derksen, A., & Small, D. M. (1991). Plasma clearance of emulsified triolein in conscious rats: Effects of phosphatidylcholine species, cholesterol content, and emulsion surface physical state. *Experimental Physiology, 76*, 39–52.

Delzenne, N., Blundell, J., Brouns, F., Cunningham, K., De Graaf, K., Erkner, A., … Westerterp-Plantenga, M. (2010). Gastrointestinal targets of appetite regulation in humans. *Obesity Reviews, 11*, 234–250.

Dobbins, W. O. (1970). An ultrastructural study of the intestinal mucosa in congenital β-lipoprotein deficiency with particular emphasis on intestinal absorptive cells. *Gastroenterology, 50*, 195–210.

Ellrichmann, M., Kapelle, M., Ritter, P. R., Holst, J. J., Herzig, K. H., Schmidt, W. E., … Meier, J. J. (2008). Orlistat inhibition of intestinal lipase acutely increases appetite and attenuates postprandial glucagon-like peptide-1-(7-36)-amide-1, cholecystokinin, and peptide YY concentrations. *Journal of Clinical Endocrinology and Metabolism, 93*, 3995–3998.

Field, F. J., & Mathur, S. (1983). β-Sitosterol: Esterification by intestinal acyl coenzyme A:cholesterol acyltransferase (ACAT) and its effect on cholesterol esterification. *Journal of Lipid Research, 24*, 409–417.

Fujimoto, K., Cardelli, J. A., & Tso, P. (1992). Increased apolipoprotein A-IV in rat mesenteric lymph after lipid meal as a physiological signal for satiation. *The American Journal of Physiology, 262*, G1002–G1006.

Gilham, D., Labonté, E. D., Rojas, J. C., Jandacek, R. J., Howles, P. N., & Hui, D. Y. (2007). Carboxyl ester lipase deficiency exacerbates dietary lipid absorption abnormalities and resistance to diet-induced obesity in pancreatic triglyceride lipase knockout mice. *The Journal of Biological Chemistry, 282*, 24642–24649.

Glatz, J. F. C., & Veerkamp, J. H. (1985). Intracellular fatty acid–binding proteins. *The International Journal of Biochemistry, 17*, 13–22.

Graf, G. A., Cohen, J. C., & Hobbs, H. H. (2004). Missense mutations in ABCG5 and ABCG8 disrupt heterodimerization and trafficking. *The Journal of Biological Chemistry, 279*, 24881–24888.

Harrison, E. H. (2005). Mechanism of digestion and absoprtion of dietary vitamin A. *Annual Review of Nutrition, 25*, 87–103.

Hofmann, A. F. (2009). Bile acids: Trying to understand their chemistry and biology with the hope of helping patients. *Hepatology, 49*, 1403–1418.

Hsieh, J., Longuet, C., Maida, A., Bahrami, J., Xu, E., Baker, C. L., … Adeli, K. (2009). Glucagon-like peptide-2 increases intestinal lipid absorption and chylomicron production via CD36. *Gastroenterology, 137*, 997–1005.

Hui, D. Y., & Howles, P. N. (2005). Molecular mechanisms of cholesterol absorption and transport in the intestine. *Journal of Lipid Research, 45*, 89–98.

Hui, D. Y., Labonté, E. D., & Howles, P. N. (2008). Development and physiological regulation of intestinal lipid absorption. III. Intestinal transporters and cholesterol absorption. *American Journal of Physiology. Gastrointestinal and Liver Physiology, 294*, G839–G843.

Jensen, G. L., McGarvey, N., Taraszewski, R., Wixson, S. K., Seidner, D. L., Pai, T., … DeMichele, S. J. (1994). Lymphatic absorption of enterally fed structured triacylglycerol vs. physical mix in a canine model. *The American Journal of Clinical Nutrition, 60*, 518–524.

Kasper, H. (1970). Faecal fat excretion, diarrhea, and subjective complaints with highly dosed oral fat intake. *Digestion, 3*, 321–330.

Kayden, H. J., Karmen, A., & Dumont, A. (1963). Alterations in the fatty acid composition of human lymph and serum lipoproteins by single feeding. *The Journal of Clinical Investigation, 42*, 1373–1381.

Kendrick, J. S., Chan, L., & Higgins, J. A. (2001). Superior role of apolipoprotein B48 over apolipoprotein B100 in chylomicron assembly and fat absorption: An investigation of apobec-1 knockout and wild-type mice. *The Biochemical Journal, 356*, 821–827.

Kindel, T., Lee, D. M., & Tso, P. (2010). The mechanism of the formation and secretion of chylomicrons. *Atherosclerosis Supplements, 11*, 11–16.

Lichtenstein, A. H., & Deckelbaum, R. J. (2001). Stanol/sterol ester-containing foods and blood cholesterol levels. *Circulation, 103*, 1177–1179.

Lindquist, S., & Hernell, O. (2010). Lipid digestion and absorption in early life: An update. *Current Opinion in Clinical Nutrition and Metabolic Care, 13*, 314–320.

Liu, M., Maiorano, N., Shen, L., Pearson, K., Tajima, D., Zhang, D. M., … Tso, P. (2003). Expression of biologically active rat apolipoprotein AIV in *Escherichia coli*. *Physiology & Behavior, 78*, 149–155.

Lu, K., Lee, M. H., Hazard, S., Brooks-Wilson, A., Hidaka, H., Kojima, H., … Patel, S. B. (2001). Two genes that map to the STSL locus cause sitosterolemia: Genomic structure and specturm of mutations involving sterolin-1 and sterolin-2, encoded by ABCG5 and ABCG8, respectively. *American Journal of Human Genetics, 69*, 278–290.

Mansbach, C. M., & Siddiqi, S. A. (2010). The biogenesis of chylomicrons. *Annual Review of Physiology, 72*, 315–333.

Mansbach, C. M., II, Dowell, R. F., & Pritchett, D. (1991). Portal transport of absorbed lipids in rats. *The American Journal of Physiology, 261*, G530–G538.

Mansbach, C. M., II, & Gorelick, F. (2007). Development and physiological regulation of intestinal lipid absorption. II. Dietary lipid absorption, complex lipid synthesis, and the intracellular packaging and secretion of chylomicrons. *American Journal of Physiology. Gastrointestinal and Liver Physiology, 293*, G645–G650.

Mansbach, C. M., II, Newton, D., & Stevens, R. D. (1980). Fat digestion in patients with bile acid malabsorption but minimal steatorrhea. *Digestive Diseases and Sciences, 25*, 353–362.

Mattson, F. H., & Volpenhein, R. A. (1972). Rate and extent of absorption of the fatty acids of fully esterified glycerol, erythritol, xylitol, and sucrose as measured in thoracic duct cannulated rats. *The Journal of Nutrition, 102*, 1177–1180.

McDonald, G. B., Saunders, D. R., Weidman, M., & Fisher, L. (1980). Portal venous transport of long-chain fatty acids absorbed from rat intestine. *The American Journal of Physiology, 239*, G141–G150.

Meier, J. J., Gethmann, A., Nauck, M. A., Götze, O., Schmitz, F., Deacon, C. F., … Holst, J. J. (2006). The glucagon-like peptide-1 metabolite GLP-1-(9-36) amide reduces postprandial glycemia independently of gastric emptying and insulin secretion in humans. *Gastroenterology, 130*, 44–54.

Nassir, F., Wilson, B., Han, X., Gross, R. W., & Abumrad, N. A. (2007). CD36 is important for fatty acid and cholesterol uptake by the proximal but not distal intestine. *The Journal of Biological Chemistry, 282*, 19493–19501.

Nissinen, M., Gylling, H., & Miettenen, T. A. (2002). Micellar distribution of cholesterol and phytosterols after duodenal sitosterol infusion. *American Journal of Physiology Gastrointestinal and Liver Physiology, 282*, G1009–G1015.

Ockner, R. K., & Manning, J. A. (1974). Fatty acid-binding protein in small intestine. Identification, isolation, and evidence for its role in cellular fatty acid transport. *Journal of Clinical Investigation, 54*, 326–338.

Peretti, N., Sassolas, A., Roy, C. C., Deslandres, C., Charcosset, M., Castagnetti, J., … Levy, E. (2010). Guidelines for the diagnosis and management of chylomicron retention disease based on a review of the literature and the experience of two centers. *Orphanet Journal of Rare Diseases, 5*, 24.

Porter, H. P., Saunders, D. R., Tytgat, G., Brunster, O., & Rubin, C. E. (1971). Fat absorption in bile fistula man. A morphological and biochemical study. *Gastroenterology, 60*, 1008–1019.

Reboul, E., Goncalves, A., Comera, C., Bott, R., Nowicki, M., Landrier, J. F., … Borel, P. (2011). Vitamin D intestinal absorption is not a simple passive diffusion: Evidences for involvement of cholesterol transporters. *Molecular Nutrition & Food Research, 55*, 691–702.

Roy, C. C., Levy, E., Green, P. H. R., Sniderman, A., Letarte, J., Buts, J. P., … Deckelbaum, R. J. (1987). Malabsorption, hypocholesterolemia, and fat-filled enterocytes with increased intestinal apoprotein B. *Gastroenterology, 92*, 390–399.

Shim, J., Moulson, C. L., Newberry, E. P., Lin, M. H., Xie, Y., Kennedy, S. M., … Davidson, N. O. (2009). Fatty acid transport protein 4 is dispensable for intestinal lipid absorption in mice. *Journal of Lipid Research*, *50*, 491–500.

Siddiqi, S. A., Siddiqi, S., Mahan, J., Peggs, K., Gorelick, F. S., & Mansbach, C. M., II. (2006). The identification of a novel endoplasmic reticulum to Golgi SNARE complex used by the prechylomicron transport vesicle. *The Journal of Biological Chemistry*, *281*, 20974–20982.

Tai, K., Hammond, A. J., Wishart, J. M., Horowitz, M., & Chapman, I. M. (2010). Carbohydrate and fat digestion is necessary for maximal suppression of total plasma ghrelin in healthy adults. *Appetite*, *55*, 407–412.

Takada, T., & Suzuki, H. (2010). Molecular mechanisms of membrane transport of vitamin E. *Molecular Nutrition & Food Research*, *54*, 616–622.

Talmud, P. J., Lloyd, J. K., Muller, D. P. R., Collins, D. R., Scott, J., & Humphries, S. (1988). Genetic evidence from two families that the apolipoprotein B gene is not involved in abetalipoproteinemia. *The Journal of Clinical Investigation*, *82*, 1803–1806.

Velasquez, O. R., Place, A. R., Tso, P., & Crissinger, K. D. (1994). Developing intestine is injured during absorption of oleic acid but not its ethyl ester. *Journal of Clinical Investigation*, *93*, 479–485.

Ways, P. O., Paramentier, C. M., Kayden, H. D., Jones, J. W., Saunders, D. R., & Rubin, C. E. (1967). Studies on the absorptive defect for triglyceride in abetalipoproteinemia. *Journal of Clinical Investigation*, *46*, 35–46.

Wetterau, J. R., Aggerbeck, L. P., Bouma, M. E., Eisenberg, C., Munck, A., Hermier, M., … Gregg, R. E. (1992). Absence of microsomal triglyceride transfer protein in individuals with abetalipoproteinemia. *Science*, *258*, 999–1001.

Whitcomb, D. C., & Lowe, M. E. (2007). Human pancreatic digestive enzymes. *Digestive Diseases and Sciences*, *52*, 1–17.

CHAPTER 11

Dietary Fiber

*Joanne L. Slavin, PhD, RD**

Fiber is not an essential nutrient in the usual way we consider essential nutrients. Tube-fed patients have survived on liquid diets devoid of fiber for many years. Additionally, traditional cold-fish based diets consumed in the Arctic region contained little plant-based material and thus little fiber. Unlike most nutrients, the benefits of fiber are linked to its lack of digestion and absorption in the upper gastrointestinal tract. In the colon, fiber may survive transit and increase stool size directly, or it may be fermented by intestinal bacteria and used for their growth and proliferation. Fermentation of dietary fiber in the colon decreases pH, promotes growth of healthy microbiota, and produces short-chain fatty acids that play a role in disease prevention. Short-chain fatty acids are also absorbed in the colon and are a potential energy source. Therefore fiber is not just an inert substance that travels through the digestive tract, but plays many roles in digestion and absorption. Additionally, dietary fiber intake has been linked to the prevention and management of many diseases.

DEFINITION OF FIBER

Crude fiber is a term used to describe the residue of plant food left after sequential extraction with solvent, dilute aqueous acid, and dilute aqueous alkali, as done in the Weende method of proximate analysis developed by William Henneberg and Fredrick Stohmann in 1864. Large fractions of the hemicelluloses, lignan, and cellulose are lost in this process and thus are not included in the crude fiber measurements reported in food composition tables. In contrast to crude fiber, there is no generally agreed upon definition or method of analysis for dietary fiber. Hugh Trowell defined dietary fiber as "the residue derived from plant cell walls that is resistant to hydrolysis by human alimentary enzymes." As such, Trowell's definition included the plant cell polysaccharides (cellulose and hemicelluloses) and lignan but did not include other plant cell components (mucilages, storage polysaccharides, and algal polysaccharides) that are not hydrolyzed by human digestive enzymes. Hence Trowell (1978) subsequently redefined dietary fiber as "the plant polysaccharides and lignin which are resistant to hydrolysis by the digestive enzymes of man." This definition essentially described the same components as the "unavailable carbohydrate" being measured at the time by the methods of Southgate (1969). In the United States, the U.S. Food and Drug Administration (FDA) first addressed dietary fiber in 1987, ruling that the amount of dietary fiber listed on foods or supplements be determined through the use of what is now known as the AOAC (Association of Official Analytical Chemists) Method 985.29 or comparable methods, all of which measure nonstarch polysaccharides, lignin, and some resistant starch in plant foods (AOAC, 2007). If applied to animal foods or whole diets, resistant carbohydrates from animal sources would also be measured by these methods.

SOME CURRENT DEFINITIONS OF DIETARY FIBER

Numerous definitions for dietary fiber have subsequently been suggested or adopted by various scientific and regulatory agencies. Some specify a physiological definition of dietary fiber, whereas others rely more on a prescribed analytical method. In 1985 Health and Welfare Canada defined dietary fiber as "the endogenous components of plant material in the diet which are resistant to digestion by enzymes produced by humans" (Health and Welfare Canada, 1985). This definition allows inclusion of water-soluble gums, mucilages, and pectic substances, and nonnutritive fiber-associated substances, such as phytates, cutins, proteins, lectins, and waxes. But it excludes indigestible materials formed during food processing, such as Maillard reaction products. In 1987 the Expert Panel on Dietary Fiber of the Life Sciences Research Office (LSRO, Bethesda, MD) proposed a definition of dietary fiber that included nonstarch polysaccharides and lignin but excluded fiber-associated substances found in the plant cell wall as well as indigestible compounds formed during cooking or processing (Pilch, 1987). Both definitions exclude non–plant derived compounds, such as chitan, chitosan, and chondroitin sulfate, and synthetic carbohydrate polymers. The Codex Alimentarius Commission, the joint food standards program of the United Nations Food and Agriculture Organization (FAO) and the World Health Organization (WHO), adopted an official definition of dietary fiber in 2009.

*This chapter is a revision of the chapter contributed by Joanne R. Lupton, PhD, and Nancy D. Turner, PhD, for the second edition.

Dietary fibre means carbohydrate polymers with ten or more monomeric units, which are not hydrolysed by the endogenous enzymes in the small intestine of humans and belong to the following categories:

- Edible carbohydrate polymers naturally occurring in the food as consumed,
- carbohydrate polymers, which have been obtained from food raw material by physical, enzymatic or chemical means and which have been shown to have a physiological effect of benefit to health as demonstrated by generally accepted scientific evidence to competent authorities,
- synthetic carbohydrate polymers which have been shown to have a physiological effect or benefit to health as demonstrated by generally accepted scientific evidence to competent authorities.

(Codex Alimentarius Commission, 2009, p. 46)

In 2001 the Institute of Medicine (IOM) Panel on the Definition of Dietary Fiber proposed a new set of working definitions for fiber in the food supply. They distinguished between fiber that occurs naturally in plant foods (lignin, cellulose, beta-glucans, hemicelluloses, pectins, gums, inulin and oligofructose, and resistant starch) and isolated or synthetic fibers that may be added to foods or used as dietary supplements (psyllium, chitin and chitosan, fructooligosaccharides, polydextrose and polyols, and resistant dextrins).

Dietary Fiber consists of nondigestible carbohydrates and lignin that are intrinsic and intact in plants.
Functional Fiber consists of isolated, nondigestible carbohydrates that have beneficial physiological effects in humans.
Total Fiber is the sum of *Dietary Fiber* and *Functional Fiber* (IOM, 2001, p. 2)

Neither the Codex nor the IOM definitions have been formally adopted by the FDA in the United States. The European Union adopted a definition similar to the Codex definition as of 2008. The FDA continues to require food labels to report "dietary fiber" based on measurements made with approved AOAC methods that measure nonstarch polysaccharides, lignin, and some resistant starch as a component of total carbohydrate.

CONTROVERSIES IN DEFINING DIETARY FIBER

Fiber definitions and measurement continue to be debated. As can be gleaned from the sampling of definitions just discussed, most definitions suggest that fiber is plant material not digested by mammalian enzymes. But some scientists consider limiting fiber to "plant material" to be too restrictive. Some would include chitosan, which forms the exoskeleton of crustaceans, or certain heat-treated animal proteins that are not readily digestible by mammalian enzymes and thus reach the large intestine relatively intact. Others include "resistant starch" in their definition of fiber. Although it is not truly indigestible by mammalian enzymes, resistant starch may not be digested and absorbed in the small intestine, and thus it can have characteristics similar to those of fiber under certain circumstances. Resistant starches occur in some foods naturally, but resistant starch may also result from manufacturing or food processing. Whether oligosaccharides present in beans and other vegetables (raffinose, stachyose, and verbacose) and the fructan polysaccharides and oligosaccharides in vegetables and fruits, such as onions and artichokes, should be considered dietary fiber is also controversial. The alcohol precipitation steps used in fiber analytical techniques excludes these substances, yet they have some biological effects similar to those of other nondigested polysaccharides.

Another point of discussion is whether dietary fiber has to be intact in the food to be characterized as fiber or whether it can be extracted from food, or even manufactured, and still be called dietary fiber. The basis for this argument is that most of the data describing physiological effects and potential health benefits from fiber were generated using high-fiber foods. Whether the same benefits would come from consuming isolated or manufactured fibers is unknown. Certain isolated fibers, such as oat bran and psyllium, are particularly effective in lowering serum lipids, but most other isolated fibers have not been extensively studied so their physiological effects are largely unknown.

Carbohydrate chemists would prefer a chemical rather than a physiological definition of fiber, as well as a simple, universally accepted, analytical method for dietary fiber to simplify compliance with and enforcement of fiber labeling laws. Methods should be suitable for the analysis of any food or food component to determine how much fiber it contains. However, because the range of fibers in foods varies greatly, it is impossible to find a simple, universally accepted method to measure fiber.

CHEMICAL AND PHYSICAL CHARACTERIZATION OF DIETARY FIBER

Properties of dietary fiber depend on the primary and secondary structure of the fiber molecules themselves, as well as on the location of the fiber components within the food and how the food material is prepared or processed.

COMPONENTS OF DIETARY FIBER

The botanical categories of fiber are cellulose, hemicelluloses, pectic substances, gums, mucilages, algal polysaccharides, and lignin. With the exception of lignin (a polyphenol), all fibers are complex, nonstarch polysaccharides. They differ from each other in the sugar residues making up the polysaccharide and in the arrangement of the residues. The principal residues in fibers are glucose, galactose, mannose, and certain pentoses. A description of the structure and bonds found in various fiber types and other information about each of the carbohydrate components of dietary fiber is presented in Chapter 4 (see Table 4-2 and Figure 4-13). If animal foods or processed foods containing animal products are analyzed by standard methods for measuring dietary fiber, chitan, chitosans, and glycosaminoglycans will also be included as dietary fiber.

Cellulose

Cellulose is widely distributed in the plant kingdom and is the major component of dietary fiber. It is the most abundant carbohydrate structural material in nature and is the major component of most plant cell walls. It also is the only truly "fibrous" fiber. Cellulose is a polymer of glucose with a β(1,4) linkage between glucose molecules, a linkage that is not hydrolyzed by amylase or α-glucosidases.

Hemicelluloses

Hemicelluloses include a wide variety of branched heteropolysaccharides, which contain both pentoses and hexoses. Hemicelluloses tend to be relatively small polymers (50 to 200 saccharide units) and to have branches that usually consist of more than two sugars. Hemicelluloses include xyloglucans, glucuronoxylans, arabinoxylans, glucomannans, and galactomannans. Although these compounds are called hemicellulose, they are chemically unrelated to cellulose. The name most likely originated from the similarity in the solubility properties of hemicelluloses and cellulose. Both are insoluble in water and dilute acid; hemicelluloses, however, are more soluble in dilute alkali and also are more easily hydrolyzed by dilute acid than is cellulose.

Lignin

Lignin, the main noncarbohydrate component of dietary fiber, is formed by the polymerization of phenolic compounds during plant growth. Lignin is associated with the cellulose of plant cell walls, resulting in their strength and rigidity. When the lignin concentration is high, the plant tissues become lignified or woody. Lignin is very hydrophobic and resistant to enzymatic breakdown.

Beta-Glucans

Beta-glucans are linear unbranched polymers of β-D-glucose residues connected by mixed linkages. Oats and barley are rich cereal sources of beta-glucans with mixed β(1,3) and β(1,4) linkages. Beta-glucans from baker's yeast and some mushrooms (e.g., shiitake), on the other hand, contain mixed β(1,3) and β(1,6) linkages. The different linkages of glucose residues in the various beta-glucans have significant effects on the solubility and physiological activity of these fiber components. Beta-glucans from oats and barley are highly soluble, whereas those from yeast have a low viscosity and low solubility in water.

Pectins

Pectic substances, or pectins, are water-soluble polysaccharides found in the cell wall and in spaces between cells. The main chains are predominantly composed of galacturonic acid residues linked α(1,4) with some L-rhamnose residues linked α(1,2). The galacturonic acid residues are partially methylated, and the degree of methylation varies. Pectins contain short branches or side chains made up of various pentoses and hexoses and derivatized sugars. Pectins are the most widespread soluble dietary fiber in foods. They are isolated from apple pomace or citrus peels and are widely used as gelling agents, thickening agents, and stabilizers in foods.

Gums and Mucilages

The terms *gum* and *mucilage* are often used interchangeably. In some cases gums and mucilages are distinguished by their function or source in the plant. Gums are usually substances that are secreted in response to injury, as in the collection of gum arabic from cuts in the bark of acacia trees. Mucilages are cell wall components or reserve nonstarch polysaccharides that serve as an energy store for the plant or germinating seed. An example of a mucilage is psyllium, which comes from the seed coat of plantago seeds. Psyllium is obtained by mechanical milling of the outer layer of the seed and is often referred to as psyllium husk. It has a xylan backbone substituted with arabinose and some uronic acids. Psyllium is commonly used as a fiber supplement and laxative (stool softener and bulker).

In most cases the term *gum* is used generally to refer to all plant polysaccharides that can be hydrated. Water-soluble plant gums are widely used as thickening agents and emulsifiers. Examples of so-named gums are the soluble galactomannans (i.e., mannose polymers with galactose side chains) found in legume seeds. Two of these, guar gum and locust bean (karob) gum, are widely used in ice cream as stabilizers to prevent ice crystal growth. Although actually plant mucilages, these polysaccharides are often called gums. The term *mucilage* is sometimes used for plant polysaccharides that are highly soluble and yield solutions with reduced viscosity. Seed mucilages such as psyllium and flaxseed gums would be classified as mucilages by this second approach to naming as well as on the basis of their function in the plant. In general, gums can be thought of as tacky, whereas mucilages are slimy.

Algal Polysaccharides

Algal polysaccharides are extracted from algae and represent a diverse group of fibers. Like the plant gums and mucilages, many algal polysaccharides are used by the food industry as thickeners, binders, and emulsifiers. Carrageenans are a family of linear sulfated polysaccharides that are extracted from red algae. Carrageenans are made up of repeating sulfated and nonsulfated galactose and anhydrogalactose units joined by alternating α(1,3) and β(1,4) linkages. Agar is a mixture of agarose, a linear polymer of repeating units of D-galactose and 3,6-anhydro-L-galactose, with some sulfated residues, and a lesser amount of smaller molecules called agaropectins. Agar is extracted from red algae. Alginates are linear polymers of D-mannuronate and its C5 epimer, α-L-glucuronate, linked β(1,4); they are extracted from brown algae.

Inulin

Inulin or fructans are polymers of fructofuranose residues linked β(2,1) with predominantly linear chains, often with a terminal sucrose disaccharide unit. Fructans serve as storage polysaccharides in certain plants, especially members of the Compositae family, such as chicory and Jerusalem artichokes, which accumulate fructans in their roots and tubers, respectively. The most common industrial source of inulin is chicory, but wheat, onions, bananas, garlic, and leeks are more important dietary sources.

Chitin, Chitosan, and Glycosaminoglycans

Chitin is the second most abundant polysaccharide in nature after cellulose. Chitin is an unbranched polymer of *N*-acetyl-D-glucosamine residues linked β(1,4); some of the sugar residues are deacetylated. The mostly deacetylated form of chitin is called chitosan. Chitin is the principal component of the cell walls of fungi (mushrooms), the exoskeletons of arthropods (e.g., crustaceans and insects), the radulas of mollusks (e.g., snails), and the beaks of cephalopods (e.g., squid). Chitan is isolated from the shells of crabs, shrimp, and crawfish, and it is used as an additive to thicken and stabilize foods. Glycosaminoglycans (or mucopolysaccharides) are linear polysaccharide chains of repeating disaccharide units made up of hexose units linked in any combination of β(1,4), β(1,3), and α(1,4). Glycosaminoglycans include chondroitin sulfate, dermatan sulfate, heparan sulfate, heparin, and hyaluronan. They are rich in uronic acid and sulfated residues and thus are highly negatively charged. Most glycosaminoglycans are covalently linked to proteins, forming proteoglycans. Proteoglycans and hyaluronic acid are found in the cellular plasma membranes and extracellular matrices of tissues of higher animals.

Resistant Starch

Resistant starch is starch that is not digested and absorbed in the small intestine and thus passes into the large intestine, where it is a substrate for fermentation by the colonic bacteria. Starch may be resistant to the action of α-amylase because of physical inaccessibility, crystalline state, or chemical modifications and cross-linkages. The properties of resistant starch are described in Chapters 4 and 8.

PRIMARY STRUCTURE

The primary structure of fiber includes the number and sequence of monosaccharide residues in the backbone chain and side chains, any substituents on the monosaccharide residues, and the positions of the bonds linking the residues. The stereochemistry of the glycosidic bonds, as well as the particular sugar units involved in these linkages, affect structure and digestibility. Arrangement of the sugar residues in the polysaccharide is often very important to the physiological effects of the fiber. Branching and substitutions on the primary carbohydrate chain can be major determinants of physical properties. The degree of methoxylation or sulfation of certain fibers also affects the physiological properties of the fiber. For example, if the galacturonic acid residues in pectin are methoxylated, there are no anionic groups available for binding calcium or trapping water. This will not affect the gel-forming properties of pectin as long as there are sufficient unmethoxylated portions of the molecule to form the gel. However, if methoxylation is randomly distributed throughout the molecule, a significant impact on gel-forming ability can occur.

SECONDARY STRUCTURE

In addition to the primary structure of fiber, the molecule's secondary structure also can affect digestibility. For example, the α(1,4) glucose linkage in starch is readily cleaved by mammalian enzymes. However, modification of the same starch molecule to produce a different three-dimensional organization may render it resistant to human digestive enzymes. In other words, the packing or arrangement of the molecule can restrict access of enzymes to the bonds they normally hydrolyze. This is why starch can become "resistant" to enzymatic hydrolysis and act like dietary fiber. Thus, raw starches, such as raw potato and banana starch, and retrograded starch in cooked and cooled food products are resistant to pancreatic amylase and thus reach the colon relatively intact. This characteristic is the basis behind some arguments that resistant starch should be included in the definition of fiber.

PHYSICAL FACTORS

In addition to the chemistry of the fiber molecules themselves, where fiber components are located within the plant and whether fiber is extracted from the plant and then added to the diet or is eaten as part of the intact plant material may have significant physiological consequences. If the fiber is contained within an intact plant cell, the cell wall must first be disrupted for the physiological effects of the particular fibers to be exerted. Resistance to breakage of the cell wall depends on the structure of the cell wall and its degree of lignification. The number of plant cells per particle ingested (particle size) also may determine the accessibility of the cell wall to digestive enzymes (Slavin, 2003), as may cooking, processing, and mastication of the food (Bjorck et al., 1994).

PHYSIOLOGICAL CHARACTERIZATION OF DIETARY FIBER

Fibers are also categorized by their physiological effects. Dietary fiber has conventionally been categorized as soluble or insoluble because of analytical approaches as well as the belief that solubility of fiber was a good predictor of its physiological effects. Although all fibers hold water to some degree, the soluble fibers have a greater holding capacity and may form gels and viscous solutions. In general, the structural fibers (cellulose, lignin, and some hemicelluloses) are insoluble in water, nonviscous, and poorly fermentable and thus contribute to increased stool bulk. In contrast, the gel-forming fibers (gums, mucilages, beta-glucans, algal polysaccharides, most pectins, and the remaining hemicelluloses) are soluble in water, viscous, and fermentable. Of total dietary fiber intake, approximately 20% to 30% is water soluble and 70% to 80% is water insoluble (Marlett and Cheung, 1997).

Although these generalizations are useful, there are many exceptions to these generalizations. Insoluble fiber is also fermented to some extent, and soluble fiber may be nonviscous. Gum arabic, for example, is a soluble fiber that does not form a viscous solution. Furthermore, some fibers, such as psyllium and oat bran, have physiological benefits attributed to both soluble and insoluble fibers. In addition, the approach of assigning physiological properties to soluble or insoluble fiber does not facilitate the evaluation of the effects of the fiber provided by mixed diets. Thus classification of fiber by water solubility has fallen into disfavor. The current trend is to no longer characterize fibers based on solubility, but to characterize them based on their functionality, which depends more on viscosity and fermentability.

MAJOR PHYSIOLOGICAL EFFECTS OF FIBER AND STRUCTURE–FUNCTION RELATIONSHIPS

The role that fiber plays within the upper and lower gastrointestinal tract depends on the fiber's physical and chemical attributes. The following sections describe the various effects fibers may have within the gastrointestinal tract segments, as well as how the chemical nature of the fiber contributes to these results.

EFFECTS OF FIBER IN THE STOMACH AND SMALL INTESTINE

Effects of fiber in the upper gastrointestinal tract may include effects on gastric emptying, satiety, and absorption of nutrients from the small intestine.

Gastric Emptying and Satiety

The viscosity of polysaccharides and their ability to form gels in the stomach may slow gastric emptying. Therefore gel-forming fibers may further contribute to a feeling of satiety by maintaining a feeling of fullness for a longer period after a meal (IOM, 2002). In contrast, fibers that do not form gels, such as wheat bran and cellulose, have little effect on the rate at which the meal exits from the stomach.

One of the neurological pathways involved in satiety is the feeling of satiety or fullness that is produced by distention or physical fullness of the stomach. Because fibers are resistant to digestion in the stomach, the bulk they add to the diet produces a feeling of fullness. Therefore, even though caloric intake may be similar, distention resulting from an increased fiber intake leads to a greater feeling of satiety (French and Read, 1994). Fiber includes a wide range of compounds, and although fiber generally affects satiety, not all fibers are equally effective in changing satiety (Slavin and Green, 2007). Typically a large dose of fiber is required, such as 10 g or more in a serving of food (an amount not naturally occurring in a single serving of food). Viscous fibers, such as guar gum, oat bran, and psyllium, are generally more effective, although insoluble fibers, such as wheat bran and cellulose, also are known to alter satiety. Willis and associates (2009) compared the satiety response of different fibers by feeding subjects a low-fiber (1.6 g fiber) or one of four high-fiber (8.0 to 9.6 g fiber) muffins at breakfast. The high-fiber muffins contained corn bran, resistant starch, barley beta-glucans, or polydextrose. Muffins containing resistant starch and corn bran had the most positive impact on satiety, whereas muffins containing polydextrose had little effect compared to the low-fiber muffin.

Generally, whole foods that naturally contain fiber are satiating. Flood-Obbagy and Rolls (2008) compared the effect of fruit in different forms on energy intake and satiety at a meal. Results showed that eating an apple reduced lunch energy intake by 15% compared to control. Fullness ratings differed significantly after preload consumption, with apple being the most satiating, followed by applesauce, then apple juice, then the control food. The addition of a pectin fiber to the apple juice did not alter satiety. However, addition of other fibers to drinks has been shown to affect satiety. Pelkman and colleagues (2007) added low doses of a gelling pectin-alginate fiber to drinks and measured satiety. The drinks were consumed twice a day over 7 days, and energy intake at the evening meal was recorded. The 2.8 g dose of pectin alginate caused a 10% decrease in energy intake at the evening meal. Thus the results indicated that high-fiber foods are more satiating and that certain isolated fibers affect satiety whereas others do not. Clinical studies are needed to assess the effectiveness of isolated fibers on satiety, because there are no measures of fiber chemistry (solubility, structure, etc.) that can predict a fiber's effect on satiety.

Effects on Absorption from the Small Intestine

Polysaccharides that produce a viscous solution can delay and even interfere with the absorption of nutrients such as carbohydrates, lipids, and proteins from the small intestine. The reasons for this effect on absorption include delayed gastric emptying, entrapment of nutrients in the gel-like structure, interference with micelle formation, and decreased access of enzymes to the nutrients. Fiber-rich foods may also contain lipase inhibitors. In addition, the mixing of intestinal contents appears to be impeded by the presence of viscous polysaccharides.

Positive benefits of delayed nutrient absorption include an improvement of glucose tolerance and a lowering of serum cholesterol levels. Delayed absorption of carbohydrate results in a lower postprandial glucose level. In general, the more viscous the fiber, the greater the effect on blood glucose, although data on this topic are conflicting (Slavin, 2008). When glucose is absorbed in small amounts over an extended period, such as seen when a meal contains viscous fibers, the insulin response is theoretically attenuated (Pick et al., 1996). Because high amounts of glucose appear to trigger sustained insulin secretion, and because insulin secretion stimulates 3-hydroxy-3-methylglutaryl coenzyme A (HMG-CoA) reductase activity, high blood glucose concentrations promote cholesterol biosynthesis. Therefore fiber may also reduce plasma cholesterol levels via its effect on glucose tolerance. Because of the flattened glucose curves seen with ingestion of viscous fibers, these fibers are often recommended for diabetics, who typically have lipid profiles that indicate an elevated risk of cardiovascular disease, to give both better glucose tolerance and improved lipid profiles.

Certain viscous fibers have been shown to lower serum cholesterol both in laboratory animals and in humans. These fibers include guar gum, pectin, psyllium, and oat bran. Bean products also produce this effect. In contrast, wheat bran and cellulose do not lower plasma cholesterol. The mechanism by which fibers lower serum cholesterol appears to be multifactorial, or alternatively, different fibers may work by different mechanisms. The major hypotheses are summarized in Table 11-1. These hypotheses include the binding of bile acids to fiber, which then interferes with their enterohepatic recirculation. By this hypothesis, more bile acids are excreted in the feces, requiring additional synthesis of bile acids from cholesterol in the liver, thus lowering the body's cholesterol pool. Another possible consequence of the binding of bile acids to fiber is that they would be less available for emulsification and micelle formation, which in turn could interfere with the absorption of cholesterol and triacylglycerols.

TABLE 11-1 Possible Mechanisms by Which Fibers Lower Serum Cholesterol

MECHANISM	EFFECT
Delayed gastric emptying	Fiber affects the entrance of chyme into the small intestine. This in turn may affect the rate of carbohydrate and lipid absorption, which influences insulin secretion and lipoprotein formation.
Interference with digestive enzymes	Viscous fibers may sequester lipids, proteins, and carbohydrates from digestive enzymes, thereby impairing their absorption.
Interference with micelle formation	Fibers may bind to the bile acids or interfere with micelle formation, impairing the absorption of cholesterol, bile acids, and lipids.
Interference with mixing of intestinal contents	Fibers may interfere with micelle formation and with the ability of digestive enzymes to hydrolyze lipids, proteins, and starch.
Inhibition of cholesterol biosynthesis	Fermentation of fiber in the colon results in the production of propionate, a short-chain fatty acid. Once absorbed through the portal vein, this short-chain fatty acid is thought to inhibit HMG-CoA reductase activity, the rate-limiting enzyme for cholesterol biosynthesis.

Large amounts of dietary fiber may interfere with mineral bioavailability. Because the ionized groups on polysaccharides are usually negatively charged, the tendency of dietary fiber is to bind cations such as calcium, magnesium, sodium, and potassium. This may limit the absorption of these minerals from the small intestine. This is not generally considered a public health concern, but it may be pertinent in certain cases when individuals have very high-fiber diets and low intakes of minerals such as calcium and magnesium. Some data suggest that inulin can actually enhance absorption of calcium (Scholz-Ahrens et al., 2007). The practical concern that fiber intake may negatively impact mineral status in humans appears unwarranted.

EFFECTS OF FIBER IN THE LOWER INTESTINE

Effects of fiber in the large intestine include those due to the fermentation of fiber by the colonic microflora and those due to the increase in fecal bulk, including the dilution of harmful compounds. Dietary fiber also affects transit time through the lower gut.

Effects of Fiber Fermentation in the Large Intestine

Fiber is metabolized by the colonic microflora in an anaerobic process with the production of short-chain fatty acids, hydrogen, carbon dioxide, and biomass (Figure 11-1). Fiber may be fermented to different amounts and types of short-chain fatty acids (such as acetate, propionate, and butyrate), each of which has specific properties. Foods containing dietary fiber composed of hemicellulose, pectin, or resistant starch provide highly fermentable substrates, whereas those with a high cellulose content provide less fermentable substrates. Currently, there is no evidence that a relationship exists between the quantity of fiber consumed and its fermentability (IOM, 2002).

The short-chain fatty acids are the major carbon products of fermentation. Acetate is rapidly absorbed from the colonic lumen into the portal blood and then goes to the liver before entering the general circulation. Acetate is used as an energy source by most nonhepatic tissues in the body. Propionate, like acetate, is also rapidly absorbed and enters

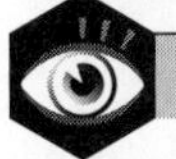

NUTRITION INSIGHT

Cholesterol Manipulation

Elevated serum cholesterol can be the result of both genetic and dietary problems. Many consumers would like to lower their serum cholesterol with foods. Different components of foods are known to lower serum cholesterol. These components include sterols, stanols, soluble fiber, soy products, and vegetable protein. Many mechanisms for how soluble fibers lower serum lipids have been suggested, including slowing nutrient absorption and trapping cholesterol and excreting it in feces. In addition, the short-chain fatty acid propionate may lower cholesterol levels. Clinical studies suggest that inclusion of soluble fibers such as oat bran, barley bran, and psyllium in the diet can reduce serum cholesterol as well as alter the lipoprotein profile.

Thinking Critically

1. What is the expected effect on serum cholesterol of including cellulose-containing foods in the diet?
2. What are some potential mechanisms by which a viscous, gel-forming fiber could reduce serum cholesterol?

the portal vein, by which it is transported to the liver. In contrast to acetate, however, propionate is used by the liver. Some studies show that propionate inhibits HMG-CoA reductase activity. Butyrate is unique in that it is the preferred energy source for colonocytes (epithelial cells lining the colon). Colonocytes metabolize butyrate to CO_2, which in part spares the use of glucose. Butyrate may also be incorporated into membrane lipids (Wong et al., 2008).

As a fiber is fermented to short-chain fatty acids, the pH of the luminal contents decreases. This is significant because many bacterial reactions are pH-sensitive. For example, the bacterial enzyme responsible for forming secondary bile acids from primary bile acids (7α-dehydroxylase) is inactivated below a pH of 6.5. Colonic contents often can reach this pH when fiber is being fermented.

Effects of Fiber on Dilution of Harmful Compounds and on Fecal Bulking

Different fibers have different bulking properties, depending on their degree of fermentation. Naturally, as a fiber is fermented, it is no longer available to contribute directly to fecal bulk. But fermentation can increase bacterial mass due to the growth and proliferation of bacteria when they are provided with fermentable substrates. The increase in bacterial mass also results in increased water retention and fecal weight. Compounds that may affect the colonocytes and are subject to dilution by dietary fibers and increased fecal volume include bile acids, diacylglycerols, long-chain fatty acids, and ammonia.

Colonic Epithelial Cell Proliferation, Differentiation, and Apoptosis

The cells lining the colon are only one epithelial cell deep. Unlike the case with the small intestine, no villi are found in the large intestine. Instead, the colonic mucosa consists of crypts that are depressions in an otherwise smooth surface epithelium. Cells are formed toward the base of the crypt and migrate upward, making several divisions in transit. A cell differentiates as it reaches the upper part of the crypt and eventually is exfoliated and excreted by way of the feces. This process takes from 3 to 30 days, depending on the location of the cell within the colon.

During the progression of normal healthy cells to colonic tumors, the normal controls on cell division are lost. Through a series of genetic changes, cells continue to divide as they migrate higher up the crypt, instead of differentiating. They may accumulate at the top of the crypt and form polyps, which then may become tumors. Tumors may invade down through the crypt and into the underlying muscle area. Because changes in colonic crypt cell proliferation precede

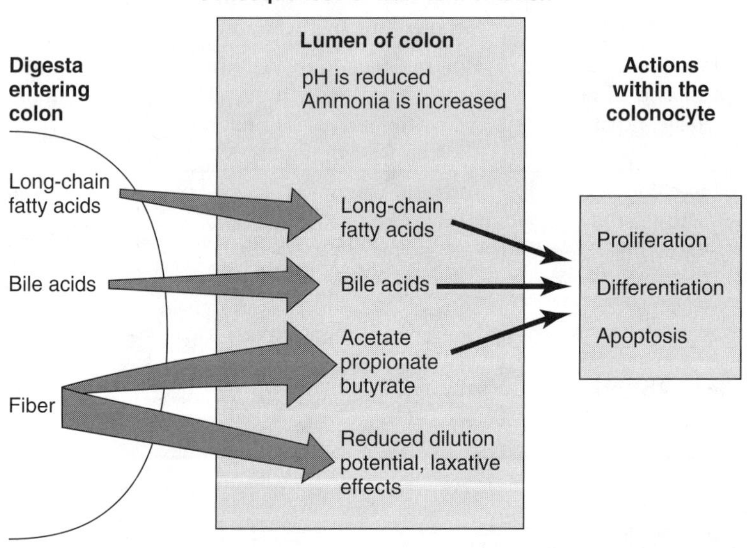

FIGURE 11-1 Intestinal contents entering the colon are fermented by bacteria, which increases the amount of short-chain fatty acids and reduces pH. As fiber is fermented, its mass is reduced as the fecal stream passes through the colon. Therefore, because the mass of fiber decreases while the mass of short-chain fatty acids increases, and the mass of bile acids and long-chain fatty acids remains the same but has less fiber with which to associate, the concentrations of short-chain fatty acids, as well as long-chain fatty acids and bile acids, increase in the fecal stream. Luminal pH and these molecules affect colonocyte proliferation, differentiation, and apoptosis. Absorption of these molecules can be concentration-dependent, making their concentration within the fecal milieu a key determinant of cell cycle activity.

CLINICAL CORRELATION

Ulcerative Colitis

Ulcerative colitis occurs predominantly in the distal colon (Chapman et al., 1994), a segment of the colon that is more dependent on butyrate oxidation as its metabolic fuel supply than is the proximal colon. In fact, Mortensen and Clausen (1996) proposed that ulcerative colitis is an energy-deficiency disease. The results of Scheppach and colleagues (1992) indicate that supplying butyrate by enemas containing short-chain fatty acids induces remission of colitis.

Thinking Critically

Patients receiving parenteral feeding for extended periods often develop ulcerative colitis. What would you recommend to alleviate this condition?

and accompany neoplasia, an upregulation of cell proliferation in the colon is considered an important marker for colon tumorigenesis. Other surrogate markers for colon cancer include a downregulation of cell differentiation and colon cell death (apoptosis) (Chang et al., 1997). Agents or dietary components that stimulate cells to divide are considered to promote cancer, because dividing cells are much more vulnerable to attack by carcinogens. In contrast, dietary factors that result in a more quiescent proliferative pattern or enhance differentiation or apoptosis are considered to protect against colon cancer. Dietary fiber is thought to decrease cell proliferation, although human data on this effect are lacking. High fiber intakes have been associated with a reduction in colon cancer incidence (Bingham et al., 2003).

Transit Time and Constipation

Colonic motility is the largest determinant of overall gastrointestinal transit times. The average emptying time of the stomach is 2 to 5 hours, and that of the small intestine is 3 to 6 hours; but the time required for residue from a particular meal to make its way through the lower portion of the gastrointestinal tract is much longer, on the order of 40 to 70 hours (Hillemeier, 1995). Dietary fiber has been described as "normalizing" total gut transit time to 1 to 3 days. In patients fed liquid diets, fast transit with resulting diarrhea is a clinical problem, and added fiber can improve fecal composition and slow transit. When transit time is prolonged, difficulty passing fecal matter is encountered, resulting in constipation. Fibers are effective in binding water and speeding transit and are the active ingredient in many laxative products (Slavin, 2008). Constipation is a persistent condition in which defecation is difficult or infrequent. Most cases of constipation are attributed to unknown causes, and many individuals can be effectively treated by increasing hydration, exercise, and fiber intake.

EFFECTS OF FIBER ON WHOLE-BODY ENERGY STATUS

Because fibers may be fermented to short-chain fatty acids, which can be absorbed from the colon and used for metabolism, the concept that dietary fiber contributes no energy is clearly wrong. However, assigning a caloric value to dietary fiber is difficult. The best estimate of energy generated by fiber fermentation in humans is 6.2 to 10.4 kJ/g (1.5 to 2.5 kcal/g) of fiber (IOM, 2002), compared with 16.7 kJ/g (4.0 kcal/g) for starch.

RECOMMENDATIONS FOR FIBER INTAKE AND TYPICAL INTAKES

In establishing the Dietary Reference Intakes (DRIs), the IOM (2002) recommended an Adequate Intake (AI) of 14 g of fiber for each 1,000 kcal of energy consumed for all individuals from 1 year of age throughout their lives. On the basis of median energy intakes, this equates to 25 g/day for women and 38 g/day for men ages 19 to 50 years. The AI was set at 21 g/day and 30 g/day, respectively, for women and men age 51 and older based on lower median energy intakes for older adults. There are no data suggesting that pregnant or lactating women would benefit from increased fiber intake; yet because energy intakes increase for these two groups, the recommended AIs are 28 g/day and 29 g/day for pregnant and lactating women, respectively.

Recommendations are not provided for infants younger than 1 year. An AI was not developed for this age group because milk, which contains no fiber, is the primary recommended food source through 6 months of age and there are no data on fiber intake in infants. AIs for children were based on median energy intakes and are similar for boys and girls through 8 years of age. Once children reach 9 years of age, variations in the average energy requirement between boys and girls are sufficient to justify differences in the recommended AIs.

Unfortunately, American women and men consume an average of only about 15 g of fiber per day, which is far short of the suggested AI levels (Slavin, 2008). However, it is possible to meet the recommended AI levels without drastically altering food choices (IOM, 2002). Many times, the limitation that prevents people from meeting these goals is that they do not know which foods provide desirable levels of dietary fiber. Food sources of fiber include whole grain products, legumes, vegetables, and dried fruits. A short list of foods is provided in the box, "Food Sources

CLINICAL CORRELATION

Short-Bowel Patients

Some diseases require the removal of segments of the small intestine, leaving patients with only a short segment of the bowel remaining, with or without a preserved colon. In many of these patients, only half the calories consumed are absorbed, making dietary manipulation critical if they are to consume enough food to prevent the need for parenteral nutritional support. In those patients with a functional colon, energy recovery through microbial fermentation can contribute significantly to total energy availability. Mortensen and Clausen (1996) noted that an increase in carbohydrate consumption from 20% to 60% of total caloric intake provided patients with an additional 465 kcal/day, which was about 30% of the total energy absorbed. Unfortunately, there was no additional energy availability with similar diet modifications in patients without a functional colon.

Thinking Critically

What types or sources of fiber would you suggest that short-bowel patients with a functional colon include in their diet? Why?

DRIs Across the Life Cycle: Dietary Fiber

	Adequate Intakes (AIs), g Dietary Fiber per Day
Infants	
0 through 12 mo	(none set)
Children	
1 through 3 yr	19
4 through 8 yr	25
Males	
9 through 13 yr	31
14 through 18 yr	38
19 through 50 yr	38
≥51 yr	30
Females	
9 through 18 yr	26
19 through 50 yr	25
≥51 yr	21
Pregnant	28
Lactating	29

Data from IOM. (2002) Dietary, functional, and total fiber. In *Dietary Reference Intakes for energy, carbohydrate, fiber, fat, fatty acids, cholesterol, protein, and amino acids.* Washington, DC: The National Academies Press.

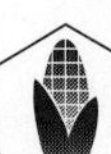

FOOD SOURCES OF TOTAL DIETARY FIBER

Breads and Grains
1.4 g per 1 piece cornbread
2.1 g per 1 slice pumpernickel bread
0.6 g per 1 slice white bread
1.9 g per 1 slice whole wheat bread
1.7 g per ½ cup brown rice
0.3 g per ½ cup white rice

Cereals
8.8 g per ½ cup Kellogg's All Bran Original
1.0 g per 1 cup Kellogg's Product 19
7.3 g per 1 cup Kellogg's Raisin Bran
3.3 g per 1 cup General Mills Wheat Chex
0.3 g per 1 ¼ cups General Mills Rice Chex
5.5 g per 2 biscuits shredded wheat
4.0 g per 1 cup oatmeal

Fruits
3.3 g per 1 apple, with skin
3.7 g per 2 figs, dried, uncooked
3.1 g per 1 orange
3.0 g per 5 prunes, dried, uncooked
4.0 g per ½ cup raspberries

Vegetables and Legumes
1.1 g per ½ cup broccoli, raw
1.2 g per ½ cup cauliflower, raw
1.2 g per ½ cup corn, sweet, yellow
5.6 g per ½ cup cowpeas, common, cooked
0.35 g per ½ cup iceberg lettuce, raw
6.6 g per ½ cup kidney beans
4.4 g per ½ cup green peas, young
7.7 g per ½ cup pinto beans
2.3 g per 1 potato, baked, with flesh
1.25 g per ½ cup yellow squash, cooked

Data from USDA, ARS. (2011). *USDA National Nutrient Database for Standard Reference, Release 24.* Retrieved from http://www.ars.usda.gov/ba/bhnrc/ndl

of Total Dietary Fiber," to demonstrate differences in fiber contents of similar types of foods. To acquire more information, readers should refer to the U.S. Department of Agriculture (USDA), Agricultural Research Service (ARS) National Nutrient Database for Standard Reference, Release 24 (USDA, ARS, 2011), which provides the dietary fiber content of most foods commonly consumed in the United States. The major sources of dietary fiber in the typical American diet are white flour and potatoes, not because they are concentrated fiber sources but because they are widely consumed (Slavin, 2008).

DIETARY FIBER INTAKE AND DISEASE

The incidences of heart disease, colon cancer, and obesity in populations consuming a Western diet are typically much higher than those observed in most developing countries. This is partly because of lower intake of fiber-rich foods. As described previously, the presence of fiber in the diet can have a considerable impact on many diseases and appears to promote a healthier gastrointestinal tract. Therefore all people should strive to include a variety of fiber-rich foods in their diets to prevent disease onset and to at least minimize the severity of disease once it has developed.

LIMITATIONS OF EXISTING KNOWLEDGE OF FIBER AND HEALTH

Many difficulties are associated with the study of fiber intake and health and with interpretation of the results of published studies. The major problem is that of defining what type of fiber is being consumed and then adequately describing how much is being consumed and how much is utilized within the intestinal tract. In addition, it is difficult to separate the effect of a change in dietary fiber from the accompanying changes in nutrient density and nutrient intake that accompany the addition of fiber sources to the diet. Comparisons of high-fiber versus low-fiber diets usually indicate an alteration in the caloric density of the diet that often results in a lower intake of energy sources and other nutrients unless the bulk quantity of diet consumed is increased. In addition, a high-fiber diet may imply the intake of additional biologically active compounds such as phytochemicals that are not present in the low-fiber diet. For studies of the effects of fiber per se, experimental diets should be designed to contain the same amount of all nutrients and nonnutrient compounds other than the fiber sources chosen for comparison. The simplest design involves use of purified fiber sources, but purified fiber sources may not have the same effect as intact food sources. Therefore much more research will be required under tightly controlled protocols before the real value of dietary fiber can be fully evaluated.

DIETARY FIBER AND CARDIOVASCULAR DISEASE

The American Dietetic Association (ADA) published a position paper on the findings of the ADA Evidence Analysis Library systematic review on the health implications of dietary fiber (Slavin, 2008). This review found fair evidence that dietary fiber from whole foods may lower blood pressure, improve serum lipids, and reduce inflammation. More recent work also supports this conclusion (Flint et al., 2009; Ruottinen et al., 2010). Other recent studies reported a range of cardiovascular benefits associated with dietary fiber. De Moura and associates (2009) evaluated the effect of applying the FDA definition of whole grains to the strength of scientific evidence that supports whole grain health claims for cardiovascular disease (CVD) risk reduction. They concluded that when studies of individual whole grains (barley, oats, or rye) that did not explicitly define whole grains in the manuscript were considered together with studies that added bran and germ with whole grains, there was sufficient evidence for a CVD-related health claim.

DIETARY FIBER AND OBESITY PREVENTION

The position paper of the ADA on the health implications of dietary fiber represents a systematic review of evidence (Slavin, 2008), which led to the conclusion that dietary fiber from whole foods provides bulk, promotes satiety, and may lead to weight loss. Three recent prospective studies and two cross-sectional studies provide additional support for the role of dietary fiber in obesity prevention. Du and associates (2010) found that total fiber and cereal fiber were inversely associated with subsequent increases in weight and waist circumference. Fruit and vegetable fiber was also inversely associated with waist circumference change, but not with weight change. In a prospective cohort study, Tucker and Thomas (2009) found that weight decreased by 0.25 kg and percent body fat decreased by 0.25% for each 1 gram increase in total fiber consumed.

DIETARY FIBER AND TYPE 2 DIABETES

The ADA position paper on the health implications of dietary fiber concluded that limited evidence suggested that "diets providing 30 to 50 g fiber per day from whole food sources consistently produce lower serum glucose levels compared to a low fiber diet" (Slavin, 2008). Hopping and colleagues (2010) examined the association between dietary fiber and type 2 diabetes in a large multiethnic cohort in Hawaii over a 14-year period. Both men and women in the top quintile of dietary fiber intake from grains had a 10% reduction in diabetes risk; whereas men, but not women, in the highest quintile of fiber intake from vegetables had a 22% reduction in diabetes risk.

DIETARY FIBER AND BOWEL HEALTH

In developed countries, chronic constipation is a common disorder for adults and children. Dietary fiber from whole foods increases stool weight and improves transit time, thereby reducing constipation. The ADA systematic review of the health implications of dietary fiber concluded that there was a lack of data examining the impact of fiber from whole foods on outcomes in gastrointestinal diseases. This may be due to the complexity and cost of these studies (Slavin, 2008).

DIETARY FIBER AND MICROBIOTA

Evidence that the intestinal microbiota is linked with overall health is emerging (Davis and Milner, 2009). The adult human gut contains 100 trillion microbial organisms, which are referred to as the microbiota. Although the importance of the microbiota has been accepted for diseases of the large intestine, it is now thought that the microbiota may play a role in obesity and other chronic diseases.

Prebiotics are defined as "a non-digestible food ingredient that beneficially affects the host by selectively stimulating the growth and/or activity of one or a limited number of bacteria in the colon, and thus improves host health" (De Vrese and Schrezenmeir, 2008). Readily fermentable oligosaccharides such as fructooligosaccharides and galactooligosaccharides are generally accepted as prebiotics and are often added to infant formula and other food products.

Probiotics are defined viable microorganisms, sufficient amounts of which reach the intestine in an active state and thus exert positive health effects (De Vrese and Schrezenmeir, 2008). Synbiotics are combinations of both probiotics and prebiotics. The idea of using probiotics to suppress and displace harmful bacteria has been around for more than a century. In 1906 Henry Tissier of the Pasteur Institute recommended the administration of bifidobacteria to infants suffering from diarrhea, claiming that bifidobacteria would supersede the putrefactive bacteria causing the disease. He showed that bifidobacteria were predominant in the gut of breast-fed infants, and encouraging the growth of bifidobacteria was the rationale for adding prebiotics to infant formula. Displacement of harmful bacteria in the intestine by the orally administered "beneficial" ones may improve microbial balance and health.

Recommended intakes of dietary fiber can provide prebiotics to the diet. Also, by observing guidelines for dairy food consumption and choosing yogurt or other fermented dairy products, probiotics will be included in the diet.

Some of the proposed health benefits of prebiotics and probiotics include reduction in diarrhea incidence, improvements in gut health, elimination of allergies, and prevention of infections. It is accepted that the gut microflora have a potential role in immune function, but studies showing an improvement in immunity with consumption of either prebiotics or probiotics are limited. Despite the continued interest in enhancing the gut environment, there are no cohort studies in which fecal samples have been collected and higher levels of bifidobacteria or lactobacillus in the feces linked to improved health status.

A systematic review of randomized controlled trials evaluating the relationship between probiotics and constipation concluded that until more data are available, the use of probiotics for the treatment of constipation should be considered investigational (Chmielewska and Szajerska, 2010). Probiotics may play a role in preventing and treating acute diarrhea in both children and adults, although results are inconsistent (Cummings, 2009). A systematic review and meta-analysis of probiotics in the treatment of irritable bowel syndrome found that probiotics could potentially play a role in irritable bowel syndrome treatment, but results of trials are inconsistent and many questions remain on the type of probiotics, dose, and whether certain subgroups of patients are more likely to benefit from probiotics (Hoveyda et al., 2009).

A review of studies of the effects of prebiotics on immune function, infection, and inflammation showed mixed results (Lomax and Calder, 2009a). Ten trials involving infants and children mostly reported benefits on infectious outcomes, whereas in 15 adult trials, little effect was seen. A similar review of the literature was conducted on studies of probiotic administration (Lomax and Calder, 2009b). Overall, the data for effects of probiotics have been mixed, with large species and strain differences in the results.

THINKING CRITICALLY

Dietary fiber consists of a number of different groups of compounds, with each group also consisting of a variety of different individual polymers. One group of compounds is called pectins or pectic substances.

1. Where in the plant would you expect to find pectins?
2. Give a general description of the chemical structure of pectins.
3. Describe three types of physiological effects (e.g., delayed gastric emptying) that pectins may have and explain, if possible, the physical or chemical characteristics of the fiber that permit or facilitate each physiological effect.

REFERENCES

Association of Official Analytical Chemists. (2007). In W. Horwitz, & G. Latimer Jr. (Eds.), *Official methods of analysis* (18th ed., Rev. 2). Gaithersburg, MD: AOAC International.

Bingham, S. A., Day, N. E., Luben, R., Ferrari, P., Slimani, N., Norat, T., … European Prospective Investigation into Cancer and Nutrition. (2003). Dietary fibre in food and protection against colorectal cancer in the European Prospective Investigation into Cancer and Nutrition (EPIC): An observational study. *Lancet, 361*, 1496–1501.

Bjorck, I., Granfeldt, Y., Liljeberg, H., Tovar, J., & Asp, N. G. (1994). Food properties affecting the digestion and absorption of carbohydrates. *The American Journal of Clinical Nutrition, 59*, 699S–705S.

Chang, W. C. Chapkin, R. S., & Lupton, J. R. (1997). Predictive value of proliferation, differentiation and apoptosis as intermediate markers for colon tumorigenesis. *Carcinogenesis, 18*, 721–730.

Chapman, M. A., Grahn, M. F., Boyle, M. A., Hutton, M., Rogers, J., & Williams, N. S. (1994). Butyrate oxidation is impaired in the colonic mucosa of sufferers of quiescent ulcerative colitis. *Gut, 35*, 73–76.

Chmielewska, A., & Szajerska, H. (2010). Systematic review of randomized controlled trials: Probiotics for functional constipation. *World Journal of Gastroenterology, 16*, 69–75.

Codex Alimentarius Commission. (2009). *Joint FAO/WHO Food Standards Programme (2009) 32nd session: Report of the 30th session of the Codex Committee on Nutrition and Foods for Special Dietary Uses (CCNFSDU).* (ALINORM 09/32/26) Retrieved from ftp://ftp.fao.org/codex/Circular_letters/CXCL2008/cl08_35e.pdf

Cummings, J. H. (2009). Probiotics: Better health from "good" bacteria. *Nutrition Bulletin, 34*, 198–202.

Davis, C. D., & Milner, J. A. (2009). Gastrointestinal microflora, food components and colon cancer prevention. *The Journal of Nutritional Biochemistry, 20*, 743–752.

De Moura, F. F., Lewis, K. D., & Falk, M. C. (2009). Applying the FDA definition of whole grains to the evidence for cardiovascular disease health claims. *The Journal of Nutrition, 139*, 2220S–2226S.

De Vrese, M., & Schrezenmeir, J. (2008). Probiotics, prebiotics, and synbiotics. *Advances in Biochemical Engineering/Biotechnology, 111*, 1–66.

Du, H., van der A, D. L., Boshuizen, H. C., Forouhi, N. G., Wareman, N. J., Halkjar, J., … Feskens, E. J. M. (2010). Dietary fiber and subsequent changes in body weight and waist circumference in European men and women. *The American Journal of Clinical Nutrition, 91*, 329–336.

Flint, A. J., Hu, F. B., Glyn, R. J., Jensen, M. K., Franz, M., Sampson, L., & Rimm, E. B. (2009). Whole grains and incident hypertension in man. *The American Journal of Clinical Nutrition, 90*, 493–498.

Flood-Obbagy, J. E., & Rolls, B. J. (2008). The effect of fruit in different forms on energy intake and satiety at a meal. *Appetite, 52*, 416–422.

French, S. J., & Read, N. W. (1994). Effect of guar gum on hunger and satiety after meals of differing fat content: Relationship with gastric emptying. *The American Journal of Clinical Nutrition, 59*, 87–91.

Health and Welfare Canada. (1985). *Report of the Expert Advisory Committee on Dietary Fibre.* Ottawa, ON: Minister of Supply and Services Canada.

Hillemeier, C. (1995). An overview of the effects of dietary fiber on gastrointestinal transit. *Pediatrics, 96*, 997–999.

Hopping, B. N., Erber, E., Grandinetti, A., Verheus, M., Kolonel, L. N., & Maskarinec, G. (2010). Dietary fiber, magnesium, and glycemic load alter risk of type 2 diabetes in a multiethnic cohort in Hawaii. *The Journal of Nutrition, 140*, 68–74.

Hoveyda, N., Heneghan, C., Mahtani, K. R., Perera, R., Roberts, N., & Glasziou, P. (2009). A systematic review and meta-analysis: Probiotics in the treatment of irritable bowel syndrome. *BMC Gastroenterology, 9*, 15.

Institute of Medicine. (2001). *Dietary Reference Intakes: Proposed definition of dietary fiber.* Washington, DC: National Academy Press.

Institute of Medicine. (2002). Dietary, functional, and total fiber. In *Dietary Reference Intakes for energy, carbohydrate, fiber, fat, fatty acids, cholesterol, protein, and amino acids* (pp. 7-1–7-69). Washington, DC: The National Academies Press.

Lomax, A. R., & Calder, P. C. (2009a). Probiotics, immune function, infection and inflammation: A review of the evidence from studies conducted in humans. *Current Pharmaceutical Design, 15*, 1428–1516.

Lomax, A. R., & Calder, P. C. (2009b). Prebiotics, immune function, infection and inflammation: A review of the evidence. *The British Journal of Nutrition, 101*, 633–638.

Marlett, J. A., & Cheung, T. F., (1997). Database and quick methods of assessing typical dietary fiber intakes using data for 228 commonly consumed foods. *Journal of the American Dietetic Association, 97*, 39–48.

Mortensen, P. B., & Clausen, M. R. (1996). Short-chain fatty acids in the human colon: Relation to gastrointestinal health and disease. *Scandinavian Journal of Gastroenterology, 31*(Suppl. 216), 132–148.

Pelkman, C. I., Navia, J. L., Miller, A. E., & Pohle, R. J. (2007). Novel calcium-gelled pectin beverage reduced energy intake in non-reducing overweight and obese women: Interaction with dietary restraint status. *The American Journal of Clinical Nutrition, 86*, 1595–1602.

Pick, M. E., Hawrysh, Z. J., Gee, M. I., Toth, E., Garg, M. L., & Hardin, R. T. (1996). Oat bran concentrate bread products improve long-term control of diabetes: A pilot study. *Journal of the American Dietetic Association, 96*, 1254–1261.

Pilch, S. (1987). *Physiological effects and health consequences of dietary fiber*. Bethesda, MD: Life Sciences Research Office, Federation of American Societies for Experimental Biology.

Ruottinen, S., Lagstrom, H. K., Niinikoski, H., Ronnemaa, T., Saarinen, M., Pahtala, K. A., … Simell, O. (2010). Dietary fiber does not displace energy but is associated with decreased serum cholesterol concentrations in healthy children. *The American Journal of Clinical Nutrition, 91*, 651–661.

Scheppach, W., Sommer, H., Kirchner, T., Paganelli, G. M., Bartram, P., Christl, S., … Kasper, H. (1992). Effect of butyrate enemas on the colonic mucosa in distal ulcerative colitis. *Gastroenterology, 70*, 211–215.

Scholz-Ahrens, K. E., Ada, P., Marten, B., Weber, P., Timm, W., Acil, Y., … Schrezenmeir, J. (2007). Prebiotics, probiotics, and synbiotics affect mineral absorption, bone mineral content, and bone structure. *The Journal of Nutrition, 137*, 838S–846S.

Slavin, J. (2003). Why whole grains are protective: Biological mechanisms. *The Proceedings of the Nutrition Society, 62*, 129–134.

Slavin, J., & Green, H. (2007). Dietary fibre and satiety. *Nutrition Bulletin, 32*(Suppl. 1), 32–42.

Slavin, J. L. (2008). Position of the American Dietetic Association: Health implications of dietary fiber. *Journal of the American Dietetic Association, 108*, 1716–1731.

Southgate, D. A. (1969). Determination of carbohydrates in foods. II. Unavailable carbohydrates. *Journal of the Science of Food and Agriculture, 20*, 331–335.

Trowell, H. (1978). The development of the concept of dietary fiber. *The American Journal of Clinical Nutrition, 31*, S3–S11.

Tucker, L. A., & Thomas, K. S. (2009). Increasing total fiber intake reduces risk of weight and fat gains in women. *The Journal of Nutrition, 139*, 576–581.

U.S. Department of Agriculture, Agricultural Research Service. (2011). USDA National Nutrient Database for Standard Reference, Release 24. Retrieved from http://www.ars.usda.gov/ba/bhnrc/ndl

Willis, H. J., Eldridge, A. L., Beiseigel, J., Thomas, W., & Slavin, J. L. (2009). Greater satiety response with resistant starch and corn bran in human subjects. *Nutrition Research, 29*, 100–105.

Wong, J. M., de Souza, R., Kendall, C. W., Eman, A., & Jenkins, D. J. (2008). Colonic health: Fermentation and short chain fatty acids. *Journal of Clinical Gastroenterology, 40*, 235–243.

RECOMMENDED READINGS

Institute of Medicine. (2001). *Dietary Reference Intakes: Proposed definition of dietary fiber*. Washington, DC: National Academy Press.

Institute of Medicine. (2002). Dietary, functional, and total fiber. In *Dietary Reference Intakes for energy, carbohydrate, fiber, fat, fatty acids, cholesterol, protein, and amino acids* (pp. 7-1–7-69). Washington, DC: The National Academies Press.

UNIT IV

Metabolism of the Macronutrients

After the products of digestion are absorbed across the intestinal epithelium and enter the circulation, they are delivered to various tissues for use. The metabolism of the macronutrients by different tissues of the body is the subject of this unit. Metabolism is a term used to describe the sum of the processes by which a particular substance is handled by the living body; this includes the chemical changes occurring in cells by which energy is provided for vital processes and activities and the processes by which the body assimilates new tissue. The metabolic processes involved in the synthesis of macromolecules such as proteins, glycogen, various lipids, and nucleic acids are called anabolic pathways or anabolism. The metabolic processes involved in the breakdown of organic compounds to CO_2 and H_2O with release of energy (which may be captured as reducing equivalents or as nucleotide triphosphate bonds) are described as catabolic pathways or catabolism. Other pathways that connect anabolism and catabolism are described as amphibolic pathways; these include pathways that serve both catabolic and anabolic purposes, such as the citric acid cycle and oxidative phosphorylation.

Nutrients are needed for the formation of the structural and functional components of tissues. Proteins, phospholipids, cholesterol, glycosaminoglycans, and nucleic acids are important structural components of cell membranes, cellular organelles, and connective tissues. In addition to these obviously structural components of the body, numerous proteins and small, nonprotein organic molecules are distributed in the body fluids, including the intracellular fluid, extracellular fluid, and plasma. These tissue components have important functions and also are essential. All these body components must increase during growth, reproduction, and repair of injured tissues. In addition, the body must have nutrients for maintenance—for replacement of constituents lost during the normal processes of metabolism and tissue remodeling. The chemical components of the human body are not static but are all in a state of constant turnover (breakdown or catabolism followed by resynthesis or anabolism). For example, proteins are broken down and resynthesized, and in the process some of the amino acids are oxidized and must be replaced via the dietary supply. Small amounts of nutrients, as well as degradation products from nutrient utilization in the body, are lost from the body in the urine or via secretion in the bile and excretion in the feces. Thus the body requires nutrients for the formation of new tissues and for the replacement or maintenance of existing ones. The processes involved in the synthesis of glycogen, glycosaminoglycans, lipids, proteins, and nonprotein, nitrogen-containing compounds are discussed in this unit.

The body, of course, must have a source of energy, and dietary macronutrients serve this purpose. Cells within the body are able to use glucose, fatty acids, ketone bodies (derived from fatty acids, especially during starvation), amino acids, and other gluconeogenic (and ketogenic) precursors, such as glycerol, lactate, and propionate, as cellular fuels. Energy substrates that are taken in beyond the amount the body is able to consume immediately are converted to glycogen or fat for storage. The body's capacity for storage of glycogen is very limited. Triacylglycerol storage in adipose tissue is the major way in which animals and humans store energy, and the body's capacity for this is very large, perhaps unlimited. Therefore the body uses macronutrients in the diet as fuels and converts excess substrates to stored fuels, mainly triacylglycerol, which can be broken down when exogenous fuels are not available. These stored fuels serve an important function in providing fuels between meals and during strenuous exercise, in protecting lean body mass from immediate catabolism in the absence of food, and in extending the length of time an individual can survive with an inadequate caloric intake. The processes involved in the storage and utilization of fuels are described in this unit.

The intake of energy from carbohydrates, proteins, and fats from the diet should balance the overall needs of the body for energy and growth. Although carbohydrates, proteins, and lipids are all important components of the diet, specific compounds within these classes may be classified as essential or nonessential components, depending upon whether the body is able to synthesize them. Even for compounds that the body is able to synthesize, the body may not be able to synthesize them in sufficient amounts. For example, although carbohydrates make up a large proportion of healthy diets, the actual minimum requirement for carbohydrate per se is probably quite low. Certain cells or tissues of the body do have an absolute requirement for glucose as a fuel, but the liver is able to synthesize glucose from other sugars and from gluconeogenic substrates such as the carbon chains of amino acids or the glycerol backbone of triacylglycerols. Likewise, the body is able to synthesize the other various sugar units required for glycoprotein, glycosaminoglycan, and nucleic acid synthesis. We could say that the diet must provide either a source of glucose or a source of gluconeogenic substrate.

Protein is required in ample amounts because it serves as the source of indispensable amino acids and as a source of available nitrogen for synthesis of proteins and numerous other essential compounds, including purine and pyrimidine bases of nucleic acids, neurotransmitters, hormones such as thyroid hormone and epinephrine, creatine phosphate, carnitine, porphyrins, 1-carbon fragments of the folate coenzyme system, and small peptides such as glutathione and carnosine. Eleven of the 20 amino acids commonly found in proteins are considered indispensable or semi-indispensable for humans. Although the nine so-called nonessential or dispensable amino acids are not strictly indispensable, because the body can synthesize their carbon chains from intermediates in glucose metabolism or from other amino acids, the diet still must contain a sufficient total amount of amino acids to supply amino groups for synthesis of all the dispensable amino acids.

Dietary fat is not essential as a fuel because the body can convert carbon chains of amino acids or sugars into fatty acids and glycerol phosphate and hence triacyglycerol and other lipids. However, certain fatty acids cannot be synthesized completely in the body. The body requires an exogenous source of the polyunsaturated fatty acids; fatty acids in both the n-6 (e.g., linoleate) and the n-3 (e.g., linolenate, docosahexaenoic acid) classes must be provided by the diet. These polyunsaturated fatty acids play important structural roles in membrane phospholipids and skin ceramides and serve as precursors for synthesis of eicosanoids.

MAJOR METABOLIC PATHWAYS FOR MACRONUTRIENT METABOLISM

Glycolysis: Glucose → Pyruvate (or Lactate)
Gluconeogenesis: Lactate/Amino acids/Glycerol → Glucose
Pentose phosphate pathway: Glucose → 5-C sugars → 6-C and 3-C sugars
Glycogenolysis: Glycogen → Glucose-P or Glucose
Glycogenesis: Glucose or Glucose-P → Glycogen
Pyruvate dehydrogenase complex: Pyruvate → Acetyl-CoA
Citric acid cycle: Acetyl-CoA → 2 CO_2
Protein synthesis: Amino acids → Protein
Protein degradation: Protein → Amino acids
Amino acid catabolism: Amino acids → CO_2 + H_2O + urea or ammonia
Fatty acid synthesis: Acetyl-CoA → Palmitate
β-Oxidation: Fatty acyl-CoA → Acetyl-CoA
Triacylglycerol synthesis: Fatty acyl-CoAs + Glycerol 3-P → Triacylglycerol
Lipolysis: Triacylglycerol → Fatty acids + Glycerol
Ketogenesis: Acetyl-CoA → Acetoacetate
Ketone body oxidation: Acetoacetate → Acetyl-CoA
CoA, Coenzyme A; *P*, $-HPO_3^-$

CHAPTER 12

Carbohydrate Metabolism: Synthesis and Oxidation

Mary M. McGrane, PhD

COMMON ABBREVIATIONS

AMPK adenosine monophosphate (AMP)-activated protein kinase
ChREBP carbohydrate response element binding protein
CoA coenzyme A
F2,6P2 fructose 2,6-bisphosphate
GLUT glucose transporter
GSK3 glycogen synthase kinase 3
IRS insulin receptor substrate
P_i inorganic phosphate, HPO_4^{2-}
6PF2K/F2,6Pase bifunctional enzyme, 6-phosphofructo-2-kinase/fructose-2,6-biphosphatase
PKA protein kinase A (cAMP-activated protein kinase)
PtdIns 3-kinase phosphatidylinositol 3-kinase
SGLT sodium/glucose cotransporter

Carbohydrates present in food provide an average of 50% (range of about 32% to 70%) of the energy in the American diet, and the recommended intake range, or Acceptable Macronutrient Distribution Range (AMDR), is 45% to 65% of calories (Institute of Medicine [IOM], 2002). Carbohydrates, consumed as disaccharides, oligosaccharides, and polysaccharides, are digested, absorbed, and transported through the body primarily as glucose, although fructose and galactose are present as well. Glucose is the primary metabolic fuel in humans in the postprandial state due to the abundance of carbohydrate in the diet, the capacity of all tissues to catabolize it, and the limited capacity for glucose storage in the body.

Some specialized cell types such as red blood cells are completely dependent on glucose for their energy needs, and it is critical for the body to maintain a glucose supply for these tissues. To maintain blood glucose within its strictly regulated concentration range (4 to 6 mmol/L) during periods in which glucose is not being absorbed from the gastrointestinal tract, the body is able to produce glucose by breakdown of body glycogen stores and by endogenous biosynthesis of glucose from nonhexose precursors. The balance among glucose oxidation, glucose biosynthesis, and glucose storage is dependent upon the hormonal and nutritional state of the cell, the tissue, and the whole organism.

Aspects of carbohydrate metabolism considered in this chapter include glucose transport, catabolism of glucose by glycolysis to pyruvate, the oxidative decarboxylation of pyruvate to acetyl-CoA by the pyruvate dehydrogenase complex, the further metabolism of acetyl-CoA by the citric acid cycle, glucose production by gluconeogenesis, glycogen metabolism, and more specialized pathways such as the pentose phosphate pathway and oligosaccharide chain synthesis. Some processes occurs in all cells, whereas others predominantly occur in specific tissues.

OVERVIEW OF TISSUE-SPECIFIC GLUCOSE METABOLISM

Tissue-specific differences in the pathways of glucose oxidation, glucose storage, glucose biosynthesis, and the utilization of glucose for the synthesis of other biomolecules are summarized in Figure 12-1 for liver, muscle, brain, and red blood cells. Pathways in the various tissues are coordinated to meet the metabolic challenges of the whole body.

LIVER

The liver plays the central role in glucose homeostasis in the body, because it can both remove and produce blood glucose. In liver parenchymal cells (hepatocytes), glucose can be oxidized for energy, stored as glycogen, or partially catabolized to provide carbons for the biosynthesis of fatty acids or amino acids. When glucose supply is low, the liver can produce glucose by glycogen degradation or by de novo synthesis and release this glucose into the bloodstream. The liver plays an important role in cycling carbon from glycolysis in muscle or other tissues back to glucose by taking up lactate, pyruvate, and alanine and using these carbon chains for gluconeogenesis. The hepatocyte also has the ability to utilize glucose for NADPH and ribose 5-phosphate production via the pentose phosphate pathway. Production of NADPH by the pentose phosphate pathway provides a necessary source of energy for synthesis of fatty acids and cholesterol from glucose. Other tissues, such as adipose tissue, skeletal and cardiac muscle, and brain, respond to blood glucose changes by altering their internal usage, but they do not contribute to whole-body glucose homeostasis by releasing glucose to the blood as the liver does.

MUSCLE

In skeletal muscle and heart, glucose can be completely oxidized or it can be stored in the form of glycogen. Although glycogen is degraded in muscle and cardiac cells, the glucose 6-phosphate produced is oxidized without leaving the cell. Glucose is not released to the circulating blood from either skeletal or cardiac muscle.

The metabolic needs of cardiac tissue differ from those of skeletal tissue. The heart has a continuous need for energy to conduct regular contractions, and glucose metabolism in cardiac tissue is aerobic at all times. In contrast, skeletal muscle can function metabolically with insufficient oxygen, or anaerobically, for limited periods. When functioning anaerobically or partially anaerobically, skeletal muscle converts glucose to lactate and releases it into the bloodstream.

ADIPOSE TISSUE

Adipose tissue presents another metabolic paradigm. In adipose cells, glucose can be partially degraded by glycolysis to provide glycerol for triacylglycerol synthesis. It can also be completely oxidized for energy. Under conditions of high carbohydrate intake, the acetyl-CoA produced during glucose oxidation can be channeled to de novo fatty acid synthesis for storage of fat. In humans, however, liver is much more active in de novo fatty acid synthesis than is adipose tissue. Under conditions of energy need, adipose cells release metabolic fuel in the form of free fatty acids to the circulating blood supply. Additionally, under these conditions, adipocytes conduct an abbreviated gluconeogenesis, referred to as glyceroneogenesis, to produce glycerol for triacylglycerol synthesis. This allows fine-tuned regulation of free fatty acid release because some free fatty acids from lipolysis are reesterified to triacylglycerols and are not released from the adipocyte. This cycle ensures that excess free fatty acids do not go into the circulation.

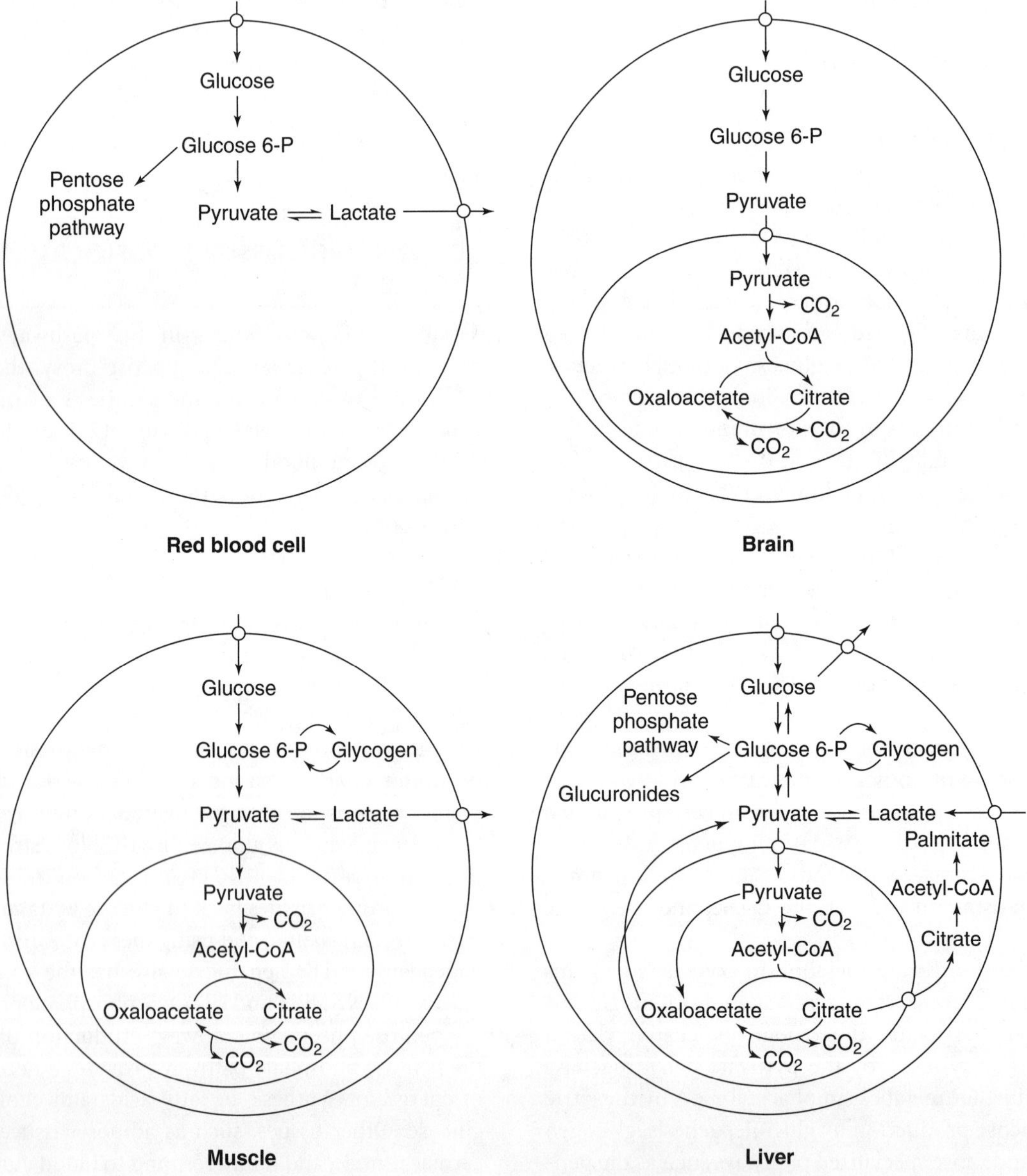

FIGURE 12-1 Overview of glucose metabolism in selected cell types.

BRAIN AND OTHER GLYCOLYTIC TISSUES

The brain, which is completely dependent upon glucose for its energy needs under normal dietary conditions, is capable of completely oxidizing glucose to CO_2 and H_2O via glycolysis and the citric acid cycle. The brain requires a continuous supply of glucose from the blood, because there is little storage of glucose in the form of glycogen in the brain. Red blood cells, on the other hand, have a limited ability to metabolize glucose because they lack mitochondria. In red blood cells, glucose is metabolized to lactate, and lactate is released to the circulation. Other specialized cells are also primarily glycolytic because of a relative lack of mitochondria or limited blood or oxygen supply relative to their rates of metabolism; these include leukocytes, white muscle fibers, cells of the testis, the renal medulla, and some cells of the cornea, lens, and retina of the eye.

TRANSPORT OF GLUCOSE ACROSS CELL MEMBRANES

Glucose is taken up into cells by glucose transporters. Most tissues contain facilitated glucose transporters, whereas the small intestinal absorptive cells (enterocytes) couple glucose and Na^+ uptake.

FACILITATED TRANSPORT OF GLUCOSE: THE GLUT TRANSPORTERS

Cellular uptake of blood glucose occurs by a facilitated transport process. Facilitated glucose uptake is mediated by a family of structurally related glucose transport proteins that have specific tissue distributions. Five isoforms of the glucose transporter have been well studied: glucose transporter type 1 (GLUT1) in red blood cells and brain, GLUT2 in liver and pancreas, GLUT3 in brain, GLUT4 (insulin-responsive) in skeletal and cardiac muscles and adipose tissue, and GLUT5 in the small intestine. Although different glucose transporters predominate in specific tissues, most tissues contain more than one isoform. These glucose transporters are encoded by genes in the *SLC2A* family of solute carriers. The demands of glucose uptake vary depending on the tissue involved and the physiological environment of the cell. The glucose transporter isoforms serve different functions to meet these variable demands. Glucose is taken up by cells in an insulin-independent manner in liver and certain extrahepatic tissues, such as brain and red blood cells, and in an insulin-dependent manner by cells in muscle and adipose tissue.

GLUT2

GLUT2 is a low-affinity glucose transporter that is localized primarily in the liver and the beta cells of the pancreas. To a lesser extent, it is found in the small intestine and kidneys. GLUT2 has a high K_m for glucose and is a key transport protein involved in responding to elevated blood glucose in humans. In liver, because of the expression of GLUT2, maximal glucose uptake occurs when blood glucose levels are high, such as after a carbohydrate-containing meal. In the pancreatic beta cell, glucose uptake via GLUT2 signals that the blood glucose concentration has increased and begins the process by which the beta cell responds to elevated blood glucose with secretion of insulin into the bloodstream. In the pancreas, glucose is transported into the beta cell where it is rapidly phosphorylated to glucose 6-phosphate by a high K_m glucokinase. The increase in glycolysis and oxidative metabolism of glucose increases the ATP/ADP ratio leading to a series of intracellular changes that result in the fusion of insulin-containing storage vesicles with the cell membrane and the release of insulin to the bloodstream (Figure 12-2). The combined action of GLUT2 and glucokinase allows the pancreatic beta cell to "sense" the blood glucose concentration and respond by increased secretion of insulin (Postic et al., 2001). In the small intestine and kidney tubules, GLUT2 is involved in glucose absorption and reabsorption, respectively, across the basolateral membranes of the epithelial cell barriers of these two tissues.

Expression of the gene for GLUT2, *SLC2A2,* is regulated in a tissue-specific manner. In liver, *SLC2A2* expression does not appear to be regulated by dietary carbohydrate or insulin, and GLUT2 levels in liver have not been found to change consistently in response to altered metabolic states. However,

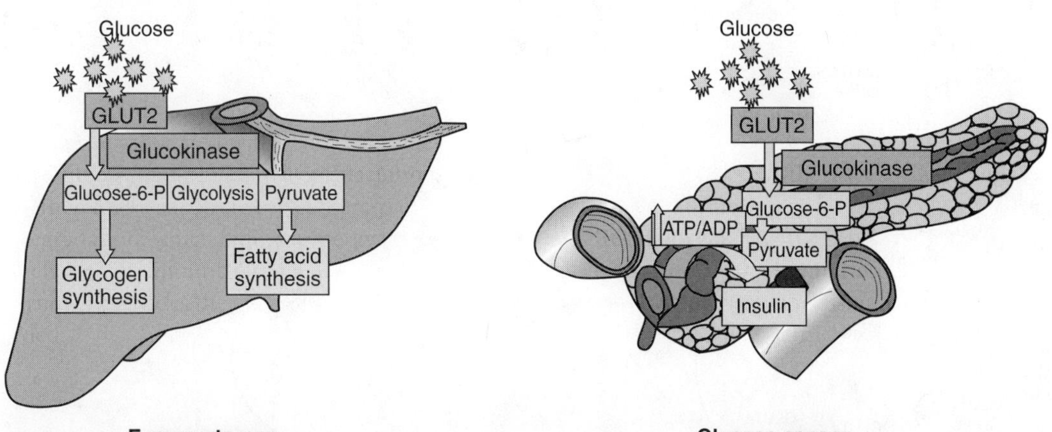

FIGURE 12-2 The combined actions of low-affinity (high K_m) GLUT2 and glucokinase produce "glucose sensing" in (1) the liver for energy storage and (2) the pancreatic beta cell for insulin secretion. The GLUT2/glucokinase system is very active in both tissues when blood glucose levels are high.

SCL2A2 gene expression in pancreatic beta cells is decreased when blood glucose levels are low. Conversely, a rise in blood glucose levels increases *SCL2A2* messenger RNA (mRNA) and protein levels in pancreatic beta cells. *SCL2A2* knockout mice are unable to sense glucose concentrations in the blood and exhibit impaired insulin secretion. This was rescued by reexpression of the *SCL2A2* gene in pancreatic cells, which restored insulin secretion by the pancreas (Thorens, 2002).

GLUT4

GLUT4 is present primarily in skeletal and cardiac muscle and in white and brown adipose tissue and is the only insulin-responsive glucose transporter. GLUT4 is encoded by the *SLC2A4* gene. GLUT4 has a unique physiological role in whole-body glucose homeostasis. In effect, GLUT4 mediates the second-tier response to elevated blood glucose. In skeletal and cardiac muscle and adipose tissue, insulin stimulates a rapid translocation of preformed GLUT4 from intracellular vesicles in the cytosol to the plasma membrane of the cell surface (Czech, 1995). By increasing the concentration of glucose transporters at the cell surface, insulin increases the capacity for glucose uptake. Insulin signaling is known to activate AS160 (Akt substrate of 160 kDa), which is a Rab GTPase-activating protein, and TC10, which is a GTP-binding protein, both of which are required for insulin-stimulated GLUT4 translocation (Miinea et al., 2005). When insulin levels fall, GLUT4 is returned to the intracellular vesicular system by endocytosis. In unstimulated muscle and adipose cells, approximately 90% of GLUT4 is intracellular (Ishiki and Klip, 2005). Upregulation of GLUT4 translocation is disrupted in individuals with insulin resistance due to accumulation of intramyocellular lipid that interferes with insulin signaling (Petersen and Shulman, 2006).

Exercise can also stimulate GLUT4 translocation to the plasma membrane in skeletal muscle, but this involves a different signaling pathway than that initiated by insulin (Uldry and Thorens, 2004). Exercise induces the cumulative effects of numerous inputs, including adenosine monophosphate (AMP)-activated protein kinase (AMPK) and increased cytosolic calcium (Ca^{2+}) levels as major factors. There may be distal convergence between the insulin and exercise signaling pathways regulating GLUT4 translocation in skeletal muscle (Cartee and Funai, 2009).

In addition to affecting the translocation of existing GLUT4 molecules to the plasma membrane, fasting, refeeding, and insulin level can also affect the expression of new GLUT4 molecules. Fasting or type 2 diabetes leads to a significant decrease in *SLC2A4* mRNA and GLUT4 protein in adipocytes. This decrease can be reversed by carbohydrate refeeding or insulin treatment. A depletion in *SLC2A4* mRNA and protein results in a decrease in the vesicular GLUT4 pool that is available for translocation to the plasma membrane. The decrease in *SLC2A4* gene expression and the decrease in insulin-stimulated GLUT4 translocation both contribute to the decrease in glucose uptake in adipocytes with insulin deprivation (Figure 12-3).

Expression of the *SLC2A4* gene has also been investigated in skeletal muscle. Because the red and white muscle fiber types have different insulin sensitivities and GLUT4 concentrations, it has been difficult to determine the hormonal responsiveness of the *SLC2A4* gene in skeletal muscle. Most studies indicate that *SLC2A4* expression in muscle is not decreased in patients with insulin resistance/type 2 diabetes. This is surprising because skeletal muscle is responsible for at least 50% of glucose uptake from the blood after a carbohydrate-containing meal, whereas adipose tissue

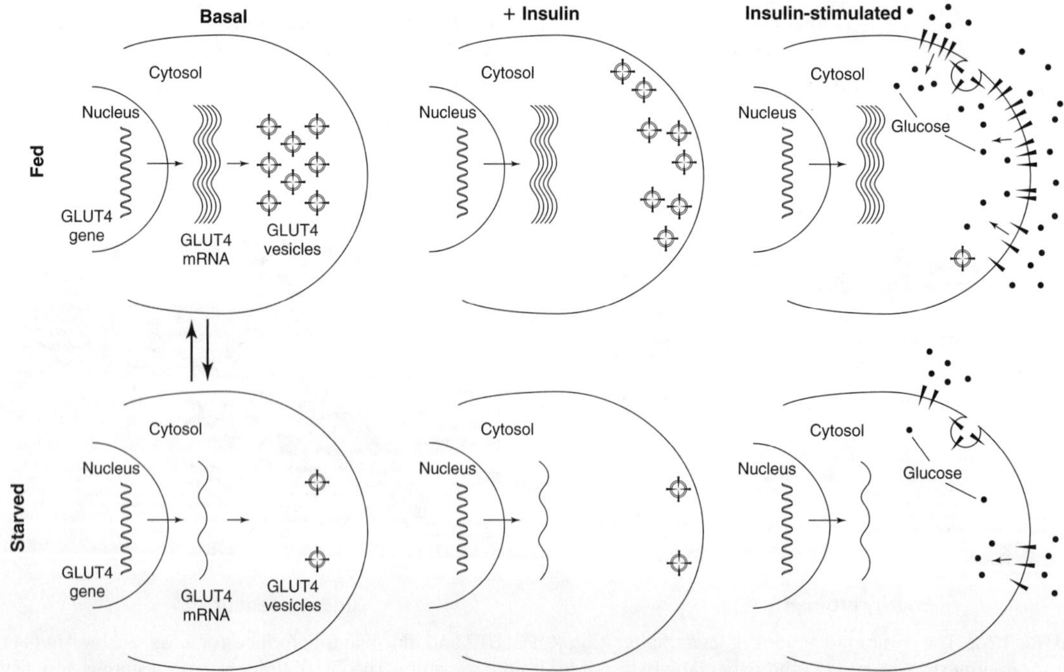

FIGURE 12-3 Effect of insulin on expression and translocation of the GLUT4 glucose transporter in adipocytes.

is responsible for much less. Studies in mice in which the *SLC2A4* gene was selectively ablated in specific tissues, such as skeletal muscle and adipose tissue, indicated that there is "cross talk" between these two tissues, such that a decrease in adipose GLUT4 level (and therefore glucose uptake) decreases glucose uptake in skeletal muscle (Minokoshi et al., 2003).

GLUT1 and GLUT3

GLUT1 and GLUT3 are both high-affinity glucose transporters. GLUT1 is abundant in the brain, placenta, and fetal tissues. In these tissues, GLUT1 mediates glucose uptake across a blood–tissue barrier (e.g., the blood–brain barrier). GLUT1 is also found at low levels in erythrocytes and most other tissues and may be involved in the underlying constitutive glucose uptake of the whole organism. Under fasting conditions, GLUT1 is present at the plasma membrane of cells in muscle and adipose tissue at a higher relative abundance than that for GLUT4. Because GLUT1 cell surface abundance is not affected by insulin, however, GLUT4 becomes the dominant glucose transporter present on the cell membrane of muscle cells and adipocytes during insulin-stimulated states. GLUT3 is present at high levels in brain and placenta and is also found in skeletal muscle (mainly slow twitch fibers) and sperm. Because both GLUT1 and GLUT 3 have a low K_m for glucose and transport glucose even when circulating levels are low, these two glucose transporters appear to be responsible for basal glucose transport in most tissues of the body.

GLUT5

GLUT5 is found primarily in the jejunum of the small intestine, but is also present in some other tissues, including kidney and sperm. GLUT5 can transport fructose but does not appear to contribute significantly to glucose transport in humans.

ACTIVE UPTAKE OF GLUCOSE: SODIUM-DEPENDENT GLUCOSE TRANSPORT

Exceptions to facilitated glucose uptake occur in the brush border membrane of the small intestinal absorptive cells and the renal proximal tubules, where glucose is taken up into the epithelial cells by an active symport process mediated by the sodium/glucose cotransporter (SGLT1), which is encoded by the gene *SLC5A1*. In this active symport, glucose is moved into the cell by a transport protein that first binds Na^+. The energy for glucose uptake is provided by the Na^+,K^+-ATPase, which maintains a low intracellular Na^+ concentration. Glucose, after entry into the epithelial cell, dissociates from the transport protein. (See Chapters 7 and 8 for more discussion of glucose transport in the intestine.)

GLYCOLYSIS

At the cellular level, the breakdown of glucose for energy can be divided into two major pathways based on the intracellular location of the enzymatic machinery involved and on the ability of different cell types to perform the enzymatic reactions. The first of these pathways is glycolysis, the anaerobic breakdown of glucose to pyruvate. The enzymes involved in glycolysis are present in the cytosol of all cell types. The second pathway is the citric acid cycle, in which acetyl-CoA is completely oxidized to CO_2 and H_2O. Flux through the citric acid cycle and most of the ATP production from aerobic metabolism of glucose requires donation of electrons to the mitochondrial electron transport chain and ultimately to molecular oxygen as the terminal electron acceptor. Because the citric acid cycle and electron transport both occur in mitochondria, the aerobic oxidation of glucose only occurs in cells that possess mitochondria. Glycolysis and the citric acid cycle are linked by the pyruvate dehydrogenase reaction, which also takes place in the mitochondria of the cell. As a result of glycolysis, the pyruvate dehydrogenase reaction, and the citric acid cycle, energy is conserved in the chemical form of ATP, with ATP synthesis occurring both by substrate-level phosphorylation and by electron transport linked to oxidative phosphorylation.

The series of enzymatic reactions that together constitute the glycolytic pathway convert one 6-carbon molecule of glucose to two 3-carbon molecules of pyruvate. All cells of the human body can catabolize glucose to this extent. The metabolic fate of pyruvate, however, is variable and depends on the cell type and the availability of oxygen. When pyruvate cannot be oxidized due to lack of mitochondria or oxygen, pyruvae is reduced to lactate. Some tissues such as red blood cells produce lactate from glucose even under aerobic conditions because of their lack of mitochondria. White or glycolytic muscle fibers have a limited blood supply and a low abundance of mitochondria and are dependent on anaerobic glycolysis for ATP production during intense work. However, most tissues, under aerobic conditions, can oxidize pyruvate to acetyl-CoA and CO_2 via the pyruvate dehydrogenase reaction in the mitochondria, followed by complete oxidation of acetyl-CoA to CO_2 and H_2O via the citric acid cycle coupled to electron transport/oxidative phosphorylation.

The series of enzymatic reactions that make up the glycolytic pathway are subdivided into two stages, as shown in Figure 12-4: (1) the priming of glucose, which requires ATP expenditure to generate phosphorylated intermediates; and (2) the production of reducing equivalents and the synthesis of ATP. The enzymes that catalyze the reactions of glycolysis are present in the cell cytosol, organized into multienzyme complexes that function together to channel the intermediates from one enzyme to another so that they do not become diluted in the cytosol. The glycolytic enzymes are associated with cellular structures such as actin filaments, microtubules, or the outer membranes of mitochondria (Lehninger et al., 1993).

INITIAL STEPS OF GLYCOLYSIS: THE PRIMING OF GLUCOSE

The series of enzymatic reactions that make up glycolysis begins with the substrate glucose, which enters the cell by carrier-mediated transport, or with glucose 6-phosphate,

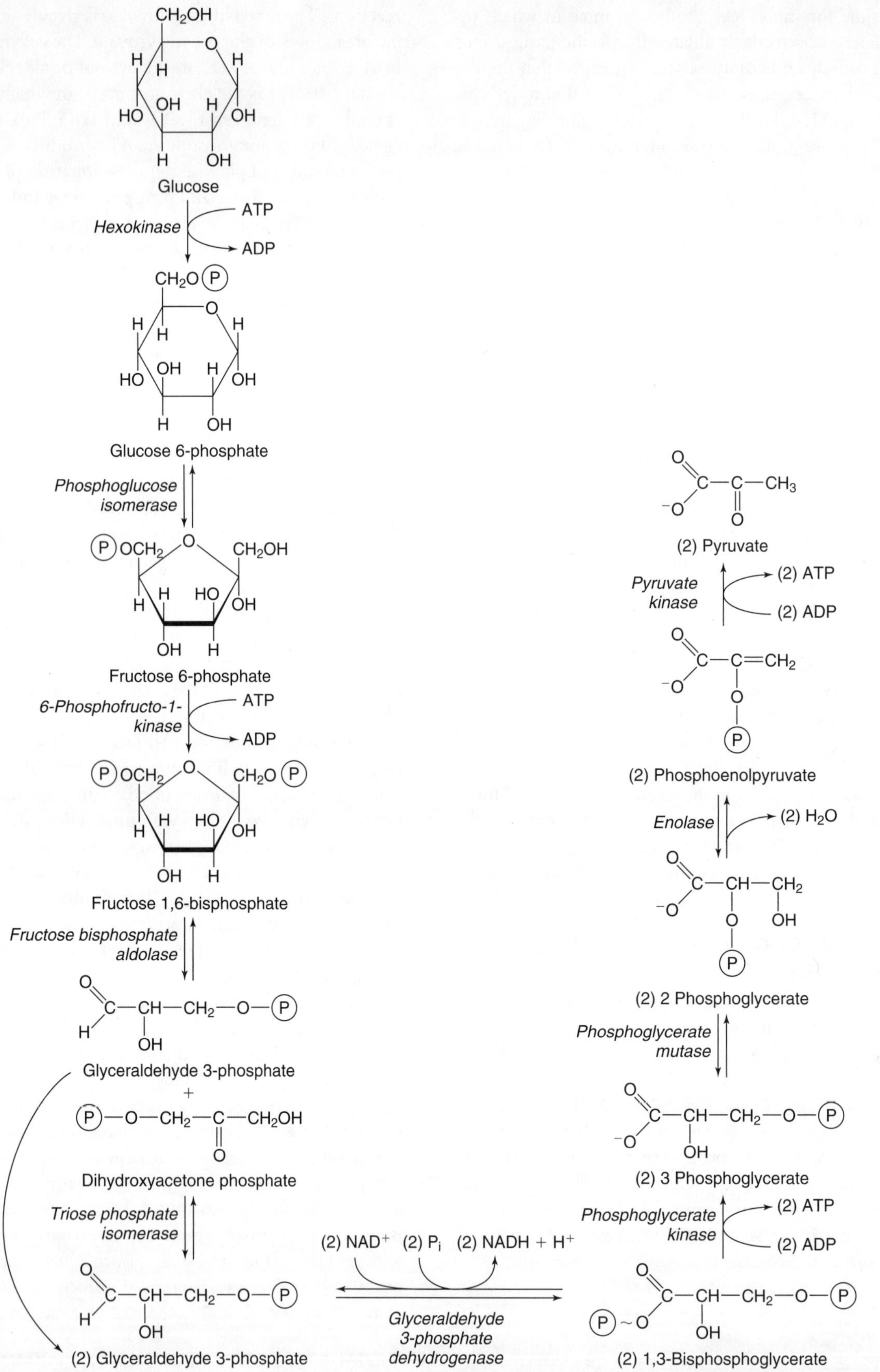

Glucose

Hexokinase — ATP → ADP

Glucose 6-phosphate

Phosphoglucose isomerase

Fructose 6-phosphate

6-Phosphofructo-1-kinase — ATP → ADP

Fructose 1,6-bisphosphate

Fructose bisphosphate aldolase

Glyceraldehyde 3-phosphate

+

Dihydroxyacetone phosphate

Triose phosphate isomerase

(2) Glyceraldehyde 3-phosphate

(2) NAD$^+$ (2) P_i (2) NADH + H$^+$

Glyceraldehyde 3-phosphate dehydrogenase

(2) 1,3-Bisphosphoglycerate

Phosphoglycerate kinase — (2) ADP → (2) ATP

(2) 3 Phosphoglycerate

Phosphoglycerate mutase

(2) 2 Phosphoglycerate

Enolase — (2) H_2O

(2) Phosphoenolpyruvate

Pyruvate kinase — (2) ADP → (2) ATP

(2) Pyruvate

FIGURE 12-4 The glycolytic pathway for conversion of glucose to pyruvate. *P* represents a phosphate substituent, PO_3^{2-}.

which is generated from glycogen degradation. For glucose that is transported into the cell, glucose is rapidly phosphorylated to glucose 6-phosphate in the following reaction:

$$\text{Glucose} + \text{ATP} \xrightarrow{Mg^{2+}} \text{Glucose 6-phosphate} + \text{ADP}$$

It should be noted that glucose 6-phosphate from glycogen does not require the hexokinase reaction. In skeletal muscle, glucose 6-phosphate from glycogen breakdown is a major substrate for glycolysis.

The mechanism of glucose phosphorylation involves the transfer of the γ phosphate from ATP to the C6 of glucose. This essentially irreversible reaction sequesters glucose within the cell because the phosphorylated form of glucose does not readily cross the plasma membrane. This phosphorylation reaction is catalyzed by hexokinase in most cell types and by glucokinase (hexokinase IV) in liver cells and pancreatic beta cells. In all cells, the product of this reaction, glucose 6-phosphate, can be broken down in the subsequent enzymatic steps of the glycolytic pathway. However, under anabolic conditions the production of glucose 6-phosphate is also the first step in the addition of glucose to the glucose polymer, glycogen, which is synthesized and stored mainly in liver and muscle tissue. In addition to glycolysis and glycogen synthesis, glucose 6-phosphate is also metabolized by the pentose phosphate pathway. This pathway provides cells with reducing equivalents in the form of NADPH and with ribose 5-phosphate for nucleotide synthesis.

Hexokinase, which catalyzes the initial phosphorylation of glucose when it enters the cell, has different tissue-specific isoenzyme forms. Isoenzymes are different molecular forms of an enzyme that catalyze the same reaction but differ in kinetics, regulatory mechanisms, and/or tissue localization. In humans, hexokinase I predominates in skeletal muscle and other extrahepatic tissues. Hexokinase I has a low K_m for glucose (less than 0.1 mmol/L) relative to blood glucose concentrations (4 to 6 mmol/L). (The K_m is the concentration of substrate at which the enzymatic reaction occurs at half-maximal velocity or, in other words, the concentration of substrate at which the enzyme is half-saturated with substrate.) In skeletal muscle, the activity of hexokinase I is coordinated with that of the low K_m glucose carrier GLUT4, which specifically transports glucose in the direction of its concentration gradient in response to insulin stimulation. Conversion of glucose to glucose 6-phosphate by hexokinase I maintains low intracellular glucose levels to favor glucose entry. However, hexokinase I is allosterically inhibited by its product, glucose 6-phosphate. This negative feedback ensures that glucose 6-phosphate does not build up in the cell. Thus the combined actions of GLUT4 and hexokinase I maintain a balance between glucose uptake and glucose phosphorylation.

Glucokinase (hexokinase IV), on the other hand, is the major hexokinase isoform in liver parenchymal cells and in the pancreatic beta cells. In contrast to hexokinase I, glucokinase has a low affinity for glucose, with a K_m of approximately 10 mM. In addition, glucokinase is not inhibited by glucose 6-phosphate. The activity of glucokinase is linked to that of the high K_m glucose transporter GLUT2, which is the major glucose carrier in liver cells and pancreatic beta cells. Because GLUT2 and glucokinase are not saturated at physiological glucose concentrations and because glucokinase is not inhibited by its product glucose 6-phosphate, they are able to respond to marked changes in blood glucose concentration. Thus GLUT2 and glucokinase in liver and the pancreatic beta cells allow uptake of glucose in proportion to its plasma concentration and the rapid conversion of this glucose to glucose 6-phosphate when blood glucose concentrations are elevated (e.g., after a carbohydrate-containing meal). Hepatocytes and pancreatic beta cells differentially regulate expression of the glucokinase gene by use of different promoters, different transcription start sites, and alternative splicing to generate glucokinase isoforms that have different N-terminal sequences (Magnuson and Jetton, 1993; Postic et al., 2001). Use of different gene promoters allows regulation of liver glucokinase in response to insulin and glucagon while pancreatic glucokinase is regulated in response to blood glucose concentration. This allows the liver to maintain blood glucose levels in the normal physiological range and the pancreas to sense elevations in blood glucose concentrations and respond with insulin secretion

The second enzymatic reaction in glycolysis is the isomerization of glucose 6-phosphate (an aldose) to fructose 6-phosphate (a ketose), catalyzed by phosphoglucose isomerase.

$$\text{Glucose 6-phosphate} \xleftrightarrow{Mg^{2+}} \text{Fructose 6-phosphate}$$

In this reaction, there is an intramolecular shift of a hydrogen atom, changing the location of the double bond. Phosphoglucose isomerase functions close to equilibrium, and therefore the reaction is reversible under intracellular conditions.

6-Phosphofructo-1-kinase catalyzes the next irreversible step in the glycolytic pathway, the phosphorylation of fructose 6-phosphate to fructose 1,6-bisphosphate:

$$\text{Fructose 6-phosphate} + \text{ATP} \xrightarrow{Mg^{2+}} \text{Fructose 1,6-bisphosphate} + \text{ADP}$$

The 6-phosphofructo-1-kinase reaction utilizes a second molecule of ATP and is the first committed step in glycolysis. Unlike glucose 6-phosphate, fructose 1,6-bisphosphate cannot be used directly as substrate for alternative pathways such as glycogen synthesis. The 6-phosphofructo-1-kinase reaction is highly regulated by allosteric modifiers and is one of the major determinants of the rate of glycolytic conversion of glucose to pyruvate. It is also regulated by changes in gene expression. In humans, there are three isoenzymes of 6-phosphofructo-1-kinase, each encoded by a separate gene. Hepatic mRNA levels of the 6-phosphofructo-1-kinase gene *(PFK)* are increased in response to carbohydrate refeeding after a fast (Granner and Pilkis, 1990), but in skeletal muscle there are no changes in expression of the *PFK* gene with either diabetes, insulin treatment, or exercise (Vestergaard, 1999).

The next reaction involves the division of the 6-carbon sugar diphosphate, fructose 1,6 bisphosphate, to two 3-carbon phosphorylated intermediates. The aldol cleavage reaction is catalyzed by aldolase as follows:

Fructose 1,6-bisphosphate ↔ Dihydroxyacetone phosphate + Glyceraldehyde-3-phosphate

Glyceraldehyde 3-phosphate is in the direct path of glycolysis, but dihydroxyacetone phosphate is not. Dihydroxyacetone phosphate is isomerized to glyceraldehyde 3-phosphate via the action of triose-phosphate isomerase. The net result of the aldolase and triose-phosphate isomerase reactions is the production of two molecules of glyceraldehyde 3-phosphate. The series of reactions that converts one molecule of glucose to two molecules of glyceraldehyde 3-phosphate constitutes the first phase of glycolysis in which the chemical energy of ATP is used to generate phosphorylated intermediates. The dihydroxyacetone phosphate produced by the aldolase reaction may also be reduced to glycerol 3-phosphate and used for synthesis of glycerolipids; this is a particularly important source of glycerol 3-phosphate for triacylglycerol synthesis in small intestinal enterocytes and in adipocytes.

GENERATION OF REDUCING EQUIVALENTS AND SUBSTRATE-LEVEL SYNTHESIS OF ATP

The second stage of glycolysis generates reducing equivalents and ATP. Reducing equivalents in the form NADH are produced by the reaction catalyzed by glyceraldehyde 3-phosphate dehydrogenase:

Glyceraldehyde 3-phosphate + NAD^+ + P_i ↔ 1,3-Bisphosphoglycerate + NADH + H^+

This reaction incorporates inorganic phosphate (P_i) to produce a high-energy phosphate bond in 1,3-bisphosphoglycerate. The second product of the reaction, NADH, provides reducing equivalents for the energy conversion of electron transport and production of ATP by oxidative phosphorylation. This is the only glycolytic reaction that generates reducing equivalents for electron transport. It is important to note that the coenzyme NAD^+ is present in limited amounts in the cytosol. For this reason, the NAD^+ used in the glyceraldehyde 3-phosphate reaction needs to be regenerated in the cytosolic compartment so that NAD^+ availability does not limit glycolysis.

The acyl-phosphate bond of 1,3-bisphosphoglycerate has a high-energy phosphoryl transfer potential that is used to generate ATP in the next reaction of glycolysis. This is the conversion of 1,3-bisphosphoglycerate to 3-phosphoglycerate:

1,3-Bisphosphoglycerate + ADP ↔ 3-Phosphoglycerate + ATP

The enzyme that catalyzes this reaction is phosphoglycerate kinase. This is the first reaction in glycolysis that generates ATP. The formation of ATP by transfer of the phosphate group from 1,3-bisphosphoglycerate to ADP is a substrate-level phosphorylation.

The next step in the glycolytic pathway is the conversion of 3-phosphoglycerate to 2-phosphoglycerate, catalyzed by phosphoglycerate mutase. The mechanism of this enzymatic reaction is complex and involves a phosphoenzyme intermediate. The end products of this reaction are 2-phosphoglycerate and the regenerated phosphoenzyme. The overall series of reactions can be summarized as follows:

Enzyme-phosphate + 3-Phosphoglycerate ↔ Enzyme + 2,3-Bisphosphoglycerate

Enzyme + 2,3-Bisphosphoglycerate ↔ Enzyme-phosphate + 2-Phosphoglycerate

A second glycolytic intermediate with a high-energy phosphate bond is generated when 2-phosphoglycerate is converted to phosphoenolpyruvate via a dehydration reaction catalyzed by enolase.

2-Phosphoglycerate ↔ Phosphoenolpyruvate + H_2O

The phosphoenolpyruvate generated by the enolase reaction is substrate for the last reaction of glycolysis, the conversion of phosphoenolpyruvate to pyruvate with the generation of ATP.

$$\text{Phosphoenolpyruvate} + \text{ADP} \xrightarrow{Mg^{2+}, K^{+}} \text{Pyruvate} + \text{ATP}$$

This reaction is catalyzed by pyruvate kinase and is the second substrate-level phosphorylation step that occurs in glycolysis. The pyruvate kinase reaction is essentially irreversible under intracellular conditions. This enzyme is highly regulated by allosteric and covalent modification, much like 6-phosphofructose-1-kinase, as is discussed in subsequent text of this chapter.

FURTHER METABOLISM OF PYRUVATE

Pyruvate produced by glycolysis can be metabolized in different ways, depending upon the availability of oxygen and the metabolic state of the cell. Pyruvate may enter the mitochondrion where it is converted to acetyl-CoA in a complex series of reactions catalyzed by the multienzyme pyruvate dehydrogenase complex. Acetyl-CoA so produced can enter the citric acid cycle for complete oxidation to CO_2 and H_2O, or it can exit the mitochondria as citrate and be used for fatty acid or sterol synthesis in certain cell types (see Chapter 16 for a discussion of de novo lipogenesis from glucose). In the absence of sufficient oxygen or in cells lacking mitochondria, pyruvate has a different fate; it is reduced to lactate by the cytosolic enzyme lactate dehydrogenase.

Pyruvate + NADH + H^+ ↔ Lactate + NAD^+

Metabolism of glucose by this anaerobic pathway may occur in active skeletal muscle, and lactate can build up when molecular oxygen becomes insufficient to meet the metabolic need for aerobic metabolism. Pyruvate is also reduced to lactate in red blood cells, which do not have mitochondria. The reduction of pyruvate to lactate generates NAD^+ from NADH. This replaces the NAD^+ that was reduced in the glyceraldehyde 3-phosphate dehydrogenase reaction of glycolysis. Therefore these two reactions balance the utilization and regeneration of NAD^+ so that glycolysis can continue. Per glucose molecule, two molecules of NAD^+ are reduced in the glyceraldehyde 3-phosphate dehydrogenase reaction, and two molecules of NAD^+ are regenerated in the reduction of pyruvate to lactate. The lactate formed in this process can be recycled to the liver to regenerate glucose via gluconeogenesis. Heart muscle is also able to take up lactate and use it as a fuel for ATP production. Under conditions of heavy physical activity, the heart may take up lactate released by exercising skeletal muscle and use it as a fuel.

In the presence of sufficient molecular oxygen and in cells with mitochondria, reducing equivalents (NADH + H^+) produced by the glyceraldehyde 3-phosphate dehydrogenase reaction can be shuttled to the mitochondria by the reduction of metabolic intermediates in the cytosol, regenerating NAD^+ in this compartment. The reduced intermediate is shuttled across the inner mitochondrial membrane with subsequent oxidation, thereby regenerating NADH + H^+ from NAD^+ in the mitochondria. NADH in the mitochondria is an electron donor, transferring reducing equivalents to Complex I (NADH dehydrogenase complex) in the series of oxidation–reduction reactions of electron transport (see Chapter 21, Figure 21-4). Under these conditions, the reduction of pyruvate to lactate is not required for the regeneration of NAD^+ in the cytosol.

ATP EQUIVALENTS PRODUCED BY GLYCOLYSIS

The total ATP produced from the reactions of glycolysis can be calculated. In this pathway, one molecule of glucose is converted to two molecules of pyruvate. Two molecules of ATP are used to prime glucose; however, four molecules of ATP are produced by substrate-level phosphorylation in the second phase, yielding a net increase of two molecules of ATP. Because one less ATP is consumed when glucose 6-phosphate from glycogen breakdown is the initial substrate for glycolysis, a net of three molecules of ATP are produced per glucose moiety from glycogen that undergoes glycolysis. In addition, two molecules of NADH are produced in the glyceraldehyde 3-phosphate dehydrogenase reaction in the cytosol of the cell. The energy gain can be summarized as follows:

$$\text{Glucose} + 2\ \text{ATP} + 2\ \text{NAD}^+ + 4\ \text{ADP} + 2\ \text{P}_i \rightarrow 2\ \text{Pyruvate} + 2\ \text{ADP} + 2\ \text{NADH} + 2\ \text{H}^+ + 4\ \text{ATP} + 2\ \text{H}_2\text{O}$$

or a net of

$$\text{Glucose} + 2\ \text{NAD}^+ + 2\ \text{ADP} + 2\ \text{P}_i \rightarrow 2\ \text{Pyruvate} + 2\ \text{NADH} + 2\ \text{H}^+ + 2\ \text{ATP} + 2\ \text{H}_2\text{O}$$

If pyruvate is reduced to lactate to regenerate NAD^+, the only net yield of ATP is the substrate-level production of two ATP per glucose molecule (or three ATP per glucose moiety from glycogen breakdown). Under aerobic conditions, NADH provides electrons to carrier molecules in the mitochondria of the cell, and these reactions release sufficient energy for the production of two to three molecules of ATP per pair of electrons by oxidative phosphorylation. The total amount of ATP generated from NADH depends upon the mechanism by which reducing equivalents from NADH enter the mitochondria. Therefore the net production of ATP from glycolysis is six to eight molecules of ATP from the catabolism of one molecule of glucose to two molecules of pyruvate (or seven to nine molecules of ATP from one molecule of glucose 6-phosphate generated from glycogen breakdown). Even though the overall energy transfer of the glycolytic series of enzymatic reactions is exergonic and a portion of this energy is stored as the high-energy phosphate bond of ATP, glucose is only partially oxidized by the process of glycolysis. Glycolysis provides only a minor percentage of the total ATP produced when all steps involved in the complete oxidation of glucose to CO_2 and H_2O are considered (see subsequent text on mitochondrial oxidation of pyruvate).

METABOLISM OF MONOSACCHARIDES OTHER THAN GLUCOSE

In addition to glucose, monosaccharides obtained from ingestion of common foods include fructose, galactose, and, in lesser amounts, mannose, all of which are converted to intermediates in glycolysis. A brief description of the entry of fructose and the other monosaccharides into the glycolytic sequence of enzymatic reactions in the liver is presented in Figure 12-5.

FRUCTOSE

Fructose is a major sweetening agent in the human diet and is especially high in the American diet because of a high intake of sucrose and high fructose corn syrup in sweetened products. It is present as a monosaccharide in honey, fruit, commercially produced high fructose corn syrup, and many vegetables. In addition, fructose is one of the residues in the disaccharide sucrose, which is common table sugar (cane or beet). Sorbitol, present in many fruits and vegetables, is also converted to fructose in the liver via the sorbitol dehydrogenase reaction. Although the end products of fructose catabolism are similar to those of glucose, fructose does not elicit the same glucose-induced hormonal response after absorption (i.e., a large increase in insulin secretion from the pancreas).

In contrast to glucose, which is metabolized by all tissues of the body with only 30% to 40% of glucose intake being metabolized by the liver, fructose is metabolized mainly by the liver. The liver has a high level of glucokinase, which does not phosphorylate fructose, and a relatively low level of hexokinase. However, liver has a relatively high concentration of fructokinase, an enzyme that catalyzes the phosphorylation of fructose at C1 to generate fructose 1-phosphate. Therefore the initial product in liver is fructose 1-phosphate rather than the fructose 6-phosphate.

$$\text{Fructose} + \text{ATP} \xrightarrow{\text{Mg}^{2+}} \text{Fructose 1-phosphate} + \text{ADP}$$

Similar to glycolysis, the next step in what is referred to as fructolysis is the aldolase reaction that hydrolyses the 6-carbon fructose to two 3-carbon intermediates. The liver has predominantly aldolase B, which hydrolyzes fructose

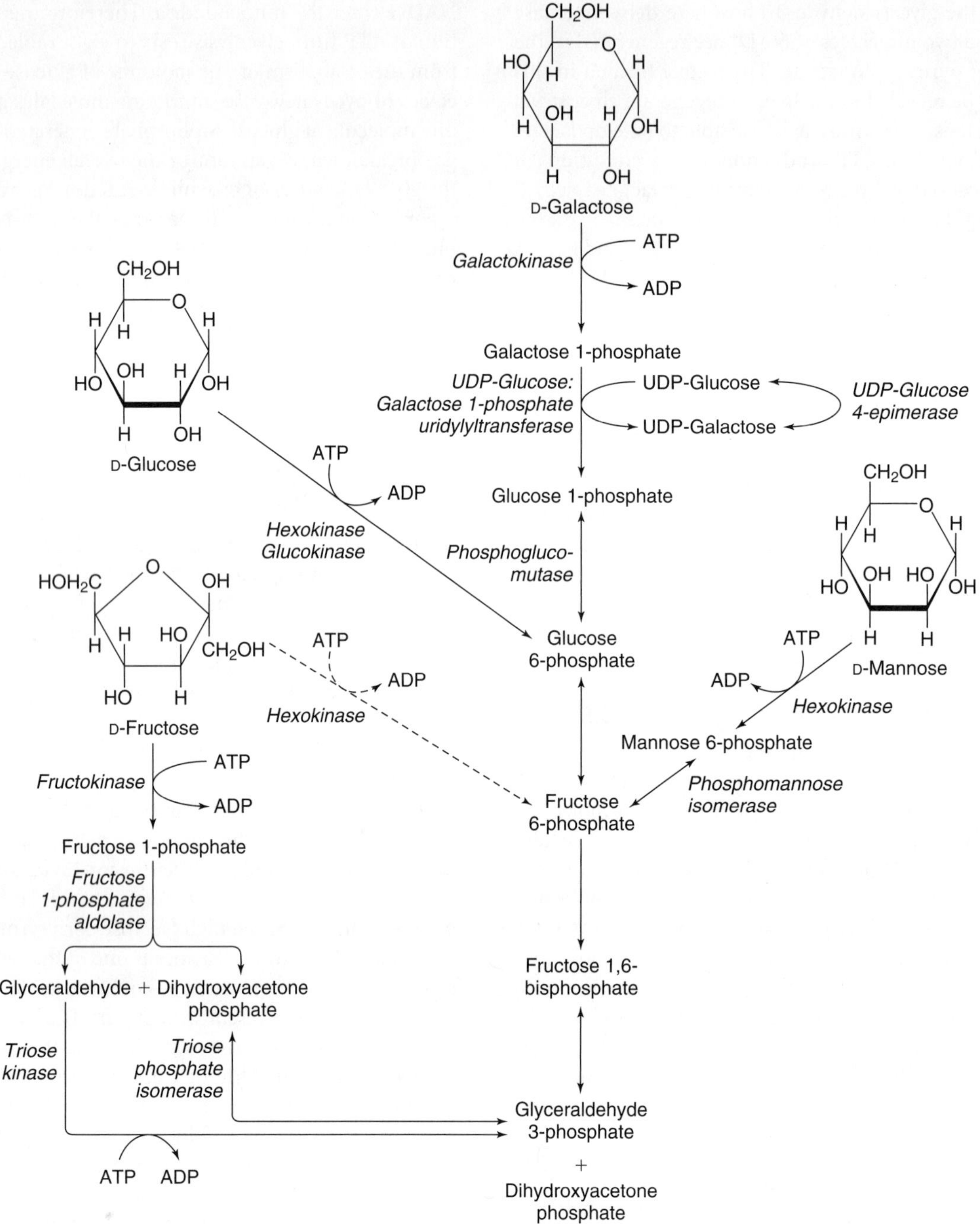

FIGURE 12-5 Conversion of absorbed monosaccharides to glycolytic intermediates in the liver.

1-phosphate as well as the glycolytic intermediate fructose 1,6-diphosphate. Therefore aldolase B (fructose 1-phosphate aldolase) continues the catabolism of fructose by hydrolyzing fructose 1-phosphate to dihydroxyacetone phosphate and glyceraldehyde.

$$\text{Fructose 1-phosphate} \leftrightarrow \text{Dihydroxyacetone phosphate} + \text{Glyceraldehyde}$$

Glyceraldehyde is then phosphorylated to glyceraldehyde 3-phosphate by glyceraldehyde kinase.

$$\text{Glyceraldehyde} + \text{ATP} \xrightarrow{Mg^{2+}} \text{Glyceraldehyde 3-phosphate} + \text{ATP}$$

Dihydroxyacetone phosphate produced from the hydrolysis of fructose 1-phosphate is converted to glyceraldehyde 3-phosphate by triose-phosphate isomerase, the enzyme that catalyzes the same conversion of triose phosphates in the glycolytic breakdown of glucose. Overall, one molecule of fructose is converted to two molecules of glyceraldehyde 3-phosphate. Glyceraldehyde 3-phosphate is then substrate for further glycolytic conversion.

The majority of the triose phosphates generated from fructose are catabolized to pyruvate, which is then converted to lactate or further catabolized via the pyruvate dehydrogenase complex and the citric acid cycle. This is due, in part, to the fact that fructolysis bypasses the phosphofructo-1-kinase

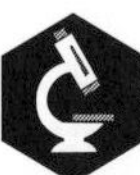

CLINICAL CORRELATION

Fructose Intolerance and Essential Fructosuria

Two genetic defects in fructose metabolism are known: fructose intolerance and essential fructosuria (Van den Berghe, 1995). Fructose intolerance is caused by an autosomal recessive defect in the liver fructose 1-phosphate aldolase (aldolase B) gene. The symptoms of hereditary fructose intolerance are absent in infancy if the infant is breast-fed. However, the introduction of sweetened milk formulas or the later introduction of fruits and vegetables provokes the symptoms of this disorder due to exposure to fructose. The deficiency in aldolase B leads to the buildup of fructose 1-phosphate and the depletion of P_i for ATP production in liver. The accumulation of fructose 1-phosphate blocks both glycogenolysis, owing to inhibition of glycogen phosphorylase by fructose 1-phosphate, and gluconeogenesis, owing to inhibition of the fructose bisphosphatase aldolase and phosphoglucose isomerase reactions in the reversal of glycolysis (Van den Berghe, 1995). Furthermore, the depletion of P_i and ATP leads to a series of imbalances, including the inhibition of protein synthesis, that cause liver cell damage and a decline in liver function.

In contrast to fructose intolerance, the symptoms of essential fructosuria are essentially those of a "nondisease" (Van den Berghe, 1995). Essential fructosuria is caused by a defect in fructokinase, which is normally found in liver, kidney, and intestinal mucosa. This relatively harmless disorder results in the excretion of fructose in the urine, as well as some metabolism of fructose to fructose 6-phosphate by hexokinase in adipose and muscle tissue.

Thinking Critically

In normal individuals, the capacity of the liver to phosphorylate fructose (fructokinase activity) greatly exceeds the liver's capacity to split fructose 1-phosphate (aldolase B activity). Why is a deficiency of fructokinase a less serious genetic defect than a deficiency of fructose 1-phosphate aldolase? Consider what happens to fructose in each case and what effect this has on hepatic metabolism.

step, which is highly regulated and normally plays a major role in regulating glycolytic flux. Alternatively, to a lesser extent, the triose phosphates from fructose can be metabolized via gluconeogenic reactions to glucose or glycogen. Overall, because fructolysis provides the liver with an abundance of pyruvate, metabolites of the citric acid cycle, such as citrate and malate, also build up. Citrate can be transported from the mitochondria and converted to acetyl-CoA via the action of citrate lyase in the cytosol; acetyl-CoA then serves as a precursor for fatty acid or cholesterol synthesis (as discussed in Chapters 16 and 17). Overall, a long-term increase in fructose or sucrose consumption can lead to increased hepatic lipogenesis (Shafrir, 1991). These lipids are then secreted from the liver as components of lipoprotein particles, causing hyperlipidemia and increased lipid storage in adipose tissue, or retained in the liver if lipogenesis is in excess of lipoprotein export. In the latter scenario, nonadipose lipid accumulation can result in hepatic steatosis and be a major contributor to nonalcoholic fatty liver disease. A recent study has shown that children with fatty liver (detected by sonogram) consume diets that are high in fructose (Mager et al., 2010).

Although fructose is normally metabolized in the liver, skeletal muscle also has the capacity for fructose catabolism. In skeletal muscle, the catabolism of fructose closely resembles that of glucose; fructose is phosphorylated to fructose 6-phosphate by the action of hexokinase, similar to the conversion of glucose to glucose 6-phosphate by the same enzyme. The fructose 6-phosphate is further metabolized via glycolysis in the muscle, being converted to fructose 1,6-bisphosphate, which is then hydrolyzed by aldolase A (fructose 1,6-bisphosphate aldolase, the predominant form of aldolase in skeletal muscle) to glyceraldehyde 3-phosphate and dihydroxyacetone phosphate. The muscle isozyme of aldolase, aldolase A, hydrolyzes only fructose 1,6-diphosphate and not fructose 1-phosphate.

In men, fructose is the major fuel utilized by a specialized cell type, spermatozoa. Cells in the seminal vesicles can synthesize fructose from glucose. Fructose synthesis involves an NADPH-dependent reduction of glucose to sorbitol, followed by an NAD^+-dependent oxidation of sorbitol to fructose. Fructose is taken up by sperm cells and oxidized completely to CO_2 and H_2O by fructolysis and the citric acid cycle.

GALACTOSE

Another dietary monosaccharide, galactose, is derived from the digestion of lactose, a disaccharide of galactose and glucose. Lactose is the major carbohydrate in milk. In liver, galactose is phosphorylated by galactokinase as follows:

$$\text{Galactose} + \text{ATP} \xrightarrow{Mg^{2+}} \text{Galactose 1-phosphate} + \text{ADP}$$

Galactose 1-phosphate then undergoes a conversion to its epimer glucose 1-phosphate through the action of uridine diphosphate (UDP)-glucose:galactose 1-phosphate uridylyltransferase. In this reaction, UDP serves as a hexose carrier, and the two substrates for this reaction are galactose 1-phosphate and UDP-glucose. UDP-glucose:galactose 1-phosphate uridylyltransferase catalyzes the transfer of the uridyl group from UDP-glucose to galactose 1-phosphate, generating a molecule of free glucose 1-phosphate and UDP-galactose as the end products. UDP-galactose is then converted back to UDP-glucose by UDP-galactose 4-epimerase. Glucose 1-phosphate is an intermediate that can be channeled to glycogen synthesis under conditions that favor glucose storage. Under conditions that favor glucose utilization for energy, however, glucose 1-phosphate is converted to

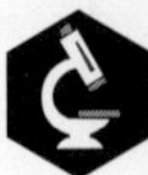

CLINICAL CORRELATION

Hereditary Defects in Galactose Metabolism

Three inborn errors in galactose metabolism have been characterized. These are due to rare autosomal recessive defects in either galactokinase, UDP-glucose:galactose 1-phosphate uridylyltransferase, or UDP-glucose-4-epimerase. Because galactose consumption is high during infancy, the clinical symptoms of these metabolic defects are exhibited early.

Galactokinase deficiency leads to the excretion of most of the ingested galactose or its conversion to the reduced metabolite galactitol because galactose is not phosphorylated to galactose 1-phosphate due to the defect. In newborn infants, galactitol concentrates in the lens, and the accumulation of galactitol results in the development of cataracts (Gitzelmann, 1995).

With UDP-glucose:galactose 1-phosphate uridylyltransferase deficiency, galactose 1-phosphate and galactose build up and galactitol is produced. This deficiency occurs in two forms: near-complete lack of the enzyme (classic galactosemia) and partial lack of the enzyme. Classic galactosemia affects the liver, kidney, and brain, as well as the eye, and can be life-threatening.

The third inborn error of galactose metabolism, caused by UDP-glucose 4-epimerase deficiency, also occurs in a mild and a severe form. Severe epimerase deficiency is very rare, and the symptoms are similar to those of classical galactosemia.

glucose 6-phosphate in the reversible phosphoglucomutase reaction:

$$\text{Glucose 1-phosphate} \leftrightarrow \text{Glucose 6-phosphate}$$

Glucose 6-phosphate can then be used by the liver cell for glycolysis or dephosphorylated to glucose by the enzyme glucose 6-phosphatase for release to the circulating blood.

MANNOSE

Mannose is the end product of digestion of various polysaccharides in the diet. But mannose is also produced intracellularly by the catabolism of high-mannose and complex glycans of glycoproteins by exoglucosidases in the lysosome (Winchester, 2005). The monosaccharides so produced are then transported across the lysosomal membrane to the cytosol by diffusion and carrier-mediated transport. In the liver, mannose is phosphorylated by hexokinase at the C6 position, generating mannose 6-phosphate:

$$\text{Mannose} + \text{ATP} \xrightarrow{Mg^{2+}} \text{Mannose 6-phosphate} + \text{ADP}$$

The mannose 6-phosphate so produced is converted to fructose 6-phosphate by phosphomannose isomerase. Therefore mannose can be converted to the glycolytic intermediate fructose 6-phosphate.

GLUCONEOGENESIS

The series of enzymatic reactions that make up the gluconeogenic pathway produces glucose from pyruvate, lactate, and glycerol and from other nonhexose precursors, especially amino acid carbon chains. The biosynthesis of glucose involves an essential reversal of glycolysis; however, the enzymatic reactions are not all a direct reversal of those of glycolysis. Enzyme reactions specific to gluconeogenesis bypass the irreversible steps of glycolysis. Furthermore, unlike glycolysis, gluconeogenesis does not occur in all cell types—it occurs primarily in liver and to a lesser extent in kidney because these two tissues are the only ones that express significant levels of glucose 6-phosphatase. In addition to having the enzymes that catalyze the reversible steps of glycolysis, liver and kidney also have glycerol kinase activity, which allows glycerol to serve as a gluconeogenic (or glycolytic) substrate, entering the gluconeogenic pathway at the level of dihydroxyacetone phosphate.

THE LIVER IS THE CENTRAL GLUCONEOGENIC ORGAN

The endogenous synthesis of glucose by the body is critical for the maintenance of blood glucose for those tissues that are dependent upon glucose for their energy needs. In humans, in the absence of dietary carbohydrate intake, liver glycogen is depleted within 18 hours. After this time, the liver must synthesize glucose from nonhexose precursors to maintain blood glucose levels. The liver is the central gluconeogenic tissue of the human body and responds to low blood glucose by releasing glucose produced by glycogen breakdown or glucose produced by gluconeogenesis into the blood for transport to other tissues. Some gluconeogenesis produces new glucose (i.e., from amino acid carbon chains) to replace glucose completely oxidized by tissues, whereas gluconeogenesis using lactate serves to recycle incompletely oxidized glucose carbon chains.

Although gluconeogenesis also occurs in the kidney, the kidney is smaller than the liver and contributes less to circulating glucose. Overall, the liver contributes approximately 90% of gluconeogenically derived glucose, whereas the kidney contributes approximately 10%. However, after a 14- to 16-hour overnight fast, the liver contributes approximately 75% to 80% of glucose released into the circulation and the kidneys release the remaining 20% to 25% (Gerich, 2010). As the length of the fast continues, the kidneys make a larger percentage contribution to circulating blood glucose levels, accounting for up to 45%. Increased gluconeogenesis is coupled to increased renal ammoniagenesis and nitrogen excretion with prolonged fasting (Wahren and Ekberg, 2007). The brain and skeletal muscle as well as some other extrahepatic tissues have some capacity to convert gluconeogenic substrates to glucose 6-phosphate for use for glycogen synthesis, but these tissues are not able to produce blood glucose because they lack glucose 6-phosphatase. The liver is also important in recycling lactate and amino acids such as alanine released by active skeletal muscle and nonoxidative tissues back to glucose.

It should be noted that the gluconeogenic pathway is not active until after birth because the levels of hepatic phosphoenolpyruvate carboxykinase are very low until the neonatal period. Within a few hours after birth, phosphoenolpyruvate carboxykinase activity increases several-fold and the gluconeogenic pathway becomes viable in the newborn that no longer is deriving glucose from the mother. In the human neonate, the brain is dependent on glucose for its energy needs and therefore is dependent on gluconeogenically derived glucose during times of carbohydrate deprivation. The premature infant is prone to hypoglycemia due to small glycogen stores and the delay in induction of phosphoenolpyruvate carboxykinase activity after birth.

THE GLUCONEOGENIC PATHWAY

The gluconeogenic pathway is shown in Figure 12-6. The three irreversible steps of glycolysis must be reversed using a different enzyme-catalyzed step.

Conversion of Pyruvate to Phosphoenolpyruvate

The first step in gluconeogenesis from pyruvate or lactate that bypasses an irreversible glycolytic reaction is the conversion of pyruvate to phosphoenolpyruvate. This involves the activity of two enzymes, pyruvate carboxylase and phosphoenolpyruvate carboxykinase. Pyruvate is transferred from the cytosol to the mitochondrial compartment where it is a substrate for mitochondrial pyruvate carboxylase. (Pyruvate also can be generated by transamination of alanine in the mitochondrion itself.) In the mitochondrion, pyruvate is carboxylated to produce oxaloacetate. One molecule of ATP is hydrolyzed to ADP + P_i in this reaction, making this reaction irreversible. Pyruvate carboxylase is a biotin-dependent enzyme in which the covalently bound coenzyme functions as the carboxyl group carrier. The reaction can be described in two stages as follows:

$$\text{Enzyme-biotin} + \text{ATP} + HCO_3^- \leftrightarrow \text{Enzyme-biotin-}CO_2 + \text{ADP} + P_i$$

$$\text{Enzyme-biotin-}CO_2 + \text{Pyruvate} \leftrightarrow \text{Enzyme-biotin} + \text{Oxaloacetate}$$

In addition to the requirement for biotin as a coenzyme, this reaction also requires acetyl-CoA as a positive allosteric activator. When acetyl-CoA builds up from fatty acid β-oxidation in liver, it becomes available for activation of pyruvate carboxylase. Activation of pyruvate carboxylase promotes the conversion of pyruvate to oxaloacetate, an important step in gluconeogenesis. Under some conditions, such as starvation or a very low carbohydrate diet, this oxaloacetate may be needed to replenish citric acid cycle intermediates so that there is sufficient oxaloacetate to condense with acetyl-CoA. Thus conversion of pyruvate to oxaloacetate is important both for gluconeogenesis and for anaplerosis (the replenishment of citric acid cycle intermediates).

In the second enzymatic step in glucose biosynthesis from pyruvate, oxaloacetate is converted to phosphoenolpyruvate. This reaction is catalyzed by phosphoenolpyruvate carboxykinase. One molecule of the high-energy compound, guanosine triphosphate (GTP), is hydrolyzed in this reaction, as follows:

$$\text{Oxaloacetate} + \text{GTP} \xrightarrow{Mg^{2+}} \text{Phosphoenolpyruvate} + CO_2 + \text{GDP}$$

Although this is a reversible reaction, it is essentially irreversible in the cell because phosphoenolpyruvate is rapidly utilized.

In human liver, phosphoenolpyruvate carboxykinase is present in approximately equal concentrations in the mitochondria and the cytosol of the hepatocyte. Oxaloacetate is metabolized differently depending upon whether it is the substrate for the mitochondrial or cytosolic enzyme and whether it is derived from pyruvate or lactate.

When the gluconeogenic precursor is lactate, it must first be converted to pyruvate by lactate dehydrogenase, a reaction that generates NADH in the cytosol. Pyruvate then enters the mitochondrion and is converted to oxaloacetate by pyruvate carboxylase. Oxaloacetate is converted to phosphoenolpyruvate by mitochondrial phosphoenolpyruvate carboxykinase, and phosphoenolpyruvate can be transported across the mitochondrial membrane to the cytosol, where the remaining enzymes for gluconeogenesis are located. The lactate dehydrogenase reaction provides the required cytosolic NADH for a distal gluconeogenic step, the reversal of the glyceraldehyde 3-phosphate dehydrogenase reaction. Without this provision of cytosolic NADH, gluconeogenesis using the mitochondrial phosphoenolpyruvate carboxykinase route cannot continue.

A more complex process occurs when pyruvate is the gluconeogenic precursor, because mitochondrial reducing equivalents must be shuttled to the cytosol to support gluconeogenesis. Pyruvate enters the mitochondrion and is converted to oxaloacetate by pyruvate carboxylase, but oxaloacetate as such cannot traverse the mitochondrial membrane. Either malate or aspartate formed from oxaloacetate can leave the mitochondria. In the cytosol, malate, either directly from the mitochondria or generated by cytosolic fumarase from the fumarate released from aspartate during ureagenesis (see Chapter 14, Figure 14-11), is converted back to oxaloacetate by cytosolic malate dehydrogenase, with the concomitant reduction of NAD^+ to NADH. Oxaloacetate is then available as substrate for cytosolic phosphoenolpyruvate carboxykinase and cytosolic NADH has been provided. In effect, the shuttling of reducing equivalents as malate or aspartate moves potential NADH from the mitochondrion to the cytosol, providing the required NADH for the glyceraldehyde 3-phosphate dehydrogenase reaction as well as carbon substrate for gluconeogenesis.

Regardless of whether mitochondrial or cytosolic phosphoenolpyruvate carboxykinase is used, the successive actions of pyruvate carboxylase and phosphoenolpyruvate carboxykinase effectively bypass the pyruvate kinase reaction. Overall, these two reactions result in the net hydrolysis of one molecule each of ATP and GTP, which is equivalent

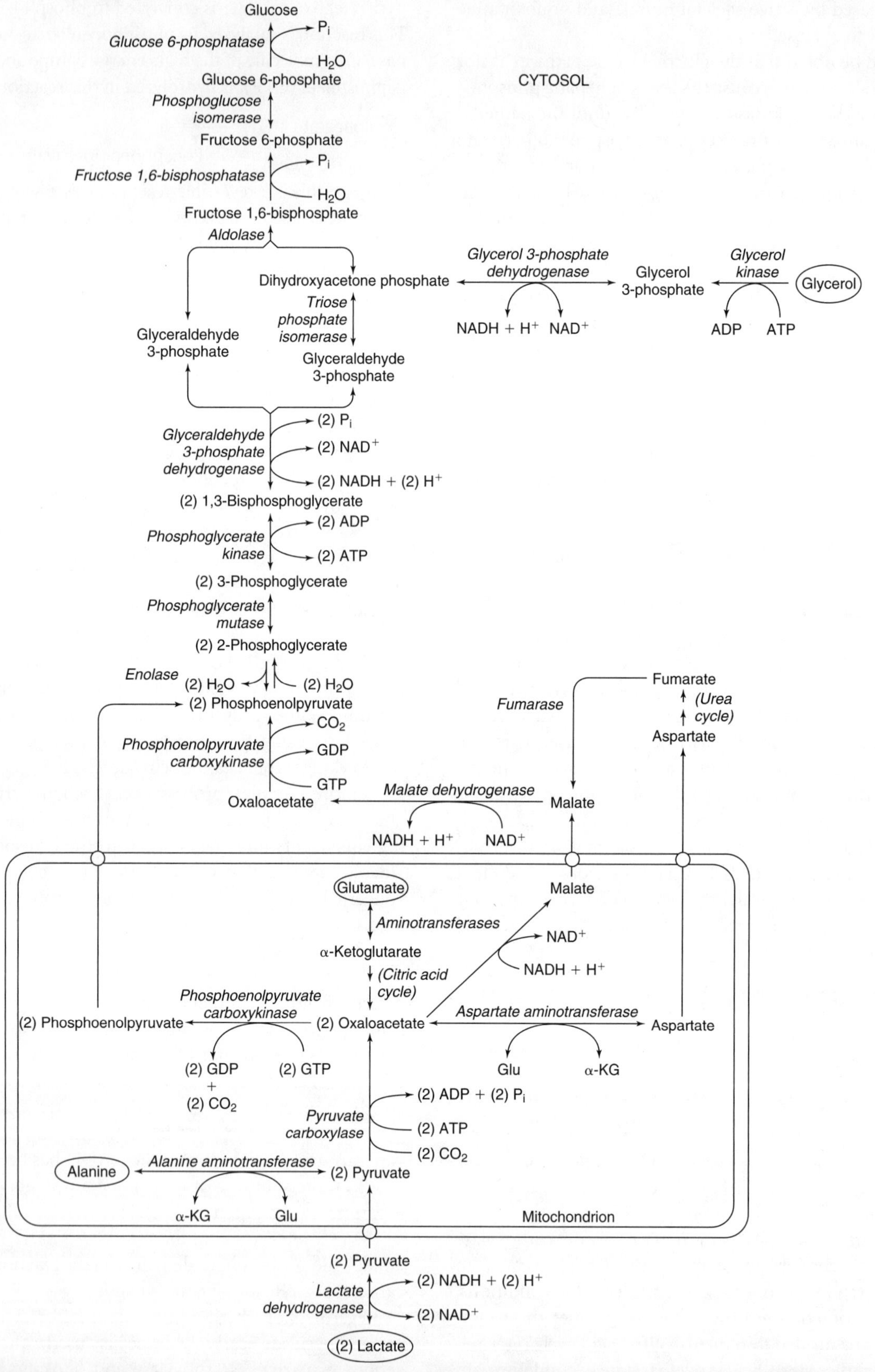

FIGURE 12-6 Gluconeogenesis from pyruvate, other precursors of phosphoenolpyruvate, and glycerol. Numbers in parentheses indicate the number of molecules of substrates and products for conversion of two molecules of lactate to one molecule of glucose in the cytosol via intermediate formation of pyruvate, oxaloacetate, and phosphoenolpyruvate. Other routes for synthesis and metabolism of oxaloacetate/phosphoenolpyruvate are shown.

to the energy cost of two molecules of ATP, because one ATP is required to convert GDP back to GTP.

Conversion of Fructose 1,6-Bisphosphate to Fructose 6-Phosphate

The second bypass reaction that is unique to gluconeogenesis is that catalyzed by fructose 1,6-bisphosphatase, as follows:

$$\text{Fructose 1,6-bisphosphate} + H_2O \rightarrow \text{Fructose 6-phosphate} + P_i$$

This reaction reverses the 6-phosphofructo-1-kinase reaction and is essentially irreversible under intracellular conditions. It should be noted that inorganic phosphate, not ATP, is generated from the bisphosphatase reaction.

Conversion of Glucose 6-Phosphate to Glucose

The terminal catalytic step in gluconeogenesis is the conversion of glucose 6-phosphate to glucose. This reaction provides free glucose for transport from the liver. The reaction is catalyzed by glucose 6-phosphatase and is essentially irreversible, as follows:

$$\text{Glucose 6-phosphate} + H_2O \rightarrow \text{Glucose} + P_i$$

The glucose 6-phosphatase reaction bypasses the glucokinase or hexokinase reaction. Glucose 6-phosphatase is important in both gluconeogenesis and glycogen breakdown because glucose 6-phosphate is produced in both of these pathways. Tissues that do not synthesize this enzyme do not have the ability to release glucose to the circulation, with the exception of glucose residues at branch points in glycogen, which can be released from glycogen as free glucose by the debranching enzyme discussed later in this chapter.

Glucose 6-phosphatase has a unique intracellular location. It is a membrane-bound enzyme in the endoplasmic reticulum (ER). Glucose 6-phosphatase activity is the result of the combined action of a glucose 6-phosphate translocase that moves glucose 6-phosphate into the lumen of the ER, the catalytic subunit that is responsible for the phosphohydrolase activity, and lastly, the glucose and P_i transporters that move the end products of the reaction back to the cytosol (Nordlie et al., 1993).

Energy Cost of Gluconeogenesis

Overall, the endogenous synthesis of glucose requires energy in the form of ATP. Six molecules of ATP/GTP and two molecules of NADH (i.e., a total of 12 ATP equivalents) are used for the synthesis of one molecule of glucose from two molecules of pyruvate. If lactate is the starting substrate for gluconeogenesis, the oxidation of lactate to pyruvate will generate NADH and the overall energy cost for conversion of two molecules lactate to glucose will be six ATP equivalents. In the liver, ATP to support gluconeogenesis is usually generated by the oxidation of fatty acids or by the partial oxidation of amino acid carbon chains, depending on fuel availability.

THE CORI AND ALANINE CYCLES

There is a metabolic connection between the liver and the tissues that depend on glucose for their energy needs. Both lactate and alanine generated in extrahepatic tissues can be carried in the circulation to the liver, where they serve as substrates for hepatic gluconeogenesis. The glucose produced from these precursors can be transported from the liver and carried back to extrahepatic tissues for glycolytic catabolism and energy generation. This occurs in two well-defined cycles: the Cori cycle and the alanine cycle, which are both shown in Figure 12-7 for muscle. Because the glucose carbon is recycled in both cases, these cycles do not require a net input of gluconeogenic substrate to the body.

In the Cori cycle, lactate generated from pyruvate, the end product of glycolysis, is released from tissues such as muscle

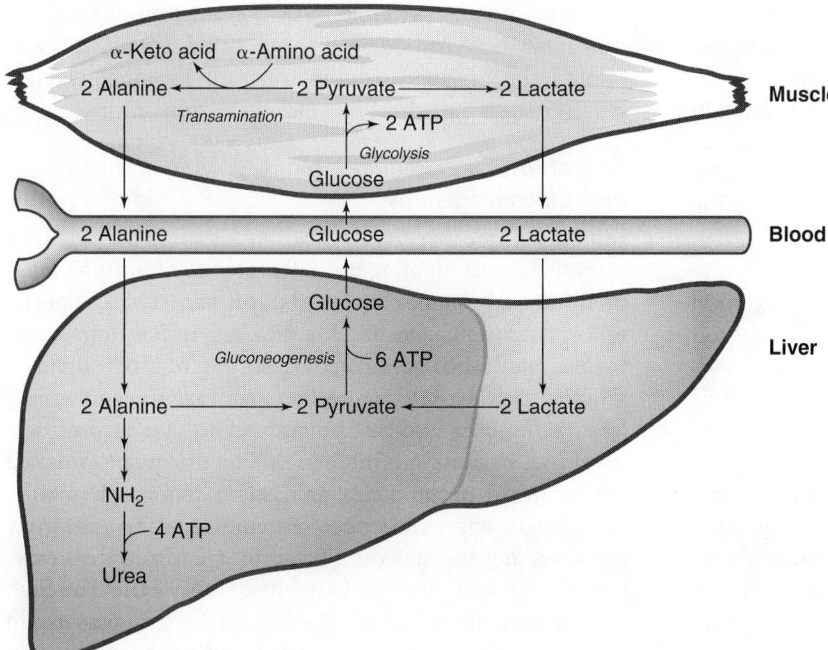

FIGURE 12-7 The Cori cycle (lactate–glucose cycle) and the alanine cycle (alanine–glucose cycle). Lactate from anaerobic metabolism of glucose is taken to the liver, where it may be used for gluconeogenesis to replenish plasma glucose. Pyruvate and amino groups leave tissues as alanine. The alanine is taken up by the liver where the pyruvate may be used for gluconeogenesis and the amino group may be converted to urea for excretion. Thus glucose may be converted to pyruvate (lacate, alanine) in tissues dependent on anaerobic metabolism, and the released lactate or alanine can be converted back to glucose in the liver and recycled back to the tissue via the blood.

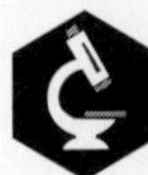

CLINICAL CORRELATION

Inherited Deficiencies in Gluconeogenic Enzymes

In humans, defects in both the cytosolic and the mitochondrial forms of phosphoenolpyruvate carboxykinase occur as rare, inherited autosomal recessive disorders. Defects in mitochondrial phosphoenolpyruvate carboxykinase are more common than ones in cytosolic phosphoenolpyruvate carboxykinase. A deficiency in either isoenzyme leads to hypoglycemia and lactic acidosis because sufficient glucose is not produced from pyruvate, lactate, or amino acid precursors. Therefore individuals with this disorder are dependent upon glycogenolysis for glucose during a fast and become hypoglycemic when glycogen is depleted. The symptoms of this disorder usually present early in life. The hypoglycemia can cause seizures, coma, or lethargy. Typically, this disorder is associated with progressive neurological damage (Buist, 1995). Other symptoms include hepatomegaly, kidney dysfunction, and cardiomyopathy. This disorder can be fatal.

Inherited fructose 1,6-bisphosphatase deficiency results in impaired gluconeogenesis from any of its precursors, including glycerol, lactate, and alanine. This disorder usually presents within the first few days of life, although in milder cases, presentation can be in early childhood. Symptoms of this disorder are similar to those described for phosphoenolpyruvate carboxykinase deficiency, that is, hypoglycemia and lactic acidosis. Fructose 1,6-bisphosphatase deficiency, however, does not result in neurodegenerative disorders as does phosphoenolpyruvate carboxykinase deficiency.

One of the most common genetic diseases to affect carbohydrate metabolism in humans is Von Gierke disease, which is caused by an autosomal recessive genetic defect in glucose 6-phosphatase. This defect results in a block in release of glucose 6-phosphate from liver as glucose. Individuals with this disease have impaired gluconeogenesis because glucose 6-phosphate cannot be converted to glucose. This defect also affects hepatic glucose export from the breakdown of glycogen. Because the glucose 6-phosphate is "trapped" in the liver, excessive accumulation of glycogen is observed.

Thinking Critically

Would defects in gluconeogenesis affect the recycling of glucose carbon by the lactate–glucose and alanine–glucose cycles? How would this affect the amount of "new" glucose that needs to be supplied by the diet to patients with these defects? Explain.

or red blood cells and is transported to the liver. In the liver, lactate is converted back to pyruvate by lactate dehydrogenase, and pyruvate can be used to synthesize glucose by gluconeogenesis. Gluconeogenically derived glucose is then secreted by the liver and recirculated through the blood to muscle or red blood cells for glycolysis.

A second cycle, the alanine cycle, involves the circulation of alanine from skeletal muscle to the liver. In muscle, alanine is generated from the transamination of glycolytically derived pyruvate and released. Liver cells take up the alanine and transaminate it to pyruvate, which serves as substrate for hepatic gluconeogenesis. Gluconeogenically derived glucose is then recycled from the liver back to muscle tissue. In the alanine cycle, unlike the Cori cycle, the NADH generated in skeletal muscle during glycolysis is not used to reduce pyruvate to lactate; therefore the NADH is available for mitochondrial electron transport and ATP production, assuming oxygen is sufficient.

REGULATION OF GLYCOLYSIS AND GLUCONEOGENESIS

In liver, the interconnected series of enzymatic reactions that constitute the glycolytic and gluconeogenic pathways are regulated in concert to ensure that cellular energy needs are met and that blood glucose levels are maintained. The mechanisms by which these pathways are regulated are complex. They include mechanisms for rapid or short-term regulation (e.g., regulation of enzyme activities by allosteric effectors or covalent modification such as phosphorylation) and mechanisms for long-term regulation by changes in the concentration of the proteins themselves. Although the complete pathway for gluconeogenesis is present only in liver and kidney, the opposing reactions of glycolysis and gluconeogenesis are also regulated in other tissues in which one or more of the gluconeogenic enzymes are present.

HORMONAL REGULATION OF GLYCOLYSIS AND GLUCONEOGENESIS

In response to nutrient and physiological stimuli, hormones mediate both short- and long-term regulation of substrate cycle enzymes. Insulin, glucagon, epinephrine, and glucocorticoids are the predominant hormones that regulate enzymes in carbohydrate metabolism.

Role of Insulin in Regulation of Glycolysis and Gluconeogenesis

When blood glucose levels are elevated, such as occurs after a carbohydrate-containing meal, the anabolic hormone insulin is secreted from the beta cells of the pancreas. The portal vein carries blood draining the digestive tract and pancreas to the liver, thereby ensuring the transport of pancreatic hormones including insulin directly to the liver sinusoids along with the absorbed monosaccharides. In the postabsorptive state, the insulin concentration is approximately threefold greater in the portal vein than in the peripheral blood. At these levels, approximately 180 pmol/L, insulin effectively decreases hepatic glucose production and also increases hepatic glycogen storage (see subsequent text). Although insulin does not stimulate glucose uptake by liver, insulin does upregulate glucokinase and signal increased glycogen storage and glycolysis at the same time that it decreases glycogenolysis and gluconeogenesis. The net result is increased glucose metabolism and decreased glucose production and release from the liver. There are also indirect effects of insulin on hepatic glucose metabolism. One indirect effect is due to insulin's inhibition of lipolysis in adipose tissue so that free fatty acid levels are decreased in the circulation and glucose is utilized by the hepatocytes for energy. The second indirect effect on liver glucose metabolism is due to insulin's ability to inhibit glucagon secretion by pancreatic beta cells (Cherrington et al., 2007). In skeletal muscle and adipose tissue, insulin stimulates glucose uptake via increased translocation of GLUT4 to the cell surface. Overall, insulin acts to decrease blood glucose levels primarily by increasing the uptake of glucose and its oxidation or storage as glycogen by liver and extrahepatic tissues and by decreasing glucose production and release by the liver.

Tissue responses to insulin depend on expression of insulin receptors and the presence of insulin signal transduction pathways. The insulin receptor is a member of the receptor tyrosine kinase family, a diverse group of glycoprotein transmembrane receptors with a cytoplasmic domain that has tyrosine kinase activity. The initiation of tyrosine kinase activity results in autophosphorylation of tyrosine residues in the β subunits of the receptor at three specific tyrosine residues: Tyr1158, Tyr1162, and Tyr1163. The tyrosine kinase activity of the insulin receptor increases with the degree of phosphorylation of these tyrosine residues and enables the insulin receptor tyrosine kinase domain to phosphorylate target proteins in the cytosol and the membrane. The phosphotyrosine residues of the insulin receptor are recognized by phosphotyrosine-binding domains of adaptor proteins, such as members of the insulin receptor substrate (IRS) family. The phosphorylation of these IRS proteins converts them to docking molecules that bind other downstream signaling proteins that have Src homology 2 (SH2) domains. The SH2 domain is a conserved region of approximately 100 amino acids that binds phosphotyrosine residues such as those on IRS proteins. The activated IRS or adaptor proteins then activate or inhibit various downstream molecules with SH2 domains and their related signaling pathways. Insulin signaling pathways are described in more detail in Chapter 19 (see Figure 19-6).

Relative to carbohydrate metabolism, insulin signaling leads to the activation or inhibition of enzyme activities, as well as to the activation or inhibition of the expression of metabolic genes. A major outcome of the phosphorylation of IRS proteins is the recruitment of phosphatidylinositol 3-kinase (PtdIns 3-kinase) to the inner face of the plasma membrane via binding of its SH2 domain to the IRS phosphotyrosine residues. PtdIns 3-kinase phosphorylates phosphatidylinositol 4,5-bisphosphate [PtdIns(4,5)P_2] and generates PtdIns(3,4,5)P_3, an important phospholipid second messenger that is involved in many of the metabolic effects of insulin (Kim and Novak, 2007). A key downstream effector of PtdIns(3,4,5)P_3 is the serine/threonine kinase Akt (also known as protein kinase B), which is recruited to the plasma membrane. Activation of Akt also requires the protein kinase 3-phosphoinositide-dependent protein kinase (PDK) and mammalian target of rapamycin complex 2 (mTORC2), which both phosphorylate and hence activate Akt. Once active, Akt leaves the membrane and enters the cytoplasm where it leads to the phosphorylation and activation or inactivation of its downstream target proteins.

With regard to glycolysis and gluconeogenesis, two key downstream targets are the forkhead box class O transcription factors (FoxOs) and phosphodiesterase (PDE). Phosphorylation of FoxO by Akt results in its nuclear exclusion so that it is inactive as a transcription factor; this causes expression of genes encoding gluconeogenic enzymes such as phosphoenolpyruvate carboxykinase and glucose 6-phosphatase to be suppressed by insulin. In addition, by activating phosphodiesterase, the enzyme that degrades cAMP, insulin specifically counters the glucagon–cAMP signaling pathway. This includes inhibiting cAMP-activated protein kinase A (PKA)–mediated phosphorylation of pyruvate kinase; producing more fructose 2,6-bisphosphate (F2,6P2), which is a positive regulator of glycolysis and a negative regulator of gluconeogenesis (described in subsequent text); and inhibiting PKA-mediated activation of cAMP-response element binding protein (CREB), a transcription factor that increases transcription of gluconeogenic genes. These effects of insulin signaling are discussed further in Chapter 19 (see Figure 19-8).

Insulin signaling via the PtdIns 3-kinase/Akt route also results in activation of the mammalian target of rapamycin complex 1 (mTORC1), which also promotes expression of glycolytic genes. In addition, insulin signaling via PtdIns 3-kinase/Akt has effects on glycogen synthesis and lipogenesis. Akt phosphorylation inhibits glycogen synthase kinase 3 (GSK3), and this favors glycogen synthesis as is discussed in a subsequent section of this chapter. Insulin also induces the transcription factor sterol regulatory element binding protein 1c (SREBP-1c) that stimulates lipogenesis in liver (Laplante and Sabatini, 2010).

Glucose and insulin signaling also result in the dephosphorylation of carbohydrate response element binding protein (ChREBP), promoting both the entry of this transcription factor into the nucleus and its binding to response elements in the promoters of certain glycolytic and lipogenic genes, including those encoding liver-type pyruvate kinase (PKLR), acetyl-CoA carboxylase, and fatty acid synthase. During starvation, activation of PKA and AMPK maintain ChREBP in an inactive state via diminished DNA binding capacity and subcellular compartmentalization mechanisms.

Role of Glucagon in Regulation of Glycolysis and Gluconeogenesis

When blood glucose levels are low, as in fasting or starvation, the alpha cells of the pancreas respond by releasing the polypeptide hormone glucagon to the bloodstream. In humans, liver is the main target for glucagon action. Glucagon promotes increased blood glucose levels by increasing hepatic glucose production via enhanced glycogenolysis and gluconeogenesis.

Glucagon receptors are integral membrane proteins that span the lipid bilayer of the plasma membrane. Binding of glucagon to a glucagon receptor on the cell surface results in a conformational change in the receptor, and this conformational change triggers GTP–GDP exchange and the release of the α-subunit of the G stimulatory (G_s) protein. This activated α-subunit in turn activates adenylate cyclase, which converts ATP to cAMP, the intracellular second messenger. The level of cAMP in the cell regulates the activity of PKA. When cAMP is low, PKA exists as an inactive heterotetrameric complex containing two regulatory subunits and two catalytic subunits. When cAMP binds to the regulatory subunits, the catalytic subunits are released in active form.

Activated PKA is responsible for the phosphorylation and consequent activation or inactivation of a variety of proteins involved in glycogen, glucose, and lipid metabolism. Gluconeogenesis is increased in liver by PKA-mediated phosphorylation and inhibition of pyruvate kinase; by phosphorylation of the bifunctional 6-phosphofructo-2-kinase/fructose-2,6-biphosphatase, resulting in decreased production of F2,6P2, the allosteric activator of glycolysis and inhibitor of gluconeogenesis; and by phosphorylation of the transcription factor CREB, resulting in increased cAMP-response element (CRE)-mediated transcription of gluconeogenic enzymes glucose 6-phosphatase and phosphoenolpyruvate carboxykinase. In general, glucagon stimulates increased hepatic glucose output and is a counterregulatory hormone to insulin, as are the glucocorticoids and epinephrine. In addition to stimulation of gluconeogenesis, glucagon signaling via cAMP/PKA stimulates hepatic glucose output by stimulating glycogenolysis. As is discussed in a subsequent section of this chapter, PKA activates phosphorylase kinase (and inhibits the phosphatase), leading to phosphorylation and activation of glycogen phosphorylase, turning on glycogen breakdown.

Role of Catecholamines and Glucocorticoids in Regulation of Glycolysis and Gluconeogenesis

Glucocorticoids and epinephrine are also released in response to decreased blood glucose. Glucocorticoids are steroid hormones produced in the adrenal cortex that are permissive for the action of other hormones such as glucagon. Epinephrine and norepinephrine are catecholamines synthesized from tyrosine and produced mainly by the chromaffin cells of the adrenal medulla and the postganglionic fibers of the sympathetic nervous system.

The response of a given tissue to catecholamines depends on the predominance of specific adrenergic receptor types on the cell surface. The adrenergic receptors are grouped into α (α_1, α_2) and β (β_1, β_2, β_3) subtypes, and tissue distribution of these receptors varies. Epinephrine stimulation of β-receptors increases glycogenolysis and gluconeogenesis in liver, as well as lipolysis in adipose tissue and muscle. Epinephrine stimulation of α_1-receptors results in increased glycogenolysis, whereas stimulation of α_2-receptors results in decreased lipolysis.

The β-adrenergic receptors, like glucagon receptors, are G_s-protein coupled receptors that, when activated, stimulate the production of cAMP and activation of PKA. The β-adrenergic receptors are more widespread than glucagon receptors and are present in muscle and adipose tissue as well as liver. Liver cells respond to both glucagon and epinephrine; the cAMP signal is the accumulated total produced by stimulation of both the glucagon and the β-adrenergic receptors. The effects of cAMP on carbohydrate metabolism were summarized for glucagon signaling.

Catecholamine binding to α_1- and α_2-adrenergic receptors has different effects. Activation of the α_1-adrenergic receptor stimulates phospholipase C on the cytoplasmic face of the plasma membrane by a GTP-binding protein mechanism similar to that for activation of adenylate cyclase. Phospholipase C hydrolyzes phosphatidylinositol 4,5-bisphosphate [PtdIns(4,5)P2], present in the plasma membrane, to release inositol 1,4,5-triphosphate [$Ins(1,4,5)P_3$] and diacylglycerol. Diacylglycerol, in turn, stimulates protein kinase C. Protein kinase C has numerous substrates in the cell, some of which are key enzymes in hepatic glycogen metabolism, as described later in this chapter. IP_3 stimulates the release of Ca^{2+} from the ER, and calcium efflux activates the calcium/calmodulin-dependent protein kinase, as well as other enzymes. The calcium/calmodulin-dependent protein kinase catalyzes the phosphorylation and inactivation of pyruvate kinase, contributing to the diminution of the glycolytic rate (Pilkis and Claus, 1991).

Activation of α_2-adrenergic receptors does not play a significant role in carbohydrate metabolism, although they are involved in decreasing lipolysis. The activated α_2-receptor stimulates a series of intracellular events similar to those initiated by the β-adrenergic receptors, except that an inhibitory (rather than a stimulatory) GTP-binding protein (G_i) is released and becomes associated with adenylate cyclase. G_i protein binding inhibits adenylate cyclase and leads to an overall decrease in intracellular cAMP levels.

Glucocorticoids are steroid hormones that are secreted in response to many types of physical or mental stress. Like other steroid hormones, glucocorticoids do not bind to plasma membrane receptors and thereby initiate a series of intracellular events but rather traverse the lipid bilayer of the plasma membrane and enter the cell. Within the cytoplasm of the cell, glucocorticoids bind to their cognate receptors and subsequently enter the nucleus as activated ligand-receptor complexes. In the nucleus, the activated receptors take on the role of transcription factors and bind to regulatory regions of target genes, thereby increasing or decreasing expression of these responsive genes, many of which encode metabolic enzymes. One of the functions of glucocorticoids is to suppress insulin signaling. Suppression of insulin signaling, in turn, stimulates gluconeogenesis in the liver, inhibits uptake of glucose in muscle and adipose tissue, stimulates lipolysis in adipose tissue, and stimulates mobilization of amino acids from extrahepatic tissues. These responses ensure increased availability of both glucose and fatty acids as fuels for the body during physical and mental stress situations.

REGULATION OF GLYCOLYSIS AND GLUCONEOGENESIS: SUBSTRATE CYCLES

Regulation of glycolysis and gluconeogenesis occurs mainly by changes in the activity of enzymes that catalyze the irreversible steps of the two pathways. The irreversible steps of glycolysis are catalyzed by glucokinase (or hexokinase), 6-phosphofructo-1-kinase, and pyruvate kinase. The "reversal" of these steps in the gluconeogenic pathway is catalyzed by glucose 6-phosphatase, fructose 1,6-bisphosphatase, and pyruvate carboxylase plus phosphoenolpyruvate carboxykinase.

The fine-tuned regulation of glycolysis and gluconeogenesis in liver can be understood by examining the functional concept of the substrate cycle. A substrate cycle consists of two opposing enzymatic reactions, with the potential to continuously cycle substrate and product (Figure 12-8). If this occurs in glucose metabolism, energy is lost and there is no net movement of product in either the glycolytic or the gluconeogenic direction. In liver, three substrate cycles exist due to the essentially irreversible reactions of glycolysis coupled with those of gluconeogenesis: the reaction catalyzed by glucokinase coupled with that catalyzed by glucose 6-phosphatase; the reaction catalyzed by 6-phosphofructo-1-kinase coupled with that catalyzed by fructose 1,6-bisphosphatase; and the reaction catalyzed by pyruvate kinase coupled with that catalyzed by pyruvate carboxylase and phosphoenolpyruvate carboxykinase. The paired enzymes of each specific substrate cycle are regulated in a coordinated fashion so that the stimulation of one is accompanied by the inhibition of the other. Although both enzymes function simultaneously, one functions at a higher and the other at a lower percentage of its maximum activity. This coordinated regulation allows for a magnification of the regulatory effect and decreases the potential for futile cycling of substrate and product (Pilkis and Claus, 1991).

In the liver, the rates of the enzymatic reactions in one substrate cycle are usually coordinated with the rates of other substrate cycle enzymes in the same pathway. For example, when blood glucose levels are low, glucagon levels increase and insulin levels decrease, resulting in an overall decrease in the insulin-glucagon ratio in the blood. This activates (by different mechanisms) phosphoenolpyruvate carboxykinase, fructose 1,6-bisphosphatase, and glucose 6-phosphatase and also inhibits pyruvate kinase, 6-phosphofructo-1-kinase, and glucokinase. These changes favor gluconeogenesis, which contributes to reestablishing normal blood glucose levels. Conversely, a high-carbohydrate diet, particularly following a fast, stimulates the release of insulin and decreases the release of glucagon from the pancreas. The rise in the insulin-glucagon ratio causes an increase in the activity of the glycolytic enzymes of the respective substrate cycles, with a concomitant decrease in the specific enzymes of gluconeogenesis. This response favors glucose utilization for energy or the synthesis of other biomolecules such as fatty

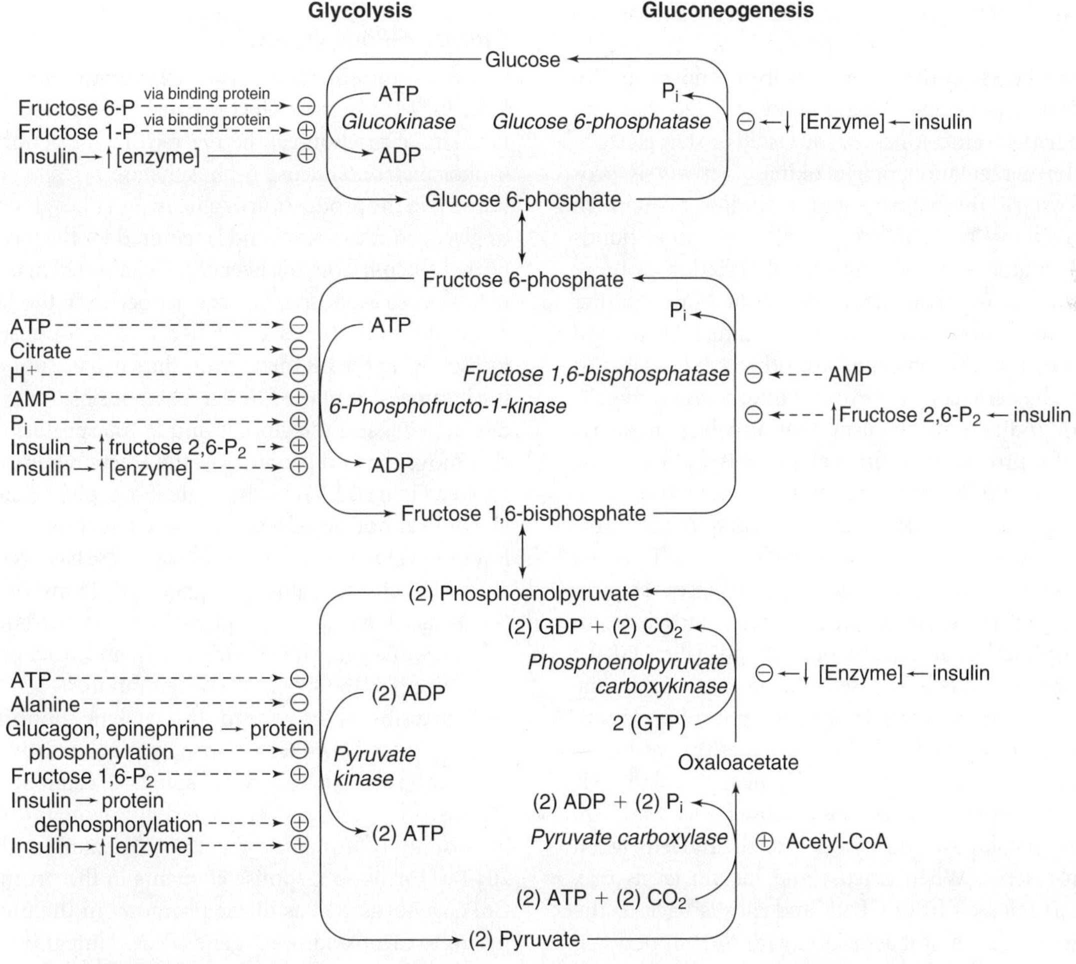

FIGURE 12-8 Substrate cycles and major points of regulation of glycolysis and gluconeogenesis in liver.

acids. Clearly, this coordinated regulation allows the liver to respond to changes in the diet with altered enzymatic activity at each substrate cycle, which in turn determines the overall glycolytic or gluconeogenic rate of the tissue.

COORDINATED REGULATION OF THE ACTIVITY OF HEPATIC GLUCOKINASE AND GLUCOSE 6-PHOSPHATASE

In liver, a substrate cycle is established between the actions of glucokinase and glucose 6-phosphatase. Similarly, the actions of hexokinase and glucose 6-phosphatase constitute a substrate cycle in kidney. Restricting glucose phosphorylation under conditions where gluconeogenesis (and hence glucose 6-phosphatase) is active limits glucose/glucose 6-phosphate futile cycling.

Glucokinase and Glucokinase Regulatory Protein

Glucokinase is present in both hepatocytes and pancreatic beta cells. These two cell types regulate expression of the tissue-specific glucokinase gene *GCK* by use of different promoters, different transcription start sites, and alternate splicing to generate glucokinase isoforms that have different N-terminal sequences (Magnuson and Jetton, 1993, Postic et al., 2001). Use of different gene promoters allows regulation of liver glucokinase in response to insulin and glucagon, whereas pancreatic glucokinase is regulated in response to blood glucose concentration. In liver, insulin stimulates transcription of *GCK,* and glucagon inhibits transcription of the *GCK* gene. This mechanism provides long-term regulation of glucokinase concentration in liver, and promotes higher levels of hepatic glucokinase in the well-fed state and low levels of hepatic glucokinase in the fasted or starved state.

Shorter-term regulation of glucokinase activity is provided by allosteric mechanisms and a binding protein. In general, glucokinase has a high K_m for glucose and responds to increases in glucose uptake by phosphorylation of more glucose to glucose 6-phosphate, as mentioned in an earlier section. Although glucokinase is not modified by its end product, glucose 6-phosphate, as are other hexokinases, it is subject to allosteric control by other intermediary metabolites by an indirect mechanism that involves allosteric regulation of a protein that binds glucokinase, glucokinase regulatory protein (GKRP) (Brocklehurst et al., 2004).

Whereas glucose phosphorylation occurs in the cytoplasm, GKRP is located in the nucleus of the cell. When GKRP is active and binds glucokinase, glucokinase is sequestered in the nucleus where it can no longer participate in glucose phosphorylation. On the other hand, when GKRP is inactive, glucokinase is released and is localized to the cytoplasm where it is active in glucose phosphorylation. Inhibition of glucokinase by GKRP is competitive with glucose. When the glucose supply is ample, most glucokinase is present in the cytoplasm of cells. As glucose levels diminish, GKRP binds glucokinase and moves it to the nucleus when it is held in reserve. When glucose and insulin levels rise, glucokinase is released from GKRP and moves back to the cytoplasm where much of it associates with the bifunctional 6-phosphofructo-2-kinase/fructose-2,6-biphosphatase.

This indirect regulation of glucokinase involves direct regulation of the affinity of GKRP for glucokinase by allosteric regulators, fructose 6-phosphate and fructose 1-phosphate (Figure 12-9). Fructose 6-phosphate is present in the cell in equilibrium with glucose 6-phosphate because of the reversibility of the phosphoglucose isomerase reaction. The affinity of GKRP for glucokinase is increased by fructose 6-phosphate, which sequesters glucokinase in the nucleus to restrict glucose phosphorylation; thus glucokinase activity is inhibited by fructose 6-phosphate. Therefore fructose 6-phosphate is a negative feedback metabolite that signals the cell that glucokinase activity should decrease to prevent the buildup of glucose 6-phosphate. Conversely, fructose 1-phosphate decreases the affinity of GKRP for glucokinase, which releases glucokinase to enter the cytoplasm and participate in glucose phosphorylation; so glucokinase activity is stimulated by fructose 1-phosphate (Nordlie et al., 1999; de la Iglesia et al., 1999). Fructose 1-phosphate is present in the liver parenchymal cell only when fructose is being metabolized; therefore when fructose is available, the negative feedback inhibition of glucokinase is released. Overall, the availability of fructose, most often from dietary sucrose, can be coordinated indirectly with increased uptake of glucose via this relief of inhibition of glucokinase activity. This may contribute to increased channeling of acetyl-CoA to lipogenesis when high-fructose diets are consumed.

Glucose 6-Phosphatase

Glucose 6-phosphatase is present primarily in the liver and kidneys. Thus in these gluconeogenic tissues, the glucokinase/hexokinase reaction can be reversed by the action of glucose 6-phosphatase. Glucose 6-phosphatase is responsible for the last step in the production of glucose by either gluconeogenesis or glycogen breakdown and is required for the terminal transport of glucose from the liver cell. As indicated in the preceding text, glucose 6-phosphatase activity occurs in the ER and is the result of the combined action of a glucose 6-phosphate translocase (T_1) in the ER membrane, the catalytic subunit (CU) on the luminal side of the ER that is responsible for the phosphatase activity, and the glucose and P_i transporters (T_2 and T_3) that move the end products of the reaction back to the cytosol (see Figure 12-9). Without glucose 6-phosphatase activity, glucose cannot be released to the circulation in response to low blood glucose. Glucose 6-phosphatase has a relatively high K_m for its substrate, glucose 6-phosphate (3 mmol/L). Because the intracellular glucose 6-phosphate concentration is about 0.2 mmol/L, the rate of this enzymatic reaction primarily depends upon the substrate concentration.

Expression of the gene for the catalytic subunit of glucose 6-phosphatase *(G6PC)* is strongly regulated by hormones. Expression of glucose 6-phosphatase catalytic subunit is increased by glucocorticoids and glucagon and is repressed by insulin (Onuma et al., 2009; Yabaluri and Bashyam, 2010). Hormone response elements in the promoter of the *G6PC* gene, as well as in the promoter of the phosphoenolpyruvate carboxykinase 1 gene *(PCK1)* integrate various signals to achieve changes in the levels of these enzymes and

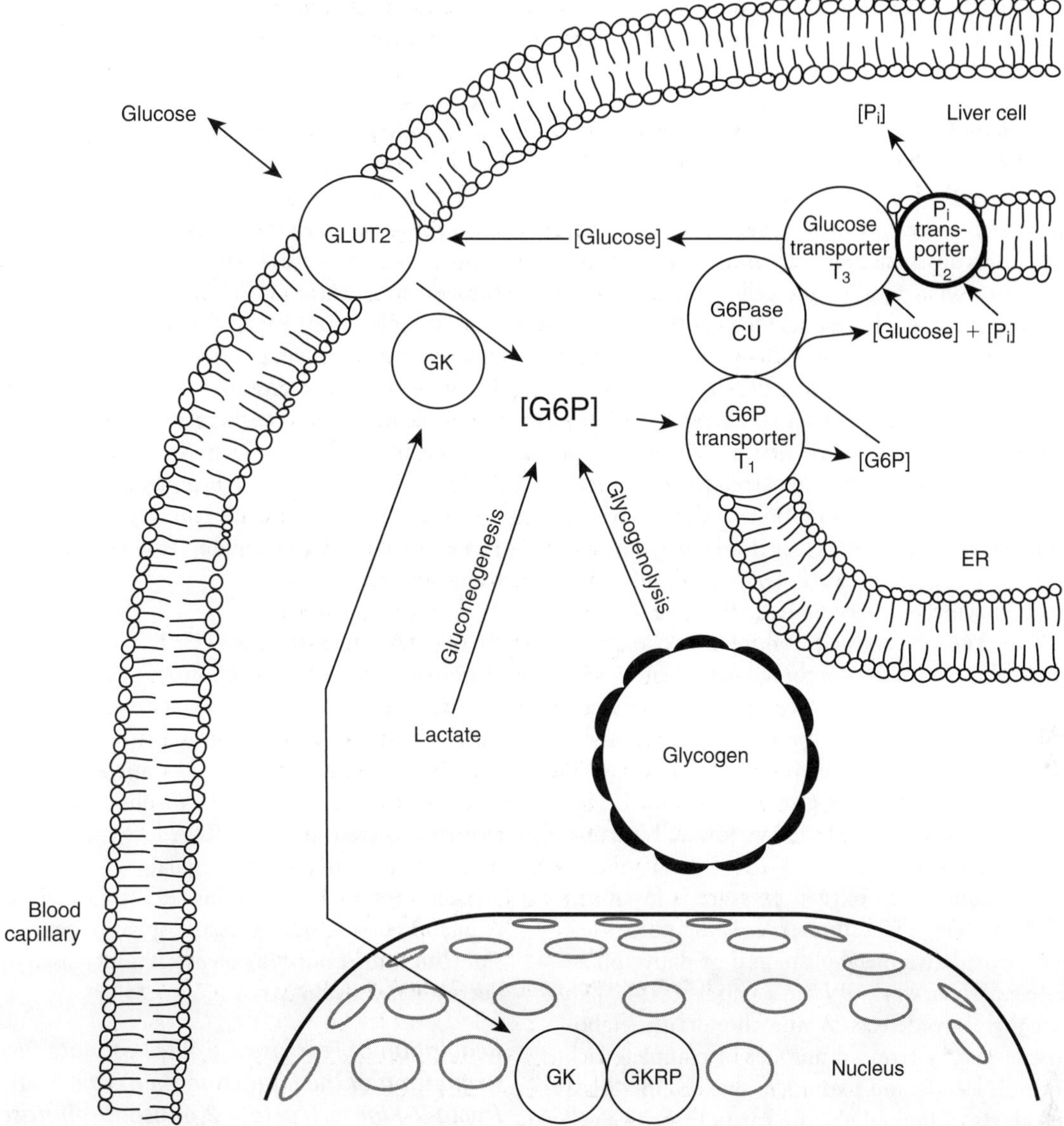

FIGURE 12-9 Diagram of the initial steps in glucose uptake and the terminal steps in glucose secretion from the liver parenchymal cell. Highlighted are GLUT2, the glucose transporter that conducts glucose import or export depending on the blood and cellular glucose concentrations; glucokinase (*GK*), the enzyme that is sequestered in the nucleus by the inhibitory protein, glucokinase regulatory protein (*GKRP*), under conditions of low glucose and high fructose 6-phosphate but is released from GKRP to the cytoplasm in the presence of fructose-1-phosphate or high glucose concentrations; and the multi-subunit glucose 6-phosphatase, which is associated with the endoplasmic reticulum (*ER*) and is made up of a catalytic subunit (*CU*) and at least three translocase (*T*) subunits that are involved in the import of glucose 6-phosphate into the ER and the export of glucose and P_i from the ER. Also shown are sources of glucose 6-phosphate (*G6P*), from either gluconeogenesis or glycogenolysis. (Used with permission of Annual Reviews, from Nordlie, R. C., Foster, J. D., & Lange, A. J. (1999). Regulation of glucose production by the liver. *Annual Review of Nutrition, 19*, 379–406; permission conveyed through Copyright Clearance Center, Inc.)

hence to maintain the plasma glucose concentration within a narrow range. *G6PC* contains elements for binding of the glucocorticoid receptor, hepatic nuclear factor 4α (HNF 4α), CREB, FoxO1 or FoxO3, and other proteins. FoxO may be the major stimulatory factor for *G6PC* expression (Matsumoto et al., 2007); the transcriptional activity of FoxO1 is inhibited by insulin signaling through PtdIns 3-kinase/Akt. Insulin also inhibits CREB-regulated transcriptional coactivator 2 (CRTC2) activation and stimulates its degradation, thus blocking CREB/CRTC2-mediated transcriptional activation of *G6PC*. Thus, the level of glucose 6-phosphatase is relatively low in the fed state but increases during fasting when gluconeogenesis and glycogen breakdown need to occur in the liver to maintain plasma glucose homeostasis.

REGULATION OF 6-PHOSPHOFRUCTO-1-KINASE AND FRUCTOSE 1,6-BISPHOSPHATASE

In liver, the central regulatory site in glycolysis and gluconeogenesis is the substrate cycle established by the 6-phosphofructo-1-kinase and fructose 1,6-bisphosphatase reactions. This substrate cycle is also present in other tissues such as kidney and muscle. Short-term regulation of this substrate cycle is critically important.

Allosteric Regulation of 6-Phosphofructo-1-kinase and Fructose 1,6-Bisphosphatase

The reaction catalyzed by 6-phosphofructo-1-kinase is the first committed step in glycolysis. It is subject to allosteric regulation by numerous metabolites that signal the energy level, pH, and hormonal status of the cell. Positive regulators of 6-phosphofructo-1-kinase include AMP, inorganic phosphate, and F2,6P2 (described in subsequent text); negative regulators include ATP, hydrogen ions, and citrate. ATP, AMP, and P_i signal the energy state of the cell; hydrogen ions signal the pH of the cell; citrate, the first metabolite of the citric acid cycle, signals the availability of sources of fuel; and F2,6P2 signals the insulin-glucagon ratio.

The gluconeogenic enzyme fructose 1,6-bisphosphatase is also allosterically regulated. AMP is a strong allosteric inhibitor of this enzyme, as are F2,6P2 and possibly fructose 1,6-bisphosphate. There is a synergistic inhibition of fructose 1,6-bisphosphatase by the combined action of F2,6P2 and AMP (Pilkis and Claus, 1991). When fuel for the citric acid cycle and oxygen are sufficient for oxidative phosphorylation, ATP levels in the cell are high, 6-phosphofructo-1-kinase is inhibited, and the rate of glycolysis is slow. Under the same conditions, AMP and P_i levels are low and fructose 1-6-bisphosphatase is active.

On the other hand, when oxygen pressure is low (e.g., hypoxia) or when ATP expenditure exceeds the mitochondrial capacity for oxidative metabolism and oxidative phosphorylation (e.g., when work is near or above VO_{2max} in muscle, when there are defects in mitochondrial metabolism, or in tissues with a reduced number or complete lack of mitochondria), lactate and hydrogen ions are increased as the end products of limited glucose catabolism. The cell releases lactate and hydrogen ions into the blood, which, when in excess, can cause lactic acidosis. However, because hydrogen ions inhibit 6-phosphofructo-1-kinase activity, the glycolytic rate can be controlled to protect against lactate buildup.

A third inhibitory metabolite, citrate, signals the cell that substrates for the citric acid cycle, both oxaloacetate and acetyl-CoA, are plentiful. Under these conditions, citrate is transported from the mitochondria to the cytosol, where it allosterically inhibits 6-phosphofructo-1-kinase, thereby decreasing the rate of glycolysis and sparing glucose. With excess carbohydrate consumption, the citrate produced is channeled to fatty acid synthesis in the cytosol of the hepatocyte, with further synthesis to triacylglycerols for export in very-low-density lipoproteins (VLDLs) (see Chapter 16).

The allosteric regulator F2,6P2 is a potent activator of 6-phosphofructo-1-kinase and an inhibitor of fructose 1,6-bisphosphatase. The level of hepatic F2,6P2 is increased by carbohydrate feeding or insulin administration. Overall, when insulin levels increase, F2,6P2 levels rise and the rate of the 6-phosphofructo-1-kinase reaction is increased, thereby stimulating glycolysis. In contrast, when glucagon or epinephrine levels are elevated, F2,6P2 levels are low and fructose 1,6-bisphosphatase activity is increased, resulting in an increase in gluconeogenesis. Regulation of the 6-phosphofructo-1-kinase/fructose-1,6-bisphosphatase substrate cycle by F2,6P2 is central in determining the overall flux of carbon to either glycolysis or gluconeogenesis in the liver. The end products, fructose 1,6-bisphosphate or fructose 6-phosphate, have positive feed-forward effects on subsequent substrate cycles in either the glycolytic or gluconeogenic direction. When 6-phosphofructo-1-kinase activity is increased by F2,6P2, the increase in product, fructose 1,6-bisphosphate, allosterically activates pyruvate kinase by a feed-forward mechanism. Conversely, when fructose 1,6-bisphosphatase activity is increased by a decrease in F2,6P2, more fructose 6-phosphate is produced. Fructose 6-phosphate is rapidly converted to glucose 6-phosphate, thereby providing increased substrate for glucose 6-phosphatase.

Regulation of Gene Expression

Expression of the 6-phosphofructo-1-kinase gene (*PFK*) in the liver is increased in response to carbohydrate refeeding after a fast, and this response can be partially blocked by the administration of cAMP. Hepatic *PFK* mRNA levels are also increased in response to insulin treatment of diabetic animals. Therefore *PFK* mRNA levels in liver appear to be determined by the counterregulatory signals of insulin and glucagon (Granner and Pilkis, 1990). Little is known about regulation of fructose 1,6-bisphosphatase gene (*FBP*) expression, but some evidence suggests it is increased by cAMP and decreased by insulin.

Regulation of Fructose 2,6-Bisphosphate Production: Regulation of the Bifunctional Enzyme 6-Phosphofructo-2-Kinase/Fructose 2,6-Bisphosphatase

The bifunctional enzyme 6-phosphofructo-2-kinase/fructose 2,6-bisphosphatase catalyzes both the synthesis and the breakdown of the allosteric factor F2,6P2. The discovery of F2,6P2 as an allosteric molecule in 1980 significantly advanced our understanding of the regulation of key enzymes involved in glucose metabolism. In liver, F2,6P2 is a major regulatory molecule, controlling the overall direction of carbon flux toward either glycolysis or gluconeogenesis (Pilkis et al., 1990).

The carbohydrate content of the diet controls insulin and glucagon concentrations in the blood, which in turn regulate the production of F2,6P2. The 6-phosphofructo-2-kinase activity of the bifunctional enzyme is responsible for F2,6P2 production, whereas the fructose 2,6-bisphosphatase activity of the bifunctional enzyme is responsible for F2,6P2 removal. The bifunctional enzyme is regulated by glucagon, insulin, and glucose, which promote changes in the phosphorylation state of the enzyme. After a carbohydrate-containing meal, circulating blood glucose levels increase and stimulate insulin secretion from the beta cells of the pancreas. Glucose, via a downstream metabolite, xylulose 5-phosphate, activates phosphoprotein phosphatase 2A, a ubiquitous cytoplasmic serine/threonine phosphatase, which dephosphorylates Ser32 of the liver bifunctional enzyme (Dentin et al., 2006; Okar et al., 2004). Insulin also activates a phosphatase that dephosphorylates the bifunctional enzyme, further promoting the dephosphorylation of the bifunctional enzyme and therefore an increase in its kinase activity. This favors F2,6P2 synthesis from fructose 6-phosphate and ATP. Overall, when glucose and insulin levels increase, F2,6P2 levels rise and the rate of the 6-phosphofructo-1-kinase reaction is increased, thereby stimulating glycolysis, as shown in Figure 12-10, *A*.

Conversely, as an individual begins to fast, circulating insulin levels decrease and the alpha cells of the pancreas respond to low blood glucose by secreting glucagon. Glucagon initiates an increase in intracellular cAMP and therefore activates PKA, which phosphorylates the bifunctional enzyme at Ser32. This alters the conformation of the bifunctional enzyme, decreasing the 6-phosphofructo-2-kinase activity and increasing the fructose 2,6-bisphosphatase activity. This rapidly decreases F2,6P2 levels in liver, which releases the inhibition of fructose 1,6-bisphosphatase and favors gluconeogenesis (see Figure 12-10, *B*). Both the 6-phosphofructo-2-kinase and the fructose 2,6-bisphosphatase reactions are also inhibited by the end products of their respective reactions, F2,6P2 and fructose 6-phosphate.

Thus the numerous blood-borne signals of nutrient status are integrated within the cell by changes in the concentration of F2,6P2 as a single signal (Okar et al., 2004). Overall, the predominant factors that determine F2,6P2 levels in liver are the concentration of fructose 6-phosphate and the phosphorylation state of the bifunctional enzyme.

Studies done in rat liver indicate that in the fed state, fructose 6-phosphate levels are in the 0.1 to 0.2 μmol/g range, and the bifunctional enzyme is in the dephosphorylated state. In this conformation, the 6-phosphofructo-2-kinase reaction is favored by a decrease in the K_m for its substrate, fructose 6-phosphate. Under these conditions, the intracellular substrate concentration is significantly higher than the K_m, maximizing the rate of F2,6P2 production. During fasting (or diabetes) the bifunctional enzyme becomes phosphorylated at Ser32, which activates the fructose 2,6-bisphosphatase and inhibits the 6-phosphofructo-2-kinase. The conformational change induced at the active site of 6-phosphofructo-2-kinase increases the K_m for substrate, fructose 6-phosphate. At the same time, during fasting, intracellular levels of fructose 6-phosphate decrease to below the K_m, and the rate of F2,6P2 production is concomitantly slowed (Pilkis et al., 1995). Fructose 6-phosphate is also a substrate for 6-phosphofructo-1-kinase; however, the rate of this reaction is two to three orders of magnitude greater than that of the 6-phosphofructo-2-kinase reaction. Therefore the shunting of fructose 6-phosphate to F2,6P2 production occurs at a much slower rate, and the amount of glycolytic fuel used for the synthesis of this regulatory molecule is small.

In addition to the role of 6-phosphofructo-2-kinase/fructose 2,6-bisphosphatase in regulation of intracellular F2,6P2 levels, the bifunctional enzyme has other regulatory roles in glucose metabolism. The dephosphorylated bifunctional enzyme can form protein–protein interactions with glucokinase in the cytosol (Okar et al., 2004). This coordinates the first step of glycolysis with the rate of the 6-phosphofructo-1-kinase reaction: the dephosphorylated bifunctional enzyme increases F2,6P2 levels and thus 6-phosphofructo-1-kinase activity; it also binds to glucokinase, thus activating glucose 6-phosphate formation.

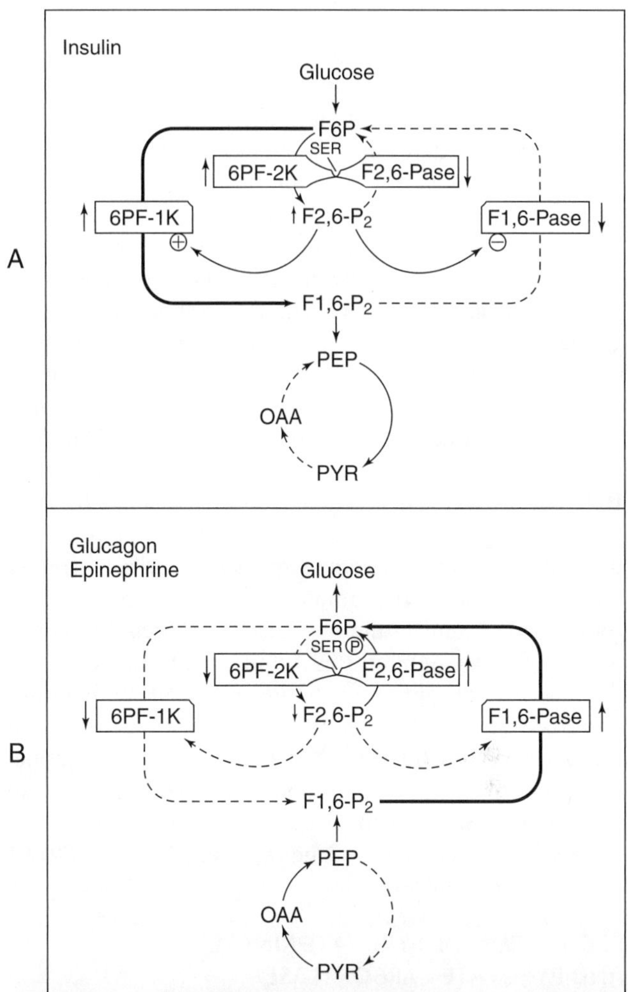

FIGURE 12-10 Regulation of the bifunctional enzyme 6-phosphofructo-2-kinase (*6PF-2K*)/fructose 2,6-bisphosphatase (*F2,6-Pase*) by phosphorylation (**B**, glucagon or catecholamines) and dephosphorylation (**A**, insulin), and the allosteric regulation of 6-phosphofructo-1-kinase (*6PF-1K*) and fructose 1,6-bisphosphatase (*F1,6-Pase*) by fructose 2,6-bisphosphate (*F2,6-P_2*). *F6P,* Fructose 6-phosphate; *SER,* serine residue; *PEP,* phosphoenolpyruvate; *OAA,* oxaloacetate; *PYR,* pyruvate; *P,* $-PO_3^{2-}$.

In addition to the short-term regulation of 6-phosphofructo-2-kinase/fructose 2,6-bisphosphatase described above, this bifunctional enzyme is regulated at the level of gene expression. There are different 6-phosphofructo-2-kinase/fructose 2,6-bisphosphatase (PFKFB) isoenzymes, which have specific catalytic properties, tissue distributions, and responses to regulatory molecules. Four genes have been identified in mammals encoding the different isoenzymes;

they are called *PFKFB1* (liver/muscle isoenzyme), *PFKFB2* (heart isoenzyme), *PFKFB3* (brain/placenta isoenzyme), and *PFKFB4* (testis isoenzyme) (Rider et al., 2004). Each of the *PFKFB* genes is located on a different chromosome. The *PFKFB1* gene contains three promoters (L, M, and F) in its 5′ regulatory sequence. The L promoter is active in liver, adipose tissue, and skeletal muscle; the M promoter is active in a number of tissues and is predominant in muscle; and the F promoter is active primarily in fetal tissues, fibroblasts, and proliferating cells. In the fasted state, the downstream actions of glucagon are to inhibit hepatic transcription from the L promoter of the *PFKFB1* gene and to decrease the stability of the mRNA produced after activation at this promoter. Refeeding (or insulin treatment of a diabetic) increases *PFKFB1* mRNA levels in liver within 24 to 48 hours (Lemaigre and Rousseau, 1994). Insulin and glucocorticoids control the *PFKFB1* gene, which has a glucocorticoid response unit (GRU) located in the first intron of the coding sequence of the gene (rather than in the upstream promoter-regulatory domain). Glucocorticoids stimulate the nuclear glucocorticoid receptor, whereas glucagon inhibits this stimulation. Insulin increases the rate of transcription of the *PFKFB1* gene, and glucose also has a positive stimulatory effect on the L promoter of the *PFKFB1* gene (Rider et al., 2004). Nutrient and hormonal conditions that increase the amount of *PFKFB1* mRNA also increase the amount of enzyme and increase the hepatic levels of F2,6P2, whereas those conditions that decrease *PFKFB1* mRNA and protein levels decrease hepatic F2,6P2 levels.

REGULATION OF PYRUVATE KINASE AND PYRUVATE CARBOXYLASE/ PHOSPHOENOLPYRUVATE CARBOXYKINASE

The final substrate cycle involves pyruvate kinase activity in the glycolytic direction and the combined actions of pyruvate carboxylase and phosphoenolpyruvate carboxykinase in the gluconeogenic direction. This substrate cycle is particularly important in liver, kidney, and adipose tissue.

Pyruvate Kinase

Pyruvate kinase catalyzes the conversion of phosphoenolpyruvate to pyruvate in the last enzymatic step of glycolysis. The pyruvate kinase reaction is an important site of hormonal and nutritional regulation in glycolysis. In the liver, the momentum of glycolysis is maintained by pyruvate kinase under conditions that increase 6-phosphofructo-1-kinase activity, because the end product of the 6-phosphofructo-1-kinase reaction, fructose 1,6-bisphosphate, is a positive allosteric regulator of pyruvate kinase. Pyruvate kinase is also allosterically inhibited by ATP and alanine. At physiological concentrations of substrate (phosphoenolpyruvate) and inhibitors (ATP and alanine), pyruvate kinase would be completely inhibited without the stimulatory effect of fructose 1,6-bisphosphate.

In the liver, pyruvate kinase is also regulated by phosphorylation. It is a substrate for both PKA, induced by the interaction of glucagon with glucagon receptors or of epinephrine with β-adrenergic receptors, and the calcium/calmodulin-dependent protein kinase, induced by epinephrine interaction with α_1-adrenergic receptors. Phosphorylation of pyruvate kinase decreases the activity of the enzyme by decreasing its affinity (increasing its K_m) for its substrate, phosphoenolpyruvate, thereby slowing the rate of glycolysis. The reversal of this response is initiated by an increase in the insulin-glucagon ratio, which decreases cAMP and thus decreases PKA activity, resulting in the dephosphorylation of pyruvate kinase and activation of the enzyme. The presence of substrate also promotes pyruvate formation, because in the presence of fructose 1,6-bisphosphate, the PKA-dependent phosphorylation of the enzyme is inhibited. It should be noted that the phosphorylated form of pyruvate kinase is less readily stimulated by fructose 1,6-bisphosphate and more readily inhibited by ATP and alanine. Conversely, in the dephosphorylated state, pyruvate kinase is more sensitive to allosteric activators and less sensitive to allosteric inhibitors, promoting conversion of phosphoenolpyruvate to pyruvate when insulin levels and substrate are high. Four pyruvate kinase isoenzymes have been characterized: the M_1 form is the predominant form in muscle, heart, and brain; the M_2 form is found in fetal tissue and in most adult tissues; the L′ (or R) form is the major form in red blood cells; and the L form is the major form in liver but is also present in kidney and the small intestine. Two pyruvate kinase (PK) genes have been isolated that code for the four isoenzymes identified. The *PKLR* and *PKM2* genes encode the L and L′ isoenzymes and the M_1 and M_2 isoenzymes, respectively, of PK. The *PKLR* gene has two promoters, which regulate two distinct transcription start sites, generating two unique first exons in the pyruvate kinase transcripts. The *PKM2* gene, on the other hand, is alternatively spliced so that the mRNAs contain either the ninth (M_1) or the tenth (M_2) exon, each expressed with the aforementioned tissue specificity (Noguchi and Tanaka, 1993).

In liver, regulation of the *PKLR* gene involves both direct nutrient and indirect hormonal effects. Importantly, pyruvate kinase is also considered a lipogenic enzyme, because in the presence of excess carbohydrate intake, glucose (or fructose) can be converted to fatty acids. As such, the hepatic *PKLR* gene is regulated in a manner similar to other lipogenic genes. Refeeding fasted rats a high-carbohydrate diet increases pyruvate kinase mRNA levels in liver, and this stimulation is dependent on the presence of insulin. Dietary fructose also increases pyruvate kinase mRNA levels, and it does so more rapidly than glucose and without the insulin requirement. Glucose stimulation of pyruvate kinase mRNA abundance in liver appears to require the catabolism of glucose to glucose 6-phosphate or another downstream metabolite, suggesting that insulin may be required because insulin stimulates the transcription of the glucokinase gene and hence glucose 6-phosphate production. Dietary glycerol is also a potent stimulator of *PKLR* gene expression in liver. It is possible that a downstream metabolite, common to glucose, fructose, and glycerol, is the regulatory intermediate involved in controlling *PKLR* gene expression.

The first glucose response element to be identified in the promoter region of a gene was in the *PKLR* gene. Two repeated DNA sequences of six nucleotides in length, referred to as "E box motifs," are required for glucose/insulin responsiveness of the *PKLR* gene when tested in cell culture or whole animal experimental models (Vaulont and Kahn, 1993). The transcription factor that binds the E box domains of the *PKLR* gene to signal the presence of increased glucose, or an increase in the concentration of a metabolite of glucose, is ChREBP (Uyeda and Repa, 2006). ChREBP is regulated at two different levels: its entry into the nucleus of the cell and its binding to the DNA of the *PKLR* gene. These processes, in turn, are regulated by both a glucose metabolite and cAMP. There are two functional PKA phosphorylation sites in ChREBP; phosphorylation of Ser196 causes impaired nuclear localization of ChREBP, and phosphorylation of Thr666 causes loss of ChREBP DNA binding. Thus PKA-dependent phosphorylation of ChREBP results in a decreased rate of *PKLR* gene transcription (Kawaguchi et al., 2001).

As mentioned previously, the predominant mRNA isoform in liver encodes the L form of pyruvate kinase. This liver isoform is also expressed in kidney and small intestine. All three of these tissues are major sites of fructose metabolism, and liver and kidney are major sites of glycerol metabolism. It stands to reason that expression of pyruvate kinase would be regulated by dietary fructose and glycerol in those tissues involved in their metabolism. Consistent with this assumption, refeeding a high-fructose diet to fasted rats increased expression of the L-isoform of pyruvate kinase in kidney and in the small intestine, whereas refeeding a high-glycerol diet increased expression in kidney alone. However, a high-glucose diet did not increase expression of the L-isoform of pyruvate kinase in either kidney or the small intestine (Noguchi and Tanaka, 1993).

Pyruvate Carboxylase and Phosphoenolpyruvate Carboxykinase

The gluconeogenic enzymes that oppose pyruvate kinase are pyruvate carboxylase and phosphoenolpyruvate carboxykinase. Pyruvate carboxylase is positively regulated by a buildup of acetyl-CoA in the mitochondria, which signals the need for more oxaloacetate. However, it is the cytosolic phosphoenolpyruvate carboxykinase reaction that is rate-determining for gluconeogenesis. Changes in the rate of the phosphoenolpyruvate carboxykinase reaction are not due to allosteric or covalent modification of the enzyme; rather, it is the enzyme concentration itself that is highly regulated. The enzyme concentration is determined by regulation of the gene that encodes phosphoenolpyruvate carboxykinase (*PCK1*).

Expression of phosphoenolpyruvate carboxykinase is high in the gluconeogenic tissues, liver and kidney. It is also expressed in adipose tissue and at lower levels in the intestinal epithelium and mammary gland. Transcription of the *PCK1* gene is controlled by a promoter–regulatory domain that is composed of a complex network of interrelated DNA response elements that are affected by nutrients, hormones, and tissue-specific transcription factors (Gurney et al., 1994). Regulatory elements that have been identified within the 5′-promoter region of *PCK1* are cAMP response elements, the thyroid hormone regulatory element, the glucocorticoid regulatory element, the insulin regulatory element, and the peroxisome proliferator-activated receptor regulatory element.

In liver, *PCK1* mRNA and phosphoenolpyruvate carboxykinase enzyme activity are both present in highest levels in the hepatocytes surrounding the portal vein. Many other gluconeogenic enzymes and urea cycle enzymes are also more abundant in the periportal than the perivenous hepatocytes.

Expression of phosphoenolpyruvate carboxykinase is highly regulated by diet and hormones. It is well documented that fasting increases *PCK1* mRNA levels, and that refeeding a high-carbohydrate diet decreases *PCK1* mRNA abundance in liver (Hanson and Reshef, 1997; Sutherland et al., 1966). In the fasted state, both the transcription rate of the *PCK1* gene and the stability of the *PCK1* mRNA are increased by cAMP. Peroxisome proliferator-activated receptor gamma coactivator 1 (PGC1) is a critical activator of *PCK1* gene expression and of gluconeogenesis overall (Yoon et al., 2001; Rhee et al., 2003). PGC1 expression is induced synergistically by the combined actions of cAMP and glucocorticoids. PGC1 interacts with and coactivates both the glucocorticoid receptor and the liver-specific transcription factor HNF4α to mediate increased *PCK1* gene expression (Yoon et al., 2001). Insulin is the dominant negative regulator of *PCK1* gene expression and inhibits *PCK1* expression upon meal intake. Insulin administration will inhibit cAMP- or glucocorticoid-stimulated increases in the rate of transcription of this gene during periods of fasting or stress. These gluconeogenic genes contain an insulin response element to which FoxO transcription factors bind in the absence of insulin, activating gene transcription. Insulin secretion triggers the phosphorylation of FoxO via the PtdIns 3-kinase/Akt pathway, and this inactivates FoxO by excluding it from the nucleus. Although the effects of carbohydrate refeeding could be mediated by insulin alone, glucose decreased *PCK1* mRNA levels by decreasing the transcription rate and the stability of the mRNA in hepatocytes cultured in the absence of insulin (Kahn et al., 1989). Therefore the inhibition of *PCK1* gene expression imposed by refeeding a high-carbohydrate diet may be due to effects of both insulin signaling and the concentration of glucose or a glucose metabolite on the *PCK1* promoter. Another important potential mediator of insulin regulation of the *PCK1* gene is the liver X receptor that is involved in carbohydrate and lipid metabolism in liver and other tissues.

In addition to the role of phosphoenolpyruvate carboxykinase in hepatic and renal gluconeogenesis, it is less well known that phosphoenolpyruvate carboxykinase functions in two other metabolic pathways: (1) glyceroneogenesis, an abbreviated version of gluconeogenesis that can produce the glycerol backbone for triacylglycerol synthesis in adipose tissue when glucose is not available; and (2) cataplerosis, the removal of citric acid cycle intermediates, primarily excess oxaloacetate, to supply other needs and/or to maintain flux through the citric acid cycle without buildup of intermediates. Disruption of expression of the *PCK1* gene in liver leads to fatty liver due to decreased hepatic cataplerosis and citrate accumulation. In contrast, decreased expression of the *PCK1*

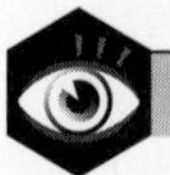

NUTRITION INSIGHT

Differential Multigene Expression Patterns

Currently, high throughput methodology is available, via microarray analysis and related transcriptomics methods, to screen the entire human genome for differential gene expression in response to specific nutrient and hormonal stimuli, as well as under different health status conditions. This has allowed for significant advances in our understanding of gene expression patterns that occur in specific tissues such as liver, skeletal muscle, and adipose tissue under conditions such as obesity and type 2 diabetes, and in response to nutrients, such as sugars and fatty acids. In addition, there have been rapid advances in determining genetic variants via whole genome association (WGA) studies that identify genes and genetic loci that are linked to complex syndromes like type 2 diabetes. The advances made by these transcriptomics and genomics approaches are extensive.

In terms of environmental effects on gene expression and related metabolism, epigenetics also plays a significant role. For example, genetic susceptibility and environmental insults can combine to increase the risk of type 2 diabetes. Specifically, intrauterine growth retardation has been associated with increased risk of developing type 2 diabetes; this is linked to epigenetic factors that are chemical modifications of specific genes of glucose metabolism. Epigenetic modification of the genome is stable and is a mechanism that allows the propagation of gene expression patterns from one generation of cells to the next via histone modification and DNA methylation. Two genes that are disrupted in type 2 diabetes have been identified as regulated by transcriptional repression due to epigenetic mechanisms during intrauterine growth retardation. These genes are the GLUT4 (*SLC2A4*) gene that is repressed in skeletal muscle and the pancreatic duodenal homeobox-1 (*Pdx1*) gene that is repressed in the pancreas. Repression of the GLUT4 gene results in insulin resistance in skeletal muscle, and repression of the *Pdx1* gene leads to decreased glucose-stimulated insulin secretion from the beta cells of the pancreas (Pinney and Simmons, 2010).

gene in adipose tissue of rodent models led to lipoatrophy, due to decreased adipose glyceroneogenesis.

The role of glyceroneogenesis in adipose tissue is very significant. In the fasting state, when blood glucose levels are low, glyceroneogenesis is an important source of de novo glycerol 3-phosphate for reesterification of free fatty acids in the adipocytes. Lipolysis in white adipose tissue produces free fatty acids for release into the circulation to meet energy needs of the body. However, if this lipolysis is not carefully regulated, the levels of released free fatty acids can become too high and have negative metabolic consequences. Therefore lipolysis is counterregulated by fatty acid reesterification back to triacylglycerols, and reesterification is dependent on adequate glyceroneogenesis, which in turn is dependent on the correct regulation of phosphoenolpyruvate carboxykinase expression in adipose tissue. According to Beale and colleagues (2004), approximately 30% to 40% of fatty acids released via lipolysis are reesterified back to triacylglycerols without leaving the adipocytes, and this process is intensified in the fasted state. Oversecretion of free fatty acids leads to the ectopic accumulation of fat in other tissues and is a central component leading to metabolic syndrome, insulin resistance, and eventually type 2 diabetes. In animal models, the thiazolidinedione, an antidiabetes drug, has been shown to stimulate phosphoenolpyruvate carboxykinase expression and glyceroneogenesis in adipose tissue, decreasing the rate of free fatty acid release from adipocytes (Tordjman et al., 2003).

These multiple metabolic roles of phosphoenolpyruvate carboxykinase in different tissues and conditions, such as fasting or refeeding, requires a complex set of regulatory processes. In addition to the complex regulatory domain that was described earlier for expression of the *PCK1* gene in gluconeogenic tissues, there is a second regulatory or enhancer region that comprises one peroxisome proliferator–activated receptor gamma (PPAR γ response element [PPRE]) (Duplus et al., 2003). Interestingly, deletion of the PPRE in the *PCK1* gene in mouse models led to decreased expression of the *PCK1* gene only in white adipose tissue, with an attendant decrease in white adipose tissue mass. This causes increased levels of free fatty acids, with attendant ectopic lipid accumulation and related insulin resistance. In large genome-wide scans, variants of the *PCK1* gene, along with those of many other genes, have been linked to type 2 diabetes.

In addition to these normal metabolic roles for phosphoenolpyruvate carboxykinase in liver and adipose tissue, additional work has been done to test the role of phosphoenolpyruvate carboxykinase expression in tissues that normally do not express the *PCK1* gene. In mice that were engineered to overexpress the *PCK1* gene in skeletal muscle, increased glyceroneogenesis in muscle and a corresponding accumulation of triacylglycerols in muscle were observed. This additional fuel in the skeletal muscle of *PCK1* overexpressing mice resulted in increased exercise capacity and endurance, presumably due to the increased local fuel availability (Hanson and Hakimi, 2008).

LIVER COMPARTMENTALIZATION OF GLUCONEOGENIC ENZYMES

In liver, the catabolism of glucose via glycolysis occurs at a low rate under aerobic conditions when glucose levels in the blood are not high. Gluconeogenesis, on the other hand, proceeds at a higher rate. It is interesting that there is a gradient of gluconeogenic enzyme activity, compartmentalized to different zones in the liver. These zones arise in functional subdivisions of the liver that are defined by the microcirculation of the tissue. The smallest functional unit of the liver is the acinus, and each acinus is circumscribed by the terminal

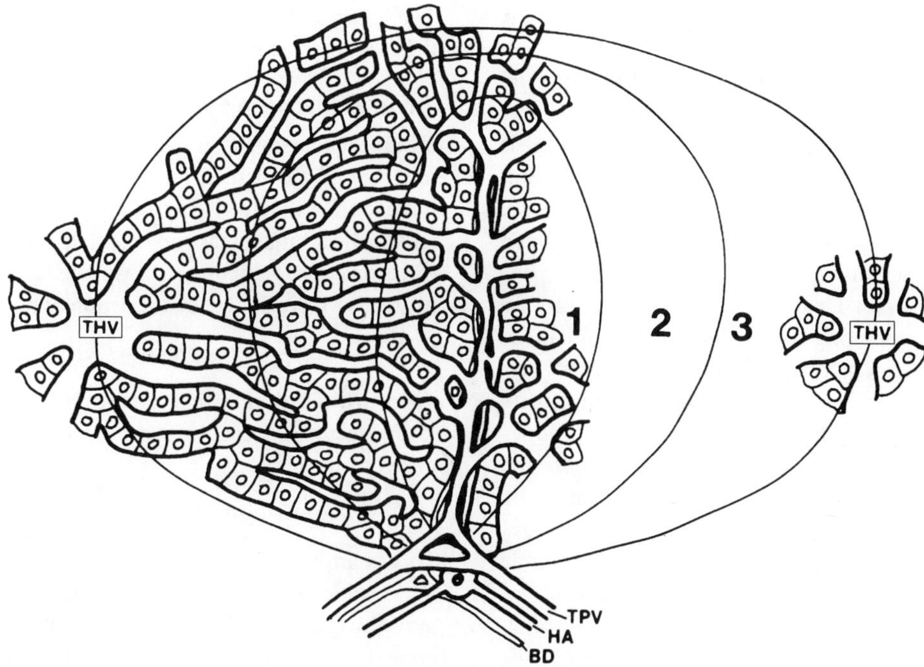

FIGURE 12-11 Hepatic acinus. The acinus is the three-dimensional structure that forms the microvascular units of hepatic lobules. The acinar axis is formed by the terminal portal venule (*TPV*), the hepatic arteriole (*HA*), and the bile ductule (*BD*). The perfusion of the acinus is unidirectional from the acinar axis to the acinar periphery where two or more terminal hepatic venules (*THV*) empty the acinus. The arbitrary division of the acinus into functional zones is represented by *1* (periportal), *2*, and *3* (perivenous). (From Gumucio, J. J., & Chianale, J. [1988]. Liver cell heterogeneity and liver function. In I. M. Arias, W. B. Jakoby, H. Popper, D. Schachter, & D. A. Shafritz [Eds.], *The liver: Biology and pathobiology* [2nd ed., pp. 931–947]. New York: Raven Press.)

hepatic venule at the periphery and a terminal portal venule and a terminal hepatic arteriole at the center (Figure 12-11). The portal vein supplies approximately 70% of the blood that comes to the liver, and the hepatic artery supplies the rest. Blood leaves the acinus via the terminal branches of the hepatic veins.

The hepatocytes that surround the incoming portal venule are referred to as periportal cells, and those that surround the outgoing central hepatic venule are referred to as perivenous cells. Distinct metabolic zones occur between these regions of afferent and efferent blood flow (Jungermann, 1992). At the proximal side of the circulatory supply to the liver acinus, the cells are receiving oxygen and nutrient-rich blood from the hepatic artery and portal vein, respectively. As the blood traverses the cell population, it becomes relatively depleted of oxygen and nutrients as it moves toward the hepatic terminal venule. It is generally accepted that the activity of gluconeogenic and urea cycle enzymes is higher in hepatocytes at the periportal side of the liver acinus. There is some debate as to whether the limited glycolysis that occurs in liver is more predominant in perivenous cells or is less compartmentalized overall than is gluconeogenesis. Because perivenous cells receive blood with a somewhat lower oxygen tension than do periportal hepatocytes, perivenous cells are thought to be more dependent upon glycolysis. It is documented that the low K_m glucose transporter GLUT1 is localized to a layer of cells surrounding the terminal hepatic venule. The high affinity of GLUT1 for glucose assures that perivenous cells take up glucose to provide for increased glycolysis. GLUT2, on the other hand, is distributed evenly across the liver acinus.

The compartmentalization of specific enzymes and transporters of glucose metabolism appears to be due to localized gene expression. The pattern of gene expression and compartmentalization changes with alterations in dietary state. For example, the periportal to perivenous ratios of the activities of phosphoenolpyruvate carboxykinase, fructose 1,6-bisphosphatase, and glucose 6-phosphatase decrease with fasting. These decreases in the periportal to perivenous ratios are due to increases in gluconeogenic enzyme activity in the perivenous cells during a fast, when total hepatic glucose output increases. Under these conditions, gluconeogenesis is activated in the larger hepatocyte population, and compartmentalization is decreased.

GLYCOGEN METABOLISM

Glucose is stored in liver and muscle tissue as glycogen, a branched-chain polymer of glucose. In humans, liver has the capacity to store glycogen up to approximately 10% of its weight. Skeletal muscle, on the other hand, has a more limited capacity to store glycogen, to approximately 1% of its weight. Because the overall mass of skeletal muscle is much greater than that of liver, however, the total amount of muscle glycogen is usually more than double the amount of liver glycogen. Low concentrations of glycogen are also found in the kidneys, the glial cells of the brain, and in red and white blood cells. Glycogen is also stored in the uterus during pregnancy, to nourish the growing embryo (Campbell et al., 2006).

Glycogen stores in liver and muscle serve different purposes in fuel metabolism, and glycogen metabolism is regulated somewhat differently in the two tissues. Glycogen is stored during the postprandial state for future use when blood glucose levels decrease. When blood glucose levels decline, the body's first line of defense is to degrade hepatic glycogen by cleaving off glucose units as glucose phosphate in the process called glycogenolysis. The liver secretes glucose into the blood to maintain circulating blood glucose levels for those tissues that are dependent upon glucose for energy. Skeletal muscle, on the other hand, utilizes glucose 6-phosphate produced by glycogenolysis for glycolysis and ATP production within the same cell. Skeletal muscle does not have the glucose 6-phosphatase enzyme necessary for removal of the phosphate from the glucose phosphate formed during glycogenolysis, so the glucose 6-phosphate generated by muscle glycogenolysis is retained in the myocyte (muscle fiber).

GLYCOGEN SYNTHESIS

The glycogen polymer is a linear array of glucose residues linked by α(1,4)-glycosidic bonds, with branch points formed by glucose units linked to the main chain by α(1,6)-glycosidic linkages. The branching structure of the molecule is not random; branch points are found approximately every fourth glucose residue along the linear chains of the polymer. The series of enzymes that catalyze the steps of glycogen synthesis is responsible for the specificity of this structure.

Steps in Glycogen Synthesis

Assuming that glycogen synthesis starts with uptake of glucose into the cell, the first enzymatic reaction in glycogen synthesis is the same as that in glycolysis, the glucokinase reaction in liver and the hexokinase reaction in skeletal muscle. The product of these reactions, glucose 6-phosphate, is further metabolized to glucose 1-phosphate by the action of phosphoglucomutase.

$$\text{Glucose 6-phosphate} \leftrightarrow \text{Glucose 1-phosphate}$$

The third reaction in this series prepares glucose for storage as glycogen. This reaction is catalyzed by glucose 1-phosphate uridylyltransferase.

$$\text{Glucose 1-phosphate} + \text{UTP} \rightarrow \text{UDP-glucose} + \text{PP}_i$$

This is an energy-requiring step, but it is made essentially irreversible by the hydrolysis of one of the end products, pyrophosphate (PP_i), to two molecules of inorganic phosphate (P_i). This reaction is catalyzed by pyrophosphatase:

$$\text{PP}_i + \text{H}_2\text{O} \rightarrow 2\text{P}_i$$

Glycogen synthase catalyzes the addition of single glucosyl residues to a growing polymer of glycogen. The substrates for this reaction are glycogen and UDP-glucose (Figure 12-12). The glucose moiety is added to the glycogen polymer by

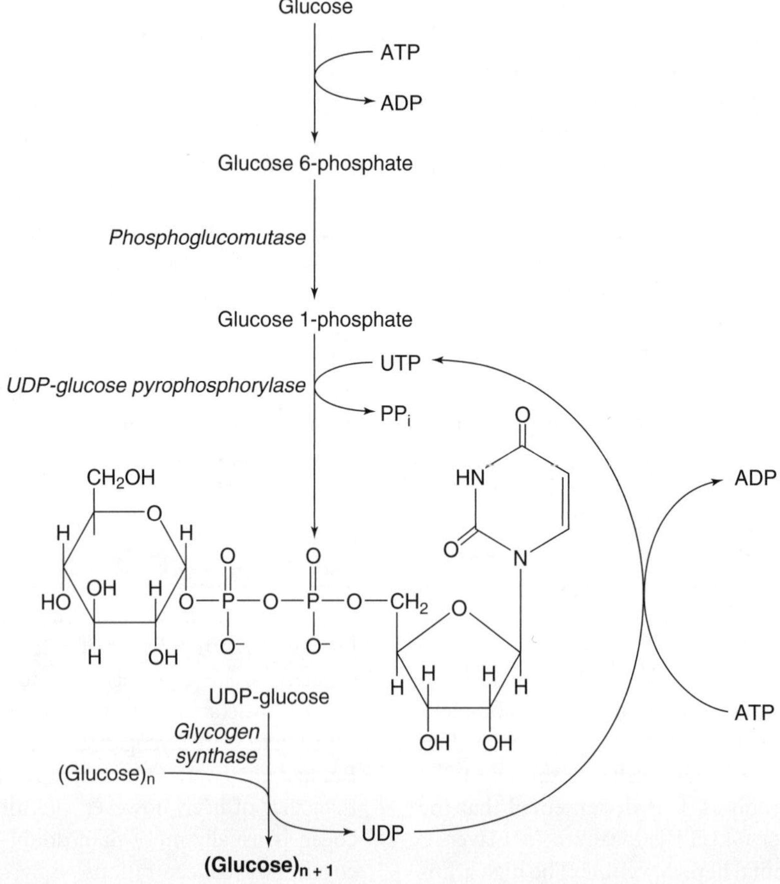

FIGURE 12-12 Addition of glucosyl residues to the linear α(1,4)-linked chains of glycogen.

forming an α(1,4)-glycosidic linkage between C1 of the "activated" glucose and C4 of the terminal glucose of a linear chain of the glycogen polymer. For each new glycogen molecule, a primer is required for the attachment of the first molecule of glucose. The protein glycogenin serves this function; the first glucose moiety in a nascent chain is attached to a specific tyrosine residue in glycogenin. Glycogen synthase then forms a complex with glucose-bound glycogenin, and extension of the polysaccharide chain is autocatalyzed by the glucosyltransferase activity of glycogenin until the linear glycogen chain reaches eight units in length (Smythe and Cohen, 1991). The nascent glycogen chain then becomes the substrate for glycogen synthase. The glycogen synthase reaction can be represented as follows:

$$(\text{Glucose})_n + \text{UDP-glucose} \rightarrow (\text{Glucose})_{n+1} + \text{UDP}$$

Because of the UTP requirement for glycogen synthesis, an "ATP equivalent" is required for the glycogen synthase reaction. When added to the ATP used in the glucokinase reaction, this generates an overall energy expenditure of two molecules of ATP for the addition of one glucose unit to the glycogen polymer.

Glycogen synthase specifically catalyzes the addition of the glucose moiety in the α(1,4) orientation; it is not involved in branching. A second enzyme, 1,4-α-glucan branching enzyme, is involved in the formation of branch points in the growing glycogen polymer. This branching enzyme catalyzes the transfer of an oligosaccharide chain of approximately seven glucose residues from the nonreducing end (i.e., from the outer terminal glucosyl residue) of a linear glycogen segment to an interior C6 of a glucose residue at least 4 units away from the last branch site, thereby creating a new branch site (Figure 12-13). The new branch linkage is an α(1, 6)-glycosidic bond.

Role of Gluconeogenesis in Glycogen Formation

There is an interesting paradox in the synthesis of glycogen in liver. A significant amount of glycogen synthesis in liver is dependent on gluconeogenically derived substrate rather than on glucose entering the hepatocyte directly by facilitated transport. In humans, approximately one third of the glucose 6-phosphate utilized for glycogen synthesis in liver is gluconeogenically derived (McGarry et al., 1987). It is postulated that the indirect route of glycogen synthesis in liver utilizes lactate from extrahepatic tissues such as skeletal muscle and red blood cells. In the absorptive phase, it appears that a certain amount of dietary glucose may be metabolized to lactate in extrahepatic tissues, with the lactate being recirculated to the liver where it becomes a substrate for gluconeogenesis. In the absorptive state, other substrates present in the portal blood, such as amino acids, are also potential sources of gluconeogenic carbon for glycogen synthesis. Thus, in the liver, gluconeogenically derived glucose 6-phosphate is used for glycogen synthesis even in the fed state when blood glucose is elevated. In contrast, muscle cells directly utilize glucose for synthesis of glycogen.

GLYCOGENOLYSIS

The glycogen polymer may contain as many as 100,000 glucose units in its highly branched structure. In humans, the liver is completely depleted of glycogen by 24 hours of fasting. The degradation of this complex molecule begins at the nonreducing ends of the multiple branches and involves the phosphorolysis of single glucose units by glycogen phosphorylase, an enzyme that uses pyridoxal 5′-phosphate as a cofactor. In the glycogen phosphorylase reaction, the α(1,4)-glycosidic bond is attacked by inorganic phosphate (P_i), generating glucose 1-phosphate and a shortened glycogen polymer (Figure 12-14).

$$(\text{Glucose})_n + P_i \rightarrow (\text{Glucose})_{n-1} - \text{Glucose 1-phosphate}$$

The phosphorylase reaction is repeated successively until the fourth glucose unit from a branch point is reached. Then the bifunctional debranching enzyme (4-α-D-glucanotransferase/amylo-α[1,6]glucosidase) comes into play. It catalyzes the transfer of three of the four glucose units to the closest nonreducing end, where they are attached in a new α(1,4)-glycosidic linkage. The debranching enzyme also has α(1,6)-glucosidase activity and removes the remaining glucose by hydrolysis of the α(1,6)-linkage at the branch point; this glucosyl residue at the branch point is released as free glucose (see Figure 12-14). The remaining linear array is now the substrate for continued glycogen phosphorylase activity.

The product of the glycogen phosphorylase reaction, glucose 1-phosphate, is converted to glucose 6-phosphate by

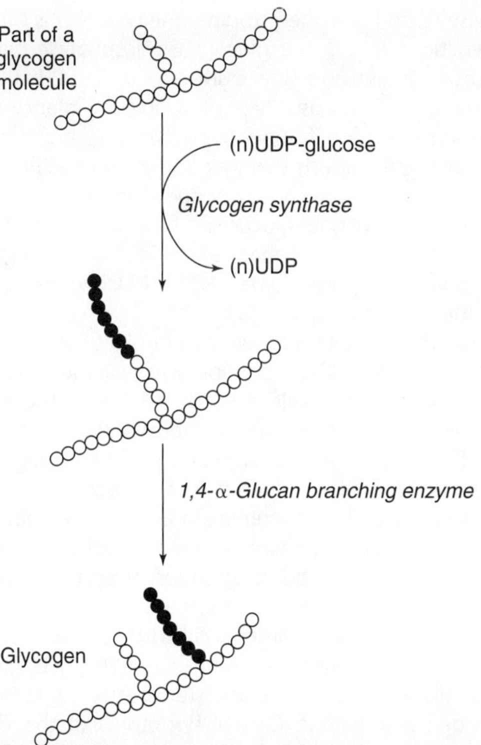

FIGURE 12-13 Pictorial illustration of the growth of glycogen chains and the role of the branching enzyme in the translocation of linear segments of growing chains to create α(1,6)-linkages and hence new branch points.

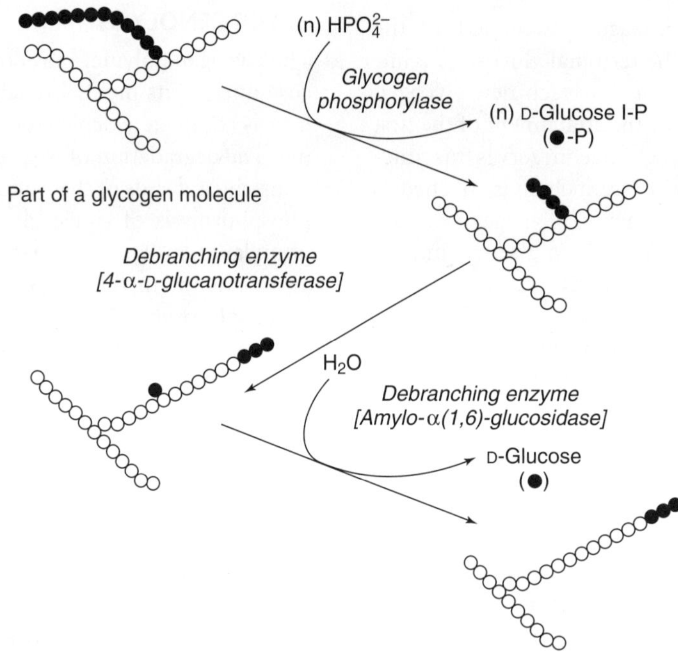

FIGURE 12-14 Pictorial illustration of the breakdown of glycogen by glycogen phosphorylase and the activities of the debranching enzyme.

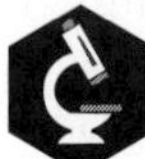

CLINICAL CORRELATION

Glycogen Storage Diseases

Loss of function mutations in several genes encoding proteins involved in glycogen metabolism cause various forms of glycogen storage diseases. A lack of glucose 6-phosphatase in liver, kidney, and intestinal mucosa causes Von Gierke disease (type I glycogen storage disease). This is caused by a genetic defect in the glucose 6-phosphatase gene that occurs as an autosomal recessive trait in 1 of 200,000 people. This deficiency usually presents in early infancy and the symptoms include fasting hypoglycemia, hepatomegaly, and recurrent acidosis (Dunger and Holton, 1994). Inborn errors of metabolism can occur due to genetic mutations of the gene that encodes glucose 6-phosphatase enzyme (type Ia), the glucose 6-phosphatase translocase (type Ib), or the phosphate transporter (type Ic). Individuals with this disease lack the ability to respond to low blood glucose by releasing glucose from either glycogenolysis or gluconeogenesis. This particularly affects the liver's ability to maintain glucose balance in the body by releasing glucose from either of these two metabolic sources. The symptoms of this disease can be modified by providing dietary carbohydrate throughout the day so that low blood glucose does not occur.

Another cause of glycogen storage disease is an impairment in glycogen phosphorylase function. Mutations in both the liver-type and muscle-type glycogen phosphorylase genes occur as rare autosomal recessive disorders. In liver, the metabolic disorder is called Hers disease (type VI) and presents in childhood. In this condition, liver glycogen accumulates because the first step in the degradation of glycogen is impaired. Clinical symptoms of this disorder include hypoglycemia, hepatomegaly (which develops slowly), and some growth delay (Fernandes and Chen, 1995). In muscle, the metabolic disorder is referred to as McArdle disease (type V), which usually presents in adult life, when progressive muscle weakness occurs; however, hepatomegaly and fasting hypoglycemia do not occur in McArdle disease. Individuals with this disease accumulate glycogen in muscle tissue and are exercise intolerant because glucose cannot be released from glycogen to meet the increased energy demand of physical activity. There are also genetic disorders in the phosphorylase kinase gene that lead to phosphorylase kinase deficiency in liver and muscle. Phosphorylase kinase deficiency is more common than glycogen phosphorylase deficiency and is inherited as an X chromosome–linked recessive trait. This disorder causes a lack of phosphorylation and hence activation of glycogen phosphorylase. Symptoms associated with this disorder are similar to those for glycogen phosphorylase deficiency.

A mutation in the gene that encodes "debranching enzyme" also occurs in the human population. The disorder is referred to as Cori disease (type III), in which glycogen accumulates in liver and muscle in the form of branched short chains. Cori disease usually presents in infancy with symptoms of fasting hypoglycemic convulsions, hepatomegaly, and myopathy (Dunger and Holton, 1994). However, the hypoglycemia and hepatomegaly usually abate by puberty.

Thinking Critically

1. Explain the underlying metabolic basis for development of (1) hypoglycemia, (2) lactic acidosis, and (3) hypertriglyceridemia in patients with glycogen storage disease type I.
2. What effect does treatment of patients with glycogen storage disease type I with frequent ingestion of carbohydrate throughout the day (and during the night via infusion of carbohydrate into the gut through a nasogastric tube) have on the overproduction of lactate and triacylglycerol? Explain.

phosphoglucomutase. In muscle tissue, the glucose 6-phosphate produced in this reaction is broken down via the glycolytic pathway to produce ATP for muscle contraction. In liver, where there is significant glucose 6-phosphatase activity and glycolysis is inhibited under the hormonal conditions that favor hepatic glycogenolysis, most glucose 6-phosphate is converted to free glucose, which is transported out of the liver cells to maintain plasma glucose levels.

REGULATION OF GLYCOGENESIS AND GLYCOGENOLYSIS

The regulatory mechanisms affecting glycogen synthesis and degradation have been extensively studied but are still incompletely understood. Glycogen synthase and glycogen phosphorylase are regulated enzymes in glycogen synthesis and degradation, respectively. As for glycolysis and gluconeogenesis, there is reciprocal regulation of glycogen synthase and glycogen phosphorylase as a consequence of the hormone-mediated phosphorylation/dephosphorylation of these two enzymes by various kinases and a phosphatase. Glycogen synthase is less active when phosphorylated, whereas glycogen phosphorylase is more active when phosphorylated.

The anabolic hormone insulin stimulates glycogen synthesis in liver and muscle in the absorptive state. Glucagon, on the other hand, stimulates glycogen degradation in liver when blood glucose levels decline. Epinephrine promotes glycogen degradation in both the liver and skeletal muscle. In the liver, both β-adrenergic and α-adrenergic receptors mediate the response to epinephrine via different signal transduction mechanisms. In skeletal muscle there are no glucagon receptors, but β-adrenergic receptors are stimulated by epinephrine, inducing the cAMP cascade of signaling events.

Regulation of Glycogen Synthase

Liver and muscle express different isozymes of glycogen synthase. Liver expresses the enzyme encoded by gene *GYS2*, and a muscle expresses the enzyme encoded by *GYS1*. The liver enzyme expression is restricted to the liver, whereas the muscle enzyme is widely expressed. Glycogen synthase is regulated by both covalent modification and allosteric effectors.

Regulation of Glycogen Synthase by Phosphorylation/Dephosphorylation

Glycogen synthase can exist in either a more active unphosphorylated (*a*) form or a less active phosphorylated (*b*) form (Jensen and Lai, 2009). The less active phosphorylated form has less affinity for substrate UDP-glucose and is less sensitive to allosteric activation by glucose 6-phosphate.

Glycogen synthase has many potential phosphorylation sites and is the target of multiple protein kinases. Multisite phosphorylation converts the enzyme from the *a* to the *b* form, decreasing its activity (Figure 12-15). It is unclear

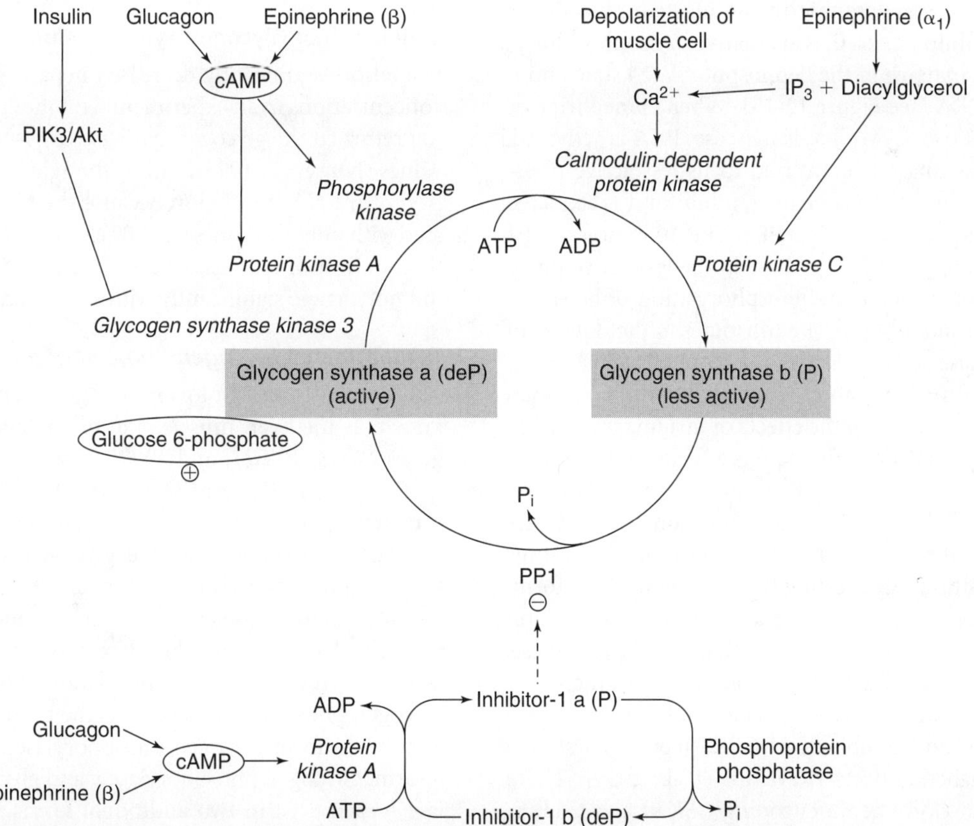

FIGURE 12-15 Regulation of glycogen synthase by phosphorylation/dephosphorylation and allosteric effectors. Phosphorylated and dephosphorylated proteins are indicated by *P* and *deP*, respectively. Allosteric activators and inhibitors are indicated by + and –, respectively.

which sites are key for glycogen synthase inhibition although Ser7, Ser641, and Ser645 seem to be involved. The various protein kinases are activated as the result of different intracellular signal transduction pathways responding to different hormonal and nutrient signals. The protein kinases that can phosphorylate glycogen synthase include PKA, which is activated in response to epinephrine or glucagon signaling; GSK3, which is regulated by insulin; phosphorylase kinase, which itself is phosphorylated by PKA; the calmodulin-dependent protein kinase, which is regulated by calcium binding to calmodulin; protein kinase C, which is activated by diacylglycerol (α_1 adrenergic receptor activation); and casein kinases I and II, which prime glycogen synthase for further phosphorylation. Thus, in response to fasting or exercise, the phosphorylation and hence inhibition of glycogen synthase is promoted by glucagon (liver) or catecholamines (liver and skeletal muscle) that signal via cAMP activation of PKA and phosphorylation of Ser7, Ser10, Ser641, Ser645, and Ser649, as well as by the action of GSK3 phosphorylation of Ser641, Ser645, and Ser649. In the fed state, insulin signaling inhibits GSK3 as well as countering cAMP signaling via activation of phosphodiesterase (PDE3), favoring maintenance of glycogen synthase in its active dephosphorylated state.

Glycogen synthase is dephosphorylated and converted back to the *a* form by the glycogen-associated protein phosphatase type 1 (PP1). PP1, in turn, is regulated by inhibitor-1, present in certain tissues and well characterized in skeletal muscle. The inhibitor decreases PP1 activity, thereby maintaining glycogen synthase in the inactive phosphorylated state. Inhibitor-1, itself, is also active in the phosphorylated state and inactive in the dephosphorylated state and is regulated via PKA (see Figure 12-15). When epinephrine or glucagon levels rise, cAMP levels increase, PKA is activated, and glycogen synthase is converted to its less active phosphorylated *b* form. At the same time, inhibitor-1 is activated by phosphorylation and inhibits PP1. The inhibition of PP1 activity maintains glycogen synthase in the less active phosphorylated *b* form. Therefore phosphorylation of both glycogen synthase and inhibitor-1 contributes to the slowing of glycogen synthase activity in response to cAMP.

GSK3 has been shown to be a signal transduction molecule that mediates many of the effects of insulin, growth factors, and nutrients. Currently there is a focus on the role of GSK3 in a number of disease states, including insulin resistance and type 2 diabetes (Jope and Johnson, 2004). GSK3 phosphorylates three Ser residues at the carboxyl terminus of glycogen synthase, converting the enzyme to the *b* form. Insulin signaling inactivates GSK3 and results in conversion of glycogen synthase to the *a* form so that glycogen synthesis is promoted. Increased expression and activity of the *GSK3* gene has been reported in type 2 diabetic subjects and obese animal models, and inhibitors of GSK3 have been shown to have antidiabetic effects (Rayasam et al., 2009). There are two human *GSK3* genes encoding *GSK3α* and *GS3Kβ*, which have similar functions. Although glycogen synthase (*GYS1*) gene expression is not changed in skeletal muscle of persons with type 2 diabetes, *GSK3* expression is increased. Higher levels of GSK3 would favor greater inhibition of glycogen synthase and therefore decreased glycogen storage in skeletal muscle of persons with type 2 diabetes (Nikoulina et al., 2002).

Regulation of Glycogen Synthase by Allosteric Mechanisms

As shown in Figure 12-15, allosteric activation of glycogen synthase by glucose 6-phosphate facilitates upregulation of glycogen synthesis when blood glucose levels are elevated. Although glucose 6-phosphate can alter the activity of either glycogen synthase *a* or *b*, the sensitivity of glycogen synthase to glucose 6-phosphate activation is increased significantly when glycogen synthase is in the more active dephosphorylated *a* state. The association of glucose 6-phosphate with glycogen synthase increases both glycogen synthase activity and its affinity for substrate UDP-glucose; it also protects the enzyme against phosphorylation by altering the conformation of the enzyme such that it is a better substrate for PP1 than the kinases.

Glycogen synthase is strongly inhibited by the glycogen content of the tissue. Glycogen content decreases the affinity of glycogen synthase for UDP-glucose and promotes the phosphorylation of glycogen synthase. Thus tissue glycogen stores serve as a strong feedback inhibitor when they are replete (Nielsen et al., 2001). This mechanism may play a major role in determining the tissue capacity for glycogen storage.

Regulation of Glycogen Synthase Concentration

Starvation significantly decreased hepatic glycogen synthase concentrations in an experimental rat model, whereas refeeding returned the glycogen synthase concentration to control values (Nur et al., 1995). This is thought to be due to regulation of mRNA translation because the *GYS2* mRNA associated with polyribosomes was 90% lower in liver of starved rats than in liver of fed rats, whereas the total *GYS2* mRNA level did not change significantly with starvation and refeeding.

Regulation of Glycogen Phosphorylase

There are three isoforms of glycogen phosphorylase, known as the liver, muscle, and brain isoforms encoded by genes *PYGL*, *PYGM*, and *PYGB*, respectively (Lockyer and McCracken, 1991; Ferrer-Martinez et al., 2004). This allows for tissue-specific regulation of glycogen phosphorylase. Glycogen phosphorylase, like glycogen synthase, is regulated by phosphorylation and by allosteric regulators. Glycogen phosphorylase exists as a dimer, and a single residue in each glycogen phosphorylase monomer (Ser14) is the target for reversible phosphorylation. Phosphorylation of glycogen phosphorylase converts the unphosphorylated less active *b* form of glycogen phosphorylase to its more active *a* form. Glycogen phosphorylase *a* and glycogen phosphorylase *b* each exist in two additional forms, a T (tense) inactive state and an R (relaxed) state. Phosphorylation favors the active R state. Thus glycogen phosphorylase *b* is normally in the inactive T state, whereas glycogen phosphorylase *a* is normally in the active R state. The shift between the R and T states can be regulated by allosteric effectors, but the sensitivity of the different isozymes to various effectors differs.

Glycogen phosphorylase contains a glycogen binding domain that allows the enzyme to covalently bind to the glycogen chain at some distance from the catalytic site, and this may allow the enzyme to initiate cleavage of the terminal glucose moieties when it is activated. Most of the glycogen phosphorylase in the cell exists bound to glycogen granules.

Regulation of Glycogen Phosphorylase by Phosphorylation/Dephosphorylation

Glycogen phosphorylase is subject to covalent modification by phosphorylation, and this phosphorylation is catalyzed by phosphorylase kinase (Figure 12-16). Phosphorylation at a single serine residue causes a conformational change of the enzyme to the more active glycogen phosphorylase *a* form.

The phosphorylation of glycogen phosphorylase is regulated by the activation of phosphorylase kinase. The gene that encodes the catalytic subunit (gamma) of phosphorylase kinase, *PHKG*, is highly regulated in a tissue-specific manner. In muscle, the expression of *PHKG* determines the rate of expression of the genes encoding the regulatory subunits of phosphorylase kinase (O'Mahony and Walsh, 2002). This ensures that all of the subunits are expressed in a coordinated way such that production of excess free catalytic subunit, which would cause excess activation of glycogen phosphorylase and excess glycogen breakdown, is prevented.

Phosphorylase kinase is phosphorylated and activated by PKA in response to increased intracellular cAMP. In the presence of cAMP, inhibitor-1 is phosphorylated and active; it inhibits phosphoprotein phosphatase, thereby preventing dephosphorylation of glycogen phosphorylase to its less active form. Both glucagon and β-adrenergic receptor activation leads to activation of adenylate cyclase and the resulting increase in intracellular cAMP. Thus an increase in cAMP concentration in response to hormonal signaling initiates a cascade involving sequential phosphorylation and activation of protein kinase A, phosphorylase kinase, and glycogen phosphorylase. In muscle, epinephrine acting via β-adrenergic receptors is the most important signal that stimulates cAMP-mediated activation of PKA. In liver, glucagon binding to its receptors is the major hormonal stimuli for hepatic glycogenolysis although epinephrine can also stimulate the mobilization of glycogen in liver. In humans, the response to epinephrine involves both epinephrine

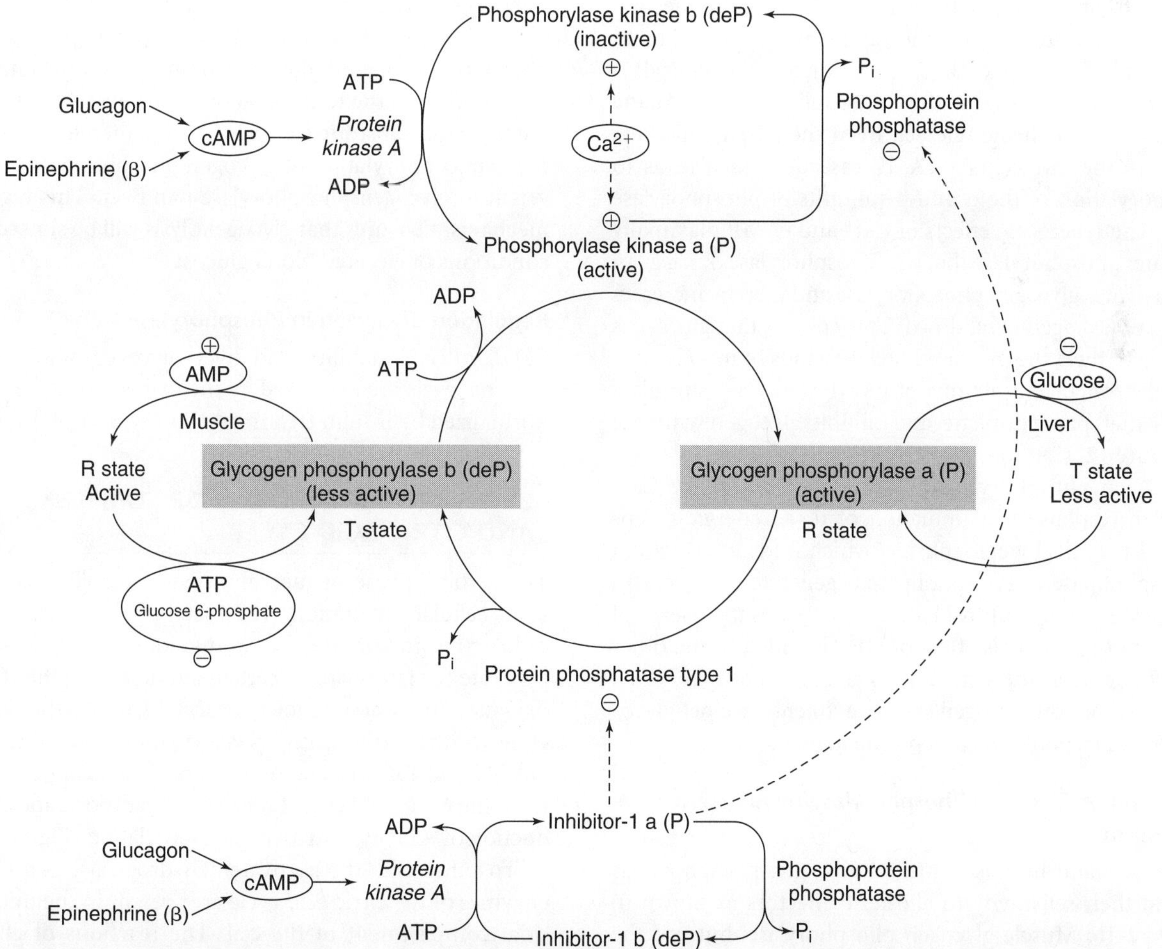

FIGURE 12-16 Regulation of glycogen phosphorylase by phosphorylation/dephosphorylation and allosteric effectors. Phosphorylated and dephosphorylated proteins are indicated by *P* and *deP*, respectively. Allosteric activators and inhibitors are indicated by + and –, respectively.

stimulation of the pancreatic alpha cells to secrete glucagon, which can then stimulate the liver glucagon receptors, and epinephrine stimulation of β-adrenergic receptors on liver and muscle cells.

Phosphorylase kinase is also regulated by a Ca^{2+}-calmodulin regulatory mechanism. Phosphorylase kinase has a complex molecular structure and consists of four subunits. The γ subunit is catalytic and the α, β, and δ subunits are regulatory. The α and β subunits are phosphorylated by PKA in the activation process. The δ subunit is a Ca^{2+}-binding protein, calmodulin. Calmodulin is an intracellular Ca^{2+} receptor and it is found in different locations in the cell, either unbound or in association with different enzymes. The calmodulin subunit of phosphorylase kinase binds Ca^{2+} when there is Ca^{2+} influx into the cytosol of the cell. This induces a conformational change that activates phosphorylase kinase. Phosphorylation of the α and β subunits by PKA makes phosphorylase kinase more sensitive to further stimulation by calcium. Maximal activation of phosphorylase kinase is achieved by phosphorylation of the α and β subunits, plus Ca^{2+} binding to the calmodulin subunit.

The importance of regulation by Ca^{2+} concentration can be seen in skeletal muscle cells, where nerve impulses in muscle contraction depolarize the cell membrane and stimulate Ca^{2+} efflux from the sarcoplasmic reticulum to the cytosol. The efflux of Ca^{2+} stimulates phosphorylase kinase by Ca^{2+} binding to the calmodulin subunit. At the same time, epinephrine released from the adrenal medulla stimulates the intracellular cAMP cascade, which leads to phosphorylation of the α and β subunits of phosphorylase kinase. The synergistic effects of Ca^{2+} and cAMP maximally stimulate phosphorylase kinase. Phosphorylase kinase, in turn, activates glycogen phosphorylase and thereby increases the rate of glycogen breakdown. This ensures that glucose is available to meet the increased fuel demands of muscle contraction. Concurrent actions of cAMP and Ca^{2+} stimulate kinases that phosphorylate and inhibit glycogen synthase (see Figure 12-15).

Glycogen phosphorylase can also be activated by Ca^{2+} release in response to stimulation of α_1-adrenergic receptors on liver cells by epinephrine, which leads to activation of phospholipase C. Phospholipase C generates Ins(1,4,5)P_3 and diacylglycerol, and Ins(1,4,5)P_3 stimulates the release of Ca^{2+} from the ER. This effect of Ca^{2+} is added to the other effects of epinephrine signaling on glycogen phosphorylase, as well as those on glycogen synthase, to enhance net glycogenolysis in response to epinephrine in liver.

Regulation of Glycogen Phosphorylase by Allosteric Mechanisms

The muscle and liver isozymes of glycogen phosphorylase differ in their sensitivity to allosteric effectors as shown in Figure 12-16. Muscle glycogen phosphorylase, but not the liver isoenzyme, has a nucleotide binding site; when AMP binds to this site on muscle glycogen phosphorylase *b*, it converts the muscle enzyme to the R state. ATP and glucose 6-phosphate compete with AMP for binding to this site, so glycogen phosphorylase *b* stays in the inactive T form when the muscle has adequate ATP and glucose 6-phosphate. This allosteric modification of muscle glycogen phosphorylase by ATP and AMP is a faster mechanism (milliseconds) of regulation than is hormone-induced phosphorylation of the enzyme (seconds to minutes). In general, these two mechanisms function in an ordered sequence. For example, in muscle contraction, glycogen phosphorylase *b*, but not glycogen phosphorylase *a*, is allosterically stimulated by AMP. When resting muscle begins to contract and AMP levels increase, this rapidly stimulates phosphorylase *b*. As muscle contraction continues, however, epinephrine stimulation of the cAMP-induced protein kinase cascade increases the concentration of phosphorylase *a*, thereby continuing the breakdown of glycogen regardless of the AMP concentration. Conversely, in the resting state, the phosphorylase *b* form predominates and ATP and glucose 6-phosphate levels are high. Under these conditions, AMP binding to phosphorylase *b* is inhibited and there is also no stimulation of phosphorylase *a* formation by epinephrine, resulting in inactivation of glycogenolysis when muscle is at rest.

The liver isozyme of glycogen phosphorylase is allosterically regulated by glucose and not by the AMP/ATP ratio. Glucose can bind to an allosteric site on hepatic glycogen phosphorylase *a*, and glucose binding causes the enzyme to transition from the R to the T form, inactivating it and making it a good substrate for PP1. Glucose therefore stimulates the dephosphorylation of glycogen phosphorylase *a* to convert it to glycogen phosphorylase *b* in liver. This regulatory mechanism ensures that glycogenolysis will be slowed under conditions of elevated blood glucose.

Regulation of Glycogen Phosphorylase Gene Expression

PYGL mRNA stability and liver glycogen phosphorylase enzyme levels are decreased by the diabetic state and can be normalized by insulin treatment (Rao et al., 1995).

PYRUVATE DEHYDROGENASE COMPLEX AND CITRIC ACID CYCLE

The aerobic phase of macronutrient catabolism is referred to as cellular respiration. The metabolic stages involved in cellular respiration are the production of acetyl-CoA from pyruvate (or fatty acids or certain amino acids); the complete oxidation of the acetyl moiety of acetyl-CoA via the citric acid cycle with substrate level ATP formation and formation of NADH and $FADH_2$; the utilization of reducing equivalents from the citric acid cycle for electron transport; and the production of ATP by oxidative phosphorylation (Figure 12-17).

Together with the pyruvate dehydrogenase complex, the enzymes of the citric acid cycle are present in the mitochondrial compartment of the cell. The reactions of glycolysis take place in the cytosol of the cell; therefore pyruvate produced as the end product of glycolysis needs to be translocated to the mitochondria. Pyruvate is transported across

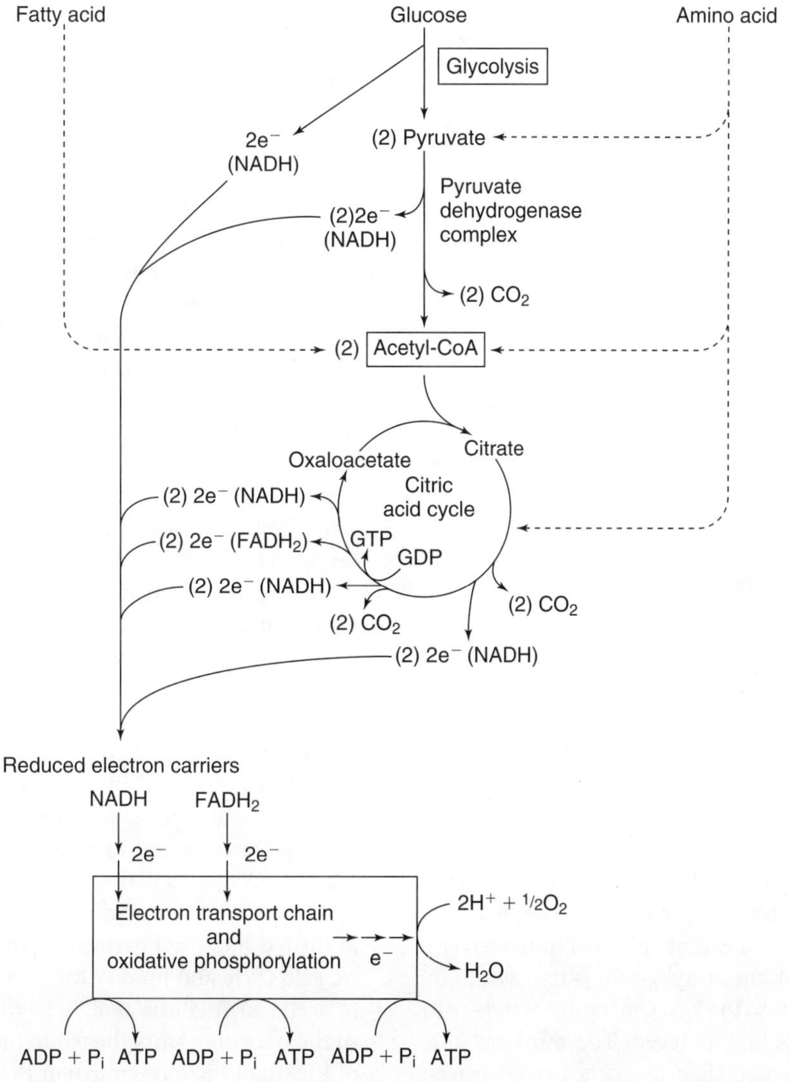

FIGURE 12-17 Complete oxidation of pyruvate in the mitochondria via the pyruvate dehydrogenase complex (oxidative decarboxylation), the citric acid cycle, the electron (e^-) transport chain, and oxidative phosphorylation.

the inner mitochondrial membrane by a monocarboxylate carrier and is then converted to acetyl-CoA by the pyruvate dehydrogenase complex. The acetyl-CoA so produced then enters the citric acid cycle. Although the complete citric acid cycle functions only in the mitochondria, it should be noted that some enzymes of the citric acid cycle also have cytosolic forms (i.e., cytosolic aconitase, isocitrate dehydrogenase, fumarase, and malate dehydrogenase) and that particular citric acid cycle enzymes in the mitochondria may play other roles in metabolism.

PYRUVATE DEHYDROGENASE COMPLEX

The pyruvate dehydrogenase complex, associated with the mitochondrial inner membrane of mammalian cells, catalyzes the conversion of pyruvate to acetyl-CoA. The overall reaction involves the activity of three individual enzymes, the activities of which are coordinated by association in a multienzyme complex. The complex includes pyruvate dehydrogenase (E_1), dihydrolipoyl transacetylase (E_2), and dihydrolipoyl dehydrogenase (E_3) (see Chapter 24, Figure 24-11). There are multiple molecules of each of the three enzymes in the large pyruvate dehydrogenase complex. The overall reaction is essentially irreversible and converts the 3-carbon intermediate, pyruvate, to acetyl-CoA. Acetyl-CoA, in turn, can be either oxidized via the citric acid cycle or used for fatty acid or isoprenoid/cholesterol/steroid synthesis, as discussed in Chapters 16 and 17.

The pyruvate dehydrogenase complex in mammals contains several different coenzymes derived primarily from the B vitamin family. These coenzymes include thiamin diphosphate (TDP), derived from thiamin; flavin adenine dinucleotide (FAD), derived from riboflavin; coenzyme A (CoA), derived from pantothenic acid; nicotinamide adenine dinucleotide (NAD), derived from niacin; and lipoate. These coenzymes perform specific functions in the activity of the three individual enzymes of the pyruvate dehydrogenase complex. These coenzymes are discussed in Chapters 24 and 26.

The first reaction of the multienzyme series is the decarboxylation of pyruvate, catalyzed by pyruvate dehydrogenase

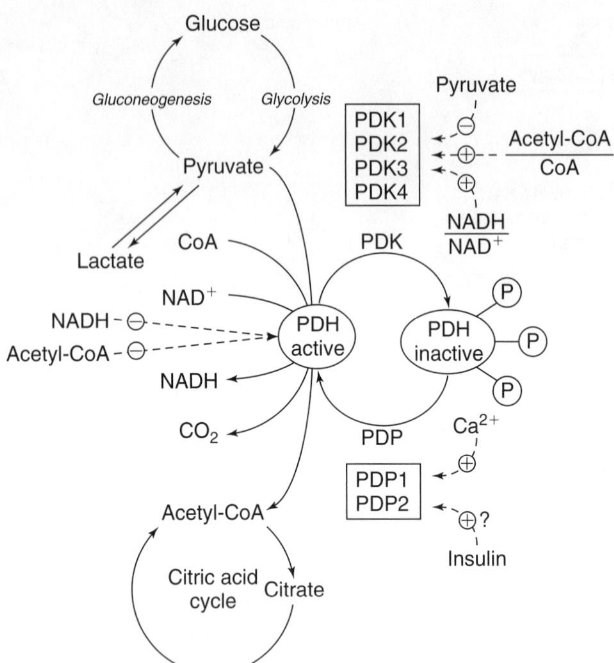

FIGURE 12-18 Regulation of the activity of the pyruvate dehydrogenase complex (PDH) by allosteric regulators and by phosphorylation/dephosphorylation by pyruvate dehydrogenase kinase (PDK) and pyruvate dehydrogenase phosphatase (PDP). Positive regulators are indicated by + and negative regulators are indicated by – signs.

(E_1), requiring the coenzyme TDP. The two electrons and the acetyl group are then transferred by E_1 to lipoate, which is attached to the second enzyme, dihydrolipoyl transacetylase (E_2). In the next reaction, the acetyl group is transferred by a transesterification reaction to CoA, generating acetyl-CoA; concomitantly, lipoate is fully reduced. The third enzyme, dihydrolipoyl dehydrogenase (E_3), transfers two hydrogen atoms from reduced lipoate to the coenzyme FAD bound to E_3, generating $FADH_2$ and regenerating the oxidized form of lipoate on E_2. A subsequent oxidation–reduction reaction transfers the hydrogen atoms of $FADH_2$ to NAD^+, forming NADH + H^+. Overall, the net reaction is the conversion of pyruvate + NAD^+ + CoA to acetyl-CoA + CO_2 + NADH + H^+.

Because the reaction catalyzed by the pyruvate dehydrogenase complex converts pyruvate to the nongluconeogenic acetyl-CoA, the enzymes of the complex are tightly regulated. The pyruvate dehydrogenase complex is regulated primarily by end product inhibition and by covalent modification, as illustrated in Figure 12-18 (Behal et al., 1993). The products of the component enzyme reactions, acetyl-CoA and NADH, act as negative feedback inhibitors of their respective reactions; acetyl-CoA inhibits E_2 and NADH inhibits E_3. Covalent modification of the multienzyme complex involves the phosphorylation and inactivation of E_1 by a specific protein kinase, pyruvate dehydrogenase kinase, which is bound to the enzyme complex. The activity of pyruvate dehydrogenase kinase is also regulated by allosteric effectors. The end product inhibitors acetyl-CoA and NADH activate the pyruvate dehydrogenase kinase, whereas pyruvate, free CoA, and NAD^+ inhibit this kinase and hence E_1 phosphorylation. Therefore when the mitochondrial [NADH]/[NAD^+] or [acetyl-CoA]/[CoA] ratio is maintained relatively high by the oxidation of fatty acids for energy, the production of acetyl-CoA from pyruvate is restrained via inhibition of the activity of the pyruvate dehydrogenase complex, via both phosphorylation and allosteric regulators. This allows tissues, such as the heart, to "spare" glucose and utilize fatty acids or ketone bodies for energy needs.

Four isozymes of pyruvate dehydrogenase kinase (PDK1-PDK4) are expressed in human tissues, with unique tissue distributions (Sugden and Holness, 2006). PDK2 is the most widely distributed. It is the major isoform in liver and kidney and is also expressed at high levels in skeletal muscle and heart. PDK4 is mainly expressed in skeletal muscle and heart. PDK1 and PDK3 have a more restricted expression pattern, with PDK1 high in heart and PDK3 highest in testis and lung. These kinases have the ability to phosphorylate sites on pyruvate dehydrogenase E_1, and phosphorylation renders E_1 and hence the pyruvate dehydrogenase complex inactive. Phosphorylation is reversible by action of pyruvate dehydrogenase phosphatase. Two isoforms of pyruvate dehydrogenase phosphatase (PDP) are expressed in humans; these are much lower in skeletal muscle than in heart, liver, kidney, and brain. Expression of PDK2 and PDK4 are suppressed by insulin, increased by glucocorticoids, and increased by PPARα ligands. PDK2 is more sensitive to negative regulation by pyruvate and to positive regulation by NADH and acetyl-CoA than is PDK4.

The pyruvate dehydrogenase complex is relatively active in the fed state, and pyruvate carbon is directed into the citric acid cycle and lipid synthesis via conversion of pyruvate to acetyl-CoA (Burri et al., 2010; Jeoung and Harris, 2010). In the transition from the fed to the starved state, expression of PDK4 and to a lesser extent PDK2 is induced in a tissue-specific manner. Increased expression of PDK results in increased phosphorylation and thus inhibition of the pyruvate dehydrogenase complex. Inhibition of pyruvate dehydrogenase then decreases glucose/pyruvate entry into the citric acid cycle as acetyl-CoA. The inhibition of the pyruvate dehydrogenase complex in liver, muscle, and other tissues prevents them from catabolizing glucose and gluconeogenic precursors during starvation. Metabolism shifts toward fat oxidation, which helps minimize muscle protein breakdown to supply gluconeogenic precursors while conserving available glucose for use by the brain and other obligate glycolytic tissues.

The use of glucose as a fuel or the conversion of glucose to fatty acids for storage requires flux through the pyruvate dehydrogenase reaction in the fed state. The regulation of pyruvate flux to acetyl-CoA despite relatively high acetyl-CoA and NADH concentrations depends largely on the ability of pyruvate to act as a potent negative allosteric effector of PDK, thus blocking its inhibitory phosphorylation of pyruvate dehydrogenase. The high concentrations of pyruvate produced when glucose is abundant are thus able to promote pyruvate's own further oxidative decarboxylation to acetyl-CoA, allowing flux of acetyl-CoA into the

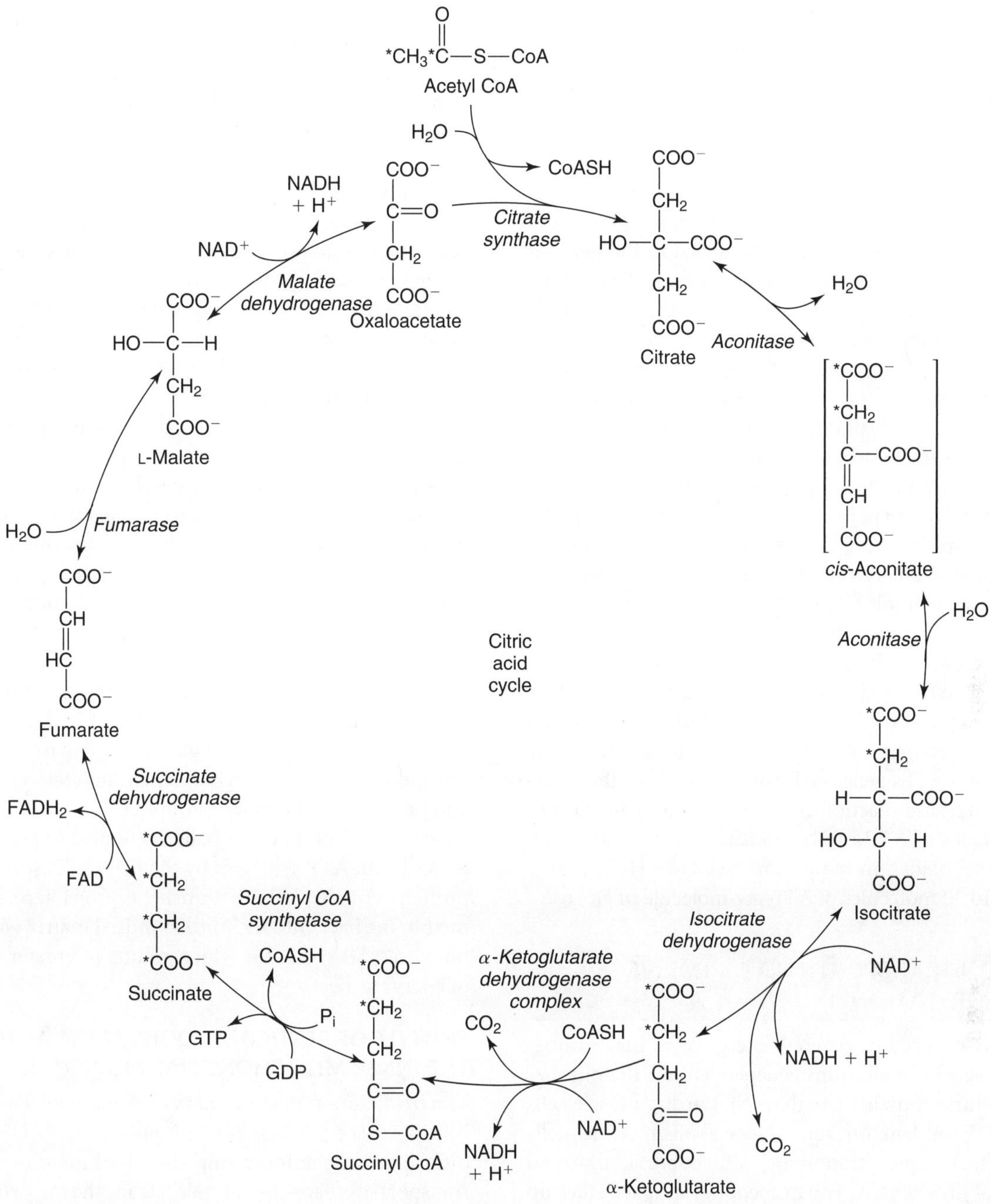

O
*CH_3*C—S—CoA
Acetyl CoA
H_2O
CoASH
Citrate synthase
COO^- CH_2 HO—C—COO^- CH_2 COO^-
Citrate
Aconitase
H_2O
*COO^- *CH_2 C—COO^- CH COO^-
cis-Aconitate
Aconitase
H_2O
*COO^- *CH_2 H—C—COO^- HO—C—H COO^-
Isocitrate
Isocitrate dehydrogenase
NAD^+
NADH + H^+
CO_2
*COO^- *CH_2 CH_2 C=O COO^-
α-Ketoglutarate
α-Ketoglutarate dehydrogenase complex
CoASH
NAD^+
NADH + H^+
CO_2
*COO^- *CH_2 CH_2 C=O S—CoA
Succinyl CoA
Succinyl CoA synthetase
CoASH
P_i
GDP
GTP
*COO^- *CH_2 *CH_2 *COO^-
Succinate
Succinate dehydrogenase
FAD
$FADH_2$
COO^- CH HC COO^-
Fumarate
Fumarase
H_2O
COO^- HO—C—H CH_2 COO^-
L-Malate
Malate dehydrogenase
NAD^+
NADH + H^+
COO^- C=O CH_2 COO^-
Oxaloacetate
Citric acid cycle

FIGURE 12-19 The oxidation of acetyl-CoA and generation of reducing equivalents and ATP equivalents by the citric acid cycle. Although these reactions result in the net oxidation of the acetyl group to two CO_2, the specific carbon atoms lost as CO_2 in a single (first) round of the cycle are derived from oxaloacetate. The carbons denoted by the asterisks are those from the acetyl moiety of acetyl-CoA. Because succinate and fumarate are symmetrical molecules, C1 and C2 cannot be distinguished from C3 and C4 once these intermediates are formed. The carbons from the acetyl moiety (now in succinate, fumarate, malate, or oxaloacetate) will be lost in subsequent rounds of the cycle.

citric acid cycle for oxidation for energy. When glucose is being used as a fuel, pyruvate acts as a feed-forward regulator of PDK/pyruvate dehydrogenase complex to ensure flux to acetyl-CoA. The negative effect of pyruvate on PDK (and hence its positive effect on pyruvate dehydrogenase complex) also allows for citrate synthesis and its use for lipogenesis when the acetyl-CoA formed from pyruvate enters the citric acid cycle along with anaplerotic substrates that generate oxaloacetate.

CITRIC ACID CYCLE

The metabolic fate of acetyl-CoA varies, depending upon dietary carbohydrate intake, the energy level of the cell, and the cell type. To meet the energy needs of the cell, acetyl-CoA can be completely oxidized by the enzymes of the citric acid cycle (Figure 12-19). If the energy needs of the cell have been met, an alternative route for acetyl-CoA utilization is for the biosynthesis of fatty acids in liver and other lipogenic tissues. Only the oxidation of acetyl-CoA via the citric acid cycle is considered in this chapter; other fates of acetyl-CoA are discussed in Chapters 16, 17, and 19. This cycle is also referred to as the *tricarboxylic acid (TCA) cycle* or the *Krebs cycle*, after Sir Hans Krebs who proposed this pathway in 1937.

The condensation of acetyl-CoA and oxaloacetate to form citrate marks the beginning of one round of the citric acid cycle, and the regeneration of oxaloacetate marks the completion. The energy transferred in the catabolism of acetyl-CoA via the citric acid cycle is carried in the reduced coenzymes and in GTP produced by substrate level phosphorylation (see Figure 12-19). For each molecule of acetyl-CoA that enters the cycle, two molecules of CO_2 are formed from the acetyl moiety, and reducing equivalents are produced in the form of three molecules of NADH and one molecule of $FADH_2$. From one molecule of NADH entering the electron transport chain, a maximum of three molecules of ATP are produced by oxidative phosphorylation. $FADH_2$ generates a maximum of two molecules of ATP by oxidative phosphorylation. Therefore the reducing equivalents produced in one round of the citric acid cycle generate a maximum of 11 molecules of ATP. To this can be added the molecule of ATP equivalent (i.e., GTP) produced by substrate-level phosphorylation at the succinyl-CoA synthetase step. Taken together, a maximum of 12 molecules of ATP are produced as a result of the complete oxidation of the acetyl moiety from acetyl-CoA through the citric acid cycle. If the maximum of 3 ATPs generated from pyruvate in the pyruvate dehydrogenase reaction is added to this, a maximum of 15 molecules of ATP can be produced as a result of the mitochondrial oxidation of pyruvate to $CO_2 + H_2O$. This is equivalent to 30 molecules of ATP per molecule of glucose.

ELECTRON TRANSPORT AND OXIDATIVE PHOSPHORYLATION

The capacity of a cell to generate energy from macronutrients under aerobic conditions is dependent on the number of mitochondria contained by that cell. Cardiac muscle cells are highly dependent on aerobic metabolism; these cells contain a high concentration of mitochondria, more so than skeletal muscle cells. The mitochondrial space takes up approximately 50% of the total cytoplasmic volume in cardiac muscle cells. Liver cells contain a similarly high concentration of mitochondria. The amount of oxygen consumed by various tissues in the human adult varies depending upon the mitochondrial respiratory capacity of the tissue and upon physiological activity. Skeletal muscle uses approximately 30% of consumed oxygen at rest, but with heavy exercise skeletal muscle may use more than 86% of consumed oxygen. The brain and abdominal tissues also consume large percentages of oxygen at rest.

STRUCTURE OF THE MITOCHONDRION

To understand the enzymatic reactions that occur during electron transport with concomitant oxidative phosphorylation and ATP production, it is important to understand the cellular physiology that makes it possible. This requires a description of the structure of mitochondria, which are organelles found within the cytoplasm of cells. Mitochondria have a membrane structure that effectively divides the mitochondrion into functional subcompartments. There is an outer membrane and an inner membrane, with numerous invaginations referred to as cristae; between these two membranes is the intermembrane space. Notably, in cells with a high rate of cellular respiration such as cardiac muscle cells, the cristae are more numerous. The space inside the inner membrane is the matrix that contains the enzymes of the pyruvate dehydrogenase complex and the citric acid cycle. Associated with the inner membrane are most of the enzymes involved in electron transport and oxidative phosphorylation, as well as carrier proteins for metabolic intermediates that are transported between the cytosol and the mitochondrial matrix. The outer membrane is permeable because it contains large, channel-forming proteins called porins. In effect, the intermembrane space is similar in composition to the cytosolic space because the outer membrane is so permeable. The inner membrane is much less permeable than the outer membrane to metabolic intermediates and nucleotides. Consequently, it is the inner membrane that effectively separates the mitochondrial and cytosolic domains of the cell. This inner membrane is not permeable to oxaloacetate, NADH, or NAD^+, but it does have transporters for malate/α-ketoglutarate, aspartate/glutamate, phosphoenolpyruvate, pyruvate, citrate/malate, ATP, ADP, and phosphate. The movement of H^+ across the inner mitochondrial membrane normally is coupled to electron transfer and with ATP synthesis by the F_1F_0-ATPase. Uncoupling proteins are also able to transfer protons across the inner membrane back into the mitochondrial matrix without coupling to ATP synthesis, which results in greater dissipation of energy as heat.

SHUTTLE OF REDUCING EQUIVALENTS ACROSS THE INNER MITOCHONDRIAL MEMBRANE

The oxidation–reduction pairs that are involved in electron transport (i.e., NAD^+/NADH and FAD/$FADH_2$) cannot diffuse across the inner mitochondrial membrane. Specific transport mechanisms compensate for the impermeability of this membrane to these cofactors. The transport of reducing equivalents (protons and electrons) from the cytosol to the mitochondrial matrix is accomplished via substrate shuttles. The most active of these shuttle systems is the malate–aspartate shuttle. Malate carries reducing equivalents, which were generated as NADH in the cytosol and then used to reduce oxaloacetate to malate in the cytosol, to the mitochondrial matrix. In the mitochondrion, NADH is regenerated by conversion of malate back to oxaloacetate, which can then be transaminated to aspartate and exit from the mitochondrion. Cytosolic and mitochondrial isozymes of malate dehydrogenase catalyze the interconversion of malate and oxaloacetate. The malate–aspartate shuttle functions primarily in liver, heart muscle, and kidney. NADH can be oxidized by the mitochondrial respiratory chain regardless of whether it is regenerated in the mitochondrial matrix from cytosolic reducing equivalents or generated within the mitochondrial matrix by the citric acid cycle and other reactions.

In skeletal muscle and brain, another NADH shuttle mechanism occurs. This is the glycerol 3-phosphate shuttle, which transports electrons by the inner membrane flavoprotein glycerol 3-phosphate dehydrogenase rather than by the transfer of organic compounds. Dihydroxyacetone phosphate, substrate for the cytosolic glycerol 3-phosphate dehydrogenase, accepts two reducing equivalents from NADH, producing glycerol 3-phosphate and NAD^+ in the cytosol. Another isozyme of glycerol 3-phosphate dehydrogenase, located on the outer face of the inner mitochondrial membrane, transfers two reducing equivalents from glycerol 3-phosphate in the intermembrane space, via an FAD coenzyme, to ubiquinone within the inner mitochondrial membrane. The glycerol 3-phosphate shuttle is different from the malate–aspartate shuttle in that the reducing equivalents are transferred from ubiquinone to complex III (the cytochrome bc_1 complex), thereby bypassing the NADH dehydrogenase complex of the electron transport chain and leading to the synthesis of a maximum of only two molecules of ATP rather than the three molecules possible when electrons enter the chain at the level of NADH (see Chapter 21, Figure 21-4).

Another critical transport step that occurs at the inner mitochondrial membrane is the transfer of adenine nucleotides by the adenine nucleotide translocator. In this case, cytosolic ADP produced in the hydrolysis of ATP is exchanged across the inner membrane for ATP produced by oxidative phosphorylation. This exchanger provides ADP as substrate for oxidative phosphorylation at the same time as it removes the product from the mitochondrial compartment.

Although the focus of the preceding discussion has been on the flow of reducing equivalents into the mitochondria, other shuttles carry potential reducing equivalents from the mitochondrial compartment into the cytosol for use in reductive synthetic processes. The transfer of substrate as well as reducing equivalents from the mitochondria to the cytosol is discussed in Chapter 14 for gluconeogenesis from amino acids and in Chapters 16 and 17 for lipogenesis from acetyl-CoA.

ELECTRON TRANSPORT

The electron transport chain is another example of a pathway channeling metabolic intermediates in a series of linked enzymatic reactions. These are oxidation–reduction reactions, in which electrons are passed through protein complexes that have numerous redox centers with increasingly greater affinity for electrons (or increased standard reduction potential). The protein complexes involved in electron transport are integral membrane proteins, with cofactors that can freely diffuse across the inner membrane. At three distinct steps (at complexes I, III, and IV), the free energy generated from electron transport is used to pump protons from the mitochondrial matrix to the intermembrane space between the inner and outer membranes; this establishes an electrochemical gradient across the inner mitochondrial membrane. The amount of energy trapped in the proton gradient at each step is sufficient to drive the synthesis of the gamma phosphate bond in one molecule of ATP (30.5 kJ, or 7.3 kcal). The three electron transfer steps where this occurs are the reduction of flavin mononucleotide by NADH in complex I, the reduction of cytochrome c_1 by cytochrome *b* in complex III, and the reduction of molecular oxygen by cytochrome a_3 in complex IV (cytochrome *c* oxidase). These oxidation–reduction reactions produce sufficient energy to effectively pump protons from the mitochondrial matrix to the intermembrane space. A proton concentration gradient is established, which changes the pH (rendering the matrix more alkaline) and electrical charge (rendering the matrix more negative) across the inner mitochondrial membrane.

The movement of electrons via a series of oxidation–reduction reactions that make up the electron transport chain in the inner membrane of the mitochondrion is a specific example of energy transfer in linked, exergonic reactions. The large free energy generated from this process can produce ATP. The question remains: What is the mechanism by which energy generated by electron transport is coupled to the production of ATP? The accepted mechanism is derived from the chemiosmotic theory, which postulates that the proton-motive force generated from the proton concentration difference across the inner mitochondrial membrane conserves energy for ATP production. ATP is produced when the movement of protons down their concentration gradient releases this energy. Protons return to the matrix via specific proton pores in the membrane. The pore or channel through which protons move is provided by a subunit structure of the mitochondrial ATP synthase that spans the inner membrane.

This mitochondrial ATP synthase is an F-type ATPase, which is characterized as an ATP-dependent proton pump. Generally, F-type ATPases utilize the energy of ATP hydrolysis to move protons against a concentration gradient. The reverse, however, occurs in oxidative phosphorylation when protons move back into the mitochondrial matrix through the channel provided by the F_0 subunit of ATP synthase. This spontaneous flow of protons releases energy for the synthesis of ATP from enzyme-bound ADP and P_i. The latter enzymatic reaction is catalyzed by the second ATP synthase subunit (F_1), which is on the interior side of the inner mitochondrial membrane.

Therefore the three sites in electron transport that pump protons to the intermembrane space generate the electrochemical energy for ATP synthesis. The electrochemical energy difference generated across the inner mitochondrial membrane is referred to as the proton-motive force. It is the amount of free energy available to do work when protons flow passively back into the mitochondrial matrix. The electrochemical energy generated by each of complexes I, III, and IV is sufficient for and coupled to ATP synthesis. Therefore three molecules of ATP are generated from the oxidation–reduction reactions initiated by NADH entry into the electron transport chain. Only two molecules of ATP are generated from $FADH_2$, which donates electrons to oxidized ubiquinone, bypassing the oxidation–reduction reactions of

CLINICAL CORRELATION

Inherited Mitochondrial Respiratory Chain Disorders

Mitochondrial respiratory chain disorders are among the most common inherited metabolic diseases, with biochemical defects arising from mutations in either the mitochondrial genome or the nuclear genome. Inheritance patterns due to mutations in the nuclear genome may be either recessive or dominant, but metabolic disease due to mutations in the mitochondrial genome are always dominant because the zygote derives its mitochondria and hence its mitochondrial DNA from the ovum.

Mitochondrial DNA is circular and encodes 13 proteins, which are synthesized in this compartment of the cell. All of these proteins are components of the respiratory chain. They include seven subunits of complex I, one subunit of complex III, three subunits of cytochrome C oxidase, and two subunits of the ATP synthase (Bindoff and Turnbull, 1994). The mitochondrial genome also has 24 RNA-encoding genes that encode two large ribosomal RNA subunits and 22 transfer RNAs. The other mitochondrial proteins and RNAs are encoded by the nuclear genome and are transported into the mitochondria after their synthesis.

Disorders of mitochondrial oxidative phosphorylation lead to decreased ATP production for energy. Such disorders can become apparent under metabolic stress such as exercise. Typical biochemical signs are the elevation of plasma lactate levels and abnormal excretion of organic acids in the urine.

complex I and the energy derived there. Approximately 40% of the energy from electron transport is conserved in the form of ATP; the remaining energy is dissipated as heat. (See Chapter 21 for more about electron transport and oxidative phosphorylation.)

ATP EQUIVALENTS PRODUCED FROM THE COMPLETE OXIDATION OF GLUCOSE

The total amount of ATP produced from the complete oxidation of glucose to CO_2 and H_2O can be summarized at this point. In glycolysis, the conversion of one molecule of glucose to two molecules of pyruvate produces a net gain of two molecules of ATP from substrate-level phosphorylation. Reducing equivalents (two molecules of NADH) are also generated in the glyceraldehyde 3-phosphate dehydrogenase reaction. These reducing equivalents generate a maximum of four to six molecules of ATP after translocation of electrons to the mitochondrion (depending on the mode of transport across the inner membrane of the mitochondrion). Therefore, under aerobic conditions in those cells with mitochondria, six to eight molecules of ATP are produced as a result of the breakdown of one molecule of glucose to two molecules of pyruvate. The pyruvate dehydrogenase reaction in the mitochondrion generates reducing equivalents as well; two molecules of NADH are produced from the conversion of two molecules of pyruvate to two molecules of acetyl-CoA. Therefore this step generates up to six molecules of ATP from electron transport and oxidative phosphorylation.

Another 24 molecules of ATP are generated in the mitochondria from oxidation of two acetyl moieties by the citric acid cycle coupled with the electron transport chain and oxidative phosphorylation. These ATPs are derived from one substrate-level ATP equivalent, three NADH, and one $FADH_2$ formed per acetyl moiety that is completely oxidized by the citric acid cycle. Overall, the total energy generated from the complete oxidation of one molecule of glucose to six molecules of CO_2 and H_2O is as much as 36 to 38 molecules of ATP.

OTHER PATHWAYS OF CARBOHYDRATE METABOLISM

There are several other secondary pathways of carbohydrate metabolism that do not involve the central anabolic and catabolic pathways described above. These pathways serve more specialized functions related to the generation of coenzymes, nucleotides, glycoproteins, glycolipids, and glucuronides, as described later.

PENTOSE PHOSPHATE PATHWAY

The pentose phosphate pathway serves as a secondary pathway of glucose oxidation, a source of reducing equivalents in the form of NADPH, and a means of generation of 5-carbon sugar phosphates, particularly ribose 5-phosphate. The pentose phosphate pathway is also called the hexose monophosphate shunt or the phosphogluconate pathway. The first three steps of the pathway shown in Figure 12-20 are involved in the oxidation of glucose 6-phosphate to ribulose 5-phosphate, which can be transformed to ribose 5-phosphate or xylulose 5-phosphate.

NADPH is formed in the first and third steps, which are catalyzed by glucose 6-phosphate dehydrogenase and phosphogluconate dehydrogenase, respectively. Glucose 6-phosphate dehydrogenase is regulated by the $NADP^+$ concentration (substrate availability), and the need for NADPH regeneration determines flux through this pathway. Glucose 6-phosphate dehydrogenase is considered a lipogenic enzyme because the NADPH generated by the pentose phosphate pathway is required for synthesis of fatty acids, cholesterol, and other sterols. The tissues most heavily involved in fatty acid and cholesterol biosynthesis (mammary gland, adipose tissue, liver, adrenal cortex, and testis) are rich in pentose phosphate pathway enzymes. The gene that encodes glucose 6-phosphate dehydrogenase (*G6PD*) is regulated by fasting and refeeding and by dietary fatty acids in the liver, consistent with the important role of the encoded enzyme in lipogenesis in liver (Stabile et al., 1996). The pentose phosphate pathway is also active in red blood cells, which require NADPH for reduction of glutathione. Reduced glutathione is

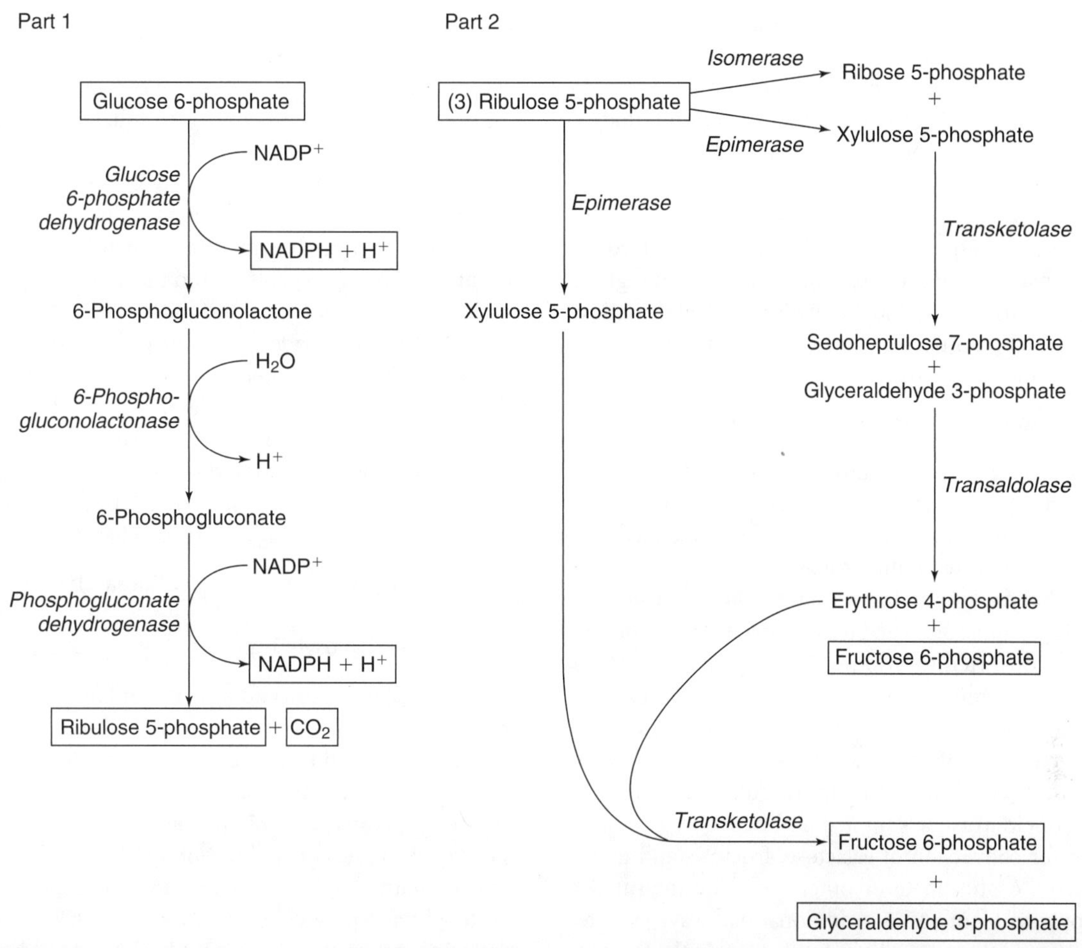

FIGURE 12-20 The pentose phosphate pathway. Oxidation of glucose occurs in part 1 of the pathway. Part 2 of the pathway shows the rearrangement of three molecules of ribulose 5-P to re-form glycolytic intermediates, fructose 6-phosphate and glyceraldehyde 3-phosphate. Although not shown, all of the reactions in Part 2 are reversible. They have been shown going in one direction only to make it easier to see how the pentose phosphate pathway can accomplish the net oxidation of glucose.

needed for maintenance of redox state and thus the integrity of the red blood cell membrane. Without adequate NADPH, the red blood cell membrane lyses and hemolytic anemia results. Oxidation of glucose by the pentose phosphate pathway occurs in the cytosol and does not require mitochondria.

The ribulose 5-phosphate produced from glucose 6-phosphate by the first three steps of the pentose phosphate pathway serves as a source of ribose 5-phosphate, which can be formed by isomerization of ribulose 5-phosphate. Ribose 5-phosphate is essential for the biosynthesis of nucleotides and nucleic acids, including ATP, coenzyme A, NAD, NADP, FAD, RNA, and DNA. If the cell needs the pentose phosphates produced from glucose 6-phosphate, the pathway may stop at the level of the pentose phosphates. Alternatively, a series of reversible reactions can convert excess ribose 5-phosphate and xylulose 5-phosphate to the glycolytic intermediates fructose 6-phosphate and glyceraldehyde 3-phosphate, as shown in part 2 of Figure 12-20. Fructose 6-phosphate and glyceraldehyde 3-phosphate can reenter glycolysis or be converted to glucose 6-phosphate and enter other pathways of glucose metabolism. These sugar rearrangements also allow for degradation of ribose 5-phosphate from nucleotide degradation. Because the reactions involved in these sugar rearrangements are freely reversible, cells that need pentose phosphates also can form them by conversion of glycolytic intermediates to pentoses without net oxidation of glucose to CO_2 and without NADPH production.

Although only C1 of glucose 6-phosphate is lost as CO_2 in the pentose phosphate pathway, net oxidation of glucose can occur if both parts 1 and 2 of the pathway, as shown in Figure 12-20, are operative. This occurs when the need for NADPH is greater than the need for ribose 5-phosphate. If six molecules of glucose 6-phosphate are oxidized to six molecules of pentose 5-phosphate, and these pentoses are further rearranged to form four molecules of fructose 6-phosphate and two molecules of glyceraldehyde 3-phosphate (the equivalent of five molecules of hexose), net conversion of one molecule of glucose to six molecules of CO_2 will have occurred with net production of 12 molecules of NADPH.

FORMATION OF SUGAR DERIVATIVES FOR SYNTHESIS OF GLUCURONIDES, LACTOSE, AND OTHER CARBOHYDRATES

Various sugars and sugar derivatives are formed from glucose phosphate. These sugar derivatives have a variety of functions in the body, including serving as substrates for glucuronidation pathways; for synthesis of glycosaminoglycans, glycoproteins, and glycolipids; and for lactose synthesis by the mammary gland. The amount of glucose that is consumed by these pathways is generally small relative to the amount that is catabolized via glycolysis and the citric acid cycle.

Glucuronide formation is an important pathway of glucose consumption in the liver. UDP-glucose, formed by reaction of glucose 1-phosphate with UTP, is oxidized to UDP-glucuronate. UDP-glucuronate serves as the glucuronosyl donor in various detoxification and elimination reactions in which conjugates of glucuronate and nonpolar acceptor molecules are formed.

$$\text{UDP-glucuronate} + \text{R-OH} \rightarrow \text{R-O-Glucuronate} + \text{UDP}$$

Many drugs, such as the anti-AIDS drug 3′-azido-2′-3′-dideoxythymidine (AZT) or the over-the-counter drug acetaminophen, and endogenous compounds, such as bilirubin, are conjugated with glucuronate to form more polar compounds that are more readily excreted in the urine and bile. UDP-glucuronate also can be converted to glucuronate, which can be converted to xylulose 5-phosphate, a pentose phosphate pathway intermediate. In most species other than primates, glucuronate is a substrate for ascorbic acid synthesis (see Chapter 27). Because humans and other primates lack one of the enzymes in this pathway, gulonolactone oxidase, ascorbic acid must be supplied in the diet.

Pathways for conversion of galactose, fructose, and mannose to glucose 6-phosphate or other glycolytic intermediates are shown in Figure 12-5. Additional pathways exist to form a number of other sugar derivatives, many in the form of nucleotide diphosphate sugars. These include GDP-L-fucose from GDP-mannose; UDP-*N*-acetylglucosamine, UDP-*N*-acetylgalactosamine, and CMP-*N*-acetylneuraminic acid (one of the sialic acids) from glucose phosphate or fructose phosphate; dTDP-rhamnose from glucose phosphate; and UDP-galactose from galactose 1-phosphate or UDP-glucose. The addition of an *O*-linked *N*-acetylglucosamine monosaccharide to a serine or threonine residue of a protein is a common, although poorly understood, reversible posttranslational modification that appears to play a regulatory function.

The disaccharide lactose is synthesized by the lactating mammary gland. The mammary enzyme lactose synthase is induced by release of the hormone prolactin. UDP-galactose and glucose are substrates; a glycosidic bond is formed between galactose and glucose to form β-galactosyl(1,4)glucose, commonly known as lactose.

SYNTHESIS OF GLYCOSAMINOGLYCANS AND PROTEOGLYCANS

Glycosaminoglycan chains are long, unbranched, heteropolysaccharide chains made up largely of disaccharide repeating units, with a hexosamine and a uronic acid commonly found in the repeating structure. Sugar residues in many glycosaminoglycans are sulfated, with the sulfate groups being linked either to hydroxyl groups of the sugar residues or to amino groups of the hexosamine residues. Both the carboxylate groups of the uronic acid units and the sulfate groups of the sulfated sugars are ionized and responsible for the high overall negative charge associated with these compounds. Six classes of glycosaminoglycans are recognized: hyaluronate, chondroitin sulfate, dermatan sulfate, heparin, heparan sulfate, and keratan sulfate. Most of these are found covalently attached to protein in proteoglycan and are present mainly in the extracellular matrix of tissues. Exceptions include hyaluronate, which is not known to be covalently bound to protein, and the heparin that is found as an intracellular component of mast cells.

The oligosaccharide chains of glycosaminoglycans contain sugars linked to other sugars by glycosidic bonds. Chondroitin sulfate, dermatan sulfate, heparin, heparan sulfate, and keratan sulfate chains are synthesized in the lumen of the ER by transfer of glycosyl units from nucleotide diphosphate (NDP) derivatives (such as UDP) to the nonreducing end of an acceptor sugar or oligosaccharide chain.

$$\text{NDP-sugar (Donor)} + \text{Sugar or Oligosaccharide (Acceptor)}$$

$$\rightarrow \text{Glycosyl-O-glycose (Glycoside)} + \text{NDP}$$

Conversely, hyaluronic acid is synthesized in association with the plasma membrane using UDP-glucuronate and UDP-*N*-acetylglucosamine as precursors; sugar units are added to the reducing end of the chain by hyaluronan synthase.

Proteoglycans are high-molecular-weight polyanionic substances that consist of many different glycosaminoglycan chains linked covalently to a protein core. Because proteoglycans may contain as much as 95% carbohydrate, their properties tend to resemble those of polysaccharides more than those of proteins. The polysaccharide chains (glycosaminoglycan chains) of proteoglycans are assembled by the sequential action of a series of glycosyltransferases in the lumen of the ER. These glycosyltransferases catalyze the transfer of a monosaccharide from an NDP-sugar to the appropriate acceptor, either the nonreducing end of another sugar or an amino acid side chain on a polypeptide. In chondroitin sulfate proteoglycan formation, for example, sugar units are added to the core protein to form a tetrasaccharide linkage region followed by alternate addition of the characteristic repeating *N*-acetylgalactosamine and glucuronate units of chondroitin sulfate and by sulfation of the *N*-acetylgalactosamine residues on either C4 or C6.

Proteoglycans are found in such tissues as cartilage, tendons, ligaments, aorta, skin, blood vessels, and heart valves. Proteoglycans are usually found together with fibrous proteins, such as collagen and elastin, in the extracellular matrix. The network of proteoglycans and the cross-linked fibers of collagen or elastin provide the extracellular matrix with tensile strength, as is found in tendons, or elasticity, as is found in ligaments. In addition, an intricate attachment is formed between cells and the proteoglycans of extracellular matrix. Integrins, integral membrane proteins of the cell, have an extracellular domain that binds members of a family of adhesion proteins, and these adhesion proteins also bind to proteoglycans. Therefore integrins and the extracellular adhesion proteins attach cells to the surrounding proteoglycans of the extracellular matrix. Common adhesion proteins are fibrin and laminin.

Chondroitin sulfate is the most abundant class of glycosaminoglycans in the body. Most chondroitin sulfate chains consist of between 60 and 100 sugar residues made up mainly of alternating *N*-acetylgalactosamine and glucuronate units. A typical chondroitin sulfate proteoglycan has about 100 chondroitin sulfate chains attached to the protein core. These chondroitin sulfate proteoglycans are abundant in cartilage, tendons, ligaments, and aorta.

Although hyaluronate chains are not covalently attached to proteins, hyaluronate can serve as a central strand around which proteoglycan molecules are organized. Hyaluronate chains can be very long (approximately 10^6 sugar residues). Because of its large molecular weight and anionic character, hyaluronate holds large volumes of water and serves as an effective lubricant and shock absorbent. It is found predominantly in the synovial fluid of the joints and the vitreous humor of the eye.

SYNTHESIS OF GLYCOPROTEINS

Glycoproteins are defined as proteins that contain one or more saccharide chains (usually less than 12 to 15 sugar residues per chain) that lack serial repeat units and that are bound covalently to the polypeptide chain. This definition distinguishes them from the carbohydrate-rich proteoglycans. Glycoproteins are found in cell membranes with the oligosaccharide portion of the glycoprotein on the external face of the plasma membrane. The carbohydrate portion of glycoproteins can range from 1% to 70% of the glycoprotein by weight. The carbohydrate chains are covalently linked to glycoproteins by *N*- or *O*-glycosyl bonds. A variety of monosaccharide units that are linked by either α- or β-glycosidic bonds result in the diversity of oligosaccharide moieties that are found in glycoproteins.

Glycosylation of proteins occurs in the ER and Golgi apparatus. Glycosylation alters the properties of proteins, and the oligosaccharide structures also act as recognition signals for various aspects of protein targeting and for cellular recognition of proteins and of other cells. The *O*-linked oligosaccharides are synthesized in the Golgi apparatus by serial addition of monosaccharide units to a completed polypeptide chain. The sugar residues are added by a series of glycosyltransferases. This process begins with transfer of a sugar such as *N*-acetylgalactosamine from UDP-*N*-acetylgalactosamine to a serine or threonine residue on the polypeptide. This is then followed by stepwise addition of other sugars.

The *N*-linked oligosaccharides are synthesized somewhat differently and usually contain a core structure made up of mannose and *N*-acetylglucosamine residues. *N*-glycosylation begins in the ER and is completed in the Golgi apparatus. This common core is preassembled as a dolichol-linked oligosaccharide before incorporation into the polypeptide. First, *N*-acetylglucosamine from UDP-*N*-acetylglucosamine is attached to dolichol phosphate to form *N*-acetylglucosaminylpyrophosphoryldolichol, with release of UMP. The addition of other core sugars occurs and, in the final step, the core oligosaccharide is transferred from the dolichol pyrophosphate to an asparagine residue in the polypeptide chain. After synthesis and transfer of the specific core region, extensive processing of the oligosaccharide chain occurs in the Golgi apparatus. Processing involves removal of some of the core oligosaccharide's sugar units followed by addition of other sugar residues to the remaining core oligosaccharide; these Golgi reactions are catalyzed by glycosyltransferases and do not require the participation of dolichol intermediates.

Glycoproteins are important components of cell membranes where the oligosaccharide portion of the glycoprotein is on the external face of the plasma membrane. Glycoproteins make up a major part of the mucus secreted by epithelial cells. Many secreted proteins such as follicle-stimulating hormone, chorionic gonadotropin, and luteinizing hormone are glycoproteins, and many plasma proteins such as immunoglobulins, prothrombin, plasminogen, and ceruloplasmin are also glycoproteins. A well-characterized erythrocyte glycoprotein called glycophorin is widely studied as a model of plasma membrane glycoproteins. The glycophorin C complex in human erythrocyte membranes regulates the stability and mechanical properties of the plasma membrane. Components of the glycophorin C complex are implicated in ion channel clustering, cytoskeletal organization, cell signaling, and cell proliferation (Chishti, 1998). The oligosaccharide component of glycoproteins also marks soluble glycoproteins in the plasma for continued circulation or degradation by the liver. A specific unit of the oligosaccharide, a sialic acid residue at the terminus of the oligosaccharide chain, marks glycoproteins for continued circulation; the loss of this sialic acid residue results in the uptake of the asialoglycoprotein and its degradation by the liver. Liver contains asialoglycoprotein receptors that recognize, bind, and internalize glycoproteins that lack terminal sialic acid residues.

SYNTHESIS OF GLYCOLIPIDS

Sphingoglycolipids are glycosyl derivatives of sphingolipids. Structure and synthesis of the glycosphingolipids, including glucocerebrosides, galactocerebrosides, globosides, and gangliosides, are discussed in Chapters 4, 6, and 17. The more complex globosides and gangliosides contain glucose and/or galactose as well as additional sugars such as L-fucose, *N*-acetylgalactosamine, and sialic acids (e.g., *N*-acetylneuraminic acid).

Another important glycolipid is glycosylphosphatidylinositol (GPI), which anchors a variety of proteins to the exterior surface of the plasma membrane. The core GPI is synthesized on the luminal side of the ER from phosphatidylinositol, UDP-*N*-acetylglucosamine, dolichol phosphate mannose, and phosphatidylethanolamine. The core GPI structure is modified by the addition of a variety of additional sugar residues, which vary with the protein to which the GPI attaches. Target proteins in the ER become attached to preformed GPI when the amino group of the GPI phosphoethanolamine moiety nucleophilically attacks a specific residue of the protein near its C-terminus, resulting in a transamidation reaction that releases a 20- to 30-amino acid residue C-terminal peptide and attaches GPI to the new C-terminal amino acid residue of the target protein. These GPI-anchored proteins are found on the exterior surface of the plasma membrane of cells; the fatty acids of GPI are inserted into the lipid membrane to provide the anchor.

DIETARY REFERENCE INTAKES AND TYPICAL INTAKES OF CARBOHYDRATES

The IOM set a Recommended Dietary Allowance (RDA) for carbohydrate for the first time in 2002 (IOM, 2002). The Estimated Average Requirement (EAR) was based on the minimum amount of glucose consumed by the brain under circumstances of adequate energy intake. The amount of glucose required by the central nervous system to prevent an increase in the plasma concentrations of acetoacetate and β-hydroxybutyrate was estimated to be approximately 100 g/day. The estimated utilization of glucose by the brain of children from 1 year onward is similar to that of adults, so the EAR was set as 100 g/day of carbohydrate for all groups except infants, for whom Adequate Intakes (AIs) are based on dietary intake. The RDA was set using a coefficient of variation of 15% [100 g/day + 2(15)] to yield an RDA of 130 g/day for children and adults. Furthermore, an Acceptable Macronutrient Distribution Range (AMDR) was also set for total digestible carbohydrate based on the role of carbohydrates as a source of energy to maintain body weight. The AMDR for children and adults is 45% to 65% of total calories. The *Report of the Dietary Guidelines Advisory Committee on the Dietary Guidelines for Americans 2010,* based on a systematic review of the current literature, concluded that macronutrient proportions of the diet are not related to weight loss (U.S. Department of Agriculture [USDA], 2010). A diet that is less that 45% of calories as carbohydrates was judged to be of no benefit for long-term (12 months) weight loss. Based on this conclusion, along with evidence that diets that are less than 45% calories as carbohydrate may pose health risks, the committee concluded that low-carbohydrate diets should not be recommended for weight loss or maintenance.

DRIs Across the Life Cycle: Digestible Carbohydrates (Starches and Sugars)

	g Carbohydrate per Day (RDA)
Infants, 0 through 6 mo	60 (AI)
6 through 12 mo	95 (AI)
Children, all age groups	130
Males, all age groups	130
Females, all age groups	130
Pregnant	175
Lactating	210

Data from IOM. (2002). *Dietary Reference Intakes for energy, carbohydrate, fiber, fat, fatty acids, cholesterol, protein, and amino acids.* Washington, DC: The National Academies Press.

AI, Adequate Intake; *DRI,* Dietary Reference Intake; *RDA,* Recommended Dietary Allowance.

Although it is recognized that humans can adapt to a diet that contains essentially no carbohydrate by using amino acids and glycerol (from fat) for gluconeogenesis, this adaptation involves increased production of β-hydroxybutyric and acetoacetic acids. The plasma concentration of these keto acids (ketone bodies) is normally very low, even after an overnight fast, but the ketone body concentrations rise markedly during adaptation to starvation. Similar increases in keto acid concentrations have been observed in children with epilepsy being treated for extended periods with "ketogenic diets" (Vining, 1999; Swink et al., 1997). The long-term effects of elevated ketone body concentrations are not known. It is possible that they could have some adverse effects on bone mineral density, cholesterol levels, development and function of the central nervous system, one's general sense of well-being, or glycogen stores.

According to the National Health and Nutrition Examination Survey (NHANES, 1999–2008) in 2007–2008, the average daily energy intake was 2,504 and 1,771 calories for adult men and women, respectively. For women, 50.5% of total caloric intake was in the form of carbohydrates, and for men, 47.9% was carbohydrate intake. Therefore, according to the most recent United States population food intake data, adult men and women are consuming carbohydrates within the AMDR range of 45% to 65% of total calories. Over the 10-year period from 1999 to 2008 energy intake was relatively stable, as there were no statistically significant changes in total energy intake in either men or women in any ethnic group. However, there were trends in macronutrient intakes; average carbohydrate intake decreased and average protein intake increased in both men and women over this period.

An increment of 35 g/day was added to the adult EAR to establish the EAR for pregnant women. This increment was

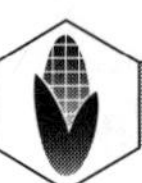

FOOD SOURCES OF CARBOHYDRATES

Grains
17 to 23 g per ½ cup grains (rice, barley, couscous, bulgur, buckwheat)
38 to 40 g per 12 oz soda (carbonated, sweetened)
20 g per ½ cup pasta or noodles
22 to 46 g per 1 cup ready-to-eat cereals
21 to 30 per 2 oz bread (roll, bun, croissant)

Fruits
13 to 20 g per ½ cup fruit, unsweetened, canned or frozen
25 to 38 g per ½ cup fruit, sweetened, canned or frozen
17 to 22 g per ¾ cup fruit juice

Vegetables
17 to 29 g per ½ cup legumes (white, navy, kidney, garbanzo beans)
11 to 16 g per ½ cup potatoes, sweet corn, mixed vegetables, green peas

Data from USDA, Agricultural Research Service. (2010). *USDA National Nutrient Database for Standard Reference, Release 23.* Retrieved from http://www.ars.usda.gov/ba/bhnrc/ndl

based on the newborn infant brain weight (~380 g) and the daily glucose consumption rate of adults (8.64 g/100 g brain) to yield a glucose requirement of the fetal brain at the end of pregnancy of 32.5 g/day. For lactating women, the EAR was set as the adult EAR plus an increment of 60 g based on the lactose content of human milk (74 g/L) times the volume of milk secreted (0.78 L/day). Therefore the EARs of carbohydrate for pregnant and lactating women are 135 and 160 g/day, respectively. The RDAs were set as the EAR + 30%, as for adults.

The IOM (2002) set AIs for infants based on the average intake of carbohydrate consumed from human milk and complementary foods. These AIs were calculated as the carbohydrate (lactose) content of human milk (74 g/L) times the intake of milk (0.78 L/day) for infants from 0 to 6 months of age, and as the carbohydrate intake from human milk (0.78 L/day times 0.6 L/day) plus the intake from complementary foods (51 g/day) for older infants. Therefore the AIs are 60 and 95 g/day of carbohydrate for 0- to 6- and 7- to 12-month-old infants, respectively.

The IOM (2002) considered setting Tolerable Upper Intake Levels (ULs) for high glycemic index carbohydrates and for sugars but did not do so because of the lack of a critical mass of evidence. However, the IOM committee highlighted a need for more research to elucidate the health effects from ingesting high versus low glycemic index carbohydrates and the possible effects of sugars and energy density on energy expenditure, food intake, and weight reduction. Although a UL was not set, a maximal intake level of 25% or less of energy from added sugars was suggested based on the decreased intake of some micronutrients by American subpopulations who exceed this level of sugar intake. The National Health and Nutrition Examination Survey (NHANES III) data indicated that added sugar intakes are particularly high in young adults, especially in males, being as high as 57 teaspoons (228 g or 912 kcal) per day for male adolescents.

THINKING CRITICALLY

1. A patient complained of muscle cramps and was unable to perform strenuous exercise. He had elevated levels of creatine phosphokinase, adolase, and myoglobin in his blood. The release of enzymes and other proteins from muscle cells is indicative of muscle cell damage. He was diagnosed with type V glycogen storage disease (McArdle disease), which is caused by an absence of muscle glycogen phosphorylase.
   a. Would you expect glycogen to accumulate in the muscle of this patient? Why or why not?
   b. Would you expect lactate to accumulate in the muscle or blood of this patient during exercise? Why or why not?
   c. What fuels would you expect this patient to use during exercise?
2. Hereditary galactosemia is a rare defect in which the enzyme galactose 1-phosphate uridylyltransferase is not synthesized in functional form. An infant with feeding difficulties, vomiting, liver enlargement, and convulsions was tested for reducing sugars in the urine. A test for reducing sugars was positive, but a specific test of D-glucose was negative. Hereditary galactosemia was suspected and confirmed by the complete absence of galactose 1-phosphate uridylyltransferase in erythrocytes (and presumably all other cells) from this patient.
   a. What would a tolerance curve (a plot of plasma glucose concentration versus time after the test dose) have looked like if plasma glucose had been measured after a test dose of D-galactose? After a test dose of lactose?
   b. Would any sugar or sugar derivative be present in the patient's plasma or tissues in excess concentration? If so, what specific sugar(s) or sugar derivative(s)?
   c. For an individual with an intestinal lactase deficiency (lactose intolerance), how would your answers to questions a and b differ from those given above? Explain.

REFERENCES

Beale, E. G., Hammer, R. E., Antoine, B., & Forest, C. (2004). Disregulated glyceroneogenesis: PCK1 as a candidate diabetes and obesity gene. *Trends in Endocrinology and Metabolism, 15*, 129–135.

Behal, R. H., Buxton, D. B., Robertson, J. G., & Olson, M. S. (1993). Regulation of the pyruvate dehydrogenase multienzyme complex. *Annual Review of Nutrition, 13*, 497–520.

Bindoff, L. A., & Turnbull, D. M. (1994). Defects of the mitochondrial respiratory chain. In J. B. Holton (Ed.), *The inherited metabolic diseases* (2nd ed., pp. 265–295). London: Churchill Livingstone.

Brocklehurst, K. J., Davies, R. A., & Agius, L. (2004). Differences in regulatory properties between human and rat glucokinase regulatory protein. *The Biochemical Journal, 378*, 693–697.

Buist, N. R. M. (1995). Disorders of gluconeogenesis. In J. Fernandes, J.-M. Saudubray, & G. van den Berghe (Eds.), *Inborn metabolic diseases: Diagnosis and treatment* (pp. 101–106). Berlin: Springer-Verlag.

Burri, L., Thoresen, G. H., & Berge, R. K. (2010). The role of PPARα activation in liver and muscle. *PPAR Research 2010*, pii 542359.

Campbell, N. A., Williamson, B., & Heyden, R. J. (2006). *Biology: Exploring life*. Boston: Pearson Prentice Hall.

Cartee, G. D., & Funai, K. (2009). Exercise and insulin: Convergence or divergence at AS160 and TBC1D1? *Exercise and Sport Sciences Reviews, 37*, 188–195.

Cherrington, A. D., Moore, M. C., Sindelar, D. K., & Edgerton, D. S. (2007). Insulin action on the liver in vivo. *Biochemical Society Transactions, 35*, 1171–1174.

Chishti, A. H. (1998). Function of p55 and its nonerythroid homologues. *Current Opinion in Hematology, 5*, 116–121.

Czech, M. P. (1995). Molecular actions of insulin on glucose transport. *Annual Review of Nutrition, 15*, 441–471.

de la Iglesia, N., Veiga-daCunha, M., Van Schaftingen, E., Guinovart, J. J., & Ferrer, J. C. (1999). Glucokinase regulatory protein is essential for the proper subcellular localization of liver glucokinase. *FEBS Letters, 456*, 332–338.

Dentin, R., Denechaud, P. D., Benhamed, F., Girard, J., & Postic, C. (2006). Hepatic gene regulation by glucose and polyunsaturated fatty acids: A role for ChREBP. *The Journal of Nutrition, 136*, 1145–1149.

Dunger, D. B., & Holton, J. B. (1994). Disorders of carbohydrate metabolism. In J. B. Holton (Ed.), *The inherited metabolic diseases* (2nd ed., pp. 21–65). London: Churchill Livingstone.

Duplus, E., Benelli, C., Reis, A. F., Fouque, F., Velho, G., & Forest, C. (2003). Expression of the phosphoenolpyruvate carboxykinase gene in human adipose tissue: Induction by rosiglitazone and genetic analyses of the adipocyte-specific region of the promoter in type 2 diabetes. *Biochimie, 85*, 1257–1264.

Fernandes, J., & Chen Y.-T. (1995). Carbohydrate metabolism: Glycogen storage diseases. In J. Fernandes, J.-M. Saudubray, & G. van den Berghe (Eds.), *Inborn metabolic diseases: Diagnosis and treatment* (pp. 71–131). Berlin: Springer-Verlag.

Ferrer-Martinez, A., Marotta, M., Baldan, A., Haro, D., & Gomez-Foix, A. (2004). Chicken ovalbumin upstream promoter-transcription factor I represses the transcriptional activity of the human muscle glycogen phosphorylase promoter in C2C12 cells. *Biochimica et Biophysica Acta, 1678*, 157–162.

Gerich, J. E. (2010). Role of the kidney in normal glucose homeostasis and in the hyperglycaemia of diabetes mellitus: Therapeutic implications. *Diabetic Medicine, 27*, 136–142.

Gitzelmann, R. (1995). Disorders of galactose metabolism. In J. Fernandes, J.-M. Saudubray, & G. van den Berghe (Eds.), *Inborn metabolic diseases: Diagnosis and treatment* (pp. 87–92). Berlin: Springer-Verlag.

Granner, D. K., & Pilkis, S. J. (1990). The genes of hepatic glucose metabolism. *The Journal of Biological Chemistry, 265*, 10173–10176.

Gurney, A. L., Park, E. A., Liu, J., Giralt, M., McGrane, M. M., Patel, Y. M., … Hanson, R. W. (1994). Metabolic regulation of gene transcription. *The Journal of Nutrition, 124*, 1533S–1539S.

Hanson, R. W., & Hakimi, P. (2008). Born to run: The story of the PEPCK-Cmus mouse. *Biochimie, 90*, 838–842.

Hanson, R. W., & Reshef, L. (1997). Regulation of phosphoenolpyruvate carboxykinase (GTP) gene expression. *Annual Review of Biochemistry, 66*, 581–611.

Institute of Medicine, Food and Nutrition Board. (2002). *Dietary Reference Intakes for energy, carbohydrate, fiber, fat, fatty acids, cholesterol, protein and amino acids.* Washington, DC: The National Academies Press.

Ishiki, M., & Klip, A. (2005). Minireview: Recent developments in the regulation of glucose transporter-4 traffic: New signals, locations, and partners. *Endocrinology, 146*, 5071–5078.

Jensen, J., & Lai, Y. C. (2009). Regulation of muscle glycogen synthase phosphorylation and kinetic properties by insulin, exercise, adrenaline and role in insulin resistance. *Archives of Physiology and Biochemistry, 115*, 13–21.

Jeoung, N. H., & Harris, R. A. (2010). Role of pyruvate dehydrogenase kinase 4 in regulation of blood glucose levels. *Korean Diabetes Journal, 34*, 274–283.

Jope, R. S., & Johnson, G. V. (2004). The glamour and gloom of glycogen synthase kinase-3. *Trends in Biochemical Sciences, 29*, 95–102.

Jungermann, K. (1992). Zonal liver cell heterogeneity. *Enzyme, 46*, 5–7.

Kahn, C. R., Lauris, W., Koch, S., Crettaz, M., & Granner, D. K. (1989). Acute and chronic regulation of phosphoenolpyruvate carboxykinase mRNA by insulin and glucose. *Molecular Endocrinology, 3*, 840–845.

Kawaguchi, T., Takenoshita, M., Kabashima, T., & Uyeda, K. (2001). Glucose and cAMP regulate the L-type pyruvate kinase gene by phosphorylation/dephosphorylation of the carbohydrate response element binding protein. *Proceedings of the National Academy of Sciences of the United States of America, 98*, 13710–13715.

Kim, S. K., & Novak, R. F. (2007). The role of intracellular signaling in insulin-mediated regulation of drug metabolizing enzyme gene and protein expression. *Pharmacology & Therapeutics, 113*, 88–120.

Laplante, M., & Sabatini, D. M. (2010). mTORC1 activates SREBP-1c and uncouples lipogenesis from gluconeogenesis. *Proceedings of the National Academy of Sciences of the United States of America, 107*, 3281–3282.

Lehninger, A. L., Nelson, D. L., & Cox, M. M. (1993). Glycolysis and the catabolism of hexoses. In *Principles of biochemistry* (2nd ed., pp. 400–439). New York: Worth Publishers.

Lemaigre, F. P., & Rousseau, G. G. (1994). Transcriptional control of genes that regulate glycolysis and gluconeogenesis in adult liver. *The Biochemical Journal, 303*, 1–14.

Lockyer, J. M., & McCracken, J. B. (1991). Identification of a tissue-specific regulatory element within the human muscle glycogen phosphorylase gene. *The Journal of Biological Chemistry, 266*, 20262–20269.

Mager, D. R., Patterson, C., So, S., Rogenstein, C. D., Wykes, L. J., & Roberts, E. A. (2010). Dietary and physical activity patterns in children with fatty liver. *European Journal of Clinical Nutrition, 64*, 628–635.

Magnuson, M. A., & Jetton, T. L. (1993). Tissue-specific regulation of glucokinase. In C. D. Berdanier & J. L. Hargrove (Eds.), *Nutrition and gene expression* (pp. 143–167). Boca Raton, FL: CRC Press.

Matsumoto, M., Pocai, A., Rossetti, L., Depinho, R. A., & Accili, D. (2007). Impaired regulation of hepatic glucose production in mice lacking the forkhead transcription factor Foxo1 in liver. *Cell Metabolism, 6*, 208–216.

McGarry, J. D., Kuwajima, M., Newgard, C. B., Foster, D. W., & Katz, J. (1987). From dietary glucose to liver glycogen: The full circle round. *Annual Review of Nutrition, 7*, 51–73.

Miinea, C. P., Sano, H., Kane, S., Sano, E., Fukuda, M., Peränen, J., … Lienhard, G. E. (2005). AS160, the Akt substrate regulating GLUT4 translocation, has a functional Rab GTPase-activating protein domain. *The Biochemical Journal, 391*, 87–93.

Minokoski, Y., Kahn, C. R., & Kahn, B. B. (2003). Tissue-specific ablation of the GLUT4 glucose transporter or the insulin receptor challenges assumptions about insulin action and glucose homeostasis. *The Journal of Biological Chemistry, 278*, 33609–33612.

Nielsen, J. N., Derave, W., Kristiansen, S., Ralston, E., Ploug, T., & Richter, E. A. (2001). Glycogen synthase localization and activity in rat skeletal muscle is strongly dependent on glycogen content. *The Journal of Physiology, 531*, 757–769.

Nikoulina, S. E., Ciaraldi, T. P., Mudaliar, N., Carter, L., Johnson, K., & Henry, R. R. (2002). Inhibition of glycogen synthase kinase 3 improves insulin action and glucose metabolism in human skeletal muscle. *Diabetes, 51*, 2190–2198.

Noguchi, T., & Tanaka, T. (1993). Dietary and hormonal regulation of L-type pyruvate kinase gene expression. In C. D. Berdanier & J. L. Hargrove (Eds.), *Nutrition and gene expression* (pp. 143–167). Boca Raton, FL: CRC Press.

Nordlie, R. C., Bode, A. M., & Foster, J. D. (1993). Recent advances in hepatic glucose 6-phosphatase regulation and function. *Proceedings of the Society for Experimental Biology and Medicine, 203*, 274–285.

Nordlie, R. C., Foster, J. D., & Lange, A. J. (1999). Regulation of glucose production by the liver. *Annual Review of Nutrition, 19*, 379–406.

Nur, T., Sela, I., Webster, N. J., & Madar, Z. (1995). Starvation and refeeding regulate glycogen synthase gene expression in rat liver at the posttranscriptional level. *The Journal of Nutrition, 125*, 2457–2462.

Okar, D. A., Wu, C., & Lange, A. J. (2004). Regulation of the regulatory enzyme, 6-phosphofructo-2-kinase/fructose-2, 6-bisphosphatase. *Advances in Enzyme Regulation, 44*, 123–154.

O'Mahony, A. M., & Walsh, D. A. (2002). Differentiation-dependent mechanisms of transcriptional regulation of the catalytic subunit of phosphorylase kinase. *The Biochemical Journal, 362*, 199–211.

Onuma, H., Oeser, J. K., Nelson, B. A., Wang, Y., Flemming, B. P., Scheving, L. A., … O'Brien, R. M. (2009). Insulin and epidermal growth factor suppress basal glucose-6-phosphatase catalytic subunit gene transcription through overlapping but distinct mechanisms. *The Biochemical Journal, 417*, 611–620.

Petersen, K. F., & Shulman, G. I. (2006). Etiology of insulin resistance. *The American Journal of Medicine, 119*, S10–S16.

Pilkis, S. J., & Claus, T. H. (1991). Hepatic gluconeogenesis/glycolysis: Regulation and structure/function relationships of substrate cycles. *Annual Review of Nutrition, 11*, 465–515.

Pilkis, S. J., Claus, T. H., Kurland, I. J., & Lange, A. J. (1995). 6-Phosphofructo-2-kinase/fructose-2,6- bisphosphatase: A metabolic signaling enzyme. *Annual Review of Biochemistry, 64*, 799–835.

Pilkis, S. J., El-Maghrabi, M. R., & Claus, T. H. (1990). Fructose-2,6-bisphosphate in control of hepatic gluconeogenesis: From metabolites to molecular genetics. *Diabetes Care, 13*, 582–599.

Pinney, S. E., & Simmons, R. A. (2010). Epigenetic mechanisms in the development of type 2 diabetes. *Trends in Endocrinology and Metabolism, 21*, 223–229.

Postic, C., Shiota, M., & Magnuson, M. A. (2001). Cell-specific roles of glucokinase in glucose homeostasis. *Recent Progress in Hormone Research, 56*, 195–217.

Rao, P. V., Pugazhenthi, S., & Khandelwal, R. L. (1995). The effects of streptozotocin-induced diabetes and insulin supplementation on expression of the glycogen phosphorylase gene in rat liver. *The Journal of Biological Chemistry, 270*, 24955–24960.

Rayasam, G. V., Tulasi, V. K., Sodhi, R., Davis, J. A., & Ray, A. (2009). Glycogen synthase kinase 3: More than a namesake. *British Journal of Pharmacology, 156*, 885–898.

Rhee, J., Inooue, Y., Yoon, J. C., Puigserver, P., Fan, M., Gonzales, F. J., & Spiegelman, B. M. (2003). Regulation of hepatic fasting response by PPAR gamma coactivator-1alpha (PGC-1): Requirement for hepatocyte nuclear factor 4 alpha in gluconeogenesis. *Proceedings of the National Academy of Sciences of the United States of America, 100*, 4012–4017.

Rider, M. H., Bertrand, L., Vertommen, D., Michels, P. A., Rousseau, G. G., & Hue, L. (2004). 6-Phosphofructo-2-kinase/fructose-2,6-bisphosphatase: Head-to-head with a bifunctional enzyme that controls glycolysis. *The Biochemical Journal, 381*, 561–579.

Shafrir, E. (1991). Metabolism of disaccharides and monosaccharides with emphasis on sucrose and fructose and their lipogenic potential. In M. Gracey, N. Kretchmer, & E. Rossi (Eds.), *Sugars in nutrition. Nestle Nutrition Workshop Series, Vol. 25.* (pp. 131–152). New York: Raven Press.

Smythe, C., & Cohen, P. (1991). The discovery of glycogenin and the priming mechanism for glycogen biogenesis. *European Journal of Biochemistry/FEBS, 200*, 625–631.

Stabile, L. P., Hodge, D. L., Klautky, S. A., & Salati, L. M. (1996). Posttranscriptional regulation of glucose-6-phosphate dehydrogenase by dietary polyunsaturated fat. *Archives of Biochemistry and Biophysics, 332*, 269–279.

Sugden, M. C., & Holness, M. J. (2006). Mechanisms underlying regulation of the expression and activities of the mammalian pyruvate dehydrogenase kinases. *Archives of Biochemistry and Biophysics, 112*, 139–149.

Sutherland, C., O'Brien, R. M., & Granner, D. K. (1996). New connections in the regulation of PEPCK gene expression by insulin. *Philosophical Transactions of the Royal Society of London. Series B, Biological Sciences, 351*, 191–199.

Swink, T. D., Vining, E. P., & Freeman, J. M. (1997). The ketogenic diet. *Advances in Pediatrics, 44*, 297–329.

Thorens, B. (2002). A gene knockout approach in mice to identify glucose sensors controlling glucose homeostasis. *Pflügers Archiv: European Journal of Physiology, 445*, 482–490.

Tordjman, J., Chauvet, G., Quette, J., Beale, E. G., Forest, C., & Antoine, B. (2003). Thiazolidinediones block fatty acid release by inducing glyceroneogenesis in fat cells. *The Journal of Biological Chemistry, 278*, 18785–18790.

Uldry, M., & Thorens, B. (2004). The SLC2 family of facilitated hexose and polyol transporters. *Pflügers Archiv: European Journal of Physiology, 447*, 480–489.

United States Department of Agriculture. (2010). *Report of the Dietary Guidelines Advisory Committee on the dietary guidelines for Americans.* Retrieved from http://www.cnpp.usda.gov/DGAs2010-DGACReport.htm

Uyeda, K., & Repa, J. J. (2006). Carbohydrate response element binding protein, ChREBP, a transcription factor coupling hepatic glucose utilization and lipid synthesis. *Cell Metabolism, 4*, 107–110.

Van den Berghe, G. (1995). Disorders of fructose metabolism. In J. Fernandes, J.-M. Saudubray, & G. van den Berghe (Eds.), *Inborn metabolic diseases: Diagnosis and treatment* (pp. 95–99). Berlin: Springer-Verlag.

Vaulont, S., & Kahn, A. (1993). Transcriptional control of metabolic regulation genes by carbohydrates. *The FASEB Journal, 8*, 28–36.

Vestergaard, H. (1999). Studies of gene expression and activity of hexokinase, phosphofructokinase and glycogen synthase in human skeletal muscle in states of altered insulin-stimulated glucose metabolism. *Danish Medical Bulletin, 46*, 13–34.

Vining, E. P. (1999). Clinical efficacy of the ketogenic diet. *Epilepsy Research, 37*, 181–190.

Wahren, J., & Ekberg, K. (2007). Splanchnic regulation of glucose production. *Annual Review of Nutrition, 27*, 329–345.

Winchester, B. (2005). Lysosomal metabolism of glycoproteins. *Glycobiology, 15*, 1R–15R.

Yabaluri, N., & Bashyam, M. D. (2010). Hormonal regulation of gluconeogenic gene transcription in the liver. *Journal of Biosciences, 35*, 473–484.

Yoon, J. C., Puigserver, P., Chen, G., Donovan, J., Wu, Z., Rhee, J., … Speigelman, B. M. (2001). Control of hepatic gluconeogenesis through the transcriptional coactivator PGC-1. *Nature, 413*, 131–138.

CHAPTER 13

Protein Synthesis and Degradation

Tracy G. Anthony, PhD, and Margaret McNurlan, PhD

COMMON ABBREVIATIONS

DNA	deoxyribonucleic acid
eEF	eukaryotic elongation factor
eIF	eukaryotic initiation factor
eRF	eukaryotic release factor
ER	endoplasmic reticulum
ERAD	endoplasmic reticulum–associated degradation
hnRNA	heterogeneous nuclear RNA
IGF	insulin-like growth factor
IL	interleukin
mRNA	messenger ribonucleic acid
rRNA	ribosomal ribonucleic acid
tRNA	transfer ribonucleic acid
TNF	tumor necrosis factor
UPR	unfolded protein response

Proteins present in food provide an average of 15% of the energy in the American diet. Proteins are unique among the macronutrients in that they contain nitrogen, which comprises about 16% of the mass of protein. Proteins are digested to amino acids in the gastrointestinal tract and enterocytes, and the amino acids are taken up into the circulation and transported throughout the body. Within the body tissues, amino acids are used to synthesize proteins and peptides as well as some other specialized small molecules. Although amino acids released in the process of protein turnover can be reused, an input of amino acids from the diet is needed to replace those that are degraded or metabolized to other compounds and those that are post-translationally modified in an irreversible manner (e.g., 3-methylhistidine).

Protein synthesis occurs on ribosomes located in the cytosol, either free or bound to the endoplasmic reticulum (ER). Protein synthesis is required for synthesis of new tissue during times of growth and pregnancy and for synthesis of milk proteins during lactation. Protein synthesis is also necessary for maintenance of existing tissue. The maintenance function of protein synthesis encompasses the replacement of proteins that are degraded each day as well synthesis of new or additional amounts of regulatory proteins when needed. Body proteins are degraded by intracellular enzymes, particularly by the proteolytic subunits of protein-digesting bodies called proteasomes and by acid hydrolases in the lysosomes of cells. Furthermore, proteins that are secreted or lost into the gastrointestinal tract undergo proteolysis by the digestive enzymes. Turnover of body proteins is important for replacement of damaged proteins and also for the regulation of amounts of various proteins.

PROTEIN TURNOVER

During any day an adult human makes and degrades about 300 g of protein. In contrast, the typical intake of protein from the diet in those consuming Western diets is approximately one third of that amount, or 100 g. This means that the body not only processes the dietary protein that is taken in but also degrades about three times as much body protein. Therefore approximately 400 g of protein is broken down to amino acids by digestion plus protein degradation over the course of each day. Amino acids are used to resynthesize about 300 g of body protein; most of the remaining amino acids are catabolized.

OVERVIEW OF PROTEIN TURNOVER

The interchange between body protein and the pool of free amino acids is depicted schematically in Figure 13-1. The process by which body protein is continually degraded and resynthesized is called protein turnover, a term used collectively to include both protein synthesis and protein degradation.

The tripeptide glutathione (γ-glutamylcysteinylglycine) is unusual in that its synthesis accounts for a large amount of the body's cysteine flux. As for amino acids in proteins, most of the amino acids in glutathione are returned to the amino acid pool upon glutathione turnover. Glutathione synthesis is catalyzed by cytosolic enzymes, not by the ribosomal machinery, and is discussed further in Chapter 14.

In addition to serving as substrates for protein synthesis, amino acids also are degraded to provide compounds that can enter central pathways of fuel metabolism, and small amounts are converted to nonprotein compounds. For most adults who are in protein balance, the amount of amino acids degraded is essentially equivalent to the amount in the

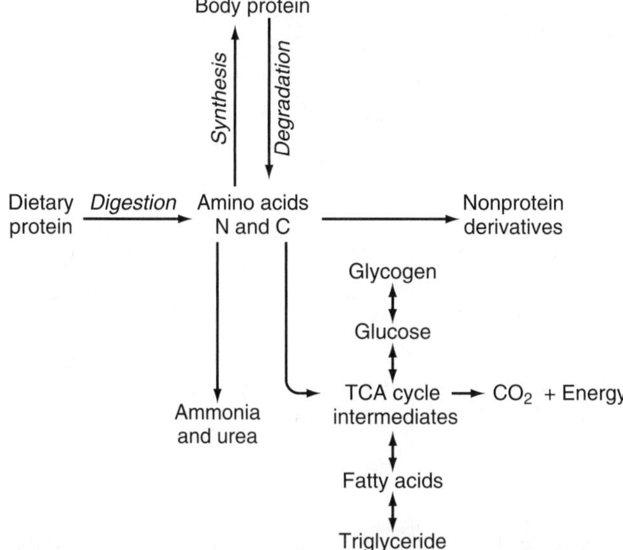

FIGURE 13-1 Overview of protein and amino acid metabolism. Amino acids are incorporated primarily into protein or degraded to provide energy. In general, the synthesis of nonprotein compounds does not consume quantitatively important amounts of amino acids. Degradation of amino acids involves removal of the nitrogen and catabolism of the carbon skeleton.

diet. The degradative pathways are also shown schematically in Figure 13-1. Degradation involves the removal of nitrogen, primarily as urea and ammonia, and the catabolism of the carbon skeleton. The end result of the degradation of the carbon skeleton of amino acids is the provision of energy either directly or through the formation of compounds such as glucose and fatty acids, which can then be stored or metabolized to provide energy. The pathways for the oxidative metabolism of amino acids and nitrogen excretion are discussed in detail in Chapter 14, but it is important to understand the integrated nature of protein metabolism that is represented by Figure 13-1. The needs of the body regulate the flux of amino acids through these possible pathways; that is, whether amino acids are used for the synthesis of protein, oxidized for energy, or used to form glucose.

There are also pathways within the body for conversion of amino acids to end products other than protein. These reactions are depicted in Figure 13-1 as nonprotein derivatives. Nonprotein derivatives include compounds such as purine and pyrimidine bases, neurotransmitters such as serotonin, nonpeptide hormones such as catecholamines, and other specialized compounds such as carnitine. Because the amounts of amino acids irreversibly consumed in the synthesis of nonprotein compounds are normally much smaller than those consumed either by protein synthesis or by amino acid oxidation, these pathways often are ignored in the assessment of protein turnover and nitrogen balance. However, the amounts of some of these compounds that are synthesized can be substantial (e.g., creatine, heme, and nucleic acids), and for some amino acids, synthesis of these nonprotein compounds can represent a significant portion of total amino acid utilization during periods of protein deprivation.

SYNTHESIS AND DEGRADATION OF PROTEIN IN RELATION TO PROTEIN BALANCE

The pathways shown in Figure 13-1 can be simplified to focus specifically on the interactions of amino acids with body protein through protein synthesis and protein degradation (Figure 13-2). In this simplified scheme, all the tissue and circulating proteins are considered together, and likewise the free amino acid pool is reduced to a single, homogeneous pool, rather than the complex arrangements of pools in blood, individual tissues, and subcellular compartments that are known to exist. This simplification has proved helpful in conceptualizing and developing methods for measuring the exchange of amino acids between the free amino acid pool and the protein pool.

This simple model in Figure 13-2 highlights the exchange of free amino acids with body protein through the processes of protein synthesis and protein degradation, and also the entry and exit of amino acids by dietary intake and oxidation. Essential amino acids enter the body free pool from the digestion and absorption of dietary protein (I) and from the degradation of body protein (D). Removal of amino acids from the free pool occurs either by the synthesis of protein (S) or through excretion (E) via oxidation to CO_2 with the concurrent excretion of nitrogen, mainly as ammonia and urea. If the amounts of free amino acids in the pool are constant, then the sum of the processes that remove amino acids (protein synthesis and catabolism) is equal to the sum of the processes by which amino acids enter the free pool (from protein degradation and dietary protein intake).

$$S + E = D + I = Q$$

Q, the sum of the rates of either entry or exit from the free amino acid pool, has been termed the flux rate. This is sometimes also known as the rate of appearance, R_a, or rate of

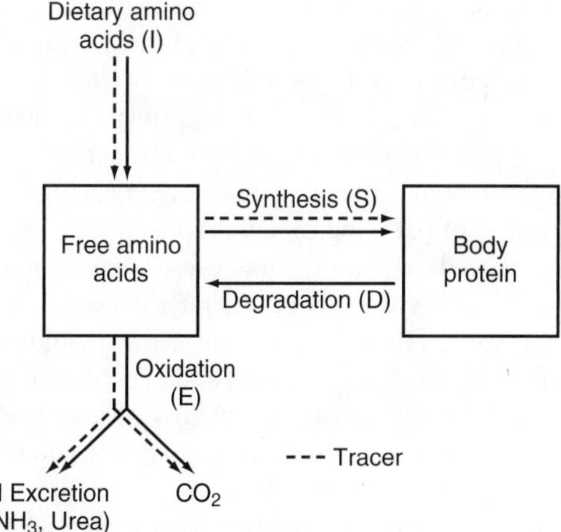

FIGURE 13-2 Protein turnover. The complexity of body protein and free amino acid pools is simplified in this two-compartment model, which can be used to assess kinetic data from labeled tracers (shown as dashed lines). In this model, amino acids enter a free amino acid pool via the diet (*I*, for intake) or from the degradation of body protein (*D*). Amino acids leave the free amino acid pool through protein synthesis (*S*) and oxidation (*E*, for excretion).

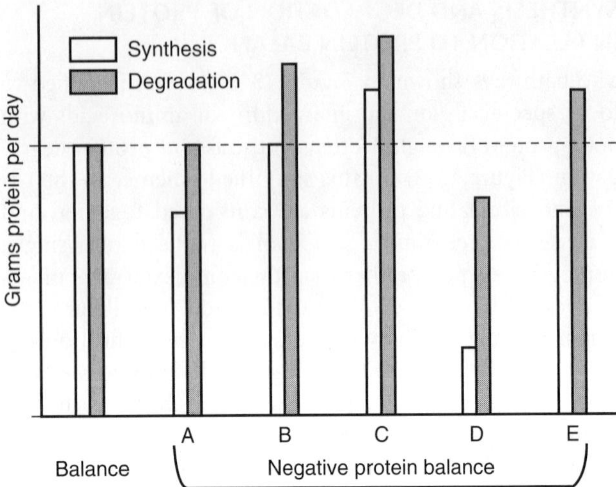

FIGURE 13-3 Five ways of achieving negative nitrogen balance. Negative nitrogen balance (degradation > synthesis) arises from changes in either protein synthesis (*A*) or protein degradation (*B*), or from changes in both synthesis and degradation (*C, D, E*). Similarly, positive balance (synthesis > degradation) arises whenever synthesis exceeds degradation. This can occur with changes in the rates of synthesis or degradation or with changes in both.

disappearance, R_d. In an adult in nitrogen equilibrium or protein balance, nitrogen intake (I) is equal to nitrogen excretion (E), and protein synthesis (S) is equal to protein degradation (D). For an individual to be in positive nitrogen balance, there must be net protein synthesis or accretion (S > D), whereas there must be net protein degradation or loss for an individual to be in negative nitrogen balance (S < D).

From the aforementioned relationships, it is clear that protein is retained in the body when synthesis exceeds degradation, and that protein is lost from the body when degradation exceeds synthesis. As shown in Figure 13-3, loss of body protein can occur from a decrease in the synthesis of protein with no change in protein degradation (Figure 13-3, *A*), an increase in the degradation with no change in protein synthesis (Figure 13-3, *B*), from either an increase (Figure 13-3, *C*) or a decrease (Figure 13-3, *D*) in both synthesis and degradation with protein degradation exceeding protein synthesis, or from an increase in degradation along with a decrease in synthesis (Figure 13-3, *E*). In a number of pathological conditions, body protein degradation exceeds synthesis, with both protein synthesis and degradation rates elevated over the rates in healthy individuals. In the case of infection in malnourished children, body protein is lost, but both synthesis and degradation rates are depressed. In early starvation, net loss of lean body mass is due to an increase in protein degradation along with a decrease in protein synthesis.

Likewise, positive protein balance can be achieved by increases in protein synthesis, by decreases in protein degradation, or with changes in both protein synthesis and degradation, such that synthesis exceeds degradation. For example, in children recovering from burn injury, both the rates of protein synthesis and degradation were increased, but the increase in synthesis was larger than the increase in protein degradation (Borsheim et al., 2010; also see Figure 13-12 later in this chapter). Although the illustration of protein turnover in Figure 13-2 is presented in terms of whole-body protein, the balance between the processes of synthesis and degradation also determines the net protein balance at the level of individual tissues or organs and for individual proteins. Examples of this type of regulation are discussed later in this chapter.

TABLE 13-1 Turnover Rates of Enzymes in Rat Liver*

ENZYME	CELLULAR COMPARTMENT	$t_{1/2}$	k_d (% per day)
Ornithine decarboxylase	Cytosol	11 minutes	91
5-Aminolevulinate synthetase	Cytosol	20 minutes	50
5-Aminolevulinate synthetase	Mitochondria	72 minutes	14
Hydroxymethylglutaryl CoA reductase	Endoplasmic reticulum	4.0 hours	4.2
Phosphoenolpyruvate carboxykinase	Cytosol	5.0 hours	3.3
Alanine-glyoxylate aminotransferase	Cytosol	3.5 days	0.20
Arginase	Cytosol	4.0 days	0.17
NAD^+ nucleosidase	Endoplasmic reticulum	16 days	0.04

Data from Waterlow, J. C., Garlick, P. J., & Milward, D. J. (1978). *Protein turnover in mammalian tissues and in the whole body* (pp. 490–492). Amsterdam: North-Holland Publishing.
*Turnover rates are expressed as half-lives ($t_{1/2}$, the time to replace half the molecules originally present) and fractional turnover rates (k_d, percent turned over per day).

PROTEIN TURNOVER AND ADAPTATION

Protein turnover allows the body to degrade and replace proteins that are oxidized, damaged, misfolded, or otherwise nonfunctional. It also allows the body to change the relative amounts of different proteins to respond to changes in nutritional and physiological conditions. Individual proteins vary in their rate of turnover, as shown in Table 13-1 for several examples of individual liver proteins. Relatively high rates of turnover of regulatory proteins allow for more rapid adaptation in the levels of these proteins in response to changing conditions. Levels of proteins with very slow turnover rates, such as collagen with a half-life of approximately 300 days, remain relatively constant.

At the level of individual tissues, higher turnover rates are associated with a more rapid cellular turnover rate (e.g., epithelial cells of small intestine) or the capacity of a tissue to

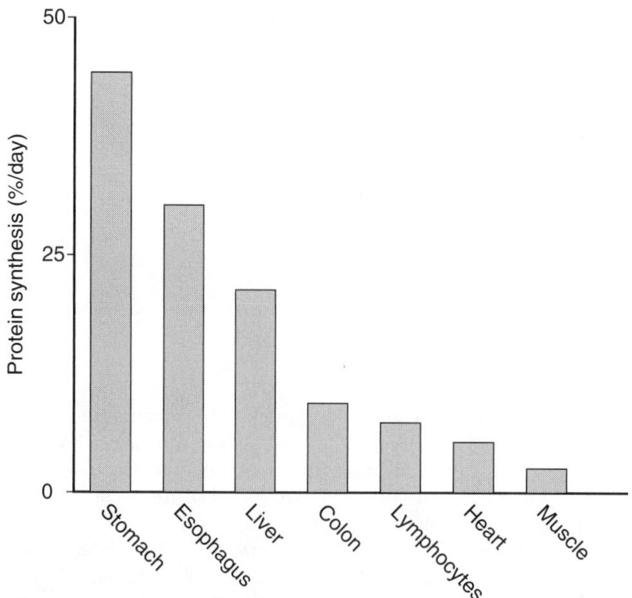

FIGURE 13-4 Fractional rates of protein synthesis in a range of human tissues. Rates of protein synthesis, assessed from the incorporation of L-[1-^{13}C]leucine or L-[$^{2}H_5$]phenylalanine into tissue protein, are expressed as a fractional rate; that is, as the percentage of the protein pool that is synthesized each day. (Data from Garlick, P. J., McNurlan, M. A., Essén, P., & Wernerman, J. [1994]. Measurement of tissue protein synthesis rates in vivo: A critical analysis of contrasting methods. *The American Journal of Physiology, 266,* E287–E297.)

respond more rapidly to changes in the environment (e.g., liver). The turnover rates for a selection of human tissues are shown in Figure 13-4. The high rates of protein synthesis in the stomach and esophagus reflect both the secretory function and the rapid replacement of cells of the gastric and esophageal mucosa. The liver also has a relatively high rate of turnover, which facilitates adaptation to changes such as alterations in nutrient intake. By contrast, the rate of protein synthesis is relatively slower in muscle tissue, and changes in protein composition of this tissue in response to altered conditions (e.g., work-induced hypertrophy) occur more slowly.

In response to altered demands or changes in the environment, tissues can respond both by altering the overall rates of protein synthesis and degradation and by changing the spectrum of individual proteins being made. This adaptation allows the body to meet continuously changing demands such as those associated with growth and development, health and illness, and pregnancy and lactation. Protein turnover is therefore a substrate cycle; there is continual synthesis and degradation, which requires energy but accomplishes no net change in amount of protein. The benefit is that protein turnover provides the capacity for rapid adaptation when needed.

PROTEIN SYNTHESIS

The most inclusive definition of protein synthesis describes the processes required for a gene to be transcribed, processed, translated, folded, and modified and localized, if necessary, to generate a fully functional protein. Each process comprises multiple steps, and regulation can occur at one or more of the steps within each process, as outlined in Figure 13-5. Major advances in understanding the regulation of protein synthesis at the molecular level have been made in the last two decades. Furthermore, with whole genome sequences now available for a growing number of different organisms, including rodents and humans, new information clarifying and extending our current understanding of the regulation of protein synthesis is accumulating at a faster rate than ever before. The revelation that the human genome contains approximately 30,000 genes, only about twice as many as found in invertebrates, has caused the scientific community to reevaluate the influence of the genome in determining animal variety and organismal complexity. It is now believed that the regulation of protein synthesis is the driver in determining cellular diversity. In eukaryotic cells, the ability to express biologically active or functional proteins comes under major regulation at several points: deoxyribonucleic acid (DNA) transcription, ribonucleic acid (RNA) processing, messenger RNA (mRNA) stability, mRNA translation, and posttranslational protein modifications and folding. Because of their complexity, only a basic overview of the processes involved in protein synthesis and its regulation are given in this chapter.

DNA TRANSCRIPTION

DNA transcription (i.e., RNA synthesis) comprises the first level at which the translation of the DNA code into functional products can be regulated. Transcription is the mechanism by which a template strand of DNA is accessed and used to generate different classes of RNA. In eukaryotes, classes of RNA made from DNA templates include:

1. Messenger RNAs (mRNAs), which are used by the translational machinery to determine the order of amino acids incorporated into an elongating polypeptide during the process of mRNA translation.
2. Transfer RNAs (tRNAs), which carry individual amino acids to the mRNA template, thereby allowing correct insertion of amino acids into the growing polypeptide chain.
3. Ribosomal RNAs (rRNAs), which are assembled with numerous ribosomal proteins to form the ribosomes, and which, in eukaryotic cells, include (designated by centrifugal sedimentation size) the 28S, 5S, and 5.8S rRNAs that are associated with the large (60S) ribosomal subunit and the 18S rRNA that is associated with the small (40S) ribosomal subunit.
4. Regulatory RNAs such as microRNAs (miRNAs) and endogenous small interfering RNAs (siRNAs), which decrease protein expression by increasing mRNA degradation or reducing mRNA translation.
5. Small nuclear RNAs (snRNAs) and small nucleolar RNAs (snoRNAs), which are involved in modifying other RNAs within the nucleus.
6. Other RNAs, including Piwi-interacting RNAs (piRNAs), antisense RNAs, and long noncoding RNAs, all of which can play diverse roles in regulating gene expression.

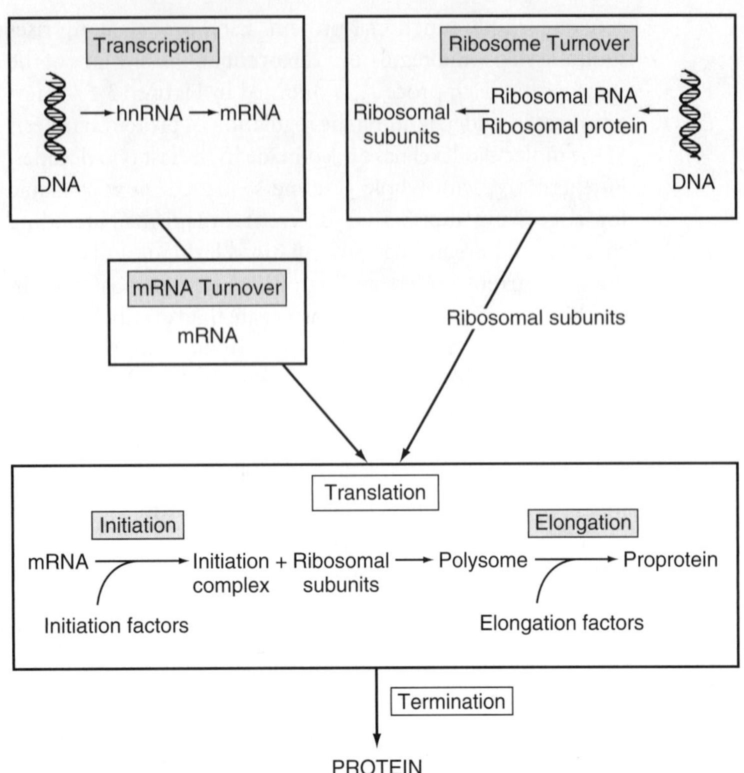

FIGURE 13-5 Protein synthesis. The scheme shows the processes involved in the synthesis of protein. The boxes all denote points of regulation. Transcription of DNA produces heterogeneous nuclear RNA (*hnRNA*), much of which is processed into messenger RNA (*mRNA*). mRNA undergoes continuous synthesis and degradation, shown as mRNA turnover. Ribosomal subunits cycle between subunits and polyribosomes. Both ribosomal RNA (*rRNA*) and ribosomal proteins also undergo synthesis and degradation. Translation of mRNA into protein involves the processes of initiation and elongation, which are regulated by initiation and elongation factors. The final step in protein formation is termination, the separation of the protein from the polyribosome.

RNA Polymerases

RNA synthesis, as illustrated in Figure 13-6, is catalyzed by a family of enzymes called RNA polymerases (RNAPs). RNAP requires a DNA template to synthesize RNA. Transcription of the different classes of RNAs in eukaryotes is carried out by three different RNAPs. RNAP I synthesizes the rRNAs that comprise the major RNA components of ribosomes. RNAP II synthesizes mRNA precursors and most miRNAs and snRNAs. RNAP III synthesizes the tRNAs, 5S rRNA, and other small RNAs. All RNAPs contain a core group of proteins that make up the basic enzymatic unit required for transcription to proceed. In addition, multisubunit protein cofactors have been identified that associate with the various RNAP core proteins to increase enzyme stability and regulate transcriptional activity.

Messenger RNA synthesis by RNAP II occurs in three stages: initiation, elongation, and termination. Transcription initiation results in the binding of the RNA polymerase to the transcription start site on a single strand of template DNA. Following this is the elongation step, in which the hallmark event is the addition of ribonucleotides to the elongating RNA. Termination causes dissociation of RNAP II from the DNA template and release of unprocessed (or partially processed) mRNA, which is called pre-mRNA.

Regulation of Transcription by Transcription Factors

The most complex controls observed in eukaryotic genes are those that regulate the expression of the genes encoding mRNAs (i.e., the protein-encoding genes). Eukaryotic genes contain a basic structure consisting of coding exons and noncoding introns, which are transcribed, plus untranscribed regulatory regions, especially promoter regions upstream of the transcription start site. Genes may also contain additional sequence domains, present in both transcribed and nontranscribed regions, that also regulate transcription.

Short nucleotide sequences within the DNA template that regulate the rate of RNA synthesis are called *cis*-acting elements. *Cis*-elements that facilitate the initiation of transcription are of two types, termed promoters and enhancers. Promoters are sequences that closely precede the transcription start site and increase the ability of RNAP II to recognize the site at which initiation begins. Almost all eukaryotic genes contain core promoters of two types that are termed CCAAT boxes and TATA boxes, names that are based on their conserved nucleotide sequences (see Figure 13-6). In addition to core promoters, proximal and distal promoter sequences enhance RNAP II activity even further. Enhancer elements are regulatory sequences that activate one or more genes in a cluster. These *cis*-elements can be located either upstream or downstream of the transcription start site. Other regulatory sequences inhibit or downregulate transcription and are called repressor domains. The number and type of *cis*-elements vary among genes.

Proteins that bind *cis*-elements are termed *trans*-acting factors, or, more commonly, transcription factors. Transcription factors are DNA-binding proteins that can enhance or repress gene expression. Recent estimates

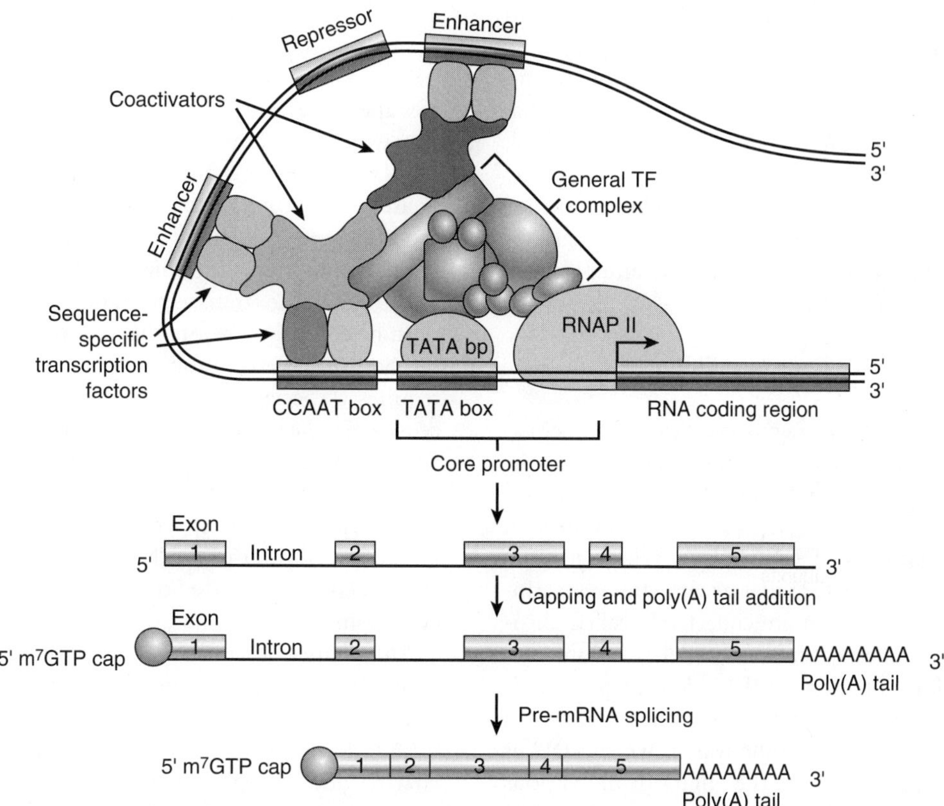

FIGURE 13-6 The basics for RNA synthesis and assembly of an mRNA transcript. *Top,* A protein called RNA polymerase II (*RNAP II*) synthesizes mRNA. Sequences in the DNA (*cis*-elements) direct RNAP II binding to the promoter region of DNA as well as the binding of DNA-binding proteins called transcription factors to activate or repress the synthesis of RNA by RNAP II. *Middle,* After transcription, the transcript is processed for mRNA translation via capping and polyadenylation. *Bottom,* After RNA splicing, the RNA species is edited by the spliceosome to form an mRNA species that contains only coding exons. This capped, polyadenylated, and spliced RNA is the mRNA that leaves the nucleus for translation in the cytoplasm.

suggest there are 1,700 to 1,900 transcription factors in humans (Vaquerizas et al., 2009). Transcription factors bind proximal or distal promoter regions, whereas still others interact with enhancer or repressor elements. For example, a family of proteins identified as TF (for general transcription factors regulating RNAP) interact with the TATA box, and the protein identified as C/EBP (for CCAAT/enhancer binding protein) binds to the CCAAT box element. When binding *cis*-elements, a transcription factor often pairs up with a second DNA-binding protein. When the second DNA-binding protein is identical, a homodimer is formed; when the second DNA-binding protein is different, a heterodimer is formed. The absolute numbers, ratios, and combinations of transcription factors that interact with regulatory sequences on DNA all impact control of RNA synthesis. This along with the presence of multiple *cis*-acting elements for each template strand of DNA results in a diverse array of binding sites for different regulatory proteins, revealing substantial combinatorial complexity. It also affords a means of coordinately regulating a number of genes. For example, the pathway for the synthesis of cholesterol (see Chapter 17) involves at least 23 enzymes, and many of the genes for enzymes in this pathway are regulated by a family of transcription factors called sterol regulatory element binding proteins (SREBPs). Another family of transcription factors responsible for coordinate regulation of genes are the retinoic acid (RAR) and 9-*cis*-retinoic acid (RXR) nuclear receptors that are activated by the binding of vitamin A derivatives and are involved in regulation of differentiation (see Chapter 30).

Regulation of Transcription by Coactivators and Corepressors

Protein cofactors that interact with DNA-binding proteins but not the DNA itself further influence the rate of RNA synthesis by altering the three-dimensional arrangement of the general transcription apparatus at target gene promoters. These proteins are called transcriptional cofactors and serve as either coactivators or corepressors. The biological activity of some transcriptional cofactors is sensitive to nutritional status. For example, the peroxisome proliferator-activated receptor-gamma coactivator (PGC) 1 family of transcriptional cofactors are activated under conditions of nutrient deprivation. Expresson of PGC1 in liver increases with fasting and plays an important role in the regulation of gluconeogenesis by binding to and coactivating transcription factors such as hepatic nuclear factor (HNF) 4α, forkhead box class O (FoxO) 1, and the glucocorticoid receptor to coordinate the expression of rate-limiting gluconeogenic genes (Liang et al., 2009). Diverse protein–protein and protein–DNA combinations that result from transcriptional cofactors yield multiple layers of regulation and control, producing the phenotypic diversity seen among eukaryotic organisms and across tissues. Though this is important for development and coordination of complex biological systems, it also contributes to disease complexity and response variation to environmental stimuli.

Regulation of Transcription by Chromatin Organization

Protein expression can also be regulated at the level of chromatin, which is a complex structure consisting of eukaryotic DNA packaged with histone proteins. Although a primary function of chromatin is compaction of DNA, chromatin is much more dynamic than was thought years ago. The changes in chromatin structure that accompany transcriptional activation or repression are collectively called chromatin remodeling. Chromatin is remodeled before and during transcription initiation (by ATP-dependent remodeling proteins) and during transcript elongation. Much evidence now demonstrates that the way in which DNA is wrapped around histones affects the ability of the various transcription factors and RNA polymerases to access specific genes and to activate transcription from them. The physical interaction of DNA with histones can be modified in two major ways. First, the addition of methyl groups to the DNA at cytosine residues can render a region of DNA less transcriptionally active. Second, posttranslational modification of histones can change the physical shape of the nucleosomes (the basic structural unit of chromatin), altering accessibility of DNA to the transcriptional apparatus. The types of covalent modifications that histones undergo include acetylation, methylation, ubiquitination, phosphorylation, and sumoylation. Different histone modifications function in different ways, and multiple modifications may occur at the same time. Importantly, these DNA–protein modifications can be passed on to subsequent generations, resulting in inheritable traits and conditions. The result is an entire field of research called epigenetics, defined as the study of gene expression that results from means other than changes to the DNA sequence itself.

PRE-mRNA PROCESSING AND EXPORT

Newly transcribed pre-mRNA undergoes significant posttranscriptional processing as illustrated in Figure 13-6. First, the 5′ end of an eukaryotic mRNA is "capped" with a 7-methylguanosine residue (m^7GTP). The covalently attached m^7GTP molecule serves to protect the mRNA from exonucleases and more importantly is recognized by specific proteins of the translational machinery (Wilkie et al., 2003). Signals near the end of the template DNA strand denote the site for cleavage of the nascent pre-mRNA strand by an endonuclease and for polyadenylation at the 3′ end of the cut. All mature eukaryotic mRNAs, except histone mRNAs, have a 3′ poly(A) tail, which is a stretch of 20 to 250 adenosine residues added by polyadenylate polymerase. The poly(A) tail protects mRNA from degradation by exonucleases and serves as a binding region for poly(A)-binding protein, which functions in the circularization of mRNA during translation. The pre-mRNA also undergoes a process that excises the introns of the primary transcript and joins the exons to generate a mature mRNA product. This process of intron removal and exon ligation is called RNA splicing. It may begin before transcription of the gene is complete and must be completed before the mature mRNA is exported to the cytoplasm. Except for rare self-splicing introns, splicing requires a specialized RNA–protein complex called a spliceosome. Spliceosomes are multicomponent ribonucleoprotein complexes containing several small nuclear RNAs and more than 100 other proteins. This ribonucleoprotein complex assembles at the splice sites as the nascent pre-mRNA is transcribed. Mature mRNAs in association with ribonucleoproteins are exported through the nuclear pores into the cytoplasm.

Differential processing of the pre-mRNA and variations in nucleocytoplasmic transport can affect the amount of mature mRNA in the cytoplasm. Incompletely processed mRNA is not exported from the nucleus. The level of the enzyme glucose-6-phosphate dehydrogenase (G6PD) is regulated at the level of pre-mRNA processing. G6PD is the first and rate-determining step of the pentose phosphate pathway, which serves an important role in carbohydrate metabolism and NADPH synthesis. Studies have shown that whereas the rate of G6PD transcription is constant irrespective of nutritional status (e.g., starvation versus refeeding), the amount of mature (spliced) G6PD mRNA is reduced during fasting and increased during refeeding. Splicing coactivator proteins modulate the efficiency of splicing of the nascent G6PD transcript, resulting in unspliced, partially spliced, and fully spliced forms. The balance of these forms influences the cytosolic G6PD mRNA level, and consequently G6PD protein level (Salati et al., 2004).

Some genes have alternative splicing sites, which allow production of multiple mRNAs from a single gene. By altering the pattern of exons and introns from a single primary transcript that are spliced, biologically different proteins can arise from a single gene, increasing genetic diversity. Nearly three quarters of human multi-exon genes undergo tissue-specific patterns of alternative splicing. Alternative splicing also can occur at specific developmental stages. Less common means of producing different proteins from the same gene use alternative cleavage sites to change the C-terminus of the protein and RNA editing to change the nucleotide sequence of coding region of the mRNA (e.g., C to U editing of apolipoprotein B (apo B) mRNA to yield apo B-48 instead of apo B-100).

STABILITY OF mRNA

Changes in the cellular abundance of a particular mRNA species can occur as a result of changes in mRNA stability, as well as because of changes in DNA transcription or pre-mRNA processing. When the degradation of a particular mRNA is reduced, that mRNA accumulates and hence the total amount of protein translated from that mRNA may increase. On the other hand, when the degradation of an mRNA is increased, less mRNA remains and less of the corresponding protein may be translated. The stability of a given mRNA transcript is determined by a variety of factors, including the presence or absence of the mRNA cap and the length of the poly(A) tail. For many mRNAs, stability or degradation is also regulated by the presence of specific sequence elements in the mRNA, usually in the 3′ untranslated region (UTR), that can bind specific RNA-binding proteins or form base pairs with miRNA or other RNA species.

Regulation of mRNA Stability by RNA-Binding Proteins

A classic example of how mRNA stability is regulated through protein–mRNA interactions is found in iron metabolism. Transferrin receptor (TfR) mRNA expression is tightly linked to intracellular iron levels (Mullner and Kuhn, 1988). The 3′ UTR of TfR mRNA contains sequences called iron responsive elements (IrREs), which form stem–loop secondary structures that are susceptible to cleavage by RNA degrading enzymes (RNases). Under conditions of low iron, the stability of TfR mRNA is enhanced by the masking of these IrREs by iron regulatory proteins (IrRPs). Because the association of IrRPs with IrREs protects the mRNA from RNase cleavage, the transferrin receptor mRNA levels rise. Under conditions of high iron, the IrRE-binding activity of IrRPs is inactivated, allowing for increased TfR mRNA degradation.

Many mRNAs contain AU-rich elements (AREs) that are targets of specialized RNA-binding proteins (ARE-RBPs). AREs are typically present in the 3′ UTR of mRNAs but are also found in 5′ UTR and in coding regions of some mRNAs. Some ARE-RBPs are stabilizing factors, whereas others are destabilizing factors. An example of this type of regulation is the regulation of renal glutaminase expression in response to acidosis (Ibrahim et al., 2008). The 3′ UTR of glutaminase mRNA contains AU sequences that function as pH-response elements to which several ARE-RBPs bind to variably stabilize or destabilize the glutaminase mRNA. When the pH of the cell drops, translocation of HuR (a stabilizing ARE-RBP) from the nucleus allows it to bind and stabilize glutaminase mRNA, resulting in increased glutaminase expression that enables ammonium ion production by the kidney for excretion of excess acid.

Regulation of mRNA Stability by miRNA

Another common mechanism regulating mRNA stability is through the base pairing of miRNAs to the 3′ UTR of mRNA. Currently there are over 500 known mammalian genes that encode miRNAs, and each miRNA is capable of repressing hundreds of genes (Williams, 2008). Transcription of miRNA genes in the nucleus results in formation of primary miRNA, which are relatively short transcripts (~1 kb) that fold to form short hairpin structures. The primary miRNA is first processed in the nucleus by Drosha (a double-stranded RNA-specific ribonuclease) into a short hairpin structure called pre-miRNA. Following transport into the cytoplasm, pre-miRNA is further processed by a protein complex called Dicer, resulting in formation of short (20- to 30-nucleotide) RNA duplexes. After Dicer processing, the miRNA duplex is unwound and the mature miRNA strand binds to an argonaute protein to form the core component of the effector complex that mediates miRNA function. This complex is known as the RNA-induced silencing complex (RISC) (Pratt and MacRae, 2009). Usually only one strand of the mi-RNA duplex is loaded into the RISC complex; this tends to be the strand in which the 5′ end is less stably base-paired to its complement. The base pairing of miRNA within RISC to the 3′ UTR of a target mRNA promotes cleavage of the mRNA by ribonucleases, resulting in mRNA degradation. One of the four argonaute proteins in humans is an active endonuclease and can cleave mRNAs to which it binds with extensive complementarity. However, most miRNAs form base pairs with their mRNA targets with imperfect complementarity and repress the translation of their mRNA targets without endonucleolytic cleavage. Translational repression, however, commonly leads to mRNA destabilization and mRNA degradation by other machinery of the cell.

The fact that miRNAs are small, can be rapidly transcribed, and do not need to be translated into protein to act gives miRNAs some advantages as regulators. Recent studies suggest that miRNAs may be important in the regulation of adaptive responses to nutritional stress or changes in environmental conditions (Strum et al., 2009).

TRANSLATION OF mRNA

If the cellular abundance of all proteins was determined by the amount of mRNAs, the relationship between molar protein and mRNA levels would be linear. However, the correlation between mRNA levels and protein abundance in a single cell is poor, emphasizing the fact that changes in mRNA translation and protein turnover also play large roles in the regulation of cellular protein abundance. In the past decade, exploration regarding the control of gene expression at the level of mRNA translation has moved beyond uncovering basic details and toward development of novel means to treat and cure diseases such as cancer (Barnhart and Simon, 2007).

Regulation of mRNA translation includes changes that alter the overall protein biosynthetic capacity of the cell (i.e., ribosome biogenesis), changes that alter the amount of protein synthesized per mRNA molecule (i.e., translational efficiency), and changes in mRNA localization. Whereas changes in ribosome biogenesis impact the synthesis of all cellular proteins, changes in translational efficiency can either alter global protein synthesis or target the translation of a specific subset of mRNAs (e.g., ATF4).

Regulation of Translation by Regulating the Localization of mRNAs

Although not well understood, it is known that mRNAs in the cytoplasm can be packaged into transient, dynamic structures known as stress granules and processing bodies.

The mRNA in these structures is not being actively translated. Stress granules contain mainly stalled preinitiation complexes, whereas processing bodies are associated with mRNA decay or degradation. The mRNAs in these structures can be cycled back into polysomes when cellular conditions change.

Regulation of Translation by Regulation of Ribosome Biogenesis

Ribosome biogenesis describes the making and assembling of ribosomal proteins and rRNAs into the 40S and 60S ribosomal subunits. Expression of the genes encoding the numerous constituents of ribosomes requires transcription by all three classes of RNAPs (Mayer and Grummt, 2006). A signaling network in yeast named target of rapamycin (TOR) is identified as critical in controlling ribosomal protein gene expression and coordinating the relative activity of all three RNAPs to achieve the proper stoichiometry of ribosomal components. Both nutrients and stress can influence mammalian TOR (mTOR) signaling, linking ribosomal capacity to nutrient availability and other environmental cues. Conditions of rapid growth require enhanced ribosome production, and increased levels of ribosomes have been observed in growing tumors (Belin et al., 2009). Ribosomal protein mRNAs all contain a *cis*-regulatory element consisting of several pyrimidines at the 5′ end. This terminal oligopyrimidine (TOP) tract is also present in mRNA translation elongation factors and poly(A)-binding protein. Feeding a protein-containing meal maximally enhances TOP mRNA translation, whereas amino acid deficiency completely abrogates translation of TOP mRNAs (Anthony et al., 2001). This exaggerated "all-or-none" binary control mechanism suggests that in the repressed state, translation is blocked. A number of studies have implicated the phosphatidylinositol 3-kinase (PtdIns3K) and mTOR signaling pathways in the activation of TOP mRNAs during high growth conditions, but consensus on the mechanism underlying this regulatory process has not been reached. The regulation of translational capacity provides the organism with an ability to adapt to chronic or sustained conditions of change.

Translational Efficiency

Translational efficiency refers to the rate at which protein is translated from a particular mRNA. In contrast to changes in the ribosomal machinery or translational capacity, changes in translational efficiency can be accomplished as needed without delay because the mRNA and all the protein synthetic machinery is already present. Factors that can alter translational efficiency include nutrient intake, hypoxia, hormones, and exercise.

The translation of mRNA, or polypeptide synthesis, is a highly organized and multicomponent pathway that, like RNA synthesis, can be divided into three stages: (1) initiation, (2) elongation, and (3) termination. During the initiation step, the small (40S) ribosomal subunit is recruited to a selected mRNA and joined with the large (60S) ribosomal subunit to form an 80S ribosome poised at the start codon, AUG. During elongation, tRNA delivers covalently bound amino acids to the ribosome according to the order dictated by the mRNA coding region, and peptide bonds are created to link the amino acids together. The termination step consists of stop codon recognition and dissociation of the ribosomal subunits from the mRNA. Each of these steps is regulated by separate categories of protein factors called eukaryotic initiation factors (eIFs), eukaryotic elongation factors (eEFs), and eukaryotic release factors (eRFs), respectively. Most of the protein factors regulating translation have multiple subunits and contain binding sites for interaction with other translation factors as well as for association with the ribosome. In addition, several are enzymes that catalyze essential reactions involved in translation. The functions of several of these proteins are regulated to stimulate or inhibit translation.

Control of Translation Initiation: Formation of Preinitiation Complex and Its Regulation by eIF2α Phosphorylation

The majority of translational control lies at the initiation step, which is summarized in Figure 13-7. This step can be further subdivided into three events that determine overall initiation activity. The first event involves assembly of a ternary complex (TC) consisting of the initiating tRNA (specifically, a particular initiator methionyl-tRNA, or Met-tRNA$_i$) bound to the protein factor eIF2 in association with GTP (guanosine 5′-triphosphate). eIF2 is a guanine nucleotide-binding protein (i.e., G-protein) made of α, β, and γ subunits. eIF2 exists either in an active GTP-bound state or in an inactive GDP (guanosine 5′-diphosphate)-bound form. Only when eIF2 is in the GTP-bound form can the TC bind the small ribosomal subunit. Following TC formation, the TC and other protein factors (e.g., eIF1, eIF3, eIF5) bind to the 40S ribosomal subunit to form the 43S preinitiation complex and eIF2–GDP is released (Lorsch and Dever, 2010).

Regeneration of the eIF2–GTP from eIF2–GDP is catalyzed by eIF2B, a guanine nucleotide exchange factor (GEF). The GEF activity of eIF2B is regulated primarily by phosphorylation of eIF2 on its α subunit, which increases its binding affinity to several eIF2B subunits, stalling eIF2B GEF activity. Phosphorylation of eIF2 is catalyzed by a family of four kinases, each responsive to a distinct set of environmental stressors. The mammalian eIF2α kinases are heme-regulated inhibitor (HRI), which is sensitive to heme deprivation; double-stranded RNA-dependent protein kinase (PKR), which is activated by a viral infection; PKR-like endoplasmic reticulum resident kinase (PERK), which is activated by misfolded proteins or other stress in the ER; and general control nonderepressible kinase 2 (GCN2), which is activated by conditions of amino acid deprivation (Wek et al., 2006). Another way in which the GEF activity of eIF2B is modulated is by the binding of the protein factor eIF5 to eIF2, sequestering eIF2 away from eIF2B, thus preventing guanine nucleotide exchange (Singh et al., 2006).

Generally speaking, reduced eIF2B GEF activity reduces TC formation and causes an overall slowing of mRNA translation. At the same time, reduced GEF activity and thus reduced TC increases the ability of the ribosome to reinitiate mRNA translation at start codons located after the first

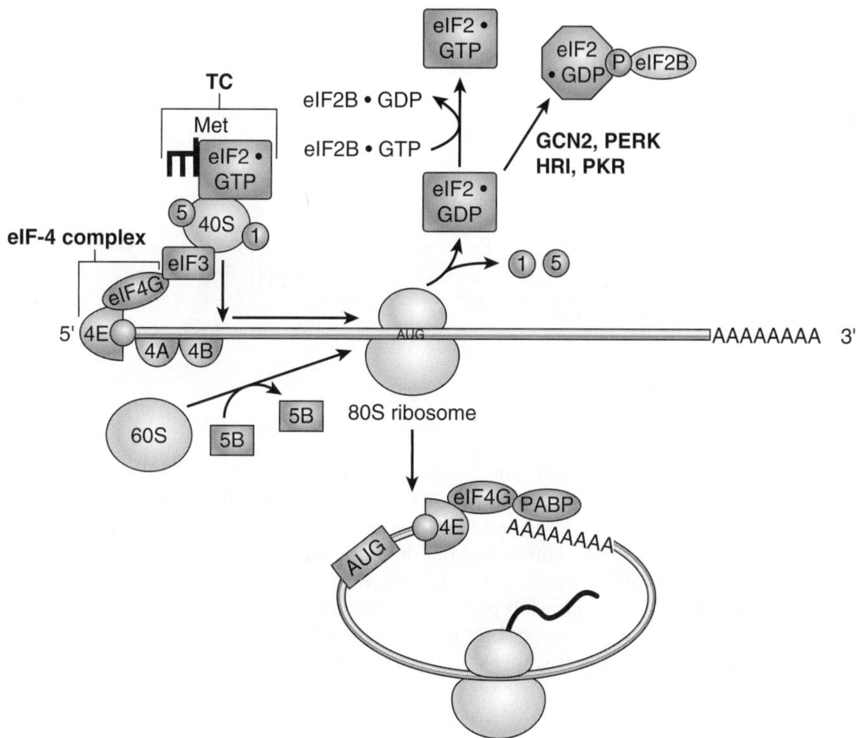

FIGURE 13-7 The pathway of initiation of eukaryotic mRNA translation. First, eukaryotic initiation factor (*eIF*) 2 binds to GTP and the initiating Met-tRNA$_i$ to form the ternary initiation complex (*TC*). TC then binds to the 40S ribosomal subunit to form the 43S preinitiation complex. The mRNA to be translated is selected by the eIF4 group of translation factors, which includes the mRNA cap binding protein eIF4E and the scaffold protein eIF4G. eIF4G is important for bringing the preinitiation complex into proximity with the mRNA. eIF4G also has a role in mRNA circularization by binding the poly(A)-binding protein (*PABP*). The eIF4 complex melts mRNA secondary structure close to the cap to generate a ribosome binding site. The 43S preinitiation complex then binds to the mRNA near the cap structure by interaction of a central domain of eIF4G with eIF3. The 43S preinitiation complex moves along the mRNA in the 5′ to 3′ direction until it finds a start codon (AUG). During AUG start codon recognition by the 43S preinitiation complex, the 60S ribosomal subunit joins the 40S to form a competent 80S ribosome, releasing several initiation factors including eIF2 with bound GDP. eIF2B, a guanine nucleotide exchange factor (GEF), facilitates exchange of GDP for GTP on eIF2 to allow subsequent TC formation. When eIF2 is phosphorylated, the GEF activity of eIF2B is stalled, however, repressing mRNA translation initiation.

AUG in the mRNA. Some mRNAs contain start codons and associated ORFs that are 5′ (upstream) of the main ORF. Translation initiation at an upstream ORF (uORF) generally inhibits translation of the main downstream ORF because ribosomes are not competent to reinitiate at the downstream AUG. However, in the presence of reduced TC, initiation may not occur at the uORF, allowing delayed initiation to occur at the downstream AUG. This mechanism permits enhanced translation of specific mRNAs (some encoding proteins that help the cell deal with the imposed stress) under conditions of overall suppression of translation. This type of gene-specific translation will be covered in greater detail in subsequent text about stress responses.

Control of Translation Initiation: Association of the 40S Ribosomal Subunit with mRNA by Cap-Dependent Recognition and Its Regulation by eIF4E Binding Protein Phosphorylation

The second event in translation initiation subject to major regulation involves the binding of the 43S preinitiation complex to the selected mRNA. This event requires eIF3 and several other initiation factors collectively called eIF4 (or eIF4F). One of the proteins in this group, named eIF4E, selects the mRNA to be translated by binding its 5′-m^{7}GTP cap structure. A second member of the eIF4 group, called eIF4G, functions as a scaffold to bring the small ribosomal subunit and the mRNA close to each other. eIF4G accomplishes this task by binding both eIF4E, which is bound to the mRNA cap, and eIF3, which is associated with the 40S ribosomal subunit in the preinitiation complex. A family of repressor proteins known as the eIF4E-binding proteins (4E-BPs) can prevent the interaction of eIF4G and eIF4E and thereby inhibit the 40S ribosome from binding mRNA. The repressor activity of the 4E-BP is regulated by phosphorylation, with increased phosphorylation reducing its affinity to associate with eIF4E. A second function of eIF4G is to associate with poly(A)-binding protein, which results in 5′,3′-circularization of mRNA, as shown in the lower part of Figure 13-7. Circularization of mRNA is believed to be important for stabilizing recruited 40S ribosomal subunits and for efficient recycling of terminating ribosomes for another round of translation of the same mRNA (Wilkie et al., 2003). After the eIF4 complex has brought the 43S preinitiation complex and mRNA together, the small ribosomal subunit moves along the mRNA toward the 3′ end scanning for

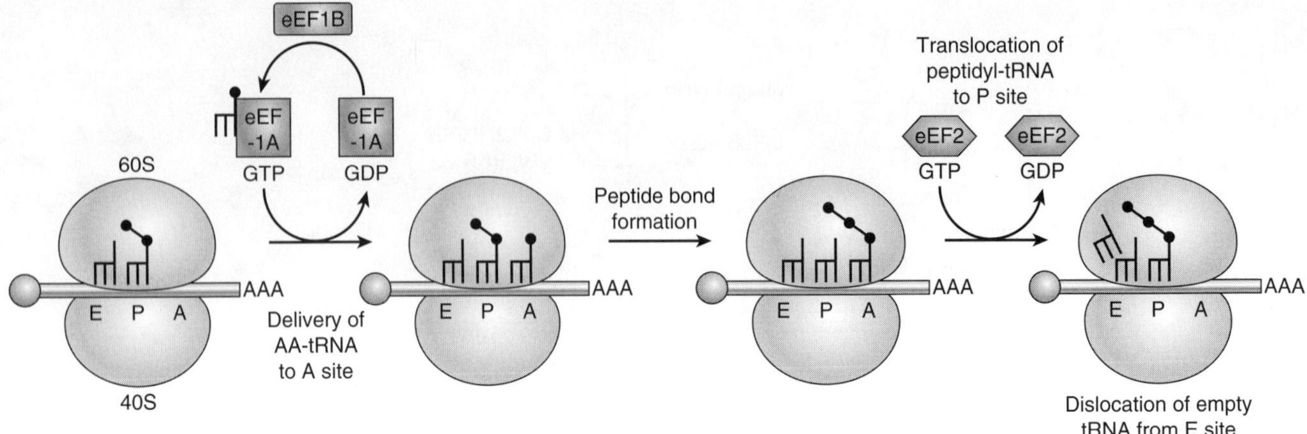

FIGURE 13-8 The pathway of elongation of eukaryotic mRNA translation. Eukaryotic elongation factor (eEF) 1A (eEF1A) bound to GTP delivers an aminoacylated tRNA to the A-site of the ribosome. When the appropriate codon–anticodon interaction occurs, GTP is hydrolyzed and eEF1A is released from the ribosome bound to GDP. eEF1B functions to regenerate the GTP-bound form of eEF1A. The growing peptide chain in site P is joined to the new amino site in site A by a peptidyl transferase that is a component of the 60S ribosomal subunit. The protein factor eEF2 promotes movement of the ribosome along the mRNA (translocation) so that the growing peptide is again shifted from the A site to the P site, the uncharged tRNA left in the P site upon peptide bond formation shifts to the E site, and the uncharged tRNA formerly in the E site exits the ribosome. GDP spontaneously dissociates from eEF2 so it can be recycled.

the start codon. Scanning is facilitated by eukaryotic initiation factor eIF4A, which functions as an ATP-dependent helicase to unwind mRNA secondary structure in the 5′ UTR.

Start Codon Recognition, Large Subunit Engagement, and eIF2 Recycling

Start codon recognition halts scanning and triggers a number of events that commit the ribosome to begin translation at that point on the mRNA. eIF1, eIF2, eIF5, and eIF5B play key roles in these events. First, eIF1 is released from the small ribosomal subunit, denoting recognition of the correct AUG start codon (Cheung et al., 2007). In addition, upon AUG recognition, GTP hydrolysis on eIF2 is triggered, an event aided by eIF5. The final event involves eIF5B-mediated joining of the 60S large ribosomal subunit with the 40S small ribosomal subunit on the mRNA to form an 80S ribosome along with release of eIF2–GDP and other initiation factors. eIF2–GDP must be converted back to eIF2–GTP before it can participate in another round of initiation.

Non-Cap-Dependent Translation Initiation

Eukaryotic mRNA translation initiation is largely cap-dependent, meaning that the association of the preinitiation complex with the eIF4 complex at the 5′-m^{7}GTP cap is required. However, for some mRNAs the preinitiation complex binds to an internal ribosome entry site (IRES) that is downstream of the 5′ cap. The IRES is a highly structured *cis*-element in the 5′ UTR that associates with specific proteins and some eIFs to bring the ribosome and mRNA together without the need for cap binding and eIF4 complex formation. This method of translation initiation may be important in conditions that require the translation of specific mRNAs under conditions in which overall mRNA translation is suppressed.

Polypeptide Synthesis: Elongation and Its Regulation

After initiation, the polypeptide is assembled with the amino acid sequence being specified by the mRNA sequence, as illustrated in Figure 13-8. This process requires substantial metabolic energy, with two molecules of GTP cleaved for every added amino acid. The elongation step of mRNA translation involves fewer protein factors than the initiation step, but the eEFs required are considered the workhorses of protein synthesis on the ribosome. During initiation, the Met-tRNA$_i$ is base-paired with the mRNA start codon in a location named the peptidyl or "P" site within the ribosome. The protein factor eEF1A with bound GTP then delivers the next correct aminoacyl–tRNA to the ribosome at the aminoacyl or "A" site, beginning the process of elongation. Upon correct codon–anticodon interaction, GTP is hydrolyzed and eEF1A with bound GDP is released from the ribosome. A second factor, a GEF named eEF1B, assists in regenerating active eEF1A–GTP, ensuring continued deliverance of aminoacyl–tRNAs to the ribosome. With delivery of an aminoacyl–tRNA into the A site, peptide bond formation proceeds, joining the amino group of the aminoacyl–tRNA in the A site to the carboxyl group of the aminoacyl–tRNA in the P site with release of water. Peptide bond synthesis is catalyzed by a peptidyl transferase that is part of the 60S ribosomal subunit. A third and final factor, named eEF2, facilitates movement of the ribosome along the mRNA, resulting in translocation of the peptidyl–tRNA from the A site to the P site and movement of the unloaded tRNA in the P site to the "E site," where it can exit the ribosome. The energy required for the ribosome to rachet forward on the mRNA is provided by GTP hydrolysis, catalyzed by eEF2. A GEF is not needed to regenerate eEF2–GTP because eEF2 has low affinity for GDP which spontaneously dissociates.

All three eEFs are subject to phosphorylation in mammalian cells. Phosphorylation of eEF1A stimulates elongation activity, whereas phosphorylation of its GEF, eEF1B, on several subunits has no reported influence on elongation rates. On the other hand, eEF2 is inactivated by phosphorylation. Phosphorylation of eEF2 does not impact the ability of the ribosome to hydrolyze GTP but instead reduces the affinity of eEF2 for the ribosome (Carlberg et al., 1990). Phosphorylation of eEF2 occurs in response to stimuli that either increase energy demand or reduce its supply. This likely serves to slow down protein synthesis and thus conserve energy under such circumstances (Andersen et al., 2003). Examples of conditions that increase eEF2 phosphorylation include intense exercise, alcohol intake, ischemia, and denervation.

Termination

The final step in translation, that of termination, occurs when one of the three stop codons (UAA, UAG, UGA) is positioned in the A site of the ribosome. This event is recognized by the protein eRF1, which binds to the ribosome and, in a GTP-dependent fashion, catalyzes the cleavage of the bond between the nascent peptide and the tRNA, thereby releasing the newly translated protein. A second release factor called eRF3 stimulates eRF1 activity in the presence of GTP.

POSTTRANSLATIONAL MODIFICATIONS AND FOLDING OF PROTEINS

Cotranslational and posttranslational modifications are essential steps for the trafficking, activation, regulation, and ultimately the degradation of proteins. In fact, there are probably only a small number of proteins that do not undergo some type of chemical change during or following their synthesis. Chaperone-mediated regulation of protein folding and a host of posttranslational modifications occur either cotranslationally or posttranslationally. Many posttranslational modifications occur in steps at specific locations in the cell as the protein is trafficked to its correct destination. Likewise, posttranslational modifications are involved in the irreversible conversion of pro-proteins into their active or functional forms.

The N-terminal methionine residue is removed from many proteins, and other proteins are cleaved to produce active peptides, remove targeting sequences that are no longer needed, or remove inhibitory prosequences for activation of the protein. Other common modifications include, but are not limited to, disulfide bond formation, glycosylation, acetylation, and fatty acylation. Some proteins require the addition of a cofactor such as heme or biotin. Despite the widespread presence of protein modifications in nature, much remains unknown about how these alterations affect the activity of each individual protein. This is mostly because a singular type of modification imparts different functions, depending on the target protein. For example, *N*-linked glycosylation may stabilize the folding process of one polypeptide, allow another protein to play an important role in cell–cell recognition, or protect a lysosomal membrane protein from degradation by lysosomal proteases. The mechanisms for these and other protein modifications during and following translation is varied and complex. Mutations in genes encoding proteins involved in protein modifications are among the causes of inherited disease. For example, mutations in several genes encoding proteins involved in the glycosylation of alpha-dystroglycan have been identified as a cause of one group of muscular dystrophies (Muntoni et al., 2008).

TRAFFICKING OF PROTEINS TO THEIR DESTINATIONS

Except for a few proteins encoded by mitochondrial DNA that are synthesized within the mitochondrial matrix (i.e., 13 subunits of the respiratory complexes), all protein synthesis occurs in conjunction with cytosolic ribosomes. Cytosolic proteins and those targeted for the mitochondria, peroxisomes, or nucleus are completely synthesized in the cytosol. Some proteins, however, have N-terminal signal sequences that temporarily stop translation of the polypeptide until the signal sequence is recognized by and bound by a signal recognition particle that in turn binds to a receptor on the cytosolic face of the ER membrane. These proteins are then cotranslationally translocated into the lumen of the ER or inserted into the membrane of the ER.

Importation of Proteins into Nucleus, Mitochondria, and Peroxisomes

Ribosomes synthesizing a protein without a signal sequence for import into the ER do not bind to the ER and continue cytosolic synthesis until the polypeptide is completed. Chaperone proteins present in the cytosol help the protein fold properly or help maintain it in an unfolded or loosely folded state until it is transported to the correct compartment. Many proteins synthesized in the cytosol remain in the cytosol. However, some proteins completely synthesized in the cytosol are destined for the nucleus, mitochondria, or peroxisomes. Nuclear proteins have nuclear localization signals that target them for active transport through pores in the nuclear envelope; these proteins may be transported in folded form. Mitochondrial proteins (except for the few that are encoded by mitochondrial DNAs and synthesized within the mitochondria) have a signal sequence that is recognized by a chaperone that targets the protein to receptors on the outer membrane of a mitochondrion. Various factors and receptors as well as ATP hydrolysis are involved in the translocation of proteins to the outer or inner membranes, matrix, or intermembrane space of the mitochondria. Mitochondrial proteins are transported across membranes in unfolded form and need new chaperones to refold on the other side. Peroxisomal import involves a system that can facilitate transport of folded and oligomeric proteins. Peroxisomal import of proteins is mediated by cycling receptors that shuttle between the cytosol and the peroxisomal lumen and that depend upon ATP and ubiquitin.

Trafficking of Proteins from the ER to the Golgi Apparatus and to the Vesicular System

At least one third of translated proteins in eukaryotic genomes are molecules that are destined for the vesicular compartments, including the ER lumen. These include those

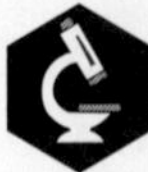

CLINICAL CORRELATION

Protein Misfolding: The Basis of Cystic Fibrosis and Alzheimer Disease

All the information for protein folding is contained in the polypeptide sequence. Because the rate of the folding process is significantly faster than the rate of translation, the folding process must be regulated to hold back the polypeptide from folding until all of the relevant sequence is available and to prevent hydrophobic regions in the newly synthesized polypeptide from intermolecular aggregation. Folding mediators or chaperones are proteins responsible for sequestering nascent polypeptides and mediating folding. Some of these chaperones (holdases) are involved in sequestering nascent polypeptides on the ribosomes. They bind to short, linear sequences with hydrophobic character as they emerge from the ribosomes, maintaining them in an extended state until productive folding can occur. This prevents premature folding that may lead to incorrectly folded aggregates. Other chaperones (foldases) are multimeric complexes that act as "cages" to isolate a molecule of folding polypeptide to prevent any intermolecular encounters so that it folds on itself.

Researchers now understand that proteins must pass through partially folded states in which they are delicately poised between folding all the way to the correct state and becoming seriously stuck as a result of premature entanglement with other molecules. Misfolding of a protein can lead to its degradation (too little of the protein) or to its aggregation (formation of toxic deposits of excessive quantities of wrongly folded proteins). This insight has opened the way to understanding some aspects of a range of human diseases.

Cystic fibrosis is the most common fatal genetic disease in humans, affecting approximately 1 in 2,000 live births among populations of whites of Northern European descent. The autosomal recessive disorder is due to lack of a protein that regulates the transport of the chloride ion across cell membranes. The most common mutation underlying cystic fibrosis (~70% of the disease alleles; >90% of CF patients) is a deletion of Phe508 in the N-terminal region of this approximately 160-kDa protein. The deletion of this single amino acid acts to hinder the dissociation of the chloride ion transport regulator protein (cystic fibrosis transmembrane conductance regulator, CFTR) from one of its chaperones. This prevents the final steps for normal folding of CFTR, and therefore normal amounts of active CFTR are not produced. Interestingly, the ΔPhe508 mutant protein, if folded into a native state, is functional under physiological conditions. The problem is that nearly all of the newly synthesized protein is shunted to the degradation pathway before it has an opportunity to form functional chloride channels in the ER membrane. The trapped, partially folded protein is subsequently degraded.

Misfolding or folding too slowly can also lead to inappropriate association of partially folded chains, giving rise to cellular pathologies due to the formation of insoluble aggregates rather than from a lack of native protein. Some diseases known as amyloidoses, of which Alzheimer disease is the best-known example, are characterized by the accumulation of plaques of insoluble protein in the extracellular tissue. Different proteins, each associated with a different disease, act as the building blocks of these plaques. Alzheimer disease is characterized by the accumulation of plaques of insoluble β-amyloid in the brain. Normally, the body processes amyloid precursor protein by hydrolysis into soluble amyloid-β peptide fragments that are mainly 40 or 42 amino acids in length. Under certain circumstances, these peptides aggregate into long filaments that then form the insoluble β-amyloid that makes up the neuritic plaque in patients with Alzheimer disease. The implication of misfolding of the amyloid β-peptides as a basis of Alzheimer disease is strongly supported by the finding that premature or early-onset Alzheimer disease is due to mutations in the amyloid precursor protein.

proteins that are targeted for insertion into membranes, including ER and Golgi membranes as well as the plasma membrane, and those that are targeted to be secreted by the cell (Dancourt and Barlowe, 2010). During elongation, these classes of proteins are first targeted via the signal recognition particle, which is located in approximately the first 30 translated amino acids, to the ER for completion of synthesis. In the ER, both cotranslational and posttranslational modifications, such as the initial steps of *N*-glycosylation and disulfide bond formation, occur on the nascent polypeptides, which are then correctly folded. Classical chaperone proteins (e.g., binding protein BiP) and nonclassical chaperones such as those necessary for folding of *N*-glycosylated proteins (calnexin and calreticulin) function as a quality control system (Hoseki et al., 2010). Unfolded or misfolded polypeptides linger in the ER lumen for a time, awaiting proper assembly. Proteins unable to be correctly folded are dislocated from the ER and targeted for degradation in the cytosol by the proteasome, a process described in greater detail later in this chapter.

Before transit to intracellular organelles or the cell surface, newly synthesized proteins are packaged into vesicles for transport to the Golgi apparatus. The Golgi apparatus is a major location for sorting proteins to different destinations, and many proteins synthesized in the ER are trafficked to the Golgi apparatus. Retrograde transport from the Golgi apparatus back to the ER recycles vesicle membrane proteins and lipids and also returns escaped ER-resident proteins that mistakenly found their way into the Golgi apparatus. The delivery of cargo between the two subcellular spaces is dynamic and in constant flux.

Once in the Golgi apparatus, proteins are further modified, sorted, and trafficked via the *trans*-Golgi–endosomal network. *N*-Glycosylation begun in the ER is completed and *O*-glycosylation of proteins occurs in the Golgi apparatus. Phosphorylation of a mannose residue of *N*-linked oligosaccharides of glycoproteins that are destined for lysosomes also occurs in the Golgi.

The sorting of diverse proteins into vesicles for transport from the ER or Golgi complex is facilitated by protein sorting receptors and by a diverse set of vesicular transmembrane proteins that bind specific carbohydrate or protein motifs on cargo proteins. Protein sorting receptors also assist in ER quality control by recognizing only fully folded and assembled proteins for delivery to the Golgi apparatus. In particular, in the Golgi complex, some proteins are directed to the lysosome, some to the plasma membrane, and some to specialized secretory vesicles.

Delivery of proteins from the ER and Golgi apparatus to these various pathways is coordinated by a complex network of cytosolic and membrane proteins. Rab GTPases control docking of vesicles on target membranes. Conversion of cytosolic Rab–GDP to Rab–GTP, catalyzed by a specific membrane-embedded GEF, induces a conformational change in Rab that enables it to interact with a surface protein on a particular transport vesicle and insert an isoprenoid anchor into the vesicle membrane. Once Rab–GTP is tethered to the vesicle surface, it interacts with a Rab effector that docks the vesicle on the appropriate membrane. Paired sets of soluble *N*-ethylmaleimide-sensitive factor attachment protein receptors (SNAREs) are key components responsible for membrane fusion between post-Golgi transport vesicles and the plasma membrane or the endosomal pathway (Chaineau et al., 2009). After Rab-mediated docking of a vesicle on its target membrane, the interactions of cognate vector-SNAREs and target-SNAREs brings the two membranes close enough that they can fuse.

The Unfolded Protein or ER Stress Response

ER homeostasis requires that the capacity of the protein-folding apparatus remains in balance with the demand. This balance can be disrupted by environmental stress (e.g., glucose starvation or disturbance of Ca^{2+} homeostasis during hypoxia), genetic mutations in proteins requiring ER assembly (e.g., cystic fibrosis transmembrane conductance regulator), or malfunctions in the folding machinery itself. When the balance becomes disrupted, unfolded or misfolded proteins accumulate. In the crowded environment of the cell, unfolded proteins are a danger because they may aggregate and become toxic. This buildup of "cellular trash" initiates an adaptive mechanism, termed the *unfolded protein response* (UPR) or *ER stress response*, which is summarized in Figure 13-9 (Schroder and Kaufman, 2005). The UPR encompasses three distinct processes. First, the global rate of protein synthesis is slowed down to reduce the ER protein-folding load. Second, ER resident chaperones are transcriptionally induced to increase the folding capacity in these organelles. Third, a protein degrading system named ER-associated degradation (ERAD) is initiated to help clear the accumulating cellular waste. Activation of ERAD is important for the degradation of unfolded proteins through the ubiquitin–proteasome pathway (Kincaid and Cooper,

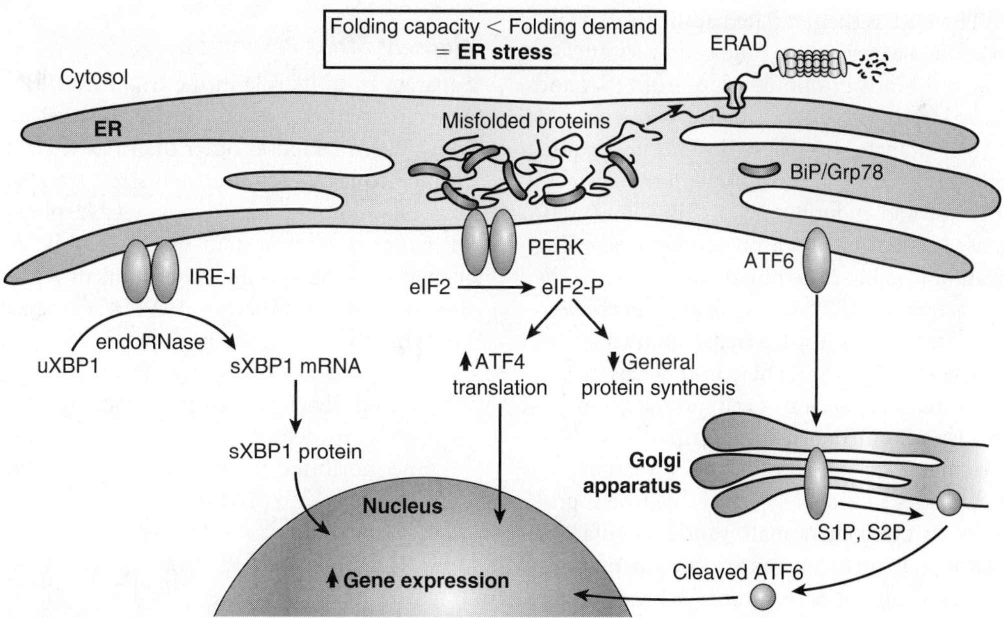

FIGURE 13-9 The functional components of the mammalian unfolded protein response (endoplasmic reticulum [*ER*] stress response). An imbalance between protein folding demand and protein folding capacity imposes stress on the ER resulting in a tripartite response. First, the expression of genes necessary for stress alleviation are increased by promoting specific mRNA translation, which is mediated by PERK activation and increased translation of the transcription factor ATF4, and by promoting DNA binding of transcription factors originating from proteins associated with the ER membrane (i.e., sXBP1 and ATF6). Second, general protein synthesis is inhibited to reduce the load on the folding apparatus. Third, ER-associated degradation (*ERAD*) is increased via molecular chaperones guiding unfolded or misfolded proteins from the ER to the 26S proteasome. Both the general reduction in protein synthesis and the upregulation of mRNA-specific translation (e.g., of ATF4) occur in association with the phosphorylation of eIF2 by the protein kinase, *PERK*.

2007). If the ER stress cannot be alleviated by these three processes, then cellular pathways will be activated to induce programmed cell death.

ER stress activates a set of three signaling pathways or branches that promote cell survival by reducing misfolded protein levels. Each of these branches is initiated by activation of transmembrane proteins with domains in the ER lumen. How these three luminal sensors are initially activated is unclear, although it appears to involve the dissociation of molecular chaperones normally bound to the luminal domain of each protein.

The first UPR branch is activated by the eIF2 kinase called PERK (PKR-like ER-localized eIF2α kinase). PERK induces phosphorylation of the translation factor eIF2, resulting in a shutdown of mRNA translation at the initiation step. This response blocks new synthesis of proteins and prevents further accumulation of unfolded proteins that form toxic aggregates. At the same time, increases in the phosphorylation of eIF2 allow for the increased translation of specific mRNAs that encode DNA-binding proteins, such as activating transcription factor 4 (ATF4). ATF4 promotes the transcription of stress-remediation genes (e.g., amino acid transporters, antioxidant molecules) as well as genes that are linked to coordinating programmed cell death. The upregulation of ATF4 mRNA translation in the face of global translational repression is a synchronized process in which delayed formation of TC, due to the inhibitory phosphorylation of eIF2 by an eIF2α kinase (e.g., PERK), results in the ribosome scanning past one or more uORFs. In the case of the ATF4 mRNA, which possesses two uORFs, translation of the full-length ATF4 ORF is then initiated at the third AUG. Increased ATF4 protein expression is followed by its nuclear translocation where it binds promoter regions of DNA and signals for increased transcription of stress-response genes.

The second UPR branch is activated by inositol requiring enzyme 1 (IRE1), a bifunctional transmembrane protein possessing both kinase and endoribonuclease functions. Activation of its kinase activity initiates a proapoptotic signaling cascade via activation of c-Jun N-terminal kinase (JNK). The endoribonuclease activity of IRE1 results in the nonconventional splicing of the mRNA for Xbp1, a transcriptional activator that upon internal splicing is brought to the nucleus to bind DNA elements to increase expression of cell survival genes.

The third and least-studied arm of the tripartite UPR is ATF6, a transcription factor that upon release from chaperones in the ER, migrates to the Golgi apparatus where proteolytic cleavage of its cytosolic domain produces an active transcription factor that turns on the expression of genes encoding molecular chaperones. All three UPR branches elicit both prosurvival and proapoptotic signals, and how the UPR coordinates these activities to make life or death decisions is a subject of much continued study. The duration of UPR branch signaling contributes in part to cell fate after ER stress (Lin et al., 2007) as does differential activation of individual UPR branches (Lin et al., 2009).

In addition to accumulation of protein, recent studies report that intracellular accumulation of saturated fatty acids and cholesterol, as seen in obesity and atherosclerosis, results in ER stress (Hotamisligil, 2010). ER stress, in turn, leads to the suppression of insulin receptor signaling, which can promote insulin resistance and diabetes (Ozcan et al., 2004). Although cellular stress is certainly a major activator of the UPR, not only harmful events trigger the UPR. To the contrary, recent studies show that normal cell processes associated with increased secretory protein production are coupled with activation of UPR components. For example, terminal differentiation of a B lymphocyte into a mature antibody-secreting plasma cell requires the ER to assemble and ship out large quantities of antibodies with remarkable efficiency. This task requires expansion of the ER protein-folding capacity during B cell differentiation (Todd et al., 2008).

Loss of PERK function is also detrimental to health. Mice with a functionally disrupted PERK gene demonstrate massive apoptosis of the exocrine pancreas a few weeks after birth, destroying the insulin-producing beta cells (Zhang et al., 2002). The early steps of insulin biosynthesis occur in the ER, and the pancreatic beta cell has a highly developed and active ER. The inability to phosphorylate eIF2 in the beta cell leads to an inability to properly regulate folding capacity during times of high glucose intake, sending the cell into apoptotic pathways. As such, patients with a similar defect in the *EIF2AK3* gene, which encodes the human form of the eIF2 kinase PERK, suffer from Wolcott-Rallison syndrome, a severe form of neonatal or early infancy insulin-dependent diabetes that is also characterized by multiple defects in bone formation and growth retardation (Delepine et al., 2000).

Nutrient Stress Responses

Separate from its role in the tripartite UPR, the eIF2/ATF4 signaling pathway is responsive to other stress conditions in which eIF2 kinases other than PERK are activated. These include conditions of nutrient stress. In response to limitation of essential amino acids, GCN2 phosphorylates eIF2 to reduce general protein synthesis while at the same time increasing gene-specific translation of ATF4 (Sikalidis and Stipanuk, 2010). Increased ATF4 expression upregulates genes involved in amino acid metabolism, amino acid transport, and redox homeostasis, in an attempt to correct the amino acid deficiency. Animals lacking GCN2 are not able to cope with dietary essential amino acid deprivation and become moribund within days of feeding a leucine-devoid diet (Anthony et al., 2004).

MOLECULAR MECHANISMS OF PROTEIN DEGRADATION

Once a protein is made, it is immediately a target for degradation. Some proteins, such as collagen and hemoglobin, are relatively resistant to degradation and therefore turn over slowly. Other proteins are readily degraded, especially those that have an acute regulatory function. Cellular proteins that are damaged in some way or that have errors in amino acid sequence are also targeted for rapid degradation.

Protein degradation, or proteolysis, in eukaryotic cells is accomplished by a large number of specific and nonspecific proteases. The two major intracellular protein degradation pathways in eukaryotes are the ubiquitin–proteasome pathway and autophagy–lysosomal system. In general, the ubiquitin–proteasome system mainly degrades the intracellular proteins, whereas the autophagy–lysosomal system mainly degrades membrane and endocytosed proteins. Investigations of the pathways directing protein degradation have proved that these processes are complicated and exquisitely controlled. The molecular steps that make up each proteolysis pathway are currently receiving much attention, but many details remain unknown. This is in part due to the fact that there are multiple systems involved in the targeting and turnover of body proteins, each differentially activated according to tissue and physiological context and sometimes coordinately activated.

The regulation of protein degradation can impact a specific protein or the overall bulk amount of protein in a tissue or cell. Inhibitor of NFκB (IκB) is an example of a regulatory protein that is specifically regulated by changes in its rate of degradation. IκB acts as a negative regulator of nuclear factor kappa B (NFκB), which is a transcription factor activated by oxidative stress and inflammatory conditions. When complexed with IκB, NFκB is sequestered in the cytoplasm and cannot enter the nucleus to promote gene transcription. Upon exposure of a cell to injurious stimuli, such as free radicals, IκB is targeted for degradation by the ubiquitin–proteasome pathway, allowing NFκB to migrate to the nucleus and alter gene expression. Increased intake of specific nutrients such as n-3 fatty acids, vitamin E, flavonoids, isoflavones, β-carotene, and selenium are thought to exhibit antiinflammatory properties in part by reducing the degradation of IκB, lowering NFκB activity (Ravasco et al., 2010). Examples of global increases in the degradation of proteins are the bulk losses of tissue protein that occur in response to fasting, sepsis, denervation, and thermal injury (Mitch and Goldberg, 1996). In some of these situations of more global proteolysis, activation of more than one degradative system occurs (Solomon et al., 2000).

UBIQUITIN–PROTEASOME PATHWAY

The ubiquitin–proteasome pathway is present in both the nucleus and the cytoplasm of eukaryotic cells and plays an essential role in the degradation of soluble proteins. This pathway is also responsible for the regulated degradation of many short-lived proteins, including those required for the control of cell growth and proliferation, cell differentiation, immune and inflammatory responses, apoptosis, and metabolic adaptation. The ubiquitin–proteasome pathway also carries out housekeeping functions in basal protein turnover and the elimination of abnormal proteins that are miscoded, misfolded, mislocalized, damaged, or otherwise rendered inoperative. The ubiquitin–proteasome pathway also degrades myofibrillar proteins and so plays a critical role in the control of muscle mass.

Components of the Ubiquitin–Proteasome Pathway

As illustrated in Figure 13-10, the ubiquitin–proteasome pathway is made up of three sequential processes: (1) recognition of a protein substrate for degradation, (2) covalent addition of a polyubiquitin chain to mark the protein for degradation, and (3) proteolysis of the protein by a 2,500-kDa complex called the proteasome.

Recognition of Target Protein

The recognition of a protein as a target for degradation appears to depend on certain structural changes in the target protein. Known signals include the exposure of specific amino acid sequences that are normally buried, posttranslational modifications such as phosphorylation or hydroxylation, binding to or release from a ligand, interaction with an adaptor protein or chaperone, and specific damage incurred to the protein such as oxidation or nitrosylation. Mechanisms for recognition are diverse and vary for different proteins, involving E3 ubiquitin ligases or adaptor proteins. How proteins are recognized for degradation is linked to their normal rates of turnover or degradation.

Polyubiquitination of Target Protein

Once a protein has been identified as a substrate for degradation, it is covalently tagged with ubiquitin. Ubiquitin, a 9-kDa protein so-named because of its presence in all cell types. Ubiquitin is made up of 76 amino acids including a C-terminal glycine and a lysine residue at position 48. Ubiquitin is covalently attached to the protein destined for degradation in a series of three reactions or steps catalyzed by enzymes known as E1 (ubiquitin-activating enzyme), E2 (ubiquitin-conjugating enzyme), and E3 (ubiquitin-ligating enzyme) (Paul, 2008). There are a few isoforms of E1, multiple isoforms of E2, and a very large number of E3 enzymes, allowing for much tissue and substrate-specific regulation of this process. For example, in skeletal muscle, the ubiquitin protein ligases MuRF1 and MAFBx are upregulated in catabolic conditions such as sepsis and exhaustive aerobic exercise (Kim et al., 2010; Murton et al., 2009).

In the first step of the ubiquitination process, a molecule of ubiquitin is activated by binding to E1 in an ATP-dependent reaction, and the ubiquitin moiety is then transferred to an E2. Both E1s and E2s have active site cysteine residues that form thioesters with the C-terminal glycine of ubiquitin. Finally, the ubiquitin attached to E2 is transferred to a lysine residue on the substrate protein; E3 mediates formation of the ubiquitin–substrate complex. Additional ubiquitins are similarly added to the monoubiquitinated substrate by forming isopeptide bonds between the C-terminal glycine of the ubiquitin molecule being added and lysine 48 of the ubiquitin molecule previously added. A chain of at least four ubiquitin molecules is required for polyubiquitinated proteins to be readily recognized and targeted to the proteasome for destruction. (Ubiquitin tags with fewer ubiquitin units or with linkages that involve other lysine residues in ubiquitin can also serve cell signaling functions or mark receptor proteins for trafficking to lysosomes.)

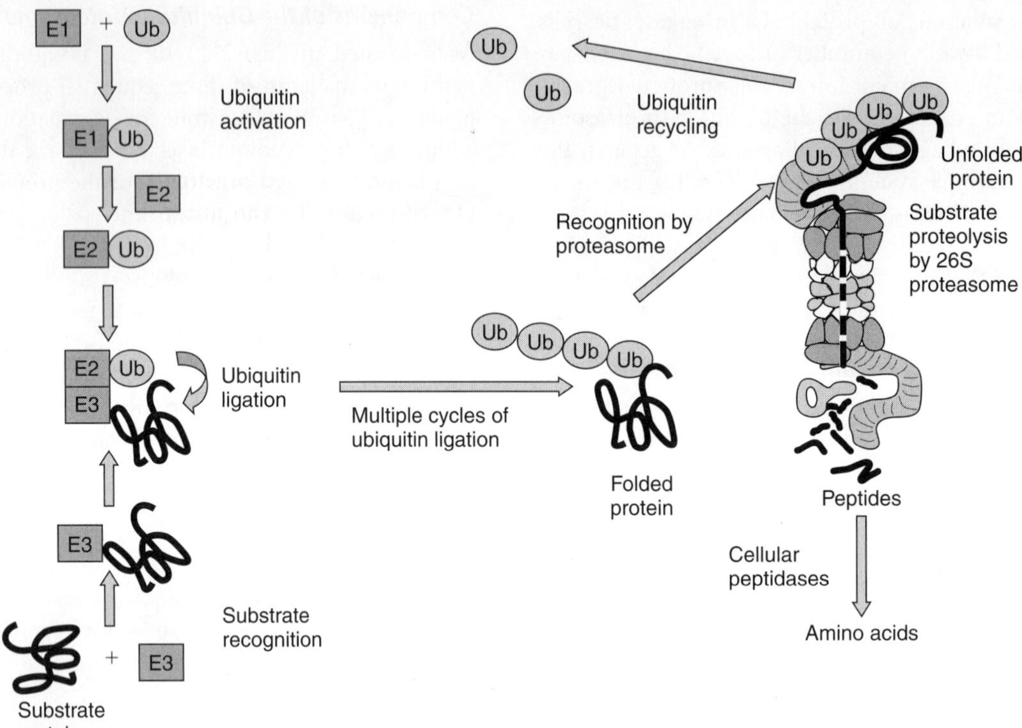

FIGURE 13-10 Major steps in the degradation of a protein by the ubiquitin–proteasome pathway. The protein substrate for degradation is recognized by a ubiquitin ligase *E3*, and ubiquitin (*Ub*) is activated by a ubiquitin activating E1 and then transferred to a ubiquitin conjugating *E2*. An *E3-E2*–substrate complex forms and *Ub* is transferred from the *E2* (in some cases, after transfer to *E3*) to the substrate to form a polyubiquitin chain attached to the protein substrate. The polyubiquitin-tagged protein is recognized by the 26S proteasome and is degraded in an ATP-dependent manner to small peptides, which are released and further hydrolyzed by intracellular peptidases.

Proteins can also have their ubiquitin molecules removed by deubiquitinating enzymes, proteases that are key effectors of the ubiquitin-proteasome system. There are nearly 100 deubiquitinating enzymes that counter the activity of E3 ligases in regulatory pathways, modify ubiquitin chain length, and recycle ubiquitin at the proteasome.

Degradation of Polyubiquitinated Target Protein

The actual degradation of ubiquitinated proteins takes place within an inner chamber of the 26S proteasome, but the ubiquitin molecules are first released so they can be reused. The proteasome is a large, multisubunit complex that consists of a core proteolytic complex with regulatory complexes attached to one or both ends. The core or 20S complex is composed of four stacked ringlike structures of seven subunits each, which together form a barrel-like structure. Rings composed of α-subunits form the outer rings, whereas rings composed of β-subunits form the inner two rings. None of the α-subunits have proteolytic activity, but they do play an important role in preventing access to the central proteolytic chamber when the proteasome is not activated. The central cavity of the barrel-like structure contains six proteolytic sites, contributed by three separate catalytic subunits of each of the two β rings. These catalytic subunits are all classified as N-terminal threonine hydrolases because the N-terminal threonine acts as the nucleophilic catalyst, but the three different subunits in each ring differ in their preference for cleaving peptide bonds immediately after basic, hydrophobic, or acidic residues. Of the three main proteolytic activities, "trypsin-like" activity is assigned to the β2 subunit; "chymotrypsin-like" activity is assigned to the β5 subunit, and "caspase-like" activity is assigned to the β1 subunit. The regulatory complex is made up of 19 or more subunits, including six ATPases and one deubiquitinase (isopeptidase). The 19S regulatory cap functions to recognize polyubuquitinated proteins plus certain nonubiquitinated proteins, to remove the polyubiquitin chain, to unfold protein substrates in an ATP-dependent manner, to open the gate formed by the α subunits of the core particle that otherwise prevents protein from entering the catalytic chamber, and to translocate unfolded substrates to the inner chamber of the core for degradation. The core complex hydrolyzes incoming substrate into peptide fragments of approximately 3 to 30 amino acid residues. These peptide products are released from the proteasome and are further hydrolyzed by other proteases and aminopeptidases in the cell.

Regulation of Proteolysis by the Proteasome

Regulation of proteasomal protein degradation occurs on several levels. Generally, regulation of substrate selection and polyubiquitination determines the rate of substrate degradation. Substrate recognition is regulated by features that uniquely specify the targeted protein for polyubiquitination. These modifications include phosphorylation, hydroxylation of a proline residue, unmasking of a degradation signal contained in the primary sequence, or association with ancillary proteins. Regulated degradation of specific classes of substrates may be achieved by altering ubiquitin-substrate complex formation. For example, it was recently discovered that longevity associated with caloric restriction in animal models is regulated by the activity of E3 ubiquitin ligase, WWP1. Overexpression of this protein increased life span in worms by 20%, whereas suppressing its expression in diet-restricted animals decreased the life span (Carrano et al., 2009). In other cases, altering deubiquitinating enzyme activity can regulate normal and disease processes. For example, the deubiquitinating enzyme A20 was observed to downregulate NFκB activation and proinflammatory gene expression (Boone et al., 2004).

The ubiquitin–proteasome pathway can be regulated at the level of proteasome activity, such as by increased or decreased expression of proteasome subunits. An example of an overall increase in capacity of the ubiquitin–proteasome pathway is the acceleration of muscle degradation in cancer cachexia, which has been associated with increased expression of ubiquitin and proteasome subunits and with increased proteasomal proteolytic activity (Schwartz and Ciechanover, 2009). A special example of change in proteasome activity that results from changes in the expression level of particular proteasomal subunits is the change in proteasomal catalytic specificity induced by interferon γ. Special proteasome subunits are expressed upon induction by interferon γ, resulting in formation of immunoproteasomes that generate different patterns of cleavage products. It is thought that these proteasomes are involved in regulating the production of antigenic peptides (8 to 9 amino acids in length) or in presentation of antigens by major histocompatibility complex (MHC) class I molecules (Kloetzel, 2004).

Proteasomal Degradation of ER/Golgi Associated Substrates: ER-Associated Degradation

Although proteasomes are not present in the ER, proteins synthesized in the ER also undergo turnover and degradation. ER-associated degradation (ERAD) directs ubiquitin-mediated degradation of a variety of ER-associated misfolded and normal proteins (Vembar and Brodsky, 2008). As such, ERAD is a major quality control pathway of the cell as well as a major component of the unfolded protein, or ER stress, response discussed earlier. Proteins located in the ER lumen or membrane that are targeted for destruction are retrotranslocated (or dislocated) from the ER into the cytosol where the ubiquitin-conjugating enzymes and proteasomes are located. ERAD is conducted in four steps, namely (1) substrate recognition and targeting, (2) retrograde transport into the cytosol, (3) ubiquitination, and (4) proteasomal degradation.

Translocation of misfolded substrates plays a particular role in quality control pathways. Substrate selection is mediated by the various molecular chaperones located in the ER. These proteins couple substrate recognition and delivery to the retrotranslocon by interacting with one or more targeting factors. For example, the removal of certain mannose sugars from misfolded glycoproteins by ER and/or Golgi α mannosidases yield *N*-glycan degradation signals, promoting binding of the protein to a targeting protein that guides the substrate protein to the retrotranslocation channel complex (Hoseki et al., 2010). The retrotranslocation channel is made up of several proteins, including members of the Derlin family of proteins, an E3 ubiquitin ligase such as HRD1, and the ATPase p97. The targeting proteins either form a complex with or become an integral part of the retrotranslocation channel, thus delivering their substrate proteins. The targeted and translocated proteins are polyubiquitinated in the cytosol (usually by an ER-membrane E3 ubiquitin ligase with a cytosolic catalytic domain) as they are translocated. Various models have been proposed to explain how ERAD substrates are retrotranslocated, particularly those that are large or remain folded, but consensus remains elusive and current evidence suggests more than one mechanism may exist. Two points of agreement are: (1) a complex of proteins that includes an ATP-hydrolyzing enzyme (e.g., p97 in mammals) uses energy to help extract the targeted polypeptide, and (2) the addition of a polyubiquitin chain onto the target protein is necessary for complete dislocation into the cytosol (Jarosch et al., 2002). Dysfunction in any of the steps can result in the toxic buildup of cellular protein waste. Examples of human diseases linked to ERAD dysfunction include cystic fibrosis, Parkinson disease, and Alzheimer disease.

AUTOPHAGY–LYSOSOMAL SYSTEM

In contrast to the ubiquitin–proteasome pathway, the autophagy–lysosomal system is restricted to the cytoplasm. The lysosomal system is also less selective in targeting specific proteins for breakdown, degrading a much wider spectrum of substrates that include longer-lived proteins and whole cellular organelles. Intracellular material is taken up by autophagy whereas extracellular material is taken up by endocytosis, as illustrated in Figure 13-11. The endocytic or autophagic vesicles containing engulfed material subsequently fuse with a membrane-enclosed acidic compartment called the lysosome. Lysosomes contain a variety of hydrolytic enzymes that degrade proteins and other substances in the engulfed endocytosed material. Lysosomes are budded off from the membrane of the Golgi apparatus and are dispersed throughout the cytosol, but they also form more gradually from late endosomes.

Endocytosis

Extracellular components, including plasma membrane components, enter the lysosomal system via endocytosis. In the process of endocytosis, vesicles form inward at the plasma membrane, internalizing membrane receptors and enclosing bound cargo and/or a portion of the extracellular milieu. Mechanisms of endocytosis include both receptor-mediated endocytosis and general endocytosis (macropinocytosis and phagocytosis). Once the vesicles are pinched off from the plasma membrane, they are delivered to "early" or "sorting" endosomes. These early sorting endosomes guide their cargo through the endosomal network toward later endocytic compartments. Some molecules are recycled back to the plasma membrane, whereas others are delivered

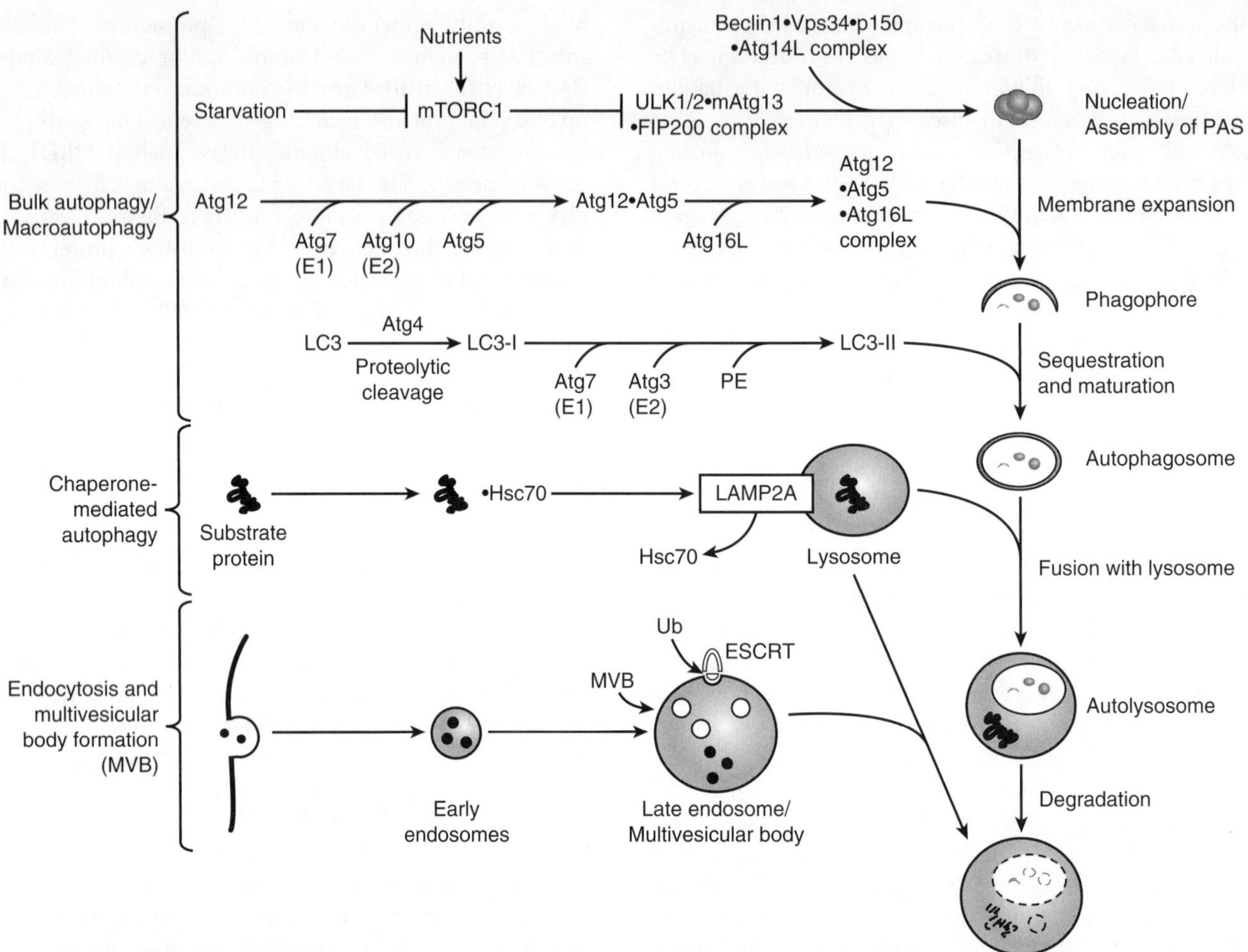

FIGURE 13-11 Degradation of intracellular and extracellular proteins by the autophagy and endocytosis. Macroautophagy is involved in the sequestering of intracellular material into double-membrane vesicles called autophagosomes. The outer membrane of the autophagosome eventually fuses with a lysosome, delivering contents and the inner membrane components to the lysosome for degradation. Chaperone-mediated autophagy is mediated by the Hsc70 chaperones that recognize the lysosomal membrane protein LAMP2A, facilitating delivery of associated proteins to the lysosome. Endocytosis involves the uptake of plasma membrane components and extracellular material into endosomes, which then fuse with lysosomes. Membrane components of the endosomes can be selectively degraded by a system that involves tagging of the selected protein with ubiquitin (*Ub*) and their clustering and uptake as small vesicles within the endosome (now called a multivesicular body, *MVB*). The uptake of membrane components into the MVB is facilitated by the endosomal sorting complex required for transport (*ESCRT*). The MVB then fuses with a lysosome for degradation of the contents of the MVB. See text for more details.

to late endosomes/lysosomes. Substrates released inside the endosomes end up in the lumen of the lysosome when late endosomes fuse with lysosomes or mature into lysosomes. The membrane components of late endosomes and lysosomes remain in the membrane when fusion occurs, but these can be internalized by multivesicular body formation.

Membrane proteins and receptor-bound cargo are targeted for degradation via the formation of multivesicular bodies (see Figure 13-11). Small internal vesicles or bodies are formed when cargo-rich patches of the endosomal membrane bud inward and are cleaved to yield intraluminal vesicles. Because late endosomes contain many of these small vesicles, late endosomes are often called multivesicular bodies. When internalized receptors and other cargo or membrane proteins are destined for lysosomal degradation, they are ubiquitinated and then sorted by the endosomal sorting complex required for transport (ESCRT). The ESCRT proteins recognize ubiquitinated proteins within endosomal membranes and facilitate their sorting to multivesicular bodies. The ESCRT proteins are necessary for vesicle formation (Hurley, 2008). Multivesicular bodies ultimately fuse with lysosomes, releasing their contents, including the small internal vesicles, into the lysosome where both the membranes and any contents of these small vesicles are further broken down. Within lysosomes, degradation of proteins is carried out by acid proteases called cathepsins.

Chaperone-Mediated Autophagy

Selected cytosolic proteins may be directly translocated across the lysosomal membrane in a chaperone-mediated manner in a process called chaperone-mediated autophagy

(CMA). Cargo is first selected for CMA through its interaction with a heat shock cognate protein known as Hsc70, which is a constitutively expressed member of the heat-shock protein 70-kDa family of cytosolic chaperones. The protein substrate–Hsc70 complex binds to the lysosome-associated membrane protein (LAMP) 2A, which drives LAMP2A multimerization into a protein complex necessary for substrate translocation. The protein substrate is then deubiquitinated, unfolded, and translocated across the membrane, with the assistance of an internal chaperone inside the lysosome. CMA thus allows for highly selective lysosomal degradation of specific proteins.

Bulk Macroautophagy

Macroautophagy is a mechanism in which intracellular components (e.g., portions of the cytoplasm, old or damaged organelles) are segregated from the rest of the cytoplasm by a limiting membrane that seals to form a double-membrane vesicle called an autophagosome. Macroautophagy is commonly simply called autophagy, although it is distinctly different than CMA. Macroautophagy can be further divided into bulk phase macroautophagy and selective autophagy.

Autophagy is initiated by the nucleation of an isolation membrane that then elongates and closes on itself to form an autophagosome. The exact origin of the isolation membrane is uncertain; it does not bud off from existing vesicles but is newly formed, perhaps from the ER or an ER-associated structure. The circular isolation membrane flattens and matures into a double-membrane cuplike structure that continues to expand and surround targeted cellular material. As the double-membrane structure matures into a vesicular compartment, the cellular material is engulfed.

Nucleation and membrane expansion into an autophagic vacuole is regulated by a set of autophagy-related genes (*Atg*, or atrogene) that encode Atg proteins. Many of these atrogenes and atrogene products are named as the mammalian orthologs of the yeast proteins (i.e., mATG13, with "m" designating mammalian), whereas other mammalian homologs have been given specific names (e.g., ULK, FIP200, and LC3-I, which are the functional orthologs of yeast Atg1, Atg17, and Atg8, respectively). The nucleation or activation of isolation membrane formation depends on mTOR complex 1 (mTORC1) regulation of the Ulk1/2•mAtg13•FIP200 complex and the Beclin 1:class III PtdIns3K complex known as Vps34. When fuel availability is high, mTORC1 is active and catalyzes inhibitory phosphorylation of the Ulk1/2•mAtg13•FIP200 complex. When fuel and amino acid availability are low and mTORC1 does not inhibit Ulk1/2, Ulk1/2 is active and catalyzes activating phosphorylations of the Ulk1/2•mAtg13•FIP200 complex. Vps34 binds to Atg14L and p150 and facilitates the recruitment of other components to the preautophagosomal structure (PAS).

Expansion and closure of the autophagosomal membrane requires two ubiquitin-like conjugation systems. Atg12 and LC3 are ubiquitin-like modifiers that are conjugated to Atg5 and phosphatidylethanolamine (PE), respectively. In the process of attachment of Atg12 to Atg5, Atg7 acts as an E1-like enzyme, activating Atg12, and Atg10 acts as an E2-like conjugating enzyme, transferring Atg12 to Atg5, as summarized in Figure 13-11. Subsequently, the Atg12-Atg5 conjugate associates with Atg16L to form a large multimeric protein complex that acts as a ubiquitin ligase for formation of LC3-PE. The LC3-PE conjugation system requires the proteolytic cleavage of LC3 by Atg4 protease to form LC3-I with a C-terminal glycine. LC3-I is activated by Atg7 (E1), transferred to Atg3 (E2), and then conjugated to PE by the Atg12-Atg5-Atg16L complex that acts as an E3 ligase. The LC3-I-PE conjugate is commonly called LC3-II. This resulting LC3-II is recruited into the forming autophagosomal membrane where it plays an essential role in expansion and closure.

Once formed, the autophagosome interacts with the endocytic pathway in a process termed maturation. In this process the autophagosome fuses with a lysosome to form an autolysosome. This process releases both the inner membrane of the autophagosome and its contents inside the lysosome (Nakatogawa et al., 2009). These components are degraded by the lysosomal enzymes, as are those taken up by endocytosis. The simple molecules that result from degradation of these components in the lysosome are transported back into the cytosol for use by the cell.

The autophagy-lysosomal system is believed to be present in all tissues, and its induction plays a key role in cell survival under stressful conditions. High level induction of autophagic proteolysis occurs under conditions of protein or energy deprivation, or both. In these situations, macroautophagy provides a major source of amino acids to the cell, particularly in the early neonatal period just after birth during which activation of macroautophagy is essential for life (Kuma et al., 2004). A number of signaling pathways are involved in the regulation of macroautophagy in response to nutrient deprivation and a variety of other stress conditions.

Selective Macroautophagy

The incorporation of LC3-II into the autophagosomal membrane facilitates both selective macrophagy and bulk macroautophagy. Selective substrates with an LC3-II interacting motif are recognized by the autophagosomal membranes for preferential degradation. Many of these direct substrates serve as receptors or adaptors for additional molecules or organelles. For example, p62 interacts with ubiquitinated proteins as well as with LC3-II, and serves to direct ubiquitinated proteins to the autophagosome for lysosomal degradation. NIX is a mitochondrial protein that interacts with LC3-II and may be involved in autophagy of mitochondria. The protein p62 and other adaptor proteins that associate with both ubiquitinated proteins and LC3-II or other autophagosomal markers appear to be involved in selective clearance of misfolded and aggregated proteins under conditions of proteotoxic stress (Wong et al., 2008). Selective macroautophagy is a relatively new area of investigation and much remains to be learned about its mechanisms and functions.

CROSSTALK BETWEEN THE UBIQUITIN–PROTEASOME PATHWAY AND THE AUTOPHAGY-LYSOSOMAL SYSTEM

For many years, the ubiquitin–proteasome pathway and the autophagy–lysosomal system were regarded as independent degradative pathways with few or no points of interaction. Accumulating evidence now shows that these two processes overlap in function (Korolchuk et al., 2010). For example, a number of studies demonstrate that impairment of proteasome activity upregulates autophagy. Explanations for the compensatory increase involve activation of ER stress and the PERK-ATF4 arm of the UPR, which leads to increased expression of atrogenes. On the other hand, impairment of autophagy leads to reduced ubiquitin–proteasome function, suggesting that an accumulation of undigested material prevents ubiquitinated proteins from being degraded by the proteasome. Finally, the coordinated induction of both pathways is reported under conditions leading to muscle atrophy, such as starvation and cachexia. In these situations, the expression of the forkhead box class O (FoxO) family of transcription factors is identified as controlling both the expression of several ubiquitin ligases and several atrogenes (J. Zhao et al., 2008). Inhibition of FoxO transcription factors is thus an attractive possibility as a target for development of drugs that could preserve or restore muscle mass under conditions of muscle wasting.

INTRACELLULAR NEUTRAL CYSTEINE PROTEASES: CALPAINS AND CASPASES

A third mechanism of cellular protein degradation that is important to human health and disease is the limited proteolysis of specific proteins by two groups of enzymes, the calpains and the caspases. In contrast to the lysosomal cathepsins, calpains and caspases are active at neutral pH. Although they are distinct families of proteolytic enzymes, calpains and caspases cleave many of the same target proteins (Liu et al., 2006). In general, much of the proteolysis catalyzed by these enzymes is regulatory in nature. However, calpains and caspases play important roles in the turnover of specific muscle fiber proteins, making them accessible to the ubiquitin–proteasome system for complete degradation. Dysregulated activation of these proteins is a component of the pathologies associated with a number of degenerative diseases.

Calpains

Calpains are a family of widely expressed calcium-dependent, nonlysosomal cysteine endoproteases (Sorimachi et al., 2010). Some of the calpains are ubiquitously expressed (i.e., calpains 1, 2, 5, 7, 10, 13 and 15), whereas others are restricted to specific tissues or organs (i.e., calpains 3, 8, 9, 6, 11, and 12). Activation of calpains involves autolytic processing in the presence of Ca^{2+}. Mammalian calpains are also regulated by an endogenous inhibitor protein, calpastatin, which has four inhibitory domains, each of which can bind one molecule of calpain. The mechanism by which calpastatin regulates calpain activity in living cells is not well understood. Calpain activation is implicated in basic cellular processes such as signal transduction and cytoskeletal dynamics as well as in tissue specific functions such as muscle fiber homeostasis.

The two best characterized calpains are μ-calpain (calpain 1) and m-calpain (calpain 2), which perform limited proteolysis on their substrates. Proteolytic substrates include cytoskeletal proteins, microtubule-associated proteins, growth factor receptors, and protein kinase C. The protein fragments that result from hydrolysis by calpains may be active substituents or may be fragments that will then be degraded by another proteolytic system. Calpain 3, a third well-studied calpain, is highly expressed in skeletal muscle and has been found to be downregulated in different atrophic situations, suggesting it may function in conjunction with E3 ubiquitin ligase to mediate sarcomere remodeling and maintenance in mature muscle cells (Murphy, 2010). Experimental evidence suggests that overactivation of calpains following loss of Ca^{2+} homeostasis is associated with a variety of degenerative conditions and processes such as Alzheimer disease, cataract formation, myocardial infarction, multiple sclerosis, various muscular dystrophies, and stroke (Bartoli and Richard, 2005).

Caspases

Caspases are cysteine-dependent aspartate-specific proteases, and this is the basis of the contraction that serves as their name. Like calpains, they have a cysteine residue at the active site. Caspases prefer to cleave peptide bonds that involve the α-carboxyl group of an aspartate residue. Caspases are often divided into three subfamilies based on amino acid sequence homology, which roughly corresponds with function (Pop and Salvesen, 2009). Class I and III caspases have long N-terminal prodomains and are initiator caspases; class I caspases (human caspases 2, 8, 9, and 10) are apoptosis activators, whereas class III caspases (human caspases 1, 4, 5, and 14) are inflammatory mediators. Class II caspases (human caspases 3, 6, and 7) have shorter prodomains and are apoptosis executioner caspases.

Caspases exist as inactive procaspases in cells. Activation and maturation involve cleavage of the prodomains and linker sequences to release the large and small subunits that are part of the procaspase, formation of heterodimers of these two subunits, and combination of two heterodimers to form heterotetramers. The so-called initiator caspases are activated by dimerization, which is facilitated by their recruitment to oligomeric activation platforms that assemble in response to apoptotic or inflammatory (pyroptotic) stimuli. The so-called effector or executioner caspases require proteolytic cleavage by an upstream caspase (i.e., an initiator caspase) to remove the linker peptide between the large and small subunits of their catalytic domain. Caspase activation may be followed by a maturation process that involves autoproteolytic cleavages (e.g., trimming of the prodomain or cleavage of the intersubunit linker). These maturation events can affect the physiological function of the caspase and are considered important for generating caspase stability and signaling downstream regulatory events.

EXTRACELLULAR METALLOPROTEASES

Proteins such as collagen and elastin in the extracellular matrix and proteins secreted in the extracellular matrix (e.g., cytokines, chemokines, and growth factors) also undergo turnover. A large superfamily of metal-requiring proteases is involved in cleavage of these extracellular matrix and nonmatrix proteins. This superfamily of zinc-dependent metalloproteases includes the matrix metalloproteinases (MMPs) and the disintegrin and metalloproteinases without (ADAMs) or with (ADAMTSs) thrombospondin motifs. These metalloproteinases are either secreted or anchored to the cell membrane by transmembrane regions, which confines their catalytic activities to membrane proteins or proteins within the secretory pathway or extracellular space. Some of the secreted proteases bind to the extracellular matrix components by specific regions, such as the thrombospondin motifs of the ADAMTSs. The regulation of metalloprotease activity is complex and occurs at various levels (van der Jagt et al., 2010). In particular, regulation occurs at the levels of transcription, secretion, proenzyme activation (e.g., by extracellular matrix metalloproteinase inducer), and inhibition by endogenous inhibitors (e.g., tissue inhibitors of metalloproteases and β-macroglobulins).

Extracellular substrates of the metalloproteases include the matrix components, nonmatrix components, and ectodomains of cell surface proteins. Thus they are necessary for tissue remodeling because they break down proteins in the extracellular matrix that provide structural support for cells. In addition, they are important regulators of the functions of various biologically active molecules such as membrane receptors, proinflammatory cytokines, chemokines, growth factors, and serine proteinase inhibitors. As such, these proteases play important roles in many physiological and pathological processes including embryonic development, inflammation, immunity, chronic wounds, arthritis, periodontitis, cardiovascular disease, and cancer (Shiomi et al., 2010).

ROLE OF HORMONES AND CYTOKINES IN REGULATION OF PROTEIN TURNOVER

Each step in the synthesis or degradation of protein is a potential site of regulation. Some steps of protein synthesis and degradation are controlled through the action of mediators such as hormones and cytokines. Although these mediators do not act in isolation, an understanding of the individual actions of hormones and cytokines is necessary for understanding the coordinated regulation involved in the responses of protein turnover to feeding, growth, and injury.

ANABOLIC HORMONES

Growth hormone and insulin are both considered to be anabolic in that reduced circulating levels of these hormones are associated with loss of body protein or decreased growth.

Insulin

Normally, the blood insulin concentration increases with feeding and decreases with fasting, and the rise and fall of insulin levels are associated with cyclic responses of carbohydrate, fat, and protein metabolism between anabolism and catabolism. An inability to mount an anabolic response to the influx of nutrients is accompanied by a loss of body protein, and individuals who lack insulin because of diabetes lose body protein. Measurements in animal models show that insulin stimulates the synthesis of protein, although some human studies suggest that provision of amino acids is also required for this response. The most consistent finding in human and animal studies is that protein degradation is inhibited by insulin both in the whole body and in skeletal muscle (De Feo, 1996; Garlick et al., 1998).

The mechanism for the acute action of insulin to stimulate protein synthesis in responsive tissues (e.g., skeletal muscle, fat) involves multiple intracellular signaling cascades that culminate in activation of the initiation step of mRNA translation. The precise way in which insulin inhibits protein degradation also depends on the tissue or cell type. For example, in skeletal muscle, insulin inhibits the ubiquitin–proteasome proteolytic pathway as well as activation of caspases (Wang et al., 2006), whereas in the liver, autophagy is increased by insulin deficiency and suppressed by hyperinsulinemia and insulin resistance (Liu et al., 2009).

Growth Hormone and IGF-1

Growth hormone is primarily known to promote longitudinal growth in children and adolescents. Growth hormone levels are higher in children, especially during growth spurts, and children are dwarfed when growth hormone is absent. Growth hormone is also used illegally by some athletes to boost performance. Growth hormone is secreted by the pituitary gland and acts by binding to its cell surface receptor, initiating signal transduction that results in the expression of genes involved in lipid metabolism and anabolic processes. One of the proteins whose synthesis is induced by growth hormone is insulin-like growth factor 1 (IGF-1), which is produced by the liver as an endocrine hormone as well as in target tissues in a paracrine/autocrine fashion. The effects of growth hormone on protein anabolism include increased protein synthesis and decreased breakdown at the whole body level and in skeletal muscle (Moller et al., 2009). Many of the protein anabolic effects of growth hormone are mediated by IGF-1 and insulin. IGF-1 largely reproduces the effects of growth hormone and is superior to insulin in terms of stimulating protein synthesis in both normal and catabolic subjects, but is similar to insulin in terms of inhibiting protein breakdown (Clemmons, 2009). The protein anabolic actions of IGF-1 occur by the binding of the peptide hormone to cell surface receptors and activation of a PtdIns3K signal transduction cascade to increase mRNA translation initiation via the activity of mTORC1. Activation of PtdIns3K also reduces proteasomal degradation by promoting nuclear exclusion and/or protein degradation of the FoxO transcription factors, which regulate the transcription of genes encoding E3 ubiquitin ligases.

Testosterone

In addition to insulin and growth hormone/IGF-1, the male sex hormone testosterone also promotes protein synthesis, particularly in muscle. Testosterone can also reduce protein degradation by suppressing expression of E3 ubiquitin ligases such as muscle atrophy F-box (MAFbx, also called atrogin-1) (W. Zhao et al., 2008). Low levels of testosterone are associated not only with a lack of lean body mass but also with an increase in adipose tissue. In older individuals with low or low-normal testosterone levels, replacement of testosterone increases muscle mass and strength by increasing protein anabolism and reducing protein catabolism (Dillon et al., 2010). The increase in muscle mass is also associated with an increase in the number of satellite cells (myogenic stem cells that can fuse with muscle fibers) (Bhasin et al., 2006). Synthetic testosterone-like compounds, classed as anabolic steroids, are also capable of promoting the retention of body protein and, similar to human growth hormone, are used illicitly by some athletes as performance-enhancing agents.

CATABOLIC HORMONES

The stress hormones cortisol and glucagon are often elevated in the plasma after injury or during infection. Infusion of these hormones together mimics stress, causing loss of body protein.

Glucagon

Glucagon promotes gluconeogenesis from amino acids and lactate. The ratio of glucagon to insulin is an important factor in both acute regulation (such as after a meal) and long-term regulation (such as with prolonged dietary deprivation). At physiological levels, glucagon is not known to have a direct effect on tissue or whole-body protein synthesis, but elevated glucagon does interfere with the ability of insulin to inhibit protein degradation (Rooyackers and Nair, 1997).

Cortisol

Cortisol, from the adrenal cortex, is a glucocorticoid hormone that has a catabolic effect similar to that of glucagon. In skeletal muscle, cortisol decreases protein synthesis and increases protein degradation. Rates of muscle protein synthesis are reduced by glucocorticoids both by downregulating ribosomal S6 kinase activity and inhibiting formation of the eIF4 complex (Shah et al., 2000). Studies using differentiated myotubes in culture have also shown that enhanced muscle protein degradation following treatment with glucocortocoids involves activation of the ubiquitin–proteasome pathway, mediated by nuclear translocation of the FoxO transcription factor family. The FoxOs have been shown to increase expression of the E3 ubiquitin ligases, muscle ring finger-1 protein (MuRF1) and MAFbx/Atrogin-1 (Glass, 2010). In the liver, the synthesis of several liver proteins is actually increased by elevated cortisol, such as enzymes involved in amino acid oxidation. This action facilitates conversion of amino acids derived from muscle breakdown into energy-yielding compounds or gluconeogenic precursors. Glucocorticoids can also cause muscle atrophy by inhibiting the muscle production of IGF-1 and increasing the muscle production of myostatin, two growth factors exhibiting opposite effects on muscle mass.

Myostatin

An emerging key negative regulator of muscle mass is the secreted growth factor, myostatin. Myostatin is a transcription factor of the transforming growth factor β family, and it is a potent inducer of muscle wasting. Specifically, myostatin inhibits insulin and IGF-1 signaling, causing downregulation of protein synthesis by activating the mTORC1 signaling cascade while at the same time increasing expression of atrophy-related genes by preventing the phosphorylation of FoxO transcription factors so that FoxO can remain in the nucleus and promote transcription of genes encoding muscle-specific E3 ubiquitin ligases (McFarlane et al., 2008). Thus, myostatin promotes muscle protein degradation and, at the same time, suppresses overall protein synthesis. In addition, myostatin inhibits the activation of satellite cells (muscle stem cells) and inhibits myoblast proliferation. This function has been demonstrated by deletion or inactivation of myostatin in animals; lack of myostatin results in a hypermuscular phenotype. As such, the development of antibodies or inhibitors of myostatin is receiving great attention as potential drugs to limit cachexia, sarcopenia, and loss of muscle mass in various human diseases.

Cytokines

Cytokines are peptides produced by cells of the immune system in response to injury, infection, or inflammation. Cytokines can have large effects on protein metabolism, but the regulation of protein metabolism by cytokines is complex and not clearly understood.

High circulating levels of proinflammatory cytokines, particularly interleukin 1β (IL1β) and tumor necrosis factor α (TNFα), are associated with protein wasting, particularly in skeletal muscle. The inhibitory effects of TNFα and IL1β on skeletal muscle protein synthesis are mediated indirectly by changes in the growth hormone/IGF-1 system and also by glucocorticoid secretion via stimulation of the central nervous system/pituitary/adrenal axis. Administration of TNFα induces MuRF1 mRNA expression, activating the ubiquitin–proteasome pathway (Adams et al., 2008). Cytokines such as TNFα may further induce muscle loss by affecting the ability of precursor cells to differentiate into mature muscle cells. Muscle differentiation is under the control of several transcription factors including NFκB. Elevated levels of TNFα are accompanied by sustained NFκB activity, resulting in both altered transcription and epigenetic silencing of myofibrillar genes (Bakkar and Guttridge, 2010).

In the liver, inflammatory cytokines such as IL1β, IL6, and TNFα increase synthesis of the acute phase proteins, which are required for resolution of inflammation, and promote gluconeogenesis, which delivers systemic glucose to the body. Increased production of urea occurs, due to the increased use of amino acid carbon chains for gluconeogenesis and the inhibitory effects of cytokines on muscle protein synthesis. At the same time, cytokines reduce IGF-1 synthesis and growth hormone receptor mRNA levels.

RESPONSES OF PROTEIN TURNOVER TO NUTRIENT SUPPLY

Protein balance is highly responsive to nutritional status, particularly as it relates to the provision of amino acids. At the whole body level, food intake stimulates protein synthesis and decreases protein degradation, resulting in a net positive balance of body protein. Insufficient and/or incomplete nutrition has the opposite effect, increasing protein degradation and/or decreasing protein synthesis, resulting in a net negative protein balance. In individual tissues, the mechanisms by which rates of protein synthesis and degradation are altered by nutrient supply are guided by the regulatory controls that dominate in each tissue. Some of these control points are highlighted in the following sections.

ANABOLIC RESPONSES TO EATING

Nutrient intake affects protein synthesis at the level of initiation of mRNA translation. In most tissues, both insulin and dietary amino acids are necessary to maximally stimulate mRNA translation following a meal. This is accomplished at two main steps. First, phosphorylation of eIF2 is relieved, allowing the TC to form and bind the 40S ribosome to form the preinitiation complex. Second, formation of the mRNA cap-binding complex eIF4 is promoted, facilitating selection and binding of mRNA to the ribosome. The amount of essential amino acids in a meal has a major influence on the amplitude and duration of protein synthesis in response to feeding. Furthermore, the addition of essential amino acids or leucine alone to protein meals further increases protein synthesis, at least in the short term. Longer-term studies have yet to consistently demonstrate positive changes in body composition by this mode of intervention (Balage and Dardevet, 2010). In addition to amino acid composition, digestibility of individual dietary proteins can vary, altering the delivery of amino acids to the portal and peripheral blood. An example of how the particular protein being consumed might alter the timing and duration of feeding-induced anabolism comes from a study in which healthy adults ingested a single meal that contained either casein or whey protein (Boirie et al., 1997). Plasma amino acid levels at 1 to 2 hours after the meal as well as the stimulation of protein synthesis rates were highest for subjects who ate the whey protein meal, but elevated plasma amino acid levels were maintained longer in those subjects who ate the casein meal. The more slowly absorbed casein meal also promoted greater net protein deposition over a 7-hour period, suggesting that a sustained period of hyperaminoacidemia may promote a greater amount of protein synthesis.

It is clear that food intake also decreases overall protein degradation in addition to stimulating protein synthesis. The mechanisms by which this is accomplished within the whole animal are tissue-specific. Amino acid intake is known to reduce macroautophagy and hence lysosomal proteolysis in liver (Kanazawa et al., 2004). In skeletal muscle, the ubiquitin–proteasome pathway is the major proteolytic system responsible for both insulin and amino acid–induced changes in protein degradation. Food intake results in reduced expression of components of the ubiquitin pathway and of proteasomal subunits, with the combination of insulin and amino acids having an additive suppressive effect. As for the human study mentioned above (Boirie et al., 1997), animal studies have also shown that changes in protein degradation in response to a meal usually lag behind changes in protein synthesis. For example, although feeding stimulated muscle protein synthesis over the first 4 hours after a meal in rats, no suppressive effect on either total or proteasome-dependent proteolysis or the rate of ubiquitination of muscle proteins was detected until 10 hours after feeding (Kee et al., 2003).

BRIEF FASTING VERSUS PROLONGED STARVATION

As the body moves from the absorptive period following a meal (also known as the postprandial period) to the postabsorptive period before the consumption of the next meal, nitrogen balance changes from net accumulation to net loss. The hormonal changes associated with fasting include a reduction in the circulating level of insulin and an increase in the level of glucagon. As the fasting period extends into early starvation and the body's stores of glycogen are exhausted, the body adapts to use amino acids from muscle protein and glycerol derived from body fat to help meet the needs for glucose production. Thus amino acids are mobilized from muscle and redirected to provide substrates for gluconeogenesis as well as maintenance of protein synthesis in liver and other tissues. Increased mobilization of body protein for glucose production is evidenced by a relatively high excretion of urinary nitrogen during early starvation. The net loss of muscle protein, or change in protein balance, is due to both an increase in protein degradation and a reduction in protein synthesis.

During longer-term starvation, whole body protein degradation rates decline to spare body protein stores. The synthesis of ketone bodies (e.g., acetoacetate, β-hydroxybutyrate) from fatty acids released by adipose lipolysis provides an additional fuel, and this helps the body conserve amino acids by reducing the requirements for new glucose synthesis. These later adaptations are reflected in the output of nitrogen, which is decreased from approximately 12 g in early starvation to approximately 3 g nitrogen per day by several weeks of starvation (Cahill,

1976). If prolonged starvation is left unmitigated and if adipose depots are depleted, body protein is again mobilized for energy by means of an increase in muscle protein degradation. This final increase in the degradation of body protein cannot be sustained for long; if feeding does not occur, death ensues.

Human studies have demonstrated distinct differences in protein metabolism between lean and obese subjects undergoing total starvation (Elia et al., 1999). During short-term starvation, both protein turnover and amino acid oxidation increased more in lean individuals than in obese individuals. During prolonged starvation, the rate of protein loss and percent energy derived from amino acid oxidation were up to threefold less in the obese as compared to the lean. In addition, the contribution of protein to net glucose production was reduced in the obese to about half of that in lean persons. Thus larger fat stores are advantageous for survival in starvation.

MALNUTRITION

Prolonged undernutrition of energy and protein (see Chapters 15, 19, and 23) shares many of the same characteristics as starvation, but these develop over a longer time frame. In protein-energy malnutrition, circulating levels of insulin decrease and those of glucagon increase. Growth hormone is elevated, but the level of IGF-1 is depressed. Thyroid hormone level is reduced, with a similar conservation of energy and amino acids as is seen in starvation. The oxidation of amino acids is reduced, as is protein turnover (both synthesis and degradation).

In children, a reduction in food intake is accompanied by a cessation of growth. Chronic malnutrition results in both stunting (reduction in height for age) and wasting (reduction in weight for height). Nutrient deprivation also results in reductions of particular proteins. Albumin concentration often is reduced, as scarce amino acids are directed to more essential proteins. This selective reduction in albumin may be mediated at least partly by a reduction in albumin gene expression in the absence of insulin. Because circulating levels of albumin respond to nutritional intake, albumin concentration has been used to assess nutritional status, but the relation of albumin levels to nutritional status often is confounded by the fall in albumin associated with injury or disease.

The data in Figure 13-12 demonstrate the reduction in protein synthesis and degradation in malnourished children in Jamaica (Golden et al., 1977). These children were studied at sequential time points as they recovered. During recovery from malnutrition, both synthesis and degradation were accelerated compared with measurements made either when the children were malnourished or after they had recovered from malnutrition. This increased synthesis and degradation was associated with catch-up growth (i.e., growth rates that are more rapid than normal). When children recovering from protein-energy malnutrition reached more appropriate weights and heights for age, their growth slowed to more age-appropriate rates.

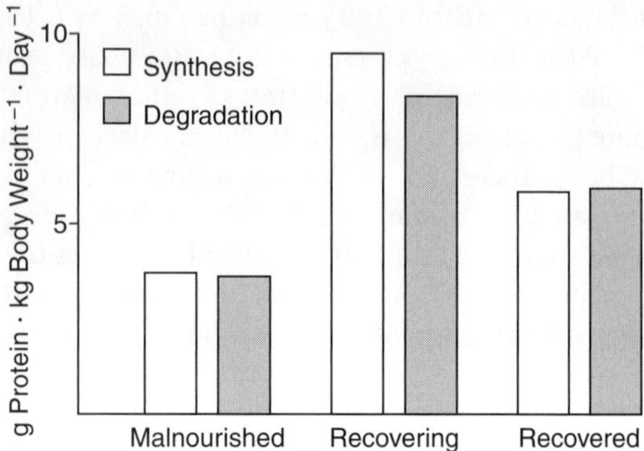

FIGURE 13-12 Rates of protein synthesis and degradation in children with malnutrition, during the recovery process (*recovering*), and when recovery was complete (*recovered*). The rates of protein synthesis and degradation, expressed in grams of protein · kilogram of body weight^{-1} · day^{-1}, were assessed with [^{15}N]glycine. (Data from Golden, M. H. N., Waterlow, J. C., & Picou, D. [1977]. Protein turnover, synthesis and breakdown before and after recovery from protein-energy malnutrition. *Clinical Science and Molecular Medicine, 53*, 473–477.)

PROTEIN TURNOVER IN GROWTH AND EXERCISE

During periods of growth as well as during exercise-induced muscle hypertrophy, net protein deposition occurs. In general, this is a consequence of an increase in protein synthesis that is greater than the increase in protein degradation that occurs at the same time. The increase in protein degradation allows tissue remodeling to occur in conjunction with growth or hypertrophy.

NORMAL GROWTH

Growth is an anabolic process that occurs over a much longer period than do the acute responses to the intake of nutrients. Although the overall process of growth includes a net increase in the amount of body protein, this is often accompanied by significant remodeling so that protein degradation is also elevated. The capacity for growth can be seen in the difference in turnover rates between growing children and adults. In newborn infants, fractional rates of whole body protein synthesis are about twice those in adults.

Increased protein synthesis throughout growth is accomplished with increased levels of RNA in the tissue, including both mRNA and rRNA, so that the capacity of the body to make protein is increased. Growth is under the influence of hormones, primarily growth hormone and IGF-1. The capacity for growth may also include responses to other anabolic agents that do not occur in the adult. For example, insulin has the capacity to stimulate protein synthesis in the young, but this anabolic response to insulin is diminished in the nongrowing adult.

In addition to an acceleration of the overall process of turnover and the positive balance between protein synthesis and degradation, growth and development also involve the selective accumulation of specific proteins at appropriate periods of development. At puberty and during pregnancy and lactation, for example, appropriate hormone concentrations are increased by the selective transcription of the appropriate genes. These hormones, in turn, provide for further alterations in protein metabolism.

EXERCISE

A similar phenomenon with increases in both synthesis and degradation associated with protein accumulation can occur in specific tissues under certain conditions, an example being work-induced hypertrophy of muscle in response to exercise. Even in adults and the aged, increased use of muscle, particularly in the form of resistance exercise, stimulates hypertrophy. Following weight-bearing exercise, rates of protein synthesis in human muscle increase relative to rates of protein degradation, and this results in net positive protein balance (Glynn et al., 2010). Most of the molecular events regulating these processes were initially discovered using animal models and are now confirmed in both male and female human subjects. In skeletal muscle, resistance exercise stimulates protein synthesis by increasing mTORC1 signaling to its downstream effectors, ribosomal protein S6 kinase and 4E-BP, leading to formation of the active eIF4 complex.

Whereas resistance exercise clearly activates muscle hypertrophy, endurance exercise does not. Depending on the mode, length, and intensity of aerobic exercise, as well as the training status of the subjects, human studies show a reduction, no change, or a small increase in muscle protein synthesis after endurance exercise.

The mechanisms controlling rates of protein breakdown during and following exercise remain poorly defined in human muscle, but several studies have reported activation of the ubiquitin–proteasome pathway (e.g., MAFbx, MuRF1) in both weight-bearing and endurance (aerobic) exercise. Endurance exercise also has been shown to elevate the activity of calpains and metalloproteinases.

Protein synthesis stimulated by exercise is synergistically enhanced by feeding of amino acids (and in particular leucine), whereas co-ingestion of carbohydrate helps to attenuate the rise in muscle protein breakdown. Whereas some researchers debate the optimal timing of feeding, most human studies agree that consumption immediately following exercise is an effective means to enhance muscle recovery and protein gains. The amount of protein can influence the degree of anabolism, but only to a point; studies testing more than 15 to 20 g of high-quality protein do not show additional anabolic benefit. Interest in the role of the specific amino acid composition of the protein is another active area of study. Though some studies claim improved muscle protein synthesis by consuming whey versus other complete proteins after exercise, others do not. Currently, no long-term studies demonstrate differential changes in body composition or muscle mass by consuming different high-quality proteins in combination with exercise.

PROTEIN LOSS WITH DISUSE, INJURY, AND DISEASE

Loss of body protein accompanies muscle disuse as well as many disease states, such as trauma, cancer, and infection. Immobilization contributes to muscle loss in healthy individuals and in those with critical illnesses. In hypermetabolic disease states, the normal adaptation to preserve lean body mass does not occur and the rate of muscle catabolism remains high. In these cases, the mobilized amino acids pass into the bloodstream for transport to the liver, where they are available for gluconeogenesis and for the synthesis of acute-phase proteins after injury or during illness.

SARCOPENIA AND DISUSE

In healthy humans, skeletal muscle mass begins to decline in the fourth or fifth decade of life. This slow but progressive loss of muscle mass with advancing age reduces muscle quantity and quality, leading to a gradual decline in strength and mobility. As locomotion becomes less frequent, disuse can exacerbate age or disease-related protein losses. Even in younger persons, protein can be lost from individual tissues during disuse. For example, loss of muscle tissue is apparent during immobilization, such as that accompanying recovery from bone fracture. This disuse atrophy is associated with decreased synthesis of muscle protein with little change in protein degradation. This allows protein degradation to dominate even though it is not enhanced (Phillips et al., 2009).

At the level of muscle protein balance, recent findings suggest that loss of skeletal muscle mass with aging is not due to chronic changes in protein synthesis or breakdown, but instead to a delay and/or resistance of muscle protein synthesis stimulation by feeding and exercise. This, in combination with an increased risk of malnourishment in older persons, highlights an important role for nutrition and exercise intervention to prevent and delay loss of muscle mass and function. Resistance training in combination with essential amino acid–containing nutrition is presently considered the best candidate to attenuate, prevent, or ultimately reverse age-related muscle wasting and weakness.

BURNS, SURGERY, AND SEPSIS

Conditions such as burn injury, surgery, and systemic infection or sepsis are all accompanied by a set of metabolic responses that are often collectively referred to as stress responses. Stress responses include increased energy expenditure, loss of body protein, and the synthesis of acute-phase proteins. Amino acids are mobilized from the skeletal muscle through decreased protein synthesis along with accelerated degradation, channeling these substrates to support increased production of acute-phase proteins by the liver. These responses are in part mediated by the concerted actions of stress hormones (glucagon, cortisol, and epinephrine) and by production of cytokines. At the level of the whole body, there is protein hypercatabolism, with degradation increased more than synthesis, so that there is net loss of body protein. This whole-body response is a composite of different responses in different tissues, however, with loss of skeletal muscle protein playing a dominant role. After surgery or in sepsis, in contrast to the suppression of protein synthesis in skeletal muscle, protein synthesis in liver is actually increased. The sepsis-stimulated increase in hepatic protein synthesis has been associated with increases in the total RNA content, the content of eIF2, and phosphorylation of ribosomal protein S6 kinase (Cooney et al., 2000).

Accelerated protein degradation in the muscle during burn injury, surgery, and sepsis is promoted by elevated circulating levels of cortisol (glucocorticoid) and the cytokines TNFα, IL1β, and IL6. Although multiple proteolytic processes play a role in the loss of muscle mass during these conditions, the ubiquitin–proteasome pathway is the most active in the degradation of myofibrillar proteins. Higher levels of stress hormones are also associated with a failure of normal anabolic responses such as the ability of insulin to reduce the rate of protein degradation and to stimulate the rate of protein synthesis (Lang et al., 2007). Resistance to another anabolic hormone, growth hormone, also occurs in burn, trauma, and sepsis. Growth hormone secretion is normally associated with elevated levels of IGF-1. In sepsis, however, levels of IGF-1 are reduced despite normal or elevated levels of growth hormone. In addition to reduced levels of IGF-1, burn and sepsis are associated with alterations in the regulatory IGF-1–binding proteins, the IGFBPs, leading to reduced bioavailability of IGF-1 as a result of increased cytokine activity. This effective reduction in IGF-1 facilitates the upregulation of MuRF1 and MAFbx also leading to increased degradation of protein.

Burn patients also have reduced levels of testosterone. When testosterone or synthetic derivatives are administered to burn patients, both children and adults show improved protein balance, which is due to reduced protein degradation, not to a stimulation of protein synthesis as would be expected from testosterone replacement therapy in healthy subjects. On the other hand, giving growth hormone to patients with critical illness to overcome growth hormone resistance and stimulate an anabolic response has been less successful and is associated with increased morbidity and mortality.

Muscle wasting is part of the response to stress and may be viewed as beneficial in that amino acids are mobilized from expendable to essential tissues to provide substrate for more vital functions such as the synthesis of acute phase proteins. However, the longer this state continues, the more detrimental it becomes. Nutritional support therefore becomes obligatory in long-term critical illness, and there is much active research on strategies for optimizing nutrition in a particular condition and efforts to combine nutrition with anabolic agents. For example, the preoperative feeding of amino acids can result in positive whole body protein balance after surgery (Schricker et al., 2008), and the provision of oxandrolone, a weak analog of testosterone, to burned children and adults improves body mass accretion and wound healing (Miller and Btaiche, 2009).

CANCER

In catabolic conditions such as cancer, the loss of body protein can be due in part to the anorexia that accompanies the disease. However, some forms of cancer, such as small cell cancer of the lung, are associated with loss of body protein even when nutrients are supplied. This wasting condition is called cachexia. Loss of skeletal muscle in cancer patients results from a depression in protein synthesis combined with an increase in protein degradation. The decrease in protein synthesis is due to a reduced formation of the eIF4 complex, increased phosphorylation of eIF2, and a slowing of elongation. The mechanism for increased protein degradation is mostly due to increased expression and activity of the ubiquitin–proteasome pathway, although activation of the lysosomal system is reported and increased activity of calpains is observed in tumor-bearing animals (Tisdale, 2009). Increases in inflammatory cytokines such as IL1β, IL6, interferon-gamma, and TNFα and tumor factors such as proteolysis-inducing factor (PIF) are also associated with these responses. PIF-induced cachexia is mediated by increased phosphorylation of eIF2 by the kinase PKR, leading to upregulation of the transcription factor NFκB. Urinary levels of PIF generally correlate with atrophy, and antagonists to PIF prevent muscle loss in cancer patients (Tisdale, 2010).

Rapid proliferation of the tumor can also contribute to loss of muscle protein in the cancer patient by sequestering available substrate (amino acids) away from healthy tissues to support malignant growth. Dysregulated growth of cells can occur at the level of mRNA translation, contributing to both cancer formation and cancer progression. Increased expression of eIF2 and mTOR have been observed in both benign and malignant tumors. In addition, overexpression of certain eIFs, such as eIF4E, enhances cell proliferation and is related to tumor progression. Studies in human cancer cell lines have shown that blocking eIF function by antisense RNA or overexpression of an inhibitory protein can suppress cellular transformation and tumor growth (Hagner et al., 2010).

Current and novel methods of killing cancerous growth are increasingly targeting the molecular regulation of protein turnover. Inhibitors of the ubiquitin–proteasome system are currently being explored as anticancer therapies. A key example of success in this area is the protesome inhibitor, bortezomib, which has shown some efficacy in treating multiple myeloma, a B-cell malignancy with historically poor prognosis (Shah and Orlowski, 2009). Modulating autophagy in cancer cells is also showing promise as a novel therapeutic strategy. Depending on the cancer cell type, either inhibiting or inducing autophagy can sensitize cancer cells to other chemotherapy agents (Dalby et al.,

2010). Tumor growth can also be blocked nutritionally by amino acid–depleting enzymes such as asparaginase, which depletes blood levels of asparagine (and, to a lesser extent, glutamine). Leukemic cells do not synthesize asparagine in amounts adequate to support their enhanced rate of growth and so depend on an exogenous source. As it turns out, asparaginase is also a very effective inhibitor of protein synthesis by increasing eIF2 phosphorylation via activating GCN2 (Bunpo et al., 2009). However, side effects of asparaginase, such as liver dysfunction or immunosuppression, can limit overall efficacy.

The challenge of retarding loss of body protein by nutritional means in cancer patients must be considered in terms of the effects on both body tissue and the tumor. The challenge is to devise feeding regimens or cancer treatments that block growth in the tumor but not in healthy tissues.

CURRENT CHALLENGES IN PROTEIN METABOLISM

The preservation of body protein in aging and during chronic illness is a current challenge in the field of protein metabolism. It is important to understand the underlying mechanisms and to develop treatments to reverse the loss of body protein, either by nutritional means or by combining specific nutritional regimens with anabolic agents.

An understanding of the molecular mechanisms involved in protein processing may lead to new therapies. Investigations into stress responses have delineated both hormonal mechanisms and those involving cytokines such as TNF-α. The link to cytokines has led to treatment modalities that include antibodies to either a cytokine or its receptor, but researchers are only beginning to understand the interplay of hormones with each other and with cytokines. Many degenerative neuromuscular diseases, including Parkinson disease, Alzheimer disease, various muscular dystrophies, and even prion-associated diseases, appear to be associated with defects in the ability of the ER to regulate the tasks of protein synthesis, protein folding, and protein breakdown. Inhibition of proteasome-associated proteolysis is also providing new lines of investigation for retarding loss of body protein and for novel forms of cancer therapy.

Feeding regimens can alter the course of disease progression, and more beneficial regimens would be helpful. Although early parenteral nutrition does not completely prevent the loss of body protein associated with stresses such as surgery, it clearly does attenuate the loss of body protein compared to that observed when nutrition is not provided. The amino acids that are supplied help preserve body tissue and may facilitate beneficial responses by the body such as the synthesis of acute-phase proteins, activation of the immune system, or synthesis of specific proteins involved in wound healing. Provision of anabolic agents (such as insulin; oxandrolone; or propranolol, a beta blocker drug that attenuates the release of catecholamines) in conjunction with adequate nutrition has been demonstrated to be more effective than nutrition alone in preventing the loss of body protein (Herndon and Tompkins, 2004).

Increasingly, the focus in catabolic illness is not only on the provision of adequate nutrition but also on altering nutrition to address the particular problems associated with different diseases. For example, patients with severe liver disease may benefit from the provision of nutrition enriched with branched-chain amino acids. As the capacity of the liver to degrade amino acids such as methionine, phenylalanine, and tyrosine is diminished, plasma levels of these amino acids rise, whereas concentrations of branched-chain amino acids, which are degraded in the periphery, fall. Enhancing the supply of branched-chain amino acids may help correct the amino acid imbalance caused by the liver disease. Another example is the use of glutamine-enriched nutrition in both critically ill patients and in patients after surgery. Glutamine is released from muscle tissue in response to stress, and provision of glutamine-containing nutritional regimens to surgical patients reduces negative nitrogen balance and may reduce infections and complications (Novak et al., 2002). Both glutamine and arginine have been used in conjunction with adequate nutrition to stimulate the immune system and to promote healing. Ongoing research seeks to understand how protein metabolism is altered by disease states and how nutrition may be employed for benefit.

Lastly, increased understanding of the genes that regulate muscle cell differentiation also has the potential to lead to better therapies for the loss of protein. The identification of novel genes that control muscle growth represent potential targets for gene-based therapy to prevent muscle loss. The expansion of research tools including transgenic animals, genomics, and proteomics is contributing to enhanced understanding of the way body protein is regulated, and each addition to our understanding has the potential to provide clinical benefit for conditions in which body protein is lost.

THINKING CRITICALLY

1. The steady-state concentration of a protein is a function of its rate of synthesis and its rate of degradation. List factors or points of regulation that might affect the rate of synthesis of a functional protein.
2. Regulatory proteins typically have a rapid degradation rate. Why is this a useful property for a regulatory protein? How does this affect the ability of the cell to effect a change in protein concentration?
3. Protein synthesis is regulated by nutrient intake at the level of translation initiation via both mTORC1 and eIF2 kinases. Describe the mechanisms involved.
4. Describe how protein turnover responds to intake of a mixed meal. Describe how it responds to starvation. Identify important points and mechanisms of regulation of protein turnover to achieve these changes.

REFERENCES

Adams, V., Mangner, N., Gasch, A., Krohne, C., Gielen, S., Hirner, S., … Labeit, S. (2008). Induction of MuRF1 is essential for TNF-alpha-induced loss of muscle function in mice. *Journal of Molecular Biology, 384*, 48–59.

Andersen, G. R., Nissen, P., & Nyborg, J. (2003). Elongation factors in protein biosynthesis. *Trends in Biochemical Sciences, 28*, 434–441.

Anthony, T. G., McDaniel, B. J., Byerley, R. L., McGrath, B. C., Cavener, D. R., McNurlan, M. A., & Wek, R. C. (2004). Preservation of liver protein synthesis during dietary leucine deprivation occurs at the expense of skeletal muscle mass in mice deleted for eIF2 kinase GCN2. *The Journal of Biological Chemistry, 279*, 36553–36561.

Anthony, T. G., Reiter, A. K., Anthony, J. C., Kimball, S. R., & Jefferson, L. S. (2001). Deficiency of dietary EAA preferentially inhibits mRNA translation of ribosomal proteins in liver of meal-fed rats. *American Journal of Physiology. Endocrinology and Metabolism, 281*, E430–E439.

Bakkar, N., & Guttridge, D. C. (2010). NF-kappaB signaling: A tale of two pathways in skeletal myogenesis. *Physiological Reviews, 90*, 495–511.

Balage, M., & Dardevet, D. (2010). Long-term effects of leucine supplementation on body composition. *Current Opinion in Clinical Nutrition and Metabolic Care, 13*, 265–270.

Barnhart, B. C., & Simon, M. C. (2007). Taking aim at translation for tumor therapy. *The Journal of Clinical Investigation, 117*, 2385–2388.

Bartoli, M., & Richard, I. (2005). Calpains in muscle wasting. *The International Journal of Biochemistry & Cell Biology, 37*, 2115–2133.

Belin, S., Beghin, A., Solano-Gonzalez, E., Bezin, L., Brunet-Manquat, S., Textoris, J., … Diaz, J. J. (2009). Dysregulation of ribosome biogenesis and translational capacity is associated with tumor progression of human breast cancer cells. *PLoS One, 4*, e7147.

Bhasin, S., Calof, O. M., Storer, T. W., Lee, M. L., Mazer, N. A., Jasuja, R., … Dalton, J. T. (2006). Drug insight: Testosterone and selective androgen receptor modulators as anabolic therapies for chronic illness and aging. *Nature Clinical Practice. Endocrinology & Metabolism, 2*, 146–159.

Boirie, Y., Dangin, M., Gachon, P., Vasson, M. P., Maubois, J. L., & Beaufrere, B. (1997). Slow and fast dietary proteins differently modulate postprandial protein accretion. *Proceedings of the National Academy of Sciences of the United States of America, 94*, 14930–14935.

Boone, D. L., Turer, E. E., Lee, E. G., Ahmad, R. C., Wheeler, M. T., Tsui, C., … Ma, A. (2004). The ubiquitin-modifying enzyme A20 is required for termination of Toll-like receptor responses. *Nature Immunology, 5*, 1052–1060.

Borsheim, E., Chinkes, D. L., McEntire, S. J., Rodriguez, N. R., Herndon, D. N., & Suman, O. E. (2010). Whole body protein kinetics measured with a non-invasive method in severely burned children. *Burns, 36*, 1006–1012.

Bunpo, P., Dudley, A., Cundiff, J. K., Cavener, D. R., Wek, R. C., & Anthony, T. G. (2009). GCN2 protein kinase is required to activate amino acid deprivation responses in mice treated with the anti-cancer agent l-asparaginase. *The Journal of Biological Chemistry, 284*, 32742–32749.

Cahill, G. F., Jr. (1976). Starvation in man. *Clinics in Endocrinology and Metabolism, 5*, 397–415.

Carlberg, U., Nilsson, A., & Nygard, O. (1990). Functional properties of phosphorylated elongation factor 2. *European Journal of Biochemistry/FEBS, 191*, 639–645.

Carrano, A. C., Liu, Z., Dillin, A., & Hunter, T. (2009). A conserved ubiquitination pathway determines longevity in response to diet restriction. *Nature, 460*, 396–399.

Chaineau, M., Danglot, L., & Galli, T. (2009). Multiple roles of the vesicular-SNARE TI-VAMP in post-Golgi and endosomal trafficking. *FEBS Letters, 583*, 3817–3826.

Cheung, Y. N., Maag, D., Mitchell, S. F., Fekete, C. A., Algire, M. A., Takacs, J. E., … Hinnebusch, A. G. (2007). Dissociation of eIF1 from the 40S ribosomal subunit is a key step in start codon selection in vivo. *Genes & Development, 21*, 1217–1230.

Clemmons, D. R. (2009). Role of IGF-I in skeletal muscle mass maintenance. *Trends in Endocrinology and Metabolism, 20*, 349–356.

Cooney, R. N., Kimball, S. R., Maish, G., 3rd, Shumate, M., & Vary, T. C. (2000). Effects of tumor necrosis factor-binding protein on hepatic protein synthesis during chronic sepsis. *The Journal of Surgical Research, 93*, 257–264.

Dalby, K. N., Tekedereli, I., Lopez-Berestein, G., & Ozpolat, B. (2010). Targeting the prodeath and prosurvival functions of autophagy as novel therapeutic strategies in cancer. *Autophagy, 6*, 322–329.

Dancourt, J., & Barlowe, C. (2010). Protein sorting receptors in the early secretory pathway. *Annual Review of Biochemistry, 79*, 777–802.

De Feo, P. (1996). Hormonal regulation of human protein metabolism. *European Journal of Endocrinology, 135*, 7–18.

Delepine, M., Nicolino, M., Barrett, T., Golamaully, M., Lathrop, G. M., & Julier, C. (2000). EIF2AK3, encoding translation initiation factor 2-alpha kinase 3, is mutated in patients with Wolcott-Rallison syndrome. *Nature Genetics, 25*, 406–409.

Dillon, E. L., Durham, W. J., Urban, R. J., & Sheffield-Moore, M. (2010). Hormone treatment and muscle anabolism during aging: Androgens. *Clinical Nutrition, 29*, 697–700.

Elia, M., Stubbs, R. J., & Henry, C. J. (1999). Differences in fat, carbohydrate, and protein metabolism between lean and obese subjects undergoing total starvation. *Obesity Research, 7*, 597–604.

Garlick, P. J., McNurlan, M. A., Bark, T., Lang, C. H., & Gelato, M. C. (1998). Hormonal regulation of protein metabolism in relation to nutrition and disease. *The Journal of Nutrition, 128*, 356S–359S.

Glass, D. J. (2010). Signaling pathways perturbing muscle mass. *Current Opinion in Clinical Nutrition and Metabolic Care, 13*, 225–229.

Glynn, E. L., Fry, C. S., Drummond, M. J., Dreyer, H. C., Dhanani, S., Volpi, E., & Rasmussen, B. B. (2010). Muscle protein breakdown has a minor role in the protein anabolic response to essential amino acid and carbohydrate intake following resistance exercise. *American Journal of Physiology. Regulatory, Integrative and Comparative Physiology, 299*, R533–R540.

Golden, M. H. N., Waterlow, J. C., & Picou, D. (1977). Protein turnover, synthesis and breakdown before and after recovery from protein-energy malnutrition. *Clinical Science and Molecular Medicine, 53*, 473–477.

Hagner, P. R., Schneider, A., & Gartenhaus, R. B. (2010). Targeting the translational machinery as a novel treatment strategy for hematologic malignancies. *Blood, 115*, 2127–2135.

Herndon, D. N., & Tompkins, R. G. (2004). Support of the metabolic response to burn injury. *Lancet, 363*(9424), 1895–1902.

Hoseki, J., Ushioda, R., & Nagata, K. (2010). Mechanism and components of endoplasmic reticulum-associated degradation. *Journal of Biochemistry, 147*, 19–25.

Hotamisligil, G. S. (2010). Endoplasmic reticulum stress and the inflammatory basis of metabolic disease. *Cell, 140*, 900–917.

Hurley, J. H. (2008). ESCRT complexes and the biogenesis of multivesicular bodies. *Current Opinion in Cell Biology, 20*, 4–11.

Ibrahim, H., Lee, Y. J., & Curthoys, N. P. (2008). Renal response to metabolic acidosis: Role of mRNA stabilization. *Kidney International, 73*, 11–18.

Jarosch, E., Taxis, C., Volkwein, C., Bordallo, J., Finley, D., Wolf, D. H., & Sommer, T. (2002). Protein dislocation from the ER requires polyubiquitination and the AAA-ATPase Cdc48. *Nature Cell Biology*, *4*, 134–139.

Kanazawa, T., Taneike, I., Akaishi, R., Yoshizawa, F., Furuya, N., Fujimura, S., & Kadowaki, M. (2004). Amino acids and insulin control autophagic proteolysis through different signaling pathways in relation to mTOR in isolated rat hepatocytes. *The Journal of Biological Chemistry*, *279*, 8452–8459.

Kee, A. J., Combaret, L., Tilignac, T., Souweine, B., Aurousseau, E., Dalle, M., … Attaix, D. (2003). Ubiquitin-proteasome-dependent muscle proteolysis responds slowly to insulin release and refeeding in starved rats. *The Journal of Physiology*, *546*, 765–776.

Kim, H. J., Jamart, C., Deldicque, L., An, G. L., Lee, Y. H., Kim, C. K., … Francaux, M. (2011). ER-stress markers and ubiquitin-proteasome pathway activity in response to 200-km run. *Medicine and Science in Sports and Exercise*, *43*, 18–25.

Kincaid, M. M., & Cooper, A. A. (2007). ERADicate ER stress or die trying. *Antioxidants & Redox Signaling*, *9*, 2373–2387.

Kloetzel, P. M. (2004). Generation of major histocompatibility complex class I antigens: Functional interplay between proteasomes and TPPII. *Nature Immunology*, *5*, 661–669.

Korolchuk, V. I., Menzies, F. M., & Rubinsztein, D. C. (2010). Mechanisms of cross-talk between the ubiquitin-proteasome and autophagy-lysosome systems. *FEBS Letters*, *584*, 1393–1398.

Kuma, A., Hatano, M., Matsui, M., Yamamoto, A., Nakaya, H., Yoshimori, T., … Mizushima, N. (2004). The role of autophagy during the early neonatal starvation period. *Nature*, *432*, 1032–1036.

Lang, C. H., Frost, R. A., & Vary, T. C. (2007). Regulation of muscle protein synthesis during sepsis and inflammation. *American Journal of Physiology. Endocrinology and Metabolism*, *293*, E453–E459.

Liang, H., Balas, B., Tantiwong, P., Dube, J., Goodpaster, B. H., O'Doherty, R. M., … Ward, W. F. (2009). Whole body overexpression of PGC-1alpha has opposite effects on hepatic and muscle insulin sensitivity. *American Journal of Physiology. Endocrinology and Metabolism*, *296*, E945–E954.

Lin, J. H., Li, H., Yasumura, D., Cohen, H. R., Zhang, C., Panning, B., … Walter, P. (2007). IRE1 signaling affects cell fate during the unfolded protein response. *Science*, *318*, 944–949.

Lin, J. H., Li, H., Zhang, Y., Ron, D., & Walter, P. (2009). Divergent effects of PERK and IRE1 signaling on cell viability. *PLoS One*, *4*, e4170.

Liu, H. Y., Han, J., Cao, S. Y., Hong, T., Zhuo, D., Shi, J., … Cao, W. (2009). Hepatic autophagy is suppressed in the presence of insulin resistance and hyperinsulinemia: Inhibition of FoxO1-dependent expression of key autophagy genes by insulin. *The Journal of Biological Chemistry*, *284*, 31484–31492.

Liu, M. C., Akle, V., Zheng, W., Dave, J. R., Tortella, F. C., Hayes, R. L., & Wang, K. K. (2006). Comparing calpain- and caspase-3-mediated degradation patterns in traumatic brain injury by differential proteome analysis. *The Biochemical Journal*, *394*, 715–725.

Lorsch, J. R., & Dever, T. E. (2010). Molecular view of 43 S complex formation and start site selection in eukaryotic translation initiation. *The Journal of Biological Chemistry*, *285*, 21203–21207.

Mayer, C., & Grummt, I. (2006). Ribosome biogenesis and cell growth: mTOR coordinates transcription by all three classes of nuclear RNA polymerases. *Oncogene*, *25*, 6384–6391.

McFarlane, C., Sharma, M., & Kambadur, R. (2008). Myostatin is a procachectic growth factor during postnatal myogenesis. *Current Opinion in Clinical Nutrition and Metabolic Care*, *11*, 422–427.

Miller, J. T., & Btaiche, I. F. (2009). Oxandrolone treatment in adults with severe thermal injury. *Pharmacotherapy*, *29*, 213–226.

Mitch, W. E., & Goldberg, A. L. (1996). Mechanisms of muscle wasting. The role of the ubiquitin-proteasome pathway. *New England Journal of Medicine*, *335*, 1897–1905.

Moller, N., Vendelbo, M. H., Kampmann, U., Christensen, B., Madsen, M., Norrelund, H., & Jorgensen, J. O. (2009). Growth hormone and protein metabolism. *Clinical Nutrition*, *28*, 597–603.

Mullner, E. W., & Kuhn, L. C. (1988). A stem-loop in the 3′ untranslated region mediates iron-dependent regulation of transferrin receptor mRNA stability in the cytoplasm. *Cell*, *53*, 815–825.

Muntoni, F., Torelli, S., & Brockington, M. (2008). Muscular dystrophies due to glycosylation defects. *Neurotherapeutics*, *5*, 627–632.

Murphy, R. M. (2010). Calpains, skeletal muscle function and exercise. *Clinical and Experimental Pharmacology & Physiology*, *37*, 385–391.

Murton, A. J., Alamdari, N., Gardiner, S. M., Constantin-Teodosiu, D., Layfield, R., Bennett, T., & Greenhaff, P. L. (2009). Effects of endotoxaemia on protein metabolism in rat fast-twitch skeletal muscle and myocardium. *PLoS One*, *4*, e6945.

Nakatogawa, H., Suzuki, K., Kamada, Y., & Ohsumi, Y. (2009). Dynamics and diversity in autophagy mechanisms: Lessons from yeast. *Nature Reviews. Molecular Cell Biology*, *10*, 458–467.

Novak, F., Heyland, D. K., Avenell, A., Drover, J. W., & Su, X. (2002). Glutamine supplementation in serious illness: A systematic review of the evidence. *Critical Care Medicine*, *30*, 2022–2029.

Ozcan, U., Cao, Q., Yilmaz, E., Lee, A. H., Iwakoshi, N. N., Ozdelen, E., … Hotamisligil, G. S. (2004). Endoplasmic reticulum stress links obesity, insulin action, and type 2 diabetes. *Science*, *306*, 457–461.

Paul, S. (2008). Dysfunction of the ubiquitin-proteasome system in multiple disease conditions: Therapeutic approaches. *Bioessays*, *30*, 1172–1184.

Phillips, S. M., Glover, E. I., & Rennie, M. J. (2009). Alterations of protein turnover underlying disuse atrophy in human skeletal muscle. *Journal of Applied Physiology*, *107*, 645–654.

Pop, C., & Salvesen, G. S. (2009). Human caspases: Activation, specificity, and regulation. *The Journal of Biological Chemistry*, *284*(33), 21777–21781.

Pratt, A. J., & MacRae, I. J. (2009). The RNA-induced silencing complex: A versatile gene-silencing machine. *The Journal of Biological Chemistry*, *284*, 17897–17901.

Ravasco, P., Aranha, M. M., Borralho, P. M., Moreira da Silva, I. B., Correia, L., Fernandes, A., … Camilo, M. (2010). Colorectal cancer: Can nutrients modulate NF-kappaB and apoptosis? *Clinical Nutrition*, *29*, 42–46.

Rooyackers, O. E., & Nair, K. S. (1997). Hormonal regulation of human muscle protein metabolism. *Annual Review of Nutrition*, *17*, 457–485.

Salati, L. M., Szeszel-Fedorowicz, W., Tao, H., Gibson, M. A., Amir-Ahmady, B., Stabile, L. P., & Hodge, D. L. (2004). Nutritional regulation of mRNA processing. *The Journal of Nutrition*, *134*, 2437S–2443S.

Schricker, T., Meterissian, S., Lattermann, R., Adegoke, O. A., Marliss, E. B., Mazza, L., … Wykes, L. (2008). Anticatabolic effects of avoiding preoperative fasting by intravenous hypocaloric nutrition: A randomized clinical trial. *Annals of Surgery*, *248*, 1051–1059.

Schroder, M., & Kaufman, R. J. (2005). The mammalian unfolded protein response. *Annual Review of Biochemistry*, *74*, 739–789.

Schwartz, A. L., & Ciechanover, A. (2009). Targeting proteins for destruction by the ubiquitin system: Implications for human pathobiology. *Annual Review of Pharmacology and Toxicology*, *49*, 73–96.

Shah, J. J., & Orlowski, R. Z. (2009). Proteasome inhibitors in the treatment of multiple myeloma. *Leukemia*, *23*, 1964–1979.

Shah, O. J., Anthony, J. C., Kimball, S. R., & Jefferson, L. S. (2000). Glucocorticoids oppose translational control by leucine in skeletal muscle. *American Journal of Physiology. Endocrinology and Metabolism*, *279*, E1185–E1190.

Shiomi, T., Lemaître, V., D'Armiento, J., & Okada, Y. (2010). Matrix metalloproteinases, a disintegrin and metalloproteinases, and a disintegrin and metalloproteinases with thrombospondin motifs in non-neoplastic diseases. *Pathology International*, *60*, 477–496.

Sikalidis, A. K., & Stipanuk, M. H. (2010). Growing rats respond to a sulfur amino acid-deficient diet by phosphorylation of the alpha subunit of eukaryotic initiation factor 2 heterotrimeric complex and induction of adaptive components of the integrated stress response. *The Journal of Nutrition*, *140*, 1080–1085.

Singh, C. R., Lee, B., Udagawa, T., Mohammad-Qureshi, S. S., Yamamoto, Y., Pavitt, G. D., & Asano, K. (2006). An eIF5/eIF2 complex antagonizes guanine nucleotide exchange by eIF2B during translation initiation. *The EMBO Journal*, *25*, 4537–4546.

Solomon, V., Madihally, S., Yarmush, M., & Toner, M. (2000). Insulin suppresses the increased activities of lysosomal cathepsins and ubiquitin conjugation system in burn-injured rats. *The Journal of Surgical Research*, *93*, 120–126.

Sorimachi, H., Hata, S., & Ono, Y. (2010). Expanding members and roles of the calpain superfamily and their genetically modified animals. *Experimental Animals*, *59*, 549–566.

Strum, J. C., Johnson, J. H., Ward, J., Xie, H., Feild, J., Hester, A., … Waters, K. M. (2009). MicroRNA 132 regulates nutritional stress-induced chemokine production through repression of SirT1. *Molecular Endocrinology*, *23*, 1876–1884.

Tisdale, M. J. (2009). Mechanisms of cancer cachexia. *Physiological Reviews*, *89*, 381–410.

Tisdale, M. J. (2010). Are tumoral factors responsible for host tissue wasting in cancer cachexia? *Future Oncology*, *6*, 503–513.

Todd, D. J., Lee, A. H., & Glimcher, L. H. (2008). The endoplasmic reticulum stress response in immunity and autoimmunity. *Nature Reviews. Immunology*, *8*, 663–674.

van der Jagt, M. F., Wobbes, T., Strobbe, L. J., Sweep, F. C., & Span, P. N. (2010). Metalloproteinases and their regulators in colorectal cancer. *Journal of Surgical Oncology*, *101*, 259–269.

Vaquerizas, J. M., Kummerfeld, S. K., Teichmann, S. A., & Luscombe, N. M. (2009). A census of human transcription factors: Function, expression and evolution. *Nature Reviews. Genetics*, *10*, 252–263.

Vembar, S. S., & Brodsky, J. L. (2008). One step at a time: Endoplasmic reticulum-associated degradation. *Nature Reviews. Molecular Cell Biology*, *9*, 944–957.

Wang, X., Hu, Z., Hu, J., Du, J., & Mitch, W. E. (2006). Insulin resistance accelerates muscle protein degradation: Activation of the ubiquitin-proteasome pathway by defects in muscle cell signaling. *Endocrinology*, *147*, 4160–4168.

Wek, R. C., Jiang, H. Y., & Anthony, T. G. (2006). Coping with stress: eIF2 kinases and translational control. *Biochemical Society Transactions*, *34*, 7–11.

Wilkie, G. S., Dickson, K. S., & Gray, N. K. (2003). Regulation of mRNA translation by 5′- and 3′-UTR-binding factors. *Trends in Biochemical Sciences*, *28*, 182–188.

Williams, A. E. (2008). Functional aspects of animal microRNAs. *Cellular and Molecular Life Sciences*, *65*, 545–562.

Wong, E. S., Tan, J. M., Soong, W. E., Hussein, K., Nukina, N., Dawson, V. L., … Lim, K. L. (2008). Autophagy-mediated clearance of aggresomes is not a universal phenomenon. *Human Molecular Genetics*, *17*, 2570–2582.

Zhang, P., McGrath, B., Li, S., Frank, A., Zambito, F., Reinert, J., … Cavener, D. R. (2002). The PERK eukaryotic initiation factor 2 alpha kinase is required for the development of the skeletal system, postnatal growth, and the function and viability of the pancreas. *Molecular and Cellular Biology*, *22*, 3864–3874.

Zhao, J., Brault, J. J., Schild, A., & Goldberg, A. L. (2008). Coordinate activation of autophagy and the proteasome pathway by FoxO transcription factor. *Autophagy*, *4*, 378–380.

Zhao, W., Pan, J., Wang, X., Wu, Y., Bauman, W. A., & Cardozo, C. P. (2008). Expression of the muscle atrophy factor muscle atrophy F-box is suppressed by testosterone. *Endocrinology*, *149*, 5449–5460.

CHAPTER 14

Amino Acid Metabolism

*Margaret E. Brosnan, PhD, and John T. Brosnan, DPhil, DSc**

This discussion of amino acid metabolism focuses on the metabolism of the 20 α-amino (or -imino, in the case of proline) α-carboxylic acids that are the precursors for protein synthesis. Many other compounds in the body, perhaps as many as 300, also could be considered amino acids, because this term can be used more broadly to describe any compound with an amine group and an acidic group. For example, other amino acids are formed when some of the 20 amino acids used for protein synthesis undergo limited posttranslational modification to form derivatized residues that are released as free amino acids during proteolysis; these include *N*-methylhistidine, γ-carboxyglutamate, hydroxyproline, and hydroxylysine. In addition, some serine is specifically converted to selenocysteine cotranslationally. A number of other amino acids (including citrulline, ornithine, γ-aminobutyrate, homocysteine, and taurine) are formed during metabolism of specific amino acids. In addition, these and other amino acid derivatives, including some that are not synthesized by mammalian tissues, are consumed in the diet.

The 20 amino acids required for protein synthesis include some for which the carbon chains cannot be synthesized in the body (essential, or indispensable, amino acids) and others for which the carbon skeletons can be made from common intermediates in metabolism (nonessential, or dispensable, amino acids). The nutritional requirement for protein is actually a requirement for the indispensable (essential) amino acids and a source of nitrogen for synthesis of dispensable (nonessential) amino acids, as is discussed in more detail in Chapter 15. Most of the nitrogen for the synthesis of dispensable amino acids must be provided by α-amino groups of amino acids, because the body has a limited ability to incorporate inorganic nitrogen (i.e., NH_3, or NH_4^+) into amino acids. The indispensable amino acids for humans include leucine, isoleucine, valine, lysine, threonine, tryptophan, phenylalanine, methionine, and histidine. Tyrosine and cysteine are termed semiessential because they can be synthesized only if their indispensable amino acid precursors (phenylalanine and methionine, respectively) are provided. Many, but not all, of these indispensable amino acids can be made from their keto acid or hydroxy acid analogs if these are fed instead of the amino acids; this is possible because of widespread transamination reactions in mammalian tissues that convert keto acids to the respective amino acids. In practice, food proteins provide all 20 amino acids, but the body can adjust the proportions by transferring nitrogen to nonessential carbon skeletons and by catabolizing excess amino acids. The reactions involved in moving amino groups among carbon skeletons, removing amino groups for nitrogen excretion and using the carbon skeleton for gluconeogenesis and other functions, and using amino acids for synthesis of essential compounds such as neurotransmitters are described in this chapter.

OVERVIEW OF AMINO ACID METABOLISM

An overview of amino acid metabolism is shown in Figure 14-1. The free amino acid pool is shown in the center of this figure; free amino acid pool is the term used to describe the amino acids that exist in the body in free form at any moment and to distinguish these free amino acids from those that exist in peptide or polypeptide/protein form. The size of this free amino acid pool in human adults is approximately 150 g, and the flux of amino acids through this pool typically amounts to 400 to 500 g per day (Jungas et al., 1992; Bergstrom et al., 1974).

As can be seen by arrows leading toward the free amino acid pool (see Figure 14-1), there are three major sources of amino acids, as follows:

1. Digestion of endogenous proteins and peptides secreted or sloughed off into the gastrointestinal tract and absorption of the resulting amino acids into the circulation (~75 g/day)
2. Dietary protein which is digested in the gastrointestinal tract and absorption of the resulting amino acids into the circulation (~100 g/day depending on diet)
3. Intracellular protein turnover or degradation (~230 g/day)

These processes are discussed in Chapters 9 and 13.

As shown by the arrows leading away from the free amino acid pool, the major metabolic fates of amino acids include (1) their use for protein synthesis, (2) their use as precursors for the synthesis of numerous nonprotein nitrogenous molecules, and (3) their catabolism with excretion of nitrogen and use of carbon chains as energy substrates. Note that the amino acids incorporated into proteins may eventually reenter the amino

*This chapter is a revision of the chapter contributed by Martha H. Stipanuk, PhD, and Malcolm Watford, DPhil, for the second edition.

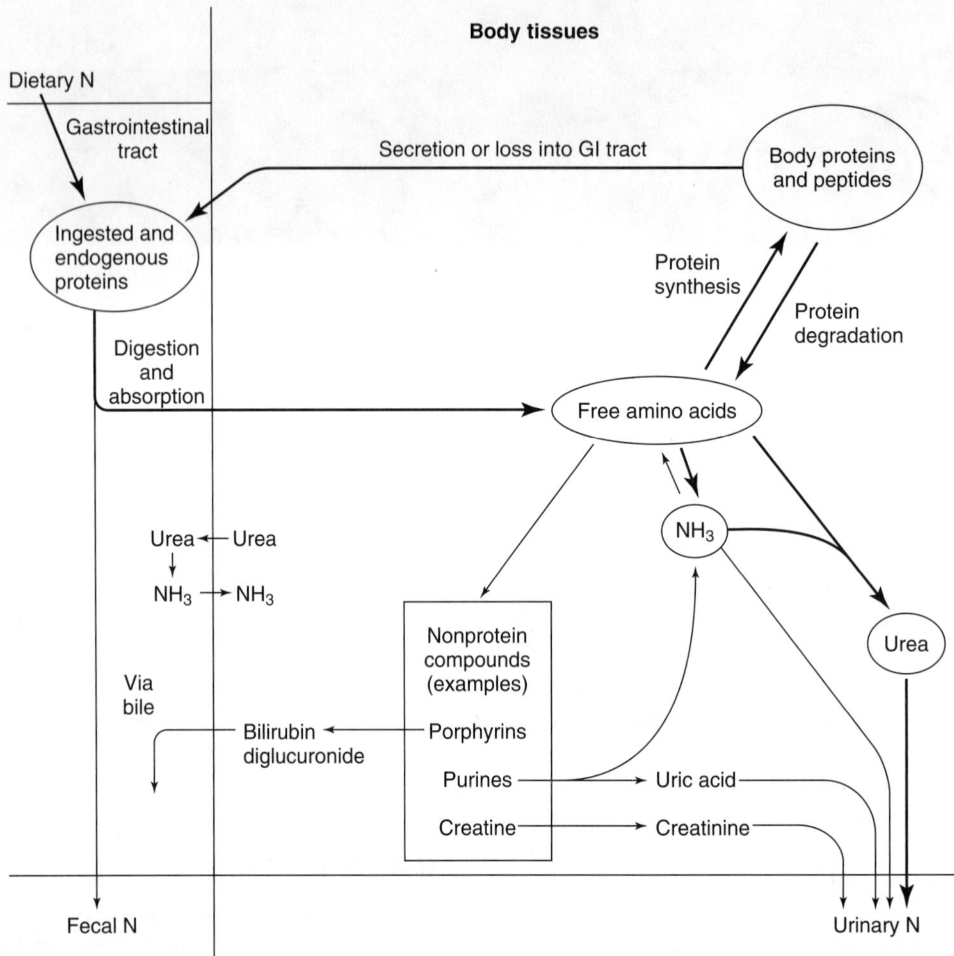

FIGURE 14-1 Schematic outline of the flow of nitrogen through the body. Major routes of nitrogen movement are indicated by the heavy lines.

acid pool as a result of protein degradation and become available for reutilization, but those amino acids that were irreversibly modified or used for synthesis of nonpeptide metabolites, or that underwent oxidative catabolism, will for the most part no longer exist as proteinogenic amino acids.

The utilization of amino acids for protein synthesis was discussed in Chapter 13. Catabolism of amino acids with the use of their carbon chains as fuels is described in the present chapter. These two fates of amino acids account for most of the amino acids that move through the amino acid pool. Although only small quantities of amino acids are involved, the very important role of amino acids in the synthesis of some other nonprotein compounds with specialized functions is also described in this chapter. The considerable chemical diversity of amino acid side chains affords much greater metabolic versatility than exists for the other macronutrients. It is hardly surprising that amino acids or their metabolic derivatives play such an important role in the regulation of cell function (e.g., as neurotransmitters). Similarly, it may be noted that three of the four known gaseous signaling molecules (ethylene in plants, nitric oxide, and hydrogen sulfide, but not carbon dioxide) are derived from amino acids or their derivatives. Synthesis of dispensable amino acids, a process that is often simply the reverse of their catabolism and that involves catabolism of another amino acid to provide the α-amino group, is also described.

In discussing the metabolism of amino acids in the body, it is important to recognize that amino groups can be transferred from one carbon skeleton to another by a number of reactions. Hence the fate of amino groups and carbon skeletons must be considered somewhat separately, and the amino acid via which nitrogen enters a particular cell may be the same as or different from the amino acid that carries the nitrogen out of the cell. For example, glutamine or glutamate catabolism by the small intestine can result in release of the carbon chain as CO_2 and pyruvate, lactate, or alanine, and release of the nitrogen as alanine, ammonia, or both. The small intestine also converts glutamine to citrulline and proline, which contain both carbon and the α-amino nitrogen from glutamine or glutamate.

Finally, it is important to emphasize a critical difference between the metabolism of amino acids and that of the other macronutrients. We have no mechanism for storing excess dietary amino acids. This contrasts with our stores of glycogen and triacylglycerol. Ingestion of excess lysine, for example, does not result in storage of the excess. Of course, dietary amino acids are used for protein synthesis but the proteins synthesized are produced for their specific functions and in the quantities required for their specific functions. In certain situations proteolysis can provide amino acids for specific purposes; an example is gluconeogenesis during starvation. However, this involves the breakdown of functional proteins, and it always come with a cost. An important physiological consequence of this lack of a store of amino acids is that dietary amino acids in excess of those needed for protein synthesis and other functions are very promptly metabolized. Another is the well-known importance of ingestion of meals that contain adequate quantities of all of the indispensable amino acids because protein synthesis requires that all 20 of the canonical amino acids be simultaneously available.

AMINO ACID POOLS AND TRANSPORT

Free amino acids are found, at varying concentrations, in extracellular fluids (e.g., plasma, interstitial fluid, and cerebrospinal fluid) and inside cells. Within cells, amino acids are compartmentalized and concentrations vary between different compartments (e.g., cytosol, mitochondria, lysosomes). Table 14-1 shows amino acid concentrations in human muscle and plasma. It is evident there is considerable variability between the concentrations of individual amino acids. For example, glutamine concentration in muscle is almost 20 mmol/L, whereas that of tyrosine is only 0.1 mmol/L. In addition, the intracellular/extracellular concentration gradient can be quite high for some amino acids; for example, the difference is about seventyfold for glutamate. Finally, it should be noted that taurine, a nonprotein amino acid, is among those with the highest intracellular concentration, and it displays a more than 200-fold concentration gradient between muscle and plasma. Establishment and maintenance of such intracellular pools and gradients require amino acid transporters, both at the plasma membrane and in intracellular membranes. Indeed, Christensen (1990) has pointed out that, in addition to the tissue-specific expression of metabolic enzymes, interorgan fluxes of amino acids require the tissue-specific expression of amino acid transporters.

As discussed in Chapter 9, amino acids taken up from the gastrointestinal tract are released by intestinal mucosal cells into the portal circulation. Distinct transport proteins with overlapping specificities are responsible for the uptake and release of amino acids from cells. A number of transport systems for amino acids have been categorized in mammalian cells (Hyde et al., 2003; Christensen, 1990) as summarized in Table 14-2. The Human Genome Project has classified 298 known solute carrier (SLC) systems into 43 families of proteins, and amino acid carriers fall into a number of these different families (see Table 14-2) (Hediger et al., 2004). Major systems for the transport of small aliphatic amino acids include Na^+-dependent system A (*SLC38A1*, *SLC38A2*, and *SLC38A3*) and ASC (*SLC7A10*), and the Na^+-independent system L (*SLC7A5* and *SLC7A8*). Other, more restricted systems transport glutamine, acidic amino acids, basic amino acids, and imino acids. In general, the amino acid transport systems carry several amino acids across the cell membrane, and the transport of a particular amino acid is subject to competitive inhibition by other amino acids that share the same transport system.

Amino acid transport is subject to short- and long-term regulation. Although many of the amino acid transporters have now been identified (Hyde et al., 2003), relatively little is known about their regulation. System A has been studied most extensively, particularly in hepatocytes and hepatoma cells, in which it is subject to a variety of regulatory signals. System A activity is rapidly increased in response to glucagon or epidermal growth factor (EGF) by mechanisms that involve hyperpolarization of the cell membrane by changes in Na^+/H^+ exchange. In addition, system A is sensitive to pH changes. In response to acidosis, there is evidence that amino acid transport into the

TABLE 14-1 Concentrations of Free Amino Acids in Human Muscle and Plasma

AMINO ACID	PLASMA (EXTRACELLULAR)	SKELETAL MUSCLE (INTRACELLULAR)
	mmol/L	
Alanine	0.33	2.34
Arginine	0.08	0.51
Asparagine	0.05	0.47
Citrulline	0.03	0.04
Cysteine	0.11	0.18
Glycine	0.21	1.33
Glutamate	0.06	4.38
Glutamine	0.57	19.45
Histidine	0.08	0.37
Isoleucine	0.06	0.11
Leucine	0.12	0.15
Lysine	0.18	1.15
Methionine	0.02	0.11
Ornithine	0.06	0.30
Phenylalanine	0.05	0.07
Proline	0.17	0.83
Serine	0.12	0.98
Taurine	0.07	15.44
Threonine	0.15	1.03
Tyrosine	0.05	0.10
Valine	0.22	0.26

Values are mean values for 21 healthy subjects who were studied after an overnight fast. Data from Bergstrom, J., Furst, P., Noree, L.-O., & Vinnars, E. (1974). Intracellular free amino acid concentration in human muscle tissue. *Journal of Applied Physiology, 36*, 693–697.

TABLE 14-2 The Human Genome Organization Nomenclature for Solute Carrier Gene Families That Code for Amino Acid Transporters

GENE FAMILY	GENERAL DESCRIPTION OF TRANSPORT SYSTEM SERIES	FUNCTIONAL NAMES
SLC1	High-affinity glutamate and neutral amino acid transporter family	ASCT (ASC), EAAT (X_{AG}^-)
SLC3	Heavy subunits of the heteromeric amino acid transporters	rBAT, 4F2hc
SLC6	Sodium- and chloride-dependent neurotransmitter transporter family (for GABA, taurine, betaine transporters)	GlyT (gly), PROT (L-proline), CRTR or CT1 (creatine), TauT (taurine, β-ala), ATB$^{0,+}$ (B$^{0,+}$), SBAT (large neutral amino acids), NTT (neutral amino acids), B^{0}AT (B^0), SIT (IMINO)
SLC7	Cationic amino acid transporter/glycoprotein–associated amino acid transporter family; the light subunits of the heteromeric amino acid transporters	CAT(y$^+$), LAT(L), y$^+$LAT(y$^+$L), b$^{0,+}$AT (b$^{0,+}$), Asc (asc), xCT (x_c^-), AGT (XAT2)
SLC15	Proton–oligopeptide symporters	Pept (oligopeptide), PHT (peptide/histidine)
SLC16	Monocarboxylate transporter family (including aromatic amino acids)	TAT1 (T)
SLC36	Proton-coupled amino acid transporter family (for small neutral amino acids)	PAT (Iminoacid)
SLC38	System A and N, sodium-coupled neutral amino acid transporter family	SNAT (A and N)
SLC43	Sodium-independent, system L–like amino acid transporter family	LAT (LAT)
SLC17	Vesicular glutamate transporter family	VGLUT
SLC18	Vesicular amine transporter family	VMAT
SLC32	Vesicular inhibitory amino acid transporter family	VIAAT

Data from Hediger, M. A., Romero, M. F., Peng, J.-B., Rolfs, A., Takanaga, H., & Bruford, E. A. (2004). The ABCs of solute carriers: Physiological, pathological and therapeutic implications of human membrane transport proteins. *Pflügers Archive: European Journal of Physiology, 447*, 465–468; Hyde R., Taylor, P. M., & Hundal, H. S. (2003). Amino acid transporters: Roles in amino acid sensing and signaling in animal cells. *The Biochemical Journal, 373*, 1–18. A complete list is available at www.bioparadigms.org/slc/menu.asp.
HUGO, Human Genome Organization; *SLC*, solute carrier.

liver may be decreased, with a resultant decrease in urea synthesis (Boon et al., 1994).

System A is also subject to long-term regulation by changes in the amount of transporter protein. System A can be induced by insulin in most cell types and by either insulin or glucagon in liver cells. This apparent paradox of induction of system A in liver by two opposing hormones probably is explained by the increased hepatic uptake of amino acids required in response to food intake (when protein synthesis and catabolism of excess exogenous amino acids predominate in the liver) and in response to starvation or diabetes (when amino acids from muscle protein degradation are taken up and catabolized by the liver as gluconeogenic precursors).

Dipeptides and tripeptides are transported into cells by two proton-linked carriers: Pept1 (*SLC15A1*), found in the intestine and possibly the kidney, and Pept2 (*SLC15A2*), expressed in kidney, brain, mammary gland, and lung (Pinsonneault et al., 2004; Adibi, 2003). In addition, urea is transported by two distinct urea transporters, UT1 (*SLC14A1*) and UT2 (*SLC14A2*), which are found in many tissues and highly expressed in the kidney, where they play an important role in concentrating urine.

Several genes coding for amino acid transporters have been shown to contain amino acid response elements (AAREs), which are responsible for transcriptional upregulation of the expression of these genes under conditions of amino acid starvation (Palii et al., 2004; Fernandez et al., 2003). These include the sodium-coupled neutral amino acid transporter system A gene (*SNAT2*, or *SLC38A2*), the arginine/lysine transporter (y$^+$) gene (*CAT-1*, or *SLC7A1*), and the cystine/glutamate transporter (x_c^-) light subunit gene (*xCT*, or *SLC7A11*). Transcription factors that belong to the ATF (activating transcription factor) and C/EBP (CCAAT/enhancer binding protein) families appear to be involved in binding to the AARE or AARE-like sequences in these genes.

Transport of amino acids between intracellular compartments also plays important metabolic roles. The mitochondrial glutamate/aspartate transporters (AGC1 [*SLC25A12*] and AGC2 [*SLC25A13*]) release aspartate to the cytosol in exchange for glutamate and a proton. These transporters are a key component of the malate/aspartate shuttle for the oxidation of cytosolic NADH, such as is produced during glycolysis or during ethanol metabolism, and the transport of reducing equivalents into the mitochondria. AGC2 in the liver plays a critical role in movement of substrates for the

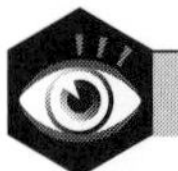

NUTRITION INSIGHT

Potential Role of the Microbiome in the Nitrogen Economy of the Body

The human gastrointestinal tract is home to some 10^{14} microorganisms, ten times the number of somatic cells in our bodies. The composite bacterial genome, the microbiome, contains at least 100 times as many genes as the human genome. Many of the genes are involved in bacterial housekeeping, whereas others are specific to life in the gut (e.g., adhesion to the mucosal layer). The microbiota and their human host form what is referred to as a superorganism because their metabolic functions are integrated. It has proved difficult to study the various functions of individual members of the microbiota, because some 80% of its members cannot easily be cultured, separately or in combination. Many of the bacteria, especially those in the colon, are located in the lumen and can be sampled in the feces. Some, however, are associated with the mucus layer, especially in the small intestine, and cannot be easily sampled in humans (Wikoff et al., 2009).

Although many species found in the gastrointestinal tract have not been identified elsewhere, these unique species belong to well-known phyla, mainly Bacteroidetes and Firmicutes. Within these phyla, the composition of the microbiota can vary depending on host genetics, sex, age, diet, and antibiotic treatment. For example, obese people or animals tend to have higher levels of Firmicutes and lower levels of Bacteroidetes compared with their lean counterparts (Bäckhed, 2009).

It is known that germ-free animals need a higher energy content in their diet than conventional animals because some members of the microbiota can catabolize normally unusable energy sources (e.g., various fibers and resistant starch) to produce short-chain fatty acids that can be absorbed from the colon. The microbiota also appears to be involved in maturation of the gastrointestinal tract and immune function early in life. It is also well established that urea synthesized in the liver can reach the intestine where it can be catabolized by the microbiota. Some of the ammonia that results is absorbed and returned to the liver by the portal circulation; some of this ammonia can be incorporated into amino acids (via the glutamate dehydrogenase and glutamine synthetase reactions) or back into urea in the liver (Jackson, 1995).

Whether the microbiota can mitigate changes in dietary amino acid intake (e.g., catabolizing some of the excess amino acids in a high-protein diet or synthesizing and releasing amino acids when protein intake is low) is not known. The question of whether changes in microbiota composition and function may explain differences in the nitrogen economy of different people remains to be answered. Clearly, bacteria can respond to changes in amino acid availability to induce degradative or synthetic enzymes; but whether these are used solely by the bacteria themselves for their growth and proliferation, with eventual excretion as bacterial mass in the feces, or whether synthesis or degradation of amino acids by the microbiota affects the pool of amino acids entering the host's circulation is not known (Metges et al., 2006).

urea cycle and gluconeogenesis, pathways that occur partly in the mitochondria and partly in the cytosol. The mitochondrial ornithine/citrulline transporter (ORNT1, encoded by *SLC25A15*) is required for transport of citrulline out of the mitochondria in exchange for transport of ornithine into the mitochondria as a fundamental part of the urea cycle. Another example of transport of amino acids across membranes of intracellular organelles is the transport of amino acids produced by proteolysis out of lysosomes. Mutations of the genes encoding the subunits of the x_c^- system impair the transport of cystine out of lysosomes, resulting in the disease called cystinosis.

AMINO ACIDS AS SIGNALING AGENTS

In addition to being substrates for protein synthesis and other processes, amino acids also play regulatory roles through signal transduction pathways. They are known to regulate such diverse functions as taste, protein synthesis and degradation, and insulin secretion.

MAMMALIAN TARGET OF RAPAMYCIN

Circulating branched-chain amino acid levels increase markedly after a protein-rich meal. It appears that this postprandial increase in the levels of the branched-chain amino acids, especially leucine, is an anabolic signal, increasing net protein synthesis. Both an increase in protein synthesis and a decrease in intracellular proteolysis appear to result from activation of the mammalian target of rapamycin complex 1 (mTORC1), a serine/threonine protein kinase that is known to be activated by insulin and IGF-1 as well as by amino acids. Although the receptors and signaling pathways for insulin and growth factors have been reasonably well elucidated, the precise mechanism or protein involved in sensing leucine (and certain other amino acids) has not been identified. The effect of leucine on protein synthesis has been best studied in skeletal muscle. Leucine activates mTORC1 and, as a consequence, the downstream targets of mTORC1, S6K1 (ribosomal protein S6 kinase) and 4E-BP (eukaryotic initiation factor 4E binding protein), are phosphorylated. The phosphorylation of these and other mTORC1 targets facilitates the assembly of the initiation complex and also stimulates other aspects of protein synthesis (Proud, 2007). An important feature of this regulatory mechanism is that it is not limited to a single messenger RNA (mRNA); rather, it enhances the synthesis of a broad range of proteins and therefore plays an important role in whole-body protein metabolism (Kimball and Jefferson, 2006). Leucine and other amino acids also act, via mTOR, to decrease intracellular proteolysis. This has been best studied for autophagic hepatic proteolysis, where a mixture of leucine, phenylalanine, and tyrosine are most effective in reducing protein degradation by autophagy (Meijer, 2008).

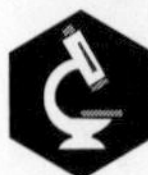

CLINICAL CORRELATION

Two Inheritable Diseases of Cystine Transport

The disulfide formed from two molecules of cysteine is called cystine. Folding of many proteins involves formation of cysteine-cysteine linkages, and these covalently-linked cysteine residues are released as cystine during protein hydrolysis. Also, cysteine can be oxidized nonenzymatically to its disulfide. Transport of cystine requires particular transport systems that are different than those for cysteine. Two inheritable diseases due to loss-of-function mutations in cystine transport systems are cystinosis and cystinuria.

Cystinosis: Cystinosis is a rare, autosomal recessively inherited disorder caused by a defect in the ubiquitous CTNS gene that encodes the lysosomal cystine transporter protein commonly called cystinosin. In cystinosis, free cystine accumulates to 15 to 1,000 times normal concentrations in the lysosomes. The cystine forms intracellular crystals that cause cellular damage. The rate of cystine accumulation and tissue damage varies among tissues. The reason for this variability is unknown but may be related to different rates of lysosomal protein degradation.

Children born with cystinosis appear normal at birth, but signs of the renal tubular Fanconi syndrome (e.g., failure of the kidney to reabsorb small molecules properly) develop, usually when the child is between 6 and 12 months of age. The renal glomerular damage progresses and children typically require dialysis or transplantation by 6 to 12 years of age. Plasma cystine concentrations and the intestinal absorption of cystine are normal in individuals with cystinosis, unlike in the disorder known as cystinuria (see later and Chapter 9). Urinary cystine levels are slightly elevated due to the renal damage, but the cystine levels are no more elevated than those of other amino acids. Damage to the cornea and the thyroid gland occur at a later age than the renal damage.

Oral cysteamine (β-mercaptoethylamine) has been used successfully to lower the cystine content of cystinotic cells. Cysteamine is taken up into the lysosomes where it reacts with cystine to form cysteine and the cysteine-cysteamine mixed disulfide. Cysteine can be transported out of the lysosome by other amino acid transporters. The cysteine-cysteamine mixed disulfide resembles lysine structurally and is transported across cystinotic lysosomal membranes in a carrier-mediated fashion by the intact lysine transporter. Diagnosis and initiation of cysteamine treatment should occur as early as possible in order to prevent the early renal damage.

Cystinuria: High concentrations of cystine are found in urine of patients with cystinuria, an inheritable disease of cystine and dibasic amino acid (ornithine, arginine, lysine) transport across the brush border membranes of the small intestinal mucosa and the renal tubules. Mutations causing cystinuria may occur in either the *SLC3A1* or *SLC7A9* genes that encode the two subunits of this dimeric transporter. Cystine transport across these membranes is due to the presence of system x_c^-, and this system is responsible for reabsorption of cystine and dibasic amino acids from the renal filtrate so they can be returned to the plasma. Cystine is poorly soluble, and its accumulation in the renal filtrate during the process of urine formation causes cystine stones to form in the renal tubules. Cystine precipitates at concentrations higher than its aqueous solubility limit (1 mmol/L). Prevention of cystine stone formation is attempted by increased fluid intake and by alkalinizing the urine to make the cystine more soluble. Intestinal uptake of free cystine is also decreased, but plasma amino acid levels are normal because amino acids and peptides can be taken up by other amino acid and peptide transporters.

The effects of leucine on protein synthesis and degradation are attenuated by rapamycin, an inhibitor of mTORC1.

Cells also display a coordinated response to intracellular amino acid deprivation, the GCN2 (general control nonderepressible) pathway. The physiologically appropriate response to amino acid limitation is to suppress global mRNA translation while permitting translation of a specific subset of genes that are required for ameliorating the amino acid depletion. In this case the intracellular detection of amino acid deprivation is indirect, via the levels of uncharged transfer RNAs (tRNAs) that increase with amino acid limitation. The accumulation of uncharged tRNAs activates GCN2, a protein kinase that in turn phosphorylates and inactivates the α subunit of eukaryotic initiation factor 2 (eIF2α). This in turn suppresses global mRNA translation but permits translation of a specific transcription factor, ATF4 (activating transcription factor 4), which acts in the nucleus to increase expression of genes for amino acid transport and aminoacyl tRNA synthesis. In this way global mRNA translation is suppressed while there is increased expression of genes that may increase cellular amino acid levels and permit synthesis of essential proteins (Kilberg et al., 2005).

TASTE

Recent work has clearly established that the umami taste is one of the fundamental tastes, in addition to the sweet, sour, salty, and bitter tastes. Full activation of umami taste receptors requires the interaction of two coagonists with the umami receptor, glutamate (in the form of its sodium salt) and a nucleotide monophosphate (GMP or IMP). The umami taste brought about by either of these agonists alone is rather weak, but there is a remarkable synergy between them, which may be accounted for by the finding that GMP greatly enhances glutamate binding to the taste receptor. Many protein-rich foods are rich in both glutamate and these nucleotides and it has been proposed that the umami taste permits animals to recognize protein food sources. However, this attractive hypothesis has not been definitively established (Beauchamp, 2009).

TWO THEMES IN AMINO ACID METABOLISM

Amino acids differ from glucose and fatty acids in that they all contain nitrogen. Because each amino acid has one or more individual pathways for metabolism, it is difficult to

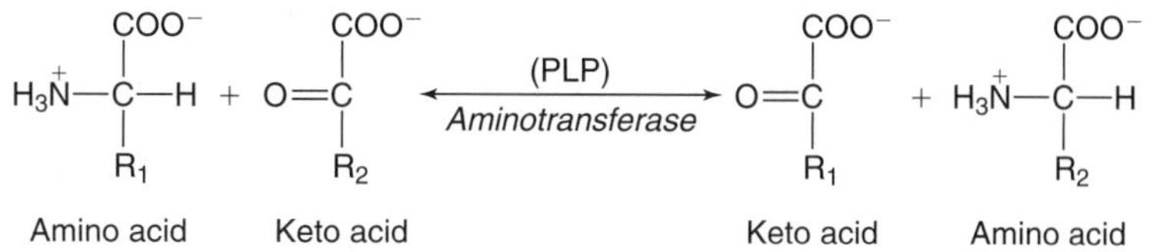

$$\underset{\text{Amino acid}}{H_3\overset{+}{N}-\underset{R_1}{\overset{COO^-}{C}}-H} + \underset{\text{Keto acid}}{O=\underset{R_2}{\overset{COO^-}{C}}} \xrightleftharpoons[\text{Aminotransferase}]{\text{(PLP)}} \underset{\text{Keto acid}}{O=\underset{R_1}{\overset{COO^-}{C}}} + \underset{\text{Amino acid}}{H_3\overset{+}{N}-\underset{R_2}{\overset{COO^-}{C}}-H}$$

FIGURE 14-2 Example of a transamination reaction. The amino acid substrate is converted to a keto acid product, whereas the keto acid cosubstrate is converted to an amino acid product. *PLP,* Pyridoxal 5′-phosphate.

present a simplified scheme for amino acid metabolism. This is particularly true for the metabolism of the amino acid carbon skeletons. Therefore amino acid metabolism will be considered as two themes, a nitrogen theme and a carbon theme.

NITROGEN THEME: REACTIONS INVOLVED IN THE TRANSFER, RELEASE, AND INCORPORATION OF NITROGEN

Some general types of reactions that are involved in the movement of amino groups and fixation of inorganic nitrogen (NH_3 or NH_4^+) are described first, followed by a summary of the fate of the carbon skeletons released by amino acid catabolism. This is followed by a discussion of specific metabolic pathways for each amino acid or related group of amino acids. Finally, the pathways for excretion of nitrogen from the body are summarized. The reader should also refer to Chapter 25 for a discussion of the roles vitamin B_6, vitamin B_{12}, and folate coenzymes play in many of the reactions of amino acid metabolism.

Transamination

The α-amino group may be moved from one carbon chain to another by transamination reactions to form the respective amino and keto acids. Transamination is the most general route for removing nitrogen from an amino acid and transferring it to another carbon skeleton. The transfer of the amino group from an amino acid to a keto acid to form another amino acid is catalyzed by aminotransferases, which are pyridoxal 5′-phosphate (PLP)–dependent enzymes. The general reaction catalyzed by an aminotransferase is shown in Figure 14-2. Most physiologically important aminotransferases have a preferred amino acid/keto acid substrate and use α-ketoglutarate/glutamate as the counter keto acid/amino acid; an example is aspartate aminotransferase, which accepts aspartate or oxaloacetate as substrate and uses glutamate or α-ketoglutarate as cosubstrate. Alanine, aspartate, glutamate, tyrosine, serine, valine, isoleucine, and leucine are actively transaminated in human tissues. Histidine, phenylalanine, methionine, cysteine, glutamine, asparagine, threonine, and glycine also may undergo transamination in human tissues, but these amino acids are metabolized primarily by other types of reactions under normal physiological conditions. In contrast, lysine, proline, tryptophan, and arginine do not participate directly in transamination reactions in mammalian tissues; intermediates in the degradation pathways of lysine, proline, tryptophan, and arginine may, however, undergo transamination for transfer of the amino group. Because α-ketoglutarate is used widely as the acceptor of amino groups in transamination reactions, the α-amino groups of numerous amino acids are funneled through glutamate in the process of amino acid catabolism. Aspartate aminotransferase and alanine aminotransferase are widespread in tissues, and these enzymes allow the movement of amino groups between glutamate/α-ketoglutarate and aspartate/oxaloacetate or alanine/pyruvate.

Deamination

A limited number of reactions in the body are capable of direct deamination of amino acids to release ammonia and form a keto acid. The major reaction in the body in which α-amino groups are released as ammonia is catalyzed by glutamate dehydrogenase. As shown in Figure 14-3, glutamate dehydrogenase brings about the interconversion of glutamate with α-ketoglutarate and ammonia. Glutamate dehydrogenase is mitochondrial and exhibits high activity in liver, kidney cortex, and brain. The fates of the products released by glutamate dehydrogenase are tissue-specific. In liver, the ammonia is mainly incorporated into urea; in the kidney, it can be excreted as urinary ammonium; in the brain, the reaction favors glutamate formation in some cells and ammonia production in others; the ammonia is then incorporated into glutamine.

That glutamate dehydrogenase plays a central role in the release of ammonia from many amino acids represents a paradox, because it is absolutely specific for glutamate. However, the combination of a transamination reaction with the glutamate dehydrogenase reaction results in the release of

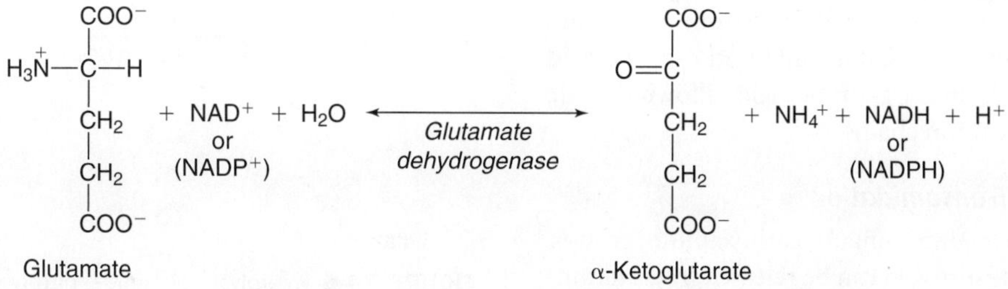

$$\underset{\text{Glutamate}}{H_3\overset{+}{N}-CH(COO^-)-CH_2-CH_2-COO^-} + NAD^+ \text{ or } (NADP^+) + H_2O \xrightleftharpoons{\text{Glutamate dehydrogenase}} \underset{\alpha\text{-Ketoglutarate}}{O=C(COO^-)-CH_2-CH_2-COO^-} + NH_4^+ + NADH \text{ or } (NADPH) + H^+$$

FIGURE 14-3 Interconversion of glutamate and α-ketoglutarate plus ammonia by glutamate dehydrogenase.

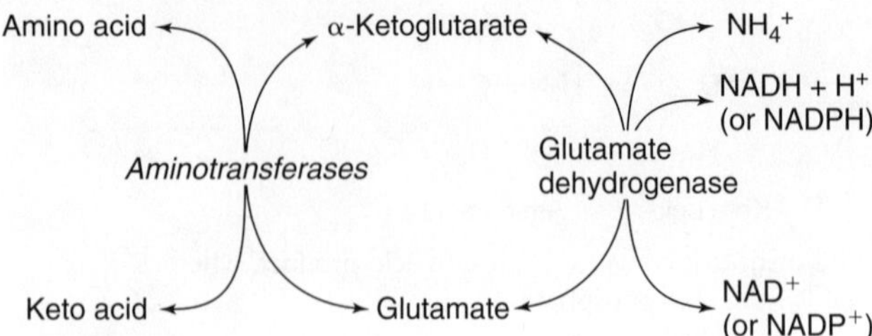

FIGURE 14-4 The equilibrium nature of aminotransferases and glutamate dehydrogenase activities in brain, liver, and kidney maintain ammonia, amino acid, and keto acid levels.

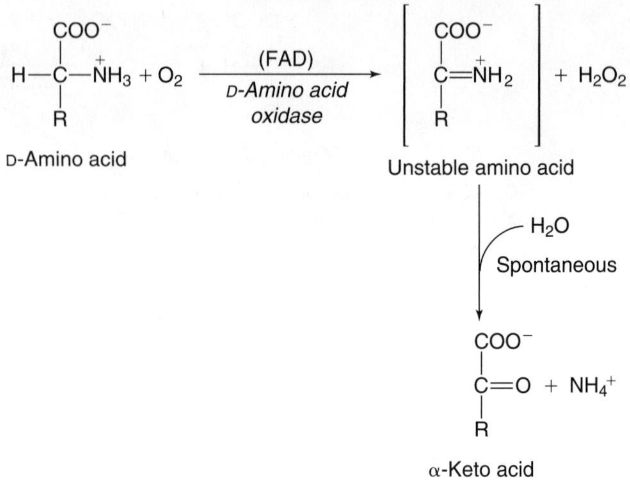

ammonia from any amino acid that undergoes transamination. For example, the combination of alanine aminotransferase with glutamate dehydrogenase removes ammonia from alanine. The combined reaction of these two enzymes is the same as that catalyzed by an alanine dehydrogenase, although no such enzyme occurs in mammals.

Figure 14-4 shows the effect of combining an aminotransferase with glutamate dehydrogenase. Specific reactions in the metabolism of individual amino acids also give rise to free ammonia from the α-amino nitrogen. In particular, ammonia is released from histidine by histidine ammonia lyase (commonly called histidase), from methionine in the process of transsulfuration (in the reaction catalyzed by cystathionine γ-lyase, commonly called cystathionase), from glycine by the glycine cleavage system, and from serine or threonine by serine–threonine dehydratase. In some tissues that lack significant glutamate dehydrogenase activity, such as skeletal muscle, the purine nucleotide cycle can function to release ammonia from adenosine via adenosine deaminase, with the subsequent resynthesis of adenosine using nitrogen obtained from aspartate (Lowenstein, 1972). The net effect of this purine nucleotide cycle is the release of the amino group from aspartate (or indirectly from glutamate following transamination of glutamate with oxaloacetate to form aspartate) as ammonia and with salvage of the aspartate (or glutamate) carbon chain.

L-Amino acid oxidase activity is very low in mammals and is likely of little importance in amino acid catabolism in humans. However, some foodstuffs contain small amounts of D-amino acids, and these appear to be degraded mainly by D-amino acid oxidase, which is expressed at high levels in the kidney (D'Aniello et al., 1993). The overall reaction catalyzed by amino acid oxidase is shown in Figure 14-5. D-Amino acid oxidase is located in peroxisomes; the occurrence of catalase in these organelles provides a means of detoxifying the hydrogen peroxide produced by D-amino acid oxidase. Once a keto acid is formed from a D-amino acid, the keto acid can be transaminated by an L-amino acid aminotransferase to form an L-amino acid, allowing some use of D-amino acid carbon chains.

Deamidation and Transamidation

Glutamine and asparagine contain carboxamide groups, from which the amide nitrogen can be released by glutaminase or asparaginase. The reaction catalyzed by glutaminase is shown in Figure 14-6. The hydrolysis of glutamine to glutamate and ammonia occurs in many tissues and is catalyzed by phosphate-activated glutaminase, which is located in the mitochondria. In most cells, the liberated ammonia is released from the cell without further modification. The glutaminase of liver is a different isozyme from that found in most other tissues; in the liver, the ammonia generated by this reaction may be used by the carbamoyl phosphate synthetase 1 reaction and incorporated into urea. In a similar reaction catalyzed by asparaginase, asparagine is deamidated to yield aspartate plus ammonia. Transfer of the amide group from glutamine also plays an important role in synthetic reactions, including the synthesis of purine and pyrimidine nucleotides, NAD+, and amino sugars, as is discussed later in this chapter.

$$\underset{\text{D-Amino acid}}{H{-}C(COO^-)(R){-}\overset{+}{N}H_3} + O_2 \xrightarrow[\text{D-Amino acid oxidase}]{(FAD)} \underset{\text{Unstable amino acid}}{\left[(COO^-)(R)C{=}\overset{+}{N}H_2 \right]} + H_2O_2$$

$$\xrightarrow[\text{Spontaneous}]{H_2O} \underset{\alpha\text{-Keto acid}}{(COO^-)(R)C{=}O} + NH_4^+$$

FIGURE 14-5 Oxidative deamination of a D-amino acid by D-amino acid oxidase.

Incorporation of Ammonia into the α-Amino Pool

Although most of the interconversions and metabolism of amino acids and other nitrogenous compounds within the body occur with organic forms of nitrogen, primarily amino and amide groups, some reactions can use ammonia. Glutamate dehydrogenase (see Figure 14-3), which was discussed as the mitochondrial enzyme responsible for release of α-amino nitrogen as ammonia, can also function in the reverse direction to incorporate ammonia into glutamate and hence into

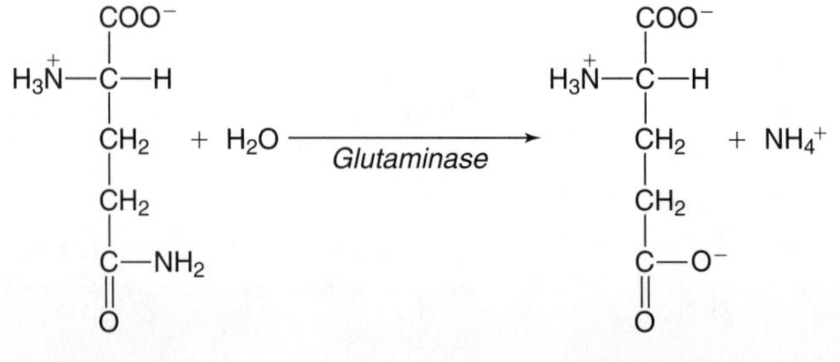

$$\underset{\text{Glutamine}}{H_3\overset{+}{N}{-}CH(COO^-){-}CH_2{-}CH_2{-}C({=}O){-}NH_2} + H_2O \xrightarrow{\text{Glutaminase}} \underset{\text{Glutamate}}{H_3\overset{+}{N}{-}CH(COO^-){-}CH_2{-}CH_2{-}C({=}O){-}O^-} + NH_4^+$$

FIGURE 14-6 Hydrolysis of amide nitrogen from glutamine by glutaminase.

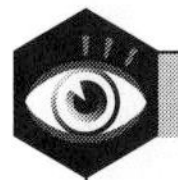

NUTRITION INSIGHT

Functional Roles for D-Amino Acids

One of the most extraordinary advances in amino acid metabolism over the past decade has been the discovery of a functional role for D-serine. D-Amino acids have long been recognized as constituents of the cell walls of some bacteria, and their occurrence in mammalian tissues has been attributed to this source. The existence of a mammalian D-amino acid oxidase has also been understood in terms of the need to catabolize these D-amino acids of bacterial origin. However, new information has made it clear that D-serine plays an important role in brain function by virtue of its role as a coagonist for the *N*-methyl-D-aspartate (NMDA) subtype of glutamate receptors and that D-amino acids are synthesized in the body.

The NMDA subtype of glutamate receptors plays a crucial role in synaptic plasticity and memory. The NMDA receptor is unique in that it requires glutamate and glycine as coagonists for activation. It is now appreciated that D-serine can activate at the glycine site, and it is thought that either glycine or D-serine may act as the coagonist in different situations (Boehning and Snyder, 2003). Mammalian brain, including human brain, contains a PLP-containing serine racemase that can convert L-serine to D-serine; this enzyme is found in astrocytes. The release of D-serine from these cells together with glutamate from presynaptic neurons results in the activation of NMDA receptors on postsynaptic neurons (Boehning and Snyder, 2003).

It has been suggested that D-serine may be an effective therapy for patients suffering from schizophrenia (Yang and Svensson, 2008). D-Aspartate has also been found to occur at significant concentrations in a number of endocrine tissues, in particular the adrenal gland, although no function has yet been definitively ascribed to it (Furuchi and Homma, 2005). Clearly, the occurrence and possible physiological functions of D-amino acids represents a revolution in our thinking on amino acid metabolism as well as an intriguing research front. Could there be other D-amino acids that exert physiological functions but whose roles have not yet been uncovered? The recent identification of D-alanine in beta cells of the rat pancreas raises the possibility of a role for this amino acid in insulin secretion (Morikawa et al., 2007). Further research will be required to answer this and other questions regarding the physiological roles played by D-amino acids.

Thinking Critically

You are interested in exploring the potential role of D-amino acids. As a first step you decide to determine which D-amino acids may be produced in the body from their corresponding L-amino acid. How would you go about doing this?

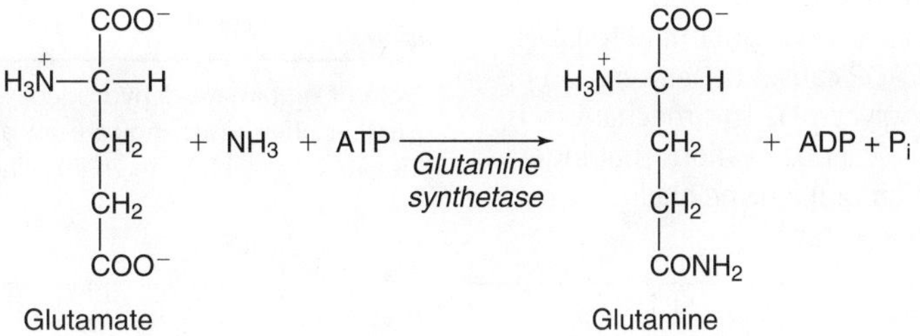

$$\underset{\text{Glutamate}}{{}^{-}OOC-CH_2-CH_2-CH(\overset{+}{N}H_3)-COO^{-}} + NH_3 + ATP \xrightarrow[\text{synthetase}]{\text{Glutamine}} \underset{\text{Glutamine}}{H_2NOC-CH_2-CH_2-CH(\overset{+}{N}H_3)-COO^{-}} + ADP + P_i$$

FIGURE 14-7 Synthesis of glutamine from glutamate and NH_3 by glutamine synthetase.

the α-amino nitrogen pool. This enzyme catalyzes a near-equilibrium reaction in tissues with high activity (particularly the liver) and can operate to either incorporate ammonia into or release it from the α-amino acid pool. The direction of flux depends on the provision and removal of reactants.

Incorporation of Ammonia into Glutamine as an Amide Group

A second major ammonia-fixing reaction in the body is the synthesis of glutamine from glutamate and ammonia; this ATP-requiring reaction is catalyzed by glutamine synthetase and involves the addition of ammonia to form a carboxamide group from the γ-carboxyl group of glutamate (Figure 14-7). Glutamine, which has two nitrogenous groups, plays an important role in the transfer of nitrogen between cells and tissues, and glutamine synthetase activity is particularly high in muscle, adipose tissue, lung, brain, and the perivenous parenchymal cells of the liver (i.e., the cells closest to the terminal hepatic venules by which blood exits the liver; see Chapter 12, Figure 12-11).

Asparagine synthetase catalyzes a similar reaction by which asparagine is synthesized from aspartate, but this enzyme can use either ammonia or glutamine as the substrate for the amidation reaction. Compared to the glutamine synthetase reaction, the asparagine synthetase reaction plays a minor role in overall nitrogen transfer in the body.

Incorporation of Ammonia into Carbamoyl Phosphate for Formation of Urea Cycle Intermediates and Urea

Although it does not result in incorporation of inorganic nitrogen into the amino acid pool (other than into the guanidinium group of arginine), carbamoyl phosphate synthetase 1 incorporates ammonia into carbamoyl phosphate for addition to ornithine for citrulline production (Figure 14-8). Carbamoyl phosphate synthetase 1 is found in the

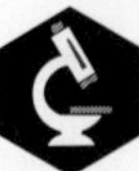

CLINICAL CORRELATION

Glutamate Dehydrogenase and the Hyperinsulinism/Hyperammonemia Syndrome

It has long been known that insulin secretion is increased by ingestion of a protein-rich meal. Leucine plays a critical role in this phenomenon through its ability to activate glutamate dehydrogenase (GDH) in the pancreatic beta cells. Insulin secretion is sensitive to the beta cell ATP/ADP ratio. Increased ATP/ADP closes an ATP-gated K^+ channel, resulting in membrane depolarization that causes an influx of Ca^{2+} into the cytosol. The consequently increased Ca^{2+} level stimulates insulin secretion. Although glucose metabolism is the principal source of beta cell ATP and hence the principal effector of insulin secretion, amino acid oxidation, particularly that of glutamate and glutamine, can also contribute to the increased ATP/ADP ratio. Unlike hepatic GDH, beta cell GDH does not function close to its thermodynamic equilibrium but is poised to act in the direction of glutamate oxidation. Leucine, an allosteric activator of GDH, further increases GDH activity and hence ATP production.

The importance of beta cell GDH in insulin secretion was highlighted by the discovery of the hyperinsulinism/hyperammonemia (HI/HA) syndrome, the second most common form of congenital hypoglycemia. GTP is an allosteric inhibitor of GDH. However, children with the HI/HA syndrome have a GDH mutation in which GTP is a much weaker inhibitor. The result is a gain-of-function mutation (i.e., one that results in a marked increase in GDH activity) (Stanley, 2009). Oxidation of both glutamate and glutamine is increased, because decreased glutamate levels will diminish the end-product inhibition of glutaminase and allow the glutaminase reaction to feed additional glutamate to GDH. The resulting increase in ATP/ADP causes hypersecretion of insulin with consequent hypoglycemia. This mechanism is entirely consistent with the clinical observations that ingestion of a protein-rich meal or an oral leucine challenge can provoke hypoglycemia in these patients.

Thinking Critically

GDH is highly active in the liver, in fact so active that its reaction is poised very close to thermodynamic equilibrium. Would you expect the gain-of-function mutation of GDH to bring about significant alterations in hepatic metabolism? Explain.

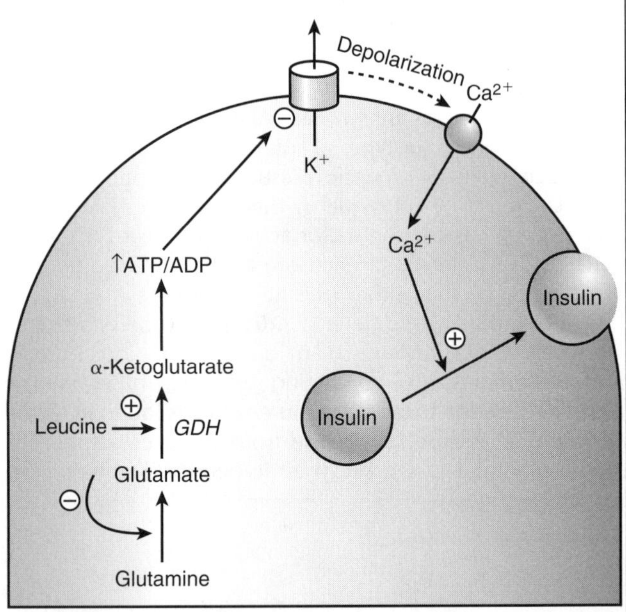

Role of glutamate dehydrogenase in insulin secretion. The encircled positive signs indicate an activation whereas the encircled negative signs indicate an inhibition.

$$NH_3 + CO_2 + 2\,ATP \xrightarrow[\textit{Carbamoyl phosphate synthetase 1}]{N\text{-Acetylglutamate}} H_2N{-}\overset{O}{\overset{\|}{C}}{-}O{-}\overset{O}{\overset{\|}{P}}(O^-){-}O^- + 2\,ADP + P_i$$

Carbamoyl phosphate

FIGURE 14-8 Synthesis of carbamoyl phosphate from NH_3 and CO_2 in mitochondria of hepatocytes and enterocytes.

mitochondria of liver and small intestinal cells. *N*-Acetylglutamate is an obligatory activator for carbamoyl phosphate synthetase 1. Within the liver, this citrulline is produced as an integral part of the urea cycle, but in the intestine the citrulline may be released into the circulation for further metabolism to arginine in the kidney. The urea cycle is discussed more completely in a later section, "Nitrogen Excretion."

CARBON THEME: METABOLISM OF THE CARBON CHAINS OF AMINO ACIDS

The use of amino acids as fuel requires the removal of the amino group and the conversion of the carbon chain to an intermediate that can enter the central pathways of fuel metabolism. The processes of amino acid catabolism, excretion of nitrogen as urea or ammonia, conversion of amino acid carbon chains to glucose or other fuels, and the eventual complete oxidation of the amino acid carbon skeleton are all metabolically interrelated.

Catabolism of Amino Acid Carbon Chains

The rate of amino acid catabolism varies with amino acid supply. When amino acids are abundant, as after a meal or during conditions of net proteolysis (e.g., in uncontrolled diabetes, hypercatabolic states, or starvation), the extent of amino acid catabolism increases markedly. Conversely, when the diet is adequate in energy but deficient

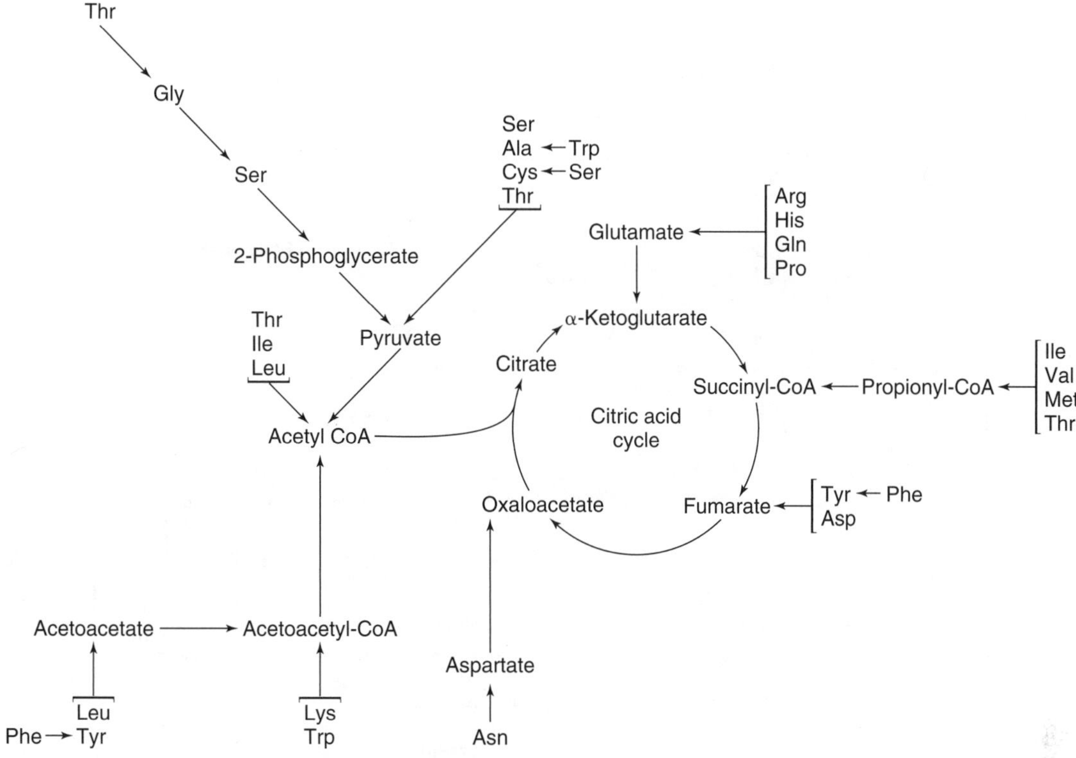

FIGURE 14-9 Formation of amphibolic intermediates from the carbon skeletons of amino acids.

in amino acids, the catabolism of amino acids is reduced significantly.

The points at which the carbon skeletons of various amino acids enter central pathways of catabolism are shown in Figure 14-9. The carbon skeletons of most amino acids are metabolized to glycolytic or citric acid cycle intermediates. Once the carbon skeleton of an amino acid enters central pathways of fuel metabolism, it may be further oxidized for energy or used for synthesis of other compounds, such as dispensable amino acids, glucose and glycogen, cholesterol, or triacylglycerols.

It is often stated that amino acids are oxidized in the liver, which is the major site of amino acid catabolism and urea production. In addition, similar statements are made about amino acid catabolism in other tissues, such as glutamine oxidation in the small intestine or branched-chain amino acid oxidation in the muscle. Such statements seem to imply that the amino acids are completely oxidized to CO_2 and H_2O. Jungas and colleagues (1992) calculated that the amount of energy that would be produced by complete catabolism of amino acids at a rate equivalent to their net uptake by the liver would exceed the total energy used by the liver. Thus amino acids not used for protein or peptide synthesis in the liver are only partially oxidized within the liver, and the carbon skeletons are converted to glucose, glycogen, carbon chains of dispensable amino acids, lipids, and small amounts of ketone bodies for use by various tissues. Like the liver, many other tissues that utilize amino acids for energy do not completely catabolize them.

Amino acids are quantitatively important as a fuel for the liver, small intestine, and other specialized cells, such as reticulocytes and cells of the immune system. It has been estimated that liver derives at least half of its ATP requirement from the partial oxidation of amino acids, and that the small intestinal jejunum may derive up to 80% of its fuel needs from amino acids. The intestinal jejunum uses glutamine, glutamate, and aspartate taken up from the luminal contents (digesta), as well as arterial glutamine (Reeds and Burrin, 2001). Although branched-chain amino acid oxidation occurs, at least partially, in muscle, nonprotein fuels are quantitatively much more important for muscle; muscle releases nitrogen primarily as glutamine and alanine (Darmaun and Dechelotte, 1991; Elia and Livesey, 1983). The kidneys consume large amounts of glutamine and significant but lesser amounts of glycine (Tizianello et al., 1982). The kidneys also release serine. The net uptake of amino acids by the liver (from the arterial and portal circulation) differs substantially from the dietary input. In particular, the uptakes of alanine and serine are high, whereas net uptakes of aspartate, glutamate, and the branched-chain amino acids are very low, and the liver may actually exhibit net glutamate release. Although the gastrointestinal tract extracts large amounts of glutamine from the circulation and also metabolizes dietary glutamine (and glutamate), there is evidence that human liver also takes up considerable amounts of glutamine (Watford, 2000; Elia, 1993; Felig et al., 1973).

Gluconeogenesis from Amino Acids

In the liver, amino acid catabolism is accompanied by both ureagenesis and gluconeogenesis, which is the synthesis of glucose from nonglucose precursors. Amino acids are an important source of carbon skeletons for gluconeogenesis.

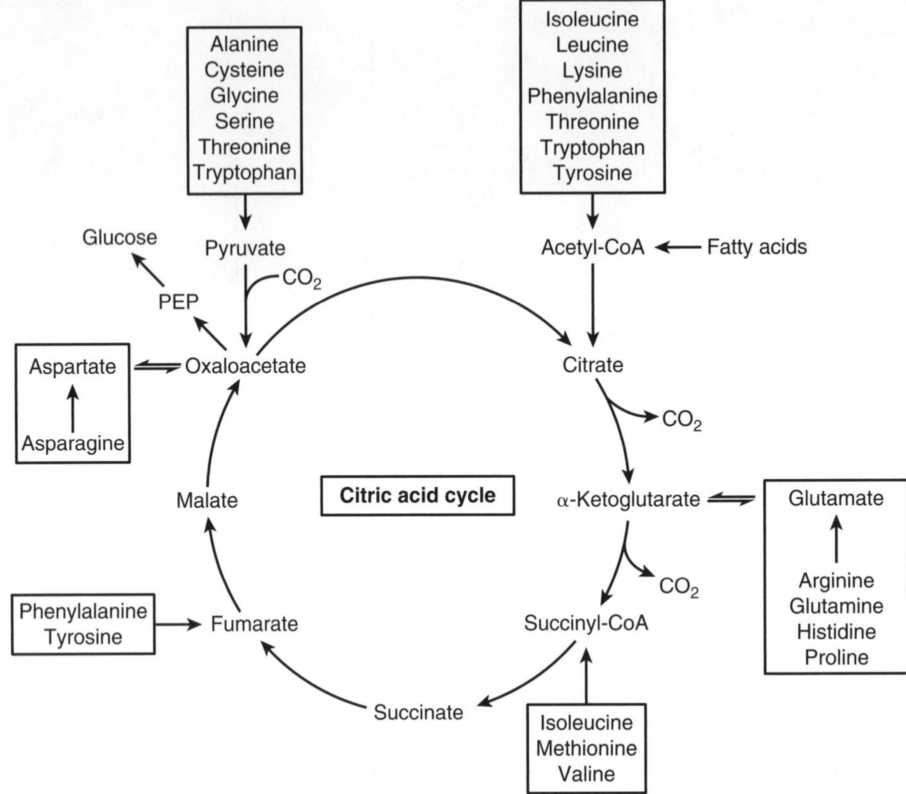

FIGURE 14-10 The metabolic relationship of amino acids to the citric acid (Krebs) cycle determines whether they are glucogenic or not.

Although gluconeogenesis in the liver has traditionally been considered to operate predominantly during fasting or starvation in response to hypoglycemia and breakdown of muscle protein, it is now apparent that gluconeogenesis also functions postprandially while amino acids are being absorbed and processed. Estimates of glucose synthesis from amino acid carbon in the fed human are 50 to 60 g of glucose per 100 g of protein partially oxidized (Jungas et al., 1992). Therefore ureagenesis and gluconeogenesis can be viewed as operating together to produce glucose (or glycogen), urea, and CO_2 from amino acids whenever the liver is processing amino acids.

It is important to understand why many amino acids are glucogenic whereas others (i.e., leucine and lysine) are not. Although gluconeogenesis is a critical metabolic pathway, in some ways it may be regarded as a threat to the citric acid cycle. This is because gluconeogenesis withdraws a molecule of oxaloacetate from the cycle. If this continued to take place without any compensation, it is evident that the citric acid cycle would cease to function, with lethal consequences. Gluconeogenesis may occur only from those amino acids that, in their metabolism, produce intermediates of the cycle that may be converted to oxaloacetate, thus providing an additional cycle intermediate and permitting the withdrawal of a molecule for gluconeogenesis. The provision of new cycle intermediates is referred to as "anaplerosis." The metabolism of leucine or lysine does not have an anaplerotic effect. Although carbon from these amino acids enters the citric acid cycle as acetyl-CoA, which reacts with oxaloacetate to produce citrate, this reaction does not expand the pool of cycle intermediates. One intermediate (oxaloacetate) is used up to produce another (citrate); it does not provide an additional molecule of cycle intermediate (Figure 14-10).

A general overview of the processes by which the liver converts amino acid carbon chains to the "universal fuel" glucose and simultaneously incorporates the nitrogen groups into urea for excretion is shown in Figure 14-11. This scheme demonstrates that when a balanced mixture of amino acids is being oxidized, most of the glucogenic carbon will be carried out of the mitochondria as aspartate, which is also the immediate donor of one of the two nitrogens for urea synthesis.

Energetics of Amino Acid Oxidation

Jungas and colleagues (1992) detailed the processes involved in amino acid oxidation in liver and calculated that the partial oxidation of dietary amino acids provides sufficient energy to support the ATP requirements for synthesis of both glucose and urea; hence the liver does not depend on oxidation of fuels other than amino acids to provide ATP to support these processes. On the basis of the detailed calculations of Jungas and colleagues (1992), complete oxidation of 1 g of meat protein by the body yields a net gain of approximately 195 mmol of ATP (an average of 21.5 moles of ATP per mole of amino acids). They also estimated that on a whole-body basis, approximately 35% of this net ATP production results from amino acid oxidation in muscle and small intestine, 60% from oxidation of the glucose generated

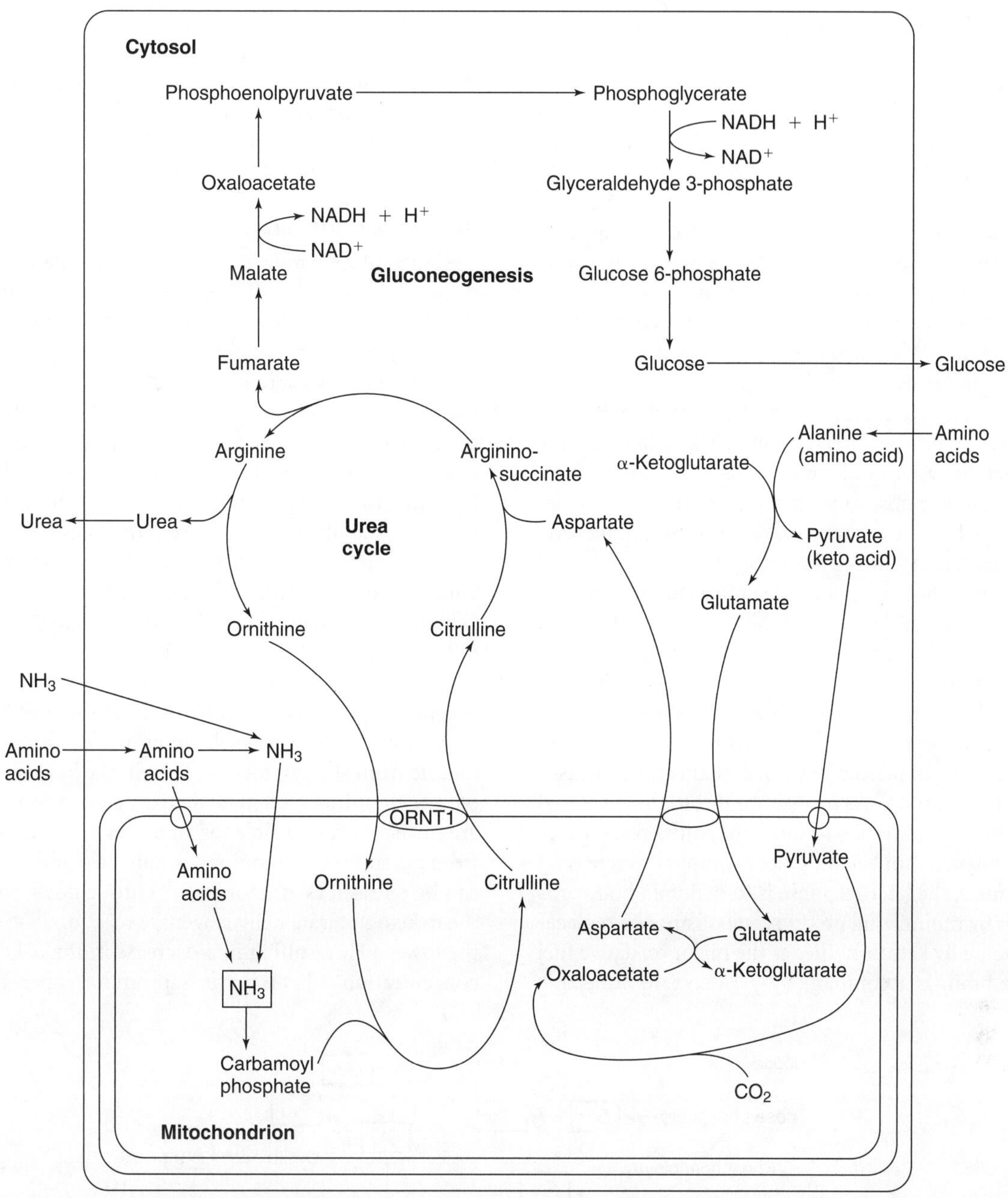

FIGURE 14-11 Metabolism of amino acids by the liver, including the partial oxidation of amino acids, gluconeogenesis, and ureagenesis. Although not shown in the figure, α-ketoglutarate generated in the mitochondria can be transported from the mitochondria to replenish the cytosolic α-ketoglutarate pool.

by hepatic gluconeogenesis, and 5% from oxidation of acetoacetate generated from amino acid carbon chains.

Regulation of Amino Acid Oxidation and Gluconeogenesis

The linked pathways of amino acid oxidation, gluconeogenesis, and ureagenesis are predominantly expressed in the periportal parenchymal cells (cells that surround the terminal portal venule and hepatic arteriole by which blood enters the liver) rather than in the perivenous cells. These processes are active in both the fed (protein-containing meal) and the starved states. Glucagon, glucocorticoids, and thyroid hormones all increase the rates of amino acid catabolism as well as ureagenesis and gluconeogenesis in the liver, whereas insulin may decrease these metabolic processes. Many amino acid catabolic enzymes exhibit greater activity under conditions that result in higher rates of amino acid catabolism. Some of these changes involve responses to hormonal signals, whereas others seem to be specific responses to high concentrations of amino acid substrates. Glucocorticoids, catecholamines, and cytokines—which are elevated during stress, infection, and trauma—play a role in increasing net muscle protein breakdown and thus the availability of amino acids to the liver for gluconeogenesis.

In the fed state, dietary glutamine, glutamate, and aspartate (which together account for ~20% of dietary protein) are metabolized within the enterocyte with the resultant production of alanine. In addition, the portal-drained viscera also extract glutamine from the arterial circulation, even during protein feeding, and metabolize this to alanine. Therefore the portal blood contains higher amounts of alanine but lower amounts of glutamine, glutamate, and aspartate when compared with the amino acid pattern of dietary protein. Because the intestine catabolizes glutamine, glutamate, and aspartate to alanine, which is subsequently released and taken up by the liver, the gluconeogenic potential of amino acid carbon chains is largely conserved despite the intestine's use of these amino acids as fuels (Watford, 1994). Uptake of alanine by the liver exceeds gut release (with additional alanine originating from the muscle and other tissues), whereas hepatic uptake of branched-chain amino acids is substantially less than gut output, such that the systemic blood levels of valine, leucine, and isoleucine rise in response to protein ingestion. There is a net uptake of these branched-chain amino acids by extrahepatic tissues (muscle, brain) during the absorptive period.

In the starved state, large amounts of glutamine and alanine are released from muscle, and these can be used as fuels or substrates for gluconeogenesis. The increases in hepatic removal of alanine and in hepatic gluconeogenesis in early starvation or uncontrolled diabetes are probably related to a rise in glucagon levels and a fall in insulin levels. A rise in the concentrations of plasma branched-chain amino acids is noted in early starvation and probably is due to the decreased insulin levels of starvation. Although the initial response to starvation is to maintain hepatic glucose output by increasing gluconeogenesis, the later response is to maintain body protein reserves by minimizing protein catabolism. The replacement of glucose by ketone bodies as the major oxidative fuel used by the brain is accompanied by a decrease in hepatic gluconeogenesis and urinary nitrogen excretion (particularly as urea, such that the ratio of ammonium to urea in the urine markedly increases in prolonged starvation). The availability of ketone bodies as a fuel for muscle and other tissues seems to contribute to protein conservation by limiting amino acid (alanine) availability for gluconeogenesis.

Acid–Base Considerations of Amino Acid Oxidation

Amino acid oxidation generates nonvolatile or fixed acids, primarily sulfuric acid (SO_4^{2-} + 2 H^+) from catabolism of the sulfur-containing amino acids methionine and cysteine. The body can compensate for some of this excess fixed anion by increasing its excretion of dietary phosphate as $H_2PO_4^-$ (titratable acidity) or by consuming HCO_3^- (bicarbonate) generated from the metabolism of dietary carboxylate anions (e.g., malate or citrate). The kidney excretes additional acid by generating NH_3 from glutamine (and to a lesser extent glycine) catabolism and then excreting it as NH_4^+ (net acid). This latter process also produces HCO_3^- (net base) from the amino acid carbon skeleton and releases it into the renal vein, thus regenerating any HCO_3^- that was consumed in the initial buffering of the hydrogen ions. Note that ureagenesis in the liver is not capable of adjusting acid–base balance, because the process consumes both HCO_3^- and NH_4^+.

Metabolic acidosis results in an increased release of glutamine from skeletal muscle. Within the kidney, the actions of mitochondrial glutamate dehydrogenase and glutaminase are primarily responsible for an increase in NH_3 production from glutamine. Glutamine contains two amine groups that can be released as ammonia. In acute acidosis, flux through the α-ketoglutarate dehydrogenase reaction is stimulated by the lower pH, resulting in a decrease in the α-ketoglutarate concentration which in turn promotes operation of the

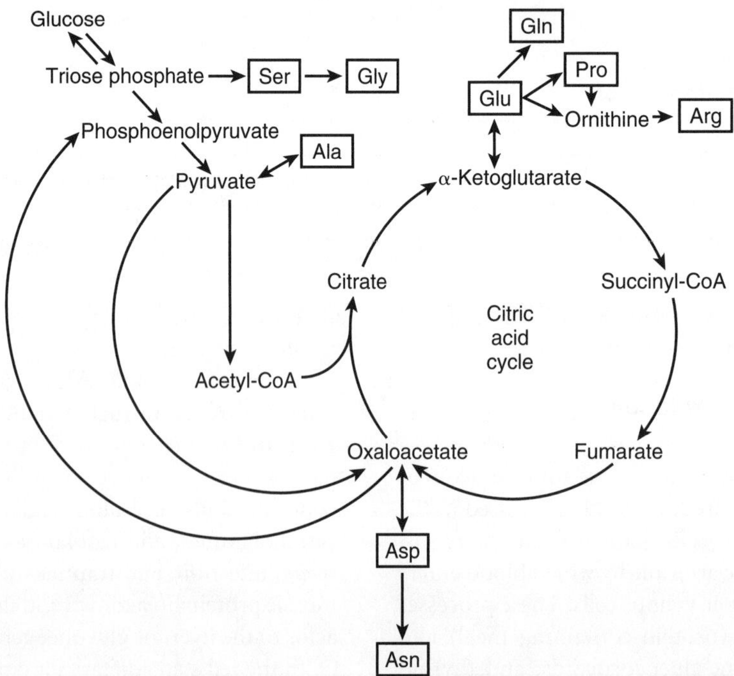

FIGURE 14-12 Synthesis of dispensable amino acids from the carbon skeletons of amphibolic intermediates.

glutamate dehydrogenase reaction in the direction of glutamate conversion to α-ketoglutarate plus NH_3. The glutamate/glutamine carbon skeleton is then further metabolized to bicarbonate and, in some species, glucose. Longer-term regulation during metabolic acidosis involves increased synthesis of the key kidney enzymes, such as glutaminase and phosphoenolpyruvate carboxykinase, and key transporters, such as the SNAT3 (*SLC38A3*) glutamine transporter (Ibrahim et al., 2008; Busque and Wagner, 2009). The increased expression of these proteins appears to be mediated mainly by an increase in mRNA stability through the presence of pH-response elements in their mRNAs. During acidosis, the association of RNA-binding proteins with these pH-responsive elements serves to stabilize the mRNAs, leading to increased levels of expression.

SYNTHESIS OF DISPENSABLE AMINO ACIDS

For the synthesis of the carbon chains of dispensable amino acids, glucose or glucogenic substrates (such as the carbon skeletons of most amino acids) are required. Pyruvate or other three-carbon glycolytic intermediates serve as substrates for synthesis of alanine, serine, and glycine. Oxaloacetate, a 4-carbon α-keto acid, is the carbon skeleton of aspartate and asparagine. The 5-carbon α-keto acid, α-ketoglutarate, or its metabolites, provides the carbon skeleton for glutamate, glutamine, proline, and arginine (Figure 14-12). Nitrogenous groups are added to these carbon chains by direct transamination of pyruvate, 3-phosphohydroxypyruvate, oxaloacetate, and α-ketoglutarate with other amino acids; by amidation of glutamate and aspartate; and by the formation of metabolites of pyrroline 5-carboxylate (Figure 14-13), as is discussed in more detail in the section on proline and arginine. The synthesis of dispensable amino acids frequently involves the cooperation of a number of tissues. This is referred to as interorgan amino acid metabolism.

INTERORGAN AMINO ACID METABOLISM

Many metabolic processes and pathways involve more than one organ. This is particularly evident in amino acid metabolism. Such interorgan traffic requires the presence of the appropriate enzymes in the different tissues as well as tissue-specific expression of transporters that permit the release of a pathway intermediate from one tissue and its uptake by another. Free amino acids are the principal vehicles for this interorgan metabolism, but small peptides may also play a minor role and proteins, particularly albumin, play a substantial role. The liver of the well-nourished adult human produces some 20 g of albumin per day, and in steady state conditions, a comparable quantity of albumin is catabolized, largely by fibroblasts. Therefore each day some 20 g of free amino acids are made available to extrahepatic tissues as a result of albumin turnover. Interorgan amino acid metabolism is often identified by measuring arteriovenous (A-V) differences across organs of interest. It should be appreciated that the A-V difference is often quite small compared with the arterial or venous amino acid concentrations, so that it is susceptible to appreciable analytical errors. In this regard it should be emphasized that many small uptakes or outputs of amino acids across tissues have probably not been identified; in general, the ones we know of tend to be relatively large.

Across the fed gut there is, of course, a substantial outflow of amino acids as a result of protein digestion and the subsequent amino acid absorption. There is also an uptake of arterial glutamine and a marked outflow of alanine and citrulline. The carbon and nitrogen in alanine have different metabolic

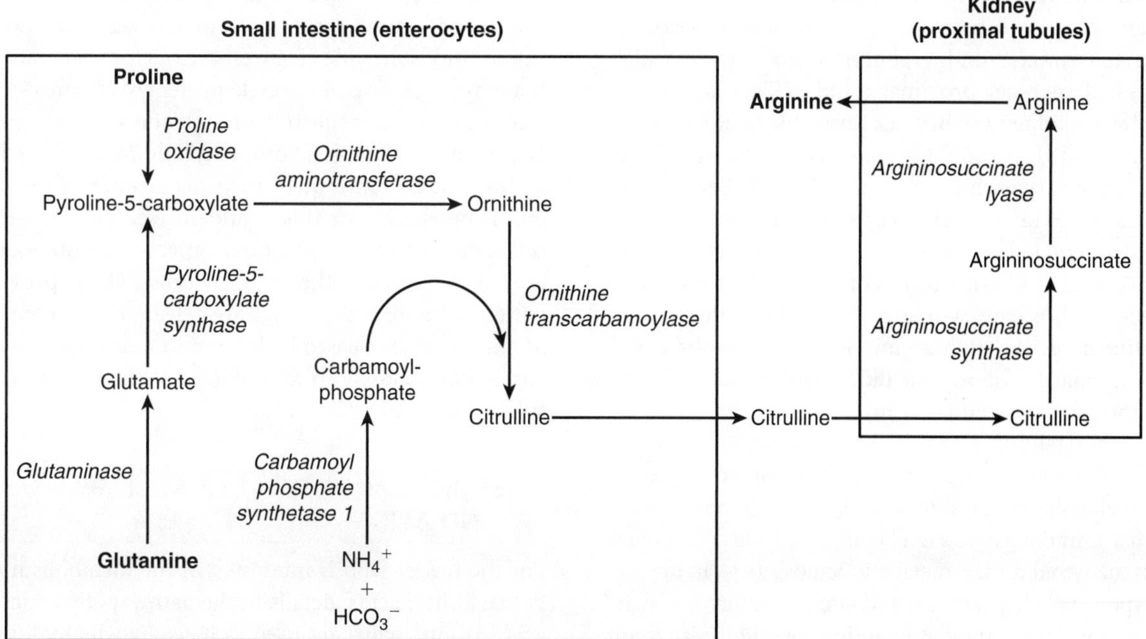

FIGURE 14-13 Intestinal/renal axis for the endogenous synthesis of arginine in adult animals.

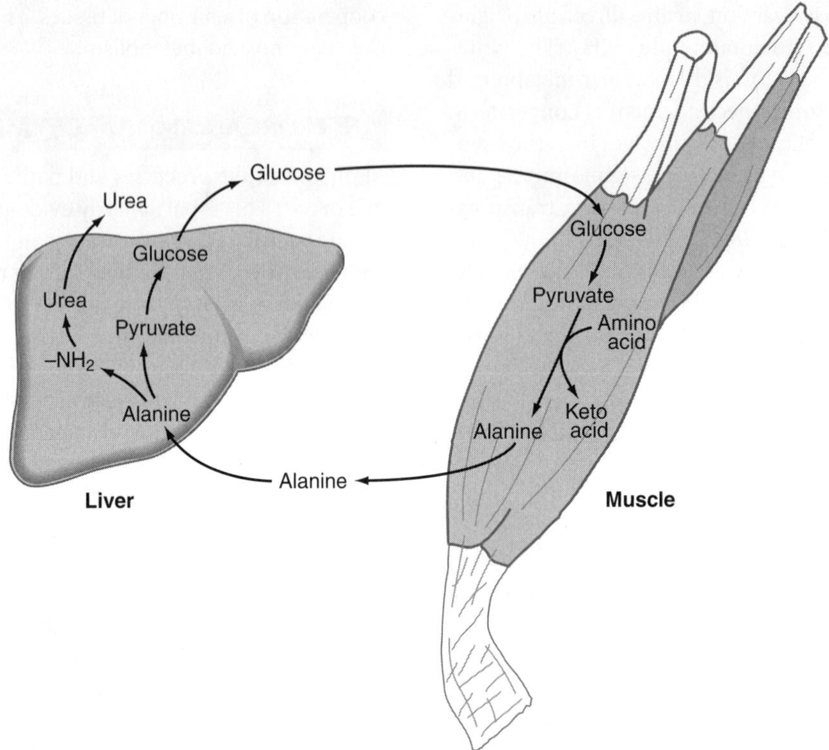

FIGURE 14-14 The glucose–alanine cycle for amino group transport. The carbon chain is cycled between glucose and pyruvate.

origins. The carbon skeleton arises from pyruvate produced by intestinal glycolysis, whereas the nitrogen is provided from glutamine catabolism. The citrulline arises from both proline and glutamine metabolism and requires the expression, in enterocytes, of a particular set of enzymes. These include proline oxidase, glutaminase, and pyrroline-5-carboxylate synthase, as well as a number of enzymes usually associated with the urea cycle: carbamoyl phosphate synthetase 1, *N*-acetylglutamate synthase, and ornithine transcarbamoylase. Citrulline released by the intestine is removed by the kidney and converted to arginine by the action of argininosuccinate synthase and argininosuccinate lyase which are expressed in renal proximal tubules. This arginine is released by the kidney and becomes available to other tissues (see Figure 14-13). It should be emphasized that metabolic processes may vary with developmental stage (Bertolo and Burrin, 2008). Figure 14-13 reflects the situation in adult animals. In neonatal animals, glutamine is a poor precursor for arginine synthesis because of very low expression of pyrroline-5-carboxylate synthase. In addition, the neonatal intestine expresses both argininosuccinate synthase and argininosuccinate lyase so that the entire pathway of arginine synthesis occurs in this organ.

Kidneys also take up glycine and convert it to serine, which is released. Kidneys take up glutamine to facilitate the excretion of metabolically produced acids as their ammonium salts. Renal ammoniagenesis is a highly adaptable process that increases manyfold during metabolic acidosis (e.g., in uncontrolled type 1 diabetes mellitus) and after ingestion of a high-protein diet when substantial quantities of sulfuric acid are produced from the catabolism of the sulfur-containing amino acids. The kidney acquires its glutamine from muscle and liver, both of which produce glutamine via glutamine synthetase.

Skeletal muscle is a major site for the oxidation of a substantial fraction of dietary branched-chain amino acids. It also releases substantial quantities of alanine and glutamine. As in the intestine, the carbon and nitrogens of alanine have different origins. Much of the nitrogen is provided from the branched-chain amino acids, whereas the carbon skeleton arises from glucose via glycolysis (see Figure 14-14). Glutamine is released from muscle as a result of the catabolism of a variety of amino acids, in particular glutamate, aspartate, valine, and isoleucine (Figure 14-15). Upon starvation there is a marked increase in muscle proteolysis to provide amino acids to the liver as substrates for gluconeogenesis. However, alanine and glutamine comprise fully 50% of the released amino acids, even though their occurrence in muscle protein is nowhere near this abundant (see Table 14-1). Their release in such large quantities reflects a substantial amino acid metabolism within muscle cells, which provides the pattern of amino acids that are released. The composition of amino acids released by human muscle during starvation corresponds closely to that of amino acids taken up by the splanchnic tissues (Felig, 1975).

METABOLISM OF THE DISPENSABLE AMINO ACIDS

For the reader who is interested in the metabolism of individual amino acids, details of the pathways by which amino acid carbon chains are used as fuels, by which amino acids are used for synthesis of numerous nonprotein compounds,

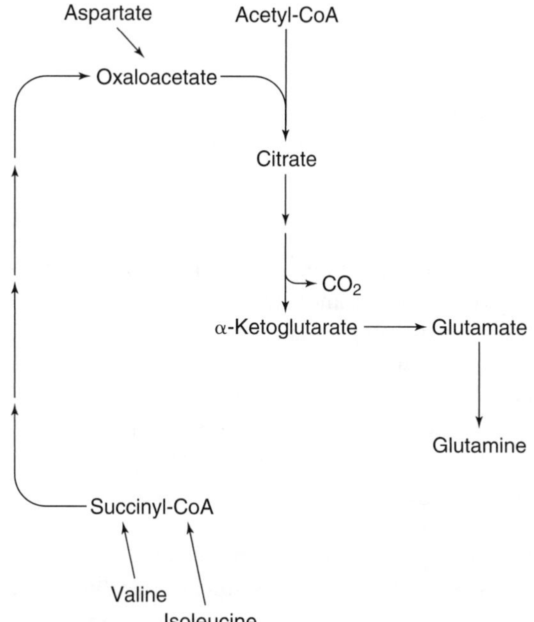

FIGURE 14-15 Proposed pathway for the de novo synthesis of glutamine in skeletal muscle. The carbon-chain precursors are aspartate and branched-chain amino acids.

and by which dispensable amino acids are synthesized are discussed in the subsequent sections, beginning with a discussion of the dispensable amino acids. To the extent possible, an effort has been made to describe the pathways and interorgan fluxes that are most significant in humans.

ALANINE

The only reactions that use alanine in mammalian tissues are those involving its incorporation into proteins and its participation in transamination. In skeletal muscle, liver, and small intestine, alanine aminotransferase catalyzes a reaction close to equilibrium, and alanine flux increases when a high-carbohydrate diet is ingested and tissues are using glucose as a major fuel (Yang et al., 1986).

As already mentioned, alanine is a major amino acid that is released from muscle and small intestine. The muscle normally releases large quantities of alanine in the postabsorptive, or basal, state, and this release of alanine from muscle is increased during early starvation. However, the release of alanine by muscle is reduced when branched-chain amino acids from a protein-containing meal are abundantly available as a fuel for muscle, in which case glutamine is the major amino acid released by muscle. The carbon skeleton of alanine is derived primarily from glucose in muscle; the nitrogen (as well as a small amount of the carbon in alanine) is derived from catabolism of branched-chain and other amino acids in muscle. The catabolism of dietary glutamate, aspartate, and glutamine, together with arterial glutamine, in the enterocytes of the small intestine results in the synthesis and release of lactate, pyruvate, and alanine. Because the enterocytes only partially oxidize the amino acids they use as fuels, the gluconeogenic potential of the amino acids is conserved within the body (Watford, 1994).

Alanine is removed from the circulation primarily by the liver, which uses the alanine for ureagenesis and gluconeogenesis (Jungas et al., 1992; Felig, 1975). Alanine alone accounts for more than 25% of the total amino acids, and hence nitrogen, removed from the blood by the liver. It should be noted, however, that most of the production of alanine in muscle, especially during exercise when glycolytic activity is high, does not represent a net contribution of alanine to body glucose, because most of the pyruvate for alanine synthesis in muscle is derived from glycolysis of glucose. The role of the glucose–alanine cycle in transporting nitrogen to the liver for ureagenesis is shown in Figure 14-14. This cycle transports nitrogen out of the muscle but does not generate any new gluconeogenic substrates. In contrast, the synthesis and release of glutamine by skeletal muscle does represent the provision of new gluconeogenic substrate (Nurjhan et al., 1995). Although not definitively known, because of problems in sampling the portal vein in humans, there is evidence that approximately 30% to 40% of the glutamine removed by the splanchnic bed (portal-drained viscera) is taken up directly by the liver (Elia, 1993; Felig et al., 1973). As indicated previously, intestinal glutamine catabolism also results in the synthesis of alanine, which is then taken up by the liver for gluconeogenesis.

GLUTAMATE, GLUTAMINE, AND ASPARTATE

Glutamate, glutamine, and aspartate play central roles in nitrogen metabolism within the body.

Roles of Glutamate, Glutamine, and Aspartate in the Movement of Amino Acid Nitrogen and Carbon in the Body

Glutamate and aspartate are involved in numerous reactions, such as the transfer of α-amino acid nitrogen in the synthesis of dispensable amino acids, purines, and pyrimidines. Most glutamate and aspartate metabolism is intracellular, and the turnover of the plasma pools is relatively slow (Battezzati et al., 1995). Glutamine, in contrast, not only plays a major role in intracellular metabolism (e.g., pyrimidine and purine synthesis), but also is the major transport form of nitrogen among tissues via the circulation.

Glutamate and aspartate are interconvertible with two citric acid cycle intermediates, α-ketoglutarate and oxaloacetate, respectively. Hence, like alanine, they have carbon skeletons that play central roles as amphibolic intermediates (serving both anabolic and catabolic purposes) in metabolism. Aspartate aminotransferase catalyzes the interconversion of aspartate and oxaloacetate, and the two isozymes of aspartate aminotransferase, cytosolic and mitochondrial, are important in the movement of carbon and reducing equivalents across mitochondrial membranes by the malate–aspartate shuttle. In addition, during ureagenesis and gluconeogenesis in the liver, as shown in Figure 14-11, aspartate carries carbon and reducing equivalents for hepatic gluconeogenesis as well as nitrogen for ureagenesis from the mitochondria to the cytosol. Glutamate and α-ketoglutarate are interconverted by a number of other aminotransferases, especially alanine aminotransferase and branched-chain aminotransferase, in addition to aspartate aminotransferase. In some tissues, glutamate is also interconverted with its keto acid via the mitochondrial glutamate dehydrogenase reaction (see Figure 14-3).

In addition to the α-carboxylic acid group, aspartate and glutamate (or aspartic acid and glutamic acid) possess a second carboxylic acid group. The β-carboxylic acid group of aspartate and the γ-carboxylic acid group of glutamate can be amidated to form amino acids with carboxamide groups; these amino acids are asparagine and glutamine, respectively. Their synthesis was described previously in the discussion of the assimilation of inorganic nitrogen (see Figure 14-7).

Glutamine catabolism occurs predominantly by the hydrolysis of the amide group from the carboxamide, a process called deamidation. A mitochondrial enzyme, glutaminase, catalyzes the reaction, which results in the production of glutamate and ammonia (see Figure 14-6). Asparagine catabolism occurs in the same manner in a reaction catalyzed by asparaginase; aspartate and ammonia are released. Glutamine also plays an important role as an amide group donor for synthesis of compounds such as nucleotides and amino sugars. The reaction involved in the donation of glutamine's carboxamide nitrogen is called a transamidation reaction. Transamidation reactions result in the conversion of glutamine to glutamate.

Tissue-Specific Metabolism of Glutamine

Glutamine is the most abundant free α-amino acid in the body, which contains approximately 80 g of free glutamine; more than 95% of this is located intracellularly. The branched-chain amino acids are a major source of carbon and nitrogen for glutamine synthesis (as well as of nitrogen for alanine synthesis) by muscle. In addition to branched-chain amino acids, there is evidence that muscle also takes up some glutamate from the circulation. During the fed state, large amounts of dietary branched-chain amino acids are taken up and catabolized in the muscle. During times of net proteolysis, the branched-chain amino acids from muscle proteins are catabolized within this tissue. In both cases, the released glutamine effectively transports carbon and nitrogen that originated from the branched-chain amino acids to other tissues, such as small intestine, immune cells, kidney, and liver.

The source of the carbon skeleton for net glutamine synthesis in muscle is not firmly established, but the propionyl-CoA derived from valine and isoleucine metabolism may be carboxylated to yield succinyl-CoA. This product is then converted to oxaloacetate, which in turn may condense with acetyl-CoA to form citrate, and citrate can be converted to α-ketoglutarate, as shown in Figure 14-15. This can be transaminated to glutamate (probably in concert with the transamination of a branched-chain amino acid to form a branched-chain keto acid) and amidated to form glutamine by glutamine synthetase (using ammonia released from glutamate or other amino acids). Thus glutamine seems to transport branched-chain amino acid carbons as well as nitrogen out of the muscle. Net synthesis of glutamine also occurs in the lungs, adipose tissue, brain, and, under certain conditions, in the liver.

In the healthy individual, the major site of glutamine catabolism is the small intestine, where glutamine is the principal respiratory fuel of enterocytes during the postabsorptive state (Reeds and Burrin, 2001). The catabolism of glutamine in the intestine results in the production of CO_2, alanine, pyruvate, and lactate from the carbon skeleton of glutamine, and of ammonia and alanine from the amide and amino groups. Proline and citrulline are additional products of intestinal glutamine/glutamate catabolism.

Thymocytes, lymphocytes, and macrophages all use glutamine as the principal respiratory fuel, and these cells show increased rates of glutamine utilization when they are activated. In these cells of the immune system, the major carbon end product is aspartate, with little or no production of alanine, proline, or citrulline.

Glutamine plays an important role in acid–base balance and is taken up by the kidney during metabolic acidosis. The kidney uses the glutamine to produce ammonia, bicarbonate, and glucose, which allows the excretion of acid and conservation of important cations. In the liver, glutamine is taken up and catabolized in periportal cells, with the resultant production of urea and glucose, whereas perivenous cells synthesize glutamine for release into the circulation.

Roles of Aspartate and N-Acetylglutamate in Urea Synthesis

In the urea cycle (see Figure 14-11), aspartate donates an α-amino group to citrulline to form argininosuccinate. This nitrogen, together with a nitrogen from ammonia that is directly contributed via carbamoyl phosphate, is ultimately released as urea. Hence aspartate serves as a direct donor of α-amino nitrogen to the urea cycle, with release of the aspartate carbon chain as fumarate, but carbamoyl phosphate serves as a direct donor of inorganic nitrogen to the urea cycle. Both nitrogen donors funnel nitrogen that originated in various dietary and endogenous amino acids into the urea cycle for ultimate excretion from the body. As discussed in the preceding text (see Figure 14-11), the fumarate derived from aspartate metabolism in the urea cycle is a carrier of both carbon and reducing equivalents that can be used in gluconeogenesis from amino acid carbon skeletons.

PROLINE AND ARGININE

Proline and arginine share the same 5-carbon skeleton with glutamate and ornithine, and glutamate and ornithine are key intermediates in the metabolism of proline and arginine.

Proline and Arginine Synthesis and Degradation

The dispensability of proline and arginine in the adult (Bertolo and Burrin, 2008) is related to the body's ability to synthesize these two amino acids from glutamate or α-ketoglutarate and amino groups. These interrelationships are illustrated in Figure 14-16. The role of the intestine in the endogenous synthesis of arginine was discussed in the section "Interorgan Amino Acid Metabolism."

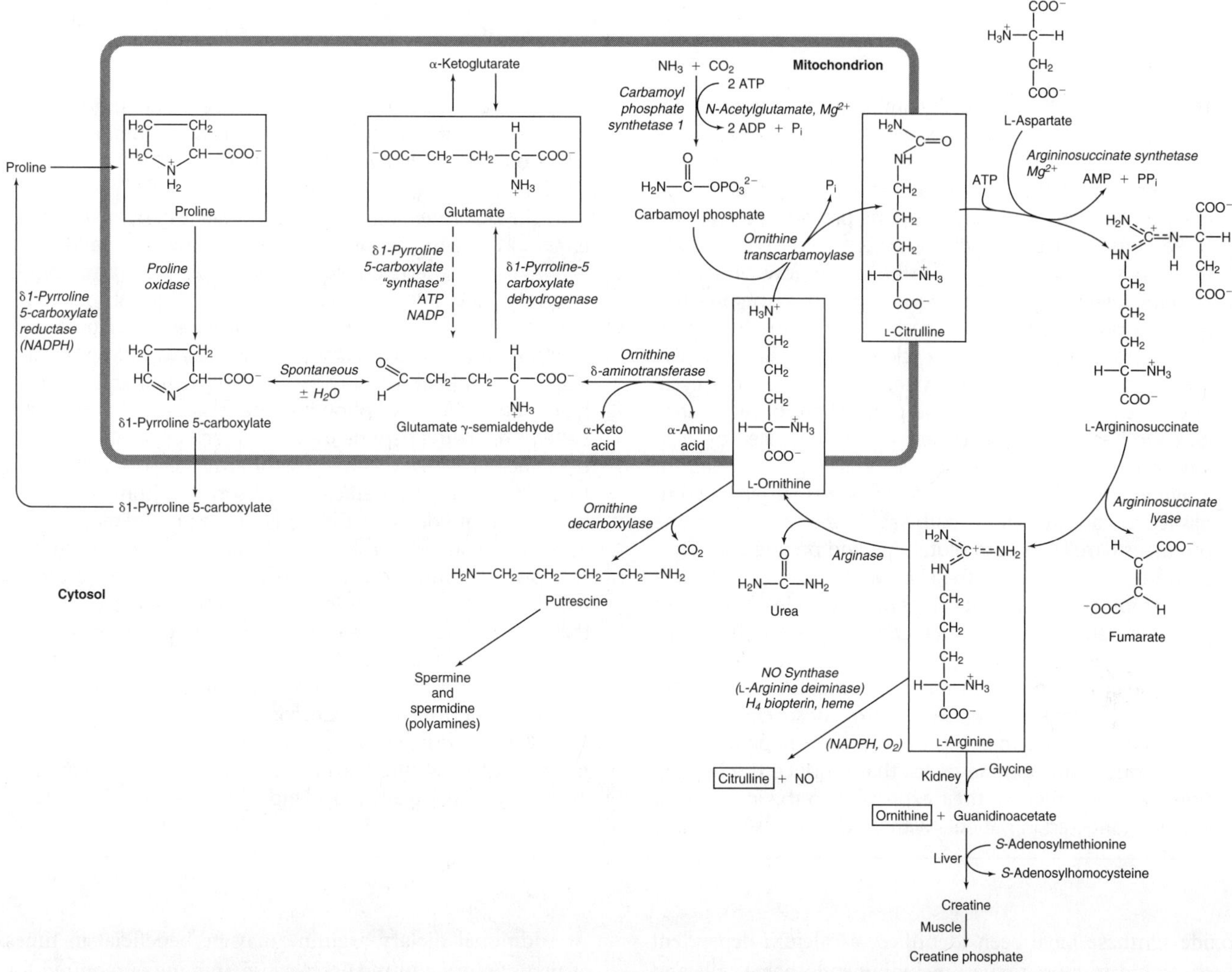

FIGURE 14-16 Reactions involved in the metabolism of arginine and proline, illustrating the interconversion of the 5-carbon skeletons and α-amino groups of glutamate, ornithine, citrulline, arginine, and proline.

The intestine of adult animals is also capable of net synthesis of proline, which depends on the presence of adequate activities of pyrroline 5-carboxylate synthase and pyrroline-5-carboxylate dehydrogenase.

The rate of arginine synthesis in the adult has been estimated to be about 25 mmol/day (Castillo et al., 1994), and arginine synthesis seemed adequate to meet arginine requirements of adults who consumed an arginine-devoid diet for several days (Carey et al., 1987). In adult subjects, the rate of de novo synthesis of arginine did not change in response to changes in arginine intake or need, but the rate of its catabolism (formation and oxidation of ornithine) was diminished in subjects with low arginine intakes; catabolism rather than synthesis seems to be regulated to conserve arginine when its availability is low (Beaumier et al., 1995).

Use of the Guanidinium Group of Arginine in the Synthesis of Creatine, Nitric Oxide, and Urea

The guanidinium group of arginine is crucial for synthesis of urea, nitric oxide, and creatine (Grillo and Colombatto, 2004; Morris, 2004; Cynober et al., 1995). In the liver, which has a complete urea cycle, arginine is formed from ornithine, carbamoyl phosphate, and the amino group of aspartate. The terminal guanidinium group of arginine is cleaved in the final step of the urea cycle to release its amidino portion as urea and to replenish the ornithine used as the starting substrate. Thus the urea cycle consumes nitrogen and bicarbonate but does not result in net synthesis of arginine. In the urea cycle, urea essentially is synthesized by forming and cleaving the amidino portion of the guanidinium group of arginine.

Some of the arginine made in the kidney is used for synthesis of guanidinoacetate, which then goes to the liver to be used for creatine synthesis. The amidino group of arginine is transferred to glycine to form guanidinoacetate in a reaction catalyzed by L-arginine:glycine amidinotransferase (Edison et al., 2007).

Arginine is also the substrate for nitric oxide synthase, which forms nitric oxide (NO) and citrulline. Nitric oxide is an effector molecule that is produced by cells of the immune system, including macrophages, which use it for cytotoxicity, and endothelial cells, which produce it as a vasodilator of smooth muscle in blood vessels. Two general types of nitric

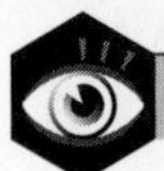

NUTRITION INSIGHT

Amino Acid Supplementation

The availability of high-quality amino acids in large quantities has permitted their use for the supplementation of diets (Jones and Heyland, 2008). Two examples of genetic diseases that are treated with amino acid supplementation are urea cycle disorders and lysinuric protein intolerance.

Patients with urea cycle disorders, except those due to arginase deficiency, tend to have very low circulating arginine levels. Arginine is derived both from the diet and from de novo synthesis in the body. Arginine is synthesized from ornithine by urea cycle enzymes. Although the liver has a functional urea cycle, the hepatic urea cycle does not result in net arginine production, because arginine synthesis within the cycle is exactly balanced by arginine breakdown. Hence the liver is not a net source of arginine. De novo synthesis of arginine is largely accomplished by an interorgan pathway whereby the intestine produces citrulline (from glutamine and proline), which is converted to arginine in the kidney. The intestine and kidney exhibit appreciable activities of urea cycle enzymes. In particular, enterocytes contain carbamoyl phosphate synthetase, *N*-acetylglutamate synthase, and ornithine transcarbamoylase; the cells of renal proximal tubules contain argininosuccinate synthetase and argininosuccinate lyase. The urea cycle enzymes expressed in extrahepatic tissues are products of the same genes that produce the hepatic urea cycle enzymes, so their expression in the intestine or kidney is affected in patients with urea cycle disorders just as is their expression in the liver. Hence de novo arginine synthesis becomes impaired and circulating arginine levels fall. Arginine supplementation is therefore part of the standard treatment of these patients (Brusilow, 1984).

Lysinuric protein intolerance also results in hypoargininemia. In this case the disorder is caused by a mutation in *SLC7A7*, the gene encoding a cationic amino transporter (y^+LAT1) that is responsible for the intestinal absorption and the renal reabsorption of lysine, arginine, and citrulline. It might be expected that such a disorder would be lethal because of impaired absorption of the essential amino acid lysine, but lysine absorption by other amino acid transport systems or via the peptide transport mechanism appears to be sufficient. However, the loss of arginine and ornithine to the urine due to inefficient reabsorption from the glomerular filtrate depletes the body of urea cycle intermediates, with consequent hyperammonemia upon ingestion of a protein-containing meal. In the case of lysinuric protein intolerance, supplementation with arginine or ornithine will not be effective because of their poor absorption. Instead, patients are given supplements with oral citrulline, which, being a neutral amino acid, enters on a different transporter. Citrulline is then converted to arginine in the kidney and possibly other tissues. Long-term treatment of patients with oral citrulline has been used to treat a number of patients, particularly in Finland (Tanner et al., 2007).

oxide synthase have been identified: a calcium-dependent form found in most tissues, including endothelial cells and neurons; and a calcium-independent inducible form found in cells that are stimulated by inflammatory cytokines (e.g., macrophages). Analogs of arginine such as *N*-monomethyl arginine are effective inhibitors of nitric acid synthase and can be used to lower nitric oxide production.

Although the amidino portion of arginine's guanidinium group is used for urea synthesis, creatine synthesis, and nitric oxide synthesis, none of these processes consumes the 5-carbon skeleton of arginine. The citrulline or ornithine released by arginine guanidinium group metabolism can be recycled back to arginine or, alternatively, used for proline synthesis or catabolized to α-ketoglutarate.

Other Requirements for Arginine and Proline

The 5-carbon skeleton of arginine is a substrate for polyamine synthesis (Cynober et al., 1995). Arginase is present in many extrahepatic tissues, where it produces the ornithine needed as a substrate for polyamine synthesis. The major polyamines include putrescine, spermidine, and spermine. These compounds are found in all tissues, where they play important roles in cell growth and division. Their synthesis is described in a subsequent section of this chapter about the role of methionine as the donor of aminopropyl groups for polyamine synthesis.

Additional dietary arginine may be beneficial in times of tissue injury and repair, because arginine is required for synthesis of nitric oxide (an effector molecule produced in response to cytokines/inflammation), polyamines (mediators of cell growth and tissue repair), and proline (needed for collagen synthesis and fibrogenesis). In this context, dietary arginine might be considered as a conditionally indispensable amino acid in states of tissue injury and repair.

GLYCINE AND SERINE

Glycine and serine play very important roles in nitrogen homeostasis and in one-carbon metabolism, as illustrated in Figure 14-17.

Glycine Degradation by the Glycine Cleavage System

Glycine is degraded by an enzyme complex known as the glycine cleavage system. The glycine cleavage system requires tetrahydrofolate (THF) and NAD^+, and it degrades glycine to CO_2 and ammonia, with formation of N^5,N^{10}-methylene-THF and NADH. In mammals, the expression of this enzyme system is restricted to liver, kidney, and brain astrocytes; it is located on the inner mitochondrial membrane of these cells. The importance of the glycine cleavage system in humans is well established from cases of inheritable metabolic disease that result in absent or very low glycine cleavage system activity in the tissues that normally express this activity.

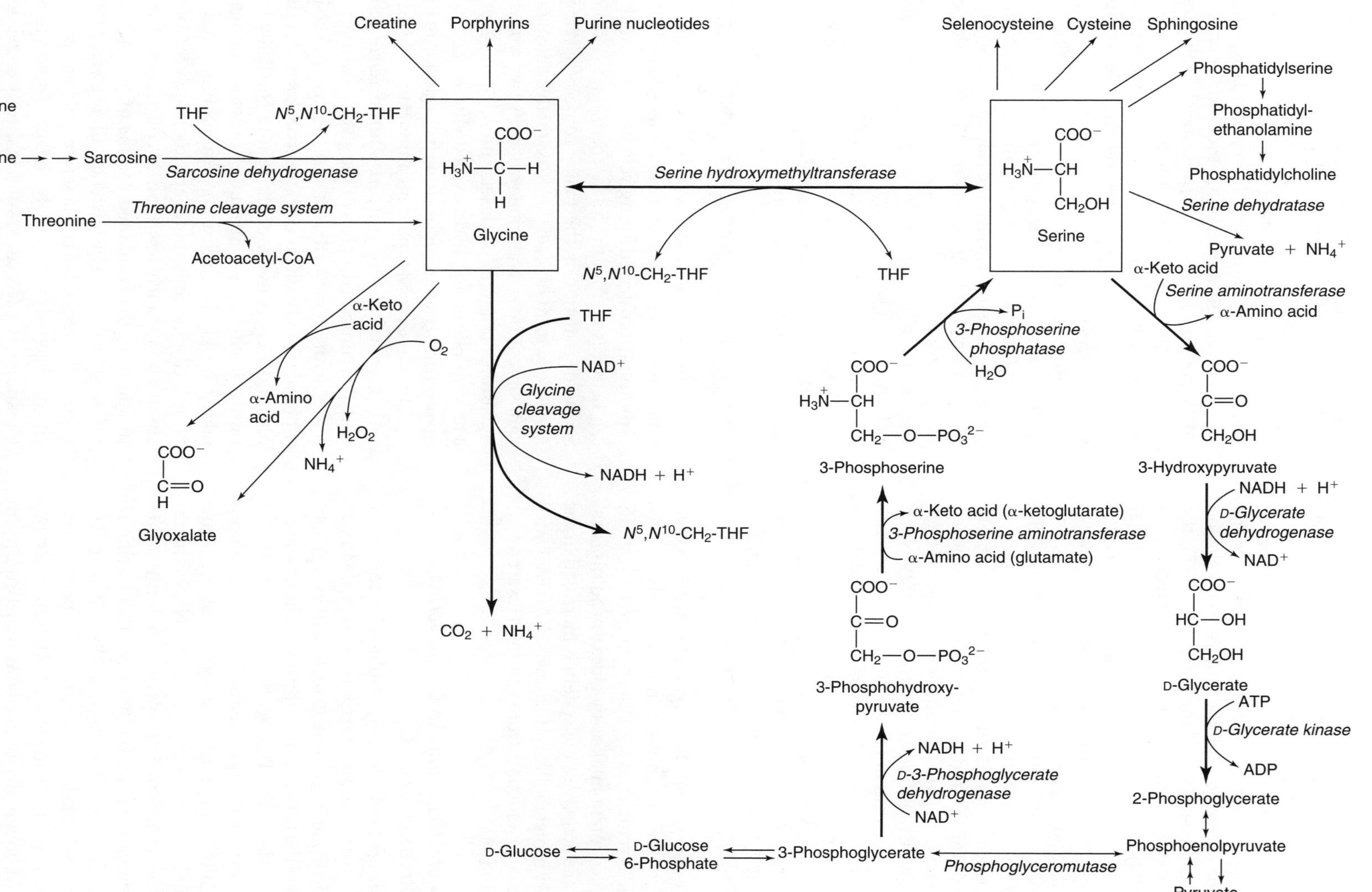

FIGURE 14-17 Reactions of glycine and serine metabolism. Major pathways of glycine and serine metabolism are indicated by the heavy lines.

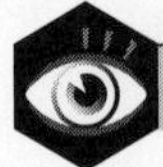

NUTRITION INSIGHT

Amino Acids as Precursors for "Gasotransmitters"

Recently, considerable attention has been paid to the role of gases, such as nitric oxide (NO) and hydrogen sulfide (H_2S), as signaling molecules. The first gas to play such a role was ethylene but it did not attract too much attention because it only occurs in ripening fruits. When nitric oxide was reported to be endothelium-derived relaxing factor (EDRF) (for review, see Moncada et al., 1991), the spotlight was firmly focused on small gaseous molecules of possible physiological importance. The third signaling gas to be reported was carbon monoxide, and most recently a fourth was reported to be hydrogen sulfide (for review, see Gadalla and Snyder, 2010). Although ethylene is synthesized from *S*-adenosylmethionine, it is a plant product and will not be discussed here.

Nitric oxide is synthesized by a family of nitric oxide synthases that uses NADPH and oxygen to convert arginine to nitric oxide and citrulline. The citrulline is recycled back to arginine in the tissues (Wu and Brosnan, 1992). Nitric oxide is produced by cells of the immune system, including macrophages, which use it for cytotoxicity, and endothelial cells, which produce it as a vasodilator of smooth muscle in blood vessels (EDRF). Three general types of nitric oxide synthase (NOS) have been identified: two calcium-dependent forms found in most tissues, including endothelial cells (eNOS, or NOS3) and neurons (nNOS, or NOS1), and a calcium-independent inducible form found in cells such as macrophages that are stimulated by inflammatory cytokines (iNOS, or NOS2). One major effect of nitric oxide is vasodilation with a fall in blood pressure. When large amounts of nitric oxide are produced by iNOS during sepsis, blood pressure can fall catastrophically (Lange et al., 2009). Analogs of arginine, such as *N*-monomethyl arginine, are effective inhibitors of NOS and might be used to lower nitric oxide production in some patients.

Hydrogen sulfide is produced from cysteine by desulfhydration reactions catalyzed by the transsulfuration enzymes, cystathionine β-synthase and cystathionine γ-lyase (for a recent review, see Gadalla and Snyder, 2010). Most hydrogen sulfide exists as HS^- at physiological pH, but a portion of it does exist in the gaseous form H_2S. Hydrogen sulfide apparently plays a role as a physiologically important vasodilator, and it is produced in the brain in response to neuronal excitation (Dominy and Stipanuk, 2004). Much work remains to understand the functions of hydrogen sulfide, the scope of its actions, and its potential pharmacological applications.

These defects give rise to nonketotic hyperglycinemia, a condition in which glycine accumulates in body fluids. In rats, the activity of the glycine cleavage system in liver is rapidly stimulated by high protein intakes, by glucagon administration, or by Ca^{2+}; the activity of the system is increased in the kidneys of rats with metabolic acidosis, which is associated with net ammonia production from glycine (Ewart et al., 1992; Lowry et al., 1985).

Interconversion of Glycine and Serine via Serine Hydroxymethyltransferase

Serine and glycine are freely interconvertible via the enzyme serine hydroxymethyltransferase. Serine hydroxymethyltransferase is a PLP-dependent enzyme. It uses THF as a cosubstrate and transfers the C3 of serine, which is at the oxidation level of formaldehyde, to the THF acceptor to form N^5,N^{10}-methylene-THF. In this reaction, serine is the major donor of one-carbon units to the folate coenzyme system. In the reverse reaction, the one-carbon group of N^5,N^{10}-methylene-THF can be transferred to glycine to form serine. Hence this enzyme allows the synthesis of either serine or glycine, provided that the other amino acid is available. The serine hydroxymethyltransferase reaction also permits serine catabolism via conversion to glycine with further catabolism of glycine. Although glycine contains only two carbon atoms, it can be considered glucogenic because of its ability to be converted to serine and hence to glucose.

Both mitochondrial and cytosolic forms of serine hydroxymethyltransferase are found in tissues. The mitochondrial serine hydroxymethyltransferase is distributed widely in tissues and seems to be involved mainly in serine catabolism to glycine plus N^5,N^{10}-methylene-THF. The one-carbon unit transferred from glycine to N^5,N^{10}-methylene-THF can be released from the folate coenzyme system as formate. Serine degradation is the major route of glycine synthesis. A cytosolic form of serine hydroxymethyltransferase is abundant only in liver and kidney of humans, with some activity also being found in skeletal muscle (Girgis et al., 1998). The cytosolic serine hydroxymethyltransferase seems to be involved in net synthesis of serine from glycine in these tissues.

Glycine seems to play an important role in nitrogen–carbon transfer among organs and in renal ammoniagenesis. The combined action of the glycine cleavage system and serine hydroxymethyltransferase allows conversion of two molecules of glycine to one molecule each of serine, ammonia, and CO_2 (Cowan et al., 1996). This allows the kidney to use glycine as a contributor to net ammoniagenesis (by taking up glycine, releasing serine, and excreting ammonium). Glycine contributes approximately 5% of the urinary ammonium, much less than is contributed by glutamine. In addition, the combined actions of glycine cleavage and serine hydroxymethyltransferase allow glycine to potentially supply all three carbons (via serine and hydroxypyruvate) for gluconeogenesis in liver. Glycine, in addition to alanine and glutamine, is released by muscle during starvation, and the renal uptake of glycine is increased in prolonged starvation.

Serine Synthesis from Glycolytic Intermediates

In addition to being synthesized from glycine via serine hydroxymethyltransferase, serine can be synthesized from the glycolytic intermediate 3-phosphoglycerate via an NAD^+-linked dehydrogenase that converts this intermediate to 3-phosphohydroxypyruvate. The latter then undergoes transamination with glutamate to 3-phosphoserine, followed by the irreversible removal of the phosphate by a phosphatase. This cytosolic pathway from 3-phosphoglycerate is distributed widely and is considered the major pathway of serine synthesis de novo in mammals. Once serine is formed from glycolytic intermediates, it can be converted to glycine via serine hydroxymethyltransferase, permitting de novo synthesis of glycine as well.

Other Routes of Glycine Synthesis

Glycine can be produced from metabolism of betaine (or its precursor, choline) by successive removal of the methyl groups from the amine group of betaine. This leads to sequential formation of dimethylglycine, monomethylglycine (sarcosine), and ultimately glycine, via transfer of the first methyl group to homocysteine to form methionine and donation of the second and third methyl groups to the folate coenzyme system to form N^5,N^{10}-methylene-THF. These reactions are catalyzed by betaine:homocysteine methyltransferase, dimethylglycine dehydrogenase, and sarcosine dehydrogenase, respectively. Direct methylation of glycine also occurs; this is catalyzed by glycine *N*-methyltransferase, which transfers the methyl group from *S*-adenosylmethionine to glycine to form sarcosine (see subsequent section on methionine and cysteine catabolism).

Other Pathways of Serine Degradation

As discussed previously, serine degradation can be accomplished by conversion of serine to glycine by serine hydroxymethyltransferase, followed by catabolism of glycine by the glycine cleavage system. Serine also can be degraded by other routes. Transamination of serine to yield 3-hydroxypyruvate is a major route of serine degradation in human liver; the serine-pyruvate aminotransferase is located in peroxisomes of human liver (Xue et al., 1999). The 3-hydroxypyruvate can be further converted to glycerate and phosphorylated to 2-phosphoglycerate, an intermediate in glycolysis and gluconeogenesis. In some species, serine (as well as threonine) is degraded by a cytosolic enzyme called serine (threonine) dehydratase, which increases markedly in liver of rats fed high-protein diets. Serine dehydratase catalyzes the deamination of serine to pyruvate plus ammonia. The activity of serine dehydratase is reported to be low in human liver (Ogawa et al., 1989), and it seems unlikely that serine deamination to pyruvate is quantitatively significant in human liver. The relative roles of various pathways of serine synthesis and degradation, however, remain to be clarified for human tissues.

Essential Roles of Glycine in the Synthesis of Nonprotein Compounds

Glycine is a substrate for synthesis of purine nucleotides, porphyrins, creatine, one-carbon fragments for the folate coenzyme system, glutathione, and glycine-conjugated bile acids. The glycine cleavage system is involved in the donation of one-carbon units to the folate coenzyme system, as shown in Figure 14-17. Glycine is incorporated intact into purine nucleotides. Delta-aminolevulinate, a precursor of porphyrins, is synthesized from glycine and succinyl-CoA with the α-carbon and the α-amino group of glycine retained in the porphobilinogen, but with the carboxyl carbon lost as CO_2. Some of the glycine nitrogen is lost when porphobilinogen is converted to porphyrinogen in the process of porphyrin and heme synthesis. Glycine is used by the kidney in the synthesis of guanidinoacetate, a precursor of creatine phosphate. Both the glycine carbons and nitrogen remain in creatine phosphate or its elimination product, creatinine. Glycine is used to conjugate bile acids in the liver, and glycine-conjugated bile acids are secreted in the bile. Other compounds also can form glycine conjugates; the best-known example is the conjugation of glycine with benzoic acid to form hippuric acid, which is excreted in the urine. The conjugation of benzoic acid with glycine facilitates the excretion of nitrogen from the body (as glycine), and this is presumed to be the basis of its therapeutic effect in patients with hyperammonemia.

Essential Roles of Serine in the Synthesis of Nonprotein Compounds

Serine is a precursor for synthesis of one-carbon fragments for the folate coenzyme system, for synthesis of phospholipids and sphingosine, and for synthesis of cysteine and selenocysteine. The C3 of serine is the major source of one-carbon fragments for the folate coenzyme system via the reaction catalyzed by serine hydroxymethyltransferase (see Figure 14-17 and Chapter 25). This reaction also results in the conversion of serine to glycine.

Serine is used in the production of phosphatidylserine, phosphatidylethanolamine, and phosphatidylcholine (see Chapter 16, Figure 16-18). Thus serine serves as the precursor of choline. The details of the conversion are not well established, but phosphatidylserine undergoes decarboxylation to phosphatidylethanolamine, followed by transfer of three methyl groups from *S*-adenosylmethionine to form phosphatidylcholine. Because choline can be degraded to betaine, sarcosine, and glycine, this synthetic route provides another way to produce glycine from serine or from dietary choline or betaine. Serine, along with palmitoyl-CoA, is used for the synthesis of the amino alcohol sphingosine, which is a component of ceramide and other sphingolipids (see Chapter 16, Figure 16-23).

Serine is the precursor of the carbon chain of both cysteine and selenocysteine. The incorporation of the three-carbon chain of serine into cysteine is accomplished enzymatically in the methionine transsulfuration pathway, by which the sulfur of methionine is transferred to serine to form cysteine (see Figure 14-22). The use of the carbon chain of serine for synthesis of selenocysteine is accomplished in a very different manner. A limited number of proteins contain the modified amino acid selenocysteine in specific location(s). This amino acid is named selenocysteine because it has the structure of cysteine, but the sulfur is replaced by selenium.

Unlike other modified amino acid residues found in proteins, selenocysteine is formed by cotranslational rather than by posttranslational modification of an amino acid residue. Serine esterified to a specific tRNA that contains an anticodon complementary to the stop codon UGA (uracil-guanine-adenine) is the substrate for selenocysteine synthesis. In certain mRNAs, this triplet acts as a codon for selenocysteine rather than as a termination sequence. (See Chapter 39 for details of selenocysteine synthesis.) Proteins also may contain selenomethionine residues at random locations owing to incorporation of selenomethionine in place of methionine; this replacement reflects dietary intake of selenomethionine and not its specific synthesis and specific incorporation into proteins.

CATABOLISM OF INDISPENSABLE AMINO ACIDS

THREONINE

Threonine may be catabolized in humans by cytosolic threonine (serine) dehydratase (L-threonine ammonia-lyase, threonine deaminase) or by mitochondrial threonine dehydrogenase, as shown in Figure 14-18. In the case of threonine dehydratase, the α-ketobutyrate formed is converted, by either pyruvate dehydrogenase or the branched-chain keto acid dehydrogenase, to propionyl-CoA, which enters the citric acid cycle (Paxton et al., 1986). Threonine dehydrogenase produces 2-amino-3-ketobutyrate, which can be converted, by 2-amino-3-ketobutyrate coenzyme A ligase, to glycine and acetyl-CoA (Edgar and Polak, 2000). Bacteria, fungi, and plants contain a third enzyme, threonine aldolase, which converts threonine to glycine and acetaldehyde. This enzyme is present at low activity in mouse liver. However, the human homolog of threonine aldolase is a nontranscribed pseudogene (Edgar, 2005).

The relative importance of the dehydrogenase pathway and the dehydratase pathway varies with the animal species studied. Pigs appear to use the dehydrogenase pathway for about 80% of their threonine oxidation and to increase flux through that pathway when threonine intake is increased (Ballevre et al., 1990). In contrast, in rat hepatocytes, about 65% of threonine oxidation occurs through threonine dehydratase (House et al., 2001), and both threonine dehydratase activity and threonine transport are increased in response to glucagon. For the human, the general consensus is that threonine dehydrogenase activity is very low and does not respond to physiological situations such as changes in threonine intake or hormone levels (Darling et al., 2000). Threonine dehydratase is responsible for about 90% of threonine oxidation and is responsive to threonine ingestion.

It should be noted that threonine concentration in plasma is not as well protected as is that for several other indispensable amino acids such as lysine. For example, threonine kinetics in humans showed increased oxidation between intakes of 20 and 80 mg threonine·kg^{-1}·day^{-1} but no further increase above an intake of 100 mg·kg^{-1}·day^{-1}, and no decrease in oxidation occurred at intakes of 3 or 10 mg threonine·kg^{-1}·day^{-1}, amounts that are probably below the dietary requirement (Zhao et al., 1986). Consequently, plasma threonine levels fell when intake was dropped below 10 mg·kg^{-1}·day^{-1} and rose markedly when intake was increased above 80 mg·kg^{-1}·day^{-1}.

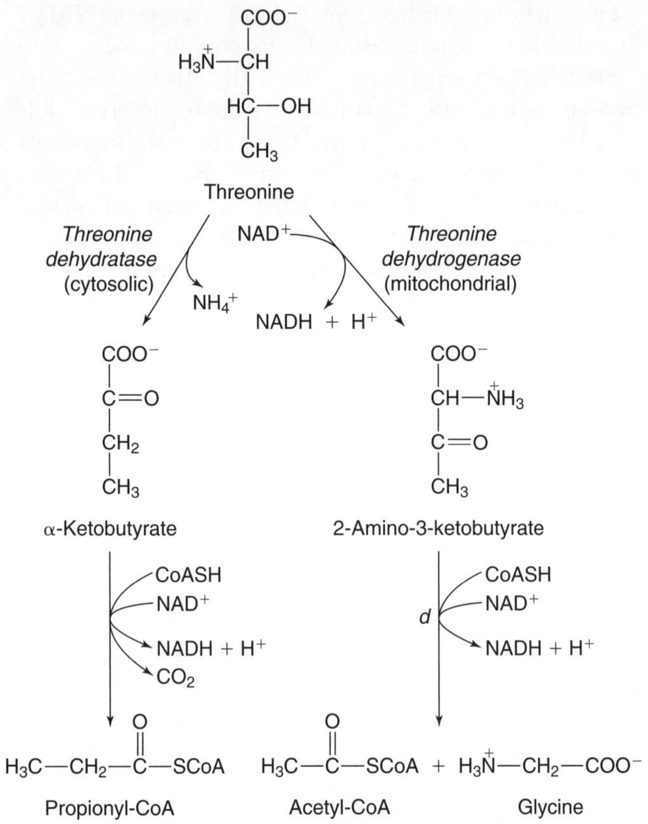

FIGURE 14-18 Catabolism of threonine in human liver.

It is probable that humans and animals do not usually experience marked changes in threonine intake. There is at most a twofold difference in threonine content of plant-based low threonine proteins and animal-based high threonine proteins, unlike the fivefold difference seen in lysine content. In addition, the intestine buffers threonine intake by using large amounts of it for mucin synthesis. About 20% to 30% of the amino acid residues in intestinal mucins are threonine.

HISTIDINE

The first step in histidine degradation involves the nonoxidative deamination of L-histidine to give *trans*-urocanic acid and ammonia by histidine ammonia-lyase, more commonly called histidase (Figure 14-19). Histidase activity is located only in the liver and in the surface layer (stratum corneum) of the skin. In the skin, the breakdown of histidine stops with the production of urocanic acid, which is an ultraviolet-absorbing compound that plays an important protective role.

In the liver, histidase is a cytosolic enzyme, with a K_m for L-histidine of approximately 2 mmol/L. The urocanate formed from histidine is converted to imidazolepropionic acid by urocanase, which adds water across the double bond between the α and β carbons of urocanate. Imidazolonepropionic

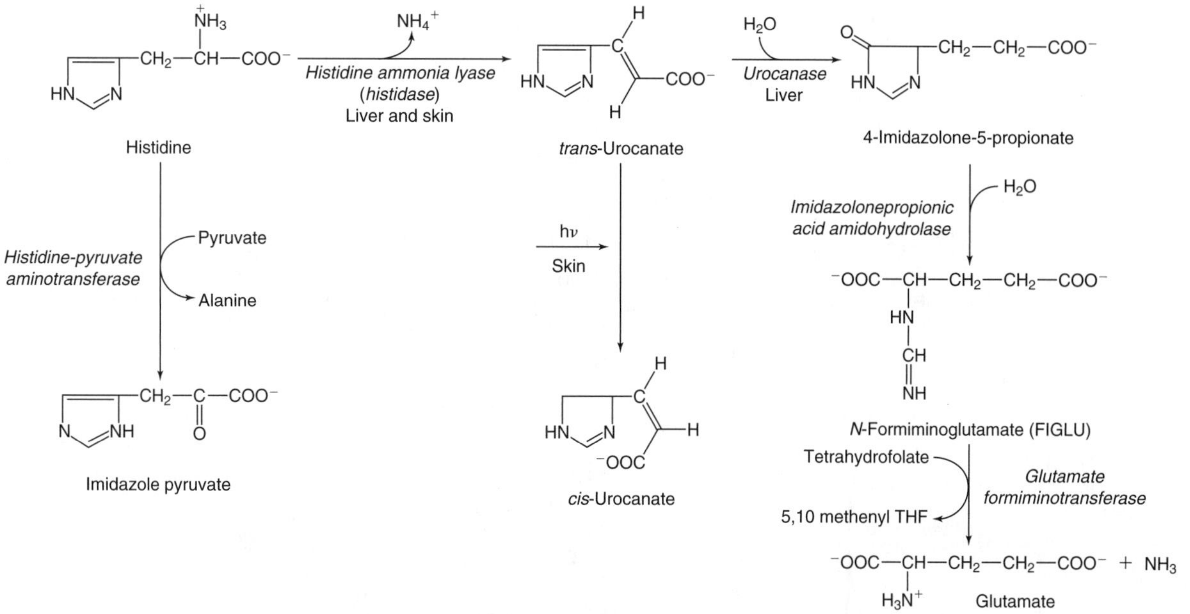

FIGURE 14-19 Catabolism of histidine in mammalian cells. Ultraviolet irradiation (270 to 320 nm) is indicated by *hv*.

acid amidohydrolase splits the imidazole ring of imidazolepropionic acid to give *N*-formiminoglutamate (FIGLU), an intermediate in one-carbon biochemistry. FIGLU donates its formimino group to THF to give formimino-THF and glutamate; the reaction is catalyzed by the bifunctional liver enzyme, glutamate formiminotransferase-cyclodeaminase. The cyclodeaminase activity converts formimino-THF to ammonia and 5,10-methenyl-THF. Thus a one-carbon group from histidine enters the de novo pathway for methyl group synthesis. This reaction is very sensitive to the folate status of the cell because THF is a cosubstrate. Deficiency of folate causes a markedly increased excretion of FIGLU in the urine.

Histidinemia is an inherited autosomal recessive disease that results from a deficiency of histidase; it is thought to be a relatively benign disorder (Lam et al., 1996), which may be recognized by an elevation in plasma histidine. Because the histidase pathway is blocked, histidine must be transaminated to give imidazolonepyruvic acid, which can be further metabolized to imidazolelactic acid and imidazoleacetic acid. The latter metabolites can be observed in urine of patients with histidinemia. The enzyme activity responsible is referred to as histidine-pyruvate aminotransferase, which may be identical to another enzyme, such as serine-pyruvate aminotransferase or phenylalanine-pyruvate aminotransferase (Noguchi et al., 1976). Because aminotransferase reactions are generally reversible in vivo, histidine can be synthesized from imidazolonepyruvic acid if this keto acid is available in the liver cell.

The histidine catabolic pathway in liver is regulated at the level of histidase; transcription of the hepatic histidase gene is induced by glucagon, glucocorticoids, and estrogen. Hepatic histidase also increases in animals fed high levels of high-quality protein, but not histidine alone; the type and amount of protein consumed alter histidase gene expression through changes in the plasma glucagon level (Tovar et al., 2002). Histidine aminotransferase is also induced in response to injection of glucagon and cortisol, but it is not induced in rats fed a high-protein diet (Morris et al., 1973).

METHIONINE AND CYSTEINE

Methionine and cysteine are known as sulfur-containing amino acids because they both contain a sulfur atom. Cysteine has a sulfhydryl group, whereas methionine contains sulfur in a thioether linkage. These two amino acids are related in that cysteine can be synthesized in the body from the sulfur atom of methionine and the dispensable amino acid serine.

Role of Methionine as the Donor of Methyl Groups

Many tissues are able to methylate DNA, RNA, polysaccharides, other small molecules, and various proteins, but it is thought that only the liver can carry out the quantitatively major methylations required for synthesis of creatine and for synthesis of phosphatidylcholine from phosphatidylethanolamine (Mudd et al., 2007). The universal methyl donor, *S*-adenosylmethionine (SAM), is formed from methionine and ATP by methionine adenosyltransferase, isozyme 2A (MAT2A), found in many tissues. Although MAT2A has a low K_m for methionine, it is inhibited by SAM, so excess SAM is not formed unless it is needed. Methylation of cytosine residues in CpG islands in DNA (i.e., short stretches of DNA that have a high frequency of CG nucleotide sequences, with the "p" indicating the nucleotides are connected by a phosphodiester bond) is known to affect transcription, as does methylation of particular lysine and arginine residues in certain histones (i.e., proteins closely associated with DNA). Both CpG methylation and histone modifications are classified as epigenetic modifications, which are modifications that can affect heritable traits but do not involve changes in the underlying DNA sequence.

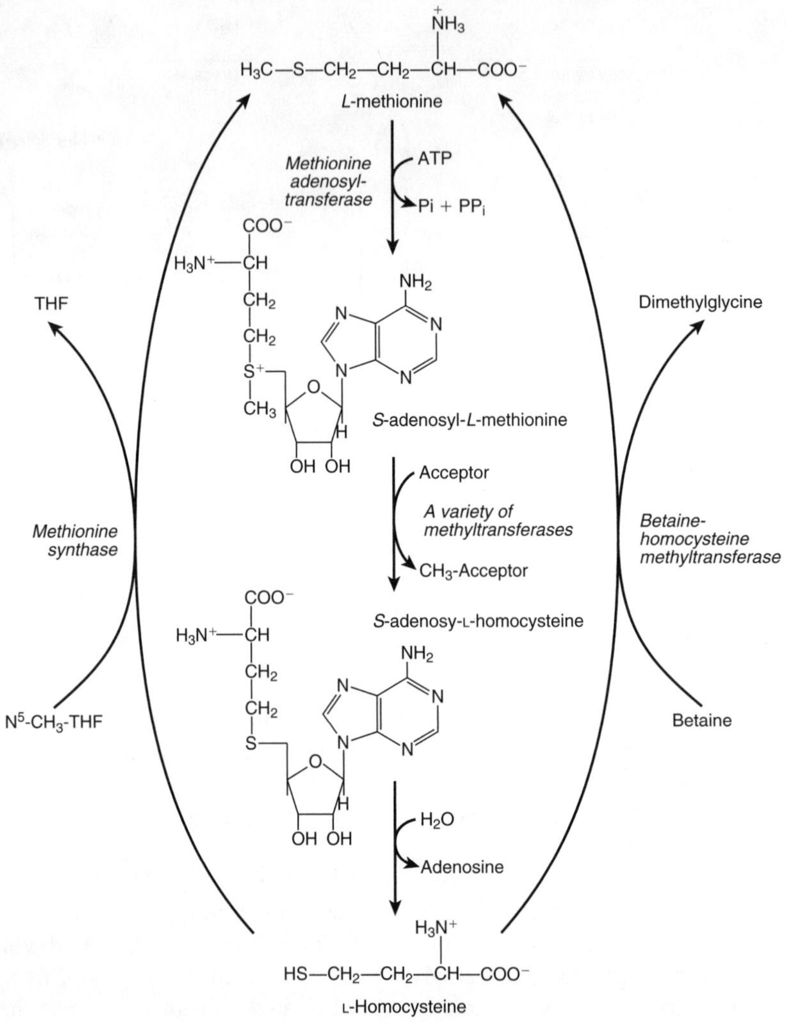

FIGURE 14-20 Pathways of methionine transmethylation to methylate DNA, RNA, and many other substrates and remethylation to conserve the cell's methionine potential. *THF,* Tetrahydrofolate.

A recent bioinformatics study predicts 208 methyltransferases in the human genome (Petrossian and Clarke, 2010). Once the methyl group is transferred to a substrate by the appropriate methyltransferase, the *S*-adenosylhomocysteine (SAH) that results is rapidly hydrolyzed to homocysteine and adenosine (Figure 14-20). Most methyl transferases, other than glycine *N*-methyltransferase, are inhibited by an elevated SAM/SAH ratio so that any problem with SAH hydrolysis could interfere with numerous methylation reactions.

Homocysteine may be remethylated to methionine by a widespread enzyme, N^5-methyl-THF:homocysteine methyltransferase (methionine synthase) or by a liver-specific betaine-homocysteine methyltransferase. Although the remethylation of homocysteine allows the body to use methyl groups from choline (betaine) or from de novo synthesis via the folate coenzyme system (N^5-CH_3-THF), these methyl groups are first incorporated into methionine before they are used for general methylation reactions. Thus SAM serves as the immediate methyl donor for the numerous methylation reactions that occur in the body. In male subjects fed methionine-adequate diets, approximately 40% of the homocysteine formed per transmethylation cycle underwent remethylation to methionine (Storch et al., 1990). The extent of remethylation increased in subjects fed methionine-deficient diets. Only if the methionine concentration is sufficient, as indicated by the SAM concentration, is cystathionine β-synthase activated so homocysteine can enter the transsulfuration pathway, as described later.

Role of Methionine as the Donor of Aminopropyl Groups for Polyamine Synthesis

Spermidine and spermine are intracellular organic cations called polyamines that are essential for proper cellular function (Agostinelli et al., 2010). Each polyamine has positively charged nitrogens (three for spermidine, four for spermine), separated by a hydrophobic chain of methyl groups. Their molecular structures permit very specific interactions with macromolecules, such as nucleic acids, proteins, and phospholipids. Polyamines are synthesized from the diamine putrescine by sequential addition of an aminopropyl group from decarboxylated SAM (Figure 14-21). The byproduct of polyamine synthesis, methylthioadenosine, is converted to adenine and methylthioribose-1-phosphate, which can be efficiently salvaged. The sulfur atom, methyl carbon, and ribose chain in the methylthioribose moiety are reincorporated

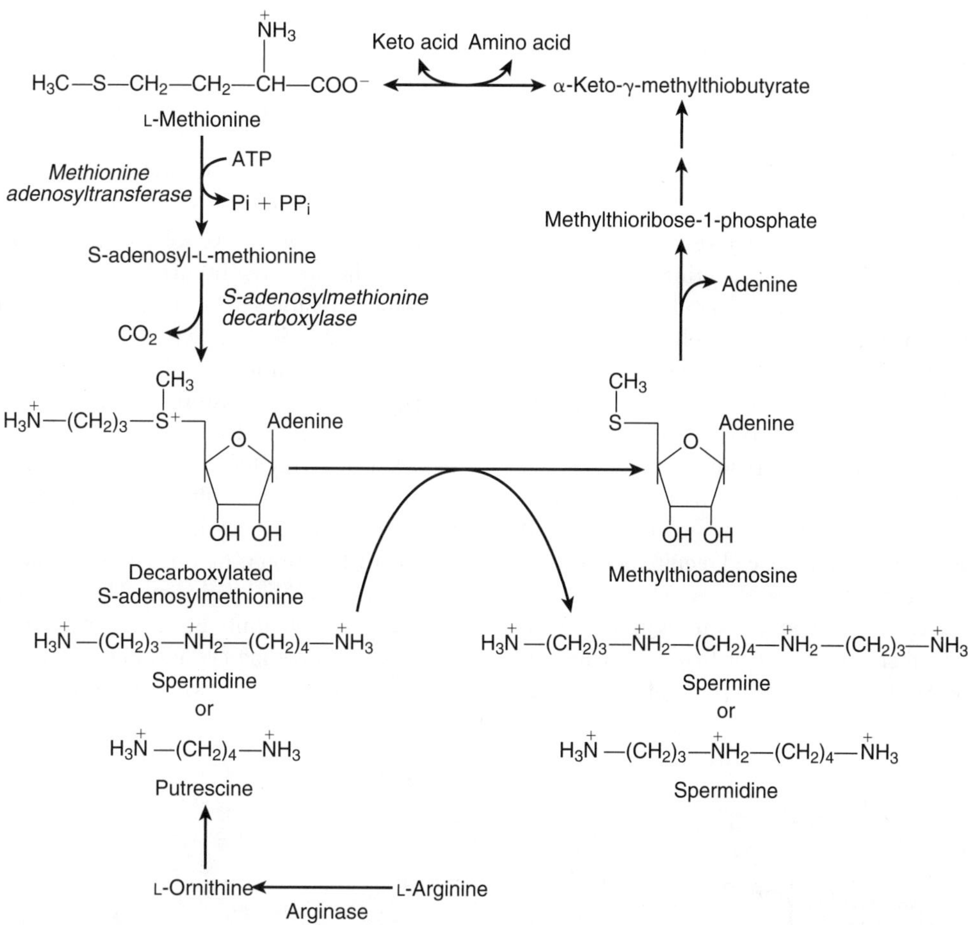

FIGURE 14-21 Synthesis of polyamines from arginine and methionine, and salvage of the methylthioribose moiety of *S*-adenosylmethionine by resynthesis of methionine.

into methionine by a series of reactions in which α-keto-γ-methylthiobutyrate is formed and then transaminated to methionine in the final step (Pirkov et al., 2008).

Methionine Catabolism and Cysteine Synthesis

Methionine is a dietary essential amino acid and is used in humans to synthesize cysteine and taurine, the other sulfur-containing amino acids that are considered to be conditionally essential. An increase in the methionine concentration triggers its degradation in liver, which occurs by a combination of the transmethylation and transsulfuration pathways. The degradation of methionine thus involves the transfer of methionine sulfur to serine to form cysteine. Excess cysteine is subsequently catabolized to taurine and to pyruvate and sulfate (Figure 14-22). Thus the pathways of methionine metabolism function in methylation of many molecules, for polyamine synthesis, and for synthesis of cysteine and, ultimately, of cysteine metabolites. The multiple functions of methionine in metabolism account for the complex regulation of some of the enzymes involved.

The first step in methionine catabolism is the transfer of an adenosyl group from ATP to the sulfur of methionine to give SAM, a reaction catalyzed by methionine adenosyltransferase (MAT). In liver there are two isoenzymes of MAT. MAT1A is liver-specific and MAT2A occurs in many tissues. MAT1A is actually activated by its product, SAM, an example of feedback activation. Thus as more methionine enters the liver, more SAM is formed. In the case of methionine degradation, SAM is substrate for hepatic glycine *N*-methyltransferase, which converts glycine to sarcosine, a nontoxic product that is rapidly converted back to glycine by sarcosine dehydrogenase, with the methyl group entering the mitochondrial one-carbon pool. Unlike most methyltransferases, glycine *N*-methyltransferase has a relatively high K_m for SAM and is only weakly inhibited by its product, SAH (Takata et al., 2003). These kinetic characteristics of glycine *N*-methyltransferase allow it to regulate the SAM concentration and to dispose of excess methyl groups.

The SAH that is generated by transfer of the methyl group subsequently is hydrolyzed by *S*-adenosylhomocysteine hydrolase to release homocysteine and adenosine. For methionine catabolism to occur, the homocysteine must be converted to cysteine by the transsulfuration pathway: remethylation of homocysteine does not result in removal of methionine but rather in its regeneration. The first enzyme in the transsulfuration pathway, cystathionine β-synthase is a heme-containing, PLP-requiring enzyme that condenses homocysteine with serine to give cystathionine. Cystathionine β-synthase is activated severalfold by binding of SAM to its C-terminal domain (Martinov et al., 2000). This regulation ensures that the more methionine, and therefore SAM, there is in the cell, the more cystathionine β-synthase activity there will be to remove it. This step commits the methionine molecule to degradation via the transsulfuration pathway. Cystathionine is cleaved by cystathionine γ-lyase to release α-ketobutyrate and ammonia as products of the homocysteine moiety, and cysteine, which contains the sulfur from homocysteine and the carbon chain and nitrogen donated by serine. Therefore transsulfuration allows cysteine to be synthesized from serine and a sulfur atom cleaved from methionine; it also degrades methionine. The carbon skeleton of methionine, α-ketobutyrate, is oxidatively decarboxylated to propionyl-CoA, which enters the citric acid cycle at the level of succinyl-CoA. Because transsulfuration permits methionine to serve as the precursor of cysteine sulfur, the sulfur amino acid requirement can be met either by methionine alone or by a mixture of methionine and cysteine. Studies in young men have indicated that approximately 50% of the total sulfur amino acid requirement can be supplied as cysteine (Storch et al., 1990).

Methionine also can be degraded by transamination to its keto acid and further catabolism of that keto acid, but this does not appear to be a substantial route of methionine degradation at physiological or even high physiological concentrations. Therefore methionine degradation depends almost entirely on the transmethylation and transsulfuration pathways, with transfer of the sulfur to cysteine.

Inborn Errors of Methionine Metabolism

A number of inborn errors of sulfur amino acid metabolism have served to verify the steps in the methionine metabolic pathway in humans. Inborn errors (e.g., the C677T polymorphism in the N^5,N^{10}-methylene-THF reductase gene) or vitamin deficiencies (e.g., folate, vitamin B_{12}) that limit the removal of homocysteine, either by remethylation to methionine or by transsulfuration, result in elevated levels of homocysteine in the blood and urine. A mildly elevated level of plasma homocysteine is considered a risk factor for vascular disease and neural tube defects (Guba et al., 1996). More severe forms of homocysteinemia/homocystinuria are caused by loss-of-function mutations in genes such as cystathionine β-synthase, N^5,N^{10}-methylene-THF reductase, methionine synthase, and vitamin B_{12} coenzyme synthesis. Mutations in the gene encoding cystathionine β-synthase are the most common. In patients with inheritable metabolic disease

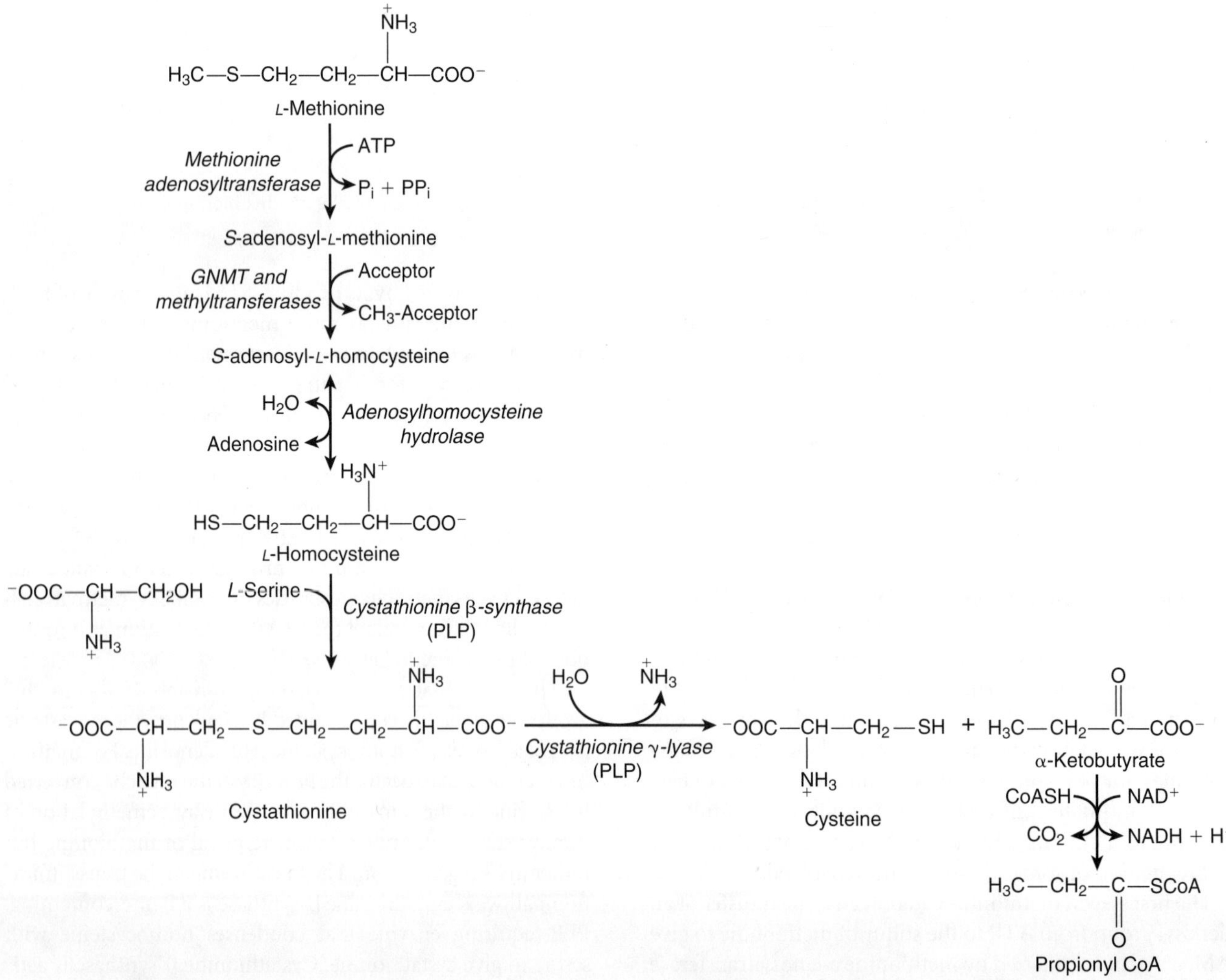

FIGURE 14-22 Catabolism of methionine in mammalian cells. Note that catabolism requires the transmethylation pathway followed by the transsulfuration pathway to give cysteine. *GNMT,* Glycine *N*-methyltransferase.

associated with homocystinuria, numerous abnormalities are observed, including premature thromboembolic and atherosclerotic disease and mental deficiencies. Some cases can be treated by vitamin supplementation (e.g., vitamin B_6 for defects in cystathionine β-synthase) if there is residual enzyme activity. Treatment by restriction of methionine intake and supplementation with betaine is used to lower the homocysteine level in homocystinuric patients. The diet should also contain sufficient cysteine because cysteine synthesis will be impaired in patients with homocystinuria.

Cysteine Catabolism and Inorganic Sulfur Production

The catabolism of cysteine results in production of several essential compounds, including taurine, sulfate, and reduced inorganic sulfur (Stipanuk, 2004). Formation of these metabolites is accomplished by the pathways shown in Figure 14-23. Taurine and inorganic sulfate are considered the main end products of cysteine catabolism and are excreted in the urine. Taurine and inorganic sulfate have important functions in the body, however, and should not be viewed simply as end products for sulfur excretion. A major pathway for cysteine catabolism involves the dioxygenation of cysteine to cysteinesulfinate by cysteine dioxygenase, followed by the metabolism of cysteinesulfinate to either taurine or pyruvate plus sulfate. Cysteine is also metabolized by desulfhydration to yield hydrogen sulfide. Although reduced forms of inorganic sulfur are readily oxidized to sulfate, hydrogen sulfide appears to have important regulatory/signaling functions as well. The activated form of sulfate, 3′-phosphoadenosine-5′-phosphosulfate (PAPS), serves as the substrate for sulfation of a number of molecules. Many structural compounds are sulfated. In particular, proteoglycans such as chondroitin sulfate contain oligosaccharide chains with many sulfated sugar residues. In addition, many compounds of both endogenous and exogenous origin are excreted as sulfoesters; sulfoesters of steroid hormones and of the drug acetaminophen are examples.

The sulfur of cysteine is also essential as a source of unoxidized sulfur for synthesis of iron–sulfur clusters for iron–sulfur proteins, for modification of specific uridine residues in tRNAs, and for molybdopterin coenzyme biosynthesis (Shi et al., 2010; Noma et al., 2009).

Role of Cysteine in the Synthesis of Taurine

Taurine or 2-aminoethanesulfonic acid is also a sulfur-containing amino acid, albeit not an α-carboxylic acid. Taurine is synthesized in liver from cysteine by a three-step pathway, shown in Figure 14-23. Cysteine dioxygenase oxidizes cysteine to cysteinesulfinate which is then decarboxylated to hypotaurine by cysteinesulfinate decarboxylase, a PLP-containing enzyme. Hypotaurine is rapidly further oxidized to taurine, but it is not clear whether this is an enzyme-catalyzed reaction. Cysteine dioxygenase is robustly regulated in response to dietary protein or sulfur amino acid intake via a cysteine-mediated inhibition of its polyubiquination and hence degradation by the 26S proteasome (Stipanuk et al., 2006). Taurine is not known to be a dietary essential nutrient in adults but infants have a lower capacity for synthesis.

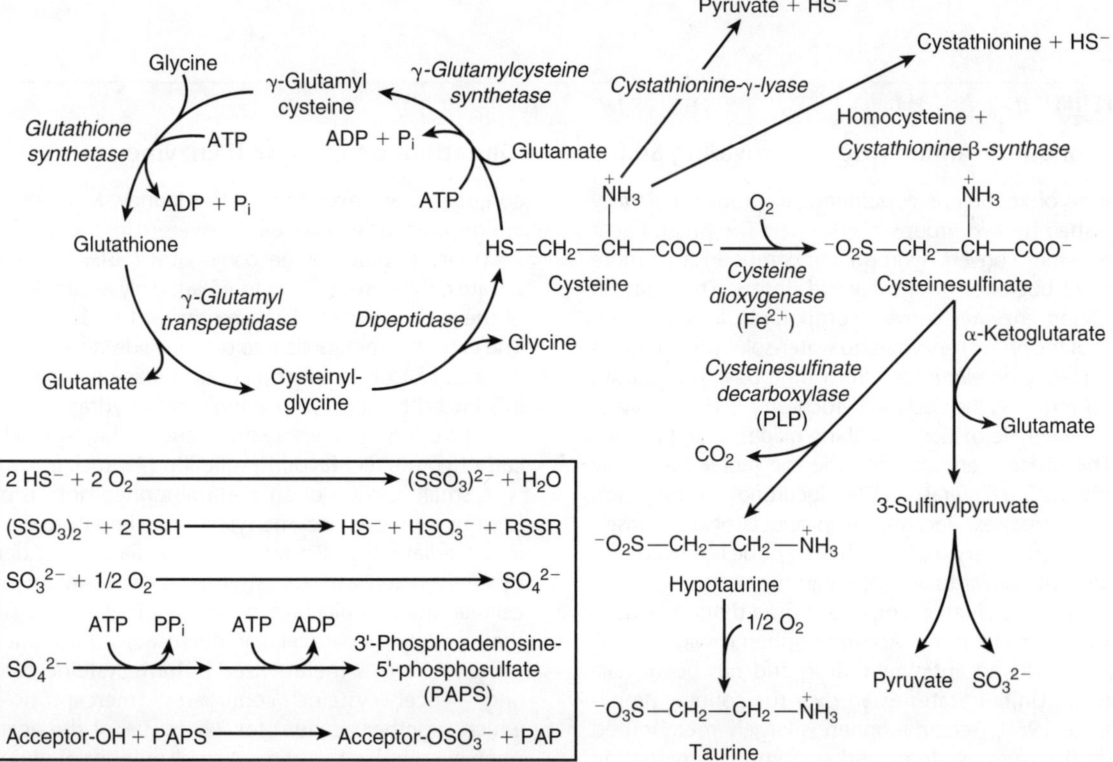

FIGURE 14-23 Pathways of cysteine and inorganic sulfur metabolism, including synthesis of taurine and glutathionine and cysteine catabolism.

Taurine is present at high concentrations in human milk and is added to infant formulas in the United States. Dietary intake of taurine can be substantial for a person on an omnivorous diet, but taurine is present mainly in animal foods. Strict vegan diets contain very little taurine, leading some to refer to taurine as a "carninutrient" (McCarty, 2004).

Taurine, like glycine, is used for the conjugation of bile acids in the liver (see Chapter 7 for the role of bile acids in digestion and absorption). Taurine is also required for two novel modifications of uridines in several mammalian mitochondrial tRNAs (e.g., 5-taurinomethyl-uridine in mitochondrial tRNAs for tryptophan and leucine), and taurine is important in removal of hypochlorite produced by activated neutrophils by formation of taurine chloramine (Suzuki et al., 2001; Schuller-Levis and Park, 2004). A number of other possible functions of taurine have been suggested, including its function as an organic osmolyte.

Both sulfate and taurine are excreted in the urine, but sulfate normally accounts for more than 80% of the total sulfur excreted. The inorganic sulfate produced from methionine and cysteine sulfur largely accounts for the acidogenic potential of protein-containing diets (Bella and Stipanuk, 1995).

Role of Cysteine in the Synthesis of Glutathione

A large amount of available cysteine is used for synthesis of γ-glutamylcysteinylglycine, as illustrated in Figure 14-23; this tripeptide is better known as glutathione (GSH). The normal turnover of GSH in adults has been estimated to be 40 mmol/day, which is slightly greater than the estimated normal turnover of cysteine in protein (Fukagawa et al., 1996). A large part of the normal GSH turnover is related to its role as a reservoir of cysteine and as a means of transporting cysteine. The enzyme γ-glutamyltranspeptidase is located on the outer surface of the plasma membrane of cells in extrahepatic tissues such as kidney and lung, and it can hydrolyze the γ-glutamyl linkage of GSH to yield cysteinylglycine (with or without transpeptidation of glutamate to another amino acid). If transpeptidation occurs, the γ-glutamyl amino acid can be transported into the cell. The cysteinylglycine dipeptide can be hydrolyzed to cysteine and glycine, either extracellularly or intracellularly by dipeptidases. Therefore cysteine may be released into the plasma or provided to peripheral tissues by hepatic GSH synthesis and extrahepatic GSH hydrolysis.

GSH has a reactive sulfhydryl group and can readily form disulfides with itself (oxidized glutathione or GSSG) or mixed disulfides with other thiol compounds (GSSR). The ratio of GSH to GSSG in most cells markedly favors the reduced state and GSH serves as a supply of reducing equivalents. GSH is involved in protection of cells from oxidative damage because of its role in reducing hydrogen peroxide and organic peroxides via glutathione peroxidases and because of its ability to inactivate free radicals through hydrogen donation. These processes result in oxidation of GSH to GSSG (White et al., 1994). GSSG and GSH can be interconverted via the glutathione reductase reaction, which uses $NADP^+$/NADPH as the oxidant–reductant; hence GSH plays a role in maintenance of the cellular redox state.

GSH also serves as cosubstrate for several reactions, including certain steps in leukotriene synthesis and melanin polymer synthesis. GSH is the substrate for a group of enzymes, the glutathione *S*-transferases, which form GSH

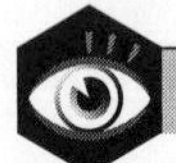

NUTRITION INSIGHT

Role of Sulfur Amino Acids in Providing Sulfate and Glutathione for Phase II Enzymes

Metabolism of xenobiotic compounds or drugs is normally accomplished by two groups of enzymes. The phase I activating enzymes convert hydrophobic compounds to more hydrophilic, but often more reactive, forms. The phase II detoxification enzymes convert compounds, including the products of the phase I enzymes, to water-soluble conjugates that can readily be eliminated from the body. The phase I activating enzymes include the cytochrome P450 family of enzymes, aldehyde oxidase, xanthine oxidases, and peroxidases. The phase II enzymes include the multigene family of glutathione S-transferases, UDP-glucuronosyltransferases, and sulfotransferases. Because the products of the phase I enzymes are often very reactive, they must be removed rapidly to prevent cellular toxicity, cell injury, or carcinogenesis.

Acetaminophen is an example of a drug that undergoes detoxification in the body. Acetaminophen is widely used as an analgesic and antipyretic drug and has been marketed in the United States as an over-the-counter preparation since 1960. Acetaminophen is largely metabolized by phase II enzyme systems and undergoes conjugation with glucuronate and sulfate in the liver. These nontoxic conjugates are excreted by the kidney. Most of an acetaminophen dose can be recovered in the urine within 24 hours as glucuronide conjugates (~50% to 65%) and sulfate conjugates (~30% to 45%). Only approximately 1% of the dose is excreted in the urine as free acetaminophen. The extent of metabolism to glucuronide versus sulfate conjugates, but not total conjugation, has been shown to be influenced by diet, with a high-carbohydrate, low-protein diet favoring glucuronidation and a high-protein, low-carbohydrate diet favoring sulfation (Pantuck et al., 1991).

A small fraction of an acetaminophen dose is metabolized by a phase I enzyme system to a hepatotoxic reactive intermediate. If this reactive intermediate is not detoxified by conjugation with glutathione, it can covalently bind to cellular macromolecules or cause other injurious effects that lead to hepatocellular necrosis. Glutathione conjugates are further metabolized to form cysteine conjugates and *N*-acetylcysteine conjugates (mercapturic acids), which together account for 2% to 3% of the acetaminophen excreted in the urine. A small amount of glutathione-derived conjugates may also be excreted in the bile.

conjugates from a variety of acceptor compounds, including various xenobiotics (foreign compounds such as drugs and carcinogens). These conjugates are normally degraded by γ-glutamyl transpeptidase and cysteinylglycine dipeptidase to yield the cysteinyl derivatives, which may be acetylated using acetyl-CoA to become mercapturic acids, which are excreted in the urine.

PHENYLALANINE AND TYROSINE

Phenylalanine and tyrosine are closely related aromatic amino acids. Tyrosine is formed by the hydroxylation of phenylalanine. This conversion is also the first step in phenylalanine degradation.

Conversion of Phenylalanine to Tyrosine

The catabolism of phenylalanine and tyrosine primarily occurs in the liver, but tyrosine is an important precursor for synthesis of several essential compounds in other tissues. As shown in Figure 14-24, phenylalanine is converted to tyrosine by phenylalanine hydroxylase, which is a tetrahydrobiopterin-dependent, mixed-function oxidase that hydroxylates phenylalanine at the C4 of the aromatic ring. This reaction is the first step in phenylalanine degradation and also is the step that allows phenylalanine to serve as a dietary precursor of tyrosine (Clarke and Bier, 1982). The reverse reaction does not occur, so tyrosine cannot totally replace phenylalanine in the diet; only approximately 50% to 70% of the total phenylalanine and tyrosine requirement can be provided as tyrosine (Pencharz et al., 2007).

The conversion of phenylalanine to tyrosine and hence phenylalanine catabolism is regulated by changes in the activity of phenylalanine hydroxylase. The activity of phenylalanine hydroxylase activity is regulated by changes in the enzyme's phosphorylation state (Doskeland et al., 1996) and by effects of phenylalanine on the enzyme's conformation (Bjorgo et al., 2001). Phosphorylation of a serine residue in a regulatory domain of the enzyme activates phenylalanine hydroxylase by increasing its specific activity. The potency of phenylalanine as an activator of phenylalanine hydroxylase is greater for the phosphorylated form of the enzyme. An increase in the phenylalanine concentration induces conformational changes that favor tetramer formation and high-affinity phenylalanine binding. The tetrameric form of phenylalanine hydroxylase exhibits cooperative binding of phenylalanine. Therefore either an increase in phenylalanine concentration (high-protein diet) or an increase in the circulating glucagon level will increase phenylalanine hydroxylase activity. In the rat, phosphorylation of the enzyme is catalyzed by both cAMP-dependent protein kinase and calcium/calmodulin-dependent protein kinase.

The absence of phenylalanine hydroxylase activity is the basis of the inherited metabolic disease, phenylketonuria (PKU); PKU is the most common disease caused by a deficiency of an enzyme of amino acid metabolism, and infants are routinely screened at birth for this defect (Erlandsen et al., 2003). Children with an absence of phenylalanine hydroxylase accumulate high levels of phenylalanine in

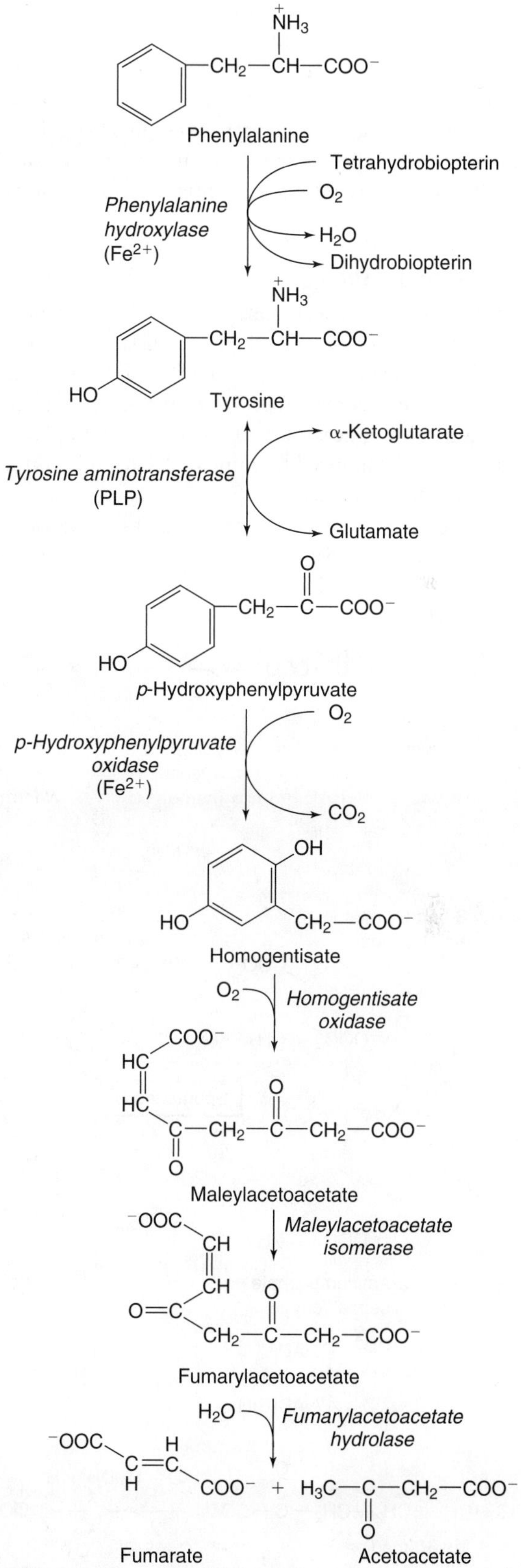

FIGURE 14-24 Metabolism of phenylalanine and tyrosine.

their tissues and also metabolize some phenylalanine via abnormal routes such as transamination. In normal individuals, transamination of phenylalanine plays a very small role, because the K_m for phenylalanine transamination is much higher than normal hepatic phenylalanine concentrations. The keto acid of phenylalanine, phenylpyruvate, and its products phenyl-lactate and phenylacetate accumulate in body fluids and are excreted in the urine of individuals with PKU who are not treated with a low-phenylalanine, but adequate-tyrosine, diet. It should be noted that in patients with PKU, tyrosine is a dietary essential amino acid because it cannot be synthesized.

Tyrosine Catabolism

Tyrosine is primarily catabolized via transamination to *p*-hydroxyphenylpyruvate (see Figure 14-24). Tyrosine aminotransferase is expressed only in the liver, has a short half-life, and is subject to regulation by a number of hormones, including insulin, glucagon, and glucocorticoids. The keto acid is further metabolized to homogentisate and ultimately to fumarate plus acetoacetate.

The role of the tyrosine transamination pathway in phenylalanine and tyrosine catabolism is demonstrated by alcaptonuria, an inborn error of metabolism that results from a deficiency of homogentisate oxidase. Individuals with alcaptonuria excrete almost all ingested tyrosine and phenylalanine as homogentisate in their urine. If urine that contains homogentisate is allowed to stand or if alkali is added, it gradually turns dark as the homogentisate is oxidized to a melanin-like product. This darkening of the urine led to early recognition of this disease, and alcaptonuria was the first condition to be identified as an inborn error of metabolism. Alcaptonuria and other inborn errors of metabolism have provided much information about amino acid metabolism in humans.

TRYPTOPHAN

Catabolism of Tryptophan in Liver and Synthesis of NAD(P)

Tryptophan is degraded primarily in the liver, by a pathway shown in Figure 14-25. The first step in the catabolic pathway is an oxygenation that opens the five-member ring of the indole nucleus of tryptophan to yield *N*-formylkynurenine. This reaction is catalyzed in the liver by tryptophan dioxygenase (also called tryptophan pyrrolase). Hepatic tryptophan dioxygenase is a heme-containing enzyme with a very

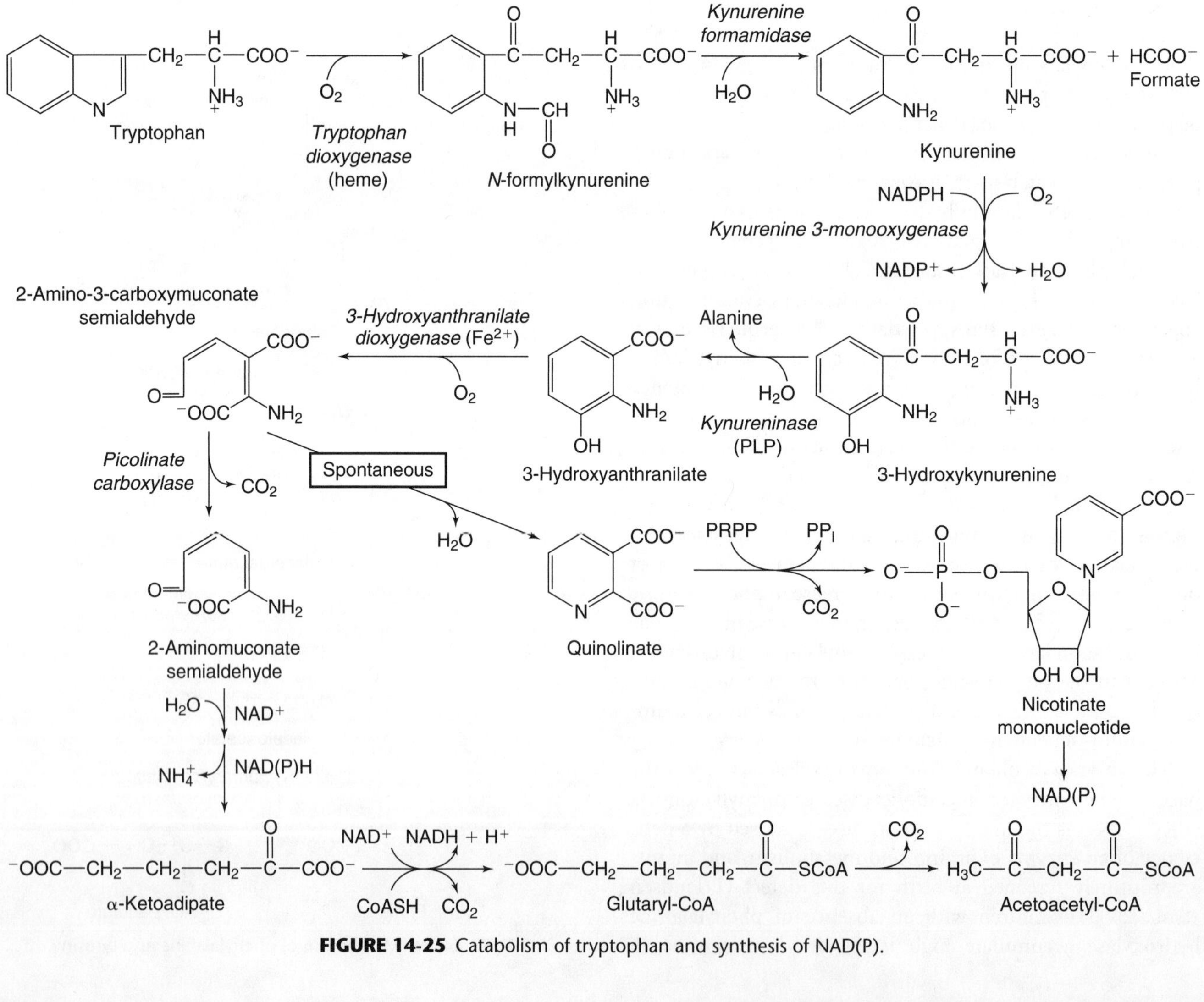

FIGURE 14-25 Catabolism of tryptophan and synthesis of NAD(P).

short half-life and it is highly regulated. Glucagon and other hormones such as glucocorticoids increase the amount of the enzyme; high levels of nicotinamide nucleotide coenzymes can inhibit the enzyme; and tryptophan can stabilize the enzyme against proteolysis, resulting in greater steady state levels of the enzyme protein.

The hydrolytic removal of formate from *N*-formylkynurenine by kynurenine formamidase yields kynurenine. The formate can enter the one-carbon pool by conversion to 10-formyl-THF. Kynurenine-3-monooxygenase, an NADPH-dependent enzyme, hydroxylates kynurenine on the benzene ring to give 3-hydroxykynurenine, which is converted to 3-hydroxyanthranilate and alanine by kynureninase, a PLP-dependent enzyme. 3-Hydroxyanthranilate-3,4-dioxygenase, which requires Fe^{2+} as a cofactor, catalyzes the oxidative ring opening of 3-hydroxyanthranilate to yield 2-amino-3-carboxymuconate semialdehyde, an intermediate that sits at a branch point. Ring closure and decarboxylation can occur spontaneously to give quinolinic acid, which can then be converted to nicotinic acid ribonucleotide by quinolinic acid phosphoribosyltransferase. The nicotinic acid ribonucleotide is further converted to NAD^+ and $NADP^+$. Alternatively, 2-amino-3-carboxymuconate-6-semialdehyde decarboxylase (picolinate carboxylase) will catalyze decarboxylation of the branch point intermediate to give 2-aminomuconate-6-semialdehyde. In humans, most of the 2-aminomuconate semialdehyde formed in this reaction is further oxidized to acetoacetyl-CoA and CO_2.

The pathway for further oxidation of 2-aminomuconate semialdehyde involves its conversion via poorly understood reactions to α-ketoadipate, which is oxidatively decarboxylated to glutaryl-CoA. Glutaryl-CoA is ultimately converted to acetoacetyl-CoA by a sequence of reactions that are similar to those involved in the metabolism of the α-aminoadipate that is formed in lysine catabolism (Figure 14-26). Glutaric aciduria type I results from a deficiency of glutaryl-CoA dehydrogenase; when patients with this inborn error of metabolism are treated with dietary restrictions of both tryptophan and lysine, the urinary excretion of glutarate is decreased (Yannicelli et al., 1994). This, along with the observed patterns of metabolite excretion, suggests that metabolism of tryptophan via kynurenine, 3-kynurenine, 2-amino-3-carboxymuconate semialdehyde, and glutaryl-CoA is the major route of tryptophan catabolism under normal conditions.

Thus 7 of the 11 carbon atoms in the tryptophan carbon skeleton are ultimately funneled into central pathways of energy metabolism as pyruvate (alanine) and acetylacetyl-CoA. The formation of alanine by kynureninase would be glucogenic, and the formation of acetoacetyl-CoA from 2-aminomuconate semialdehyde in the major branch of the catabolic pathway is ketogenic. The other four carbon atoms are lost as formate and CO_2.

Although the pathway shown in Figure 14-25 represents the main pathway for tryptophan catabolism in the human, several side reactions can occur. Kynurenine or 3-hydroxykynurenine can be transaminated by kynurenine aminotransferase to give kynurenic acid or xanthurenic acid, respectively, compounds that are excreted in the urine. Loss of kynurenine, kynurenic acid, 3-hydroxykynurenine, or xanthurenic acid in the urine represents a loss of both gluconeogenic and ketogenic precursors; the basal excretion of these tryptophan catabolites normally accounts for approximately 3% to 6% of the ingested tryptophan (Leklem, 1971). A deficiency of vitamin B_6 results in decreased kynureninase activity and increased excretion of kynurenine, 3-hydroxykynurenine, kynurenic acid, and xanthurenic acid in the urine. During pregnancy, increased urinary excretion of these same tryptophan metabolites is observed; this seems to result from a pregnancy-specific decrease in kynureninase activity that is not related to a vitamin B_6 deficiency (van de Kamp and Smolen, 1995).

Metabolism of Tryptophan by the Kynurenine Pathway in Nonhepatic Tissues

Whereas tryptophan dioxygenase is present in liver and is involved in the major pathway of tryptophan catabolism, the enzyme indoleamine 2,3-dioxygenase is ubiquitous in nonhepatic tissues, such as placenta, lung, and intestine, and it also catalyzes the conversion of tryptophan to *N*-formylkynurenine from which it can be converted to kynurenine. Indoleamine 2,3-dioxygenase is inducible by the proinflammatory cytokine, interferon-γ, and accelerated tryptophan degradation is observed concomitant to cellular immune activation (Wirleitner et al., 2003; Maes et al., 2002). In fact, active indoleamine dioxygenase depletes tryptophan from local tissues and promotes formation of bioactive kynurenine pathway metabolites. Activation of indoleamine dioxygenase appears to play a role in promotion of the immune tolerance involved in situations such as prevention of fetal rejection and rendering a host tolerant to a cancerous lesion (King and Thomas, 2007). Depletion of circulating tryptophan may also lead to reduced serotonin production, which may contribute to the development of anxiety and depression in individuals with chronic disease and in women in the early weeks following childbirth. Indoleamine dioxygenase is present in the lens of the eye where the tryptophan catabolites, kynurenine and 3-hydroxykynurenine glucoside, bind to lens proteins to form yellow and fluorescent adducts (Takikawa et al., 2001). These adducts are responsible for the yellowing of the lens with age.

LYSINE

Lysine does not participate in classical transamination reactions so it cannot be replaced by its keto acid in the diet, as can many other amino acids. Lysine catabolism occurs by the saccharopine pathway or by the pipecolate pathway.

Saccharopine Pathway

Most degradation of lysine occurs by way of the saccharopine pathway (see Figure 14-26), which is present in liver mitochondria of mammals (Scislowski et al., 1994). This pathway involves the reaction of the ε-amino group of lysine with the carbonyl group of α-ketoglutarate to form saccharopine; the reaction is catalyzed by lysine-α-ketoglutarate

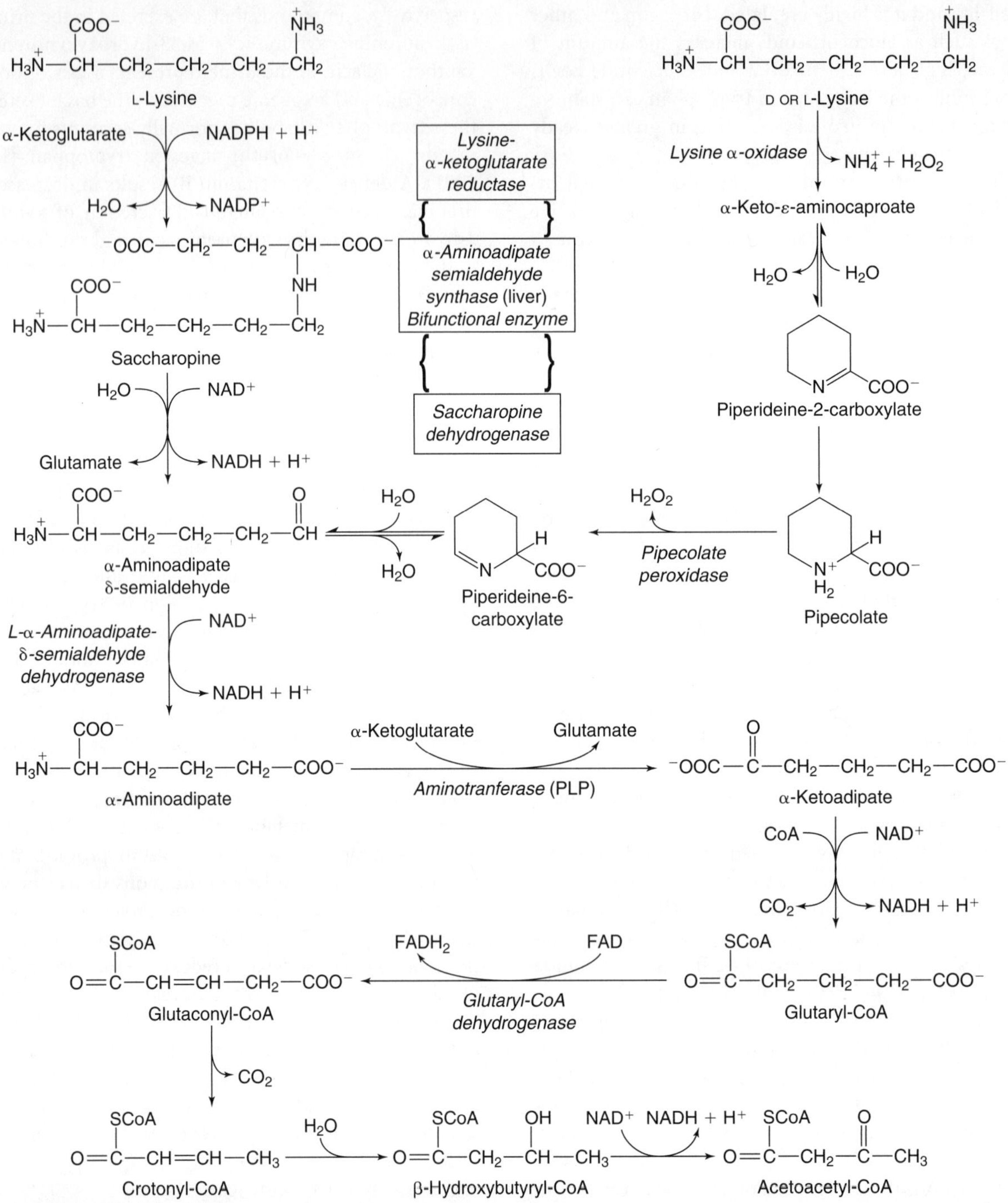

FIGURE 14-26 Catabolism of L-lysine, initiated by the bifunctional enzyme, α-aminoadipate semialdehyde synthase and minor pathway for oxidation of D (or L)-lysine.

reductase, using NADPH as cofactor. The saccharopine is further metabolized to α-aminoadipic semialdehyde plus glutamate by saccharopine dehydrogenase, with reduction of NAD^+. The net effect of these two reactions is to incorporate the ε-amino group of lysine into the α-amino nitrogen pool via glutamate. The α-aminoadipate semialdehyde is oxidized to α-aminoadipate by α-aminoadipate semialdehyde dehydrogenase with the reduction of NAD^+. The amino group of the α-aminoadipate is transferred to α-ketoglutarate by aminoadipate aminotransferase to give glutamate and α-ketoadipate. The α-ketoadipate, which is a higher homolog of α-ketoglutarate, is oxidized to glutaryl-CoA and ultimately to acetoacetyl-CoA; these final steps of lysine catabolism are analogous to those involved in the final steps of tryptophan catabolism (see Figure 14-26).

The formation and dehydrogenation of saccharopine are catalyzed by a bifunctional protein (α-aminoadipic semialdehyde synthase), which contains active sites for lysine-α-ketoglutarate reductase and saccharopine dehydrogenase on the same protein (Sacksteder et al., 2000). A rare inborn error of metabolism in which both activities are deficient results in hyperlysinemia and excretion of lysine and smaller amounts of saccharopine in the urine (Divry et al., 1991). The saccharopine pathway is regulated by changes in the activity of α-aminoadipate semialdehyde synthase, which is increased in animals fed diets high in lysine or protein (increased amount of enzyme protein) and in rats treated with glucagon (increased activity state) (Scislowski et al., 1994).

Pipecolate Pathway

Although not sufficient to compensate for deficiency in the saccharopine pathway, the pipecolate pathway of lysine degradation may play a role, especially in nonhepatic tissues, such as brain (Praphanphoj et al., 2001), and particularly for the nonphysiological stereoisomer, D-lysine (Broquist, 1991). The α-amino group of lysine can be released as ammonia by a lysine α-oxidase reaction with formation of a cyclic derivative, piperideine-2-carboxylate, which is reduced to form pipecolate, a cyclic imino acid. The pipecolate is oxidized by pipecolate peroxidase, which is found in peroxisomes in human liver, brain, and kidney. Pipecolate accumulates in individuals with peroxisomal disorders (Steinberg et al., 2006). The oxidation of pipecolate by pipecolate peroxidase yields hydrogen peroxide and piperideine-6-carboxylate, which is hydrolyzed spontaneously to α-aminoadipate semialdehyde, an early intermediate in the saccharopine pathway of lysine catabolism. Hence the two pathways converge, and the process of lysine catabolism is completed by the same series of reactions.

BRANCHED-CHAIN AMINO ACIDS

The three branched-chain amino acids, leucine, isoleucine, and valine, make up a considerable part of dietary protein (20% to 30% of all amino acids). If the level in the diet is more than is required for protein synthesis, the excess must be degraded because high levels of branched-chain amino acids are toxic (Harris et al., 2005).

Catabolism of Branched-Chain Amino Acids

Catabolism begins by transamination of the amino acids with α-ketoglutarate, catalyzed by branched-chain amino acid aminotransferase to form the corresponding branched-chain α-keto acids, as shown in Figure 14-27. Both mitochondrial and cytosolic forms of branched-chain aminotransferase exist in the brain, but only the mitochondrial form is widespread in other human tissues (Sweatt et al., 2004). Both isoenzymes are capable of using all three branched-chain amino or α-keto acids as substrate. Based on enzyme level and tissue mass, skeletal muscle has the highest capacity for branched-chain amino acid transamination in humans. Liver, brain, and kidney may also contribute significantly (Suryawan et al., 1998).

The branched-chain α-keto acids formed as a result of transamination are oxidized via a mitochondrial branched-chain keto acid dehydrogenase complex to CO_2, NADH, and the branched-chain acyl-CoAs. The branched-chain keto acid dehydrogenase complex is similar to the pyruvate and α-ketoglutarate dehydrogenase complexes and is composed of three enzymes known as E1, E2, and E3 (see Chapter 12, Figure 12-18). As the first irreversible step in their catabolism, this is the most important regulatory enzyme in the catabolic pathways of the branched-chain amino acids. In the rat, much of the keto acid of valine formed by heart muscle is released into the circulation to be further metabolized in the liver, whereas most of the keto acid of leucine is fully oxidized in heart muscle (Letto et al., 1990). The oxidative decarboxylation of all three branched-chain keto acids in humans probably occurs predominantly in muscle, liver, kidney, and brain (Suryawan et al., 1998).

The branched-chain acyl-CoAs are further oxidized by specific branched-chain acyl-CoA dehydrogenases to form the corresponding α,β-unsaturated compounds (see Figure 14-27). Catabolism of valine and isoleucine continues through several steps to produce propionyl-CoA from valine and both propionyl-CoA and acetyl-CoA from isoleucine. Release of β-hydroxyisobutyrate from muscle and heart has been observed in animals; this valine catabolite can be converted to glucose in the liver (Letto et al., 1986). The branched-chain acyl-CoA formed from leucine, isovaleryl-CoA, is oxidized to β-methylcrotonyl-CoA by isovaleryl-CoA dehydrogenase, followed by a biotin-dependent carboxylation step to convert β-methylcrotonyl-CoA to β-methylglutaconyl-CoA. β-Methylglutaconyl-CoA hydratase adds a water to give β-hydroxy-β-methylglutaryl-CoA (HMG-CoA) that is split by HMG-CoA lyase to give acetoacetate and acetyl-CoA. Complete oxidation of leucine yields 39 mol ATP per mol of leucine, slightly more than that yielded by complete oxidation of glucose. Much of the branched-chain amino acid nitrogen is carried out of muscle as alanine and glutamine (Darmaun and Dechelotte, 1991).

The branched-chain keto acid dehydrogenase complex is subject to feedback regulation by high ratios of $NADH/NAD^+$ and acyl-CoA/CoA and is also regulated by phosphorylation/dephosphorylation. The activity state of the branched-chain keto acid dehydrogenase complex is regulated by the phosphorylation state of specific serine residues of the E1 component of the complex, which in turn is regulated by the relative activities of a specific mitochondrial kinase and phosphatase (Harris et al., 2004). The complex is inactive in its phosphorylated state. In animals, adaptation to higher-protein diets results in the association of less kinase with the branched-chain keto acid dehydrogenase complex, which favors the dephosphorylated, active state. Short-term regulation of the complex is achieved by inhibition of the branched-chain keto acid dehydrogenase kinase by branched-chain keto acids (especially by α-ketoisocaproate), which are the substrates for the branched-chain keto acid dehydrogenase complex. This mechanism allows leucine to regulate its own catabolism or tissue concentrations and thus to self-limit its positive effects on protein accretion (increased protein synthesis, decreased protein degradation, and increased insulin secretion).

An inborn error of branched-chain amino acid metabolism, called maple syrup urine disease because of the odor of the urine, results from mutations affecting different subunits of the mitochondrial branched-chain keto acid dehydrogenase complex. A thiamine-responsive form of maple syrup urine disease is due to mutations in the gene for the

E2 subunit (Chuang et al., 2004). Plasma and urinary levels of branched-chain amino acids and their α-keto acids are elevated. Small amounts of α-hydroxy acids (formed by reduction of α-keto acids) are also found in the urine of patients with this inborn error. This rare inborn error is associated with severe neurological symptoms if not diagnosed early and treated with a protein-modified diet. Defects in branched-chain amino acid metabolism that affect a number of the other intermediary steps also have been identified in human patients (Gibson et al., 1994).

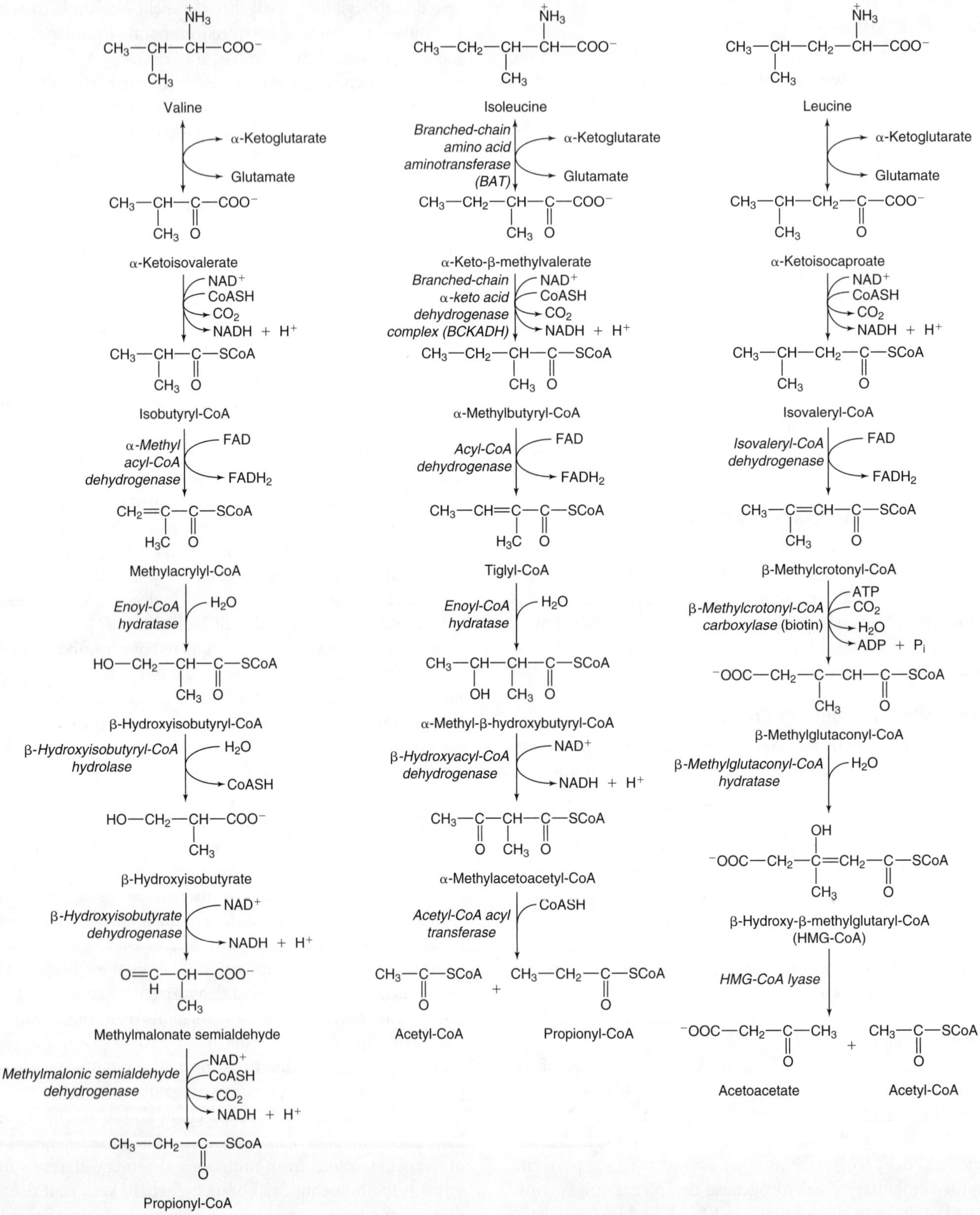

Valine: $CH_3-CH(CH_3)-CH(NH_3^+)-COO^-$
- *Branched-chain amino acid aminotransferase (BAT)*: α-Ketoglutarate → Glutamate
- α-Ketoisovalerate: $CH_3-CH(CH_3)-C(=O)-COO^-$
- *Branched-chain α-keto acid dehydrogenase complex (BCKADH)*: NAD^+, CoASH → CO_2, NADH + H^+
- Isobutyryl-CoA: $CH_3-CH(CH_3)-C(=O)-SCoA$
- *α-Methyl acyl-CoA dehydrogenase*: FAD → $FADH_2$
- Methylacrylyl-CoA: $CH_2=C(H_3C)-C(=O)-SCoA$
- *Enoyl-CoA hydratase*: H_2O
- β-Hydroxyisobutyryl-CoA: $HO-CH_2-CH(CH_3)-C(=O)-SCoA$
- *β-Hydroxyisobutyryl-CoA hydrolase*: H_2O → CoASH
- β-Hydroxyisobutyrate: $HO-CH_2-CH(CH_3)-COO^-$
- *β-Hydroxyisobutyrate dehydrogenase*: NAD^+ → NADH + H^+
- Methylmalonate semialdehyde: $O=C(H)-CH(CH_3)-COO^-$
- *Methylmalonic semialdehyde dehydrogenase*: NAD^+, CoASH → CO_2, NADH + H^+
- Propionyl-CoA: $CH_3-CH_2-C(=O)-SCoA$

Isoleucine: $CH_3-CH_2-CH(CH_3)-CH(NH_3^+)-COO^-$
- *Branched-chain amino acid aminotransferase (BAT)*: α-Ketoglutarate → Glutamate
- α-Keto-β-methylvalerate: $CH_3-CH_2-CH(CH_3)-C(=O)-COO^-$
- *Branched-chain α-keto acid dehydrogenase complex (BCKADH)*: NAD^+, CoASH → CO_2, NADH + H^+
- α-Methylbutyryl-CoA: $CH_3-CH_2-CH(CH_3)-C(=O)-SCoA$
- *Acyl-CoA dehydrogenase*: FAD → $FADH_2$
- Tiglyl-CoA: $CH_3-CH=C(H_3C)-C(=O)-SCoA$
- *Enoyl-CoA hydratase*: H_2O
- α-Methyl-β-hydroxybutyryl-CoA: $CH_3-CH(OH)-CH(CH_3)-C(=O)-SCoA$
- *β-Hydroxyacyl-CoA dehydrogenase*: NAD^+ → NADH + H^+
- α-Methylacetoacetyl-CoA: $CH_3-C(=O)-CH(CH_3)-C(=O)-SCoA$
- *Acetyl-CoA acyl transferase*: CoASH
- Acetyl-CoA $CH_3-C(=O)-SCoA$ + Propionyl-CoA $CH_3-CH_2-C(=O)-SCoA$

Leucine: $CH_3-CH(CH_3)-CH_2-CH(NH_3^+)-COO^-$
- α-Ketoglutarate → Glutamate
- α-Ketoisocaproate: $CH_3-CH(CH_3)-CH_2-C(=O)-COO^-$
- NAD^+, CoASH → CO_2, NADH + H^+
- Isovaleryl-CoA: $CH_3-CH(CH_3)-CH_2-C(=O)-SCoA$
- *Isovaleryl-CoA dehydrogenase*: FAD → $FADH_2$
- β-Methylcrotonyl-CoA: $CH_3-C(CH_3)=CH-C(=O)-SCoA$
- *β-Methylcrotonyl-CoA carboxylase* (biotin): ATP, CO_2 → H_2O, ADP + P_i
- β-Methylglutaconyl-CoA: $^-OOC-CH_2-C(CH_3)-CH-C(=O)-SCoA$
- *β-Methylglutaconyl-CoA hydratase*: H_2O
- β-Hydroxy-β-methylglutaryl-CoA (HMG-CoA): $^-OOC-CH_2-C(OH)(CH_3)=CH_2-C(=O)-SCoA$
- *HMG-CoA lyase*
- Acetoacetate $^-OOC-CH_2-C(=O)-CH_3$ + Acetyl-CoA $CH_3-C(=O)-SCoA$

FIGURE 14-27 Catabolism of the branched-chain amino acids

NEUROACTIVE AMINES, HORMONES, AND PIGMENTS FORMED FROM AMINO ACIDS BY SPECIALIZED CELL TYPES

SYNTHESIS OF γ-AMINOBUTYRIC ACID FROM GLUTAMATE IN NEURONS

The conversion of glutamate to γ-aminobutyric acid (GABA) is catalyzed by glutamate decarboxylase, which releases the α-carboxyl group as CO_2, as shown in Figure 14-28. GABA is removed by transamination with α-ketoglutarate to yield glutamate and succinate semialdehyde; the succinate semialdehyde is then oxidized to succinate, which can be used to regenerate α-ketoglutarate via citric acid cycle enzymes. The cycling of α-ketoglutarate to glutamate to GABA to succinate and back to α-ketoglutarate is called the GABA shunt. Nerve terminals and neurons also may use glutamine for synthesis of glutamate (and hence GABA) because neurons have high glutaminase activity. Some of the glutamate and GABA released by neurons is taken up by glial cells, which have high glutamine synthetase activity, and is used in the resynthesis of glutamine.

NEUROTRANSMITTER FUNCTION OF GLUTAMATE, GABA, AND GLYCINE

In the central nervous system, glutamate is a major excitatory neurotransmitter, whereas GABA and glycine are inhibitory neurotransmitters, glycine mainly in spinal cord and brainstem and GABA in other parts of the brain. Glutamate exerts its actions through receptors that function as ligand-gated cation channels, such as NMDA receptors and AMPA receptors (both of which are named for drugs that function as agonists for the specific receptors). The receptors for glycine and GABA are also ligand-gated channels, but they are anion channels selectively permeable to chloride. When these channels are open, the membrane potential becomes more negative (hyperpolarized) rather than depolarized as occurs when excitatory cation channels are opened. A neuron inhibited by hyperpolarization requires a more intense depolarization than is otherwise required to trigger an action potential.

CONVERSION OF TRYPTOPHAN TO SEROTONIN AND MELATONIN

Tryptophan is converted to serotonin, an important neurotransmitter that may also have functions outside the central nervous system (Peters, 1991). Serotonin synthesis involves the hydroxylation of tryptophan at C5 by a mixed-function oxygenase that uses tetrahydrobiopterin as a cosubstrate, followed by decarboxylation of the resulting 5-hydroxytryptophan

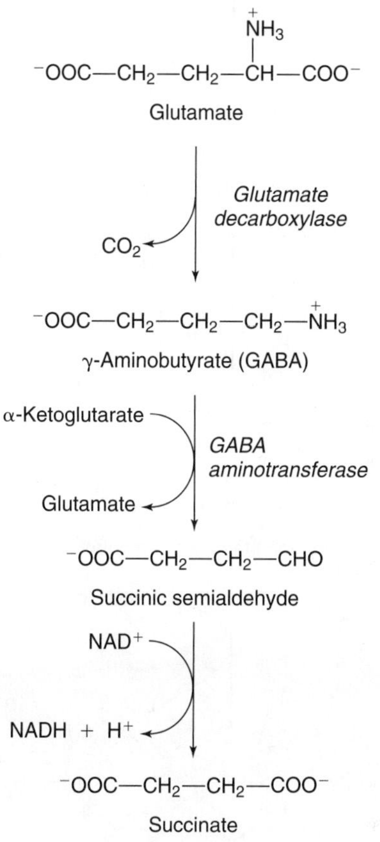

$^{-}OOC—CH_2—CH_2—CH(\overset{+}{N}H_3)—COO^{-}$

Glutamate

↓ Glutamate decarboxylase ($\rightarrow CO_2$)

$^{-}OOC—CH_2—CH_2—CH_2—\overset{+}{N}H_3$

γ-Aminobutyrate (GABA)

↓ GABA aminotransferase (α-Ketoglutarate → Glutamate)

$^{-}OOC—CH_2—CH_2—CHO$

Succinic semialdehyde

↓ (NAD^+ → NADH + H^+)

$^{-}OOC—CH_2—CH_2—COO^{-}$

Succinate

FIGURE 14-28 Synthesis and degradation of γ-aminobutyric acid (GABA).

CLINICAL CORRELATION

Two Genetic Disorders of Neurotransmitter Degradation

In the central nervous system, GABA and glycine are inhibitory neurotransmitters, with glycine functioning mainly in spinal cord and brainstem and GABA in other parts of the brain. Nonketotic hyperglycinemia and GABA transaminase deficiency are genetic disorders that cause accumulation of these inhibitory neurotransmitters.

Nonketotic hyperglycinemia is an autosomal recessive disorder that results in a biochemical defect in one of the components of the glycine cleavage system complex, causing the accumulation of large quantities of glycine in all body tissues. Most patients show severe neurological abnormalities, including lethargy, hypotonia, myoclonic jerks, and apnea, often progressing to coma and death. Those who regain spontaneous respiration develop intractable seizures and profound mental retardation.

GABA transaminase deficiency is a very rare autosomal recessive disorder associated with seizures, hypotonia, and profound psychomotor retardation. GABA transaminase has the highest activity in liver, followed by kidney, brain, and pancreas, with lower levels in a few other tissues. Deficiency of the enzyme has been reported to cause an accumulation of GABA in tissues, plasma, cerebrospinal fluid, and urine. Because cultured skin fibroblasts do not contain GABA transaminase, they cannot be used to diagnose a deficiency condition, but the enzyme is present in chorionic villus tissue and in cultured lymphocytes, and these tissues are available for diagnostic use.

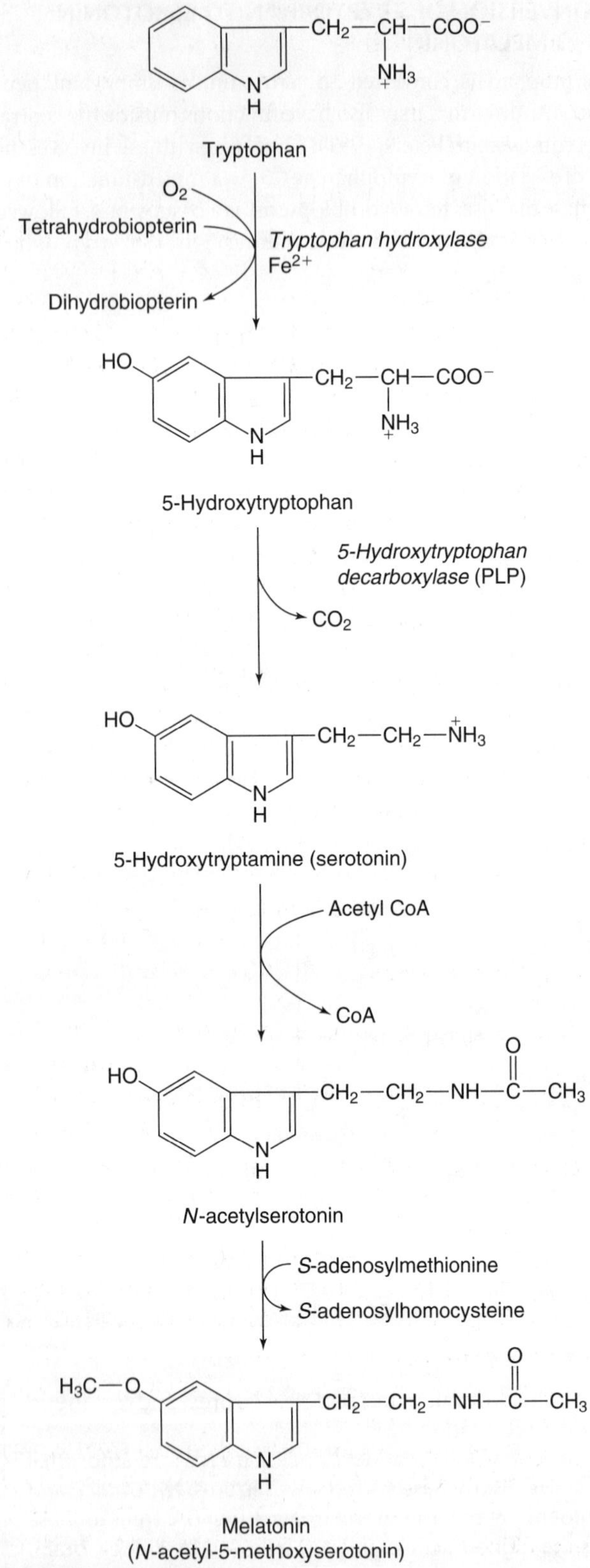

Tryptophan

O_2

Tetrahydrobiopterin

Dihydrobiopterin

Tryptophan hydroxylase
Fe^{2+}

5-Hydroxytryptophan

5-Hydroxytryptophan decarboxylase (PLP)

CO_2

5-Hydroxytryptamine (serotonin)

Acetyl CoA

CoA

N-acetylserotonin

S-adenosylmethionine

S-adenosylhomocysteine

Melatonin
(*N*-acetyl-5-methoxyserotonin)

FIGURE 14-29 Synthesis of serotonin and melatonin from tryptophan.

by a PLP–dependent enzyme to give 5-hydroxytryptamine (serotonin), as shown in Figure 14-29. Tryptophan hydroxylase is not normally saturated with substrate, and increased uptake of tryptophan by a tissue can result in increased serotonin synthesis. Serotonergic neurons have an active reuptake mechanism, and they can inactivate the serotonin by oxidation to 5-hydroxyindoleacetic acid. The inactive metabolites and their conjugates are excreted in the urine. Serotonin is methylated and acetylated to form melatonin (N-acetyl-5-methoxytryptamine) in the pineal gland and, perhaps, other tissues. Melatonin production in the pineal gland is elevated during the dark phase of the daily cycle and is believed to play a role in maintenance of daily and seasonal rhythms.

ROLE OF TYROSINE IN THE SYNTHESIS OF NEUROACTIVE AMINES, HORMONES, AND PIGMENTS

In catecholamine-producing neurons and chromaffin cells of the adrenal medulla, tyrosine is hydroxylated to 3,4-dihydroxyphenylalanine (DOPA) by tyrosine hydroxylase, which is a tetrahydrobiopterin-dependent enzyme similar to phenylalanine hydroxylase (Eisenhofer et al., 2003; Dix et al., 1987). DOPA is further metabolized to various products, depending on the tissue (Figure 14-30). In specific regions of the brain, DOPA is decarboxylated to dopamine, which functions as a neurotransmitter. Decreased production of dopamine is the cause of Parkinson disease. In noradrenergic neurons, DOPA is converted to dopamine and further hydroxylated to norepinephrine. Norepinephrine is the chemical transmitter at most sympathetic postganglionic nerve endings. Norepinephrine is synthesized by the noradrenergic neurons and stored in vesicles in the termini of the axons; these cells also have an active mechanism for reuptake of norepinephrine. In chromaffin cells in the adrenal medulla, dopamine and norepinephrine also are produced, but most of the norepinephrine is methylated (by a methyltransferase that uses SAM) to epinephrine, the major hormone secreted by the adrenal medulla of humans. Epinephrine, norepinephrine, and dopamine, collectively called catecholamines, are stored in the chromaffin cells in vesicles (granules) and are subsequently released from these vesicles into the blood. Inactivation of catecholamines is accomplished by the reactions catalyzed by monoamine oxidase and catechol-*O*-methyltransferase and by conjugation of catecholamines with sulfate or glucuronate.

In melanin-producing cells (melanocytes), DOPA formed by tyrosine hydroxylase is oxidized by tyrosinase to form dopaquinone and various derivatives of dopaquinone. These compounds condense to form melanins or dark pigments, which are contained in cellular organelles called melanosomes. Melanins are a family of high-molecular-weight polymers that contain various metabolites of dopaquinone and, in the case of reddish pigments, cysteine. Melanins are concentrated in the skin, hair, and parts of the eye and brain. Genetic disorders in melanin synthesis are responsible for albinism.

Tyrosine residues in the protein thyroglobulin serve as precursors of thyroid hormones. Thyroglobulin in the thyroid gland contains iodinated aromatic amino acids derived from tyrosine. Posttranslational iodination and coupling of tyrosine residues in thyroglobulin is followed by release of triiodothyronine (T_3) and thyroxin (T_4) from the thyroid gland after proteolysis of thyroglobulin (see Chapter 38).

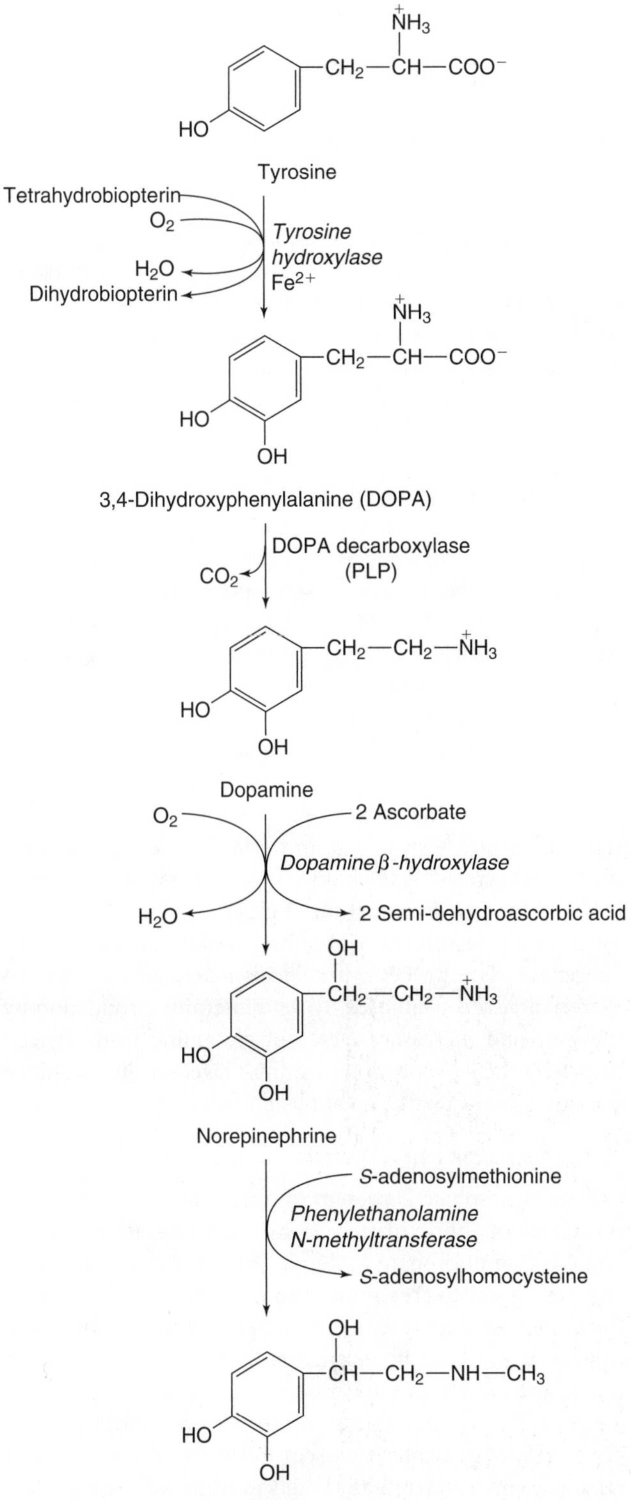

Tyrosine

Tetrahydrobiopterin, O_2 → H_2O, Dihydrobiopterin — *Tyrosine hydroxylase* Fe^{2+}

3,4-Dihydroxyphenylalanine (DOPA)

DOPA decarboxylase (PLP) → CO_2

Dopamine

O_2, 2 Ascorbate → H_2O, 2 Semi-dehydroascorbic acid — *Dopamine β-hydroxylase*

Norepinephrine

S-adenosylmethionine → *S*-adenosylhomocysteine — *Phenylethanolamine N-methyltransferase*

Epinephrine

FIGURE 14-30 Synthesis of catecholamines from tyrosine.

NITROGEN EXCRETION

The major end products of amino acid catabolism in humans are CO_2, H_2O, and urea, with a small amount of ammonia. Because energy is required for urea synthesis and urea has a heat of combustion of 151.6 kcal per mole, the net physiological fuel value mammals can gain from dietary protein is less than would be predicted based on complete oxidation of absorbed amino acids. In adults in nitrogen balance, nitrogen excretion as urea approximates the daily intake of nitrogen from protein. Urine also contains smaller amounts of other nitrogenous end products formed from catabolism of amino acids or of nonprotein compounds formed from amino acids (Table 14-3). Although most of the body's loss of nitrogen occurs via the urine, nitrogen is also lost via the feces (including loss of remnants from digestion of dietary and endogenous proteins in the gastrointestinal tract and endogenous nitrogenous compounds excreted by the liver in the bile) and via loss of proteins and other nitrogenous compounds in the hair, nails, sloughed-off skin, various bodily secretions, and blood losses.

TABLE 14-3 Major Nitrogen-Containing Components of Normal Human Urine

EXCRETED NITROGEN END PRODUCT	(g N/24 hr)
Urea	10–15*
Creatinine	0.3–0.8
NH_3, NH_4^+	0.4–1.0
Uric acid	0.1–0.2
Amino acids	0.1–0.2
Other nitrogen	0.2–0.8†
TOTAL NITROGEN	12–18

*Urea N depends heavily on the amount of dietary protein and may vary from less than 2 g to more than 20 g per day.
†Other N includes trace amount of proteins, δ-aminolevulinic acid, porphobilinogen, 5-hydroxyindole acetic acid, catecholamine metabolites, and tryptophan metabolites.

INCORPORATION OF NITROGEN INTO UREA BY THE UREA CYCLE IN THE LIVER

The urea cycle was first described by Hans Krebs and Kurt Henseleit in 1932, based on experiments in which they found that ornithine stimulated urea synthesis by rat liver without itself being utilized in the process. In mammals, a complete urea cycle functions only in liver, the major site of urea synthesis. (Some urea cycle enzymes are expressed in the intestine, kidney, and other tissues, where they play a role in the synthesis of citrulline, arginine, and ornithine, as discussed in the preceding text in this chapter.) The urea cycle is shown in Figures 14-11 and 14-16. The pathway begins with the incorporation of ammonia and carbon dioxide into carbamoyl phosphate by the mitochondrial enzyme carbamoyl phosphate synthetase 1. The carbamoyl phosphate then combines with ornithine to form citrulline, which exits from the mitochondria in exchange for ornithine via the ornithine transporter 1 (ORNT1) carrier (Indiveri et al., 1992). In the cytosol, argininosuccinate synthetase and argininosuccinate lyase effectively add a nitrogen (from aspartate) to the citrulline to produce arginine. The arginine is then hydrolyzed by arginase, thereby liberating urea and ornithine; ornithine reenters the mitochondria to begin a new cycle.

The urea cycle is subject to both short- and long-term regulation. The first step, catalyzed by carbamoyl phosphate synthetase 1, can be activated by *N*-acetylglutamate (Watford, 2003). Although *N*-acetylglutamate levels always change in parallel with changes in the rate of urea synthesis, *N*-acetylglutamate does not control flux through the cycle. Rather, changes in *N*-acetylglutamate levels allow changes in flux through the cycle to occur at relatively constant ammonia levels. Therefore increased rates of amino acid catabolism result in increased levels of both ammonia and *N*-acetylglutamate, and the *N*-acetylglutamate stimulates carbamoyl phosphate synthetase 1 activity to effectively buffer the ammonia levels. With an increase in carbamoyl phosphate synthesis, flux through the rest of the urea cycle also increases because all the subsequent enzymes have K_m values that are below or near the physiological concentrations of their substrates and thus are unsaturated with substrate at physiological substrate concentrations.

Long-term regulation is brought about by adaptive changes in the amounts of urea cycle enzymes. Conditions that result in high rates of urea synthesis (high-protein diets and hypercatabolic states) are accompanied by increases in the activities of all the urea cycle enzymes, whereas conditions that result in low rates of urea synthesis (low-protein diets) result in decreased activities of the urea cycle enzymes. Although the enzymes of the urea cycle appear to be coordinately regulated, the mechanisms involved in regulation of different enzymes vary. Regulation occurs both by changes in the rate of protein degradation and by changes in the rate of enzyme synthesis, with changes in protein synthesis being primarily due to changes in the rate of gene transcription (Takiguchi and Mori, 1995).

For each molecule of urea, one nitrogen is derived from ammonia via the carbamoyl phosphate synthetase 1 reaction; the second nitrogen is donated to the urea cycle from the α-amino nitrogen of aspartate, with the carbon chain of aspartate being released as fumarate. In the postabsorptive state, the principal extrahepatic sources of nitrogen used for ureagenesis are glutamine and alanine, which are released by muscle, and ammonia from the portal blood. Glutamine is largely taken up by the intestine, and glutamine nitrogen is released back into the portal blood as citrulline, alanine, proline, and ammonia. The ammonia delivered to the liver via the portal blood originates predominately from glutamine catabolism in the small intestinal absorptive cells (enterocytes) and from bacterial metabolism of urea in the lumen of the large intestine. It is estimated that nearly 25% of the urea that is synthesized by the liver over the course of a day is broken down to ammonia in the large intestine and returned to the liver as ammonia for reincorporation into urea. Alanine and ammonia are readily removed by the liver. Alanine can be transaminated to pyruvate, and the pyruvate can be carboxylated to alanine and then transaminated to aspartate, as shown in Figure 14-11.

In the fed state, most amino acids that reach the liver can serve as precursors for ureagenesis. The immediate sources of hepatic ammonia funneling into the urea cycle have been estimated to include ammonia taken up from the portal blood (33%); glutamine deamidation in the liver (6% to 13%); release of α-amino nitrogen from glutamate by the glutamate dehydrogenase–catalyzed reaction in the liver, with the amino groups of various amino acids being transferred to glutamate via transamination (20%); and direct catabolism of certain amino acids such as glycine to release ammonia (33% to 40%) (Meijer et al., 1990). A variety of amino acids, especially alanine, contribute amino groups to aspartate (via the coupled activities of alanine or another aminotransferase and aspartate aminotransferase), with glutamate being the direct donor of the amino group to oxaloacetate to form aspartate. These α-amino groups are funneled into the urea cycle to provide the second nitrogen atom for urea synthesis.

EXCRETION OF AMMONIUM BY THE KIDNEY

Ammonia excretion usually is low, because most ammonia is incorporated into urea. However, in metabolic acidosis (resulting from diabetic ketosis, lactic acidosis, or excess protein catabolism), the urinary output of ammonium is increased. The production and excretion of strong acids (such as acetoacetic, β-hydroxybutyric, lactic, and sulfuric acids, which exist as anions at physiological pH) requires the coexcretion of a cation. Excretion of ammonia as the cation ammonium (NH_4^+) allows the body to conserve cations such as Na^+, K^+, and Ca^{2+}, facilitates the excretion of excess H^+, and has the net effect of conserving bicarbonate ion (HCO_3^-), which serves as an important buffer. The ammonia that is excreted by the kidney is generated predominantly in the kidney by deamidation of glutamine by glutaminase, followed by deamination of glutamate by glutamate dehydrogenase. The process of acidosis-increased ammonium excretion also is facilitated by net glutamine production by the liver and increased release of glutamine from skeletal muscle. A small proportion of ammoniagenesis in the kidney is accomplished by the metabolism of glycine.

EXCRETION OF CREATININE

Creatine phosphate is present in muscle cells at a high concentration of approximately 25 mmol per kg. Both creatine and creatine phosphate undergo spontaneous loss of water and cyclization to creatinine, and this creatinine is excreted from the body in the urine. Approximately 1.7% (~12 mmol) of the total body creatine is replaced each day by synthesis from glycine, arginine, and *S*-adenosylmethionine. The rate of creatinine formation reflects the amount of creatine/creatine phosphate present in the muscle mass and is relatively constant from day to day in adults who are not losing or gaining muscle mass. Because of this relation, creatinine excretion has been used to estimate the completeness of 24-hour urine collections, as a basis for normalizing urinary concentrations of various metabolites, and to estimate the lean body mass of individuals; however, the contribution of meat intake to creatinine excretion can limit the usefulness of urinary creatinine for these purposes. Because the renal tubules do not reabsorb creatinine, its excretion also can be used to calculate the volume of plasma filtered by the kidneys, and this is used as a measure of renal function.

THINKING CRITICALLY

1. Consider the essential amino acid histidine. List at least four possible fates or roles that histidine plays in metabolism (i.e., what can happen to histidine in the body?). Consider both general fates of amino acids and specific fates of histidine.
2. Alanine serves as a major means of moving carbon (pyruvate) and nitrogen (amino group) from the muscle to the liver for gluconeogenesis and urea synthesis, respectively. Using relatively common reactions, sketch a scheme for conversion of alanine carbon to pyruvate (or glucose, if you wish) and of alanine nitrogen to urea. Consider a scheme that would allow alanine to serve as the original (to the liver) source of both nitrogens that enter the urea cycle to form one molecule of urea. You may wish to start with two molecules of alanine so that you have two nitrogens for your one molecule of urea.
3. In total parenteral nutrition, the gut is bypassed in supplying nutrients. What effect might this have on the synthesis of dispensable amino acids? On amino acid requirements?

REFERENCES

Adibi, S. A. (2003). Regulation of expression of the intestinal oligopeptide transporter (Pept-1) in health and disease. *The American Journal of Physiology, 285*, G779–G788.

Agostinelli, E., Marques, M. P. M., Calheiros, R., Gil, F. P. S. C., Tempera, G.,Viceconte, N., … Toninello, A. (2010). Polyamines: Fundamental characters in chemistry and biology. *Amino Acids, 38*, 393–403.

Bäckhed, F. (2009). Changes in intestinal microflora in obesity: Cause or consequence? *Journal of Pediatric Gastroenterology and Nutrition, 48*, S56–S57.

Ballevre, O., Cadenhead, A., Calder, A. G., Rees, W. D., Lobley, G. E., Fuller, M. F., & Garlick, P. J. (1990). Quantitative partition of threonine oxidation in pigs: Effect of dietary threonine. *The American Journal of Physiology, 259*, E483–E491.

Battezzati, A., Brillon, D. J., & Matthews, D. E. (1995). Oxidation of glutamic acid by the splanchnic bed in humans. *The American Journal of Physiology, 269*, E269–E276.

Beauchamp, G. K. (2009). Sensory and receptor responses to umami: An overview of pioneering work. *The American Journal of Clinical Nutrition, 96*(Suppl), 723S–727S.

Beaumier, L., Castillo, L., Ajamik, A. M., & Young, V. R. (1995). Urea cycle intermediate kinetics and nitrate excretion at normal and "therapeutic" intakes of arginine in humans. *The American Journal of Physiology, 269*, E884–E896.

Bella, D. L., & Stipanuk, M. H. (1995). Effects of protein, methionine, or chloride on acid-base balance and on cysteine catabolism. *The American Journal of Physiology, 269*, E910–E917.

Bergstrom, J., Furst, P., Noree, L.-O., & Vinnars, E. (1974). Intracellular free amino acid concentration in human muscle tissue. *Journal of Applied Physiology, 36*, 693–697.

Bertolo, R. F., & Burrin, D. G. (2008). Comparative aspects of tissue glutamine and proline metabolism. *The Journal of Nutrition, 138*, 2032S–2039S.

Bjorgo, E., de Carvalho, R. M. N., & Flatmark, T. (2001). A comparison of kinetic and regulatory properties of the tetrameric and dimeric forms of wild-type and Thr427-Pro mutant human phenylalanine hydroxylase: Contribution of the flexible hinge region Asp425-Gln429 to the tetramerization and cooperative substrate binding. *European Journal of Biochemistry/FEBS, 268*, 997–1005.

Boehning, D., & Snyder, S. H. (2003). Novel neural modulators. *Annual Review of Neuroscience, 26*, 105–131.

Boon, L., Blommaart, P. J., Meijer, A. J., Lamers, W. H., & Schoolwerth, A. C. (1994). Acute acidosis inhibits liver amino acid transport: No primary role for the urea cycle in acid-base balance. *The American Journal of Physiology, 267*, F1015–F1020.

Broquist, H. P. (1991). Lysine-pipecolic acid metabolic relationships in microbes and mammals. *Annual Review of Nutrition, 11*, 435–448.

Brusilow, S. W. (1984). Arginine, an indispensable amino acid for patients with inborn errors of urea synthesis. *The Journal of Clinical Investigation, 74*, 2144–2148.

Busque, S. M., & Wagner, C. A. (2009). Potassium restriction, high protein intake, and metabolic acidosis increase expression of the glutamine transporter SNAT3 (Slc38a3) in mouse kidney. *The American Journal of Physiology Renal Physiology, 297*, F440–F450.

Carey, G. P., Kime, Z., Rogers, Q. R., Morris, J. G., Hargrove, D., Buffington, C. A., & Brusilow, S. W. (1987). An arginine-deficient diet in humans does not evoke hyperammonemia or orotic aciduria. *The Journal of Nutrition, 117*, 1734–1739.

Castillo, L., Sanchez, M., Chapman, T. E., Ajami, A., Burke, J. F., & Young, V. R. (1994). The plasma flux and oxidation rate of ornithine adaptively decline with restricted arginine intake. *Proceedings of the National Academy of Sciences of the United States of America, 91*, 6393–6397.

Christensen, H. (1990). Role of amino acid transport and countertransport in nutrition and metabolism. *Physiological Reviews, 70*, 43–77.

Chuang, J. L., Wynn, R. M., Moss, C. C., Song, J., Li, J., Awad, N., Mandel, H., & Chuang, D. T. (2004). Structural and biochemical basis for novel mutations in homozygous Israeli maple syrup urine disease patients. *The Journal of Biological Chemistry, 279*, 17792–17800.

Clarke, J. T. R., & Bier, D. M. (1982). The conversion of phenylalanine to tyrosine in man: Direct measurement by continuous intravenous tracer infusions of L-[ring-$^2H_5$]phenylalanine and L-[1-^{13}C]tyrosine in the postabsorptive state. *Metabolism, 31*, 999–1005.

Cowan, G. J., Willgoss, D. A., Bartley, J., & Endre, Z. H. (1996). Serine isotopomer analysis by ^{13}C-NMR defines glycine-serine interconversion in situ in the renal proximal tubule. *Biochimica et Biophysica Acta, 1310*, 32–40.

Cynober, L., Le Boucher, J., & Vasdson, M.-P. (1995). Arginine metabolism in mammals. *The Journal of Nutritional Biochemistry, 6*, 402–413.

D'Aniello, A., Vetere, A., & Petrucelli, L. (1993). Further study on the specificity of D-amino acid oxidase and of D-aspartate oxidase and time course for complete oxidation of D-amino acids. *Comparative Biochemistry and Physiology. B. Comparative Biochemistry, 105B*, 731–734.

Darling, P. B., Grunow, J., Rafii, M., Brookes, S., Ball, R. O., & Pencharz, P. B. (2000). Threonine dehydrogenase is a minor degradative pathway of threonine catabolism in adult humans. *American Journal of Physiology, Endocrinology and Metabolism, 278*, E877–E884.

Darmaun, D., & Dechelotte, P. (1991). Role of leucine as a precursor of glutamine alpha-amino nitrogen in vivo in humans. *The American Journal of Physiology, 260*, E326–E329.

Divry, P., Vianey-Liaud, C., & Mathieu, M. (1991). Inborn errors of lysine metabolism. *Annales de Biologie Clinique, 49*, 27–35.

Dix, T. A., Kuhn, D. M., & Benkovic, S. J. (1987). Mechanism of oxygen activation by tyrosine hydroxylase. *Biochemistry, 26*, 3354–3361.

Dominy, J. E., & Stipanuk, M. H. (2004). New roles for cysteine and transsulfuration enzymes: Production of H_2S, a neuromodulator and smooth muscle relaxant. *Nutrition Reviews, 62*, 348–353.

Doskeland, A. P., Martinez, A., Knappskog, P. M., & Flatmark, T. (1996). Phosphorylation of recombinant human phenylalanine hydroxylase: Effect on catalytic activity, substrate activation and protection against non-specific cleavage of the fusion protein by restriction protease. *The Biochemical Journal, 313*, 409–414.

Edgar, A. J. (2005). Mice have a transcribed L-threonine aldolase/GLY 1 gene, but the human GLY 1 gene is a non-processed pseudogene. *BMC Genomics, 6*, 32.

Edgar, A. J., & Polak, J. M. (2000). Molecular cloning of the human and murine 2-amino-3-ketobutyrate coenzyme A ligase cDNAs. *European Journal of Biochemistry, 267*, 1805–1812.

Edison, E. E., Brosnan, M. E., Meyer, C., & Brosnan, J. T. (2007). Creatine synthesis: Production of guanidinoacetate by the rat and human kidney in vivo. *American Journal of Physiology. Renal Physiology, 293*, F1799–F1804.

Eisenhofer, G., Tian, H., Holmes, C., Matsunaga, J., Roffler-Tarlov, S., & Hearing, V. J. (2003). Tyrosinase: A developmentally specific major determinant of peripheral dopamine. *The FASEB Journal, 17*, 1248–1255.

Elia, M. (1993). Glutamine metabolism in human adipose tissue in vivo. *Clinical Nutrition, 12*, 51–53.

Elia, M., & Livesey, G. (1983). Effects of ingested steak and infused leucine on forelimb metabolism in man and the fate of the carbon skeletons and amino groups of branched-chain amino acids. *Clinical Science, 64*, 517–526.

Erlandsen, H., Patch, M. G., Gamez, A., Straub, M., & Stevens, R. C. (2003). Structural studies on phenylalanine hydroxylase and implications toward understanding and treating phenylketonuria. *Pediatrics, 112*, 1557–1565.

Ewart, H. S., Jois, M., & Brosnan, J. T. (1992). Rapid stimulation of the hepatic glycine-cleavage system in rats fed on a single high-protein meal. *The Biochemical Journal, 283*, 441–447.

Felig, P. (1975). Amino acid metabolism in man. *Annual Review of Nutrition, 44*, 933–955.

Felig, P., Wahren, J., & Raf, L. (1973). Evidence of interorgan amino acid transport by blood cells in man. *Proceedings of the National Academy of Sciences of the United States of America, 70*, 1775–1779.

Fernandez, J., Lopez, A. B., Wang, C., Mishra, R., Zhou, L., Yaman, I., … Hatzolgou, M. (2003). Transcriptional control of the arginine/lysine transporter, Cat-1, by physiological stress. *The Journal of Biological Chemistry, 278*, 50000–50009.

Fukagawa, N. K., Ajami, A. M., & Young, V. R. (1996). Plasma methionine and cysteine kinetics in response to an intravenous glutathione infusion in adult humans. *The American Journal of Physiology, 270*, E209–E214.

Funuchi, T., & Homma, H. (2005). Free D-aspartate in mammals. *Biological & Pharmaceutical Bulletin, 28*, 1566–1570.

Gadalla, M. M., & Snyder, S. H. (2010). Hydrogen sulfide as a gasotransmitter. *Journal of Neurochemistry, 113*, 14–26.

Gibson, K. M., Lee, C. F., & Hoffmann, G. F. (1994). Screening for defects of branched-chain amino acid metabolism. *European Journal of Pediatrics, 153*, S62–S67.

Girgis, S., Nasrallah, I. M., Suh, J. R., Oppenheim, E., Zanetti, K. A., Mastri, M. G., & Stover, P. J. (1998). Molecular cloning, characterization and alternative splicing of the human cytoplasmic serine hydroxymethyltransferase gene. *Gene, 210*, 315–324.

Grillo, M. A., & Colombatto, S. (2004). Arginine revisited: Mini review article. *Amino Acids, 26*, 345–351.

Guba, S. C., Fink, L. M., & Fonseca, V. (1996). Hyperhomocysteinemia: An emerging and important risk factor for thromboembolic and cardiovascular disease. *American Journal of Clinical Pathology, 105*, 709–722.

Harris, R. A., Joshi, M., & Jeoung, N. H. (2004). Mechanisms responsible for regulation of branched-chain amino acid catabolism. *Biochemical and Biophysical Research Communications, 313*, 391–396.

Harris, R. A., Joshi, M., Jeoung, N. H., & Obayashi, M. (2005). Overview of the molecular and biochemical basis of branched-chain amino acid catabolism. *The Journal of Nutrition, 135*, 1527S–1530S.

Hediger, M. A., Romero, M. F., Peng, J.-B., Rolfs, A., Takanaga, H., & Bruford, E. A. (2004). The ABCs of solute carriers: Physiological, pathological and therapeutic implications of human membrane transport proteins. *Pflügers Archiv: European Journal of Physiology, 447*, 465–468.

House, J. D., Hall, B. N., & Brosnan, J. T. (2001). Threonine metabolism in isolated rat hepatocytes. *American Journal of Physiology. Endocrinology and Metabolism, 281*, E1300–1307.

Hyde, R., Taylor, P. M., & Hundal, H. S. (2003). Amino acid transporters: Roles in amino acid sensing and signaling in animal cells. *The Biochemical Journal, 373*, 1–18.

Ibrahim, H., Lee, Y. J., & Curthoys, N. P. (2008). Renal response to metabolic acidosis: Role of mRNA stabilization. *Kidney International, 73*, 11–18.

Indiveri, C., Tonazzi, A., & Palmieri, F. (1992). Identification and purification of the ornithine/citrulline carrier from rat liver mitochondria. *European Journal of Biochemistry/FEBS, 207*, 449–454.

Jackson, A. A. (1995). Salvage of urea-nitrogen and protein requirements. *The Proceedings of the Nutrition Society, 54*, 535–547.

Jones, N. E., & Heyland, D. K. (2008). Pharmaconutrition: A new emerging paradigm. *Current Opinion in Gastroenterology, 24*, 215–222.

Jungas, R. L., Halperin, M. L., & Brosnan, J. T. (1992). Quantitative analysis of amino acid oxidation and related gluconeogenesis in humans. *Physiological Reviews, 72*, 419–448.

Kilberg, M. S., Pan, Y. X., Chen, H., & Leung-Pineda, V. (2005). Nutritional control of gene expression: How mammalian cells respond to amino acid limitation. *Annual Review of Nutrition, 25*, 59–85.

Kimball, S. R., & Jefferson, L. S. (2006). New functions for amino acids: Effects on gene transcription and translation. *The American Journal of Clinical Nutrition, 83*(Suppl), 500S–507S.

King, N. J. C., & Thomas, S. R. (2007). Molecules in focus: Indoleamine 2,3-dioxygenase. *The International Journal of Biochemistry & Cell Biology, 39*, 2167–2172.

Lam, W. K., Cleary, M. A., Wraith, J. E., & Walter, J. H. (1996). Histidinaemia: A benign metabolic disorder. *Archives of Disease in Childhood, 74*, 343–346.

Lange, M., Enkhbaatar, P., Nakano, Y., & Traber, D. L. (2009). Role of nitric oxide in shock: The large animal perspective. *Frontiers in Bioscience, 14*, 1979–1989.

Leklem, J. E. (1971). Quantitative aspects of tryptophan metabolism in humans and other species: A review. *The American Journal of Clinical Nutrition, 24*, 659–672.

Letto, J., Brosnan, J. T., & Brosnan, M. E. (1990). Oxidation of 2-oxoisocaproate and 2-oxoisovalerate by the perfused rat heart: Interactions with fatty acid oxidation. *Biochemistry and Cell Biology, 68*, 260–265.

Letto, J., Brosnan, M. E., & Brosnan, J. T. (1986). Valine metabolism: Gluconeogenesis from 3-hyroxyisobutyrate. *The Biochemical Journal, 240*, 909–912.

Lowenstein, J. M. (1972). Ammonia production in muscle and other tissues: The purine nucleotide cycle. *Physiological Reviews, 52*, 383–414.

Lowry, M., Hall, D. E., & Brosnan, J. T. (1985). Increased activity of renal glycine-cleavage-enzyme complex in metabolic acidosis. *The Biochemical Journal, 231*, 477–480.

Maes, M., Verkerk, R., Bonaccorso, S., Ombelet, W., Bosmans, E., & Sharpe, S. (2002). Depressive and anxiety symptoms in the early puerperium are related to increased degradation of tryptophan into kynurenine, a phenomenon which is related to immune activation. *Life Sciences, 71*, 1837–1848.

Martinov, M. V., Vitvitsky, V. M., Mosharov, E. V., Banerjee, R., & Ataullakhanov, F. I. (2000). A substrate switch: A new mode of regulation in the methionine metabolic pathway. *Journal of Theoretical Biology, 204*, 521–532.

McCarty, M. F. (2004). Sub-optimal taurine status may promote platelet hyperaggregability in vegetarians. *Medical Hypotheses, 63*, 426–433.

Meijer, A. J. (2008). Amino acid regulation of autophagosome formation. *Methods in Molecular Biology, 445*, 89–109.

Meijer, A. J., Lamers, W. H., & Chamuleau, R. A. F. M. (1990). Nitrogen metabolism and ornithine cycle function. *Physiological Reviews, 70*, 701–749.

Metges, C. C., Eberhard, M., & Petzke, K. J. (2006). Synthesis and absorption of intestinal microbial lysine in humans and non-ruminant animals and impact on estimated average requirement of dietary lysine. *Current Opinion in Clinical Nutrition and Metabolic Care, 9*, 37–41.

Moncada, S., Palmer, R. M. J., & Higgs, E. A. (1991). Nitric oxide: Physiology, pathophysiology, and pharmacology. *Pharmacological Reviews, 43*, 109–142.

Morikawa, A., Hamase, K., Ohgusu, T., Etoh, S., Tanaka, H., Koshiishi, I., ... Zaitsu, K. (2007). Immunohistochemical localization of D-alanine to beta-cells in rat pancreas. *Biochemical and Biophysical Research Communications, 355*, 872–876.

Morris, M. L., Lee, S.-C., & Harper, A. E. (1973). A comparison of the responses of mitochondrial and cytosol histidine-pyruvate aminotransferases to nutritional and hormonal treatments. *The Journal of Biological Chemistry, 248*, 1459–1465.

Morris, S. M., Jr. (2004). Enzymes of arginine metabolism. *The Journal of Nutrition, 134*, 2743S–2747S.

Mudd, S. H., Brosnan, J. T., Brosnan, M. E., Jacobs, R. L., Stabler, S. P., Allen, R. H., ... Wagner, C. (2007). Methyl balance and transmethylation fluxes in humans. *The American Journal of Clinical Nutrition, 85*, 19–25.

Noguchi, T., Okuno, E., & Kido, R. (1976). Identity of isoenzyme 1 of histidine-pyruvate aminotransferase with serine-pyruvate aminotransferase. *The Biochemical Journal, 159*, 607–613.

Noma, A., Sakaguchi, Y., & Suzuki, T. (2009). Mechanistic characterization of the sulfur-relay system for eukaryotic 2-thiouridine biogenesis at tRNA wobble positions. *Nucleic Acids Research, 37*, 1335–1352.

Nurjhan, N., Bucci, A., Stumvoll, M., Bailey, G., Bier, D. M., Toft, I., ... Gerich, J. E. (1995). Glutamine: A major gluconeogenic precursor and vehicle for interorgan carbon transport in man. *The Journal of Clinical Investigation, 95*, 272–277.

Ogawa, H., Gomi, T., Konishi, K., Date, T., Nakashima, H., Nose, K., ... Fujioka, M. (1989). Human liver serine dehydratase: cDNA cloning and sequence homology with hydroxyamino acid dehydratases from other sources. *The Journal of Biological Chemistry, 264*, 15818–15823.

Palii, S. S., Chen, H., & Kilberg, M. S. (2004). Transcriptional control of the human sodium-coupled neutral amino acid transporter system A gene by amino acid availability is mediated by an intronic element. *The Journal of Biological Chemistry, 279*, 3463–3471.

Pantuck, E. J., Pantuck, C. B., Kappas, A., Conney, A., & Anderson, K. E. (1991). Effects of protein and carbohydrate content of diet on drug conjugation. *Clinical Pharmacology and Therapeutics, 50*, 254–258.

Paxton, R., Scislowski, P. W. D., Davis, E. J., & Harris, R. A. (1986). Role of branched-chain 2-oxo acid dehydrogenase and pyruvate dehydrogenase in 2-oxobutyrate metabolism. *The Biochemical Journal, 234*, 295–303.

Pencharz, P. B., Hsu, J. W.-C., & Ball, R. O. (2007). Aromatic amino acid requirements in healthy human subjects. *The Journal of Nutrition, 137*, 1576S–1578S.

Peters, J. C. (1991). Tryptophan nutrition and metabolism: An overview. In R. Schwarcz, S. N. Young, & R. R. Brown (Eds.), *Kynurenine and serotonin pathways* (pp. 345–358). New York: Plenum Press.

Petrossian, T. C., & Clarke, S. (2010). Uncovering the human methyltransfersome. *Molecular & Cellular Proteomics 2011, 10*(1), M110.000976.

Pinsonneault, J. K., Nielsen, C. U., Sadee, W. (2004). Genetic variants of the humans H^+/dipeptide transporter PEPT2: Analysis of haplotype functions. *The Journal of Pharmacology and Experimental Therapeutics, 311*, 1088–1096.

Pirkov, I., Norbeck, J., Gustafsson, L., & Albers, E. (2008). A complete inventory of all enzymes in the eukaryotic methionine salvage pathway. *The FEBS Journal, 275*, 4111–4120.

Praphanphoj, V., Sacksteder, K. A., Gould, S. J., Thomas, G. H., & Geraghty, M. T. (2001). Identification of the α-aminoadipic semialdehyde dehydrogenase-phosphopantetheinyl transferase gene, the human ortholog of the yeast *LYS5* gene. *Molecular Genetics and Metabolism, 72*, 336–342.

Proud, C. G. (2007). Amino acids and mTOR signalling in anabolic function. *Biochemical Society Transactions, 35*, 1187–1190.

Reeds, P. J., & Burrin, D. G. (2001). Glutamine and the bowel. *The Journal of Nutrition, 131*, 2505S–2508S.

Sacksteder, K. A., Biery, B. J., Morrell, J. C., Goodman, B. K., Geisbrecht, B. V., Cox, R. P., ... Geraghty, M. T. (2000). Identification of the alpha-aminoadipic semialdehyde synthase gene, which is defective in familial hyperlysinemia. *American Journal of Human Genetics, 66*, 1736–1743.

Schuller-Levis, G. B., & Park, E. (2004). Taurine and its chloramine: Modulators of immunity. *Neurochemical Research, 29*, 117–126.

Scislowski, P. W. D., Foster, A. R., & Fuller, M. F. (1994). Regulation of oxidative degradation of l-lysine in rat liver mitochondria. *The Biochemical Journal, 300*, 887–891.

Shi, R., Proteau, A., Villarroya, M., Moukadri, I., Zhang, L., Trempe, J. F., ... Cygler, M. (2010). Structural basis for Fe-S cluster assembly and tRNA thiolation mediated by IscS protein-protein interaction. *PLoS Biology, 8*, e1000354.

Stanley, C. A. (2009). Regulation of glutamate metabolism and insulin secretion by glutamate dehydrogenase in hypoglycaemic children. *The American Journal of Clinical Nutrition, 90*, 862S–866S.

Steinberg, S. J., Dodt, G., Raymond, G. V., Braverman, N. E., Moser, A. B., & Moser, H. W. (2006). Peroxisome biogenesis disorders. *Biochimica et Biophysica Acta, 1763*, 1733–1748.

Stipanuk, M. H. (2004). Sulfur amino acid metabolism: Pathways for production and removal of homocysteine and cysteine. *Annual Review of Nutrition, 24*, 539–577.

Stipanuk, M. H., Dominy, J. E., Lee, J.-I., & Coloso, R. M. (2006). Mammalian cysteine metabolism: New insights into regulation of cysteine metabolism. *The Journal of Nutrition, 136*, 1652S–1659S.

Storch, K. J., Wagner, D. A., Burke, J. F., & Young, V. R. (1990). [1-^{13}C;methyl-$^{2}H_3$]methionine kinetics in humans: Methionine conservation and cystine sparing. *The American Journal of Physiology, 258*, E790–E798.

Suryawan, A., Hawes, J. W., Harris, R. A., Shimomura, Y., Jenkins, A. E., & Hutson, S. M. (1998). A molecular model of human branched-chain amino acid metabolism. *The American Journal of Clinical Nutrition, 68*, 72–81.

Suzuki, T., Suzuki, T., Wada, T., Saigo, K., & Watanabe, K. (2001). Novel taurine-containing uridine derivatives and mitochondrial human diseases. *Nucleic Acids Research, 1*(Suppl), 257–258.

Sweatt, A. J., Wood, M., Suryawan, A., Wallin, R., Willingham, M. C., & Hutson, S. M. (2004). Branched-chain amino acid metabolism: Unique segregation of pathway enzymes in organ systems and peripheral nerves. *American Journal of Physiology. Endocrinology and Metabolism, 286,* E64–E76.

Takata, Y., Huang, Y., Komoto, J., Yamada, T., Konishi, K., Ogawa, H., ... Takusagawa, F. (2003). Catalytic mechanism of glycine *N*-methyltransferase. *Biochemistry, 42,* 8394–8402.

Takiguchi, M., & Mori, M. (1995). Transcriptional regulation of genes for ornithine cycle enzymes. *The Biochemical Journal, 312,* 649–659.

Takikawa, O., Littlejohn, T. K., & Truscott, R. J. W. (2001). Indoleamine 2,3-dioxygenase in the human lens, the first enzyme in the synthesis of UV filters. *Experimental Eye Research, 72,* 271–277.

Tanner, L. M., Näntö-Salonen, K., Venetoklis, J., Kotilainen, S., Niinikoski, H., Huoponen, K., & Simmell, O. (2007). Nutrient intake in lysinuric protein intolerance. *Journal of Inherited Metabolic Disease, 30,* 716–721.

Tizianello, A., Deferrari, G., Garibotto, G., Robaudod, C., Acquarone, N., & Ghiggeri, G. M. (1982). Renal ammoniagenesis in an early stage of metabolic acidosis in man. *The Journal of Clinical Investigation, 69,* 240–250.

Tovar, A. R., Ascencio, C., & Torres, N. (2002). Soy protein, casein, and zein regulate histidase gene expression by modulating serum glucagons. *American Journal of Physiology, Endocrinology and Metabolism, 283,* E1016–E1022.

van de Kamp, J. L., & Smolen, A. (1995). Response of kynurenine pathway enzymes to pregnancy and dietary level of vitamin B-6. *Pharmacology, Biochemistry, and Behavior, 51,* 753–758.

Watford, M. (1994). Glutamine metabolism in rat small intestine: Synthesis of three-carbon products in isolated enterocytes. *Biochimica et Biophysica Acta, 1200,* 73–78.

Watford, M. (2000). Glutamine and glutamate metabolism across the liver sinusoid. *The Journal of Nutrition, 130,* 983S–987S.

Watford, M. (2003). The urea cycle. *Biochemistry and Molecular Biology Education, 31,* 289–297.

White, A. C., Thannickal, V. J., & Fanburg, B. L. (1994). Glutathione deficiency in human disease. *The Journal of Nutritional Biochemistry, 5,* 218–226.

Wikoff, W. R., Anfora, A. T., Liu, J., Schultz, P. G., Lesley, S. A., Peters, E. C., & Siuzdak, G. (2009). Metabolomics analysis reveals large effects of gut microflora on mammalian blood metabolites. *Proceedings of the National Academy of Sciences of the United States of America, 106,* 3698–3703.

Wirleitner, B., Neurauter, G., Schrocksnadel, K., Frick, B., & Fuchs, D. (2003). Interferon-gamma-induced conversion of tryptophan: Immunologic and neuropsychiatric aspects. *Current Medicinal Chemistry, 10,* 1581–1591.

Wu, G., & Brosnan, J. T. (1992). Macrophages can convert citrulline into arginine. *The Biochemical Journal, 281,* 45–48.

Xue, H. H., Sakaguchi, T., Fujie, M., Ogawa, H., & Ichiyama, A. (1999). Flux of the L-serine metabolism in rabbit, human, and dog livers. *The Journal of Biological Chemistry, 274,* 16028–16033.

Yang, C. R., & Svensson, K. A. (2008). Allosteric modulation of NMDA receptor via elevation of brain glycine and D-serine: The therapeutic potentials for schizophrenia. *Pharmacology & Therapeutics, 120,* 317–332.

Yang, R. D., Matthews, D. E., Bier, D. M., Wen, Z. M., & Young, V. R. (1986). Response of alanine metabolism in humans to manipulation of dietary protein and energy intakes. *The American Journal of Physiology, 250,* E39–E46.

Yannicelli, S., Rohr, F., & Warman, M. L. (1994). Nutrition support for glutaric acidemia type I. *Journal of the American Dietetic Association, 94,* 183–191.

Zhao, X., Wen, Z.-M., Meredith, C. N., Matthews, D. E., Bier, D. M., & Young, V. R. (1986). Threonine kinetics at graded threonine intakes in young men. *The American Journal of Clinical Nutrition, 43,* 795–802.

RECOMMENDED READINGS

Jungas, R. L., Halperin, M. L., & Brosnan, J. T. (1992). Quantitative analysis of amino acid oxidation and related gluconeogenesis in humans. *Physiological Reviews, 72,* 419–448.

Leser, T. D., & Molbak, L. (2009). Better living through microbial action: The benefits of the mammalian gastrointestinal microbiota on the host. *Environmental Microbiology, 11,* 2194–2206.

Morris, S. M., Jr. (2002). Regulation of enzymes of the urea cycle and arginine metabolism. *Annual Review of Nutrition, 22,* 87–105.

Stipanuk, M. H. (2004). Sulfur amino acid metabolism: Pathways for production and removal of homocysteine and cysteine. *Annual Review of Nutrition, 24,* 539–577.

Watford, M. (2003). The urea cycle. *Biochemistry and Molecular Biology Education, 31,* 289–297.

CHAPTER 15

Protein and Amino Acid Requirements

*Crystal L. Levesque, PhD, and Ronald O. Ball, PhD**

COMMON ABBREVIATIONS

BV	biological value
DAAO	direct amino acid oxidation
IAAO	indicator amino acid oxidation
NPU	net protein utilization
PDCAAS	protein digestibility–corrected amino acid score
PEM	protein energy malnutrition
PER	protein efficiency ratio
P/E ratio	energy from protein/total energy in diet, expressed as fraction or percentage

The dietary requirement for protein represents the need for the amino acids that constitute it and, in fact, dietary protein can be replaced by mixtures of amino acids. It might seem then that a measure of the amount of each amino acid needed for metabolic processes (i.e., maintenance and growth) would define the need for protein. However, because 11 out of 20 of the amino acids can be synthesized de novo, not all amino acids need to be provided in the amounts that are actually used for anabolic processes. Some amino acids can be synthesized from common intermediates of metabolism if amino acids that can donate an amino group are available. Thus the diet does not need to provide all amino acids in the exact amounts used by cells. Rather, the total amount of protein or total amino acids provided by the diet is an important consideration along with the requirements for specific amounts of particular amino acids.

CLASSIFICATION OF DISPENSABLE AND INDISPENSABLE AMINO ACIDS

The 20 amino acids required for protein synthesis have been divided into two categories: (1) indispensable (or essential), and (2) dispensable (or nonessential). The term *dispensable* may be preferred over the term *nonessential* because all the amino acids found in protein are metabolically essential, even though some are dispensable in the diet.

INDISPENSABLE AMINO ACIDS

Borman and colleagues (1946) defined an indispensable amino acid as "one which cannot be synthesized by the animal organism, out of materials ordinarily available to the cells, at a speed commensurate with the demands for normal growth" (p. 593). Humans do not possess the pathways for the synthesis of nine amino acids from compounds ordinarily available to cells: histidine, isoleucine, leucine, lysine, methionine, phenylalanine, threonine, tryptophan, and valine (Box 15-1). Thus these nine amino acids are always indispensable.

SEMIDISPENSABLE, CONDITIONALLY INDISPENSABLE, AND DISPENSABLE AMINO ACIDS

The other eleven amino acids (alanine, arginine, asparagine, aspartate, cysteine, glutamate, glutamine, glycine, proline, serine, and tyrosine) can be synthesized by cells from materials ordinarily available to the cells. However, the extent of synthesis of some of these amino acids depends upon the dietary supply of particular precursor amino acids or the biosynthetic capacity of the organism. In addition, the amount of an amino acid needed may vary under specific circumstances such as injury or parenteral feeding. These factors have led to subclassifications of the dispensable amino acids and the use of the terms *semiessential, conditionally indispensable,* and *truly dispensable* (Reeds, 2000; Institute of Medicine [IOM], 2005).

Semidispensable Amino Acids

Cysteine, or its disulfide cystine, and tyrosine are considered semiessential because their synthesis depends upon an adequate dietary supply of an indispensable amino acid precursor. Cysteine can be synthesized in the body from serine and the sulfur group of methionine. Tyrosine can be formed in the body by the hydroxylation of phenylalanine. Both of these syntheses are irreversible; therefore a lack of tyrosine in the diet can be compensated by an excess of phenylalanine, but the reverse is not true: excess tyrosine cannot compensate for a deficiency of phenylalanine. Likewise, methionine cannot be synthesized from cyst(e)ine. Each of these semiessential amino acids must be considered along with its indispensable amino acid precursor when evaluating indispensable amino acid intake for adequacy; both the sum and the proportion

*This chapter is a revision of the chapter contributed by Martha H. Stipanuk, PhD, for the second edition.

BOX 15-1 An Acronym for the Indispensable Amino Acids: PVT TIM HALL

Acronyms or initialisms can be used to abbreviate names or identify groups of common items such as the indispensable amino acids. They are typically created by using the first letter of each important word. In the case of protein, the initialism PVT TIM HALL uses the letters of each of the 10 indispensable amino acids.

P – phenylalanine
V – valine
T – threonine
T – tryptophan
I – isoleucine
M – methionine
H – histidine
A – arginine*
L – lysine
L – leucine

*Although arginine can be synthesized in sufficient quantities by adult humans, it is indispensable in babies and young children as well as in species that do not use the urea cycle for removal of excess nitrogen (e.g., birds).

of methionine and cyst(e)ine or of phenylalanine and tyrosine must be taken into account. The requirements for methionine and cysteine and for phenylalanine and tyrosine are referred to as total sulfur amino acids and total aromatic amino acids, respectively.

Conditionally Indispensable Amino Acids

Arginine, proline, glutamine, and glycine are considered to be conditionally indispensable from a dietary viewpoint because the rate at which they are provided by endogenous synthesis may fall below the rate at which they are used. In a state of rapid growth, such as in the neonate, the essentiality of these amino acids is much more dependent on their rates of de novo synthesis. For example, in neonatal piglets, arginine is synthesized primarily in the small intestine from proline and citrulline, but the gut synthesis of arginine is insufficient to meet the whole body arginine demand (Urschel et al., 2007). Conditions that affect gut metabolism and function (i.e., intestinal disease, gut atrophy, or parenteral nutrition) can also affect the requirement for arginine as well as proline. Dramatic decreases in both arginine and proline synthesis occurred when piglets were fed parenterally, demonstrating the conditional essentiality of arginine and proline during total parenteral nutrition when amino acids bypass the gut, limiting synthesis of proline and citrulline (Bertolo et al., 2003).

During critical illness, glutamine is used as a fuel for the immune system and gastrointestinal tract with increased uptake of glutamine by immune cells, the intestinal mucosa, and the kidney. Although large amounts of glutamine are released from the muscle, the increased demand for glutamine during critical illness may not be met sufficiently by an increase in synthesis, such that glutamine often becomes conditionally indispensable (Wischmeyer, 2008). Further contributing to a deficiency in glutamine during critical illness can be a decline in total body muscle tissue with progressing disease state. Glutamine-supplemented total parenteral nutrition reduced infection rate and incidence of pneumonia in critically ill patients in a large double-blind, randomized clinical trial in France (Déchelotte et al., 2006).

The rate of endogenous glycine production during recovery (catch-up growth) from severe childhood malnutrition may be less than the rate of glycine utilization (Badaloo et al., 1999). There are suggestions that glycine may similarly behave as an indispensable amino acid in infants (especially premature infants), who have a limited capacity for glycine synthesis (Jackson et al., 1981).

In preterm infants, cysteine, tyrosine, glutamine, arginine, proline, and glycine are typically considered conditionally indispensable because of their low endogenous synthesis. Courtney-Martin and colleagues (2010) demonstrated that the total sulfur amino acid requirement in preterm infants could be met by methionine alone. This suggests that cysteine may not be a conditionally indispensable amino acid in preterm infants. High plasma phenylalanine and excretion of abnormal metabolites of phenylalanine were observed when phenylalanine was added to commercial total parenteral nutrition solutions fed to neonatal piglets (Wykes et al., 1994), suggesting a low conversion of phenylalanine to tyrosine in neonatal piglets. Interestingly, the mean tyrosine requirement in parenterally fed neonates was three to four times higher than that supplied by commercial total parenteral nutrition solutions (Roberts et al., 2001). Some of these conditionally essential amino acids may need to be present in higher concentrations in formulations used for enteral or parenteral feeding, particularly of preterm infants.

Truly Dispensable Amino Acids

Alanine, aspartate, asparagine, glutamate, and serine are classified as truly dispensable amino acids. There are no known cases in which these amino acids need to be present in the diet. As long as the total protein (amino acid) requirement is met, these amino acids can be synthesized from common metabolic intermediates (e.g., pyruvate, oxaloacetate, and α-ketoglutarate) and amino groups from other amino acids.

REQUIREMENT FOR PROTEIN (AMINO ACIDS)

The requirement for protein must be stated in such a way that the total need for protein (amino acids) and the need for individual indispensable or semidispensable amino acids are both considered. Usually, this is done by stating a total requirement for protein with a consideration of protein quality that relates to the level of indispensable amino acids in the protein sources. In general, the requirements for amino acids or protein are the sum of the physiological requirements for net tissue accretion during growth and pregnancy or for milk secretion during lactation and the requirements for tissue maintenance. Maintenance needs represent the largest fraction of the protein/amino acid requirement and nearly all of the requirement for adults. During growth and in pregnancy, when protein synthesis is greater than protein degradation, the use of amino acids for protein accretion is a major component of the requirements.

TABLE 15-1 Obligatory Nitrogen Losses in Healthy Adults on Protein-Free Diets

	NITROGEN ($mg \cdot kg^{-1} \cdot day^{-1}$)	PROTEIN ($g \cdot kg^{-1} \cdot day^{-1}$)	PROTEIN (g/day for 70-kg adult man)
Urinary N	32	0.2	14
Fecal N	11	0.07	4.9
Integumental and miscellaneous losses of N	5	0.03	2.1
Sum of obligatory losses	48	0.3	21
N balance of adults consuming ≤5 mg $N \cdot kg^{-1} \cdot day^{-1}$	−48	−0.3	−21

Based on data summarized by Rand, W. M., Pellett, P. L., & Young, V. R. (2003). Meta-analysis of nitrogen balance studies for estimating protein requirements in healthy adults. *The American Journal of Clinical Nutrition, 77*, 109–127.

Likewise, in lactation, the needs of the mammary gland for milk protein synthesis become a large component of requirements.

PROTEIN (AMINO ACID) REQUIREMENT FOR MAINTENANCE

Maintenance is the state in which there is no net change in body protein mass. Although protein degradation returns amino acids to the free amino acid pool for use in protein synthesis, some irreversible loss of amino acids occurs such that there is a dietary requirement for amino acids at maintenance. Even when there is no change in body protein mass, amino acids or proteins are lost due to irreversible modification of amino acids, loss of proteins through the epithelia, loss of amino acids in the urine, use of amino acids for synthesis of nonprotein substances, and oxidation of amino acids as fuels (see Chapters 5, 9, 13, and 14). Except for the first months of life, maintenance requirements account for the major proportion of the dietary protein needs of children, adolescents, and adults. For example, the proportion of the total requirement due to maintenance is approximately 80% at 1 to 3 years and more than 98% by age 18 years.

The maintenance requirement can be defined as the dietary intake needed to replace the obligatory losses of amino acids. Maintenance requirements can be estimated using the factorial method to add up obligatory losses of protein or nitrogen and then to adjust this for an estimate of the efficiency of utilization of dietary protein to replace these obligatory losses. Alternatively, maintenance requirements can be determined by the nitrogen balance technique.

Obligatory Losses of Proteins and Amino Acids

Estimation of the magnitude of obligatory amino acid and nitrogen losses is usually done by feeding protein-free diets to adults and measuring the loss of nitrogen from the body in the urine and feces, as well as cutaneous and miscellaneous losses. The association between obligatory nitrogen losses of individuals adapted to protein-free diets (i.e., ≤ 5 mg $N \cdot kg^{-1} \cdot day^{-1}$, or ≤ 2.2 g $protein \cdot kg^{-1} \cdot day^{-1}$) and the magnitude of the negative nitrogen balance experienced by these subjects is illustrated in Table 15-1. It should be noted, however, that obligatory nitrogen losses are expected to be somewhat higher in individuals consuming protein in their diets; this is especially true for losses due to amino acid catabolism.

Because dietary intake can vary enormously, the body must have mechanisms to adjust the rate of amino acid disposal according to the supply, and the major mechanism is the modulation of amino acid oxidation. This adaptive component changes only slowly with a sustained change in intake, as illustrated by the pattern of urinary nitrogen excretion by subjects switched from a diet containing adequate protein to one providing only a minimal level of protein; an example is shown in Figure 15-1. Thus obligatory losses will be affected by prior intake as well as by current intake unless a period of adaptation to the new intake is allowed before measurement of losses.

The major loss of amino acids is due to oxidation, or catabolism. Even when dietary intake is less than the requirement, a residual rate of amino acid catabolism occurs, and although small in comparison with the rate in normal diets, amino acid catabolism remains the major route of obligatory loss. When amino acids are catabolized, the nitrogen is excreted in the urine, mainly as urea and to a lesser extent as ammonium. Amino acid catabolism therefore is commonly assessed by measuring the amount of nitrogen excreted in the urine (as urea and ammonium). Urinary nitrogen losses also include amino acids that are irreversibly modified after incorporation into proteins (i.e., methylhistidine, hydroxylysine) as well as very small amounts of amino acids that escape renal reabsorption.

Obligatory fecal nitrogen loss represents nitrogen released from the body into the gastrointestinal tract but not reabsorbed; the sources of obligatory nitrogen lost via the gut are proteins secreted into the gastrointestinal tract in the salivary, gastric, pancreatic, hepatic (bile) and intestinal secretions and proteins of cells shed from the gastrointestinal epithelium. Most of the endogenous proteins released into the gastrointestinal tract are digested and reabsorbed, but about 20% of the endogenous proteins (particularly proteins such as mucin that are inherently resistant to proteolysis) escape digestion and pass into the large intestine where they are used by the gastrointestinal microflora. Accurate measurement of obligatory losses of amino acids from the gastrointestinal tract has raised considerable debate, and although the protein-free diet method is most commonly used, no one method is without limitations (Stein et al., 2007).

Dermal losses of protein (skin, hair, nails), sweat, sputum, nasal fluids, menstrual fluids, seminal fluids, and

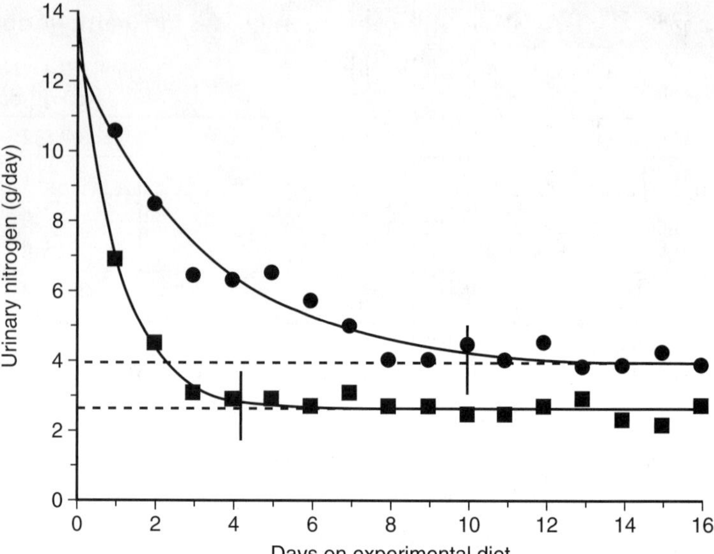

FIGURE 15-1 Time course of changes in the urinary nitrogen excretion of two subjects on changing, at day 0, from a high to a minimal level of protein intake. The vertical lines at 4.2 and 10.0 days represent the time it took the subject to reach a new plateau or stable rate of urinary nitrogen excretion. (Data from Rand, W. M., Young, V. R., & Scrimshaw, N. S. [1976]. Change of urinary nitrogen excretion in response to low-protein diets in adults. *The American Journal of Clinical Nutrition, 29,* 639–644.)

breath ammonia represent integumental and miscellaneous losses that collectively account for the loss of approximately 0.03 g protein·kg^{-1}·day^{-1}.

Synthesis of essential substances such as hormones, neurotransmitters, pyrimidines, and purines makes up the final route of obligatory amino acid loss. The contribution of the synthesis of nonprotein compounds to the daily requirement for protein and amino acids is typically small but still significant. As these nonprotein compounds are degraded in the normal process of turnover, their metabolites or end products are excreted in the urine or feces or lost in bodily secretions and thus are included with the urinary, fecal, and integumental and miscellaneous losses of N.

As summarized in Table 15-1, the sum of obligatory nitrogen losses in adults amounts to 48 mg N·kg^{-1}·day^{-1}. Using the general conversion factor of 6.25 g protein per g of nitrogen, the obligatory protein loss is 0.3 g protein·kg^{-1}·day^{-1}. The amount of protein required to maintain N equilibrium is much greater than the sum of the obligatory losses, however, because the efficiency with which absorbed amino acids are used for protein synthesis is not 100%. The efficiency of dietary protein utilization is about 50% (47% for adults and 58% for children), as determined from the slope of N balance response curves. This means that 0.5 g N is retained per 1 g N consumed. Thus (0.3/0.5) g protein·kg^{-1}·day^{-1}, or 0.6 g protein·kg^{-1}·day^{-1}, would be required to replace losses measured under the protein-free condition, and even more might be required in practice because obligatory losses are higher with normal diets than with protein-free diets. (With regard to this issue, note that the average protein requirement determined by nitrogen balance studies is about 0.66 g protein·kg^{-1}·day^{-1}.)

Protein (Amino Acid) Requirements for Nitrogen Equilibrium or Maintenance

The nitrogen balance method, in which the difference between nitrogen intake and nitrogen losses is determined, is the basis of current estimates of maintenance requirements of adults. Use of the nitrogen balance method is not a perfect measure of protein requirements because the body can maintain nitrogen equilibrium over a wide range of intakes. In cases of low intake of protein, N balance may be achieved only at the expense of the loss of significant lean body mass. Therefore the protein or amino acid "requirement" is usually defined as the minimum intake consistent with nitrogen equilibrium (no change in body protein mass).

Considering only the major fluxes of amino acids, the following equations apply to an individual in nitrogen (N) equilibrium or zero N balance:

- Supply of amino acid N to free amino acid pool = Removal of amino acid N from free amino acid pool
- Amino acid N intake + Amino acid N from endogenous protein degradation = Amino acid N used for protein synthesis + Amino acid catabolism
- Amino acid intake = Amino acid catabolism
- Amino acids used for protein synthesis = Amino acids liberated by degradation of endogenous proteins

Nitrogen balance data have been used by both the IOM (2005) and the World Health Organization (WHO, 2007) as well as many other groups for estimating protein requirements. For nonpregnant, nonlactating adults in nitrogen equilibrium, the nitrogen intake required for balance represents the requirement for maintenance. The average requirement of adults for protein was based on a meta-analysis of published nitrogen balance studies, as illustrated in Figure 15-2 (Rand et al., 2003). For each study, the lowest continuing intake of dietary protein that was sufficient to achieve body nitrogen equilibrium was considered as the individual requirement. The median nitrogen requirement derived from the meta-analysis was 105 mg·kg^{-1}·day^{-1}, and this value, along with the conversion factor of 6.25 g protein per g of nitrogen, was used to set the average requirement for protein at 0.66 g·kg^{-1}·day^{-1} for men and women (≥19 years of age). Maintenance requirements of children aged 6 months to 18 years are similar to those of adults on a per unit body weight basis.

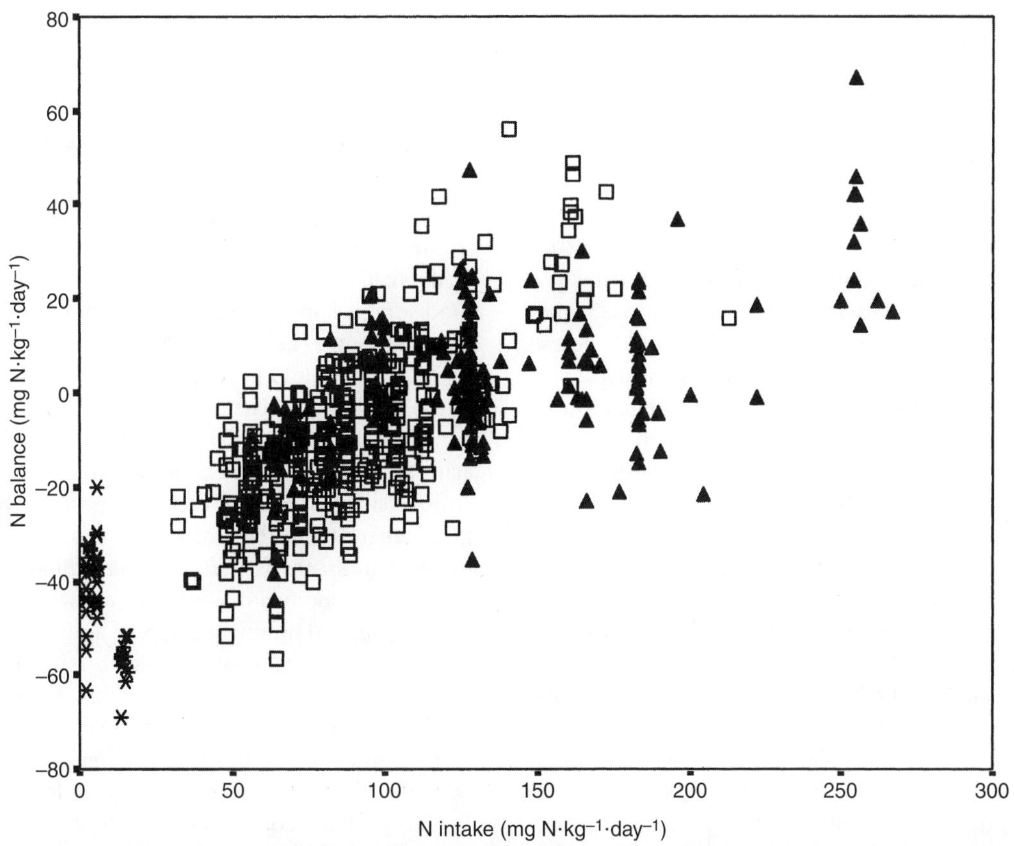

FIGURE 15-2 Relation between individual nitrogen balances, corrected for dermal and miscellaneous losses, and nitrogen intake in healthy adults. Each point represents an individual's observed response to a specific intake. The median nitrogen requirement is the intake needed for zero balance; this was determined to be approximately 105 mg·kg^{-1}·day^{-1}. (From Rand, W. M., Pellett, P. L., & Young, V. R. [2003]. Meta-analysis of nitrogen balance studies for estimating protein requirements in healthy adults. *The American Journal of Clinical Nutrition, 77*, 109–127, with permission from the American Society for Clinical Nutrition.)

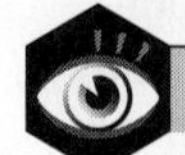

NUTRITION INSIGHT

Does Muscular Work Require the Breakdown of Muscle Protein for Fuel?

Justus Liebig, in his influential *Animal Chemistry* published in 1840, stated that protein broke down during the release of energy, with the nitrogenous fraction being converted to urea and excreted by the kidney, so that the total amount of work performed (both internally and externally) was proportional to the nitrogen excreted. These points were tested by two Swiss physiologists, Adolf Fick and Johannes Wislicenus, in 1866 (Carpenter, 1994). Using themselves as subjects, Fick and Wislicenus spent a day walking up a steep mountain path carrying urine collection equipment. From noon the day before the climb and until 6 hours after the climb, Fick and Wislicenus ate only cakes from starch paste fried in fat. Both men excreted approximately 5.6 g of N during a 14-hour period including the 8-hour climb plus the 6-hour period after the climb. Relying on the concurrent studies of Sir Edward Frankland on the heat of oxidation of organic materials and of James Prescott Joule in establishing the mechanical equivalent of heat, they calculated that the urinary N was equivalent to the breakdown of approximately 35 g of protein, and that 35 g of protein would be equivalent to approximately 154 kcal, or a work equivalent of 65×10^3 kg-m. The net external work required to ascend the 1,956-m path was calculated to be approximately 139×10^3 kg-m. Even without considering the energy required for basal or internal work or a correction for incomplete efficiency of the muscle in converting chemical energy to work, the quantity of protein metabolized was clearly insufficient to have provided the energy needed for their climb. Therefore Fick and Wislicenus (1866) concluded that the burning of protein could not be the only source of muscular power, and although their conclusion was not immediately accepted, we now know this to be true.

PROTEIN (AMINO ACID) REQUIREMENTS FOR GROWTH, PREGNANCY, AND LACTATION

The additional protein above the maintenance requirement that is needed for growth and pregnancy is usually estimated based on tissue protein accretion corrected for the efficiency of dietary protein utilization. Similarly, protein requirements for lactation are based on milk protein secretion corrected for efficiency of dietary protein utilization.

The protein needs for growth are an important component of the protein requirement of infants, children, and adolescents. A newborn infant deposits about 0.55 g protein·kg^{-1}·day^{-1}; this rate of protein deposition gradually decreases to about 0.11 g·kg^{-1}·day^{-1} by age 18 months, and then to less than 0.06 g·kg^{-1}·day^{-1} by age 3 years (WHO, 2007). Using an efficiency of dietary protein utilization of 58%, the protein requirements for growth would be 0.95, 0.19, and 0.10 g·kg^{-1}·day^{-1} at ages 1 month, 18 months, and 3 years, respectively. By adding the growth requirement to an assumed maintenance requirement of 0.66 g protein·kg^{-1}·day^{-1}, the total protein requirement would be 1.61, 0.83, and 0.76 g·kg^{-1}·day^{-1} at age 1 month, 18 months, and 3 years, respectively. Thus during the first 2 months of life, an infant's requirement for growth exceeds the infant's requirement for maintenance with almost 60% of the newborn's protein requirement being for growth. The proportion of the total protein requirement needed for growth decreases to about 22% at 18 months and then to 12% or less by 3 years, remaining in the range of 0% to 12% throughout the remainder of childhood and adolescence.

Protein is deposited in fetal and maternal tissues during pregnancy. The Food and Agriculture Organization (FAO) of the United Nations, the WHO, and the United Nations University (UNU) arms of the United Nations system used estimates of 0, 1.9, and 7.4 g/day for amounts of protein deposited during the first, second, and third trimesters of pregnancy, based on a mean gestational weight gain of 13.8 kg (WHO, 2007). The efficiency of dietary protein intake for protein accretion during pregnancy was conservatively set at 0.42, yielding additional protein requirements of 4.5 and 17.7 g/day for the second and third trimesters, respectively. It should be noted that maintenance requirements also increase during pregnancy on a g/day basis due to the increase in total body mass. The IOM (2005) used a similar approach in estimating needs during pregnancy but averaged total protein accretion during gestation over the second and third trimesters (5.4 g/day). They used this average, along with an efficiency of 0.43, to set the need for additional protein at 12.6 g/day for protein accretion during pregnancy. Based on a reference weight of 57 kg, this corresponds to an increase of 0.22 g·kg^{-1}·day^{-1} or a total protein requirement of $0.66 + 0.22 = 0.88$ g·kg^{-1}·day^{-1} during the later two trimesters.

The additional amino acid requirements for lactation derive primarily from the quantity and composition of the protein and amino acids secreted in the milk. The IOM (2005) based the increase in protein requirement for lactating women on an average output of 10 g protein per day in the milk (g N × 6.25) and the adult efficiency of protein utilization of 0.47, yielding an increased protein requirement of 21 g protein per day, or 0.39 g·kg^{-1}·day^{-1}. Adding the lactation requirement to the maintenance requirement, the total protein requirement for lactating women is $0.39 + 0.66 = 1.05$ g·kg^{-1}·day^{-1}. The FAO/WHO/UNU (WHO, 2007) used a similar approach but made separate recommendations for the first 6 months and second 6 months of breast-feeding. Based on estimates of milk protein content and milk volume, along with correction for an efficiency of 0.47, WHO set the average increase in requirement for protein at 15 g/day for the first 6 months and at 10 g/day for the second 6 months, assuming partial breast-feeding during the second 6 months (WHO, 2007).

CONSIDERATION OF PROTEIN QUALITY

The degree to which a food protein, if consumed in an amount that meets the requirement for total protein, is able to meet the requirements for all of the indispensable amino acids is called its *protein quality*. Protein quality of a particular food source is influenced by the amino acid composition of the food source (i.e., the composition of amino acids making up the protein) and the digestibility of the protein contained in the food source. The digestibility determination for a protein source includes assessment of the availability of amino acids for absorption and thus accounts for modifications of amino acids that prevent their absorption. Availability refers to whether or not the amino acid can be used in the body for protein synthesis (i.e., whether amino acids have been irreversibly modified in a way that allows absorption but not entrance into common pathways of amino acid metabolism). Different individual proteins (e.g., casein, gelatin) or different food proteins (e.g., milk proteins, soy proteins), which are actually mixtures of proteins, are not identical in terms of their amino acid composition and hence are not identical in their ability to replace losses or support net protein accretion.

The protein requirements established by the IOM and the FAO/WHO/UNU are based on nitrogen balance studies in which subjects were fed high-quality proteins or protein mixtures. In setting the Dietary Reference Intakes (DRIs) for the populations of the United States and Canada, the IOM (2005) did not include an adjustment for protein quality, because it was assumed that these North American populations consume varied diets with both high-quality and complementary proteins, such that protein quality is not of concern for most of the population. However, recommended intakes would need to be higher for populations or individuals consuming diets in which the overall protein quality is not high. The FAO/WHO/UNU (WHO, 2007) made their recommendations with provisions for additional adjustments for protein quality when appropriate. The topic of protein quality is considered in more detail later in this chapter.

DRIs FOR PROTEIN

Requirements for protein are the amounts of dietary protein that will meet the needs of the organism for maintenance and for protein accretion during growth and pregnancy or milk production during lactation. Safe requirement levels or recommended intakes are conventionally set as the average requirement plus 2 standard deviations (SD) based on between-individual variance so that the recommended intake should cover the needs of 97.5% of the population. For protein requirements, the coefficient of variation is typically about 12.5%, so the actual recommended intakes are about 25% (2 × 12.5) higher than the average requirement.

The IOM (2005) set DRIs for protein intake of various age and sex groups. In the DRIs Across the Life Cycle box, the Estimated Average Requirement (EAR) and Recommended

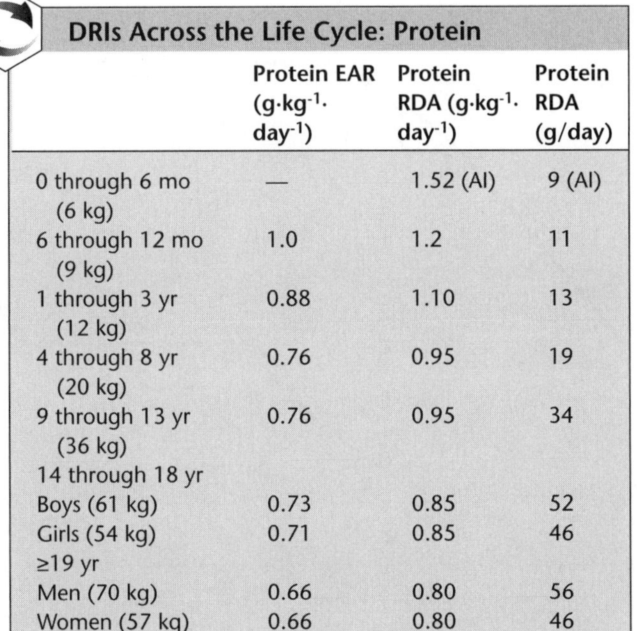

DRIs Across the Life Cycle: Protein

	Protein EAR ($g \cdot kg^{-1} \cdot day^{-1}$)	Protein RDA ($g \cdot kg^{-1} \cdot day^{-1}$)	Protein RDA (g/day)
0 through 6 mo (6 kg)	—	1.52 (AI)	9 (AI)
6 through 12 mo (9 kg)	1.0	1.2	11
1 through 3 yr (12 kg)	0.88	1.10	13
4 through 8 yr (20 kg)	0.76	0.95	19
9 through 13 yr (36 kg)	0.76	0.95	34
14 through 18 yr			
Boys (61 kg)	0.73	0.85	52
Girls (54 kg)	0.71	0.85	46
≥19 yr			
Men (70 kg)	0.66	0.80	56
Women (57 kg)	0.66	0.80	46
Pregnant women	0.88	1.1	71
Lactating women	1.05	1.3	71

Data from IOM. (2005). *Dietary Reference Intakes for energy, carbohydrate, fiber, fat, fatty acids, cholesterol, protein, and amino acids.* Washington, DC: The National Academies Press. *AI,* Adequate Intake; *DRI,* Dietary Reference Intake; *EAR,* Estimated Average Requirement; *RDA,* Recommended Dietary Allowance.

Dietary Allowance (RDA) are shown as g protein$\cdot kg^{-1} \cdot day^{-1}$, and RDAs are also given as g/day for reference size males and females (e.g., 70-kg man and 57-kg woman). Thus the RDA for protein is 0.8 $g \cdot kg^{-1} \cdot day^{-1}$ for adults, or 46 g/day for the 57-kg reference woman and 56 g/day for the 70-kg reference man.

There is considerable debate whether the requirement for protein is higher in elderly adults. The IOM (2005) and the FAO/WHO/UNU (WHO, 2007) concluded that the lack of demonstrated improvement in biochemical indicators of protein sufficiency or measured nitrogen balance with higher protein intakes suggests that the requirement for protein does not increase with age. However, it was noted that the protein to energy ratio for diets of the elderly needs to be higher than for younger individuals because of the decreased energy expenditure of the elderly, despite no change in their protein requirement per se.

For infants, the IOM (2005) did not determine an EAR/RDA, but an Adequate Intake (AI) was set based on the known adequacy of breast milk for infants. The AI for infants up to 6 months of age, set by the IOM, is based on the average volume of milk intake (0.78 L/day) and the average protein content of human milk during the first 6 months of lactation (11.7 g/L) and is 9 g/day. The AI can be stated as 1.5 $g \cdot kg^{-1} \cdot day^{-1}$, based on a reference weight of 6 kg for 2- to 6-month-old infants. A similar estimate based on milk plus complementary food intake is the basis of the AI for infants during the second 6 months of life. The FAO/WHO/UNU (WHO, 2007) has calculated safe protein intakes for infants based on estimates of their maintenance

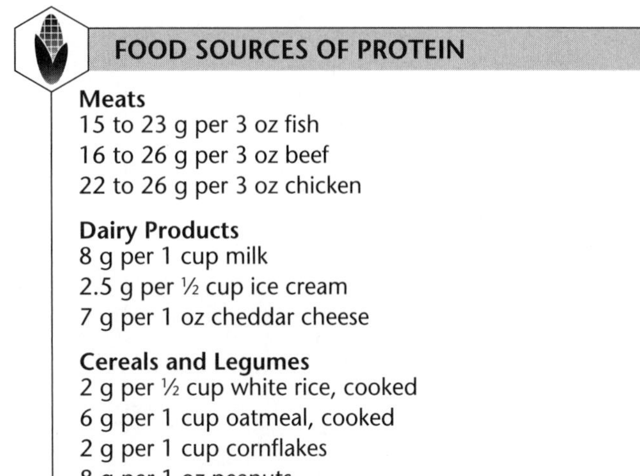

FOOD SOURCES OF PROTEIN

Meats
15 to 23 g per 3 oz fish
16 to 26 g per 3 oz beef
22 to 26 g per 3 oz chicken

Dairy Products
8 g per 1 cup milk
2.5 g per ½ cup ice cream
7 g per 1 oz cheddar cheese

Cereals and Legumes
2 g per ½ cup white rice, cooked
6 g per 1 cup oatmeal, cooked
2 g per 1 cup cornflakes
8 g per 1 oz peanuts
8 g per ½ cup black beans
9 g per ½ cup tofu

Eggs
6 g per 1 egg

Data from U.S. Department of Agriculture, Agricultural Research Service. (2011). *USDA National Nutrient Database for Standard Reference, Release 24.* Washington, DC: USDA/ARS. Retrieved from www.ars.usda.gov/ba/bhnrc/ndl/

requirements (0.58 g protein$\cdot kg^{-1} \cdot day^{-1}$ from nitrogen balance studies) and growth requirements (protein deposition adjusted for an efficiency of 0.66), with the average requirement increased by 2 SD, to yield safe levels ranging from 1.8 g protein$\cdot kg^{-1} \cdot day^{-1}$ (for the 1-month-old) to 1.1 g protein$\cdot kg^{-1} \cdot day^{-1}$ (for the 6-month-old infant).

REQUIREMENTS FOR INDIVIDUAL AMINO ACIDS

Protein is made up of all the indispensable and dispensable amino acids; therefore the expression of protein requirements must also include a consideration of the supply of indispensable amino acids that cannot be synthesized in the body. Over the course of the last century, several approaches have been developed and applied to the determination of amino acid requirements, resulting in refinements in our ability to precisely estimate these requirements for humans. Essentially two approaches have been used to assess amino acid requirements: empirical analysis of dose response and factorial method.

AMINO ACID REQUIREMENTS BASED ON EMPIRICAL ANALYSIS OF DOSE RESPONSES

The empirical analysis of dose responses measures a physiological response (i.e., growth rate, nitrogen balance, or amino acid oxidation) at graded intakes of protein or amino acid. The nitrogen balance technique has been used to determine protein requirements for maintenance, and the criterion of nitrogen balance also provided the basis of the first quantitative estimates of the amino acid needs of human adults. However, direct amino acid oxidation or indicator amino acid oxidation has been used as the response criterion in more recent studies. Regardless of the response criterion, a range

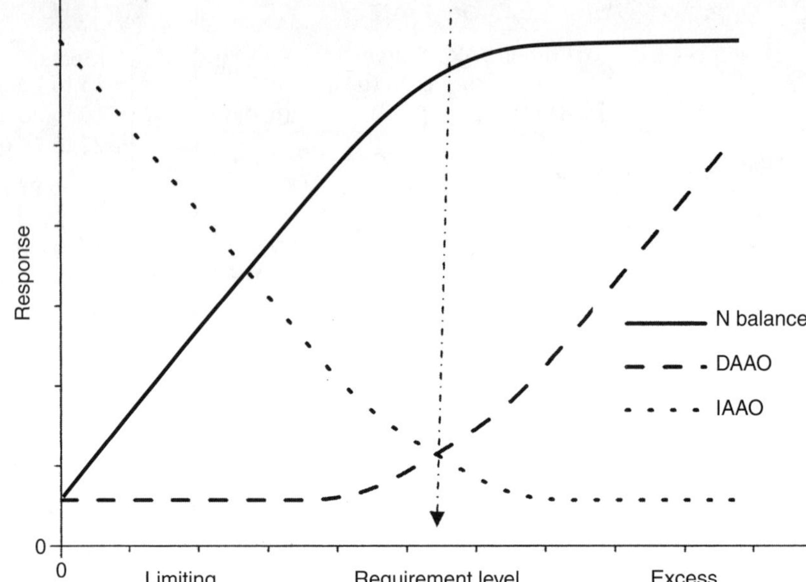

FIGURE 15-3 General patterns of metabolic responses to graded intakes of an indispensable amino acid. *DAAO,* Direct amino acid oxidation; *IAAO,* indicator amino acid oxidation. (Modified from Pencharz, P. B., & Ball, R. O. [2003]. Different approaches to define individual amino acid requirements. *Annual Review of Nutrition, 23,* 101–116.)

of amino acid levels greater than and less than the requirement (six or more levels) should be tested in each individual subject. The basal diet must be adequate in all other amino acids and energy, as well as in all other essential nutrients, such that the amount of the amino acid being tested is the only factor that limits the extent of protein synthesis.

Depending on the approach used to determine an indispensable amino acid requirement, three different patterns of response are possible; these are illustrated in Figure 15-3. One pattern is that seen when either nitrogen balance in the adult or growth in a growing animal or child is plotted against amino acid intake. Nitrogen balance or growth will increase as the intake of the limiting indispensable amino acid (i.e., test amino acid) increases up until the requirement amount is reached, at which point nitrogen balance or growth will plateau. A second pattern is seen for the indicator amino acid oxidation (IAAO) method where oxidation of the indicator amino acid is high when amino acids are not being used maximally for protein synthesis but decreases to a plateau once the requirement of the limiting amino acid for protein synthesis has been met. For nitrogen balance, growth, and IAAO, once the requirement is reached the measured response will plateau despite the addition of higher levels of protein or limiting amino acid. A third pattern occurs when oxidation of a test amino acid is measured directly, called the direct amino acid oxidation (DAAO) method. In this case, oxidation of the test amino acid remains low with little change until the requirement is approached or met, after which its oxidation increases progressively as intake is further increased. A similar pattern may be observed by following the plasma level of the test amino acid; the level of the test amino acid will begin to increase once intake exceeds the requirement. When lines are drawn for the slope of the two phases (change and plateau) of the response curve, the crossover point or breakpoint of the two lines is used to determine the requirement level as illustrated in Figure 15-3.

Estimates of Indispensable Amino Acid Requirements by Nitrogen Balance Studies

In nitrogen balance experiments, the rate of body nitrogen retention is estimated as the difference between the dietary nitrogen intake and the sum of the losses in urine and feces and by other routes (integumental and miscellaneous). Nitrogen balance is based on the premise that protein or lean body tissue is the major nitrogen-containing component in the body; thus nitrogen loss or gain equates to protein loss or gain. It is assumed that body nitrogen increases in the growing child and remains constant in the adult (WHO, 2007). As described previously, it is generally presumed that the protein requirement of an adult is achieved when the individual is in zero nitrogen balance (i.e., nitrogen equilibrium). Infants, children, pregnant women, and individuals recovering from disease states in which lean body mass was lost should be in positive nitrogen balance, reflecting net deposition of protein.

Nitrogen balance studies were used to obtain the first estimates of the amino acid requirements of human adults. Rose and colleagues, in a series of nitrogen balance studies in the 1940s, determined the amino acid requirements of young men (see Rose, 1957). First, men were given diets devoid of a single amino acid so as to establish which amino acids were dispensable and which were indispensable. Eight amino acids were determined to be indispensable. In these studies, removal of histidine from the diet did not lead to a negative nitrogen balance; this was interpreted to mean that histidine was dispensable, and this conclusion was only reversed much later by longer-term experiments. Rose and colleagues then conducted a series of quantitative studies in which they gave each subject a succession of diets with different concentrations of the amino acid under investigation. From the changes in nitrogen balance that ensued, they attempted to identify the intake of each amino acid that was required for nitrogen equilibrium to be achieved. Similar experiments were conducted on young women, but using more subjects and with several improvements in experimental procedures (Leverton et al., 1959). The results of these early experiments in determining the amino acid requirements of men and women formed the basis of the international estimates of adult amino acid requirements (WHO, 1985) that were widely used before 2000.

One of the greatest challenges with the nitrogen balance method is accurate measurement of nitrogen losses. Due to difficulties in measuring integumental and miscellaneous losses, they are not always included in the calculation of nitrogen balance. Not accounting for integumental and miscellaneous losses results in underestimation of nitrogen loss. Urinary and fecal nitrogen can be measured relatively accurately; however, incomplete measurement of food spillage and food residues results in overestimation of nitrogen intake. The tendency to overestimate intake and to underestimate losses both contribute to the tendency of nitrogen balance studies to underestimate protein or amino acid requirements (WHO, 2007). This means that a subject apparently receiving sufficient amino acid (or protein) to maintain nitrogen equilibrium may actually be in negative nitrogen balance and need more of the amino acid (or protein) to maintain true nitrogen equilibrium.

A further problem with the nitrogen balance approach, especially in short-term studies, may arise through the implicit assumption that a subject in nitrogen equilibrium must also be in amino acid equilibrium. This is not necessarily so. Histidine, for example, is stored in the form of the peptide carnosine (β-alanylhistidine). Carnosine, in experimental animals at least, is depleted during dietary histidine deficiency. This allows obligatory losses of histidine to be met for a time without loss of body protein, despite an inadequate histidine intake. There may also be a potential to adapt to an indispensable amino acid deficiency through modification of the amino acid composition of the body protein pool as a whole. Of course, it is not possible to modify the amino acid composition of any of the body's proteins, but it is possible to vary the relative amounts of the various proteins. Because proteins have different amino acid compositions, there is the potential to adapt, at least temporarily, to a deficiency of one amino acid by depleting the body of proteins rich in that amino acid. This also happens in histidine deficiency, in which hemoglobin, which is very rich in histidine, can be gradually depleted. The mechanism of this adaptation is not known. However, this ability of the body to use endogenous sources of histidine explains why histidine was not identified as an indispensable amino acid in the early balance studies (Rose, 1957; Leverton, 1959).

Estimates of Indispensable Amino Acid Requirements by Amino Acid Oxidation Studies

Both direct and indirect amino acid oxidation are based on the principle that there is no storage of amino acids; therefore amino acids not used for protein synthesis are oxidized. In both direct and indirect methods, the oxidation of an amino acid that is labeled with ^{13}C in the α-carboxyl group is assessed. The ^{13}C is released to the body bicarbonate pool in an early step of the amino acid's committed degradation pathway, and its oxidation is measured by the appearance of labeled $^{13}CO_2$ in the breath.

In DAAO, it is the amino acid of interest (i.e., the test amino acid) that is labeled. Thus, application of the DAAO method is limited to amino acids whose α-carboxyl group is irreversibly released early in the degradation pathway. In the DAAO method, the test amino acid is labeled and its content in the diet is varied. As long as the level of the test amino acid remains below the requirement for protein synthesis, it will be efficiently incorporated into protein with little excess for oxidation. Once the requirement is exceeded, the excess test amino acid will be oxidized, giving rise to a rapid increase in the amount of labeled $^{13}CO_2$ in the breath.

In the IAAO method, a separate indispensable amino acid is labeled (i.e., an indicator amino acid) and its oxidation is measured. The indicator amino acid is another indispensable amino acid present in adequate amounts while intake of the test amino acid is altered. When intake of the test amino acid is low and protein synthesis is limited by a lack of the test amino acid, the excess indicator amino acid (i.e., that not used for protein synthesis) will be oxidized. As the intake of the test amino acid is increased, incorporation of the indicator amino acid, as well as all other non-test amino acids, into protein will increase, such that oxidation of the indicator amino acid to $^{13}CO_2$ will decrease. The IAAO method is not dependent upon release of the carboxyl carbon of the test amino acid and thus can be used to assess the requirement of any indispensable amino acid. Phenylalanine has been found to be the most responsive and accurate of the indispensable amino acids for use as the indicator amino acid in determining amino acid requirements (Levesque et al., 2010).

Adult Requirements for Indispensable Amino Acids and Indispensable Amino Acid Requirement Patterns

There has been considerable debate over the most appropriate requirement estimates for indispensable amino acids in adults. However, extensive reviews (Young, 1986; Millward, 1988; Fuller and Garlick, 1994) of the original nitrogen balance studies by Rose (1957) and Irwin and Hegsted (1971) all conclude that previous estimates (WHO, 1985) based on nitrogen balance were too low. The greatest concern with these early studies was the lack of measurement of miscellaneous nitrogen losses, resulting in low estimates of the indispensable amino acid requirements for achieving nitrogen balance. The current FAO/WHO/UNU (WHO, 2007) and IOM (2005) estimates of indispensable amino acid requirements (mg amino acid·kg^{-1}·day^{-1}) are based primarily on amino acid oxidation studies. As shown in Table 15-2, the current estimates of requirements for 6 out of 10 of the indispensable amino acids are close to double the previous 1985 estimates.

The estimates of amino acid requirements can be used to generate safe intakes for individual indispensable amino acids and for generation of the pattern or amounts of

TABLE 15-2 Requirements and Reference Patterns for Indispensable Amino Acids in Adults and Comparison to Previous Estimates

	Estimated Average Requirement (mg amino acid·kg^{-1}·day^{-1})			Adult Reference Pattern for Dietary Protein* (mg amino acid/g protein)		
	2007 FAO/WHO/UNU†	2005 IOM‡	1985 FAO/WHO/UNU§	2007 FAO/WHO/UNU	2005 IOM	1985 FAO/WHO/UNU
Histidine	10	11	8–12	15	17	15
Isoleucine	20	15	10	30	23	15
Leucine	39	34	14	59	52	21
Lysine	30	31	12	45	47	18
Methionine + Cysteine	15	15	13	22	23	20
Phenylalanine + Tyrosine	25	27	14	38	41	21
Threonine	15	16	7	23	24	11
Tryptophan	4	4	3.5	6	6	5
Valine	26	19	10	39	29	15
Total indispensable amino acids	184	172	93.5	277	262	141

*Calculated as the individual indispensable amino acid requirement (mg amino acid·kg^{-1}·day^{-1}) divided by the requirement for total protein (0.66 g protein·kg^{-1}·day^{-1}).

†WHO. (2007). *Protein and amino acid requirements in humans: Report of Joint FAO/WHO/UNU Expert Consultation.* WHO Technical Series 935. Geneva: FAO.

‡IOM. (2005). *Dietary Reference Intakes: Energy, carbohydrate, fiber, fat, fatty acids, cholesterol, protein, and amino acids.* Washington, DC: The National Academies Press.

§WHO. (1985). *Energy and protein requirements: Report of a Joint FAO/WHO/UNU Expert Consultation.* WHO Technical Report Series 724. Geneva: WHO.

indispensable amino acids needed in a protein source for it to meet both the dietary protein and the indispensable amino acid requirements. In order for the required amount of dietary protein to meet all amino acid needs, it must contain the indispensable amino acid in amounts equal to or greater than the required pattern. The requirement patterns for indispensable amino acids are also shown in Table 15-2. Even based on the highest requirement pattern, only 27% of the total amino acids in the dietary protein need to be indispensable amino acids. If the pattern of the dietary protein mixture of a population has an inadequate amount of one or more indispensable amino acids, adjustments should be made to increase the total protein requirements of that population to allow intake of a sufficient amount of the limiting indispensable amino acids. Thus for lower-quality protein mixtures, higher total protein intakes will be needed. Another approach, of course, would be to improve the quality of the protein mixture by using a mixture of complementary proteins or adding a small amount of high-quality protein to the mixture.

Estimates of Indispensable Amino Acid Requirements of Children and of Pregnant and Lactating Women by the Factorial Method

As with setting protein requirements, the requirements for indispensable amino acids in children, pregnant women, and lactating women were based on the factorial approach and include a component for both maintenance and growth or milk secretion. The factorial method is the approach in which the relevant components of the requirement (maintenance, growth, accretion of maternal tissues and growth of the fetus during pregnancy, and milk secretion during lactation) are estimated separately and then added to set the requirement. Although this approach ostensibly provides a logical system for determination of requirements, the direct estimation of the component requirements is difficult. This is particularly true during pregnancy, where direct estimates of protein and amino acid requirements for fetal growth are largely unknown. For example in school-aged children, the factorial estimate for total sulfur amino acids (15 mg·kg^{-1}·day^{-1}) and lysine (30 mg·kg^{-1}·day^{-1}) were similar to the mean requirement determined by IAAO (13 and 35 mg·kg^{-1}·day^{-1}, respectively) (Turner et al., 2006; Elango et al., 2007). However, the factorial estimate for total branched-chain amino acids (85 mg·kg^{-1}·day^{-1}) in school-aged children was significantly lower than the mean requirement based on IAAO (147 mg·kg^{-1}) (Mager et al., 2003).

To estimate the indispensable amino acid requirements of children, the IOM (2005) used the factorial method. The maintenance requirements for children were based on the EARs for indispensable amino acids in adults. To this was added the requirements for accretion of protein, which were based on the amino acid composition of body proteins and an estimated efficiency of utilization of amino acids derived from the diet (0.58). Safe intakes

TABLE 15-3 Average Requirements for Indispensable Amino Acids in Children and Adults

	Daily Intake of Indispensable Amino Acids in Breast-fed Infants	Amino Acid Requirement Determined by Factorial Method					Adult Requirement
		Age in Years					
	BIRTH TO 6 MONTHS	0.5	1–2	3–10	11–14	15–18	>18
		(mg amino acid·kg^{-1}·day^{-1})					
Histidine	20	22	15	12	12	11	10
Isoleucine	52	36	27	23	22	21	20
Leucine	90	73	54	44	44	42	39
Lysine	65	64	45	35	35	33	30
Methionine + Cysteine	31	31	22	18	17	16	15
Phenylalanine + Tyrosine	88	59	40	30	30	28	25
Threonine	41	34	23	18	18	17	15
Tryptophan	16	9.5	6.4	4.8	4.8	4.5	4.0
Valine	51	49	36	29	29	28	26

Data from WHO. (2007). *Protein and amino acid requirements in humans: Report of Joint FAO/WHO/UNU Expert Consultation.* WHO Technical Series 935. Geneva: FAO.

for infants were based on adequate intakes from breast milk during the first 6 months and from breast milk and complementary foods during the second 6 months. FAO/WHO/UNU (WHO, 2007) used a similar approach to estimate indispensable amino acid requirements of children and infants. However, to estimate the amino acid requirements of infants from 6 months to 1 years of age, the FAO/WHO/UNU applied the factorial method instead of simply relying on the amino acid composition and intake volume of human milk. Table 15-3 shows the indispensable amino acid intake of breast-fed infants and the indispensable amino acid requirements of children from 6 months to 18 years of age.

To set amino acid requirements for pregnant and lactating women, both the IOM (2005) and FAO/WHO/UNU (WHO, 2007) added an increment to the maintenance requirement of adults to support tissue accretion during pregnancy and milk production during lactation. Incremental requirements were based on the amino acid composition of human tissues for pregnant women and on the amino acid composition of human milk for lactating women, with these amounts being corrected for an efficiency of utilization of 0.42 or 0.43 for pregnancy and 0.47 for lactation.

For estimation of protein quality, age-specific requirement patterns can be used. As for the adult indispensable amino acid requirements, division of the requirements for indispensable amino acids by the requirement for total protein for each age group will yield an age-specific requirement pattern for evaluation of protein quality (WHO, 2007). The IOM also used the indispensable amino acid content of human milk proteins to derive an adequate intake pattern for assessing the quality of protein mixtures in infant diets.

FACTORS THAT AFFECT AMINO ACID REQUIREMENTS

Protein and amino acid requirements of healthy individuals are affected by several important factors, energy intake being one of the most important. In addition, the approaches used to set protein requirements do not address all of the metabolic functions of amino acids, do not consider the possibility of microbial synthesis of amino acids using dietary nitrogen, and do not consider the role of bioactive peptides or proteins consumed as part of the diet.

DIETARY ENERGY

Perhaps the most important dietary factor affecting protein utilization is dietary nonprotein energy (carbohydrate and fat). If energy is insufficient, amino acids will be used as a fuel rather than for protein synthesis. When amino acids are oxidized as a fuel, most of their carbon enters the citric acid cycle and other central pathways of fuel metabolism via pyruvate, oxaloacetate, α-ketoglutarate, or acetyl-CoA (see Chapter 14, Figure 14-9). The ability of amino acids to substitute for other energy sources is important, for example, in starvation, when body protein is depleted to provide amino acids both as precursors for important synthetic pathways and as a source of glucose and other energy-yielding substrates. However, when energy is available in other forms, either from body glycogen and fat or from dietary carbohydrate and fat, the need for net breakdown of body protein with oxidation of amino acids is diminished.

Dietary energy, in the form of carbohydrate or fat, has a profound effect on protein utilization in both the growing and the adult states. With generous intakes of nonprotein energy, in excess of immediate energy needs, amino acid oxidation is minimized and amino acids are utilized with maximum efficiency. In adults, the effect is typically to spare 2 mg of nitrogen for each kcal added to a nutritionally adequate basal diet, which is associated with an increase in lean body mass that accompanies the deposition of body fat. In growing animals, the magnitude of the effect is similar, or even greater, and diminishes as the highest levels of energy intake are approached. Thus excess energy has the effect of lowering apparent amino acid requirements for maintenance in adults and for normal growth in children. Conversely, when carbohydrate and fat intakes are limited, amino acid oxidation rises and apparent amino acid requirements are increased. This means that amino acid requirements cannot be stated without reference to the provision of other nutrients, particularly carbohydrate and fat. Deficiencies of many other nutrients, such as vitamins and minerals, also can limit the utilization of dietary protein. In published estimates of requirements, it is assumed that other nutrients are also provided at the appropriate levels and that adult subjects are not gaining weight.

POSSIBLE CONTRIBUTION OF MICROBIAL SYNTHESIS OF AMINO ACIDS

It is normally assumed that the indispensable amino acids can be derived only from the diet. However, this may not be entirely true. Evidence from both human and animal studies indicates that some amino acids synthesized by gastrointestinal microorganisms may be absorbed. Whether this route makes a significant net contribution to meeting human requirements is dependent on the source of the nitrogen used for microbial synthesis (Libao-Mercado et al., 2009). If nitrogenous substrates that are unavailable to the host (e.g., urea, ammonia) or amino acids from indigestible protein are used to synthesize new indispensable amino acids, then a net positive contribution occurs. However, if amino acids from the diet or endogenous proteins secreted into the digestive tract are used to synthesize microbial amino acids, then no net positive contribution to the host's amino acid supply occurs unless surplus dispensable or excess indispensable amino acids not specifically needed are used to synthesize needed indispensable amino acids (Metges et al., 2006).

Although there is very limited data on the nutritional contribution of amino acids synthesized by the microflora, the quantity of microbial lysine used for whole body lysine homeostasis in humans has been estimated to range from 12 to 68 $mg \cdot kg^{-1} \cdot day^{-1}$ (Metges et al., 1999; Jackson et al., 2004). However, microbial protein was found to be almost exclusively synthesized from dietary and endogenous protein sources and hence contributed minimally to net new amino acid synthesis (Libao-Mercado et al., 2009). Regardless of the magnitude of the contribution of microbial amino acid synthesis to whole body homeostasis, current recommended amino acid requirements (WHO, 2007) are based primarily on data from amino acid oxidation studies, which actually reflect the total need for absorbed indispensable amino acids including contributions of both diet and the microbiota (Metges et al., 2006). Thus, the true dietary requirements for indispensable amino acids might be somewhat lower than the amino acid requirements based on amino acid oxidation.

IS THE CRITERION OF ADEQUACY TOO LIMITED?

As we have seen, amino acid requirements may be derived in a number of different ways. It is perhaps not surprising that these should yield rather different estimates. However, most have been based on some measure of body protein status. In considering maintenance requirements, for example, it has been assumed that the requirement is that amount needed to preserve the total protein or amino acid content of the body. This may be too limited a definition on which to base dietary recommendations. We need to ask if there are aspects of health and well-being that would benefit from amounts of protein or individual amino acids that are greater than those that are needed simply to maintain protein homeostasis. Is the diet optimal for protein-related health such as immune function, bone health, or growth in height?

Higher tryptophan intakes are associated with greater synthesis of nicotinamide adenine dinucleotide (NAD), and higher sulfur amino acid intakes are associated with greater synthesis of glutathione and taurine. However, the relation of dietary supply to optimal production or tissue concentrations of these nonprotein metabolites is not considered by current methods used for establishing amino acid and protein requirements and allowances. In addition, it is possible that intakes of specific dispensable amino acids affect metabolic state and health. For example, arginine supplements have been shown to enhance aspects of immune function and to have beneficial effects on wound healing, possibly due to the function of arginine in the formation of nitric oxide and polyamines. Likewise, glutamine, another amino acid normally considered dispensable, may improve recovery from injury or disease. This may relate to the fact that glutamine is a major fuel for rapidly proliferating cells, including lymphocytes. There is, however, little reliable evidence for any beneficial effect of higher habitual protein intakes on mortality, morbidity, and longevity.

Although the question of whether protein intakes somewhat greater than those needed for maintenance would be beneficial to health of adults has not been studied to any extent, it does seem clear that the optimum level of protein is not likely to be lower than the current EAR. In a study designed to evaluate the safe level of protein that had been set by FAO/WHO in 1973, young men were fed egg protein at a level of 0.59 $g \cdot kg^{-1} \cdot day^{-1}$ for 12 weeks (Garza et al., 1977). Four of the six subjects were in negative nitrogen balance and experienced loss of lean body mass (based on total body potassium measurements and creatinine excretion). Two of the six subjects exhibited an excessive rise in serum aspartate aminotransferase and alanine aminotransferase, which rapidly fell to normal levels when the subjects were switched to a diet higher in protein. These findings suggest that 0.59 g of high-quality $protein \cdot kg^{-1} \cdot day^{-1}$ is not adequate for long-term maintenance of most healthy young men, and that the current estimate of the adult EAR for protein (0.66 $g \cdot kg^{-1} \cdot day^{-1}$)

is close to the actual requirement, despite the limitations of nitrogen balance studies.

PHYSIOLOGICAL EFFECTS OF INTACT DIETARY PROTEINS AND PEPTIDES

Although dietary requirements for protein are correctly viewed as requirements for the amino acids contained in the proteins, there are some examples of intact peptides and proteins that are of nutritional significance, such as the immunoglobulins and lactoferrin passed to the infant's gastrointestinal tract in mother's milk. Other bioactive proteins, such as retinol-binding protein, transforming growth factor, and epidermal growth factor, may also be derived from maternal milk. It is also possible that certain peptides resulting from the incomplete hydrolysis of dietary proteins may sufficiently resemble bioactive peptides as to mimic their function in the body. Proteins in the diet also include antigens, toxins, and proteins with antinutritional effects such as the trypsin inhibitors in a number of legumes. Some of these exert their effects in the gut lumen; others are absorbed. All of these could be important in determining the extent to which protein nutriture may amount to more than simply the provision of amino acids and nitrogen.

FOOD PROTEINS AND PROTEIN QUALITY

The purpose of determining amino acid requirements is to ensure adequate protein and amino acid nutrition. Intake of the requirement level of protein will be sufficient only if the ingested protein also contains sufficient amounts of each of the indispensable amino acids. Thus estimates of the capacity of food sources to supply both the protein and the required indispensable amino acids are necessary for practical application of amino acid requirements. This has led to a variety of approaches for assessing protein quality.

Growth assays in rats, and chicks, were traditionally used to assess protein quality of food sources. An assay called the protein efficiency ratio (PER) was based on the grams of weight gain per gram of protein consumed. The PER provided a measure of the availability of the protein source to support metabolic processes. Similarly, other variations of rat growth assay such as net protein utilization (NPU) and biological value (BV) describe the efficiency with which nitrogen intake (NPU) or nitrogen actually absorbed (BV) is used to support a gain in body nitrogen (rather than simply weight gain). Although the rat is a reasonable surrogate for estimating the digestibility of amino acids from food sources, the amino acid requirement pattern of the growing rat is dominated by growth, whereas maintenance processes are the predominant demand for amino acids in humans. Also, the specific types and amounts of different proteins vary in rats and humans. For example, the proteins present in hair or fur are high in sulfur-containing amino acids. Thus the profile of required amino acids is different between rats and humans: a food source relatively low in sulfur-containing amino acids that would receive a low PER when fed to rapidly growing rats might supply adequate sulfur-containing amino acids to meet the maintenance requirement of adult humans. The PER approach using the rapidly growing rat tends to underestimate the value of vegetable proteins and overestimate the value of animal proteins for adults. Furthermore, biological assays of protein quality are only meaningful when they are determined for whole diets. There is no simple way to use the information from rat bioassays to predict the effects that result from combinations of various food proteins, which often improves the overall protein quality of the diet.

In 1985 the FAO/WHO concluded that a combined amino acid scoring/digestibility measurement should replace the traditional growth assays in evaluation of protein quality (FAO, 1985). A joint FAO/WHO expert consultation group recommended that the protein digestibility–corrected amino acid score (PDCAAS) serve as the standard for protein quality evaluation (FAO, 1991). This method involves the use of reference amino acid patterns, and these are now typically derived by dividing best estimates of individual indispensable amino acid requirements by the best estimate of the total protein requirement, as was done for the adult requirement patterns shown in Table 15-2. It should be noted that protein quality says nothing about the total amount of protein in the food source under study or about the ratio of protein to energy in the food, both of which are also important factors. Protein quality is essentially a measure of the extent to which all indispensable amino acids will be met by the food or food mixture if a sufficient amount of it were eaten to meet the protein requirement and assuming that the diet contains sufficient energy from fat and carbohydrates. The score reflects the relative availability of the indispensable amino acid present in lowest abundance relative to its requirement. This amino acid is called the first limiting amino acid, and it defines the protein quality score.

PROTEIN DIGESTIBILITY–CORRECTED AMINO ACID SCORE

Determination of the amino acid composition of the protein or protein mixture and determination of the digestibility of the protein are necessary before the PDCAAS can be calculated. FAO/WHO/UNU (WHO, 2007) recommends use of age-specific amino acid requirement patterns for the reference pattern.

The amino acid score (AAS) is the proportion of the limiting amino acid from a test protein expressed as a percentage of the content of the same amino acid in a reference pattern of essential amino acids. It can be calculated as follows:

AAS (%) = [(mg of limiting amino acid in 1 g of test protein or test protein mixture) / (mg of same amino acid in 1 g of recommended reference pattern)] × 100%

The PDCAAS is the proportion of the limiting amino acid from a test protein expressed as a percentage of the content of the same amino acid in a reference pattern of essential amino acids, corrected for the digestibility of the test protein as measured in a rat fecal digestibility study. It can be calculated as follows:

$$\text{PDCAAS (\%)} = \text{AAS (\%)} \times \text{digestibility (fraction)}$$

Thus both the AAS and the PDCAAS are determined by the amino acid present in the test protein (or available from the test protein) in lowest abundance relative to the requirement pattern. If none of the amino acids in the protein is below the reference pattern, the quality of the protein is 100%, never more than 100% even though the calculated value may be above 100%.

Amino Acid Score

The concept of the amino acid score was initially devised by Block and Mitchell (1946) where the concentration of each amino acid in the test protein was expressed as a proportion of the corresponding concentration in the reference protein. At that time, egg protein was used as the reference protein because it had been found to be unsurpassable in its ability to support growth in animals, and thus was known to be a high-quality protein. However, it cannot be assumed that the amino acid pattern of egg protein closely matches the "ideal" amino acid pattern. In fact, the amino acid pattern of egg contains some indispensable amino acids in excess relative to the actual amino acid requirement, and use of an egg protein pattern underestimates the true quality of some proteins. One of the improvements proposed by FAO/WHO/UNU (WHO, 1985) was to use an amino acid reference pattern based on human amino acid requirements rather than egg protein for the PDCAAS. A subsequent report (FAO, 1991) further proposed that the scoring pattern be based on the requirement pattern of preschool children because at that time satisfactory adult values were not available. However, the most recent report (WHO, 2007) suggested that age-specific patterns be used.

Table 15-4 demonstrates the calculation of the amino acid score for two common food protein sources (rice and wheat flour) using either the egg amino acid pattern or the current FAO/WHO/UNU amino acid requirement pattern for a human adult (see Table 15-2). As shown in Table 15-4, lysine is identified as the limiting amino acid in both rice and wheat because it is present at less than 100% of the requirement pattern and is the amino acid present at the lowest percentage of its requirement pattern. Thus the calculated percentage for lysine defines the amino acid score for these two protein sources regardless of which of the two reference patterns was used. Note that when the amino acid score is based on the egg amino acid pattern, however, both rice and wheat flour would be considered of lower quality (55% and 40% amino acid scores for rice and wheat flour, respectively) than when based on the human amino acid requirement pattern (85% and 62% amino acid scores for rice and wheat flour, respectively), illustrating the now-known fact that use of the egg protein pattern results in underestimation of protein quality for humans. Based on comparison with the human amino acid requirement pattern, rice would be considered a good-quality protein source because its amino acid score is 85, which means it meets a high proportion of the limiting amino acid requirement.

Another important point to remember is that protein quality provides no information about the total amount of protein in the food; a food could have a very small amount of a very-high-quality protein and thus have a high amino acid score but be relatively unimportant as a dietary source of protein.

Digestibility

Digestibility, as the name suggests, measures the digestion and absorption of protein and amino acids from the digestive tract. Apparent protein digestibility (d), expressed as the fraction of amino acid intake that is absorbed, is conventionally described as

$$d = (I - F) / I$$

where I is the protein or nitrogen intake and F is fecal nitrogen or protein excretion, with both measured in the same units (i.e., g/day). This is called apparent digestibility in recognition of the fact that the fecal nitrogen output does not consist entirely of undigested dietary matter but includes nitrogen from endogenous sources (i.e., secretions and sloughed intestinal cells). By deducting this endogenous component, which can be estimated by measuring fecal nitrogen in individuals consuming protein-free diets, a value for the true digestibility of the dietary protein can be derived. True digestibility is higher than apparent digestibility because of this correction. Digestibility is often reported as the percentage of protein amino acid intake that is absorbed. As illustrated in Table 15-5, the true digestibility of most animal proteins such as milk, meat, and eggs is high, between 90% and 99%. However, many plant proteins, especially when eaten raw, are less digestible (70% to 90%), partly because they are contained within cell walls that are resistant to mammalian digestive enzymes and are broken down only by the gastrointestinal microflora. Additionally, some dietary proteins, such as legumes, contain antinutritional factors such as trypsin inhibitors that affect digestibility.

Practical Application of Amino Acid Score and PDCAAS

Table 15-6 demonstrates the calculation of amino acid scores of proteins for two different food sources (peanut butter and wheat bread) as well as for a mixture of the two protein sources (peanut butter sandwich). Comparison of the amino acid composition of peanut butter and white bread to the FAO/WHO/UNU requirement pattern indicated that the only amino acid in either food source at relative levels below the reference pattern was lysine. The amino acid score for peanut butter was 87% and that for white wheat bread was 37%. Amino acid scores are not additive, and in general the amino acid composition of the components of the mixture should be determined for the mixture as a whole and then compared to the reference pattern. Both the amino

TABLE 15-4 Amino Acid Requirement Pattern and Amino Acid Score of Various Food Sources Based on Either an Egg or Requirement Scoring Pattern

	Amino Acid Pattern				Amino Acid Score*			
					Rice		Wheat Flour	
AMINO ACID	FAO/WHO/UNU REFERENCE PATTERN FOR ADULTS†	EGG PROTEIN‡	RICE PROTEIN‡	WHEAT FLOUR PROTEIN‡	COMPARED TO REQUIREMENT PATTERN FOR ADULT§	COMPARED TO EGG PROTEIN PATTERN¶	COMPARED TO REQUIREMENT PATTERN FOR ADULT§	COMPARED TO EGG PROTEIN PATTERN¶
	mg indispensable amino acid per g protein				% of pattern			
Histidine	15	24	25	21	160	101	141	88
Isoleucine	30	63	44	41	147	70	137	65
Leucine	59	88	87	70	147	99	119	80
Lysine	45	70	38	28	**85**	**55**	**62**	40
Methionine + cysteine	22	58	39	39	176	67	178	68
Phenylalanine + tyrosine	38	99	85	81	223	86	213	82
Threonine	23	51	35	34	152	68	146	66
Tryptophan	6	15	12	12	200	80	200	80
Valine	39	68	61	47	156	90	121	69

*Amino acid score (%) = amino acid concentration food protein source/amino acid concentration reference protein × 100. The lowest of the proportions (in bold) identifies the limiting amino acid and defines the score. The amino acid score is calculated using either the adult human amino acid requirement pattern or the egg amino acid pattern as the reference protein.

†WHO. (2007). *Protein and amino acid requirements in humans: Report of Joint FAO/WHO/UNU Expert Consultation*. WHO Technical Series 935. Geneva: FAO.

‡Food and Agriculture Organization of the United Nations. (1980). *Amino acid content of foods and biological data on proteins*. FAO Food and Nutrition Series No. 24.

§Calculated by dividing amino acid pattern (mg amino acid/g protein) of rice or wheat flour by the FAO/WHO/UNU amino acid scoring pattern for adults (mg amino acid/g protein) and then multiplying the product by 100. See Table 15-2 for origin of scoring pattern.

¶Calculated by dividing amino acid pattern (mg amino acid/g protein) of rice or wheat flour by the amino acid pattern of egg protein (mg amino acid/g protein) and then multiplying the product by 100.

TABLE 15-5 Protein Digestibility Values

PROTEIN SOURCE	TRUE DIGESTIBILITY (%)
Egg	97
Milk, cheese	95
Meat, fish	94
Peanut butter	95
Soy protein isolate	95
Soy flour	86
Wheat, refined	96
Wheat, whole	86
Rice, polished	88
Corn, whole	87
Millet	79
Maize	85
Oatmeal	86
Peas, mature	88
Beans	78
Indian rice and bean diet	78
American mixed diet	96

Data from FAO. (1991). *Protein quality evaluation: Report of Joint FAO/WHO Expert Consultation.* FAO Food and Nutrition Paper #51. Rome: FAO.

acid amounts and the total protein amounts of the components can be added; then the sum for each amino acid can be divided by the sum for total protein in the mixture to obtain the overall amino acid pattern for the mixture. Finally, this pattern can then be compared to the reference or requirement pattern to obtain an amino acid score for the mixture. Only in cases in which the same amino acid is the first limiting amino acid of each protein in the mixture is it possible to obtain the amino acid score for the mixture by multiplying the amino acid score for each component by its fractional contribution to the total amount of protein in the mixture and then adding the products. Thus for calculation of the amino acid score of the peanut butter sandwich, the amino acid contents and the protein contents of the 2 tbsp of peanut butter and the 2 slices of bread can be added together and the total for each individual amino acid can then be divided by the total amount of protein, as shown in Table 15-7 (example uses the reference pattern for human adults). Alternatively, in this case where the same amino acid is limiting in both components of the mixture, one can determine the proportion of the total protein provided by peanut butter (8.0 g/11.8 g = 0.68) and by bread (3.8 g/11.8 g = 0.32) and then calculate an amino acid score for the sandwich: (87% × 0.68) + (37% × 0.32) = 71%.

The calculation of the PDCAAS is essentially the same as the calculation shown in Table 15-6 with the addition of a digestibility correction for the amino acid scores. Using the protein digestibility values in Table 15-5 for peanut butter (95%) and refined wheat (96%), the PDCAAS for peanut butter is 87% × 0.95 = 83%, and that for white bread is 38% × 0.96 = 36%. Because the digestibility of peanut and wheat proteins is high, the PDCAAS is only slightly lower than the uncorrected AAS. Note that the whole protein digestibility value is used to calculate the PDCAAS because digestibility values for the individual indispensable amino acids in various proteins are not widely determined.

Another example is shown in Table 15-7. This second example demonstrates amino acid complementation and calculation of amino acid score in a mixture of proteins with different limiting amino acids. In this case, rice, red beans, and milk are used as the sources of protein. As shown by the calculated amino acid scores in Table 15-7, rice is first limiting in lysine, red beans are first limiting in sulfur amino acids, and milk provides a complete protein compared to the FAO/WHO/UNU (WHO, 2007) adult reference pattern. To determine the amino acid score for the mixture, the mg of each amino acid provided by 1 g of protein in the food protein is multiplied by the fractional contribution of each food protein to the protein mixture. The amounts of each amino acid provided by each food are then added to obtain the total amino acid pattern for the mixture (mg amino acid per g total protein in the mixture). Note that this example involves a mixture defined by the proportion of the total protein derived from each source rather than the amount of the total food in the mixture. Comparison of the amino acid pattern of the total mixture to the reference pattern yields an amino acid score for the mixture.

To determine the amino acid content of a mixture providing 50% protein from rice and 50% protein from beans:

Lysine from rice: 39 mg/g protein × 0.5 = 19.5 mg/g protein

Lysine from beans: 75 mg/g protein × 0.5 = 37.5 mg/g protein

Total lysine from mixture: 19.5 mg/g protein + 37.5 mg/g protein = 57 mg/g protein

Sulfur amino acids from rice: 44 mg/g protein × 0.5 = 22 mg/g protein

Sulfur amino acids from beans: 20 mg/g protein × 0.5 = 10 mg/g protein

Sulfur amino acids from mixture: 22 mg/g protein + 10 mg/g protein = 32 mg/g protein, and so on for remaining amino acids

Thus in a 50:50 mixture of rice protein and bean protein, the rice supplies 19.5 mg lysine and the beans supply 37.5 mg lysine, for a total lysine content of 57 mg lysine/g protein in the mixture. The mixture also supplies 32 mg sulfur amino acids, 37 mg threonine, and 12 mg tryptophan per g protein.

Each of these values is then compared to the reference pattern:

Lysine: (57 mg/g protein) / (45 mg/g protein) × 100% = 127%

TABLE 15-6 Sample Calculation of Amino Acid Score for Peanut and Wheat Proteins and a Mixture of the Two Proteins (Peanut Butter Sandwich)

	Peanut Butter			White Bread (Wheat)			Peanut Butter Sandwich			WHO (2007) Reference Pattern for Adults
	mg AMINO ACID per g PROTEIN	mg AMINO ACID per 2 TBSP OR mg AMINO ACID per 8 g of PROTEIN	AMINO ACID SCORE (%)	mg AMINO ACID per g PROTEIN	mg AMINO ACID per 2 SLICES OR mg AMINO ACID per 3.8 g PROTEIN	AMINO ACID SCORE (%)	mg AMINO ACID per g PROTEIN	mg AMINO ACID per SANDWICH OR mg AMINO ACID per 11.8 g PROTEIN	AMINO ACID SCORE (%)	mg AMINO ACID per g PROTEIN
Histidine	30	240		18	68		26	308		15
Isoleucine	40	320		34	129		38	449		27
Leucine	77	616		62	236		72	852		54
Lysine	39	312	87	17	65	38	32	377	71	45
Methionine + cysteine (sulfur amino acids)	24	192		36	137		28	336		22
Phenylalanine + tyrosine (aromatic amino acids)	108	864		64	243		94	1107		40
Threonine	30	240		24	91		28	331		23
Tryptophan	12	96		10	38		11	134		6
Valine	46	368		38	144		43	512		36

Amino acid scores were calculated only for amino acids present below the requirement; all others would be 100%. In the unique case where the same amino acid is the first limiting amino acid of each protein in a mixture, the amino acid score for each component multiplied by its fractional contribution to the total mixture can be added. In this case where lysine is first limiting in both bread and peanut, peanut butter contributes 8 g/11 g or 68% of the total protein in the sandwich and bread contributes 3.8 g/11.8 g or 32% of the total protein in the sandwich. The amino acid score for the sandwich = (87% × 0.68) + (37% × 0.32) = 59% + 12% = 71%.

TABLE 15-7 Illustration of the Concept of Amino Acid Complementation and Calculation of Amino Acid Scores for Mixtures of Proteins*

	RICE PROTEIN	RED BEAN PROTEIN	MILK PROTEIN	Mixture (% of Protein)‡ 50:50 RICE/ BEANS†	67:33 RICE/MILK†	33:33:33 RICE/ BEANS/ MILK†	FAO/WHO/UNU (WHO, 2007) REFERENCE PATTERN FOR ADULTS
	mg AMINO ACID/g PROTEIN						
Lysine	39	75	80	57	53	65	45
Sulfur amino acids	44	20	30	32	39	31	22
Threonine	44	34	37	39	42	38	23
Tryptophan	11	10	12	10.5	11	11	6
Limiting amino acid	Lysine	Sulfur amino acids	None	None	None	None	
Score (%)	87	90	100	100	100	100	

*For this table, only lysine, sulfur amino acids (methionine + cysteine), threonine, and tryptophan were considered because they are the only amino acids that are commonly limiting in typical foods. Lysine is first limiting for rice and sulfur amino acids are first limiting for red beans. Milk provides a complete protein compared to the reference pattern for human adults.
‡Fractional composition of the mixtures refers to the food protein component, not to the entire food.
†The correct method for calculating the amino acid score for a mixture of proteins is shown above: the amino acids in each component of the mixture must be multiplied by the fractional contribution of each respective food to total protein. The amino acid contributions of each component of the total protein mixture are added to calculate the overall pattern of the mixture (mg amino acid/g of protein). This pattern is then compared to the 2007 FAO/WHO/UNU reference pattern to determine the amino acid score of the mixture.

Sulfur amino acids: (32 mg/g protein) / (22 mg/g protein) × 100% = 145%, and so on for the remaining amino acids

For each amino acid the score is greater than 100, and thus the given amino acid score for the mixture is 100%. This illustrates the principle of complementation; rice alone has an amino acid score of 87% (lysine), and red beans alone have an amino acid score of 90% (sulfur amino acids), but a 50:50 mixture of these two proteins has a better score (100%) than either protein alone. If PDCAAS had been used here, the digestibility correction (0.88 for rice, 0.78 for beans) would have been applied to the individual food protein amino acid patterns before they were added together. Thus the PDCAAS of rice is 76% and the PDCAAS of beans is 71%. Application of digestibility corrections to the mixture likewise lowers the calculated scores for lysine and other amino acids, but the complementation of rice and bean proteins is such that, even with digestibility corrections, all amino acids in this particular mixture are still available at levels above the reference pattern and the final PDCAAS is still 100%. The complementation of rice and beans is an example of the general principle of combining cereals, which typically are limiting in lysine, with legumes, which typically are limiting in sulfur amino acids but higher in lysine, to generate complete protein mixtures.

Table 15-7 also shows the calculated amino acid score for a 67:33 mixture of rice protein and milk protein and a 33:33:33 mixture of rice protein, bean protein, and milk protein, based on the reference pattern for human adults. These examples all show that when mixtures of proteins are consumed, complementation may occur such that the amino acid score for the mixture of proteins may be higher than that of any of the individual proteins. This suggests that protein quality is most likely to be a concern when a very limited variety of protein sources is consumed, particularly when the major dietary staple contains a small amount of total protein and the staple protein has a low amino acid score. In these cases, complementation of proteins (i.e., corn and beans) or supplementation of the diet with a small amount of high-quality protein (i.e., milk or meat) can be of significant benefit.

Limitations of PDCAAS for Assessment of Protein Quality

There are a number of limitations of the PDCAAS. First, the reference pattern is restricted to the eight indispensable amino acids. As discussed previously, some dispensable amino acids become indispensable under certain physiological conditions, and thus their contribution to the nutritional quality of a protein source becomes important but is not considered in calculating the PDCAAS value.

Second, PDCAAS values greater than 100% are truncated to 100% because it is assumed that there is no additional nutritional benefit; however, where a high-quality protein is used to supplement the amino acid composition of a lower-quality protein, the additional value of the extra amino acids is not accounted for unless calculations are made for each potential mixture as illustrated in the examples shown in Tables 15-6 and 15-7 (Schaafsma, 2005).

Reeds and colleagues (2000) suggested identifying the score of proteins for their ability to satisfy the nitrogen and amino acid requirement but also for their capacity to complement another protein deficient in one or more amino acids. For example, meat and milk proteins are high in lysine, threonine, and sulfur amino acids, which are conversely limiting in vegetable proteins. Based on the suggestion of Reeds and colleagues (2000) the score for milk protein would be 128 (lysine), 123 (threonine), and 120 (methionine and cysteine), demonstrating the value of milk as a complement to vegetable proteins.

Third, the use of fecal losses to determine crude protein digestibility has limitations (Schaafsma, 2005; Humayun et al., 2007). As previously discussed, digestibility depends on the difference between intake and fecal excretion, (I − F)/I. When excretion (F) is reduced, the calculated digestibility is increased. Large intestinal microflora use food protein and amino acids that exit the terminal ileum for fuel and synthesis of microbial protein. In the process, food amino acids may be converted to non–amino acid nitrogenous compounds that are absorbed from the large intestine (e.g., ammonia). If these non–amino acid nitrogenous compounds are absorbed, they disappear from the gastrointestinal tract but are largely unused for body protein synthesis. This tends to decrease amino acid excretion (F), thus making digestibility appear to be increased.

Ileal digestibility is considered a more accurate reflection of the true availability of protein and amino acids from foods because amino acid disappearance (F) is based on the residual amino acids present in the terminal ileum (see Chapter 9). However, within the digestive tract, endogenous proteins (i.e., mucin, digestive enzymes) are secreted into the stomach and small intestine. Measurement of ileal digestibility without accounting for amino acids derived from endogenous secretions leads to an underestimation of the true digestibility, because measured ileal amino acids consist of food amino acids plus endogenous amino acids (i.e., value for F increased). In pigs, collection of ileal digesta is typically accomplished by surgical implantation of a cannula in the terminal ileum; however, collection of digesta in humans is much more challenging.

Fourth, the PDCAAS approach is based on the assumption that the digestibility of crude protein equals the digestibility of each individual amino acid. A single protein digestibility correction factor based on measured nitrogen digestibility is used. The assumption that the digestibility value for nitrogen represents the digestibility value for individual amino acids may not always hold true. For example, the overall apparent protein digestibility of casein was 76%, but the apparent digestibility of individual indispensable amino acids in casein ranged from 76% for threonine to 92% for lysine (Declaire et al., 2009).

In addition, aspects of food processing and inherent characteristics of diets (i.e., fiber, antinutritional factors) can affect amino acid availability. In these cases, PDCAAS based on reported values may overestimate the available amino acid content of foods. Heat processing may cause chemical alterations, such as reactions between amino acids and carbohydrates, that decrease amino acid availability. For example, heating peas reduces the availability of lysine from 88.8% to 54.8% (Moehn et al., 2005).

ADVANCES IN PROTEIN QUALITY EVALUATION

As the population continues to grow, a major challenge will be ensuring an adequate supply of quality protein sources for human consumption (Reeds et al., 2000). Consequently, an area of active research is the development of rapid and reliable methods to assess the digestibility and availability of amino acids.

Use of Pigs to Assess Digestibility

Pigs are an excellent animal model for digestibility in humans because the anatomy and physiology of the pig gastrointestinal tract is very similar to humans, they are a meal-eating species, and they do not practice coprophagy (consumption of feces) (Schaafsma, 2005). The digestibility of amino acids from foods is similar between humans and pigs (Rowan et al., 1994) and there are extensive data for the digestibility of protein and amino acids from traditional and nontraditional protein sources in pigs. However, standardization of digestibility terminology and assessment of individual amino acid digestibility rather than only protein or nitrogen digestibility will be necessary to maximize the potential use of the pig model.

Ileal digestibility, rather than fecal digestibility, has become the standard for evaluation of protein quality in swine nutrition. Ileal digestibility has been further categorized as apparent, standard, and true ileal digestibility, based on the extent to which values are corrected for endogenous amino acid losses. True ileal digestibility most accurately reflects the actual bioavailability of amino acids for metabolic processes, but accurate measurement of endogenous losses is not easy (Stein et al., 2007). Inherent characteristics of foods (i.e., fiber or antinutritional factors) can significantly affect endogenous losses, but the most common measure of endogenous losses (protein-free diets) does not account for changes in endogenous secretions due to inherent food characteristics. Dietary fiber can increase endogenous secretions as well as reduce digestion of both dietary and endogenous protein and absorption of the component amino acids; both processes result in the recovery of more amino acids in the terminal ileum, thus increasing ileal amino acid excretion and reducing the calculated ileal digestibility value. Correction of apparent digestibility values for endogenous amino acids determined in subjects fed a protein-free diet would result in an undercorrection of the endogenous component in the ileal fluid and hence an overestimation of the true digestibility value in the case of the fiber-rich protein source.

Digestibility measures may not account for some types of loss of amino acid availability. For example, heat processing can render amino acids, particularly lysine, metabolically unavailable, but these altered amino acids may still be absorbed and would not reduce the measured digestibility. In this case, digestibility overestimates the true amino acid bioavailability.

Determination of Metabolic Availability

Recent developments with the use of stable isotopes and IAAO have the potential to advance protein quality evaluation (Elango et al., 2009). Metabolic availability evaluates whole body utilization of amino acids rather than just disappearance from the gut. The IAAO method is based on the principle that amino acids are either used for protein synthesis or are oxidized. Because the method essentially measures the change in whole body protein synthesis with changes in availability of amino acids, it should account for all losses of amino acids and thus be a measure of the true bioavailability of amino acids from foods. Metabolic availability has been used to determine the availability of lysine, threonine, and sulfur amino acids in a number of food ingredients in animals and humans. Metabolic availability has the significant advantage that it can be measured directly in human subjects. It can also be used to assess changes in amino acid availability due to age or physiological state (Levesque et al., 2010).

TYPICAL INTAKES OF PROTEIN AND AMINO ACIDS AND SIGNIFICANCE OF PROTEIN TO ENERGY RATIOS

According to survey data collected by the U.S. Department of Agriculture (http://www.ars.usda.gov), the mean intake of dietary protein by 30- to 50-year-old adults in the United States was 103 g/day for men and 70 g/day for women (National Health and Nutrition Examination Survey, 2007-2008). Overall, protein intake of adults ranged from approximately 27 g/day for some elderly women to 190 g/day for some young men. Median protein intakes for young individuals ranged from 15 g/day for infants aged 0 to 6 months and 50 g/day for children aged 1 to 3 years to 97 g/day and 65 g/day for males and females (aged 14 to 18 years), respectively (Continuing Survey of Food Intake by Individuals 1994-1996, 1998). In a nutrition survey of adults in the United Kingdom, protein intake of adults was found to be similar to that reported for the United States: 88 ± 32 g/day for men and 64 ± 17 g/day for women (mean ± SD) (Henderson et al., 2003).

The protein to energy (P/E) ratio, expressed as the percentage or fraction of total energy that is derived from protein, is a useful calculation. According to the CSFII (1994–96, 1998; data for all individuals), the median percentage of total energy from protein consumed in the United States from 1994 to 1998 was 15.1% (IOM, 2005). This, however, ranged from a median of 8.8% for 0- to 6-month-old infants to 16% for adults, with intermediate values of 10.4% for 7- to 12-month-old infants and 14% for children 1 to 18 years of age. Although the median percentage of total energy from protein was 16% for adults, protein intake as a percentage of energy ranged from low values of approximately 9% to high values of approximately 24%. Food intake data for the United Kingdom gave P/E values, expressed as a percentage, of 14.2% for omnivores and 12.7% for vegetarians (Millward and Jackson, 2003).

Because protein EARs and RDAs are defined as a constant function of body weight (kg), variation in basal metabolic rate and variation in the level of energy expenditure will affect the percentage of energy that needs to be supplied as protein. If calculations are made based on the DRIs for protein and the estimated energy requirements (EERs), the percentage of total energy needed in the form of protein increases with age, is higher for females than males, and is higher for small compared with large adults at any age; it also decreases with an increase in physical activity and hence energy intake. Therefore the breast-fed infant is able to satisfy a high demand for protein by consuming large quantities of food with very low protein levels. Because the energy requirement per kilogram is very high during infancy and decreases with age at a greater rate than does the protein requirement per kilogram, the P/E ratio of the requirements for infants is relatively low and increases with age.

This concept is illustrated in Figure 15-4. By using adult weights representative of those in developed countries, Millward and Jackson (2003) calculated desirable P/E ratios for population groups of various ages and at three levels of physical activity. They then compared these with the protein-quality adjusted P/E ratios of four diets: the diet of adult omnivores in the United Kingdom; the diet of adult vegetarians (meat-free) in the United Kingdom; the average diet of India; and the average diet of West Bengal (a state in eastern India). Assuming that approaches to determining protein requirements and protein quality are correct and that the energy density or bulk of the diet does not limit consumption to the extent that the diet fails to satisfy energy requirements, this figure indicates that protein deficiency would most likely occur in elderly sedentary women and would least likely occur in moderately active young children, the opposite of what has often been assumed. Adolescent females would also be a vulnerable group.

Unadjusted P/E ratios for various foods, along with P/E ratios adjusted for the food protein's PDCAAS, are given in Table 15-8 (Millward and Jackson, 2003). The majority of the world's population live in developing countries where plants constitute the major source of proteins, with wheat, rice, and maize accounting for the bulk of the cereal intake. Digestibility and availability of plant proteins ranges from 50% to 90%, because of resistant plant cell walls, antinutritional factors, and effects of processing and heat treatment. Lysine is the most important limiting amino acid in cereal-based diets, and estimates of BV depend heavily on the level of lysine in the scoring pattern that is applied. Note that the P/E ratios drop markedly for many staple cereals and root vegetables when they are corrected for protein quality. Millward and Jackson (2003) calculated an average P/E ratio of 0.111 for India, but the P/E ratio was lower for certain states within India (e.g., 0.088 in West Bengal). Food balance data sheets from the FAO for the period 1961-1992 show P/E ratios of 0.080 for Sierra Leone and 0.084 for Bangladesh. If adjusted for protein quality (digestibility and biological value), the ratios for West Bengal, Sierra Leone, and Bangladesh each fall to less than 0.070. Therefore both the quantity and the quality of protein are limiting features of many cereal-based diets.

Although the exact interpretation of the type of calculation illustrated in Figure 15-4 can be debated, two conclusions are clear. First, food supplies or diets with adjusted

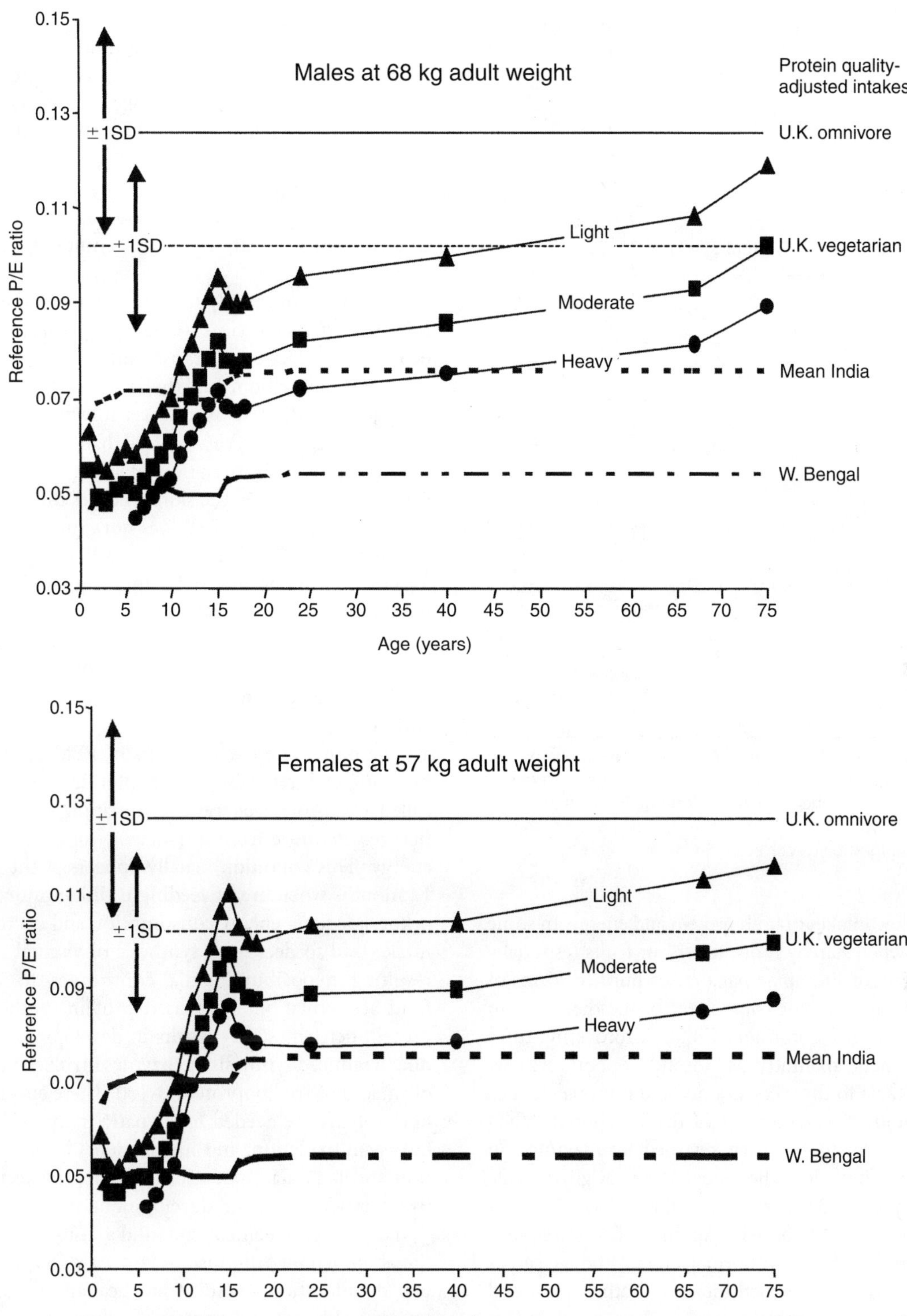

FIGURE 15-4 Reference P/E ratios (energy from protein/total energy in diet), expressed as a fraction (i.e., kcal from protein/total kcal from food), for men and women compared with the adjusted P/E ratios of diets. (From Millward, D. J., & Jackson, A. A. [2003]. Protein/energy ratios of current diets in developed and developing countries compared with a safe protein/energy ratio: Implications for recommended protein and amino acid intakes. *Public Health Nutrition, 7*, 387–405.)

P/E ratios of less than 0.07 are likely to be suboptimal for a substantial fraction of any population, and this will be especially true for individuals with low energy expenditures who need higher P/E ratios. Second, any population with a low energy intake is at greater risk of protein deficiency because protein will be used as a fuel when energy from fat and carbohydrate is insufficient.

In addressing needs of populations of protein-energy malnourished individuals, it is often the bulk and low energy density of the habitual diet or the lack of an adequate quantity of food

TABLE 15-8 Protein/Energy Ratios of Foods

	P/E RATIO	PDCAAS-ADJUSTED P/E RATIO
	kcal FROM PROTEIN/ TOTAL kcal	
Beef	0.660	0.660
Egg	0.340	0.340
Cow's milk	0.194	0.194
Breast milk	0.060	0.060
Soy	0.388	0.349
Wheat	0.166	0.089
Maize	0.135	0.071
Improved variety of maize (variety o2 or o2s2)	0.140	0.102
Potatoes	0.097	0.079
Rice	0.072	0.047
Yam	0.061	0.045
Cassava	0.034	0.019
Cassava-soy mix (90% kcal from cassava/10% kcal from soy)	0.069	0.059

Data from Millward, D. J., & Jackson, A. A. (2003). Protein/energy ratios of current diets in developed and developing countries compared with a safe protein/energy ratio: Implications for recommended protein and amino acid intakes. *Public Health Nutrition, 7*, 387–405.
PDCAAS, Protein digestibility–corrected amino acid score.

that results in low intakes of both protein and energy. In some cases, such as when starchy roots, tubers, or fruits (especially cassava, plantain, or Ethiopian banana) or purified forms of starch or sugar are a major component of the diet, protein density of the diet is a constraint. Children recovering from severe protein-energy malnutrition, infection, or both, are particularly vulnerable to these constraints, and improvement in the quality, not just the quantity, of the diet is required. When children whose growth has been retarded by malnutrition are switched to a nutritious diet, their fractional growth rate may then reach 2% to 3% per day, and the amino acid needs for this rapid rate of body protein gain may increase requirements to two or three times the normal levels. Although catch-up growth requires an increased intake of both protein and energy, the percentage increase for protein is greater than that for energy. For children recovering from protein-energy malnutrition, infection, or other stress, diets with up to 12% of calories from protein may be appropriate (Badaloo et al., 1999).

EFFECTS OF INADEQUATE PROTEIN INTAKE AND ASSESSMENT OF PROTEIN STATUS

Protein-energy malnutrition (PEM) is common in both children and adults throughout the world. FAO estimates that 13.6% (925 million) of the world population is undernourished, with 98% located in developing countries (FAO, 2010). Of these, 175 million (19%) are underweight, 347 million (37.5%) have stunted growth, and 92.5 million (10%) die before the age of 5 years, all of which are symptoms of PEM. More than 90% of the undernourished population lives in Asia (65%) and Africa (27%). In developed countries, PEM occurs primarily as a secondary complication of illnesses that impair the body's ability to absorb or use nutrients or to compensate for nutrient losses.

The most commonly used method to clinically evaluate protein status is the measurement of plasma proteins. Serum or plasma albumin and transferrin are the best measures of protein malnutrition, but the levels of these two proteins may also be affected by disease, infection, injury, or iron deficiency. Because the skin and hair are rapidly growing tissues, physical examination of these tissues is useful. In protein malnutrition, the skin becomes thinner and appears dull, whereas the hair first does not grow and then may fall out or show color changes. Over a longer period, a loss of lean body mass occurs. In infants and children, borderline inadequate protein intake is reflected in failure to grow in length or height and in increased vulnerability to infections. Mid-upper-arm muscle circumference (or diameter) has been used as a measure of protein nutritional status in children.

The more severe expressions of PEM are typically seen in young children (also see Chapter 23). Kwashiorkor, also called wet protein-energy malnutrition, is a form of PEM that results more from a deficiency of protein rather than energy. This condition usually appears at the age of about 12 months when breast-feeding is discontinued. In kwashiorkor, adequate energy consumption and decreased protein intake lead to decreased synthesis of visceral proteins. The resulting hypoalbuminemia contributes to extravascular fluid accumulation. Decreased protein synthesis in severe protein deficiency also results in development of fatty liver due to reduced synthesis of enzymes involved in lipid metabolism and of apolipoprotein B-100. These enzymes and apolipoproteins are needed for hepatic triglyceride export and fatty acid oxidation, and impairments in lipoprotein secretion and fatty acid oxidation underlie the accumulation of liver triacylglycerol and development of fatty liver.

The liver enlargement and fluid accumulation can distend the abdomen and disguise weight loss. Dry or peeling skin, hair discoloration, anemia, diarrhea, and fluid and electrolyte disorders are also commonly observed in children with kwashiorkor. In developed countries, kwashiorkor-like secondary PEM is observed primarily in patients who have been severely burned or who have had trauma or sepsis.

HOW MUCH PROTEIN IS TOO MUCH PROTEIN?

Although a Tolerable Upper Intake Level (UL) for protein has not been set by the IOM (2005), caution should be exercised in terms of very high levels of protein intake. An

CLINICAL CORRELATION

Protein-Energy Malnutrition

Protein-energy malnutrition (PEM) is currently the most common deficiency disease in the world. As its name implies, PEM is a macronutrient deficiency disease resulting from an inadequate intake and/or utilization of protein and calories. Often the energy deficiency is more important than the protein deficiency, because proper protein utilization by the body depends on adequate energy intake. PEM ranges from mild to moderate forms, where the only obvious symptoms are inadequate growth in children, to the severe forms, kwashiorkor and marasmus, which can lead to death. PEM is often associated with micronutrient deficiencies; a diet that is lacking in calories and protein is also likely to be lacking in micronutrients. PEM is also associated with infections, which can increase nutrient requirements and/or decrease absorption and utilization of nutrients in the diet. Although adults can have PEM, it is most commonly seen in early childhood. This is partly because of a young child's relatively higher needs for protein and calories per kilogram body weight compared to older children or adults. Young children also have more parasitic and infectious diseases that can reduce appetite and food intake, decrease absorption and utilization of nutrients, and increase nutrient losses and requirements.

The classic theory of PEM is illustrated in the following diagram, along with some examples of diets that might result in kwashiorkor or marasmus.

All forms of PEM can be treated with a diet high in protein and calories. The more severe forms are life-threatening and usually require hospitalization to treat the dehydration, electrolyte disturbance, and infections that often accompany severe PEM. Micronutrient deficiencies also need to be identified and treated. Although the immediate cause of PEM is an inadequate diet, it is important to remember that the underlying causes include poverty, inequity in food distribution, unsanitary conditions, and lack of knowledge. These underlying causes must be corrected if PEM is to be prevented. Even in developed countries, PEM is sometimes observed because of neglect or inadequate feeding of young children or substitution of low-protein products (e.g., rice milk) for milk or infant formula.

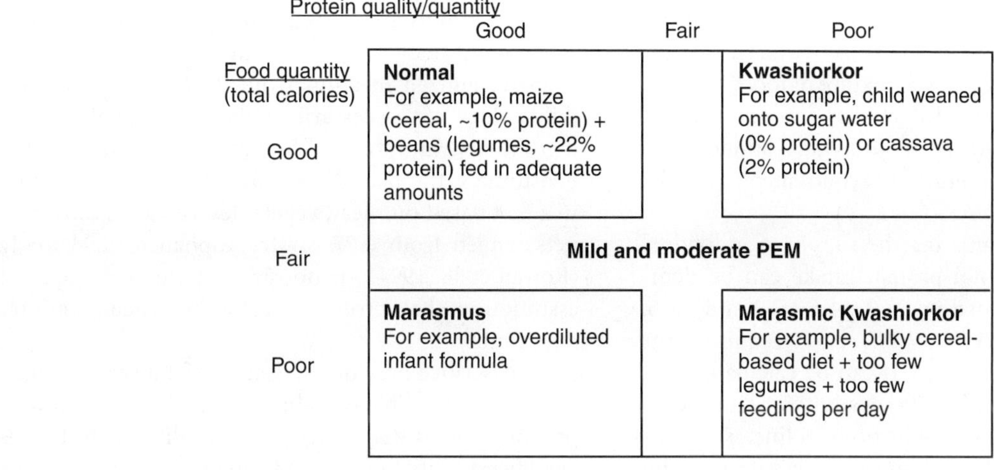

all-meat diet that provided 20% to 35% of energy as protein was consumed by explorers, trappers, and hunters during winters in northern America. These men survived exclusively on pemmican, a concentrated food made by mixing lean dried meat (powdered jerked bison or caribou meat) with melted fat (Stefansson, 1944). A 1930 report described a study of two men, both Arctic explorers, who ate a meat-only diet for an entire year while living in a temperate climate (New York City) and under medical supervision. The diet was made up of muscle, liver, kidney, brain, bone marrow, bacon, and fat from beef, lamb, veal, pork, and chicken. The diet provided about 21% of energy as protein, 78% of energy as fat, and less than 2% of energy as carbohydrate (McClellan and Du Bois, 1930). These men lost weight during the first week, due to a shift in the water content of the body while it adjusted itself to the low-carbohydrate diet, but their weights remained constant thereafter. No ill effects of the all-meat diet were evident, but total acidity of the urine and calcium loss in the urine were both increased above control levels (mixed diet), and ketoaciduria was present throughout the study period. No evidence of renal hypertrophy or damage was observed.

Protein intakes exceeding 30% of calories (diets made up of essentially all meat or all animal products) have been described for the Masai of southern Kenya and northern Tanzania (~30% to 35% of calories as protein), the Ache hunters in the forests of eastern Paraguay (~39% of calories as protein), and Inuit on the east coast of Greenland studied in the mid-1930s (45% of calories as protein), as summarized by Speth (1989). Ill effects from consuming large portions of lean meat (more than 45% of calories as protein) have been reported, including a condition known as "rabbit starvation" that resulted in death of early American explorers who ate rabbit meat, which contains very little fat (Speth and Spielmann, 1983). Animal studies have clearly demonstrated that renal hypertrophy and damage occurs with very high protein intakes, and high protein intakes have adverse effects on patients with renal failure. In general, it seems wise to avoid protein intakes of greater than 250 g/day or more than 40% of energy.

No ULs have been set for intakes of individual amino acids, but available information about hazards of high intakes of amino acids was summarized by the IOM (2005). There is no reason to believe that levels of amino acids consumed as part of food proteins, even at high protein intakes near about 40% of energy, are of concern. However, caution should be used with either amino acid or protein supplements and with additives that contain amino acids (e.g., aspartame).

THE NEED FOR ADDITIONAL RESEARCH IN NUTRITIONAL SCIENCE

The physiological requirement is for a mixture of indispensable amino acids plus aminonitrogen for the synthesis of dispensable amino acids. However, because requirements for amino acids are normally met by a mixture of food proteins, requirements and recommended intakes are expressed in terms of dietary protein rather than individual amino acids. Greater consideration of amino acid requirements, supply, and availability is needed.

The importance of evaluating the supply of individual amino acids as well as total protein intake can be demonstrated using the information in Tables 15-2 and 15-6. Based on the 2007 FAO/WHO/UNU adult requirements for amino acids (see Table 15-2), it can be calculated that the average requirement of a 70-kg adult for indispensable amino acids (mg/day) would be histidine, 700; isoleucine, 1,400; leucine, 2,730; lysine, 2,100; sulfur amino acids, 1,050; aromatic amino acids, 1,750; threonine, 1,050; tryptophan, 280; and valine, 1,820. Similarly, the average protein requirement of a 70-kg adult would be (0.66 $g \cdot kg^{-1} \cdot day^{-1} \times 70$ kg =) 46 g per day. The peanut butter sandwich described in Table 15-6 supplies 11.8 g of total protein, which is about 26% of the daily requirement for protein, so it might be presumed that four peanut butter sandwiches a day would provide all the necessary protein for a 70-kg adult. However, on an individual amino basis, four peanut butter sandwiches would supply only 72% [(377 × 4)/2,100] of the daily lysine requirement, and the requirement for lysine would not be met. At the same time, four peanut butter sandwiches would provide 253% [(1,107 × 4)/1,750] of the total aromatic amino acids requirement, an amount in large excess of the requirement.

One limitation of current protein data is the widespread use of the conversion factor of 6.25 to convert nitrogen to protein. This conversion factor is an average value that is used in the calculation of protein content of foods and the protein gains or losses in nitrogen balance studies. This average conversion factor may be substantially in error, however, when applied to particular foods. The amino acid composition of individual proteins varies, resulting in different percentages of nitrogen in different proteins. That this would occur is obvious if one simply considers that the nitrogen content of tyrosine is 77 mg/g, whereas that of arginine is 322 mg/g. It must be noted, too, that not all the nitrogen in food is in the form of amino acids. Substances such as nitrates, amides, urea, amino sugars, and nucleic acids may account for a significant proportion of the total nitrogen in some foods, and these components affect the relationship between nitrogen and protein contents. As an example, the actual factor for milk is 6.38 g protein per g N, and that for wheat is 5.7 g protein per g N. The 6.25 average factor underestimates the protein content of milk and overestimates the protein content of wheat. Such underestimation or overestimation of total protein can affect the adequacy of diets planned using these data. Underestimation or overestimation of total protein also leads to overestimation or underestimation, respectively, of amino acid scores.

Similarly, the digestibility of nitrogen converted to protein digestibility by the 6.25 conversion factor is assumed to be equivalent to amino acid digestibility. It has long been recognized in animal nutrition that protein digestibility does not necessarily reflect individual amino acid digestibility. In a study of human subjects with established ileostomies, the ileal digestibility of essential amino acids in a diet based on meat, vegetables, cereal, and dairy products ranged from 0.77 for tryptophan to 0.94 for lysine (Rowan et al., 1994), demonstrating the inadequacy of the assumption that protein digestibility equals amino acid digestibility.

As described previously, ileal digestibility is a better measure of the true bioavailability of amino acids from food protein sources than is fecal digestibility. A shift to use of ileal digestibility to evaluate protein quality is an important advancement in human nutrition. However, ileal digestibility still has limitations. The influence of heat damage or fiber on amino acid bioavailability may not be accounted for by application of digestibility estimates. Errors in protein quality evaluation have a greater impact in situations of minimal variety in protein sources, a predominance of low-quality proteins in the diet, and/or marginal intakes of total protein, situations that exist in many developing countries. On the other hand, the high consumption by adolescents of fast foods and snack foods, which are more likely to supply proteins and amino acids damaged by heat (Seiquer et al., 2006), and the recommendation to increase consumption of dietary fiber, which may alter protein digestion and absorption in the small intestine (U.S. Department of Health and Human Services, *www.healthierus.gov/dietaryguidelines*), also underscore the need to develop new techniques, such as metabolic availability, to measure true amino acid bioavailability.

THINKING CRITICALLY

1. Choose a protein source (maize, cassava, rice, yams, or spinach) and look up its macronutrient composition and amino acid composition in the USDA National Nutrient Database for Standard Reference (U.S. Department of Agriculture, Agricultural Research Service. [2011]. *USDA National Nutrient Database for Standard Reference, Release 24*. Retrieved from *www.ars.usda.gov/ba/bhnrc/ndl).* From this information, determine (a) the first-limiting amino acid in the protein according to the WHO/FAO/UNU adult reference pattern; (b) the percentage of food calories that are provided by protein in the food, assuming a fuel value of 4 kcal per gram of protein; (c) the number of cups of the food an adult would need to consume each day to meet all of the WHO/FAO/UNU adult allowances for indispensable amino acids; (d) the number of cups a 63-kg adult would need to eat to meet all of the adult RDA for protein (without consideration of quality or amino acid composition); (e) whether it would be reasonable for a 63-kg woman with an average energy expenditure of 2,200 kcal/day to meet her needs for protein by a diet in which this protein source is the main staple and no supplement of protein-rich food is provided?
2. Currently, dietary recommendations and food labeling focus on the total protein content of the food. (a) What are the limitations of reliance on total protein without consideration of quality? (b) What additional information would be needed to ensure that one's diet is meeting recommendations for indispensable amino acid intake? (c) How important would it be to have information for all indispensable amino acids versus some subset of indispensable amino acids? (d) If you were going to provide information about just one or a few of the indispensable amino acids, which one or few would you choose?

REFERENCES

Badaloo, A., Boyne, M., Reid, M., Persaud, C., Forrester, T., Millward, D. J., & Jackson, A. A. (1999). Dietary protein, growth and urea kinetics in severely malnourished children and during recovery. *The Journal of Nutrition, 129*, 969–979.

Bertolo, R. F. P., Brunton, J. A., Pencharz, P. B., & Ball, R. O. (2003). Arginine, ornithine and proline interconversion is dependent on small intestinal metabolism in neonatal piglets. *American Journal of Physiology. Endocrinology and Metabolism, 284*, E915–E922.

Block, R. J., & Mitchell, H. H. (1946). The correlation of the amino-acid composition of proteins with their nutritive value. *Nutrition Abstracts and Reviews, 16*, 249–278.

Borman, A., Wood, T. R., Black, H. C., Anderson, E. G., Oesterling, M. J., Wormack, M., & Rose, W. C. (1946). The role of arginine in growth with some observations on the effects of argininic acid. *The Journal of Biological Chemistry, 166*, 585–594.

Carpenter, K. J. (1994). *Protein and energy: A study of changing ideas in nutrition*. New York: Cambridge University Press.

Courtney-Martin, G., Moore, A. M., Ball, R. O., & Pencharz, P. B. (2010). The addition of cysteine to the total sulfur amino acid requirement as methionine does not increase erythrocytes glutathione synthesis in the parenterally fed human neonate. *Pediatric Research, 67*, 320–324.

Déchelotte, P., Hasselmann, M., Cynober, L., Allaouchiche, B., Coëffier, M., Hecketsweiler, B., … Bleichner, G. (2006). L-Alanyl-L-glutamine dipeptide-supplemented total parenteral nutrition reduces infectious complications and glucose intolerance in critically ill patients: The French controlled, randomized, double-blind, multicenter study. *Critical Care Medicine, 34*, 598–604.

Declaire, A., Bos, C., Tomé, D., & Moughan, P. (2009). Ileal digestibility of dietary protein in the growing pig and adult human. *The British Journal of Nutrition, 102*, 1752–1759.

Elango, R., Humayun, M. A., Ball, R. O., & Pencharz, P. B. (2007). Lysine requirement of healthy school-age children determined by the indicator amino acid oxidation method. *The American Journal of Clinical Nutrition, 85*, 360–365.

Elango, R., Ball, R. O., & Pencharz, P. B. (2009). Amino acid requirements in humans: With a special emphasis on the metabolic availability of amino acids. *Amino Acids, 37*, 19–27.

Fick, A., & Wislicenus, J. (1866). On the origin of muscular power. *The Philosophical Magazine* (4th series), *31*, 485–503.

Food and Agriculture Organization of the United Nations. (1985). *Protein quality evaluation: Report of Joint FAO/WHO Expert Consultation.* WHO Technical Series #724. Geneva: WHO.

Food and Agriculture Organization of the United Nations. (1991). *Protein quality evaluation in human diets. Report of Joint FAO/WHO Expert Consultation.* FAO Food and Nutrition Paper 51. Rome: FAO.

Food and Agriculture Organization of the United Nations. (2010). *The state of food insecurity in the world. Addressing food insecurity in protracted crisis. Economic and Social Development.* Department Food and Agriculture Organization of the United Nations. Rome: FAO.

Fuller, M. F., & Garlick, P. J. (1994). Human amino acid requirements: Can the controversy be resolved? *Annual Review of Nutrition, 14*, 217–241.

Garza, C., Scrimshaw, N. S., & Young, V. R. (1977). Human protein requirements: A long-term metabolic nitrogen balance study in young men to evaluate the 1973 FAO-WHO safe level of egg protein intake. *The Journal of Nutrition, 107*, 335–352.

Henderson, L., Gregory, J., Irving, K., & Swan, G. (2003). *The National Diet and Nutrition Survey: Adults aged 19 to 64 years. Vol. 2. Energy, protein, carbohydrate, fat and alcohol intake*. London: Office for National Statistics and Food Standards Agency.

Humayun, M. A., Elango, R., Moehn, S., Ball, R. O., & Pencharz, P. B. (2007). Application of the indicator amino acid oxidation technique for the determination of metabolic availability of sulfur amino acids from casein versus soy protein isolate. *The Journal of Nutrition, 137*, 1874–1879.

Institute of Medicine. (2005). *Dietary Reference Intakes: Energy, carbohydrate, fiber, fat, fatty acids, cholesterol, protein, and amino acids*. Washington, DC: The National Academies Press.

Irwin, M. I., & Hegsted, D. M. (1971). A conspectus of research on amino acid requirements of man. *The Journal of Nutrition, 101*, 539–566.

Jackson, A. A., Gibson, N. R., Bundy, R., Hounslow, A., Millward, D. J., & Wootton, S. A. (2004). Transfer of ^{15}N from oral lactose-ureide to lysine in normal adults. *International Journal of Food Sciences and Nutrition, 55*, 455–462.

Jackson, A. A., Shaw, J. C. L., Barber, A., & Golden, M. H. N. (1981). Nitrogen metabolism in preterm infants fed human donor breast milk: The possible essentiality of glycine. *Pediatric Research, 15*, 1454–1461.

Leverton, R. M., Waddill, F. S., & Skellenger, M. (1959). The urinary excretion of five essential amino acids by young women. *The Journal of Nutrition*, *67*, 19–28.

Levesque, C. L., Moehn, S., Pencharz, P. B., & Ball, R. O. (2010). Review of advances in metabolic bioavailability of amino acids. *Livestock Science*, *133*, 4–9.

Libao-Mercado, A. J. O., Zhu, C. L., Cant, J. P., Lapierre, H., Thibault, J. N., Sève, B., … de Lange, C. F. M.(2009). Dietary and endogenous amino acids are the major contributors to microbial protein in the upper gut of normally nourished pigs. *The Journal of Nutrition*, *139*, 1088–1094.

Mager, D., Wykes, L. J., Ball, R. O., & Pencharz, P. B. (2003). Branched-chain amino acid requirements in school-aged children determined by indicator amino acid oxidation (IAAO). *The Journal of Nutrition*, *133*, 3540–3545.

McClellan, W. S., & Du Bois, E. F. (1930). Clinical calorimetry: XLV. Prolonged meat diets with a study of kidney function and ketosis. *The Journal of Biological Chemistry*, *87*, 651–668.

Metges, C. C., Eberhard, M., & Petzke, K. J. (2006). Synthesis and absorption of intestinal microbial lysine in humans and non-ruminant animals and impact on human estimated average requirement of dietary lysine. *Current Opinion in Clinical Nutrition and Metabolic Care*, *9*, 37–41.

Metges, C. C., El-Khoury, A. E., Henneman, L., Petzke, K. J., Grant, I., Shahinaze, B., Pereira, P. P., Ajami, A. M., Fuller, M. F., & Young, V. R. (1999). Availability of intestinal microbial lysine to lysine homeostasis in human subjects. *American Journal of Physiology. Endocrinology and Metabolism*, *277*, E597–E607.

Millward, D. J. (1988). Metabolic demand for amino acids and the human dietary requirement: Millward and Rivers (1988) revisited. *The Journal of Nutrition*, *128*(12 Suppl.), 2563S–2576S.

Millward, D. J., & Jackson, A. A. (2003). Protein/energy ratios of current diets in developed and developing countries compared with a safe protein/energy ratio: Implications for recommended protein and amino acid intakes. *Public Health Nutrition*, *7*, 387–405.

Moehn, S., Bertolo, R. F., Pencharz, P. B., & Ball, R. O. (2005). Development of the indicator amino acid oxidation technique to determine the availability of amino acids from dietary protein in pigs. *The Journal of Nutrition*, *135*, 2866–2870.

Rand, W. M., Pellett, P. L., & Young, V. R. (2003). Meta-analysis of nitrogen balance studies for estimating protein requirements in healthy adults. *The American Journal of Clinical Nutrition*, *77*, 109–127.

Reeds, P., Schaafsma, G., Tomé, D., & Young, V. (2000). Summary of the workshop with recommendations. *The Journal of Nutrition*, *130*, 1874S–1876S.

Reeds, P. J. (2000). Dispensable and indispensable amino acids for humans. *The Journal of Nutrition*, *130*, 1835S–1840S.

Roberts, S. A., Ball, R. O., Moore, A. M., Filler, R. M., & Pencharz, P. B. (2001). The effect of graded intake of glycyl-L-tyrosine on phenylalanine and tyrosine metabolism in parenterally fed neonates with an estimation of the tyrosine requirement. *Pediatric Research*, *49*, 111–119.

Rose, W. C. (1957). The amino acid requirements of adult man. *Nutrition Abstracts and Reviews*, *27*, 631–647.

Rowan, A. M., Moughan, P. J., Wilson, M. N., Maher, K., & Tasman-Jones, C. (1994). Comparison of the ileal and faecal digestibility of dietary amino acids in adult humans and evaluation of the pig as a model animal for digestion studies in man. *British Journal of Nutrition*, *71*, 29–42.

Schaafsma, G. (2005). The protein digestibility-corrected amino acid score (PDCAAS)—A concept for describing protein quality in foods and food ingredients: A critical review. *Journal of AOAC International*, *88*, 988–994.

Seiquer, J., Díaz-Aquacil, J., Delgado-Andrada, C., López-Fríaz, M., Hoyos, A. M., Galdó, G., & Navarro, M. P. (2006). Diets rich in Maillard reaction products affect protein digestibility in adolescent males ages 11-14 y. *The American Journal of Clinical Nutrition*, *83*, 1082–1088.

Speth, J. D. (1989). Early hominid hunting and scavenging: The role of meat as an energy source. *Journal of Human Evolution*, *18*, 329–343.

Speth, J. D., & Spielmann, K. A. (1983). Energy source, protein metabolism, and hunter-gatherer subsistence strategies. *Journal of Anthropological Archaeology*, *2*, 1–31.

Stefansson, V. (1944). Pemmican. *Military Surgeon*, *95*, 89–98.

Stein, H. H., Séve, B., Fuller, M. F., Moughan, P. J., & de Lange, C. F. M. (2007). Invited review: Amino acid bioavailability and digestibility in pig feed ingredients: Terminology and application. *Journal of Animal Science*, *85*, 172–180.

Turner, J. M., Humayun, M. A., Elango, R., Rafii, M., Langos, V., Ball, R. O., & Pencharz, P. B. (2006). Total sulfur amino acid requirement of healthy school-aged children as determined by indicator amino acid oxidation technique. *The American Journal of Clinical Nutrition*, *83*, 619–623.

Urschel, K. L., Evans, A. R., Wilkinson, C. W., Pencharz, P. B., & Ball, R. O. (2007). Parenterally fed neonatal piglets have a low rate of endogenous arginine synthesis from circulating proline. *The Journal of Nutrition*, *137*, 601–606.

Wischmeyer, P. (2008). Glutamine: Role in critical illness and ongoing clinical trials. *Current Opinion in Gastroenterology*, *24*, 190–197.

World Health Organization. (1985). *Energy and protein requirements: Report of a Joint FAO/WHO/UNU Expert Consultation.* WHO Technical Report Series 724. Geneva: World Health Organization.

World Health Organization. (2007). *Protein and amino acid requirements in humans: Report of Joint FAO/WHO/UNU Expert Consultation.* WHO Technical Series 935. Geneva: FAO.

Wykes, L. J., House, J. D., Ball, R. O., & Pencharz, P. B., (1994). Amino acid profile and aromatic amino acid concentration in total parenteral nutrition: effect on growth, protein metabolism and aromatic amino acid metabolism in the neonatal piglet. *Clinical Science (Lond)*, *87*, 75–84.

Young, V. R. (1986). Nutritional balance studies: Indication of human requirements or adaptive mechanism. *The Journal of Nutrition*, *116*, 700–703.

RECOMMENDED READINGS

Elango, R., Ball, R. O., & Pencharz, P. B. (2009). Amino acid requirements in humans: With a special emphasis on the metabolic availability of amino acids. *Amino Acids*, *37*, 19–27.

Millward, D. J. (2003). An adaptive metabolic demand model for protein and amino acid requirements. *The British Journal of Nutrition*, *90*, 249–260.

Millward, D. J., & Jackson, A. A. (2003). Protein/energy ratios of current diets in developed and developing countries compared with a safe protein/energy ratio: Implications for recommended protein and amino acid intakes. *Public Health Nutrition*, *7*, 387–405.

Pencharz, P. B., & Ball, R. O. (2003). Different approaches to define individual amino acid requirements. *Annual Review of Nutrition*, *23*, 101–116.

Rand, W. M., Pellett, P. L., & Young, V. R. (2003). Meta-analysis of nitrogen balance studies for estimating protein requirements in healthy adults. *The American Journal of Clinical Nutrition*, *77*, 109–127.

Stein, H. H., Sève, B., Muller, F., Moughan, P., & de Lange, C. F. M. (2007). Invited review: Amino acid bioavailability and digestibility in pig feed ingredients: Terminology and application. *Journal of Animal Science*, *85*, 172–180.

CHAPTER 16

Metabolism of Fatty Acids, Acylglycerols, and Sphingolipids

Hei Sook Sul, PhD

COMMON ABBREVIATIONS

ACP	acyl carrier protein
AMPK	5′-AMP–activated protein kinase
cAMP	3′-5′-cyclic adenosine monophosphate
CoA	coenzyme A (also abbreviated as CoA-SH to show reactive sulfhydryl group)
CPT	carnitine palmitoyltransferase
HMG-CoA	hydroxymethylglutaryl-coenzyme A
HSL	hormone sensitive lipase
PPAR	peroxisome proliferator–activated receptor
SREBP	sterol regulatory element binding protein
VLDL	very-low-density lipoproteins

BIOLOGICAL ROLES FOR LIPIDS

There are four major and a multitude of minor roles for lipids in living organisms. Major roles include serving as an energy source or fuel, structural components of membranes, lubricants (especially of the body surfaces), and signaling molecules. These four major functions require specific classes of lipids that differ in general structure. Each class contains numerous members with small but substantial structural differences. These lipid structures and their characteristics are discussed in Chapter 6.

Acylglycerols are the major lipids in the body. Lipids in the form of triacylglycerol play a critical role in metabolism as the primary form of stored energy in the mammalian body. Approximately 85% of the energy stored in the body of a 70-kg normal-weight man is in the form of triacylglycerol, primarily stored in adipose tissue. Triacylglycerol in the diet provides a concentrated source of energy. Triacylglycerol in milk is important for supplying calories to the newborn infant. When the caloric content of the diet exceeds the immediate energetic requirements of the individual, carbohydrates (and to some extent amino acids) may be converted to fatty acids and esterified to glycerol to form triacylglycerol. Triacylglycerol is a very efficient chemical form for storing energy because it contains approximately 9 kcal compared to approximately 4 kcal/g for carbohydrate and protein. In addition, triacylglycerol is advantageous because it can be stored in a relatively anhydrous form requiring about 0.1 g of water per gram of fat, whereas carbohydrate and protein require about 4 g of water per gram of glycogen or protein. Conversion of carbohydrate and protein to triacylglycerol is regulated by diet; the conversion is high in the fed state, especially if the diet is rich in carbohydrate, and is low in the fasting state. Storage of triacylglycerol also is high in the fed state and low in the fasting state, regardless of the composition of the diet.

The principal structural role of lipids is in the membranes—both the plasma membrane and subcellular membranes. A lipid bilayer constitutes the external boundary of every mammalian cell. Similarly, lipid membranes form the boundaries of numerous subcellular organelles. The principal components of the lipid bilayer are acylglycerols, phospholipids, sphingolipids, and cholesterol, the proportions of which vary with the membrane type.

Lipids also play an important role in lubrication and conditioning of body surfaces. Most sebaceous glands, which are microscopic, are found in skin and the mucous membranes of external orifices of the mammalian body. These glands secrete a lipid product composed of triacylglycerol, squalene, and wax esters. This secretion lubricates mucous membranes and conditions skin and hair. Some larger modified sebaceous glands have specific functions. The meibomian glands in the eyelids, for example, provide lubricant and protection for the surface of the eye.

Lipids are important signaling molecules, both outside and inside cells. Sex hormones, adrenocortical hormones, and vitamin D are derived from cholesterol and play important extracellular signaling roles. Eicosanoids derived from arachidonic acid hydrolyzed from membrane phospholipids, and platelet-activating factor which is a phospholipid-like compound, are also important in extracellular signaling. Inside cells, fatty acids alone or compounds derived from them can be ligands for transcription factors, such as the peroxisome proliferator–activated receptors, to regulate transcription of specific genes. In addition, diacylglycerol and molecules derived from phospholipids and sphingolipids are involved in the transmission of signals from the plasma membrane to enzymes in the cytosol or other subcellular compartments and to proteins that regulate the expression of specific genes in the nucleus. In this chapter, synthesis and oxidation of fatty acids and acylglycerols as well as sphingolipids are discussed. Cholesterol and lipoprotein metabolism and transport are discussed in Chapter 17.

OVERVIEW OF FATTY ACID AND TRIACYLGLYCEROL METABOLISM

Fat or triacylglycerol metabolism involves a series of hydrolysis and reesterification processes in the body. Free fatty acids are transported across membranes, but triacylglycerols are the major form of lipid in the large lipoprotein complexes in the circulation and in the lipid droplets present inside cells that store fat. Although the processes involved in fatty acid and triacylglycerol metabolism are described in detail in this chapter, a brief overview helps to place these pathways within the context of whole body metabolism. To illustrate these processes, the major aspects of lipid metabolism following intake of a carbohydrate- and fat-containing meal are shown in Figure 16-1, *A*. Dietary fat is digested in the small intestine and the products are converted back to triacylglycerols in the small intestinal absorptive cells where they are also incorporated into chylomicrons that are released into the lymphatic circulation and eventually the blood. When dietary carbohydrate is high, the liver synthesizes fatty acids de novo. These fatty acids as well as fatty acids returned to the liver by lipoprotein remnants are reesterified to triacylglycerol and incorporated into very-low-density lipoproteins (VLDLs) that are released by the liver into the venous circulation. The chylomicrons and VLDLs are acted upon by extracellular lipoprotein lipase in the capillaries of various tissues, in particular by adipose tissue lipoprotein lipase in the postprandial state. The fatty acids released from the triacylglycerol are taken up by adipose tissue where they are reesterified and stored as triacylglycerol. Reesterification can also occur in muscle for storage of fatty acids as intramyocellular triacylglycerol (IMTG). Fatty acids are also oxidized to CO_2 and H_2O by skeletal muscle; although resting muscle will be using mainly glucose as fuel in the postprandial period, working muscle will still use fatty acids as fuel. Glycerol (released from hydrolysis of chylomicron triacylglycerol) and the cholesterol-rich lipoprotein remnants (chylomicron remnants and the intermediate- and low-density lipoproteins, IDL and LDL, formed from VLDL) remain in the circulation and are subsequently taken up by the liver. The liver is able to convert glycerol to glycerol 3-phosphate and use it for esterification of fatty acids or as a glycolytic/gluconeogenic intermediate.

During fasting or exercise, free or nonesterified fatty acids are released from the triacylglycerol stores in adipose tissue and are used as fuel by many tissues. Figure 16-1, *B*, illustrates the important role of adipose tissue as a source of free fatty acids. The triacylglycerol in lipid droplets in the adipocytes is hydrolyzed to fatty acids and glycerol, both of which are released into the venous circulation. These free fatty acids are subsequently oxidized by muscle and other tissues in a process known as β-oxidation. The glycerol is taken up by liver, as in the fed state. Although chylomicrons are not present in the fasting state, VLDL are still synthesized by the liver from lipids returned to the liver in the LDL and IDL and are available as a substrate for lipoprotein lipase in extrahepatic tissues, especially in the muscle. In prolonged starvation, the release of fatty acids is large and some of these will be used for ketone body synthesis in the liver. Ketone bodies in the circulation then serve as an additional lipid fuel for various tissues.

SYNTHESIS OF PALMITATE FROM ACETYL-CoA

The primary anatomical sites for synthesis of fatty acids are the liver and adipose tissue. In humans, the extent and the contribution of each of these tissues to de novo lipogenesis are still debated (Nye et al., 2008; Schutz, 2004). The lipogenic pathway may be suppressed by the high fat content of the modern diet (~34% of total energy), and de novo lipogenesis may not contribute greatly to triacylglycerol biosynthesis in most individuals consuming western diets. However, low but regulated rates of lipogenesis still may be critical for overall control of metabolism in humans. The substrates and intermediates in pathways of lipid synthesis and oxidation are mainly thioesters of fatty acids and coenzyme A (CoA). As discussed in subsequent text, malonyl-CoA, the product of the acetyl-CoA carboxylase reaction, inhibits fatty acid transport into mitochondria, thereby controlling fatty acid metabolism. In addition, de novo lipogenesis may also contribute to glycemic control by diverting excess glucose to fat. Furthermore, in some physiological and pathophysiological conditions, de novo lipogenesis may play a quantitatively significant role. For example, developmental needs for lipid in the fetus may be met by de novo lipogenesis, the rate of which is extremely high in premature infants. De novo lipogenesis also contributes significantly to hypertriglyceridemia and hepatic steatosis. Some of the metabolic abnormalities in untreated type 1 diabetes mellitus arise from the impaired fatty acid synthesis caused by low insulin levels. Another calorically important site of fat synthesis is the lactating mammary gland, in which medium-chain fatty acids are synthesized and esterified to glycerol for milk fat. Branched-chain fatty acids for conditioning body surfaces are synthesized in sebaceous and other more specialized glands.

TRANSFER OF ACETYL-CoA FROM INSIDE THE MITOCHONDRIA TO THE CYTOSOL

Fatty acid synthesis requires acetyl-CoA units as building blocks for fatty acids. The enzymes that catalyze the reactions for fatty acid synthesis are cytosolic. This localization is important because it separates the processes of fatty acid synthesis from those of fatty acid oxidation (mitochondrial). Although the enzymes that catalyze the reactions in these two pathways are different, the substrate of one pathway is the product of the other and vice versa. Because the reactions occur in different compartments, the strategy for regulating these competing processes is different from that used in gluconeogenesis and glycolysis, in which most of the competing reactions are in the same compartment. Therefore fatty acid

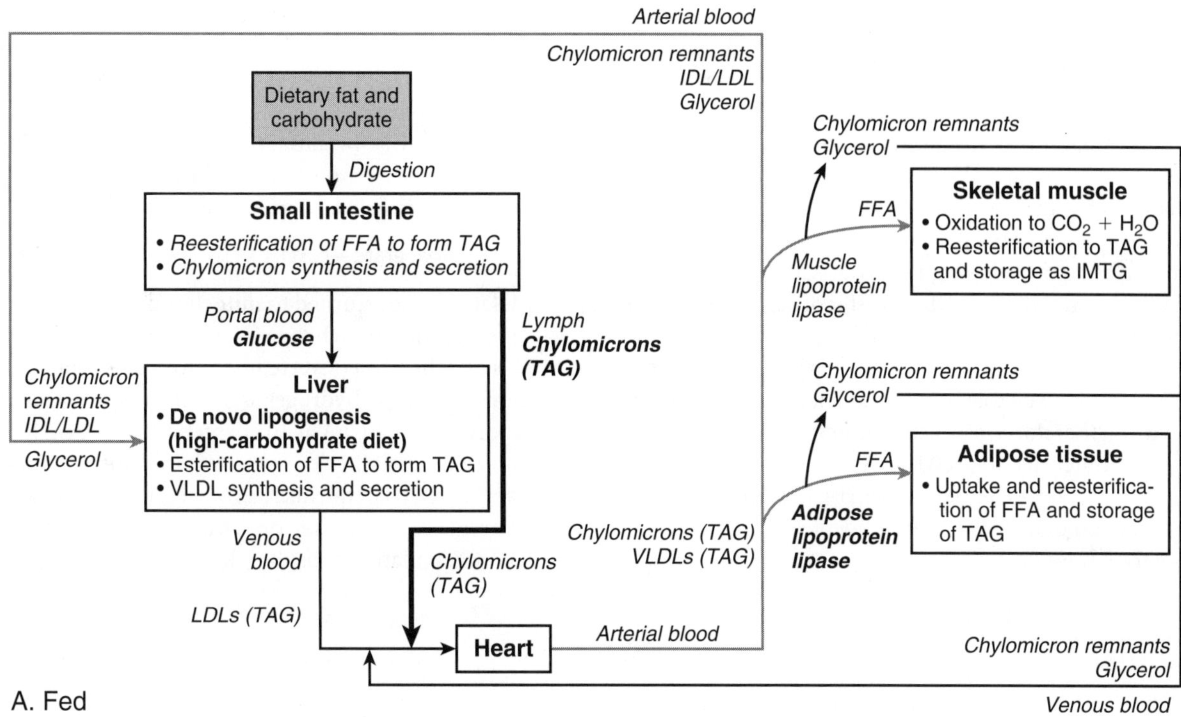

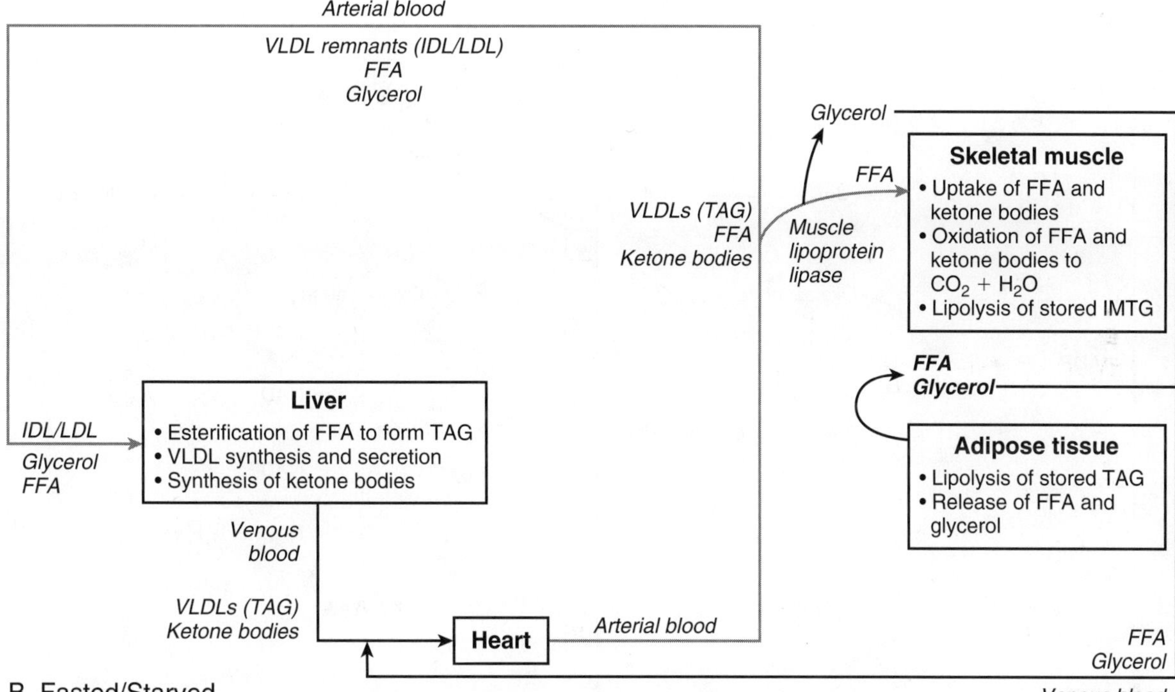

FIGURE 16-1 Overview of free fatty acid and triacylglycerol metabolism. **A,** Following intake of a carbohydrate- and fat-containing meal, fatty acids from the diet as well as fatty acids synthesized de novo from excess carbohydrate are targeted to the adipose tissue for storage. **B,** During fasting or exercise, lipid stores in the adipose tissue are the major source of plasma free fatty acids, which are an important source of fuel for various tissues. *FFA,* Free fatty acid; *IDL,* intermediate-density lipoprotein; *LDL,* low-density lipoprotein; *TAG,* triacylglycerol; *VLDL,* very-low-density lipoprotein.

synthesis is regulated by provision of cytosolic substrate and by the phosphorylation and allosteric control of acetyl-CoA carboxylase, the key regulatory enzyme of fatty acid synthesis. On the other hand, fatty acid oxidation is regulated primarily by control of the rate of uptake of fatty acid substrates by the mitochondria, which depends on the inhibition of carnitine palmitoyltransferase 1 (CPT1) by malonyl-CoA.

The substrate for fatty acid synthesis, acetyl-CoA, is formed from pyruvate in the mitochondria. The inner mitochondrial membrane is impermeable to acetyl-CoA and does not contain a carrier to transport the acetyl-CoA into the cytosol. When production of acetyl-CoA from pyruvate is high, the rate of formation of citrate catalyzed by citrate synthase in the citric acid cycle also is elevated, resulting in the accumulation of intramitochondrial citrate. Under these conditions, citrate can be translocated to the cytosol in exchange for a dicarboxylate anion, probably malate, by the tricarboxylate anion carrier in the inner mitochondrial membrane, as shown in Figure 16-2. Citrate, therefore, serves as the intermediary for the transfer of acetyl-CoA from mitochondria to cytosol. As described in subsequent text of this chapter, citrate as a feed-forward activator of acetyl-CoA carboxylase plays a key role in regulating fatty acid synthesis. In the cytosol, therefore, fatty acid synthesis actually starts by cleavage of citrate back to acetyl-CoA.

Cytosolic citrate is cleaved to acetyl-CoA and oxaloacetate in a reaction that is catalyzed by adenosine triphosphate (ATP)–citrate lyase.

$$\text{Citrate} + \text{CoA} + \text{ATP} + H_2O \rightarrow \text{Acetyl-CoA} + \text{Oxaloacetate} + \text{ADP} + P_i$$

Oxaloacetate formed in the cytosol cannot be returned to the mitochondria because the mitochondrial membrane lacks the necessary transporter. However, oxaloacetate can be reduced to malate by cytosolic malate dehydrogenase.

$$\text{Oxaloacetate} + \text{NADH} + H^+ \leftrightarrow \text{Malate} + \text{NAD}^+$$

Malate can be returned to mitochondria on a tricarboxylate anion carrier in exchange for another molecule of citrate. Malate can then be converted back to oxaloacetate by mitochondrial malate dehydrogenase. This cycle results in the net transport of acetyl-CoA at an energetic cost of 1 mole of ATP per mole of acetyl-CoA translocated. In addition, it results in transfer of NADH equivalents formed in the cytosol to the mitochondria, where they can contribute to the generation of ATP via oxidative phosphorylation.

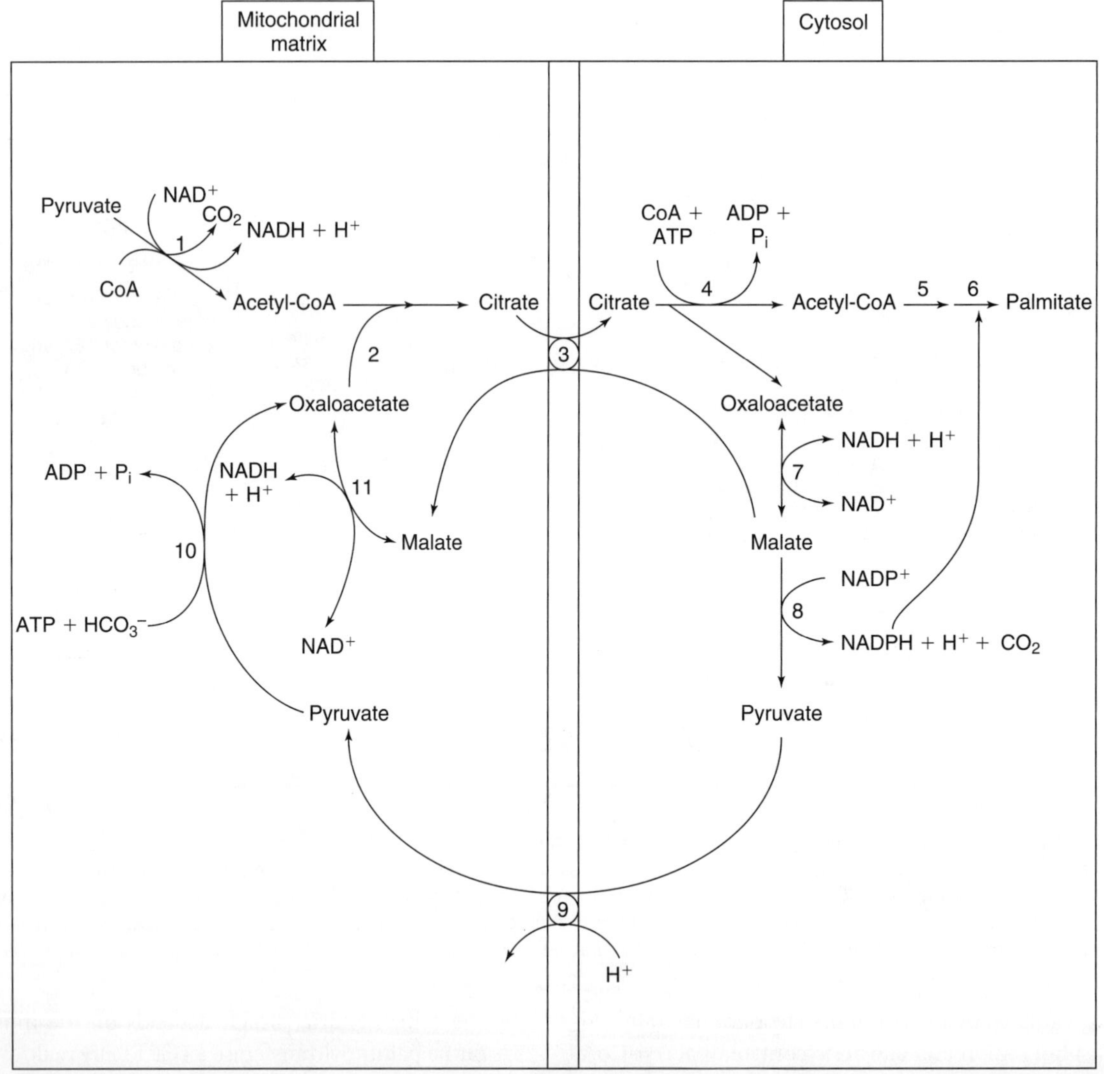

FIGURE 16-2 A schematic diagram of the pathways involved in the synthesis of fatty acids. *1,* Pyruvate dehydrogenase; *2,* citrate synthase; *3,* tricarboxylate transporter; *4,* ATP-citrate lyase; *5,* acetyl-CoA carboxylase; *6,* fatty acid synthase; *7,* malate dehydrogenase; 8, malic enzyme; *9,* pyruvate transporter; *10,* pyruvate carboxylase; *11,* malate dehydrogenase.

Alternatively, or perhaps in addition, malate generated by reduction of oxaloacetate in the cytosol can, in turn, be oxidized to pyruvate and carbon dioxide by malic enzyme in the cytosol. The pyruvate can then be returned to the mitochondria. Oxidation of malate to pyruvate by the malic enzyme requires $NADP^+$ as the electron acceptor and generates NADPH. As discussed in subsequent text, NADPH is the required electron donor for the reductive step in fatty acid biosynthesis. This longer cycle is then completed in the mitochondria by the ATP-dependent carboxylation of pyruvate to oxaloacetate that is catalyzed by pyruvate carboxylase. The malic enzyme cycle thus translocates 1 mole of acetyl-CoA and generates 1 mole of NADPH per 2 moles of ATP expended. By this pathway, reducing equivalents from cytosolic NADH are transferred to NADP to form NADPH, which can be used directly for fatty acid synthesis in the cytosol along with NADPH produced by the pentose phosphate pathway.

CONVERSION OF ACETYL-CoA TO MALONYL-CoA

The next reaction in the synthesis of fatty acids is catalyzed by acetyl-CoA carboxylase and involves an ATP-dependent carboxylation of acetyl-CoA to malonyl-CoA. This is the first committed step in fatty acid synthesis and is highly regulated. Like pyruvate carboxylase, acetyl-CoA carboxylase utilizes bicarbonate as a source of carbon dioxide, has a two-step reaction mechanism, and requires a covalently bound biotin.

$$HCO_3^- + ATP + \text{Biotin-enzyme} \rightarrow \text{Carboxybiotin-enzyme} + ADP + P_i$$

$$\text{Carboxybiotin-enzyme} + \text{Acetyl-CoA} \rightarrow \text{Malonyl-CoA} + \text{Biotin-enzyme}$$

$$\text{NET: Acetyl-CoA} + HCO_3^- + ATP \rightarrow \text{Malonyl-CoA} + ADP + P_i$$

In the first step, the biotin, which is bound to a specific lysine residue of the enzyme, is carboxylated with the energy furnished by the hydrolysis of ATP (biotin carboxylation). In the second step (transcarboxylation), the activated, biotin-bound carboxyl group is transferred to acetyl-CoA, regenerating enzyme-bound biotin and synthesizing malonyl-CoA. Both of these reactions are catalyzed by a single polypeptide chain that also contains a domain for the covalently linked biotin. In biotin deficiency, the acetyl-CoA carboxylase reaction is impaired, and thus fatty acid synthesis from acetyl-CoA is decreased. (See Chapter 26 for further discussion of biotin-dependent carboxylation.)

Acetyl-CoA carboxylase is regulated by an array of control mechanisms, thereby permitting the rate of fatty acid synthesis to fluctuate in response to physiological and developmental conditions (Sul and Smith, 2008; Wakil and Abu-Elheiga, 2009). At the same time, malonyl-CoA, the product of acetyl-CoA carboxylase, is a potent inhibitor of carnitine palmitoyltransferase 1 (CPT1), an enzyme that controls transport of long-chain fatty acids into mitochondria for oxidation (as discussed in subsequent text). Therefore acetyl-CoA carboxylase reciprocally regulates fatty acid synthesis and oxidation. There are two isoforms of acetyl-CoA carboxylase: ACC1 is for acetyl-CoA synthesis in lipogenic tissues (i.e., liver and adipose tissue), whereas ACC2 present in muscle and other tissues is for formation of malonyl-CoA for regulating fatty acid oxidation. The activity of acetyl-CoA carboxylase is stimulated by citrate, an allosteric activator, and inhibited by long-chain acyl-CoA, an allosteric inhibitor. In the fed state, production of cytosolic citrate is increased and the concentration of long-chain acyl-CoA is low, resulting in activation of acetyl-CoA carboxylase. Conversely, during starvation, the long-chain acyl-CoA level increases and the cytosolic citrate level decreases, resulting in inhibition of fatty acid synthesis. Activation of lipolysis in the adipose tissue gives rise to the increase in long-chain acyl-CoA concentration, and the lack of excess anaphlerotic substrate (e.g., pyruvate, oxaloacetate) for citrate formation in the mitochondrial citric acid cycle gives rise to the lack of cytosolic citrate. These allosteric mechanisms thus represent examples of feed-forward (citrate) and feedback (long-chain acyl-CoA) regulation of acetyl-CoA carboxylase as shown in Figure 16-3.

Acetyl-CoA carboxylase also is regulated by covalent modification (Brownsey et al., 2006; Saggerson, 2008), as shown in Figure 16-3. Up to seven serine residues in acetyl-CoA carboxylase can be phosphorylated. The phosphorylated enzyme is less active, less sensitive to the stimulatory effects of citrate, and more sensitive to the inhibitory action of long-chain acyl-CoA. A number of different protein kinases catalyze phosphorylation of acetyl-CoA carboxylase and do so at different specific serine residues on the enzyme. 5′-AMP–activated protein kinase (AMPK) is the physiologically important kinase that phosphorylates acetyl-CoA carboxylase. When the cellular energy state is low, with increased intracellular AMP levels, AMPK is allosterically activated by AMP. AMPK is also activated by phosphorylation by upstream kinases such as LKB1, and phosphorylation of AMPK is promoted by AMP (Steinberg and Kemp, 2009). Activated AMPK in turn phosphorylates acetyl-CoA carboxylase resulting in a decrease in its activity.

In liver, glucagon is an important effector increasing production of 3′-5′-cyclic adenosine monophosphate (cAMP). Catecholamines can also increase production of cAMP. An increase in cAMP in turn activates protein kinase A (see Figure 16-3). There may be a potential physiological role for protein kinase A in the hormone-mediated inactivation of acetyl-CoA carboxylase. However, regulation of acetyl-CoA carboxylase activity by protein kinase A–mediated phosphorylation is somewhat smaller in magnitude than that by AMPK-mediated phosphorylation. It is also possible that protein kinase A regulation of acetyl-CoA carboxylase may not occur via direct phosphorylation of this enzyme.

In addition to regulation by allosteric and phosphorylation–dephosphorylation mechanisms, acetyl-CoA carboxylase also is regulated by changes in the number of molecules present in the cell. The concentration of the enzyme is low in the liver of starved animals and high in the liver of fed animals, especially if the diet is high in carbohydrate. The acetyl-CoA carboxylase protein concentration in cells is controlled primarily by changes in the rate of transcription of the acetyl-CoA carboxylase gene. In this regard, in

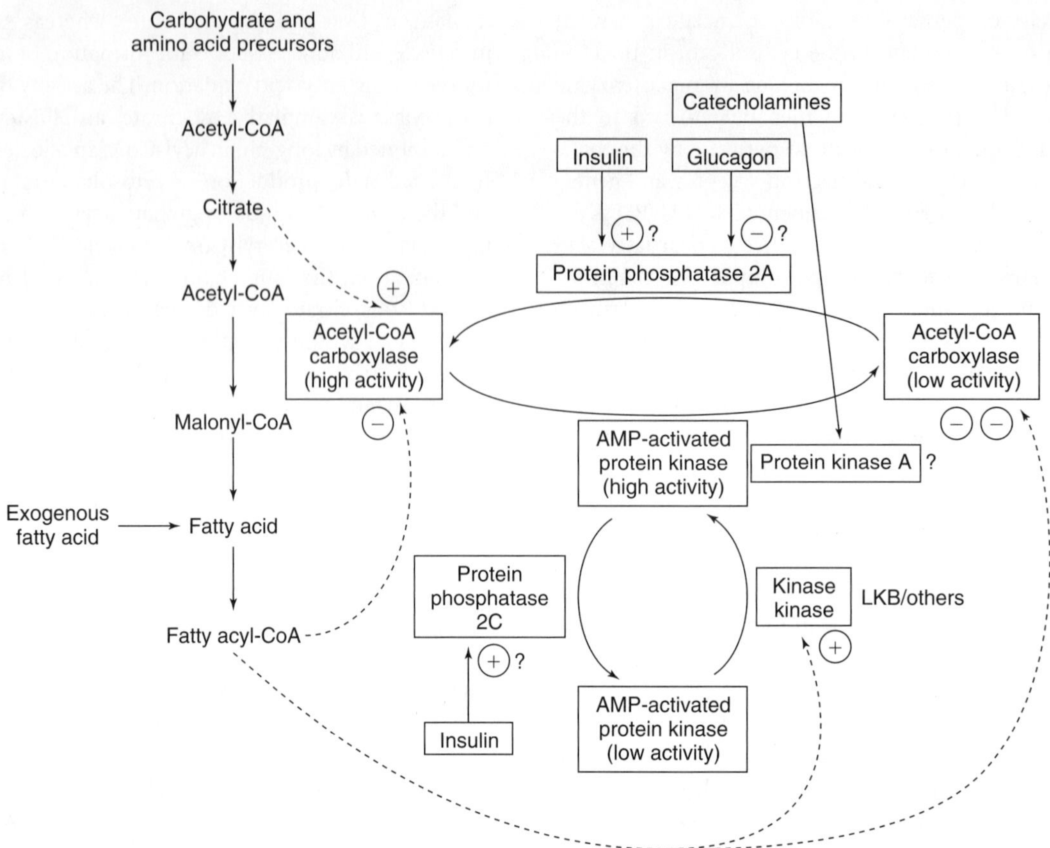

FIGURE 16-3 Model for the regulation of acetyl-CoA carboxylase. Acetyl-CoA carboxylase is phosphorylated and converted to a less active form by AMP-activated protein kinase. The latter enzyme is phosphorylated and activated by a kinase. Arrows with dotted lines indicate either positive (+) or negative (–) allosteric effects of fatty acyl-CoA on the specified enzyme. Extent of allosteric inhibition is indicated by the number of (–) symbols. The phosphatases that inactivate AMP-activated protein kinase or activate glucagon/catecholamine inhibition of this step have not been demonstrated definitively.

addition to acetyl-CoA carboxylase, transcription of many of the enzymes involved in fatty acid synthesis are coordinately regulated. These transcriptionally regulated enzymes include ATP-citrate lyase, which hydrolyzes citrate to provide the cytosolic acetyl-CoA that is used as a substrate for acetyl-CoA carboxylase and fatty acid synthase, and malic enzyme and some of the enzymes in the pentose phosphate pathway that generate the NADPH required for fatty acid synthase. Transcription of these enzymes is high in the fed state (especially if the diet is high in carbohydrate) and low in the fasting state. Fat, especially polyunsaturated fatty acids in the diet, decreases transcription. Changes in circulating insulin and glucagon, as well as changes in glucose levels, participate in the transcriptional regulation of lipogenic enzymes, including acetyl-CoA carboxylase. Insulin and glucose increase, whereas glucagon and catecholamines (via cAMP) decrease, the rate of transcription of acetyl-CoA carboxylase. When glucose levels are elevated in the fed state, insulin signaling via the insulin/phosphatidylinositol 3-kinase/Akt pathway results in activation of sterol regulatory element binding protein (SREBP) 1c, a basic helix-loop-helix transcription factor that resides at the ER but, upon cleavage, becomes a mature transcription factor and translocates to the nucleus to activate lipogenic gene transcription in the fed state. SREBP1c is expressed predominantly in the lipogenic tissues and SREBP1c gene transcription is itself suppressed in the fasted state but induced by high carbohydrate feeding. Liver X receptor (LXR), a ligand activated nuclear hormone receptor, activates transcription of SREBP1c as well as lipogenic enzymes in the fed state. LXR also increases transcription of another basic helix-loop-helix transcription factor, carbohydrate response element binding protein (ChREBP), which mediates transcriptional activation of lipogenic enzymes by glucose (Wong et al., 2009, Wong and Sul, 2010). The function of SREBP is discussed in more detail in Chapter 17.

SYNTHESIS OF PALMITATE FROM MALONYL-CoA, ACETYL-CoA, AND NADPH BY FATTY ACID SYNTHASE

The second and final committed step in fatty acid synthesis is catalyzed by a multifunctional polypeptide, fatty acid synthase, which catalyzes all the reactions shown in Figure 16-4 and which contains an acyl carrier protein (ACP) domain with a 4′-phosphopantetheine prosthetic group. The substrates for the synthesis of one palmitate molecule by fatty acid synthase are 7 molecules of malonyl-CoA, 1 of acetyl-CoA, 14 of NADPH, and 14 of H^+. The products are 1 molecule of

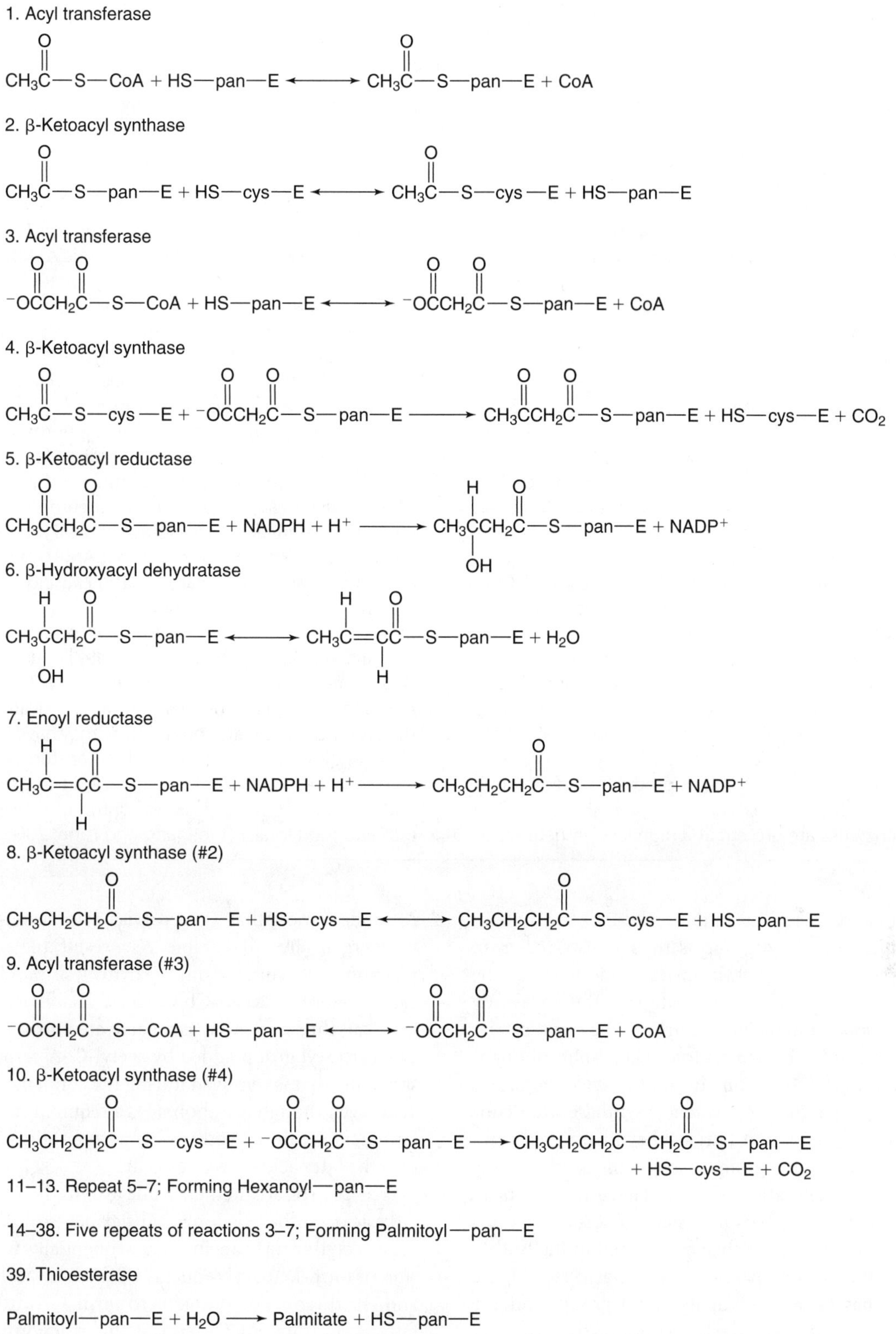

1. Acyl transferase

$$CH_3\overset{O}{\overset{\|}{C}}—S—CoA + HS—pan—E \longleftrightarrow CH_3\overset{O}{\overset{\|}{C}}—S—pan—E + CoA$$

2. β-Ketoacyl synthase

$$CH_3\overset{O}{\overset{\|}{C}}—S—pan—E + HS—cys—E \longleftrightarrow CH_3\overset{O}{\overset{\|}{C}}—S—cys—E + HS—pan—E$$

3. Acyl transferase

$$^{-}O\overset{O}{\overset{\|}{C}}CH_2\overset{O}{\overset{\|}{C}}—S—CoA + HS—pan—E \longleftrightarrow {}^{-}O\overset{O}{\overset{\|}{C}}CH_2\overset{O}{\overset{\|}{C}}—S—pan—E + CoA$$

4. β-Ketoacyl synthase

$$CH_3\overset{O}{\overset{\|}{C}}—S—cys—E + {}^{-}O\overset{O}{\overset{\|}{C}}CH_2\overset{O}{\overset{\|}{C}}—S—pan—E \longrightarrow CH_3\overset{O}{\overset{\|}{C}}CH_2\overset{O}{\overset{\|}{C}}—S—pan—E + HS—cys—E + CO_2$$

5. β-Ketoacyl reductase

$$CH_3\overset{O}{\overset{\|}{C}}CH_2\overset{O}{\overset{\|}{C}}—S—pan—E + NADPH + H^+ \longrightarrow CH_3\overset{H}{\underset{OH}{C}}CH_2\overset{O}{\overset{\|}{C}}—S—pan—E + NADP^+$$

6. β-Hydroxyacyl dehydratase

$$CH_3\overset{H}{\underset{OH}{C}}CH_2\overset{O}{\overset{\|}{C}}—S—pan—E \longleftrightarrow CH_3\overset{H}{C}{=}\underset{H}{C}\overset{O}{\overset{\|}{C}}—S—pan—E + H_2O$$

7. Enoyl reductase

$$CH_3\overset{H}{C}{=}\underset{H}{C}\overset{O}{\overset{\|}{C}}—S—pan—E + NADPH + H^+ \longrightarrow CH_3CH_2CH_2\overset{O}{\overset{\|}{C}}—S—pan—E + NADP^+$$

8. β-Ketoacyl synthase (#2)

$$CH_3CH_2CH_2\overset{O}{\overset{\|}{C}}—S—pan—E + HS—cys—E \longleftrightarrow CH_3CH_2CH_2\overset{O}{\overset{\|}{C}}—S—cys—E + HS—pan—E$$

9. Acyl transferase (#3)

$$^{-}O\overset{O}{\overset{\|}{C}}CH_2\overset{O}{\overset{\|}{C}}—S—CoA + HS—pan—E \longleftrightarrow {}^{-}O\overset{O}{\overset{\|}{C}}CH_2\overset{O}{\overset{\|}{C}}—S—pan—E + CoA$$

10. β-Ketoacyl synthase (#4)

$$CH_3CH_2CH_2\overset{O}{\overset{\|}{C}}—S—cys—E + {}^{-}O\overset{O}{\overset{\|}{C}}CH_2\overset{O}{\overset{\|}{C}}—S—pan—E \longrightarrow CH_3CH_2CH_2\overset{O}{\overset{\|}{C}}—CH_2\overset{O}{\overset{\|}{C}}—S—pan—E + HS—cys—E + CO_2$$

11–13. Repeat 5–7; Forming Hexanoyl—pan—E

14–38. Five repeats of reactions 3–7; Forming Palmitoyl—pan—E

39. Thioesterase

$$Palmitoyl—pan—E + H_2O \longrightarrow Palmitate + HS—pan—E$$

FIGURE 16-4 The component reactions of fatty acid synthase. The abbreviations HS–cys–E and HS–pan–E indicate an enzyme-bound cysteine residue and an enzyme-bound 4′-phosphopantetheine group, respectively.

palmitate, 8 of CoA, 7 of CO_2, 14 of NADP, and 6 of H_2O. The reaction is complex in two ways. First, the fatty acid is built up by the serial addition of two-carbon fragments to a growing chain. Second, after each addition, the added carbons are reduced, dehydrated, and reduced again. The process then repeats itself—condensation, reduction, dehydration, and reduction—until a 16-carbon fatty acid (palmitate) has been formed and is released from the enzyme.

The first step in this complicated process involves an acyl transferase activity that transfers the acetyl moiety of

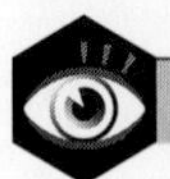

NUTRITION INSIGHT

Malonyl-CoA, AMPK, and Regulation of Food Intake

Obesity, a major health issue in modern society, is a disorder of energy imbalance in which energy intake exceeds energy expenditure. As discussed in Chapter 22, many neuromodulators as well as peripheral signals, including leptin, are involved in the control of food intake. Malonyl-CoA is a critical metabolite in fatty acid metabolism in peripheral tissues. It is an intermediate of fatty acid synthesis and provides acetyl groups to the growing fatty acid chain. It also regulates fatty acid oxidation by inhibiting transport of fatty acids into the mitochondria via carnitine palmitoyltransferase 1 (CPT1). There may be separate pools of malonyl-CoA for fatty acid synthesis and CPT1 inhibition. Malonyl-CoA generated by cytosolic acetyl-CoA carboxylase 1 is used for fatty acid synthesis, whereas malonyl-CoA produced by the acetyl-CoA carboxylase 2 isoform, which is associated with the outer mitochondrial membrane, inhibits CPT1. Recently, malonyl-CoA has been implicated in the regulation of food intake. Pharmacological inhibition of fatty acid synthase activity, which causes accumulation of malonyl-CoA, resulted in reduced food intake in rodents (Loftus et al., 2000). Genetic knockout of fatty acid synthase specifically in the hypothalamus of mice or adeno-associated virus-mediated overexpression of malonyl-CoA decarboxylase in the hypothalamus also increased malonyl-CoA concentration in brain and decreased food intake (Chakravarthy et al., 2007; He et al., 2006). Conversely, genetic knockout of acetyl-CoA carboxylase 2 in mice, which would block production of malonyl-CoA, increased food intake (Abu-Elheiga et al., 2003). The lipogenic enzymes are present at a high level in neurons in many brain regions, including hypothalamic neurons that regulate feeding behavior. Malonyl-CoA may act as a signal of energy status for the brain, causing changes in neuropeptide levels and thereby decreasing food intake.

AMP-activated protein kinase (AMPK), which is known to be an energy sensor for cells, may also be involved in the control of food intake. Hypothalamic AMPK is activated by fasting and inhibited by refeeding. Direct injection of an AMPK activator AICAR (5-aminoimidazole 4-carboxamide riboside) into the hypothalamus or expression of an activated mutant form of AMPK in the hypothalamus increased food intake, whereas a dominant-negative inhibitory mutant of AMPK decreased food intake in mice (Minokoshi et al., 2004). Interestingly, the adipose tissue hormone leptin has been suggested to stimulate dephosphorylation and inactivation of AMPK in the hypothalamus, and the decrease in AMPK activity can, in turn, change neuropeptide levels to regulate food intake. These effects of AMPK on food intake are also consistent with the fact that AMPK phosphorylates and inhibits acetyl-CoA carboxylase, causing a decrease in malonyl-CoA levels. Interestingly, high fructose sweeteners used in the processed foods and soft drinks may increase food intake. Fructose bypasses the rate-limiting step of glycolysis and uses a rapid ATP-requiring reaction, depleting ATP with a compensatory rise in AMP to activate the AMPK/malonyl-CoA pathway. Thus fructose may have the opposite effect of glucose on food intake. Further studies are needed to clarify the circumstantial evidence linking malonyl-CoA and/or AMPK to hypothalamic control of energy metabolism and food intake (Wolfgang and Lane, 2008).

acetyl-CoA to a serine residue in the acyltransferase domain of the enzyme. The acetyl group is then transferred from the serine residue in the acyltransferase domain to the 4′-phosphopantetheine if the sulfhydryl of the covalently linked 4′-phosphopantetheine group in the acyl carrier protein domain of the enzyme is free. The 4′-phosphopantetheine group of the ACP domain of fatty acid synthase is described in Chapter 26. The β-ketoacyl synthase (the "condensing enzyme") activity of fatty acid synthase then catalyzes transfer of the acetyl group to a cysteine residue at the active site of the condensation reaction. The serine residue in the acyl transferase domain is now free to accept a malonyl group. The malonyl group is then transferred to the sulfhydryl group of the phosphopantetheine side arm (see Figure 16-4), which has been freed of its acetyl group, and the enzyme is poised to carry out the first condensation reaction.

During the condensation reaction, the methylene carbon of the malonyl-phosphopantetheine form of the enzyme attacks the carbonyl group of the acetyl moiety in the active site of the β-ketoacyl transferase, forming the acetoacetyl-phosphopantetheine form of the enzyme and releasing the carboxyl group at C2 of the malonyl moiety as CO_2. The energy for this reaction is provided by coupling condensation of the acetyl and malonyl groups with decarboxylation. A condensation that started with two acetyl-CoAs would be energetically unfavorable. As a result, the energy for this reaction really comes from the hydrolysis of ATP during the carboxylation of acetyl-CoA to form malonyl-CoA; malonyl-CoA can thus be viewed as an activated form of acetyl-CoA. The carboxyl group added by acetyl-CoA carboxylase is the same one that is removed during the condensation reaction. Thus even though bicarbonate is a required substrate for the fatty acid synthesis pathway, incorporation of bicarbonate into the fatty acid does not occur.

The phosphopantetheine side arm in the ACP domain of fatty acid synthase is long and flexible, so that its attached acetoacetyl group can interact sequentially with the active sites of the β-ketoacyl reductase, β-hydroxyacyl dehydratase, and enoyl reductase domains to form a 4-carbon saturated fatty acyl group. At the end of this reaction sequence, the butyryl moiety remains attached to the phosphopantetheinyl moiety, but it is then transferred to the cysteine residue in the active site of the β-ketoacyl synthase domain. This leaves the sulfhydryl of the phosphopantetheinyl moiety free to receive a new malonyl-CoA moiety from the serine residue in the acyltransferase domain. The next cycle of condensation, reduction, dehydration, and reduction then forms a 6-carbon saturated fatty-acyl group (hexanoyl) attached to

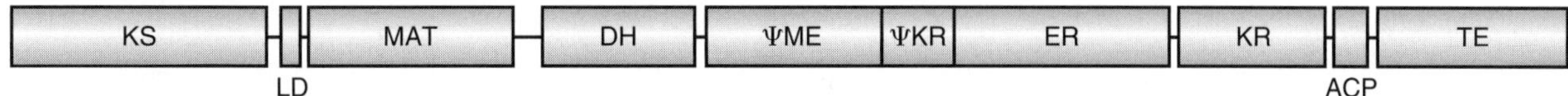

FIGURE 16-5 The domain organization of mammalian fatty acid synthase. Seven functional domains are indicated: *KS,* β-ketoacyl synthase; *MAT,* malonyl/acetyltransferase, or acyltransferase; *DH,* β-hydroxyacyl dehydratase; *ER,* enoyl reductase; *KR,* β-ketoacyl reductase; *ACP,* acyl carrier protein; *TE,* thioesterase. Other domains are also shown: *LD,* linker domain; *ΨME,* pseudo-methyltransferase; *ΨKR,* pseudo-ketoreductase.

the phosphopantetheine side arm. The hexanoyl group is transferred to the active site cysteine residue of the β-ketoacyl synthase domain, and another malonyl group is condensed, reduced, dehydrated, and reduced. After seven cycles, the growing acyl chain reaches 16 carbons, and a thioesterase activity in the thioesterase domain of fatty acid synthase cleaves the free fatty acid from the enzyme (see Figure 16-4).

As mentioned previously, all of the reactions required for fatty acid synthesis from acetyl-CoA and malonyl-CoA are catalyzed by a single polypeptide (i.e., fatty acid synthase) that contains all activities in separate domains. The multifunctional fatty acid synthase can provide a greater efficiency by channeling intermediates from one active site to the next rather than relying on diffusion of intermediates between separate enzymes. In addition, the amounts of each enzyme can be regulated simultaneously by controlling expression of a single gene. Mammalian fatty acid synthase is synthesized as an inactive monomer of about 270 kDa (Figure 16-5). The active enzyme is an intertwined head-to-head homodimer of two fatty acid synthase monomers that has an X shape, with each of the two lateral clefts of the X defining a reaction chamber (Maier et al., 2008). One complete set of domains for progressive elongation of the fatty acid chain is present in each of the lateral clefts.

Similar to acetyl CoA carboxylase, fatty acid synthase activity is low in the fasted state but increases drastically in the fed state, especially when the diet is rich in carbohydrate. However, neither allosteric nor phosphorylation–dephosphorylation mechanisms appear to contribute significantly to these changes in fatty acid synthase activity. The major regulation is at the level of protein concentration as a consequence of changes in gene transcription by the previously described mechanism involving several transcription factors, including SREBP-1c (Wong and Sul, 2010).

SYNTHESIS OF FATTY ACIDS OTHER THAN PALMITATE

The product of the reaction catalyzed by fatty acid synthase is exclusively palmitate, a 16-carbon saturated fatty acid. However, saturated and unsaturated fatty acids with 18 or more carbon atoms are abundant in animal tissues. For example, more than 50% of the human adipose tissue triacylglycerol molecules contain one or more fatty acids of 18 carbons in length. Acyl chain length and the degree of saturation can influence membrane function, and membrane polyunsaturated long-chain fatty acids serve as precursors for biologically active signaling molecules such as eicosanoids. Therefore, although a variety of fatty acids are provided by the diet, the capacity to modify and elongate fatty acid chains before esterification is required to maintain specific fatty acid composition in cells. Elongases and desaturases are regulated primarily by changes in the transcription of genes encoding these enzymes. Many specialized organs, such as mammary and sebaceous glands, synthesize fatty acids with shorter acyl chains and branched acyl chains. The de novo synthesis of these specialized fatty acids requires separate enzymes and enzyme systems.

ELONGATION OF FATTY ACIDS

Fatty acids can be elongated in two-carbon steps. Elongation of fatty acids occurs in the endoplasmic reticulum (ER), mitochondria, and peroxisomes. In general, the enzyme systems for elongation are not well understood, but the ER elongation system is the most active and most studied. The ER elongation system uses both saturated and unsaturated fatty acyl-CoAs as substrates. The individual reactions are analogous to those catalyzed by fatty acid synthase, except that long-chain acyl-CoAs are used as primers rather than acetyl-CoA, and different gene products catalyze the individual reactions. The sequence of reactions is condensation, reduction, dehydration, and reduction. In the ER, malonyl-CoA is the elongating group, and NADPH is the electron donor. The initial rate-controlling step of a condensation reaction is referred to as elongation of very-long-chain fatty acids (ELOVL), and there are at least seven ELOVL enzymes that prefer either saturated and monounsaturated fatty acids or polyunsaturated fatty acids (Guillou et al., 2010). The mitochondrial elongation system appears to use acetyl-CoA as the elongating unit and NADH or NADH plus NADPH as electron donors. The mitochondrial elongation system is not a simple reversal of fatty acid oxidation involving two-carbon units (β-oxidation) because flavoenzymes are not involved in catalysis for either the first or the second reduction in each cycle. Fatty acid elongation in peroxisomes is even less understood but may produce very-long-chain fatty acids of 24 to 36 carbons in length.

DESATURATION OF FATTY ACIDS

Monounsaturated fatty acids are formed by direct oxidative desaturation of preformed long-chain saturated fatty acids in reactions catalyzed by a complex of enzymes located in the ER. The first double bond introduced into a saturated acyl chain is generally in the Δ9 position. The Δ9 desaturase complex (also called stearoyl-CoA desaturase, SCD) uses saturated fatty acids with 14 to 18 carbons; stearate is the most active. This complex, which is sometimes called a mixed function oxidase, uses two electrons and

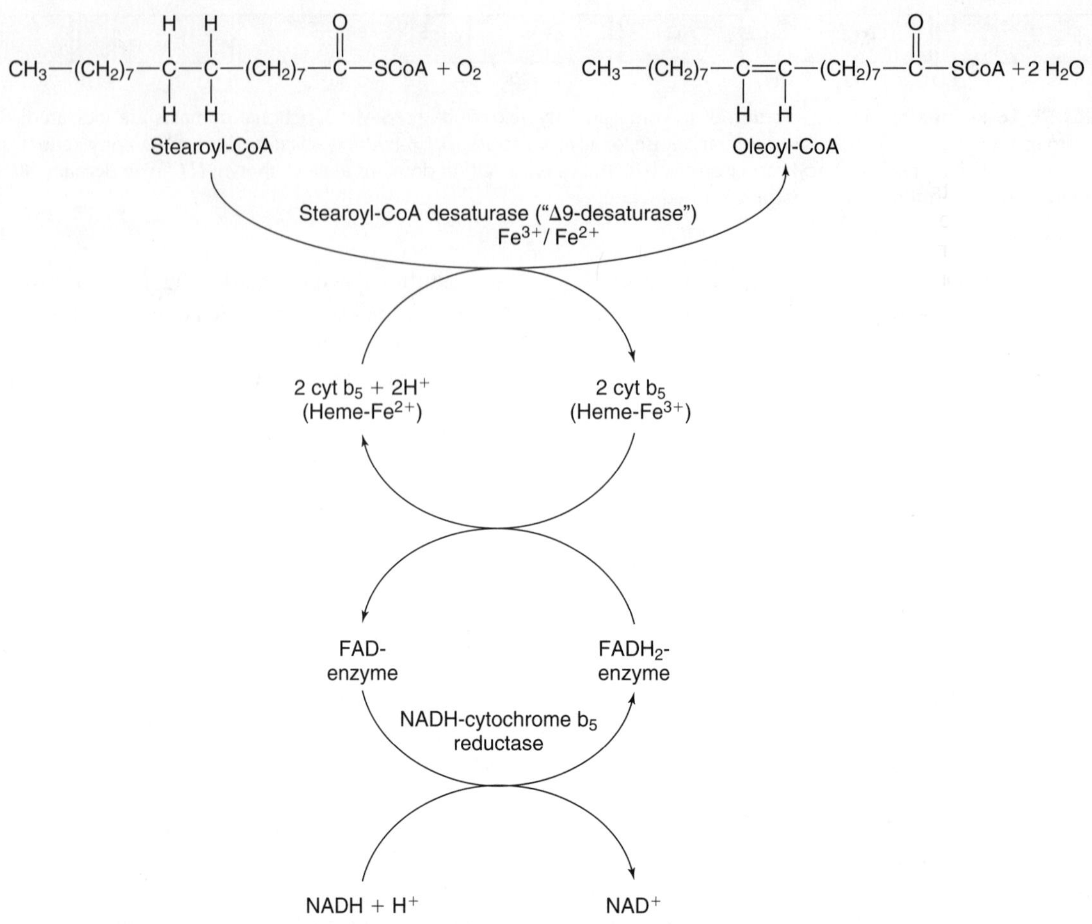

FIGURE 16-6 Stearoyl-CoA desaturase reaction.

two protons donated by NADH (+ H^+), two electrons and two protons from the fatty acid, and oxygen (as an electron acceptor) to generate the unsaturated fatty acid and two water molecules, as shown in Figure 16-6. The substrates and products are the acyl-CoA derivatives of the fatty acid. Electrons donated by NADH are passed via $FADH_2$ to the heme iron of cytochrome b_5, reducing it to the ferrous form, in a reaction catalyzed by NADH:cytochrome b_5 reductase. Cytochrome b_5 then donates two electrons to the nonheme iron of the desaturase component, reducing it to the ferrous form. This form then interacts with molecular oxygen and the fatty acyl-CoA to form water and the unsaturated fatty acyl-CoA. The desaturase activity regulates the overall reaction. Multiple forms of Δ9 desaturase are present with differing tissue distributions and regulation. The activity of SCD1, the isozyme present mostly in liver and adipose tissue, is controlled by diet and hormones in much the same manner as are the activities of the lipogenic enzymes, mainly by regulation of enzyme concentration.

Polyunsaturated fatty acids, usually containing double bonds interrupted by methylene groups, are produced in mammalian tissues. By using the enzymatic mechanism just described for desaturation at the Δ9 position by Δ9 desaturase, mammalian cells can further introduce double bonds into long-chain fatty acids at the Δ5 and Δ6 positions by Δ5 and Δ6 desaturases. However, due to the lack of Δ12 and Δ15 desaturases, double bonds cannot be introduced beyond the Δ9 position (i.e., at the third or sixth carbon from the methyl end, which is equivalent to a double bond at the twelfth or fifteenth carbon from the carboxyl end of an 18-carbon fatty acid). As a consequence, linoleate (18:2, Δ9, Δ12), an n-6 fatty acid, or α-linolenate (18:3, Δ9, Δ12, Δ15), an n-3 fatty acid, cannot be synthesized in humans, and they or longer chain members of the n-3 or n-6 classes must be provided in the diet. These fatty acids are essential for the synthesis of polyunsaturated fatty acids such as arachidonate (20:4, Δ5, Δ8, Δ11, Δ14) and eicosapentaenoate (20:5, Δ5, Δ8, Δ11, Δ14, Δ17). An alternating desaturation and elongation produces arachidonate and eicosapentaenoate from linoleate and α-linolenate, respectively.

18:2, Δ 9, Δ 12 (Linoleate) → 18:3, Δ 6, Δ 9, Δ 12 →
20:3 Δ 8, Δ 11, Δ 14 → 20:4, Δ 5, Δ 8, Δ 11, Δ 14
(Arachidonate)

18:3, Δ 9, Δ 12, Δ 15 (α-Linolenate) →
18:4, Δ 6, Δ 9, Δ 12, Δ 15 → 20:4, Δ 8, Δ 11, Δ 14, Δ 17 →
20:5, Δ 5, Δ 8, Δ 11, Δ 14, Δ 17 (Eicosapentaenoate)

Multiple desaturation and elongation reactions, plus a retroconversion step by peroxisomal β-oxidation, are involved in synthesis of docosahexaenoate (22:6, Δ4, Δ7, Δ10, Δ13, Δ16, Δ19) from α-linolenate. (See Chapters 6 and 18 for

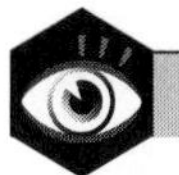

NUTRITION INSIGHT

Endocannabinoids for the Control of Food Intake and Lipid Metabolism

Cannabinoid receptors are molecular targets of Δ^9-tetrahydrocannabinol (THC), the principle active compound for the psychotropic effects of marijuana. In humans there are endogenous ligands for cannabinoid receptors, and these so-called endocannabinoids are polyunsaturated fatty acid derivatives, *N*-arachidonoylethanolamine (anandamide) and 2-arachidonoylglycerol. There also are other *N*-acylethanolamides, such as oleoylethanolamide, palmitoylethanolamide and docosatetraenoylethanolamide, that belong to the same group of metabolites produced from the membrane phospholipids. These latter compounds do not serve as ligands themselves but regulate the action of the endocannabinoid ligands. Endocannabinoids exert various central and peripheral effects mainly by activating the membrane cannabinoid receptors that are coupled to G proteins to affect signal transduction molecules, including adenylate cyclase and certain ion channels and kinases (Maccarrone et al., 2010).

Because THC stimulates appetite and increases body weight in wasting syndromes, cannabinoid receptors and endocannabinoids could be predicted to control energy balance. The endocannabinoids control food intake via both central and peripheral mechanism and stimulate fat synthesis and accumulation. Cannabinoid receptors and the enzymes involved in the synthesis and degradation of the two endocannabinoids may be attractive targets for the management of obesity. However, the psychiatric side effects of the newly developed cannabinoid receptor antagonists have dampened the enthusiasm for their application in the therapy of obesity. A better understanding of cannabinoid receptors and how central and peripheral signals are integrated into behavioral and metabolic responses may help to develop compounds that have the desired selective actions (Ligresti et al., 2009).

further discussion of essential fatty acids and fatty acid nomenclature.)

SYNTHESIS OF MEDIUM-CHAIN FATTY ACIDS

Medium-chain fatty acids are synthesized in mammary gland and are present as triacylglycerol in milk. Mammary gland has the same fatty acid synthase as does liver. Therefore fatty acid synthase purified from either tissue can synthesize palmitate because the thioesterase activity of fatty acid synthase is specific for 16-carbon acyl groups. However, secretory cells of the mammary gland also contain a second thioesterase that is specific for medium-chain fatty acids. This enzyme interacts with growing acyl chains on the fatty acid synthase and cleaves them from fatty acid synthase when they are 8 to 12 carbons in length.

PRODUCTION OF SIMPLE BRANCHED-CHAIN FATTY ACIDS

Sebaceous glands and certain related glands, such as the meibomian glands in the eyelids, synthesize fatty acids with one-carbon side chains. The "normal" fatty acid synthase carries out these reactions using unusual substrates. For example, propionyl-CoA can be used as a primer for fatty acid synthase rather than acetyl-CoA, and the resulting fatty acid will have a methyl branch at the C2 (i.e., the αC) position. Methyl groups also can be inserted at other positions along the fatty acid chain. Although it has a lower affinity for the condensing enzyme than does malonyl-CoA, methylmalonyl-CoA can be used as an elongating group if the concentration of malonyl-CoA is lower than that of methylmalonyl-CoA. In sebaceous glands, propionyl-CoA is converted to methylmalonyl-CoA in a reaction catalyzed by acetyl-CoA carboxylase. Acetyl-CoA carboxylase uses both acetyl-CoA and propionyl-CoA equally efficiently so the relative concentrations of malonyl-CoA and methylmalonyl-CoA depend on the relative concentrations of acetyl-CoA and propionyl-CoA. In sebaceous glands, a soluble malonyl-CoA decarboxylase keeps malonyl-CoA levels low. The mechanism for generating high levels of propionyl-CoA in sebaceous glands is not known.

SYNTHESIS OF TRIACYLGLYCEROL

Triacylglycerols are esters of glycerol and three molecules of fatty acids. The substrates for this pathway are glycerol 3-phosphate and fatty acyl-CoAs, and the fatty acyl groups (i.e., fatty acids) are esterified to the three alcohol groups on glycerol.

SOURCES OF GLYCEROL 3-PHOSPHATE FOR TRIACYLGLYCEROL SYNTHESIS

Two reactions catalyze formation of glycerol 3-phosphate. First, dihydroxyacetone phosphate, a glycolytic (and gluconeogenic) intermediate, can be reduced to glycerol 3-phosphate. NADH is the electron donor in the reaction catalyzed by glycerol 3-phosphate dehydrogenase. This reaction is freely reversible, also allowing glycerol 3-phosphate to enter the glycolytic or gluconeogenic pathways under certain conditions.

$$\text{Dihydroxyacetone phosphate} + \text{NADH} + \text{H}^+ \leftrightarrow \text{Glycerol 3-phosphate} + \text{NAD}^+$$

Second, in some tissues such as liver, but not appreciably in adipose or muscle tissues, glycerol can be phosphorylated to glycerol 3-phosphate in a reaction catalyzed by glycerol kinase.

$$\text{Glycerol} + \text{ATP} \rightarrow \text{Glycerol 3-phosphate} + \text{ADP}$$

SOURCES OF FATTY ACIDS FOR TRIACYLGLYCEROL SYNTHESIS

Fatty acids to be used for synthesis of triacylglycerol comprise fatty acids from de novo synthesis and those from hydrolysis of triacylglycerols in the cell, as well as fatty acids taken up from the circulation. The fatty acids taken up from the circulation may be free fatty acids (mainly released by lipolysis and associated with plasma albumin) or fatty acids generated locally from circulating lipoproteins (by the action of lipoprotein lipases localized on the endothelium of the capillaries within the tissue). These fatty acids from the plasma are taken up by the cell either by passive diffusion or by plasma membrane fatty acid transporters, such as fatty acid translocase (FAT/CD36), fatty acid transport proteins (FATPs), or plasma membrane fatty acid binding protein (FABPpm) (Glatz et al., 2010; Su and Abumrad, 2008). Because of their hydrophobic properties, once inside the cell, long-chain fatty acids are bound to fatty acid binding proteins (FABPs) to be transferred from membrane to membrane within the cell (Storch and Corsico, 2008).

ACTIVATION OF FATTY ACIDS BY COENZYME A THIOESTER FORMATION

Before esterification to glycerol or transport to the mitochondria for oxidation, fatty acids must be activated to their CoA derivatives. This reaction is catalyzed by fatty acyl-CoA synthetase (also called fatty acyl-CoA ligase or fatty acid thiokinase). Different isoforms of fatty acyl-CoA synthetase are present in the membranes of mitochondria, ER, and peroxisomes, where fatty acids are used for either esterification or oxidation (Ellis et al., 2010). One of the proposed fatty acid transporters FATP also has intrinsic fatty acyl-CoA synthetase activity and may function to trap fatty acids in the cell and thereby facilitate fatty acid transport.

The ATP-dependent fatty acyl-CoA synthetase reaction has three steps. In the first step, fatty acid reacts with ATP to form a fatty acyl-AMP intermediate plus pyrophosphate. In the second step, the acyl moiety is transferred to coenzyme A and AMP is generated. As written, the reactions are freely reversible: one high-energy bond is cleaved between PP_i and AMP, and one is formed between the fatty acid and CoA.

(1) Fatty acid + ATP ↔ Fatty acyl-AMP + PP_i

(2) Fatty acyl-AMP + CoA ↔ Fatty acyl-CoA + AMP

In the third step, the reaction is driven in the direction of formation of fatty acyl-CoA by a ubiquitous pyrophosphatase that rapidly cleaves pyrophosphate to inorganic phosphate.

(3) $PP_i + H_2O \rightarrow 2\ P_i$

NET: Fatty acid + ATP + CoA + H_2O →
Fatty acyl-CoA + AMP + 2 P_i

As will be shown in other pathways in this chapter, the hydrolysis of pyrophosphate is a relatively common mechanism for driving reactions to completion.

ESTERIFICATON OF FATTY ACIDS

The glycerol 3-phosphate reaction pathway for the synthesis of triacylglycerols starts with fatty acyl-CoA and glycerol 3-phosphate, as shown in Figure 16-7. The acyl group of a fatty acyl-CoA is transferred to the *sn*-1 position of glycerol 3-phosphate in the reaction catalyzed by glycerol 3-phosphate acyltransferase. This is the first committed step in glycerolipid biosynthesis.

(1) Glycerol 3-phosphate + Fatty acyl-CoA →
1-Acylglycerol 3-phosphate + CoA

The 1-acylglycerol 3-phosphate (lysophosphatidic acid) is esterified by a second molecule of fatty acyl-CoA to form 1,2-diacylglycerol 3-phosphate (phosphatidic acid). The enzyme that catalyzes this reaction is 1-acylglycerol 3-phosphate acyltransferase. Although their distinctive roles are not clear, several isoforms for each of these acyltransferases have been found (Wendel et al., 2009; Takeuchi and Reue, 2009).

(2) 1-Acylglycerol 3-phosphate + Fatty acyl-CoA →
1,2-Diacylglycerol 3-phosphate + CoA

Usually, the *sn*-1 position of the glycerol backbone is esterified with a saturated fatty acid, whereas the *sn*-2 position is esterified with an unsaturated fatty acid. However, the fatty acid composition of lipids in the diet influences the fatty acid composition of triacylglycerol in adipose tissue.

In the third reaction of this pathway, 1,2-diacylglycerol 3-phosphate is dephosphorylated to 1,2-diacylglycerol and inorganic phosphate. The enzyme that catalyzes this reaction is 1,2-diacylglycerol 3-phosphate phosphatase (also called phosphatidic acid phosphohydrolase).

(3) 1,2-Diacylglycerol 3-phosphate → 1,2-Diacylglycerol + P_i

Up to this point the reactions of triacylglycerol synthesis are the same as those leading to synthesis of phospholipids, some of which use 1,2-diacylglycerol 3-phosphate as substrate and some of which use 1,2-diacylglycerol. The final reaction for triacylglycerol synthesis involves acylation of diacylglycerol to form triacylglycerol. This reaction is catalyzed by 1,2-diacylglycerol acyltransferase, which is particularly active in intestine, liver, and adipose tissue.

(4) 1,2-Diacylglycerol + Fatty acyl-CoA →
Triacylglycerol + CoA

Dihydroxyacetone phosphate also can be used in the first acylation of fatty acyl-CoA. The first reaction, catalyzed by a dihydroxyacetone acyltransferase, which is present in ER and also in peroxisomes, forms 1-acyl dihydroxyacetone as the product. This compound is then reduced by 1-acyl dihydroxyacetone reductase with NADPH as the electron donor and 1-acylglycerol 3-phosphate and NADP as products. The remaining steps are the same as outlined for the glycerol 3-phosphate pathway. The role of this second pathway in phosphatidic acid biosynthesis is not clear. It is generally accepted that 1-acyl dihydroxyacetone phosphate is an intermediate in the synthesis of alkyl and alkenyl lipids, a process that occurs exclusively in peroxisomes.

REGULATION OF TRIACYLGLYCEROL SYNTHESIS

Glycerolipid biosynthesis occurs mostly in ER. The enzymes reside on the ER membrane. Because these enzymes are membrane-bound, their characterization has been difficult,

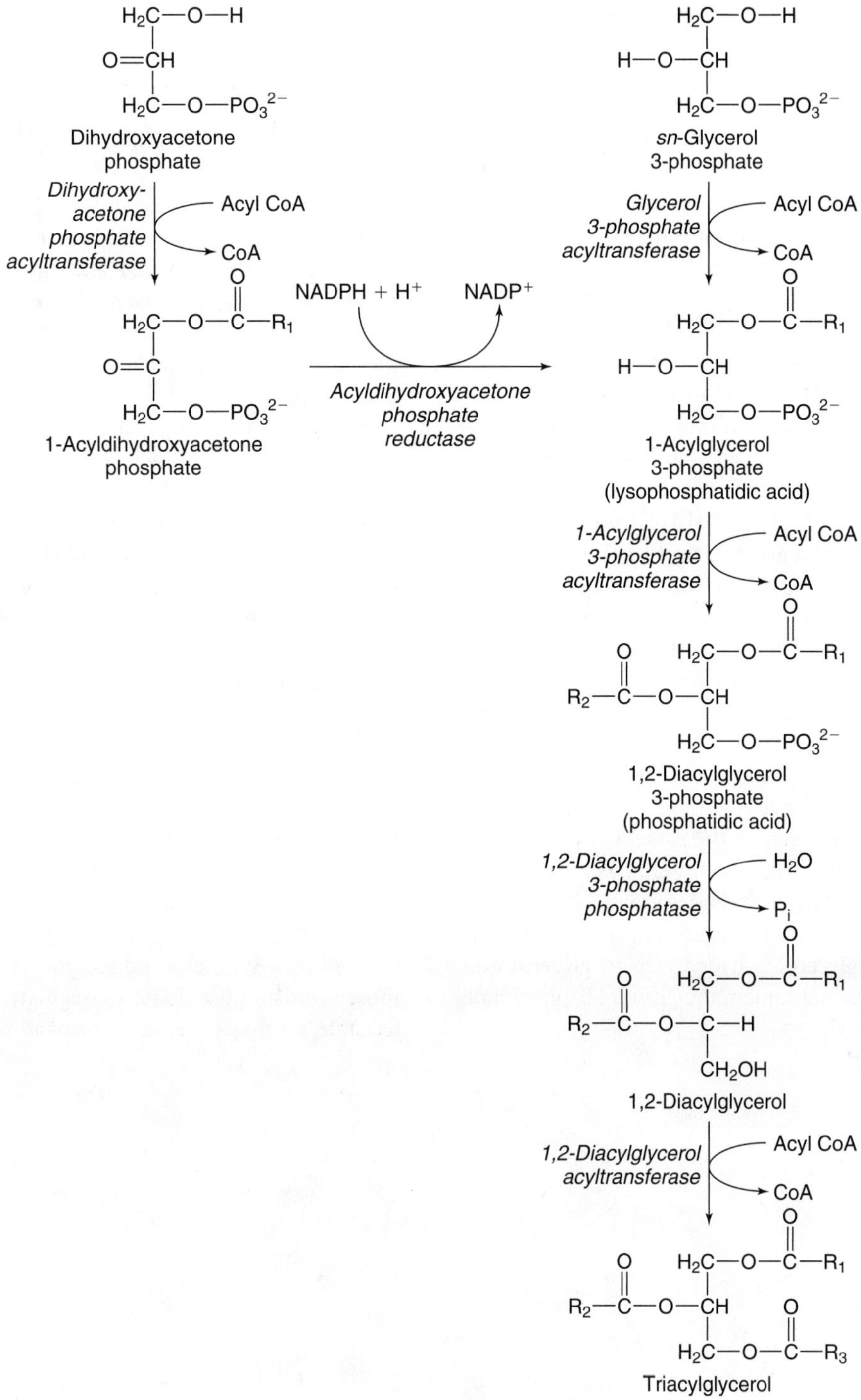

FIGURE 16-7 Triacylglycerol biosynthesis.

and their regulation is largely unknown. It is presumed that 1,2-diacylglycerol 3-phosphate phosphatase may be a rate-controlling step in triacylglycerol synthesis, and that the enzyme activity is regulated via translocation of the enzyme from the cytosol to the ER where it becomes active. The reaction catalyzed by 1,2-diacylglycerol acyltransferase is a unique step in triacylglycerol synthesis that is not involved in phospholipid synthesis. Glycerol 3-phosphate acyltransferase also may be a regulatory step. An isoform of glycerol 3-phosphate acyltransferase, with characteristics different from those of the form present in ER, is present in mitochondrial membrane. The mitochondrial enzyme is expressed mostly in lipogenic tissues (the liver and adipose tissue) and is regulated by nutritional changes as described earlier for the enzymes involved in fatty acid synthesis (Wendel et al., 2009; Dircks and Sul, 1999). During the fasting state, the activity of glycerol 3-phosphate acyltransferase is very low; in the fed state, especially on a high carbohydrate diet, enzyme activity increases. Regulation is at the transcriptional level.

TRANSPORT OF TRIACYLGLYCEROL IN VLDL

Much of the triacylglycerol synthesized in the liver is destined for export to extrahepatic tissues, especially to adipose tissue where it is stored. Triacylglycerol is not soluble in water, so special arrangements must be made to permit its transport in the blood. Lipoproteins perform this function. The triacylglycerols synthesized in liver are packaged into lipoproteins in liver and secreted into the blood as VLDLs, as described in more detail in Chapter 17.

ESTERIFICATION OF FATTY ACIDS TO 2-MONOACYLGLYCEROL IN THE INTESTINE AND THEIR TRANSPORT IN CHYLOMICRONS

Synthesis of triacylglycerol in enterocytes (intestinal cells) follows a somewhat different pathway than that just described for liver and adipose tissue and is discussed in Chapter 10. The major products of the hydrolysis of triacylglycerol in the lumen of the intestine are unesterified fatty acids and 2-monoacylglycerol. These compounds are taken up by enterocytes and recombined to form triacylglycerol. The triacylglycerol is then packaged into the core of a specific type of lipoprotein, chylomicrons, to be secreted into the lymph; ultimately, the chylomicrons enter the bloodstream at the thoracic duct. In the first reaction of triacylglycerol resynthesis in enterocytes, 2-monoacylglycerol reacts with fatty acyl-CoA to form diacylglycerol (2-monoacylglycerol acyltransferase). The next step is the same as that in other tissues and is catalyzed by the same enzyme, diacylglycerol acyltransferase (Mansbach and Siddiqi, 2010). The 2-monoacylglycerol pathway is dominant in enterocytes, but because some triacylglycerol is hydrolyzed to glycerol and fatty acids in the intestinal lumen, the glycerol 3-phosphate pathway also is essential.

HYDROLYSIS OF TRIACYLGLYCEROL IN LIPOPROTEINS, UPTAKE OF FATTY ACIDS, AND UTILIZATION OF FATTY ACIDS FOR ENERGY OR STORAGE AS TRIACYLGLYCEROL

Whether triacylglycerols are synthesized in the liver or intestine, they are transported in triacylglycerol-rich lipoprotein particles. Fatty acids released from the triacylglycerol in these lipoprotein particles (VLDL and chylomicrons) are taken up by extrahepatic tissues such as muscle, where they provide a source of oxidizable fatty acids, and adipose tissue, where they are reconverted to triacylglycerol and stored in the unilocular lipid droplet of the adipocyte until needed.

Lipoprotein lipase facilitates uptake of fatty acids by hydrolyzing plasma triacylglycerols in the circulating lipoproteins. As illustrated in Figure 16-8, lipoprotein lipase is localized on the luminal face of the endothelial cells that form the "walls" of capillaries. The enzyme is synthesized by myocytes (muscle cells) or adipocytes (adipose cells) and secreted into the interstitial space (Wang and Eckel, 2009). It then is taken up at the interstitial (basal) side of the endothelial cells, transported across those cells, secreted, and bound to the plasma side of the luminal surface, where it is bound to GPIHBP1 (glycosylphosphatidylinositol-anchored HDL-binding protein 1) (Beigneux et al., 2009). As discussed in more detail in Chapter 17, triacylglycerol in lipoproteins is hydrolyzed by lipoprotein lipase, producing unesterified fatty acids. The unesterified fatty acids cross the endothelial cells by an uncertain mechanism (by diffusion or by a protein-mediated transport) and are taken up by adipocytes or myocytes. Synthesis and secretion of lipoprotein lipase in muscle and adipose tissue are regulated differentially. In the fed state, synthesis and secretion of adipose tissue lipoprotein

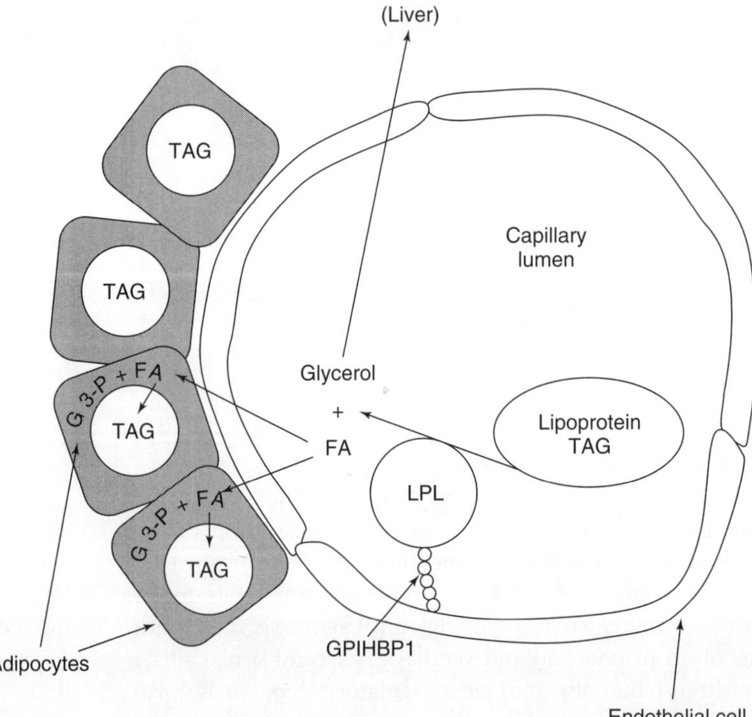

FIGURE 16-8 Model for hydrolysis of lipoprotein-bound triacylglycerol (*TAG*) and uptake of fatty acid (*FA*) into adipocytes resulting in assimilation of TAG for storage. Hydrolysis of FA from TAG-rich lipoproteins by lipoprotein lipase (*LPL*) bound to the capillary endothelial surface via sulfated proteoglycans is shown. Released FA are then taken up by adipocytes and reesterified to TAG for storage. *GPIHBP1,* Glycosylphosphatidylinositol-anchored HDL-binding protein 1.

lipase are increased, which favors storage. During a shortage of energy (such as overnight fasting or exercise), adipose lipoprotein lipase is decreased whereas muscle lipoprotein lipase is increased, thus favoring the use of lipoprotein triacylglycerols as fuel. Inside adipocytes, the fatty acids are activated to their CoA derivatives, esterified to form triacylglycerol via the glycerol 3-phosphate pathway, and stored as a lipid droplet in those cells. Inside myocytes the fatty acids are used primarily for oxidation, but they can also be converted to triacylglycerols and be stored as intramyocellular droplets in muscle.

MOBILIZATION OF STORED TRIACYLGLYCEROL

Triacylglycerols are stored in cytoplasmic lipid droplets in adipocytes and to a lesser extent in most cell types. Stored triacylglycerol in adipocytes can be hydrolyzed and the fatty acids are released to the circulation for use by other organs as fuels when needed, such as during starvation or exercise. Lipid lipases catalyze the release of fatty acids from the triacylglycerol stored as lipid droplets in the adipocytes. Hormone-sensitive lipase (HSL) is classically known to act at the surface of the triacylglycerol droplet and hydrolyzes fatty acids at the *sn*-1 and *sn*-3 positions. However, HSL hydrolyzes diacylglycerol more efficiently than triacylglycerol and recently adipose triacylglycerol lipase, which prefers triacylglycerol, has been identified (Duncan et al., 2007). Thus it is now believed that adipose triacylglycerol lipase acts on triacylglycerol to generate diacylglycerol, which is then the substrate for HSL. The 2-monoacylglycerol generated by HSL is subsequently substrate for monoacylglycerol lipase, which is present at high activity and hydrolyzes fatty acids at the *sn*-2 position.

There is a normal substrate (futile) cycling between triacylglycerol and fatty acids in the adipocyte. In regulation of adipocyte lipolysis, HSL is regulated by a phosphorylation–dephosphorylation mechanism. Lipid droplets are coated with lipid-droplet associated proteins (Walther and Farese, 2009) that are important for triacylglycerol mobilization. One of these, perilipin, is involved in regulation of adipose triacylglycerol lipase activity; perilipin is also regulated by phosphorylation–dephosphorylation.

In the fed state, the insulin level in the blood rises and brings about dephosphorylation and inactivation of HSL in adipocytes, as shown in Figure 16-9. Inactivation of adipose triacylglycerol lipase activity by perilipin dephosphorylation also plays an important role. Fat mobilization from adipose tissue is therefore decreased. In addition, insulin promotes uptake of glucose into the adipocyte. Because the rate of glycolysis is limited by the rate of uptake of glucose, the enhancement of glucose uptake ensures a steady production of triose phosphate sugars and hence glycerol 3-phosphate. Thus, as a consequence of the inactivation of hormone-responsive lipases and the availability of glycerol 3-phosphate in fed animals, fatty acids produced by lipolysis in the adipose tissue are mainly reesterified in the fed state.

On the other hand, in the fasting state, stored triacylglycerol in adipose tissue is the major source of energy. HSL and perilipin are phosphorylated by protein kinase A, which is activated by increased intracellular cAMP. In isolated rat adipocytes, glucagon, which rises during starvation, is a potent stimulator of fat mobilization. In humans, however, epinephrine and norepinephrine play the major role in increasing intracellular cAMP levels in adipose tissue and thus the phosphorylation and activation of adipose HSL. This leads to the accelerated hydrolysis of triacylglycerol (see Figure 16-9). HSL is present in the cytosol of adipocytes and translocates to the surface of lipid droplets upon hormonal stimulation. Phosphorylation of both HSL and perilipin is necessary for HSL translocation and for HSL activation. The antilipolytic action of insulin mentioned earlier is due, to a large extent, to insulin-mediated phosphorylation and activation of phosphodiesterase, which lowers the cAMP levels and hence reduces phosphorylation of HSL and perilipin. In addition to activation of HSL, the decrease in insulin levels during starvation inhibits glucose uptake by adipose tissue and therefore production of triose phosphate. This, then, reduces the rate of fatty acid reesterification. Thus when production of fatty acids increases due to activation of HSL during starvation and reesterification of fatty acids is low, release of fatty acids to the blood proceeds at a high rate. Once in the blood, nonesterified fatty acids are bound noncovalently to albumin and transported in that form to other tissues, primarily destined for oxidation but also for VLDL and ketone body formation in the liver. Glycerol produced in adipose tissue during triacylglycerol hydrolysis also is released to the blood and is transported to the liver for reutilization. Unlike in adipose tissue, fatty acids from hydrolysis of intramuscular triacylglycerol are not released to blood but are used as a fuel source within muscle when needed such as during exercise. Paradoxically, in patients who are obese or have type 2 diabetes, intramuscular triacylglycerol deposition may be increased and contribute to insulin resistance.

OXIDATION OF FATTY ACIDS

Long-chain fatty acids are supplied to most tissues via the circulation. Free fatty acids released by adipose lipolysis are insoluble in water and circulate largely noncovalently bound to albumin. The concentration of free fatty acids varies from 0.3 to 2.0 mmol/L in plasma; levels are high during starvation and low in the postprandial period. Long-chain fatty acids are also obtained by tissues such as muscle from the action of lipoprotein lipase on the triacylglycerol in circulating lipoproteins (VLDL and chylomicrons). Chylomicrons contain absorbed fat from a meal, whereas VLDLs are primarily synthesized by the liver. Transport of triacylglycerol in chylomicrons and VLDLs is discussed in more detail in Chapter 17 (also see Figure 16-1).

Fatty acids are taken up into cells by diffusion or plasma membrane fatty acid transporters and once inside the cell are bound to a fatty acid–binding protein (Glatz et al., 2010). Most tissues use fatty acids as fuel, but, as for triacylglycerol

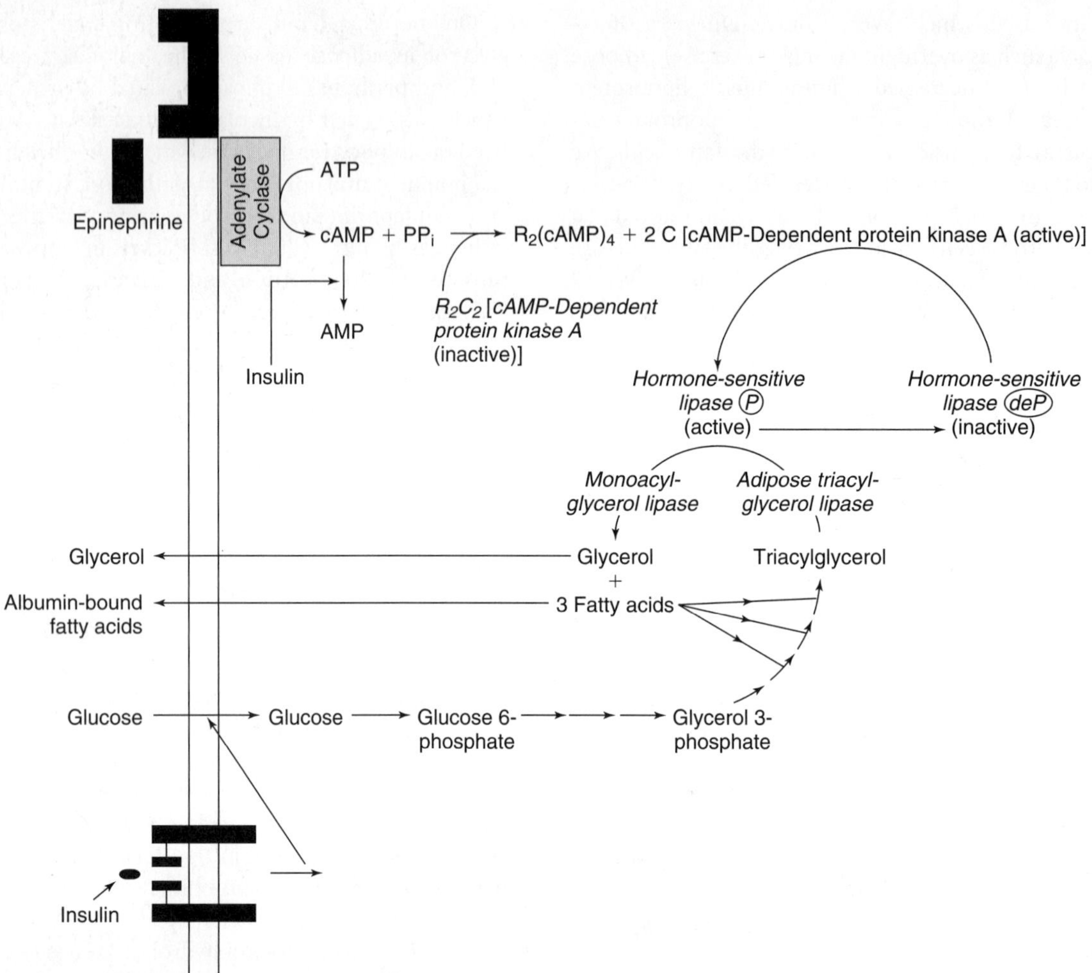

FIGURE 16-9 Role of hormones in regulation of synthesis and hydrolysis of stored triacylglycerol in adipose tissue. Insulin promotes triacylglycerol synthesis by promoting glucose uptake via upregulation of GLUT4. Insulin also decreases lipolysis by activating phosphodiesterase that removes cAMP, which promotes the dephosphorylation and hence inactivation of hormone-sensitive lipase. Epinephrine and norepinephrine stimulate cAMP formation by adenylate cyclase, which leads to activation of protein kinase A and hence the phosphorylation and activation of hormone-sensitive lipase. Protein kinase A also phosphorylates perilipin, which results in activation of adipose triacylglycerol lipase. R and C represent the regulatory and catalytic subunits of cAMP-dependent protein kinase A.

synthesis, fatty acids must be activated to a fatty acyl-CoA by fatty acyl-CoA synthetase before they can be oxidized for energy production. The oxidation of fatty acids in the cell occurs primarily in the mitochondria by the process called β-oxidation.

Fatty acid utilization in various tissues varies according to physiological conditions. With rapid mobilization of fatty acids in adipose tissue causing an increase in the level of plasma nonesterifed fatty acids, fatty acid oxidation is high in muscle and liver during starvation. The converse is true in the fed state. During exercise, fatty acid oxidation in muscle also increases. Although circulating fatty acid levels during exercise may remain the same, delivery of fatty acids increases with higher blood flow. However, certain tissues do not use fatty acids as a fuel even when the circulating concentration is high. For example, fatty acid transport to the brain is limited by the blood–brain barrier, and red blood cells are not able to oxidize fatty acids because they lack mitochondria.

ROLE OF CARNITINE IN TRANSPORT OF ACYL GROUPS FROM CYTOSOL TO MITOCHONDRIA

Oxidation of fatty acids occurs mainly in the mitochondrial compartment, but neither nonesterified long-chain fatty acids nor their fatty acyl-CoA derivatives can diffuse across the inner mitochondrial membrane. Entry of the acyl groups is catalyzed by a "carnitine" cycle, as shown in Figure 16-10.

Acyl Group Translocation

On the outer mitochondrial membrane, an enzyme called carnitine palmitoyltransferase 1 (CPT1) catalyzes the transfer of long-chain acyl groups from CoA to carnitine.

$$\text{Fatty acyl-CoA} + \text{Carnitine} \leftrightarrow \text{Fatty acylcarnitine} + \text{CoA}$$

Carnitine–palmitoylcarnitine translocase catalyzes transport of the acylcarnitine across the impermeable inner mitochondrial membrane in exchange for free carnitine. On the inner surface of the inner mitochondrial membrane,

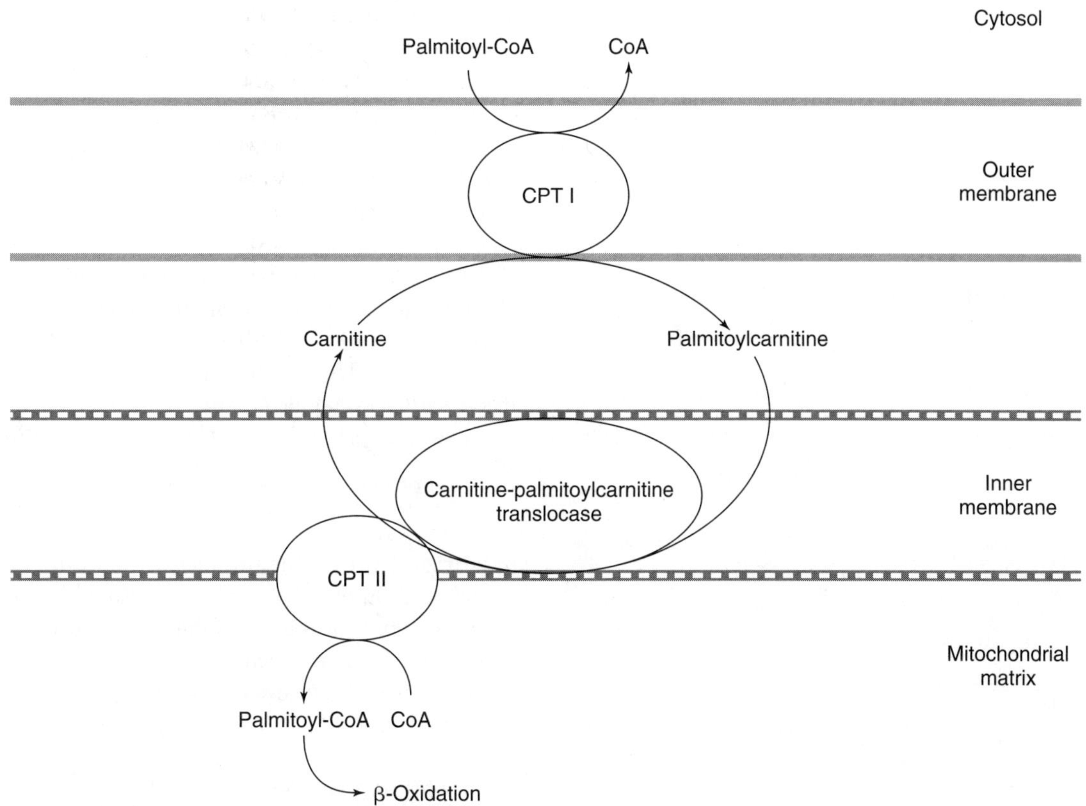

FIGURE 16-10 Transport of long-chain fatty acyl-CoA into mitochondria. *CPT,* Carnitine palmitoyl transferase.

carnitine palmitoyltransferase 2 (CPT2) catalyzes the reesterification of acylcarnitines to form acyl-CoA esters.

$$\text{Fatty acylcarnitine} + \text{CoA} \leftrightarrow \text{Fatty acyl-CoA} + \text{Carnitine}$$

The free carnitine is again available for exchange with acylcarnitine, allowing the process of fatty acid translocation to continue. Rapid oxidation of the fatty acyl-CoA in the β-oxidation pathway likely provides the driving force to keep everything moving in the same direction through these largely freely reversible reactions. Both saturated and unsaturated long-chain fatty acids are metabolized via this pathway.

Regulation of Fatty Acid Translocation

In the fed state, the rate of lipolysis in adipose tissue is low, and the concentration of plasma free fatty acids and hence their availability for β-oxidation in other tissues is also low. In liver, the rate of production of malonyl-CoA and its intracellular concentration are elevated in the fed state, because acetyl-CoA carboxylase, the key regulatory enzyme in de novo lipogenesis, is activated by insulin. Malonyl-CoA, by potently inhibiting CPT1, limits entry of fatty acyl-CoA into the mitochondrial compartment and consequently depresses β-oxidation. This reciprocal regulatory mechanism minimizes substrate (futile) cycling by ensuring that the opposing processes of β-oxidation and fatty acid biosynthesis are not activated simultaneously. As mentioned previously, in nonlipogenic tissues such as skeletal and cardiac muscle where the ACC2 form of acetyl-CoA carboxylase is expressed, malonyl-CoA functions mainly as an inhibitor of CPT1. With increasing AMP levels during exercise, phosphorylation and inhibition of acetyl-CoA carboxylase by AMPK will decrease malonyl-CoA production to increase fatty acid transport into the mitochondrial compartment for oxidation. In these tissues, malonyl-CoA is converted back to acetyl-CoA by a reaction catalyzed by malonyl-CoA decarboxylase (Saggerson, 2008) in order to tightly regulate malonyl-CoA concentration. (Although most fatty acids from the diet or endogenous synthesis are long-chain fatty acids, it should be noted that fatty acids shorter than 12 carbons do not require CPT activity for mitochondrial entry.)

MITOCHONDRIAL β-OXIDATION

The function of mitochondrial fatty acid oxidation is primarily to supply energy. Fatty acids are oxidized by a series of reactions that overall are the reverse of those catalyzed by fatty acid synthase. The two processes, however, are catalyzed by different enzymes, have different subcellular localizations, and have a number of chemical differences (Eaton, 2002). Instead of the condensation, reduction, dehydration, and reduction involved in fatty acid synthesis, the β-oxidation cycle involves oxidation, hydration, oxidation, and cleavage, catalyzed by four enzymes, as shown in Figure 16-11. The intermediates of β-oxidation, however, have not been detected in cells. It is probable that the product of one reaction is transferred directly to the next enzyme. In fact, several steps in β-oxidation are catalyzed by a multifunctional enzyme. β-Oxidation occurs in two-carbon increments, as with fatty acid synthesis.

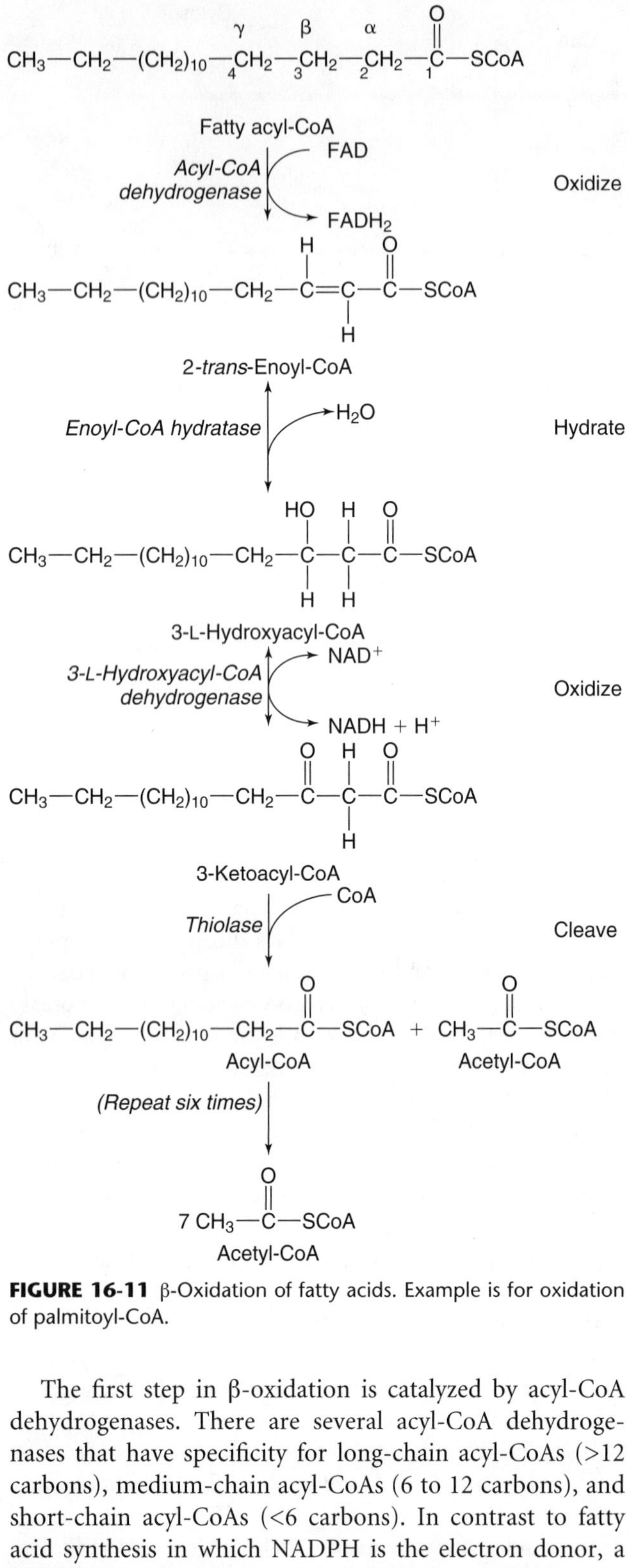

$CH_3—CH_2—(CH_2)_{10}—CH_2(\gamma, 4)—CH_2(\beta, 3)—CH_2(\alpha, 2)—C(=O)(1)—SCoA$

Fatty acyl-CoA

Acyl-CoA dehydrogenase (FAD → $FADH_2$) — Oxidize

$CH_3—CH_2—(CH_2)_{10}—CH_2—CH=CH—C(=O)—SCoA$

2-*trans*-Enoyl-CoA

Enoyl-CoA hydratase (H_2O) — Hydrate

$CH_3—CH_2—(CH_2)_{10}—CH_2—CH(OH)—CH_2—C(=O)—SCoA$

3-L-Hydroxyacyl-CoA

3-L-Hydroxyacyl-CoA dehydrogenase (NAD^+ → $NADH + H^+$) — Oxidize

$CH_3—CH_2—(CH_2)_{10}—CH_2—C(=O)—CH_2—C(=O)—SCoA$

3-Ketoacyl-CoA

Thiolase (CoA) — Cleave

$CH_3—CH_2—(CH_2)_{10}—CH_2—C(=O)—SCoA + CH_3—C(=O)—SCoA$

Acyl-CoA Acetyl-CoA

(Repeat six times)

$7\ CH_3—C(=O)—SCoA$

Acetyl-CoA

FIGURE 16-11 β-Oxidation of fatty acids. Example is for oxidation of palmitoyl-CoA.

The first step in β-oxidation is catalyzed by acyl-CoA dehydrogenases. There are several acyl-CoA dehydrogenases that have specificity for long-chain acyl-CoAs (>12 carbons), medium-chain acyl-CoAs (6 to 12 carbons), and short-chain acyl-CoAs (<6 carbons). In contrast to fatty acid synthesis in which NADPH is the electron donor, a tightly but noncovalently linked flavin adenine dinucleotide (FAD) is the electron acceptor in the first reaction of β-oxidation.

$$\text{Acyl-CoA} + \text{Enzyme-FAD} \rightarrow \text{2-}trans\text{-Enoyl-CoA} + \text{Enzyme-FADH}_2$$

FAD is used as the electron acceptor because the ΔG of this reaction is not sufficient to drive production of NADH. The $FADH_2$ generated in this first reaction of β-oxidation donates its electrons to the FAD prosthetic group of electron-transferring flavoprotein, which in turn transfers its electrons to ubiquinone in the electron transfer chain. Oxidation of each mole of $FADH_2$ generates a maximum of 2 moles of ATP. Separate acyl-CoA dehydrogenases encoded by different genes catalyze the oxidation of long-, medium-, and short-chain fatty acids.

The next three steps in β-oxidation are catalyzed by a mitochondrial trifunctional protein that has enoyl-CoA hydratase, 3-hydroxyacyl-CoA dehydrogenase, and 3-ketoacyl-CoA thiolase activities. The second step in β-oxidation is catalyzed by the enoyl-CoA hydratase activity and involves hydration of the *trans* double bond created by the first oxidation.

$$\text{2-}trans\text{-Enoyl-CoA} + H_2O \leftrightarrow \text{L-3-Hydroxyacyl-CoA}$$

Hydration of the double bond is stereospecific; L-3-hydroxyacyl-CoA is the product when a *trans* double bond is hydrated. Enoyl-CoA hydratase also hydrates *cis* double bonds; this produces the D-isomer of 3-hydroxyacyl-CoA.

In the third step, a dehydrogenase that is specific for the L-isomer of hydroxyacyl-CoA catalyzes a second oxidation step. NAD is the electron acceptor. Oxidation of each mole of NADH by the electron transport chain yields a maximum of 3 moles of ATP. (See Chapter 21, Figure 21-4, for reactions involved in transfer of electrons through the electron transport chain.)

$$\text{L-3-Hydroxyacyl-CoA} + \text{NAD} \leftrightarrow \text{3-Ketoacyl-CoA} + \text{NADH} + H^+$$

In the final step of each two-carbon cycle of β-oxidation, 3-ketoacyl-CoA thiolase (acetyl-CoA acyltransferase 2) catalyzes the thiolytic cleavage of the 3-ketoacyl-CoA to acetyl-CoA plus an acyl-CoA that is two carbons shorter.

$$\text{3-Ketoacyl-CoA} + \text{CoASH} \rightarrow \text{Acetyl-CoA} + \text{Acyl-CoA (n-2)}$$

DEFICIENCIES IN β-OXIDATION

Deficiencies in each of the enzymes in the β-oxidation pathway, including specific short-, medium-, and long-chain fatty acyl-CoA dehydrogenase deficiencies, cause disorders in metabolic adaptation during starvation owing to an impairment of fatty acid oxidation. The most common deficiency is that of medium-chain fatty acyl-CoA dehydrogenase, an inherited metabolic disorder (Scriver et al., 2004). Intermediates of fatty acid oxidation accumulate and result in increased levels of related plasma and urinary metabolites, especially during conditions such as fasting and infection when the rate of lipolysis is increased. Accumulation of some intermediates, such as dicarboxylic acids, is due to the metabolic block of fatty acid oxidation in general. Dicarboxylic acids can be formed by ω-oxidation of fatty acids, which is normally a minor pathway, converting $–CH_3$ group to first $–CH_2OH$ that subsequently is oxidized to –COOH. Accumulation of some others, such as *cis*-4-decanoic acid, phenylpropionylglycine, octanoyl carnitine, and *cis*-4-decenoylcarnitine, is unique to deficiency of medium-chain fatty acyl-CoA dehydrogenase.

CLINICAL CORRELATION

Defects in Fatty Acid Transport Into Mitochondria for Oxidation

Genetic disorders in any of the enzymes in the carnitine cycle, including carnitine palmitoyltransferases 1 and 2 (CPT1 and CPT2) and carnitine-acylcarnitine translocase (see Figure 16-10), block oxidation of long-chain fatty acids because of impaired transport of long-chain fatty acids into the mitochondrial matrix (Scriver et al., 2004). There are two tissue-specific isoforms of CPT1 encoded by separate genes: the liver form is expressed mainly in liver and kidney, and the muscle form is expressed in muscle and heart. Conversely, there appears to be only one form of CPT2.

Reported cases of CPT1 deficiency involve defects of liver metabolism: enlarged fatty livers, hypoketotic hypoglycemia, and possibly coma during fasting. Neither muscle weakness nor cardiomyopathy was associated with CPT1 deficiency. Although the molecular basis of CPT1 deficiency has not been elucidated, the finding that patients diagnosed with this genetic defect mainly have liver defects suggests that only the liver isoform of CPT1 is defective.

CPT2 deficiency can take two distinct clinical forms. Classical CPT2 deficiency in adults affects primarily fatty acid metabolism in skeletal and/or cardiac muscle. In these patients, long-chain acylcarnitine translocated across the inner mitochondrial membrane is not reconverted to acyl-CoAs. The accumulated long-chain acylcarnitine species are then transported from the mitochondria and into plasma. Under normal conditions, fuel metabolism is still adequate. During sustained exercise or starvation, however, in which fatty acid oxidation is important quantitatively, patients experience cramps and fatigue. Although the CPT2 deficiency primarily affects muscle, defects in CPT2 also occur in other tissues. The manifestation of a severe infantile form of CPT2 deficiency is hypoketotic hypoglycemia with cardiomyopathy; it is usually fatal. In the adult-onset form, there is a partial deficiency of CPT2 activity. In the more severe infantile form, CPT2 activity is less than 10% of normal. CPT2 in a patient with an infantile form of the disease was shown to have an arginine-to-cysteine substitution at amino acid residue 631; this variant CPT2 has decreased CPT2 activity.

Carnitine deficiency causes a similar impairment of fatty acid oxidation, but fatty acid oxidation in this case can be restored by administering carnitine. Carnitine in the diet is absorbed in the intestine. In addition, human tissues can synthesize carnitine de novo, mostly in liver and kidney. Endogenous synthesis normally meets the metabolic need, provided the diet contains sufficient lysine and methionine (precursors) and ascorbic acid, vitamin B_6, niacin, and iron (cofactors) for the biosynthesis. (Synthesis of carnitine is discussed in Chapter 27 and outlined in Figure 27-11.) Carnitine deficiency is rare in adults. However, patients undergoing kidney dialysis or those with organic aciduria may lose large amounts of carnitine; they and patients receiving long-term parenteral nutrition may exhibit carnitine deficiency. Carnitine deficiency also may occur in neonates, particularly in premature infants.

Thinking Critically

1. Why does hypoketotic hypoglycemia occur in CPT1 deficiency?
2. What dietary recommendations would you make for patients with CPT1 or CPT2 deficiency?
3. Why are the symptoms of CPT1 and CPT2 deficiencies more severe during starvation?
4. What changes in plasma carnitine and acylcarnitine levels could be used to distinguish between CPT1 and CPT2 deficiencies?

Carnitine supplementation has been used to treat patients with medium-chain acyl-CoA dehydrogenase deficiency. Although the supplementation does not correct the underlying defect, it may help remove potentially toxic acyl-CoA intermediates by promoting formation of acylcarnitines. In patients with this deficiency, nonketotic hypoglycemia can be provoked by fasting during the first two years of life. Avoidance of fasting and administration of glucose in acute episodes of hypoglycemia are recommended. Deficiencies in enzymes of β-oxidation cause muscle weakness and hypoglycemia, as does a deficiency in CPT2.

PEROXISOMAL β-OXIDATION

Peroxisomes also carry out β-oxidation, and some fatty acids, including very-long-chain fatty acids, are preferentially oxidized in peroxisomes. However, β-oxidation of very-long-chain fatty acids in peroxisomes generally does not proceed past reduction of acyl-CoA to octanoyl-CoA. Further oxidation of octanoyl-CoA to acetyl-CoA occurs in the mitochondria. Peroxisomes do not contain an energy-coupled electron transport system to generate ATP but use flavin oxidases and release energy as heat.

Fatty acid oxidation can be increased upon treatment with synthetic ligands of lipid-activated peroxisomal proliferator–activated receptors (PPARs), which belong to the nuclear hormone receptor family. Physiological ligands may include certain fatty acids or eicosanoids. PPAR ligands not only induce the expression of some of the enzymes in peroxisomal β-oxidation, including acyl-CoA oxidase that catalyzes the first step in peroxisomal fatty acid oxidation, but also cause the proliferation of peroxisomes in the liver of rodents. As discussed in subsequent text of this chapter, diagnosis of peroxisome defects such as Zellweger syndrome can be based on measurement of the concentrations of very-long-chain fatty acids (Wanders et al., 2010).

ENERGY YIELD FROM β-OXIDATION OF PALMITATE

For each cycle of β-oxidation—oxidation, hydration, oxidation, and cleavage—an acyl-CoA is shortened by two carbons, and one molecule each of $FADH_2$, NADH, hydrogen ion, and acetyl-CoA are produced. Therefore, for the oxidation of palmitate, which requires seven cycles of β-oxidation, the balanced equation is:

$$\text{Palmitoyl-CoA} + 7\ \text{CoASH} + 7\ \text{FAD} + 7\ \text{NAD}^+ + 7\ H_2O \rightarrow 8\ \text{Acetyl-CoA} + 7\ \text{FADH}_2 + 7\ \text{NADH} + 7\ H^+$$

Each $FADH_2$ yields a maximum of 2 ATPs as it passes its electrons down the electron transport chain; each NADH yields a maximum of 3 ATPs. Therefore oxidation of palmitoyl-CoA as shown in the preceding equation yields a maximum of 35 ATPs. As noted in Chapter 12, the complete oxidation of acetyl-CoA to CO_2, H_2O, and CoA yields a maximum of 12 ATPs. In sum, the complete oxidation of palmitoyl-CoA yields 131 ATPs. Two high-energy bonds are used up in the activation of palmitate to palmitoyl-CoA because ATP is split into AMP and PP_i, which is further hydrolyzed to $2P_i$. The complete oxidation of palmitate to CO_2 and H_2O thus yields a net maximum of 129 moles of ATP per mole of palmitate.

Living cells are remarkably efficient at capturing the energy available in foodstuffs. The standard free energy for the complete oxidation of palmitate is about 9,800 kJ/mol (2,344 kcal/mol). The standard free energy for the hydrolysis of ATP is 30.5 kJ/mol (7.3 kcal/mol). Therefore palmitate oxidation in the living cell, if it were under standard conditions (1 atm pressure, 1 mol/L concentration of substrates), would conserve a maximum of 129 × 30.5, or 3,935 kJ/mol (940 kcal/mol) in ATP. This represents a very respectable efficiency of approximately 40%. However, if the free energy changes are calculated under the conditions that exist in vivo, the energy conservation is actually closer to 80%.

ADDITIONAL REACTIONS REQUIRED FOR β-OXIDATION OF UNSATURATED FATTY ACIDS

Unsaturated fatty acids are abundant in nature and are also degraded via β-oxidation. Most of the double bonds in natural monounsaturated and polyunsaturated fatty acids are in the *cis* configuration. For the purpose of this discussion, it is convenient to place these fatty acids into two classes: ones with double bonds that extend from odd-numbered (e.g., Δ9 of oleic acid or Δ9 of linoleic acid) and ones with double bonds that extend from even-numbered (e.g., Δ12 of linoleic acid) carbons in the fatty acid chain. Neither of these double bonds is a natural intermediate in β-oxidation, so auxiliary enzymes must rearrange the double bonds to permit complete oxidation. The simplest of these rearrangements involves double bonds extending from odd-numbered carbons, as is summarized in Figure 16-12. Oleoyl-CoA (9-*cis*-octadecenoyl-CoA) undergoes three rounds of β-oxidation to form 3-*cis*-dodecenoyl-CoA. This intermediate is not a substrate for either of the dehydrogenases or enoyl-CoA hydratase. This problem is circumvented by isomerization of the double bond to yield 2-*trans*-dodecenoyl-CoA. The auxiliary enzyme that catalyzes this reaction is 3-*cis*,2-*trans*-enoyl-CoA isomerase (enoyl-CoA isomerase); this enzyme also isomerizes 3-*trans*-enoyl-CoA to its 2-*trans*-enoyl-CoA isomer. This reaction allows β-oxidation to continue, but in the fourth cycle of β-oxidation, the first dehydrogenase step catalyzed by acyl-CoA dehydrogenase is omitted. Therefore complete oxidation of oleate (18:1) yields 1 less $FADH_2$—or 2 less ATPs—than complete oxidation of stearate (18:0).

The oxidation of linoleate, as summarized in Figure 16-13, proceeds like that of oleate, including the isomerase step just described, for four cycles plus the first dehydrogenase reaction of the fifth cycle. At this point the product is 2-*trans*,4-*cis*-decadienoyl-CoA. This intermediate is not a substrate for the enoyl-CoA hydratase or for the β-hydroxyacyl-CoA dehydrogenase. This potential block to β-oxidation is circumvented by two reactions catalyzed by auxiliary enzymes. First, 2-*trans*,4-*cis*-decadienoyl-CoA is reduced to 3-*trans*-decenoyl-CoA. This reaction utilizes NADPH as the electron donor and is catalyzed by 2,4-dienoyl-CoA reductase. The product of this reaction, 3-*trans*-decenoyl-CoA, is not a substrate for the enzymes of β-oxidation and must be isomerized to 2-*trans*-decenoyl-CoA, which is a substrate for the enoyl-CoA hydratase. The isomerization of 3-*trans*-enoyl-CoA to its 2-*trans*-enoyl-CoA is catalyzed by 3-*cis*,2-*trans*-enoyl-CoA isomerase. β-Oxidation then continues to complete the fifth cycle and three more complete cycles as shown in Figure 16-13. In the oxidation of linoleate, one $FADH_2$ (2 ATPs) is lost in the third cycle, as with oleate. The fifth cycle utilizes both dehydrogenases, generating both $FADH_2$ and NADH. However, the utilization of 1 NADPH balances the production of 1 NADH, meaning that 3 potential ATPs are lost. Overall then, the complete oxidation of linoleate (18:2) generates 5 less ATPs than that of stearate (18:0).

Although most naturally occurring unsaturated fatty acids contain *cis* double bonds, small amounts of *trans* fatty acids with conjugated double bonds are found in cow's milk fat. During hydrogenation of polyunsaturated fatty acids by rumen microorganisms, the double bonds are isomerized from the *cis* to the *trans* configuration. In the chemical process of hydrogenation used in the manufacture of margarine and other hydrogenated vegetable fats, considerable amounts of *trans* fatty acids are introduced. Although they have a lower affinity for isomerases than *cis* fatty acids, *trans* fatty acids are substrates for the enoyl-CoA isomerases. Dietary *trans* fatty acids produced by the chemical hydrogenation of polyunsaturated fatty acids seem to have effects similar to, or potentially worse than, saturated fatty acids in promoting atherosclerosis. (See Chapter 17 for a discussion of dietary fat and cardiovascular disease.)

β-OXIDATION OF FATTY ACIDS WITH AN ODD NUMBER OF CARBONS OR WITH METHYL SIDE CHAINS TO GENERATE PROPIONYL-CoA

Fatty acids of odd-chain length are not synthesized in animals and therefore are not commonly found in meat. However, small amounts of odd-chain fatty acids are found in vegetables. The β-oxidation of straight-chain fatty acids containing an odd number of carbons requires three auxiliary enzymes, as shown in Figure 16-14. Oxidation proceeds as described in the preceding text for other saturated fatty acids until the last step of the last cycle, producing $FADH_2$,

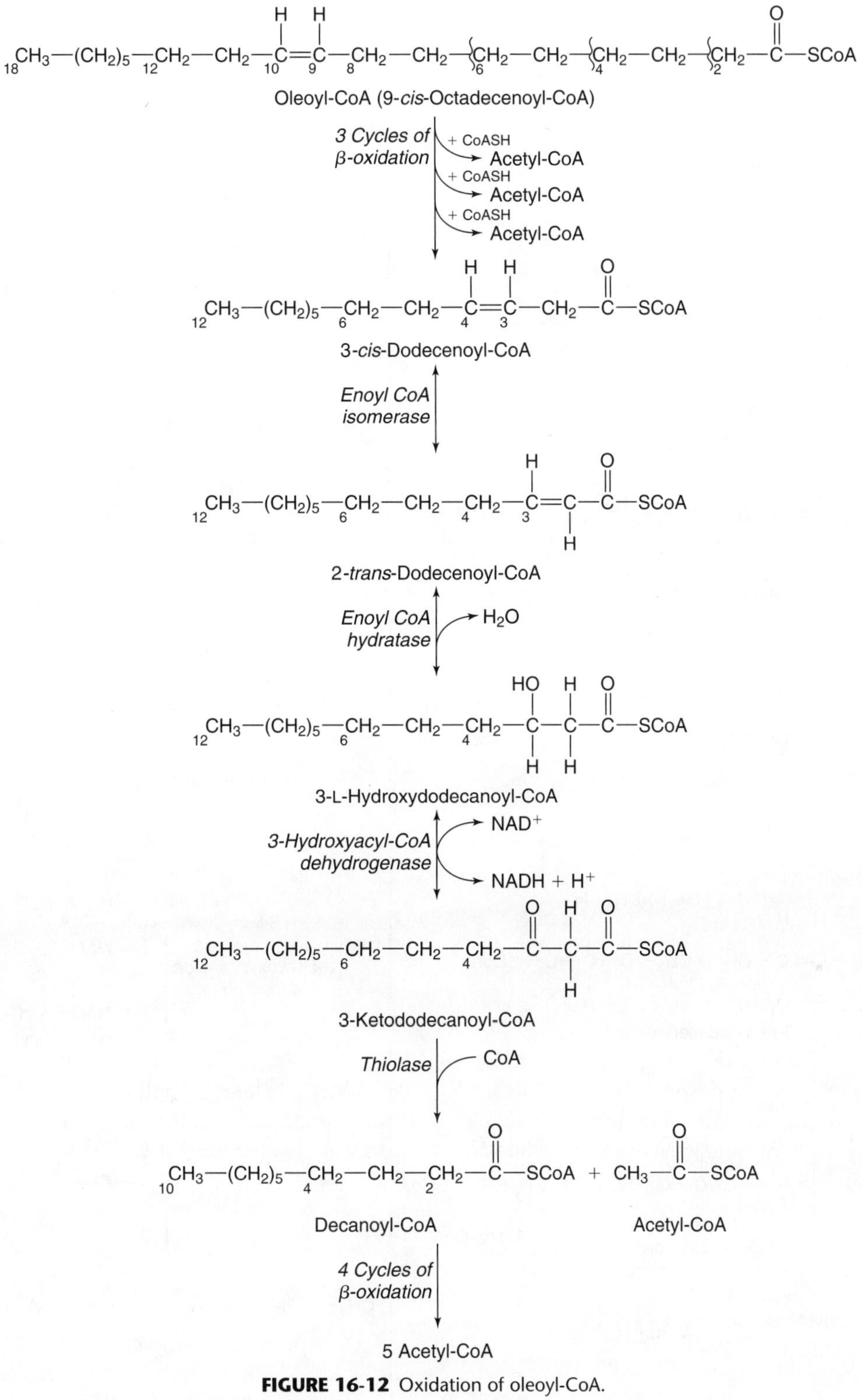

$$\overset{18}{CH_3}-(CH_2)_5-\overset{12}{CH_2}-CH_2-\overset{10}{CH}=\overset{9}{CH}-\overset{8}{CH_2}-CH_2-\overset{6}{CH_2}-CH_2-\overset{4}{CH_2}-CH_2-\overset{2}{CH_2}-\overset{O}{\overset{\|}{C}}-SCoA$$

Oleoyl-CoA (9-*cis*-Octadecenoyl-CoA)

3 Cycles of β-oxidation (+ CoASH → Acetyl-CoA; + CoASH → Acetyl-CoA; + CoASH → Acetyl-CoA)

$$\overset{12}{CH_3}-(CH_2)_5-\overset{6}{CH_2}-CH_2-\overset{4}{CH}=\overset{3}{CH}-CH_2-\overset{O}{\overset{\|}{C}}-SCoA$$

3-*cis*-Dodecenoyl-CoA

Enoyl CoA isomerase

$$\overset{12}{CH_3}-(CH_2)_5-\overset{6}{CH_2}-CH_2-\overset{4}{CH_2}-\overset{3}{CH}=CH-\overset{O}{\overset{\|}{C}}-SCoA$$

2-*trans*-Dodecenoyl-CoA

Enoyl CoA hydratase (H_2O)

$$\overset{12}{CH_3}-(CH_2)_5-\overset{6}{CH_2}-CH_2-\overset{4}{CH_2}-\overset{HO}{\overset{|}{C}}H-CH_2-\overset{O}{\overset{\|}{C}}-SCoA$$

3-L-Hydroxydodecanoyl-CoA

3-Hydroxyacyl-CoA dehydrogenase (NAD^+ → $NADH + H^+$)

$$\overset{12}{CH_3}-(CH_2)_5-\overset{6}{CH_2}-CH_2-\overset{4}{CH_2}-\overset{O}{\overset{\|}{C}}-CH_2-\overset{O}{\overset{\|}{C}}-SCoA$$

3-Ketododecanoyl-CoA

Thiolase (CoA)

$$\overset{10}{CH_3}-(CH_2)_5-\overset{4}{CH_2}-CH_2-\overset{2}{CH_2}-\overset{O}{\overset{\|}{C}}-SCoA + CH_3-\overset{O}{\overset{\|}{C}}-SCoA$$

Decanoyl-CoA Acetyl-CoA

4 Cycles of β-oxidation

5 Acetyl-CoA

FIGURE 16-12 Oxidation of oleoyl-CoA.

NADH, and acetyl-CoA in each cycle. However, the product of the final cleavage reaction is 1 acetyl-CoA and 1 propionyl-CoA instead of 2 acetyl-CoA molecules. Propionyl-CoA is more abundantly generated by metabolism of certain amino acids (valine, isoleucine, threonine, and methionine), as described in Chapter 14, than by fatty acid oxidation. Propionyl-CoA is carboxylated to D-methylmalonyl-CoA in an ATP-dependent reaction catalyzed by propionyl-CoA carboxylase. The reaction mechanism is similar to that for acetyl-CoA carboxylase. The enzyme methylmalonyl-CoA racemase catalyzes the isomerization of the D-isomer to the L-isomer, and L-methylmalonyl-CoA is isomerized to succinyl-CoA in a reaction catalyzed by methylmalonyl-CoA mutase. Succinyl-CoA is an intermediate in the citric acid cycle. Unlike acetyl-CoA, which is the final product of β-oxidation of fatty acids containing an even number of

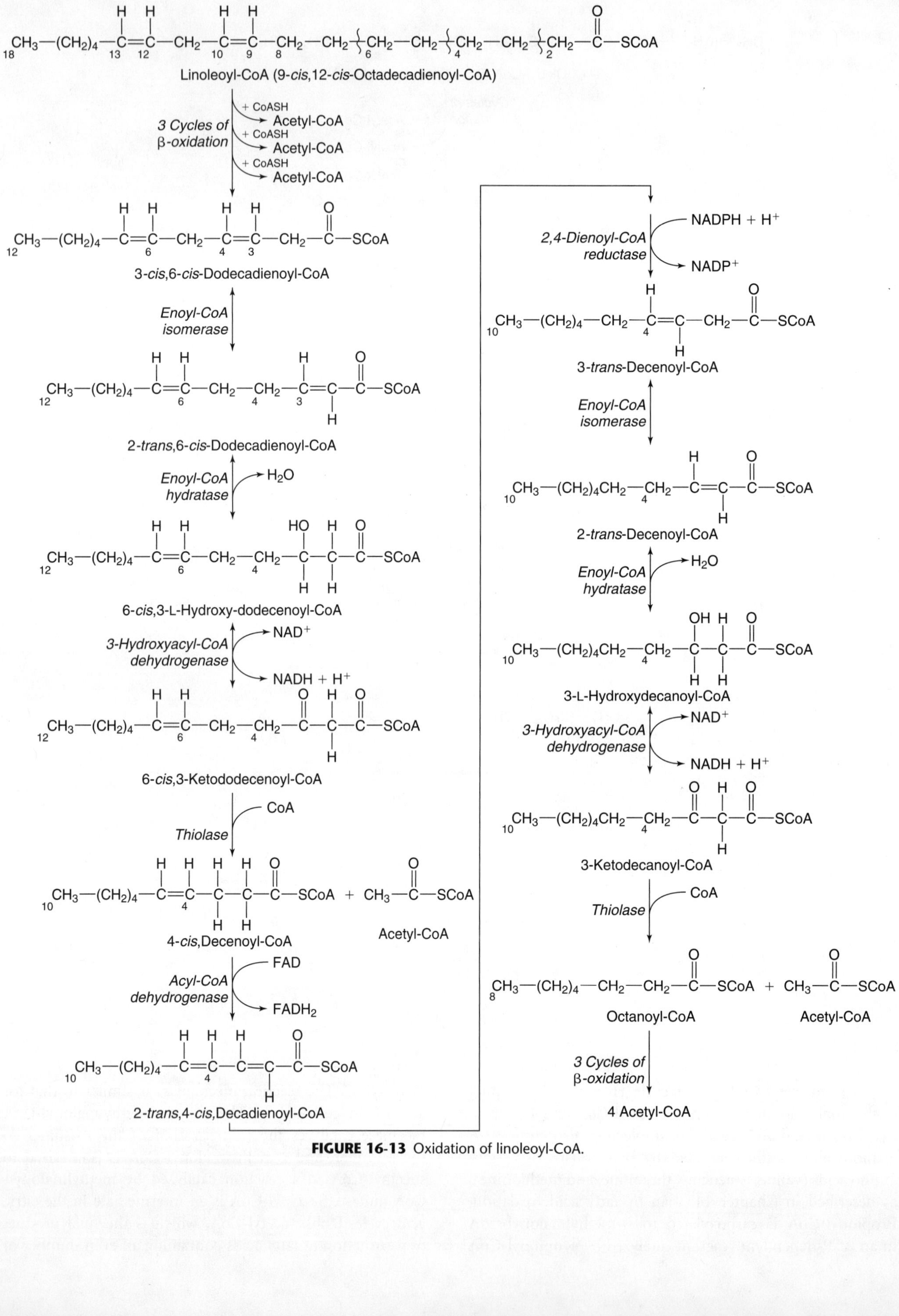

Linoleoyl-CoA (9-*cis*,12-*cis*-Octadecadienoyl-CoA)

3 Cycles of β-oxidation (+ CoASH → Acetyl-CoA; + CoASH → Acetyl-CoA; + CoASH → Acetyl-CoA)

3-*cis*,6-*cis*-Dodecadienoyl-CoA

Enoyl-CoA isomerase

2-*trans*,6-*cis*-Dodecadienoyl-CoA

Enoyl-CoA hydratase (H_2O)

6-*cis*,3-L-Hydroxy-dodecenoyl-CoA

3-Hydroxyacyl-CoA dehydrogenase (NAD^+ → $NADH + H^+$)

6-*cis*,3-Ketododecenoyl-CoA

Thiolase (CoA)

4-*cis*,Decenoyl-CoA + Acetyl-CoA

Acyl-CoA dehydrogenase (FAD → $FADH_2$)

2-*trans*,4-*cis*,Decadienoyl-CoA

2,4-Dienoyl-CoA reductase ($NADPH + H^+$ → $NADP^+$)

3-*trans*-Decenoyl-CoA

Enoyl-CoA isomerase

2-*trans*-Decenoyl-CoA

Enoyl-CoA hydratase (H_2O)

3-L-Hydroxydecanoyl-CoA

3-Hydroxyacyl-CoA dehydrogenase (NAD^+ → $NADH + H^+$)

3-Ketodecanoyl-CoA

Thiolase (CoA)

Octanoyl-CoA + Acetyl-CoA

3 Cycles of β-oxidation

4 Acetyl-CoA

FIGURE 16-13 Oxidation of linoleoyl-CoA.

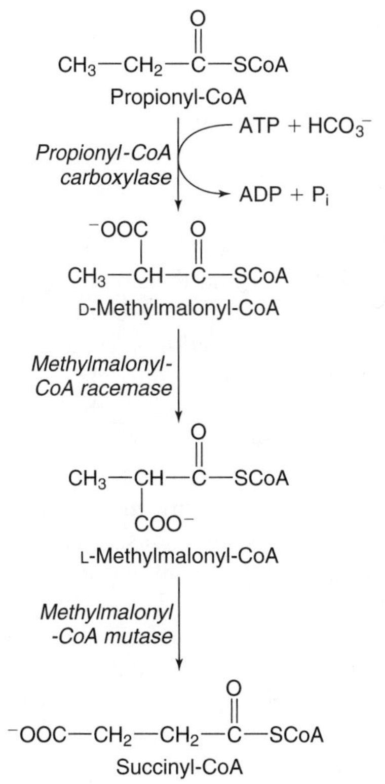

$CH_3—CH_2—C(=O)—SCoA$
Propionyl-CoA
Propionyl-CoA carboxylase
ATP + HCO_3^-
ADP + P_i
$^-OOC—CH(CH_3)—C(=O)—SCoA$
D-Methylmalonyl-CoA
Methylmalonyl-CoA racemase
$CH_3—CH(COO^-)—C(=O)—SCoA$
L-Methylmalonyl-CoA
Methylmalonyl-CoA mutase
$^-OOC—CH_2—CH_2—C(=O)—SCoA$
Succinyl-CoA

FIGURE 16-14 Propionate metabolism.

carbons, succinyl-CoA can be converted to phosphoenolpyruvate and hence to glucose. Therefore fatty acids with an odd number of carbons, especially propionic acid, can be considered gluconeogenic. Methylmalonyl-CoA mutase requires deoxyadenosylcobalamin, a derivative of vitamin B_{12}, as a cofactor. Individuals who are deficient in vitamin B_{12} have impaired conversion of methylmalonyl-CoA to succinyl-CoA and excrete methylmalonate in their urine.

Odd- or even-numbered fatty acids that contain methyl side chains are oxidized by the usual β-oxidation scheme. A methyl side chain on the carbon does not interfere with β-oxidation. The products of the thiolytic cleavage are propionyl-CoA and chain-shortened acyl-CoA. The latter continues through additional cycles of β-oxidation, and the propionyl-CoA is metabolized to succinyl-CoA.

FORMATION OF KETONE BODIES FROM ACETYL-CoA IN THE LIVER AS A FUEL FOR EXTRAHEPATIC TISSUES

In muscle and other nonhepatic tissues in any nutritional state, and in the liver in the well-fed state, acetyl-CoA formed during the β-oxidation of fatty acids is oxidized to CO_2 and H_2O in the citric acid cycle. When the rate of mobilization of fatty acids from adipose depots is accelerated, as for example during starvation, the liver converts acetyl-CoA generated from fatty acid oxidation into ketone bodies: acetoacetate and 3-hydroxybutyrate. The rate of formation of ketone bodies is directly proportional to the rate of fatty acid β-oxidation. Therefore when the rate of mobilization of fatty acids from adipose tissue is high, hepatic oxidation of fatty acids with production of acetoacetate and 3-hydroxybutyrate is high. Ketone bodies are "water-soluble" metabolites of fatty acids that are readily transported to other organs for oxidation to CO_2 and H_2O.

SYNTHESIS OF ACETOACETATE AND 3-HYDROXYBUTYRATE IN LIVER MITOCHONDRIA

Ketone bodies are synthesized in mitochondria. This is important because production of acetyl-CoA, the substrate for synthesis of ketone bodies, occurs in the mitochondria via β-oxidation of fatty acids. Furthermore, initial steps for the de novo synthesis of cholesterol use some of the same reactions, but the enzymes for synthesis of cholesterol precursors are present in the cytosol of the liver as discussed in Chapter 17. Differential localization permits independent regulation of ketone body production and cholesterol synthesis.

The first step in ketone body synthesis is condensation of two molecules of acetyl-CoA to form acetoacetyl-CoA (Figure 16-15). This reaction is catalyzed by the reversible acetoacetyl-CoA thiolase.

$$\text{Acetyl-CoA} + \text{Acetyl-CoA} \leftrightarrow \text{Acetoacetyl-CoA} + \text{CoA}$$

The second step involves condensation of a third molecule of acetyl-CoA with acetoacetyl-CoA to form 3-hydroxy-3-methylglutaryl-CoA (HMG-CoA). This reaction is catalyzed by HMG-CoA synthase.

$$\text{Acetyl-CoA} + \text{Acetoacetyl-CoA} \rightarrow \text{3-Hydroxy-3-methylglutaryl-CoA} + \text{CoA}$$

In the third step of ketone body synthesis, HMG-CoA is cleaved to acetoacetate and acetyl-CoA in a reaction catalyzed by HMG-CoA lyase.

$$\text{3-Hydroxy-3-methylglutaryl-CoA} \rightarrow \text{Acetoacetate} + \text{Acetyl-CoA}$$

Both acetoacetate and 3-hydroxybutyrate are considered ketone bodies because they are rapidly interconverted via a reaction catalyzed by 3-hydroxybutyrate dehydrogenase. This NAD-requiring enzyme catalyzes a reversible reaction in which the concentrations of the products are nearly in thermodynamic equilibrium with NAD^+ and NADH in the mitochondria. Both acetoacetate and 3-hydroxybutyrate circulate in the blood. The ratio of their concentrations reflects the molar ratio of NAD to NADH in liver mitochondria.

$$\text{Acetoacetate} + \text{NADH} + \text{H}^+ \leftrightarrow \text{3-Hydroxybutyrate} + \text{NAD}^+$$

Of the two "ketone bodies," only one is a keto compound. So, how did these compounds become known as ketone bodies? Acetoacetate spontaneously undergoes decarboxylation to form acetone in the blood. When the plasma concentration of ketone bodies is very high—as in untreated diabetics—sufficient acetone accumulates in the blood to be detectable by breath odor. This led early investigators to give the name "ketone bodies" to the chemically uncharacterized material that accumulated in the blood of diabetics. The name has been retained even though we now know that acetone is only a minor component and 3-hydroxybutyrate, a non-keto compound, is the major component.

OXIDATION OF KETONE BODIES IN EXTRAHEPATIC TISSUES

The liver produces ketone bodies, but it cannot utilize them because it lacks the mitochondrial enzyme, succinyl-CoA:3-keto acid (3-oxoacid) CoA transferase, required for activation of acetoacetate to acetoacetyl-CoA. This results in the net flow of ketone bodies from the liver to extrahepatic tissues for use as a fuel. The plasma concentration of fatty acids (albumin-bound) can increase from approximately 0.5 mmol/L in the fed state to 2 mmol/L in the fasting state. During prolonged starvation, plasma glucose concentration can decrease from 5.5 mmol/L to 3.5 mmol/L. The plasma concentration of ketone bodies is about 0.01 mmol/L in the fed state and 0.1 mmol/L after an overnight fast, but the concentration of ketone bodies can reach 2 mmol/L after 3 days of starvation or more than 5 mmol/L after a week of starvation. At these increased concentrations, ketone bodies become significant fuels. In extrahepatic tissues such as muscle, ketone bodies are an important source of energy, especially when fatty acid mobilization has been activated. The brain also requires a large and constant source of energy. In the fed state, the brain depends exclusively on glucose for energy, because the blood–brain barrier limits uptake of long-chain fatty acids and the circulating level of ketone bodies is low in the fed individual. During starvation, however, ketone body concentration is elevated in the plasma and acetoacetate and 3-hydroxybutyrate become important energy sources for the brain, sparing the limited sources of glucose. In untreated type 1 diabetes mellitus, ketosis (i.e., ketonemia and ketonuria) can occur. Because acetoacetic and 3-hydroxybutyric acids are moderately strong acids, ketonuria causes loss of sodium ions, metabolic acidosis, and severe dehydration and can result in coma and death.

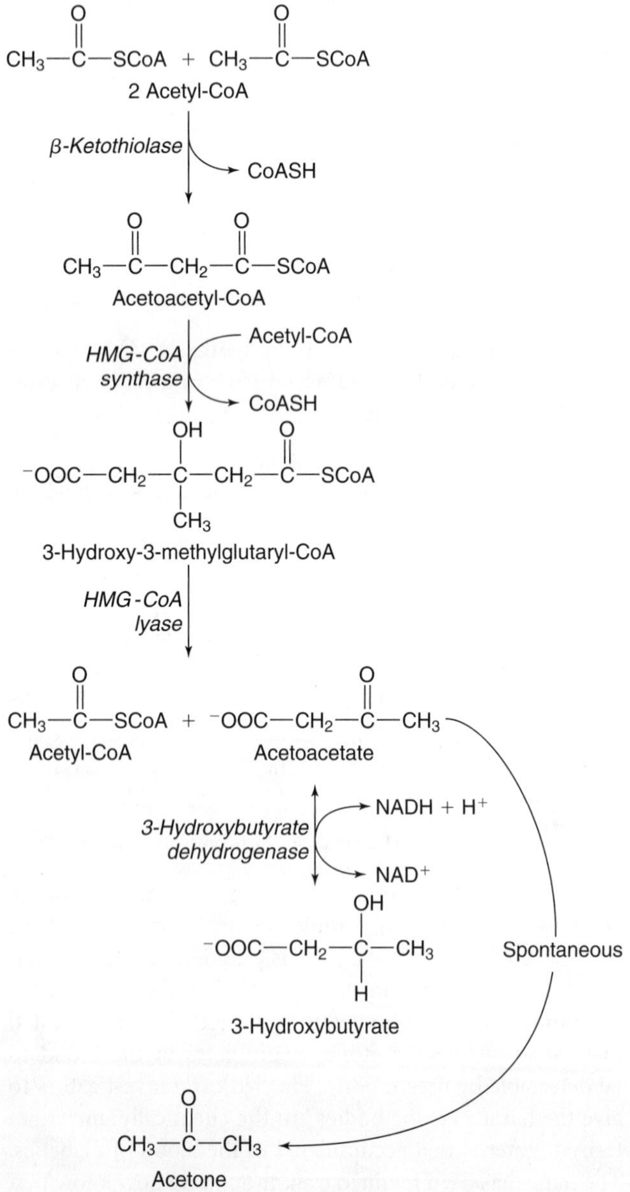

Both 3-hydroxybutyrate and acetoacetate diffuse into extrahepatic tissues along their concentration gradients. The rates of their metabolism are related directly to their concentrations in the blood, which, in turn, are proportional to the rate of release of fatty acids from adipose tissue. The reaction pathway is shown in Figure 16-16.

3-Hydroxybutyrate must be converted to acetoacetate before it can be used. The same enzyme that catalyzes interconversion of 3-hydroxybutyrate and acetoacetate in liver, 3-hydroxybutyrate dehydrogenase, also does so in extrahepatic tissues. In extrahepatic tissues, acetoacetate is activated to acetoacetyl-CoA in a reaction catalyzed by succinyl-CoA:3-keto acid CoA transferase.

Acetoacetate + Succinyl-CoA → Acetoacetyl-CoA + Succinate

Acetoacetyl-CoA is then cleaved to two molecules of acetyl-CoA by the action of acetoacetyl-CoA thiolase.

Acetoacetyl-CoA ↔ 2 Acetyl-CoA

The reactions of ketone body metabolism are localized in mitochondria, so that the acetyl-CoA that is formed enters the citric acid cycle and is oxidized to CO_2 and water.

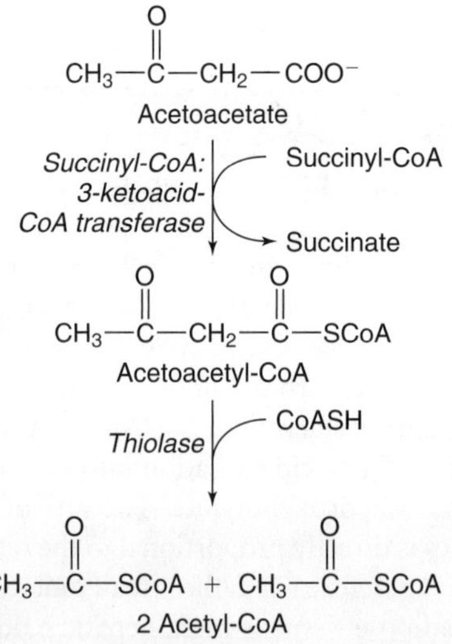

FIGURE 16-15 Ketone body formation.

FIGURE 16-16 Ketone body metabolism.

ENERGY YIELD FROM OXIDATION OF PALMITATE VIA THE KETONE BODY PATHWAY

Conversion of acetyl-CoA to ketone bodies before further oxidation is associated with some additional energy cost beyond direct use of acetyl-CoA by the tissue, but ketone body synthesis allows the acetyl units to be used as fuel by extrahepatic tissues instead of the liver. Oxidation of palmitoyl-CoA to acetyl-CoA in the liver yields 8 acetyl-CoA, 7 $FADH_2$, and 7 NADH and therefore a maximum of 35 moles of ATP per mole of palmitoyl-CoA—as described for β-oxidation previously in this chapter. An additional 96 moles of ATP can be generated from the oxidation of the 8 moles of acetyl-CoA generated from the ketone bodies in the mitochondria of extrahepatic tissues (i.e., by the citric acid cycle and oxidative phosphorylation). However, ketone body utilization in extrahepatic tissues requires additional energy expenditure because the conversion of acetoacetate to 2 acetyl-CoAs utilizes the equivalent of 1 ATP (succinate + CoA + GTP → succinyl-CoA + GDP + P_i). The acetoacetyl-CoA thiolase–catalyzed synthesis of 2 acetyl-CoAs from 1 acetoacetyl-CoA utilizes the energy released in the cleavage of the four-carbon ketone body to drive synthesis of the second molecule of CoA derivative. The NADH used to reduce acetoacetate to 3-hydroxybutyrate in the liver is recovered in the extrahepatic organs when the 3-hydroxybutyrate is converted back to acetoacetate via the same reaction. Thus the net result is utilization of 1 mole of ATP per mole of ketone body. Because there are 4 molecules of acetoacetyl group per molecule of palmitoyl-CoA, oxidation of palmitoyl-CoA via ketone body formation costs 4 moles of ATP per mole of palmitoyl-CoA, resulting in the net production of a maximum of 127 moles of ATP instead of 131 moles of ATP per mole of palmitoyl-CoA oxidized (or 125 instead of 129 moles per mole of palmitate oxidized).

Why has this apparently wasteful pathway of ketone body formation been preserved during evolution? A simple explanation is that the brain cannot metabolize fatty acids and therefore needs ketone bodies as a fuel during prolonged starvation. Moreover, by generating ketone bodies, the liver does not completely use the energy derived from fatty acids but distributes it as ketone bodies for other tissues to use during metabolic adaptation to starvation or stress (or other dietary conditions, such as high protein/low carbohydrate diets, that cause production and utilization of ketone bodies).

PHOSPHATIDIC ACID AND DIACYLGLYCEROL AS PRECURSORS OF THE COMMON PHOSPHOLIPIDS

Glycerophospholipids are a diverse class of amphipathic lipids that are also commonly described as phospholipids or phosphoglycerides. The common phospholipids are the diacylphospholipids, which contain acyl groups esterified to the *sn*-1 and *sn*-2 positions of the glycerol moiety and an alcohol linked to the phosphate in the *sn*-3 position by a phosphodiester bond. The amphipathic nature of phospholipids makes them suitable for their roles as components of membranes and as surfactants. In eukaryotic phospholipids, the most common alcohols are choline, ethanolamine, serine, glycerol, and inositol. The number of different molecular species of phospholipids is enormous because the long-chain fatty acyl groups in the *sn*-1 or *sn*-2 positions vary in length and degree of unsaturation. Synthesis of triacylglycerols and phospholipids follows a common pathway up to the phosphatidic acid or diacylglycerol stage (see Figure 16-7). In this section, the reactions that occur in higher animals are described (Vance and Vance, 2008). Most of the reactions occur in the ER, as do those of triacylglycerol biosynthesis.

SYNTHESIS OF PHOSPHATIDYLCHOLINE

Phosphatidylcholine (lecithin) is the most abundant phospholipid in eukaryotic cells. It may be synthesized using choline as a substrate or by methylation of the ethanolamine moiety of phosphatidyl ethanolamine.

Choline Kinase Pathway

The synthesis of phosphatidyl choline using choline and diacylglycerol as substrates is shown in Figure 16-17.

Choline from the diet is phosphorylated to phosphocholine by choline kinase. Choline kinase also uses ethanolamine

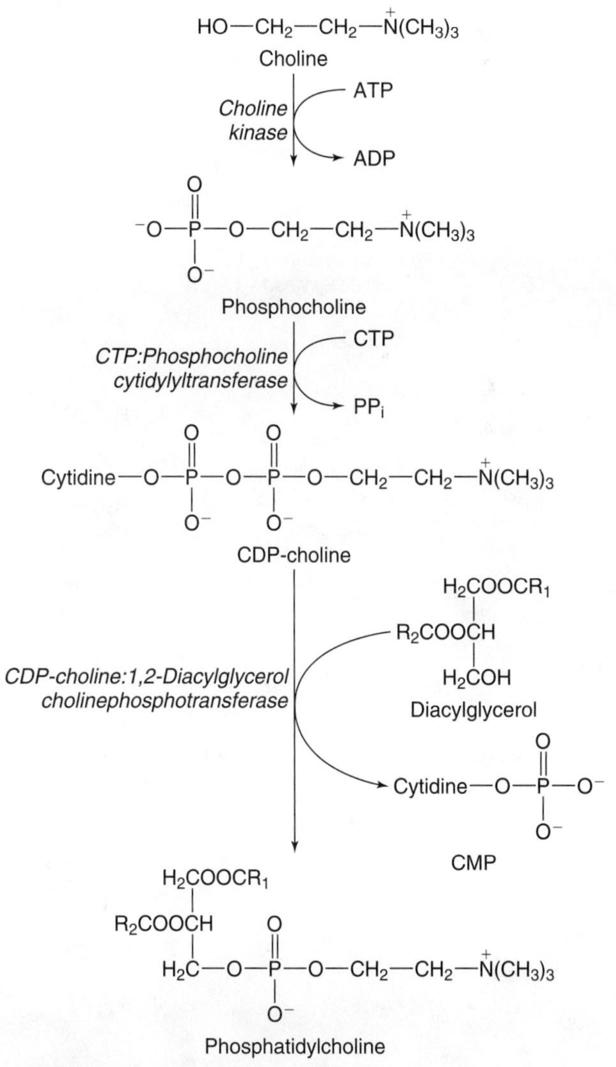

$HO—CH_2—CH_2—\overset{+}{N}(CH_3)_3$
Choline
Choline kinase (ATP → ADP)
$^{-}O—P(=O)(O^{-})—O—CH_2—CH_2—\overset{+}{N}(CH_3)_3$
Phosphocholine
CTP:Phosphocholine cytidylyltransferase (CTP → PP_i)
$Cytidine—O—P(=O)(O^{-})—O—P(=O)(O^{-})—O—CH_2—CH_2—\overset{+}{N}(CH_3)_3$
CDP-choline
CDP-choline:1,2-Diacylglycerol cholinephosphotransferase (H_2COOCR_1 / R_2COOCH / H_2COH Diacylglycerol → $Cytidine—O—P(=O)(O^{-})—O^{-}$ CMP)
H_2COOCR_1 / R_2COOCH / $H_2C—O—P(=O)(O^{-})—O—CH_2—CH_2—\overset{+}{N}(CH_3)_3$
Phosphatidylcholine

FIGURE 16-17 Phosphatidylcholine synthesis from choline and diacylglycerol. $R_1COO–$ and $R_2COO–$ represent fatty acids esterified to the glycerol backbone.

as a substrate. This lack of substrate specificity suggests that it is not a regulatory step but may serve as a means of trapping choline inside the cell.

$$\text{Choline} + \text{ATP} \rightarrow \text{Phosphocholine} + \text{ADP}$$

Phosphocholine then reacts with cytidine triphosphate (CTP) to yield the activated form of choline, cytidine diphosphate (CDP)–choline and pyrophosphate. The enzyme CTP:phosphocholine cytidylyltransferase catalyzes this reaction. The pyrophosphate is rapidly degraded to two inorganic phosphates by the ubiquitous pyrophosphatase. As noted previously, this ensures that the reaction will proceed in the direction of CDP-choline synthesis.

$$\text{Phosphocholine} + \text{CTP} \rightarrow \text{CDP-Choline} + \text{PP}_i$$

$$\text{PP}_i + H_2O \rightarrow 2\ \text{P}_i$$

The step catalyzed by CTP:phosphocholine cytidylyltransferase is the main regulatory point in this pathway. CTP:phosphocholine cytidylyltransferase is found in both soluble and membrane fractions. The enzyme requires phospholipid for activity, and translocation between the phospholipid-rich ER membrane and the phospholipid-poor cytosol is a regulatory mechanism. Diacylglycerol and phosphatidylcholine are potential feed-forward (positive) and feedback (negative) regulators of CTP:phosphocholine cytidylyltransferase activity, respectively.

In the final reaction in this pathway, CDP-choline reacts with diacylglycerol to form phosphatidylcholine in a reaction catalyzed by CDP-choline:1,2-diacylglycerol cholinephosphotransferase. The enzyme catalyzing this reaction is localized in the ER and does not appear to be limiting for phosphatidylcholine synthesis.

$$\text{CDP-choline} + \text{Diacylglycerol} \rightarrow \text{Phosphatidylcholine} + \text{CMP}$$

Phosphatidylethanolamine Methylation Pathway

Phosphatidylcholine also is formed from phosphatidylethanolamine, as shown in the lower half of Figure 16-18. The three methyl groups are donated by *S*-adenosylmethionine in

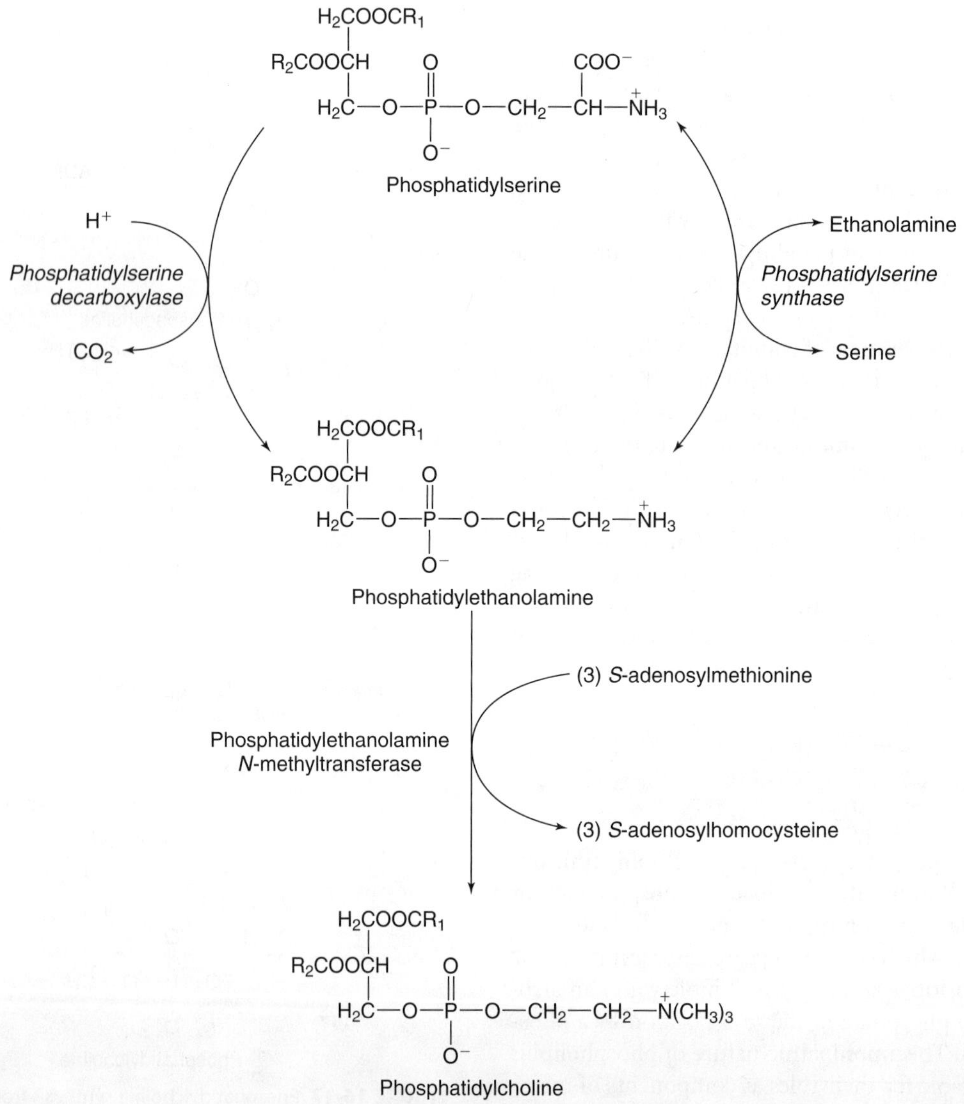

H_2COOCR_1 / R_2COOCH / $H_2C{-}O{-}P(=O)(O^-){-}O{-}CH_2{-}CH(COO^-){-}\overset{+}{N}H_3$
Phosphatidylserine

H^+
Phosphatidylserine decarboxylase
CO_2

Ethanolamine
Phosphatidylserine synthase
Serine

H_2COOCR_1 / R_2COOCH / $H_2C{-}O{-}P(=O)(O^-){-}O{-}CH_2{-}CH_2{-}\overset{+}{N}H_3$
Phosphatidylethanolamine

(3) *S*-adenosylmethionine
Phosphatidylethanolamine *N*-methyltransferase
(3) *S*-adenosylhomocysteine

H_2COOCR_1 / R_2COOCH / $H_2C{-}O{-}P(=O)(O^-){-}O{-}CH_2{-}CH_2{-}\overset{+}{N}(CH_3)_3$
Phosphatidylcholine

FIGURE 16-18 Synthesis of phosphatidylcholine from phosphatidylethanolamine and interconversion of phosphatidylserine and phosphatidylethanolamine. *R_1COO–* and *R_2COO–* represent fatty acid chains esterified to the glycerol backbone.

a series of three reactions catalyzed by phosphatidylethanolamine *N*-methyltransferase.

3 *S*-adenosylmethionine + Phosphatidylethanolamine →
3 *S*-adenosylhomocysteine + Phosphatidylcholine

Sources of Choline

Normal diets provide sufficient choline. In humans, choline cannot be synthesized directly but is produced indirectly via the foregoing phosphatidylethanolamine *N*-methyltransferase reaction. The metabolic pathways involving choline, methionine, and folate are closely interrelated. The three methyl groups of choline can be made available for one-carbon metabolism upon conversion of choline to betaine. One-carbon metabolism is discussed in detail in Chapter 25. In malnutrition, when stores of choline, methionine, and folate are depleted, or if choline is not included in total parenteral nutrition, choline may become deficient. Carbohydrate loading, because it enhances hepatic triacylglycerol synthesis, also increases the amount of choline required; more phosphatidylcholine is needed for lipoprotein synthesis and secretion. In choline deficiency, biosynthesis of phosphatidylcholine is inhibited, causing development of fatty liver.

SYNTHESIS OF PHOSPHATIDYLETHANOLAMINE

Three possible pathways exist for phosphatidylethanolamine synthesis. The first and most prevalent pathway for synthesis of phosphatidylethanolamine is de novo synthesis. This pathway involves phosphorylation of ethanolamine, which is catalyzed by choline kinase, the same enzyme that is involved in the synthesis of phosphatidylcholine. The remainder of the pathway is also similar to the de novo pathway for synthesis of phosphatidylcholine (see Figure 16-17). Ethanolamine reacts with CTP to produce its activated form, CDP-ethanolamine, in a reaction catalyzed by CTP:phosphoethanolamine cytidylyltransferase. CDP-ethanolamine:1,2-diacylglycerol ethanolaminephosphotransferase then catalyzes the reaction of CDP-ethanolamine with diacylglycerol to form phosphatidylethanolamine.

In addition, there are two pathways for synthesis of phosphatidylethanolamine via modification of preexisting phospholipids. These two pathways are shown in Figure 16-18. First, phosphatidylserine decarboxylase catalyzes the decarboxylation of phosphatidylserine to form phosphatidylethanolamine.

Phosphatidylserine + H^+ → Phosphatidylethanolamine + CO_2

The second route involves an exchange reaction with phosphatidylserine in which phosphatidylserine reacts with ethanolamine to form phosphatidylethanolamine and serine. The reaction is catalyzed by phosphatidylserine synthase (see Figure 16-18).

Phosphatidylserine + Ethanolamine →
Phosphatidylethanolamine + Serine

SYNTHESIS OF PHOSPHATIDYLSERINE

Phosphatidylserine constitutes only 5% to 15% of phospholipids in cells. Although the CDP-diacylglycerol pathway, similar to that described in the next section for phosphatidylglycerol, is used in the de novo synthesis of phosphatidylserine in bacteria, the enzyme catalyzing the reaction of CDP-diacylglycerol and serine does not appear to be present in mammalian tissue. Instead, phosphatidylethanolamine or phosphatidylcholine reacts with serine to undergo base exchange to form phosphatidylserine and ethanolamine or choline (phosphatidylserine synthase).

SYNTHESIS OF PHOSPHATIDYLGLYCEROL AND DIPHOSPHATIDYLGLYCEROL (CARDIOLIPIN)

Synthesis of phosphatidylglycerol begins with the reaction of CTP with phosphatidic acid to form CDP-diacylglycerol and pyrophosphate. This reaction is catalyzed by CDP-diacylglycerol synthase. Cleavage of the resulting pyrophosphate drives the reaction toward completion.

Phosphatidic acid + CTP → CDP-diacylglycerol + PP_i

$PP_i + H_2O \rightarrow 2\ P_i$

In the next reaction, CDP-diacylglycerol reacts with *sn*-glycerol 3-phosphate to form phosphatidylglycerol phosphate and CMP, as shown in Figure 16-19. The reaction is catalyzed by glycerophosphate phosphatidyltransferase.

CDP-diacylglycerol + *sn*-Glycerol 3-phosphate →
Phosphatidylglycerol phosphate + CMP

In the second step, phosphatidylglycerol phosphate phosphatase catalyzes hydrolysis of phosphate from phosphatidylglycerol phosphate to form phosphatidylglycerol.

Phosphatidylglycerol phosphate → Phosphatidylglycerol + P_i

Another molecule of CDP-diacylglycerol may react with phosphatidylglycerol to form diphosphatidylglycerol (cardiolipin) and CMP (see Figure 16-19, reaction catalyzed by phosphatidate phosphatidyltransferase). In eukaryotes, cardiolipin is synthesized exclusively in the mitochondria and is particularly enriched in the inner mitochondrial membrane. Cardiolipin is rich in unsaturated 18-carbon fatty acids such as oleate and linoleate.

Phosphatidylglycerol + CDP-diacylglycerol →
Diphosphatidylglycerol + CMP

SYNTHESIS OF PHOSPHATIDYLINOSITOL

As shown in Figure 16-20, CDP-diacylglycerol is also an intermediate in the synthesis of phosphatidylinositol in a reaction localized in the ER and catalyzed by phosphatidylinositol synthase.

Inositol + CDP-diacylglycerol → Phosphatidylinositol + CMP

The inositol phospholipids are constituents of membranes and represent 10% of the phospholipids in cells and tissues. A small portion (1% to 3%) of the phosphatidylinositols are phosphorylated. Phosphatidylinositol phosphates play key roles in signaling and are precursors to the important intracellular second messengers, diacylglycerol and inositol polyphosphates, as described in subsequent text of this chapter.

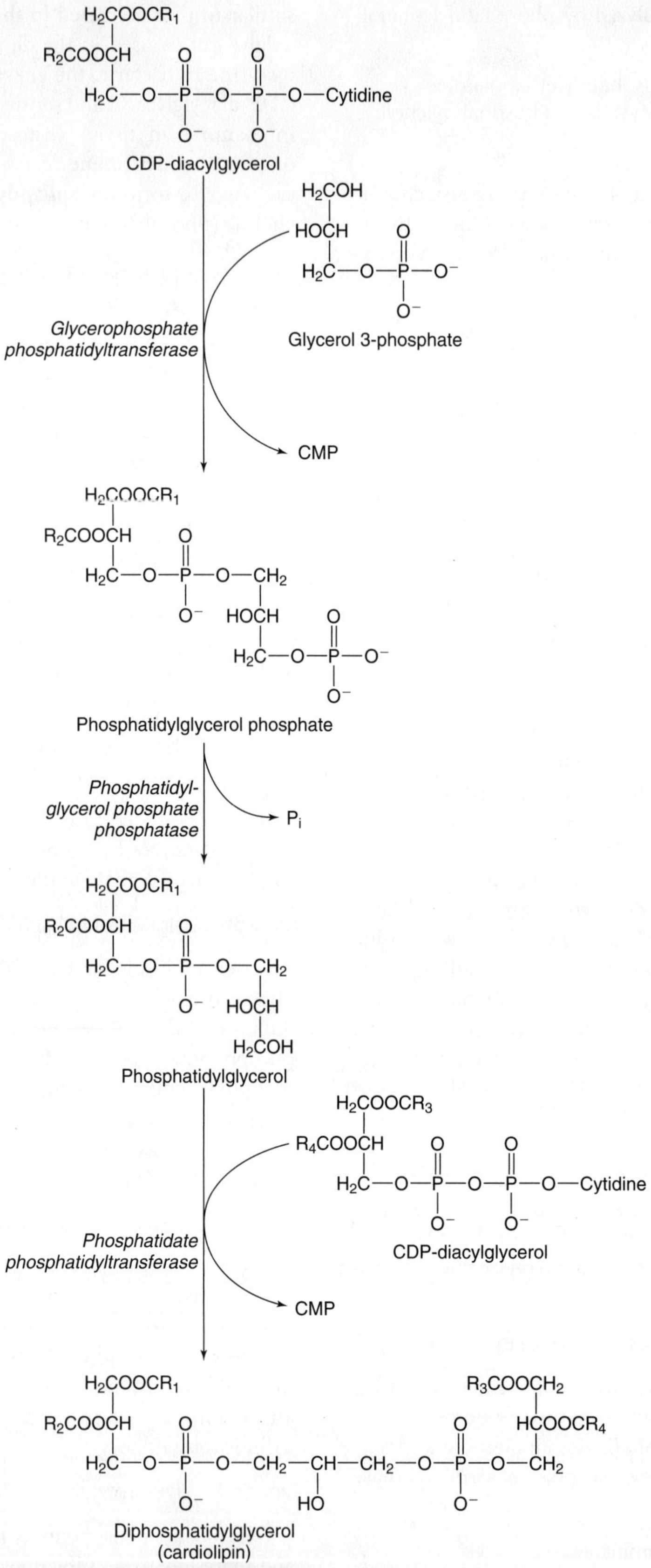

FIGURE 16-19 Synthesis of phosphatidylglycerol and cardiolipin. R_1COO–, R_2COO–, R_3COO–, and R_4COO– represent fatty acids esterified to the glycerol backbone.

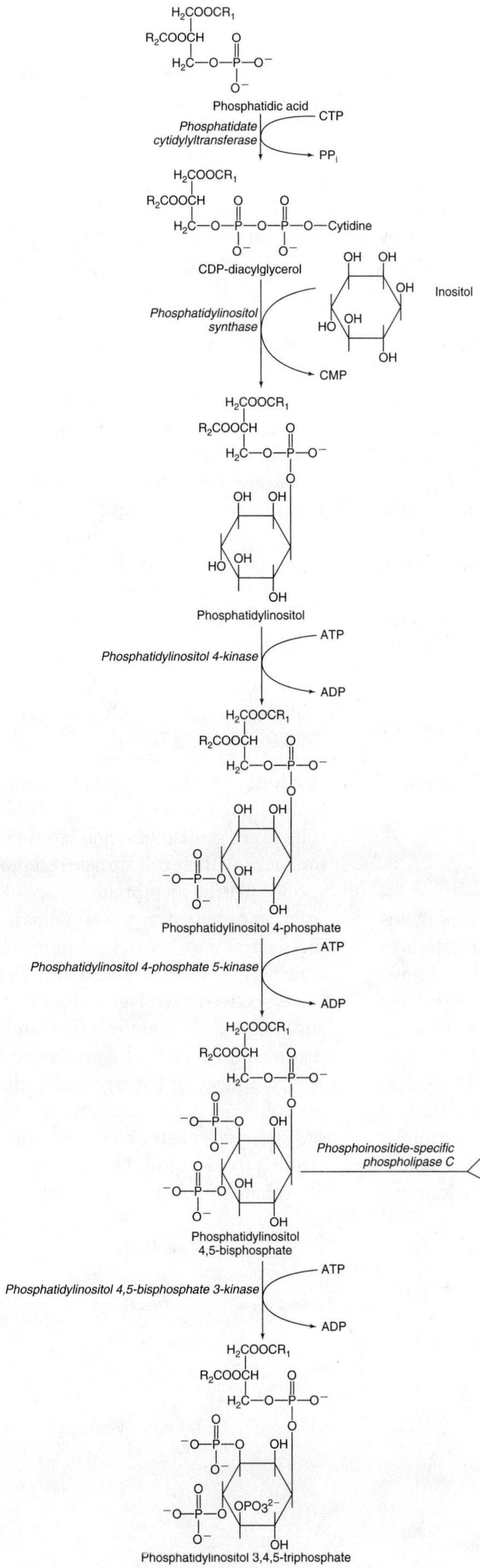

FIGURE 16-20 Inositol phospholipid synthesis.

As shown in Figure 16-20, phosphatidylinositol phosphate, phosphatidylinositol bisphosphate, and phosphatidylinositol triphosphate are formed by the sequential addition of phosphate as catalyzed by various ATP-dependent reactions catalyzed by phosphatidylinositol kinases. Furthemore, phosphatidylinositides can undergo rapid interconversions catalyzed by complex sets of phosphatidylinositol kinases and lipid phosphatases. For example, a key signaling molecule, phosphatidylinositol 3,4,5-triphosphate is formed by phosphorylation of phosphatidylinositol 4,5-bisphosphate catalyzed by phosphatidylinositol 4,5-bisphosphate 3-kinase, commonly known as phosphatidylinositol 3-kinase. The reverse reaction, dephosphorylation of phosphatidylinositol 3,4,5-triphosphate to phosphatidylinositol 4,5-phosphate, is catalyzed by a phosphatidylinositol phosphate phosphatase, PTEN (phosphatase and tensin homolog). Phosphatidylinositol 3-kinase mediates insulin and growth factor signaling and thus controls cell survival, growth, and differentiation. The importance of phosphoinositide signaling in cell function is demonstrated by diseases that are associated with mutations in the enzymes involved in phosphatidylinositol metabolism: both phosphatidylinositol 3-kinase and PTEN are among the proteins that are most frequently altered in cancer, and these enzymes are targets for development of therapeutics. Several inositol polyphosphates with more than three phosphates can be derived from the inositol triphosphate released by the hydrolysis of phosphatidylinositol bisphosphate catalyzed by phospholipase C. The additional phosphorylations of inositol triphosphate to form polyphosphates are catalyzed by kinases that use free inositol polyphosphates as substrates.

REMODELING OF PHOSPHOLIPIDS IN SITU

The phospholipid composition of different cellular membranes is usually specific for each organelle. Differences involve both the fatty acyl groups in the *sn*-1 and *sn*-2 positions and the alcohol base in the *sn*-3 position. In general, the *sn*-1 position of phospholipids contains saturated fatty acids, whereas the *sn*-2 position contains unsaturated fatty acids. However, dietary content of fatty acids influences fatty acid composition of phospholipids. The specificity of insertion of fatty acids at the *sn*-1 and *sn*-2 positions is usually determined by the specificities of glycerol 3-phosphate acyltransferase and 1-acylglycerol 3-phosphate acyltransferase. An additional mechanism for generating and/or maintaining these specific compositions is to remove acyl groups from phospholipids through the action of phospholipases and to reesterify with a specific acyl group. The abundance of polyunsaturated fatty acids at the *sn*-2 position is due to phospholipid remodeling. The alcohol bases also can be rearranged when a specific phospholipase generates diacylglycerol or phosphatidic acid.

The phospholipases that cleave acyl groups or alcohol bases can be categorized into five groups, based on the specific phospholipid bond that they attack, as illustrated in Figure 16-21. Phospholipases A1, A2, and B are acyl hydrolases. Phospholipase A1 cleaves the ester bond between the *sn*-1 position and its acyl group, generating 2-acylglycerol 3-phospholipid. Phospholipase A2 attacks the ester bond between the *sn*-2 position and its acyl group, generating 1-acylglycerol 3-phospholipid. Phospholipase B cleaves the ester bonds at either the *sn*-1 or *sn*-2 position but is relatively rare. Phospholipases C and D are phosphodiesterases. Phospholipase C cleaves the bond between the *sn*-3 position and the phosphate (glycerophosphate bond) and encompasses a family of enzymes that generate diacylglycerol and the free phosphorylated alcohol as products. Phospholipase D attacks the bond between the alcohol base and the glycerol phosphate.

GENERATION OF SIGNALING MOLECULES BY REGULATED PHOSPHOLIPASES

In addition to the remodeling of molecular species of membrane lipids, some of the phospholipases play important roles in cell signaling. When certain hormones or growth factors occupy their cell surface receptors, a phosphoinositide-specific plasma membrane phospholipase C is activated. The reaction catalyzed by phospholipase C generates the second messengers inositol 1,4,5-triphosphate and diacylglycerol, which cause Ca^{2+} release and activation of protein kinase C, respectively (see Figure 16-20). Inositol polyphosphates and diacylglycerol are recycled, and recycling accomplishes two purposes. First, it ends the action of the second messenger, and second, it regenerates the substrates upon which phospholipases can act. Specific phosphatases act on inositol polyphosphates to remove the phosphates, ultimately yielding free inositol. The diacylglycerol can be converted to phosphatidic acid via the action of diacylglycerol kinase, or

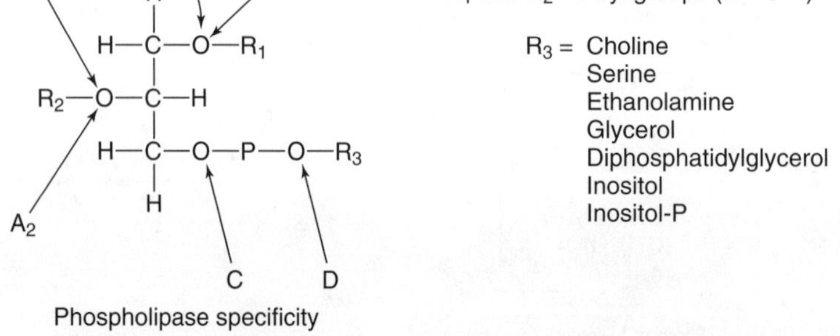

R_1 and R_2 = Acyl groups (R—C(=O)—)

R_3 = Choline
Serine
Ethanolamine
Glycerol
Diphosphatidylglycerol
Inositol
Inositol-P

Phospholipase specificity

FIGURE 16-21 Phospholipase specificity.

it can react with CDP-inositol to form phosphatidylinositol or with other compounds activated with CDP to yield other phospholipids. Lithium, a drug that is used to treat bipolar disorders, exerts its therapeutic effects by inhibiting hydrolysis of inositol monophosphate to inositol. This depletes the intracellular supply of inositol and therefore interrupts the phosphatidylinositol signaling pathway, which is presumably hyperactive in bipolar disorders.

Phospholipase A2 also can be activated by extracellular stimuli, including local mediators, by a receptor-mediated process. Arachidonic acid released by phospholipase A2 can be used for synthesis of prostaglandins and thromboxanes via the cyclooxygenase pathway and for synthesis of leukotrienes via the lipoxygenase pathway (see Chapter 18 for further discussion of these eicosanoids).

SYNTHESIS OF ETHER-LINKED GLYCEROLPHOSPHOLIPIDS

A second group of glycerophospholipids are those that contain an ether-linked alkyl or alkenyl group.

There are two major classes of ether-linked lipids in the cells. Glycerol ethers have *O*-alkyl groups; plasmalogens have *O*-alk-1-enyl groups. In each case, the ether linkage is to the *sn*-1 position. Some ether-linked lipids have potent biological activity. Platelet activating factor, 1-alkyl-2-acetyl-*sn*-glycerol 3-phosphocholine, for example, causes aggregation of blood platelets at concentrations as low as 0.01 nmol/L. Plasmalogens, the other class of ether-linked lipids, constitute approximately 5% to 20% of the phospholipids of cell membranes. Although the exact biological functions of these compounds are not known, their importance is suggested by the symptoms of plasmalogen deficiency (Zellweger syndrome) described in subsequent text. Plasmalogen is especially abundant in nervous tissue and in the membranes of the myelin sheath; for example, ethanolamine plasmalogen may represent as much as 80% of phospholipids in the myelin sheath membranes. High levels of choline plasmalogens are found in heart tissue.

Plasmalogens are synthesized using a fatty acid and dihydroxyacetone phosphate (instead of glycerol 3-phosphate) to form 1-acyldihydroxyacetone phosphate as the initial step. The ether-linked group is donated by a fatty alcohol. The fatty alcohol is produced from an acyl-CoA in a reaction that requires NADPH. This reaction involves an aldehyde intermediate and is catalyzed by a membrane-associated acyl-CoA reductase.

(1) Acyl-CoA + NADPH + H^+ → Fatty aldehyde + $NADP^+$ + CoA

(2) Fatty aldehyde + NADPH + H^+ → Fatty alcohol + $NADP^+$

As shown in Figure 16-22, the first reaction in the synthesis of ether-linked lipids is catalyzed by the dihydroxyacetone phosphate acyltransferase that was described in the section on synthesis of triacylglycerol.

Dihydroxyacetone phosphate + Fatty acyl-CoA → 1-Acyldihydroxyacetone phosphate + CoA

In triacylglycerol synthesis, the next step is reduction of the keto group to a hydroxyl group to form lysophosphatidic acid. In ether–lipid synthesis, the next step is an exchange reaction with a fatty alcohol to produce 1-alkyldihydroxyacetone phosphate in a reaction catalyzed

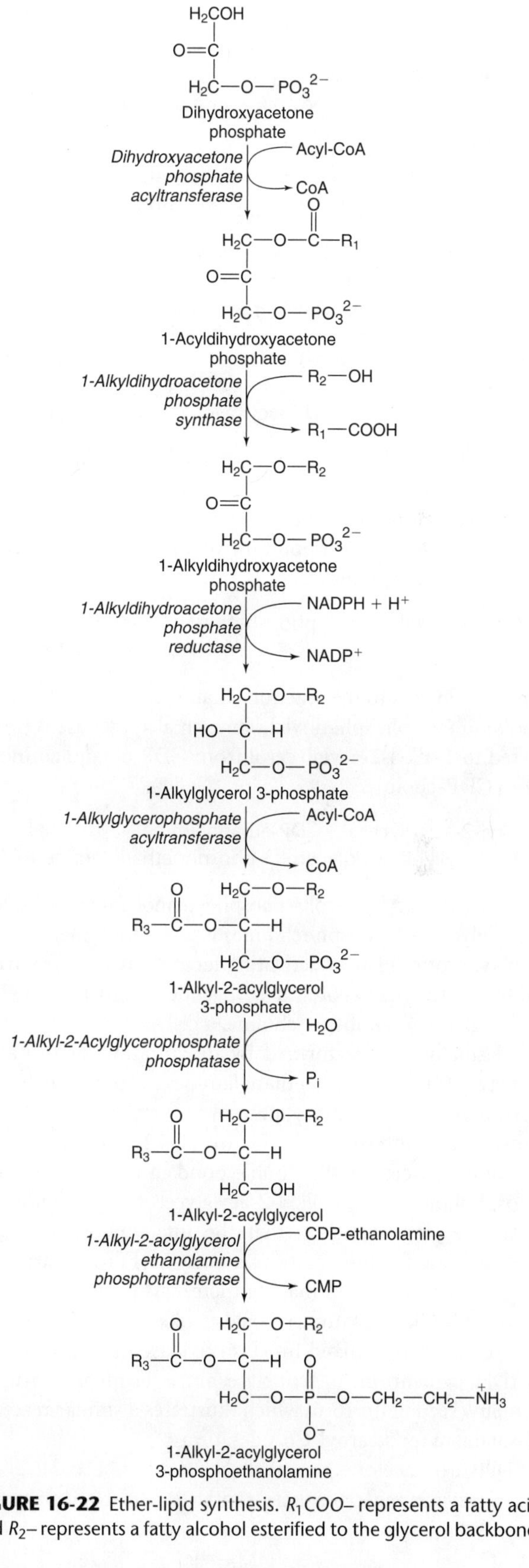

Dihydroxyacetone phosphate
Dihydroxyacetone phosphate acyltransferase (Acyl-CoA → CoA)
1-Acyldihydroxyacetone phosphate
1-Alkyldihydroacetone phosphate synthase (R_2—OH → R_1—COOH)
1-Alkyldihydroxyacetone phosphate
1-Alkyldihydroacetone phosphate reductase (NADPH + H^+ → $NADP^+$)
1-Alkylglycerol 3-phosphate
1-Alkylglycerophosphate acyltransferase (Acyl-CoA → CoA)
1-Alkyl-2-acylglycerol 3-phosphate
1-Alkyl-2-Acylglycerophosphate phosphatase (H_2O → P_i)
1-Alkyl-2-acylglycerol
1-Alkyl-2-acylglycerol ethanolamine phosphotransferase (CDP-ethanolamine → CMP)
1-Alkyl-2-acylglycerol 3-phosphoethanolamine

FIGURE 16-22 Ether-lipid synthesis. R_1COO– represents a fatty acid and R_2– represents a fatty alcohol esterified to the glycerol backbone.

by 1-alkyldihydroxyacetone phosphate synthase, which is specific for a substrate with a ketone functional group.

1-Acyldihydroxyacetone phosphate + Fatty alcohol → 1-Alkyldihydroxyacetone phosphate + Fatty acid

The next reaction is a reduction of the keto group of alkyldihydroxyacetone phosphate to yield alkylglycerol 3-phosphate. This reaction is catalyzed by NADPH-dependent alkyldihydroxyacetone phosphate reductase. This reductase is capable of reducing both acyl and alkyl analogs of dihydroxyacetone phosphate.

1-Alkyldihydroxyacetone phosphate + NADPH + H^+ → 1-Alkylglycerol 3-phosphate + $NADP^+$

In the next reaction, the alkyl analog of phosphatidic acid is synthesized by adding an acyl group to the *sn*-2 position. This reaction is catalyzed by 1-alkylglycerol phosphate acyltransferase.

1-Alkylglycerol 3-phosphate + Acyl-CoA → 1-Alkyl-2-acylglycerol 3-phosphate + CoA

The next step in this pathway creates an alkylacylglycerol by dephosphorylation. This compound represents a branch point in ether–lipid synthesis in much the same way as diacylglycerol is at a branch point for synthesis of triacylglycerol and glycerophospholipids.

1-Alkyl-2-acylglycerol 3-phosphate + H_2O → + 1-Alkyl-2-acylglycerol + P_i

Next, analogous to the reactions that form phosphatidylethanolamine or phosphatidylcholine, an alcohol base is transferred to 1-alkyl-2-acylglycerol from CDP-ethanolamine or from CDP-choline.

1-Alkyl-2-acylglycerol + CDP-ethanolamine → 1-Alkyl-2-acylglycerol 3-phosphoethanolamine + CMP

The 1-alkyl-2-acylglycerol 3-phosphoethanolamine (or 1-alkyl-2-acylglycerol 3-phosphocholine) is a glycerol ether with an *O*-alkyl group. Platelet activating factor is synthesized from 1-alkyl-2-acetylglycerol and CDP-choline and is 1-alkyl-2-acetyl-glycerol 3-phosphocholine.

Plasmalogens are formed by desaturation of the alkyl moiety of the phosphoethanolamine or phosphocholine derivative of 1-alkyl-2-acylglycerol to form an *O*-alk-1-enyl substituent (not shown in Figure 16-22). The enzymatic reaction that creates the double bond in the glycerol ether phospholipid (e.g., 1-alkyl-2-acylglycerol 3-phosphoethanolamine) is unusual in that the intact phospholipid is the substrate for the desaturase. Fatty acyl groups are usually desaturated before making them part of more complex lipids. Δ1-Alkyl desaturase behaves like a typical acyl-CoA desaturase; it is a mixed function oxidase that requires O_2, NADH, cytochrome b_5 reductase, and a terminal desaturase protein (see Figure 16-6, which illustrates a similar reaction mechanism for stearoyl-CoA desaturase).

Dihydroxyacetone phosphate acyltransferase and 1-alkyldihydroxyacetone phosphate synthase, which catalyze the first two reactions in ether–lipid biosynthesis, are localized in peroxisomes. One of the manifestations of Zellweger syndrome, a block in peroxisome biogenesis, is decreased tissue plasmalogen levels, and these deficiencies may contribute to pathological features of this disease, including profound neurological deficits and death within the first year of life. Some types of β-oxidation of fatty acids, including oxidation of very-long-chain fatty acids, polyunsaturated fatty acids, and dicarboxylic fatty acids, occur in peroxisomes. Patients with Zellweger syndrome therefore show both accumulation of very-long-chain fatty acids and decreased plasmalogen levels.

SYNTHESIS OF SPHINGOLIPIDS

The backbone of sphingolipids is a sphingoid long-chain base, the most common of which is sphingosine. Ceramide, the simplest sphingolipid, consists of a sphingoid base to which a fatty acid is attached at C2 by an amide linkage. Sphingolipids also contain a hydrophilic moiety, usually phosphocholine (as in sphingomyelin) or one or more sugar residues (as in cerebrosides and gangliosides).

Sphingolipids play both structural and regulatory roles. After glycerophospholipids, the most abundant lipids in membranes are sphingolipids. Sphingolipids are thought to be localized in membrane rafts that are microdomains for signal transduction and protein sorting. Sphingolipids are particularly abundant in the white matter of the central nervous system. Ceramide and sphingosine play important physiological roles in intracellular signaling (Bartke and Hannun, 2009; Kim et al., 2009; Lahiri and Futerman, 2007; Fyrst and Saba, 2010). Numerous gangliosides are displayed on the external face of mammalian cells and probably play roles in recognition of other cells and basement membranes. Many bacteria have developed specific adhesion mechanisms that recognize and result in their binding to specific gangliosides. Further evidence for the importance of these compounds is that inherited mutations in enzymes in the pathway for degradation of sphingolipids result in the accumulation of specific gangliosides, cerebrosides, and ceramides. These lipid accumulations account for the pathologies of several lipid storage diseases.

SYNTHESIS OF CERAMIDE, THE PRECURSOR OF MOST MAMMALIAN SPHINGOLIPIDS

Enzymes involved in the synthesis of ceramide, shown in Figure 16-23, are localized in the ER.

In the first reaction, palmitoyl-CoA reacts with serine to form 3-keto-dihydrosphingosine. This reaction requires pyridoxal 5′-phosphate (vitamin B_6 coenzyme) for decarboxylation and is catalyzed by serine palmitoyltransferase.

Palmitoyl-CoA + Serine → 3-Keto-dihydrosphingosine + CoA + CO_2

The next reaction is a reductase that requires NADPH and converts the keto group at C3 of the long-chain base to a hydroxyl, forming dihydrosphingosine (sphinganine).

3-Keto-dihydrosphingosine + NADPH + H^+ → Sphinganine + $NADP^+$

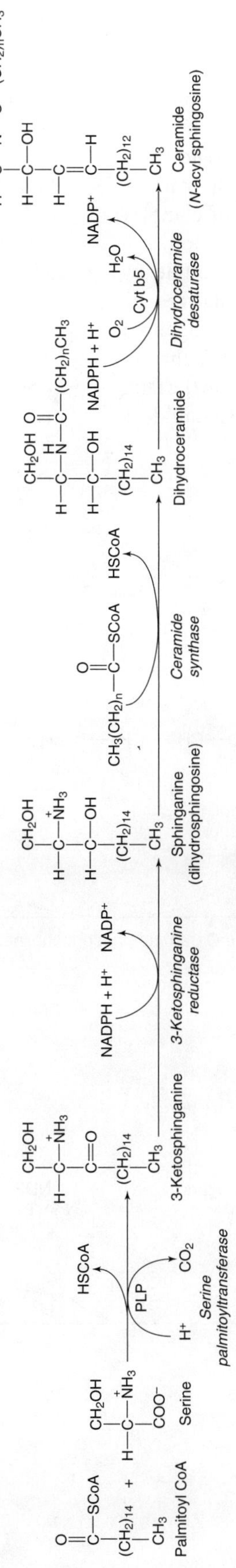

FIGURE 16-23 Ceramide synthesis.

Addition of a long-chain acyl group to sphinganine to produce dihydroceramide is catalyzed by ceramide synthase.

Sphinganine + Fatty acyl-CoA → Dihydroceramide + CoA

Fumonisins are inhibitors of ceramide synthase and are produced by fungi. They were originally discovered in search for food contaminants that cause various pathologies such as cancer and birth defects. By inhibiting ceramide synthase activity, fumonisins not only block formation of complex sphingolipids but also cause sphinganine accumulation.

Finally, dihydroceramide is converted to ceramide by the introduction of a 4,5-*trans*-double bond catalyzed by dihydroceramide Δ4-desaturase (also called sphingolipid Δ4-desaturase). Although the reaction needs further characterization, it requires cytochrome b_5 and is similar to the fatty acid Δ9-desaturase reaction (see Figure 16-23). Ceramide is the precursor of all complex sphingolipids (note structural similarity of ceramide with diacylglycerol).

SYNTHESIS AND FUNCTION OF SPHINGOMYELIN

Whereas ceramide is synthesized de novo in the ER, further metabolism of ceramide to sphingomyelin and glycosphingolipids occurs mainly in the Golgi apparatus. Sphingomyelin is the only major sphingolipid that contains phosphate. As shown in the upper half of Figure 16-24, sphingomyelin is synthesized when ceramide reacts with phosphatidylcholine to form sphingomyelin and diacylglycerol.

Ceramide + Phosphatidylcholine → Sphingomyelin + Diacylglycerol

Sphingomyelin is in the plasma membrane of most mammalian cells and is a major component of the myelin sheath

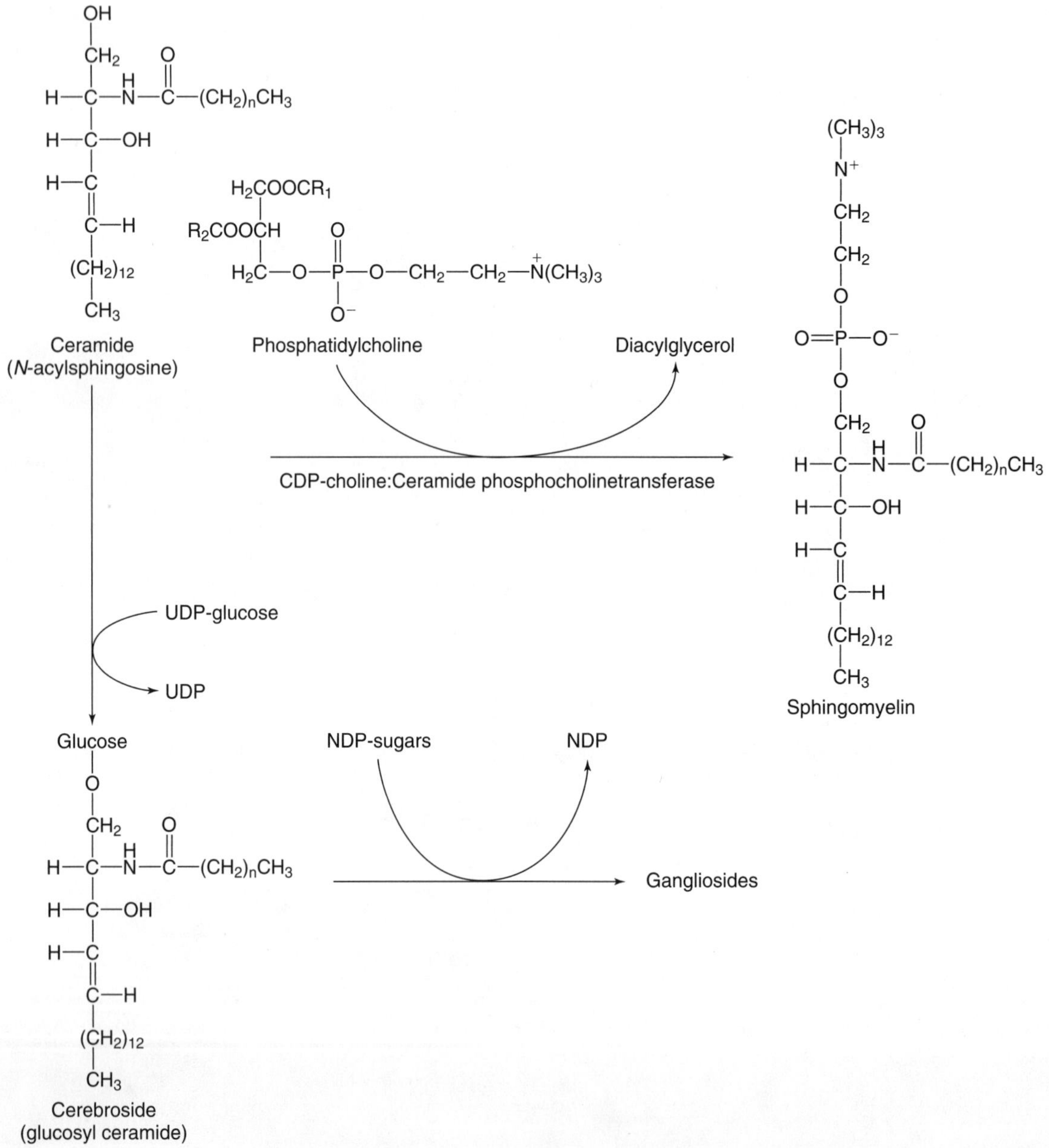

FIGURE 16-24 Sphingolipid synthesis from ceramide.

that surrounds nerve cells. Sphingomyelin is hydrolyzed by sphingomyelinase to produce ceramide and phosphocholine. Ceramide is hydrolyzed by ceramidase to produce the sphingoid base, sphingosine. Both ceramide and sphingosine can be phosphorylated to become ceramide-1-phosphate and sphingosine-1-phosphate, respectively. Ceramide, sphingosine, ceramide-1-phosphate, and sphingosine-1-phosphate act as second messengers in a signaling cascade regulating cell growth and differentiation, cell functions, and programmed cell death. Ceramide and sphingosine-1-phosphate often have countering functions. These signals can be produced by turnover of sphingomyelin and glycosphingolipids but can also be synthesized de novo. Patients with Niemann-Pick disease types A and B accumulate sphingomyelin because of genetic defects in acid sphingomyelinase that hydrolyze sphingomyelin to ceramide and phosphocholine. (Although patients with Niemann-Pick disease type C also accumulate sphingomyelin, but these patients have genetic defects in cholesterol transport. See Chapter 17.)

SYNTHESIS AND DEGRADATION OF GLYCOSPHINGOLIPIDS

Cerebrosides, galactosylceramide and glucosylceramide, which contain monosaccharide attached to C1 of ceramide by a β-glycosidic linkage, are intermediates in the synthesis of more complex gangliosides. As shown in Figure 16-24, they are formed by the reaction of ceramide with uridine diphosphate (UDP)-galactose or UDP-glucose to form the corresponding cerebroside.

$$\text{Ceramide} + \text{UDP-glucose} \rightarrow \text{Cerebroside} + \text{UDP}$$

Gangliosides are created by adding one or more sugars to the nonreducing end of the carbohydrate moiety of cerebroside or of the growing carbohydrate chain. Specific glycosyl transferases catalyze these reactions. The sugar donors are nucleotide diphosphate sugars. The "terminal" sugar of all gangliosides is *N*-acetylneuraminic acid (sialic acid).

Specific acid exoglycosidases localized in lysosomes degrade plasma membrane–bound and extracellular gangliosides. The pathway for this sequential removal of sugars has been worked out based on the metabolic consequences of known genetic defects in humans that are often manifested in childhood. In Tay-Sachs, Fabry, Sandhoff, and Gaucher diseases, specific gangliosides accumulate because degradation of a specific ganglioside is blocked whereas synthesis and the initial steps of degradation occur at normal rates. Abnormal accumulations of these lipids, particularly in nervous tissues, cause the pathologies of these diseases, including mental retardation.

Lysosomal defects in acid ceramidase (Farber disease) and acid sphingomyelinase (Niemann-Pick disease types A and B) result in tissue accumulation of ceramide and sphingomyelin, respectively, and metabolic disturbances. Acid ceramidase catalyzes the hydrolysis of ceramide to release sphingosine and long-chain fatty acid. Acid sphingomyelinase catalyzes the degradation of sphingomyelin to form ceramide plus phosphocholine. All of these defects are lysosomal disorders of sphingolipid catabolism. Nonlysosomal ceramidases and sphingomyelinases, which have optimal activity at neutral or slightly alkaline pH, probably are involved in turnover of ceramide and sphingomyelin, respectively, for cell signaling.

THINKING CRITICALLY

1. List possible fates of acetyl-CoA in metabolism. Try to list as many different general fates as you can (e.g., synthesis of fatty acids would be one item on the list).
2. Carnitine deficiency due to a genetic defect in its synthesis or transport may result in recurrent muscle cramping and severe muscle weakness.
   a. Muscle carnitine levels are very low in patients with these defects, and pathological accumulation of triacylglycerol droplets in muscle is common. Would you expect that fatty acid β-oxidation would be impaired in patients with carnitine deficiency? Why? How might this be related to muscle weakness?
   b. Replacement of normal dietary fat by triacylglycerols containing medium-chain (9- or 10-carbon) fatty acids has proven effective in some cases. Why would this therapy be expected to work?
   c. How might carnitine deficiency account for the triacylglycerol accumulation in the muscles? Would the lipid accumulate in the cytosol or mitochondria of the cells? Why?
3. Inherited defects that impair the β-oxidation of fatty acids at different stages of the chain-shortening process have been identified. A long-chain acyl-CoA dehydrogenase, a medium-chain acyl-CoA dehydrogenase, and a short-chain acyl-CoA dehydrogenase are required to attach acyl-CoA chains of greater than 12 carbons, 6 carbons to 12 carbons, and 4 carbons to 6 carbons, respectively. Patients with one of these defects generally do well simply by avoiding prolonged periods of starvation.
   a. Medium-chain acyl-CoA deficiency was first recognized in 1982 and is now thought to be a relatively common inheritable metabolic disease. If a patient with a defect in the medium-chain acyl-CoA dehydrogenase is starved, the patient will develop hypoglycemia and have symptoms including vomiting, lethargy, and frequently coma. Hypoglycemia would normally be accompanied by an elevation in ketone body production, but this does not occur in these patients. Why do these patients fail to generate ketone bodies as an alternative fuel?
   b. What is a likely cause of the hypoglycemia?

REFERENCES

Abu-Elheiga, L., Oh, W., Kordari, P., & Wakil, S. J. (2003). Acetyl-CoA carboxylase 2 mutant mice are protected against obesity and diabetes induced by high-fat/high-carbohydrate diets. *Proceedings of the National Academy of Sciences of the United States of America, 100*, 10207–10212.

Bartke, N., & Hannun, Y. A. (2009). Bioactive sphingolipids: Metabolism and function. *Journal of Lipid Research, 50*, S91–S96.

Beigneux, A. P., Weinstein, M. M., Davies, B. S., Gin, P., Bensadoun, A., Fong, L. G., & Young, S. G. (2009). GPIHBP1 and lipolysis: An update. *Current Opinion in Lipidology, 20*, 211–216.

Brownsey, R. W., Boone, A. N., Elliott, J. E., Kulpa, J. E., & Lee, W. M. (2006). Regulation of acetyl-CoA carboxylase. *Biochemical Society Transactions, 34*, 223–227.

Chakravarthy, M., Zhu, Y., Lopez, M. M., Yin, L., Wozniak, D. F., Coleman, T., … Semenkovich, C. F. (2007). Brain fatty acid synthase activates PPARalpha to maintain energy homeostasis. *The Journal of Clinical Investigation, 117*, 2539–2552.

Dircks, L. & Sul, H. S. (1999). Acyltransferases of de novo glycerophospholipid biosynthesis. *Progress in Lipid Research, 38*, 461–479.

Duncan, R. E., Ahmadian, M., Jaworski, K., Sarkadi-Nagy, E., & Sul, H. S. (2007). Regulation of lipolysis in adipocytes. *Annual Review of Nutrition, 27*, 79–101.

Eaton, S. (2002). Control of mitochondrial β-oxidation flux. *Progress in Lipid Research, 41*, 197–239.

Ellis, J. M., Frahm, J. L., Li, L. O., & Coleman, R. A. (2010). Acyl-coenzyme A synthetases in metabolic control. *Current Opinion in Lipidology, 21*, 212–217.

Fyrst, H., & Saba, J. D. (2010). An update on sphingosine-1-phosphate and other sphingolipid mediators. *Nature Chemical Biology, 6*, 489–497.

Glatz, J. F. C., Luiken, J. F. P., & Bonen, A. (2010). Membrane fatty acid transports as regulators of lipid metabolism: Implications for metabolic disease. *Physiological Reviews, 90*, 367–417.

Guillou, H., Zadravec, D., Martin, P. G. P., & Jacobsson, A. (2010). The key roles of elongases and desaturases in mammalian fatty acid metabolism: Insights from transgenic mice. *Progress in Lipid Research, 49*, 186–199.

He, W., Lam, T. K., Obici, S., & Rossetti, L. (2006). Molecular disruption of hypothalamic nutrient sensing induces obesity. *Nature Neuroscience, 9*, 227–233.

Kim, R. H., Takabe, K., Milstien, S., & Spiegel, S. (2009). Export and functions of sphingosine-1-phosphate. *Biochimica et Biophysica Acta, 1791*, 692–696.

Lahiri, S., & Futerman, A. H. (2007). The metabolism and function of sphingolipids and glycosphingolipids. *Cellular and Molecular Life Sciences, 64*, 2270–2284.

Ligresti, A., Petrosino, S., & di Marzo, V. (2009). From endocannabinoid profiling to endocannabinoid therapeutics. *Current Opinion in Chemical Biology, 13*, 321–331.

Loftus, T. M., Jaworsky, D. E., Frehywot, G. L., Townsend, C. A., Ronnett, G. V., Lane, M. D., & Kuhajda, F. P. (2000). Reduced food intake and weight in mice treated with fatty acid synthase inhibitors. *Science, 288*, 2379–2381.

Maccarrone, M., Gasperi, V., Catani, M. V., Diet, T. A., Dainese, E., Hansen, H. S., & Avigliano, L. (2010). The endocannabinoid system and its relevance for nutrition. *Annual Review of Nutrition, 30*, 423–440.

Maier, T., Leibundgut, M., & Ban, N. (2008). The crystal structure of a mammalian fatty acid synthase. *Science, 321*, 1315–1322.

Mansbach, C. M., & Siddiqi, S. A. (2010). The biogenesis of chylomicrons. *Annual Review of Physiology, 72*, 315–333.

Minokoshi, Y., Alquier, T., Furukawas, N., Kim, Y. B., Lee, A., Xue, B., Mu, J., Foufelle, F., Ferre, P., Birnbaum, M. J., Stuck, B. J., & Kahn, B. B. (2004). AMPK-kinase regulates food intake by responding to hormonal and nutrient signals in the hypothalamus. *Nature, 428*, 569–572.

Nye, C., Kim, J., Kalhan, S. C., & Hanson, R. W. (2008). Reassessing triglyceride synthesis in adipose tissue. *Trends in Endocrinology and Metabolism, 19*, 356–361.

Saggerson, D. (2008). Malonyl-CoA, a key signaling molecule in mammalian cells. *Annual Review of Nutrition, 28*, 253–272.

Schutz, Y. (2004). Concept of fat balance in human obesity revisited with particular reference to de novo lipogenesis. *International Journal of Obesity, 28*, S3–S11.

Scriver, C. R., Beaudet, A. L., Sly, W. S., Valle, D., Childs, B., Kinzler, K. W., & Vogelstein, B. (2004). *Metabolic and Molecular Bases of Inherited Disease* (8th ed.). New York: McGraw Hill.

Steinberg, G. R., & Kemp, B. E. (2009). AMPK in health and disease. *Physiological Reviews, 89*, 1025–1078.

Storch, J., & Corsico, B. (2008). The emerging functions and mechanisms of mammalian fatty acid binding proteins. *Annual Review of Nutrition, 28*, 73–95.

Su, X., & Abumrad, N. A. (2008). Cellular fatty acid uptake: A pathway under construction. *Trends in Endocrinology and Metabolism, 20*, 72–77.

Sul, H. S., & Smith, S. (2008). Fatty acid synthesis in eukaryotes. In V. Vance & J. Vance (Eds.), *Biochemistry of lipids, lipoproteins and membranes* (5th ed., pp. 155–190). New York: Elsevier.

Takeuchi, K., & Reue, K. (2009). Biochemistry, physiology, and genetics of GPAT, AGPAT, and lipin enzymes in triglyceride synthesis. *American Journal of Physiology. Endocrinology and Metabolism, 296*, E1195–E1209.

Vance, D. E., & Vance, J. E. (Eds.). (2008). *Biochemistry of lipids, lipoproteins and membranes* (5th ed.). New York: Elsevier.

Wakil, S. J., & Abu-Elheiga, L. A. (2009). Fatty acid metabolism: Target for metabolic syndrome. *Journal of Lipid Research, 50*, S138–S143.

Walther, T. C., & Farese, R. V., Jr. (2009). The life of lipid droplets. *Biochimica et Biophysica Acta, 1791*, 459–466.

Wanders, R. J. A., Ferdinandusse, S., & Kemp, B. S. (2010). Peroxisomes, lipid metabolism and lipotoxicity. *Biochimica et Biophysica Acta, 1801*, 272–280.

Wang, H., & Eckel, R. H. (2009). Lipoprotein lipase: From gene to obesity. *American Journal of Physiology. Endocrinology and Metabolism, 297*, E271–E288.

Wendel, A. A., Lewin, T. M., & Coleman, R. A. (2009). Glycerol-3-phosphate acyltransferases: Rate limiting enzymes of triacylglycerol biosynthesis. *Biochimica et Biophysica Acta, 1791*, 501–506.

Wolfgang, M. J., & Lane, M. D. (2008). Hypothalamic malonyl-coenzyme A and the control of energy balance. *Molecular Endocrinology, 22*, 2012–2020.

Wong, R. H. F., Chang, I., Hudak, C. S. S., Hyun, S., Kwan, H. Y., & Sul, H. S. (2009). A role of DNA-PK in metabolic response to insulin. *Cell, 136*, 1056–1072.

Wong, R. H. F., & Sul, H. S. (2010). Insulin signaling in fatty acid and fat synthesis: A transcriptional perspective. *Current Opinion in Pharmacology, 10*, 684–691.

RECOMMENDED READING

American Society for Biochemistry and Molecular Biology. (2009). Special 50th anniversary supplement to the *Journal of Lipid Research. Journal of Lipid Research, 50*(Suppl. 1).

CHAPTER 17

Cholesterol and Lipoproteins: Synthesis, Transport, and Metabolism

Hei Sook Sul, PhD, and Judith Storch, PhD

COMMON ABBREVIATIONS

ABCA1	ATP-binding cassette transporter A1
ACAT	Acyl-CoA cholesterol acyltransferase
AMPK	AMP-activated protein kinase
apo A-I	apolipoprotein A-I
apo B	apolipoprotein B
apo C-II	apolipoprotein C-II
apo E	apolipoprotein E
CETP	cholesteryl ester transfer protein
HDL	high-density lipoprotein
HMG-CoA	3-hydroxy-3-methylglutaryl coenzyme A
HSL	hormone-sensitive lipase
IDL	intermediate-density lipoprotein
LCAT	lecithin:cholesterol acyltransferase
LDL	low-density lipoprotein
LDLR	LDL (apo B-100/apo E) receptor
LPL	lipoprotein lipase
PLTP	phospholipid transfer protein
SCAP	SREBP cleavage-activating protein
SRE	sterol regulatory element
SREBP	sterol regulatory element–binding protein
VLDL	very-low-density lipoprotein

Cholesterol is a sterol molecule with critical biological importance. It is an essential structural component of cell membranes, affecting their stability and permeability. Cholesterol also is essential as the precursor of the sex and adrenal steroid hormones and of the bile acids that play important roles in lipid digestion and absorption. Oxidized metabolites of cholesterol, called oxysterols, are also important regulators of lipid metabolic pathways. Moreover, isoprenoids, intermediates in the cholesterol biosynthetic pathway, are used for production of small amounts of molecules that have important biological functions. These include dolichol, which is required for glycoprotein synthesis, and ubiquinone (coenzyme Q), which is involved in electron transport in mitochondria. Isoprenoids also are used for posttranslational farnesylation or geranylgeranylation (called prenylation) of a variety of proteins including the membrane-associated heterotrimeric G proteins and the small GTP-binding proteins. Cholesterol itself is also used for modification of specific proteins. The covalently attached isoprenoid or cholesterol moieties serve in most cases as anchors for targeting proteins to certain membrane compartments or submembrane domains.

OVERVIEW OF CHOLESTEROL METABOLISM

Cholesterol is provided by foods of animal origin. In addition to dietary sources, de novo synthesis of cholesterol occurs in all nucleated cells. Synthesis and disposal of cholesterol must be tightly regulated both to meet cellular cholesterol needs and to prevent excess cholesterol accumulation. Abnormal deposition of cholesterol and cholesterol-rich lipoproteins in the coronary arteries eventually leads to atherosclerosis, a major contributory factor to cardiovascular diseases.

An overview of major aspects of cholesterol metabolism and transport by lipoproteins is shown in Figure 17-1. Cholesterol is transported in the plasma lipoprotein fractions. Transport of dietary cholesterol to the tissues is mediated initially by chylomicrons and subsequently by very-low-density lipoproteins (VLDLs) after the liver reincorporates cholesterol from chylomicron remnants into these new lipoprotein particles. Tissues remove triacylglycerol from lipoproteins, as discussed in Chapter 16, converting them into lipoprotein remnants that are removed by the liver. Much of the VLDL remnants (also called intermediate-density lipoproteins, or IDLs) are further metabolized to cholesterol-rich low-density lipoproteins (LDLs), which are taken up by most tissues as a source of cholesterol. Cholesterol excretion largely occurs via cholesterol efflux to form high-density lipoproteins (HDLs) which deliver cholesterol to tissues through exchange of cholesteryl esters for triacylglycerol molecules from other lipoprotein fractions, ultimately transferring the cholesterol to the LDL pool. LDL is mainly removed by the liver, and the liver secretes both cholesterol and bile acids synthesized from cholesterol into the lumen of the small intestine via the bile. To the extent that the cholesterol and bile acids are not completely reabsorbed, there is some net excretion of cholesterol in the feces. Each of these steps in cholesterol metabolism is discussed in this chapter.

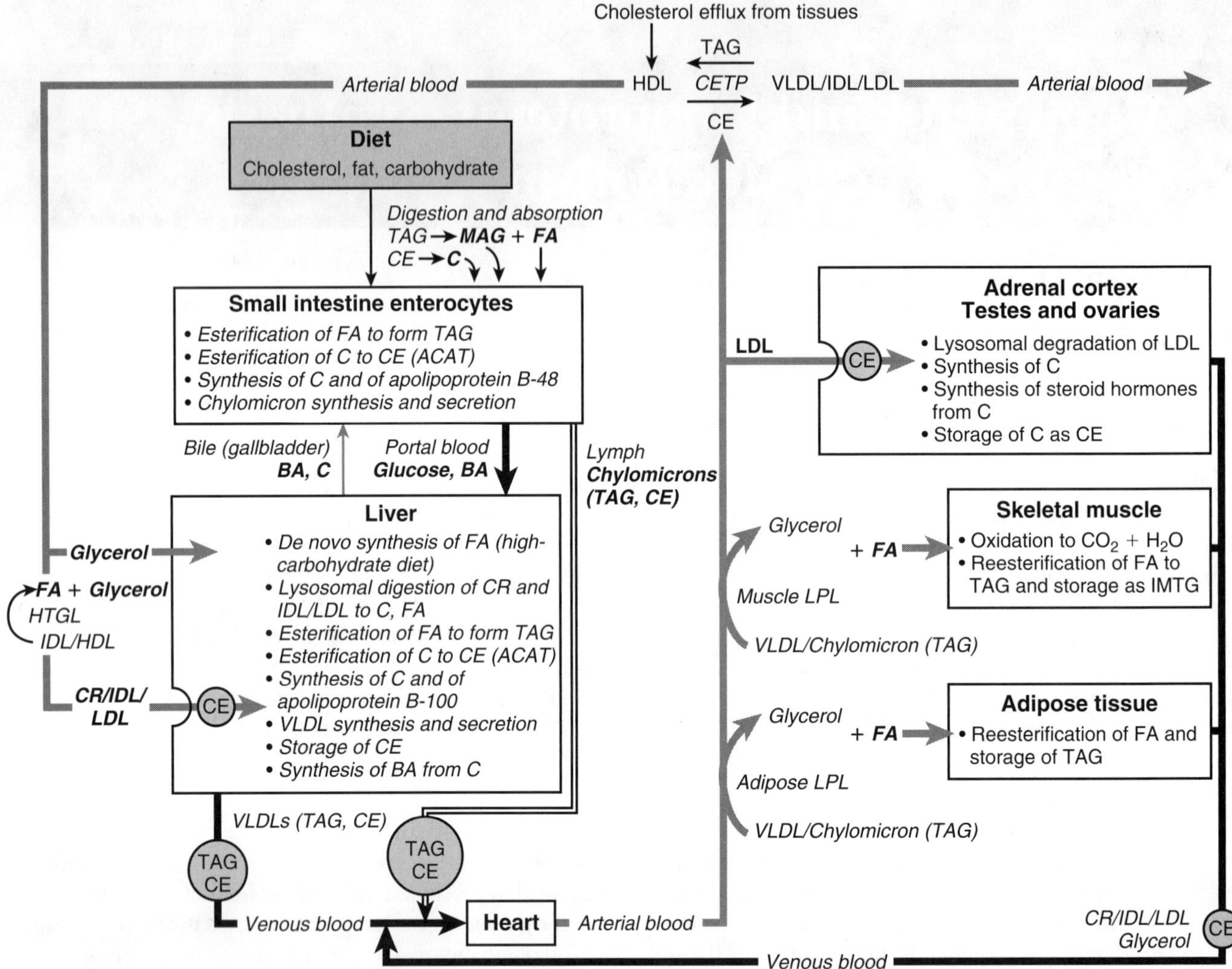

FIGURE 17-1 Overview of cholesterol synthesis and lipoprotein secretion. Cholesterol (*C*) is obtained from the diet or is synthesized by tissues, especially by the liver and intestine. The enzyme *ACAT* in the endoplasmic reticulum of cells converts C to cholesteryl esters (*CE*). The intestine and the liver secrete CE along with triacylglycerol (*TAG*) in large lipoprotein complexes known as chylomicrons (apo B-48–containing) and VLDL (apo B-100–containing), respectively. The chylomicrons and VLDL are reduced in size because of hydrolysis of TAG in these lipoproteins by lipoprotein lipase (*LPL*) associated with the capillary endothelium of various tissues. Adipose tissue and muscle have the highest concentrations of LPL and play an important role in removal of TAG from circulating lipoproteins. The action of LPL to remove core TAG is followed by loss of some surface components and the conversion of chylomicrons to chylomicron remnants (*CR*) and of VLDL to VLDL remnants called intermediate density lipoproteins (*IDL*) and to cholesterol-rich low-density lipoproteins (*LDL*). The liver has a similar enzyme called hepatic triglyceride lipase (*HTGL*) that acts on these remnants, as well as on high-density lipoproteins (*HDL*), to remove additional TAG. In addition, following HDL formation via cholesterol efflux from the tissues, there is exchange of CE from HDL for TAG from other lipoproteins, ultimately funneling CE to LDL for shipment to the liver for excretion. Receptor-mediated uptake of LDL by the LDL receptor (*LDLR*), which is an apo B-100/apo E receptor, is a major means of delivery of C to tissues. Almost all cells take up LDL but the largest number of these LDLRs are in the liver. LDLRs are also abundant in tissues involved in steroid hormone synthesis (adrenal cortex, testes, ovaries). LDL and other remnants taken up by the liver or other tissues are trafficked to the lysosomes where hydrolytic enzymes release free C into the cytosol. In the liver this C derived from receptor-mediated endocytosis of plasma lipoprotein remnants along with C synthesized in the liver can be secreted in VLDL, converted to bile acids (*BA*), secreted as free C in the bile, or stored in the liver as CE droplets. The major route for C excretion from the body is by the biliary secretion of BA and C followed by their excretion in the feces. Loss is small, however, due to the efficient reabsorption of BA into the portal blood (i.e., the enterohepatic circulation).

SYNTHESIS OF CHOLESTEROL AND ISOPRENOIDS

More than half of the cholesterol in the body is biosynthesized rather than absorbed from dietary sources. Quantitatively, the liver and intestine are the major sites of cholesterol synthesis, although synthesis occurs in all nucleated cells, including the skin, adrenal cortex, and gonads. Cholesterol intake from the diet is approximately 0.5 g/day, whereas cholesterol from synthesis is approximately 1 g/day. The enzymes of cholesterol synthesis are extramitochondrial, thus separating cholesterol synthesis from the

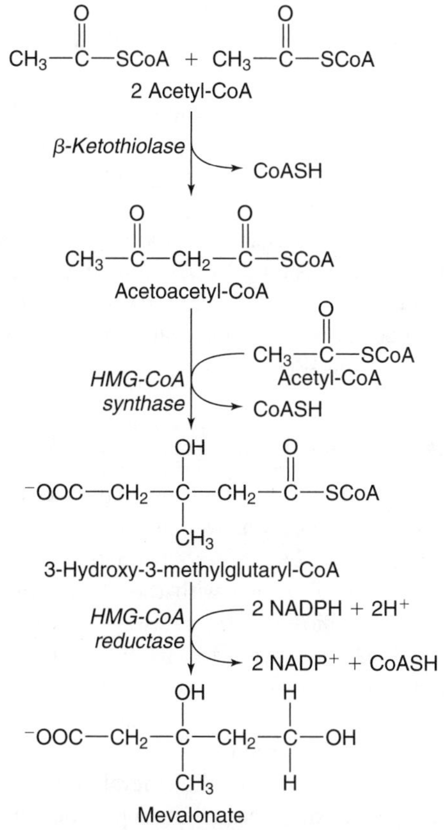

$CH_3{-}C({=}O){-}SCoA + CH_3{-}C({=}O){-}SCoA$

2 Acetyl-CoA

β-Ketothiolase → CoASH

$CH_3{-}C({=}O){-}CH_2{-}C({=}O){-}SCoA$

Acetoacetyl-CoA

HMG-CoA synthase ← $CH_3{-}C({=}O){-}SCoA$ Acetyl-CoA → CoASH

$^{-}OOC{-}CH_2{-}C(OH)(CH_3){-}CH_2{-}C({=}O){-}SCoA$

3-Hydroxy-3-methylglutaryl-CoA

HMG-CoA reductase ← 2 NADPH + $2H^+$ → 2 $NADP^+$ + CoASH

$^{-}OOC{-}CH_2{-}C(OH)(CH_3){-}CH_2{-}CH_2{-}OH$

Mevalonate

FIGURE 17-2 Mevalonate biosynthesis.

processes of fatty acid oxidation and ketone body metabolism. Cholesterol synthesis occurs in the cytosol, mainly in association with the smooth endoplasmic reticulum (ER) of the cell. Acetyl-CoA is a substrate for cholesterol synthesis, and this must be transferred from the mitochondrial matrix to the cytosol as citrate, as in lipogenesis. Mevalonate and squalene are key intermediates in the synthetic pathway.

CHOLESTEROL SYNTHESIS: CONVERSION OF ACETYL-CoA TO MEVALONATE IN THE CYTOSOL

The first steps in cholesterol biosynthesis result in the synthesis of mevalonate, a 6-carbon compound, from acetyl-CoA, as shown in Figure 17-2. Synthesis of the key intermediate 3-hydroxy-3-methylglutaryl coenzyme A (HMG-CoA) follows the same pathway described in Chapter 16 for the synthesis of ketone bodies, except that it occurs in the cytosol instead of the mitochondria, catalyzed by enzymes localized to the ER membrane. Two molecules of acetyl-CoA condense to form acetoacetyl-CoA (acetyl-CoA:acetoacetyl-CoA acetyltransferase). Another molecule of acetyl-CoA then condenses with a molecule of acetoacetyl-CoA to form HMG-CoA, a reaction catalyzed by HMG-CoA synthase. HMG-CoA is converted to mevalonate (see Figure 17-1) by HMG-CoA reductase, which is anchored in the ER membrane with its active site located in a long carboxyl terminal domain in the cytosol:

$$\text{HMG-CoA} + 2\ \text{NADPH} + 2\ H^+ \rightarrow \text{Mevalonate} + 2\ \text{NADP}^+ + \text{CoA}$$

This NADPH-requiring enzyme catalyzes the committed step in isoprenoid synthesis. The conversion of HMG-CoA to mevalonate is the main regulated step in cholesterol biosynthesis, and HMG-CoA reductase is regulated by several mechanisms, as described in the material that follows.

CHOLESTEROL SYNTHESIS: SYNTHESIS OF SQUALENE AND ISOPRENOIDS FROM MEVALONATE

Conversion of mevalonate to "active" isoprenoid units (5-carbon units) occurs as summarized in Figure 17-3. Mevalonate is converted to 3-phospho-5-pyrophosphomevalonate by three sequential phosphorylations.

(1) Mevalonate + ATP → 5-Phosphomevalonate + ADP

(2) 5-Phosphomevalonate + ATP → 5-Pyrophosphomevalonate + ADP

Synthesis of isopentenyl pyrophosphate from 5-pyrophosphomevalonate involves transient formation of a phosphorylated intermediate, 3-phospho-5-pyrophosphomevalonate and decarboxylation of the 5-pyrophosphomevalonate to form isopentenyl pyrophosphate.

(3) 5-Pyrophosphomevalonate + ATP → Isopentenyl pyrophosphate + CO_2 + ADP + P_i

Squalene, and thus the sterol molecule, is built from multiple isopentenyl groups, as shown in Figure 17-4. The reaction sequence involves condensation of two 5-carbon molecules to form one of 10 carbons. A third 5-carbon molecule is added to form a 15-carbon intermediate. Two 15-carbon intermediates are linked to form the 30-carbon squalene:

$$\text{5-C} \rightarrow \text{10-C} \rightarrow \text{15-C} \rightarrow \text{30-C}$$

Formation of the 10-carbon geranyl pyrophosphate involves two enzymatic reactions. First, isopentenyl pyrophosphate isomerase catalyzes the isomerization of isopentenyl pyrophosphate to dimethylallyl pyrophosphate (as shown in Figure 17-3). Then one molecule of each of these two activated isoprenes condenses. As shown in Figure 17-4, C1 of one isoprene bonds with C5 of the other (head-to-tail) to form geranyl pyrophosphate.

Isopentenyl pyrophosphate + Dimethylallyl pyrophosphate → Geranyl pyrophosphate + PP_i

In a mechanistically similar reaction, a third 5-carbon isopentenyl pyrophosphate condenses with geranyl pyrophosphate—in a head-to-tail manner—to form farnesyl pyrophosphate. Farnesyl pyrophosphate is a precursor of cholesterol, dolichol, ubiquinone, and the isoprenyl groups on a number of proteins and thus represents a branch-point in the synthesis of steroid and isoprenoid compounds.

Squalene synthase, the next step in cholesterol biosynthesis, is the committed step in sterol biosynthesis. This enzyme catalyzes the head-to-head condensation of two farnesyl pyrophosphates to form an intermediate, presqualene pyrophosphate. Presqualene pyrophosphate then undergoes

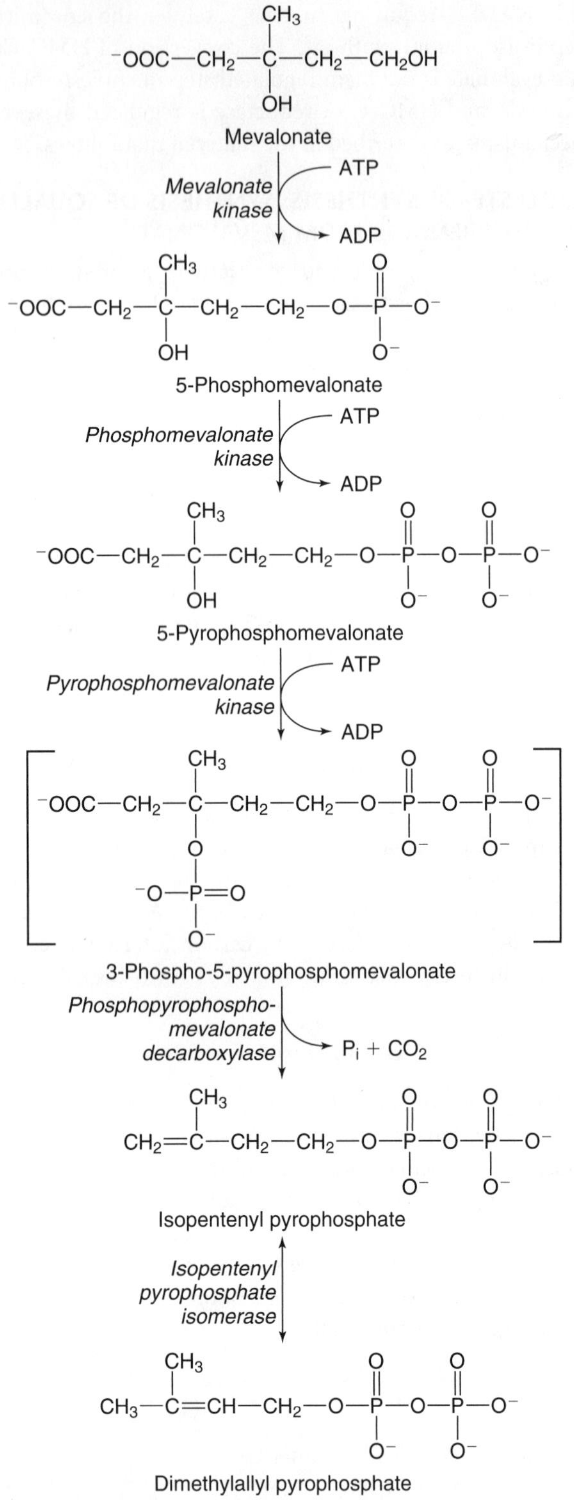

$^-OOC-CH_2-C(CH_3)(OH)-CH_2-CH_2OH$

Mevalonate

Mevalonate kinase (ATP → ADP)

$^-OOC-CH_2-C(CH_3)(OH)-CH_2-CH_2-O-PO_3^{2-}$

5-Phosphomevalonate

Phosphomevalonate kinase (ATP → ADP)

$^-OOC-CH_2-C(CH_3)(OH)-CH_2-CH_2-O-P(=O)(O^-)-O-P(=O)(O^-)-O^-$

5-Pyrophosphomevalonate

Pyrophosphomevalonate kinase (ATP → ADP)

$[^-OOC-CH_2-C(CH_3)(O-PO_3^{2-})-CH_2-CH_2-O-P(=O)(O^-)-O-P(=O)(O^-)-O^-]$

3-Phospho-5-pyrophosphomevalonate

Phosphopyrophosphomevalonate decarboxylase ($\rightarrow P_i + CO_2$)

$CH_2{=}C(CH_3)-CH_2-CH_2-O-P(=O)(O^-)-O-P(=O)(O^-)-O^-$

Isopentenyl pyrophosphate

Isopentenyl pyrophosphate isomerase

$CH_3-C(CH_3){=}CH-CH_2-O-P(=O)(O^-)-O-P(=O)(O^-)-O^-$

Dimethylallyl pyrophosphate

FIGURE 17-3 Synthesis of isoprenoid units.

NADPH-dependent reduction and pyrophosphate elimination to form squalene.

In Chapter 16, we noted that activation of fatty acids to their acyl-CoA derivatives involves hydrolysis of ATP to AMP and PP_i. Ubiquitous pyrophosphatases in cells then rapidly degrade PP_i to two inorganic phosphates. This same biochemical mechanism is used to drive to completion several of the intermediate reactions in isoprenoid and cholesterol biosynthesis.

CHOLESTEROL SYNTHESIS: SYNTHESIS OF LANOSTEROL AND CHOLESTEROL FROM SQUALENE

Several further rearrangements, with lanosterol as one of the intermediates, convert the 30-carbon squalene to the 27-carbon cholesterol. The conversion of squalene to lanosterol requires two enzymes, squalene epoxidase, which incorporates an oxygen atom from O_2 and uses NADPH as the source of reducing equivalents, and oxidosqualene:lanosterol cyclase, which converts the 30-carbon molecule into a structure with four rings. Lanosterol is further converted to cholesterol by a series of reactions that involves 19 steps and requires O_2 and NADPH.

REGULATION OF CHOLESTEROL SYNTHESIS

Cholesterol synthesis is tightly regulated in cells. Cholesterol synthesis in the cell, as well as cholesterol uptake via the LDL receptor (LDLR) as described later, is under negative feedback control. Along with the LDLR, the enzymes in the cholesterol biosynthetic pathway—HMG-CoA synthase, HMG-CoA reductase, farnesyl diphosphate synthase, and squalene synthase—are regulated coordinately at the transcriptional level. The primary target for regulation, however, is HMG-CoA reductase. HMG-CoA reductase is under negative feedback control by mevalonate, its immediate product, and by the eventual main product, cholesterol. The principal mechanism of regulation involves changes in the number of enzyme molecules per cell, which results from regulation at several levels ranging from transcription of the gene to stability of the protein. This enzyme also is inhibited by a class of drugs called statins, which are potent competitive inhibitors with inhibitor constants (K_i values) in the nanomolar range, that are used therapeutically for lowering plasma cholesterol levels.

ROLE OF STEROL REGULATORY ELEMENT–BINDING PROTEIN IN TRANSCRIPTIONAL RESPONSES TO CHANGES IN CHOLESTEROL LEVELS

Cholesterol itself regulates transcription of HMG-CoA reductase, as well as other enzymes involved in cholesterol homeostasis, by a mechanism that senses cellular cholesterol levels (Brown and Goldstein, 2009). Transcriptional control by cholesterol requires the presence of a sterol regulatory element (SRE) in the promoter regions of the genes where the transcription factor termed SRE-binding protein (SREBP) binds. There are three SREBPs: SREBP1a and SREBP1c, which are both encoded by the *SREBP1* gene by alternative exon usage, and SREBP2, which is encoded by the *SREBP2* gene. SREBPs induce transcription of genes coding for the enzymes involved in not only cholesterol metabolism but also fatty acid and triacylglycerol synthesis. SREBP2 is the main form that responds to cholesterol levels and activates transcription of genes encoding proteins involved in cholesterol metabolism including all the enzymes in cholesterol biosynthesis and the LDLR. SREBP1a activates genes involved in both cholesterol and fatty acid synthesis and thus may be important during cell division in meeting the need

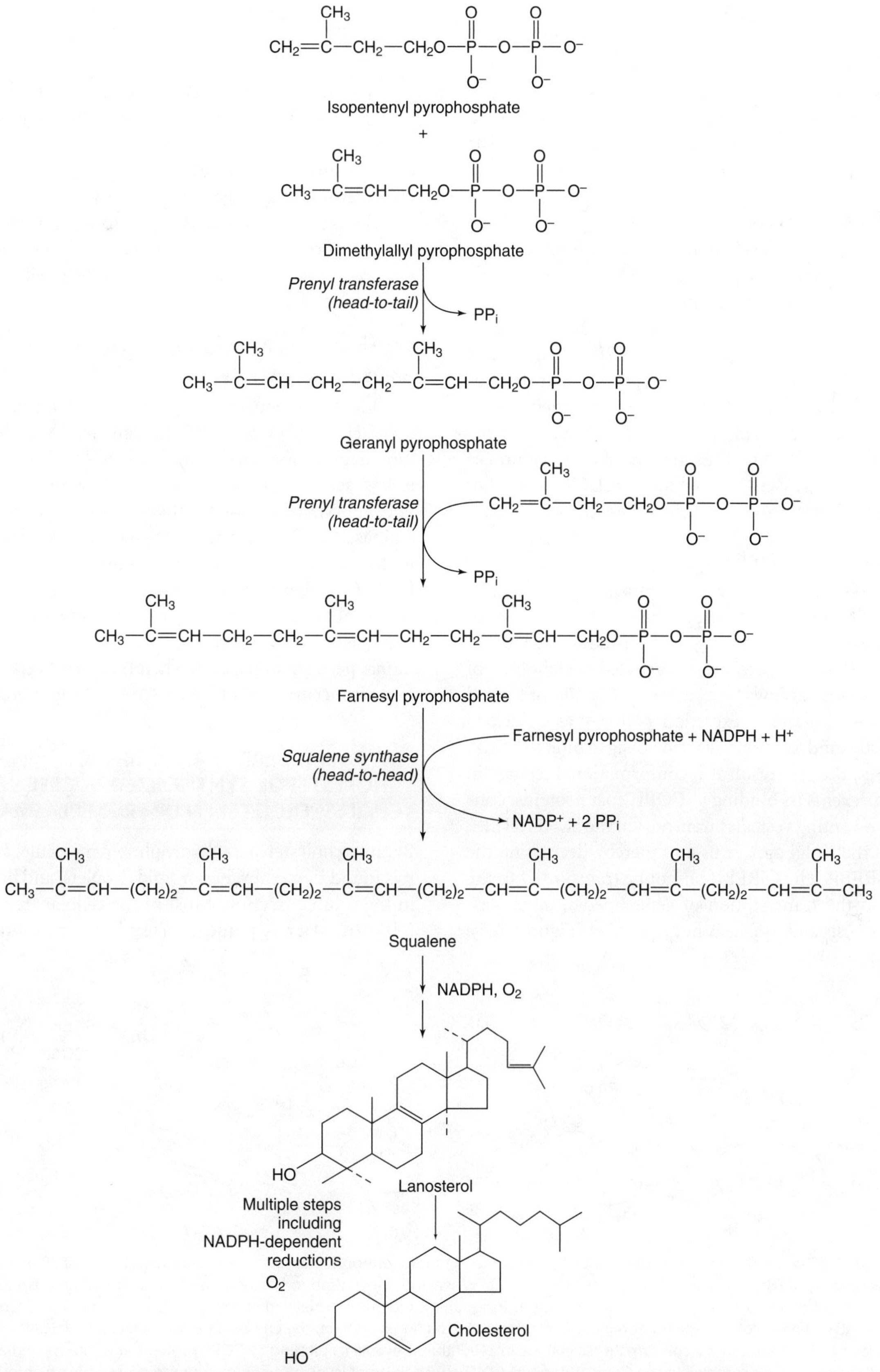

Isopentenyl pyrophosphate

+

Dimethylallyl pyrophosphate

Prenyl transferase (head-to-tail)

PP_i

Geranyl pyrophosphate

Prenyl transferase (head-to-tail)

PP_i

Farnesyl pyrophosphate

Squalene synthase (head-to-head)

Farnesyl pyrophosphate + NADPH + H^+

$NADP^+$ + 2 PP_i

Squalene

NADPH, O_2

HO

Lanosterol

Multiple steps including NADPH-dependent reductions O_2

HO

Cholesterol

FIGURE 17-4 Synthesis of squalene and cholesterol.

for increased membrane lipids. In contrast, SREBP1c expression is increased by insulin and/or feeding. SREBP1c mediates the induction of enzymes in fatty acid and triacylglycerol synthesis, as described in Chapter 16. All SREBPs contain two transmembrane helices that anchor these proteins in the ER. The N-terminal domain faces the cytosol and contains a basic helix-loop-helix leucine zipper transcription factor motif.

Low Cellular Cholesterol

When the cholesterol level in the ER membrane is low, SREBP cleavage–activating protein (SCAP) binds to a component of COPII coat proteins (proteins involved in vesicle budding from the ER). This binding mediates sequestration of the SCAP/SREBP complex in COPII-coated vesicles that leave the ER to be transported to the Golgi apparatus, where two proteases cleave SREBPs to release their N-terminal domains. The N-terminal domains can then enter the nucleus, where they bind to SREs to activate transcription of genes that encode HMG-CoA reductase, LDLR, and other enzymes of cholesterol and fatty acid metabolism.

High Cellular Cholesterol

When cholesterol level in the ER membrane is high, cholesterol directly binds SCAP, triggering SCAP to bind to an ER retention protein called Insig (insulin-induced gene). In addition, oxysterols, which are oxygenated metabolites of cholesterol present at low concentrations that are produced as part of the cholesterol excretion pathway as described below, directly bind to Insig, triggering Insig to bind to SCAP. In both cases, the end result is a conformational change in SCAP that prevents its binding to COPII coat proteins, consequently preventing vesicular transport of the SCAP/SREBP complex to the Golgi apparatus and thereby decreasing the release of SREBP. Thus SREBP cannot be transported to the nucleus, and the transcription of genes mediating cholesterol biosynthesis and uptake is not enhanced (Figure 17-5).

REGULATION OF HMG-CoA REDUCTASE DEGRADATION IN RESPONSE TO CHOLESTEROL LEVELS

The level of HMG-CoA reductase protein also is controlled by regulating its degradation. HMG-CoA reductase, which is localized in the ER membrane, contains a sterol-sensing domain similar to that in SCAP. When the ER membrane cholesterol level is high, cholesterol triggers the binding of HMG-CoA reductase to Insig through the sterol-sensing domain of reductase, causing not only ER retention but also the ubiquitination and proteosomal degradation of HMG-CoA reductase.

REGULATION OF HMG-CoA REDUCTASE BY PHOSPHORYLATION

In addition to regulation of enzyme protein levels, the activity of HMG-CoA reductase is regulated by a phosphorylation–dephosphorylation mechanism. HMG-CoA reductase is less active in the phosphorylated state. The enzyme is phosphorylated by AMP-activated protein kinase (AMPK), a kinase that is activated by an increase in cellular AMP as well as by phosphorylation by upstream kinases, such as LKB1 (Steinberg and Kemp, 2009). This phosphorylation–dephosphorylation mechanism explains why HMG-CoA reductase activity can respond rapidly to nutritional or hormonal perturbations, even when there has been little change in the concentration of HMG-CoA reductase protein.

INTRACELLULAR TRAFFICKING OF CHOLESTEROL SYNTHESIZED IN CELL VERSUS CHOLESTEROL TAKEN UP FROM PLASMA IN LDL

Because cholesterol is a hydrophobic molecule, almost all of it is found in membranes or lipid droplets, and little is found in the soluble fraction. Most of the cellular free cholesterol (60% to 80%) is found in the plasma membrane. Excess

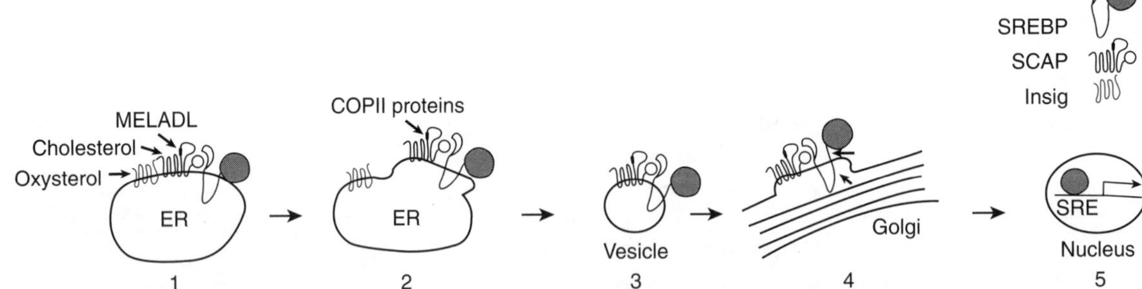

FIGURE 17-5 Cholesterol-dependent SREBP processing. (1) In the endoplasmic reticulum (ER) membrane, SREBP is associated with SREBP cleavage-activating protein (SCAP). When the concentration of cholesterol in ER membrane is high, cholesterol binds to SCAP, which allows binding to Insig, an ER retention protein, through SCAP's hexapeptide sequence (MELADL). Oxysterols, on the other hand, directly bind to Insig. In both cases, the end result is an association of SCAP with Insig, which brings about a conformational change in SCAP that prevents its binding to COPII proteins and thus movement of the SREBP/SCAP complex to the Golgi apparatus. (2) A low cholesterol level in the ER membrane causes release of Insig, which allows the SCAP/SREBP complex to bind components of COPII-coated proteins. (3) COPII vesicles form to deliver SCAP/SREBP to the Golgi. (4) In the Golgi apparatus, SREBP is cleaved at two sites (marked with arrows). (5) Mature SREBP, corresponding to the amino-terminal bHLH-ZIP domain (depicted as a filled circle), can then move to the nucleus where it can bind to sterol regulatory elements (SREs) in the promoters of various genes to increase lipid synthesis and uptake, such as those encoding HMG-CoA reductase and the LDL receptor.

cholesterol may be esterified to fatty acids and stored in lipid droplets. Cholesterol synthesized within the cell originates in the ER where it is synthesized, whereas cholesterol taken up from the plasma is brought into the endosomal–lysosomal system via LDL receptor–mediated endocytosis. Within the cell, the subcellular distribution of cholesterol is regulated by several distinct processes. There are two general mechanisms for intracellular cholesterol trafficking (Soccio and Breslow, 2004). One mechanism is through vesicular transport, in which cholesterol incorporated into membranes moves as part of membrane vesicles. The second way in which cholesterol can move from one subcellular location to another is by the monomolecular diffusion of protein-bound, or perhaps unbound, cholesterol, within the aqueous cytosol. Distinct trafficking pathways exist for cholesterol synthesized de novo and for cholesterol obtained via receptor-mediated endocytosis of LDLs.

Newly synthesized cholesterol moves from the ER primarily to the plasma membrane. A small fraction of this occurs by vesicular trafficking through the Golgi apparatus. The remainder of cholesterol movement from the ER to the plasma membrane likely occurs by nonvesicular, protein-mediated pathways, but the proteins involved are not known. Excess ER cholesterol can be esterified to form cholesteryl esters, which are stored in lipid droplets that are often found close to the ER. The cholesteryl esters in these droplets can be hydrolyzed to liberate free cholesterol when needed, and this cholesterol is thought to then be trafficked to the ER by protein-mediated diffusional transfer. Excess cholesterol in the plasma membrane can be trafficked back to the ER for esterification and storage in lipid droplets. As with transport from the ER to the plasma membrane, transport of cholesterol from the plasma membrane to the ER involves both vesicular and diffusional processes, but these do not appear to be the same steps in reverse.

As is detailed in subsequent text of this chapter, cholesteryl ester–rich LDLs are taken up by receptor-mediated endocytosis, thereby delivering exogenous cholesterol and cholesterol ester into the endosomal–lysosomal system. Acid lipases hydrolyze the cholesterol esters, liberating free cholesterol, some of which recycles back to the plasma membrane via the so-called endocytic recycling compartment that also delivers the LDL receptor back to the plasma membrane. The rest of the cholesterol remains in the endocytic vesicles, which are processed into the late endosome–lysosome (LE/LY) compartment. For exogenously derived LDL cholesterol to be used by the cell or to be involved in regulation of cholesterol-mediated homeostatic responses, the cholesterol must exit the LE/LY compartment.

Specific proteins in the LE/LY compartment are thought to be involved in the egress of cholesterol from the vesicular compartment. Evidence for a role of the Niemann-Pick type C (NPC) disease proteins (NPC1 and NPC2) in cholesterol trafficking or transport comes from abnormalities observed in patients with NPC disease. NPC disease is caused by defects in either NPC1 or NPC2, and the indistinguishable clinical phenotypes produced by defects in either protein suggest that the two proteins work together. In patients with NPC disease, unesterified cholesterol, as well as glycolipids, are trapped in the LE/LY compartment. Progression of neurological deterioration and premature death in these patients are thought to be due to both derangement in LE/LY function, which is secondary to sterol and lipid accumulation, and the absence of normal postendolysosomal metabolism of cholesterol. The transporter NPC1 has multiple membrane-spanning domains and contains a sterol-sensing domain similar to that found in several other proteins involved in cholesterol homeostasis, including SCAP and HMG-CoA reductase. NPC2 is a soluble intralysosomal protein that binds cholesterol. It has been proposed that NPC2 binds cholesterol directly following its generation from cholesterol esters by acid lipase; or it may extract membrane-bound cholesterol from internal LE/LY membranes by interacting with the LE/LY–specific phospholipid, lysobisphosphatidic acid (Storch and Xu, 2009). The cholesterol bound to NPC2 in the LE/LY lumen is proposed to then be delivered to NPC1, residing in the limiting membrane of the LE/LY, so that it can then be exported from the LE/LY compartment to other organelles (Wang et al., 2010; Peake and Vance, 2010). Cholesterol from the LE/LY compartment is trafficked primarily to the plasma membrane, with some of the cholesterol going through the Golgi apparatus before reaching the plasma membrane. A small portion of exogenously derived cholesterol moves from the LE/LY compartment directly to the ER.

Thus, whether cholesterol originates by endogenous synthesis within the cell or from vesicular uptake, the cholesterol ends up being distributed among the plasma and ER membranes and other cellular compartments. Cholesterol synthesis within the cell is regulated in response to the total cholesterol content of the cell, primarily that in the ER where SREBP2 and HMG-CoA reductase are located.

Trafficking of cholesterol to the mitochondria is also important because the mitochondria perform important steps in sterol metabolism and are necessary for synthesis of bile acids and steroid hormones. Cholesterol in mitochondria is converted into 27-hydroxycholesterol, which is the most abundant oxysterol in all tissues and which serves as an intermediate in bile acid synthesis in liver. Overall, the cholesterol content of mitochondria is relatively low, and the majority of the cholesterol is in the outer mitochondrial membrane.

SYNTHESIS OF STEROID HORMONES FROM CHOLESTEROL

At the inner mitochondrial membrane of steroidogenic cells, cholesterol is first converted into pregnenolone, the precursor of all steroid hormones. These reactions occur on the inner leaflet of the inner mitochondrial membrane. Mitochondrial cholesterol may be trafficked from the plasma membrane, from the endosomal–lysosomal compartment, or perhaps from lipid droplets. The movement of cholesterol into the mitochondria is accomplished by steroidogenic acute regulatory protein (StAR), which interacts with cholesterol and with specific outer mitochondrial membrane proteins in assembling a transport complex that moves the lipid to the inner mitochondrial membrane. The principal protein that interacts with StAR is translocator protein, TSPO (previously called peripheral-type benzodiazepine receptor). Cholesterol is passed from StAR to TSPO, which, along with other interacting proteins, moves cholesterol from the outer to the inner mitochondrial membrane (Rone et al., 2009; Mesmin and Maxfield, 2009).

SYNTHESIS OF BILE ACIDS AND OXYSTEROLS FROM CHOLESTEROL

As mentioned in Chapter 7, conversion of cholesterol to bile acids occurs exclusively in the liver. Bile acids and free cholesterol are incorporated into bile, which is destined for secretion into the proximal small intestine where the bile acids facilitate digestion and absorption of lipids. The ultimate excretion of bile acids and free cholesterol in bile is the major route for removing excess cholesterol from the body. Bile acids also have endocrine functions; they are ligands for several nuclear receptors that modulate a variety of cellular processes (Lefebvre et al., 2009).

Synthesis of bile acids involves a cascade of reactions catalyzed by enzymes located in the ER, mitochondria, cytosol, and peroxisomes. The steroid nucleus is modified in the ER and mitochondria, and the cholesterol side chain is removed in peroxisomes. The major steps of the two pathways for bile acid synthesis are shown in Figure 17-6 (Russell, 2009). In the major or "classic" pathway, the steroid nucleus modification includes 7α-hydroxylation catalyzed by cholesterol 7α-hydroxylase (CYP7A1), epimerization of the 3β-hydroxyl group (to 3α-), and saturation of the steroid nucleus. There is also a 12α-hydroxylation in the case of cholic acid synthesis, but not in chenodeoxycholic acid synthesis. These reactions precede the removal of the terminal three carbons of the cholesterol side chain by oxidative cleavage. In an alternative pathway, hydroxylation of the side chain at either the C24, C25, or C27 position to form oxysterols precedes the modification of the steroid nucleus by 7α-hydroxylation. Cholic acid and chenodeoxycholic acid are the two primary bile acids in human bile. They are conjugated with either glycine or taurine to become water soluble and are then secreted from the liver into the bile. Further modification of the primary bile acids by gut bacteria form secondary bile acids, which may be reabsorbed via the enterohepatic circulation and are thus found in the liver and bile along with the primary bile acids.

The rate of bile acid synthesis parallels the activity of CYP7A1, the main regulated step in the bile acid synthetic pathway. This step is under feedback regulation. Bile acids excreted from the liver are reabsorbed in the distal small intestine and transported back to the liver by the enterohepatic recirculation as mentioned below and in Chapter 7 (see Figure 7-9). Therefore bile acid reabsorption controls the overall rate of bile acid synthesis in the liver. Identification of farnesoid X receptor (FXR), which belongs to the nuclear receptor family, as a bile acid receptor provides a mechanism for this feedback regulation (Hageman et al., 2010). Thus gene expression for several proteins in bile acid metabolism, such as CYP7A and ileal BABP (an intestinal bile acid–binding protein that may shuttle bile acids from the apical to basolateral side of enterocytes upon reabsorption), may be controlled by FXR, either directly or indirectly. Bile acids may also regulate lipid, glucose, and energy metabolism by binding not only to FXR but also to the other nuclear hormone receptors, such as pregnane X receptor (PXR), constitutive androstane receptor (CAR), and a G protein–coupled bile acid receptor (TGR5).

Oxysterols, potent regulators of cholesterol synthesis and lipid metabolism, can be formed from cholesterol by both enzymatic and nonenzymatic reactions (Bjorkhem, 2009). The most abundant oxysterol in human plasma is 27-hydroxycholesterol. Oxysterols are ligands for another member of the nuclear hormone receptor family, liver X receptor (LXR) (Calkin and Tontonoz, 2010). The LXR response element is present in the promoter region of the *CYP7A1* gene, and LXR binding activates *CYP7A1* gene transcription in mice. Therefore regulation of *CYP7A1* transcription and bile acid synthesis in some mammals may depend on the balance between the positive LXR control and negative FXR control. The human *CYP7A1* promoter, however, does not contain an LXR-binding site and may not be a direct target of LXR. Nevertheless, LXR activates a variety of other genes involved in cholesterol and triacylglycerol metabolism. LXR activates transcription of genes encoding ATP-binding cassette transporters and other proteins involved in reverse cholesterol transport, mentioned later in this chapter. In addition, activation of the SREBP1c gene by LXR stimulates transcription of enzymes in fatty acid and triacylglycerol synthesis.

CHOLESTEROL TRANSPORT DURING ENTEROHEPATIC RECIRCULATION

Newly synthesized bile acids, along with those transported into the liver from the portal blood that drains the gastrointestinal tract, are secreted into bile for storage in the gallbladder before release into the small intestine after a meal (see Chapters 7 and 10). Cholesterol is also a component of bile, and secretion of cholesterol into bile is facilitated by the heterodimer of ABCG5/ABCG8, present at the canalicular membrane of hepatocytes. ABCG5/ABCG8 is also present on the brush border membrane of enterocytes where it secretes sterols in enterocytes back into the intestinal lumen. The rare mutation of either ABCG5 or ABCG8 causes β-sitosterolemia. Normally, plant sterol levels in plasma and tissues are very low due to the secretion of plant sterols back into the gut lumen. Patients with β-sitosterolemia absorb plant sterols efficiently, resulting in abnormally high plant sterol levels (including β-sitosterol) in plasma and tissues and deposition of sterols in the skin and arteries, which increases the risk of premature atherosclerosis (Berge et al., 2000).

Solubilization of biliary and dietary sterols in the intestinal lumen is aided by bile acids and phospholipids to form mixed micelles. Sterols are then absorbed via Niemann-Pick

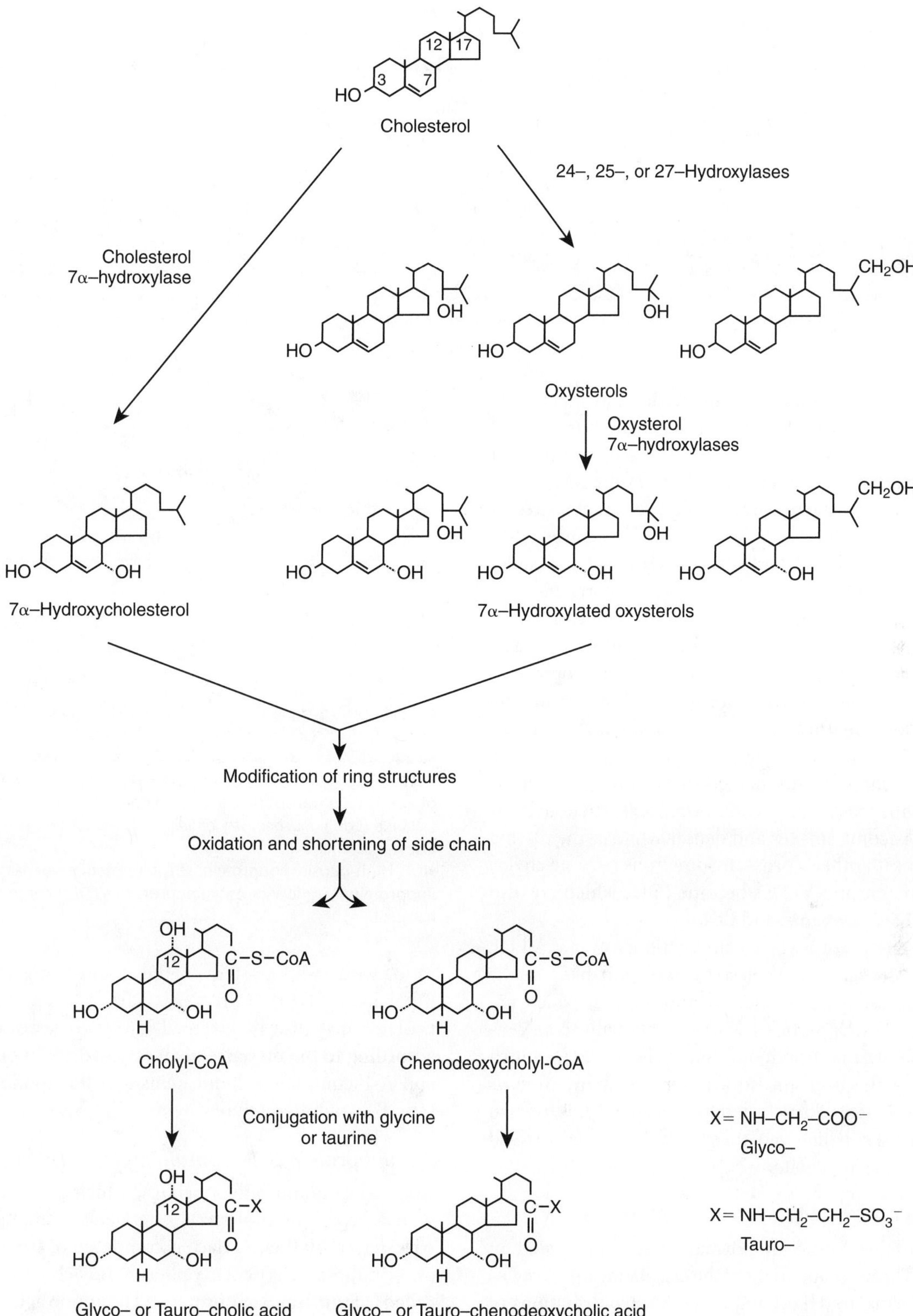

FIGURE 17-6 Synthesis of bile acids from cholesterol.

C1–like 1 protein (NPC1L1) at the apical membrane of enterocytes (Davis and Altmann, 2009; Betters and Yu, 2010). Ezetimibe, a plasma cholesterol reducing drug, inhibits intestinal absorption of cholesterol by binding to NPC1L1. Ezetimibe is used in combination with statins for lowering plasma cholesterol levels.

LIPOPROTEINS AND THEIR METABOLISM

For transport in aqueous blood plasma, the small intestine and liver package the nonpolar lipids (triacylglycerols and cholesteryl esters) in the core of large lipoprotein particles with amphipathic cholesterol and phospholipids, along

TABLE 17-1 Classification of Plasma Lipoproteins

MAJOR LIPOPROTEINS		OTHER MAJOR APOLIPOPROTEINS	DENSITY (g/mL)
Apo B-48 lipoproteins:	Chylomicrons	Apo C-II, apo C-III, apo E	<1.00
Apo B-100 lipoproteins:	VLDLs	Apo C-II, apo C-III, apo E	<1.006
	IDLs	Apo E	1.006–1.019
	LDLs	None	1.019–1.063
Apo A-I lipoproteins:	Pre-β-HDLs	None	>1.21
	α-HDLs	Apo A-II	1.063–1.21

HDL, High-density lipoprotein; *IDL,* intermediate-density lipoprotein; *LDL,* low-density lipoprotein; *VLDL,* very-low-density lipoprotein.

with certain apolipoproteins, on the surface, as mentioned in Chapters 10 and 16. The particles from the intestine are nascent chylomicrons, and those from the liver are nascent VLDLs. Chylomicrons secreted by the intestine after a fat-containing meal can have average molecular weights greater than 100 times those of the VLDLs secreted by the liver. They can contain approximately 500,000 triacylglycerol molecules and 30,000 cholesteryl ester molecules in their cores and perhaps 45,000 phospholipid molecules and 25,000 cholesterol molecules on their surfaces. Once the nascent lipoproteins enter the plasma, they pick up additional apolipoproteins (such as apo C and apo E apoproteins) from circulating HDLs to become mature chylomicrons and VLDLs. Largely because of the loss of triacylglycerol from the core of the lipoprotein complexes via the action of lipoprotein lipase associated with the capillary endothelial cells, chylomicrons and VLDLs become smaller and denser while in the plasma compartment. In other words, chylomicrons become chylomicron remnants and VLDLs become IDLs, which are also known as VLDL remnants, and LDLs.

Nascent HDLs are involved in chylomicron and VLDL metabolism as well as in cholesterol transport back to the liver. In contrast to chylomicrons and VLDLs, which are secreted as lipid-rich particles, HDLs are thought to be generated in the plasma. Apolipoprotein A-I (apo A-I), which is secreted by the liver and to a lesser extent intestine, is thought to associate with cell-derived phospholipids to form lipid-poor HDLs, which can then accumulate cell-derived cholesterol as they circulate.

TABLE 17-2 Distribution of Triacylglycerol and Cholesterol among Fasting Plasma Lipoproteins

	CHOLESTEROL	TRIACYLGLYCEROL
	mg/100 mL Plasma	
Total	176.4 ± 20 (100%)	84.9 ± 19.1 (100%)
VLDL	9.1 ± 3.7 (5.1%)	46.5 ± 12.8 (54.8%)
IDL	3.5 ± 4.3 (1.9%)	5.8 ± 6.2 (6.6%)
LDL	114.8 ± 28 (65.1%)	15.9 ± 8.8 (18.7%)
HDL	45.3 ± 11.8 (25.7%)	12.2 ± 1.6 (14.3%)

Recalculated from Fielding, P. E., & Fielding, C. J. (1996). Dynamics of lipoprotein transport in the circulatory system. In D. E. Vance & J. Vance (Eds.). *Biochemistry of lipids* (pp. 495–516). Amsterdam: Elsevier Science-NL.
HDL, High-density lipoprotein; *IDL,* intermediate-density lipoprotein; *LDL,* low-density lipoprotein; *VLDL,* very-low-density lipoprotein.

MAJOR GROUPS OF PLASMA LIPOPROTEINS

The lipoproteins found in normal plasma are listed in Table 17-1. The most abundant of the circulating lipoproteins in fasting plasma are HDLs and LDLs. The contributions of the major lipoprotein fractions to the triacylglycerol and total cholesterol content of normal plasma are shown in Table 17-2.

The plasma lipoproteins can be separated by ultracentrifugation or electrophoresis. Their names are based on their density or electrophoretic migration. Density is inversely proportional to the lipid content (% by weight) of the lipoproteins, with HDLs being denser than VLDLs, for example. In agarose gel electrophoresis, lipoprotein complexes are mainly separated on the basis of their charge-to-mass ratio, with α-lipoproteins (HDLs) migrating farther than β-particles (LDLs) or pre-β-particles (VLDLs). Plasma lipoproteins may also be grouped into two classes of particles according to the presence of an essential apolipoprotein: the apo A-I–containing lipoproteins and the apolipoprotein B (apo B)–containing lipoproteins.

Apolipoprotein A-1–Containing Lipoproteins

Apo A-I is found only in HDLs, which are small particles with a "core" of cholesteryl esters and a small amount of triacylglycerol; their surface is composed of free cholesterol, phospholipids (particularly phosphatidylcholine, commonly called lecithin), and apoproteins. The amino acid sequence of apo A-I includes a series of amphipathic helical repeats, each made up of 22 amino acids. Hydrophobic amino acids are predominantly localized to one face of the helix and turned toward the lipid core, whereas charged and other hydrophilic residues are turned out to face the aqueous medium. Apo A-I is flexible and is weakly associated with the surface of HDLs. As a result, the shape of apo A-I on the surface of HDLs can adapt as the lipid core of the particle expands. If the diameter of the HDL particles is reduced by loss of core lipids (cholesteryl esters and triacylglycerols), lipid-poor apo A-I easily dissociates from the surface of HDLs. Many HDL particles contain smaller amounts of other apolipoproteins in addition to apo A-I (i.e., apo A-II, apo A-IV, apo C-I, apo C-III, and apo E). The functions of several of these proteins are clearly established, and their mechanisms of lipid binding are similar to those described for apo A-I. In addition to being an essential structural component of HDL, apo A-I promotes desorption of free cholesterol from cell membranes and activates cholesterol esterification by the lecithin:cholesterol acyltransferase (LCAT).

Apoliprotein B–Containing Lipoproteins

The apo B–containing lipoproteins are chylomicrons, VLDLs, and their circulating lipoprotein lipolysis products (i.e., chylomicron remnants, IDLs, and LDLs). Each VLDL particle contains a single molecule of apo B-100, a large protein comprising 4,536 amino acid residues. IDLs and LDLs are formed in the circulation as lipolysis products of VLDL, and therefore these particles also contain one copy of apo B-100. Apo B-100 is synthesized only in liver and makes a single turn around the circumference of an LDL particle. As mentioned in Chapter 10, chylomicrons and their remnants contain one molecule of a shorter form of apo B called apo B-48 (2,152 amino acids in length, 48% of the mass of apo B-100). Apo B-48 is encoded by the same gene as apo B-100, but is made only in intestine where an intestine-specific cytosine deaminase converts a cytosine to a uracil, creating a premature stop codon in the apo B messenger RNA (mRNA). Other apolipoproteins adsorbed to the chylomicron and VLDL surface include the lipoprotein lipase cofactor apo C-II and the receptor ligand apo E. These increase the stability of the large particles, regulate the catabolism of chylomicron and VLDL lipids, and control the removal of partially lipolyzed chylomicron and VLDL particles (IDLs) from the circulation by receptor-mediated uptake into cells.

The large apo B-48 and B-100 polypeptides, like apo A-I, contain stretches of amphipathic helix, but these helical regions form a smaller proportion of the whole sequence in apo B than in apo A-I. Apo B-100 contains at least 11 cystine bridges, most of them in the N-terminal region. Unlike Apo A-I, Apo B does not dissociate during the metabolism of VLDL to IDL and LDL or of chylomicrons to chylomicron remnants. Apo B plays an essential role in VLDL and chylomicron secretion, and it also is important in the association of triacylglycerol-rich lipoproteins with the capillary endothelium before lipolysis. Apo B also allows for removal of apo B-100–containing lipoprotein particles from the circulation by receptor-mediated uptake. The apo B in VLDL remnants (IDLs and LDLs) recognizes the LDLR in the liver and other tissues for uptake by endocytosis. In contrast, chylomicron remnants are removed by the LDLR or LDL receptor–like protein (LRP1) by recognition of apo E. Apo B-48 lacks the C-terminal half of apo B-100 that contains the amino acid sequence that binds to the LDLR, so chylomicron remnant uptake is mediated by apo E and not by apo B. The LDLR binds apo E with higher affinity than apo B-100. Heparin sulfate proteoglycans, such as syndecan-1, may also play a role in removal of lipoprotein remnants (Stanford et al., 2009; Williams and Chen, 2010).

Plasma normally contains a relatively large amount of apo B-100 and only a very small amount of apo B-48 because chylomicrons are very rapidly cleared from the circulation by lipase-mediated catabolism and removal of chylomicron remnants by hepatic receptors. Most of the circulating apo B-100 is in LDLs, with only small amounts in IDLs and VLDLs, because VLDL particles are relatively rapidly catabolized by lipases. Some VLDL particles are removed as IDLs (i.e., VLDL remnants), but most (50% to 70%) are converted to LDL particles, which have a much longer circulation time (~2 days) than the lighter triacylglycerol-rich lipoproteins.

SYNTHESIS AND SECRETION OF TRIACYLGLYCEROL-RICH LIPOPROTEINS: CHYLOMICRONS AND VLDLS

As mentioned in Chapter 10, intestinal cells make apo B-48, the structural protein of chylomicrons. Initially the intracellular precursor of the chylomicron particle is a lipid-poor phospholipid monolayer encapsulating cholesteryl ester. The first addition of triacylglycerol to the chylomicron precursor particles, which occurs cotranslationally at the luminal side of the ER membrane, requires the microsomal triacylglycerol transfer protein (MTP) (Mansbach and Siddiqi, 2010). A second step of triacylglycerol addition, which leads to the formation of mature, triacylglycerol-rich chylomicrons, is a fusion of this dense apo B-48–containing primordial particle with a lipid-rich, protein-poor particle that does not contain apo B-48 but is composed mostly of triacylglycerols and cholesteryl esters. The importance of MTP is evident from the human disorder called abetalipoproteinemia. In this hereditary disease, mutations in the gene encoding MTP result in an inability to produce chylomicrons and VLDLs in the intestine and liver, respectively.

Nascent chylomicrons, thus assembled within the ER–Golgi apparatus, are released from the enterocyte within mature Golgi vesicles that fuse with the basolateral region of the plasma membrane. These newly secreted particles are too large to penetrate the capillary membrane. Therefore they enter the lymphatic system through the lacteals of the intestinal villi and subsequently enter the venous plasma compartment via the left thoracic lymph duct. Chylomicron secretion into the lymphatics rather than directly into the portal vein is thought to be important for delivery of dietary lipid to extrahepatic tissue without a first pass through the liver. Removal of associated toxins by lymphatic leukocytes is also thought to occur by the same lymphatic route.

The assembly of VLDL within the hepatocyte follows a similar two-step process. Initially precursor particles are assembled with a phospholipid shell containing apo B-100 surrounding a hydrophobic core of cholesteryl ester. Some triacylglycerol is added via MTP. The second step of VLDL assembly involves the addition of triacylglycerol to these precursor particles. Synthesis of apo B proteins is constant, but apo B proteins undergo degradation depending upon the availability of triacylglycerol on the luminal side of the ER.

Whereas triacylglycerol in chylomicrons originates mainly from dietary fat, some of the fatty acids in the VLDL triacylglycerol are synthesized de novo from dietary carbohydrate. VLDL triacylglycerol secretion and circulating concentrations both increase after a carbohydrate-rich meal. Other fatty acyl groups in the triacylglycerols of VLDLs originate from plasma lipoprotein remnants that are internalized by the liver or from unesterified circulating fatty acids. Thus the fatty acyl groups in chylomicron triacylglycerols reflect directly the dietary intake, whereas those in VLDL triacylglycerols represent a mixture of exogenously and endogenously derived fatty acyl chains.

CLEARANCE OF TRIACYLGLYCEROL IN CHYLOMICRONS AND VLDLS BY LIPOPROTEIN LIPASE

Because of their hydrophobicity, most of the triacylglycerol and cholesteryl esters are concentrated in the core of plasma lipoprotein particles; but this core is in rapid equilibrium with small amounts of the same lipids dissolved within the surface monolayer, which is made up mainly of phospholipid and free cholesterol. The hydrolysis of triacylglycerol of apo B–containing lipoproteins by plasma lipases or the transfer of triacylglycerol by lipid transfer proteins depletes only the surface pool of lipids. The surface lipids are replenished by equilibration from the core of the particle. The surface triacylglycerol is hydrolyzed by lipoprotein lipase (LPL), a triacylglycerol hydrolase present on the capillary endothelium of various tissues, with highest concentrations present in muscle and adipose tissues (Wang and Eckel, 2009). LPL is synthesized by the parenchymal cells of these tissues and is then secreted. The secreted LPL is transported to the vascular face of the endothelial cells within the tissue, where it is anchored by ionic interaction with heparin sulfate proteoglycans and/or by glycosylphosphatidylinositol so that its active site faces the lumen of the capillary. Only LPL present in the endothelial fraction of adipose or muscle tissue can hydrolyze the triacylglycerol present in lipoprotein particles (see Chapter 16, Figure 16-8).

Regulation of Muscle and Adipose Lipoprotein Lipase Abundance and Activity

Chylomicrons and VLDLs are the substrates for LPLs that are bound to the endothelial cell surface of adipose and muscle tissues. Much of the free fatty acid produced by lipolysis is taken up locally, although some escapes into the general circulation. During fasting, the plasma concentration of VLDL triacylglycerol (from liver) is relatively low, and chylomicron triacylglycerol (from intestine) is almost absent. LPL is regulated by nutritional and hormonal states at the transcriptional and posttranscriptional levels in a tissue-specific manner. During fasting, the expression of LPL in adipose tissue is downregulated because of the lack of insulin, whereas LPL levels in heart and other muscle tissues are maintained. LPL on the capillary endothelial surface of the heart has a higher affinity (lower K_m) for lipoprotein substrate (triacylglycerol) than does LPL in the adipose tissue. This difference in affinity of LPL for lipoprotein substrate may provide a mechanism for regulating the partitioning of lipoprotein triacylglycerol–derived fatty acids between storage in adipose tissue and oxidation in muscle tissues. According to this model, triacylglycerol hydrolysis by the vascular bed of the heart is determined mainly by the endothelial LPL abundance, because heart LPL has a low K_m and, as a result, is saturated at low circulating VLDL or chylomicron concentrations. In contrast, in adipose tissue, where the apparent K_m exceeds normal circulating triacylglycerol concentrations, triacylglycerol hydrolysis is influenced by VLDL and chylomicron concentrations as well as by LPL abundance. Thus, during starvation, when muscle LPL is relatively more abundant compared to adipose tissue LPL and when lipoprotein concentrations are relatively low, the energy needs of muscle cells (such as those of the heart) that use fatty acids from lipoprotein triacylglcerol hydrolysis as a fuel would receive priority. In the fed state, however, adipose tissue would be exposed to higher concentrations of fatty acids both because of the increase in adipose tissue endothelial LPL abundance and because of the higher concentrations of lipoproteins. The increased direction of fatty acids to the adipose tissue promotes the reesterification and storage of the fatty acids in the adipose tissue. The stored triacylglcerol in adipose tissue can be hydrolyzed to release fatty acids and glycerol during extended periods of exercise or fasting by activation of hormone-sensitive lipase (HSL) and adipose triacylglycerol lipase/perilipin in adipose tissue, as described in Chapter 16.

Role of Apolipoprotein C-II as an Activator of Lipoprotein Lipase

The hydrolysis of triacylglycerol by LPL depends on the presence of its activator, apo C-II, on the surface of chylomicron and VLDL particles. Apo C-II preferentially transfers from other lipoproteins (e.g., HDLs) to the newly secreted nascent VLDLs and chylomicrons as these particles are released into the plasma.

As the triacylglycerol of a chylomicron is hydrolyzed by LPL, the chylomicron decreases in size. This usually occurs within an hour after a meal. As the chylomicron loses its triacylglycerol core, apo C-II dissociates from its surface. After approximately 80% of the initial triacylglycerol has been lost, insufficient apo C-II remains to support LPL activity, and the chylomicron remnant is then cleared by the liver via apo E recognition. In addition, lipolysis may be modified by other proteins, such as endothelial cell–specific glycosylphosphatidylinositol-anchored HDL-binding protein 1 (GPIHBP1), apo C-III, apo A-V, and certain angiopoietin-like proteins (Beigneux et al., 2009). The chylomicron remnants contain residual triacylglycerol together with most of the cholesteryl ester that was in the initial chylomicron.

Similarly, the triacylglycerol in VLDLs is hydrolyzed by LPL, with VLDLs, IDLs, and LDLs making up a lipolysis cascade. All LDLs in the plasma are formed from the catabolism of VLDLs and IDLs, but not all VLDLs become LDLs; some are cleared as IDLs. As VLDL triacylglcyerol is catabolized, apo C-II dissociates, as it does from chylomicrons, leaving cholesterol-rich VLDL remnants (usually called IDLs) that still contain both apo B-100 and apo E. Some IDL may be internalized, but most is converted to LDL in humans by another lipase, hepatic triacylglycerol lipase (HTGL), which is present at the endothelial surface of the liver capillaries (Olivecrona and Olivecrona, 2010). HTGL is structurally related to the LPL found in muscle and adipose tissue. HTGL hydrolyzes IDL triacylglcerol, converting IDL to LDL, and it also plays an important role in hydrolyzing HDL triacylglycerol. During the process of IDL to LDL conversion, apo E also is transferred from plasma IDL to plasma HDL. Some of the IDL particles become LDLs by losing additional triacylglcyerol at the hepatocyte surface.

CHOLESTEROL UPTAKE BY LDL RECEPTOR–MEDIATED ENDOCYTOSIS AND INTRACELLULAR ESTERIFICATION OF CHOLESTEROL

Cholesterol-rich LDLs as well as VLDL remnants (IDLs) and chylomicron remnants, which have lost triacylglycerols but are rich in cholesteryl esters, are all taken up into cells via the high-affinity LDLR, which recognizes apo E and apo B-100 (Figure 17-7). The LDLR spans the plasma membrane. An extracellular domain contains the apo B-100/apo E binding site. The intracellular domain directs clustering of LDLRs into regions of the plasma membrane called clathrin-coated pits. Once the lipoprotein remnant (chylomicron remnant, IDL, or LDL) binds to the LDLR, the complex is rapidly internalized by the process of endocytosis. The receptor/remnant complex undergoes invagination within the coated pit, forming a vesicle that is pinched off to internalize the lipoprotein remnant. The clathrin coat is removed from the internalized endosomal vesicle, and the endosome is then acidified through the action of an ATP-dependent proton pump. In this acidified endosome, the lipoprotein remnant and the LDLR dissociate and sorting occurs. The endosomal membranes harboring the receptor are sorted to recycling endosomes and returned to the plasma membrane, whereas the lipoprotein remnants remain in the endosome and enter the LE/LY compartment. Acid hydrolases in the lysosome degrade the apoprotein to free amino acids and the cholesteryl esters to fatty acids and cholesterol. Movement of the free cholesterol out of the late endosomal-lysosomal compartment requires NPC1 and NPC2 proteins, as discussed previously for the intracellular trafficking of cholesterol.

Almost all mammalian cells contain LDLRs. However, the greatest number of functional LDLRs is expressed in the liver, and the majority of circulating lipoprotein remnants are eventually taken up by the liver. LDLRs also are relatively abundant in adrenal and gonadal cells. Because the circulating concentration of apo B lipoproteins exceeds that required for saturation of the high-affinity LDLRs, the rate of internalization of LDL by the liver is determined by the number of LDLRs rather than by the concentration of LDL. In contrast to LDL and IDL, chylomicron remnants are rapidly cleared by the LDLR. Familial hypercholesterolemia (FH) is caused by a mutation in the LDLR gene and is a prevalent disorder of lipoprotein metabolism. Patients with FH have very high plasma LDL levels.

Although receptor-mediated endocytosis is the predominant mechanism for uptake of lipoproteins, there are other minor processes of nonspecific (receptor-independent) uptake of intact LDL particles by the liver, especially when circulating LDL levels are high.

The free cholesterol released in the cell by lysosomal hydrolysis of LDL is esterified in the ER in a reaction catalyzed by acyl-CoA:cholesterol acyltransferase (ACAT). Esterification of cholesterol is a means to remove excess free cholesterol (Chang et al., 2009) and to either store it or secrete it in lipoproteins.

$$\text{Cholesterol} + \text{Fatty acyl-CoA} \rightarrow \text{Cholesteryl ester}$$

ACAT plays an important role in establishing the cellular free cholesterol pool that provides substrates for synthesis of bile acids or steroid hormones in liver and adrenal cortex, respectively. The cholesteryl esters formed are either

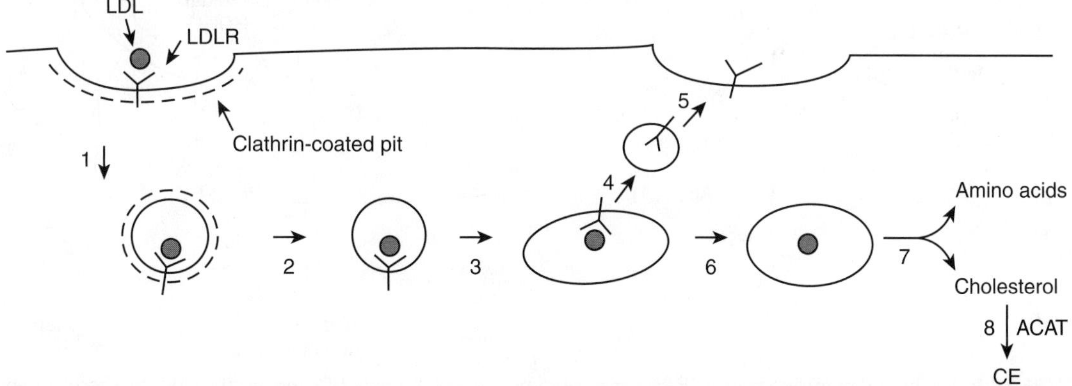

FIGURE 17-7 Receptor-mediated endocytosis of lipoproteins. When a low-density lipoprotein (*LDL*) particle binds to an LDL receptor (*LDLR*) at a clathrin-coated pit, a coated vesicle is invaginated and internalized (*1*). The vesicle is uncoated (*2*) and fuses with an endosome (*3*). In the early endosome, the LDL/LDLR complex dissociates (*4*) and budding of a transport/recycling vesicle recycles the LDLR back to the membrane (*5*). The remaining LDL-containing late endosome fuses with a lysosome (*6*), and hydrolytic enzymes in the lysosome produce amino acids as well as free cholesterol (*7*). Cholesterol is esterified to cholesteryl ester (*CE*) by acyl-CoA cholesterol acyltransferase (*ACAT*), which is an ER membrane enzyme (*8*).

deposited in the core of lipoprotein particles or in cytosolic lipid droplets. ACAT is critical for supplying cholesteryl esters as a core lipid for chylomicron and VLDL synthesis in intestine and liver, respectively, as well as in the formation of cholesteryl-ester–laden foam cells from macrophages, as is described later in this chapter. The stored cholesteryl esters are hydrolyzed by neutral cholesteryl ester hydrolase to generate free cholesterol when it is needed. There may be additional cholesteryl ester hydrolases; for example, HSL is known to function as a cholesteryl ester hydrolase in addition to its major action in diacylglycerol hydrolysis. HSL as well as perilipin, a lipid droplet surface protein that regulates HSL translocation and activation, are found on the surface of cholesteryl ester droplets in steroidogenic cells, such as adrenal cortical cells.

REVERSE CHOLESTEROL TRANSPORT AND HDLS

The apo B–containing lipoproteins, particularly LDLs, are thought to deliver several hundred milligrams of cholesterol to tissues daily. Consequently, there must be some mechanism to balance that delivery system to maintain homeostasis. HDL plays an important role in cholesterol homeostasis by transporting cholesterol from extrahepatic tissues back to liver for conversion to bile acids and excretion into the bile, a process called reverse cholesterol transport (Fielding and Fielding, 1995).

Approximately 95% of HDL in plasma consists of spherical particles with a hydrophobic lipid core; these are called α-HDLs because they migrate fast (so-called α-migration) in agarose gel electrophoresis. The hallmark of all HDLs is the presence of apo A-I. In addition to a few molecules of apo A-I, these particles also contain apo A-II, a small protein implicated in HDL turnover. A small proportion of spherical HDLs also contain other lipoproteins (including apo C-II and apo E) that can be transferred to apo B–containing lipoproteins and that are involved in the metabolism of plasma VLDL and chylomicron triacylglycerol. The remaining HDLs are very small particles (6 to 7 nm in diameter) composed of apo A-I and phospholipids, without a significant lipid core. These lipid-poor HDLs migrate slowly (so-called pre-β migration) in gel electrophoresis and are called pre-β–HDL.

Cholesterol Efflux from Tissues

The majority of pre-β–HDLs are formed from spherical α-HDL by several reactions, all of which increase the surface-to-volume ratio of the particle. Reduction of HDL core volume leads to dissociation of some of the apo A-I, probably as a complex with a small amount of phospholipid. The hydrolysis of HDL triacylglycerol by hepatic triacylglycerol lipase, the activity of plasma phospholipid transfer protein (PLTP), and a hepatic cell-surface receptor SR-BI (scavenger receptor class B type I) that selectively internalizes cholesteryl esters from HDL all probably contribute to formation of pre-β–HDL from α-HDL (Krimbou et al., 2006; Zannis et al., 2006). As shown in Figure 17-8, pre-β–HDLs (molecular mass: 65 to 70 kDa) cross the endothelium freely.

Pre-β–HDLs are enriched in the extracellular fluid of extrahepatic tissues, compared with the larger spherical

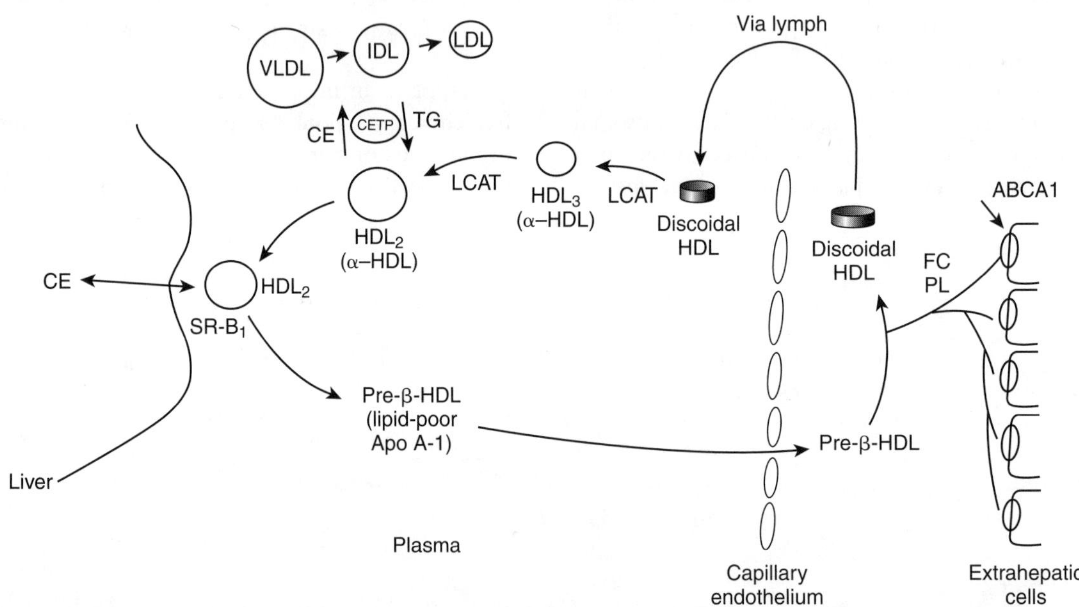

FIGURE 17-8 The high-density lipoprotein (*HDL*) cycle. Lipid-poor apo A-I (*pre-β–HDL*) passes through the vascular bed to the extravascular space and accumulates free cholesterol (*FC*) and phospholipid (*PL*) from the parenchymal cells of extrahepatic tissues via ABC-cassette transporter A1 (*ABCA1*). The discoidal HDLs that form reenter the plasma compartment via the lymph. Free cholesterol in HDL is esterified by LCAT (lecithin:cholesterol acyltransferase) as HDL discs become spheres and then larger spheres (α-HDLs from *HDL$_3$* to *HDL$_2$*). After hepatic triacylglycerol lipase (HTGL) and/or cholesteryl ester transfer protein (*CETP*) activity, cholesterol is selectively taken up by the liver via scavenger receptor-B1(*SR-B$_1$*) and pre-β–HDL or lipid-poor apo A-I is released for recycling.

α-HDLs, most of which have a molecular mass of 180 to 250 kDa, that are found in the plasma. Pre-β–HDLs are exceptionally active as acceptors of free cholesterol and phospholipids from the parenchymal cells of extrahepatic tissues. A major location from which free cholesterol in these tissues is transferred to pre-β–HDLs is at plasma membrane caveolae, microdomains of the plasma membrane that are rich in cholesterol. Free cholesterol efflux to pre-β–HDL is directly, or indirectly via phospholipid efflux, dependent on the cell membrane transporter ABCA1 (ATP-binding cassette transporter A1) and possibly ABCG1 (Yvan-Charvet et al., 2010). Cholesterol efflux is a complex process that may include both intracellular and extracellular events. Gradually, within the extracellular space, the small pre-β–HDLs become enlarged into disc-shaped nascent HDL by the continuing transfer of phosphatidylcholine and free cholesterol from cell membranes via ABCA1. In addition, apo A1 may undergo endocytosis to take up cholesterol from intracellular membranes, such as ER membrane, and then be retroendocytosed as lipidated nascent HDL (Lorkowski, 2008). Discoidal HDLs formed in these ways reenter the plasma via the main lymph trunks.

Esterification of Cholesterol in HDL and Transfer of Some Cholesteryl Ester to Apo B–Containing Lipoproteins

Within the plasma, LCAT esterifies free cholesterol with a fatty acid (e.g., linoleate) from phosphatidylcholine. This reaction preferentially uses the *sn*-2 acyl chain of phosphatidylcholine as the fatty acid (Rousset et al., 2009). The LCAT reaction is as follows:

Cholesterol + Phosphatidylcholine →
Lysophosphatidylcholine + Cholesteryl ester

Apo A-I present in the HDL particles activates plasma LCAT, probably by directly interacting with the enzyme. The hydrophobic cholesteryl ester formed then moves from the surface of the HDL into the core, a process that allows more free cholesterol to adsorb onto the surface. As the cholesteryl ester core builds up, the nascent discoidal HDL particle becomes spherical, larger, and less dense. The transfer of phospholipids from tissues is much slower than that of free cholesterol. As a result, much of the phosphatidylcholine needed for the LCAT reaction may come from transfer of phospholipids from apo B-100–containing lipoproteins (VLDLs, IDLs, and LDLs) by the reaction catalyzed in the plasma by PLTP.

Approximately one third of the cholesteryl ester made by the LCAT reaction is transferred from HDL to apo B-100–containing lipoproteins through the action of the plasma cholesteryl ester transfer protein (CETP) (Nissen, 2007). The optimal substrate of CETP (i.e., the recipient of the HDL cholesteryl ester) appears to be an apo B-100–containing particle, with a density near that of IDL/LDL, that can be taken up by the LDLR. However, some HDL-derived cholesteryl ester is also transferred to VLDL. Thus most of the cholesterol in circulating lipoproteins (e.g., LDL) is cholesteryl ester that has been produced from HDL cholesterol by the LCAT-catalyzed reaction. Triacylglycerol is moved from the apo B-100–containing particles to HDL in exchange for the cholesteryl ester. This CETP-mediated exchange would not modify the core volume of HDL appreciably, unless this was followed by hepatic lipase–mediated hydrolysis of HDL triacylglycerol. The rest of the cholesteryl ester generated by the LCAT reaction is selectively taken up from HDL by hepatocytes, and to a lesser extent by adrenal and gonadal cells via SR-BI, without the concomitant uptake of the entire HDL particle. However, SR-B1 may also play a role in cholesterol efflux to HDL from various tissues, including macrophages, by endocytosis/retroendocytosis of HDL as mentioned earlier (Marcel et al., 2008). Thus SR-B1 may mediate bidirectional exchange of cholesterol between cells and HDL. Regardless, the cholesteryl ester taken up by hepatocytes and by adrenal and gonadal cells is used for bile acid and steroid hormone synthesis, respectively.

Cholesterol Efflux is Important for Maintenance of HDL Levels

Tangier disease, caused by mutations of the ABCA1 gene, is a rare recessive genetic disorder characterized by an almost complete absence of HDL in plasma, accumulation of cholesteryl esters in macrophages, and, as a result, increased susceptibility to atherosclerosis. Infiltration of cholesteryl ester in hematopoietic organs occurs also. As discussed previously, ABCA1 appears to be necessary for the efflux of tissue cholesterol and phospholipids from extrahepatic cells into the reverse cholesterol transport pathway. When there is insufficient cholesterol efflux, as in the case of patients affected by Tangier disease, pre-β–HDL (lipid-poor apo A-I) is rapidly removed from the circulation and apo A-I is destroyed in the kidney.

POSTPRANDIAL LIPOPROTEIN METABOLISM

Meal intake results in an influx of triacylglycerols and cholesterol into plasma in the form of chylomicrons. Triacylglycerols in these chylomicrons are hydrolyzed, fatty acids are taken up by various tissues, and the chylomicron remnants are taken up by the liver. Liver also synthesizes triacylglycerols and secretes them back into the plasma as VLDL. The concentration and proportions of plasma lipoproteins following an overnight (16-hour) fast are often used as a baseline state from which the effects of postprandial lipemia can be evaluated. The proportions and types of dietary fat and carbohydrate consumed have major effects upon postprandial plasma lipid levels. The effects of a moderate meal (e.g., one third of the daily caloric requirement) can be observed over a 9- to 12-hour period postprandially as changes (from the fasting baseline) in plasma lipid concentrations and in activities of lipoprotein-metabolizing enzymes, as illustrated in (Figure 17-9). Because humans typically eat more often than every 9 hours, most people have nonfasting plasma lipid profiles for most of each day.

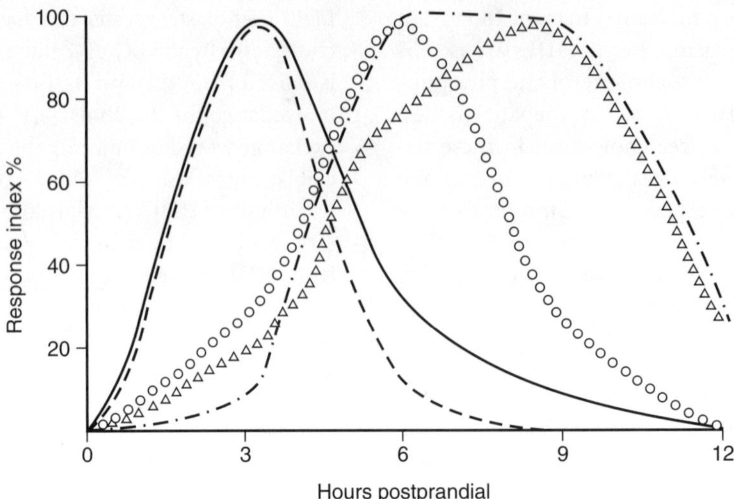

FIGURE 17-9 The postprandial response of triacylglycerol and plasma metabolic activities. Subjects were fed a moderate meal (approximately one third of daily calories) of whole foods and changes in plasma were followed over 12 hours. Shown in the figure are plasma triacylglycerol concentration (*solid line*); net exchange of cholesteryl ester in HDL for triacylglycerol, catalyzed by CETP (*dashed line*); transfer of cellular free cholesterol to plasma (*open circles*); cholesterol esterification by LCAT (*dashed-and-dotted line*); and phospholipid transfer catalyzed by PLTP (*triangles*). Values have been scaled between 0% (fasting) and 100% (peak postprandial response) to facilitate comparison among different factors. (Data from Castro, G. R., & Fielding, C. J. [1985]. Effects of postprandial lipemia on plasma cholesterol metabolism. *The Journal of Clinical Investigation, 75,* 874–882.)

CHANGES IN PLASMA TRIACYLGLYCEROL AND CHOLESTEROL CONCENTRATIONS IN RESPONSE TO A MEAL

Plasma triacylglycerol levels peak about 3 hours after a moderate meal (see solid line in Figure 17-9) although the magnitude and duration of the postprandial response depend on the fat content of the meal. After ingestion of a normal meal containing one third of the daily caloric intake, plasma triacylglycerol levels typically double by 3 hours, then decrease toward or even below fasting levels by 9 hours, and finally return to fasting levels by 12 hours after the meal.

The concentrations of circulating apo B-48 and apo B-100 proteins (as part of the triacylglycerol-rich lipoproteins) increase postprandially. However, even at peak triacylglycerol levels, apo B-48 makes up only a small part of the total apo B lipoproteins circulating within the triacylglycerol-rich lipoproteins. The greater abundance of apo B-100 than of apo B-48 in plasma is due to several factors. First, the ratio of apo B to triacylglycerol content is lower for chylomicrons than for VLDL. The triacylglycerol content of a newly secreted chylomicron is 10 to 100 times greater than that of a nascent hepatic VLDL particle, yet both lipoprotein particles contain a single apo B polypeptide. As a result, the apo B-48 to apo B-100 ratio greatly underrepresents the proportion of triacylglycerol of intestinal origin that is present in postprandial plasma. In addition, chylomicron triacylglycerol is hydrolyzed more rapidly by LPL ($t_{½}$ = 5 to 15 minutes) than is triacylglycerol in VLDL ($t_{½}$ = 1 to 5 hours). Furthermore, the apo B-48–containing chylomicron remnants are cleared rapidly by the liver, whereas the plasma concentration of apo B-100–containing LDL remains relatively high at all times.

Dietary cholesterol appears as cholesteryl ester in chylomicrons. It is retained within the chylomicron remnants and is taken up rapidly by the liver. Because of their relatively rapid clearance, chylomicrons/chylomicron remnants contain an insignificant part of total plasma cholesterol, even after a meal rich in cholesterol. Loss of free cholesterol from LDL and a comparable increase within the triacylglycerol-rich lipoprotein fractions have been observed during the postprandial response. This probably reflects mainly a passive transfer of free cholesterol, driven by the low free cholesterol content of newly secreted VLDL. There is little change postprandially in the cholesterol or triacylglycerol content of HDL.

POSTPRANDIAL CHANGES IN PLASMA LIPID METABOLISM

Adipose tissue LPL regulates fatty acid storage after a meal. After a meal, LPL activity at the endothelial surface of adipose tissue is increased. The principal factor mediating this effect is a rise in the circulating level of insulin. Insulin increases the transcription of the gene encoding LPL in the adipocyte and also stimulates the processing of polysaccharide chains in newly synthesized LPL to the trimmed state found in the secreted lipase. The low affinity (high K_m) of adipose LPL also allows it to hydrolyze more triacylglycerol with the increase in chylomicron and VLDL concentrations after a meal.

Lipemia in postprandial plasma also stimulates the activity of CETP, which exchanges VLDL triacylglycerol for HDL cholesteryl ester (see dashed line in Figure 17-9). Although the activity of CETP is increased, the concentration of CETP is not. Because the proportion of plasma triacylglycerol in

CLINICAL CORRELATION

Familial Hypercholesterolemia

Familial hypercholesterolemia (FH) is characterized by a genetic defect in the gene encoding the low-density lipoprotein receptor (LDLR), showing a dominant inheritance pattern. A variety of mutations in the LDLR gene have been identified that affect synthesis, processing, binding, or clustering of the receptor on the cell surface. The prevalence of heterozygous FH is about 1 in 500 individuals, whereas the prevalence of homozygous FH is rare, estimated at 1 in 1 million people.

Typically, patients with two mutated alleles (homozygous or compound heterozygous) have LDLR activity of less than 2% of normal, whereas patients with only one affected gene (heterozygous) have up to 25% of normal activity, depending on the nature of the mutation. The diagnosis of both homozygous and heterozygous FH is based primarily on the finding of severe elevations in plasma LDL (and consequently plasma cholesterol) levels, along with relatively normal triglyceride and HDL levels. More severe hypercholesteremia and an earlier onset of cardiovascular disease is characteristic of patients who are homozygous for the disease allele.

Total cholesterol levels in homozygous patients are usually greater than 600 mg/dL, whereas total cholesterol levels in heterozygous patients are typically higher than 250 mg/dL and increase with age. Coronary artery disease typically occurs during childhood in homozygotes, whereas it occurs early in adulthood with a prevalence of approximately 25 times that of the general population in heterozygotes.

Patients with FH often deposit cholesterol in their skin and tendons, forming nodules known as xanthomas. When cultured in lipoprotein-containing media, fibroblasts taken from either normal subjects or FH homozygotes do not express LDLRs at their cell surfaces. However, when these cells are equilibrated in vitro in lipoprotein-deficient plasma to reduce their cellular free cholesterol content, normal cells express LDLRs but cells from FH homozygotes do not. Cells from heterozygotes remove LDL at about half the normal rate. These results with fibroblasts are considered to model in vivo hepatic clearance of LDL.

Thinking Critically

What effects [direction of change (increase/decrease) and degree of change (little/moderate/major)] would you expect a null mutation of the LDLR gene to have on the following features of plasma lipid concentration and metabolism in vivo? Why?

a. Plasma cholesterol in very-low-density lipoproteins (VLDLs) and high-density lipoproteins (HDLs)
b. Extrahepatic cholesterol synthesis
c. Nonspecific uptake of LDL by the liver
d. Lecithin:cholesterol acyltransferase (LCAT) activity

acceptor lipoproteins (VLDLs, IDLs, and LDLs) increases after a meal, there is a greater likelihood, on average, that a cholesteryl ester molecule transferred from HDL to VLDL or LDL will be replaced by transfer of a triacylglycerol molecule—rather than by a cholesteryl ester molecule—from VLDL or LDL back to HDL. As a result, the net exchange of HDL cholesteryl ester mass (e.g., from HDL to VLDL) for triacylglycerol mass (e.g., from VLDL to HDL) becomes greater. By 9 hours after a meal, the flux of cholesteryl ester through CETP has usually decreased again to baseline fasting levels.

Postprandial lipemia also stimulates free cholesterol mass transfer from cells into plasma (see open circles in Figure 17-9). Increased transfer of triacylglycerol to HDL in exchange for cholesteryl ester, followed by hydrolysis of the triacylglycerol by hepatic triacylglycerol lipase, leads to a significant decrease in the size of HDL particles. If sequential plasma samples obtained during the course of postprandial lipemia are incubated in vitro with monolayers of non-liver cells, an increase in the mass transfer of free cholesterol from the cells to plasma lipoproteins is seen for plasma samples obtained 6 to 9 hours postprandially. The model shown in Figure 17-8 suggests that small, lipid-poor pre-β–HDL (generated from α-HDL) first cross the endothelium into the interstitial space of the extrahepatic tissues. "Discoidal" HDLs are then formed extravascularly from small pre-β–HDLs by accumulation of phospholipids and free cholesterol from extrahepatic cells; they accumulate in the lymph and are then returned to the plasma via the lymphatic ducts. Finally, LCAT activity (but not the plasma concentration of LCAT protein) and phospholipid transfer by PLTP also increase postprandially (see dashed-and-dotted line for LCAT activity and open triangles for PLTP in Figure 17-9). These increases normally peak after about 6 to 9 hours and favor esterification of the free cholesterol picked up by the pre-β–HDLs. Therefore postprandial lipemia is associated with stimulation of the reverse transport of cholesterol from extrahepatic tissues to the liver. This extravascular/lymphatic phase of HDL metabolism is likely to explain the 3-hour lag between the increase in net exchange of HDL cholesteryl ester for triacylglycerol (catalyzed by CETP) and the subsequent rise of LCAT activity (esterification of free cholesterol to form HDL cholesteryl ester). This lag is characteristic of postprandial lipemia. The difference in the shape of the response curves of LCAT and CETP activities (see Figure 17-9) means that the ratio of LCAT to CETP activity is increased at 6 hours postprandially compared to fasting levels. As a result, the mean diameter of HDL, which decreases early in postprandial metabolism (3 hours), increases back to its fasting value later in the postprandial period (6 hours) as LCAT-derived cholesteryl ester accumulates in the HDL.

In summary, the sequential changes that characterize postprandial lipid metabolism in plasma (see Figure 17-9) have several effects. Fatty acids in triacylglycerols are directed for storage to adipose tissue through the properties and regulation of adipose tissue LPLs. The accumulation of unstable, cholesterol-enriched remnant lipoproteins is prevented by the efficient removal of these particles by the liver. Fat-soluble vitamins are delivered efficiently to the liver as part of the chylomicron remnants. Finally, postprandial lipemia promotes reverse cholesterol transport from extrahepatic tissues to the liver by accelerating the recycling of apo A-I through pre-β–HDL. However, postprandial hyperlipemia is also considered a risk factor for atherosclerosis, as discussed next.

ATHEROSCLEROTIC CARDIOVASCULAR DISEASE

Epidemiological studies have generated an enormous database linking diets high in saturated fatty acids and cholesterol to human diseases. These observational studies have been paralleled by the rapid development of the field of lipid and lipoprotein metabolism, with studies stretching from human dietary investigations to studies of diet and atherosclerosis in transgenic and knockout mouse models of human dyslipidemia.

PATHOPHYSIOLOGY OF ATHEROSCLEROSIS

Atherosclerosis is a vascular disease characterized by fatty plaques in the intima of arteries. These plaques not only block blood flow but can rupture and precipitate blood clots within smaller arteries, thereby leading to heart attack, stroke, or peripheral vascular disease. The key event in atherogenesis is retention of apo B–containing lipoproteins in the intima of arterial walls. To carry out their role as transporters for cholesterol, the smaller apo B–containing lipoproteins move across the endothelial cells lining the blood vessels to reach the extracellular space and then normally return to the circulation. LDL is the predominant lipoprotein passing through the endothelial layer, but there is evidence that chylomicron remnants and VLDL remnants (IDLs) can do so as well. In certain focal areas of arteries, usually at branching points with disturbed blood flow, lipoproteins may be retained by the extracellular proteoglycans, which makes lipoproteins susceptible to being "modified." Modification may include oxidation of phospholipids with accumulation of lipid hydroperoxides, as well as oxidation of apo B-100. Alternatively, modified apo B–containing lipoproteins may be prone to aggregate or stick to extracellular matrix molecules in the subendothelial space. In either case, greater numbers of circulating lipoproteins will infiltrate the endothelium and be retained.

As illustrated in Figure 17-10, modification and retention of apo B–containing lipoproteins, particularly LDLs, signal endothelial cells to produce cell adhesion molecules, monocyte chemotactic proteins, and monocyte colony-stimulating factor. Together, these molecules stimulate formation,

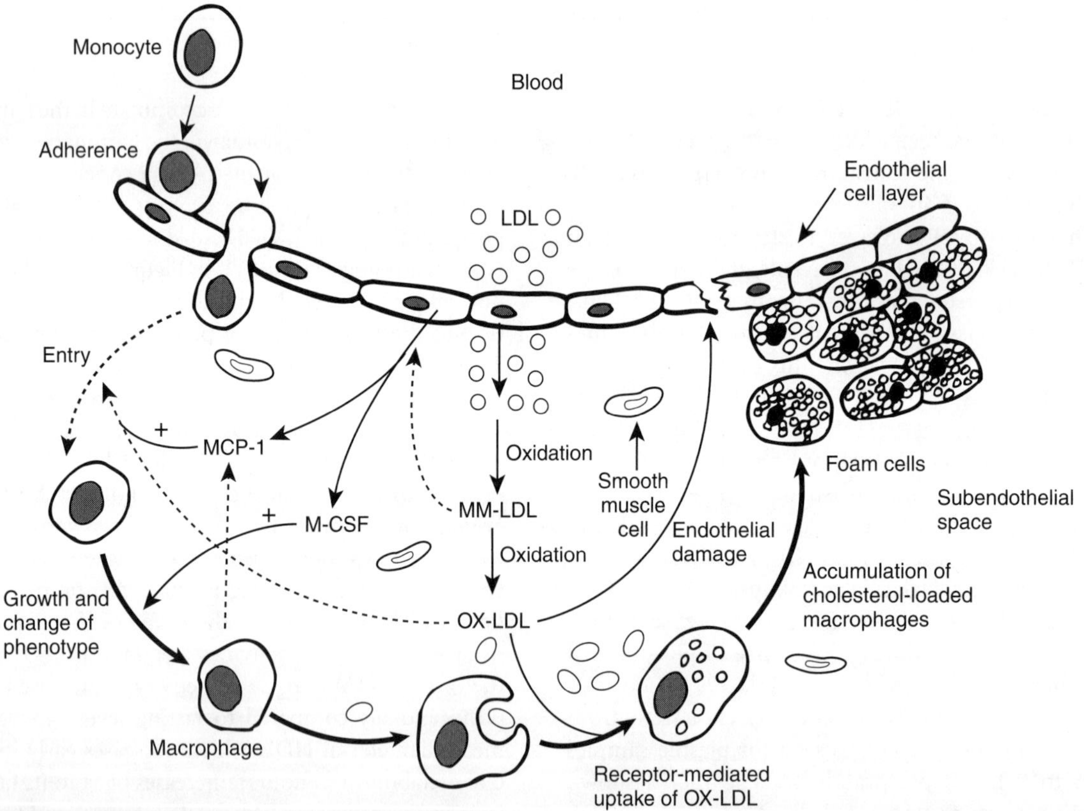

FIGURE 17-10 Depiction of the early stages of atheroma formation, including low-density lipoprotein (*LDL*) entry into the vessel wall, endothelial damage or dysfunction, LDL modification and oxidation, recruitment of monocytes into the vessel wall, and uptake of modified/oxidized LDL by monocyte-derived macrophages. *MCP-1,* Monocyte chemotactic protein; *M-CSF,* macrophage colony-stimulating factor; *MM-LDL,* lightly oxidized LDL; *OX-LDL,* oxidized LDL. (From Steinberg, D. [1991]. Antioxidants and atherosclerosis: A current assessment. *Circulation, 84,* 1420–1425.)

migration, and sequestration of monocytes at sites where lipoproteins are retained in the subendothelial space. These monocytes are then activated and perpetuate a local inflammatory response, take up modified LDLs, and transform into macrophages. The inflammatory response includes T cell recruitment, cytokine secretion, and monocyte chemotaxis. The accumulated macrophages further oxidize and internalize the retained lipoproteins, becoming lipid-laden foam cells. They also secrete growth factors that stimulate smooth muscle cell proliferation and migration. The monocytes and macrophages and the activated smooth muscle cells begin to secrete extracellular matrix molecules as well. At this point, all the components of the advanced lesion are in place and atherogenesis is well under way.

Because atherosclerosis is an inflammatory disease, markers of inflammation such as C-reactive protein are suggested to be risk factors for coronary artery disease (Libby et al., 2009; Tabas, 2010; Miller et al., 2009). Statins, mentioned in the preceding text as inhibitors of HMG-CoA reductase activity, are potent cholesterol-lowering drugs that reduce the risk of heart attack and stroke. Increasing evidence suggests that the beneficial effects of statins are due not only to their cholesterol-lowering effects but also to their direct effects on endothelial cell function, including antiinflammatory and antithrombotic effects (Zhou and Liao, 2010). This may be due to inhibition of prenylation of signaling molecules (geranylgeranylation). Recent evidence also links the statins to decreased levels of C-reactive protein, independent of the cholesterol-lowering actions of the drug.

ASSOCIATION OF PLASMA LIPIDS AND LIPOPROTEINS WITH RISK FOR ATHEROSCLEROTIC CARDIOVASCULAR DISEASE

Disorders of lipoprotein metabolism can lead to alterations in plasma cholesterol and triacylglycerol levels, and these disorders are usually associated with increased risk of cardiovascular disease. Plasma total cholesterol is strongly associated with CAD, but this association is confounded by the distribution of cholesterol among the lipoprotein classes. High total cholesterol level in blood is usually paralleled by a high plasma concentration of LDL cholesterol, and LDL-cholesterol level is a significant indicator of risk for atherosclerosis. Nevertheless, LDL is not a homogeneous class, and some types may be associated with higher risk.

Small, dense LDLs, which are commonly found in individuals with higher triacylglycerol and lower HDL cholesterol levels, have been proposed to be more atherogenic (Austin et al., 1990). Small, dense LDLs may be more atherogenic because they penetrate into the artery wall more easily or are more readily oxidized. However, it is known that the large, cholesteryl ester–enriched LDLs found in patients with familial hypercholesterolemia are also quite atherogenic. Because oxidized LDLs affect endothelial cells, convert macrophages into foam cells, and cause inflammation, oxidized LDL levels in plasma are implicated as a risk factor for coronary artery disease. In addition, the small dense lipoprotein known as lipoprotein (a) has been linked to increased risk for atherosclerotic cardiovascular disease, although the mechanism remains unclear. Lipoprotein (a) is composed of LDL with a second protein, apo(a), covalently linked to apo B. Apo(a) is a large protein that is synthesized in the liver and present only in humans. It is believed that apo(a) interacts with LDL apo B in the plasma to form lipoprotein (a). The size of apo(a) is highly variable from individual to individual (e.g., 200 to 700 kDa) due to size polymorphisms in the gene. Some evidence suggests there is an inverse correlation between apo(a) isoform size and the plasma concentration of lipoprotein (a).

Although HDLs also contain cholesterol, the HDL cholesterol level is inversely related to risk for coronary artery disease. As described previously, HDL is critical for the reverse transport of cholesterol from tissues throughout the body back to the liver. HDL appears to have protective effects against atherosclerosis. Some studies have indicated that only the larger, more cholesteryl ester–rich HDL_2 (density of 1.063 to 1.12 g/mL) is protective against coronary artery disease in comparison with HDL_3 (density of 1.12 to 1.21 g/mL), but other investigators have failed to see a difference between the two types of HDLs. HDLs may also be antiatherogenic because of their potential role in counteracting LDL oxidation (Florentin et al., 2008; Natarajan et al., 2010; Shao et al., 2010). Inhibition of LDL oxidation by HDL is usually attributed to HDL's high content of lipid-soluble antioxidants (e.g., vitamin E), the antioxidative properties of apo A-I, and the presence of several enzymes in HDL that prevent LDL oxidation or hydrolyze lipid peroxides. HDLs also may exert an antiatherogenic effect by protecting endothelial cells from dysfunction (Lowenstein and Cameron, 2010).

The role of plasma triacylglycerol level as an "independent" risk factor has been controversial (Goldberg, 2009; Yuan et al., 2007). The controversy stems from several observations, including the finding that triacylglycerols account for a minor component of lipids in vessel wall lesions, the inverse relationship between triacylglycerols and HDL cholesterol, and the lack of strong evidence of triacylglycerols as an independent predictor of disease. However, triacylglycerols may play a role in atherogenesis as a source of free fatty acids that can be converted into lipid oxidation products, such as hydroperoxides and peroxyl radicals that are bioactive in the formation of lesions. Recent data established a consistent strong relation of postprandial, or non-fasting, hypertriglyceridemia with coronary artery disease risk, and fibrate drugs that decrease plasma triacylglycerol levels can prevent coronary artery disease. So-called remnant-like particles (RLPs) are remnants of triacylglycerol-rich lipoproteins, mainly of chylomicrons and VLDLs, after the action of lipoprotein lipase in the capillary beds of adipose tissue and muscle. Plasma RLP–cholesterol level may also be a risk factor, and RLP–cholesterol and plasma triacylglycerol levels are correlated. Cholesterol transported in VLDLs along with triacylglycerols can accumulate in arterial wall macrophages. This suggests that an elevated triacylglycerol level may be a marker of increased delivery of non-LDL cholesterol to lesion sites.

CHRONIC EFFECTS OF DIETARY LIPIDS ON PLASMA LIPOPROTEINS AND LIPID METABOLISM

The major differences among diets that affect plasma lipids are the percentage of total calories consumed as fat, the proportions of saturated and polyunsaturated fatty acids (monounsaturated fatty acids being considered neutral), and the amount of dietary cholesterol. The major effects of dietary lipids on plasma lipids involve their effects on the concentrations of circulating triacylglycerol and LDL cholesterol.

EFFECTS OF TOTAL FAT

Switching from a typical American diet (~35% of calories provided by fat) to a low-fat diet, in which dietary fat has been replaced isocalorically by carbohydrate, typically increases the fasting triacylglycerol levels and decreases, probably by a CETP-mediated process, both fasting LDL and HDL cholesterol levels. Because a low-fat diet is higher in carbohydrate, the increase in serum triacylglycerol observed in individuals who switch to low-fat diets has been attributed to the influence of carbohydrate in stimulating de novo fatty acid synthesis and the secretion of triacylglycerol-rich VLDL from the liver. Because an increase in dietary fat is associated with modest increases (10% to 20%) in the levels of LPL and hepatic triacylglycerol lipase, it is also possible that corresponding decreases in lipase activities occur when individuals switch to low-fat diets and that these reductions in lipase activities contribute to the modest hypertriglyceridemia that is observed in individuals who switch to a low-fat diet. In fact, high-carbohydrate, low-fat diets, particularly when enriched in refined carbohdyrates and in conjunction with obesity, may worsen atherogenic dyslipidemia by elevating triacylglycerols, reducing HDL, and increasing small dense LDL particles in the plasma (Siri-Tarino et al., 2010).

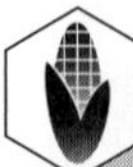

FOOD SOURCES OF DIETARY FATS AND CHOLESTEROL

Saturated Fatty Acids
Dairy fats: whole milk, cream, butter, cheese
Meat fats: pork, beef
Certain plant oils: coconut, palm, palm kernel

Monounsaturated Fatty Acids
Meat fats: pork, lamb
Nuts: macadamia, hazelnuts, pecans
Plant oils: canola, olive

Polyunsaturated Fatty Acids
n−6 (Linoleic Acid)
Nuts and seeds: walnuts, sunflower seeds, pinenuts, pecans
Plant oils: soybean, safflower, corn

n−3
Fish: sardines, salmon (eicosapentaenoic acid and docosahexaenoic acid)
Plant oils: soybean, flaxseed, canola (α-linolenic acid)

***Trans* Fatty Acids**
Hydrogenated oils: margarines and vegetable shortenings
Processed foods containing PHVO (partially hydrogenated vegetable oils)

Conjugated Linoleic Acids
Dairy fats: whole milk, cheese, butter
Ruminant meat fats: beef, lamb

Cholesterol
Meat, poultry, and fish fats: chicken, salmon, lamb, pork, crab
Eggs
Dairy fats: whole milk, butter, cheese

Data from U.S. Department of Agriculture, Agricultural Research Service. (2010). *USDA National Nutrient Database for Standard Reference, Release 23*. Retrieved from www.ars.usda.gov/ba/bhrnc/ndl.

EFFECTS OF DIETARY FAT SATURATION

The degree of dietary fat saturation is often expressed as a P/S ratio (weight of polyunsaturated fatty acids/weight of saturated fatty acids). This ratio is an approximation that does not take into account the differing effects of different polyunsaturated or of different saturated fatty acids. Linoleic (n−6) and α-linolenic (n−3) acids are the major dietary polyunsaturated fatty acids, with linoleic acid being much more abundant than α-linolenic. Similarly, though it is well known that stearic acid does not raise serum cholesterol levels, it is grouped with other saturated fatty acids that do. Typical western diets have P/S ratios of 0.6 to 0.7.

The effects of dietary fat saturation depend upon the dietary cholesterol level. For example, Hayes and Khosla (1992) showed that when cholesterol intake was low (~200 mg/day), there was no significant effect of P/S ratios (0.8 to 0.2 at constant total fat and constant monounsaturated fatty acid) on the plasma cholesterol level. In contrast, when the cholesterol intake was approximately 600 mg/day, a decrease in the P/S ratio from 0.8 to 0.2 resulted in a doubling of the fasting plasma cholesterol levels. In contrast to the elevation of plasma cholesterol levels by increased intake of saturated fatty acids, plasma triacylglycerol level was minimally affected by an increase in saturated fatty acids (with constant dietary cholesterol and total fat calories) when there was no change in body weight.

Polyunsaturated fatty acids may be of the n−6 family or the n−3 family, as described in Chapters 6 and 18. The long-chain n−3 or so-called fish oil fatty acids (i.e., eicosapentaenoic acid and docosahexaenoic acid) have been shown to decrease the risk of cardiovascular disease by lowering plasma triacylglycerol and cholesterol levels and by virtue of their metabolic conversion to antithrombotic and antiinflammatory eicosanoids (Schmitz and Ecker, 2008).

Trans-unsaturated fatty acids that arise from the chemical hydrogenation of vegetable oils to make solid fats have been shown to be atherogenic. An increase in LDL cholesterol level and a decrease in HDL cholesterol level were observed in several clinical trials in which subjects were fed *trans*-unsaturated fatty acids (Zock and Katan, 1997). When considering effects of dietary fat saturation on plasma lipid levels, *trans*-unsaturated fatty acids, with their structural similarity to saturated fatty acids, are typically thought of as akin to saturated fatty acids rather than as unsaturated fatty acids.

Monounsaturated fatty acids are found in high proportions in Mediterranean diets. Studies suggest that oils enriched in monounsaturated fatty acids contribute no negative effects on plasma lipid levels (Lecerf, 2009).

EFFECTS OF DIETARY CHOLESTEROL ON FASTING PLASMA LIPID LEVELS

In responsive individuals, increased dietary cholesterol is generally associated with increased LDL cholesterol without significant changes in the cholesterol content of other lipoprotein fractions. This effect is mediated, at least in part, by downregulation of hepatic LDLR expression. Increases in dietary cholesterol (+ 400 to 600 mg/day), at different levels of total fat and fatty acid saturation, are usually associated with approximately 20% increases in the flux of lipids through both LCAT and CETP. Because of the long circulation time of LDL ($t_{½}$ = ~2 days), even modest changes in CETP activity alone could lead to significant redistribution of cholesteryl esters among plasma lipoproteins. CETP activity could affect the circulating level of LDL cholesterol in human plasma, but more information is needed to determine the contribution of increased CETP activity relative to the contribution of decreased hepatic LDLR levels on plasma LDL cholesterol levels.

RECOMMENDATIONS AND TYPICAL INTAKES FOR DIETARY FAT

Fat is important in the diet because it is a major source of fuel for the body, it aids in the absorption of fat-soluble vitamins and carotenoids, and it provides the essential n−3 and n−6 fatty acids. The Institute of Medicine (IOM, 2005) did not establish Dietary Reference Intakes (DRIs) for total fat (except for infants) because of insufficient data for determination of the level of fat intake at which risk of inadequacy or lack of promotion of chronic disease occurs. Any increase in incremental intake of saturated fatty acids, as well as of *trans* fatty acids, appears to be associated with increased risk of coronary artery disease. The Acceptable Macronutrient Distribution Range (AMDR) for total fat is set at 20% to 35% of energy. Diets low in saturated fatty acids and as low as possible in *trans* fatty acids are advised.

Adequate Intakes (AIs) for total fat were established for infants based on the intake of fat from human milk and from complementary foods during the second half of the first year of life. The AIs are 31 g/day for infants from 0 to 6 months of age and 30 g/day for infants from 7 to 12 months of age. Therefore fat provides 55% and 40% of total energy intake for infants during the first and second 6 months of life, respectively. Human milk contains 20% to 25% of energy as saturated fatty acids, 6% of energy as n−6 fatty acids, 1% to 5% of total energy as *trans* fatty acids, 1% as n−3 fatty acids, and the remainder (~23%) as monounsaturated fatty acids.

The IOM (2005) summarized surveys of fat intake in the United States and Canada. Median total fat intake ranged from 65 to 100 g/day for men and 48 to 63 g/day for women in the United States, as determined in the Continuing Survey of Food Intakes of Individuals (U.S. Department of Agriculture, 1998). These intake ranges represent about 32% to 34% of total energy intake. Median saturated fatty acid intake ranged from 21 to 34 g/day for men and 15 to 21 g/day for women, providing about 11% to 12% of total energy in adult diets. Monounsaturated fatty acid intake ranged from 25 to 39 g/day for men and 18 to 24 g/day for women, providing about 14% of total energy. Median n−6 polyunsaturated fatty acid intake ranged from about 12 to 17 g/day for men and 9 to 11 g/day for women, contributing about 5% to 7% of total energy intake in the diets of adults. Approximately 85% to 90% of the n−6 polyunsaturated fatty acid intake was in the form of linoleic acid. Total n−3 polyunsaturated fatty acid intake was 1.3 to 1.8 g/day for men and 1.0 to 1.2 g/day for women, contributing about 0.7% of total energy intake. Approximately 90% of the n−3 polyunsaturated fatty acid intake was α-linolenic acid, with approximately 5% as docosahexaenoic acid (DHA). Rough estimates of *trans* fatty acid intake suggest that these accounted for about 2.6% of total energy intake. Estimates of the typical intake of conjugated linoleic acid (a possible bioactive compound discussed in Chapters 2 and 6) in the United States and Canada fall in the range of 0.15 to 0.33 g/day.

The IOM (2005) established AIs for the essential polyunsaturated fatty acid classes for all age and gender groups. These are described in more detail in Chapter 18. The AIs for n−6 polyunsaturated fatty acids (linoleic acid) are 17 g/day for young men and 12 g/day for young women. AIs for n−3 polyunsaturated fatty acids (e.g., α-linolenic acid) are 1.6 and 1.1 g/day for men and women, respectively.

THINKING CRITICALLY

1. A young girl was diagnosed with hypertriglyceridemia. Her plasma triacylglycerol concentration was in the range of 5 to 13 mmol/L. A normal concentration of apo C-II was observed by immunochemical analysis, but separation of proteins by two-dimensional electrophoresis revealed that the apo C-II had a low molecular mass and a high isoelectric point compared with apo C-II in control subjects. It was concluded that apo C-II was defective. The girl was placed on a low-fat diet and her plasma triacylglycerol concentration was maintained between 5.0 and 7.5 mmol/L on this diet.
   a. What lipoproteins normally contain apo C-II? What is its function in these lipoproteins?
   b. Why would a deficiency of apo C-II cause hypertriglyceridemia?

Continued

THINKING CRITICALLY—cont'd

c. What is the rationale for treatment of this patient with a low-fat diet?
d. A similar hypertriglyceridemia with chylomicronemia is observed in patients with lipoprotein lipase deficiency. Why?

2. Just after a person has eaten a meal, the digestion products of fat are absorbed and reincorporated into triacylglycerols in the enterocytes. These triacylglycerols are then incorporated into chylomicrons. Consider one single triacylglycerol molecule that has been incorporated into the triacylglycerol core of a chylomicron.
   a. What is the most likely fate of the fatty acids in this triacylglycerol molecule during the postprandial period (i.e., what is the metabolically favored method for disposal of circulating triacylglycerol in response to meal intake)?
   b. What is the most likely fate or possible fates of the glycerol backbone during this postprandial period?
   c. Draw a sketch showing the movement of the chylomicron triacylglycerol and subsequently of the fatty acids and glycerol through tissues/cells/blood to their postprandial period "end-products."
3. Sketch the path (both tissue/blood locations and metabolic pathways, including lipoprotein particles that are involved) that a cholesteryl ester molecule in a chylomicron takes on its way to uptake by the adrenal medulla. What are possible fates of cholesterol in the adrenal cortex?
4. Describe ways in which cholesterol can be removed from cells and from the body.

REFERENCES

Austin, M. A., King, M. C., Vranizan, K. M., & Krauss, R. M. (1990). Atherogenic lipoprotein phenotype. A proposed genetic marker for coronary heart disease risk. *Circulation, 82,* 495–506.

Beigneux, A. P., Weinstein, M. M., Davies, B. S., Gin, P., Bensadoun, A., Fong, L. G., & Young, S. G. (2009). GPIHBP1 and lipolysis: An undate. *Current Opinion in Lipidology, 20,* 211–216.

Berge, K. E., Tian, H., Graf, G. A., Yu, L., Grishin, N. V., Schultz, J., ... Hobbs, H. H. (2000). Accumulation of dietary cholesterol in sitosterolemia caused by mutations in adjacent ABC transporters. *Science, 290,* 1771–1775.

Betters, J. L., & Yu, L. (2010). NPC1L1 and cholesterol transport. *FEBS Letters, 584,* 2740–2747.

Bjorkhem, I. (2009). Are side-chain oxidized oxysterols regulators also in vivo? *Journal of Lipid Research, 50,* S213–S218.

Brown, M. S., & Goldstein, J. L. (2009). Cholesterol feedback: From Schoenheimer's bottle to Scap's MELADL. *Journal of Lipid Research, 50,* S15–S28.

Calkin, A. C., & Tontonoz, P. (2010). Liver X receptor signaling pathways and atherosclerosis. *Arteriosclerosis, Thrombosis, and Vascular Biology, 30,* 1513–1518.

Chang, T. Y., Li, B.-L., Chang, C. C. Y., & Urano, Y. (2009). Acyl-coenzyme A: Cholesterol acyltransferases. *The American Journal of Physiology, 297,* E1–E9.

Davis, H. R., Jr., & Altmann, S. W. (2009). Niemann-Pick C1 like 1 (NPC1L1) an intestinal sterol transporter. *Biochimica et Biophysica Acta, 1791,* 679–683.

Fielding, C. J., & Fielding, P. E. (1995). Molecular physiology of reverse cholesterol transport. *Journal of Lipid Research, 36,* 211–228.

Florentin, M., Liberopoulos, E. N., Wierzbicki, A. S., & Mikhailidis, D. P. (2008). Multiple actions of high-density lipoprotein. *Current Opinion in Cardiology, 23,* 370–378.

Goldberg, I. J. (2009). Hypertriglyceridemia: Impact and treatment. *Endocrinology and Metabolism Clinics of North America, 38,* 137–149.

Hageman, J., Herrema, H., Groen, A. K., & Kuipers, F. (2010). A role of the bile salt receptor FXR in atherosclerosis. *Arteriosclerosis, Thrombosis, and Vascular Biology, 30,* 1519–1528.

Hayes, K. C., & Khosla, P. (1992). Dietary fatty acid thresholds and cholesterolemia. *The FASEB Journal, 6,* 2600–2607.

Institute of Medicine. (2005). *Dietary Reference Intakes for energy, carbohydrate, fiber, fat, fatty acids, cholesterol, protein, and amino acids (macronutrients).* Washington, DC: National Academies of Sciences, Institute of Medicine, Food and Nutrition Board.

Krimbou, L., Marcil, M., & Genest, J. (2006). New insights into the biogenesis of human high-density lipoproteins. *Current Opinion in Lipidology, 17,* 258–267.

Lecerf, J. M. (2009). Fatty acids and cardiovascular disease. *Nutrition Reviews, 67,* 273–283.

Lefebvre, P., Cariou, B., Lien, F., Kuipers, F., & Staels, B. (2009). Role of bile acids and bile acid receptors in metabolic regulation. *Physiological Reviews, 89,* 147–191.

Libby, P., Ridker, P. M., & Hansson, G. K. (2009). Inflammation in atherosclerosis: From pathophysiology to practice. *Journal of the American College of Cardiology, 54,* 2129–2138.

Lorkowski, S. (2008). The ins and outs of lipid efflux. *Journal of Molecular Medicine, 86,* 129–134.

Lowenstein, C. J., & Cameron, S. J. (2010). High-density lipoprotein metabolism and endothelian function. *Current Opinion in Endocrinology, Diabetes, and Obesity, 17,* 166–170.

Mansbach, C. M., & Siddiqi, S. A. (2010). The biogenesis of chylomicrons. *Annual Review of Physiology, 72,* 315–333.

Marcel, Y. L., Ouimet, M., & Wang, M.-D. (2008). Regulation of cholesterol efflux from macrophages. *Current Opinion in Lipidology, 19,* 455–461.

Mesmin, B., & Maxfield, F. R. (2009). Intracellular sterol dynamics. *Biochimica et Biophysica Acta, 1791,* 636–645.

Miller, Y. I., Choi, S.-H., Fang, L., & Harkewicz, R. (2009). Toll-like receptor-4 and lipoprotein accumulation in macrophages. *Trends in Cardiovascular Medicine, 19,* 227–232.

Natarajan, P., Ray, K. K., & Cannon, C. P. (2010). High-density lipoprotein and coronary heart disease: Current and future therapies. *Journal of the American College of Cardiology, 55,* 1283–1299.

Nissen, S. E., Tardif, J.-C., Nicholls, S. J., Revkin, J. H., Shear, C. L., Duggan, W. T., ... Tuzcu, E. M. (2007). Effect of torcetrapib on the progression of coronary atherosclerosis. *New England Journal of Medicine, 356,* 1304–1316.

Olivecrona, G., & Olivecrona, T. (2010). Triglyceride lipases and atherosclerosis. *Current Opinion in Lipidology, 21,* E-Pub.

Peake, K. B., & Vance, J. E. (2010). Defective cholesterol trafficking in Niemann-Pick C-deficient cells. *FEBS Letters, 584,* 2731–2739.

Rone, M. B., Fan, J., & Papdopoulos, V. (2009). Cholesterol transport in steroid biosynthesis: Role of protein-protein interactions and implications in disease states. *Biochimica et Biophysica Acta, 1791*, 646–658.

Rousset, X., Vaisman, B., Amar, M., Sethi, A., & Remaley, A. T. (2009). Lecithin:cholesterol acyltransfease: From biochemistry to role in cardiovascular disease. *Current Opinion in Endocrinology, Diabetes, and Obesity, 16*, 163–171.

Russell, D. W. (2009). Fifty years of advances in bile acid synthesis and metabolism. *Journal of Lipid Research, 50*(Suppl), S120–S125.

Schmitz, G., & Ecker, J. (2008). The opposing effects of n–3 and n–6 fatty acids. *Progress in Lipid Research, 47*, 147–155.

Shao, B., Oda, M. N., Oram, J. F., & Heinecke, J. W. (2010). Myeloperoxidase: An oxidative pathway for generating dysfunctional high-density lipoprotein. *Chemical Research in Toxicology, 23*, 447–454.

Siri-Tarino, P. W., Sun, Q., Hu, F. B., & Krauss, R. M. (2010). Saturated fat, carbohydrate, and cardiovascular disease. *The American Journal of Clinical Nutrition, 91*, 502–509.

Soccio, R. E., & Breslow, J. L. (2004). Intracellular cholesterol transport. *Arteriosclerosis, Thrombosis, and Vascular Biology, 24*, 1150–1160.

Stanford, K. I., Bishop, J. R., Foley, E. M., Gonzales, J. C., Niesman, I. R., Witztum, J. L., & Esko, J. D. (2009). Syndecan-1 is the primary heparan sulfate proteoglycan mediating hepatic clearance of triglyceride-rich lipoproteins in mice. *The Journal of Clinical Investigation, 119*, 3236–3245.

Steinberg, G. R., & Kemp, B. E. (2009). AMPK in health and disease. *Physiological Reviews, 89*, 1025–1078.

Storch, J., & Xu, Z. (2009). Niemann-Pick C2 (NPC2) and intracellular cholesterol trafficking. *Biochimica et Biophysica Acta, 1791*, 671–678.

Tabas, I. (2010). Macrophage death and defective inflammation resolution in atherosclerosis. *Nature Reviews. Immunology, 10*, 36–46.

U.S. Department of Agriculture. (1998). *Continuing survey of food intakes of individuals (1994–1996, 1998) diet and health knowledge survey CD-ROM*. Springfield, VA: National Technical Information Service.

Wang, H., & Eckel, R. H. (2009). Lipoprotein lipase: From gene to obesity. *The American Journal of Physiology, 297*, E271–E288.

Wang, M. L., Motamed, M., Infante, R. E., Abi-Mosleh, L., Kwon, H. J., Brown, M. S., & Goldstein, J. L. (2010). Identification of surface residues on Niemann-Pick C2 essential for hydrophobic handoff of cholesterol to NPC1 in lysosomes. *Cell Metabolism, 12*, 166–173.

Williams, K. J., & Chen, K. (2010). Recent insights into factors affecting remnant lipoprotein uptake. *Current Opinion in Lipidology, 21*, 218–228.

Yuan, G., Al-Shali, K. Z., & Hegele, R. A. (2007). Hypertriglyceridemia: Its etiology, effects and treatment. *Canadian Medical Association Journal, 176*, 1113–1120.

Yvan-Charvet, L., Wang, N., & Tall, A. R. (2010). Role of HDL, ABCA1, and ABCG1 transporters in cholesterol efflux and immune responses. *Arteriosclerosis, Thrombosis, and Vascular Biology, 30*, 139–143.

Zannis, V., Chroni, A., & Krieger, M. (2006). Role of apoA-1, ABCA1, LCAT, and SR-B1 in the biogenesis of HDL. *Journal of Molecular Medicine, 84*, 276–295.

Zhou, Q., & Liao, J. K. (2010). Pleiotropic effects of statins: Basic research and clinical perspective. *Circulation Journal, 74*, 818–826.

Zock, P. L., & Katan, M. B. (1997). Butter, margarine and serum lipoproteins. *Atherosclerosis, 131*, 7–16.

RECOMMENDED READINGS

American Society for Biochemistry and Molecular Biology. (2009). Special 50th anniversary supplement to *Journal of Lipid Research. Journal of Lipid Research, 50*(Suppl. 1).

Ikonen, E. (2008). Cellular cholesterol trafficking and compartmentalization. *Nature Reviews. Molecular Cell Biology, 9*, 125–138.

Institute of Medicine. (2005). *Dietary Reference Intakes for energy, carbohydrate, fiber, fat, fatty acids, cholesterol, protein, and amino acids (macronutrients)*. Washington DC: The National Academies Press.

Steinberg, D. (2004). An interpretive history of the cholesterol controversy: Part I. *Journal of Lipid Research, 45*, 1583–1593.

Steinberg, D. (2005). Part II: The early evidence linking blood cholesterol to coronary disease in humans. *Journal of Lipid Research, 46*, 179–190.

Steinberg, D. (2005). Part III: Mechanistically defining the role of hyperlipidemia. *Journal of Lipid Research, 46*, 2037–2051.

Steinberg, D. (2006). Part IV: The 1984 Coronary Primary Prevention Trial ends it—almost. *Journal of Lipid Research, 47*, 1–14.

Steinberg, D. (2006). Part V: The discovery of the statins and the end of the controversy. *Journal of Lipid Research, 47*, 1339–1351.

Vance, D. E., & Vance, J. (Eds.). (2008). *Biochemistry of lipids, lipoproteins and membranes* (5th ed.). Amsterdam: Elsevier B. V.

Williams, K. J. (2008). Molecular processes that handle—and mishandle—dietary lipids. *The Journal of Clinical Investigation, 118*, 3247–3259.

CHAPTER 18

Lipid Metabolism: Polyunsaturated Fatty Acids

Sarah K. Orr, BSc; Chuck T. Chen, BSc; Arthur A. Spector, MD; and Richard P. Bazinet, PhD

COMMON ABBREVIATIONS

ARA	arachidonic acid	**G protein**	GTP-binding protein
DHA	docosahexaenoic acid	**LDL**	low-density lipoprotein
EPA	eicosapentaenoic acid	**PUFA**	polyunsaturated fatty acid

Essential fatty acids are polyunsaturated fatty acids (PUFAs) that are necessary for growth and normal physiological function but cannot be completely synthesized in the body. There are two classes of essential PUFAs, n−6 (omega 6) and n−3 (omega 3). They cannot be interconverted. Therefore the dietary fat intake must contain both of these classes of PUFAs to maintain good health and prevent an eventual deficiency. Plants have the ability to synthesize the first 18-carbon member of each class, linoleic acid (n−6) and α-linolenic acid (n−3), and plant products are the ultimate sources of essential fatty acids in the human food chain.

DISCOVERY OF ESSENTIAL FATTY ACIDS

Early work demonstrated that a small amount of dietary fat was necessary for laboratory rats to grow normally, remain healthy, and reproduce. Two opposing views were put forward to explain this observation. Some thought that the protective action was due entirely to the vitamin E present in the dietary fat. Others believed that, in addition to vitamin E, some component of the fat itself was an essential nutrient. This controversy was resolved in 1929 when Burr and Burr demonstrated that linoleic acid, the 18-carbon n−6 PUFA that contains two double bonds, was an essential nutrient for the rat. The syndrome produced in rats by a lack of PUFAs, called essential fatty acid deficiency, causes a cessation of growth, dermatitis, loss of water through the skin, loss of blood in the urine, fatty liver, and loss of reproductive capacity. Subsequent work showed that linoleic acid also is an essential nutrient for other mammals, including humans.

No well-defined disease occurred when experimental animals were fed a diet deficient in α-linolenic acid, the corresponding 18-carbon member of the n−3 PUFA class. Therefore it initially appeared that n−3 PUFAs were not essential nutrients and were present in the body simply because small amounts ordinarily are contained in the diet. This view gradually changed during the last 35 years because of increasing evidence that n−3 PUFAs are required for optimal visual and nervous system development (Innis, 2008). A consensus now exists that, like the n−6 class, the n−3 PUFAs are essential nutrients for humans.

STRUCTURE OF POLYUNSATURATED FATTY ACIDS

Fatty acids contain a hydrocarbon chain and a carboxyl group. All fatty acids that have two or more double bonds in the hydrocarbon chain are classified as polyunsaturated. In humans and other mammals almost all of the PUFAs present in the blood and tissues contain between 18 and 22 carbons and from two to six double bonds. The double bonds normally are three carbons apart; a carbon atom that is fully saturated (called a methylene carbon) separates them.

$$-CH{=}CH-CH_2-CH{=}CH-$$

Methylene carbon

The double bonds in all unsaturated fatty acids synthesized by plants and animals are in the *cis* configuration. This introduces a rigid 45-degree bend at each double bond in the fatty acid chain. The bent conformation reduces the tightness with which adjacent fatty acid chains can pack, producing a more mobile physical state and thereby decreasing the melting point of lipids containing unsaturated fatty acyl chains.

The PUFAs found in the body and in foods are mainly of the n−6 and n−3 classes. Figure 18-1 illustrates the chemical structures of the major n−6 and n−3 PUFAs present in humans and animals. The n−6 PUFAs are shown on the top and the n−3 PUFAs on the bottom. Although each class contains eight fatty acids, the six fatty acids shown in this figure account for more than 90% of the PUFAs present in the plasma and tissues under normal physiological conditions.

Humans and other mammals do not have the enzymes necessary to form either the n−3 or the n−6 double bonds

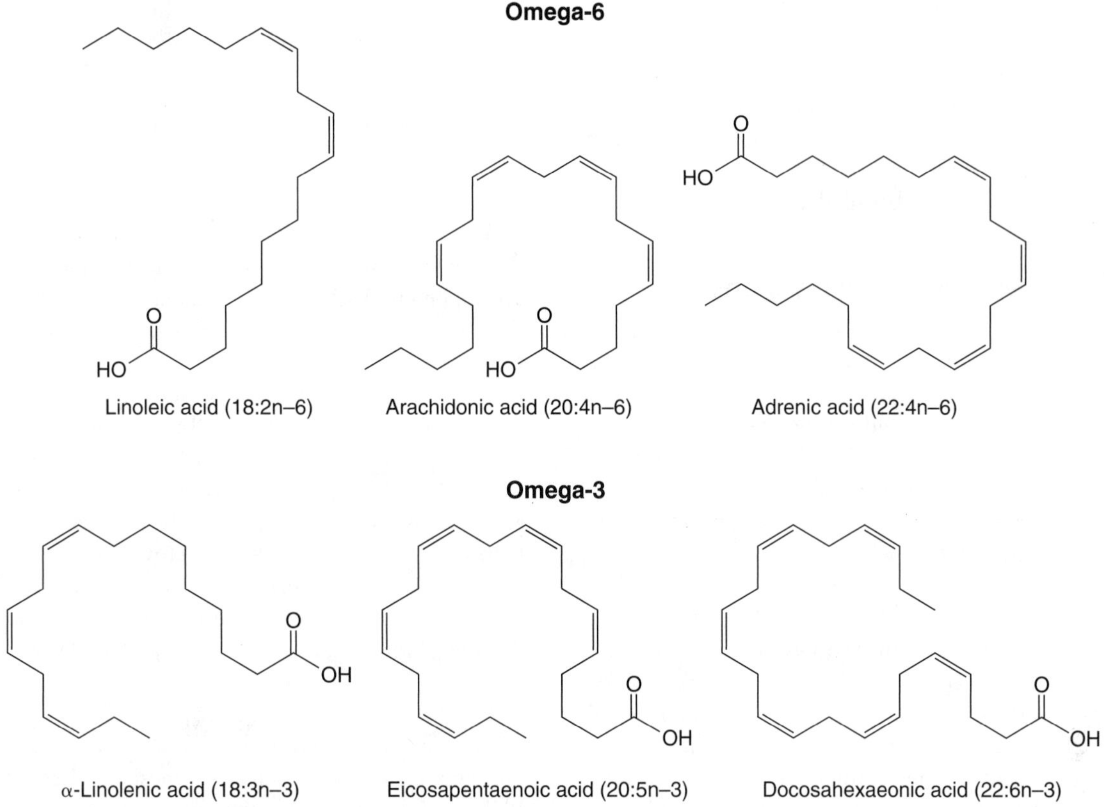

FIGURE 18-1 Structures of the most prominent n–6 and n–3 essential PUFAs.

that are present in essential fatty acids. However, plants have the capacity to synthesize PUFAs containing these double bonds; terrestrial plants can form 18-carbon n–3 and n–6 PUFAs and marine plants up to 22-carbon n–3 and n–6 PUFAs. Together, terrestrial and marine plants are the ultimate sources of essential fatty acids in the human food chain.

NOMENCLATURE OF POLYUNSATURATED FATTY ACIDS

The carbon atoms of fatty acids are numbered in two different ways. In the delta (Δ) numbering system, the carboxyl carbon is designated as carbon 1. The reverse occurs in the n– numbering system; the carbon at the methyl end of the hydrocarbon chain is designated as carbon 1. Another designation for the n– notation is ω, and both ω and n– notations are used interchangeably for numbering double bonds from the methyl end of a fatty acid. The n– notation is currently more popular and is used in this chapter.

Numbering system	CH_3 —	CH_2 —	CH_2 —	CH_2 —	CH_2 —	COOH
Omega (ω or n–)	1	2	3	4	5	6
Delta (Δ)	6	5	4	3	2	1

When the methyl end notation is used, a number is usually placed after the n– or ω to indicate the location of the first double bond in relation to the methyl carbon. For example, ω3 indicates that the first double bond is the third carbon, counting from the methyl end of the fatty acid. The designation n–3 similarly indicates that the first double bond is the third carbon from the methyl carbon, although technically it indicates that the double bond begins at carbon number "n minus 3" counting from the carboxyl carbon. In every member of the n–3 class, the double bond closest to the methyl end is located 3 carbons from the methyl end.

n–3 $CH_3—CH_2—CH{=}CH—$

In every member of the n–6 class, the double bond closest to the methyl end is located 6 carbons from the methyl end.

n–6 $CH_3—CH_2—CH_2—CH_2—CH_2—CH{=}CH—$

Fatty acids are often abbreviated as a ratio of the number of carbons to the number of double bonds (e.g., 18:0 for stearic acid). If the fatty acid is unsaturated, the location of the double bonds is also given. The location of the double bonds may be indicated by placing the location of each double bond before the number of carbons. For example, the notation for a PUFA that contains 18 carbons and two double bonds that are present at C9 and C12 is 9,12-18:2. Alternatively, the location of the double bonds for the commonly occurring PUFAs can be indicated by denoting the position of the first double bond counting from the methyl end (i.e., n–3, n–6, or n–9) because the double bonds are all methylene-interrupted. With this designation, for example, 18:3n–3 would be the same as 9,12,15-18:3. Thus, the location of a double bond in the Δ numbering system can be determined from the n– notation if the number of carbons that the fatty acid contains is known. For example, a double bond located in the n–3 position of an 18-carbon fatty acid is at C15 in the Δ nomenclature (i.e., n−3, or 18−3=15), and an n−6 double bond in an 18-carbon fatty acid is at C12 in the Δ nomenclature (i.e., 18−6=12). If the fatty acid is 18:3n−3, the double bonds will be between carbon atoms 15 and 16, 12 and 13, and 9 and 10, leaving a methylene carbon between each double bond.

The structure and nomenclature of fatty acids is described more fully in Chapter 6.

THE n−6 POLYUNSATURATED FATTY ACIDS

Linoleic acid (18:2n−6), the first member of the n−6 class, is the main PUFA synthesized by terrestrial plants. It is the most abundant fatty acid contained in the triacylglycerols of corn oil, sunflower seed oil, and safflower oil, and linoleic acid accounts for most of the n−6 PUFAs obtained from the diet. Moreover, because there is much more n−6 than n−3 PUFA in most foods that we eat, linoleic acid usually is the most abundant PUFA in the diet.

The most prominent member of the n−6 class from a functional standpoint is arachidonic acid (20:4n−6; ARA). It is the main substrate used for the synthesis of the eicosanoid biomediators, such as the prostaglandins and leukotrienes, and it is also a major fatty acid component of the inositol glycerolphospholipids. Although a small amount of ARA is present in meat and other animal products in the diet, most of the ARA contained in the body is synthesized from linoleic acid. Adrenic acid (22:4), the elongation product of ARA, accumulates in tissues that have a high content of ARA. When necessary, adrenic acid can be converted back to ARA by removal of two carbons from its carboxyl end.

THE n−3 POLYUNSATURATED FATTY ACIDS

The n−3 PUFAs are present in large amounts in the retina and certain areas of the brain. Like their n−6 counterparts, n−3 PUFAs can be structurally modified but cannot be synthesized completely in the body and ultimately must be obtained from the diet. The structures of the most important n−3 PUFAs are shown in Figure 18-1. α-Linolenic acid (18:3n−3), the 18-carbon member, is structurally similar to linoleic acid except for the presence of an additional double bond at C15. Some terrestrial plants synthesize small amounts of this fatty acid, and α-linolenic is present in soybean oil and canola oil. Larger amounts of α-linolenic acid are produced by vegetation that grows in cold water, and it is a prominent component in the food chain of fish and other marine animals. Although the intestinal mucosa can desaturate α-linolenic acid, most of the dietary intake is incorporated into the intestinal lipoproteins and absorbed by humans without structural modification.

Members of the n−3 fatty acid class that have five and six double bonds are present in fish, other marine animals, and foods that contain fish oils. The most abundant are eicosapentaenoic acid (20:5n−3; EPA) and docosahexaenoic acid (22:6n−3; DHA), which are often referred to as the fish oil fatty acids. Humans typically ingest a mixture of n−3 PUFAs, with the amount of α-linolenic acid compared to EPA and DHA depending on the relative amounts of plant products as compared with seafood and products containing fish oil in the diet. This differs from n−6 PUFA dietary intake, which is mostly in the form of linoleic acid.

HIGHLY UNSATURATED FATTY ACIDS, LONG-CHAIN PUFAs, AND VERY-LONG-CHAIN PUFAs

The terms *highly unsaturated fatty acids, long-chain PUFAs,* and *very-long-chain PUFAs* are sometimes used for PUFAs that contain four or more double bonds. These terms generally are applied to ARA (20:4n−6) and adrenic acid (22:4n−6) of the n−6 class and to EPA (20:5n−3) and DHA (22:6n−3) of the n−3 class (see Figure 18-1). The terms *highly unsaturated fatty acids, long-chain PUFAs,* and *very-long-chain PUFAs* were introduced to distinguish between the 20- and 22-carbon PUFAs, which produce most of the functional effects of essential fatty acids, and their 18-carbon precursors, which serve primarily as substrates for the synthesis of these more highly unsaturated derivatives. However, in chemistry the term *long-chain fatty acid* means any fatty acid greater than 12 carbons, thus leading to some confusion between the definitions of long-chain and very-long-chain fatty acids.

ESSENTIAL FATTY ACID METABOLISM

Humans cannot completely synthesize either n−3 or n−6 PUFAs. However, all humans, even infants, can convert the 18-carbon members of each class to the corresponding 20- and 22-carbon products (Brenna et al., 2009). It is generally agreed that the human requirement for n−6 PUFAs can be fully satisfied by synthesis from dietary linoleic acid. However, there is ongoing debate as to whether humans, especially infants, can synthesize enough 20- and 22-carbon n−3 PUFAs from α-linolenic acid for optimal growth and development of the neural and visual systems.

SYNTHESIS OF 20- AND 22-CARBON PUFAs

The synthesis of the longer, more highly unsaturated derivatives from the 18-carbon members of the n−3 and n−6 classes occurs through the pathway illustrated in Figure 18-2. Three types of reactions are involved: fatty acid chain elongation, desaturation, and β-oxidation (Sprecher, 2000). These reactions occur with both n−6 and n−3 PUFAs, but the two classes cannot be interconverted. Therefore an n−6 PUFA can be converted only to another n−6 PUFA, and likewise, an n−3 PUFA can be converted only to another n−3 PUFA. Therefore both classes of essential fatty acids are necessary in the diet. Of related interest, a gene from *Caenorhabditis elegans* encoding an n−3 desaturase, capable of converting n−6 PUFAs into n−3 PUFAs, has been isolated and transfected into mice and pigs, allowing them to synthesize n−3 PUFAs from n−6 PUFAs (Kang et al., 2004; Lai et al., 2006).

All the reactions in the PUFA metabolic pathway utilize fatty acids in the form of acyl-coenzyme A (CoA) derivatives. The complete pathway involves three elongation reactions, three desaturation reactions, and one retroconversion reaction. Fatty acids containing similar numbers of carbons and double bonds occur in the n−3 and n−6 classes

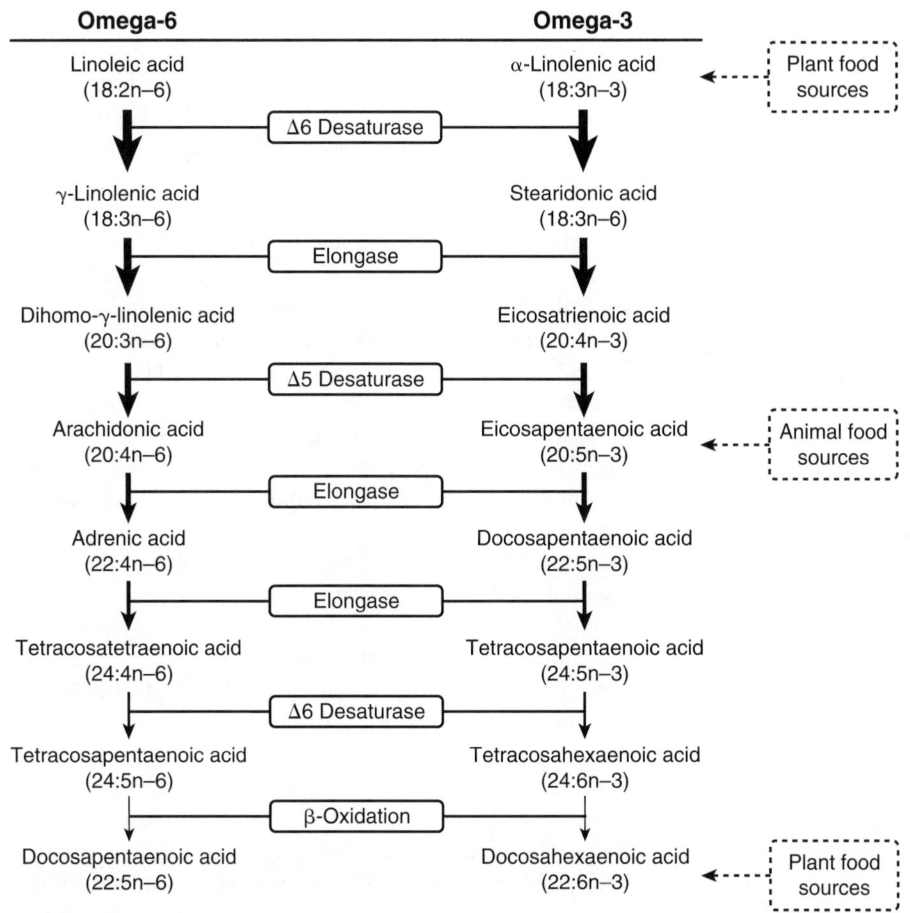

FIGURE 18-2 Pathway for the conversion of 18-carbon n−6 and n−3 essential PUFAs to their elongated and more highly unsaturated products in mammalian tissues. The fatty acids are abbreviated as number of carbons:number of double bonds, followed by the location of the first double bond counting from the methyl end. Although not evident from the figure, this enzymatic pathway only uses fatty acids in the form of fatty acyl-CoAs.

(e.g., 18:3, 20:4, and 22:5). They are positional isomers, not identical compounds. Therefore the 18:3 in the n−3 pathway is α-linolenic acid (9,12,15-18:3, or 18:3n−3), whereas the 18:3 in the n−6 pathway is γ-linolenic acid (6,9,12-18:3, or 18:3n−6). Likewise, the 20:4 and 22:5 fatty acids that occur in both pathways are isomeric pairs. The 24-carbon fatty acids present in each class are metabolic intermediates that normally do not accumulate in either the plasma or the tissues.

Although each of the seven reactions in PUFA metabolism can utilize either n−3 or n−6 PUFAs, the pathway functions differently with the two classes of essential fatty acids under normal physiological conditions. The main n−6 PUFA product normally is ARA, and the last n−6 product normally formed is 22:4. The final three reactions in the n−6 PUFA metabolic pathway—(1) elongation to a 24-carbon intermediate, (2) Δ6-desaturation of this intermediate, and (3) retroconversion to the 22-carbon end-product—only become prominent when there is an n−3 PUFA deficiency. On the other hand, n−3 PUFA metabolism does lead to formation of the final 22:6n−3 product, DHA.

Fatty Acid Elongation

Fatty acids are elongated in the endoplasmic reticulum (ER) through the mechanism illustrated in Figure 18-3. The fatty acid must be in the form of an acyl-CoA, and malonyl-CoA is the elongating agent. In the condensation reaction, which is the rate-limiting step, the free carboxyl group of malonyl-CoA is released as CO_2 and the remaining 2-carbon fragment is attached to the fatty acid carbonyl group by displacement of CoA. Finally, the carbonyl group, which is C3 in the elongated product, is reduced in a three-step process that utilizes two NADPH molecules.

The position of the double bonds does not shift relative to the methyl end when a PUFA is elongated, and their numbering remains the same in the n− or omega nomenclature. However, the numbering of the double bonds changes in the Δ nomenclature because the 2-carbon fragment that adds becomes C1 and C2 of the lengthened product. Therefore when 6,9,12-18:3 undergoes one elongation, the resulting 20-carbon fatty acid is 8,11,14-20:3. A fatty acid can undergo more than one elongation. Each elongation sequence consists of the enzymatic reactions shown in Figure 18-3 and uses two NADPH, and the fatty acid is lengthened by the addition of two carbons to the carboxyl end.

All the elongation enzymes that have been studied effectively utilize both n−3 and n−6 PUFAs. However, there are at least five different human long-chain fatty acid elongase genes, denoted ELOVL1 to ELOVL5 (Jakobsson et al., 2006). The expression of these genes is tissue dependent. Furthermore, each ELOVL enzyme has different substrate specificity, although there is some overlap. For example, ELOVL5 acts on 18- and 20-carbon fatty acids, whereas ELOVL2 and ELOVL4 act on 20- and 22-carbon fatty acids. Consequently, at least two different fatty acid elongation enzymes operating in sequence are needed to convert an 18-carbon polyunsaturated fatty acid to the 24-carbon intermediate, and the enzymes that act in one tissue may be different from those that act in another tissue. These factors make elongation a complicated process that still is not fully understood.

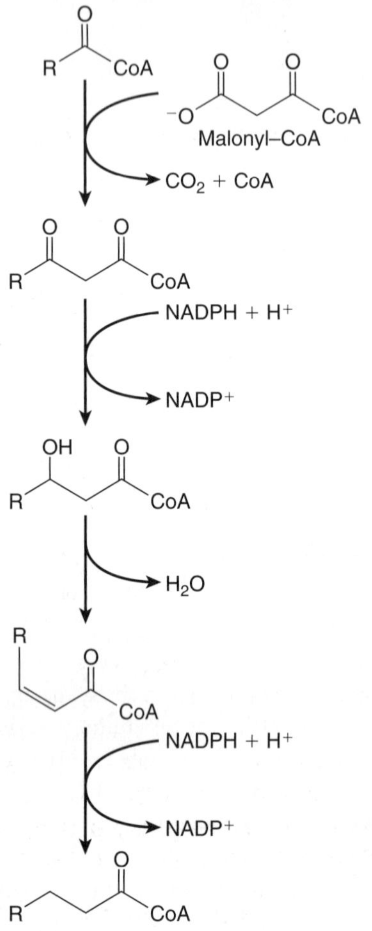

FIGURE 18-3 Mechanism of fatty acid chain elongation.

Fatty Acid Desaturation

Double bonds are inserted into fatty acids by desaturation, a process that also occurs in the ER. The double bonds that are formed are always in the *cis* configuration. There are two classes of desaturase enzymes: (1) the stearoyl-CoA desaturases (SCDs) that act on saturated fatty acids, and (2) the fatty acyl-CoA desaturases (FADSs) that act on PUFAs.

Although several genes may encode the FADS enzymes, in terms of PUFA metabolism, *FADS1* and *FADS2* are the most studied. FADS1 is the fatty acid Δ5-desaturase, and FADS2 is the fatty acid Δ6-desaturase. The genes coding for FADS1 and FADS2 are located on human chromosome 11q12-q13.1 in reverse orientation, separated by about 10,000 bp (Marquardt et al., 2000). The expression of these two genes is coordinately regulated. In addition, a third desaturase gene, *FADS3*, is located in the 11q12-q13.1 region, but the function of its gene product is unknown (Lattka et al., 2010). Figure 18-2 illustrates where the fatty acid Δ5- and Δ6-desaturases act in essential fatty acid metabolism.

Both fatty acid desaturases can utilize either n−3 or n−6 polyunsaturated fatty acyl-CoA substrates, and they both require O_2, NADH, cytochrome b_5, and cytochrome b_5 reductase. Figure 18-4 illustrates the two reactions. The desaturases act on the segment of the acyl-CoA chain between the carboxyl group and the first existing double bond. The Δ5-desaturase acts on polyunsaturated acyl-CoAs that have the first double bond at C8, inserting the new double bond at C5. This enzyme acts at only one point in the metabolic pathway, converting 20:3n−6 to ARA in n−6 PUFA metabolism and 20:4n−3 to EPA in n−3 PUFA metabolism. The Δ6-desaturase acts on polyunsaturated fatty acyl-CoA substrates that have the first double bond at C9, and inserts the new double bond at C6. There is only one fatty acid Δ6-desaturase, and this enzyme functions twice in n−3 PUFA metabolism, converting α-linolenic acid to 18:4n−3 and 24:5n−3 to 24:6n−3 (Sprecher, 2000). The Δ6-desaturase ordinarily functions only once in n−6 PUFA metabolism, converting linoleic acid to 18:3n−6. It also is capable of converting 24:4n−6 to 24:5n−6, but this

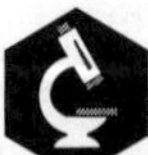

CLINICAL CORRELATION

Fatty Acid Δ6-Desaturase Deficiency

A 4-year-old girl who had persistent health problems since birth was referred to a pediatric genetic disease specialist for evaluation because of poor growth, ulcerated cornea, severe photophobia, scaly skin lesions over her arms and legs, and cracking of the skin at the corners of her mouth. Analysis of her plasma revealed abnormally low levels of ARA and DHA. A supplement of fish oil and black currant seed oil, which contains γ-linolenic acid (18:3n−6), was prescribed. This treatment corrected the deficiencies of ARA and DHA in the plasma, and many of her symptoms gradually improved. A skin biopsy subsequently was obtained and fibroblasts were grown in culture. Biochemical studies revealed that the fatty acid Δ6-desaturase activity of the fibroblasts was very low as compared with normal human skin fibroblasts (Williard et al., 2001).

Thinking Critically

1. Why was black currant seed oil prescribed instead of corn oil as a source of n−6 PUFAs for this patient?
2. Could capsules containing purified EPA ethyl ester be used instead of fish oil to effectively treat the DHA deficiency in this patient?
3. Would you expect to find an elevation in 20:3n−9 in the patient's plasma?

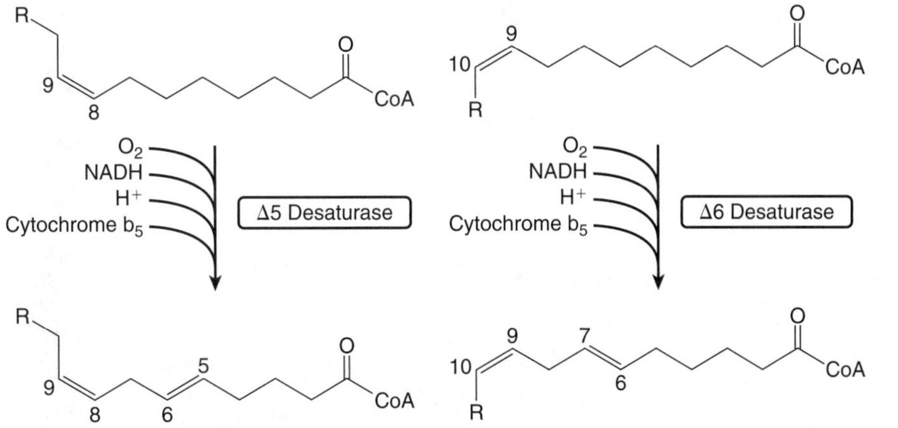

FIGURE 18-4 Positional differences in the double bonds inserted by the fatty acid Δ5- and Δ6-desaturases.

occurs to an appreciable extent only if there is a deficiency of n−3 PUFAs.

Retroconversion in the Peroxisomes

Conversion of the 24-carbon acyl-CoA intermediates to the 22-carbon end products is thought to occur through peroxisomal fatty acid oxidation, a β-oxidation system that shortens very-long-chain fatty acids. This process requires transport of the 24-carbon intermediate from the ER to the peroxisomes and, subsequently, transport of the 22-carbon product back to the ER where it is incorporated into tissue lipids. As shown in Figure 18-5, the retroconversion reaction requires O_2, FAD, NAD^+, and CoA, and it removes two carbons in the form of acetyl-CoA from the carboxyl end of the fatty acyl-CoA. The peroxisomal enzymes that catalyze this β-oxidation process are straight-chain acyl-CoA oxidase, D-bifunctional protein, and either 3-ketoacyl-CoA thiolase or sterol carrier protein X (SCP-X) (Ferdinandusse et al., 2001).

In n−3 PUFA metabolism, this process converts 24:6n−3 to DHA. The numbering of the carbons in the Δ nomenclature changes when retroconversion occurs because the carbons that were numbered 1 and 2 in the original fatty acid are removed. Therefore the C6 double bond in the 24-carbon intermediate becomes the C4 double bond of DHA, the 22-carbon product. A similar process can occur with n−6 PUFAs to produce 22:5n−6 from 24:5n−6 (see Figure 18-2). Retroconversion also appears to be responsible for the increase in C20 PUFAs when C22 PUFAs are fed (e.g., increase in arachidonate when 22:4n−6 is fed, or of EPA when 22:5n−3 is fed). Thus elongation, desaturation, and retroconversion together may enable the body to utilize whichever n−3 and n−6 PUFAs are available in the diet to produce all of the necessary members of these essential fatty acid classes.

Peroxisomal fatty acid β-oxidation is deficient in cells of patients with Zellweger syndrome, which is caused by mutations in genes encoding proteins required for biogenesis of peroxisomes. Patients with Zellweger syndrome have elevated levels of very-long-chain fatty acids (e.g., C26:0 and C26:1), high ratios of C24/C22 and C26/C22 fatty acids, and low levels of DHA because they cannot produce DHA from the C24 n−3 PUFA precursor.

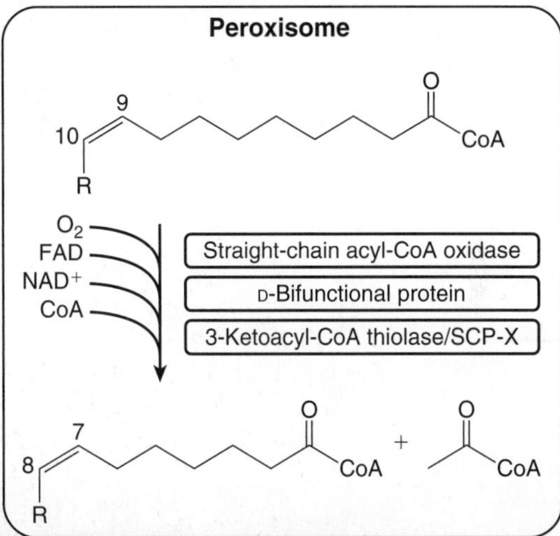

FIGURE 18-5 Retroconversion reaction that occurs in essential fatty acid metabolism. *SCP-X,* Sterol carrier protein X.

ESSENTIAL FATTY ACID COMPOSITION OF PLASMA AND TISSUE LIPIDS

Both dietary intake and metabolism influence the types of PUFAs that accumulate in the body. Western diets typically contain about 10 times more n−6 than n−3 PUFAs. Linoleic acid is the most abundant PUFA in the diet. Dietary PUFAs are incorporated into the lipids in chylomicrons produced by the small intestinal absorptive cells, and these lipoproteins are a major source of essential fatty acids for the tissues in the postprandial state. Many tissues are able to convert linoleic acid to ARA through the pathway illustrated in Figure 18-2, and linoleic acid (18:2n−6) and ARA (20:4n−6) are the main n−6 PUFAs that accumulate in the body. Very little α-linolenic acid (18:3n−3) ordinarily is present in the plasma or tissues, and unless the diet is supplemented with fish oil or n−3 PUFA ethyl esters, there also is little EPA (20:5n−3).

The levels of PUFAs present in the plasma lipids of human subjects who consumed western diets are shown in Table 18-1 (Edelstein, 1986). These data show that n−6 PUFAs accounted for 17% of the fatty acids in the plasma free fatty acid fraction, 37% of the fatty acids in phospholipids,

TABLE 18-1 Essential Fatty Acid Composition of Normal Human Plasma Lipids

		Lipoprotein Lipids		
FATTY ACID*	FREE FATTY ACID	PHOSPHOLIPIDS†	TRIACYLGLYCEROLS	CHOLESTERYL ESTERS‡
	(FRACTION OF TOTAL FATTY ACIDS, % BY WEIGHT)			
n−3				
18:3	0.71 ± 0.11	0.21 ± 0.03	1.18 ± 0.08	0.50 ± 0.06
22:6	0.34 ± 0.06	2.23 ± 0.14	0.35 ± 0.04	0.49 ± 0.08
n−6§				
18:2	15.60 ± 0.63	22.94 ± 0.57	19.54 ± 0.84	49.82 ± 1.79
20:3	0.14 ± 0.04	3.11 ± 0.12	0.36 ± 0.05	0.91 ± 0.06
20:4	1.25 ± 0.17	10.95 ± 0.45	1.64 ± 0.14	8.08 ± 0.39

Modified from data compiled by Edelstein, C. (1986). General properties of plasma lipoproteins and apoproteins. In A. M. Scanu & A. A. Spector (Eds.), *Biochemistry and biology of the plasma lipoproteins* (pp. 495–505). New York: Marcel Dekker.
*Abbreviated as ratio of number of carbons to number of double bonds.
†Phospholipids contain 0.65 ± 0.08% 20:5n−3 and 0.77 ± 0.03% 22:5n−3. The other lipid fractions contain only trace amounts (<0.3%) of these n−3 fatty acids.
‡Cholesteryl esters contain 1.07 ± 0.07% 18:3n−6, but the other lipid fractions contain only trace amounts.
§The lipids contain only trace amounts (<0.5%) of 22:4n−6 and 22:5n−6.

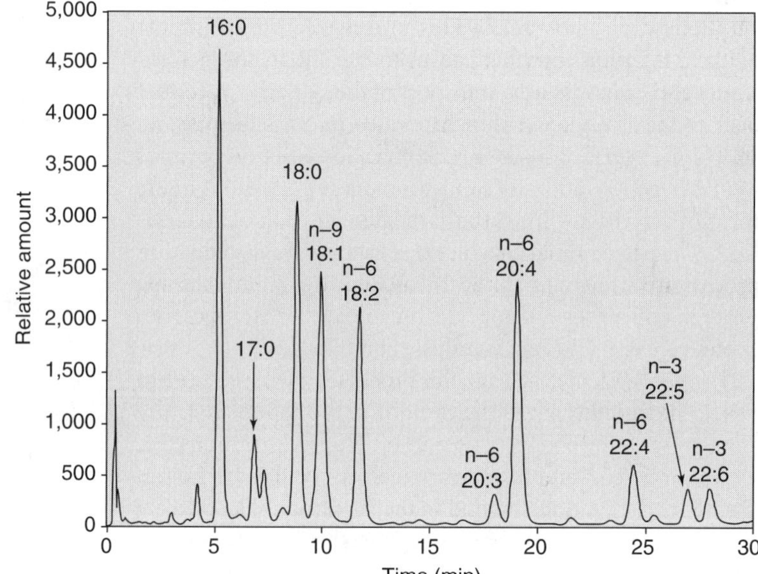

FIGURE 18-6 Fatty acid composition of the human erythrocyte as determined by gas liquid chromatography. The fatty acids are indicated as a ratio of the number of carbons to the number of double bonds. Heptadecanoic acid, 17:0, was added as an internal standard for the analysis and is not ordinarily present in erythrocyte lipids. The classes of the unsaturated fatty acids detected in the erythrocyte lipids are n–9 (18:1), n–6 (18:2, 20:3, 20:4, 22:4), and n–3 (22:5, 22:6).

22% of the fatty acids in triacylglycerols, and 59% of the fatty acids in cholesteryl esters. Linoleic acid and ARA comprised most of the n−6 PUFAs contained in these plasma lipids. In contrast to the high n−6 PUFA content, n−3 PUFAs comprised only 1% to 3% of the total fatty acids in any of the plasma lipid fractions.

The essential PUFAs in tissues are contained primarily in membrane phospholipids. Within the phospholipids, the PUFAs are located almost entirely in the *sn*-2 position (i.e., esterified to the middle carbon of the glycerol moiety). Although each phospholipid class contains a mixture of PUFAs, one or two fatty acids usually predominate in each phospholipid class. ARA is highly enriched in phosphatidylinositol, whereas linoleic acid and ARA are contained in large amounts in the choline glycerolphospholipids. The 22-carbon members, DHA and adrenic acid (22:4n−6), tend to accumulate in the ethanolamine glycerolphospholipids and phosphatidylserines, and DHA is highly enriched in the ethanolamine plasmalogens. These differences in fatty acid distribution are due primarily to the substrate specificities of the acyltransferases that incorporate acyl-CoA into the *sn*-2 position of phospholipids.

Figure 18-6 shows the fatty acid composition of normal human erythrocytes from a person consuming a typical western diet, as determined by gas-liquid chromatography. Many more n−6 than n−3 PUFAs are contained in the erythrocyte lipids. The n−6 PUFAs present are 18:2n−6, 20:3n−6, 20:4n−6, and 22:4n−6, with linoleic acid (18:2n−6) and

ARA (20:4n−6) accounting for about 80% of the total. The small amount of n−3 PUFAs are distributed almost equally between 22:5n−3 and DHA (22:6n−3).

The most notable exceptions to the general pattern of PUFAs found in plasma and tissues are those in the retina and brain. The retina and brain have a high content of n−3 PUFAs, with this being mostly DHA. Some DHA is obtained directly from the diet, and dietary DHA is an important source of DHA for the brain (Rapoport et al., 2010). The remainder is obtained by synthesis in the body from α-linolenic acid and other n−3 PUFAs that may be present in the diet. It is currently thought that the α-linolenic acid and EPA that enter the brain are rapidly β-oxidized and thus are not substrates for local DHA synthesis. Hepatocytes express the complete metabolic pathway shown in Figure 18-2 and can supply DHA to the circulation for uptake by other tissues. Many other tissues in addition to the brain do not convert α-linolenic acid to DHA and likewise depend on the circulation for a supply of DHA synthesized elsewhere in the body. For example, the retina utilizes DHA that is formed in the liver from n−3 PUFA precursors.

FUNCTIONS OF POLYUNSATURATED FATTY ACIDS

The n−3 and n−6 PUFAs are essential primarily because they are required for two important physiological processes, the synthesis of lipid biomediators and the production of membrane phospholipids that have optimal structural and signal transduction properties. Because these are fundamental processes, it is surprising that some animal cell lines can grow in culture for many passages in the absence of any detectable essential fatty acids. Many of these cell lines were derived from rodent malignant tumors that do not express the fatty acid Δ6-desaturase. Although a few biochemical functions are slightly compromised in these cells, they are viable and grow well. Therefore essential fatty acids apparently are not required for the maintenance of basic life processes in a mammalian cell. The functions of essential fatty acids appear to become necessary when cells differentiate and form multicellular organisms, in which intercellular communication, highly specialized membrane functions, and coordination of gene expression are vital. More recently, the role of n−3 PUFA derivatives in the inflammatory process has become increasingly recognized.

FUNCTIONS OF n−6 POLYUNSATURATED FATTY ACIDS

Figure 18-7 illustrates the main functions of n−6 PUFAs. These processes must operate properly for the body to function normally. Linoleic acid and ARA have membrane structural effects, especially linoleic acid in the sphingolipids that prevent water loss from the skin. In addition, ARA is the primary substrate for eicosanoid synthesis, and it is a major component of the phosphatidylinositols that are involved in membrane signal transduction. In addition, n−6 PUFAs and some of the eicosanoids are ligands for the peroxisome proliferator-activated receptors (PPARs) and thereby affect the expression of many genes involved in lipid metabolism.

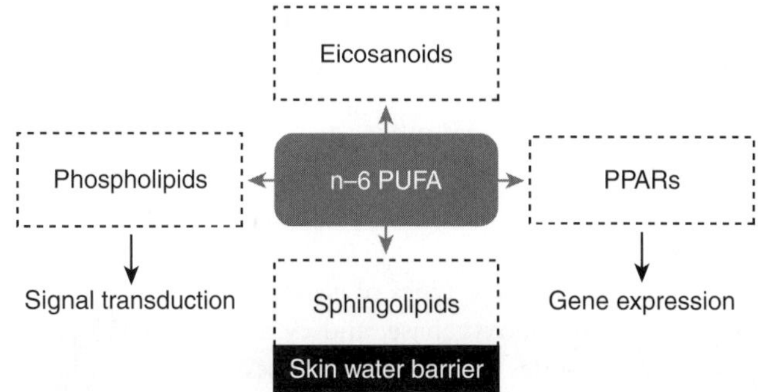

FIGURE 18-7 Physiological functions of the n−6 essential PUFAs. *PPARs,* Peroxisome proliferator–activated receptors.

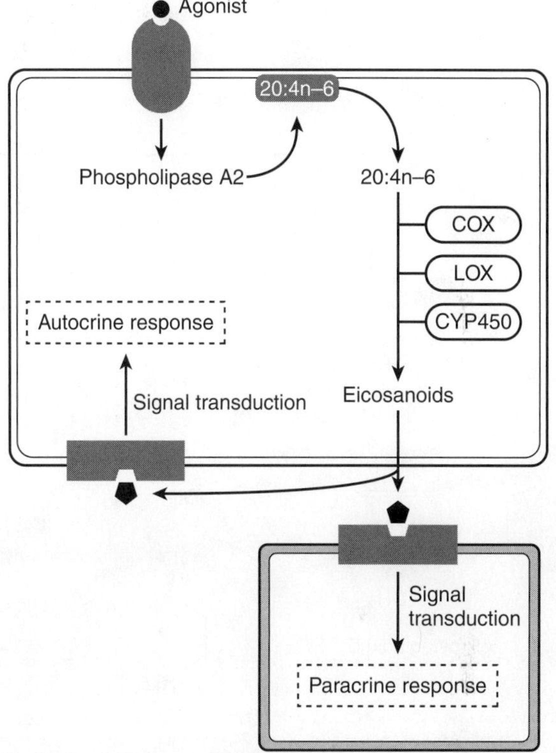

FIGURE 18-8 Synthesis and mechanism of action of n−6 eicosanoids. *COX,* Cyclooxygenase; *CYP450,* Cytochrome P450; *LOX,* lipoxygenase.

Arachidonic Acid and Eicosanoids

Eicosanoids synthesized from ARA are lipid biomediators that regulate many cellular functions. Figure 18-8 illustrates the production and action of these compounds. The binding of a cytokine or hormone to a plasma membrane receptor triggers eicosanoid production by the target cell via activation of a calcium-dependent cytoplasmic phospholipase A2. This phospholipase hydrolyzes ARA from the *sn*-2 position of intracellular membrane phospholipids, primarily choline glycerolphospholipids. The cyclooxygenase, lipoxygenase, or cytochrome P450 pathway contained in the cell converts the ARA to one or more eicosanoid products. A major function of eicosanoids is cell–cell communication. These compounds are released into the extracellular fluid and function as autocrine and paracrine mediators by binding to plasma membrane GTP-binding protein (G protein)–coupled receptors that either activate or modulate the activity of intracellular signaling pathways. Some of the responses occur very rapidly, whereas others that involve transcriptional mechanisms occur more slowly.

Figure 18-9 lists the types of eicosanoids formed by the cyclooxygenase, lipoxygenase, and cytochrome P450 pathways and illustrates the structures of several representative products. The cyclooxygenase pathway produces prostaglandins and thromboxanes. There are two cyclooxygenase isozymes, a constitutive form (COX1) and an inducible form (COX2). The structure of prostaglandin E_2 (PGE_2), one of the major prostaglandins, is shown. The subscript 2 denotes that the eicosanoid has two double bonds outside the ring structure, a characteristic of all cyclooxygenase products synthesized from ARA. Eicosanoids formed by the cyclooxygenase pathway have many physiological actions, including modulation of cardiovascular and renal function, blood coagulation, and inflammation.

Lipoxygenases convert ARA to a hydroperoxyeicosatetraenoic acid (HPETE). There are three isozymes, 5-, 12-, and 15-lipoxygenase, which differ in their positional specificity for the ARA double bonds. The HPETE then is converted to a hydroxyeicosatetraenoic acid (HETE), leukotriene, lipoxin,

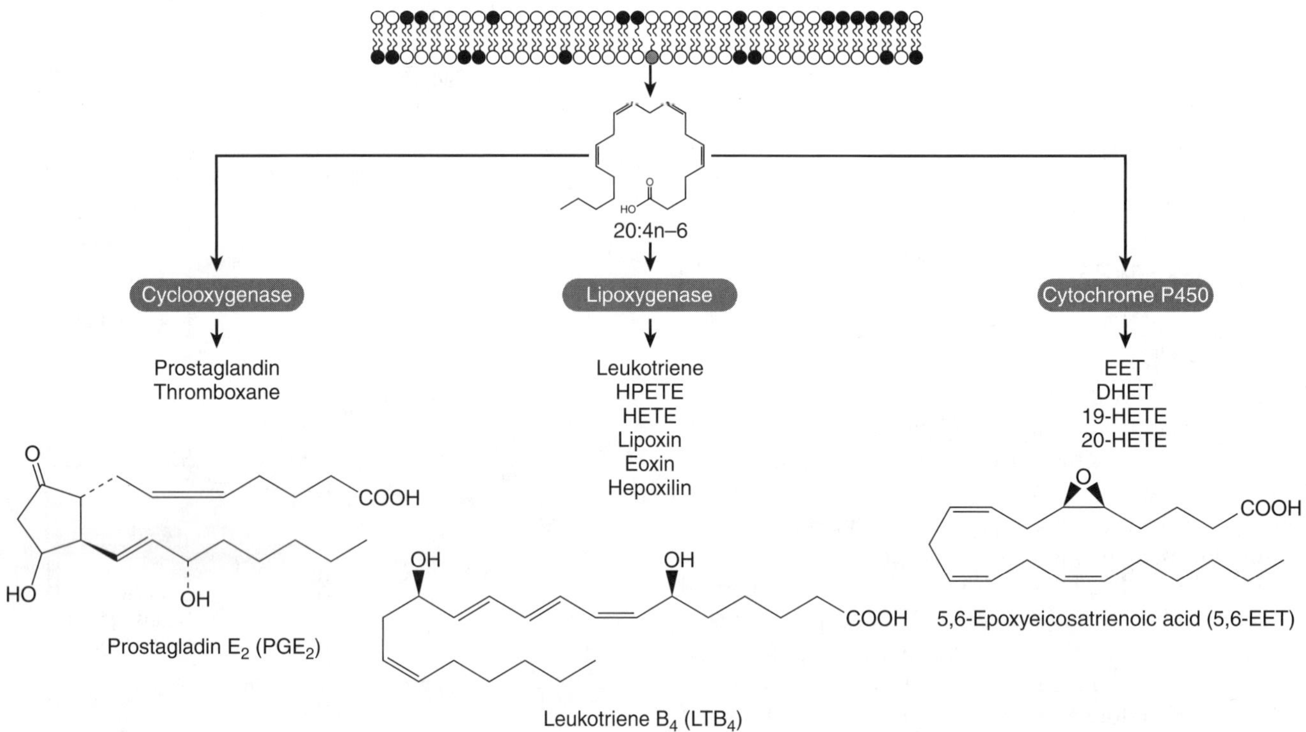

FIGURE 18-9 Pathways of eicosanoid synthesis and structures of some representative products. *DHET,* Dihydroxyeicosatrienoic acid; *EET,* epoxyeicosatrienoic acid; *HETE,* hydroxyeicosatetraenoic acid; *19-HETE,* 19-hydroxyeicosatetraenoic acid; *20-HETE,* 20-hydroxyeicosatetraenoic acid; *HPETE,* hydroperoxyeicosatetraenoic acid.

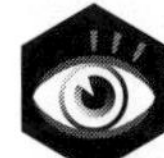

NUTRITION INSIGHT

Dietary Effects on Membrane Fatty Acid Composition

Modifying the dietary fat intake can alter the fatty acid composition of membrane phospholipids. Even the fatty acid composition of the phospholipid membranes in the heart, which one might think of as a very stable tissue, can be modified rapidly in experimental animals. The brain is the only organ that is resistant to such diet-induced change. Except for this case, the fatty acid composition of most membranes adapts to some extent to the type of fat available in the diet. This flexibility is surprising, considering the vital role that membranes play in so many cellular functions. Diet-induced changes in membrane lipid composition support the old saying that "you are what you eat." However, there are limits to the extent of change that can take place in mammalian cells. Most of the variation occurs in the relative proportions of unsaturated fatty acids. For example, if the diet is enriched in sunflower seed oil, which contains 70% linoleic acid, the n–6 PUFA content of the membrane phospholipids increases and is counterbalanced by a decrease in oleic acid. This reduction in monounsaturated fatty acid content is a compensation that protects against an excessive increase in membrane fluidity due to an overabundance of unsaturated fatty acid in the membrane phospholipids. The relative amounts of n–3 and n–6 PUFAs in membrane phospholipids also depend to some extent on the dietary intake of these essential PUFAs.

TABLE 18-2 Prostaglandin Receptors

RECEPTOR	MAIN LIGAND	SIGNAL TRANSDUCTION MECHANISM	MAJOR PHYSIOLOGICAL FUNCTIONS
DP	PGD_2	Inositol phospholipids Increases intracellular Ca^{2+}	Platelet aggregation Smooth muscle contraction
EP_1	PGE_2	Inositol phospholipids Increases intracellular Ca^{2+}	Smooth muscle contraction
EP_2	PGE_2	Adenylate cyclase Increases cAMP	Smooth muscle relaxation
EP_3	PGE_2	Adenylate cyclase Decreases cAMP	Water reabsorption Gastric acid secretion Uterine contraction
EP_4	PGE_2	Adenylate cyclase Increases cAMP	Smooth muscle relaxation
FP	$PGF_{2\alpha}$	Inositol phospholipids Increases intracellular Ca^{2+}	Smooth muscle contraction
IP	PGI_2	Adenylate cyclase Increases cAMP	Arterial smooth muscle relaxation Platelet aggregation
TP	TXA_2	Inositol phospholipids Increases intracellular Ca^{2+}	Platelet aggregation Vasoconstriction Bronchoconstriction

PG, Prostaglandin; *TX*, thromboxane.

eoxin, or hepoxilin. The structure of leukotriene B_4 (LTB_4), one of the main leukotrienes, is shown; the subscript 4 indicates the number of double bonds in the leukotriene. Lipoxygenase products function primarily in the tissue response to inflammatory stimuli.

Cytochrome P450 epoxygenases convert ARA to epoxyeicosatrienoic acids (EETs). The structure of 5,6-EET, one of the four EET positional isomers, is shown. Another class of cytochrome P450 enzymes, the ω-oxidases, insert a hydroxyl group at or near the methyl terminus of ARA. 20-HETE is the main product. Eicosanoids formed by the cytochrome P450 pathway act on small arteries and in the kidney. They modulate vascular resistance and blood pressure.

Table 18-2 lists the prostaglandin receptors, the main prostanoids that they bind, the biochemical mechanism of action, and the physiological responses that are produced. Eight different types of prostaglandin receptors have been cloned; they are all G protein–coupled receptors. Although there is some overlap in substrate specificity, each type is designated according to the main product that it binds. For example, IP is the PGI receptor, and EP is a PGE receptor. The four subtypes of EP receptors have different tissue distributions, are linked to different G proteins, and produce different functional responses.

Prostaglandin-mediated signaling is a very complicated process that can occur in different ways, depending on the type of prostaglandin and the receptor to which it binds. One mechanism is activation of adenylate cyclase. PGI_2 functions in this way. It binds to the IP receptor, which is coupled to a G_s protein. This activates adenylate cyclase, causing a large increase in cyclic adenosine monophosphate (cAMP) within the target cell. PGE_2 produces a similar response when it binds to the EP_2 receptor. However, when PGE_2 binds to the EP_3 receptor, it activates a G_i protein that reduces adenylate cyclase activity, thereby decreasing cAMP production. To further complicate matters, PGE_2 also can bind to EP_1 receptors, which are coupled to G_q proteins that activate phospholipase C. This stimulates hydrolysis of phosphatidylinositol 4,5-bisphosphate, producing an increase in the cytosolic calcium concentration.

Arachidonic Acid and Signal Transduction

Another important function of ARA is phospholipid-mediated signal transduction. In the brain, phospholipase A2 is activated by glutamatergic, serotonergic, cholinergic, and dopaminergic signaling, releasing ARA as a secondary messenger (Duncan and Bazinet, 2010). Although the direct messages relayed by the released ARA are not known, drugs that are therapeutic in bipolar disorder target this pathway, which is an active area of research (Rao et al., 2008). Furthermore, the membrane phosphatidylinositols that are involved in activation of the intracellular protein kinase C signaling pathway following activation of G_q protein–coupled receptors contain a relatively high percentage of ARA. Activation of the G_q protein in turn activates phospholipase C, which hydrolyzes phosphatidylinositol 4,5-bisphosphate into inositol 1,4,5-triphosphate and 1,2-diacylglycerol. The 1,2-diacylglycerol contains ARA and is involved in activating protein kinase C. The function of the high ARA content of the diacylglycerols released by phospholipase C is not known. The possibilities include targeting to specific membrane domains or imparting special binding properties to the diacylglycerol. Alternatively, the diacylglycerol may be hydrolyzed by a diacylglycerol lipase, releasing the ARA for eicosanoid production.

CLINICAL CORRELATION

Fish Oil for the Prevention of Coronary Thrombosis

Daily fish oil supplements are being recommended by some physicians to reduce the risk of coronary thrombosis. Patients usually take between 1 and 3 g/day, administered either in the form of fish oil capsules or capsules containing purified EPA and DHA ethyl esters.

Thinking Critically

1. How might n−3 PUFAs act to reduce the risk of coronary thrombosis?
2. Would the administration of canola oil, which contains α-linolenic acid as the only source of n−3 PUFAs, be as effective as fish oil for this purpose?

Linoleic Acid

The average requirement for n−6 PUFAs in healthy adults, 11 to 17 g/day, greatly exceeds the amount of ARA needed for the synthesis of the eicosanoid biomediators. Explanations for this discrepancy include the possibilities that other actions of ARA are also essential, that other n−6 PUFAs have essential functions, or that the current recommendations for n−6 PUFAs are overestimated. Emphasis has focused on the skin because essential fatty acid deficiency leads to a breakdown of the epidermal barrier to water loss. Linoleic acid is strongly preferred for the synthesis of two sphingolipids, acylceramide and acylglucosylceramide, which maintain the structure of the stratum corneum, the outer layer of the skin. This suggests that linoleic acid is required to impart an optimal barrier property to the skin surface sphingolipids, thereby preventing excessive water loss.

Lipoxygenase enzymes can oxygenate linoleic acid, adding oxygen at one of its double bonds. 15-Lipoxygenase is the main lipoxygenase that acts on linoleic acid in human tissues, forming the 13-hydroperoxyoctadecadienoic acid. This product is reduced to the corresponding hydroxy-derivative, 13-hydroxyoctadecadienoic acid (13-HODE). No physiological requirement for this or other oxygenated linoleic acid derivatives has been established, and it is uncertain as to whether the lipoxygenase pathway of linoleic acid metabolism has any essential function.

A decrease in the level of plasma low-density lipoproteins (LDLs) occurs when fats enriched in linoleic acid, such as corn oil or safflower oil, are substituted for dietary saturated fats. Most of the plasma cholesterol is present in LDLs which are involved in plaque formation. The decrease in LDL level reduces the risk of developing coronary heart disease. The mechanism producing the decrease in LDL level is complex and may depend more on the reduction in saturated fat intake than on a direct biochemical effect produced by linoleic acid or one of its n−6 PUFA products. Whether linoleic acid itself has any benefit in this regard is not known (Ramsden et al., 2010).

FUNCTIONS OF n−3 POLYUNSATURATED FATTY ACIDS

Two approaches have been used to investigate the functions of n−3 PUFAs. One is to determine the effects of n−3 PUFA-deficient diets in experimental animals. The other is to study humans who consume a diet high in n−3 PUFAs or are treated with dietary supplements containing either fish oil or n−3 PUFA ethyl esters. No unique functional effects have been reported for α-linolenic acid in humans or animals, except to serve as the substrate for EPA and DHA synthesis.

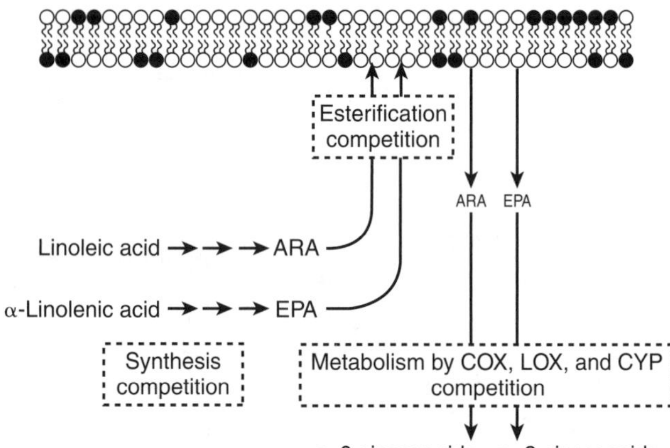

FIGURE 18-10 Competition between EPA (20:5n−3) and ARA (20:4n−6) for eicosanoid synthesis. The synthesis of both ARA and EPA requires enzymes Δ6-desaturase, elongase, and Δ5-desaturase. EPA also competes with ARA in its incorporation into the membrane phospholipids. Third, EPA competes with ARA in metabolism by cyclooxygenase (*COX*), lipoxygenase (*LOX*), and cytochrome P450 (*CYP*). Overall, EPA reduces the availability of ARA in the phospholipid membrane and the metabolism of ARA to n−6 eicosanoids.

Eicosapentaenoic Acid

Classically, EPA was considered antithrombotic and anti-inflammatory through its competitive inhibition of ARA metabolism. Competition occurs at several points in metabolism. First, the synthesis of EPA and ARA from their respective n−3 and n−6 PUFA precursors occur through the same enzymatic pathway (see Figure 18-2). Second, EPA can replace ARA in the phospholipid membrane, thus reducing the amount of ARA released by phospholipases for the production of thrombotic and proinflammatory ARA eicosanoids. Third, EPA also competes with ARA for metabolism by cyclooxygenases, lipoxygenases, and cytochrome P450 enzymes for which EPA is also a substrate. The competition mechanisms are illustrated schematically in Figure 18-10.

More recently, oxygenated derivatives of EPA have been identified and found to be potently anti-inflammatory. EPA derivatives resolvin E1 and E2 (RvE1 and RvE2) are produced following a series of enzymatic reactions, beginning

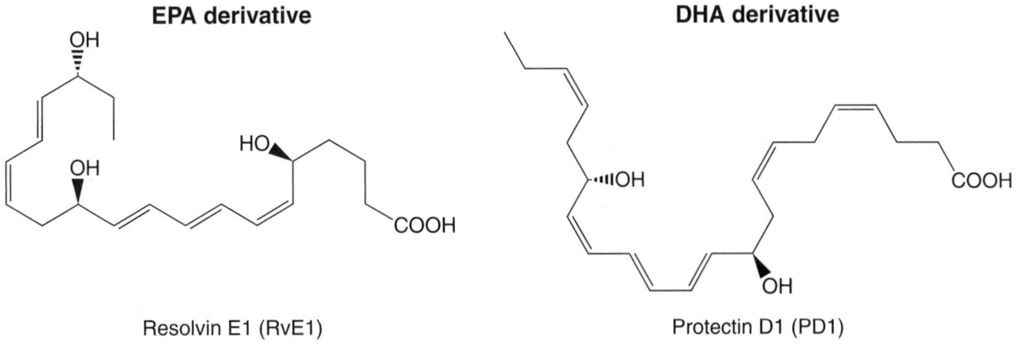

FIGURE 18-11 Structures of the EPA derivative resolvin E1 (RvE1) and the DHA derivative protectin D1 (PD1).

with the addition of an 18(R)-hydro(pero)xy group (Bannenberg and Serhan, 2010). Figure 18-11 illustrates RvE1, which is produced from EPA with the addition of three hydroxyl groups. RvE1 is known to reduce proinflammatory cytokine production, reduce inflammatory angiogenesis, stimulate phagocytosis by macrophages, and reduce neutrophil–endothelial cell interactions and the subsequent influx of immune cells to sites of inflammation. Two receptors (CMKLR1 and BLT1) through which RvE1 exerts these effects have been identified. RvE2 has not been researched beyond its identification and chemical characterization, although it is possible that RvE2 has its own unique role in the inflammatory process.

EPA produces a portion of the hypotriglyceridemic effect of fish oil, likely by increasing mitochondrial β-oxidation in the liver and thus decreasing the production of triacylglycerol (Berge et al., 1999). In addition, it probably contributes the antihypertensive effects of fish oil (Grynberg, 2005). These actions, together with its antiinflammatory and antithrombotic effects, can prevent or reduce the severity of chronic and life-threatening illnesses.

Docosahexaenoic Acid

DHA, which is highly enriched in retinal and brain phospholipids, is responsible for the visual and cognitive actions of the n−3 PUFAs. It is present in the phospholipids of cell membranes, primarily in the ethanolamine glycerolphospholipids, phosphatidylserine, and ethanolamine plasmalogens. These phospholipids are contained primarily in the inner (cytoplasmic) leaflet of the membrane lipid bilayer, so the functional effects produced by DHA most likely occur in this region of the membrane. The DHA chains contained in phospholipids are highly flexible and transition very rapidly between a large number of conformations, providing an optimal microenvironment for the function of certain proteins that are embedded in the membrane (Gawrisch et al., 2003).

Phospholipids enriched in DHA augment the response of the retina to light and enhance the transmission of the visual signal. The retinal light receptor, rhodopsin, is a G protein–coupled receptor. When rhodopsin is activated by light, the structure of the surrounding phospholipids with DHA fatty acyl chains facilitates the conformational change of rhodopsin to the metarhodopsin II state, increasing the rate of coupling to the retinal G protein. This enhances the amplification in the first stage of the visual pathway. The high DHA content of the retinal phospholipids also increases the activity of the phosphodiesterase, which is a measure of the integrated visual signal response (Mitchell et al., 2003). The need for DHA to produce optimal membrane lipid bilayer properties in the retina for the visual response is one reason why n−3 PUFAs are essential nutrients. If a similar DHA-mediated mechanism applies to G protein–coupled receptor signaling in the brain, it also may explain the cognitive benefits produced by n−3 PUFAs (Moriguchi et al., 2000). More recently, DHA has also been implicated in neuronal survival and the regulation of endocannabinoid signaling, which may also explain some of the beneficial effects of DHA in the brain (Wood et al., 2010).

Biophysical studies indicate that some phospholipids have a tendency not to form a bilayer structure. One of the alternate arrangements is a hexagonal structure, an inverted configuration in which the polar head groups of the phospholipids cluster together on the inside and the hydrocarbon chains point outward. Phosphatidylethanolamine has an increased tendency to form this type of hexagonal arrangement when it contains a high percentage of DHA. The tendency to form such a structure may affect the packing of the phospholipid head groups at the surface of the lipid bilayer and thereby change the surface properties of the membrane. This is likely to facilitate vesicle formation and membrane–vesicle fusion. Furthermore, the transient formation of a hexagonal structure in a membrane domain might allow the passage of a polar solute through the lipid bilayer by creating a temporary aqueous channel in the center of the clustered phospholipid head groups. The unique properties of phospholipids enriched in DHA might be necessary for the optimal function of membranes such as neural synapses that must rapidly respond to excitation, and this probably is another reason why n−3 fatty acids are essential.

A relationship exists between DHA and plasmalogens, a class of membrane phospholipids that contains a vinyl ether-linked fatty acid (Nagan and Zoeller, 2001). Low tissue levels of DHA occur in genetic diseases associated with plasmalogen deficiency, and mutant cell lines that are deficient in plasmalogens incorporate less than the usual amount of DHA into glycerophospholipids. The functions of plasmalogens include membrane–vesicle fusion, intracellular signal transduction, and protection against oxidant stress.

However, it is uncertain whether supplying DHA for plasmalogen synthesis is an essential function of n−3 PUFAs.

Like EPA, DHA also can be oxygenated stereospecifically, producing bioactive hydroxylated derivatives called docosanoids. These compounds are antiinflammatory and protect against brain injury due to ischemia–reperfusion (Marcheselli et al., 2003). One pathway, which is initiated by 15-lipoxygenase, produces a group of DHA derivatives that contain a 17(S)-hydroxyl group. An example of a DHA derivative produced by this lipoxygenase pathway is the antiinflammatory 10,17(S)-docosatriene known as protectin D1 (PD1), which is illustrated in Figure 18-11. A second pathway, also initiated by 15-lipoxygenase, converts DHA to D-series resolvins. Resolvins D1 through D4 have so far been identified. D-series resolvins are also potent antiinflammatory mediators, although they act through different targets than PD1. RvD1, for instance, reduces neutrophil migration to sites of inflammation and oxidative damage from neutrophil burst. A third pathway produces 14(S)-hydroxyl groups via 12-lipoxygenase. One of the characterized products is named maresin 1 (MaR1), which plays a role in resolving inflammation.

The n−3 PUFAs also decrease fatal heart arrhythmias in experimental models by modulating the conductance of ion channels in cardiac myocyte membranes (Leaf et al., 2003). The interaction of the ion channel with n−3 fatty acyl chains causes a conformational change that alters the conductance of the channel. Although this effect can be lifesaving, the modulation of ion channel conductance probably is a pharmacological action rather than an essential function of n−3 PUFAs.

REGULATION OF GENE EXPRESSION BY ESSENTIAL FATTY ACIDS

PUFAs regulate the expression of many genes involved in fatty acid and glucose metabolism (Jump, 2002; Ntambi and Bené, 2001). Dietary studies with corn oil and fish oil indicate that Δ6-desaturation must occur before either n−3 or n−6 PUFAs become transcriptionally active; in other words, linoleic acid is inactive, but its derivatives such as ARA that have undergone Δ6-desaturation are effective. Table 18-3 lists some of the genes that are regulated by the highly unsaturated forms of essential fatty acids. These genes control fatty acid synthesis, mitochondrial and peroxisomal fatty acid oxidation, saturated fatty acid desaturation, the synthesis of fatty acid binding proteins, and insulin-mediated glucose utilization.

Essential fatty acids exert their transcriptional effects by regulating the activity of three major classes of transcription factors: PPARs, liver X receptor (LXR), and sterol regulatory element binding protein (SREBP). PPARs become activated when they bind either PUFAs or their eicosanoid derivatives. Lipid binding also activates LXR, but SREBP activation occurs through an entirely different mechanism. Increases in PUFAs inhibit the proteolytic process that releases the transcription factor domain from intact SREBP. This decreases the amount of active SREBP available for transport to the nucleus. SREBP1c, the form that regulates fatty acid metabolism, is especially responsive to PUFAs. Dietary fish oil is more effective than safflower oil in suppressing SREBP1c processing, indicating that this is primarily an effect of n−3 PUFAs. These PUFAs also regulate the transcription of SREBP1c and the stability of the SREBP1c messenger RNA (mRNA).

In addition, DHA can modulate gene expression through a different mechanism. It binds to and activates the retinoid X receptor (RXR) in the brain (Mata de Urquiza et al., 2000). The activated RXR forms heterodimers with PPAR and LXR, as well as with the thyroid hormone receptor, vitamin D receptor, and retinoic acid receptor. Each of these transcription factors must form a heterodimer with RXR in order to bind to the response elements in the promoter of their target genes. Therefore DHA has the potential to exert widespread and very complex effects on gene expression in the central nervous system.

TABLE 18-3 Representative Genes Regulated by Essential Fatty Acids or Their Products

GENE	FUNCTION
Acyl-CoA oxidase (*ACOX*)	Peroxisomal fatty acid β-oxidation
Acyl-CoA synthase (*ACSL*)	Conversion of fatty acids to fatty acyl-CoA
Adipocyte fatty acid binding protein (*FABP4*)	Intracellular fatty acid transport
Cytochrome P450 4A6 (*CYP4A6*)	Fatty acid ω-oxidation
D-Bifunctional protein (*HSD17B4*)	Peroxisomal fatty acid β-oxidation
Fatty acid synthase (*FASN*)	Synthesis of saturated fatty acids from acetyl-CoA
Glucose 6-phosphate dehydrogenase (*G6PD*)	NADPH production
Liver fatty acid binding protein (*FABP1*)	Intracellular fatty acid transport
Malic enzyme (*ME1*)	NADPH production
Medium-chain acyl-CoA dehydrogenase (*ACADM*)	Mitochondrial fatty acid β-oxidation
Stearoyl-CoA desaturase (*SCD*)	Desaturation of saturated fatty acids

RECOMMENDATIONS FOR ESSENTIAL FATTY ACID INTAKE

The Institute of Medicine (IOM) is responsible for setting Dietary Reference Intake (DRI) values for Americans and Canadians. When sufficient scientific evidence is available for a given nutrient, an Estimated Average Requirement (EAR) is set, and from it a Recommended Dietary Allowance (RDA) value is derived. According to the IOM, there

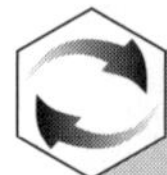

DRIs Across the Life Cycle: Polyunsaturated Fatty Acids

	n−6 PUFAs (g/day)	n−3 PUFAs (g/day)
Infants		
0 through 6 mo	4.4	0.5
7 through 12 mo	4.6	0.5
	Linoleic Acid (g/day)	**α-Linolenic Acid (g/day)**
Children		
1 through 3 yr	7	0.7
4 through 8 yr	10	0.9
Males		
9 through 13 yr	12	1.2
14 through 18 yr	16	1.6
19 through 50 yr	17	1.6
≥51 yr	14	1.6
Females		
9 through 13 yr	10	1.0
14 through 18 yr	11	1.1
19 through 50 yr	12	1.1
≥51 yr	11	1.1
Pregnant	13	1.4
Lactating	13	1.3

Data from Institute of Medicine. (2005). *Dietary Reference Intakes for energy, carbohydrate, fiber, fat, fatty acids, cholesterol, protein, and amino acids.* Washington, DC: The National Academies Press.

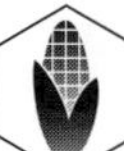

FOOD SOURCES OF ESSENTIAL FATTY ACIDS

	18:3n−3 (g)	18:2n−6 (g)
Oils		
Canola oil, 1 tbsp	1.5	3
Soybean oil, 1 tbsp	1	7
Olive oil, 1 tbsp	0.1	1
Corn oil, 1 tbsp	trace	8
Margarine, soybean oil	0.2	2
Nuts, Seeds, and Grains		
Flax seeds, 2 tbsp, ground	3	1
English walnuts, 2 tbsp	1	5
Wheat germ	0.1	1
Legumes		
Soybeans, ½ cup	0.5	4
Tofu, ½ cup	0.5	4
Rich Sources of Highly Unsaturated n−3 Fatty Acids (20:5 and 22:6)		
Cod liver oil (~21% 20:5 + 22:6)		
Salmon oil (~20% 20:5 + 22:6)		

Data from U.S. Department of Agriculture, Agricultural Research Service. (2010). *USDA National Nutrient Database for Standard Reference, Release 23.* Retrieved from www.ars.usda.gov/ba/bhnrc/ndl

is insufficient evidence to determine specific n−6 and n−3 PUFA intake levels which reduce the risk of inadequacy or chronic disease. These fatty acids, however, are recognized as essential, and deficiency disorders have been characterized. Thus Adequate Intake (AI) values have been established based on the average consumption of n−6 and n−3 PUFAs in the United States, where deficiency syndromes are virtually nonexistent.

For infants aged 0 to 6 months, AI values are based on the average total n−6 and n−3 PUFA intakes of exclusively breast-fed infants, estimated from the average concentration of these PUFAs in human milk and average milk consumption. For infants aged 7 to 12 months, AI values are based on the average intakes of total n−6 and n−3 PUFAs from both human milk and complementary foods. AI values for children, adolescents, and adults are based specifically on average linoleic and α-linolenic acid intakes. Although not considered in setting the AI values for non-infants, both EPA and DHA intakes can contribute to meeting the need for dietary n−3 fatty acids (IOM, 2005).

Upper tolerable limits were not set for essential fatty acids because of the lack of a defined level at which adverse effects can occur. Although there is some evidence suggesting that high intakes of n−3 PUFAs, particularly EPA and DHA, may impair immune response and result in prolonged bleeding times, the highest intakes of EPA and DHA reported in the United States are one fifth of the intake of Greenland Inuit and well below the daily intakes of populations (i.e., of Japan) where fish is a prominent part of the diet. The IOM did establish acceptable macronutrient distribution ranges (AMDRs) for the essential fatty acids. The AMDR for linoleic acid is 5% to 10% of energy and for α-linolenic acid is 0.6% to 1.2% of energy.

Although the IOM (2005) concluded that there is a lack of evidence to determine n−6 and n−3 PUFA intake levels that prevent chronic diseases, other bodies including the American Heart Association (AHA) and the International Society for the Study of Fatty Acids and Lipids (ISSFAL) have assembled expert panels that have established such guidelines. These guidelines are less conservative than those of the IOM, particularly in their recommended intakes of EPA and DHA for the prevention of cardiovascular disease. The AHA suggests that healthy adults consume two fish servings per week, that adults with a history of cardiovascular disease consume 1 g/day of EPA + DHA, and that those needing to lower their plasma triacylglycerol level consume 2 to 4 g/day of EPA + DHA. ISSFAL recommends that adults consume linoleic acid as 2% and α-linolenic acid as 0.7% of energy and in addition consume 500 mg of EPA + DHA per day.

ESSENTIAL FATTY ACID DEFICIENCY

An illness develops if the diet is deficient in essential fatty acids over a prolonged period. Although the dietary deficiency usually involves both classes of essential fatty acids, the n−6 PUFAs are depleted from the tissues much more rapidly than DHA. Therefore the symptoms observed when

CLINICAL CORRELATION

Triene-Tetraene Ratio in Essential Fatty Acid Deficiency

Clinicians often use the term *triene-tetraene ratio* in evaluating the essential fatty acid status of a patient. Triene and tetraene refer to the number of double bonds in polyunsaturated fatty acids. A trienoic fatty acid has three double bonds; a tetraenoic fatty acid has four. Arachidonate is the main tetraenoic fatty acid in plasma, and it normally comprises 8% to 10% of the plasma fatty acids. Because little trienoic fatty acid ordinarily is present, the triene to tetraene ratio normally is very low, about 0.1. This ratio becomes abnormally high in essential fatty acid deficiency. Because of a lack of n−6 PUFAs, the arachidonate content of the plasma decreases and is replaced by the n−9 eicosatrienoic acid (5,8,11-20:3) that is synthesized from oleic acid. This produces an increase in the triene to tetraene ratio of the plasma, and this ratio is the biomarker used to confirm the clinical diagnosis of essential fatty acid deficiency.

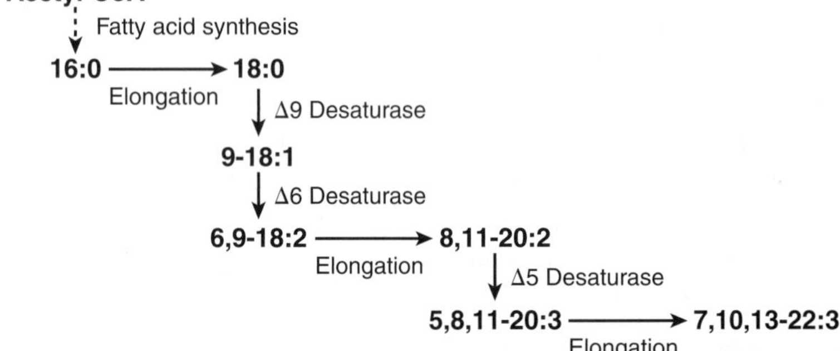

FIGURE 18-12 Pathway for the synthesis of n−9 polyunsaturated fatty acids. This enzymatic pathway can utilize fatty acids in the form of fatty acyl-CoA only. The fatty acids are abbreviated as indicated in Figure 18-2.

the disease manifests itself are likely due to a deficiency in n−6 PUFAs.

SIGNS OF n−6 POLYUNSATURATED FATTY ACID DEFICIENCY

In practical terms, essential fatty acid deficiency is caused by a dietary deficiency of linoleic acid. The diagnostic signs are dermatitis and poor wound healing. In infants and children, failure to grow is also observed in n−6 PUFA deficiency. Only a relatively small linoleic acid intake, between 3 and 5 g/day for the average adult, is sufficient to prevent this disease. Because most diets contain far more linoleic acid, often 20 g/day or more, essential fatty acid deficiency is extremely rare. It occurs primarily in patients who are not able to eat because of serious injury or major surgery and who receive total parenteral nutrition without a source of essential fatty acids for an extended period.

A biomarker that is diagnostic for essential fatty acid deficiency is a large increase in the plasma concentration of the n−9 eicosatrienoic acid (5,8,11-20:3), associated with a decrease in ARA. The pathway for the synthesis of the n−9 eicosatrienoic acid and its elongation product, 7,10,13-22:3n−9, is shown in Figure 18-12. This class of PUFAs can be completely synthesized from acetyl-CoA. Oleic acid, the most abundant monounsaturated fatty acid, is an intermediate in this pathway. The desaturation and elongation enzymes are the same as those that normally act on n−3 and n−6 PUFAs, but the fatty acid Δ6-desaturase uses appreciable quantities of oleic acid as a substrate only if there is a deficiency of linoleic acid. Therefore only very small amounts of n−9 PUFAs ordinarily are present in the plasma and tissues. The 5,8,11-20:3n−9 and 7,10,13-22:3n−9 PUFAs that are synthesized compensate to some extent by substituting for essential fatty acids in structural lipids. However, 5,8,11-20:3n−9 cannot be converted to eicosanoids, so it does not prevent the abnormalities caused by insufficient eicosanoid production. The fact that 5,8,11-20:3n−9 and 7,10,13-22:3n−9 are produced by the body as an attempt to compensate for the essential fatty acid deficiency emphasizes the importance of essential fatty acids for normal physiological function.

SIGNS OF n−3 POLYUNSATURATED FATTY ACID DEFICIENCY

Decreased visual acuity and peripheral neuropathy are the signs of an n−3 PUFA deficiency in humans. This is consistent with findings in experimental animals indicating that n−3 PUFA deficiency affects the development and function of the visual and central nervous system (Salem et al., 2001). Although it is possible that large segments of the population may be consuming less than the amount of n−3 PUFAs needed for optimal health, the frequency of an obvious n−3 PUFA deficiency disease is extremely rare for several reasons. If the diet is deficient in all essential fatty acids, the symptoms of n−6 PUFA deficiency appear first and predominate because of the longer retention of DHA in the brain and retina. In the rare case in which the dietary deficiency involves only n−3 PUFAs, some of the functional deficits are compensated by replacement with n−6 PUFAs. For example, when DHA becomes deficient, n−6 PUFAs are taken through the entire PUFA metabolic pathway shown in Figure 18-2. The n−6 analog of DHA, 22:5n−6, is produced and is incorporated into the tissue

CLINICAL CORRELATION

Oxidized Low-Density Lipoproteins and Atherosclerosis

Lipid peroxidation appears to be a key event in atherosclerosis, the disease caused by cholesterol accumulation in the arterial wall. When plasma low-density lipoproteins (LDLs) penetrate into the arterial wall, the LDLs are exposed to reactive oxygen species and undergo lipid peroxidation, forming oxidized LDL. Oxidation converts LDL into a form that can be taken up by macrophages that are attracted into the arterial wall. The cholesterol contained in the LDL cannot be degraded by the macrophages. As cholesterol builds up in the cells, it is converted to cholesteryl esters that accumulate in the macrophages as cytoplasmic lipid droplets. The lipid-filled macrophages, called foam cells, form fatty streak lesions in the arterial intima. In the process, the macrophages become activated and induce a locally damaging inflammatory reaction that eventually progresses into an atherosclerotic plaque. The plaques can increase in size and gradually obstruct the artery or they can rupture and cause thrombosis. The recognition that lipid peroxidation probably is involved in the pathogenesis of atherosclerosis suggests that antioxidants might be beneficial in preventing this disease and its most serious complications, coronary thrombosis and stroke. However, the clinical trials that have been done so far with vitamin E have been disappointing and have not demonstrated any protective effect.

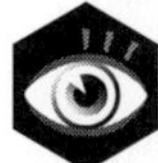

NUTRITION INSIGHT

Olive Oil in the Treatment of Hypercholesterolemia

It has been known for 50 years that replacement of dietary saturated fat with plant oils rich in linoleic acid, such as corn, sunflower seed, or safflower oil, reduces the plasma LDL-cholesterol concentration. This is considered to be a beneficial effect because LDL-cholesterol is a major risk factor for atherosclerotic cardiovascular disease. Recent studies indicate that substitution of olive oil for saturated fat produces a similar effect. Olive oil contains large amounts of oleic acid, the most abundant monounsaturated fatty acid in the plasma and tissues. Therefore it appears that the cholesterol-lowering effect of dietary fat modification results primarily from a reduction in saturated fatty acid intake rather than from any specific effect of the type of unsaturated fat that replaces it. Because of concerns about the susceptibility of LDL to lipid peroxidation and the role of oxidized LDL in atherosclerosis, there is an increasing tendency to recommend diets rich in monounsaturated fats (e.g., olive oil) rather than linoleic acid when dietary therapy is utilized in patients with hypercholesterolemia.

phospholipids that normally contain DHA. Although the structural properties of 22:5 n−6 are different from those of DHA (Eldho et al., 2003), there is enough similarity to allow the system to operate. The resulting function is not optimal, but it is sufficient to prevent a readily apparent disease phenotype.

PEROXIDATION OF POLYUNSATURATED FATTY ACIDS

Although essential fatty acids are required for normal physiological function and optimal health, they are susceptible to lipid peroxidation. This can cause tissue damage. Lipid peroxidation is a nonenzymatic process initiated when a free radical attacks the methylene carbon present between a pair of double bonds. The process is autocatalytic and is propagated by the presence of oxygen and transition metal ions such as Fe^{2+}. When a PUFA is converted to a free radical, it reacts with oxygen and attacks an adjacent PUFA. As a result, the second fatty acid also is converted to a free radical and attacks a third PUFA, and so on, continually spreading the process. Peroxidation perturbs the structural integrity of the membrane lipid bilayer. In addition, some of the radicals that are generated can attack proteins and DNA, injuring or even killing the cell. (Lipid peroxidation is discussed further in Chapter 29.)

Isoprostanes are ARA products formed by lipid peroxidation that have a prostaglandin-like structure. They are produced while the ARA is still attached to phospholipids. The isoprostane is then hydrolyzed by a phospholipase, released into the plasma, and excreted in the urine. Isoprostanes can be measured either by gas chromatography combined with mass spectrometry or by immunoassay, and they are considered to be one of the best biomarkers of in vivo oxidative stress (Montuschi et al., 2004). Similar products called neuroprostanes are formed by lipid peroxidation of DHA. This process occurs in the brain, and an increase in neuroprostanes in the cerebrospinal fluid is considered to be a biomarker of oxidative injury in the brain (Greco and Minghetti, 2004).

Tissues are protected against lipid peroxidation by antioxidants such as vitamin E and by antioxidant enzymes such as superoxide dismutase, catalase, and glutathione peroxidase. Because many tissues contain substantial quantities of essential fatty acids, it is important that they also contain an adequate supply of antioxidants as well as properly functioning antioxidant enzyme systems to protect against lipid peroxidation.

THINKING CRITICALLY

1. Linoleic acid is consumed in the diet, mainly as a component of triacylglycerols. Trace its absorption and transport through the body, its conversion to a 20-carbon PUFA, the incorporation of arachidonate into phospholipid, and the ultimate conversion of that fatty acid to TXA_2. Draw structures for some key intermediates in your scheme and note (cellular or tissue) locations when relevant.
2. What are some major differences in unsaturated fatty acid distribution between phospholipids, triacylglycerols, and cholesteryl esters found in plasma?

REFERENCES

Bannenberg, G., & Serhan, C. N. (2010). Specialized pro-resolving lipid mediators in the inflammatory response: An update. *Biochimica et Biophysica Acta, 1801*, 1260–1273.

Berge, R. K., Madsen, L., Vaagenes, H., Tronstad, K. J., Göttlicher, M., & Rustan, A. C. (1999). In contrast with docosahexaenoic acid, eicosapentaenoic acid and hypolipidaemic derivatives decrease hepatic synthesis and secretion of triacylglycerol by decreased diacylglycerol acyltransferase activity and stimulation of fatty acid oxidation. *The Biochemical Journal, 343*, 191–197.

Brenna, J. T., Salem, N., Jr., Sinclair, A. J., Cunnane, S. C., & International Society for the Study of Fatty Acids and Lipids. (2009). α-Linolenic acid supplementation and conversion to n−3 long-chain polyunsaturated fatty acids in humans. *Prostaglandins, Leukotrienes, and Essential Fatty Acids, 80*, 85–91.

Duncan, R. E., & Bazinet, R. P. (2010). Brain arachidonic acid uptake and turnover: Implications for signaling and bipolar disorder. *Current Opinion in Clinical Nutrition and Metabolic Care, 13*, 130–138.

Edelstein, C. (1986). General properties of plasma lipoproteins and apoproteins. In A. M. Scanu & A. A. Spector (Eds.), *Biochemistry and biology of the plasma lipoproteins* (pp. 495–505). New York: Marcel Dekker.

Eldho, N. V., Feller, S. E., Tristram-Nagle, S., Polozov, I. V., & Gawrisch, K. (2003). Polyunsaturated docosahexaenoic vs docosapentaenoic acid—Differences in lipid matrix properties from the loss of one double bond. *Journal of the American Chemical Society, 125*, 6409–6421.

Ferdinandusse, S., Denis, S., Mooijer, P. A. W., Zhang, Z., Reddy, J. K., Spector, A. A., & Wanders, R. J. A. (2001). Identification of the peroxisomal β-oxidation enzymes involved in the biosynthesis of docosahexaenoic acid. *Journal of Lipid Research, 42*, 1987–1995.

Gawrisch, K., Eldho, N. V., & Holte, L. L. (2003). The structure of DHA in phospholipid membranes. *Lipids, 38*, 445–452.

Greco, A., & Minghetti, L. (2004). Isoprostanes as biomarkers and mediators of oxidative injury in infant and adult central nervous system diseases. *Current Neurovascular Research, 1*, 341–354.

Grynberg, A. (2005). Hypertension prevention: From nutrients to (fortified) foods to dietary patterns. Focus on fatty acids. *Journal of Human Hypertension Suppl, 3*, S25–S33.

Innis, S. M. (2008). Dietary omega 3 fatty acids and the developing brain. *Brain Research, 1237*, 35–43.

Institute of Medicine. (2005). *Dietary Reference Intakes for energy, carbohydrate, fiber, fat, fatty acids, cholesterol, protein, and amino acids. Part 2.* Washington, DC: The National Academies Press.

Jakobsson, A., Westerberg, R., & Jacobsson, A. (2006). Fatty acid elongases in mammals: Their regulation and roles in metabolism. *Progress in Lipid Research, 45*, 237–249.

Jump, D. B. (2002). Dietary polyunsaturated fatty acids and regulation of gene transcription. *Current Opinion in Lipidology, 13*, 155–164.

Kang, J. X., Wang, J., Wu, L., & Kang, Z. B. (2004). Transgenic mice: Fat-1 mice convert n−6 to n−3 fatty acids. *Nature, 427*, 504.

Lai, L., Kang, J. X., Li, R., Wang, J., Witt, W. T., Yong, H. Y., ... Dai, Y. (2006). Generation of cloned transgenic pigs rich in omega-3 fatty acids. *Nature Biotechnology, 24*, 435–436.

Lattka, E., Illig, T., Heinrich, J., & Koletzko, B. (2010). Do FADS genotypes enhance our knowledge about fatty acid related phenotypes? *Clinical Nutrition, 29*, 277–287.

Leaf, A., Kang, J. X., Xiao, Y.-F., & Billman, G. E. (2003). Clinical prevention of sudden cardiac death by n−3 polyunsaturated fatty acids and mechanism of prevention of arrhythmias by n 3 fish oils. *Circulation, 107*, 2646–2652.

Marcheselli, V. L., Hong, S., Lukiw, W. J., Tian, X. H., Gronert, K., Musto, A., ... Bazan, N. G. (2003). Novel docosanoids inhibit brain ischemia-reperfusion-mediated leukocyte infiltration and pro-inflammatory gene expression. *The Journal of Biological Chemistry, 278*, 43807–43817.

Marquardt, A., Stor, H., White, K., & Weber, B. H. F. (2000). cDNA cloning, genomic structure, and chromosomal localization of three members of the human fatty acid desaturase family. *Genomics, 66*, 175–183.

Mata de Urquiza, M., Liu, S., Sjoberg, M., Zetterstrom, R. H., Griffiths, W., Sjovall, J., & Perlmann, T. (2000). Docosahexaenoic acid, a ligand for the retinoid X receptor in mouse brain. *Science, 290*, 2140–2144.

Mitchell, D. C., Niu, S. L., & Litman, B. J. (2003). Enhancement of G protein–coupled signaling by DHA phospholipids. *Lipids, 38*, 437–443.

Montuschi, P., Barnes, P. J., & Roberts, L. J., 2nd (2004). Isoprostanes: Markers and mediators of oxidative stress. *The FASEB Journal, 18*, 1791–1800.

Moriguchi, T., Greiner, R. S., & Salem, N., Jr. (2000). Behavioral deficits associated with dietary induction of decreased brain docosahexaenoic acid concentration. *Journal of Neurochemistry, 75*, 2563–2573.

Nagan, N., & Zoeller, R. A. (2001). Plasmalogens: Biosynthesis and functions. *Progress in Lipid Research, 40*, 199–229.

Ntambi, J. M., & Bené, H. (2001). Polyunsaturated fatty acid regulation of gene expression. *Journal of Molecular Neuroscience, 16*, 273–278.

Ramsden, C. E., Hibbeln, J. R., Majchrzak, S. F., & Davis, J. M. (2010). n−6 Fatty acid–specific and mixed polyunsaturate dietary interventions have different effects on CHD risk: A meta-analysis of randomised controlled trials. *The British Journal of Nutrition, 104*, 1586–1600.

Rao, J. S., Lee, H. J., Rapoport, S. I., & Bazinet, R. P. (2008). Mode of action of mood stabilizers: Is the arachidonic acid cascade a common target? *Molecular Psychiatry, 13*, 585–596.

Rapoport, S. I., Igarashi, M., & Gao, F. (2010). Quantitative contributions of diet and liver synthesis to docosahexaenoic acid homeostasis. *Prostaglandins, Leukotrienes, and Essential Fatty Acids, 82*, 273–276.

Salem, N., Jr., Moriguchi, T., Greiner, R. S., McBride, K., Ahmad, A., Catalan, J. N., & Slotnick, B. (2001). Alterations in brain function after loss of docosahexaenoate due to dietary restriction of n−3 fatty acids. *Journal of Molecular Neuroscience, 16*, 299–307.

Sprecher, H. (2000). Metabolism of highly unsaturated n−3 and n−6 fatty acids. *Biochimica et Biophysica Acta, 1486*, 219–231.

Williard, D. E., Nwankwo, J. O., Kaduce, T. L., Harmon, S. D., Irons, M., Moser, H. W., ... Spector, A. A. (2001). Identification of a fatty acid Δ^6-desaturase deficiency in human skin fibroblasts. *Journal of Lipid Research, 42*, 501–508.

Wood, J. T., Williams, J. S., Pandarinathan, L., Janero, D. R., Lammi-Keefe, C. J., & Makriyannis, A. (2010). Dietary docosahexaenoic acid supplementation alters select physiological endocannabinoid-system metabolites in brain and plasma. *Journal of Lipid Research, 51*, 1416–1423.

CHAPTER 19

Regulation of Fuel Utilization in Response to Food Intake

Martha H. Stipanuk, PhD

COMMON ABBREVIATIONS

AMPK	5′-AMP-activated protein kinase
cAMP	5′-cyclic AMP
CoA	coenzyme A
FoxO	forkhead box transcription factor, class O
GLUT2	glucose transporter 2
GLUT4	insulin-responsive glucose transporter 4
IGF	insulin-like growth factor
K_m	Michaelis constant
mTORC1	mammalian target of rapamycin complex 1
PKA	cAMP-activated protein kinase A
PtdIns3K	phosphatidylinositol 3-kinase
VLDL	very-low-density lipoprotein

Humans require food to maintain body tissues and health and to perform work. Food is a source of all of the nutrients, but the amount or dry weight of food that is required is largely determined by energy expenditure. The bulk of the carbohydrates, lipids, and proteins, as well as alcohol, consumed in the human diet are metabolized to provide the energy needed to support cellular and bodily functions and physical activity. Despite the need for continual metabolism of macronutrients as a source of energy, the intake of fuel from the diet is discontinuous. Vertebrates have the capacity to deal with the inevitable periods of food deprivation by storing fuel, first as glycogen and then as triacylglycerol, when food is available and then using these stored fuels during times of deprivation. To a limited extent, this same cycle functions over the feeding and fasting episodes that occur during a 24-hour period, with an important example being the use of liver glycogen stores to maintain plasma glucose levels during the overnight period.

Adults typically consume a diet of mixed foods that supplies 1,500 to 3,000 kcal per day. In the United States, approximately 15% of the energy is supplied by protein, 50% by carbohydrate, and 35% by fat, but the proportion provided by each macronutrient can vary considerably for different populations and for individuals within a population and still be adequate. The body must regulate the metabolism of the amino acids, sugars, and triacylglycerols taken up from the gastrointestinal tract during the absorptive phase to meet immediate energy needs and also to store fuel to meet energy needs during the postabsorptive period and potentially during longer periods of food deprivation. In addition, the use of some essential nutrients as fuels must be coordinately regulated with their use for other essential processes, such as the use of indispensable amino acids for protein synthesis or certain fatty acids for synthesis of membrane lipids.

In addition to the overall fuel needs of the body, the synthesis, oxidation, and storage of each of the individual macronutrients must be regulated to meet the specific needs of the various body tissues. In the context of fuel metabolism, different tissues have unique functions and metabolic pathways and also are exposed to circulating fuels in differing ways. For example, the portal blood draining the gastrointestinal tract is the major blood supply to the liver such that the glucose and amino acid supply to the liver during the absorptive period exceeds the fuel needs of the liver itself, and the liver plays a key role in modulating the mixture of circulating fuels that are supplied to the rest of the body. In addition, some tissues require specific types of fuel molecules. Red blood cells, which do not contain mitochondria, cannot obtain energy by oxidizing fatty acids, but they can generate ATP by converting glucose to lactate, which is released back into the circulation. If plasma glucose levels are not maintained, tissues dependent upon glucose as a fuel will suffer damage. Without energy, cells no longer function and eventually die, resulting in tissue injury. Lack of fuel can even result in permanent brain damage, stroke, and death. The brain is capable of using only glucose and ketone bodies as major fuels; although brain cells have mitochondria, the blood–brain barrier in key regions of the brain limits the rate of transfer of long-chain fatty acids. Thus, long-chain fatty acids are not a major fuel for the brain even when their level in the circulation is elevated (Vannucci and Hawkins, 1983). Ketone body production by the liver plays a key role in reducing brain glucose use during prolonged starvation. Thus the body must maintain a mixture of circulating fuel molecules that will meet the needs of all tissues, and this might be remarkably different from the mixture absorbed from the gastrointestinal tract following a meal or the mixture released from endogenous stores of fat and glycogen

TABLE 19-1 Tissue-Specific Metabolism

TISSUE	FUELS USED	FUELS RELEASED
Brain	Glucose Ketone bodies Lactate (when plasma concentration is elevated)	Lactate
Skeletal muscle	Glucose Free fatty acids Triacylglycerols Branched-chain amino acids Lactate	Lactate Alanine Glutamine
Heart	Free fatty acids Triacylglycerols Ketone bodies Glucose Lactate	
Liver*	Amino acids (partial oxidation) Free fatty acids Lactate Glycerol Glucose Alcohol	Glucose Ketone bodies Lactate (during absorptive phase) Triacylglycerols
Intestine†	Glucose Glutamine	Lactate Alanine
Red blood cells	Glucose	Lactate
Kidney	Glucose Free fatty acids Ketone bodies Lactate Glutamine	Glucose (renal gluconeogenesis important in prolonged starvation)
Adipose tissue	Glucose Triacylglycerols	Glycerol Free fatty acids Lactate

*The liver is also the site of galactose and fructose metabolism.
†The small intestine also releases dietary glucose, galactose, fructose, amino acids, and lipids.

during starvation. Table 19-1 summarizes the main circulating fuels that are used and released by various tissues.

Specific macronutrients may be only partially catabolized within a particular tissue, with released partially oxidized compounds consequently serving as metabolic fuels for other tissues. The production of ketone bodies produced from fatty acids by the liver, the release of branched-chain keto acids by the skeletal muscle, and the production of lactate from glucose by red blood cells are examples. At the tissue level, the definition of a fuel includes both the macromolecules absorbed from the gastrointestinal tract or released from endogenous storage reserves and some partially oxidized forms of these molecules. Thus a metabolic fuel may be defined as a circulating compound that is taken up by tissues for energy production; the major circulating fuels include glucose, triacylglycerols in lipoprotein complexes, amino acids, fatty acids, ketone bodies, lactate, and glycerol.

In this chapter, fuel utilization in the postprandial or absorptive (fed) state is compared to that in the postabsorptive (fasted) and more extreme starved state. These contrasts illustrate various regulatory processes governing macronutrient metabolism and fuel utilization. A further discussion of fuel utilization by skeletal muscle in the context of rest and exercise is the topic of Chapter 20. In preparation for describing the changes in fuel utilization that occur under these conditions, this chapter begins with a brief overview of the mechanisms used by tissues to regulate metabolism in the face of changing fuel availability or energy need.

REGULATION OF MACRONUTRIENT METABOLISM AT THE WHOLE-BODY LEVEL

Several whole-body mechanisms play an extremely important role in the regulation of fuel metabolism.

CHANGES IN NUTRIENT SUPPLY

The body must rely on food intake or its own stores for a source of glucose, fatty acids, and amino acids for use as fuels. Because food intake is not continuous but occurs as discrete meals, with varying periods between meals, the body must have mechanisms to store excess fuel for later use. Meal size and composition will influence metabolism by establishing the exogenous nutrients the body must use or store. In the absence of food intake, the body must rely on stored fuels, mainly glycogen and triacylglycerols.

Release of endocrine hormones, particularly the pancreatic hormones insulin and glucagon, responds to meal size and composition and thus plays an over-arching role in communicating the body's status with respect to influx of nutrients from the gastrointestinal tract to various tissues and in triggering metabolic remodeling of the tissue to respond appropriately to changes in nutrient supply. As discussed in Chapters 12 and 16, high insulin/low glucagon promotes lipid and carbohydrate storage, whereas low insulin/high glucagon results in stimulated adipose tissue lipolysis and hepatic glucose production. High insulin and low glucagon levels are characteristic of the postprandial state, whereas low insulin and high glucagon levels are characteristic of the fasted state.

The body has a complex system for regulation of food intake and energy expenditure that involves the central nervous system's integration of numerous signals from the gastrointestinal tract, pancreas, and adipose tissue. Output from the central nervous system stimulates changes in food intake to maintain energy balance. These include the impetus to initiate eating and also the satiety/satiation effects that promote the ending of a meal; regulation of food intake is discussed in more detail in Chapter 22.

Underlying the use of macronutrients by tissues in response to changes in nutrient availability is the metabolic flexibility of most tissues to use more than one fuel. Glucose and fatty acids are the major fuels used by tissues, and most tissues can use either glucose or fatty acids. The "glucose–fatty acid cycle," which was first proposed by Randle and associates (1963), is a helpful concept in understanding fuel flux between tissues and fuel selection by tissues. The primary tenet of the Randle cycle was that the increased provision of exogenous lipid fuels or the increased breakdown of endogenous triacylglycerol stores promotes the use of lipid fuels and, in so doing, blocks the utilization of glucose. This was based on studies with isolated heart and skeletal muscle preparations in which they found that the provision of lipid fuels (fatty acids, ketone bodies) suppressed glucose uptake and glycolysis whether or not hormones were added. Thus the glucose–fatty acid cycle drew attention to the competition between glucose and fatty acids for their oxidation in muscle. Although hormones such as insulin play important roles not only in determining nutrient availability but also in altering the metabolic capacities of tissues, Randle's observation that the utilization of one nutrient could inhibit the use of the other nutrient directly and without hormonal mediation introduced the concept of nutrient-mediated fine-tuning of fuel utilization that occurs on top of the more coarse substrate availability/hormonal effects. These observations also led to the discovery of biochemical mechanisms by which fatty acids suppressed glucose utilization and, subsequently, of mechanisms by which glucose could suppress fatty acid utilization (Hue and Taegtmeyer, 2009). Some of these mechanisms are discussed in subsequent text and in Chapters 12 and 16.

BLOOD FLOW PATTERNS

Because nutrients are carried to and from tissues via the blood, blood flow patterns and rates, as well as the form of nutrients in the blood, can affect nutrient availability. For example, the drainage of the splanchnic tissues into the portal vein, which becomes the major blood supply to the liver, exposes the liver to high concentrations of absorbed nutrients. During exercise, the increase in blood flow to the skeletal muscle results in the transport of more oxygen and blood-borne fuels to the working muscle. The transport of absorbed lipids as triacylglycerol in chylomicrons prevents the liver and other tissues from being exposed to high levels of free fatty acids during the fed state and facilitates their direction to adipose tissue for storage. Hemodynamics also affects tissue exposure to circulating hormones. For example, resting skeletal muscle is relatively insensitive to changes in circulating levels of insulin compared to working muscle.

HISTORICAL TIDBIT

The Glucose–Fatty Acid Cycle

In 1963 Philip Randle, Peter Garland, Nick Hales, and Eric Newsholme published a paper in *Lancet* in which they proposed a glucose–fatty acid cycle, which came to be commonly referred to as the "Randle cycle" (Randle et al., 1963). The primary tenet of the Randle cycle was that the increased provision of exogenous lipid fuels or the increased breakdown of endogenous triacylglycerol stores promotes the use of lipid fuels and, in so doing, blocks the utilization of glucose.

Randle and colleagues showed, in studies with isolated heart and skeletal muscle preparations, that the provision of lipid fuels (fatty acids, ketone bodies) suppressed glucose uptake and glycolysis whether or not hormones were added. Randle went on to demonstrate the role of several glycolytic enzymes in the "fine-tuning" of fuel utilization at the cellular level. In particular, Randle demonstrated the role of the products of β-oxidation in inhibition of the pyruvate dehydrogenase complex, thus blocking glucose/pyruvate oxidation when lipid fuels were being metabolized. Fatty acid or ketone body oxidation in the mitochondria results in increases in the mitochondrial ratios of acetyl-CoA/CoA and $NADH/NAD^+$, both of which strongly inhibit pyruvate dehydrogenase complex activity (Randle, 1998).

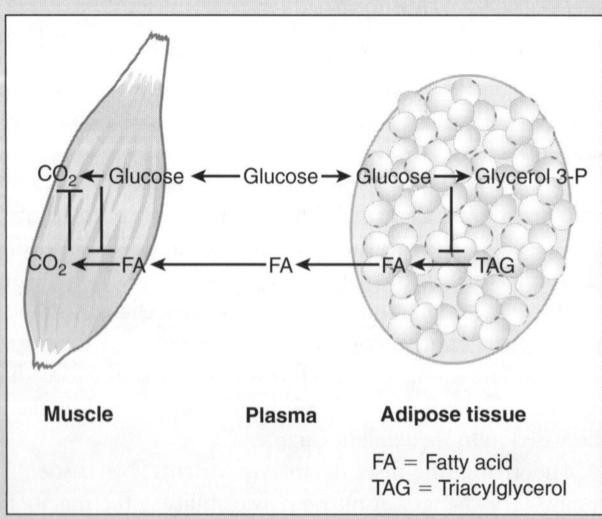

Although Randle and colleagues recognized the effects of glucose and insulin in promoting triacylglycerol storage and by blocking lipolysis and β-oxidation of fatty acids, it was more than a decade before a cellular mechanism for the reciprocal process by which glucose oxidation can block utilization of fatty acids as fuel was elucidated (McGarry et al., 1977). This mechanism involves the formation of malonyl-CoA by acetyl-CoA carboxylase when glucose is available as a fuel and the consequent inhibition of carnitine palmitoyltransferase 1 by malonyl-CoA (McGarry, 1998). In addition, metabolism of glucose by adipose tissue fosters the storage of fatty acids by providing glycerol 3-phosphate for triacylglycerol synthesis.

Today we know that the regulation of fuel utilization is complex and occurs at many levels in addition to the short-term regulation of pyruvate dehydrogenase and acetyl-CoA carboxylase (Hue and Taegtmeyer, 2009). Nevertheless, the fundamental concept of cellular coordination of metabolic fuel selection developed by Randle and colleagues made a large contribution to our current understanding of fuel utilization by various tissues.

DISTRIBUTED CONTROL

Consideration of the many factors that influence fuel utilization has led to the understanding that metabolic regulation of fuel utilization is under "distributed control" by several different processes, and that the steps that limit fuel utilization vary in response to physiological and biochemical changes. Both whole-body and cell-specific processes are involved. An excellent example of distributed control is provided by the work of Wasserman and colleagues on the regulation of glucose flux into muscle in vivo (Wasserman et al., 2011). Muscle glucose uptake is regulated by control of glucose delivery to muscle, control of membrane transport into muscle, and control of the phosphorylation of glucose within muscle. Glucose transport into muscle is regulated by translocation of the insulin-responsive glucose transporter GLUT4 to the plasma membrane. In the fasted state GLUT4 limits glucose uptake, but in the insulin-stimulated or fed state the upregulated GLUT4 glucose uptake is such that other factors become more limiting. Carbohydrate intake and hepatic glucose production are important factors affecting glucose concentrations and hence muscle glucose delivery. Glucose is phosphorylated by hexokinase, which traps glucose in the myocyte. If glucose 6-phosphate accumulates, this feedback inhibits hexokinase and slows glucose uptake and utilization. Pathways downstream of glucose phosphorylation (i.e., glycogen synthesis and glycolysis) can play a role in control of glucose uptake through their effects on glucose 6-phosphate levels.

REGULATION OF MACRONUTRIENT METABOLISM AT THE CELLULAR LEVEL

Fuel metabolism occurs at the level of individual cells in various tissues. Different tissues and even various types of cells within tissues are differentiated to serve their particular functions, and this is associated with the expression, or lack of expression, of genes encoding enzymes of different pathways, receptors for various hormones, transporters for particular substrates, particular transcription factors, and other proteins. Most tissues have some flexibility to adapt to using either glucose or fatty acids as the major fuel, and both rapid and longer-term metabolic remodeling occurs within tissues to respond to short-term changes in food intake and to longer-term dietary changes, respectively.

BIOCHEMICAL MECHANISMS OF REGULATION OF METABOLIC PATHWAYS

In describing metabolism, we often look at particular pathways as going from beginning substrate(s) through various steps to end product(s) of the pathway. Many reactions in pathways, however, are reversible and function at near equilibrium, and many intermediates or substrates are shared by various pathways and essentially link the pathways to each other. Intermediates may enter or leave pathways at any of the sequential steps. For example, oxaloacetate might be seen as a citric acid cycle intermediate that does not leave the cycle, but it also is used as a substrate for gluconeogenesis, as a partner with malate for movement of reducing equivalents out of the mitochondria, and as a precursor of aspartate by transamination. It can also be synthesized by transamination of aspartate, dehydrogenation of malate generated in the cytosol, or carboxylation of pyruvate.

Because tissues with different capabilities work together to maintain various bodily functions, it is difficult to view fuel metabolism as occurring simply within individual cells or individual tissues. For example, even the simple pathway of glycolysis in red blood cells, which appears to begin with glucose and end with lactate, actually requires the continual provision (from the intestine or liver) of glucose into the plasma and the continual removal of the lactate by the liver. Thus the utilization of glucose by red blood cells is directly linked to the control of such processes as hepatic glycogen metabolism and gluconeogenesis. The glucose–alanine cycle similarly functions to recover the carbon skeleton (pyruvate) of alanine for gluconeogenesis, recycling the glucose carbon back to muscle or other tissues. As an additional example, during prolonged starvation, the upregulation of lipolysis in adipose tissue is accompanied by increased synthesis of ketone bodies from these fatty acids by the liver and consequently increased uptake and oxidation of ketone bodies by the muscle and brain. Thus metabolic remodeling in one tissue needs to be coordinated with metabolic changes in other tissues.

Regulation of Flux through a Metabolic Pathway

The regulation of flux through a pathway is usually regulated by multiple factors, and each of those factors may in turn be regulated by multiple factors. The ultimate flux through a particular pathway under a given circumstance in the cell reflects the integrated regulation of many different steps in the pathway, with each catalyzed by a different protein, perhaps with each protein being regulated by multiple mechanisms. Flux also depends upon regulation of the uptake of substrates and the removal of intermediates or products. In most cases of macronutrient metabolism, cells have opposing pathways, as, for example, glycogenesis and glycogenolysis or glycolysis and gluconeogenesis. In general, both pathways are operating all the time and the ability to upregulate one while downregulating the other allows the cell to fine-tune the overall metabolic flux to the needs of the body. Such reciprocal and coordinated regulation is common in macronutrient metabolism. The coordinated regulation of opposing pathways is further facilitated by spatial segregation of some opposing pathways in different tissues (e.g., ketone body synthesis in liver and ketone body oxidation in extrahepatic tissues) or in different subcellular compartments (e.g., cholesterol synthesis from acetyl-CoA in the cytosol and ketone body synthesis from acetyl-CoA in the mitochondria; de novo synthesis of fatty acids in the cytosol and β-oxidation of fatty acids in the mitochondria).

Although regulation of metabolism generally involves many types of regulation at many different steps in a pathway and related pathways and processes, some changes have large effects on flux through a pathway, while other changes have little or no effect. Obviously, those that result in changes in flux are more significant physiologically, but it is not always easy to discern the consequence of an individual change in the context of the whole body. One example of a highly regulated enzyme with substantial physiological consequences for cholesterol synthesis is 3-hydroxy-3-methylglutaryl-CoA (HMG-CoA) reductase (Goldstein et al., 2006). This is an early step in the overall cholesterol synthetic pathway that is highly regulated and can exhibit a many-fold change in activity. HMG-CoA reductase is the target of the statin drugs used to treat patients with hypercholesterolemia.

Short-Term and Long-Term Regulation

In describing the regulation of the cellular capacity to perform various enzymatic reactions or other processes, we often speak of short-term and long-term regulation. As their names imply, they may be distinguished by the length of time required for bringing about changes, but this distinction does not apply absolutely. In reality, these two terms refer to two distinct mechanisms of regulation. *Short-term control* refers to changes in the specific activity of an enzyme (or transporter, transcription factor, etc.), with no change in its concentration. *Long-term control* refers to changes in the amount of enzyme (or transporter, transcription factor, etc.), with no change in its kinetic properties. The two mechanisms are not exclusive, and some proteins are subject to both short-term and long-term control in response to the same stimulus or different stimuli. In some cases, a long-term response can occur as rapidly as a short-term response; control of protein concentration is highly dependent on the half-life of the protein and new steady state concentrations are reached quickly for proteins with very short half-lives (see Chapter 13). Regardless of whether they are short-term or long-term, regulatory mechanisms must be reversible if they are to be of physiological importance. In other words, the concentration or the activity state of the protein must be able to be both upregulated and downregulated.

SHORT-TERM CONTROL OF METABOLISM

Short-term control can be brought about by a variety of mechanisms. Many specific examples are given in Chapters 12, 14, 16, and 17.

Changes in Levels of Key Metabolites or Regulators

Changes in fuel availability may bring about changes in flux through metabolic pathways. Either an altered concentration of a substrate or an altered concentration of a metabolite in the pathway can result in a change in the concentration of allosteric effectors. Short-term regulation is often related to small changes in the levels of key intermediates such as ATP and NADH. This may result simply from changes in cosubstrate or coenzyme supply. For example, a change in NADH concentration will usually be mirrored by an opposite change in NAD^+, and a change in acyl-CoA concentration likewise will result in an opposite change in the free coenzyme A (CoA) concentration. Any change in these ratios will affect flux through enzymatic reactions utilizing one of these couplets. Both allosteric activation and inhibition are also important short-term mechanisms that involve the binding of a regulatory molecule to a distinct site on an enzyme. Several examples of short-term control can be seen in the pathway for glycolysis. For example, ATP is a strong inhibitor of 6-phosphofructo-1-kinase, and this inhibition can be relieved by a second allosteric factor, such as fructose 2,6-bisphosphate in liver or AMP in muscle (see Chapter 12, Figure 12-8). Hexokinase is inhibited by glucose 6-phosphate, restricting uptake of glucose in tissues that do not express the glucokinase isoform, which is insensitive to the inhibitory effects of glucose 6-phosphate. Hepatic pyruvate kinase is stimulated by fructose 1,6-bisphosphate, which is elevated when glucose is being metabolized, and inhibited by alanine, which is an important gluconeogenic substrate during starvation (see Chapter 12, Figure 12-8). In addition, hepatic pyruvate kinase is subject to covalent modification (phosphorylation) by 5′-cyclic adenosine monophosphate (cAMP)-dependent protein kinase A (PKA); this makes it more sensitive to allosteric inhibition. The inhibition of mitochondrial uptake of long-chain fatty acids by the effects of malonyl CoA on the carnitine palmitoyltransferase 1 (CPT1) is another example of regulation by allosteric effects of small molecules; in this case a substrate or intermediate in a competing pathway, fatty acid synthesis, acts to inhibit the opposing pathway, fatty acid oxidation.

Reversible Covalent Modification of Proteins

Reversible covalent modification of proteins is another important short-term regulatory mechanism. A common type of regulatory modification is phosphorylation–dephosphorylation, catalyzed by kinases and phosphatases. Phosphorylation of proteins usually occurs on particular serine, threonine, or tyrosine residues of the proteins, resulting in activation of some proteins and in inhibition of others. Phosphorylation may affect the target protein by changing its kinetic properties, its ability to associate with other proteins, its sensitivity to allosteric effectors, or its intracellular localization. Important examples of enzymes that are controlled by phosphorylation–dephosphorylation include hormone-sensitive lipase in adipose tissue, which is activated by phosphorylation in response to catecholamines and inactivated by dephosphorylation in response to insulin (see Chapter 16, Figure 16-9); acetyl-CoA carboxylase in liver, which is activated by dephosphorylation in response to insulin, so that cytosolic acetyl-CoA is converted to malonyl-CoA (see Chapter 16, Figure 16-3); glycogen synthase, which is inactivated by phosphorylation in response to glucagon in liver (see Chapter 12, Figure 12-15); and 6-phosphofructo-2-kinase, a bifunctional enzyme that loses kinase activity while its fructose 2,6-bisphosphatase activity is enhanced in response to glucagon in liver (see Chapter 12, Figure 12-10).

Another very important phosphorylation is that of the pyruvate dehydrogenase complex, which is inactivated by phosphorylation catalyzed by a specific kinase bound to the enzyme complex. Phosphorylation (inactivation) of the pyruvate dehydrogenase complex is stimulated by acetyl-CoA and NADH and inhibited by high CoA, NAD^+, or pyruvate (see Chapter 12, Figure 12-18). These effectors influence the activity of the pyruvate dehydrogenase kinase that catalyzes the covalent modification and inactivation of the pyruvate dehydrogenase complex. The tissue-specific expression of different isoforms of pyruvate dehydrogenase kinase and phosphatase allows different tissues to respond differently in terms of pyruvate dehydrogenase complex inactivation during starvation (Sugden and Holness, 2006; Harris et al., 2002).

Thus the oxidative decarboxylation of pyruvate to acetyl-CoA is inhibited when the cell is oxidizing fatty acids or ketone bodies as fuel, playing a significant role in the suppression of glucose oxidation when fatty acids are available as a fuel (i.e., the Randle or glucose-fatty acid cycle). The mitochondrial β-oxidation of these lipid fuels generates high acetyl-CoA and NADH levels during starvation, and this is a condition in which glucose carbon needs to be conserved. In the presence of high acetyl-CoA and NADH and in the absence of insulin or excess pyruvate, the pyruvate dehydrogenase kinase will be activated and its phosphorylation of the pyruvate dehydrogenase complex will cause the complex to be inactivated. Inactivation of the pyruvate dehydrogenase complex blocks conversion of pyruvate to acetyl-CoA, thus conserving the pyruvate carbon and reducing net glucose oxidation. On the other hand, in the fed state when glucose is available as a fuel, the sensitivity of pyruvate dehydrogenase kinases to pyruvate allows regulation of the pyruvate dehydrogenase complex in response to glucose and insulin availability. When the cell is exposed to a high level of glucose, the kinase is inhibited by pyruvate and, in addition, the dephosphorylation of pyruvate dehydrogenase complex by its phosphatase is stimulated by insulin. Hence the pyruvate dehydrogenase is in its active, dephosphorylated form. This allows conversion of pyruvate to acetyl-CoA and its entrance into the citric acid cycle for oxidative metabolism as a fuel. In the liver, a lipogenic tissue, the higher activity of the pyruvate dehydrogenase complex in the fed state allows more entrance of acetyl-CoA into the citric acid cycle, with the accumulation of citrate and its ultimate use for de novo lipogenesis.

Changes in Intracellular Localization of Proteins

A somewhat different form of short-term control is the physical movement of proteins within a cell. Sequestering a protein in a subcellular compartment, which is often facilitated by other proteins that associate with the regulated protein, can remove it from the spatial location where it carries out its function. In contrast, processes that facilitate the movement of a protein to the location where it carries out its function (e.g., the movement of a transcription factor to the nucleus or a transporter to the plasma membrane) will upregulate its physiological effect. A well-known example of this is the sequestering of GLUT4 glucose transporters in intracellular vesicles until insulin activates the movement of these insulin-sensitive glucose transporters to the cell surface of myocytes and adipocytes. The increase in GLUT4 transporters in the plasma membrane increases the glucose transport capacity of these cells and can result in increased uptake and utilization of glucose by the tissue. Sometimes a combination of methods of short-term regulation are involved as, for example, in the phosphorylation of forkhead box class O (FoxO) transcription factors by Akt, which results in exclusion of FoxO from the nucleus where it would act as a transcriptional activator. Another example is the movement and activation of glucokinase and glycogen synthase within the liver in response to hormones, a process that results in these proteins becoming physically close to or removed from their substrates (Watford, 2002). In the postabsorptive state glucokinase is present within the nucleus where it is bound by a glucokinase regulatory protein together with fructose 6-phosphate. During the absorptive period in the presence of fructose 1-phosphate or high glucose, glucokinase is released from the regulatory protein and translocates to the cytosol where it is active in hepatic glucose uptake and metabolism (see Chapter 12, Figure 12-9).

LONG-TERM CONTROL OF METABOLISM

Changes in protein expression are important in the metabolic remodeling of tissues, allowing the body to adapt to sustained changes in nutrient availability or physiological state. Long-term changes can alter the overall capacity of the metabolic system to respond to change and may improve or diminish the short-term regulatory response to subsequent physiological stressors.

Changes in the amount of protein (long-term control) are brought about by changes in the synthesis and/or degradation of the protein and consequently are rather slow, often taking hours or days to occur. However, some enzymes can show these long-term changes within relatively short time-periods (less than 1 hour), which can be comparable to the timescale over which some short-term covalent modifications take place. The steady state concentrations of proteins are functions of the rates of their synthesis and degradation. Different proteins exhibit half-lives that range from a few minutes to many days. Proteins with very short half-lives not only will be degraded rapidly but also will respond rapidly to changes in the synthesis or degradation rate. Thus enzymes with short half-lives are able to establish new steady state concentrations much more quickly than proteins with long half-lives. Such proteins are ideal candidates for regulation.

In recent decades, much emphasis has been given to predicting changes in metabolism from changes in the abundance of messenger RNA (mRNA) transcripts of genes. Regulation of levels of functional proteins, however, is a much more complex process. The synthesis of a protein depends upon gene transcription, mRNA processing, mRNA stability and/or localization, and mRNA translation. Furthermore, the function or activity of a translated protein depends upon proper posttranslational modifications, folding, and trafficking to its correct location, as well as its subsequent regulation by covalent modification, allosteric effectors, or other mechanisms. The concentration of the protein also depends on the rate of degradation of the protein. Protein degradation is regulated, and most cellular proteins are degraded in a regulated manner by the ubiquitin–proteasome system. Damage to cellular proteins, such as cross-linking or oxidation of functional groups, also may affect their functions and their degradation rates.

An example of a highly regulated key enzyme of hepatic glucose metabolism is phosphoenolpyruvate carboxykinase (PEPCK). This protein has a half-life of about 6 hours and is regulated exclusively by long-term mechanisms. Most of this regulation is brought about by changes in the rate of transcription of the PEPCK gene and hence changes in the overall level of enzyme protein (see Chapter 12, Figure 12-8). The fall in circulating insulin during starvation allows the FoxO transcription factors to enter the nucleus and activate transcription of the PEPCK gene. In addition, the rise in circulating glucagon during starvation acts via cAMP to stimulate transcription of the PEPCK gene. Thus, as starvation slowly develops and as liver glycogen stores are gradually depleted, the liver is synthesizing new PEPCK and thereby increasing its capacity to carry out gluconeogenesis. Such a mechanism is highly suited to a situation such as starvation in which changes in metabolism occur over hours or days. On the other hand, this mechanism would not be suitable for rapid responses such as those needed for muscle contraction, during which short-term regulatory mechanisms are necessary to allow for compensatory responses within fractions of a second.

Long-term changes can improve or diminish short-term regulatory responses to subsequent physiological stressors. An example of how long-term adaptation can affect short-term fuel availability is illustrated by a study in which aerobically trained men were adapted to a 75% fat/5% carbohydrate diet or to a 30% fat/50% carbohydrate control diet (Pehleman et al., 2005). Adaptation to the high-fat/low-carbohydrate diet increased muscle pyruvate dehydrogenase kinase activity, which decreased pyruvate dehydrogenase activation to the "a" form, and decreased the oxidative disposal of glucose by skeletal muscle. Subsequent administration of an oral glucose load to these men resulted in decreases in pyruvate kinase activity and increases in pyruvate dehydrogenase activity, in both subjects fed the control diet and in subjects fed the high-fat/low-carbohydrate diet. However, the absolute level of pyruvate dehydrogenase "a" remained lower in men adapted to the control diet.

MANY PROTEINS ARE REGULATED BY MULTIPLE MECHANISMS

A number of key proteins/enzymes are regulated by many different mechanisms, each having a contribution to the fine-tuning of the protein's concentration, activity, or both. For example, acetyl-CoA carboxylase, which catalyzes the carboxylation of acetyl-CoA to malonyl-CoA, is regulated by changes in gene transcription, with enzyme concentration being increased in fed animals due to the influence of insulin and/or glucose on the activity of transcription factors such as sterol response element binding protein 1c (SREBP1c) and carbohydrate response element binding protein (ChREBP). Acetyl-CoA carboxylase is also regulated by phosphorylation/dephosphorylation, being

CLINICAL CORRELATION

PPARs as Therapeutic Drug Targets: Fibrates and Thiazolidinediones

Certain lipids exert transcriptional effects through binding to peroxisome proliferator–activated receptors (PPARs). The PPARs are nuclear receptors (ligand-activated transcription factors) that contribute to the regulation of energy homeostasis via their long-term transcriptional effects. The first PPAR was first discovered during the search for the molecular target of agents that increased peroxisomal numbers in rodent liver. The three members of this family are PPARα, PPARγ, and PPARδ (also known as PPARβ). Through their distinct but overlapping functions and tissue distributions, they mediate some of the long-term adaptations of the glucose–fatty acid cycle. The physiological ligands for the PPARs have been elusive. Polyunsaturated fatty acids (n–3 and n–6) and their eicosanoid oxidation products can act as ligands for PPARs. Recent work identified 1-palmitoyl-2-oleoyl-*sn*-glycerol-3-phosphocholine (a phospholipid) as a physiologically relevant ligand for PPARα (Chakravarthy et al., 2009). Because of their effects on lipid storage, lipid oxidation, and prevention of oxidative stress, the PPARs have been of interest as therapeutic targets (Wang, 2010).

PPARα is the target of the hypolipidemic fibrate drugs that induce transcription of genes involved in fatty acid uptake and mitochondrial and peroxisomal β-oxidation of fatty acids, particularly in liver, kidney, heart, and skeletal muscle. Studies in mice have shown that PPARα is induced by fasting and is required for hepatic ketogenesis (Kersten et al., 1999). This action probably requires peroxisome proliferator-activated receptor gamma coactivator 1 (PGC1α) as a coactivator. Fibrates, acting as PPARα agonists, also inhibit the hepatic synthesis of triacylglycerols and VLDL, increase expression of lipoprotein lipase, and decrease expression of apolipoprotein A-I, all of which contribute to a reduction in plasma triacylglycerol levels. By increasing expression of other proteins such as apolipoprotein A-I, fibrates also favor a rise in HDL concentrations and reverse cholesterol transport.

PPARγ is the target of thiazolidinediones (TDZs), drugs used for management of type 2 diabetes. PPARγ is expressed mainly in adipose tissue and is necessary for adipocyte differentiation. TDZs improve insulin sensitivity of obese type 2 diabetic patients in parallel with changes in fat metabolism. It is thought that TDZs cause expansion of the subcutaneous adipose tissue, allowing lipid repartitioning from the skeletal muscle and liver to adipose tissue, thus eliminating the deleterious effects of lipid on insulin signaling and glucose metabolism. TDZs may also act by influencing adipokine secretion.

phosphorylated and converted to a less active form by AMP-activated protein kinase (AMPK). In addition, acetyl-CoA carboxylase is regulated by allosteric effectors. The activity of acetyl-CoA carboxylase is increased by citrate, the cytosolic source of acetyl-CoA substrate that is present when glucose is abundant, and decreased by long-chain fatty acyl-CoAs, which are elevated during active lipolysis and β-oxidation when production of malonyl-CoA and palmitate from glucose would be undesirable. The presence of two genes encoding acetyl-CoA carboxylase 1 and 2 allow tissue-specific regulation of their expression. The first form is predominantly expressed in lipogenic tissues and is cytosolic. The second form is expressed in heart, skeletal muscle, and liver and has a unique N-terminal sequence that targets acetyl-CoA carboxylase 2 for insertion in the mitochondrial membrane. Its location near CTP1 facilitates its role in regulation of fatty acid transport into mitochondria for β-oxidation. Thus in liver of subjects consuming a high-carbohydrate diet, acetyl-CoA carboxylase 1 concentration would be high, and the enzyme would be active due to lack of phosphorylation by AMPK, to allosteric inactivation by citrate, and to lack of inactivation by long-chain acyl-CoAs.

INTEGRATIVE PATHWAYS FOR REGULATION OF MACRONUTRIENT METABOLISM AT THE CELLULAR LEVEL

Over the past decade our understanding of how metabolism is regulated at the cellular level has greatly increased. In particular, several integrative pathways have been elucidated that serve to integrate various signals and outputs. The AMP-activated protein kinase senses fuel (ATP) depletion and phosphorylates many downstream targets to correct the ATP deficit. The mammalian target of rapamycin (mTOR) pathway is involved in regulating protein synthesis, autophagy, and growth. This pathway integrates insulin and growth factor signaling, sensing of the fuel supply, and sensing of amino acid substrate availability to ensure that all of these are present before protein synthesis and growth are positively regulated by mTOR.

ROLE OF AMP-ACTIVATED PROTEIN KINASE IN THE REGULATION OF CELLULAR ATP LEVELS

Each cell must regulate its rate of ATP production (ADP phosphorylation) versus ATP consumption (ATP hydrolysis to ADP) and maintain ATP and ADP levels within a limited range. A drop in ATP serves as a signal that the cell needs to diminish its consumption of ATP and increase its production of ATP. When ADP begins to accumulate, adenylate kinase stimulates the conversion of 2 ADP to ATP + AMP. In the case of a cellular energy deficit, the ratio of AMP to ATP changes more dramatically than does the ratio of ATP to ADP, and thus the ratio of AMP to ATP is a useful indicator of the cell's energy status.

$$\text{ATP} \rightarrow \text{ADP} + \text{P}_i$$

$$2\ \text{ADP} \rightarrow \text{ATP} + \text{AMP}$$

A protein kinase that responds to changes in AMP levels is an important regulator of ATP levels at the cellular level. This kinase is called 5′-AMP-activated protein kinase, usually referred to as AMPK, or somewhat inappropriately as "AMP kinase." As shown in Figure 19-1, AMPK is phosphorylated by various upstream kinases (AMPKKs such as LKB1 and calmodulin-dependent protein kinase kinase β) and dephosphorylated by a phosphatase. The AMPKKs specifically phosphorylate residue Thr172 of the α-subunit of AMPK. When the energy status of the cell is low, as indicated by a high AMP/ATP ratio, AMPK is in its active phosphorylated state. Phosphorylation of AMPK may be regulated both by activation of an upstream AMPKK, although some of these are thought to be constitutively active, and by the allosteric regulation of the phosphorylation state of AMPK by AMP (Witczak et al., 2008; Carling et al., 2011). The allosteric regulation of AMPK by AMP involves the binding of AMP to the γ-subunit of AMPK; this appears to make AMPK a better substrate for the upstream kinases and a poorer substrate for the phosphatase. Binding of AMP at another site may also activate AMPK directly.

AMPK is activated by metabolic stresses, such as a decrease in glucose, oxygen deprivation, or an increase in energy demand (e.g., muscle exercise), that increase the AMP/ATP ratio. Once activated, AMPK acts on a number of downstream substrates to stimulate processes that lead to increased ATP production and to inhibit processes that lead to increased ATP consumption (Viollet et al., 2006; Hardie, 2008; Steinberg and Kemp, 2009). The net effect is a return of ATP, ADP, and AMP levels to the normal range. Many proteins involved in macronutrient metabolism have been shown to be downstream targets of AMPK. The downstream effects of AMPK activation include activation of the NPY/AgRP hypothalamic neurons, leading to increased food intake and decreased peripheral energy expenditure; inhibition of Rab GTPase-activating proteins, thereby permitting GLUT4 translocation to increase glucose uptake in muscle; activation of the heart isoform of 6-phosphofructo-2-kinase (6PF2K), increasing glycolysis; enhanced secretion of lipoprotein lipase (LPL) and enhanced translocation of CD36 fatty acid transporter to plasma membrane, which increase fatty acid uptake by muscle; and inhibition of acetyl-CoA carboxylase 2 (ACC2) to prevent malonyl-CoA formation, which would block transport of fatty acids into the mitochondria. All of these events serve to increase catabolic processes that generate ATP. In addition, a number of anabolic processes that would consume ATP are suppressed. Acetyl-CoA carboxylase 1 (ACC1) is inhibited in liver, leading to decreased hepatic fatty acid, triacylglycerol and VLDL synthesis. SREBP1c and hepatic nuclear factor 4 (HNF4) transcription factors are inhibited, which prevents their activation of lipogenic gene transcription. Cytosolic HMG-CoA reductase is inhibited, resulting in decreased cholesterol/isoprenoid synthesis. Glycogen synthase (GS) is inhibited, limiting the storage of glucose as glycogen. cAMP response element binding protein (CREB) regulated transcription coactivator 2 (CRTC2) is inhibited, which in turn inhibits cAMP response element (CRE)-mediated transcription

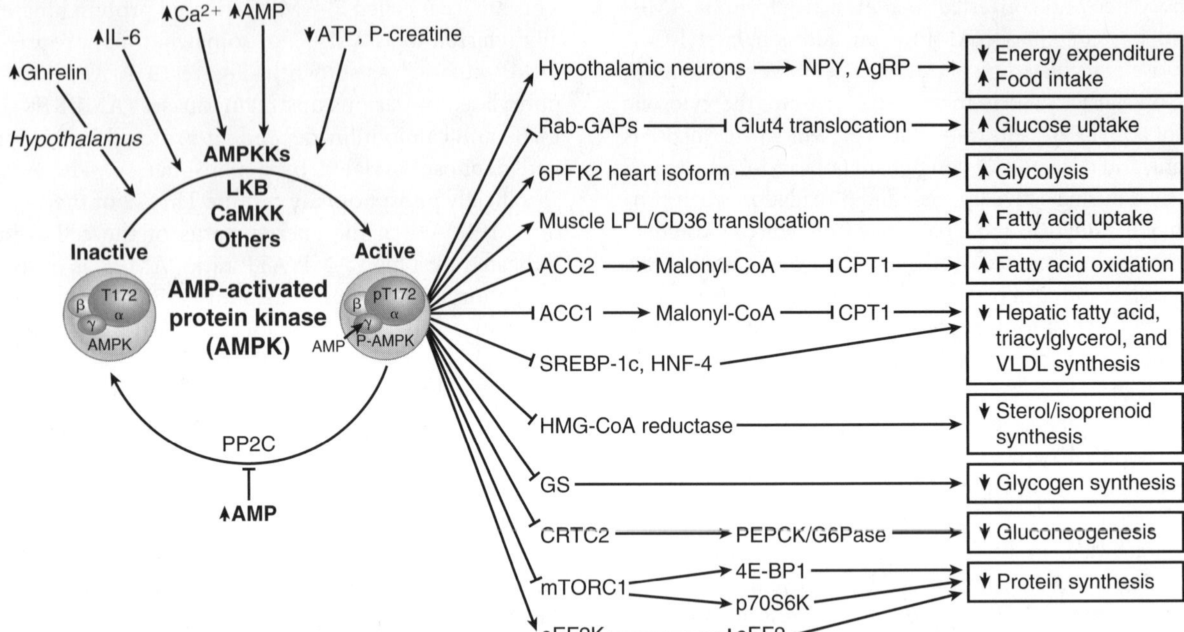

FIGURE 19-1 Role of AMP-activated protein kinase (AMPK) in the regulation of cellular ATP levels. AMP-activated protein kinase (*AMPK*) is phosphorylated by various kinases (*AMPKK*) and dephosphorylated by a phosphatase (*PP2C*) that is inhibited by AMP. When energy status of the cell is low, as indicated by a high AMP/ATP ratio, AMPK is in its active state (phosphorylated at Thr172). AMPK acts on a number of downstream substrates to stimulate processes that lead to increased ATP production and to inhibit processes that lead to increased ATP consumption. The net effect is a return of ATP and AMP levels to the normal range. Specific examples of AMPK targets are shown with —| = inhibition/deactivation and ⟶ = stimulation/activation. The direction of the arrows inside of boxes indicates the final effect on the pathway or process listed in the box. Examples include the activation of NPY/AgRP hypothalamic neurons, leading to increased food intake and decreased peripheral energy expenditure; inhibition of Rab GTPase-activating proteins (i.e., Akt substrate 160), thereby permitting GLUT4 translocation to increase glucose uptake in muscle; activation of the heart isoform of 6-phosphofructo-2-kinase (6PF2K), increasing glycolysis; enhanced secretion of lipoprotein lipase (*LPL*) and enhanced translocation of CD36 fatty acid transporter to plasma membrane, which increases fatty acid uptake by muscle; inhibition of acetyl-CoA carboxylase (*ACC2*) to prevent malonyl-CoA formation which would block transport of fatty acids into the mitochondria. Other examples include the inhibition of ACC1 in liver, leading to decreased hepatic fatty acid, triacylglycerol and VLDL synthesis; inhibition of SREBP1c and HNF4 transcription factors, which prevents their activation of lipogenic gene transcription; inhibition of cytosolic HMG-CoA reductase, resulting in decreased cholesterol/isoprenoid synthesis; inhibition of glycogen synthase (*GS*), limiting the storage of glucose as glycogen; inhibition of cAMP element binding protein (*CREB*) regulated transcription coactivator 2 (*CRTC2*) which in turn inhibits cAMP response element (*CRE*)-mediated transcription of gluconeogenic genes; stimulatory phosphorylation of tuberous sclerosis complex 2 (*TSC2*) or inhibitory phosphorylation of the mammalian target of rapamycin complex 1 (*mTORC1*), either of which will inhibit mTORC1 activity and lead to inhibition of protein synthesis and activation of autophagy (not shown); and activation of eukaryotic elongation factor 2 kinase (*eEF2K*) which will lead to inhibition of eEF2 required for protein synthesis.

of gluconeogenic genes. Stimulatory phosphorylation of tuberous sclerosis complex 2 (TSC2) or inhibitory phosphorylation of the mTOR complex 1 (mTORC1) leads to inhibition of mTORC1 serine-threonine kinase activity and thus leads to inhibition of protein synthesis and activation of autophagy. AMPK-mediated activating phosphorylation of eukaryotic elongation factor 2 kinase (eEF2K) leads to phosphorylation and inhibition of eEF2, which in turn inhibits protein synthesis. Thus the catabolism of fuels is stimulated while the synthesis and storage of fuels and proteins is inhibited whenever the cell needs to increase its ATP to ADP ratio, ensuring that the cell has energy for its essential maintenance functions, even if it must delay growth or deplete energy reserves. When cellular ATP levels are low due to lack of substrate or oxygen, AMPK activation can turn on utilization of all available fuels (i.e., glucose, fatty acids, and amino acids at the same time) in order to maintain ATP concentrations and cell survival.

THE ROLE OF mTORC1 IN INTEGRATING SIGNALS FROM INSULIN, IGF, AMINO ACIDS, AND ENERGY STATUS OF THE CELL

The mTORC1 is regulated by growth factor signaling and by nutrients. As summarized in Figure 19-2, insulin, insulin-like growth factor (IGF), and amino acids, especially leucine, promote activation of mTORC1 (Laplante and Sabatini, 2009; Dowling et al., 2010). On the other hand, a lack of fuel (high AMP/low ATP) or hypoxia (low oxygen) leads to mTORC1 inhibition, with the effects of high AMP being mediated by AMPK. The integration of these various signaling pathways at the level of mTORC1 ensures that the mTORC1 kinase can be inhibited if any

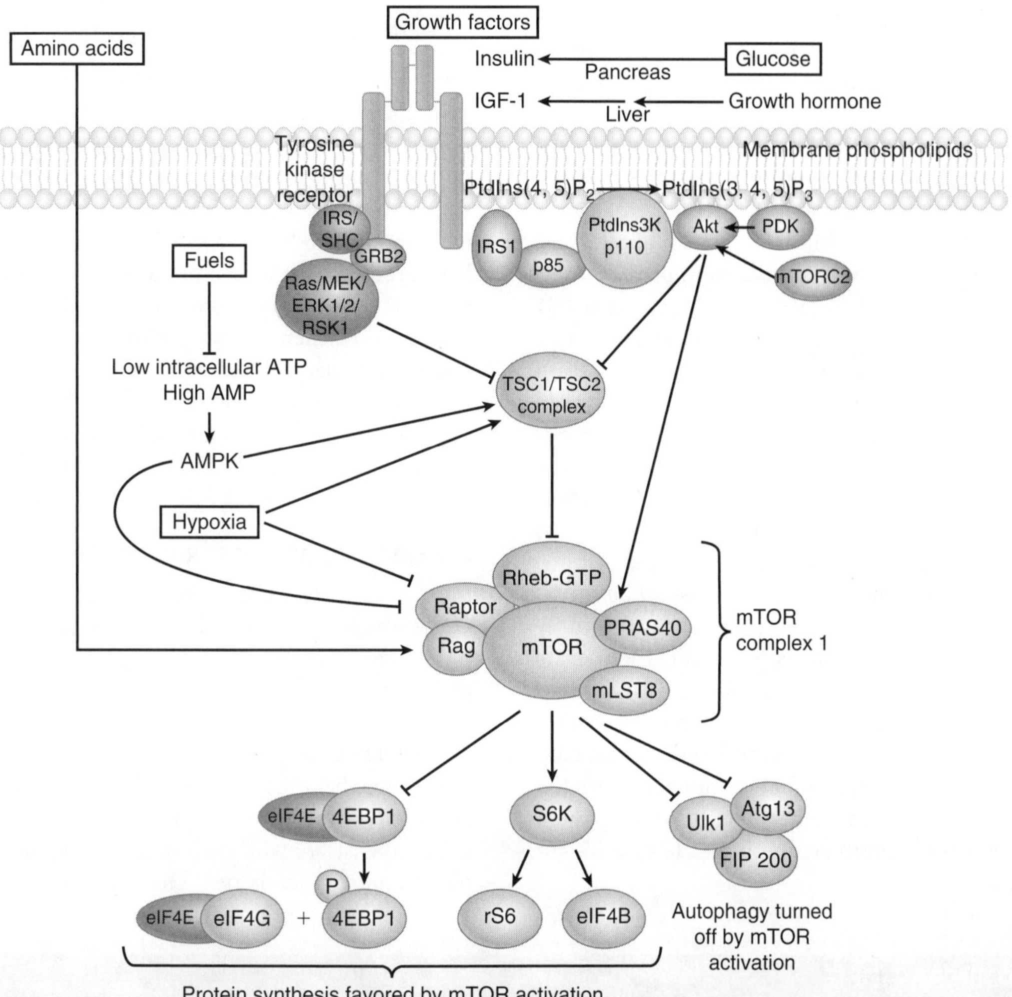

FIGURE 19-2 The role of the mammalian target of rapamycin complex 1 (mTORC1) in integrating signals from insulin, insulin-like growth factor (IGF), fuels, and energy status of the cell. The mammalian target of rapamycin complex 1 (mTORC1) is regulated by growth factor signaling and by nutrients. Insulin and IGF promote activation of mTORC1. Binding of either insulin or IGF to tyrosine kinase receptors results in activation of the phosphatidyl inositol 3-kinase (PtdIns3K)/Akt pathway, as well as of a Ras/Erk (small GTPase named for its intial discovery in rat sarcoma/extracellular ligand-regulated kinase) pathway, that leads to mTORC1 activation. Akt catalyzes an inhibitory phosphorylation of tuberous sclerosis protein 2 (TSC2), which inhibits TSC1/TSC2 GTPase activity toward Rheb-GTP, allowing the active mTORC1 to form. Akt also catalyzes a stimulatory phosphorylation of the mTORC1 complex. Either action of Akt results in activation of mTORC1. Lack of fuel (low ATP/high AMP) or hypoxia (low oxygen) leads to mTORC1 inhibition. These effects are largely mediated by their stimulatory effects on the TSC1/TSC2 complex, which acts as a GTPase of Rheb-GTP, converting Rheb-GTP to Rheb-GDP and preventing the formation of active mTORC1. AMP-activated protein kinase (AMPK) can also catalyze a direct inhibitory phosphorylation of mTORC1. Amino acids, especially leucine, activate mTORC1, by effects that appear to be mediated at the level of the complex itself and may involve the co-localization of mTOR to Rheb-GTP with involvement of Rag GTPases, type 3 PtdIns3K, and vacuolar protein sorting proteins such as Vps34. The downstream targets of mTORC1 include eIF4E-binding protein (4EBP) that regulates cap-dependent initiation of mRNA translation, rS6 kinase (S6K) that in turn phosphorylates the ribosomal S6 protein and other proteins involved in protein synthesis, and the Ulk1 and Atg13 autophagy proteins involved in triggering macroautophagy. The actions of 4EBP in blocking cap-dependent translation initiation and of Ulk1 and Atg13 in triggering autophagy are inhibited by mTORC1, whereas those of the S6K targets in promoting protein synthesis are stimulated. Thus protein synthesis and growth are stimulated when fuels, amino acids, insulin, and growth factors are all present. On the other hand, these processes are downregulated when growth factors and substrates are low or when oxygen or ATP is insufficient. Under the latter conditions, macroautophagy is stimulated, which allows cells to self-digest a portion of their cytoplasm to provide fuels and amino acids for survival.

one of these factors is absent, ensuring that protein synthesis is upregulated only when the body has plenty of substrate and fuel and is in an anabolic or growth mode. The downstream targets of mTORC1 include eIF-4E-binding protein (4EBP) that regulates cap-dependent initiation of mRNA translation; rS6 kinase (S6K) which phosphorylates the ribosomal S6 protein and other proteins involved in protein synthesis; and the Ulk1 and Atg13 autophagy proteins involved in triggering macroautophagy. The actions of 4EBP in blocking translation initiation and of

Ulk1 and Atg13 in triggering autophagy are inhibited by mTORC1 kinase activity, whereas the activity of S6K is stimulated. Thus protein synthesis and growth are stimulated when fuels, amino acids, insulin, and growth factors are present. On the other hand, these processes are downregulated when growth factors and substrates are low or when oxygen or ATP is insufficient. Under the latter conditions, macroautophagy is stimulated, which allows cells to self-digest a portion of their cytoplasm to provide fuels and amino acids for survival. More recently, mTORC1 signaling has been shown to be involved in activation or inactivation of certain transcription factors. Inactivation of mTORC1 was required in mice for the fasting-induced activation of peroxisome proliferator activated receptor alpha (PPARα), the master transcriptional activator of ketogenic genes (Sengupta et al., 2010). Activation of mTORC1 promotes the processing of SREBP1c to its active form, resulting in increased transcription of lipogenic genes; this action of mTORC1 appears to be mediated by S6K (Düvel et al., 2010). These latter results imply a role for mTORC1 in regulating lipid and carbohydrate metabolism as well as protein metabolism. This type of broad integration of regulation of metabolism makes sense in the context of humans consuming diets made up of foods that contain a mixture of macronutrients and the fact that a variety of macronutrients are needed for growth (e.g., amino acids for protein synthesis and fatty acids for membrane lipids).

THE METABOLIC FATES OF MACRONUTRIENTS

The body undergoes regular cycles of substrate utilization in the context of intermittent eating. The period immediately after meal intake is called the postprandial or absorptive period. During the absorptive period, chyme is entering the small intestine from the stomach and nutrients are being absorbed into the bloodstream and lymph. Once the stomach and small intestine have processed the meal and nutrient absorption is complete, the body enters the postabsorptive period during which it must rely on stored energy reserves, particularly on hepatic glycogen reserves for maintenance of plasma glucose levels. Normally, the postabsorptive period is interrupted by intake of another meal, but in cases of prolonged starvation the body makes further metabolic adaptations to reduce the need to catabolize muscle mass as a source of gluconeogenic substrate.

ABSORPTIVE OR POSTPRANDIAL PHASE

Most individuals eat discrete meals, and the macronutrients are absorbed, processed, and stored during the absorptive phase after a meal. During this postprandial or absorptive phase, exogenous fuels are utilized. Let's start with a person who has not eaten for 5 to 6 hours, is clearly postabsorptive, and has a fasting plasma glucose level of 4 mmol/L. Then let's have him or her eat a typical meal, perhaps containing 660 kcal provided by 90 g of carbohydrate, 30 g of protein, and 20 g of fat. As the carbohydrate is digested and glucose is absorbed, plasma glucose levels rise. The digestion and absorption of

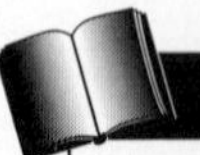

HISTORICAL TIDBIT

How mTOR Got Its Name

Rapamycin was discovered as an antifungal agent produced by a microorganism present in a soil sample taken in 1965 from the Polynesian island of Rapa Nui (Easter Island). Rapamycin has been used for its immunosuppressive effects since 1999. In the search for molecules that were affected by rapamycin, two target proteins were identified in yeast, target of rapamycin 1 (TOR1) and target of rapamycin 2 (TOR2). Both TOR1 and TOR2 were shown to regulate protein translation in yeast, and TOR2 also was found to function in cytoskeleton organization. The mammalian homolog of yeast TOR was subsequently identified and named mammalian target of rapamycin (mTOR). Thus this important protein kinase was named based on the ability of rapamycin to inhibit it rather than on its biochemical or physiological function. Rapamycin binds to a protein called FKBP12 (12-kDa-FK506-binding protein) to form a complex, and it is this complex that inhibits mTOR.

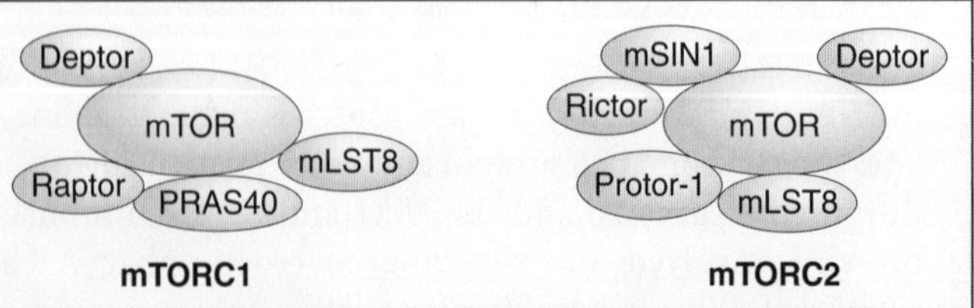

In mammals, there is only one mTOR protein, but this protein interacts with other proteins to form two complexes, mTORC1 and mTORC2, that have different functions. Both complexes have five or more protein components, with Raptor (regulatory-associated protein of mTOR) being found only in mTORC1 and Rictor (rapamycin-insensitive companion of mTOR) being found only in mTORC2. As might be assumed from these names, only mTORC1 is inhibited by rapamycin. Much has been learned about the regulation and function of mTORC1 since its discovery, and many features of its regulation by upstream signals, the targets of its protein kinase activity, and its cellular functions have been elucidated. In contrast, relatively little is known about mTORC2. However, mTORC2 appears to be the previously elusive protein that phosphorylates the serine/threonine protein kinase Akt at Ser473. This initial phosphorylation of Akt by mTORC2 stimulates a second phosphorylation of Akt by protein kinase 3-phosphoinositide-dependent protein kinase (PDK1) at Thr308, which leads to full Akt activation. The availability of rapamycin as an inhibitor of mTORC1 greatly facilitated studies of mTORC1, whereas the lack of a specific inhibitor of mTORC2 has contributed to the slow progress made so far in defining its regulation and function.

protein result in an elevation of plasma amino acid levels, and the digestion and absorption of fat result in the transport of triacylglycerols in chylomicrons. The rise in the circulating glucose level, together with other signals, triggers release of insulin and suppresses release of glucagon by the endocrine cells of the pancreas. The consequent changes in circulating insulin and glucagon levels are important hormonal signals to cells that express insulin or glucagon receptors, informing them of the body's nutritional state.

The importance of pancreatic hormones in the regulation of macronutrient metabolism is underscored by the metabolic consequences of diabetes mellitus. In acute diabetes mellitus, the lack of insulin or insulin signaling when exogenous fuels are available results in a miscommunication of fuel status to body tissues. Body tissues respond to the lack of insulin signaling as though exogenous fuels are not available, resulting in inappropriate gluconeogenesis by the liver, inappropriate lipolysis by adipose tissue, and inappropriate ketogenesis by the liver. The situation in the obese, insulin-resistant, and diabetes mellitus type 2 phenotype is more complex and involves impairments that have been described as a type of metabolic fuel inflexibility (Kelley and Mandarino, 2000; Corpelijn et al., 2009). Kelly and co-workers found that obese insulin-resistant subjects did not modulate their reliance on lipid versus glucose oxidation as did lean control subjects, such that rates of lipid oxidation remained relatively fixed in the obese subjects (Kelley et al., 1999). This resulted in less reliance on lipid oxidation during fasting (not removing the lipid fuels) and more reliance on lipid oxidation during insulin-stimulated conditions (not removing the glucose) in obese insulin-resistant subjects compared to lean subjects. Impairments in the expected rise in fat oxidation after β-adrenergic stimulation or during exercise have also been reported (Corpelijn et al., 2009). Metabolic fuel inflexibility is associated with the accumulation of lipid metabolites in skeletal muscle and increased levels of circulating adipokines. It is hypothesized that genetic determinants, lipid overflow (obesity, high fat intake, fasting), adipokines and inflammatory mediators, and lifestyle factors (diet, physical activity) all contribute to metabolic inflexibility and insulin resistance (Kotani et al., 2004; Corpelijn et al., 2009; Taube et al., 2009).

CLINICAL CORRELATION

Diabetes Mellitus

Diabetes mellitus is a chronic disease that results from a lack of secretion of insulin in sufficient amounts or from a lack of insulin stimulation of its target cells due to insulin insensitivity. Diabetes mellitus is often diagnosed by an elevated fasting plasma glucose level, by excretion of glucose in the urine, or by an abnormal glucose tolerance test. Consistent with the symptom of glucosuria, the name diabetes mellitus comes from the Greek words *diabetes,* meaning siphon and referring to the discharge of excessive amounts of urine, and *mellitus,* meaning honey and reflecting the sweet taste of the urine. Diabetes mellitus is the third leading cause of death in the United States, following heart disease and cancer. Diabetes mellitus occurs in two major forms: (1) type 1, insulin-dependent, juvenile-onset diabetes mellitus, and (2) type 2, non–insulin-dependent, maturity-onset diabetes mellitus.

In insulin-dependent diabetes mellitus (IDDM), the pancreas lacks or has defective beta cells and secretes no, or essentially no, insulin. Onset is thought to occur when 80% or more of the pancreatic beta cells have been destroyed by the immune system. Because the patients do not synthesize or secrete insulin, daily insulin injections are essential. The destruction of beta cells also results in a lack of amylin secretion and in abnormal regulation of alpha cell glucagon secretion. These hormonal abnormalities also contribute to alterations in macronutrient metabolism in patients with diabetes. The postprandial glucose concentration rises due to a lack of insulin-stimulated glucose disappearance, a lack of suppression of glucagon release by alpha cells, poorly regulated hepatic glucose production, and an increased or abnormal rate of gastric emptying after the meal.

Non–insulin-dependent diabetes mellitus (NIDDM) is a more complex disease that may be present for many years before diagnosis and that has a strong genetic component. NIDDM accounts for the majority (>80%) of the diagnosed cases of diabetes. It usually occurs after age 40 years, although it is increasingly being diagnosed in younger individuals including children, and NIDDM is often (>80%) associated with obesity. Patients with NIDDM exhibit varying levels of plasma insulin, but their tissues are resistant to its actions. Before the onset of diabetes, these patients probably maintained plasma glucose homeostasis by increasing the release of insulin in response to a glucose load. Ultimately, as insulin resistance develops, the pancreas is not able to secrete sufficient insulin to maintain plasma glucose levels and beta cell insulin granules become depleted. Insulin resistance means that insulin fails to control key functions in liver, skeletal muscle, and adipose tissue. Changes in diet, together with a loss of weight and increased physical activity, or the use of drugs that enhance insulin secretion and action often can control NIDDM without the need for exogenous insulin administration.

Thinking Critically

1. In untreated NIDDM, the plasma glucose level is high because of both reduced clearance of glucose from the plasma and increased release of glucose into the plasma. Explain how a reduced response to insulin would decrease the removal of glucose from, and increase glucose release into, the circulation.
2. In what ways are the fuel supply and hormonal signals similar in untreated diabetes mellitus and starvation? In what ways are they dissimilar?
3. Untreated IDDM is associated with high levels of ketone bodies in the circulation. Explain how the hormonal signals sensed by cells of a patient with untreated IDDM lead to diabetic ketoacidosis.

Effects of a Meal on Plasma Glucose, Insulin, and Glucagon Levels

The pancreatic endocrine cells are present in the pancreas as "islands" of cells called islets of Langerhans (Figure 19-3). The beta cells in these islets are the cells that synthesize and secrete insulin. These beta cells express the high K_m, high-capacity glucose transporter 2 (GLUT2), which can respond to an increase in plasma glucose by taking up more glucose into the cell, and the glucokinase isozyme of hexokinase, which also has a high K_m and is able to respond to the increased glucose uptake by increased formation of glucose 6-phosphate. In addition, the glucokinase isozyme is not inhibited by its product glucose 6-phosphatase and so remains active. Although glucose is by far the most potent stimulus of insulin secretion, some amino acids, some incretin hormones secreted by the gut following a meal (e.g., glucagon-like peptide 1), and parasympathetic stimulation via the vagus nerve also can stimulate insulin release in response to food intake. The further metabolism of glucose 6-phosphate results in stimulation of the pancreatic beta cells to secrete insulin. The consequent increase in ATP/ADP ratio leads to an increase in cytosolic Ca^{2+} concentration, which triggers insulin extocytosis and an increase in plasma insulin levels (Torres et al., 2009; Zitzer et al., 2006). At the same time, the high plasma glucose concentration, along with neural signals and the paracrine communication between beta and alpha cells, suppresses the

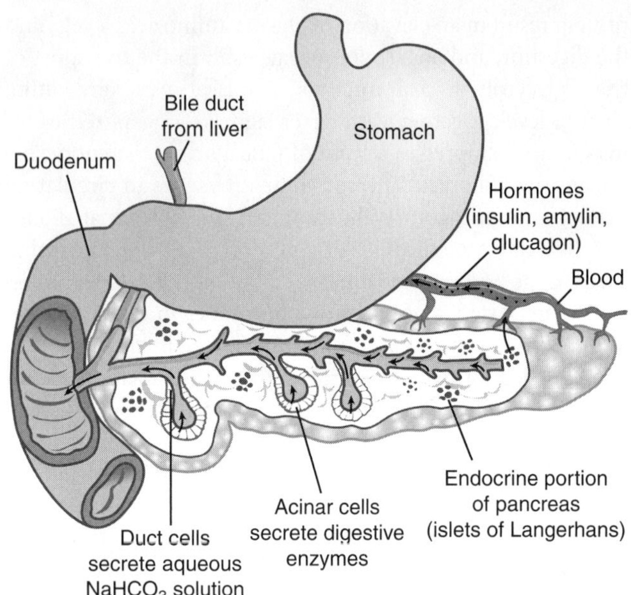

FIGURE 19-3 Diagram of pancreas. The islets of Langerhans are made up of several types of endocrine cells. The dominant types of endocrine cells in the islets are the beta cells, which secrete insulin and amylin, and the alpha cells, which secrete glucagon. The islets also contain cells that produce and secrete somatostatin, pancreatic polypeptide, and ghrelin.

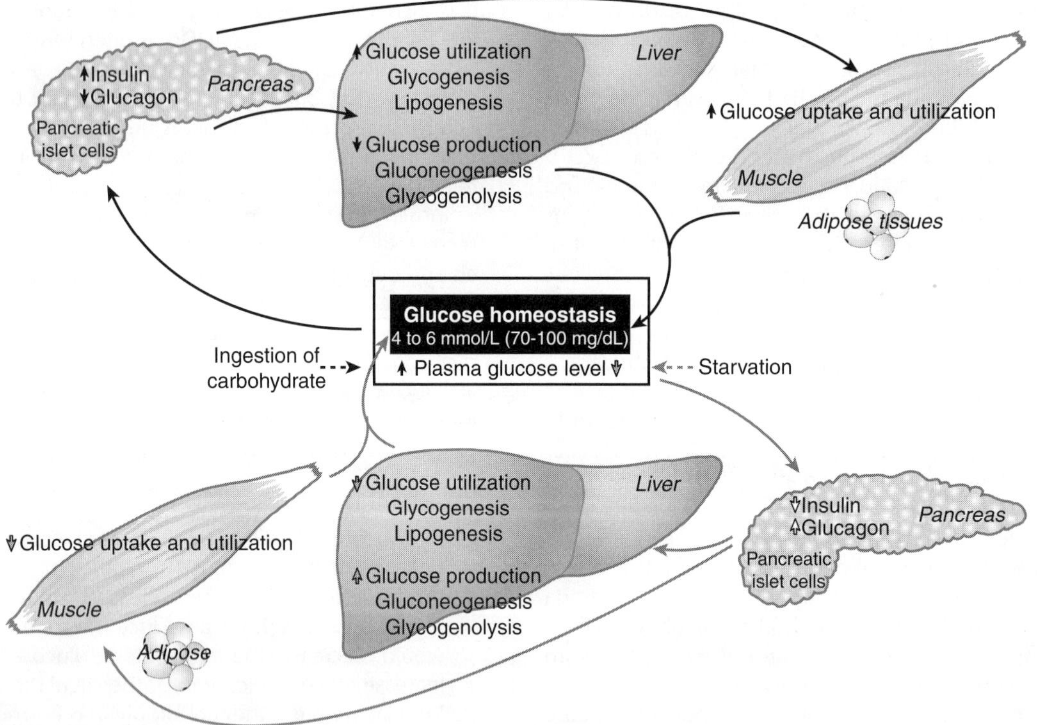

FIGURE 19-4 Maintenance of glucose homeostasis: roles of pancreas, liver, muscle, and adipose tissues. Ingestion of carbohydrate increases the plasma glucose level above its homeostatic range. This results in increased insulin and decreased glucagon secretion by the pancreas, increased glucose uptake and utilization by tissues, and decreased hepatic glucose production, which return plasma glucose to its homeostatic range *(black arrows)*. A lack of food intake (*starvation*) has the opposite effects. Starvation results in a decrease in plasma glucose. The fall in plasma glucose results in decreased insulin and increased glucagon secretion by the pancreas, decreased glucose uptake and utilization by tissues, and increased hepatic glucose production, all of which act to raise plasma glucose back to its homeostatic range (*grey arrows*).

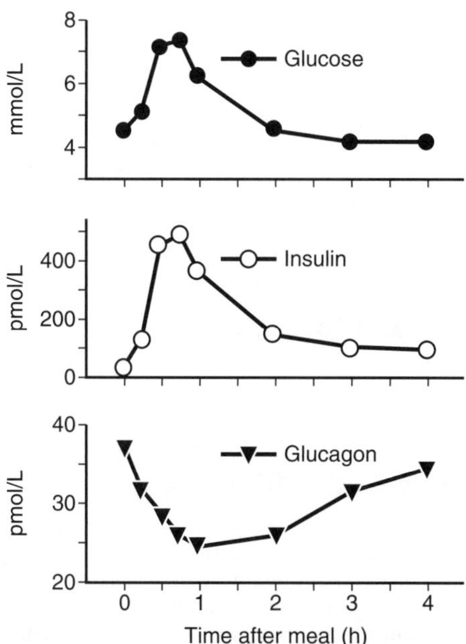

FIGURE 19-5 Changes in plasma levels of glucose, insulin, and glucagon in response to a meal. (Plotted values are from the data of Owen, O. E., Mozzoli, M. A., Boden, G., Patel, M. S., Reichard, G. A., Jr., Trapp, V., Shuman, C. R., & Felig, P. [1980]. Substrate, hormone, and temperature responses in males and females to a common breakfast. *Metabolism, 29,* 511–523.)

release of glucagon by the alpha cells, resulting in a decrease in plasma glucagon levels (Quesada et al., 2008; Gromada et al., 2007). Amylin, which is co-secreted with insulin by the beta cells, serves as a signal to the brain and can suppress glucagon secretion via the central nervous system and efferent vagal signals. Amylin also leads to a reduction in the rate of gastric emptying and thereby the rate at which glucose is absorbed from the small intestine, and also plays a role in satiety.

The major effects of ingestion of carbohydrate are summarized in the top half of Figure 19-4 and in Figure 19-5. The changes in plasma insulin and glucagon levels result in a decreased rate of gastric emptying and decreased glucose production by the liver via glycogenolysis and gluconeogenesis. The increased plasma insulin as well as high plasma glucose levels promote glucose utilization for glycogenesis and lipogenesis in the liver and increased glucose uptake and utilization in the muscle and adipose tissue. The increased glucose utilization for fuel or storage, along with the reduced glucose production by the liver, returns plasma glucose levels to a homeostatic range. When plasma glucose levels drop and glucose influx drops as the meal is completely digested and absorbed, insulin and glucagon secretions are returned to basal postabsorptive levels as well (Owen et al., 1980).

Insulin and Glucagon Signaling

Circulating insulin binds to membrane insulin receptors, which are found on essentially all cells, triggering activation of the cytoplasmic tyrosine kinase domain of the receptors. Activation of the tyrosine kinase receptor results in its autophosphorylation. The phosphorylated domain of the receptor then binds to an insulin receptor substrate (IRS) or adaptor protein, and this association in turn leads to activation or inhibition of the various downstream signaling pathways by which insulin has its effects on metabolism, as summarized in Figure 19-6 (Kim and Novak, 2007). Insulin is considered an anabolic hormone in that it increases storage of glycogen and triacylglycerols and stimulates net protein synthesis.

Circulating glucagon binds to membrane glucagon receptors, which are abundant on hepatocytes in the liver. When glucagon binds to its receptor, the conformational change triggers GTP–GDP exchange and the release of the α-subunit of the G-stimulatory (G_s) protein (Figure 19-7). The activated α-subunit in turn activates adenylate cyclase, which converts ATP to cAMP. The level of cAMP in the cell regulates the activity of PKA, which plays a major role in regulating fuel metabolism. In the fed state, glucagon levels are low and hence PKA is largely inactive and the processes activated by PKA-mediated phosphorylation are not upregulated. Thus the effects of insulin signaling dominate in the fed state, but the absence of the effects of glucagon signaling is also very important in determining the overall metabolic state, particularly in the liver.

Outcomes of Increased Insulin and Suppressed Glucagon Signaling during the Postprandial Period

The key outcomes of insulin and glucagon signaling during the postprandial or absorptive period are summarized in Figure 19-8. Many of the details of pathways summarized here are discussed in Chapters 12, 13, and 16. Glucose utilization is clearly favored, whereas glucose production is suppressed in the absorptive period. When glucose levels are elevated, insulin signaling via several arms promotes GLUT4 synthesis and translocation to the plasma membrane of adipose and muscle cells, and the GLUT4-mediated increase in glucose uptake ensures that these tissues have glucose to use as a fuel and for triacylglycerol backbone (i.e., glycerol 3-phosphate) synthesis (Klip, 2009). Although the liver does not express GLUT4, hepatocytes do express the high K_m glucose transporter (GLUT2) and the high K_m isoform of hexokinase (glucokinase) and thus respond to elevated plasma glucose levels by taking up and using more glucose, similar to the beta cells of the pancreatic islets. The liver is exposed to high concentrations of both glucose and pancreatic hormones because venous blood from both the small intestine and the pancreas drains into the portal vein, which is the main blood supply for the liver.

In addition to the effects of plasma glucose and insulin levels on glucose uptake, insulin is involved in regulating many metabolic pathways within cells. Insulin signaling results in the inhibition of glycogen synthase kinase 3 (GSK3); GSK3 is the kinase responsible for phosphorylation and inhibition of glycogen synthase. In the presence of insulin, the uninhibited glycogen synthase is thus able to synthesize glycogen from glucose, both replenishing glycogen stores and facilitating removal of excess glucose. Insulin signaling promotes lipogenic gene transcription (Mounier and Posner, 2006), and the upregulation of lipogenic enzymes favors fatty acid and

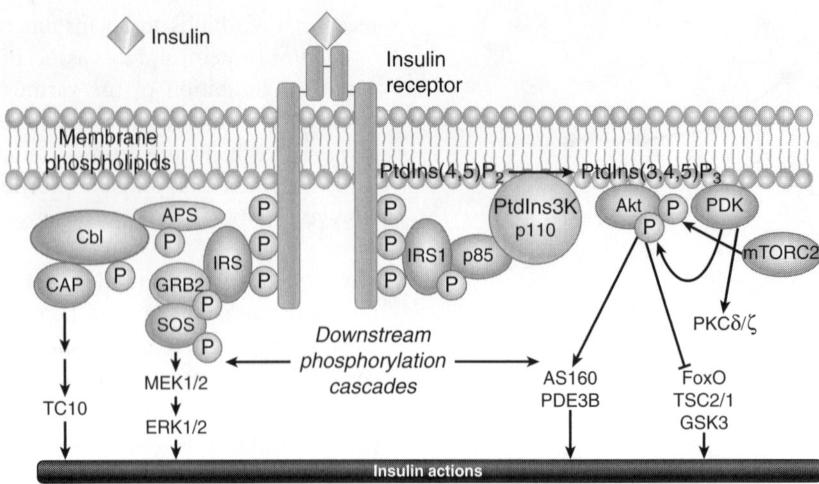

FIGURE 19-6 Insulin signaling via insulin receptors. The insulin receptor is composed of two extracellular α-subunits and two transmembrane β-subunits linked together by disulphide bonds. Binding of insulin to the α-subunit induces a conformational change resulting in the autophosphorylation of a number of tyrosine residues present in the β-subunit. These residues are recognized by phosphotyrosine-binding domains of adaptor proteins such as members of the insulin receptor substrate family (*IRS*). The activated IRS or adaptor proteins, in turn, activate or inhibit various downstream signaling pathways. Shown on the right is the recognition of phosphorylated IRS1 by the p85 regulatory subunit of phosphatidylinositol 3-kinase (*PtdIns3K*). The p85 subunit contains an Src homology 2 (*SH2*) domain that recognizes phosphorylated tyrosine residues. The catalytic subunit of PtdIns3K, p110, then phosphorylates membrane phosphatidylinositol (4,5) bisphosphate [*PtdIns(4,5)P*$_2$], leading to the formation of phosphatidylinositol (3,4,5)P$_3$ [*PtdIns(3,4,5)P*$_3$]. A key downstream effector of PtdIns(3,4,5)P$_3$ is the serine/threonine kinase Akt (also known as protein kinase B), which is recruited to the plasma membrane. Activation of Akt also requires the protein kinase 3-phosphoinositide-dependent protein kinase (*PDK*), which in combination with mTORC2 leads to the phosphorylation and activation of Akt. Once active, Akt leaves the membrane and enters the cytoplasm where it leads to the phosphorylation and activation or inactivation of its downstream target proteins. (See Figure 19-8 for more details on Akt actions.) PDK also phosphorylates and activates atypical protein kinase C family members (PKCδ/ζ). Shown on the left are two other signal transduction pathways. The interaction of IRS with adaptor complex proteins GRB2 (growth factor receptor-bound protein 2) and SOS (son of sevenless) leads to sequential activation of MEK1/2 (*MAP/ERK kinase 1/2*) and ERK1/2 (a mitogen-activated protein kinase known as extracellular signal-regulated kinase) and hence mitogenic responses in the form of gene transcription. APS (adapter protein with a PH and SH2 domain) is a Cbl-binding protein that is tyrosine phosphorylated by the insulin receptor kinase. Insulin-stimulated phosphorylation of APS leads to its association with Cbl (Casitas B-lineage lymphoma c) and with the adaptor protein CAP (Cbl-associated protein), resulting in the phosphorylation of Cbl. This pathway leads to activation of the GTP-binding protein TC10, which ultimately promotes GLUT4 (glucose transporter 4) translocation to the plasma membrane. *P,* phosphate group to indicate phosphorylated protein; ⟶ = stimulation/activation; —| = inhibition/deactivation.

triacylglycerol synthesis in the liver. Lipid storage in the adipose tissue is also favored by the insulin-mediated increase in lipoprotein lipase activity, which favors the uptake of fatty acids from circulating lipoproteins into adipocytes. In the fed state, the elevations in insulin and amino acid levels result in activation of the mTORC1 pathway, which enhances protein synthesis.

Other direct actions of insulin result in the inhibition of pathways that would promote the generation of fuels from body stores, as these are not needed when exogenous fuels are available, as illustrated in Figure 19-8. A major route by which insulin inhibits these processes is the phosphatidylinositol 3-kinase (PtdIns3K)/Akt-mediated phosphorylation of the FoxO transcription factors, which causes their exclusion from the nucleus of the cell. Thus the processes promoted by active nuclear FoxO transcription factors (e.g., gluconeogenesis, ketogenesis, VLDL synthesis, and proteolysis) are not promoted when insulin is high. In addition, insulin signaling activates phosphodiesterase, which hydrolyzes and hence removes cAMP, the second messenger of glucagon and β-adrenergic signaling. The activation of phosphodiesterase further promotes the suppression of pathways that oppose the effects of insulin on fuel utilization (e.g., glycogenolysis, lipolysis, and gluconeogenesis). Insulin signaling also suppresses autophagy, the "self-eating" of portions of the cell to provide essential substrates such as amino acids. Furthermore, the activation of lipogenesis or fatty acid synthesis by insulin results in elevation of cytosolic levels of malonyl-CoA. Malonyl-CoA acts as a strong inhibitor of fatty acid uptake by the mitochondria via inhibition of CPT1, thus blocking the utilization of fatty acids as a fuel, promoting triacylglycerol storage and utilization of glucose as a fuel.

Changes in Circulating Fuel Levels Following a Meal

Figure 19-9 shows changes in the circulating levels of other fuel molecules following intake of a meal. In addition to the transient increase in plasma glucose, the total amino acid level and the level of triacylglycerols in circulating lipoproteins are elevated compared to the fasted state. Lactate levels are increased as a consequence of increased partial oxidation of glucose as a fuel by liver, muscle, and obligate glycolytic tissues.

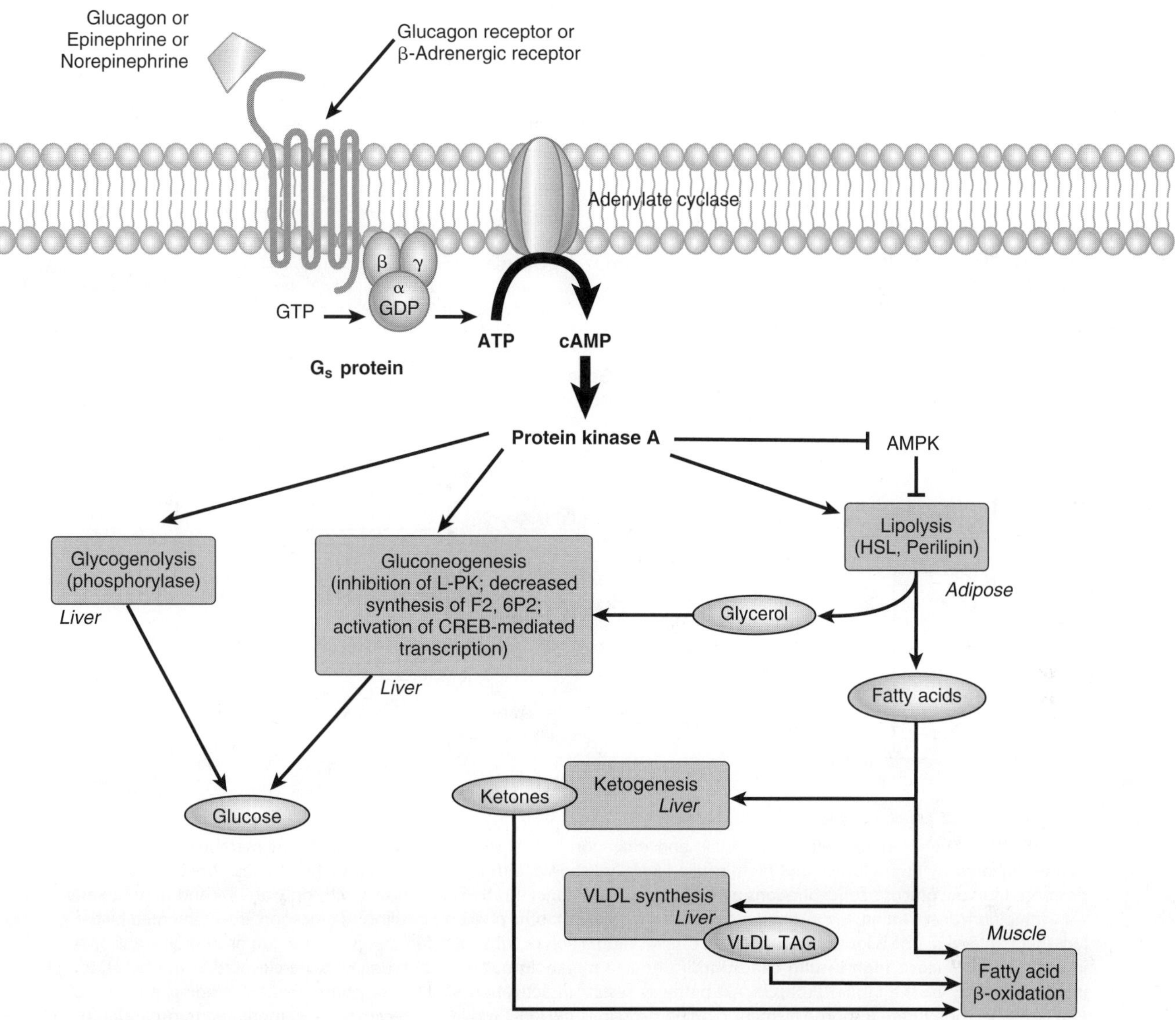

FIGURE 19-7 Glucagon and catecholamine signaling via G_s protein–coupled receptors. Glucagon receptors are transmembrane proteins. Binding of glucagon to the glucagon receptor on the cell surface results in a conformational change that triggers GTP-GDP exchange and the release of the α-subunit of the G-stimulatory (G_s) protein. This activated α-subunit in turn activates adenylate cyclase, which converts ATP to cAMP, the intracellular second messenger. The levels of cAMP in the cell regulate the activity of cAMP-activated protein kinase A (*PKA*). When cAMP is low, PKA exists as an inactive heterotetrameric complex containing two regulatory subunits and two catalytic subunits. When cAMP binds to the regulatory subunits, the catalytic subunits are released in active form. Activated PKA is responsible for the phosphorylation and consequent activation or inactivation of a variety of proteins involved in glycogen, glucose, and lipid metabolism. Glucose metabolism: PKA activates phosphorylase kinase (and inhibits the phosphatase), leading to phosphorylation and activation of glycogen phosphorylase, turning on glycogen breakdown. Gluconeogenesis is increased in liver by PKA-mediated phosphorylation of pyruvate kinase, which decreases its activity and favors retention of phosphoenolpyruvate; by phosphorylation of the bifunctional 6-phosphofructo-2-kinase/fructose-2,6-biphosphatase (*6PF2K/F2,6Pase*), resulting in decreased production of fructose 2,6-bisphosphate (*F2,6P2*), the allosteric regulator of glycolysis (+) and gluconeogenesis (–); and by phosphorylation of cAMP-response element binding protein (*CREB*), resulting in increased cAMP-response element (*CRE*)-mediated transcription of gluconeogenic enzymes such as glucose 6-phosphatase (*G6Pase*) and phosphoenolpyruvate carboxykinase (*PEPCK*). Lipid metabolism: PKA plays a critical role in the activation of lipolysis in adipose tissue via phosphorylation of hormone sensitive lipase and perilipin. The activation of lipolysis leads to release of fatty acids, which serve as fuel via β-oxidation and for production of very-low-density lipoproteins (*VLDL*) and ketone bodies in liver, both of which provide lipid fuel to muscle and other tissues. The activation of lipolysis also leads to release of glycerol, which is taken up by the liver where it is a major substrate for gluconeogenesis. In addition to activating lipolysis, PKA phosphorylates and inhibits AMP-activated protein kinase (*AMPK*) to prevent AMPK's inhibitory effects on hormone sensitive lipase, ensuring efficient lipolysis. Catecholamine receptors: Epinephrine and norepinephrine are ligands for β-adrenergic receptors, which are also G_s protein–coupled receptors that, when activated, stimulate the production of cAMP and activation of PKA. The β-adrenergic receptors are more widespread than glucagon receptors and are present in muscle and adipose tissue as well as liver. —| = inhibition/deactivation; ⟶ = stimulation/activation. Metabolic pathways or processes are shown in rectangles. Fuels or substrates for energy production or storage are shown in ovals.

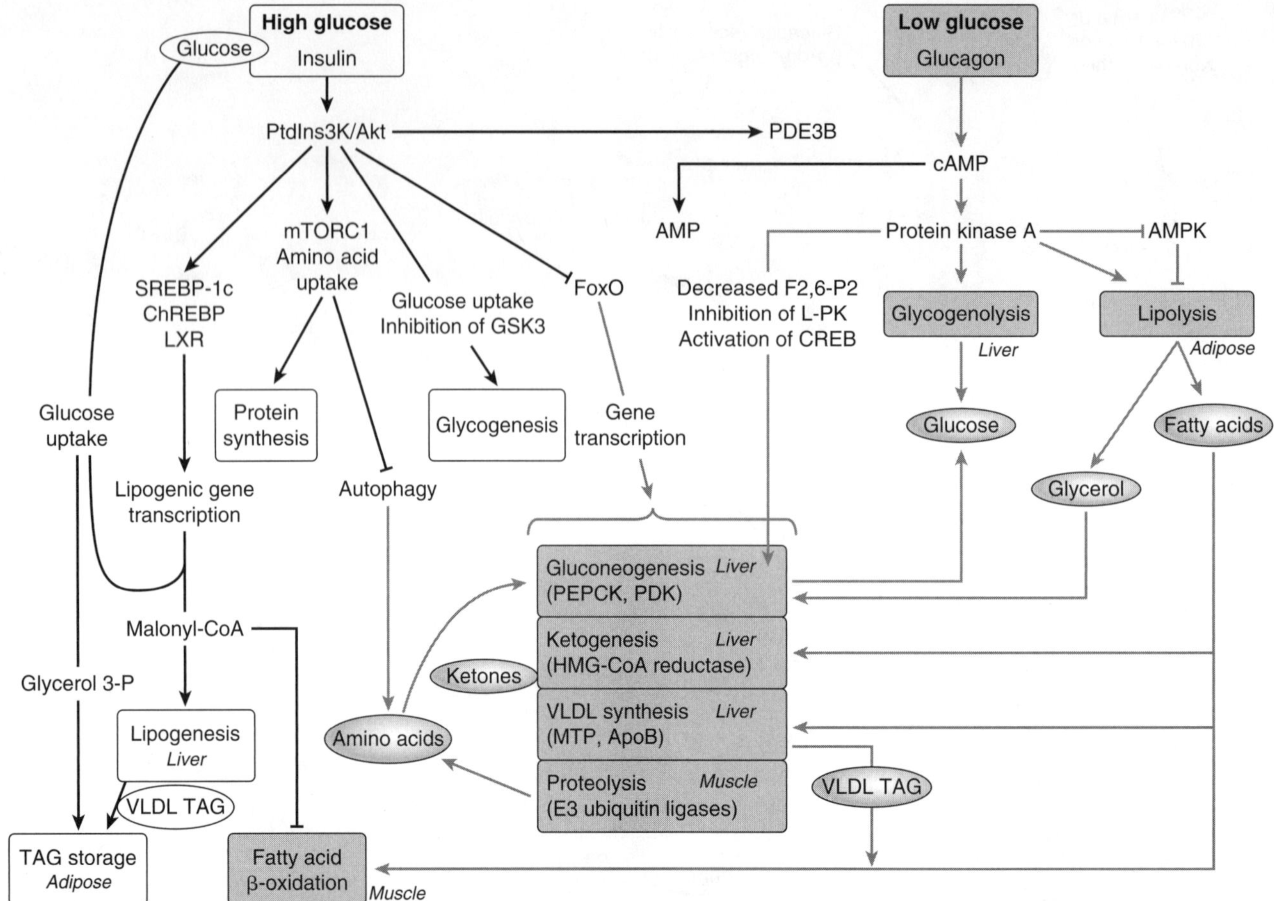

FIGURE 19-8 The integrated effects of insulin and glucagon in the regulation of macronutrient metabolism. Processes that are favored by high glucose and high insulin levels are shown with black arrows and white boxes. Processes that are promoted by low glucose concentrations and high glucagon concentrations are shown with gray arrows and gray boxes. —| = inhibition/deactivation. ⟶ = stimulation/activation. Note that the effects of insulin and glucagon are augmented by the fact that the level of one is low when that of the other is high. Fuels or substrates for energy production or storage are shown in ovals. **High glucose/high insulin condition.** Fatty acid metabolism: When glucose levels are elevated in the fed state, insulin signaling via the insulin/PtdIns3K/Akt pathway results in activation of sterol response element binding protein 1c (*SREBP1c*)-, carbohydrate response element binding protein (*ChREBP*)-, and liver X receptor (*LXR*)-mediated transcription of lipogenic genes, which along with the high glucose availability promotes hepatic lipogenesis and elevated malonyl-CoA levels that inhibit fatty acid uptake and oxidation by the mitochondria. Instead, dietary fatty acids are esterified to form triacylglycerols (*TAGs*) that are transported in very-low-density lipoproteins (*VLDL*) to the adipose tissue where lipoprotein lipase activity is elevated in response to insulin signaling. At the same time, the relative absence of glucagon- or β-adrenergic–stimulated signaling is further diminished by the activation of phosphodiesterase (*PDE3B*) by insulin/PtdIns3K/Akt signaling, which removes the cAMP second messenger. The lack of cAMP-mediated signaling thus ensures that lipolysis is diminished, and glucose utilization is further promoted by the relative lack of fatty acid fuels. Blocking of lipolysis also prevents release of glycerol as a gluconeogenic substrate for liver under conditions when glucose is not needed. Ketogenesis in the liver is inhibited both because insulin/PtdIns3K/Akt inhibits the forkhead box class O transcription factors (*FoxOs*) and the lack of glucagon/cAMP/PKA signaling decreases lipolysis to maintain a low circulating free fatty acid level. Glucose metabolism: In response to Akt signaling, the inhibitory glycogen synthase kinase 3 (*GSK3*) is inhibited and glycogen synthesis is promoted. Several arms of the insulin signaling pathway promote insulin-responsive glucose transporter (*GLUT4*) expression and translocation in adipose and muscle. Uptake and utilization of glucose as a fuel and for synthesis of the glycerol 3-phosphate backbone of triacylglycerol is favored. The absence of glucagon/cAMP/PKA signaling ensures the downregulation of glycogen breakdown. Gluconeogenesis is inhibited, both because insulin/PtdIns3K/Akt inhibits forkhead box transcription factor, class O (FoxO) and because the lack of glucagon/cAMP/PKA signaling limits the availability of glycerol and amino acids as gluconeogenic substrates and prevents the activation of cAMP response element binding protein (*CREB*) transcription factor. The lack of cAMP/PKA signaling favors glycolysis versus gluconeogenesis due to maintenance of high levels of the allosteric regulator F2,6P_2, which promotes glycolysis and inhibits gluconeogenesis. Protein metabolism: Insulin/PtdIns3K/Akt signaling promotes net protein synthesis by its stimulatory effects on the mammalian target of rapamycin complex 1 (*mTORC1*) pathway and the consequent stimulation of protein synthesis and inhibition of macroautophagy. In addition, insulin signaling via inhibition of FoxO ensures that muscle proteolysis is not activated. This also prevents amino acids being released by muscle for uptake by liver for gluconeogenesis. **Low glucose/low insulin condition.** Effects are essentially the reverse, with pathways on the left being activated and those on the right being suppressed.

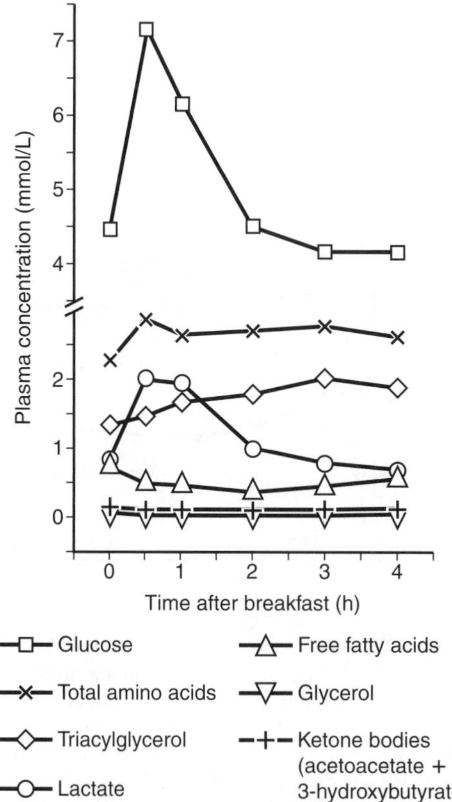

FIGURE 19-9 Changes in plasma levels of fuels after consumption of a meal. (Plotted values are from the data of Owen, O. E., Mozzoli, M. A., Boden, G., Patel, M. S., Reichard, G. A., Jr., Trapp, V., Shuman, C. R., & Felig, P. [1980]. Substrate, hormone, and temperature responses in males and females to a common breakfast. *Metabolism, 29,* 511–523.)

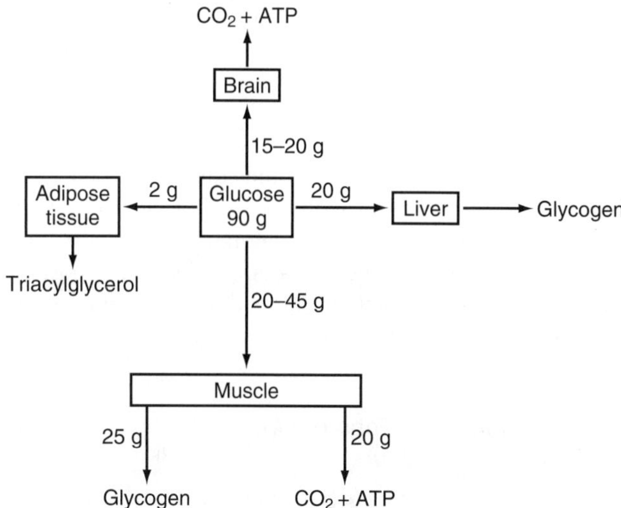

FIGURE 19-10 Fate of dietary carbohydrate (glucose) from one meal during the absorptive phase (~2 hours). Glucose provides the glycerol moiety for triacylglycerol synthesis. In addition to the fates shown, 2 to 3 g of glucose is used by the obligatory glycolytic cells.

Quantitative Aspects of Fuel Utilization by Tissues during the Postprandial State

Returning to our "typical" meal containing 660 kcal provided by 90 g of carbohydrate, 30 g of protein, and 20 g of fat, we can consider the fate of each macronutrient during the postprandial period. During the postprandial state, when both glucose and insulin levels are elevated, glucose is the major fuel that is oxidized by the body. The liver is exposed to high glucose concentrations (~15 mmol/L) in the portal blood and plays an important role in removal of glucose from the circulation. During the 2 to 3 hours following the meal, about 20 g of the glucose will be removed by the liver, and most of this will be converted to glycogen for replenishment of hepatic glycogen stores. Some may be partially catabolized to lactate and released by the liver during the absorptive period. As summarized in Figure 19-10, the remaining glucose (70 g) passes through the liver, causing peripheral plasma glucose levels to rise to 6 to 7 mmol/L. Over the next few hours, the brain will take up approximately 15 to 20 g of glucose to be oxidized directly as fuel. Obligatory glycolytic cells such as red blood cells and the renal medulla will use some glucose (4 to 5 g) but will oxidize it only to lactate. Most of the glucose, however, will be taken up in an insulin-dependent manner (due to upregulation of the GLUT4 transporter) by skeletal muscle (45 g) and adipose tissue (2 g). In skeletal muscle, approximately half will be oxidized and half stored as glycogen. In adipose tissue, most will be used for the synthesis of glycerol 3-phosphate for triacylglycerol synthesis, and a small quantity may be metabolized to lactate. During the absorptive phase, there is evidence that the net production of lactate by the liver and other tissues provides an important fuel for the kidneys, heart, and possibly colon. Consequently, 2 to 3 hours after the meal, about half of the glucose has been stored and the rest has been oxidized.

During the same period, about one third of the amino acids are used for protein synthesis, and most other amino acids undergo catabolism, providing the major energy source of the liver together with some storage of the carbon skeletons as glycogen. The increase in amino acid and insulin levels after a meal are signals for increased protein synthesis and, of about 30 g of amino acids from a meal, approximately 10 g will be converted to protein in various tissues of the body. Because there is no purely storage form of amino acids in the body, the remaining 20 g of amino acids not used for protein synthesis will be degraded. Much of the glutamine, glutamate, and aspartate in the meal (4 g) is metabolized by the intestine, with resultant production of alanine, proline, citrulline, ammonia, and lactate. Branched-chain amino acids that are not used for protein synthesis are catabolized primarily in the skeletal muscle and liver in humans. Other amino acids are partially catabolized primarily by the liver, providing the liver with its major energy source during the absorptive period and also resulting in the synthesis of approximately 7 to 9 g of glucose (which mainly is stored as glycogen) via gluconeogenesis from the carbon skeletons (Jungas et al., 1992). Gluconeogenesis is coupled to urea synthesis in the liver, resulting in excretion of nitrogen when amino acids are catabolized for use as fuel (see Chapter 14).

Lipids are absorbed more slowly, as this requires chylomicron synthesis and release into the lymphatic system before their entrance into the circulation. Because the products of fat digestion and absorption are transported in the circulation as triacylglycerols in lipoproteins, their availability to tissues is dependent upon hydrolysis of the triacylglycerol by lipoprotein lipase. The insulin-mediated increase in adipose tissue lipoprotein lipase activity favors the uptake of fatty acids from the triacylglycerol by the adipocytes, which also have plenty of glucose for synthesis of glycerol 3-phosphate backbone for reesterification of the fatty acids. Thus most of the fatty acids from dietary fat are ultimately deposited, mainly in adipose tissue (with limited amounts in liver and skeletal muscle), as stores for use when other fuels are less available.

Effects of a Meal on Food Intake and Energy Expenditure

In the fed state, various gut peptides and endocrine hormones are sensed by the brain (Zheng and Berthoud, 2008). These include amylin, pancreatic polypeptide, leptin, and several gut peptides such as cholecystokinin, protein YY, and glucagon-like peptide-1. These proteins act as satiety signals and lead to suppression of gastric emptying (regulating the entrance of digesta into the small intestine), suppression of glucagon secretion, and suppression of appetite (favoring cessation of food intake). The central nervous system also sends signals to tissues that result in some increase in energy expenditure, which requires increased oxidation of fuels, when energy intake is in excess of energy expenditure.

POSTABSORPTIVE STATE OR STARVATION

Once the nutrients in a meal have been absorbed, the body relies on endogenous sources for its energy. The endogenous stores in a 70-kg adult include a very small amount of glucose or lipid in circulating fluids (100 kcal) and the body's glycogen (~0.35 kg or 1,400 kcal) and triacylglycerol (~15 kg or 140,000 kcal) stores. Just as glucose was the major fuel during the absorptive period as a result of the availability of exogenous glucose and the metabolic response to changes in insulin and glucagon levels, we see that stored fat becomes the major fuel during starvation. Fatty acids and fatty acid-derived ketone bodies become the major cellular fuels as a consequence of both their availability (stored fat) and their increased concentrations in the plasma (due to increased lipolysis). Lipolysis is stimulated in the adipose tissue as a consequence of metabolic responses to changes in insulin/glucagon and catecholamine (epinephrine and/or norepinephrine) levels. The increased availability of fatty acids and ketone bodies as a fuel for muscle and other tissues suppresses glucose utilization, largely via inhibitory effects of fatty acid utilization on glycolytic flux and the activity of the pyruvate dehydrogenase complex.

Effects of Starvation on Plasma Glucose, Insulin, Glucagon, and Catecholamine Levels

As the body moves into the postabsorptive or fasting period, plasma glucose levels begin to fall, and this causes decreased insulin secretion and increased glucagon secretion, as illustrated in Figure 19-11. The body responds to maintain glucose homeostasis as illustrated in the lower half of Figure 19-3. The relative absence of insulin and abundance of glucagon stimulate the liver to break down glycogen and use gluconeogenic substrates for glucose synthesis, along with release of the resulting glucose into the plasma. At the same time, glucose uptake and utilization by muscle and adipose tissue are minimized, mediated by the downregulation of the insulin-responsive GLUT4 transporter and also by the increased availability of lipid fuels due to the stimulation of lipolysis in adipose tissue in the absence of insulin.

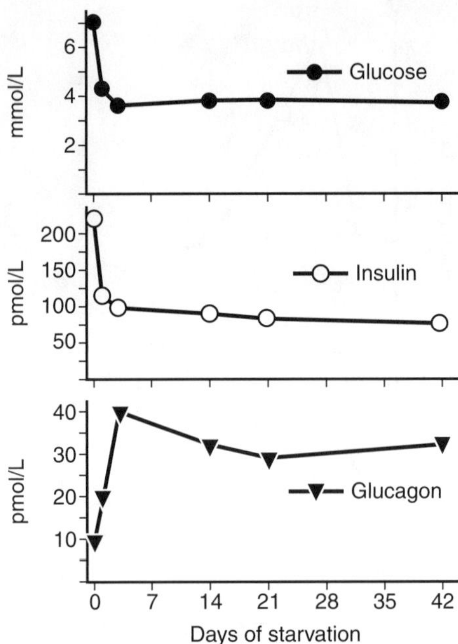

FIGURE 19-11 Changes in plasma glucose, insulin, and glucagon levels over the course of starvation. (Values are based on the data of Owen, O. E., Felig, P., Morgan, A. P., Wahren, J., & Cahill, G. F., Jr. [1969]. Liver and kidney metabolism during prolonged starvation. *The Journal of Clinical Investigation, 48,* 574–583; Marliss, E. B., Aoki, T. T., Unger, R. H., Soeldner, J. S., & Cahill, G. F., Jr. [1970]. Glucagon levels and metabolic effects in fasting man. *The Journal of Clinical Investigation, 49,* 2256–2270; Dela, F., Mikines, K. J., von Linstow, M., & Galbo, H. [1991]. Twenty-four-hour profile of plasma glucose and glucoregulatory hormones during normal living conditions in trained and untrained men. *The Journal of Clinical Endocrinology and Metabolism, 73,* 982–989.)

In addition to the absence of insulin, catecholamines released by the sympathetic nerve endings or adrenal medulla are also important regulators of lipolysis by the adipose tissue. The regulation of catecholamine levels by fasting and starvation are not well understood, but hypoglycemia is one factor that is known to enhance sympathetic nervous system activity, at least in early starvation, leading to a selective increase in adipose norepinephrine levels and/or an increase in the release of catecholamines by the adrenal medulla (Patel et al., 2002; Chan et al., 2007; Zauner et al., 2000). Catecholamine signaling through β-adrenergic receptors, which are G_s protein–coupled receptors, is analogous to glucagon signaling in that cAMP is produced as the second messenger. In humans, β-adrenergic receptors are found in adipose, muscle, and liver, so these tissues can all respond to changes in circulating catecholamine levels.

Outcomes of Suppressed Insulin and Increased Glucagon and Catecholamine Signaling during Starvation

Overall, during starvation the diminished use of glucose as a fuel along with the increased production and release of glucose by the liver maintains plasma glucose within the homeostatic range and protects tissues that are absolutely dependent upon glucose as a fuel.

As shown in Figure 19-8, the relative lack of insulin suppresses lipogenesis, protein synthesis, and glycogenesis; results in activation of FoxOs, which increase the expression of genes involved in gluconeogenesis, ketogenesis, VLDL synthesis, and proteolysis (Zhang et al., 2006); and suppresses the activation of phosphodiesterase, which hydrolyzes cAMP, thus significantly extending the half-life of cAMP and permitting its accumulation to levels that facilitate PKA activation (Kim and Novak, 2007). At the same time, the relative abundance of glucagon and catecholamines (norepinephrine/epinephrine) stimulates cAMP production. Both the increased production and the diminished hydrolysis of cAMP promote an elevation of the cellular cAMP level and thus result in strong stimulation of cAMP/PKA-mediated pathways. These cAMP/PKA-mediated pathways activate glycogenolysis and gluconeogenesis in the liver and lipolysis in the adipose tissue. Glycogenolysis and gluconeogenesis result in glucose production and release by the liver, so that plasma glucose levels are maintained. At the same time, lipolysis of triacylglycerol releases both glycerol and fatty acids into the plasma (Lafontan and Langin, 2009). Glycerol is an important substrate for hepatic gluconeogenesis during starvation. Fatty acids are used as a fuel by muscle and other tissues. In addition, fatty acids are taken up by the liver where they are partially oxidized to ketones (acetoacetate and 3-hydroxybutyrate) or packaged into triacylglycerol-rich VLDL and released as alternative fuels.

Changes in Circulating Fuel Levels during Starvation

Changes in the plasma concentrations of fuels during starvation are shown in Figure 19-12. Both glucose and total amino acid levels decrease and free fatty acid levels increase to higher steady state concentrations after 2 to 3 days of starvation (Owen et al., 1969). On the other hand, the ketone levels continue to increase over 14 to 21 days of starvation.

Quantitative Aspects of Fuel Utilization by Tissues during Prolonged Starvation

In long-term starvation (Figure 19-13), the brain is the only tissue that continues to completely oxidize glucose. However, the brain's consumption of glucose does occur at a reduced rate, and some of this is limited to lactate production (with no loss of glucose carbon). Ketone bodies provide most of the fuel to the brain during prolonged starvation. Glucose use in other tissues, such as the obligatory glycolytic tissues, is limited to glycolysis to lactate (or alanine), which conserves the gluconeogenic potential. The liver derives most of its energy from the partial oxidation of fatty acids, and most other tissues are using either fatty acids or ketone bodies as the major fuel. Carbon for de novo gluconeogenesis is provided by lipolysis and proteolysis, which provide glycerol and amino acids, respectively, as gluconeogenic substrates. As shown in Figure 19-13, the major carriers of nitrogen derived from muscle proteolysis out of the muscle are alanine and glutamine, and thus these two amino acids are the major fuels leaving the muscle. Although amino acid carbon skeletons in the form of alanine and glutamine are major gluconeogenic substrates at the level of the liver and kidney during prolonged starvation, a variety of amino acids are actually degraded to provide metabolites for replenishment of the pyruvate and α-ketoglutarate carbon chains and are the source of the amino groups present in circulating alanine and glutamine (see Chapter 14 for more about interconversions of amino acid carbon chains).

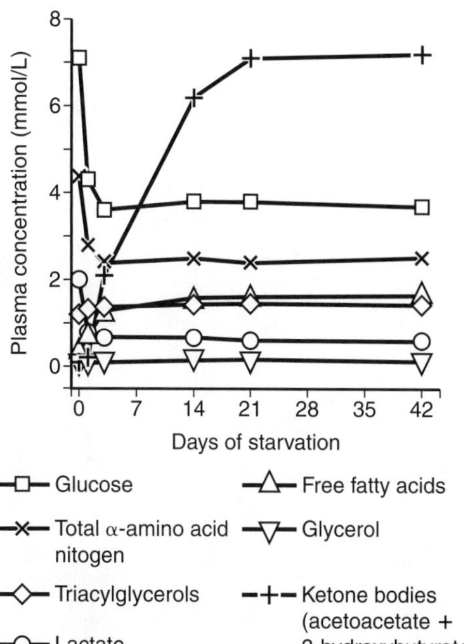

FIGURE 19-12 Changes in plasma fuel concentrations over the course of starvation. (Values are based on the data of Owen, O. E., Felig, P., Morgan, A. P., Wahren, J., Cahill, G. F., Jr. [1969]. Liver and kidney metabolism during prolonged starvation. *The Journal of Clinical Investigation, 48,* 574–583; Owen, O. E., Smalley, K. J., D'Alessio, D. A., Mozzoli, M. A., & Dawson, E. K. [1998]. Protein, fat, and carbohydrate requirements during starvation: Anaplerosis and cataplerosis. *The American Journal of Clinical Nutrition, 68,* 12–34; Markel, A., Brook, J. G., & Aviram, M. [1985]. Increased plasma triglycerides, cholesterol and apolipoprotein E during prolonged fasting in normal subjects. *Postgraduate Medical Journal, 61,* 395–400; Dela, F., Mikines, K. J., von Linstow, M., & Galbo, H. [1991]. Twenty-four-hour profile of plasma glucose and glucoregulatory hormones during normal living conditions in trained and untrained men. *The Journal of Clinical Endocrinology and Metabolism, 73,* 982–989.)

Effects of Starvation on Appetite and Energy Expenditure

During starvation there is an absence or decrease in the anorexigenic peptides and an increase in ghrelin levels. Grehlin is produced predominantly by endocrine cells in the stomach and in the pancreas, and its secretion is increased by fasting and in response to weight loss. It acts as an orexigen and augments the drive to eat. The central nervous system also

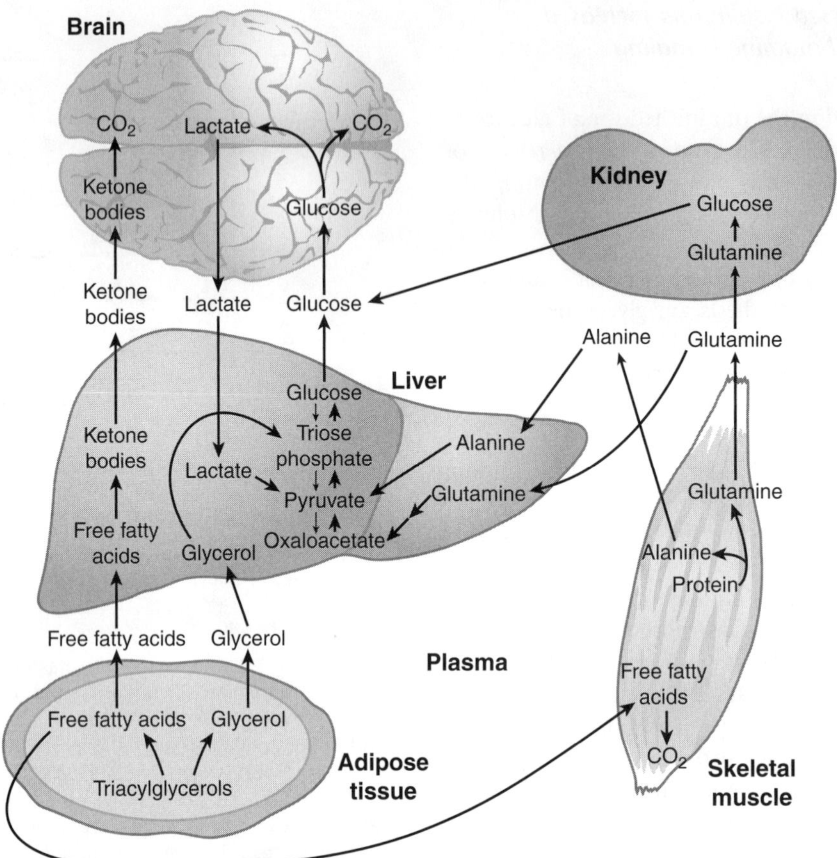

FIGURE 19-13 Fuel utilization during prolonged starvation. The only tissues utilizing glucose are the brain and the obligatory glycolytic tissues (omitted for clarity). Fatty acids have become the major fuel for tissues such as liver and muscle, and ketone bodies have replaced a considerable amount of the brain's glucose utilization. In addition, the brain has restricted some of its glucose utilization to glycolysis with the release of lactate, thereby reducing the complete oxidation of glucose to extremely low rates. Glycerol and amino acids from proteolysis provide fuel for synthesis of new glucose.

sends signals to tissues that result in some decrease in energy expenditure, which results in less oxidation of fuels, when energy intake is below energy expenditure. It should be noted, however, that ghrelin levels may actually decrease after a prolonged period of starvation, and in this case appetite may be low during the early refeeding period (Korbonits et al., 2007).

STAGES OF GLUCOSE HOMEOSTASIS DURING PROLONGED STARVATION

In the late 1960s George Cahill studied a group of obese men undergoing therapeutic starvation for 6 weeks (Cahill, 1970). This work led to the concept that glucose homeostasis could be divided into different stages (Figure 19-14). In this model of glucose homeostasis, the body maintains circulating glucose levels through five major phases, using different physiological mechanisms to regulate glucose production and utilization and to provide alternative fuels (Ruderman et al., 1976; Cahill, 2006).

Stage 1 refers to the absorptive or postprandial period when all tissues are using glucose from the diet. (If excess amino acids are available, they will also be used as fuel by some tissues.) Stages II and III refer to the postabsorptive or overnight fasting period up through about 24 hours without food, during which breakdown of hepatic glycogen stores and hepatic gluconeogenesis maintain plasma glucose levels. Stress responses, as shown in Figure 19-15, play a role in the adjustment to prolonged starvation. Although tissues other than liver are still using glucose during these stages, it is at a reduced rate, and tissues are beginning to substitute fat-derived fuels. The brain, however, is still using about 110 to 120 g of glucose per day. Although the switch of some tissues to the use of fat-derived fuels helps preserve glycogen stores, liver glycogen stores are limited and eventually, after about 24 hours of starvation, become depleted.

Once liver glycogen stores are depleted, the only source of glucose is gluconeogenesis (the synthesis of glucose from noncarbohydrate precursors). Therefore in stages IV and V of glucose homeostasis, gluconeogenesis is the only source of glucose. Although most tissues switch to oxidation of fatty acids for energy during prolonged starvation, gluconeogenesis remains essential because plasma glucose levels must be maintained to allow the brain and obligatory glycolytic tissues to function. However, gluconeogenesis is very costly in terms of substrate when endogenous reserves are considered. The major energy stores, the fatty acyl groups of the triacylglycerol in adipose tissue, do not provide substrate for gluconeogenesis. Only the glycerol backbone of the triacylglycerols and amino

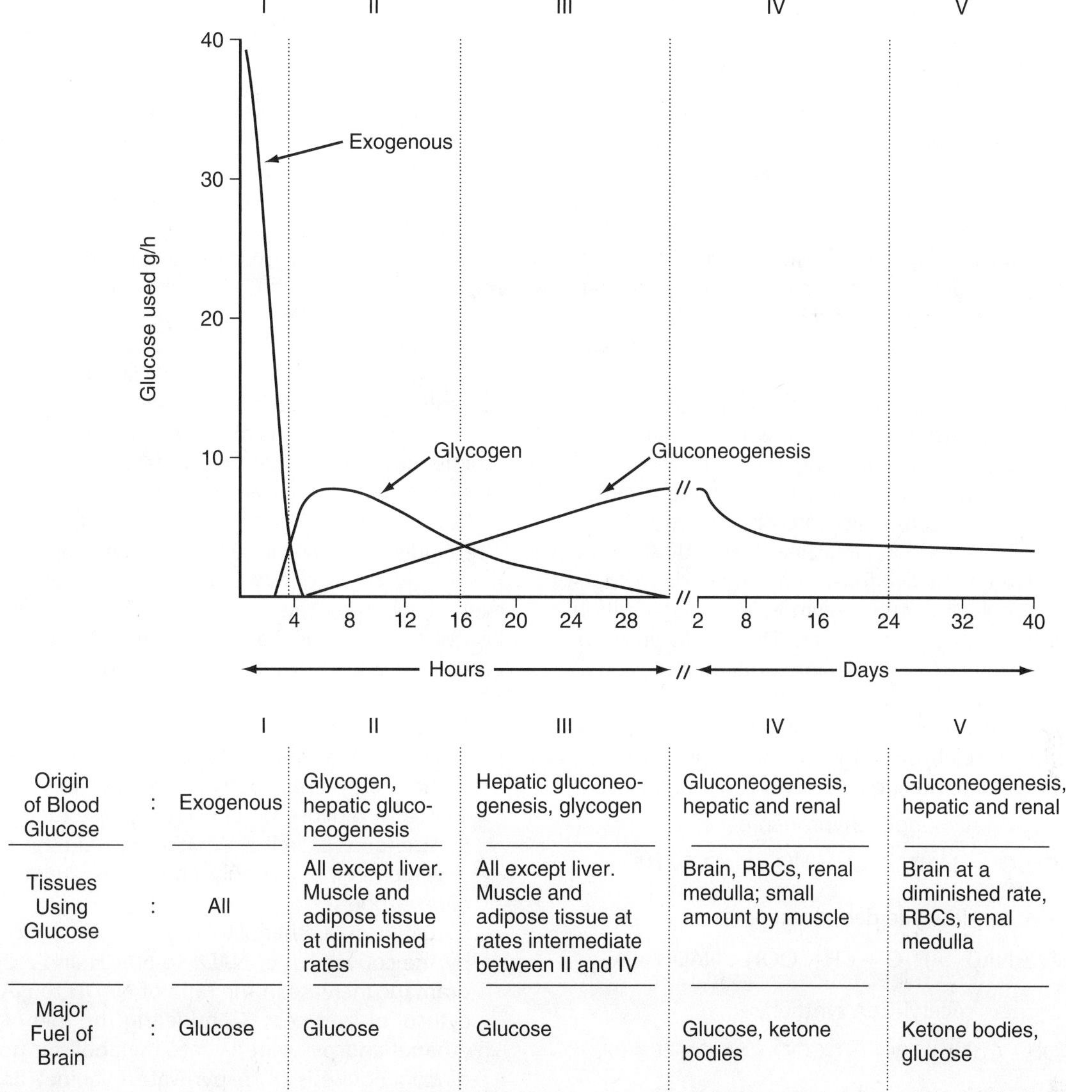

		I	II	III	IV	V
Origin of Blood Glucose	:	Exogenous	Glycogen, hepatic gluco-neogenesis	Hepatic gluconeo-genesis, glycogen	Gluconeogenesis, hepatic and renal	Gluconeogenesis, hepatic and renal
Tissues Using Glucose	:	All	All except liver. Muscle and adipose tissue at diminished rates	All except liver. Muscle and adipose tissue at rates intermediate between II and IV	Brain, RBCs, renal medulla; small amount by muscle	Brain at a diminished rate, RBCs, renal medulla
Major Fuel of Brain	:	Glucose	Glucose	Glucose	Glucose, ketone bodies	Ketone bodies, glucose

FIGURE 19-14 Glucose utilization versus time in the five phases of glucose homeostasis. Stage *I* refers to the absorptive or postprandial period; *II*, to the postabsorptive period; *III*, to early starvation; *IV*, to intermediate starvation; and *V*, to prolonged starvation. *RBCs*, Red blood cells. (From Ruderman, N. B., Aoki, T. T., & Cahill, G. F., Jr. [1976]. Gluconeogenesis and its disorders in man. In R. W. Hanson & M. A. Mehlman (Eds.), *Gluconeogenesis: Its regulation in mammalian species.* New York: John Wiley & Sons, Wiley Interscience.)

acids from body protein are available for net gluconeogenesis. The amount of glucose that can be synthesized from glycerol released by lipolysis is inadequate, so body protein must be broken down to supply amino acid carbon chains as gluconeogenic substrates. Although the principal source of amino acids for gluconeogenesis during stage II of starvation may be hepatic proteins, the source of amino acids during subsequent stages is the net proteolysis of skeletal muscle. Not all amino acid carbon will yield glucose; on average, 1.6 g of mixed amino acids from protein is required to synthesize 1 g of glucose. Therefore to keep the brain supplied with glucose at a rate of 110 to 120 g/day, the breakdown of 160 to 200 g of protein, or close to 1 kg of muscle tissue, per day would be required. This is clearly undesirable and unsustainable, and the body needs to limit glucose utilization to reduce the need for gluconeogenesis and thereby spare body protein to increase survival during prolonged starvation.

The production and use of ketone bodies as an alternative fuel for the brain is extremely important in allowing the body to limit the amount of new glucose required during prolonged starvation. Beyond 1 to 2 days of starvation (i.e., in stages IV and V of glucose homeostasis), ketone bodies become important fuels. The fall in insulin relieves its inhibition of lipolysis in adipose tissue, and the simultaneous rise in catecholamines that accompanies starvation stimulates lipolysis in adipose tissue. As the rate of lipolysis increases and more fatty acids are released into the circulation, the liver partially oxidizes fatty acids to produce ketone bodies. The liver cannot use ketone bodies as a fuel but releases them into the circulation for use by other tissues that express succinyl-CoA acetoacetate transferase and thus are able to activate acetoacetate to its CoA ester. The ketone body concentration increases markedly over several weeks of starvation, becoming increasingly important as a fuel. Many tissues, including the brain and skeletal muscle,

NUTRITION INSIGHT

Alcohol Metabolism and Hypoglycemia

Alcohol is rapidly absorbed, particularly when ingested on an empty stomach, from the stomach and small intestine. Metabolism and elimination of alcohol in a healthy adult occurs at an average rate of 0.5 to 0.75 ounce per hour, the equivalent of one 12-ounce beer, about 4 ounces of wine, or 1.5 ounces of 80-proof distilled spirits. Ethanol's acute effects are largely due to its nature as a central nervous system depressant. If too much alcohol is consumed, it depresses the nerves that control breathing, heartbeat, and the gag reflex.

Alcohol is metabolized in the liver by alcohol dehydrogenase, which catalyzes the oxidation of ethanol to acetaldehyde, and by acetaldehyde dehydrogenase, which catalyzes the further oxidation of acetaldehyde to acetate (Deitrich et al., 2007). Acetate can be activated by acetyl-CoA synthetase to yield acetyl-CoA (Yamashita et al., 2002). Some individuals have an inactive form of aldehyde dehydrogenase due to a single nucleotide polymorphism that results in an amino acid switch in the enzyme. These individuals are particularly susceptible to alcohol intoxication and alcohol-related death. Persons of Asian descent, including the Inuit and Native Americans, are more likely to have genes for the inactive form of aldehyde dehydrogenase and thus may experience alcohol poisoning at lower blood alcohol levels.

Alchohol dehydrogenase

$$CH_3CH_2OH + NAD^+ \rightarrow CH_3CHO + NADH + H^+$$

Aldehyde dehydrogenase

$$CH_3CHO + NAD^+ + H_2O \rightarrow CH_3COOH + NADH + H^+$$

Acetyl-CoA synthetase

$$CH_3COOH + CoA + ATP \rightarrow CH_3COO\text{-}CoA + AMP + PP_i$$

Pyrophosphatase

$$PP_i \rightarrow 2\ P_i$$

Toxic effects of alcohol are due to direct toxicity of ethanol and its metabolites as well as oxidative stress and metabolic changes associated with its rapid uptake and metabolism, primarily by the liver. If excess alcohol is consumed, the NAD^+ to NADH equilibrium can be pushed toward NADH. NADH inhibits isocitrate dehydrogenase and α-ketoglutarate dehydrogenase and hence metabolism of acetyl-CoA by the citric acid cycle. The consequent accumulation of acetyl-CoA results in hepatic ketogenesis, excacerbating the acidic condition that already existed due to the high lactate concentration. The processing of alcohol in the liver becomes inefficient and acetaldehyde accumulates. Acetaldehyde is reactive and particularly toxic. Acetaldehyde forms covalent bonds with various functional groups in proteins, impairing protein function. This can cause severe liver damage.

Consumption of alcohol, especially by an undernourished individual, can cause hypoglycemia due to its inhibition of gluconeogenesis. Drinking alcohol after strenuous exercise can have the same effect. This hypoglycemia can be quite dangerous, causing seizures, in addition to the other toxic effects produced by ethanol.

Thinking Critically

1. What is the normal source of glucose for maintenance of normoglycemia between meals? How might this source of glucose be affected by fasting/starvation or by strenuous exercise? What role would this play in the development of hypoglycemia subsequent to alcohol consumption?
2. Metabolism of ethanol to acetaldehyde is accompanied by the conversion of NAD^+ to NADH and a potentially dramatic increase in the ratio of NADH to NAD^+ in the cytosol of liver cells. Considering the role of NAD^+ in ethanol and pyruvate/lactate metabolism, how would gluconeogenesis from pyruvate (alanine) and lactate be affected by alcohol consumption? What role might this play in development of hypoglycemia?
3. Ketoacidosis is an additional complication of alcohol intoxication. How would hypoglycemia due to excess alcohol intake exacerbate ketogenesis?

use ketone bodies as fuels. In particular, the use of ketone bodies replaces some of the glucose required by the brain, a tissue that does not use fatty acids as a fuel. In addition, oxidation of ketone bodies reduces aerobic oxidation of glucose in the brain, such that much of the glucose used by the brain is only metabolized by the glycolysis to lactate, which conserves the glucose carbon. Thus after 4 to 6 days of starvation, utilization of plasma glucose has decreased from 5 g/hour to about 1 g/hour for complete oxidation in the brain. This reduction in net glucose consumption reduces the need for new gluconeogenic carbon and thus reduces the extent of muscle protein breakdown.

During starvation, the kidneys produce large amounts of ammonia and bicarbonate and excrete ammonium ions (NH_4^+). In prolonged starvation, ammonium excretion may be tenfold basal levels, and the amount of nitrogen excreted as ammonia may nearly equal the amount excreted as urea. The substrate for renal ammonia production is glutamine (derived from muscle proteolysis), and the carbon skeleton of glutamine is recovered as glucose through renal gluconeogenesis. Although the kidney is able to efficiently reabsorb ketone bodies, some loss of ketone bodies in the urine occurs during starvation. The excretion of ketone bodies (3-hydroxybutyrate and acetoacetate), which are strong acids and negatively charged at physiological pH, is associated with increased excretion of ammonium ions (NH_4^+) and increased ammonia production by renal glutaminase may be important in balancing ionic charge to maintain near electroneutrality of the urine.

Owen and colleagues (1998), based on extensive studies in obese subjects undergoing prolonged starvation, calculated that the minimum amount of new glucose that must be available for fuel homeostasis after 18 to 21 days of starvation was about 1 g·kg body $wt^{-1}·d^{-1}$, or 1.9 g·kg fat-free $mass^{-1}·d^{-1}$. They calculated that glycerol and amino acids each contributed approximately 20 g of glucose equivalents per day in their subjects, for a total of 40 g glucose equivalents per day for subjects weighing approximately 132 kg. Thus glycerol and certain amino acids are both important gluconeogenic substrates during starvation. Lipolysis, by making glycerol available, limits the need for protein breakdown to support gluconeogenesis during starvation. Owen and colleagues (1998) further determined that about half of the amino acids were used without being converted to glucose, suggesting a need for replenishment of anaplerotic substrates by various tissues, whereas the other half was first converted to glucose and the glucose was subsequently completely oxidized (presumably by the brain). Subjects lost lean mass and fat mass at similar rates over the course of starvation, but based on the differing water content of adipose tissue versus muscle tissue and the differing energy density of fat versus protein, fat mass provided about 90% of the energy needs during starvation whereas muscle breakdown provided the other 10%.

Gluconeogensis is also important in the recycling of lactate and alanine carbons (i.e., pyruvate carbon chains) back to glucose. During starvation, this is very important because the glycolytic tissues and to a lesser extent the brain oxidize glucose to lactate, and this lactate is recycled back to glucose by hepatic gluconeogenesis, conserving the glucose carbon. Therefore glycolytic tissues do not represent a drain on the circulating glucose pool, but they do demand continuing gluconeogenesis from lactate in liver (i.e., the Cori cycle). The energy for the synthesis of glucose within the liver is provided from the partial oxidation of fatty acids. Similarly, although alanine is quantitatively the most important amino acid taken up by the liver for glucose synthesis, the

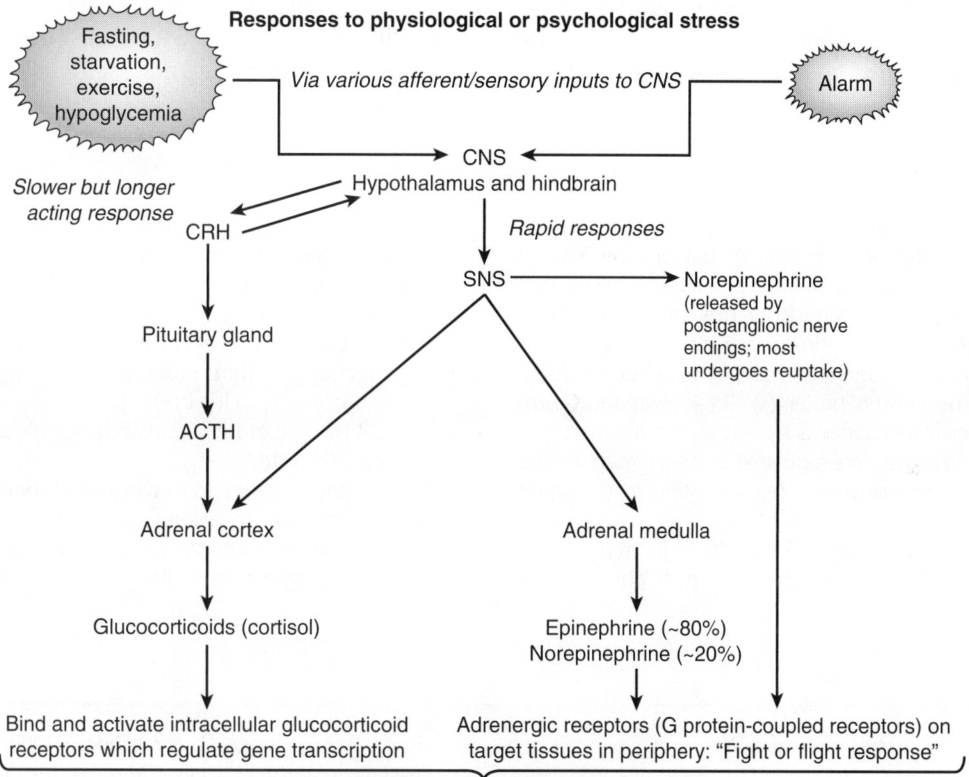

FIGURE 19-15 The central nervous system (*CNS*) and peripheral components of the body's stress response system. The release of corticotropin-releasing hormone (*CRH*) by the hypothalamus stimulates the release of adrenocorticotropic hormone (*ACTH*) by the pituitary gland and also stimulates central activation of the sympathetic nervous system (*SNS*). The SNS is rapidly activated in response to a stressor, leading to release of norepinephrine by the postganglionic neurons and epinephrine and norepinephrine by the adrenal medulla. The glucocorticoid (cortisol) level usually peaks about 15 to 30 minutes later. These hormones have effects on numerous targets including the wake–sleep, cognitive, and fear/anger centers in the brain; the growth, reproductive, and thyroid-hormone axes; and the gastrointestinal, cardiorespiratory, metabolic, and immune systems. The stress response is regulated by a negative feedback loop for glucocorticoid synthesis and by rapid uptake and/or degradation of catecholamines.

carbon skeleton of this alanine is derived primarily from glucose metabolism in extrahepatic tissues and likewise simply recycles glucose carbon via the glucose–alanine cycle (see also Chapters 12 and 14). Although important for glucose conservation, recycled glucose cannot contribute to the net amount of glucose required by the brain because net use of glucose from this pool would compromise the metabolism of a number of extrahepatic tissues and lead to hypoglycemia.

RESPONSES TO PHYSIOLOGICAL OR PSYCHOLOGICAL STRESS

In addition to starvation, macronutrient metabolism is also affected by stressors that are not associated with a lack of adequate nutrition but operate to ensure that an abundance of fuels, both glucose and fatty acids, are available for the body to respond to the situation underlying the stress. In addition, stress responses trigger the catabolism of muscle protein to ensure the availability of amino acids for synthesis of stress response proteins as well as for gluconeogenesis (see Chapter 13). Stress may be defined as a state of threatened or perceived-as-threatened homeostasis. A drop in plasma glucose due to strenuous exercise, fasting, or infection is one indicator of stress associated with activation of the body's stress response system. The body's stress response system has both central nervous system and peripheral components, as summarized in Figure 19-15. The release of corticotropin-releasing hormone (CRH) by the hypothalamus stimulates the release of adrenocorticotropic hormone (ACTH) by the pituitary gland and also stimulates central activation of the sympathetic nervous system (SNS). The principal peripheral effectors of the stress response are glucocorticoids, which are regulated by the hypothalamic–pituitary–adrenal (HPA) axis; norepinephrine, which is released from the widely distributed synapses of the sympathetic nervous system; and epinephrine, which is released by the adrenal medulla. Many of the effects of epinephrine on metabolism are mediated by β-adrenergic receptors and were discussed earlier in conjunction with starvation. In most cases, the stress response is activated rapidly and efficiently terminated within an hour or two. In cases such as acute diabetes, sepsis, or starvation, impaired insulin signaling along with an increase in glucocorticoid levels leads to muscle catabolism and muscle atrophy (Hu et al., 2009).

THINKING CRITICALLY

1. Choose one or more key proteins (enzymes, transporters, or other regulatory proteins) that are involved in macronutrient metabolism. Suggestions are GLUT4, glucokinase, glucokinase regulatory protein, phosphofructokinase, pyruvate dehydrogenase complex, glycogen phosphorylase, glycogen synthase, or acetyl-CoA carboxylase. For the chosen protein(s), list known short-term and long-term mechanisms by which the function and activity of the protein are regulated. For each mechanism, describe its potential role in fed to fasting to starvation transitions.
2. Macronutrient utilization is usually regulated to foster the oxidation of fuels that are most abundant at the time and/or that cannot be stored. Typically, this means that most tissues oxidize glucose in the postprandial state and that most tissues oxidize fatty acids in the starved state.
   a. Describe several of the most important regulatory mechanisms that underlie the use of glucose but not fatty acids in the postprandial state OR the use of fatty acids but not glucose in the starved state.
   b. Are there instances in which metabolism is altered to promote oxidation of both glucose and fatty acids at the same time? If so, what unique mechanisms play a role in allowing this to occur?

REFERENCES

Cahill, G. F., Jr. (1970). Starvation in man. *New England Journal of Medicine, 282*, 668–675.

Cahill, G. F., Jr. (2006). Fuel metabolism in starvation. *Annual Review of Nutrition, 26*, 1–22.

Carling, D., Mayer, F. V., Sanders, M. J., & Gamblin, S. J. (2011). AMP-activated protein kinase: Nature's energy sensor. *Nature Chemical Biology, 7*, 512–518.

Chakravarthy, M. V., Lodhi, I. J., Yin, L., Malapaka, R. R., Xu, H. E., Turk, J., & Semenkovich, C. F. (2009). Identification of a physiologically relevant endogenous ligand for PPARα in liver. *Cell, 138*, 476–488.

Chan, J. L., Mietus, J. E., Raciti, P. M., Goldberger, A. L., & Mantzoros, C. S. (2007). Short-term fasting-induced autonomic activation and changes in catecholamine levels are not mediated by changes in leptin levels in healthy humans. *Clinical Endocrinology, 66*, 49–57.

Corpeleijn, E., Saris, W. H., & Blaak, E. E. (2009). Metabolic flexibility in the development of insulin resistance and type 2 diabetes: Effects of lifestyle. *Obesity Research, 10*, 178–193.

Deitrich, R. A., Petersen, D., & Vasiliou, V. (2007). Removal of acetaldehyde from the body. *Novartis Foundation Symposium, 285*, 23–40.

Dowling, R. J., Topisirovic, I., Fonseca, B. D., & Sonenberg, N. (2010). Dissecting the role of mTOR: Lessons from mTOR inhibitors. *Biochimica et Biophysica Acta, 1804*, 433–439.

Düvel, K., Yecies, J. L., Menon, S., Raman, P., Lipovsky, A. I., Souza, A. L., … Manning, B. D. (2010). Activation of a metabolic gene regulatory network downstream of mTOR complex 1. *Molecular Cell, 39*, 171–183.

Goldstein, J. L., DeBose-Boyd, R. A., & Brown, M. S. (2006). Protein sensors for membrane sterols. *Cell, 124*, 35–46.

Gromada, J., Franklin, I., & Wollheim, C. B. (2007). Alpha-cells of the endocrine pancreas: 35 years of research but the enigma remains. *Endocrine Reviews, 28*, 84–116.

Hardie, D. G. (2008). AMPK: A key regulator of energy balance in the single cell and the whole organism. *International Journal of Obesity, 32*(Suppl. 4), S7–S12.

Harris, R. A., Bowker-Kinley, M. M., Huang, B., & Wu, P. (2002). Regulation of the activity of the pyruvate dehydrogenase complex. *Advances in Enzyme Regulation, 43*, 249–259.

Hu, Z., Wang, H., Lee, I. H., Du, J., & Mitch, W. E. (2009). Endogenous glucocorticoids and impaired insulin signaling are both required to stimulate muscle wasting under pathophysiological conditions in mice. *The Journal of Clinical Investigation, 119*, 3059–3069.

Hue, L., & Taegtmeyer, H. (2009). The Randle cycle revisited: A new head for an old hat. *American Journal of Physiology. Endocrinology and Metabolism, 297*, E578–E501.

Jungas, R. L., Halperin, M. L., & Brosnan, J. T. (1992). Quantitative analysis of amino acid oxidation and related gluconeogenesis in humans. *Physiological Reviews, 72*, 419–448.

Kelley, D. E., Goodpaster, B., Wing, R. R., & Simoneau, J. A. (1999). Skeletal muscle fatty acid metabolism in association with insulin resistance, obesity, and weight loss. *The American Journal of Physiology, 277*, E1130–E1141.

Kelley, D. E., & Mandarino, L. J. (2000). Fuel selection in human skeletal muscle in insulin resistance: A reexamination. *Diabetes, 49*, 677–683.

Kersten, S., Seydoux, J., Peters, J. M., Gonzalez, F. J., Desvergne, B., & Wahli, W. (1999). Peroxisome proliferator-activated receptor alpha mediates the adaptive response to fasting. *The Journal of Clinical Investigation, 103*, 1489–1498.

Kim, S. K., & Novak, R. F. (2007). The role of intracellular signaling in insulin-mediated regulation of drug metabolizing enzyme gene and protein expression. *Pharmacology & Therapeutics, 113*, 88–120.

Klip, A. (2009). The many ways to regulate glucose transporter 4. *Applied Physiology, Nutrition, and Metabolism, 34*, 481–487.

Korbonits, M., Blaine, D., Elia, M., & Powell-Tuck, J. (2007). Metabolic and hormonal changes during the refeeding period of prolonged fasting. *European Journal of Endocrinology, 157*, 157–166.

Kotani, K., Peroni, O. D., Minokoshi, Y., Boss, O., & Kahn, B. B. (2004). GLUT4 glucose transporter deficiency increases hepatic lipid production and peripheral lipid utilization. *The Journal of Clinical Investigation, 114*, 1666–1675.

Lafontan, M., & Langin, D. (2009). Lipolysis and lipid mobilization in human adipose tissue. *Progress in Lipid Research, 48*, 275–297.

Laplante, M., & Sabatini, D. M. (2009). mTOR signaling at a glance. *Journal of Cell Science, 122*, 3589–3594.

McGarry, J. D. (1998). Glucose-fatty acid interactions in health and disease. *The American Journal of Clinical Nutrition, 67*, 500S–504S.

McGarry, J. D., Mannaerts, G. P., & Foster, D. W. (1977). A possible role for malonyl-CoA in the regulation of hepatic fatty acid oxidation and ketogenesis. *The Journal of Clinical Investigation, 60*, 265–270.

Mounier, C., & Posner, B. I. (2006). Transcriptional regulation by insulin: From the receptor to the gene. *Canadian Journal of Physiology and Pharmacology, 84*, 713–724.

Owen, O. E., Felig, P., Morgan, A. P., Wahren, J., & Cahill, G. F., Jr. (1969). Liver and kidney metabolism during prolonged starvation. *The Journal of Clinical Investigation, 48*, 574–583.

Owen, O. E., Mozzoli, M. A., Boden, G., Patel, M. S., Reichard, G. A., Jr., … Felig, P. (1980). Substrate, hormone, and temperature responses in males and females to a common breakfast. *Metabolism, 29*, 511–523.

Owen, O. E., Smalley, K. J., D'Alessio, D. A., Mozzoli, M. A., & Dawson, E. K. (1998). Protein, fat, and carbohydrate requirements during starvation: Anaplerosis and cataplerosis. *The American Journal of Clinical Nutrition, 68*, 12–34.

Patel, J. N., Coppack, S. W., Goldstein, D. S., Miles, J. M., & Eisenhofer, G. (2002). Norepinephrine spillover from human adipose tissue before and after a 72-hour fast. *The Journal of Clinical Endocrinology and Metabolism, 87*, 3373–3377.

Pehleman, T. L., Peters, S. J., Heigenhauser, G. J., & Spriet, L. L. (2005). Enzymatic regulation of glucose disposal in human skeletal muscle after a high-fat, low-carbohydrate diet. *Journal of Applied Physiology, 98*, 100–107.

Quesada, I., Tudurí, E., Ripoll, C., & Nadal, A. (2008). Physiology of the pancreatic alpha-cell and glucagon secretion: Role in glucose homeostasis and diabetes. *The Journal of Endocrinology, 199*, 5–19.

Randle, P. J. (1998). Regulatory interactions between lipids and carbohydrates: The glucose fatty acid cycle after 35 years. *Diabetes/Metabolism Reviews, 14*, 263–283.

Randle, P. J., Garland, P. B., Hales, C. N., & Newsholme, E. A. (1963). The glucose fatty-acid cycle: Its role in insulin sensitivity and the metabolic disturbances of diabetes mellitus. *Lancet, 1*, 785–789.

Ruderman, N. B., Aoki, T. T., & Cahill, G. F., Jr. (1976). Gluconeogenesis and its disorders in man. In R. W. Hanson & M. A. Mehlman (Eds.), *Gluconeogenesis: Its regulation in mammalian species* (pp. 515–532). New York: Wiley Interscience.

Sengupta, S., Peterson, T. R., Laplante, M., Oh, S., & Sabatini, D. M. (2010). mTORC1 controls fasting-induced ketogenesis and its modulation by ageing. *Nature, 468*, 1100–1104.

Steinberg, G. R., & Kemp, B. E. (2009). AMPK in health and disease. *Physiological Reviews, 89*, 1025–1078.

Sugden, M. C., & Holness, M. J. (2006). Mechanisms underlying regulation of the expression and activities of the mammalian pyruvate dehydrogenase kinases. *Archives of Physiology and Biochemistry, 112*, 139–149.

Taube, A., Eckardt, K., & Eckel, J. (2009). Role of lipid-derived mediators in skeletal muscle insulin resistance. *American Journal of Physiology. Endocrinology and Metabolism, 297*, E1004–E1012.

Torres, N., Noriega, L., & Tovar, A. R. (2009). Nutrient modulation of insulin secretion. *Vitamins and Hormones, 80*, 217–244.

Vannucci, S., & Hawkins, R. (1983). Substrates for energy metabolism of the pituitary and pineal glands. *Journal of Neurochemistry, 41*, 1718–1725.

Viollet, B., Foretz, M., Guigas, B., Horman, S., Dentin, R., Bertrand, L., … Andreelli, F. (2006). Activation of AMP-activated protein kinase in the liver: A new strategy for the management of metabolic hepatic disorders. *The Journal of Physiology, 574*, 41–53.

Wang, Y. X. (2010). PPARs: Diverse regulators in energy metabolism and metabolic diseases. *Cell Research, 20*, 124–137.

Wasserman, D. H., Kang, L., Ayala, J. E., Fueger, P. T., & Lee-Young, R. S. (2011). The physiological regulation of glucose flux into muscle in vivo. *The Journal of Experimental Biology, 214*, 254–262.

Watford, M., (2002). Small amounts of dietary fructose dramatically increase hepatic glucose uptake through a novel mechanism of glucokinase activation. *Nutrition Reviews, 60*, 253–257.

Witczak, C. A., Sharoff, C. G., & Goodyear, L. J. (2008). AMP-activated protein kinase in skeletal muscle: From structure and localization to its role as a master regulator of cellular metabolism. *Cellular and Molecular Life Sciences, 65*, 3737–3755.

Yamashita, H., Fukuura, A., Nakamura, T., Kaneyuki, T., Kimoto, M., Hiemori, M., & Tsuji, H. (2002). Purification and partial characterization of acetyl-coA synthetase in rat liver mitochondria. *Journal of Nutritional Science and Vitaminology, 48*, 359–364.

Zauner, C., Schneeweiss, B., Kranz, A., Madl, C., Ratheiser, K., Kramer, L., … Lenz, K. (2000). Resting energy expenditure in short-term starvation is increased as a result of an increase in serum norepinephrine. *The American Journal of Clinical Nutrition, 71*, 1511–1515.

Zhang, W., Patil, S., Chauhan, B., Guo, S., Powell, D. R., Le, J., … Unterman, T. G. (2006). FoxO1 regulates multiple metabolic pathways in the liver: Effects on gluconeogenic, glycolytic, and lipogenic gene expression. *The Journal of Biological Chemistry, 281*, 10105–10117.

Zheng, H., & Berthoud, H. R. (2008). Neural systems controlling the drive to eat: Mind versus metabolism. *Physiology (Bethesda)*, *23*, 75–83.

Zitzer, H., Wente, W., Brenner, M. B., Sewing, S., Buschard, K., Gromada, J., & Efanov, A. M. (2006). Sterol regulatory element-binding protein 1 mediates liver X receptor-beta-induced increases in insulin secretion and insulin messenger ribonucleic acid levels. *Endocrinology*, *147*, 3898–3905.

RECOMMENDED READINGS

Hue, L., & Taegtmeyer, H. (2009). The Randle cycle revisited: A new head for an old hat. *American Journal of Physiology. Endocrinology and Metabolism*, *297*, E578–E591.

Wasserman, D. H. (2009). Four grams of glucose. *American Journal of Physiology. Endocrinology and Metabolism*, *296*, E11–E21.

CHAPTER 20

Regulation of Fuel Utilization in Response to Physical Activity

Martha H. Stipanuk, PhD

COMMON ABBREVIATIONS

AMPK AMP-activated protein kinase
CPT1 carnitine palmitoyltransferase 1
GLUT4 insulin-stimulated glucose transporter 4
IMTG intramyocellular triacylglycerol; also known as IMCL, intramyocellular lipid
RQ respiratory quotient, defined as moles CO_2 produced/moles O_2 consumed; also known as respiratory exchange ratio (RER)
VO_{2max} maximum aerobic capacity; measure of maximum volume of O_2 consumption

Skeletal muscle is the largest body compartment in humans, accounting for 40% to 50% of total body mass in an ordinary lean subject. Muscle accounts for much of the daily energy metabolism, although this varies greatly depending on the amount of physical work performed. Like most other tissues, skeletal muscle uses glucose and fatty acids as fuels and has the metabolic flexibility to vary the rates at which it uses the two different fuels. To support the high energy needs of muscle contraction, working muscle typically uses a mixture of fat and carbohydrate as fuel. The sources of the carbohydrate and lipid used by the muscle include those provided from the diet or from other tissues via the plasma and those stored within the muscle cells themselves.

MUSCLE STRUCTURE

Skeletal muscle connects the various parts of the skeleton through one or more connective tissue tendons and is the type of muscle used to produce movement or force during physical activity or exercise. During muscle contraction, skeletal muscle generates tension, which may involve shortening of the muscle (concentric contractions), lengthening of the muscle (eccentric contractions), or no change in muscle length (isometric contractions). Movement of the limbs is associated with concentric and eccentric contractions, but not with isometric contractions.

Muscle cells are called muscle fibers. Each skeletal muscle fiber is produced by the fusion of many immature myoblasts to form a multinucleated cylinder-shaped cell. The muscle fiber is contained within the cell's plasma membrane covered by an outer connective tissue sheath; the muscle fiber's plasma membrane is called the sarcolemma, and the outer layer of connective tissue is called the endomysium (Figure 20-1, *C*). The endomysium contains capillaries, nerves, and lymphatics. The sarcoplasm of each muscle fiber contains an array of cylindrical contractile filaments called myofibrils that are stacked lengthwise and run the entire length of the fiber, being connected to the cell surface membrane at each end. The nuclei are pressed against the outer edges of the fiber, adjacent to the sarcolemma. The mitochondria are located between the myofibrils, as are the intramyocellular lipid droplets and glycogen granules (Figure 20-2). At each end of the muscle fiber, the surface layer of the sarcolemma fuses with a tendon fiber, and the tendon fibers in turn collect into bundles to form the muscle tendons that then attach to bones.

Each myofibril is about 1 μm in diameter, extends along the complete length of the muscle fiber, and is composed of contractile units called sarcomeres that are attached end to end (Figure 20-1, *D*). Each sarcomere contains thick filaments (diameter of ~15 nm) that contain myosin and thin filaments (diameter of ~5 nm) that contain actin, with the thick and thin filaments overlapping in a structured way. In addition to actin and myosin, skeletal muscle sarcomeres also contain other proteins, such as troponin and tropomyosin, which are necessary for muscle contraction, and nebulin and titin, which give structure and stability to the sarcomere. In skeletal muscle, the sarcomeric subunits of one myofibril are in nearly perfect alignment with those of the myofibrils next to it. This alignment forms bands of alternating high and low refractive index that gives skeletal muscle its striated appearance.

Ten to more than 100 muscle fibers are bundled into fascicles, and each fascicle is covered by a sheath of connective tissue called perimysium (see Figure 20-1, *B*). Fascicles are, in turn, grouped together to form a muscle, which is covered by a layer of connective tissue that ensheathes the entire muscle and is continuous with the tendons (see Figure 20-1, *A*). The size, number, and arrangement of fascicles within the muscle determine the strength and range of movement of a muscle.

A. Muscle (organ)

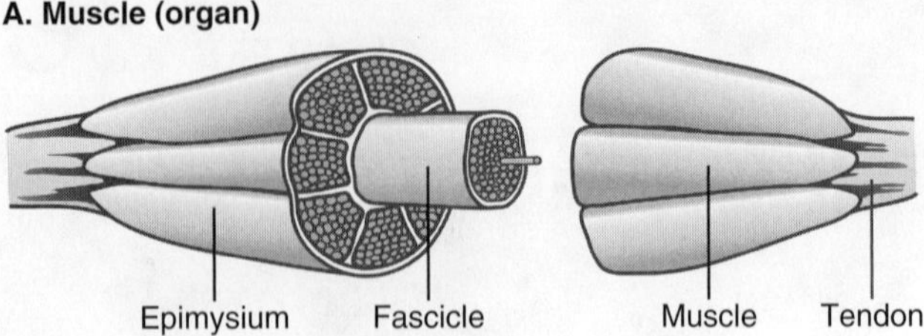

B. Fascicle (a portion of the muscle)

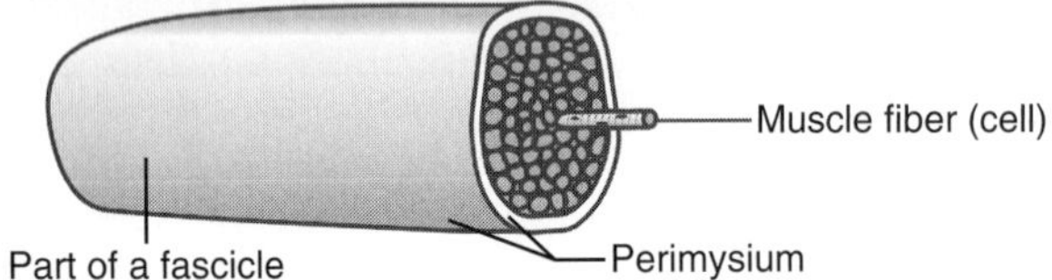

C. Muscle fiber (cell)

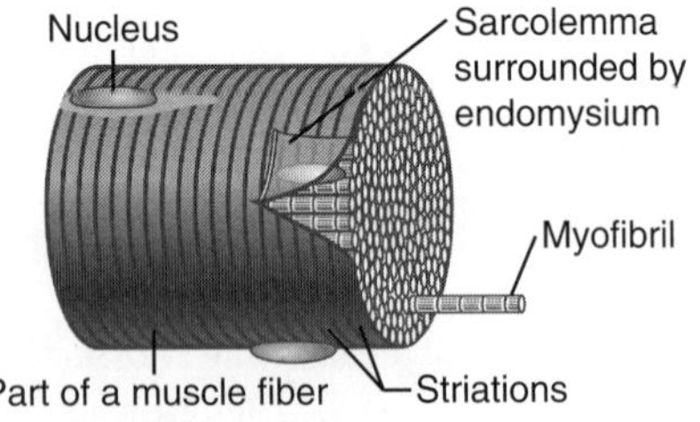

D. Sarcomere structure of myofibril

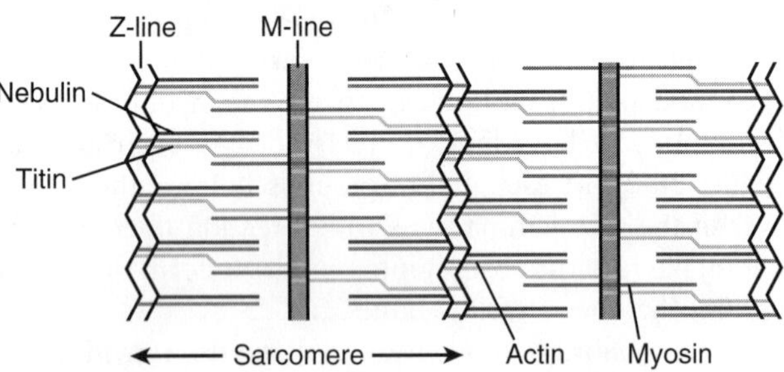

E. Motor units

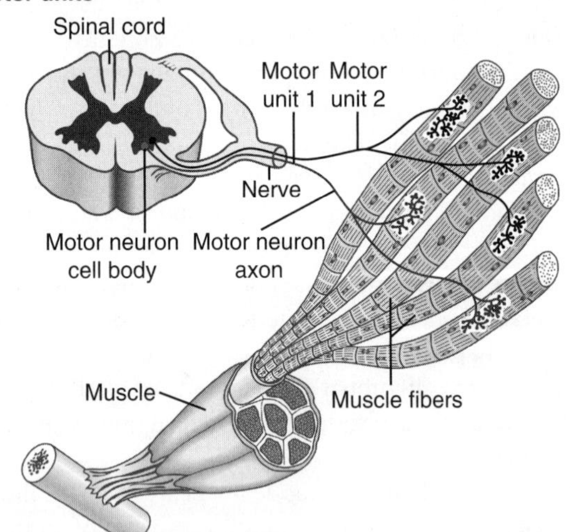

FIGURE 20-1 Structure of skeletal muscle. A muscle is made up of hundreds or thousands of muscle cells, connective tissue, blood vessels, and nerve fibers. The structure of muscle is illustrated in panels **A–E**. Skeletal muscle cells, usually called muscle fibers or myocytes, are formed when myoblasts fuse together to form long multinucleated cells. (**C**) The plasma membrane of this multinucleated muscle cell is called the sarcolemma, and the sarcolemma is surrounded by a layer of connective tissue called endomysium. The endomysium contains capillaries, nerves, and lymphatics. The contractile units within each muscle cell are the cylindrical myofibrils, and each muscle fiber (cell) contains many myofibrils. (**D**) Each myofibril is made up of thousands of sarcomeres, which are multi-protein complexes composed of the actin and myosin filament systems that are assembled in series to form a long myofibril. A muscle fiber (cell) contains hundreds of mytofibrils. Each end of each long myofibril is attached to the muscle cell surface membrane. (**B**) Ten to more than 100 muscle fibers (cells) are bundled into fascicles; each fascicle is covered by a sheath of connective tissue called perimysium. (**A**) The fascicles are further bundled to form a muscle, which is covered by a layer of connective tissue that ensheaths the entire muscle and is continuous with the tendons. (**E**) Activation of muscle fibers occurs via motor units that innervate only one type of muscle fiber.

Tunnel-like extensions of the sarcolemma, called tranverse tubules or simply T tubules, pass through the muscle fiber from one side of it to the other, forming rings around every sarcomere. The sarcoplasmic reticulum of the muscle fiber consists of tubules that run parallel to the sarcomeres from T tubule to T tubule. The sarcoplasmic reticulum serves as a repository for calcium ions (Ca^{2+}). When a signal comes from the motor nerve activating the fiber, the neurotransmitter acetylcholine is released and travels across the neuromuscular junction. The action potential then travels along the T tubules until it reaches the sarcoplasmic reticulum, where it changes the permeability of the sarcoplasmic reticulum. Once a cell is sufficiently stimulated, the cell's sarcoplasmic reticulum releases Ca^{2+}, which then interacts with the regulatory protein troponin. Calcium binding by troponin results in a conformational change in troponin that leads to the movement of tropomyosin, uncovering the myosin-binding sites on actin. In resting muscle, myosin-binding sites on actin are obscured and myosin exists in a high-energy conformational state poised to carry out a contractile cycle. When myosin binding sites on actin are exposed, myosin and actin form a crossbridge or complex, which is followed by the dissociation of inorganic phosphate (P_i) and a conformational change in myosin that propels the attached actin filament toward the center (M-line) of the sarcomere (see Figure 20-1, *D*). The actomyosin complex then releases ADP, which is followed by ATP binding to the myosin of the actomyosin complex and breaking of the crossbridges. As soon as detachment occurs, myosin splits the ATP, reversing the conformational change performed while it was attached to actin and returning myosin back to its high-energy state. Repetition of these processes allows for myosin and actin crossbridge cycling, which in turn leads to the generation of tension or fiber contraction.

MUSCLE FIBER TYPES

Individual human muscles are a mixture of muscle fiber types that are differentiated by their myosin heavy chain isoform expression (Canepari et al., 2010). A particular motor unit innervates only one type of muscle fiber within the muscle (see Figure 20-1, *E*). In fact, the muscle fiber type and myosin heavy chain (MHC) isoform expression depends on the motor neuron axon supplying that particular fiber.

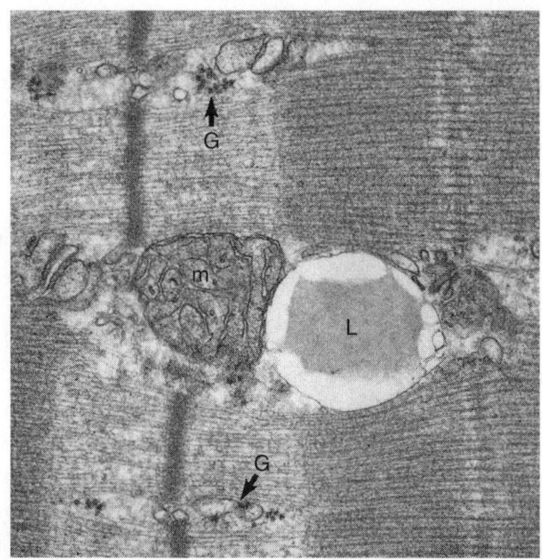

FIGURE 20-2 Electron micrograph of skeletal muscle showing mitochondria (*m*), lipid droplets (*L*), and glycogen granules (*G*).

Myosin is a motor protein that moves along actin filaments while hydrolyzing ATP. The skeletal muscles of human adults contain three isoforms of MHC: MHC-1, MHC-2A, and MHC-X, which are encoded by *MYH7, MYH2,* and *MYH1,* respectively. Rodents, but not adult humans, express MHC-2B. The myosin heavy chain isoforms are important determinants of the contractile characteristics of the muscle fibers, because the heavy chain is the portion of myosin that attaches to actin and hydrolyzes ATP. The myosin isoforms differ in their rate of release of ADP during the attachment to actin and therefore have different attachment times. Characteristics of muscle fibers that express type 1, type 2A, and type 2X MHC are given in Table 20-1. Hybrid fibers that contain type 1/2A or type 2A/2X MHC isoforms also exist in human muscles.

Type 1 fibers have the relatively slow acting myosin isoform and hence contract slowly, but they have a high capacity for oxidative metabolism (many mitochondria and hence high activities of enzymes of the citric acid cycle, of fatty acid oxidation, and of the electron transport chain), a high content of intramyocellular triacylglycerols (IMTGs), high hormone-sensitive lipase activity, and moderate glycolytic capacity. Type 2A fibers possess a more rapidly acting myosin ATPase and thus have faster contraction times than type 1 fibers. Type 2A fibers have a high glycolytic capacity but also have a moderate oxidative capacity. Type 2X fibers have the fastest acting myosin ATPase and a very high glycolytic capacity but a low oxidative capacity. These type 2X fibers contain more glycogen and much less IMTG than do the type 1 fibers.

TABLE 20-1 Characteristics of Major Skeletal Muscle Fiber Types

	TYPE 1 RED FIBERS SLOW OXIDATIVE FATIGUE RESISTANT	TYPE 2A RED FIBERS FAST OXIDATIVE FATIGUE RESISTANT	TYPE 2X WHITE FAST GLYCOLYTIC FATIGABLE
Myosin heavy chain isoform	MHC-β (gene *MCH7*)	MHC-2A (gene *MYH2*)	MHC-X (gene *MYH1*)
Myosin ATPase activity	Slow	Intermediate	Fast
Contraction velocity	Slow	Fast	Very fast
Resistance to fatigue	High	Intermediate	Low
Recruitment order	Early	Intermediate	Late
Activity used for	Aerobic (e.g., long-distance running)	Long-term aerobic plus anaerobic (e.g., middle-distance running and swimming)	Short-term anaerobic (e.g., sprinting)
Myoglobin content	High	Intermediate	Low
Generate ATP by	Aerobic system	Aerobic system	Anaerobic system
Mitochondrial density	High	Intermediate	Low
Capillary density	High	Intermediate	Low
Oxidative capacity	High	Intermediate	Low
Glycolytic capacity (glycogen phosphorylase)	Low	High	High
Creatine phosphate content	Intermediate	High	High
Glycogen content	Low	High	High
Triacylglycerol content	High	Intermediate	Low

Although all three types of fibers are found within individual muscles, the proportions of fiber types vary depending on the action of that muscle. Although a mixture of fiber types is present within skeletal muscles, only one type of muscle fiber is contained within a particular motor unit. Therefore if a weak contraction is needed, only the type 1 motor units will be activated, whereas if a stronger contraction is needed, the type 2A fibers will also be activated to assist the type 1 fibers. Type 2X fibers are activated last and are needed for maximal contractions, but these fibers tire easily. In addition to increasing the number of contractile units simultaneously activated, the intensity of the overall muscle contraction can be increased by increasing the frequency at which action potentials are sent to muscle fibers.

It has traditionally been assumed that type 2 fibers are specialized to perform sprinting exercise, whereas type 1 fibers are more suited to perform endurance exercise. In agreement with this, the better sprinters tend to have a high percentage of type 2 fibers, whereas a marathoner may have a much higher percentage of type 1 fibers. Certainly, genetic factors play a role in determining fiber type distribution. In addition, muscle fibers display a degree of plasticity that allows them to reversibly change their biochemical and morphologic properties when exposed to different functional demands. For example, strength or resistance (low repetition, high load) training can lead to an increase in the myofibrillar volume (hypertrophy) of both type 1 and type 2 fibers. High-intensity endurance (high repetition, low load) training can increase the proportion of type 1 fibers (increase in mitochondrial and capillary density), but it does not result in an increase in fiber size. It is thought that both metabolic and mechanical signals are involved in bringing about these changes (Putman et al., 2004; Hoppeler and Flück, 2002).

THE ENERGY COST OF MOVEMENT

Muscle shortening and movement are brought about by repeated formation of crossbridges between the thin (actin) and thick (myosin) filaments of the myofibrils. This process costs energy and requires hydrolysis of ATP by the myofibrillar ATPase. The contraction cycles are under nervous control. Whenever a sufficient number of nerve impulses during a limited time period arrive at the muscle fiber, the following sequence is set into action: (1) the plasma membrane is depolarized by a short-term loss of potassium ions (K^+) and uptake of sodium ions (Na^+) into the muscle fiber; (2) the formed action potential is propagated along the sarcolemma into the T tubules, where (3) the signal is transmitted to the sarcoplasmic reticulum; this then leads to (4) a rapid release of Ca^{2+} from the sarcoplasmic reticulum and a 1,000-fold increase in the cytosolic Ca^{2+} concentration. This increase in cytosolic Ca^{2+} leads to (5) crossbridge formation between the actin and myosin filaments of the myofibrils and (6) activation of the myofibrillar ATPases, which couple ATP hydrolysis with breaking the formed crossbridges. The cytosolic Ca^{2+} concentration simultaneously is reduced again by the action of the calcium ATPase in the sarcoplasmic reticulum, and the muscle is ready for the next contraction.

The myofibrillar ATPase, the Na^+, K^+-ATPase (needed to restore the membrane potential following a depolarization), and the Ca^{2+}-ATPase are all much more active during exercise than at rest, resulting in consumption of large amounts of ATP. A muscle can in seconds increase its aerobic ATP turnover rate by more than a hundredfold. The higher the exercise intensity, the more contraction cycles are needed per unit of time, the greater the amount of ATP that needs to be synthesized per unit time, and the higher the amount of fuel that needs to be oxidized. Energy expenditure of skeletal muscle therefore is greatly influenced by the increased contractile activity needed to walk, work, or run.

At rest, whole-body energy expenditure of humans is about 80 watts or 68 kcal/hour (comparable to that of a light bulb), with approximately 25% (20 watts or 17 kcal/hour) being expended in the skeletal muscles. Energy expenditure during a marathon run covering 42 km in a little over 2 hours is about 20 times resting energy expenditure (1,600 watts or 1,377 kcal/hour). Because more than 90% of the increase in energy expenditure originates from fuel oxidation in the active muscle (part is needed for the cardiovascular response), and assuming that maximally about one half of skeletal muscle mass is actively used in running a marathon, the energy expenditure of this active half of skeletal muscle can be estimated to increase by more than 130-fold (from 10 watts to 1,368 watts), as shown in Figure 20-3. Skeletal muscle must therefore have powerful mechanisms to increase the rates of ATP synthesis and fuel oxidation. In an individual running a marathon, most of the required ATP is produced by aerobic oxidation of carbohydrate and fat.

A top-class sprinter during a 100-m sprint can achieve a power output of around 3,600 watts, which is approximately 45 times the resting energy expenditure. Because more than 95% of the increase in energy expenditure originates from increased fuel metabolism in the active muscle

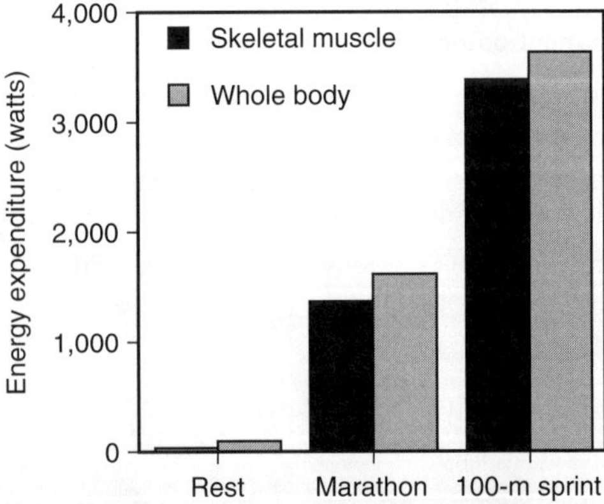

FIGURE 20-3 Whole-body and muscle energy expenditure at rest, during marathon running, and during a 100-m sprint. One watt is equivalent to 1 J/second or 2.39×10^{-4} kcal/second. One thousand watts therefore is equivalent to an energy expenditure of 0.239 kcal/second or 14 kcal/minute or 860 kcal/hour.

during a sprint, the energy expenditure of the active muscle is estimated to increase by more than 300-fold. Most of the ATP for a 100-meter sprint is produced anaerobically by net breakdown of muscle creatine phosphate and by conversion of muscle glycogen to lactate.

SKELETAL MUSCLE FUEL UTILIZATION DURING REST

Resting skeletal muscle needs less energy for maintenance per kilogram than that needed by such tissues as liver, gut, or kidney. The latter tissues not only have to take care of their own maintenance but also serve many essential functions in whole-body metabolism (e.g., digestion, absorption, fluid retention, urea synthesis, and lipoprotein synthesis) and are the sites of synthesis of many export proteins (e.g., albumin, fibrinogen, apolipoproteins, and digestive enzymes). Apart from a few muscles that are active continuously in the maintenance of posture, skeletal muscles in resting conditions have low energy expenditures. At rest, energy in the form of ATP is required for basic functions, including the maintenance of electrolyte and calcium gradients via ATP-dependent ion pumps, the maintenance of amino acid gradients (much higher intracellular than extracellular concentrations), the replacement of fuel stores lost via oxidation (glycogen and intramuscular triacylglycerols), the operation of substrate cycles (e.g., the fructose 6-phosphate/fructose 1,6-bisphosphate cycle and the triacylglycerol/free fatty acid cycle), and the maintenance of protein turnover (the continuous synthesis and breakdown of proteins). Even from the point of view of protein turnover, skeletal muscle needs less energy than abdominal tissues because the mean turnover rate of skeletal muscle protein (0.05% per hour) is lower than that of most other proteins of the human body and much lower than that of the intracellular and export proteins of liver and gut (e.g., apolipoprotein B-100, which is synthesized in the liver, with a turnover rate of 16% per hour). Therefore the need for ATP synthesis during rest is easily met by aerobic metabolism. For these reasons, skeletal muscle oxygen consumption constitutes only about 20% of whole-body oxygen consumption during resting conditions, despite the fact that the skeletal muscle compartment constitutes about 40% to 50% of body mass in a lean individual.

Skeletal muscle oxidizes a mixture of carbohydrate and fat even at rest. Although the impact of resting skeletal muscle gas exchange on the whole-body respiratory quotient (RQ) is small, measurements of the arteriovenous difference for oxygen and carbon dioxide across skeletal muscle have demonstrated the relative importance of fat and carbohydrate as fuels for the resting muscle. Himwich and Rose (1927), using such techniques in dogs, observed that the RQ of skeletal muscle in fed dogs was about 0.92, whereas the RQ of skeletal muscle in starved dogs was 0.80 and lower. The RQ is defined as moles CO_2 produced/moles O_2 consumed, and it is usually measured as volume of CO_2 produced/volume of O_2 consumed (see Chapter 21). Because an RQ of 1.00 indicates 100% carbohydrate oxidation and a value of 0.70 indicates 100% fat oxidation, it is clear that skeletal muscle at rest always oxidizes a mixture of carbohydrate and fat, even though the proportions vary substantially. This finding has been confirmed in humans on many occasions, using the same technique.

As discussed in Chapter 19, skeletal muscle of insulin-sensitive individuals is able to adapt to changes in fuel availability in response to meal intake or fasting and uses proportionately more glucose during the postprandial period and more fatty acids during the postabsorptive period. Carbohydrate is the main fuel for resting skeletal muscle in the fed situation, whereas fat oxidation accounts for two thirds or more of oxygen consumption in the postabsorptive and fasted situation. The transition from the fed to the fasted state is carefully controlled, as described in Chapters 12, 16, and 19.

Blood-borne fuels are sufficient for resting muscle. Plasma glucose is the major source of carbohydrate for oxidation in skeletal muscle at rest, particularly in the postprandial state. Plasma glucose originates from the diet in the first hours after a meal and originates from the liver in the postabsorptive or fasted state. The breakdown of liver glycogen to glucose is the major source of hepatic glucose output in the first 16 hours of fasting, whereas gluconeogenesis from glycerol and amino acids becomes the primary source of hepatic glucose output after 16 to 24 hours of fasting. The resting muscle uses mainly fatty acids during fasting, which originate from adipose tissue lipolysis and from very-low-density lipoprotein hydrolysis by muscle lipoprotein lipase. Fat oxidation by muscle is increased and carbohydrate disposal is decreased when the availability of fatty acids is increased by feeding high-fat diets or by infusion of lipids. Likewise, glucose infusion or loading can increase the muscle's utilization of glucose as fuel. Intramuscular fuels are relatively unimportant for resting muscle, so breakdown of muscle glycogen or of IMTG makes a minimal contribution to the energy needs of resting muscle.

FUEL UTILIZATION BY WORKING MUSCLE

Along with the increased energy expenditure by muscle when muscle is used to perform work, the fuel needs of muscle increase dramatically. At the onset of physical activity, signals from inside and outside the muscle fibers increase the availability of both carbohydrate and fat fuels as well as the ability to upregulate oxidation of both fuels simultaneously.

The fuel requirements of working muscle and the particular fuels that meet those energy requirements depend to a large extent on the intensity of the work being performed. The intensity of muscular work is often defined relative to a person's maximum aerobic capacity (VO_{2max}). VO_{2max} is a measure of the maximum volume of O_2 consumption. The maximal aerobic work rate is defined as 100% VO_{2max}. To exert a more intense effort, the fast glycolytic muscle fibers must be recruited. These fast glycolytic fibers function anaerobically using creatine phosphate and muscle glycogen as fuels, which is accompanied by lactate production. The extent to which an activity is primarily aerobic or primarily

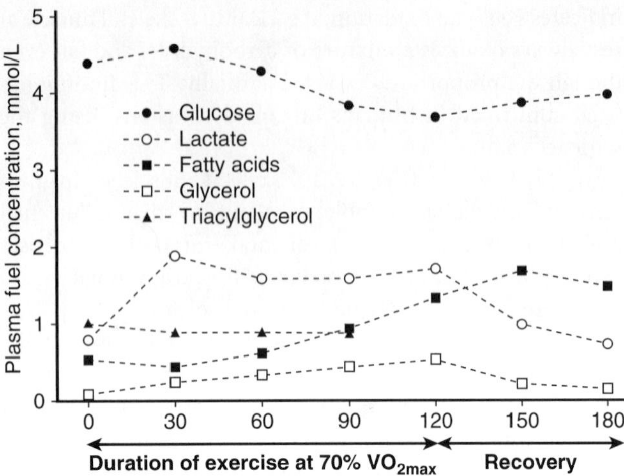

FIGURE 20-4 Plasma concentrations of fuels in healthy young male subjects in response to 120 minutes of exercise at 70% VO_{2max} followed by 1 hour of recovery. (Based on data from Hiscock, N., Fischer, C. P., Sacchetti, M., van Hall, G., Febbraio, M. A., & Pedersen, B. K. [2005]. Recombinant human interleukin-6 infusion during low intensity exercise does not enhance whole body lipolysis or fat oxidation in humans. *American Journal of Physiology. Endocrinology and Metabolism, 289,* E2–E7; Febbraio, M. A., Hiscock, N., Sacchetti, M., Fischer, C. P., & Pedersen, B. K. [2004]. Interleukin-6 is a novel factor mediating glucose homeostasis during skeletal muscle contraction. *Diabetes, 53,* 1643–1648; Whitley, H. A., Humphreys, S. M., Campbell, I. T., Keegan, M. A., Jayanetti, T. D., Sperry, D. A., ... Frayn, K. N. [1998]. Metabolic and performance responses during endurance exercise after high-fat and high-carbohydrate meals. *Journal of Applied Physiology, 85,* 418–424; Wallis, G. A., Dawson, R., Achten, J., Webber, J., & Jeukendrup, A. E. [2006]. Metabolic response to carbohydrate ingestion during exercise in males and females. *American Journal of Physiology. Endocrinology and Metabolism, 290,* E708–E715.)

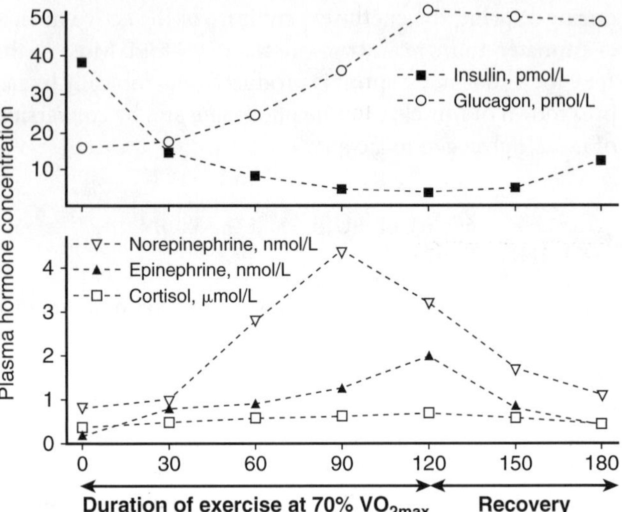

FIGURE 20-5 Plasma concentrations of hormones in healthy young male subjects in response to 120 minutes of exercise at 70% VO_{2max} followed by 1 hour of recovery. (Based on data from Hiscock, N., Fischer, C. P., Sacchetti, M., van Hall, G., Febbraio, M. A., & Pedersen, B. K. [2005]. Recombinant human interleukin-6 infusion during low-intensity exercise does not enhance whole body lipolysis or fat oxidation in humans. *American Journal of Physiology. Endocrinology and Metabolism, 289,* E2–E7; Febbraio, M. A., Hiscock, N., Sacchetti, M., Fischer, C. P., & Pedersen, B. K. [2004]. Interleukin-6 is a novel factor mediating glucose homeostasis during skeletal muscle contraction. *Diabetes, 53,* 1643–1648.)

anaerobic depends on its intensity relative to the individual's capacity for that type of physical activity.

PHYSIOLOGICAL CHANGES THAT ACCOMPANY PHYSICAL ACTIVITY

The onset of exercise results in changes in circulating hormone levels, an increase in blood flow to the working muscle, changes in muscle cytosolic Ca^{2+} concentration, and changes in the AMP/ATP ratio of the myocytes. These changes are responsible for many of the changes in fuel availability and fuel utilization that accompany an increase in physical activity.

Glucagon Increases Hepatic Glucose Production

With the onset of exercise, there is a fall in plasma glucose level (Figure 20-4). In response to the fall in the plasma glucose level, glucagon secretion from the pancreatic alpha cells increases during exercise, whereas insulin secretion from the pancreatic beta cells decreases (Figure 20-5). The increase in glucagon is the primary stimulator of hepatic glucoenogenesis during exercise. Berglund et al. (2009) showed that increasing glucagon in sedentary mice to levels similar to those seen during exercise caused a marked discharge of hepatic energy stores so that the AMP to ATP ratio increased. This increase in the AMP to ATP ratio presumably acts at least partially through activation of AMP-activated protein kinase (AMPK), as well as through allosteric mechanisms, to stimulate breakdown of glycogen in the liver. Glucagon is released from the pancreas into the portal circulation and may be largely removed by the liver before the blood reaches the arterial circulation, so that an increase in glucagon levels in the systemic circulation may not always be detected (Wasserman et al., 2011). Catecholamines do not seem to directly play an important role in increasing hepatic glucose production during exercise, although catecholamines can increase glucagon secretion. Thus during exercise, glucagon is important in stimulating hepatic glycogenolysis to maintain plasma glucose levels.

Catecholamines Stimulate Lipolysis and Use of Intracellular Fuels

The main stimuli to fat mobilization during exercise are the catecholamines, epinephrine and norepinephrine. Circulating catecholamine levels are regulated by the sympathoadrenal system. Current evidence indicates that the adrenergic stimulation of lipolysis during exercise is due mainly to circulating catecholamines rather than to sympathetic innervation of adipose tissue (Stallknecht et al., 2001; de Glisezinski et al., 2009). As shown in Figure 20-5, plasma catecholamine concentrations increase markedly with exercise (Hiscock et al., 2005; Febbraio et al., 2004). The fall in plasma insulin levels during exercise also creates a lipolytic environment and likely reinforces the effects of catecholamines. Growth hormone and glucocorticoids may also play a role, especially in prolonged exercise.

The consequence of this stimulation of adipose lipolysis during exercise is an increase in the rate of free fatty acid appearance in the plasma. The release of fatty acids into the plasma is typically two to three times that observed at rest. Because the release of free fatty acids is greater than the rate of total free fatty acid oxidation by the whole body, the plasma free fatty acid level increases above resting levels (see Figure 20-5). A portion of the free fatty acids released by adipose lipolysis can be reesterified, mainly in the liver where triacylglycerol synthesis is important for secretion of very-low-density lipoprotein (VLDL) triacylglycerol. Thus increased adipose lipolysis during exercise results in increased provision of both plasma free fatty acids (i.e., bound to albumin) and esterified fatty acids in the triacylglycerols of plasma lipoproteins.

The increased level of catecholamines also stimulates the use of the glycogen and triacylglycerol stores within the muscle fibers. Skeletal muscle fibers have β-adrenergic receptors that are activated by epinephrine and norepinephrine, and the intracellular cAMP-signaling pathway stimulates lipolysis of the IMTG and breakdown of glycogen to glucose phosphate for use by the muscle fiber. Therefore working muscle is able to use internal lipid and glycogen fuel stores and the circulating fuels supplied to the working muscle by the liver, adipose tissue, and diet.

Blood Flow to the Muscle Is Increased

Muscle blood flow is markedly increased with exercise. Local arterioles compensate for this by dilating and allowing more blood to reach the tissue, resulting in more delivery of oxygen and blood-borne fuels to working muscle as well as increased surface area for exchange due to increased capillary perfusion.

Stimulation of Muscle Contraction Results in Increases in Muscle Cytosolic Ca^{2+} Concentration and AMP/ATP Ratio

The stimulation of muscle fibers results in large increases in the cytosolic concentration of calcium ions, which in turn promotes muscle contraction. Muscle contraction and maintenance of ion fluxes require large expenditures of ATP. Thus both the cytosolic Ca^{2+} concentration and the AMP/ATP ratio are elevated in working muscle fibers. The levels of free ADP, free AMP, and P_i are particularly likely to be elevated during the first minutes of exercise before blood flow to the muscle is increased and the muscle is able to function aerobically, during prolonged endurance activity, and during work at super maximal intensities. Note that most of the AMP and ADP in muscle is bound to myosin and actin; "free" refers to the portion of these nucleoside phosphates that is not bound to proteins and hence is available for metabolic regulation.

The increase in free AMP level leads to activation of AMPK in skeletal muscle. AMPK acts as a sensor of cellular energy status and is activated by metabolic stresses, such as a decrease in substrate supply (as discussed in Chapter 19) or an increase in energy demand (such as muscle contraction), both of which increase the AMP/ATP ratio. The increases in cytosolic Ca^{2+} that accompany muscle contraction can also activate AMPK independently of adenine nucleotide changes. Once activated, AMPK acts on its downstream target proteins to alter metabolism in the working muscle to promote utilization of both glucose and fatty acids as fuels.

AMPK Overrides the Fatty Acid–Glucose Cycle and Permits Upregulation of Both Glucose and Fat Utilization

One of the targets of AMPK is the inhibitory phosphorylation of acetyl-CoA carboxylase (ACC2) to prevent malonyl-CoA formation which would block transport of fatty acids into the mitochondria. This action of AMPK essentially overrules the biochemical mechanisms involved in the glucose–fatty acid cycle, so that glucose oxidation by muscle no longer inhibits concurrent fatty acid oxidation. AMPK may also mediate enhanced secretion of lipoprotein lipase (LPL) and enhanced translocation of CD36 fatty acid transporter to the plasma membrane, both of which would favor fatty acid uptake by muscle.

AMPK Increases GLUT4 Translocation to the Sarcolemma in the Absence of Elevated Insulin Levels

Membrane transport is a primary barrier to muscle glucose uptake in the fasted, sedentary state, when myocyte membrane GLUT4 content is low. GLUT4 translocation to the muscle membrane is accelerated by muscle contraction and the intracellular signaling mechanisms (e.g., AMPK activation), resulting in increased muscle glucose uptake independent of the action of insulin. The fate of glucose extracted from the plasma is different in response to exercise than in response to insulin; the working muscle oxidizes glucose, whereas insulin-stimulated muscle primarily stores glucose.

Muscle Contraction Increases Glycogenolysis and Glycolysis in Muscle

Although glycogenolysis in muscle is upregulated by catecholamines during physical activity (i.e., cAMP/protein kinase A signaling pathway), the Ca^{2+} and AMP that result from an increased rate of muscle contraction may also promote net glycogen breakdown in muscle (see Chapter 12, Figures 12-15 and 12-16). These actions are the result of activation of calmodulin-dependent protein kinase, which inhibits glycogen synthase, and the activation of phosphorylase kinase, which activates glycogen phosphorylase and inhibits glycogen synthase. Muscle glycogen phosphorylase is also activated allosterically by AMP and inhibited by ATP. Free AMP and P_i are also important allosteric regulators of key enzymes in the pathways of glucose metabolism, stimulating the activity of 6-phosphofructo-1-kinase and inhibiting the activity of fructose 1,6-bisphosphatase. Thus increases in the concentrations of AMP and P_i in combination with the contraction-induced rise in cytosolic Ca^{+2} lead to a massive increase in the rates of glycogenolysis and glycolysis, especially when muscle is functioning anaerobically with lactate production.

CHANGES IN FUEL UTILIZATION DURING THE FIRST MINUTES OF INCREASED PHYSICAL ACTIVITY

Upon the start of physical activity, the ATP requirement for muscle contraction instantly increases to manyfold the resting level of ATP consumption, whereas the delivery of O_2 via the blood is somewhat delayed and restricts the muscle's capacity for aerobic oxidation of fuels. During this brief initial period, ATP hydrolysis is matched by resynthesis of ATP via creatine phosphate and glycogenolysis plus anaerobic glycolysis of the glucose phosphate to lactate.

The concentration of creatine phosphate in human muscle is 80 to 85 μmol/g of dry muscle—that is, some four to five times higher than the ATP concentration. The transfer of the phosphate group from creatine phosphate to ADP generated during contraction is catalyzed by the enzyme creatine kinase in the following reaction:

$$\text{Creatine phosphate} + \text{ADP} + H^+ \leftrightarrow \text{Creatine} + \text{ATP}$$

Lactate, as well as pyruvate and alanine, are released by the muscle during this period (van Hall, 2010). The initial adjustment of glycolytic rate may be the result of activation of 6-phosphofructo-1-kinase by AMP and P_i (see Chapter 12, Figure 12-8). Lactate production from pyruvate is driven by mass action due to the high concentrations of pyruvate and NADH that are generated. If exercise continues at the same workload, the muscle cells will switch to aerobic metabolism of fuels, which is accompanied by a decrease in the glycogenolytic rate and decreased lactate release. However, when workload is increased incrementally, each step of increase in workload may cause an initial period of creatine phosphate hydrolysis and lactate production from glucose phosphate obtained from muscle glycogen.

FUEL UTILIZATION BY MUSCLE FOR AEROBIC ACTIVITIES

For physical activity below the VO_{2max}, skeletal muscle uses both carbohydrate and lipid fuels. As illustrated in Figure 20-6, utilization of total fat and utilization of total carbohydrate both increase as the intensity of exercise is increased from rest or low intensity to moderate intensity (Romijn et al., 1993; van Loon et al., 2001). Oxidation of total fat increases with an increase in exercise intensity up to approximately 65% VO_{2max}, and then decreases as intensity is further increased. It has been difficult to discriminate between utilization of fatty acids derived from the action of muscle lipoprotein lipase on circulating lipoprotein triacylglycerol and utilization of intramuscular lipid stores, so these two sources are grouped together in the data used to generate Figure 20-6. Oxidation of both fatty acids and IMTGs decreases beyond 65% VO_{2max}. The mechanisms by which fat utilization is decreased at higher intensities of muscular work are not fully understood. In contrast to fat, utilization of total carbohydrate increases progressively over the whole range of exercise intensity. Although utilization of both plasma glucose and muscle glycogen stores increase progressively as exercise intensity increases from low to moderate to high, these increases are not proportionate. The contribution of muscle glycogen is much greater than that of plasma

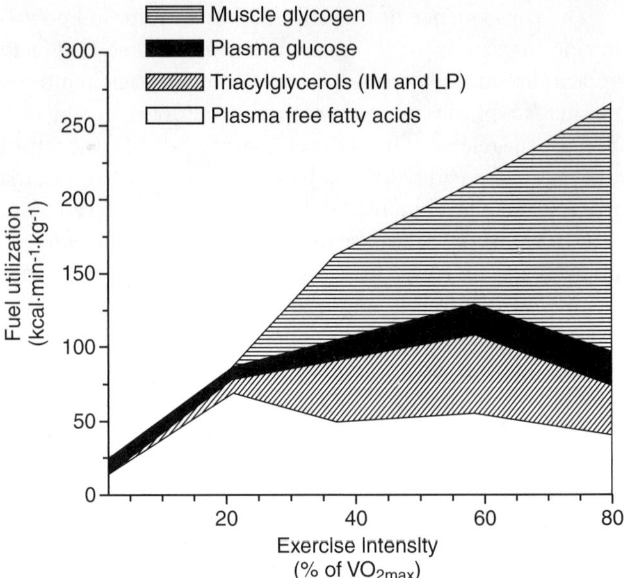

FIGURE 20-6 Utilization of fuel mixtures by the exercising muscle at different exercise intensities. Values are based on data for male cyclists who exercised while in the postabsorptive state following an overnight fast. (Data from Romijn, J. A., Coyle, E. F., Sidossis, L. S., Gastaldelli, A., Horowitz, J. F., Endert, E., & Wolfe, R. R. [1993]. Regulation of endogenous fat and carbohydrate metabolism in relation to exercise intensity and duration. *The American Journal of Physiology, 265,* E380–E391; van Loon, L. J. C., Greenhaff, P. L., Constantin-Teodosiu, D., Saris, W. H. M., Wagenmakers, A. J. M. [2001]. The effects of increasing exercise intensity on muscle fuel utilization in humans. *The Journal of Physiology, 536,* 295–304.)

glucose at work intensities above 35% VO_{2max}. At the higher work intensities, muscle glycogen provides more than half of the total energy used by the muscle.

Use of Fatty Acids by Exercising Muscle

Figure 20-7 summarizes the sources of fatty acids for muscle. The increase in fat oxidation with a shift from rest to moderate exercise intensity results mainly from increased fatty acid availability due to stimulation of lipolysis and increased blood flow to muscle (see Figure 20-7). A decrease in the plasma free fatty acid concentration during the first 15 minutes of exercise (e.g., from ~0.3 mmol/L in the fed state to ~0.15 mmol/L) is frequently observed because the muscle initially takes up fatty acids faster than fatty acids are generated by lipolysis. However, the rate of generation soon exceeds the rate of utilization by muscle, and the plasma fatty acid concentration increases up to 1.5–2.0 mmol/L. Because an increase in plasma fatty acid concentration also leads to increased uptake by the liver and incorporation of these fatty acids into triacylglycerols that are in turn incorporated into VLDL, the increase in plasma fatty acid concentrations along with greater blood flow delivers more free fatty acids and lipoprotein triacylglycerols to muscle to use as fuel during exercise.

In addition, fatty acids are mobilized from the IMTG within the muscle fibers by muscle triacylglycerol lipase, hormone-sensitive lipase (diacylglycerol lipase), and monoacylglycerol lipase. IMTG is highest in oxidative type 1 muscle

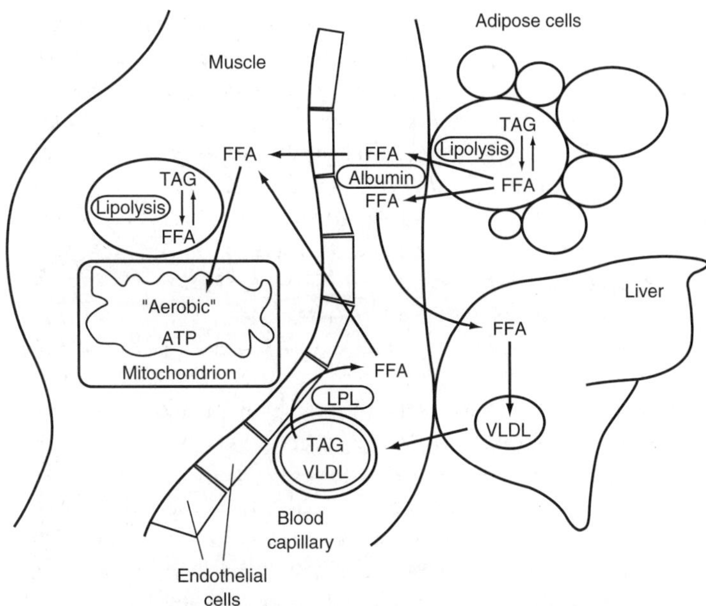

FIGURE 20-7 Sources of fatty acids for oxidation by skeletal muscle during prolonged exercise. *FFA,* Free fatty acid; *LPL,* lipoprotein lipase; *TAG,* triacylglycerol; *VLDL,* very-low-density lipoprotein.

fibers and is localized mostly adjacent to the mitochondria. The intramuscular stores of triacylglycerol are relatively small compared to those of adipose tissue; the total IMTG amounts to approximately 300 g in an adult (Jeukendrup, 2003). In the initial minutes of low and moderate aerobic exercise, muscle lipolysis of IMTG is activated by contractions in the apparent absence of increases in circulating epinephrine, perhaps due to increased Ca^{2+} levels (Watt and Spriet, 2004). As exercise continues beyond a few minutes, activation of lipolysis by epinephrine through the cAMP signaling cascade also may occur. Depletion of IMTG appears to occur almost exclusively in type 1 muscle fibers. IMTG content of muscle of male cyclists was measured before and after 120 minutes of moderate-intensity exercise (60% of VO_{2max}); the IMTG in type 1 fibers was decreased by 62% of the pre-exercise level, whereas the IMTG content of type 2 fibers was not significantly affected (van Loon et al., 2003).

In addition to an increase in fatty acid availability to the muscle as a result of fatty acid uptake from the circulation and from intracellular lipolysis of IMTG, the rate of fatty acid oxidation by muscle is upregulated in response to exercise. Biopsies of moderately trained men performing bicycle exercise (60 minutes, 65% VO_{2max}) demonstrated that the exercise period resulted in a decrease in the malonyl-CoA concentration, which was associated with, and presumably secondary to, increased activity of AMPK and inhibition of acetyl-CoA carboxylase as a result of its phosphorylation by AMPK (Roepstorff et al., 2004). The decrease in malonyl-CoA level relieves inhibition of carnitine palmitoyltransferase 1 (CPT1) facilitating entry of fatty acids into the mitochondria for β-oxidation.

The contribution of fat as fuel dominates at low work intensities and seems to peak at moderate exercise intensities (~60% VO_{2max}, as shown in Figure 20-6). The exact intensity at which fat oxidation peaks varies among individuals and typically ranges from 45% to 65% of VO_{2max}. The average maximal fat oxidation is about 0.5 g per minute (Venables et al., 2005). The control of fat oxidation appears to be distributed among the acyl-CoA synthetase activity, which activates the long-chain fatty acids; CPTI activity, which transports the long-chain fatty acid across the mitochondrial membrane; and electron transport chain capacity, by way of substrate competiton between redox equivalents produced by fat or carbohydrate oxidation (Sahlin et al., 2008).

Use of Glucose by Exercising Muscle

Figure 20-8 summarizes the sources of glucose for muscle. As a result of exercise initiation, delivery of glucose to working muscle increases. Liver glycogen breakdown and the hepatic glucose output increase at the onset of exercise. As mentioned previously, activation of AMPK is one signal responsible for upregulation of GLUT4 translocation in working muscle. The maximal contribution of plasma glucose is approximately 1 g/minute, and this seems to be limited by the rate of appearance of glucose into plasma. Exogenous carbohydrate oxidation was increased to as much as 1.7 g/minute in athletes who ingested a carbohydrate source that provided a mixture of glucose plus fructose instead of glucose only (Wallis et al., 2005; Jentjens et al., 2004). The higher rate of carbohydrate oxidation when a mixture of glucose and fructose was consumed may be due to the fact that the two sugars use different intestinal transporters for absorption such that the rate of total sugar absorption can be increased by providing both glucose and fructose (Jeukendrup, 2004).

Muscle glycogen stores also are an important source of carbohydrate during moderate exercise. Typical muscle glycogen stores in an adult are approximately 300 g when intramuscular stores are full, compared with 80 to 100 g glycogen in liver stores in the postprandial state. Muscle

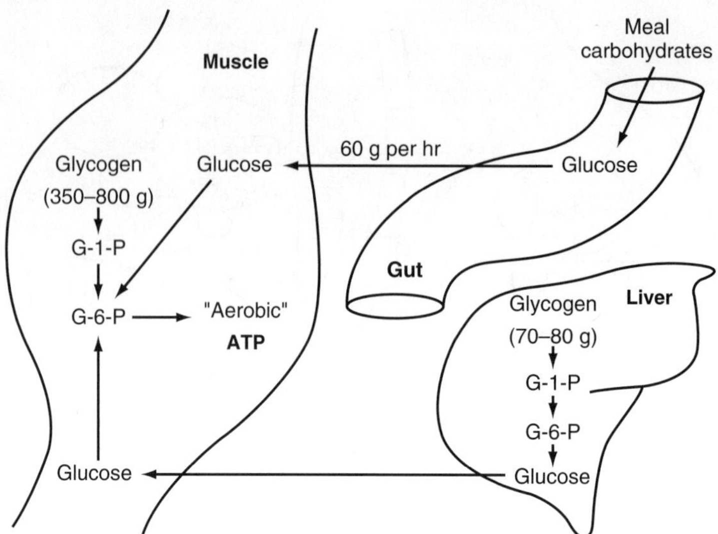

FIGURE 20-8 Sources of glucose available for oxidation by skeletal muscle during prolonged exercise.

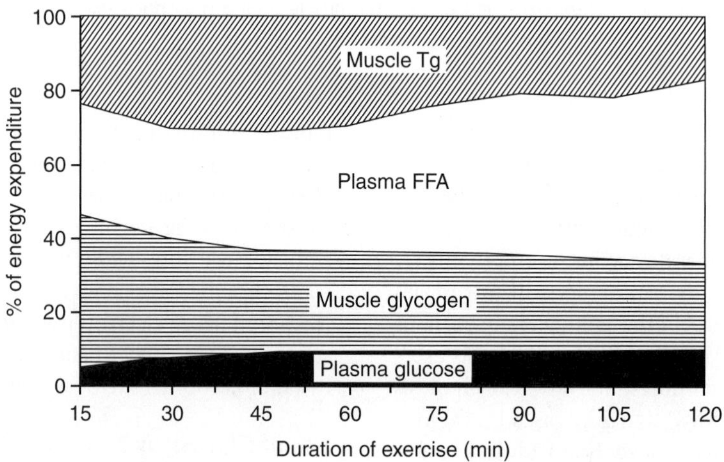

FIGURE 20-9 Relative contribution of carbohydrate and lipid fuels to energy production during 120 minutes of exercise at 65% VO_{2max} by endurance-trained cyclists who were in the postabsorptive state after a 10- to 12-hour fast. From Romijn, J. A., Coyle, E. F., Sidossis, L. S., Gastaldelli, A., Horowitz, J. F., Endert, E., & Wolfe, R. R. [1993]. Regulation of endogenous fat and carbohydrate metabolism in relation to exercise intensity and duration. *The American Journal of Physiology, 265,* E380–E391, with permission from the American Physiological Society.)

glycogen stores can vary from 50 g after strenuous exercise to 900 g in a well-fed, well-trained muscular person. Within muscle, glucose 1-phosphate generated from muscle glycogen breakdown is isomerized to glucose 6-phosphate and used along with plasma glucose. Because the muscle lacks glucose 6-phosphatase and is not able to produce much free glucose, muscle glycogen is used almost exclusively as a local fuel store and does not contribute much, if any, glucose to the circulation for maintenance of plasma glucose levels.

The extent of muscle glycogen stores appears to influence the relative utilization of fat versus carbohydrate during moderate-intensity work. The muscle of glycogen-depleted subjects oxidized more fat and had lower pyruvate dehydrogenase complex activity, lower concentrations of acetyl-CoA and acetylcarnitine, and a higher concentration of free carnitine (Roepstorff et al., 2005). Thus muscle of glycogen-depleted subjects should readily transport fatty acids into the mitochondria for oxidation. Conversely, in subjects with high muscle glycogen, the oxidative decarboxylation of pyruvate to acetyl-CoA would be favored, and this would favor malonyl-CoA synthesis and the inhibition of fatty acid transport into the mitochondria for oxidation. To a more limited extent, similar effects could presumably be accomplished by increasing plasma glucose availability during exercise by glucose infusion or provision of glucose plus fructose-containing drinks.

DEPLETION OF GLYCOGEN AFFECTS FUEL UTILIZATION IN PROLONGED EXERCISE

Despite the increased reliance on carbohydrate fuels as exercise intensity increases, these carbohydrate fuels are limited. Prolonged exercise at moderate or high intensities will ultimately lead to depletion of muscle glycogen stores and a greater reliance on lipid fuels, as illustrated in Figure 20-9.

A greater reliance on lipid fuels, however, will decrease the VO_{2max} at which one can work because optimal aerobic performance is dependent upon oxidation of both glucose and fatty acids simultaneously (see Figure 20-6).

EFFECTS OF PHYSICAL ACTIVITY ON MUSCLE ENERGY STATUS

Vastus lateralis muscle (which is located on the outer side of the thigh) of untrained volunteers performing prolonged cycle exercise (2 or 3 h at 60% VO_{2max}) exhibited depletion of creatine phosphate to 50% of the pre-exercise level and of muscle glycogen to 25% of the pre-exercise level (Green et al., 2011). In addition, muscle lactate concentration was increased to two to six times over the pre-exercise level, and the levels of free ADP and free AMP were markedly elevated. Intermittent cycling (1 or 16 cycles of cycling for 6 min at 90% VO_{2max}, with 54 min between repetitions) similarly resulted in depletion of creatine phosphate to 10% to 30% of the pre-exercise level, an increase in muscle lactate concentration to 10 to 22 times the pre-exercise level, and marked elevations in free ADP and free AMP concentrations (Green et al., 2007). Glycogen fell by about 25% during the first repetition, did not recover in the rest period between repetitions, and continued to fall with successful repetitions of cycling, reaching about 10% of the initial resting level by the end of the sixteenth repetition. During the postexercise recovery period, ATP, creatine phosphate, and glycogen levels need to be restored to resting conditions.

IMTG in type 1 muscle fibers is also depleted during physical activity, but difficulties with accurate measurement of IMTG have made it difficult to quantitate the extent of depletion. Analysis of vastus lateralis biopsies from male subjects who performed 2 to 3 h of cycling at 62% or 75% VO_{2max} indicated that IMTG was reduced to 30% to 70% of pre-exercise levels (Stellingwerff et al., 2007; de Bock et al. 2007).

FUEL UTILIZATION DURING THE POSTEXERCISE RECOVERY PERIOD

During the postexercise period, both fatty acids and glucose are taken up by muscle. The insulin sensitivity of muscle is greater when glycogen is depleted, so glucose uptake is upregulated. However, in studies of fuel utilization by endurance-trained male subjects over the 18-hour period after an exhaustive bout of exercise, plasma lipids appeared to be the major source of fuel at 1, 4, and 7 hours of recovery, even in subjects fed high-carbohydrate meals (66% of energy as carbohydrate, 21% as fat) (Kimber et al., 2003). Despite the elevation of glucose and insulin following the high-carbohydrate meal, carbohydrate oxidation and pyruvate dehydrogenase complex activation were decreased, supporting the hypothesis that glycogen resynthesis is of high metabolic priority during the postexercise period. Muscle glycogen increased significantly and progressively at 3, 6, and 18 hours of recovery. Consistent with less reliance on carbohydrate as fuel, the concentrations of acetyl-CoA, acetylcarnitine, and pyruvate all declined during recovery. No net change in the content of IMTG was observed over the course of the recovery period. Therefore plasma lipids (free fatty acids and/or lipoprotein triacylglycerol) were the major fuels used by muscle during recovery.

Repletion of IMTG stores in type 1 fibers requires a longer recovery period. In a study of trained male cyclists (van Loon et al., 2003), IMTG content was decreased by 21% by prolonged endurance cycling (3 hours at 55% VO_{2max}). During recovery, IMTG content at 24 and 48 hours postexercise was not increased in subjects consuming a carbohydrate-rich diet (24% energy from fat) but did increase in subjects consuming a higher-fat diet (39% energy from fat), reaching pre-exercise levels within 48 hours. IMTG stores were nearly replenished by 5 hours in fasted subjects (Krssak et al., 2000). It appears that IMTG accumulates largely in response to elevations of plasma free fatty acids, and, in fact, the IMTG pool is dynamic during exercise, with both lipolysis and esterification occurring concurrently (Johnson et al., 2004).

FUELS FOR SHORT BURSTS OF SUPER INTENSE PHYSICAL ACTIVITY

Recruitment of type 2X fast glycolytic fibers permits work at intensities greater than VO_{2max} for short periods of up to about 2 minutes. The major fuels for such activities are stored ATP, creatine phosphate, and muscle glycogen. Nearly all the glycogen that is used is broken down anaerobically to lactic acid. Sporting events that require short bursts of activity that depend on contraction of the glycolytic fibers include very short running, swimming, or cycling events (i.e., sprinting); track and field activities such as jumping or vaulting; many gymnastic routines; and weight lifting. Strength training is primarily an anaerobic activity that uses gravity or elastic/hydraulic forces to oppose muscle contraction. Pedaling a bicycle ergometer at heavy loads that can be maintained for no more than 1 or 2 minutes also requires use of glycolytic fibers. In addition, somewhat less intense exercise lasting upwards of about 4 minutes (e.g., a mile race) may still have a considerable anaerobic energy expenditure component.

During the first seconds of super-intense activity, creatine phosphate is used to replenish ATP, but this is followed by greater glycogen breakdown and glycolysis. Breakdown of the glycogen stores and subsequent glycolysis with formation of lactate is quantitatively the most important process for ATP production during sprinting. If the activity is performed only once, muscle creatine phosphate stores can be substantially depleted but only small changes in glycogen occur due to the short period of activity. If bursts of maximal activity are repeated many times with intervening rest pauses, there will be some replenishment of ATP and creatine phosphate during the rest periods, at least partially at the expense of glycogen stores. At the end of repeated work-rest intervals, creatine phosphate is likely to be severely depleted and glycogen is likely to be modestly reduced.

Figure 20-10 shows the use of fuels by a runner during a 10-second sprint. During the first seconds of the sprint, ATP hydrolyzed during contraction is almost instantaneously regenerated from creatine phosphate, with ATP level being reduced by about 20% and creatine phosphate by about 80%. The increase in the AMP/ATP ratio and the contraction-induced rise in cytosolic Ca^{2+} that occur during the first few seconds lead to a massive increase in the rate of glycogenolysis and glycolysis (lactate production). In approximately 4 to 5 seconds from the start of a sprint, the rate of glycolysis increases to 1,000-fold or more. Most of the energy demand of the 100-m sprint is covered by anaerobic metabolism of muscle glycogen. Even though muscle glycogen stores are not exhausted, even world class athletes begin to slow down after 80 to 100 m and cannot maintain full speed. Fatigue processes come into operation and reduce the force-generating capacity of the muscle, but the exact mechanism of fatigue during sprinting is not known. Although a 100-m sprint can be run at highest power using anaerobic fibers, an athlete running a longer 400-m sprint must deliberately reduce the maximal power output so that fatigue develops less rapidly and so that a reasonable pace can be maintained. Part of the ATP production is covered, in this case, by aerobic oxidation of glycogen (glycolysis, oxidative decarboxylation of pyruvate by the pyruvate dehydrogenase complex, and oxidation of acetyl-CoA via the citric acid cycle, coupled with the electron transport chain and oxidative phosphorylation); the contribution of aerobic oxidation rapidly increases between the start and finish of a 400-m sprint.

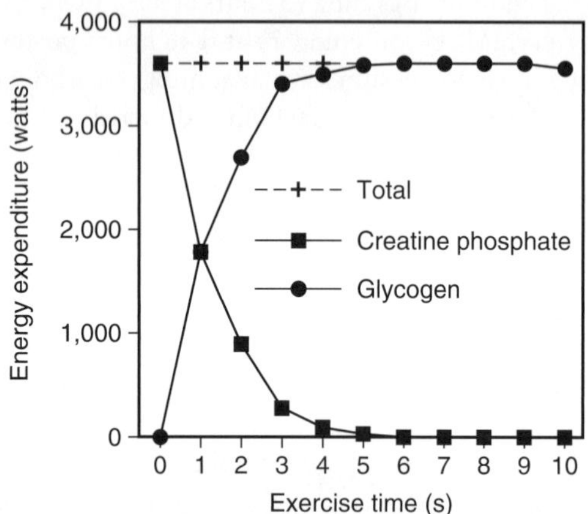

FIGURE 20-10 Utilization of creatine phosphate and muscle glycogen as fuels over the course of a 100-m sprint.

CLINICAL CORRELATION

McArdle Disease—A Disorder Affecting Muscle Fuel

McArdle disease is a metabolic myopathy characterized by exercise intolerance manifested by rapid fatigue, myalgia (muscle pain), and cramps in exercising muscles. Symptoms are precipitated by isometric exercise (e.g., weight lifting) and sustained aerobic exercise (e.g., stair-climbing and jogging) and typically are relieved by rest. McArdle disease was first diagnosed in 1951 by Brian McArdle in a patient who presented with exercise-induced myalgia and who failed to produce a rise in blood lactate during an ischemic forearm exercise test. McArdle disease was subsequently found to be caused by a deficiency of the skeletal muscle-specific isoform of glycogen phosphorylase. In most affected individuals, there is no detectable glycogen phosphorylase activity in skeletal muscle, resulting in a complete block in muscle glycogen breakdown. In addition to having a flat plasma lactate curve in response to onset of exercise, patients have elevated levels of plasma creatine kinase activity.

A number of underlying mutations in the muscle glycogen phosphorylase gene (*PYGM*) have been identified for this disease, which is inherited in an autosomal recessive manner. The disease is rare, affecting less than 1 in 100,000 in the general population. McArdle disease is one of many types of glycogen storage diseases and is classified as glycogen storage disease type V. Although patients are often not diagnosed until their second or third decade, patients have often had symptoms since childhood.

Most individuals with McArdle disease are able to improve their exercise tolerance by exploiting the "second wind" phenomenon. Pain generally occurs within a few minutes of initiating exercise. However, if at this stage the person rests until the pain subsides, the person can resume the physical activity (e.g., walking or cycling) with much better tolerance. Another adjustment the body may make in individuals with McArdle disease is to recruit more motor units, and hence a larger muscle mass, to perform a particular workload. This may partially explain observations that these patients have an abnormally high cardiac output and heart rate at a given absolute power.

In general, individuals with McArdle disease need to avoid intense anaerobic exercise and maximal aerobic exercise to prevent cramps and muscle damage. They should also avoid continuing to exercise at any activity level if they are experiencing severe pain, as this can result in muscle damage and myoglobinuria, which in turn can lead to renal failure.

Thinking Critically

1. Why would patients with McArdle disease tolerate light or moderate aerobic physical activity much better than anaerobic or intense or sustained aerobic exercise?
2. Why would the first few minutes of any exercise be difficult for an individual with McArdle disease? What is the metabolic basis of the "second wind"?
3. Would ingestion of carbohydrate immediately before exercise be of benefit? Would this be practical for patients who experience exercise intolerance during activities of daily living?
4. How does regular moderate aerobic exercise improve exercise tolerance in McArdle patients? What would happen if patients avoided exercise and became increasingly sedentary?

SKELETAL MUSCLE ADAPTATIONS IN RESPONSE TO TRAINING AND THE CONSEQUENCES FOR FUEL UTILIZATION AND PERFORMANCE

The response to training is determined largely by the mode of training (i.e., aerobic/endurance versus anaerobic/resistance/strength) and by the volume, intensity, and frequency of the contractions. Furthermore, response to training varies with individual characteristics and with degree of initial fitness. Bone mineral density tends to increase with exercise in the specific bones upon which substantial force is placed due to contraction of muscles or gravity. Muscles that are relatively untrained tend to show more substantial responses to training than do trained ones. Although most physical activities involve both dynamic and static contractions and aerobic and anaerobic metabolism, activities are usually classified based on the predominant mechanical or metabolic characteristics.

Dynamic aerobic training (e.g., jogging, biking, swimming laps) has long been known to be associated with cardiovascular adaptations (e.g., increased cardiac output and heart rate, increased gas exchange in the lungs, and increased capillary density in skeletal muscle) that improve endurance and VO_{2max}. Aerobic training also affects the characteristics of the muscle fibers themselves. One of the most important training-induced adaptations is the increase in the number of mitochondria per unit mass of skeletal muscle. This results in increased activities of enzymes involved in the citric acid cycle, oxidative phosphorylation, and β-oxidation. Aerobic training also results is an increased uptake and oxidation of fatty acids by muscle, which may be at least partially due to changes in fatty acid transport proteins (FAT/CD36 and FABPm) in the sarcolemmal and mitochondrial membranes (Talanian et al., 2010; Hawley et al., 2011). In addition, the IMTG content of muscle can be substantially greater in trained endurance athletes than in sedentary subjects (van Loon et al., 2004). Because aerobic training results in a greater reliance on fat oxidation, it reduces the rate of utilization of muscle glycogen and plasma glucose and limits the rate of lactate production during exercise of moderate to high intensity.

Resistance training (e.g., lifting weights, working with resistance bands, push-ups) enhances muscular strength and muscle mass. Although anaerobic or resistance/strength training also improves metabolic homeostasis, it appears to do this in a manner largely distinct from that of aerobic/endurance training. Resistance exercise increases the size and abundance of predominantly glycolytic fibers. However, distinct from endurance training, the activity of key oxidative enzymes and aerobic capacity are not enhanced. Thus changes in metabolic fitness may occur without changes in aerobic capacity. Resistance exercise is effective therapy for the reversal of injury or illness-induced muscle loss, as well as for the enhancement of muscle mass.

NUTRITIONAL AND ERGOGENIC AIDS TO TRAINING AND/OR PERFORMANCE

The greatest stimulus to any exercise-induced skeletal muscle adaptation is the repeated bouts of training. Use of dietary alterations or ergogenic aids might have some effects on training or performance for the elite athlete, but these are generally of little importance for the typical individual. Strategic eating and refueling, as well as a few ergogenic aids, may optimize performance and training adaptations (Kreider et al., 2010).

CARBOHYDRATE INTAKE AND GLYCOGEN LOADING

Manipulation of muscle glycogen stores during training and performance may have beneficial effects, although not all investigations have led to the same conclusions. High skeletal muscle glycogen stores exert a negative regulatory effect on both contraction- and insulin-stimulated GLUT4 translocation and modulate the expression of many exercise-induced genes. Beginning endurance exercise with low muscle glycogen stores results in a greater transcriptional activation of enzymes involved in carbohydrate metabolism, including hexokinase and pyruvate dehydrogenase complex, compared with when glycogen content is normal (Hawley and Burke, 2010; Hawley et al., 2011). However, restricting carbohydrate availability has reciprocal and pronounced effects on lipid availability, so benefits of training with low glycogen stores could be offset by the increased lipid availability to muscle. High-fat, low-carbohydrate diets decrease circulating insulin levels and downregulate the active form of pyruvate dehydrogenase complex, mainly through an increase of the diet-sensitive pyruvate dehydrogenase kinase 4 isozyme (PDK4); this decreases carbohydrate oxidation (Hawley and Burke, 2010).

Resting glycogen concentrations in human skeletal muscle range from about 10 to 23 g/kg of wet muscle, generally with greater concentrations found in highly trained athletes than in sedentary individuals. Carbohydrate loading is frequently used by athletes to enhance or supersaturate their muscle glycogen stores before competition. Carbohydrate loading leading to high glycogen content at the start of a prolonged endurance event, such as running a marathon, helps athletes maintain their pace for a longer period of time before they must slow down. In intermittent high-intensity sports involving many repeated short distance sprints, the size of the glycogen stores in the muscle determines the total distance that can be covered at full speed. Carbohydrate loading is usually done by tapering training for 2 to 3 days before competition and by consuming 200 to 300 g per day extra carbohydrate in the diet. Ingestion of a carbohydrate-rich meal about 4 hours before competition also improves performance because it helps replenish the liver glycogen stores lost during the postabsorptive period between meals.

Performance may be increased by ingestion of small amounts of carbohydrate before and during exercise. Ingestion of a carbohydrate snack 30 to 60 min before exercise may increase carbohydrate availability near the end of an intense exercise bout. When exercise lasts more than 1 hour, ingestion of sugar- and electrolyte-containing drinks helps maintain plasma glucose levels and prevents dehydration. By maintaining plasma glucose concentration, carbohydrate ingestion maintains the total glucose oxidation rate at higher values during prolonged exercise.

PROTEIN AND AMINO ACID INTAKE

In the middle of the nineteenth century, the renowned German physiologist Justus von Liebig assumed that the protein of skeletal muscle was consumed during muscular work as a fuel and believed that large quantities of meat and protein should be eaten by industrial workers to replenish the protein losses during physical exercise. This was shown to be incorrect in the late nineteenth century, when careful nitrogen balance studies failed to show increased nitrogen losses during periods of increased physical activity. Use of stable isotope studies to assess whole-body protein turnover in fed subjects have shown that net whole-body protein oxidation during periods of exercise generally do not differ from those observed in the resting state or during the postexercise period. Modest increases in plasma urea concentration and urinary urea excretion have been observed, however, during ultramarathons and during exercise in the laboratory after overnight or more prolonged fasting.

Although protein is not a major fuel during exercise, net protein synthesis in response to resistance-type exercise may be synergistically stimulated by protein or amino acid intake, depending on the timing of intake (Hawley et al., 2011). Provision of protein or amino acids very soon after resistance exercise has a significant, positive effect on muscle protein synthesis, yielding rates of muscle protein synthesis that are markedly greater than those obtained by exercise alone or that are obtained by providing a similar number of calories as carbohydrate. Pre-exercise protein or amino acid supplementation does not appear to be of much benefit, whereas provision of protein during exercise appears to allow earlier rises in the blood amino acid profile and further promote a rise in muscle protein synthesis. Leucine is a key regulator of muscle protein synthesis, and leucine-enriched amino acid mixtures or naturally leucine-enriched proteins are most effective in promoting postexercise hypertrophy.

Koopman and colleagues (2004) studied the effect of addition of protein to a carbohydrate-containing beverage on protein balance in trained male subjects who were studied after an overnight fast. Subjects were evaluated at rest before exercise, during a 6-hour period of cycling and treadmill at moderate intensity, and during a 4-hour recovery period. Combined ingestion of protein (0.25 g/kg every hour) and carbohydrate (0.7 g/kg every hour) improved net protein balance at rest as well as during exercise and postexercise recovery compared to intake of carbohydrate alone. In another study, untrained male subjects who had fasted overnight performed a 45-minute resistance exercise protocol (Koopman et al., 2005). After exercise, subjects were given a bolus of a test drink that contained carbohydrate (0.3 g/kg per hour) with or without protein (0.2 g/kg per hour) and leucine (0.1 g/kg per hour). Additional boluses of the test drink were given at 30-min intervals throughout a 6-hour postexercise period. The plasma insulin response was greater for subjects given the beverage that contained both protein and carbohydrate than in those given only carbohydrate, and it was also greater in subjects given the drink that contained carbohydrate plus both protein and leucine than in subjects given the test beverage with carbohydrate and protein. Mixed muscle fractional synthetic rate, measured over the 6-h postexercise recovery period, was highest in subjects given the beverage supplemented with both protein and leucine, intermediate in those given the beverage supplemented with protein, and lowest in those given only carbohydrate.

Although these studies suggest a role of protein ingestion during the postexercise period for subjects who exercised while fasted, it should be noted that athletes normally perform in the fed state. Benefits observed in fasted subjects may not be observed in fed subjects. Also, in general, the stimulation of net protein deposition by protein or amino acid intake is rather transitory, lasting a few hours at most, whereas the stimulation of net muscle protein synthesis by contractile activity continues after the end of the resistance-type exercise period, lasting for hours or days.

Individuals engaged in general fitness programs do not need protein intakes above the Recommended Dietary Allowance (RDA). A typical diet, which provides about 15% of total energy from protein, should easily meet the protein requirement of most individuals. It is frequently recommended that individuals who are engaged in intense training consume more than the generally recommended daily amount of protein (i.e., more than the RDA of 0.8 g per kg body weight), and there is evidence that higher protein intakes ensure faster recovery and greater training adaptations in untrained subjects. Addition of protein and or branched-chain amino acids during or after resistance training may increase protein synthesis and gains in muscle mass beyond normal adaptation. It should be noted, however, that individuals engaged in intense training will consume higher amounts of protein in their typical diets due to their increased energy expenditure and therefore will increase their intakes of both energy and protein just by their increased food intake without the use of any supplements.

WATER, CREATINE, AND CAFFEINE

Preventing dehydration during exercise or physical activity is important for performance and health, particularly in hot and humid environments. Frequent ingestion of water or sports drinks during exercise is one of the most effective ergogenic aids. Most sports drinks contain salt (electrolytes) and carbohydrates (sugars).

Creatine is often recommended to athletes as an effective ergogenic aid, particularly to those performing high intensity, intermittent exercise. Creatine supplementation during training (e.g., ~0.3 g/kg for at least 3 days followed by daily intake of 3 to 5 g thereafter) has been shown to increase muscle mass and strength, mainly due to its enabling the athlete to train harder and thereby promote greater muscle adaptation and hypertrophy during training. Creatine has been shown to increase exercise capacity in a variety of events.

Caffeine appears to improve performance in both endurance and resistance sports. The benefits may be greatest for individuals who do not regularly consume caffeinated drinks. Caffeine may exert its effects through the central nervous system or through its metabolic effects on fuel metabolism.

MUSCLE FUEL UTILIZATION AND HEALTH OUTCOMES

Physical activity has well-established effects on cardiorespiratory fitness, body composition, and insulin sensitivity. Physical activity increases energy expenditure and therefore helps to prevent and treat obesity. Physical activity and energy expenditure directly facilitate the disposal of glucose and lipid via oxidation to generate ATP to support muscle contraction. An increase in muscle mass as a result of resistance training can also enhance energy expenditure and fuel utilization. In addition, physical activity stimulates numerous adaptations in skeletal muscle and in the cardiorespiratory system (Williams et al., 2007). These changes, in turn, influence metabolism in other tissues. Different types of physical activity appear to cause different types of adaptations in skeletal muscle, and a combination of endurance and resistance exercise is generally beneficial. Acute extreme exercise often elicits an inflammatory response (Ploeger et al., 2009; Gleeson et al., 2011). Participation in regular exercise or training can reduce the resting levels of pro-inflammatory markers and blunt the inflammatory response to a single bout of acute exercise in some individuals.

Endurance exercise results in stimulation of peroxisome proliferator-activated receptor-γ coactivator 1 (PGC1), increased mitochondrial biogenesis, augmentation of oxidative capacity, increased insulin-stimulated glucose uptake by skeletal muscle, and increased glucose disposal by muscle (Wang and Sahlin, 2011; Wang et al., 2011). PGC1 is preferentially expressed in type 1 oxidative fibers, and reduced PGC1 expression is associated with obesity and type 2 diabetes mellitus (Eckardt et al., 2011). PGC1 is thought to act downstream of calcium signaling pathways to coordinate the expression of various nuclear genes, including those involved in mitochondrial biogenesis and in adaptations of the metabolic and contractile properties of muscle fibers. Increased formation of reactive oxygen species, increased secretion of cytokines and myokines, and decreased levels of certain lipid metabolites (e.g., diacylglycerol and ceramide) have been implicated in the effects of muscle activity on insulin sensitivity and metabolic disease. IMTG content of muscle has been shown to decrease during prolonged submaximal exercise (Schrauwen-Hinderling et al., 2006; Zehnder et al., 2006). In active lean individuals, the IMTG pool appears to be regularly depleted during exercise and replenished during subsequent feeding (Shaw et al., 2010). This active turnover of muscle IMTG may be responsible for maintenance of low concentrations of lipid metabolites and a high level of insulin sensitivity.

Resistance training also improves metabolic homeostasis in patients with type 2 diabetes or cardiovascular disease. In humans with type 2 diabetes mellitus, resistance training

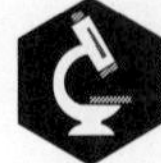

CLINICAL CORRELATION

Recommendations for Physical Activity for Health Benefits

A number of groups have established recommendations for physical activity, and more recent recommendations include a resistance/strength training component in addition to aerobic or "cardio" activities. The U.S. Department of Health and Human Services (USDHHS), the American College of Sports Medicine (ACSM), and the American Heart Association (AHA) have made recommendations for healthy adults with the goal of maintaining health and reducing risk for chronic disease. The ACSM and AHA recommended that healthy adults under age 65 years do moderately intense aerobic exercise 30 minutes a day for 5 days a week, or do vigorously intense aerobic exercise 20 minutes a day for 3 days a week and do 8 to 10 strength-training exercises with 8 to 12 repetitions of each exercise twice a week (Haskell et al., 2007). Additional strength-training repetitions were recommended for older adults. In the *2008 Physical Activity Guidelines for Americans,* the USDHHS (2008) recommended that adults get 150 minutes of moderate-intensity aerobic activity (e.g., brisk walking) every week, 75 minutes of vigorous-intensity aerobic activity (e.g., jogging or running) every week, or an equivalent mix of moderate- and vigorous-intensity aerobic activity and muscle-strengthening activities that work all major muscle groups (legs, hips, back, abdomen, chest, shoulders, and arms) performed on 2 or more days a week. Given the dose–response relationship observed between physical activity and health benefits in epidemiological studies, additional benefit may be gained from physical activity above the recommended minimum amount. The USDHHS recommends that aerobic exercise be twice the minimum recommended levels for greater health benefits. Moderate-intensity physical activity is defined as that in which one works hard enough to raise one's heart rate and break a sweat while still being able to carry on a conversation, and vigorous-intensity physical activity is defined as activity that causes rapid and hard breathing and that prevents one from saying more than a few words without pausing for breath. The recommended amounts of physical activity can be distributed throughout the day in 10-minute bouts. Most routine activities of daily living are of light intensity or less than 10 minutes of duration, but moderate- or vigorous-intensity activity, such as brisk walking to work, pushing a lawn mower, or gardening with a shovel, that is performed in bouts of 10 minutes or more can be counted toward the recommended amounts of activity.

leads to improved insulin sensitivity as indicated by a lower percentage of glycosylated hemoglobin, an increase in glucose disposal, and an improved lipid and cardiovascular disease risk profile (Zanuso et al., 2010). Improved insulin sensitivity may be the consequence of increased muscle mass or of metabolic adaptations (e.g., increases in insulin receptor, Akt, GLUT4, and glycogen synthase).

SKELETAL MUSCLE ADAPTATIONS IN RESPONSE TO DISUSE, AGING, AND DISEASE AND THE CONSEQUENCES FOR FUEL UTILIZATION AND WELL-BEING DURING NORMAL DAILY LIFE

Adaptive changes in skeletal muscle have consequences for fuel utilization, exercise tolerance, and feelings of fitness and well-being in the daily life of people. Muscle disuse (i.e., a reduction of muscular activity) for a prolonged period of time leads to a remarkable adaptation in skeletal muscle. Changes in skeletal muscle also occur as a natural consequence of aging and certain disease states.

Muscle disuse results in muscle atrophy and reduced muscular strength (Marimuthu et al., 2011; Glover and Phillips, 2010). The muscle appears to become resistant to anabolic stimuli, and muscle fibers decrease in size and contractile protein content, largely as a result of a reduction in protein synthesis. Mitochondrial content of muscle also decreases with muscle disuse. Muscle atrophy due to disuse may occur in individuals confined to bedrest due to illness, in limbs that are immobilized in a cast or sling, and in muscles that are not used due to joint pain. Resistance exercise is an effective therapy for the reversal, as well as the prevention, of muscle disuse atrophy. Exercise need not be as intense or frequent for the preservation of strength and muscle mass (i.e., prevention of atrophy) as is needed for muscle hypertrophy. Dynamic endurance exercise generally improves the oxidative capacity of muscle but has little effect on muscle mass.

A decline in skeletal muscle mass also occurs with aging. Aging-related loss of muscle mass and strength is called sarcopenia. Sarcopenia involves a decrease in muscle fiber size (atrophy) as well as a decrease in number of muscle fibers (hypoplasia) (Narici and Maffulli, 2010). Decreases in myosin concentration, selective fast fiber atrophy, loss of motor units, and an increase in hybrid fibers occur in individuals in the seventh or eighth decades of life. Because of the net motor unit denervation that occurs after about 60 years of age, a marked decrease in circumference of the type 2 fibers occurs between 60 and 80 years, with little or no decrease in the circumference of type 1 fibers. In the elderly, muscle protein synthesis shows a blunted response to anabolic stimuli, including amino acids and exercise, and the antiproteolytic effects of insulin are also blunted. Satellite cell activation and proliferation is also impaired in elderly individuals, limiting the ability of skeletal muscle to repair or replace muscle fibers. This is evidenced by a decline in the number of both type 1 and type 2 muscle fibers. The changes in muscle architecture that accompany the aging-associated remodeling of skeletal muscle result in loss of muscle force and power. In sarcopenia, muscle tissue that is lost may be replaced with fat, and an increase in fibrosis may be observed in addition to the muscle fiber atrophy. Resistance/strength training exercise appears to slow down the aging-associated decreases in muscle mass, but there may be an age limit to the benefit of resistance training. Ingestion of essential amino acid and carbohydrate immediately following resistance exercise was shown to promote greater training adaptations in elderly, untrained men, as compared to waiting until 2 hours after exercise to consume the supplement (Esmarck et al., 2001).

Maintenance of skeletal muscle structure and function requires innervation by motor neurons. Neurogenic atrophy is a severe form of muscle atrophy that results from diseases affecting the nerves that supply individual muscles (e.g., poliomyelitis, amyotrophic lateral sclerosis, and Guillain-Barré syndrome) and from some muscle diseases (e.g., muscular dystrophy, myotonic dystrophy). It may also result from compression or injury that causes temporary or permanent nerve deficit. One mechanism by which diseases of the nerves cause muscle atrophy is upregulation of myogenin expression (Macpherson et al., 2011). Myogenin, a member of the MyoD family of transcription factors, is upregulated in skeletal muscle following denervation. Myogenin in turn upregulates expression of the E3 ubiquitin ligases (i.e., MuRF1 and atrogin1) that promote muscle proteolysis.

A more generalized wasting of skeletal muscle occurs in hypermetabolic states and inflammatory states. Severe burns and generalized malnutrition, which result in elevated levels of glucocorticoids and catecholamines, result in loss of muscle tissue. Glucocorticoids can cause muscle atrophy by altering the muscle production of insulin-like growth factor 1 (IGF1) and myostatin, two growth factors exhibiting opposite effects on muscle mass. A decrease in IGF1 together with increase in myostatin inhibit satellite cells activation as well as myoblast proliferation and differentiation. In mature muscle fibers, these changes in levels of growth factors cause both downregulation of protein synthesis and stimulation of protein degradation. Inflammatory conditions, including sepsis, cachexia, and HIV-associated wasting, are also associated with generalized muscle wasting. Cytokines released by immune cells and tissues during inflammation lead to increased release of glucocorticoids and may also induce muscle degeneration by other mechanisms. Inflammation and hypercortisolemia are profound stimulants of muscle-specific proteolytic systems, and increased proteolysis is the major driving force for muscle breakdown in inflammatory conditions. Muscle loss can be rapid and severe in these states.

THINKING CRITICALLY

1. Studies of prolonged exercise in untrained subjects have shown elevations in expression of PGC1α and PDK4. What role might these proteins play in the metabolic adaptation of skeletal muscle in response to exercise? What changes would you expect to see in muscle fiber structure or metabolism?

2. Elite athletes tend to be more susceptible to common infections, perhaps due to a degree of immunosuppression. What are some hormonal, cytokine, or other changes that occur with prolonged exercise that might contribute to this situation?

REFERENCES

Berglund, E. D., Lee-Young, R. S., Lustig, D. G., Lynes, S. E., Donahue, E. P., Camacho, R. C., ... Wasserman, D. H. (2009). Hepatic energy state is regulated by glucagon receptor signaling in mice. *The Journal of Clinical Investigation, 119*, 2412–2422.

Canepari, M., Pellegrino, M. A., D'Antona, G., & Bottinelli, R. (2010). Skeletal muscle fibre diversity and the underlying mechanisms. *Acta Physiologica, 199*, 465–476.

de Bock, K., Dresselaers, T., Kiens, B., Richter, E. A., Van Hecke, P., & Hespel, P. (2007). Evaluation of intramyocellular lipid breakdown during exercise by biochemical assay, NMR spectroscopy, and Oil Red O staining. *American Journal of Physiology. Endocrinology and Metabolism, 293*, E428–E434.

de Glisezinski, I., Larrouy, D., Bajzova, M., Koppo, K., Polak, J., Berlan, M., ... Stich, V. (2009). Adrenaline but not noradrenaline is a determinant of exercise-induced lipid mobilization in human subcutaneous adipose tissue. *The Journal of Physiology, 587*, 3393–3404.

Eckardt, K., Taube, A., & Eckel, J. (2011). Obesity-associated insulin resistance in skeletal muscle: Role of lipid accumulation and physical inactivity. *Reviews in Endocrine & Metabolic Disorders, 12*(3), 163–172.

Esmarck, B., Andersen, J. L., Olsen, S., Richter, E. A., Mizuno, M., & Kjaer, M. (2001). Timing of postexercise protein intake is important for muscle hypertrophy with resistance training in elderly humans. *The Journal of Physiology, 535*, 301–311.

Febbraio, M. A., Hiscock, N., Sacchetti, M., Fischer, C. P., & Pedersen, B. K. (2004). Interleukin-6 is a novel factor mediating glucose homeostasis during skeletal muscle contraction. *Diabetes, 53*, 1643–1648.

Gleeson, M., Bishop, N. C., Stensel, D. J., Lindley, M. R., Mastana, S. S., & Nimmo, M. A. (2011). The anti-inflammatory effects of exercise: Mechanisms and implications for the prevention and treatment of disease. *Nature Reviews/Immunology, 11*, 607–615.

Glover, E. I., & Phillips, S. M. (2010). Resistance exercise and appropriate nutrition to counteract muscle wasting and promote muscle hypertrophy. *Current Opinion in Clinical Nutrition and Metabolic Care, 13*, 630–634.

Green, H. J., Duhamel, T. A., Holloway, G. P., Moule, J., Ouyang, J., Ranney, D., & Tupling, A. R. (2007). Muscle metabolic responses during 16 hours of intermittent heavy exercise. *Canadian Journal of Physiology and Pharmacology, 85*, 634–645.

Green, H. J., Duhamel, T. A., Smith, I. C., Rich, S. M., Thomas, M. M., Ouyang, J., & Yau, J. E. (2011). Muscle metabolic, enzymatic and transporter responses to a session of prolonged cycling. *European Journal of Applied Physiology, 111*, 827–837.

Haskell, W. L., Lee, I.-M., Pate, R. R., Powell, K. E., Blair, S. N., Franklin, B. A., ... Bauman, A. (2007). Physical activity and public health: Updated recommendation for adults from the American College of Sports Medicine and the American Heart Association. *Medicine and Science in Sports and Exercise, 39*, 1423–1434.

Hawley, J. A., & Burke, L. M. (2010). Carbohydrate availability and training adaptation: Effects on cell metabolism. *Exercise and Sport Sciences Reviews, 38*, 152–160.

Hawley, J. A., Burke, L. M., Phillips, S. M., & Spriet, L. L. (2011). Nutritional modulation of training-induced skeletal muscle adaptations. *Journal of Applied Physiology, 110*, 834–845.

Himwich, H. E., & Rose, M. I. (1927). The respiratory quotient of exercising muscle. *The American Journal of Physiology, 81*, 485–486.

Hiscock, N., Fischer, C. P., Sacchetti, M., van Hall, G., Febbraio, M. A., & Pedersen, B. K. (2005). Recombinant human interleukin-6 infusion during low-intensity exercise does not enhance whole body lipolysis or fat oxidation in humans. *American Journal of Physiology. Endocrinology and Metabolism, 289*, E2–E7.

Hoppeler, H., & Flück, M. (2002). Normal mammalian skeletal muscle and its phenotypic plasticity. *The Journal of Experimental Biology, 205*, 2143–2152.

Jentjens, R. L., Achten, J., & Jeukendrup, A. E. (2004). High oxidation rates from combined carbohydrates ingested during exercise. *Medicine and Science in Sports and Exercise, 36*, 1551–1558.

Jeukendrup, A. E. (2003). Modulation of carbohydrate and fat utilization by diet, exercise and environment. *Biochemical Society Transactions, 31*, 1270–1273.

Jeukendrup, A. E. (2004). Carbohydrate intake during exercise and performance. *Nutrition, 20*, 669–677.

Johnson, N. A., Stannard, S. R., & Thompson, M. W. (2004). Muscle triglyceride and glycogen in endurance exercise: Implications for performance. *Sports Medicine (Auckland, N.Z.), 34*, 151–164.

Kimber, N. E., Heigenhauser, G. J., Spriet, L. L., & Dyck, D. J. (2003). Skeletal muscle fat and carbohydrate metabolism during recovery from glycogen-depleting exercise in humans. *The Journal of Physiology, 548*, 919–927.

Koopman, R., Pannemans, D. L., Jeukendrup, A. E., Gijsen, A. P., Senden, J. M., Halliday, D., ... Wagenmakers, A. J. (2004). Combined ingestion of protein and carbohydrate improves protein balance during ultra-endurance exercise. *American Journal of Physiology. Endocrinology and Metabolism, 287*, E712–E720.

Koopman, R., Wagenmakers, A. J., Manders, R. J., Zorenc, A. H., Senden, J. M., Gorselink, M., ... van Loon, L. J. (2005). Combined ingestion of protein and free leucine with carbohydrate increases postexercise muscle protein synthesis in vivo in male subjects. *American Journal of Physiology. Endocrinology and Metabolism, 288*, E645–E653.

Kreider, R. B., Wilborn, C. D., Taylor, L., Campbell, B., Almada, A. L., Collins, R., ... Antonio, J. (2010). ISSN exercise & sport nutrition review: Research & recommendations. *Journal of the International Society of Sports Nutrition, 7*, 7.

Krssak, M., Petersen, K. F., Bergeron, R., Price, T., Laurent, D., Rothman, D. L., ... Shulman, G. I. (2000). Intramuscular glycogen and intramyocellular lipid utilization during prolonged exercise and recovery in man: A ^{13}C and ^{1}H nuclear magnetic resonance spectroscopy study. *The Journal of Clinical Endocrinology and Metabolism, 85*, 748–754.

Macpherson, P. C., Wang, X., & Goldman, D. (2011). Myogenin regulates denervation-dependent muscle atrophy in mouse soleus muscle. *Journal of Cellular Biochemistry, 112*, 2149–2159.

Marimuthu, K., Murton, A. J., & Greenhaff, P. L. (2011). Mechanisms regulating mass during disuse atrophy and rehabilitation in humans. *Journal of Applied Physiology, 110*, 555–560.

Narici, M. V., & Maffulli, N. (2010). Sarcopenia: Characteristics, mechanisms and functional significance. *British Medical Bulletin, 95*, 139–159.

Ploeger, H. E., Takken, T., de Greef, M. H., & Timmons, B. W. (2009). The effects of acute and chronic exercise on inflammatory markers in children and adults with a chronic inflammatory disease: A systematic review. *Exercise Immunology Review, 15*, 6–41.

Putman, C. T., Xu, X., Gillies, E., MacLean, I. M., & Bell, G. J. (2004). Effects of strength, endurance and combined training on myosin heavy chain content and fibre-type distribution in humans. *European Journal of Applied Physiology, 92*, 376–384.

Roepstorff, C., Halberg, N., Hillig, T., Saha, A. K., Ruderman, N. B., Wojtaszewski, J. F., Richter, E. A., & Kiens, B. (2005). Malonyl-CoA and carnitine in regulation of fat oxidation in human skeletal muscle during exercise. *American Journal of Physiology. Endocrinology and Metabolism, 288*, E133–E142.

Roepstorff, C., Vistisen, B., Roepstorff, K., & Kiens, B. (2004). Regulation of plasma long-chain fatty acid oxidation in relation to uptake in human skeletal muscle during exercise. *American Journal of Physiology. Endocrinology and Metabolism, 287*, E696–E705.

Romijn, J. A., Coyle, E. F., Sidossis, L. S., Gastaldelli, A., Horowitz, J. F., Endert, E., & Wolfe, R. R. (1993). Regulation of endogenous fat and carbohydrate metabolism in relation to exercise intensity and duration. *The American Journal of Physiology, 265*, E380–E391.

Sahlin, K., Sallstedt, E. K., Bishop, D., & Tonkonogi, M. (2008). Turning down lipid oxidation during heavy exercise—What is the mechanism? *Journal of Physiology and Pharmacology, 59*(Suppl. 7), 19–30.

Schrauwen-Hinderling, V. B., Hesselink, M. K. C., Schrauwen, P., & Kooi, M. E. (2006). Intramyocellular lipid content in human skeletal muscle. *Obesity, 14*, 357–367.

Shaw, C. S., Clark, J., & Wagenmakers, A. J.-M. (2010). The effect of exercise and nutrition on intramuscular fat metabolism and insulin sensitivity. *Annual Review of Nutrition, 30*, 13–34.

Stallknecht, B., Lorentsen, J., Enevoldsen, L. H., Bülow, J., Biering-Sørensen, F., Galbo, H., & Kjaer, M. (2001). Role of the sympathoadrenergic system in adipose tissue metabolism during exercise in humans. *The Journal of Physiology, 536*, 283–294.

Stellingwerff, T., Boon, H., Jonkers, R. A., Senden, J. M., Spriet, L. L., Koopman, R., & van Loon, L. J. (2007). Significant intramyocellular lipid use during prolonged cycling in endurance-trained males as assessed by three different methodologies. *American Journal of Physiology. Endocrinology and Metabolism, 292*, E1715–E1723.

Talanian, J. L., Holloway, G. P., Snook, L. A., Heigenhauser, G. J., Bonen, A., & Spriet, L. L. (2010). Exercise training increases sarcolemmal and mitochondrial fatty acid transport proteins in human skeletal muscle. *American Journal of Physiology. Endocrinology and Metabolism, 299*, E180–E188.

U.S. Department of Health and Human Services. (2008). *2008 physical activity guidelines for Americans*. Retrieved from www.health.gov/paguidelines

van Hall, G. (2010). Lactate kinetics in human tisssues at rest and during exercise. *Acta Physiologica, 199*, 499–508.

van Loon, L. J., Greenhaff, P. L., Constantin-Teodosiu, D., Saris, W. H. M., & Wagenmakers, A. J. M. (2001). The effects of increasing exercise intensity on muscle fuel utilisation in humans. *The Journal of Physiology, 536*, 295–304.

van Loon, L. J., Koopman, R., Manders, R., van der Weegen, W., van Kranenburg, G. P., & Keizer, H. A. (2004). Intramyocellular lipid content in type 2 diabetes patients compared with overweight sedentary men and highly trained endurance athletes. *American Journal of Physiology. Endocrinology and Metabolism, 287*, E558–E565.

van Loon, L. J., Schrauwen-Hinderling, V. B., Koopman, R., Wagenmakers, A. J., Hesselink, M. K., Schaart, G., Kooi, M. E., & Saris, W. H. (2003). Influence of prolonged endurance cycling and recovery diet on intramuscular triglyceride content in trained males. *American Journal of Physiology. Endocrinology and Metabolism, 285*, E804–E811.

Venables, M. C., Achten, J., & Jeukendrup, A. E. (2005). Determinants of fat oxidation during exercise in healthy men and women: A cross-sectional study. *Journal of Applied Physiology, 98*, 160–167.

Wallis, G. A., Rowlands, D. S., Shaw, C., Jentjens, R. L., & Jeukendrup, A. E. (2005). Oxidation of combined ingestion of maltodextrins and fructose during exercise. *Medicine and Science in Sports and Exercise, 37*, 426–432.

Wang, L., Mascher, H., Psilander, N., Blomstrand, E., & Sahlin, K. (2011). Resistance exercise enhances the molecular signaling of mitochondrial biogenesis induced by endurance exercise in human skeletal muscle. *Journal of Applied Physiology* [Epub ahead of print].

Wang, L., & Sahlin, K. (2011). *The effect of continuous and interval exercise on PGC-1α and PDK4 mRNA in type I and type II fibres of human skeletal muscle*. Oxford: Acta Physiologica [Epub ahead of print].

Wasserman, D. H., Kang, L., Ayala, J. E., Fueger, P. T., & Lee-Young, R. S. (2011). The physiological regulation of glucose flux into muscle in vivo. *The Journal of Experimental Biology, 214*, 254–262.

Watt, M. J., & Spriet, L. L. (2004). Regulation and role of hormone-sensitive lipase activity in human skeletal muscle. *The Proceedings of the Nutrition Society, 63*, 315–322.

Williams, M. A., Haskell, W. L., Ades, P. A., Amsterdam, E. A., Bittner, V., Franklin, B. A., Gulanick, M., Laing, S. T., Stewart, K. J., American Heart Association Council on Clinical Cardiology, & American Heart Association Council on Nutrition, Physical Activity, and Metabolism. (2007) Resistance exercise in individuals with and without cardiovascular disease: 2007 update: A scientific statement from the American Heart Association Council on Clinical Cardiology and Council on Nutrition, Physical Activity, and Metabolism. *Circulation, 116*, 572–584.

Zanuso, S., Jimenez, A., Pugliese, G., Corigliana, G., & Balducci, S. (2010). Exercise for the management of type 2 diabetes: A review of the evidence. *Acta Diabetologica, 47*, 15–22.

Zehnder, M., Christ, E. R., Ith, M., Acheson, K. J., Pouteau, E., Kreis, R., Trepp, R., Diem, P., Boesch, C., & Decombaz, J. (2006). Intramyocellular lipid stores increase markedly in athletes after 1.5 days lipid supplementation and are utilized during exercise in proportion to their content. *European Journal of Applied Physiology, 98*, 341–354.

RECOMMENDED READING

Wasserman, D. H., Kang, L., Ayala, J. E., Fueger, P. T., & Lee-Young, R. S. (2011). The physiological regulation of glucose flux into muscle in vivo. *The Journal of Experimental Biology, 214*, 254–262.

RECOMMENDED WEBSITE

Centers for Disease Control and Prevention. Topical information on physical activity information includes guidelines, statistics, policy, and resources. www.cdc.gov/physicalactivity/index.html

UNIT V

Energy

Energy is defined as the capacity for doing work. In the biological world, the various types of work that require energy include mechanical work, chemical work, and osmotic and electrical work. In animals and humans, the energy that sustains the various forms of biological work is derived from the carbohydrates, lipids, and proteins of the diet; this energy initially came from the sun and was stored by plants during photosynthesis at the beginning of the food chain. Some of the food energy is stored in the body as specific fuel reserves, mainly as glycogen and triacylglycerol, for use during the absence of food intake.

All forms of energy may be described as consisting of either potential or kinetic energy. For people, food is a source of potential energy. In the catabolism of carbohydrates, proteins, and lipids, some of this potential energy is stored or conserved in forms in which it can be used to support various energy-utilizing reactions. The first law of thermodynamics states that energy can be neither created nor destroyed. Some of the chemical energy available in glucose is converted in the process of catabolism to another form of chemical energy, adenosine 5′-triphosphate (ATP). The energy involved in the proton gradient produced across the inner mitochondrial membrane during electron transport is converted to chemical energy when the proton gradient is used to drive ATP synthesis. In skeletal and cardiac muscle, chemical energy involved in the energy-rich phosphate bonds of ATP is converted to mechanical energy during the process of muscle contraction. Another compound used to transfer chemical energy is NADPH, which is used to provide energy for lipid and steroid synthesis. Ultimately, most of the potential energy taken in as food is converted to and lost from the body as heat.

The second law of thermodynamics states that all processes tend to progress toward a situation of maximum entropy (disorder or randomness). Entropy can be viewed as the energy in a system that is unavailable to perform useful work. The portion of the total energy in a system that is available for useful work is called the Gibbs free energy and is usually denoted by G. The change in Gibbs free energy for a chemical reaction is defined as $\Delta G = G_{products} - G_{reactants}$. Reactions with positive free-energy changes (endergonic reactions) may be coupled to and driven by reactions that have negative free-energy changes (exergonic reactions); the sum of the ΔG values for the individual reactions in a pathway must be negative for a metabolic sequence to be thermodynamically feasible. For biochemical reactions, it is common to tabulate ΔG values as $\Delta G^{0\prime}$ values, which are ΔG values determined under standard conditions of temperature (usually 25°C), pressure (1 atm), pH (7.0), reactant concentrations (1 mol/L), and water concentration (55.6 mol/L).

Most biological work is mediated by hydrolysis of energy-rich bonds, particularly by hydrolysis of so-called high-energy phosphate bonds. These high-energy phosphate esters retain the energy in the structural, chemical, electrostatic, and resonant properties of the molecules. They release or transfer large amounts of free energy upon hydrolysis of the phosphate ester bonds because hydrolysis results in formation of products that are more stable (i.e., have more resonant forms or less electrostatic repulsion) than the high-energy phosphate substrate. The hydrolysis of simple phosphate esters, such as glucose 6-phosphate and glycerol 3-phosphate, has $\Delta G^{0\prime}$ values in the range of −1 to −3 kcal/mol. Hydrolysis of phosphoric acid anhydrides such as the β- and γ-phosphates of ATP, of enol phosphates such as phosphoenolpyruvate, and of thiol esters such as acetyl CoA is associated with $\Delta G^{\circ\prime}$ values of approximately −7.3, −14.8, and −7.7 kcal/mol, respectively.

ATP plays a central role in linking energy-producing and energy-utilizing pathways. Potential ATP "units" or "equivalents" are often counted as a means of expressing the amount of available energy, the rate at which energy can be produced and/or utilized, or the amount of energy that can be obtained from storage depots. In the cell, the hydrolysis of ATP must be balanced with the phosphorylation of adenosine diphosphate (ADP). During macronutrient catabolism, some ATP equivalents are formed as a result of substrate-level phosphorylation, but most ATP is formed in the final stages of fuel catabolism in the mitochondria. ATP is generated by the transfer of reducing equivalents to oxygen via the electron transport chain and oxidative phosphorylation driven by the proton gradient. Because of the central role of oxidative phosphorylation in conservation of chemical energy in ATP, the production of reducing equivalents, such as NADH + H^+ or $FADH_2$, by catabolic pathways and the transfer of these hydrogens (electrons and protons) to oxygen as the terminal acceptor are closely linked to overall energy expenditure by the body.

In this unit, energy nutrition is considered largely from a whole-body perspective. Nutritionists have traditionally considered the energy requirement or expenditure as being constituted by three major categories: energy for support of the normal processes of growth and maintenance (called basal metabolism), energy for the assimilation or use of dietary fuels (called specific dynamic action or thermic effect of food), and energy for physical activity. For maintenance of body weight, energy intake must be balanced by energy expenditure. If energy intake is greater than energy expenditure, excess energy will be stored as triacylglycerol in adipose tissue and lead to obesity. If energy intake is less than energy expenditure, this will result in loss of body weight and, if severe, can lead to protein-energy malnutrition.

CHAPTER 21

Cellular and Whole-Animal Energetics

Darlene E. Berryman, PhD, RD, and Matthew W. Hulver, PhD

COMMON ABBREVIATIONS

ADP adenosine 5′-diphosphate
ATP adenosine 5′-triphosphate
BEE basal energy expenditure (also known as BMR, basal metabolic rate)
EEPA energy expenditure for physical activity
$FADH_2$ flavin adenine dinucleotide (reduced)
NADPH nicotinamide adenine dinucleotide phosphate (reduced)
PAL physical activity level
RMR resting metabolic rate
RQ respiratory quotient
TEE total energy expenditure
TEF thermic effect of food

CELLULAR ENERGETICS

Total-body energy utilization is the sum of the collective energy-utilizing and energy-producing reactions occurring within individual cells throughout the body. Both energy in foods and energy expenditure by the body are typically measured in calories or joules. The various metabolic reactions that serve to sustain life are fueled by the energy released from the biological oxidation of energy-yielding nutrients in the food we consume. A fraction of the energy released from biological oxidation processes is captured in high-energy bonds in molecules, namely in the phosphate–phosphate bonds of adenosine 5′-triphosphate (ATP), which is the main energy currency of the cell. ATP is then used to fuel the various biochemical processes within cells that support basal metabolism, growth, and other essential functions.

CALORIES, JOULES, AND WATTS

Energy (amount) is generally measured in joules (SI unit), but the nutrition community still mainly uses calories. The calorie is defined as the energy needed to increase the temperature of 1 gram of water by 1° C. The joule is widely used in physics and is defined as the work or energy required to move an object with the force of 1 newton over a distance of 1 meter. One joule is equivalent to 0.2389 calories. More commonly, kilojoules (1000 joules) and kilocalories (1000 calories) are used as convenient units when referring to food calories. Sometimes, calorie is used to refer to kilocalorie when caloric values of foods are reported.

$$1 \text{ kJ} = 0.2389 \text{ kcal}$$

$$1 \text{ kcal} = 4.184 \text{ kJ}$$

The rate of energy expenditure or work rate is expressed as watts, with 1 watt equivalent to the expenditure of 1 joule of energy per second. A human climbing a flight of stairs is doing work at the rate of about 200 watts (0.200 kJ/second). Using the conversion factor for kilojoules to kilocalories, the expenditure of 200 watts is equivalent to expenditure of 0.048 kcal/second or 172 kcal/hour.

ADENOSINE TRIPHOSPHATE AND NICOTINAMIDE ADENINE DINUCLEOTIDE PHOSPHATE

Animal cells obtain energy by oxidizing food molecules. The oxidation of fuel molecules in the body is referred to as catabolism. The metabolic reactions that result in breakdown of the fuel molecules are not completely efficient and result in loss of some of the inherent energy in the fuel molecule as heat. However, a substantial portion of the energy in the fuel molecules is conserved as either ATP or the reduced form of nicotinamide adenine dinucleotide phosphate (NADPH). Whereas ATP is the main source of energy for driving most cellular functions, NADPH is used mainly to drive reactions involved in the synthesis of fatty acids and sterols and a few other reactions such as reduction of oxidized glutathione (see Chapters 12, 16, and 17). Thus ATP and NADPH serve a unique role in coupling the energy-yielding processes of catabolism to the energy-consuming reactions of cellular work.

ATP formation occurs by either substrate-level phosphorylation or by oxidative phosphorylation. In substrate-level phosphorylation, the phosphate used to phosphorylate adenosine 5′-diphosphate (ADP) comes from a phosphorylated reactive intermediate rather than inorganic phosphate, and the process is not associated with redox reactions [i.e., not with formation of reduced nicotinamide dinucleotide

(NADH) or reduced flavin adenine dinucleotide ($FADH_2$)]. Substrate-level ATP formation occurs during two steps of glycolysis, and equivalent guanosine 5′-triphosphate (GTP) formation occurs in the citric acid cycle. The overwhelming majority of ATP synthesis, however, is the result of electron transport in the mitochondria and is called oxidative phosphorylation. In oxidative phosphorylation, inorganic phosphate ($H_2PO_4^-/HPO_4^{2-}$, often abbreviated as P_i) is used to synthesize ATP from ADP, and the process is driven by redox reactions via the electron transport chain. Both pathways of ATP synthesis result in the addition of a phosphate group to ADP.

ATP is the main energy source for the majority of cellular functions, being hydrolyzed to ADP when it is consumed. ATP is often considered the energy currency of the cell, with the metabolic unit of exchange being the ATP equivalent. An ATP equivalent is defined as the conversion of ATP to ADP (or ADP to ATP). ATP is generated by energy-releasing (exothermic) processes but consumed by energy-requiring (endothermic) processes. Some reactions are driven by hydrolysis of GTP, uridine 5′-triphosphate (UTP), or creatine phosphate, but these are considered equivalent to ATP expenditure because rephosphorylation of GDP, UDP, or creatine may be accomplished by reactions coupled to the conversion of ATP to ADP. Some reactions require more energy than can be obtained from ATP hydrolysis to ADP + inorganic phosphate (P_i) and involve hydrolysis of ATP to adenosine 5′-monophosphate (AMP) + pyrophosphate (PP_i), which is further hydrolyzed to 2 P_i. This is considered equivalent to expenditure of 2 ATPs because expenditure of 2 ATPs is required for ATP resynthesis from AMP as shown in Figure 21-1.

NADPH does not donate its reducing equivalents to the electron transport chain but, rather, is directly used to drive some specific biosynthetic reactions, particularly in the synthesis of fatty acids and steroids. Because NADPH is not directly used to support ATP synthesis by oxidative phosphorylation in the mitochondria, the metabolic value of NADPH in ATP equivalents is not obvious. However, because the $NADPH/NADP^+$ couple is a much better electron donating system than the $NADH/NAD^+$ couple, NADPH may be considered to have a metabolic energy value close to 4 ATP equivalents.

Neither ATP nor NADPH can be stored, and the amounts of ATP and NADPH in cells are fairly stable. When ATP or NADPH is used to drive other reactions or processes, the product is ADP, AMP, or $NADP^+$. ATP and NADPH are then regenerated from these products via the catabolic oxidation of fuel molecules and, for ATP, the electron transport chain. The regeneration process is efficient and regulated in response to energy expenditure to maintain high intracellular ratios of ATP/ADP and of $NADPH/NADP^+$. The total content of ATP in the human body is only about 0.1 mole (0.05 kg), but the human body requires hydrolysis of about 100 to 150 moles of ATP each day. Therefore we can calculate that each ATP molecule must be recycled 1,000 to 1,500 times during a single day (equivalent to about once per minute) by the phosphorylation of ADP back to ATP.

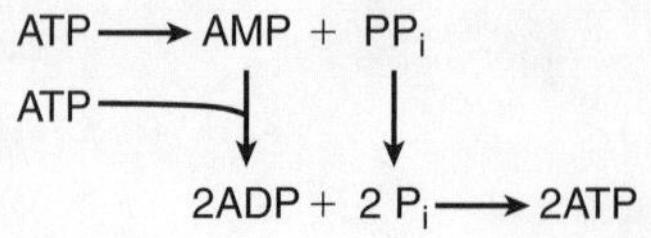

$$\mathrm{ATP} \longrightarrow \mathrm{AMP} + \mathrm{PP_i}$$
$$\mathrm{ATP} + \mathrm{AMP} \longrightarrow 2\mathrm{ADP};\quad \mathrm{PP_i} \longrightarrow 2\,\mathrm{P_i}$$
$$2\mathrm{ADP} + 2\,\mathrm{P_i} \longrightarrow 2\mathrm{ATP}$$

$$\mathrm{PP_i} = \mathrm{HP_2O_7}^{3-}$$
$$\mathrm{P_i} = \mathrm{HPO_4}^{2-}$$

FIGURE 21-1 Hydrolysis of ATP to AMP + PP_i is equivalent to hydrolysis of 2 ATP to 2 ADP + 2 P_i.

In addition to serving as the major energy currency of the cell, ATP also serves as an important allosteric effector in the regulation of metabolism. Its concentration relative to those of ADP and AMP is an index of the energy status of the cell and determines the rates of regulatory enzymes situated at key points in metabolism. AMP-activated protein kinase (AMPK) is an important sensor of intracellular AMP/ATP ratios that exerts regulatory effects on multiple ATP-producing and ATP-consuming pathways (see Figure 19-1 in Chapter 19).

METABOLIC SOURCES OF HEAT PRODUCTION

All living cells produce heat as a by-product of metabolism. Heat production within cells of an organism in the resting, postabsorptive state has two essential components: (1) obligatory and (2) regulatory (Figure 21-2).

Obligatory Heat Production

Obligatory heat production is the heat released during anabolic and catabolic reactions responsible for all cellular processes, primarily through the utilization and resynthesis of ATP molecules. At rest, the majority of the energy expended by a cell is being used to drive various molecular transport mechanisms, many of which are responsible for maintaining essential electrochemical gradients across membranes. For example, it has been estimated that the Na^+,K^+-ATPase pump reaction, which couples ATP hydrolysis to transport of K^+ into cells and movement of Na^+ out of cells, accounts for 20% to 40% of whole-body resting energy expenditure (McBride and Kelly, 1990). In highly metabolically active cell types, such as hepatocytes (liver cells), proton (H^+) pumping across the mitochondrial membrane may represent up to 30% of the energy used by the cell. At rest, other processes that contribute substantially to energy needs include reactions responsible for macromolecular synthesis and degradation (e.g., protein and phospholipid turnover) and substrate cycling (discussed later in this chapter).

Regulatory Heat Production

Regulatory heat production is important for homeothermic organisms (i.e., those that maintain a constant body temperature). Regulatory heat production is needed to maintain a constant body temperature in the face of fluctuating environmental temperature. Shivering, which is triggered

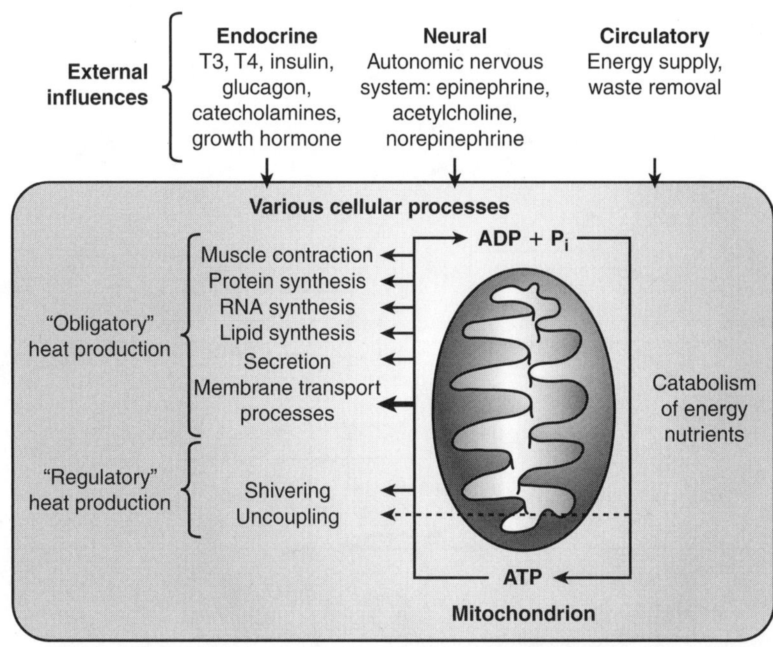

FIGURE 21-2 Nature of cellular biochemical pathways for heat production and their extracellular influences. The thicker arrow for transport processes is meant to imply that transport processes are a major contributor to ATP consumption in most cell types. The dotted arrow shows that uncoupling results in increased heat production that is not coupled with ATP synthesis because of dissipation of the proton gradient in the mitochondria.

in response to cold exposure, can involve a substantial increase in skeletal muscle contraction, which results in a significant increase in ATP turnover and subsequently increased heat production. Heat generated through uncoupling mechanisms (discussed in a subsequent section of this chapter) can also contribute significantly to regulatory heat production. Conversely, exposure to increased environmental temperature stimulates sweat production, which helps cool the body through the heat loss associated with evaporation (see Chapter 35). The processes of modulating heat production and loss confer tremendous flexibility to many species so that they may survive in many different environmental conditions.

Postprandial Heat Production and Exercise Thermogenesis

Excess heat production also occurs during the postprandial period by the reactions referred to as the thermic effect of food (TEF). During physical activity, large amounts of heat can be produced as a consequence of muscle contraction and related processes. This heat production is referred to as the energy expenditure for physical activity (EEPA). The heat production associated with food intake or physical activity can also contribute to maintenance of body temperature in a cold environment.

OXIDATION OF FUEL MOLECULES

Energy for the synthesis of ATP within cells comes mainly from the oxidation of energy-yielding molecules, which include predominantly carbohydrate and fat but also protein and alcohol (Flatt, 1985). The complete metabolic oxidation of fuel molecules to CO_2 and H_2O occurs with a similar stoichiometry to that for combustion of the fuels in a flame, but the processes involved are quite different. As summarized in Figure 21-3, catabolism of fuel molecules involves the oxidation of the fuel molecules coupled to the reduction of other molecules such as NAD(P) and FAD. Some ATP equivalents are formed by substrate-level phosphorylation (e.g., in two steps of glycolysis and in the citric acid cycle). CO_2 is formed primarily from oxidation of acetyl-CoA by the citric acid cycle with H_2O as the source of the additional oxygen needed to convert the acetyl moiety to CO_2. However, most ATP production and almost all molecular O_2 consumption occur at the level of oxidative phosphorylation in the mitochondria. The electrons carried by the reduced NADH and $FADH_2$ generated in the citric acid cycle as well as by glycolysis and β-oxidation are transferred to the mitochondrial electron transport chain, which fuels phosphorylation of ADP to yield ATP. Molecular O_2 is the terminal electron (and proton) acceptor in electron transport; O_2 is reduced to produce H_2O. In macronutrient oxidation, the release of CO_2 generally occurs at earlier stages in nutrient catabolism and thus prior to O_2 consumption and H_2O production.

The ATP yield per gram of glucose, fatty acid, or amino acid differs in proportion to the oxidation state of the different molecules. For example, carbohydrates are partially oxidized compounds, already have one oxygen atom (hydroxyl substituent) for every carbon atom, and thus yield fewer reducing equivalents per carbon atom during their catabolism. In contrast, almost every carbon atom in a fat molecule is saturated with hydrogen; therefore fat yields more reducing equivalents per carbon atom during its catabolism. Amino acids have an intermediate oxidation state in between that of fat and carbohydrate. However, because of the need to excrete the nitrogen as urea, the actual energy yield per carbon atom is similar for carbohydrates and amino acids. The following equations for the complete oxidation (requiring input of O_2) of representative macromolecules (e.g., glucose, palmitic acid, and alanine) to CO_2 and H_2O (and urea,

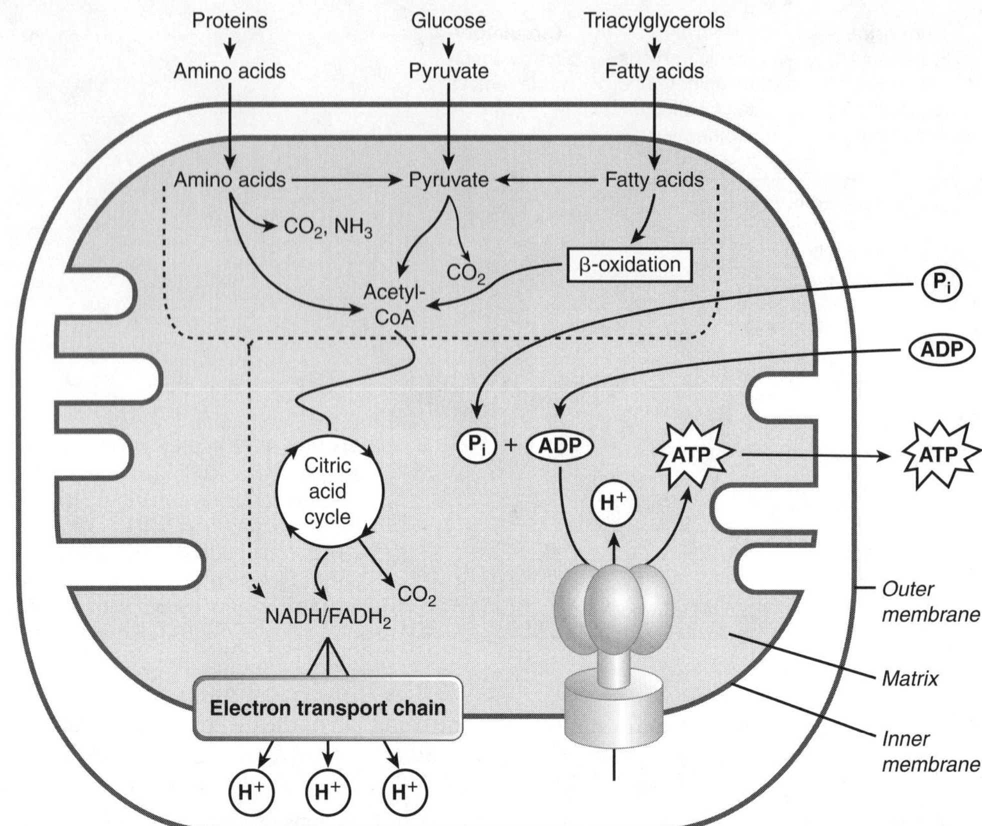

FIGURE 21-3 Main pathways of cellular and mitochondrial energy metabolism. Energy nutrients (glucose, triacylglycerols, and amino acids to a lesser degree) are transported into the mitochondrial matrix in the form of pyruvate, fatty acids, or amino/keto acids. Pyruvate and free fatty acids are oxidized through the pyruvate decarboxylase reaction and β-oxidation, respectively, to produce acetyl CoA, NADH, H^+, and $FADH_2$. The acetyl CoA is further oxidized by the citric acid cycle to produce NADH, H^+, and $FADH_2$. These reduced adenine dinucleotides are then oxidized by the electron transport chain. The proton gradient formed in the mitochondrial intermembrane space is used to drive the formation of ATP, which can then be transported out of the mitochondria to fuel other metabolic processes. Where amino acids enter this pathway depends on the specific amino acid.

in the case of alanine) illustrate the basis for the relationships among energy expenditure, O_2 consumption, CO_2 release, the respiratory quotient (RQ), and type of macronutrient oxidized as fuel.

Glucose:

$$C_6H_{12}O_6 + 6\ O_2 \rightarrow 6\ CO_2 + 6\ H_2O + 673 \text{ kcal per mole (or 3.8 kcal/g)}$$

$$\text{RQ for glucose} = 6\ CO_2/6\ O_2 = 1$$

Palmitic acid:

$$C_{16}H_{32}O_2 + 23\ O_2 \rightarrow 16\ CO_2 + 16\ H_2O + 2{,}380 \text{ kcal per mole (or 9.3 kcal/g)}$$

$$\text{RQ for palmitic acid} = 16\ CO_2/23\ O_2 = 0.7$$

Alanine:

$$2\ (C_3H_7O_2N) + 6\ O_2 \rightarrow 5\ CO_2 + 5\ H_2O + \underset{\text{Urea}}{CH_4ON_2} + 312 \text{ kcal per mole (or 3.5 kcal/g)}$$

$$\text{RQ for alanine} = 5\ CO_2/6\ O_2 = 0.83$$

Although these reactions, with the exception of urea formation, appear similar to those used to describe the combustion of organic compounds in a flame, it is important to remember that the processes of O_2 consumption and CO_2 and H_2O production do not occur simultaneously in the body as they do when these compounds are oxidized by burning. In the body, metabolism (or oxidation) of fuel molecules occurs in small and separate steps. The initial processes involve the production of CO_2 and the transfer of reducing equivalents to flavin and pyridine nucleotides. In the later steps, the reducing equivalents are transferred to the electron transport chain, which ultimately transfers the electrons and H^+ to O_2, resulting in O_2 consumption and H_2O production as well as conservation of some of the energy in the chemical bonds of ATP.

OXIDATIVE PHOSPHORYLATION

The coupling of oxidation of fuel molecules to ATP synthesis (with the exception of some substrate-level ATP formation) is localized within the mitochondria of mammalian cells, as illustrated in Figure 21-3. The specialized proteins and enzymes required for oxidative phosphorylation are specifically localized on the inner mitochondrial membrane. Oxidative phosphorylation is the process by which a molecule of inorganic phosphate

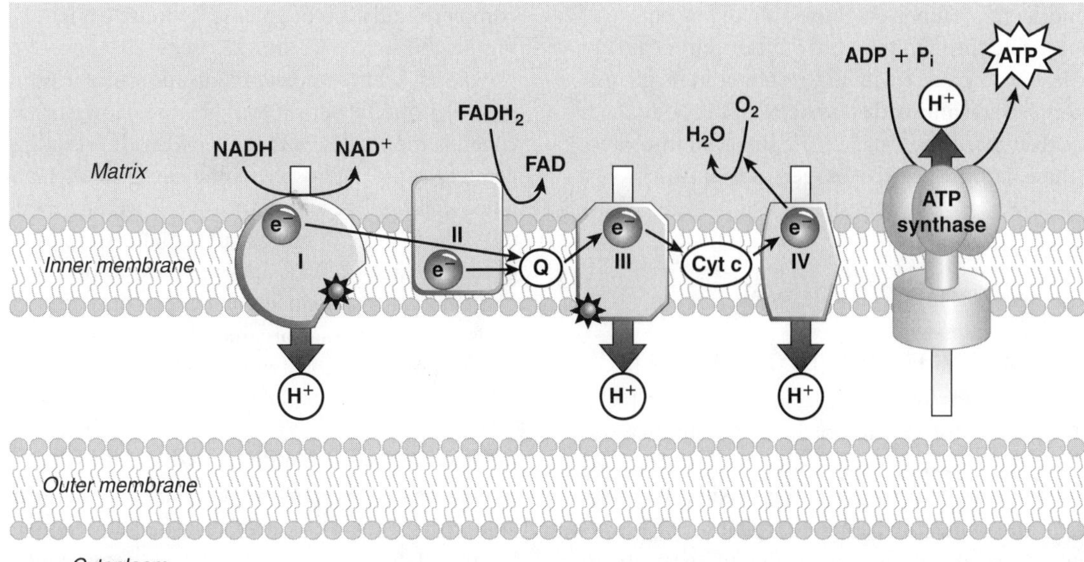

FIGURE 21-4 A general scheme for mitochondrial electron transport and oxidative phosphorylation. The transport of electrons from NADH and $FADH_2$ is accomplished by specific carrier molecules that constitute the electron transport chain. The terminal electron (and proton) acceptor is oxygen, and water is formed as a product of electron transport. The generation of the proton gradient by pumping protons out of the mitochondrial matrix is also shown. Dissipation of this proton gradient by ATP synthase is coupled to ATP synthesis. The dark stars represent major sites of superoxide radical formation.

is condensed with ADP to form ATP, a process driven by the step-by-step transfer of electrons along a chain of electron carriers termed the electron transport chain (Figure 21-4).

Phosphorylation of ADP to ATP

The synthesis of ATP during oxidative phosphorylation is linked to the release of electrons carried by the flavin and pyridine nucleotides to proteins of the electron transport chain. Hydrogen ions are pumped out of the mitochondrial matrix across the inner mitochondrial membrane at three sites along the electron transport chain to create an electrochemical gradient. This proton gradient is subsequently dissipated as protons are allowed back through the membrane by ATP synthase, which couples this process to ATP synthesis, as shown in Figure 21-4. Sufficient free energy may be collected at three sites along the electron transport chain (complexes I, III, and IV) to allow phosphorylation of ADP, yielding ATP. A maximum of three molecules of ATP can be generated from each molecule of NADH that is oxidized via donation of its pair of electrons to the electron transport chain. $FADH_2$ donates its electrons at a later step in the electron transport chain, allowing a maximum of only two molecules of ATP to be generated from each $FADH_2$ molecule.

Terminal Electron Acceptor: O_2 Consumption

Molecular oxygen serves as the terminal electron acceptor at the end of the electron transport chain. Transfer of 4 electrons plus 4 protons (H^+) to 1 molecule of O_2 results in formation of 2 molecules of H_2O. Because most fuel oxidation results in the transfer of electrons from reduced pyridine and flavin coenzymes to the mitochondrial electron transport chain, the energy yield or heat produced by oxidation of fuel molecules can be closely estimated by measuring oxygen consumption.

P/O Ratio

A frequently used index of the efficiency of oxidative phosphorylation is the P/O ratio. The P/O ratio is defined as the number of ATP molecules produced per pair of electrons traveling through the electron transport chain (or per oxygen atom that is reduced). Depending on where electrons enter the chain, the maximal P/O ratio will change (Murphy and Brand, 1987). At maximal biological efficiency, the complete oxidation of NADH yields 3 ATP molecules, and so the maximal P/O ratio for this process is 3. For the complete oxidation of $FADH_2$, the maximal P/O ratio is 2. Few direct attempts to determine the P/O ratio in intact cells have been made because of the difficulties encountered in determining the rapid turnover of ATP molecules involved in the maintenance of a cell's metabolic activities without disturbing the cell's internal milieu. Nevertheless, the physiological P/O ratio is almost certainly somewhat less than the maximal values of 3 and 2 (probably closer to 2.5 and 1.5) that are commonly used as a basis for calculating the "ATP equivalents" produced by oxidation of NADH and $FADH_2$, respectively, by the electron transport chain.

Generation of Oxygen Free Radicals

Molecular oxygen is an excellent electron acceptor, but the reduction of O_2 can produce potentially harmful intermediates. Although the transfer of 4 electrons and 4 H^+ to O_2 to produce 2 H_2O is harmless, the transfer of one electron to O_2 forms superoxide ($O_2^{\bullet-}$) and the transfer of 2 electrons forms peroxide ($O_2^{\bullet 2-}$). These anionic species each have one unpaired valence shell electron and thus are free radicals. These reactive oxygen species and their reaction products are harmful to cells. Complexes I and III of the electron transport chain have been described as the main producers of reactive oxygen species in the mitochondria; this happens because a small percentage of the electrons passing through the electron transport chain are prematurely leaked and react with O_2, resulting in its incomplete reduction. Several antioxidant systems in the body, such as superoxide dismutase and catalase, are involved in protection against these harmful reactive oxygen species (ROS).

$$O_2 + e^- \rightarrow O_2^{\bullet -} \text{ (superoxide)}$$

$$O_2 + 2e^- \rightarrow O_2^{\bullet 2-} \text{ (peroxide)}$$

NET ATP PRODUCTION FROM FUEL OXIDATION

Net ATP yield depends on the amount of energy (ATP equivalents) the cell must expend in the complete metabolism of the energy-yielding molecule and on that produced via substrate-level phosphorylation and via oxidative phosphorylation. For example, the complete oxidation of 1 molecule of glucose via glycolysis, conversion of pyruvate to acetyl-CoA, and oxidation of acetyl-CoA in the citric acid cycle (as described in Chapter 12) produces 34 ATPs by oxidative phosphorylation and 6 ATPs (or equivalent GTP) by substrate-level phosphorylation. However, 2 ATPs are consumed in glycolysis, so the net yield is 38 ATPs.

The net ATP yield may vary somewhat according to the particular tissue or pathway by which the fuel is catabolized. For example, the overall ATP yield to the body from the complete oxidation of glucose by muscle might vary depending on the source of the glucose. If the glucose comes from the blood, then complete oxidization of glucose would yield 38 moles of ATP per mole of glucose. However, if muscle glycogen is the source of the glucose, with breakdown of glycogen to glucose 1-phosphate, the complete metabolism of this glucose phosphate within the muscle would generate 39 moles of ATP per mole of glucose phosphate; the additional ATP is gained because an ATP does not need to be expended for the phosphorylation of glucose. Glycogen breakdown by glycogen phosphorylase uses inorganic phosphate for the initial phosphorylation of glucose, whereas glucose from plasma requires ATP-dependent phosphorylation by hexokinase.

EFFICIENCY OF TRAPPING FUEL ENERGY AS ATP

Not all of the free energy of dietary fuel molecules is available to the body. The fate of absorbed fuel energy is shown in Figure 21-5. Some energy is lost because of incomplete digestion and absorption of fuel molecules. In general, a small amount (usually no more than 5% to 10%) of the gross energy content of food is lost in feces because of incomplete digestion and absorption. Once absorbed, an additional 5% to 10% of the energy in food molecules is expended in the processes of transport, storage, and biochemical conversion of different fuels into appropriate storage forms (e.g., glucose is converted to glycogen, fatty acids are esterified to

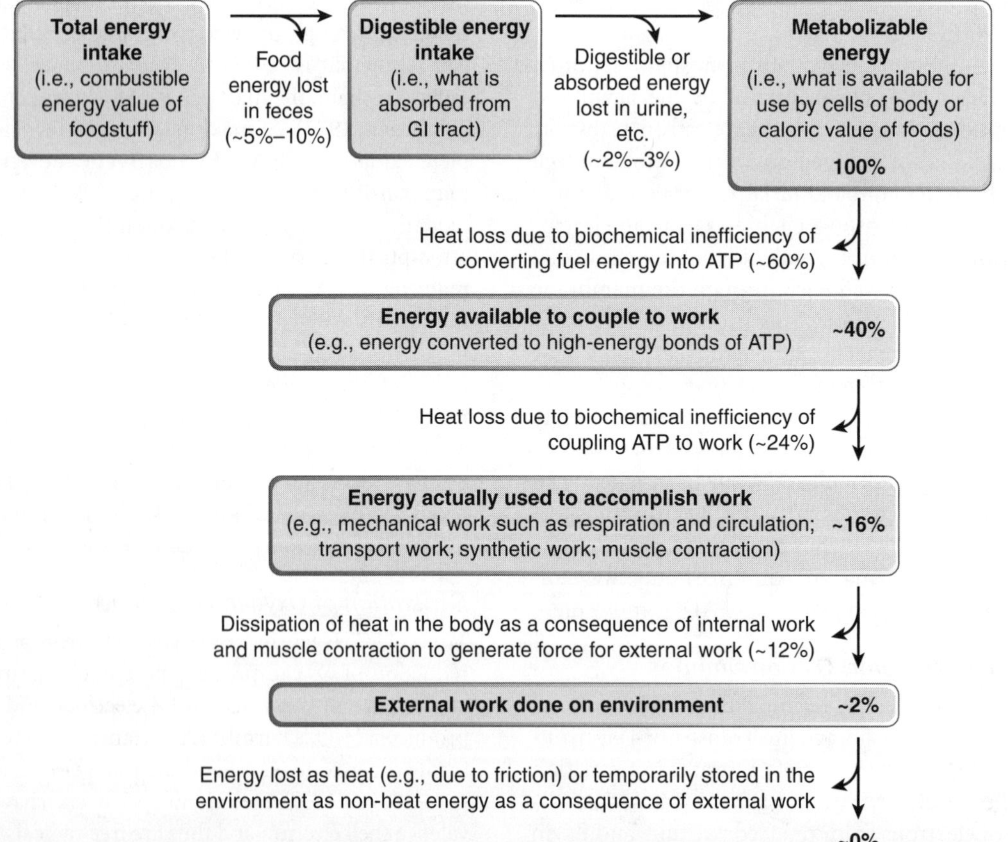

FIGURE 21-5 Conversion of fuel energy to heat and external work in an adult who has no net tissue deposition. For convenience, the metabolizable energy intake (i.e., the food energy available for use by the body) is shown as 100%. The combustible energy value of consumed food is somewhat greater than the physiological energy value of the food.

form triacylglycerols, and amino acids are utilized for tissue protein synthesis) (Acheson et al., 1984). Some absorbed energy, about 3% to 5%, is lost in the urine, feces, or other secretions due to excretion of incompletely oxidized metabolites. In particular, the excretion of urea as a waste product of amino acid catabolism results in a loss of approximately 20% of the potential energy that could have been derived from amino acid oxidation.

Theoretically the remaining absorbed energy is available for the body to use for basic processes and physical activity. This energy is called "metabolizable energy" and is shown as 100% of energy intake in Figure 21-5. This metabolizable energy is equivalent to the physiological energy values of foods that are used in reporting caloric content of foods for nutrient analysis/food tables and food product labels. Although energy values of foods are shown as 100% in Figure 21-5 to be consistent with the common practice of reporting caloric values of foods as physiological energy values, it should be noted that the total combustible energy in foods is approximately 8% higher. Thus caloric values of foods have already been corrected for losses due to incomplete digestion and absorption, the cost of excreting nitrogen as urea, and other small obligatory losses.

In theory, all of the metabolizable energy from exogenous (or stored endogenous) fuels is available for the body's use. However, the coupling of energy released by exergonic reactions with energy consumed in endergonic processes is not 100% efficient. The overall efficiency with which the metabolizable energy is used for work depends upon both the efficiency with which the chemical energy in fuel molecules is converted to ATP and the efficiency with which the chemical energy of ATP hydrolysis is converted to work. In fuel oxidation or catabolism, only about 40% to 50% of the available bond energy is conserved in the form of the high-energy phosphate bonds of ATP. Thus roughly 50% to 60% of the total energy released from oxidation of metabolic fuel is lost as heat to the environment. The remaining energy that is captured in the form of ATP is used to fuel both internal (e.g., mechanical, transport, and synthetic processes within the body) and external work (e.g., climbing up stairs). However, the energy released by ATP hydrolysis is not completely coupled to the endergonic reactions it is used to drive, so further losses of captured energy as heat occur when the ATP is consumed. The inefficiency of converting fuel energy to ATP and ATP energy to work is illustrated in Figure 21-5. The energy value of work accomplished ends up being only about 16% of the metabolizable fuel value. Most of the energy actually coupled to cellular work is ultimately lost as heat, giving rise to additional heat production associated with macronutrient oxidation. For example, the energy from ATP hydrolysis that is coupled to muscle contraction in the heart is ultimately lost as heat due to friction as the blood moves through the blood vessels. The heat released in all of these processes is used to maintain body temperature, but heat release can also raise body temperature beyond what can be regulated by vasodilation and thus increase the need for regulatory heat loss (i.e., by sweating).

To the extent that external work is performed, some energy may be transferred to the environment. Some of the energy may remain in the environment in the form of work accomplished (e.g., boxes stacked on a high shelf). This transfer of energy to the environment is relatively small for most individuals, particularly considering that even very active individuals are not performing physical work while sleeping.

Total energy expenditure = Internal heat production
+ External work performed

It should be noted that even much of the energy used for physical activity is dissipated as heat into the environment (e.g., as friction during walking). Thus in cases where humans or animals are enclosed in calorimeter chambers that allow measurement of total heat losses, these losses of heat into the environment as a result of physical work performed on the environment may be captured in addition to heat losses from the body itself.

Overall, the vast majority of the metabolizable energy that is not used for growth or an increase in body energy stores (e.g., fat depots) becomes body heat. The same occurs when body stores are metabolized as fuel in the absence of exogenous fuel intake. Thus heat production is a valid measure of fuel oxidation or energy expenditure.

UNCOUPLING OXIDATIVE PHOSPHORYLATION

The coupling of electron transfer to oxidative phosphorylation can be affected by physiological proteins called uncoupling proteins and by pharmacological agents that cause dissipation of the electrochemical gradient.

Uncoupling Protein 1 and Brown Fat

Physiological uncoupling of oxidative phosphorylation occurs in the presence of specialized uncoupling proteins within the mitochondrial membrane (Figure 21-6). Brown

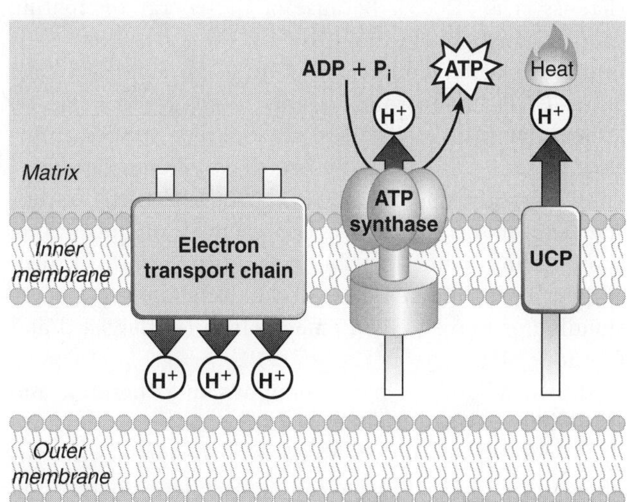

FIGURE 21-6 Uncoupling proteins (UCP) are embedded within the inner mitochondrial membrane and function to dissipate the proton gradient generated by the electron transport chain before it can be used to provide the energy for oxidative phosphorylation.

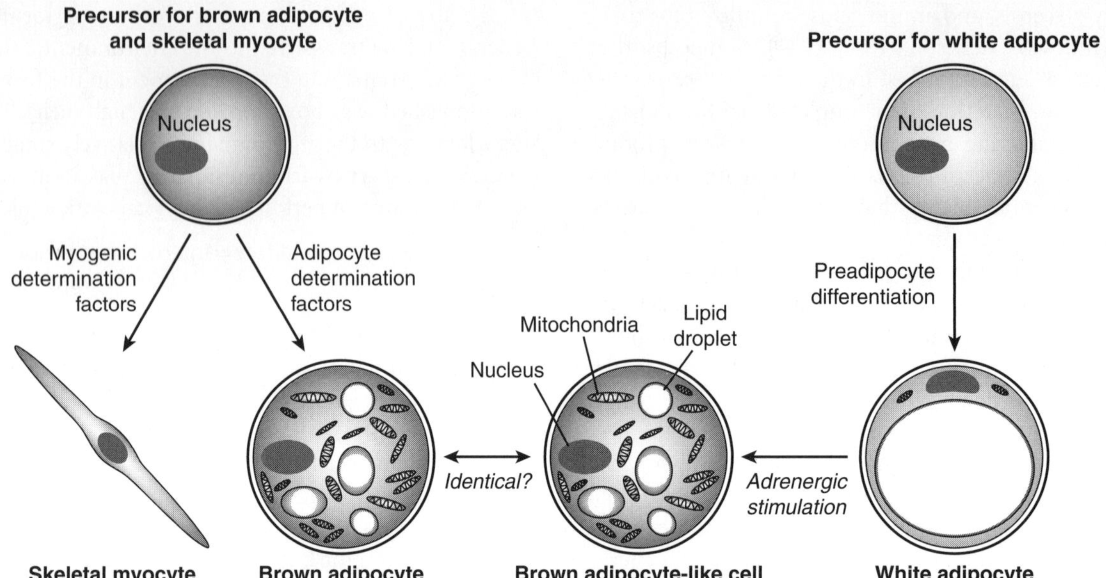

FIGURE 21-7 Brown adipocytes are multilocular (many small lipid droplets) with numerous mitochondria. Brown adipocytes (Myf5 positive) can be derived from the same precursor cells that give rise to myocytes. Cells similar to brown adipocytes (Myf5 negative) can result from transdifferentiation of white adipocytes in response to β-adrenergic stimulation. Myogenic factor 5 (Myf5) plays a role in muscle cell differentiation and is used as a marker for myogenic lineage. (Modified from Lazar, M. A. [2008]. How now, brown fat? *Science, 321*, 1048–1049.)

adipose tissue (BAT) is a site of significant uncoupling, which occurs via a unique protein in the inner mitochondrial membrane. The protein, uncoupling protein 1 (UCP1), permits the reentry of protons into the mitochondrial matrix independent of ATP synthesis, so that the potential energy generated by the proton gradient is lost as heat. UCP1 appears to be unique to brown adipocytes and mainly functions in thermogenesis, but there are other uncoupling proteins (UCP2, UCP3, UCP4, UCP5) in many tissues of the human body, and these have varying ability to uncouple and to influence thermogenesis (Krauss et al., 2005). Because of the energy-dissipating properties of uncoupling proteins, there has been great interest in better understanding their physiological role. Some UCPs may protect against oxidative damage by attenuating production of reactive oxygen species, influence signaling in pancreatic beta cells, or alter fatty acid handling or transport (Cioffi et al., 2009). A better understanding of the function and regulation of uncoupling proteins and of the distribution and function of brown adipocytes in humans is needed to facilitate our understanding of human energy metabolism (Nedergaard and Cannon, 2010).

Brown adipocytes have numerous mitochondria and small lipid droplets, and they are more metabolically active than white adipocytes. BAT specifically expresses uncoupling protein 1 (UCP1) and functions in fat oxidation and thermogenesis. As illustrated in Figure 21-7, there is now evidence that brown adipocytes are actually derived from myocyte precursor cells rather than from preadipocytes (white adipocyte precursor cells). In addition to the specific but small deposits of BAT in humans, white adipose tissue contains some proportion of brown adipocytes, which may be resident cells derived from myocyte precursors or cells derived from transdifferentiation of white adipocytes that are similar to brown adipocytes. Brown adipocytes from either type of precursor have many mitochondria and express UCP1.

BAT has long been recognized as important for maintenance of body temperature in hibernating animals, rodents, and newborn animals, including human infants. The presence of small but metabolically active BAT depots have now been identified in specific regions of adult humans (Cypess and Kahn, 2010). BAT levels have been observed to be higher in women than men, higher in individuals with lower body mass indexes, and higher in individuals with extensive cold exposure. These recent observations suggest that BAT content in adults may be relatively more important in energy expenditure and heat production than previously realized.

Pharmacological Uncoupling Agents

Pharmacological uncoupling agents are lipid-soluble weak acids that dissolve in the membrane and function as carriers for H^+. Different pharmacological agents, such as 2,4-dinitrophenol, caffeine, nicotine, and amphetamines, can affect the efficiency of the coupling of electron transfer to ATP synthesis. These agents dissipate the proton-motive force across the inner mitochondrial membrane, which is essential for driving ATP synthesis; so while electron transport from NADH and $FADH_2$ to oxygen proceeds normally, ATP synthesis is disrupted. This loss of respiratory control leads to more rapid oxidation of NADH and $FADH_2$ and increased oxygen consumption, with less regeneration of ATP from ADP but greater loss of energy as heat (Argyropoulos et al., 1998).

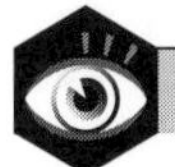

NUTRITION INSIGHT

Targeting Brown Adipose Tissue to Increase Thermogenesis as a Potential Therapeutic for Extreme Obesity

With obesity rates reaching epidemic proportions, effective treatment methods are needed. One approach is the development of pharmaceutical treatments, and a number of drugs are currently being developed and tested in clinical trials. As of 2011, only phentermine (phenyl-tertiary-butylamine) and orlistat were approved by the United States Food and Drug Administration for weight loss treatments. Phentermine promotes maintenance of high levels of catecholamines that in turn suppress appetite and hunger signals and increase peripheral energy expenditure. Orlistat blocks lipase activity in the gastrointestinal tract and thus reduces lipid absorption. Another approach for regulation of energy balance is to increase energy expenditure. Recent evidence that adults maintain potentially active brown adipose tissue (BAT) has increased interest in the possibility of selectively increasing energy expenditure through targeting thermogenesis by BAT. In response to cold, noradrenaline released from the sympathetic nervous system acts on BAT to promote the proliferation and differentiation of brown preadipocytes and to activate uncoupling protein 1 to induce thermogenesis. It might be possible to develop adrenergic receptor agonists and other drugs that mimic the normal cold response to induce an increase in brown adipocyte numbers and to promote active thermogenesis in BAT. "Magic bullets" that are safe for long-term use are likely to be difficult to find, but the possibility as well as the difficulties are illustrated by experience with 2,4-dinitrophenol. In the early 1930s, 2,4-dinitrophenol, an industrial chemical, was found to greatly increase thermogenesis by nonselectively uncoupling mitochondrial oxidation. It inhibits mitochondrial ATP synthase and reduces cellular ATP levels, while the energy from electron transport is released as heat. However, this metabolic poison was soon banned by the U.S. Food and Drug Administration because of severe hazards associated with its use, including extreme overheating and death.

SUBSTRATE CYCLING

Substrate cycling refers to sets of opposing, nonequilibrium reactions that are catalyzed by different enzymes and that are active simultaneously. At least one of the reactions is driven by the hydrolysis of ATP so the effect is a net hydrolysis of ATP along with heat production, but this occurs without a net gain in substrate or product. Because ATP is consumed in these cycles with no net change in the proportion of substrate to product, these reactions are often termed futile cycles. A specific example of a substrate cycle is the interconversion of fructose 6-phosphate and fructose 1,6-bisphosphate by 6-phosphofructo-1-kinase (a glycolytic enzyme) and fructose 1,6-bisphosphatase (a gluconeogenic enzyme), as shown in Figure 21-8. In this cycle, as in all futile cycles, ATP is expended but no net metabolism is accomplished. Excessive flux through such cycles is generally prevented by reciprocal regulatory controls, but substantial unproductive flux may still occur. Many other potentially important substrate cycles exist for carbohydrate and fat metabolism.

The relative importance of these cycles is not fully understood. One possibility is that substrate cycles allow the amplification of metabolic signals by permitting regulation of both the forward and the reverse reactions. Another possibility is that substrate cycles facilitate rapid fine-tuning of net metabolic flux. More relevant to this chapter, substrate cycling has the potential to alter energy expenditure by influencing thermogenesis, because the ATP hydrolysis used to fuel these cycles generates heat. The rates of these substrate cycles vary and can increase manyfold in response to specific conditions, such as severe burns, cold exposure, or exercise. Hormones can also radically influence the rate of substrate cycling. For example, leptin is an adipokine (more fully discussed in Chapter 22) that influences long-term energy expenditure in mammals. One manner in which leptin influences energy expenditure is by stimulating triacylglycerol and fatty acid cycling. Fatty acids released by lipolysis undergo immediate reesterification, with ATP being hydrolyzed at each cycle of reesterification due to its requirement for acyl-CoA synthesis. This leptin-induced cycling occurs primarily to dissipate

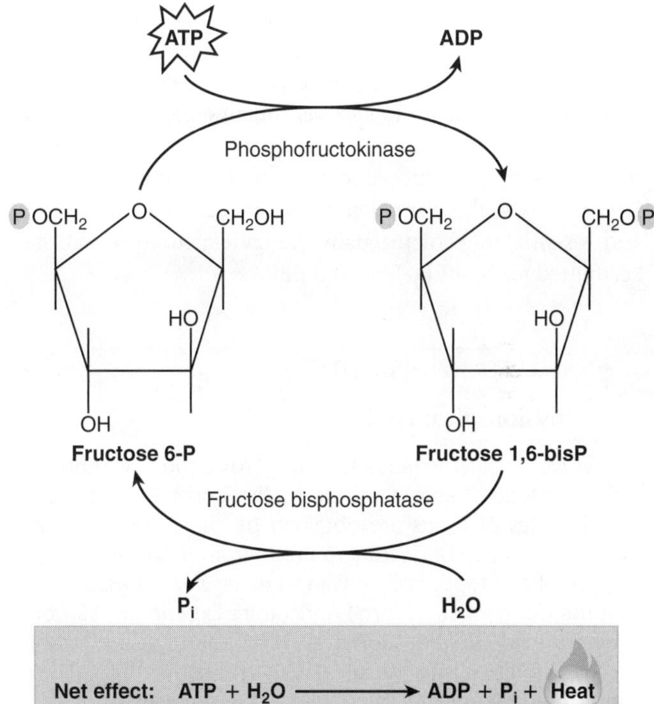

FIGURE 21-8 Example of substrate cycling. The phosphorylation of fructose 6-phosphate (fructose 6-P) to fructose 1,6-bisphosphate (fructose 1,6-bisP) requires ATP during glycolysis. The dephosphorylation of fructose 1,6-bisP, as occurs during gluconeogenesis, consumes H_2O and produces inorganic phosphate. The result of substrate cycling is no net change in substrate or product, only hydrolysis of ATP to ADP + P_i and production of heat.

energy for thermogenesis but also results in an increase in circulating fatty acids that results in a shifting of cellular fuel preference from glucose to fatty acids (Reidy and Weber, 2002). Because the rates of substrate cycling can vary within cells in response to endocrine or environmental stimuli, changes in substrate cycles could alter the efficiency of energy use and hence change the overall efficiency of metabolism and energy use by the whole body (Newsholme and Parry-Billings, 1992).

WHOLE-ANIMAL ENERGETICS

The typical energy expenditure of adults in the United States is 1,500 to 3,000 kcal/day. In adults who are not pregnant or lactating and are not gaining weight, total energy expenditure is essentially equal to total energy intake, as calculated using physiological fuel values that have been precorrected for losses in the feces and urine.

COMPONENTS OF ENERGY EXPENDITURE

There are three principal components of human energy expenditure: BEE (basal energy expenditure), TEF (thermic effect of food), and EEPA (energy expenditure of physical activity), as shown in Figure 21-9. There are also other small components of energy expenditure that may contribute to the whole, such as the energetic costs of cold adaptation. Although cold adaptation is well documented in humans (van Marken Lichtenbelt and Daanen, 2003), the majority of humans are not exposed to extremes of cold temperature. In most cases, these small components can be disregarded, and essentially all of the daily energy expenditure will be accounted for by BEE, TEF, and EEPA.

Basal Energy Expenditure

BEE is the energy expended when an individual is supine at complete rest, in the morning, after sleep, and in the post-absorptive state. BEE accounts for approximately 60% of total daily energy expenditure in individuals with sedentary lifestyles. Because it is not always possible to measure BEE under rigidly defined conditions, resting metabolic rate (RMR) is often used as an approximation of BEE. RMR is slightly higher than BEE because of the additional energy costs of arousal, posture, and being in a nonfasted state. BEE and RMR are sometimes used interchangeably even though RMR and BEE are not equivalent.

Thermic Effect of Food

TEF is the increase in energy expenditure associated with the digestion, absorption, and storage of food. It accounts

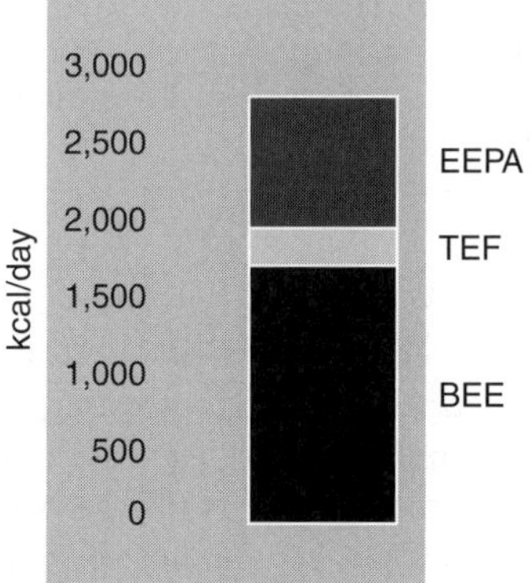

FIGURE 21-9 The components of energy expenditure in sedentary adults. *BEE,* Basal energy expenditure; *EEPA,* energy expenditure for physical activity; *TEF,* thermic effect of food.

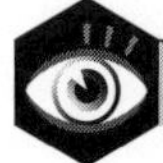

NUTRITION INSIGHT

Physiological Fuel Values

Physiological fuel value is a term used to connote the energy from a food that is available to the body. Physiological fuel values of foods are obtained by subtracting energy lost in the excreta (feces and urine) from the total energy value of the food. Wilbur Olin Atwater and his associates at the Connecticut (Storrs) Agriculture Experiment Station determined the digestibility and fuel values of a number of food materials in the late 1800s and early 1900s. They proposed the general physiological fuel equivalents of 4.0, 8.9, and 4.0 kcal/g for dietary protein, fat, and carbohydrate, respectively, for application to the mixed American diet. In the years following the publication of Atwater's work, the 4, 9, and 4 (rounded) factors became widely used in estimating the caloric value of foods.

It should be noted that factors for carbohydrate, fat, or protein in specific foods may vary considerably because of differences in digestibility or chemical composition. The general factors are intended for application to mixed diets. The carbohydrate factor is applied to total food carbohydrate, which includes nondigestible carbohydrate that is now referred to as dietary fiber. In addition, in deriving the factors, Atwater attributed all of the energy lost in the urine to excretion of protein nitrogen as urea; this is not strictly correct, but the error associated with the calculation of energy value of foods by applying Atwater's factors to diets has been estimated to be small.

In the early 1970s the data and values of Atwater were checked and confirmed by 108 digestion experiments conducted by Annabel L. Merrill and Bernice K. Watt at the U.S. Department of Agriculture (Merrill and Watt, 1973). The available energy of the diets, determined from gross energy values of food, feces, and urine, showed close agreement with calculations based on the application of average energy factors to the protein, fat, and carbohydrate in the diet. Merrill and Watt also recalculated Atwater's general factors for protein, fat, and carbohydrate, based on a typical U.S. mixed diet in 1949. They obtained average values of 4.0, 8.9, and 3.9, which were essentially the same as the general factors Atwater reported in 1899. The rounded 4, 9, and 4 factors for physiological fuel values derived by Atwater are still widely used today, more than a century later.

for approximately 5% to 15% of total daily energy expenditure of adults (Warwick, 2006; Granata and Brandon, 2002). TEF can be observed as an increase in energy expenditure that occurs over several hours following ingestion of food. Estimates of TEF are usually based on intake of a mixed diet. However, if single macronutrients are considered, TEF would theoretically differ, being highest for assimilation of protein, intermediate for assimilation of carbohydrate, and least for assimilation of fat. There is also evidence that there is modulation in TEF based on meal patterns, habits of physical activity, and degree of adiposity (de Jonge and Bray, 2002; Denzer and Young, 2003; Farshchi et al., 2004).

Energy Expenditure of Physical Activity

EEPA is the sum of the daily energy expenditure for physical movement or work. For most individuals, even those who regularly engage in purposeful exercise, the predominant component of EEPA is the energy expenditure associated with all the activities that are part of daily living. This includes occupational activities (e.g., construction work, office work, or housekeeping), leisure activities, sitting, standing, lifting, walking, talking, toe tapping, jittering, playing guitar, dancing, and shopping. Levine and colleagues have given the term *nonexercise activity thermogenesis* (NEAT) to this component of EEPA (Levine et al., 2000; Kotz and Levine, 2005). Exercise or purposeful physical activity undertaken for health or fitness (e.g., sporting events or planned resistance or endurance training) can be a significant component of EEPA for individuals who regularly engage in strenuous activities for substantial periods of time (Pacy et al., 1986).

MEASUREMENT OF ENERGY EXPENDITURE

Energy expenditure in the whole body is most often measured using the methods of direct and indirect calorimetry. Direct calorimetry measures the energy that is lost as heat. Indirect calorimetry measures the gas exchange that occurs in fuel oxidation.

Direct Calorimetry

Direct calorimetry measures the heat released from the body by directly measuring changes in the temperature of the environment surrounding the organism (usually a carefully controlled, closed environmental chamber) (Jequier and Schutz, 1983). Direct calorimetry or measurement of heat loss is a good measure of energy expenditure because fuel utilization in the body results in the loss of almost all of the energy as heat due to inefficiencies at each step of energy transfer. In addition to energy lost directly by transfer of heat to the environment, some energy or heat is lost by evaporation of water. In addition, a small amount of energy may be lost from the body as external physical work, which includes both subsequent heat transferred to the environment as a consequence of work (e.g., from friction associated with pedaling a bike) and true net work (e.g., charging of a battery accomplished by pedaling a stationary bicycle). Limitations of direct calorimetry are that it may not measure energy transfer to the environment, which is usually only a concern when the individual is engaged in high-intensity work, and that it will not measure transient heat storage in the body associated with changes in core body temperatures during measurement periods of less than 24 hours. In practice, direct calorimetry is rarely used because of the cost and complexity of the equipment and the constraints placed on the subject.

Indirect Calorimetry

Indirect calorimetry is more commonly used to measure energy expenditure. Oxygen uptake or carbon dioxide release via the lungs is measured as a surrogate for heat production. Measurement of gas exchange is relatively easy, requiring the subject to breathe in and out through a face mask or mouth piece. Indirect calorimetry is based on the knowledge that heat production in the body originates from the coupled metabolic processes involved in ATP turnover, O_2 consumption, and the conversion of fuels to CO_2 plus H_2O. Although the biological oxidation of fuel molecules does not occur in the same manner in which these organic compounds are converted to CO_2, H_2O, and heat when they are burned in a flame, the overall reaction is similar. Thus O_2 is consumed and CO_2 and heat are produced in specific amounts depending on the substrate (or mixture of substrates) oxidized. For example, the oxidation of glucose yields products with the following stoichiometry:

$$C_6H_{12}O_6 + 6\ O_2 \rightarrow 6\ H_2O + 6\ CO_2 + 673\ \text{kcal/mol}$$

The energy yields per mole of O_2 utilized and per mole of CO_2 produced have been determined experimentally for the main oxidative substrates, and these factors can be used to calculate heat production from the quantity of O_2 consumed or the quantity of CO_2 produced. As can be seen in Table 21-1, the values for O_2 consumption in kilocalories per liter are more consistent than those for CO_2 production, so O_2 consumption is usually used if only one gas is measured. In a resting subject accustomed to an average diet (providing 35% of total energy as fat, 12% as protein, and 53% as carbohydrate) who is studied in the postabsorptive state, approximately 4.83 kcal are expended for every liter of O_2 consumed. Although different amounts of oxygen are consumed during the biological oxidation of different energy-yielding foodstuffs, the multiplication of liters of O_2 consumed by 4.83 kilocalories per liter will provide an estimate of heat production to within approximately 8% of the actual value regardless of which nutrients are being oxidized.

Indirect calorimetry has the advantages of requiring relatively simple equipment and less restriction of the subject. Because the body's oxygen store is very small, measurement of oxygen consumption by indirect calorimetry can provide a rapid measure of heat production that is temporally linked to metabolic energy utilization. Indirect calorimetry also measures energy used for external work on the environment, because it does not depend on capturing the energy expenditure per se, but rather assesses the metabolic processes involved in generating the ATP that fuels the physical

TABLE 21-1 Energy and Respiratory Equivalent of Body Fuels

	Energy			Fuel/Energy/Gas Volume Relationships				
FOOD	COMPLETE OXIDATION OF FOOD COMPONENT BY BURNING (kcal/g)	"COMPLETE OXIDATION" OF ABSORBED OR STORED FUEL IN BODY* (kcal/g)	PHYSIOLOGICAL FUEL VALUE OF CONSUMED FOODSTUFF† (kcal/g)	O_2 (kcal/L)	CO_2 (kcal/L)	RQ (Vco_2/Vo_2)	O_2 (L/g)	CO_2 (L/g)
Carbohydrate	4.1	4.1	4	5.05	5.05	1.00	0.81	0.81
Protein	5.4	4.2	4	4.46	5.57	0.80	0.94	0.75
Fat	9.3	9.3	9	4.74	6.67	0.71	1.96	1.39
Alcohol	7.1	7.1	7	4.86	7.25	0.67	1.46	0.98
AVERAGE				4.83	5.89	0.82		

*N is excreted as urea, which has an energy content of 5.4 kcal/g N. All energy in urine is attributed to N excretion in this calculation, yielding a conversion factor of 7.9 kcal/g N for estimation of urinary energy from urinary N.

†Values are adjusted for digestibility (incomplete absorption) and incomplete oxidation.

RQ, Respiratory quotient.

work. On the other hand, indirect calorimetry may underestimate energy expenditure during intense exercise when rapid glycolysis with lactate production (without O_2 uptake or CO_2 production) can significantly contribute to total ATP turnover via substrate level phosphorylation. Additionally, washout or storage of CO_2 in the carbonate pool (e.g., due to increased or decreased respiration rate) can affect the accuracy of short-term measurements.

Indirect calorimetry has become a frequently used and informative tool to assess energy expenditure and substrate utilization under various physiological states or in response to interventions (e.g., pharmacological, dietary, and physical training) in humans as well as rodents. An important point to consider is how results from these studies are interpreted (Butler and Kozak, 2010). In humans, experimental data are generally presented relative to fat-free mass or lean body mass, of which skeletal muscle is the predominant constituent. This is appropriate because skeletal muscle and other tissues making up the lean body mass are metabolically more active than adipose tissues and the approximate contribution of lean body mass to total body mass is easily determined by assessment of body composition. However, in rodent research there is greater disparity in how indirect calorimetry data are presented and interpreted. This is a controversial area of discussion but nonetheless a very important consideration when interpreting rodent research and its translational relevance to humans (Butler and Kozak, 2010).

Respiratory Quotient

An additional advantage of indirect calorimetry is the ability to determine the particular fuels being oxidized. The amount of heat released per liter of O_2 consumed or CO_2 produced depends on the type of nutrient being oxidized (i.e., protein, carbohydrate, or fat). By measuring CO_2 production and urinary nitrogen excretion in addition to O_2 consumption, it is possible to determine the proportion of the different nutrients that are oxidized and thus to calculate the heat released from each nutrient class. The ratio of CO_2 produced to O_2 consumed is called the respiratory quotient (RQ), and values for different types of nutrients are given in Table 21-1.

In essence, the RQ reflects the relative amount of oxygen in the hydrocarbon fuel molecule. For example, triacylglycerol, or fat, is much more reduced than glucose or carbohydrate. A molecule of tripalmitolyglycerol ($C_{51}H_{96}O_6$) contains 0.12 oxygen atoms per carbon atom (e.g., 6 O/51 C), requires 72.5 O_2 molecules for its complete oxidation, has a low RQ of 0.70 (i.e., 51 CO_2/72.5 O_2), and is able to donate many reducing equivalents during its metabolic oxidation. On the other hand, glucose ($C_6H_{12}O_6$) is a polyhydroxy alcohol that contains 1.0 oxygen atom per carbon atom (e.g., 6 O/6 C), requires 6 molecules of O_2 for its complete oxidation, has a high RQ of 1.0 (i.e., 6 CO_2/6 O_2), and, because it is relatively more oxidized, has fewer electrons to donate to pyridine and flavin nucleotides during its catabolism to CO_2.

Indirect Calorimetry Using Doubly Labeled Water

Another indirect method was developed in the 1960s for measuring total energy expenditure (TEE) in free-living individuals over periods of 10 to 14 days (Schoeller et al., 1986). This method uses water that has been doubly labeled with the isotopes ^2H (deuterium) and ^{18}O. The principle behind the doubly labeled water method is illustrated in Figure 21-10. ^2H from the body's labeled water pool leaves as deuterated water, whereas the ^{18}O equilibrates with

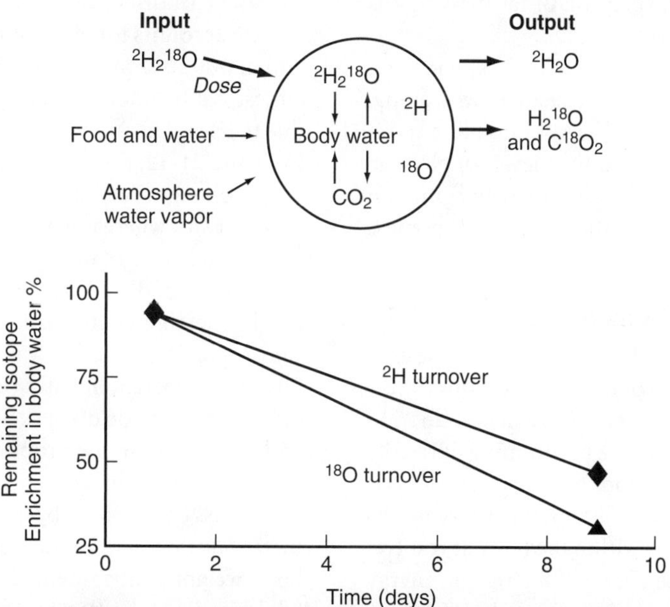

FIGURE 21-10 Model of doubly labeled water technique. Water labeled with ^2H and ^{18}O mixes with the total body water. ^2H is lost in H_2O, whereas the ^{18}O from the H_2O equilibrates with CO_2 ($CO_2 + H_2O \leftrightarrow H_2CO_3$) and is lost in both H_2O and CO_2. The difference in the rate of loss of ^2H and ^{18}O from the body water pool is related to the rate of CO_2 production from the fuel metabolized. From this analysis, energy expenditure can be determined in a free-living individual by sampling body fluids (H_2O) over time.

CO_2 via the reaction catalyzed by carbonic anhydrase ($H_2CO_3 \rightleftharpoons CO_2 + H_2O$) and thus leaves the body in both water and CO_2. The difference in the disappearance rates of the two isotopes and a measure of the size of the body water pool provide an estimate of unlabeled CO_2 production from oxidation of fuels. Oxygen consumption can then be calculated from an estimate of the RQ; RQ can be measured or estimated from diet composition and tabled values.

FACTORS INFLUENCING BASAL ENERGY EXPENDITURE

BEE is the major component of TEE for most individuals. Based on analysis of published studies in which BEE was measured for adult women and men (Ramirez-Zea, 2005), the average BEE was determined to be 1,300 ± 120 kcal/day for women (range of 880 to 1,600 kcal/day) and 1600 ± 180 kcal/day for men (range of 1,100 to 2,000 kcal/day). Under standard conditions the within-individual coefficient of variation (CV) in BEE of healthy adult humans is approximately 3% to 8% when measured on the same or different days.

Lean Body Mass

BEE is largely a function of lean body mass. Age and gender have modest effects beyond that accounted for by lean body mass (Kien and Bunn, 2008; Bosy-Westphal et al., 2003). Total daily energy expenditure declines with increasing age. It is also documented that lean body mass declines with aging, and because BEE is highly correlated with lean body mass, a decline in BEE is expected. Recent evidence indicates that not only decreases in the mass of individual organs but also a reduction in the metabolic rate of specific organs account for the reduction in BEE observed with aging (St-Onge and Gallagher, 2010). The decreased BEE is thought to be a major contributor to the expansion of fat mass that is also associated with increasing age.

Regarding other components of energy expenditure, there is no convincing evidence that TEF changes with aging. In many elderly individuals, EEPA decreases due to a more sedentary lifestyle. In people who maintain levels of physical activity, however, much of the decline in BEE with aging can be prevented, largely due to preservation of lean body mass (Poehlman and Horton, 1990).

Contribution of Individual Tissues to BEE

The O_2 consumption of individual tissues in vivo can be estimated by making measurements of the arteriovenous difference of oxygen concentration across a tissue in conjunction with measurement of blood flow. The partitioning of resting energy expenditure among the various body organ systems is shown in Figure 21-11. Brain, liver, kidney, and heart are the most metabolically active organs within the body at rest (on a per gram basis) and comprise over half the resting energy expenditure, even though they account for only 5% to 6% of body weight. These four tissues have metabolic rates that are 15 to 40 times greater than an equivalent mass of resting muscle and 50 to 100 times greater than an equivalent mass of adipose tissue. Although the energy expenditure of

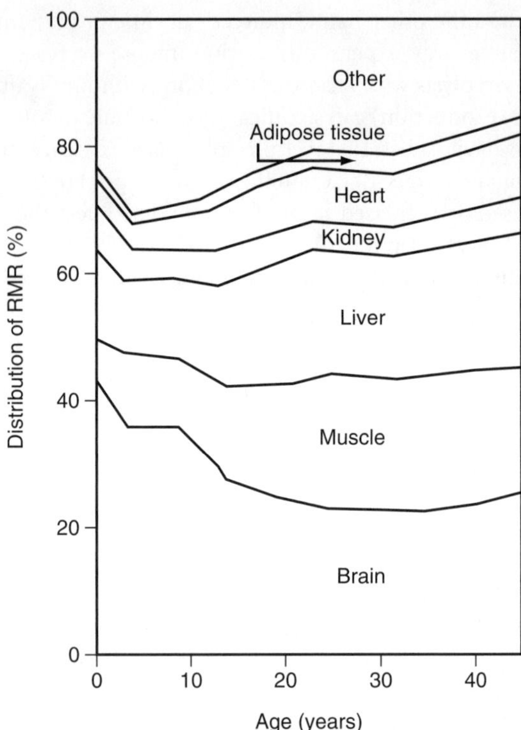

FIGURE 21-11 The contribution of energy expenditure by different organs to resting metabolic rate (*RMR*) or basal energy expenditure. Area is calculated from the product of the organ (tissue) weight and organ (tissue) metabolic rate. (Modified from Elia, M. [1992]. Organ and tissue contribution to metabolic rate. In J. M. Kinney & H. N. Tucker [Eds.], *Energy metabolism: Tissue determinants and cellular corollaries* [pp. 61–79]. New York: Raven Press Ltd.)

resting skeletal muscle is relatively low on a per gram basis, skeletal muscle represents a significant fraction of resting energy expenditure because of its large total mass. Skeletal muscle accounts for about 40% of the total adult body mass and about 20% to 25% of BEE. In infants, the brain is the largest contributor to resting or basal energy expenditure, due to its exaggerated size per unit of body weight. As shown in Figure 21-12, the resting metabolic rate per unit of organ weight changes very little throughout life for the main metabolic organs, whereas whole-body resting metabolic rate per unit of body weight decreases dramatically between infancy/early childhood and adulthood. The drop in whole-body resting metabolic rate is due, at least partly, to an increase in the proportion of the body made up of tissues with relatively low resting metabolic rates (e.g., increases in the proportion of body mass made up of skeletal muscle in men and women and an increase in the proportion of body mass contributed by adipose tissue in women), a decrease in the proportion of body mass contributed by tissues with relatively high resting metabolic rates (e.g., a marked decrease in the proportion of body weight contributed by the brain between infancy and adulthood), and a decreased need for regulatory heat production in the adult due to the larger body mass relative to surface area. (Of course, the total contribution of skeletal muscle increases dramatically during physical exercise, but this is part of the EEPA, not the BEE.)

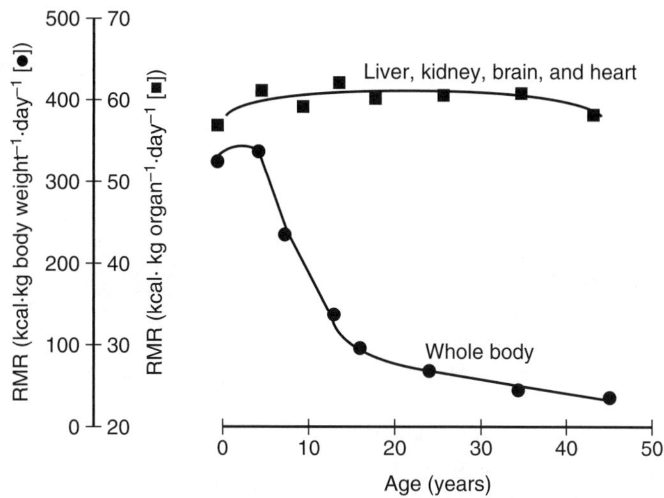

FIGURE 21-12 Changes in resting metabolic rate during growth and development. The whole-body resting metabolic rate (RMR) per kg of body weight is shown along with the metabolic rate for liver, kidney, brain, and heart combined per kg of organ weight. (Organ weight refers to the sum of the weights of liver, kidney, brain, and heart.) (Modified from Elia, M. [1992]. Organ and tissue contribution to metabolic rate. In J. M. Kinney & H. N. Tucker [Eds.], *Energy metabolism: Tissue determinants and cellular corollaries* [pp. 61–79]. New York: Raven Press Ltd.)

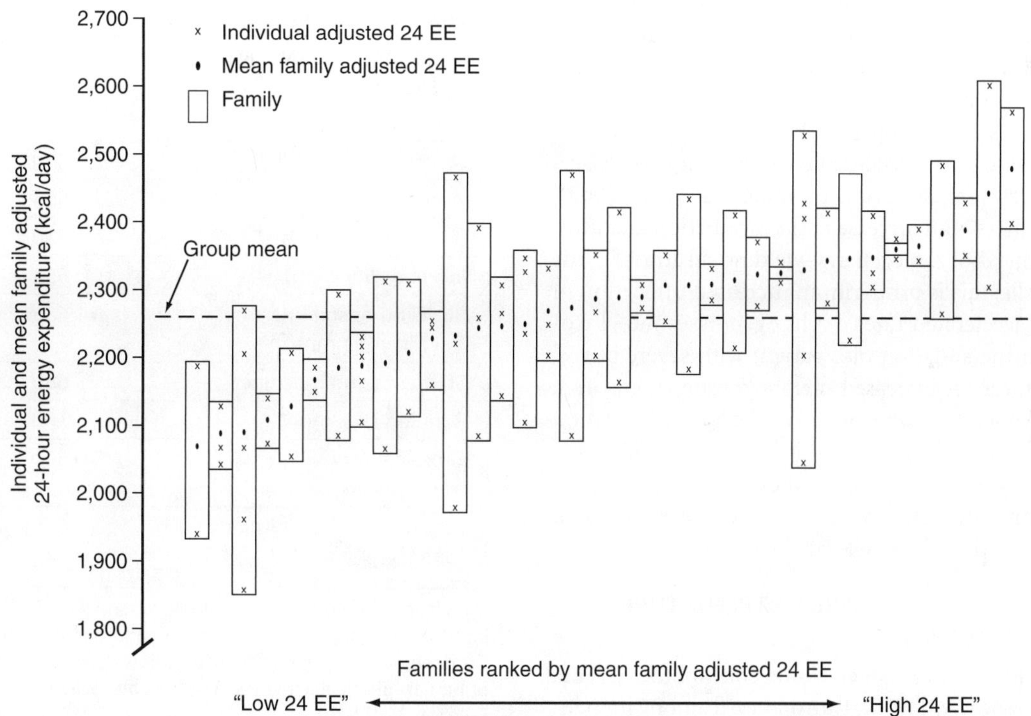

FIGURE 21-13 Individual and mean family total daily (24-hour) energy expenditure (*24 EE*) adjusted for fat-free body mass, fat mass, age, and sex. (Based on the data of Bogardus, C., Lillioja, S., Ravussin, E., Abbott, W., Zawadzki, J. K., Young, A., … & Moll, P. P. [1986]. Familial dependence of the resting metabolic rate. *New England Journal of Medicine, 315*, 96–100.)

Genetic Contribution to BEE

Figure 21-13 shows a strong tendency for 24-hour energy expenditure to aggregate closely within families compared to between families. This familial trait suggests but does not prove that metabolic rate has a strong genetic component (Bogardus et al., 1986). In a study of the heritability of BEE in monozygotic and dizygotic twins, Bouchard and colleagues (1989) observed higher correlations in monozygotic twins than in dizygotic twins, whether BEE was expressed per kg of body weight or per kg of lean body mass. These investigators suggested that an increased number of shared genes is correlated with a greater similarity in the metabolic rate, independent of body size and composition.

Physiological Factors Affecting BEE

Many neural, circulatory, and endocrine factors affect the various heat-producing reactions within cells and thus affect BEE. In particular, thyroid hormone affects BEE. Thyroid hormone affects the expression of specific proteins by altering nuclear transcription rates, thereby affecting metabolic rate and heat production. Thyroid hormone affects several components of the electron transport chain, the cell membrane Na^+,K^+-ATPase pump, and metabolism of macronutrients (Kim, 2008). These effects occur over a period of days to weeks in response to a change in thyroid hormone level. Another example of the effect of hormones is the biphasic pattern observed for BEE over the menstrual cycle, with a greater BEE observed in the luteal phase compared to the follicular phase, presumably due to elevated serum concentrations of estrogen and progesterone (Solomon et al., 1982). Although conducted in older male research participants, a recent study concluded that acute changes in sex steroid hormone concentrations did not change BEE, suggesting that the influence of sex hormones on metabolism may be more a product of the long-term direct effects on body composition (Santosa et al., 2010). However, it is important to note that these findings may be gender specific.

BEE also increases in response to various physiological stresses such as injury, fever, surgery, renal failure, burns, infections, and even starvation or malnutrition (Elia, 2000). In these cases, characteristically catecholamine and other hormone levels increase, BEE increases, and glucose and free fatty acid concentrations rise in the blood. Studies of patients with severe illnesses accompanied by fever have shown up to a 13% increase in metabolic rate for each degree Celsius increase in body temperature (Powanda and Beisel, 2003). During fever, there is an increase in the production and utilization of the metabolizable, energy-yielding substrates made available to cells; this is primarily an increased utilization of glucose from accelerated rates of glycogenolysis and gluconeogenesis. In the situation of a patient with severe burns, the body requires an increased metabolic rate to ensure a stable body temperature when much of the body's insulation is lost by the injury to skin. In addition, in most illnesses, increased energy is required as a result of the increased production of immune response agents and the subsequent energy-requiring processes associated with their actions.

TABLE 21-2 Approximate Energy Cost Above Resting Energy Expenditure of Various Forms of Physical Activity

	ENERGY BURNED PER HOUR* (kcal)
MILD TO MODERATE EXERCISE	
Walking (2–2.5 mph)	185–255
Bicycling or stationary cycling (5.5 mph)	245
Golf (walking with clubs)	270
Aerobic exercise (low impact)	275
Ballroom dancing	300
Strength training	300
Hiking (3 mph, with 20-lb backpack)	400
Treadmill walking (4 mph)	345
Tennis	425
Rowing machine (easy)	300
MODERATE TO INTENSE EXERCISE	
Jumping rope	660
Swimming	540
Walking (5 mph)	555
Bench-stepping class	610
Jogging (5.5 mph)	655
Bicycling or stationary cycling (13 mph)	655
Stair-climbing machine	680
Running (7.2 mph)	700
Cross-country skiing (5 mph)	600
Rowing machine (higher intensity)	655

Data from Ainsworth, B. E., Haskell, W. L., Leon, A. S., Jacobs, D. R., Jr., Montoye, H. J., Sallis, J. F., & Paffenbarger, R. S., Jr. (1993). Compendium of physical activities: Classification of energy costs of human physical activities. *Medicine and Science in Sports and Exercise, 25,* 71–80.

*Values are kcal/hour above resting metabolic rate for an average 70-kg subject.

mph, Miles per hour.

FACTORS INFLUENCING ENERGY EXPENDITURE FOR PHYSICAL ACTIVITY

Besides BEE, EEPA is the other major contributor to TEE. The large differences in TEE that are observed among individuals are largely due to differences in EEPA. For two adults of similar size, TEE can easily vary by as much as 1,500 or 2,000 kcal/day. The energy cost above resting energy expenditure of various forms of physical activity is shown in Table 21-2.

Physical Activity Level

Physical activity level (PAL) is a value used to classify levels of physical activity. PAL is defined as TEE/BEE, ignoring the small contribution of TEF. Figure 21-14 shows the energy expenditure above BEE for various activities and the associated PAL levels (Levine et al., 2000). Thus sitting increases TEE by only 5% compared to BEE, yielding a PAL of 1.05, whereas walking at 3 mph increases TEE by 250% above BEE to give a PAL of 3.5. Because BEE is largely a function of body size, division of TEE by BEE gives a relative measure of physical activity that is adjusted for body size.

Occupation, leisure time activities, and participation in sports or planned exercise all affect one's EEPA. PALs vary substantially among individuals engaged in different occupations, as shown in Table 21-3. To illustrate this point, consider a sedentary office worker with a daily TEE of 2,400 kcal/day, a BEE of 1,500 kcal/day, and a PAL of 1.6.

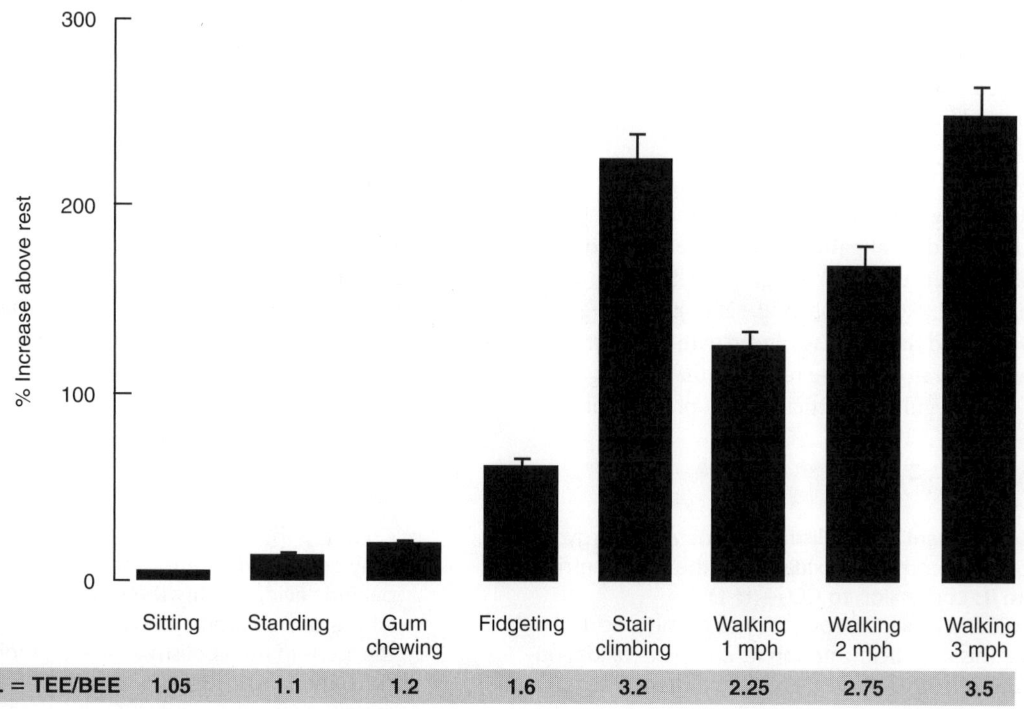

FIGURE 21-14 Energy expenditure above resting for a variety of activities. The physical activity level (*PAL*) for the period of time a person is engaging in the activity is shown below the graph.

TABLE 21-3 Prediction of Physical Activity Level on the Basis of Occupation

OCCUPATION TYPE	PAL
Chairbound or bedbound	1.2
Seated work with no option of moving around and little or no strenuous leisure activity	1.4–1.5
Seated work with discretion and requirement to move around but little or no strenuous leisure activity	1.6–1.7
Standing work (e.g., housewife, shop assistant)	1.8–1.9
Strenuous work or highly active leisure	2.0–2.4

From Black, A. E., Coward, W. A., Cole, T. J., & Prentice, A. M. (1996). Human energy expenditure in affluent societies: An analysis of 574 doubly-labelled water measurements. *European Journal of Clinical Nutrition, 50,* 72–92.
PAL, Physical activity level.

If he or she were to change occupations to achieve a PAL of 2.4, say by starting to work in agriculture or construction, EEPA could be increased by 1,200 kcal/day. Leisure time activities can also have a large impact on TEE. Consider again the same office worker. Assume he or she returns home from work, by car, at 5 PM and from then until 11 PM does little except operate the television remote control in a semirecumbent position. For these 6 hours, the average energy expenditure above resting would approximate 8%, and EEPA would be approximately 30 kcal for the evening [$0.08 \times 1{,}500\ \text{kcal}^{BEE} \times (6/24)$ hour]. Now imagine that he or she instead uses the evening time to paint a bedroom and weed the garden and also chooses to cycle home from work. The increase in energy expenditure would be equivalent to walking approximately 1 to 2 mph for the same period of leisure time (5 to 11 PM), and EEPA would be increased by approximately 560 kcal for the evening [$1.5 \times 1{,}500^{BEE} \times (6/24)$ hour]. Thus for this hypothetical office worker the variance in leisure time EEPA has the potential of increasing TEE by approximately 25%.

Environmental and Physiological Factors Affecting EEPA

EEPA is obviously affected by one's activity level, whether that is determined by preference or necessity. Because EEPA is a large component of TEE and the easiest one to increase, it is an important consideration for prevention and treatment of overweight and obesity. It is also important to recognize that there do appear to be biological influences on EEPA. Evidence suggests that EEPA is biologically regulated, has genetic determinants, and is impacted by shifts in energy balance (Thorburn and Proietto, 2000; Dulloo, 2002). Examples of physiological conditions that contribute to variations in EEPA include dietary intake, type of physical activity, training status (e.g., regularly physically active versus regularly sedentary), degree of adiposity (children and adults), metabolic health status, ethnicity, and age (Elbelt et al., 2010; Westerterp, 2008; Westerterp and Plasqui, 2004; Hollowell et al., 2009; Goran and Treuth, 2001; Soric and Misigoj-Durakovic, 2010; Camoes and Lopes, 2008; Karelis et al., 2008; Holt et al., 2007; Wickel and Eisenmann, 2006; Starling, 2001; Ekelund et al., 2005; Ekelund et al., 2004; Lovejoy et al., 2001). Regulation of energy expenditure is further addressed in Chapter 22.

FACTORS INFLUENCING TEF

Recent evidence suggests that degree of adiposity, habits of physical activity, and meal patterns modulate TEF (de Jonge and Bray, 2002; Denzer and Young, 2003; Farshchi et al., 2004; Thyfault et al., 2004; Stob et al., 2007). De Jonge and Bray (2002) reported that TEF is reduced with increasing adiposity. Several laboratories have reported that TEF is higher in humans who regularly participate in physical activity, both endurance and resistance training (Denzer and Young, 2003; Thyfault et al., 2004; Stob et al., 2007). However, effects of training on TEF may depend on whether the predominant macronutrient in the meal is carbohydrate or fat, being increased in resistance-trained men only when meals were high-carbohydrate/low-fat (Thyfault et al., 2004). Farshchi and colleagues (2004) reported that a regular meal schedule is associated with higher levels of TEF than those found with irregular meal frequency. Although the previously mentioned studies demonstrate that TEF can be altered by adiposity and different patterns of behavior, it is not clear to date whether changes in TEF over time significantly influence day-to-day energy balance and long-term changes in body composition.

THINKING CRITICALLY

1. In macronutrient catabolism to generate energy for the body, the complete oxidation of the macronutrient leads to its conversion to $CO_2 + H_2O$.
   a. Consider a molecule (or mole) of palmitic acid. Trace this fatty acid through its complete oxidation to CO_2 and H_2O. Indicate all steps where CO_2 is produced or O_2 is consumed. As appropriate, indicate steps where substrate-level ATP (or ATP equivalent) is generated and steps where electrons are transferred to NADH or $FADH_2$ for ATP generation by oxidative phosphorylation. See Chapters 12 and 16, if needed, for pathways of fatty acid β-oxidation and acetyl-CoA oxidation via the citric acid cycle. Calculate the RQ for palmitic acid oxidation.
   b. Consider a molecule (or mole) of glucose. Trace glucose through its complete oxidation to CO_2 and H_2O. Indicate all steps where CO_2 is produced or O_2 is consumed. As appropriate, indicate steps where substrate-level ATP (or ATP equivalent) is generated and steps where electrons are transferred to NADH or $FADH_2$ for ATP generation by oxidative phosphorylation. See Chapter 12, if needed, for pathways of glycolysis, conversion of pyruvate to acetyl-CoA, and acetyl-CoA oxidation via the citric acid cycle. Calculate the RQ for glucose oxidation.
   c. Compare the RQs for glucose and palmitic acid. Why are they different? For both glucose and palmitic acid, identify the steps in metabolism where carbon atoms are released as CO_2. Identify the steps in metabolism where O_2 molecules are consumed. What are the sources of the oxygen atoms incorporated into CO_2?
2. Owen et al. (1998) determined that obese subjects starved for 3 weeks lost 11.7 kg, which consisted of 5.9 kg of fat mass and 5.9 kg of fat-free mass. Assume that fat mass is 85% fat and 15% water. Assume that fat-free mass is 20% protein and 80% water.
   a. Calculate the energy yield that could be derived from the oxidation of the fat and the lean tissue.
   b. What percentage of the total energy used during starvation came from fat? From protein?
   c. We know that long-term starvation will eventually lead to death. Is it likely that fat stores would be depleted before death in an obese subject? Explain.

REFERENCES

Acheson, K. J., Ravussin, E., Wahren, J., & Jequier, E. (1984). Thermic effect of glucose in man, obligatory and facultative thermogenesis. *The Journal of Clinical Investigation*, *74*, 1572–1580.

Argyropoulos, G., Brown, A. M., Peterson, R., Likes, C. E., Watson, D. K., & Garvey, W. T. (1998). Structure and organization of the human uncoupling protein 2 gene and identification of a common biallelic variant in Caucasian and African-American subjects. *Diabetes*, *47*, 685–687.

Bogardus, C., Lillioja, S., Ravussin, E., Abbott, W., Zawadzki, J. K., Young, A., … Moll, P. P. (1986). Familial dependence of the resting metabolic rate. *New England Journal of Medicine*, *315*, 96–100.

Bosy-Westphal, A., Eichhorn, C., Kutzner, D., Illner, K., Heller, M., & Müller, M. J. (2003). The age-related decline in resting energy expenditure in humans is due to the loss of fat-free mass and to alterations in its metabolically active components. *The Journal of Nutrition*, *133*, 2356–2362.

Bouchard, C., Tremblay, A., Nadeau, A., Despres, J. P., Theriault, G., Boulay, M. R., … Fournier, G. (1989). Genetic effect in resting and exercise metabolic rates. *Metabolism*, *38*, 364–370.

Butler, A. A., & Kozak, L. P. (2010). A recurring problem with the analysis of energy expenditure in genetic models expressing lean and obese phenotypes. *Diabetes*, *59*, 323–329.

Camoes, M., & Lopes, C. (2008). Dietary intake and different types of physical activity: Full-day energy expenditure, occupational and leisure-time. *Public Health Nutrition*, *11*, 841–848.

Cioffi, F., Senese, R., de Lange, P., Goglia, F., Lanni, A., & Lombardi, A. (2009). Uncoupling proteins: A complex journey to function discovery. *BioFactors*, *35*, 417–428.

Cypess, A. M., & Kahn, C. R. (2010). The role and importance of brown adipose tissue in energy homeostasis. *Current Opinion in Pediatrics*, *22*, 478–484.

de Jonge, L., & Bray, G. A. (2002). The thermic effect of food is reduced in obesity. *Nutrition Reviews*, *60*, 295–297.

Denzer, C. M., & Young, J. C. (2003). The effect of resistance exercise on the thermic effect of food. *International Journal of Sport Nutrition and Exercise Metabolism, 13*, 396–402.

Dulloo, A. G. (2002). Biomedicine: A sympathetic defense against obesity. *Science, 297*, 780–781.

Ekelund, U., Brage, S., Franks, P. W., Hennings, S., Emms, S., Wong, M. Y., & Wareham, N. J. (2005). Physical activity energy expenditure predicts changes in body composition in middle-aged healthy whites: Effect modification by age. *The American Journal of Clinical Nutrition, 81*, 964–969.

Ekelund, U., Yngve, A., Brage, S., Westerterp, K., & Sjöström, M. (2004). Body movement and physical activity energy expenditure in children and adolescents: How to adjust for differences in body size and age. *The American Journal of Clinical Nutrition, 79*, 851–856.

Elbelt, U., Schuetz, T., Hoffmann, I., Pirlich, M., Strasburger, C. J., & Lochs, H. (2010). Differences of energy expenditure and physical activity patterns in subjects with various degrees of obesity. *Clinical Nutrition, 29*, 766–772.

Elia, M. (2000). Hunger disease. *Clinical Nutrition, 19*, 379–386.

Farshchi, H. R., Taylor, M. A., & Macdonald, I. A. (2004). Decreased thermic effect of food after an irregular compared with a regular meal pattern in healthy lean women. *International Journal of Obesity and Related Metabolic Disorders, 28*, 653–660.

Flatt, J. P. (1985). Energetics of intermediary metabolism. In J. S. Garrow & D. Halliday (Eds.), *Substrate and energy metabolism* (pp. 58–69). London: John Libbey.

Goran, M. I., & Treuth, M. S. (2001). Energy expenditure, physical activity, and obesity in children. *Pediatric Clinics of North America, 48*, 931–953.

Granata, G. P., & Brandon, L. J. (2002). The thermic effect of food and obesity: Discrepant results and methodological variations. *Nutrition Reviews, 60*, 223–233.

Hollowell, R. P., Willis, L. H., Slentz, C. A., Topping, J. D., Bhakpar, M., & Kraus, W. E. (2009). Effects of exercise training amount on physical activity energy expenditure. *Medicine and Science in Sports and Exercise, 41*, 1640–1644.

Holt, H. B., Wild, S. H., Wareham, N., Ekelund, U., Umpleby, M., Shojaee-Moradie, F., … Byrne, C. D. (2007). Differential effects of fatness, fitness and physical activity energy expenditure on whole-body, liver and fat insulin sensitivity. *Diabetologia, 50*, 1698–1706.

Jequier, E., & Schutz, Y. (1983). Long-term measurements of energy expenditure in humans using a respiration chamber. *The American Journal of Clinical Nutrition, 38*, 989–998.

Karelis, A. D., Lavoie, M. E., Messier, V., Mignault, D., Garrel, D., Prud'homme, D., & Rabasa-Lhoret, R. (2008). Relationship between the metabolic syndrome and physical activity energy expenditure: A MONET study. *Applied Physiology, Nutrition, and Metabolism, 33*, 309–314.

Kien, C. L., & Bunn, J. Y. (2008). Gender alters the effects of palmitate and oleate on fat oxidation and energy expenditure. *Obesity (Silver Spring), 16*, 29–33.

Kim, B. (2008). Thyroid hormone as a determinant of energy expenditure and the basal metabolic rate. *Thyroid, 18*, 141–144.

Kotz, C. M., & Levine, J. A. (2005). Role of nonexercise activity thermogenesis (NEAT) in obesity. *Minnesota Medicine, 88*, 54–57.

Krauss, S., Zhang, C. Y., & Lowell, B. B. (2005). The mitochondrial uncoupling-protein homologues. *Nature Reviews. Molecular Cell Biology, 6*, 248–261.

Levine, J. A., Schleusner, S. J., & Jensen, M. D. (2000). Energy expenditure of nonexercise activity. *The American Journal of Clinical Nutrition, 72*, 1451–1454.

Lovejoy, J. C., Champagne, C. M., Smith, S. R., de Jonge, L., & Xie, H. (2001). Ethnic differences in dietary intakes, physical activity, and energy expenditure in middle-aged, premenopausal women: The Healthy Transitions Study. *The American Journal of Clinical Nutrition, 74*, 90–95.

McBride, B. W., & Kelly, J. M. (1990). Energy cost of absorption and metabolism in the ruminant gastrointestinal tract and liver: A review. *Journal of Animal Science, 68*, 2997–3010.

Merrill, A. L., & Watt, B. K. (1973). *Energy values of foods—basis and derivation. USDA Agriculture Handbook #74 (revised)*. Washington, DC: U.S. Department of Agriculture.

Murphy, M. P., & Brand, M. D. (1987). Variable stoichiometry of proton pumping by the mitochondrial respiratory chain. *Nature, 329*, 170–172.

Nedergaard, J., & Cannon, B. (2010). The changed metabolic world with human brown adipose tissue: Therapeutic visions. *Cell Metabolism, 11*, 268–272.

Newsholme, E. A., & Parry-Billings, M. (1992). Some evidence for the existence of substrate cycles and their utility in vivo. *The Biochemical Journal, 285*, 340–341.

Pacy, P. J., Webster, J., & Garrow, J. S. (1986). Exercise and obesity. *Sports Medicine (Auckland, N.Z.), 3*, 89–113.

Poehlman, E. T., & Horton, E. S. (1990). Regulation of energy expenditure in aging humans. *Annual Review of Nutrition, 10*, 255–275.

Powanda, M. C., & Beisel, W. R. (2003). Metabolic effects of infection on protein and energy status. *The Journal of Nutrition, 133*, 322S–327S.

Ramirez-Zea, M. (2005). Validation of three predictive equations for basal metabolic rate in adults. *Public Health Nutrition, 8*, 1213–1228.

Reidy, S. P., & Weber, J. M. (2002). Accelerated substrate cycling: A new energy-wasting role for leptin in vivo. *American Journal of Physiology. Endocrinology and Metabolism, 282*, E312–E317.

Santosa, S., Khosla, S., McCready, L. K., & Jensen, M. D. (2010). Effects of estrogen and testosterone on resting energy expenditure in older men. *Obesity (Silver Spring), 18*, 2392–2394.

Schoeller, D. A., Leitch, C. A., & Brown, C. (1986). Doubly labeled water method: In vivo oxygen and hydrogen isotope fractionation. *The American Journal of Physiology, 251*, R1137–R1143.

Solomon, S. J., Kurzer, M. S., & Calloway, D. H. (1982). Menstrual cycle and basal metabolic rate in women. *The American Journal of Clinical Nutrition, 36*, 611–616.

Soric, M., & Misigoj-Durakovic, M. (2010). Physical activity levels and estimated energy expenditure in overweight and normal-weight 11-year-old children. *Acta Paediatrica, 99*, 244–250.

Starling, R. D. (2001). Energy expenditure and aging: Effects of physical activity. *International Journal of Sport Nutrition and Exercise Metabolism, 11*(Suppl.), S208–S217.

Stob, N. R., Bell, C., van Baak, M. A., & Seals, D. R. (2007). Thermic effect of food and beta-adrenergic thermogenic responsiveness in habitually exercising and sedentary healthy adult humans. *Journal of Applied Physiology, 103*, 616–622.

St-Onge, M.-P., & Gallagher, D. (2010). Body composition changes with aging: The cause or the result of alterations in metabolic rate and macronutrient oxidation? *Nutrition, 26*, 152–155.

Thorburn, A. W., & Proietto, J. (2000). Biological determinants of spontaneous physical activity. *Obesity Reviews, 1*, 87–94.

Thyfault, J. P., Richmond, S. R., Carper, M. J., Potteiger, J. A., & Hulver, M. W. (2004). Postprandial metabolism in resistance-trained versus sedentary males. *Medicine and Science in Sports and Exercise, 36*(4), 709–716.

van Marken Lichtenbelt, W. D., & Daanen, H. A. (2003). Cold-induced metabolism. *Current Opinion in Clinical Nutrition and Metabolic Care, 6*, 469–475.

Warwick, P. M. (2006). Factorial estimation of daily energy expenditure using a simplified method was improved by adjustment for excess post-exercise oxygen consumption and thermic effect of food. *European Journal of Clinical Nutrition, 60*, 1337–1340.

Westerterp, K. R. (2008). Physical activity as determinant of daily energy expenditure. *Physiology & Behavior, 93*, 1039–1043.

Westerterp, K. R., & Plasqui, G. (2004). Physical activity and human energy expenditure. *Current Opinion in Clinical Nutrition and Metabolic Care, 7*, 607–613.

Wickel, E. E., & Eisenmann, J. C. (2006). Within- and between-individual variability in estimated energy expenditure and habitual physical activity among young adults. *European Journal of Clinical Nutrition, 60*, 538–544.

RECOMMENDED READINGS

Cioffi, F., Senese, R., de Lange, P., Goglia, F., Lanni, A., & Lombardi, A. (2009). Uncoupling proteins: A complex journey to function discovery. *BioFactors, 35*, 417–428.

Novak, C. M., & Levine, J. A. (2007). Central neural and endocrine mechanisms of non-exercise activity thermogenesis and their potential impact on obesity. *Neuroendocrinology, 19*, 923–940.

Schoeller, D. A. (2008). Insights into energy balance from doubly labeled water. *International Journal of Obesity, 32*(Suppl. 7), S72–S75.

Schoeller, D. A. (2009). The energy balance equation: Looking back and looking forward are two very different views. *Nutrition Reviews, 67*, 249–254.

Wallace, D. C., Fan, W., & Procaccio, V. (2010). Mitochondrial energetics and therapeutics. *Annual Review of Pathology, 5*, 297–348.

Westerterp, K. R. (2010). Physical activity, food intake, and body weight regulation: Insights from doubly labeled water studies. *Nutrition Reviews, 68*, 148–154.

CHAPTER 22

Control of Energy Balance

Darlene E. Berryman, PhD, RD; Brenda M. Davy, PhD, RD; and Edward O. List, PhD*

COMMON ABBREVIATIONS

AgRP	agouti-related protein
α-MSH	alpha–melanocyte-stimulating hormone
ARC	arcuate nucleus
CCK	cholecystokinin
CNS	central nervous system
GI	gastrointestinal
GLP	glucagon-like peptide
LHA	lateral hypothalamic area
NPY	neuropeptide Y
NTS	nucleus tractus solitarius
OXM	oxyntomodulin
POMC	pro-opiomelanocortin
PP	pancreatic polypeptide
PVN	paraventricular nucleus
PYY	polypeptide YY
VMH	ventromedial hypothalamus

A typical adult human who consumes 2,500 kcal/day will ingest nearly 1 million kcal of energy in a single year. This energy is used to fuel obligatory and regulatory metabolic processes and to provide fuel for physical activity. For an individual to maintain energy balance, therefore, the 1 million kcal ingested must be balanced by equivalent energy expended. Failure to achieve energy balance results in either an increase or decrease in body energy stores. The observation that many individuals maintain a relatively constant body weight from year to year is evidence that this system works remarkably well. Nevertheless, an error of only 1% will result in a net change of more than 1 kg body weight per year. The widespread occurrence of obesity in developed countries in recent decades illustrates the impact that environmental factors, such as food availability and the demand for physical activity, can have on the regulation of energy balance. In this chapter, basic concepts of energy and nutrient balance are described and the current understanding of the control of energy intake, energy expenditure, and their interaction are reviewed.

ENERGY BALANCE

The first law of thermodynamics states that energy can be converted from one form to another, but it can be neither created nor destroyed. Thus the energy supplied and used or stored by the body must be in balance. The following equation summarizes this concept:

$$\text{Energy intake} = \text{Energy expenditure} + \text{Change in body stores of energy}$$

Energy balance, by definition, is a state in which energy intake and energy expenditure are equivalent over the period of observation such that there is no change in stores:

$$\text{Energy balance} = \text{Energy intake} - \text{Energy expenditure} = 0$$

Energy intake includes all the usable energy consumed in the form of carbohydrate, fat, protein, and alcohol and not lost in feces or urine. Energy expenditure includes the heat released for basal metabolism, physical activity, and thermic effect of food (TEF), as more fully explained in Chapter 21. As illustrated in Figure 22-1, when energy intake is not equal to energy expenditure, the energy stored in the body must be altered to balance the equation. That is, when energy intake exceeds energy expenditure, energy balance is positive and a net gain in body energy stores occurs. Conversely, when energy expenditure exceeds energy intake, energy balance is negative and a net loss in body energy stores occurs.

Estimates of total body energy stores (dry weight) are shown in Table 22-1. When an individual is in energy balance, these stores remain stable. Energy to fuel basal metabolism and everyday activity is provided by energy-yielding nutrients in food. Short-term energy needs (e.g., between meals or during exercise) are met mainly by utilization of liver or muscle glycogen reserves and some fat. However, glycogen reserves and energy-yielding substrates in the circulation represent very small storage depots and normally are exhausted within 24 hours during a fast. During prolonged fasting or during energy restriction for weight loss, significant protein is also degraded and used for energy in addition to substantial catabolism of the fat depots. Most of the triacylglycerol stored in adipose tissue is available to the body during a prolonged fast, but not all energy contained in body protein is available for use as fuel. Body proteins serve

*This chapter is a revision of the chapter contributed by John C. Peters, PhD, for the second edition.

important structural and functional purposes and therefore cannot be depleted without affecting survival of the organism.

The magnitude of change in body energy that occurs when there is an imbalance between energy intake and expenditure, of course, depends on the magnitude of the daily imbalance and the length of time for which the energy imbalance continues. Because total daily energy needs in most individuals range between 1,500 and 3,000 kcal and because the body has a large energy reserve, short-term imbalances such as those that occur from meal to meal or from day to day would not be expected to significantly change body energy stores (or body weight). However, sustained imbalances that occur over several days, weeks, or months can lead to substantial changes in body energy reserves and subsequent changes in body weight.

Gain or loss of significant amounts of body mass may in turn affect other components of the energy balance equation. Weight gain or loss is associated with gain or loss of metabolically active tissue mass, which itself results in an increase or decrease in total energy expenditure. Likewise, alterations in body mass usually affect energy intake, because food intake normally is proportional to energy expenditure. Therefore when a prolonged imbalance occurs between energy intake and energy expenditure, the resulting change in body energy stores (and body weight) is not a linear function of the energy excess or deficit; rather, it depends on the composition of the tissue mass lost or gained and the effects of those specific changes on total energy expenditure and energy intake.

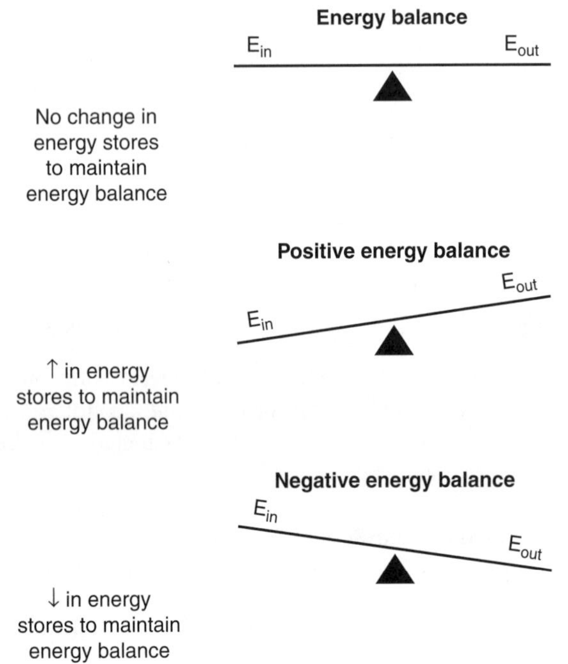

FIGURE 22-1 Schematic representation of the energy balance equation. E_{in} is the metabolizable energy intake due to the consumption of food (minus whatever is not absorbed and whatever is lost by excretion). E_{out} includes basal metabolism, physical activity (voluntary and obligatory), and thermogenesis (cold or diet induced).

NUTRIENT BALANCE

In a practical sense, people do not eat "energy"; they eat nutrients in the form of food, and the nutrients are oxidized by the body to provide energy. The predominant energy-yielding nutrients in the human diet are the macronutrients: protein, carbohydrate, and fat. Alcohol, if ingested, is also a source of energy. Because there is little net conversion of either protein or carbohydrate into fat in humans unless large excesses of protein or carbohydrate are ingested, achieving balance between energy intake and energy expenditure generally means achieving a balance for intake and oxidation of each macronutrient (Flatt and Tremblay, 2004). As illustrated in Figure 22-2, nutrient and energy balance in the adult occurs when the intake of protein, carbohydrate, and fat (and alcohol) is equivalent to the body's oxidation of each. When energy and nutrient balance are achieved, the following result:

- Carbohydrate intake = Carbohydrate oxidized
- Protein intake = Protein oxidized
- Fat intake = Fat oxidized
- Alcohol intake = Alcohol oxidized

In a typical carbohydrate-rich diet, the carbohydrate will serve as the main source of oxidizable energy. Because the body's capacity to store carbohydrate is limited, there must be a tight control to balance overall carbohydrate oxidation with carbohydrate consumption. Protein intake and protein oxidation are also typically balanced, with protein stores only significantly increasing in response to growth stimuli. Alcohol cannot be stored, so ingested alcohol must be oxidized. Thus acute changes in intake of carbohydrate, protein, or alcohol are rapidly balanced by changes in oxidation of each; the more of these nutrients you consume, the more you will oxidize.

TABLE 22-1 Energy Stores in a 30-kg Child and a 70-kg Adult Man

		30-kg Child*		70-kg Adult Man†	
ENERGY FORM	STORAGE SITE	kg	kcal	kg	kcal
Triacylglycerol	Adipose tissue	4.5	42,000	15	140,000
Protein	Muscle	1.5	6,300	6	25,000
Glycogen	Liver and muscle	0.13	500	0.35	1,400
Glucose or lipid	Body fluids	0.011	40	0.025	100

*Data from Rosenbaum, M., & Leibel, R. L. (1988). Pathophysiology of childhood obesity. *Advances in Pediatrics, 35*, 73–137.
†Data from Cahill, G. F. (1970). Starvation in man. *New England Journal of Medicine, 282*, 668–675; Frayn, K. (1996). *Metabolic regulation: A human perspective* (pp. 78–102). London: Portland Press.
All values are given as dry weights of triacylglycerol, protein, and glycogen that are available for consumption as fuel. These values are not the wet weights of tissue containing these fuels.

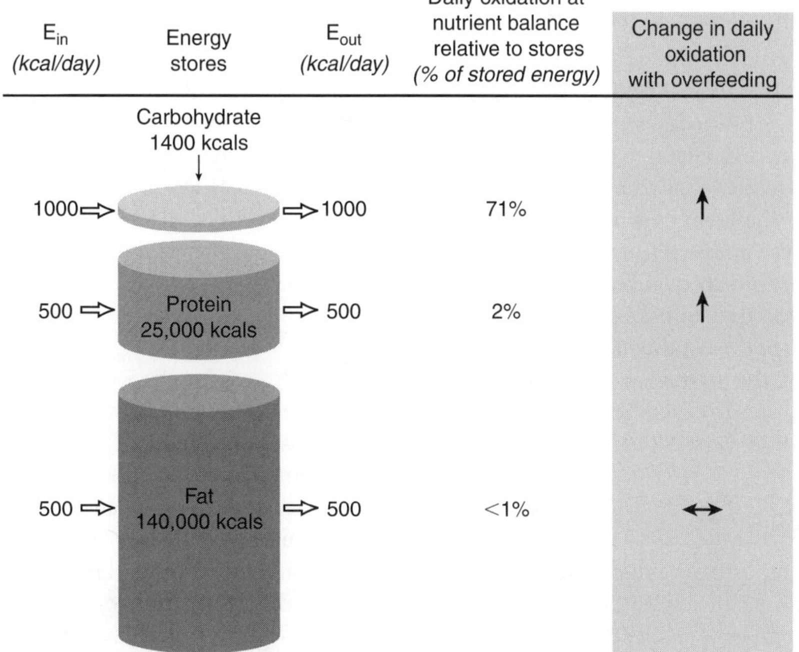

FIGURE 22-2 Schematic representation of the concept of nutrient balance. Depicted are the carbohydrate, protein, and fat energy stores in a representative 70-kg adult male who is in energy balance when consuming a 2,000-kcal diet (50% carbohydrate, 25% protein, and 25% fat). With nutrient balance and a eucaloric feeding, intake and oxidation would be equivalent for each macronutrient. Because of the much larger fat stores, the amount of fat oxidized represents only a small fraction of the percent stored. With overfeeding of a mixed diet, carbohydrate and protein oxidation would increase to compensate for the increased intake. However, the fat in the diet has lowest priority for oxidation, and consistent overfeeding would result in a positive fat balance and an increase in body fat stores.

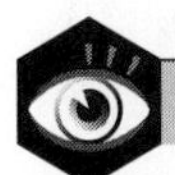

NUTRITION INSIGHT

Energetic Equivalent of Body Tissues: Implications for Weight Loss

The energetic equivalent of a given amount of body mass either gained or lost depends on its composition. Lean tissue such as muscle is about 80% water, with the remaining 20% largely consisting of protein with smaller amounts of fat and carbohydrate. In contrast, adipose tissue is only approximately 15% water, and the remainder (85%) is storage lipid with a very small amount of protein contributing to the cell structure and intracellular enzymes. Given these differences in the composition of body tissues, the amount of energy represented by a kilogram of body weight will differ accordingly.

A rough estimate of the energy provided by oxidation of fat or protein stores can be made using caloric equivalents for oxidation of stored fuels. The available energy values of stored fuels are higher than those of ingested fuels because there are no losses due to inefficient digestion and absorption nor costs related to assimilation (see Table 21-1). For example, the available energy obtained when a kilogram of muscle is broken down would be roughly 840 kcal (200 g × 4.2 kcal/g for protein). This is less than the energy that would be released by burning 1 kg of muscle tissue in a flame because some of the total chemical energy in the muscle protein is lost as incompletely oxidized organic compounds in the urine when muscle is catabolized in vivo. Urea is the major energy-containing compound excreted in the urine. Urea formation is a necessary process when amino acids from either protein stores or dietary protein are used as fuels. Urea excretion in the urine results in the loss of about 280 kcal of potential energy per 1 kg of muscle tissue that is catabolized.

Loss of a kilogram of adipose tissue (85% lipid) represents a body energy loss of about 7,905 kcal (850 g × 9.3 kcal/g). In contrast to protein, essentially all of the energy represented by stored fat can contribute to net fuel energy. Therefore a kilogram of body fat can provide nearly 10 times the amount of energy provided by a kilogram of lean tissue (7,905 kcal/kg for fat compared to 840 kcal/kg for lean tissue). The higher energy value of a kilogram of adipose tissue as compared to muscle tissue results from the lower water content of adipose tissue, the higher energy value of fat than of protein, and the absence of a need to excrete nitrogen when fat is the fuel.

These figures provide some perspective on weight loss claims appearing in the popular press. Take the example of a claim touting a 2.5-kg weight loss in a week by simply following a new diet (i.e., no exercise involved). If the weight lost was really all adipose tissue, as hoped by the dieter, the loss would represent 19,760 kcal of body energy. For the average sedentary individual only about 2,500 kcal per day, or 17,500 kcal per week, are needed to maintain body weight. It is therefore impossible to lose 2.5 kg of fat in a week by dieting alone—to lose 2.5 kg of fat, the individual would have to eat nothing for more than a week or increase energy expenditure by about 2,820 kcal/day (or some combination of the two), and this assumes that it would be possible to lose fat without an accompanying loss of muscle! Typically, loss of 1 kg of adipose tissue is accompanied by loss of 1 kg of lean body mass during prolonged starvation. To lose adipose tissue without an accompanying loss of lean body mass, a more modest restriction of calories along with increased exercise is recommended.

In contrast to the other macronutrients, fat can be stored in large amounts and fat intake is not tightly coupled to fat oxidation. As a consequence, fat stores serve as an energy buffer, and positive or negative energy balances are largely conditions of positive or negative fat balance. When excess calories are consumed in the form of a mixed diet, carbohydrate and protein that are not used to replace glycogen or body proteins will be preferentially oxidized. In contrast, any fat not oxidized will be stored in adipose tissue. For a given individual, the major factors that influence fat balance are overall caloric intake (i.e., the amount and composition of food eaten) and the total energy expenditure, especially the amount of physical activity (Peters, 2003).

RELATIVE STABILITY OF BODY WEIGHT

Body weight and body composition remain quite stable over long periods (years) in most individuals. This might suggest that body weight, body composition, or perhaps energy balance itself, is regulated much like other homeostatic systems in biology, such as plasma glucose concentration. Indeed, there are multiple overlapping physiological systems that maintain body energy homeostasis in response to variations in the supply of food energy and inconsistent patterns of energy expenditure. Two theories are commonly used to describe this tendency of adults to maintain a relatively stable body weight; these are the set point theory and the settling point theory.

SET POINT THEORY

The set point theory is based on the recognition that humans tend to maintain stable body weight over long periods, and they defend this weight against conditions that would otherwise promote weight gain or loss. For example, when humans are overfed to force weight gain, upon cessation of overfeeding they spontaneously lose weight and return toward their starting condition. Although these individuals lose weight when no longer overfed, the weight loss often is not sufficient to return them to their exact starting point (Bouchard et al., 1996). Likewise, when individuals are subjected to a weight-reducing regimen for a prolonged period, they lose weight, but they rapidly regain the lost weight when the condition of negative energy balance is relieved (Sims and Horton, 1968).

These observations in humans support the concept of a body weight set-point, such that the energy balance system in an individual is programmed to defend a particular body weight. Studies in experimental animals have also provided strong evidence of a physiological mechanism that defends a particular body weight under conditions of energy deficit or surplus (Keesey and Corbett, 1984). To alter this apparent body weight set-point, a change in the fundamental central nervous system (CNS) mechanisms regulating food intake and energy expenditure is required. For example, early animal studies showed that destruction of the ventromedial hypothalamus in the brain, the so-called satiety center, caused animals to overeat and reach a new higher body weight, which the animal then defended (i.e., a new set-point). Alternatively, destruction of the lateral hypothalamus, the so-called feeding center, resulted in reduced food intake, weight loss, and a new lower body weight or set-point that was defended. Recent studies have refined our understanding of the brain mechanisms affecting energy balance, and a number of specific hypothalamic neural networks and signaling systems that control different elements of energy intake, expenditure, and storage have been identified.

THE SETTLING POINT THEORY

Yet body weight often does not remain fixed throughout adult life, despite many years during which relative constancy is achieved. In an individual, changes in body weight over time can be in either direction. Therefore it could be more accurate to designate a particular body weight that an individual defends at a particular point in time as a settling point rather than a set-point. Settling points are determined by the different physiological, psychological, and environmental circumstances the individual may experience. For example, declining levels of physical activity encourage positive energy balance, weight gain, and thus a new, higher settling point (Hill et al., 2003). Similarly, an increase in body weight occurs in many women around the time of menopause (Sowers et al., 2007). Regardless of whether the set-point or settling point construct seems more appealing, the existence of a physiological control system that defends body weight cannot be denied based on the available evidence.

BIOLOGICAL BIAS TOWARD BODY WEIGHT GAIN

Although body weight is defended in response to challenges that either decrease or increase energy stores, this defense appears to be asymmetrical. That is, the body's defense against a gain in energy stores appears to be weaker than that protecting against a loss of energy stores. This is borne out by years of clinical experience in treating obese individuals; although a high percentage can achieve weight loss, only about 17% of individuals maintain weight losses of 10% or more (Kraschnewski et al., 2010). The bias in the energy balance control system toward promoting weight gain is also apparent in the growing prevalence of obesity among both adults and children. Today, more than one third of the U.S. population is obese, up from 25% just a decade ago, and an additional one third of the population is overweight (Flegal and Troiano, 2000; Flegal et al., 2010). The relatively weak defense against positive energy balance appears to exist whether the energy gain is provoked by increased energy intake, decreased physical activity, or both. In experimental overfeeding studies, it has been shown that the body has a limited capacity to burn off excess energy, and most of the excess is stored (Horton et al., 1995; Klein and Goran, 1993; Levine et al., 1999).

BEHAVIORAL ASPECTS OF CONTROL OF ENERGY INTAKE AND ENERGY EXPENDITURE

Energy intake is controlled by a complex system involving both behavioral and biological components. These components are interrelated in as much as food intake itself is a behavior and the biological components of the system must respond to, and indeed may be forced to adapt to, the consequences of this behavior. Ultimately, eating behavior involves the interaction and integration of genetics, neurobiology, metabolism, learning history, physical activity, and the context (e.g., physical, social, and emotional environment) in which eating takes place.

Human eating behavior is a learned habitual behavior (Savage et al., 2007). Food intake in any given circumstance is influenced by the learning history of the individual as it relates to that circumstance. Learning begins in early childhood, at which time the child develops food preferences through experience with different foods. Properties of the food itself (e.g., orosensory properties), energy content and density, and the social and cultural context in which the food is consumed can all be associated with the metabolic effects of the food to yield a learned, conditioned response.

The taste (e.g., sweet, sour), energy density, and variety of foods offered to children have been found to shape children's food preferences. Infants and young children display an innate preference for the sweet taste, and young children demonstrate preferences for foods that are energy dense (Savage et al., 2007). Offering children a wide variety of foods to choose from increases the spectrum of foods they come to prefer. All of these factors appear to contribute to ensuring that the child consumes adequate energy and sufficient essential nutrients to support proper growth and development. As the child grows older, learned food acceptance patterns and eating habits are continually reinforced and extended, so that by adulthood there is a rich experiential background that affects eating behavior at any given meal.

At any given eating occasion, the amount and composition of food an individual consumes are affected by the immediate context of consumption superimposed on the underlying biology (i.e., mechanisms controlling food intake and energy balance) and the learning history. As described earlier in the chapter, the two primary determinants of energy balance are energy intake and energy expenditure. Yet many factors influence energy intake and energy expenditure, both at individual and environmental levels. A list of some factors believed to influence energy balance behaviors is provided in Table 22-2. For example, the cost of food acquisition, the variety of foods present, food form (i.e., solid or liquid), energy density, portion size, and the number of other people present are just a few of the factors that affect short-term food and energy intake (Wansink, 2004; Rolls, 2009; Flood-Obbagy and Rolls, 2009; Herman and Polivy, 2008). With respect to energy expenditure, the design of neighborhoods and communities (i.e., the "built environment") may influence an individual's physical activity level (Saelens and Handy, 2008). Socioeconomic status and cognitive factors also play important roles in energy balance behaviors, such as an individual's perceived control over diet and physical activity behaviors and social norms (Kremers et al., 2005; Stringhini et al., 2010).

TABLE 22-2 Individual and Environmental Factors That Influence Energy Balance Behaviors: Influences on Energy Intake and Energy Expenditure

	ENERGY INTAKE	ENERGY EXPENDITURE
Individual	Dietary macronutrient composition	Sedentary behaviors
	Dietary energy density	Work-related activity
	Food form (solid, liquid)	Activities of daily living
	Palatability	Leisure time activity
	Food variety and availability	Planned exercise
	Food cost	
	Portion size	
	Sleep duration	
	Mental work	
Environmental	Dining partners	Built environment
	Food accessibility and variety	Family/social environment
	Family and home environment	

Much current research is focused on understanding the relative contribution of the modern environment to the growing prevalence of obesity in both children and adults (Cohen, 2008). Among the factors under investigation are the impacts of portion size and food advertising on food selection and intake. Short-term food and energy intake is increased when there are many palatable foods from which to choose and when the food is served in large portions (Wansink, 2004). Likewise, aggressive advertising of high-calorie foods and increased participation in sedentary behaviors have been highlighted as environmental pressures that promote excessive eating, reduced energy expenditure, and, consequently, increased risk for excessive weight gain (Peters et al., 2002). Research is also directed at investigating interrelationships between biology and energy balance behaviors. For example, the association of food intake and food reward (Neary and Batterham, 2010), decision making about food intake in an environment where many constraints on availability and many costs associated with obtaining food have been removed (Rowland et al., 2008), and sex differences in regulation of food intake induced by physical activity (Hagobian and Braun, 2010) are topics of recent investigations.

BIOLOGICAL CONTROL OF ENERGY INTAKE AND ENERGY EXPENDITURE

Underlying the complex behavioral elements are the biological mechanisms that coordinate energy intake to meet energy needs.

REGULATION OF ENERGY HOMEOSTASIS

The CNS (brain and spinal cord) orchestrates the control of energy balance via a complex homeostatic pathway that has three main parts. As illustrated in Figure 22-3, the central part of this system involves specific regions within the CNS that detect and integrate signals reflecting changes in energy availability and mediate appropriate modifications of energy intake and expenditure. Inputs or afferent signals that provide information about the periphery, including status of energy intake, energy expenditure, and available energy stores, feed into the CNS. Afferent signals can be neural or humoral. The final part involves the outputs or efferent signals from the brain that direct a coordinated response to alter energy intake and energy expenditure or change partitioning of nutrients to achieve energy homeostasis. These afferent and efferent signal pathways constitute the essential elements of a feedback scheme, conceptually similar to the functional elements of a common household heating system in which a temperature sensor is linked to a system that adjusts heat output to maintain a specific temperature.

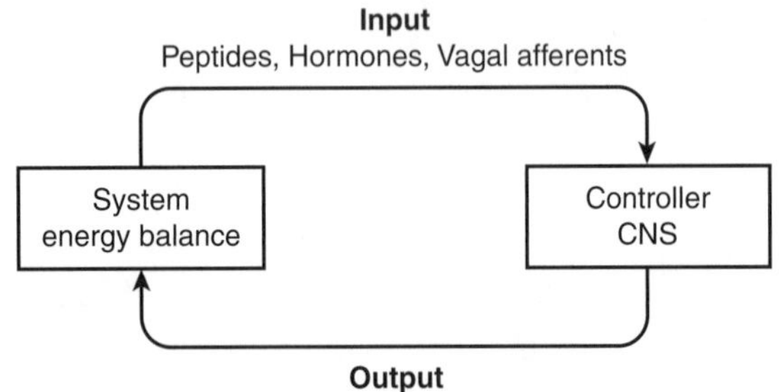

FIGURE 22-3 Simplified diagram of the regulatory circuit for control of energy balance.

CENTRAL ROLE OF THE HYPOTHALAMUS AND BRAINSTEM

Although the regulation of energy balance is complex and involves many brain centers and neuronal circuits, the hypothalamus and brainstem (Figure 22-4) play critical roles in relaying afferent signals from the peripheral tissues as well

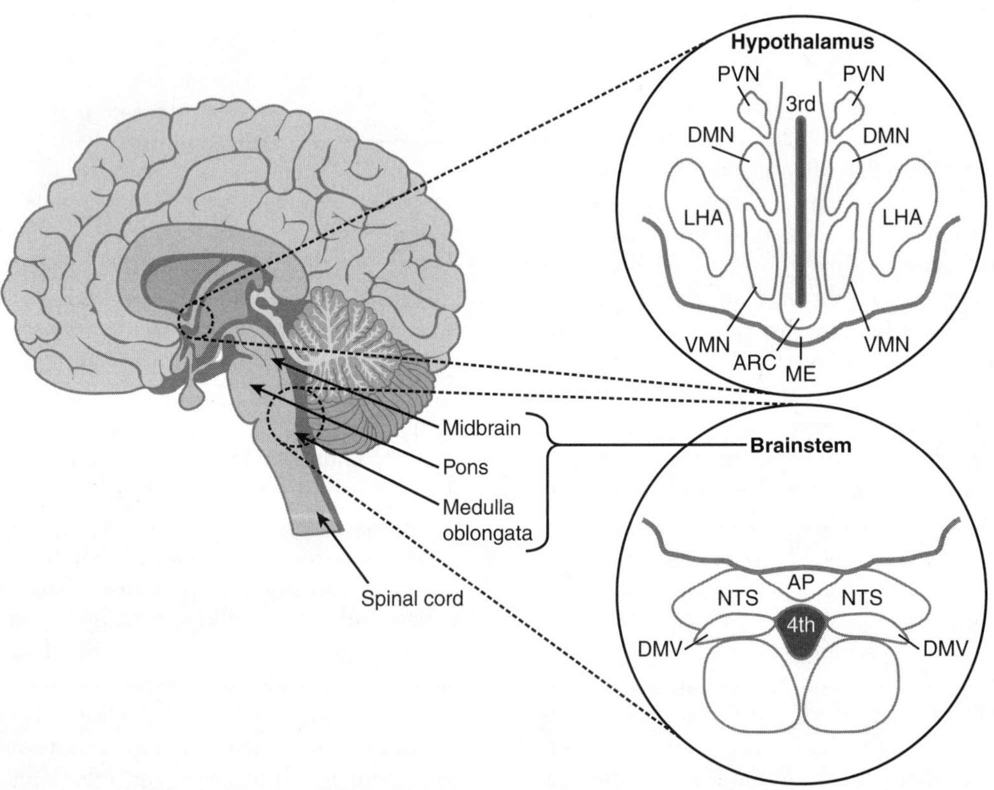

FIGURE 22-4 Diagram of the brain showing areas of the hypothalamus and brainstem involved in regulation of energy balance. Regions of the hypothalamus include the arcuate nucleus (*ARC*), dorsomedial nucleus (*DMN*), lateral hypothalamic area (*LHA*), paraventricular nucleus (*PVN*), and ventromedial nucleus (*VMN*). Areas of the brainstem, mainly located in the medulla oblongata, include the nucleus of the solitary tract (nucleus tractus solitarius) (*NTS*) and dorsomedial nucleus (*DMV*), which together are also called the dorsal motor nucleus of the vagus nerve. Also shown are the circumventricular organs that interface the systemic and cerebrospinal circulations. The median eminence (*ME*) is near the third ventricle and the ARC of the hypothalamus, and the area postrema (*AP*) is associated with the fourth ventricle and the NTS of the brainstem.

as processing efferent signals that modulate food intake and energy expenditure.

Afferent Input to the CNS

Vagal afferent fibers directly connect the gastrointestinal (GI) tract with neurons in the nucleus of the solitary tract (NTS, nucleus tractus solitarius), which is part of the brainstem. The cell bodies of these vagal afferent fibers sit just outside the CNS in a pair of ganglia called the nodose ganglia. Thus input from stretch receptors, osmoreceptors, and chemoreceptors in the GI tract is carried to the CNS via vagal afferent nerve fibers. The central processes of these neurons enter the brainstem via the NTS. The afferent signals from the GI tract are integrated by neurons of the NTS that project to, among other areas, the adjacent dorsal motor nucleus of the vagus nerve (DMV). Taste fibers also enter the solitary tract of the medulla and synapse in the NTS.

Direct Effects of Hormones and Peptides on the CNS

In addition, both the hypothalamus and the brainstem contain aggregates of specialized nervous tissue, which are called circumventricular organs because of their interface between the blood and cerebrospinal circulations. The median eminence (ME) of the hypothalamus and the area postrema (AP) of the brainstem, which are shown in Figure 22-4, are two of these circumventricular organs. The capillaries of these organs do not have typical tight junctions between the endothelial cells and have fenestrations (pores). These special areas of the brain thus have an incomplete blood–brain barrier and are thought to allow selective uptake of circulating hormones and peptides so that they can interact directly with their receptors on neurons in these areas of the brain.

Integration of Signals in the Hypothalamus

The hypothalamus is subdivided into various nuclei that include the arcuate nucleus (ARC), the paraventricular nucleus (PVN), the ventromedial nucleus (VMN), the dorsomedial nucleus (DMN), and the lateral hypothalamic area (LHA), as illustrated in Figure 22-4. These hypothalamic nuclei interconnect and interact with higher cortical centers of the brain as well as with the brainstem. Neuronal pathways between these nuclei are organized into a complex network in which orexigenic and anorexigenic circuits influence food intake and energy expenditure.

Efferent Output from the CNS

The cell bodies for the majority of parasympathetic efferent fibers that project to the upper GI tract originate in the DMV. Signals from the DMV neurons are the final step in the efferent output of the CNS to the periphery.

AFFERENT SIGNALS

Afferent signals feed into the CNS where they are integrated. These signals may be circulating nutrients, circulating hormones, or afferent nerve inputs to the brain, as shown in Figure 22-5. These signals reach brain centers either via vagal afferent fibers or, in the case of molecules that are able

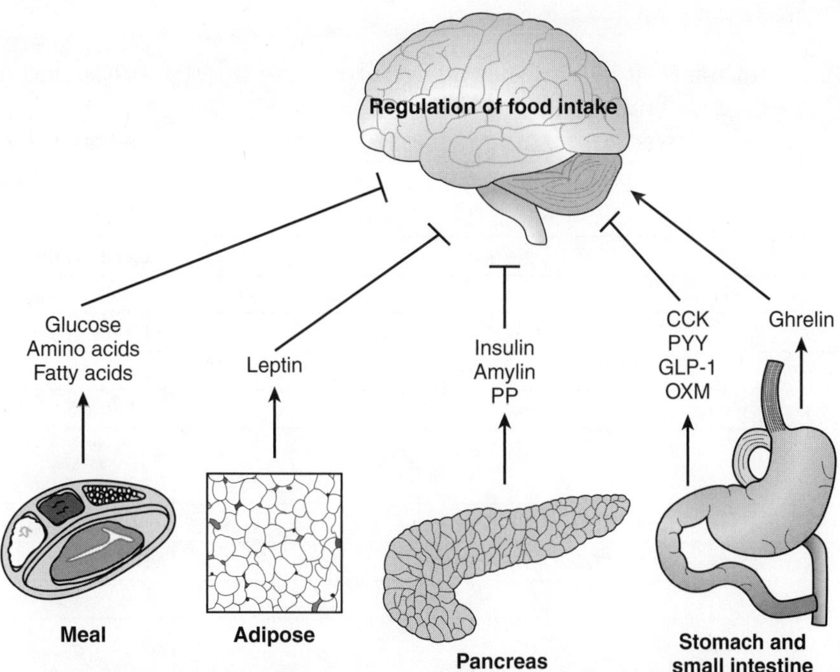

FIGURE 22-5 Afferent signals controlling energy balance. Nutrients and hormones or peptides released by the gastrointestinal tract, pancreas, and adipose tissue inform the central nervous system about the body's energy status. Signaling molecules may act on peripheral receptors with inputs to the brain being carried via the vagal afferent fibers. Nutrients and some hormones such as insulin and leptin are able to cross the blood–brain barrier and act directly on neuronal receptors within the central nervous system. Inhibitory effects on food intake are shown as ⊥, whereas the stimulatory effect of ghrelin is shown as ↑. *CCK,* Cholecystokinin; *GLP-1,* glucagon-like peptide 1; *OXM,* oxyntomodulin; *PP,* pancreatic polypeptide; *PYY,* peptide YY (3-36).

to cross the blood–brain barrier, via direct action on brain neurons (Suzuki et al., 2010). Afferent signals are considered to reflect both short-term (e.g., nutrient and gut-related signals that result from meal consumption) and long-term (e.g., signals reflecting body energy stores, mainly adipose tissue) changes in the body's energy status. These signaling pathways often overlap and involve a variety of different neurotransmitter and neuropeptide systems.

NUTRIENT SIGNALS

Various nutrient signals have been identified that inform the brain about the quantity and type of the food ingested and overall energy status. Signals derived from circulating nutrients themselves (e.g., glucose and amino acids) were among the earliest suggested mechanisms by which the food consumed informs the brain to influence appetite. For example, the glucostatic (Mayer, 1953) theory of food intake control was based on the idea that either the plasma or tissue concentration of glucose or the rate of glucose utilization serves as a feedback signal to the brain to modulate food intake. Indeed, decades after the glucostatic theory was proposed, two different types of glucose-responsive neurons, glucose-excited neurons and glucose-inhibited neurons, have been shown to be sensitive to glucose levels (Dunn-Meynell et al., 2002). Specific brain regions have been identified that sense amino acids. For example, leucine exerts an anorexigenic action by activating the mammalian target of rapamycin (mTOR) pathway in neurons within the hypothalamus (Cota et al., 2006). Likewise, regions of the hypothalamus involved in regulating food intake have been shown to sense fatty acids via a mechanism that involves AMP-activated protein kinase (AMPK) (Obici et al., 2002; Ronnett et al., 2009).

GUT-DERIVED SIGNALS

The GI tract is responsible for a wide range of mechanical and chemical signals that control food intake, hunger, and satiety. Stretch receptors in the stomach signal the brain via neural pathways about meal size, whereas a variety of other gut-derived hormones play roles in meal initiation and termination. Gut peptides act peripherally to modulate digestion and absorption of nutrients, but some also act as neurotransmitters to regulate energy balance or food intake. For the most part, these gut-derived hormones are released following a meal and act primarily to reduce meal size and lengthen the between meal interval; their net effect is to act as a brake on eating. These peptides that act to reduce meal size are considered "satiety" peptides. One gut peptide, ghrelin, is known to stimulate initiation of eating. Although many gut hormones appear to signal through the CNS to influence appetite, receptors for these hormones also are present in peripheral tissues, and these gut hormones likely have peripheral activities. It is important to note that gut-derived and other signals affecting energy balance are not generated individually and do not act in isolation. They are secreted in concert in response to meals in varying amounts that reflect the complex characteristics of the meal as well as the underlying energy balance of the organism (Table 22-3).

Providing a complete overview of the numerous GI peptides and their specific functions is beyond the scope of this

TABLE 22-3 Summary of the Major Hormones Derived from the Gut, Pancreas, and Adipocytes That Influence Energy Balance

	EFFECT OF FEEDING ON HORMONE LEVEL*	PRIMARY SITE OF SECRETION
GUT HORMONES		
PYY_{3-36}	↑	L cells in the gut
GLP-1	↑	L cells in the gut
GLP-2	–	L cells in the gut
OXM	↑	L cells in the gut
CCK	↑	I cells (small intestine)
Ghrelin	↓	Mainly X/A-like cells of the stomach
PANCREATIC HORMONES		
PP	↑	PP cells (pancreas)
Glucagon	↓	Alpha cells (pancreas)
Amylin	↑	Beta cells (pancreas)
Insulin	↑	Beta cells (pancreas)
ADIPOSE HORMONES		
Leptin	↑	Adipocytes

Data from Suzuki, K., Simpson, K. A., Minnion, J. S., Shillito, J. C., & Bloom, S. R. (2010). The role of gut hormones and the hypothalamus in appetite regulation. *Endocrine Journal, 57*, 359–372.

CCK, Cholecystokinin; *GLP-1*, glucagon-like peptide 1; *GLP-2*, glucagon-like peptide 2; *OXM*, oxyntomodulin; *PP*, pancreatic polypeptide; PYY_{3-36}, peptide YY (3-36).

*Arrows indicate whether hormone level increases (↑), decreases (↓), or does not change (–) in response to meal intake.

chapter. Brief descriptions of the actions of selected peptides are provided as examples of the roles played by these important signaling molecules in regulating energy balance.

Ghrelin

Ghrelin is a 28–amino acid hormone predominantly produced in the GI tract with highest production occurring in specialized neuroendocrine X/A-like cells of the stomach (Karra and Batterham, 2010; Neary and Batterham, 2009). Among the gut peptides identified to date that affect food intake, ghrelin is unique in that it stimulates rather than inhibits food intake. Because ghrelin levels increase during food deprivation in humans (Suzuki et al., 2010) and just before spontaneous eating in animals (Cummings et al., 2001), it is thought to signal meal initiation. Both direct and indirect administration of ghrelin to the brain stimulates feeding (Suzuki et al., 2010). Ghrelin binds to the growth hormone secretagogue receptor. Ghrelin receptors are found in the hypothalamus and other regions of the brain as well as in vagal afferent fibers. The hypothalamus is thought to be the primary site of ghrelin's effect on appetite. However, the growth hormone secretagogue receptor is also found in many other tissues, suggesting that ghrelin may play a more complex role; and the presence of ghrelin receptors in other areas of the brain suggests ghrelin also could be involved in activating some reward circuits (Neary and Batterham, 2010).

In addition to its more transient role in stimulating food intake, ghrelin is thought to have longer-lasting effects on body weight, adipose tissue metabolism, and glucose metabolism (Karra and Batterham, 2010). In humans, circulating ghrelin is negatively correlated with obesity. Lower levels are found in obese individuals and higher levels are found in leaner individuals. Ghrelin levels have been observed to decline following Roux-en-Y gastric bypass surgery in obese subjects, and this decrease in ghrelin levels may partially explain the success of this procedure (Beckman et al., 2010). Disruption of the ghrelin gene in mice results in mice that are resistant to diet-induced obesity. Ghrelin-null mice also have enhanced glucose-stimulated insulin secretion and improved insulin sensitivity (Zigman et al., 2005; Sun et al., 2006). In contrast, chronic administration of ghrelin to mice induces weight gain (Tschöp et al., 2000).

Cholecystokinin

Cholecystokinin (CCK) is the first discovered of the gut-secreted satiety peptides. The major form of CCK is a 58–amino acid peptide. CCK is released from I cells of the duodenum and jejunum into the circulation in response to certain amino acids and fatty acids from ingested food. Levels of CCK peak within 15 minutes postprandially, and CCK is active for only a short time, limiting CCK's actions to terminate an individual meal (Suzuki et al., 2010). CCK has two receptor subtypes, CCK1R and CCK2R. Both subtypes are widely distributed in the brain, including the hypothalamus and the brainstem. However, the anorectic action of CCK appears to be largely mediated via CCK1R on the afferent vagal fibers innervating the stomach and proximal intestine, which send signals to the hindbrain to reduce meal size (Suzuki et al., 2010). Disruption of vagal afferent signaling from the GI tract blocks the ability of CCK to inhibit eating. CCK has multiple biologically active forms and also has important roles in controlling gallbladder contraction, pancreatic secretion, gut motility, and gastric emptying in addition to meal termination (Badman and Flier, 2005).

Peptide YY

Peptide YY (PYY) is synthesized and secreted from specialized enteroendocrine cells, called L cells, located in the distal GI tract (ileum and colon). PYY is released into the circulation in relation to meal size. Plasma levels begin to rise within 15 minutes after the onset of eating, but they typically do not peak until after meal termination. Levels remain elevated for up to 6 hours postprandially; thus this hormone may have a greater effect on the size or timing of subsequent meals than on meal termination. PYY appears to exert its anorectic effects by binding to its receptors, which are known as Y2 receptors. Many lines of evidence suggest it acts mainly through the ARC of the hypothalamus to trigger a reduction in food intake, but there is also evidence that PYY's actions may be mediated via vagal–brainstem pathways. Food consumption, caloric load, food consistency, and nutrient composition all affect circulating PYY concentrations (Karra and Batterham, 2010). Postprandial levels of PYY appear to be reduced in obese individuals, and restoration of normal PYY levels in obese subjects reduces appetite.

PYY is a member of the PP-fold peptide family that also includes neuropeptide Y (NPY), which is produced in the ARC, and pancreatic polypeptide (PP), which is produced by PP cells of the pancreas. NPY is discussed in more detail later in this chapter. These peptides share sequence homology including several conserved tyrosine (Y) residues, thus their name. The major circulating form of PYY is $PYY_{3\text{-}36}$, which results from cleavage of the N-terminal tyrosine–proline residues from full length $PYY_{1\text{-}36}$ (Karra and Batterham, 2010).

Glucagon-like Peptide 1

Glucagon-like peptide 1 (GLP-1), like PYY, is released from the L cells of the intestine in response to meals (Neary and Batterham, 2010). It is released in proportion to calories consumed. GLP-1 exists in two forms that are designated GLP-$1_{1\text{-}37}$ and GLP-$1_{1\text{-}36}$. Additional N-terminal cleavage of the first six amino acids from both forms is required to produce biologically active GLP-$1_{7\text{-}37}$ and GLP-$1_{7\text{-}36}$, representing peptides of 31 and 30 amino acids, respectively. GLP-$1_{7\text{-}36}$ is the predominant biologically active form in circulation. GLP-1 is released from both gut and brain following meal ingestion; it reduces appetite and stimulates the sympathetic nervous system to increase energy expenditure. GLP-1 receptors are widely distributed in the CNS, including the ARC and brainstem, as well as in peripheral tissues. How GLP-1 acts on the brain is uncertain, but signaling is thought to occur primarily via vagal afferents. GLP-1, glucagon, glicentin, GLP-2, and oxyntomodulin (OXM) are all produced by posttranslational cleavage of a larger prohormone called proglucagon. Proglucagon is expressed in the pancreas, GI tract, and brain, and its proteolytic cleavage occurs in a tissue-specific manner. GLP-1, GLP-2, and oxyntomodulin are the major products in the GI tract.

Oxyntomodulin

OXM is a 37–amino acid peptide that is a potent inhibitor of food intake. Similar to GLP-1, OXM is cleaved from proglucagon and released from L cells of the intestine after a meal. The postprandial release of OXM is proportional to caloric load (Karra and Batterham, 2010). OXM appears to signal through GLP-1 receptors, although it has a much lower affinity for the receptor than does GLP-1. Administration of OXM reduces appetite and increases energy expenditure and voluntary physical activity in human subjects, which results in weight loss (Wynne et al., 2006). In rodents, OXM has been shown to suppress food intake, increase core temperature, increase heart rate, and cause weight loss (Sowden et al., 2007).

Incretins

In addition to their roles in reducing food intake, both GLP-1 and OXM belong to a class of molecules called incretins, which are defined as gut hormones that can increase the amount of insulin released from the beta cells of the pancreas (Neary and Batterham, 2010). More specifically, incretins enhance insulin secretion beyond the levels caused by glucose alone. This effect can occur even before plasma glucose levels become elevated. Incretins are thought to be responsible for the observation from glucose tolerance tests that the amount of insulin secreted is greater when glucose is given orally as opposed to intravenously. Another important gut-derived incretin not described earlier is glucose-dependent insulinotropic polypeptide. Glucose-dependent insulinotropic polypeptide is produced in K cells of the duodenum and the jejunum of the GI tract. The primary function of this peptide is as an incretin. Its potential direct role in food intake and energy expenditure is controversial (Badman and Flier, 2005).

Regardless of whether incretins have direct roles in regulating energy balance, all incretins control insulin, a satiety signal and also a long-term adiposity signal as described later, and glucose levels, a nutrient signal described previously. Thus they certainly play an indirect role in controlling food intake by increasing insulin secretion. Furthermore, because of their ability to lower plasma glucose level while promoting decreased food intake, incretin hormone–based therapies represent a novel strategy to treat type 2 diabetes (Mudaliar and Henry, 2010).

PANCREATIC ISLET-DERIVED SIGNALS

Pancreatic polypeptides are involved in the regulation of energy balance. These pancreatic polypeptides include pancreatic polypeptide (PP), insulin, and amylin, and they signal both food intake and the degree of adiposity. All three promote satiety.

Pancreatic Polypeptide

Pancreatic polypeptide (PP) contains 36 amino acids and is primarily produced by PP cells in the pancreatic islets (endocrine cells). PP belongs to the same protein family as NPY and PYY. PP is thought to reduce food intake through binding to Y4 or Y5 receptors in the brainstem and perhaps in the hypothalamus. It also appears to act via vagal afferents from the peripheral tissues to the brainstem. Circulating PP concentrations increase following food intake, and total release of PP is proportional to caloric intake. Peripheral infusion of PP in humans reduces food intake by 25% (Batterham et al., 2003). PP also has peripheral effects, including regulation of pancreatic and gastrointestinal secretory functions.

Insulin

Insulin, a hormone secreted by the beta cells of the pancreas, regulates the disposition of metabolic fuels and is more thoroughly discussed in Chapters 12 and 19. In the CNS, insulin acts as both a satiety signal and an adiposity signal. Circulating insulin levels increase rapidly in response to meal intake, especially the influx of glucose, and they also reflect body energy stores, falling in starvation. Basal insulin levels tend to reflect body adiposity, being higher in obese individuals; this may result, at least to some extent, from higher rates of insulin secretion in obese individuals due to reduced insulin sensitivity of liver, muscle, and adipose tissue. Insulin is transported into the brain via a saturable transporter and binds to neuronal insulin receptors to influence feeding behavior and energy expenditure. It is known to act on neurons in the ARC of the hypothalamus to mediate an anorexigenic response.

Amylin

Amylin is an anorectic 37–amino acid polypeptide that is released together with insulin from the beta cells of the pancreas. Amylin release closely mirrors that of insulin, with a ratio of about 1 mole of amylin per 100 moles of insulin. Like insulin, amylin secretion reflects both changes in circulating glucose level in response to meal intake and the extent of body fat stores. Amylin shows structural similarity with calcitonin. Although no amylin-specific receptors have been identified, amylin has been shown to bind to calcitonin receptors. Tissue specificity of amylin binding to the calcitonin receptor requires receptor activity-modifying proteins (RAMPs). Though the full distribution of its receptors is still being determined, amylin appears to decrease appetite largely through the area postrema (Neary and Batterham, 2010). Amylin administration activates cells in both the area postrema and the underlying NTS, and lesions to the area postrema block the ability of amylin to inhibit eating (Lutz et al., 2001). Other activities of amylin, such as its ability to inhibit gastric emptying and to inhibit glucagon secretion, combined with its anorectic effects have made amylin a drug candidate to treat obesity and type 2 diabetes. However, amylin's ability to bind to itself and form toxic amyloid fibrils has limited the therapeutic use of this protein.

ADIPOCYTE-DERIVED SIGNALS

The concept that regulation of food intake may be linked to amount of adipose tissue was first introduced by Kennedy (1953) over a half a century ago. It is only over the last two decades that research has revealed the nature of the signals that convey status of body fat depots to the brain as well as the role of this system in controlling energy balance (see Chapter 23, Figure 23-1). In addition to insulin and amylin, leptin is an important adiposity signal (Sánchez-Lasheras et al., 2010). Leptin is thought to play a substantial role in the central regulation of energy balance.

Leptin

Leptin is the protein product of the *LEP* gene, which is more commonly known as the *ob* gene. It is synthesized and secreted mainly by white adipocytes in proportion to body fat content and serves as a signal of energy sufficiency. Mice and humans lacking the *ob* gene, which encodes leptin, display spontaneous obesity. Systemic or intracerebroventricular injection of leptin into genetically obese mice or humans reduces food intake and increases energy expenditure, thereby reducing body fat. Extremely high doses of leptin also reduce food intake in nonobese animals. In general, obese individuals have high concentrations of plasma leptin, which may be the consequence of a systemic leptin resistance resulting from high sustained concentrations of leptin from enlarged adipose stores.

Leptin crosses the blood–brain barrier and binds to the B or long-form of the leptin receptor (Ob-Rb), which is widely expressed in the hypothalamus, including the ARC. Leptin binding to its receptor activates anorectic pathways and inhibits orexigenic pathways, as is discussed more thoroughly later. Leptin receptors are also found in many other tissues. A complete understanding of how leptin helps maintain energy homeostasis in humans is still emerging. The main function of leptin from an evolutionary perspective may be to signal the brain whether body fat stores are sufficient for initiation of high-energy processes, such as puberty and pregnancy (Blüher and Mantzoros, 2009).

Although leptin in general reflects adiposity and its level is about five times as high in obese as in lean individuals, leptin concentrations drop markedly during periods of short-term fasting (e.g., 22 hours), declining much faster than body fat stores are depleted (Landt et al., 2001). Such a drop in leptin levels can initiate a starvation response (Lustig, 2006).

CENTRAL NERVOUS SYSTEM INTEGRATION OF SATIETY AND ADIPOSITY SIGNALS

The brain receives and integrates the various homeostatic afferent signals about short-term and long-term energy intake. The hypothalamus is critical in relaying afferent signals from the gut and brainstem as well as processing efferent signals that modulate food intake and energy expenditure. Efferent responses ensure that there are sufficient energy stores for survival and reproduction. Nonmetabolic factors also affect the initiation and maintenance of ingestive behavior; these factors include environmental cues, rewards, cognitive factors, and emotional factors. The nonmetabolic inputs are processed mainly in the corticolimbic structures of the brain. There are interactions between the hypothalamus/brainstem pathways and the corticolimbic pathways, however, resulting in the integration of external and internal information (Zheng and Berthoud, 2008; Zheng et al., 2009). These interactions can result in the cortex and limbic system overpowering the hypothalamus into an ingestive mode, despite the presence of satiety and replete energy stores.

REGIONS OF THE BRAIN INVOLVED WITH SENSING OF NUTRIENT, SATIETY, AND ADIPOSITY SIGNALS

As mentioned previously, the hypothalamus and brainstem are key regions for sensing homeostatic input about energy balance (see Figure 22-4). Neurons within these regions contain receptors for long-term afferent signals, such as leptin and insulin, as well as circulating signals from the gut, such as ghrelin and PYY. In addition, the collection of neurons in the brainstem integrates sensory information from the abdominal organs and GI tract and taste information from the mouth (Benarroch, 2010). The brainstem neurons, including those in the area postrema and the NTS, have receptors for some of the gut-derived hormones, and they also receive input via the afferent fibers from peripheral tissues, predominantly by the vagal afferents carrying signals from the upper GI tract. In addition to these areas, there are regions of the prefrontal cortex involved in conditioned taste aversion, as well as reward centers that ultimately interact with hypothalamic nuclei. Thus many regions of the brain sense afferent signals and form a complex overlapping neural network to produce the efferent response. The integrated output of the brain centers receiving these inputs determines the nature and intensity of the efferent responses. These include efferent pathways determining hunger and food-seeking behaviors, the level of resting and activity-associated energy expenditure, and a variety of other neural and hormonal mechanisms involved in regulating growth and reproduction and energy partitioning within the body.

INTEGRATION OF AFFERENT SIGNALS IN THE ARCUATE NUCLEUS

One of the primary sites where afferent signals are integrated is the ARC of the hypothalamus (Suzuki et al., 2010). This region has been extensively studied for its ability to recognize and interpret long-term adiposity signals and some circulating gut peptides via specific receptors, such as those for insulin, leptin, and ghrelin. In addition to having receptors that bind signaling molecules that are able to cross the blood–brain barrier, the ARC receives input from neurons in other areas of the hypothalamus, including other integration centers. Neurons in the ARC also receive information from satiety signals that are relayed to the ARC from the

NUTRITION INSIGHT

Chronobiology of Energy Balance

Chronobiology refers to the time-dependent (or circadian) changes in biological functions. Indeed, there are important chronobiological aspects of energy intake and energy expenditure. Circadian rhythms are controlled and generated by the so-called master clock in the suprachiasmatic nuclei within the hypothalamus. At the molecular level, circadian clocks use clock and clock-controlled genes to generate rhythmicity and distribute temporal signals. Many molecular modifiers of energy intake and expenditure are directly or indirectly controlled by clock genes. For example, leptin secretion has a circadian rhythm with higher levels released at night. In mammals, synchronization of the master circadian clock is accomplished mainly by light stimuli. Thus sleep pattern, including how much and how regular the timing is of the sleep, could influence overall energy expenditure. In recent decades, there has been not only an increase in obesity but also a considerable decline in sleep duration (Laposky et al., 2008). However, in addition to light, food is a potent synchronizer of central and peripheral clocks. A number of recent studies in animals linking energy regulation and the circadian clock raise the possibility that the timing, frequency, and composition of food intake itself may play a significant role in weight gain. For example, mice fed a high-fat diet in the light cycle when they are normally asleep showed very different trends in body weight gain when compared to feeding during the dark cycle when they are normally active and feeding. Mice fed during the light cycle gained more weight and tended to be less active and to consume slightly more feed (Arble et al., 2009). Although systematic studies evaluating the influence of food intake patterns on the circadian system are lacking, there is some evidence that a regular eating pattern is advantageous for weight control and energy balance (Ekmekcioglu and Touitou, 2010).

hindbrain (e.g., the NTS). In addition, there is evidence that ARC neurons are directly sensitive to local levels of glucose and long-chain fatty acids in the plasma.

Within the ARC of the hypothalamus are two subpopulations of neurons involved in energy homeostasis. The first of these neuron types is sensitive to positive energy balance (e.g., energy surplus) and responds by synthesizing and secreting melanocortins, which are peptides cleaved from a precursor molecule called pro-opiomelanocortin (POMC). Most POMC neurons also express another peptide called cocaine- and amphetamine-regulated transcript (CART). Therefore these neuronal cells are called either POMC or POMC/CART neurons. The net effect of activation of POMC neurons is an increase in expression of alpha–melanocyte-stimulating hormone (α-MSH), which acts to decrease food intake via activation of the melanocortin pathway, the major neural circuit inhibiting food intake (Seeley et al., 2004). Activation of melanocortin pathways occurs via the binding of α-MSH to downstream G protein–coupled melanocortin receptors, particularly to the melanocortin receptor MC4R in the PVN of the hypothalamus.

A second neuronal cell type opposes the actions of POMC neurons. This second type of neuron secretes NPY and agouti-related protein (AgRP) when activated. Activation of the NPY/AgRP neurons results in stimulation of food intake and reduction of energy expenditure. The orexigenic effect of NPY is mediated by binding to receptors Y1R and Y5R on its target cells in other hypothalamic nuclei, including the LHA that contains orexigenic neuropeptides (melanin-concentrating hormone and orexins). AgRP, on the other hand, acts as a selective antagonist at the MC4R in the PVN, thus blocking the action of α-MSH released by the anorexigenic POMC neurons. Activation of the NPY/AgRP neurons is likely responsible for the hyperphagia that occurs in response to body fat loss. As might be expected, receptors for ghrelin, the major orexigenic peptide, are highly localized on NPY/AgRP neurons and stimulate NPY and AgRP production to promote food intake (Mondal et al., 2005).

Both the POMC and the NPY/AgRP neurons are influenced by circulating leptin and insulin. The reciprocal regulation of the activity of the NPY/AgRP and the POMC neurons under conditions of energy surfeit or energy deficit is depicted in Figure 22-6 (Stanley et al., 2005). In conditions of energy surfeit (Figure 22-6, *A*), circulating levels of leptin and insulin are elevated. These hormones interact with their receptors on the two populations of neurons to activate the POMC neurons and inhibit the NPY/AgRP neurons, resulting in increased release of α-MSH and decreased release of AgRP by the neuronal fibers projecting into the adjacent hypothalamic nuclei. Thus activation of POMC neurons (release of α-MSH) and the suppression of NPY/AgRP neurons (release of α-MSH antagonist) both result in increased binding of α-MSH to the MC4R in the PVN to activate anorexigenic pathways leading to suppression of feeding and increased energy expenditure by peripheral tissues. Because efferents from the PVN of the hypothalamus primarily play an inhibitory role in the control of food intake, PVN is considered a satiety center.

In contrast, in conditions of energy deficit (Figure 22-6, *B*), levels of insulin, leptin, and circulating nutrients are low, the POMC neurons are not activated, and the NPY/AgRP neurons are not inhibited. This results in higher levels of NPY and AgRP release but lower levels of α-MSH release. The lack of α-MSH and presence of AgRP inhibit the anorexigenic neurons in the PVN, whereas the abundance of NPY activates the orexigenic neurons in the LHA. The LHA generally plays a stimulatory role in the control of food intake and can be considered a feeding center. Activation of orexigenic neurons also leads to reduced fuel consumption and energy expenditure by peripheral tissues.

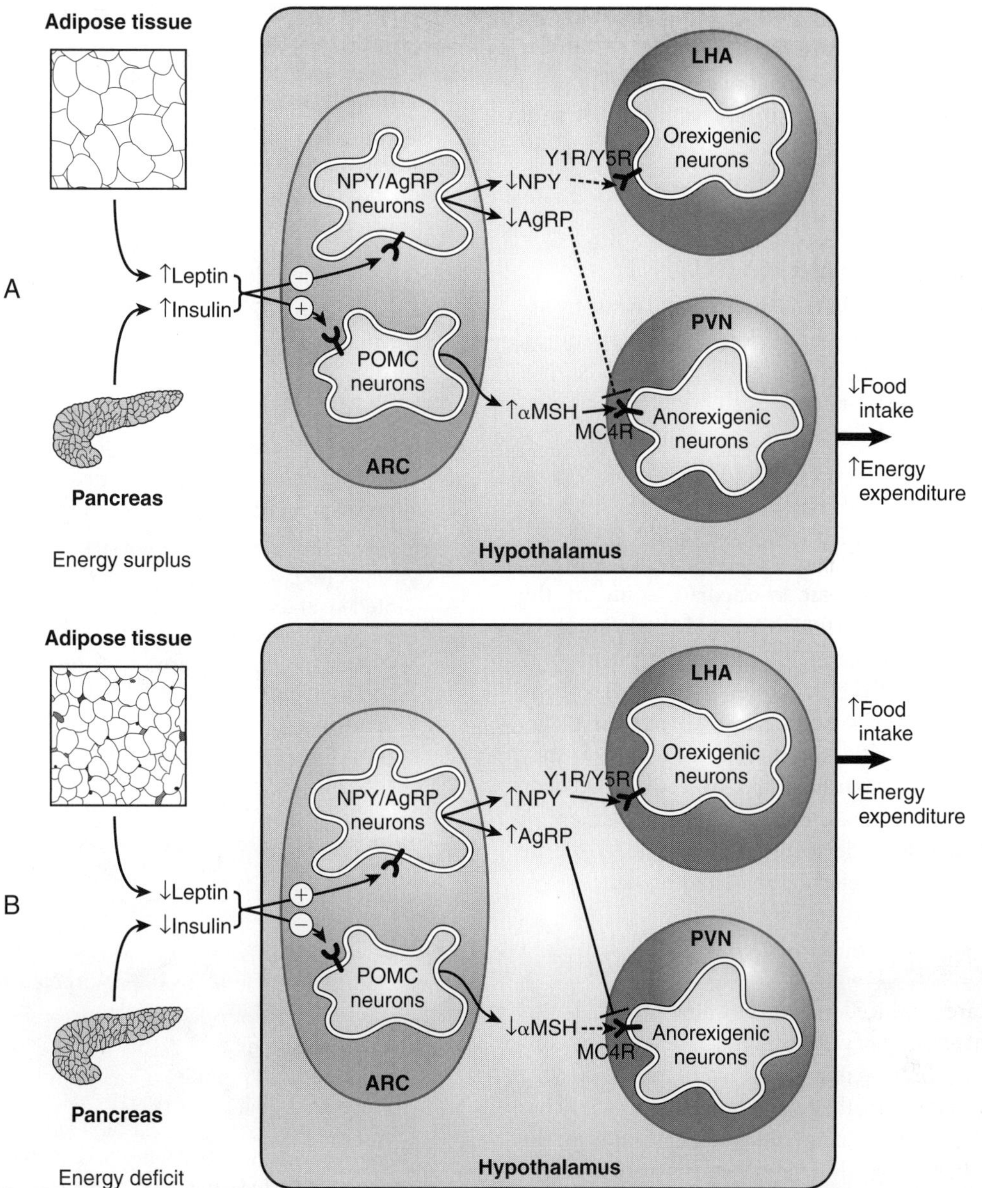

FIGURE 22-6 A, Regulation of food intake at the level of the arcuate nucleus by increased levels of insulin and leptin. Leptin and insulin are both anorexigenic and induce a decrease in food intake (i.e., anorexigenic behavior). Insulin and leptin directly diffuse into the ARC where they bind to their receptors on both NPY/AgRP and POMC neurons. Leptin and insulin promote expression of α-MSH (an anorexigenic neuropeptide) by POMC neurons but suppress expression of NPY and AgRP (orexigenic neuropeptides) by NPY/AgRP neurons. Thus binding of α-MSH to the melanocortin receptors dominates. As a consequence, activation of melanocortin anorexigenic pathways predominate, and the net result is decreased food intake and increased energy expenditure. **B**, Regulation of food intake at the level of the ARC by decreased levels of insulin and leptin, promoting orexigenic pathways. Reduced levels of insulin/leptin trigger release of NPY and AgRP, which stimulate orexigenic neurons in the lateral hypothalamus while simultaneously blocking α-MSH binding to anorexigenic neurons. The net result is increased food intake and decreased energy expenditure. *AgRP,* Agouti-related protein; *α-MSH,* alpha–melanocyte-stimulating hormone; *ARC,* arcuate nucleus; *LHA,* lateral hypothalamic area; *MC4R,* melanocortin-4 (α-MSH) receptor; *NPY,* neuropeptide Y; *POMC,* pro-opiomelanocortin; *PVN,* paraventricular nucleus; *Y1R/Y5R,* NPY receptors.

INTEGRATION OF NUTRIENT SIGNALS IN THE ARCUATE NUCLEUS

The hypothalamus is also involved in nutrient sensing, and the ARC is thought to be a primary nutrient-sensing center. Although considerable data support a role for nutrient-sensing neurons in regulating energy balance, the neuronal circuits by which this sensing occurs and how it is coupled to downstream responses are relatively uncharacterized (Blouet and Schwartz, 2010). A direct response of hypothalamic nutrient neurons to acute postprandial changes in nutrient availability has not yet been demonstrated. Nevertheless, two fuel-sensing protein kinases, known as AMPK and mTOR, appear to be important in sensing levels of fatty acids, glucose, and amino acids. These kinases have been discussed in other chapters (see Chapter 19) because of their importance in gauging energy status of peripheral tissues. Thus it appears that different organs share some commonalities in biochemical and nutrient-sensing mechanisms, albeit with tissue-specific outcomes (Ronnett et al., 2009; Steinberg and Kemp, 2009).

ROLE OF CNS NEUROTRANSMITTERS AND NEUROMODULATORS ON ENERGY BALANCE

It has long been recognized that the monoamine neurotransmitters, which include serotonin (5-hydroxytryptamine), norepinephrine, and dopamine, are involved in CNS control of feeding behavior. The monoamines are widely distributed throughout the CNS and act to enhance or diminish transmission via many pathways, affecting a variety of behaviors, including appetite and mood. For example, increased serotonin neurotransmission appears to enhance the sensitivity of brain centers to the action of satiety peptides, whereas dopaminergic pathways appear to mediate some of the reward aspects of feeding (Liebowitz and Hoebel, 2004). In addition, endogenous cannabinoid and opioid systems play an overall modulatory effect on the reward circuitry of the brain and can have orexigenic effects (Maccarrone et al., 2010). A number of other neuromodulators (Box 22-1) may also be involved in the central control of feeding behavior and energy balance in animals. Evidence for involvement of numerous compounds underscores the complexity of the system controlling eating behavior and energy balance.

BOX 22-1 Neuromodulators That Stimulate or Inhibit Food Intake

NEUROMODULATORS THAT STIMULATE FOOD INTAKE

Neuropeptide (NPY)
Galanin, galanin-like peptides
Agouti-related protein (AgRP)
Hypocretins/orexins A, B
Melanin-concentrating hormone (MCH)
Opioid peptides
Endocannabinoids
Growth hormone–releasing hormone (GHRH)
Beacon
VGF-derived peptides
Ghrelin
Prolactin

NEUROMODULATORS THAT INHIBIT FOOD INTAKE

Melanocortins (e.g., POMC, α-MSH)
Cytokines (e.g., tumor necrosis factor, interleukin 1, interleukin 6)
Cocaine-amphetamine–related transcript (CART)
Corticotropin-releasing hormone (CRH)
Neurotensin
Neuromedins B and U
Calcitonin
Acidic fibroblast growth factor
Cyclo (His-Pro) dipeptide
Oxytocin
Vasopressin
Peptide YY_{3-36}
Insulin
Leptin
Neuropeptide K
Brain-derived neurotrophic factor
Lipopolysaccharide
Prolactin-releasing peptide
Ciliary neurotrophic factor (CNTF)

Data from Liebowitz, S. F., & Hoebel, B. G. (2004). Behavioral neuroscience and obesity. In G. A. Bray & C. Bouchard (Eds.), *Handbook of obesity* (2nd ed., pp. 301–307). New York: Marcel Dekker.
MSH, Melanocyte-stimulating hormone; *POMC,* pro-opiomelanocortin.

EFFERENT SIGNALS

Efferent signals are produced by regions of the hypothalamus in response to integration of various inputs. These signals converge at sites in the brainstem and regions of the spinal cord that control the parasympathetic and sympathetic branches of the autonomic nervous system. Integrated output from the brain results in efferent signals. Efferent signals from nuclei in the brainstem (i.e., the locus coeruleus and the NTS) activate the sympathetic nervous system. Efferent signals sent via the dorsal vagal complex (NTS and DMV) of the brainstem activate the parasympathetic nervous system (vagus nerve).

Postganglionic neurons of the sympathetic system release norepinephrine as the neurotransmitter that activates adrenergic receptors on the peripheral target tissues. The adrenal medulla acts as a modified sympathetic ganglion, and the norepinephrine and epinephrine released within the medulla are discharged into the blood. Postganglionic neurons of the parasympathetic system predominantly use acetylcholine as the neurotransmitter, and acetylcholine acts on muscarinic receptors of target organs.

In addition to direct signaling via peripheral innervation of target tissues in the body, efferent signaling also occurs through neuroendocrine connections. These include the activation of the hypothalamic–pituitary–thyroid axis by release of thyrotropin-releasing hormone by the neurons of the PVN. In other cases, hormone release is modified as a response to parasympathetic nervous system activity (e.g., increased insulin release by the pancreas) or sympathetic nervous system activity (e.g., secretion of epinephrine and norepinephrine by the adrenal medulla). These hormones in turn act on target tissues that express receptors for the specific hormones as part of the response to alterations in energy balance. In response to negative energy balance, food intake is increased and energy expenditure is decreased to bring the body back into energy balance. In the case of positive energy balance, the brain signals the body to decrease food intake and increase energy expenditure.

Activities of the sympathetic and parasympathetic systems change in a reciprocal fashion with alterations in food intake and associated metabolism to regulate energy storage and energy expenditure in an opposing manner (Bray, 1991; Lustig, 2006; Blouet and Schwartz, 2010), as summarized in Figure 22-7. A surplus of energy leads to activation

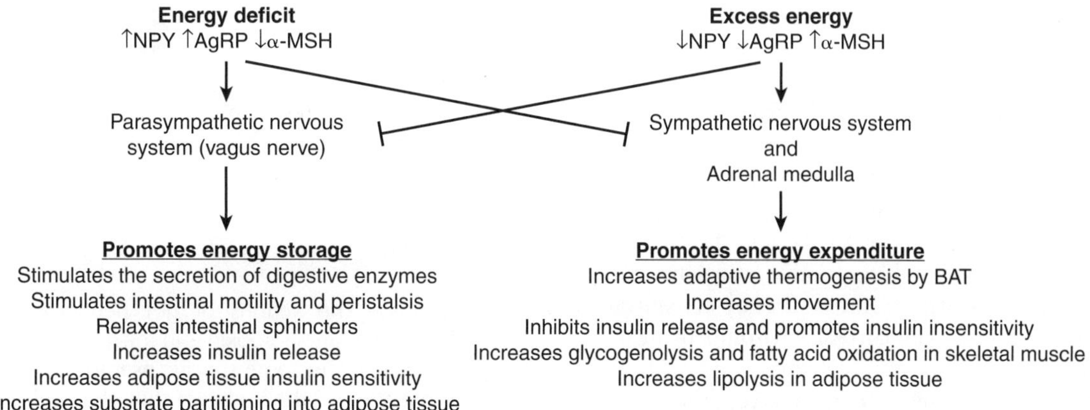

FIGURE 22-7 Efferent signals controlling energy balance. Once the various hormone and neural signals are integrated in the CNS, efferent outputs via the autonomic nervous system regulate energy storage and energy expenditure at the levels of the peripheral tissues. An energy deficit stimulates parasympathetic output to promote energy storage and inhibits sympathetic output that would promote energy expenditure. By increasing energy intake and decreasing energy expenditure, the body returns to energy balance. In contrast, an excess of energy stimulates sympathetic output to increase energy expenditure and inhibits parasympathetic output to promote food intake and energy storage. Thus when the body has surplus energy, a decrease in food intake and an increase in energy expenditure operate to bring the body back toward energy balance.

of the sympathetic nervous system, which promotes energy expenditure by increasing movement and thermogenesis, by increasing glycogenolysis and fatty acid oxidation in skeletal muscle and lipolysis in adipose tissue, and by inhibiting insulin release. These processes are largely mediated by β-adrenergic receptor activation in skeletal muscle and adipocytes and by activation of α2-adrenergic receptors on beta cells of the pancreas. On the other hand, the parasympathetic nervous system output is inhibited when the hypothalamus detects energy surplus so that food intake and energy storage are not activated. An energy deficit leads to activation of the parasympathetic nervous system (i.e., the vagus nerve) to promote energy storage by increasing digestion and absorption in the GI tract, increasing insulin secretion, increasing adipose tissue insulin sensitivity, and increasing substrate partitioning into adipose tissue. At the same time, sympathetic activity decreases during starvation to conserve energy by reducing energy expenditure. Reciprocal regulation of the sympathetic and parasympathetic systems is also seen with certain experimental manipulations. For example, administration of an appetite suppressant such as an amphetamine both decreases parasympathetic activity and hence food intake and increases sympathetic activity which increases energy expenditure. Conversely, VMH lesions increase parasympathetic activity and food intake and decrease sympathetic activity and energy expenditure.

It should be noted that although basal energy expenditure and the thermic effect of food are largely regulated by the autonomic, or involuntary, nervous system in response to outputs of the brain centers involved in controlling energy balance, the energy expenditure of physical activity is voluntary and can vary significantly. The variation depends on the type and intensity of activity chosen, the duration of the activity, the mechanical efficiency of the activity performed, and the person's body weight. Choosing to perform more physical activity is one way an individual can alter the energy balance equation.

IMPORTANCE OF DIET AND EXERCISE IN PREVENTION OF OVERWEIGHT AND OBESITY

Whether energy balance is reached at a healthy body weight is subject to a variety of other variables. Despite the elegant neural control systems described earlier for defending body weight, it is possible to override these systems through cognitive means. For example, many nonphysiological cues are involved in determining whether an individual chooses to eat; these cues range from the mere presence of food to complex social and cultural habits and circumstances (see Table 22-2). The amount eaten, although subject to the feedback systems described, can still be cognitively determined. Likewise, despite the body's ability to adjust basal and adaptive components of total energy expenditure, the amount of physical activity performed is still largely an individual cognitive choice. Therefore the overall level of energy balance achieved is still subject to many nonphysiological factors. Indeed, seasonal changes in body weight and the increase in the prevalence of obesity in the populations of most developed countries is testimony to the power of environmental and cognitive influences on eating and activity behaviors.

Work highlighting the importance of achieving nutrient balance in addition to total energy balance has improved our understanding of how environmental factors, such as changes in diet composition and changes in physical activity patterns, affect the body weight regulatory system (Flatt and Tremblay, 2004). As discussed in preceding text, acute changes in intake of alcohol, protein, or carbohydrate are rapidly balanced by changes in oxidation of each. In contrast, fat has lowest priority for oxidation, is readily stored, and hence fat oxidation is not tightly linked to fat intake. A positive fat balance is relatively easy to achieve with overconsumption of energy.

Diets high in fat are particularly problematic. Fat increases the palatability and energy density of the food consumed, which contributes to overconsumption of total energy. In turn, the excess energy intake leads to incomplete oxidation of dietary fat, and the fat not needed temporally is stored. Restricting the habitual level of physical activity reduces fat oxidation because working muscle is a major contributor to the body's total oxidation of fat. Because fat intake and oxidation are not closely linked, positive fat balance results if the decline in fat oxidation is not offset by an equivalent reduction in fat intake. The current environment in many industrialized nations, however, is characterized by the wide availability of energy-dense, high-fat foods combined with an increasingly sedentary lifestyle (Hill et al., 2003). This environment promotes maintenance of fat balance only after a large body fat mass has been gained. The best strategies for avoiding positive fat, or energy, balance are to avoid overconsumption of energy and to engage in regular physical activity.

For overweight and obese individuals who want to reduce body fat stores, negative fat balance can be brought about by underconsumption of total energy or by an increase in the level of habitual physical activity. During underconsumption of energy (i.e., caloric restriction), the supply of the metabolic fuels is not sufficient to meet the body's energy needs, so the remaining energy needs must be met by oxidation of fat from endogenous fat stores. Similarly, increased oxidation of fat stores is the predominant mechanism by which energy needs are met when the level of habitual physical activity is increased.

THINKING CRITICALLY

1. Describe the actions of gut peptides, pancreatic hormones, and adipokines in the regulation of energy balance, using some specific examples.
2. What areas of the brain are thought to play key roles in the central regulation of energy balance? What are their specific functions?
3. When energy intake is in excess, describe the homeostatic systems that lead to a decrease in food intake and an increase in energy expenditure to bring the body back toward energy balance.
4. What are some factors that might play a role in making it difficult for individuals to lose weight and/or maintain a weight loss?

REFERENCES

Arble, D. M., Bass, J., Laposky, A. D., Vitaterna, M. H., & Turek, F. W. (2009). Circadian timing of food intake contributes to weight gain. *Obesity (Silver Spring), 17*, 2100–2102.

Badman, M. K., & Flier, J. S. (2005). The gut and energy balance: Visceral allies in the obesity wars. *Science, 307*, 1909–1914.

Batterham, R. L., Le Roux, C. W., Cohen, M. A., Park, A. J., Ellis, S. M., Patterson, M., … Bloom, S. R. (2003). Pancreatic polypeptide reduces appetite and food intake in humans. *The Journal of Clinical Endocrinology and Metabolism, 88*, 3989–3992.

Beckman, L. M., Beckman, T. R., & Earthman, C. P. (2010). Changes in gastrointestinal hormones and leptin after Roux-en-Y gastric bypass procedure: A review. *Journal of the American Dietetic Association, 110*, 571–584.

Benarroch, E. E. (2010). Neural control of feeding behavior: Overview and clinical correlations. *Neurology, 74*, 1643–1650.

Blouet, C., & Schwartz, G. J. (2010). Hypothalamic nutrient sensing in the control of energy homeostasis. *Behavioral Brain Research, 209*, 1–12.

Blüher, S., & Mantzoros, C. S. (2009). Leptin in humans: Lessons from translational research. *The American Journal of Clinical Nutrition, 89*, 991S–997S.

Bouchard, C., Tremblay, A., Despres, J. P., Nadeau, A., Lupien, P. J., Moorjani, S., … Kim, S. Y. (1996). Overfeeding in identical twins: 5-Year postoverfeeding results. *Metabolism, 45*, 1042–1050.

Bray, G. A. (1991). Weight homeostasis. *Annual Review of Medicine, 42*, 205–216.

Cohen, D. A. (2008). Obesity and the built environment: Changes in environmental cues cause energy imbalances. *International Journal of Obesity, 32*, S137–S142.

Cota, D., Proulx, K., Smith, K. A., Kozma, S. C., Thomas, G., Woods, S. C., & Seeley, R. J. (2006). Hypothalamic mTOR signaling regulates food intake. *Science, 312*, 927–930.

Cummings, D. E., Purnell, J. Q., Frayo, R. S., Schmidova, K., Wisse, B. E., & Weigle, D. S. (2001). A preprandial rise in plasma ghrelin levels suggests a role in meal initiation in humans. *Diabetes, 50*, 1714–1719.

Dunn-Meynell, A. A., Routh, V. H., Kang, L., Gaspers, L., & Levin, B. E. (2002). Glucokinase is the likely mediator of glucosensing in both glucose-excited and glucose-inhibited central neurons. *Diabetes, 51*, 2056–2065.

Ekmekcioglu, C., & Touitou, Y. (2010). Chronobiological aspects of food intake and metabolism and their relevance on energy balance and weight regulation. *Obesity Reviews, 12*, 14–25.

Flatt, J. P., & Tremblay, A. (2004). Energy expenditure and substrate oxidation. In G. A. Bray & C. Bouchard (Eds.), *Handbook of obesity* (2nd ed., pp. 705–731). New York: Marcel Dekker.

Flegal, K. M., Carroll, M. D., Ogden, C. L., & Curtin, L. R. (2010). Prevalence and trends in obesity among US adults, 1999–2008. The Journal of the American Medical Association, 303, 235–241.

Flegal, K. M., & Troiano, R. P. (2000). Changes in the distribution of body mass index of adults and children in the US population. *International Journal of Obesity and Related Metabolic Disorders, 24*, 807–818.

Flood-Obbagy, J. E., & Rolls, B. J. (2009). The effect of fruit in different forms on energy intake and satiety at a meal. *Appetite, 52*, 416–422.

Hagobian, T. A., & Braun, B. (2010). Physical activity and hormonal regulation of appetite: Sex differences and weight control. *Exercise and Sport Sciences Reviews, 38*, 25–30.

Herman, C. P., & Polivy, J. (2008). External cues in the control of food intake in humans: The sensory-normative distinction. *Physiology & Behavior, 94*, 722–728.

Hill, J. O., Wyatt, H. R., Reed, G., & Peters, J. C. (2003). Obesity and the environment: Where do we go from here? *Science, 299*, 853–855.

Horton, T. J., Drougas, H., Brachey, A., Reed, G. W., Peters, J. C., & Hill, J. O. (1995). Fat and carbohydrate overfeeding in humans: Different effects on energy storage. *The American Journal of Clinical Nutrition, 62*, 19–29.

Karra, E., & Batterham, R. L. (2010). The role of gut hormones in the regulation of body weight and energy homeostasis. *Molecular and Cellular Endocrinology, 316*, 120–128.

Keesey, R. E., & Corbett, S. W. (1984). Metabolic defense of the body weight set point. In A. J. Stunkard & E. Stellar (Eds.), *Eating and its disorders* (pp. 87–96). New York: Raven Press.

Kennedy, G. C. (1953). The role of depot fat in the hypothalamic control of food intake in the rat. *Proceedings of the Royal Society of London. Series B, Biological Sciences, 140*, 578–596.

Klein, S., & Goran, M. (1993). Energy metabolism in response to overfeeding in young adult men. *Metabolism, 42*, 1201–1205.

Kraschnewski, J. L., Boan, J., Esposito, J., Sherwood, N. E., Lehman, E. B., Kephart, D. K., & Sciamanna, C. N. (2010). Long-term weight loss maintenance in the United States. *International Journal of Obesity, 34*, 1644–1654.

Kremers, S. P., Visscher, T. L., Seidell, J. C., van Mechelen, W., & Brug, J. (2005). Cognitive determinants of energy balance-related behaviours: Measurement issues. *Sports Medicine (Auckland, N.Z.), 35*, 923–933.

Landt, M., Horowitz, J. F., Coppack, S. W., & Klein, S. (2001). Effect of short-term fasting on free and bound leptin concentrations in lean and obese women. *The Journal of Clinical Endocrinology and Metabolism, 86*, 3768–3771.

Laposky, A. D., Bass, J., Kohsaka, A., & Turek, F. W. (2008). Sleep and circadian rhythms: Key components in the regulation of energy metabolism. *FEBS Letters, 582*, 142–151.

Levine, J. A., Eberhardt, N. L., & Jensen, M. D. (1999). Role of nonexercise activity thermogenesis in resistance to fat gain in humans. *Science, 283*, 212–214.

Liebowitz, S. F., & Hoebel, B. G. (2004). Behavioral neuroscience and obesity. In G. A. Bray & C. Bouchard (Eds.), *Handbook of obesity* (2nd ed., pp. 301–371). New York: Marcel Dekker.

Lustig, R. H. (2006). Childhood obesity: Behavioral aberration or biochemical drive? Reinterpreting the first law of thermodynamics. *Nature Clinical Practice. Endocrinology & Metabolism, 2*, 447–458.

Lutz, T. A., Mollet, A., Rushing, P. A., Riediger, T., & Scharrer, E. (2001). The anorectic effect of a chronic peripheral infusion of amylin is abolished in area postrema/nucleus of the solitary tract (AP/NTS) lesioned rats. *International Journal of Obesity and Related Metabolic Disorders, 25*, 1005–1011.

Maccarrone, M., Gasperi, V., Catani, M. V., Diep, T. A., Dainese, E., Hansen, H. S., & Avigliano, L. (2010). The endocannabinoid system and its relevance for nutrition. *Annual Review of Nutrition, 30*, 423–440.

Mayer, J. (1953). Glucostatic mechanism of regulation of food intake. *New England Journal of Medicine, 249*, 13–16.

Mondal, M. S., Date, Y., Yamaguchi, H., Toshinai, K., Tsuruta, T., Kangawa, K., & Nakazato, M. (2005). Identification of ghrelin and its receptor in neurons of the rat arcuate nucleus. *Regulatory Peptides, 126*, 55–59.

Mudaliar, S., & Henry, R. R. (2010). Effects of incretin hormones on beta-cell mass and function, body weight, and hepatic and myocardial function. *The American Journal of Medicine, 123*, S19–S27.

Neary, M. T., & Batterham, R. L. (2009). Gut hormones: Implications for the treatment of obesity. *Pharmacology & Therapeutics, 124*, 44–56.

Neary, M. T., & Batterham, R. L. (2010). Gaining new insights into food reward with functional neuroimaging. *Forum of Nutrition, 63*, 152–163.

Obici, S., Feng, Z., Morgan, K., Stein, D., Karkanias, G., & Rossetti, L. (2002). Central administration of oleic acid inhibits glucose production and food intake. *Diabetes, 51*, 271–275.

Peters, J. C. (2003). Dietary fat and body weight control. *Lipids, 38*, 123–127.

Peters, J. C., Wyatt, H. R., Donahoo, W. T., & Hill, J. O. (2002). From instinct to intellect: The challenge of maintaining healthy weight in the modern world. *Obesity Reviews, 3*, 69–74.

Rolls, B. J. (2009). The relationship between dietary energy density and energy intake. *Physiology & Behavior, 97*, 609–615.

Ronnett, G. V., Ramamurthy, S., Kleman, A. M., Landree, L. E., & Aja, S. J. (2009). AMPK in the brain: Its roles in energy balance and neuroprotection. *Journal of Neurochemistry, 109*(Suppl.), 1, 17–23.

Rowland, N. E., Vaughan, C. H., Mathes, C. M., & Mitra, A. (2008). Feeding behavior, obesity, and neuroeconomics. *Physiology & Behavior, 93*, 97–109.

Saelens, B. E., & Handy, S. L. (2008). Built environment correlates of walking: A review. *Medicine and Science in Sports and Exercise, 40*, S550–S566.

Sánchez-Lasheras, C., Könner, A. C., & Brüning, J. C. (2010). Integrative neurobiology of energy homeostasis-neurocircuits, signals and mediators. *Frontiers in Neuroendocrinology, 31*, 4–15.

Savage, J. S., Fisher, J. O., & Birch, L. L. (2007). Parental influences on eating behavior: Conception to adolescence. *The Journal of Law, Medicine & Ethics, 35*(1), 22–34.

Seeley, R. J., Drazen, D. L., & Clegg, D. J. (2004). The critical role of the melanocortin system in the control of energy balance. *Annual Review of Nutrition, 24*, 133–149.

Sims, E. A., & Horton, E. S. (1968). Endocrine and metabolic adaptation to obesity and starvation. *The American Journal of Clinical Nutrition, 21*, 1455–1470.

Sowden, G. L., Drucker, D. J., Weinshenker, D., & Swoap, S. J. (2007). Oxyntomodulin increases intrinsic heart rate in mice independent of the glucagon-like peptide-1 receptor. *American Journal of Physiology. Regulatory, Integrative and Comparative Physiology, 292*, R962–R970.

Sowers, M., Zheng, H., Tomey, K., Karvonen-Gutierrez, C., Jannausch, M., Li, X., … Symons, J. (2007). Changes in body composition in women over six years at midlife: Ovarian and chronological aging. *The Journal of Clinical Endocrinology and Metabolism, 92*, 895–901.

Stanley, S., Wynne, K., McGowan, B., & Bloom, S. (2005). Hormonal regulation of food intake. *Physiological Reviews, 85*, 1131–1158.

Steinberg, G. R., & Kemp, B. E. (2009). AMPK in health and disease. *Physiological Reviews, 89*, 1025–1078.

Stringhini, S., Sabia, S., Shipley, M., Brunner, E., Nabi, H., Kivimaki, M., & Singh-Manoux, A. (2010). Association of socioeconomic position with health behaviors and mortality. *The Journal of the American Medical Association, 303*, 1159–1166.

Sun, Y., Asnicar, M., Saha, P. K., Chan, L., & Smith, R. G. (2006). Ablation of ghrelin improves the diabetic but not obese phenotype of ob/ob mice. *Cell Metabolism, 3*, 379–386.

Suzuki, K., Simpson, K. A., Minnion, J. S., Shillito, J. C., & Bloom, S. R. (2010). The role of gut hormones and the hypothalamus in appetite regulation. *Endocrine Journal, 57*, 359–372.

Tschöp, M., Smiley, D. L., & Heiman, M. L. (2000). Ghrelin induces adiposity in rodents. *Nature, 407*, 908–913.

Wansink, B. (2004). Environmental factors that increase the food intake and consumption volume of unknowing consumers. *Annual Review of Nutrition, 24*, 455–479.

Wynne, K., Park, A. J., Small, C. J., Meeran, K., Ghatei, M. A., Frost, G. S., & Bloom, S. R. (2006). Oxyntomodulin increases energy expenditure in addition to decreasing energy intake in overweight and obese humans: A randomised controlled trial. *International Journal of Obesity, 30*, 1729–1736.

Zheng, H., & Berthoud, H.-R. (2008). Neural systems controlling the drive to eat: Mind versus metabolism. *Physiology, 23*, 75–83.

Zheng, H., Lenard, N. R., Shin, A. C., & Berthoud H.-R. (2009). Appetite control and energy balance regulation in the modern world: Reward-driven overrides repletion signals. *International Journal of Obesity, 33*, S8–S13.

Zigman, J. M., Nakano, Y., Coppari, R., Balthasar, N., Marcus, J. N., Lee, C. E., … Elmquist, J. K. (2005). Mice lacking ghrelin receptors resist the development of diet-induced obesity. *The Journal of Clinical Investigation, 115*, 3564–3572.

RECOMMENDED READINGS

Galgani, J., & Ravussin, E. (2008). Energy metabolism, fuel selection and body weight regulation. *International Journal of Obesity*, *32*, S109–S119.

Hill, J. O. (2006). Understanding and addressing the epidemic of obesity: An energy balance perspective. *Endocrine Reviews*, *27*, 750–761.

Schoeller, D. A. (2009). The energy balance equation: Looking back and looking forward are two very different views. *Nutrition Reviews*, *67*, 249–254.

Stefater, M. A., & Seeley, R. J. (2010). Central nervous system nutrient signaling: The regulation of energy balance and the future of dietary therapies. Annual Review of Nutrition, 30, 219–235.

CHAPTER 23

Disturbances of Energy Balance

*Darlene E. Berryman, PhD, RD, and Christopher A. Taylor, PhD, RD, LD**

COMMON ABBREVIATIONS

BMI	body mass index [weight in kg ÷ (height in m)^2]
PEM	protein-energy malnutrition
TLC	therapeutic lifestyle changes
WAT	white adipose tissue
WC	waist circumference

A stable body weight is an indicator that energy balance has been maintained. As discussed in the previous chapter, the human body has a highly complex interactive means to help sustain energy balance. Despite this, many individuals experience chronic positive or negative energy balance resulting in significant weight gain or loss, respectively. The metabolic and health consequences that occur under energy imbalance will be reviewed in this chapter.

ADIPOSE TISSUE IN ENERGY BALANCE

Adipose tissue is the major site of stored energy in the body, with fat stores serving as an energy buffer; therefore this tissue is critical to energy balance. The importance of this energy reservoir in energy balance can best be illustrated by the metabolic disturbances that accompany an extreme excess (obesity) or an extreme loss (lipoatrophy) of adipose tissue. Because excess or deficient energy storage within this tissue is central to the metabolic disturbances observed in patients with obesity and lipodystrophies, it is important first to appreciate the varied functions and complexity of adipose tissue. Although once considered relatively simple, adipose tissue is clearly a much more interactive and dynamic tissue than originally appreciated. The focus of this section will be white adipose tissue (WAT); however, as mentioned in Chapter 21, there is also a more recent appreciation that brown adipose tissue may have a significant role in energy balance as well.

PHYSIOLOGY OF WHITE ADIPOSE TISSUE

WAT is a specialized loose connective tissue characterized by numerous lipid-laden adipocytes. These adipocytes have a great capacity to expand (hypertrophy) with excess energy changing their diameter up to twentyfold. However, their ability to expand is not infinite. Excess energy intake can also promote the formation of new adipocytes from precursor cells (preadipocytes) resident in the tissue (Drolet et al., 2008). Although the relatively large adipocytes contribute a large fraction of the total adipose tissue mass (~35% to 75% depending on how much fat they contain), they only comprise about 25% of the total cell population in adipose tissue. In addition to adipocytes, WAT contains macrophages, pericytes, lymphocytes, preadipocytes, fibroblasts, endothelial cells, and blood cells. These other cell types contribute to the tissue's complexity and can influence the metabolic function of the tissue. The increased number of macrophages present in adipose tissue of obese animals or humans is an example of a case in which the tissue complexity changes the metabolic functions of the tissue (Weisberg et al., 2003).

WAT is unique in that it is not a discrete tissue but is a distributed tissue found in various depots and as a component of most organs. WAT is not a uniform tissue, and marked differences can be observed among adipose tissue located in different regions of the body. Conventionally, WAT has been classified as either subcutaneous, which is just under the skin, or as visceral (intrabdominal), which surrounds internal organs. WAT typically accounts for the majority (~70%-90%) of all WAT. Visceral adipose tissue accounts for the other 10% to 30% (Müller et al., 2011). Visceral adipose tissue can be further subdivided into intraperitoneal (e.g., omental and mesenteric WAT) and extraperitoneal/retroperitoneal (e.g., perirenal WAT) deposits, and subcutaneous adipose tissue may be described by location (e.g., femoral, gluteal, or abdominal) (Frühbeck, 2008). Differences in vascularization (blood and lymphatic circulations), neural innervations, and cell composition all contribute to the differences in various adipose depots. For example, macrophage infiltration in adipose tissue of obese individuals is more prominent in visceral depots than in subcutaneous depots (Harman-Boehm et al., 2007). There are also sex-specific patterns of fat distribution and metabolism (Lee et al., 2010). For example, women have larger femoral-gluteal subcutaneous fat depots than do men. Because of the functional differences in various depots, it is not surprising that the specific regional distribution of adipose tissue is considered to be an important

*This chapter is a revision of the chapter contributed by Martha H. Stipanuk, PhD, for the second edition.

indicator of the metabolic alterations that accompany chronic disease. Overall, excess visceral adipose tissue is associated with an increased risk of numerous comorbidities that are associated with obesity as well as overall mortality. An excess of visceral fat is known as central obesity, and individuals with excess visceral fat have an "apple shaped" body type and large waist circumference. Although visceral fat itself has been implicated in the etiology of obesity and metabolic disease, the ability of the much larger subcutaneous depots to expand to store excess energy and prevent storage of fat in visceral adipose or nonadipose tissues is also important.

FUNCTIONS OF WHITE ADIPOSE TISSUE

For many years, WAT was considered to serve three main functions: heat insulation, mechanical cushion, and most importantly, energy reservoir. Heat insulation is a main function of the subcutaneous depot. Because adipose tissue conducts heat poorly as compared to other tissues, the large subcutaneous depot under the skin can provide a layer of insulation to the entire body. Several internal depots, by surrounding internal organs, can protect those organs from trauma. All depots, albeit to varying degrees, have the capability to store or provide energy. Energy storage is a vital function of adipose tissue, and it is the largest energy reservoir in the body.

More recently, adipose tissue has been shown to have important additional functions. Specifically, adipose tissue is a potent endocrine tissue (Galic et al., 2010). Collectively, the adipocyte-derived molecules secreted by adipose tissue are referred to as adipokines. Adipokines influence a variety of body processes including insulin sensitivity, inflammation, energy balance, adipocyte differentiation, and angiogenesis (Figure 23-1). Although adipokines, by definition, are adipocyte-derived hormones or cytokines produced by adipocytes, some of these molecules may also be produced by other cell types within the adipose tissue. For example, leptin is produced solely by adipocytes, but tumor necrosis factor-α is made by both the macrophages and the adipocytes. Thus the cellular composition of the WAT can influence the proportions of adipokines produced.

Although the list of adipokines continues to grow, a full understanding of the function of most remains elusive. Proinflammatory adipokines have been implicated in the development of insulin resistance and the increased risks of type 2 diabetes and cardiovascular disease that are associated with obesity. Leptin levels may play an important role in the regulation of immune function, and lack of leptin might be involved in increased susceptibility to infection in malnourished individuals. Some of these adipokines, such as leptin, have important roles in controlling energy balance, as discussed in Chapter 22. Regardless, as adipose tissue mass is altered, adipokine production is impacted, which likely contributes to the pathogenic effects associated with obesity and lipodystrophies.

OBESITY

Obesity has become a significant public health concern in the United States and around the world. A combination of genetic, lifestyle, and environmental factors have contributed to the increased prevalence of overweight and obesity. Accumulation of body fat has serious deleterious health outcomes (McPherson, 2007). The current rates of obesity have contributed to the rise in incidence of obesity-related comorbidities, such as sleep apnea, depression, hypertension, cardiovascular disease, diabetes, and some cancers.

DEFINITION OF OBESITY

Overweight and obesity refer to an individual possessing a greater body weight than considered healthy because of excess accumulation of adipose tissue. Clinically, obesity is most commonly defined by an increased body mass index (BMI) or waist circumference (WC). BMI has historically served as the clinical marker of obesity in adults. BMI is the ratio of weight in kilograms to the square of height in meters (kg/m^2). Individuals with a BMI greater than 25 kg/m^2 are

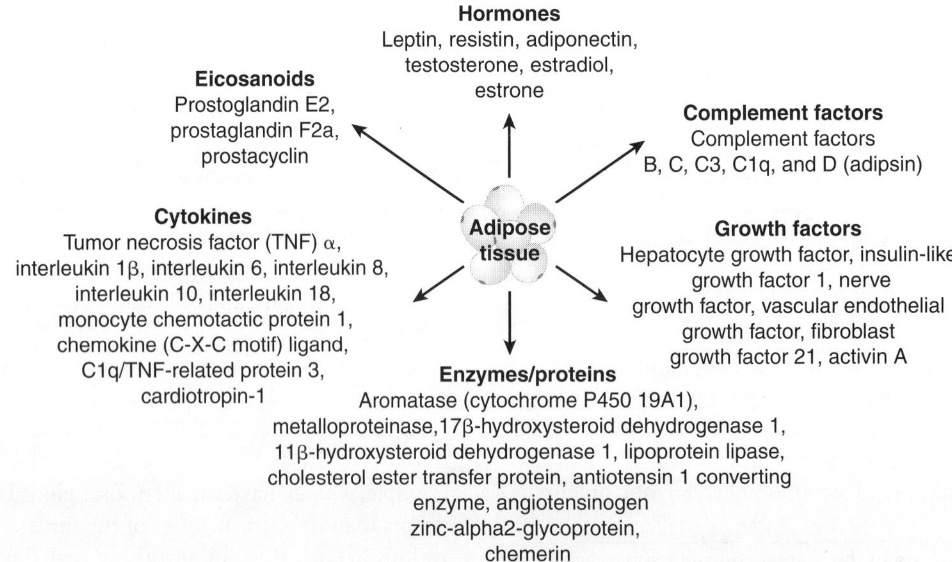

FIGURE 23-1 Adipokines grouped according to type of compound molecule.

considered overweight, and those with a BMI greater than 30 kg/m^2 are classified as obese (Table 23-1; National Institutes of Health [NIH], 1998). These categories are based on evidence that health risks are greater in individuals with a BMI of 25 kg/m^2 or greater, with risk progressively increasing as BMI increases above of 25 kg/m^2 (Figure 23-2). Although a useful screening tool to assess weight status and to monitor trends in populations, BMI cannot discern between lean mass and adipose tissue directly. It should be noted, therefore, that individuals with a greater amount of lean muscle mass may be falsely classified as overweight or obese on the basis of BMI.

In addition to high BMI values, the distribution of excess fat depots and the amount of weight gained during adulthood seem to be associated with increased risk of morbidity. Individuals who accumulate excess body fat in upper body adipose depots, particularly visceral depots, may be at greater risk of developing negative health consequences of obesity than individuals who accumulate the same amount of excess body fat in the lower body (Pouliot et al., 1994). For this reason, WC has become another clinical measure to assess obesity and determine chronic disease risk. Chronic disease risk is increased in men with a WC larger than 102 cm (>40 inches) and in women with a WC larger than 88 cm (>35 inches). The visceral location of excess adipose tissue increases risk of comorbid conditions beyond that indicated by an elevated BMI alone (World Health Organization [WHO], 1997; Pi-Sunyer, 1993). Data from many studies suggest that excess fat located in visceral depots is an independent risk factor for type 2 diabetes and cardiovascular disease (Mathieu et al., 2010).

Because of the normal changes associated with growth and puberty, assessment of obesity in children and adolescents requires that age be considered when calculating BMI.

TABLE 23-1 Definitions of Child and Adult Obesity Based on BMI

WEIGHT CATEGORY	CHILDREN* (BMI-FOR-AGE PERCENTILE)	ADULTS† (BMI)
Underweight	<5th percentile	<18.5 kg/m^2
Healthy weight	5th to 84th percentile	18.5–24.9 kg/m^2
Overweight	85th to 94th percentile	25–29.9 kg/m^2
Obese class I	≥95th percentile	30–34.9 kg/m^2
Obese class II		35–39.9 kg/m^2
Obese class III		≥40 kg/m^2

Child obesity is based on the gender-specific body mass index (BMI)–for-age percentiles from the growth charts. Adult obesity is based on BMI values (kg/m^2).

*Barlow S. E., & Expert Committee. (2007). Expert Committee recommendations regarding the prevention, assessment, and treatment of child and adolescent overweight and obesity: Summary report. *Pediatrics, 120*(Suppl. 4), S164–S192.

†NIH. (1998). Clinical guidelines on the identification, evaluation, and treatment of overweight and obesity in adults—The evidence report. *Obesity Research 6*(Suppl. 2), 51S–209S.

BMI-for-age standardized growth curves were developed to account for the trajectories of growth and development in children and adolescents (Figure 23-3). BMI-for-age categories similar to the BMI categories applied to adults are used to describe child and adolescent obesity data; the classification cutoffs are presented in Table 23-1. More recently, an examination of central, or abdominal, adiposity in children and adolescents was done to generate thresholds specific for age, gender, and race–ethnicity for assessment of obesity by measuring WC. Children and adolescents with a WC above the age and gender-specific 90th percentile are classified as obese (Fernandez et al., 2004).

PREVALENCE OF OBESITY

Obesity is increasing at an alarming rate in both developed and developing countries and in both adults and children. In 2005 the World Health Organization (WHO) estimated that more than 1.6 billion individuals older than age 14 years were overweight, with approximately one quarter of them being obese. The worldwide prevalence of obesity ranges from less than 5% of the population in rural China, Japan, and some African countries to levels as high as 80% of the adult population in the South Pacific island nation of Nauru (WHO, 2005). In the United States, the prevalence of obesity has significantly increased during the past three decades; age-adjusted rates of obesity more than doubled from 1960 (13.4%) to 2008 (33.9%). Trends in obesity among U.S. adults are presented in Figure 23-4. According to the data from the 2007–2008 National Health and Nutrition Examination Survey (NHANES), the age-adjusted prevalence of overweight or obesity in the United States was over 68%, with one third (33.8%) of U.S. adults presenting with obesity (Flegal et al., 2010). Hispanics have the highest rates of overweight, with more than three quarters with a BMI higher than 25 kg/m^2. Non-Hispanic blacks, especially females, were most likely to be classified as obese.

Overweight and obesity are more difficult to assess in children than in adults because the height and weight of growing children are constantly changing. However, all indications are that overweight and obesity are also increasing in children

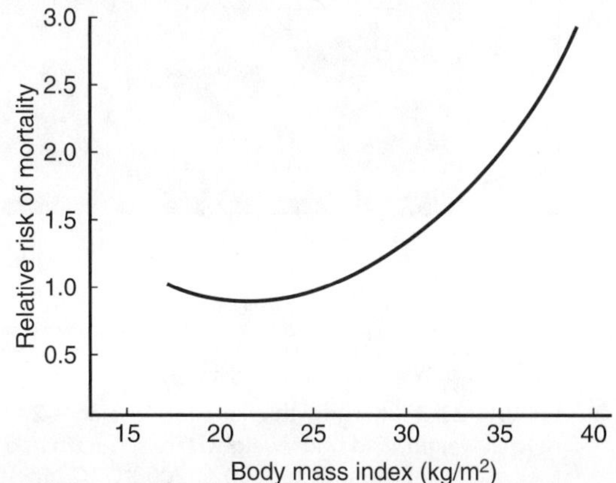

FIGURE 23-2 U-shaped relationship of body mass index (BMI) to excess mortality in adults. Relative risk was defined as 1.0 for adults with BMI between 20 and 25.

2 to 20 years: Boys
Body mass index-for-age percentiles

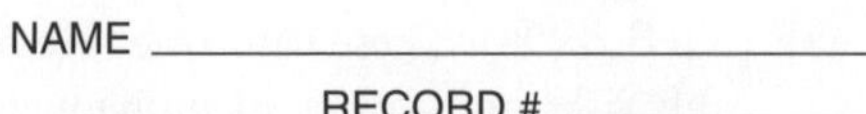

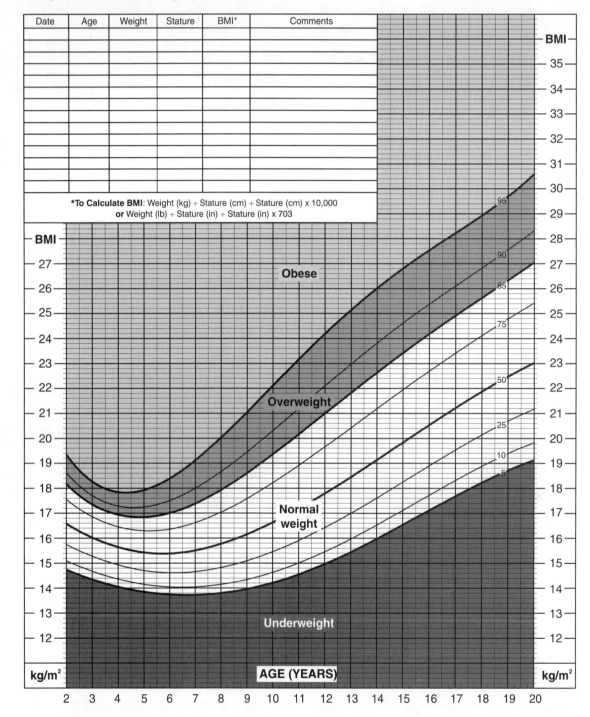

Date	Age	Weight	Stature	BMI*	Comments

***To Calculate BMI**: Weight (kg) ÷ Stature (cm) ÷ Stature (cm) x 10,000
or Weight (lb) ÷ Stature (in) ÷ Stature (in) x 703

Published May 30, 2000 (modified 10/16/00).
SOURCE: Developed by the National Center for Health Statistics in collaboration with the National Centre for Chronic Disease Prevention and Health Promotion (2000).
http://www.cdc.gov/growthcharts

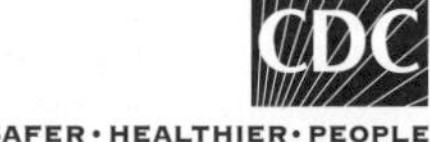

FIGURE 23-3 BMI growth charts for boys ages 2 to 20 years. Modified to add labels and shading for obese, overweight, normal weight, and underweight. (From Kuczmarski, R. J., Ogden, C. L., Guo, S. S., Grummer-Strawn, L. M., Flegal, K. M., Mei, Z., ... Johnson, C. L. [2002]. 2000 CDC growth charts for the United States: Methods and development. *Vital and Health Statistics, 11*(246), 1–190. Retrieved from *www.cdc.gov/growthcharts*)

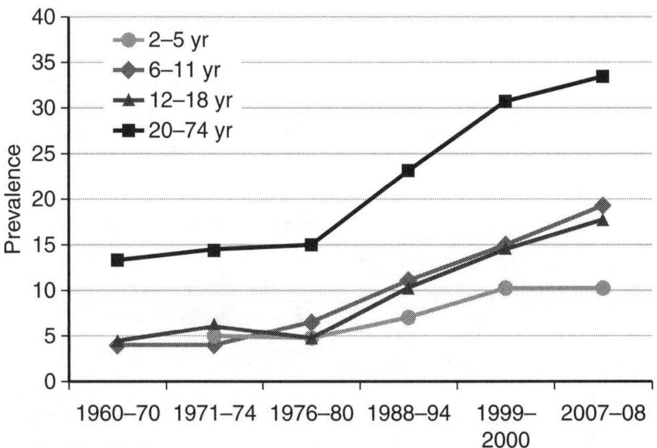

FIGURE 23-4 Changes in prevalence of overweight and obesity in American children, adolescents, and adults between 1960–70 and 2007–08. Overweight was defined as a body mass index (BMI) of 25.0 to 29.9 kg/m^2 and obesity as a BMI ≥30 kg/m^2. Child overweight was defined as being in the 85th to 94th percentile of gender-specific BMI-for-age values. Child obesity was defined as being at or above the 95th percentile of gender-specific BMI-for-age values. Values are the sum of prevalence of overweight and obesity in each age group. (Data from Ogden, O., & Carroll, M. [2010]. *Prevalence of obesity among children and adolescents: United States, trends 1963–1965 through 2007–2008;* Ogden, O., & Carroll, M. [2010]. *Prevalence of overweight, obesity, and extreme obesity among adults: United States, trends 1976–1980 through 2007–2008.* National Center for Health Statistics. Health E-Stats. Retrieved from *www.cdc.gov/nchs/fastats/overwt.htm*)

(Ogden and Carroll, 2010). Based on the 2007–2008 NHANES data, child obesity has increased twofold to fourfold since the 1960s, with 10% of children age 2 to 5 years and 20% of children age 6 to 11 years being classified as obese based on the 2007–2008 data (see Figure 23-4). Marked increases in obesity also have been observed in adolescent boys and girls, with the prevalence of obesity in 2007–2008 being more than 25% for Mexican American adolescent boys and non-Hispanic black girls. Thus the prevalence of overweight and obesity has increased in children and adolescents as well as in adults in the United States over the last several decades.

FACTORS INVOLVED IN THE DEVELOPMENT OF OBESITY

It is clear that no single event or change has caused the increased rates of obesity that have occurred over the past three decades. Because of the many genetic and environmental influences on both energy intake and energy expenditure, obesity must be considered to be a disorder with multiple causes. The gene–environment interaction is likely to explain much of the variation in body weight, and separating the genetic from the environmental determinants of obesity presents a formidable challenge for scientists. The following section addresses many of the issues underlying the increasing rates of obesity.

Genetic Factors

Early evidence for a genetic component to body weight regulation comes from studies of families, twins, and adoptees. That is, identical twins, even when raised in different environments, show similarities in body weight and body composition. Similarly, these studies reveal that body weight and composition of twins is more strongly correlated with biological parents than adoptive parents, again implicating a strong genetic influence (Silventoinen et al., 2010). In fact, some studies have suggested that genetic factors contribute anywhere from 40% to 70% to the interindividual variation in the susceptibility to obesity. Humans appear to have evolved many redundant genetic pathways to prevent starvation; fewer genes appear to be involved in prevention of excess adipose tissue mass, a problem faced by many current societies.

The role of genetics in obesity is firmly supported by examples of single gene defects (mutations, deletions, insertions) that cause obesity. As of October 2005 (the last update of the Human Obesity Gene Map), 176 cases of obesity due to single gene defects had been published worldwide, and these 176 cases involved mutations in 11 different genes (Rankinen et al., 2006). The majority of the reported cases of monogenic obesity are due to defects in the gene encoding melanocortin receptor 4. Among the other 10 genes are those encoding leptin, leptin receptor, melanocortin receptor 3, proopiomelanocortin (POMP), corticotorpin-releasing hormone receptor, and several others. Monogenic causes of obesity are clearly extremely rare and cannot explain the current obesity epidemic. Additional candidate genes have been identified from the study of patients with syndromes, such as Prader-Willi syndrome, that both are associated with obesity and show a Mendelian pattern of inheritance (i.e., due to single gene mutations). These studies have identified about 50 loci (regions of chromosomes) and the associated candidate genes that may influence susceptibility to obesity.

Common forms of obesity are thought to be influenced by several genes and are said to be multigenic. Individuals have always differed somewhat in body fat levels, and evidence from animal models, human linkage studies, twin studies, and population studies suggests that the variation in susceptibility to obesity has a genetic component. Progress in identifying genes associated with the common forms of obesity has been slow but is accelerating with advances in genotyping and genomic technology. Hundreds of promising candidates have been identified by genome-wide association scans. Two gene variants that consistently show promise are the *MC4R* (melanocortin 4 receptor) and *FTO* (fat mass and obesity-associated protein) genes. *MC4R* is expressed in the arcuate nucleus and influences feeding behavior as discussed in Chapter 22; mutations in or around this gene are the most common form of monogenic obesity, as mentioned above. Variants in *MC4R* also are strongly associated with a significant fraction of obesity cases in several populations (e.g., up to 6% of obese adults) (Tao, 2010). Many independent population-based studies report that variants in *FTO* might be responsible for up to 22% of all cases of common obesity in the general population. Interestingly, variants of this gene also show a strong association with type 2 diabetes and polycystic ovary syndrome, both of which are characterized by insulin resistance (Tan et al., 2010). The function of this gene is not fully understood and is currently under intense scientific investigation.

Behavioral and Environmental Factors

The exponential increase in the prevalence of obesity that has occurred in the United States over the last few decades cannot be solely attributed to genetic causes, suggesting a more complex milieu at work. Changes in lifestyle behaviors as well as a host of environmental factors are influencing the prevalence of obesity. Increased access to foods, especially less expensive and less healthy options, and a decline in the physical environment that supports regular physical activity both provide additional barriers to obesity prevention and treatment (Drewnowski and Darmon, 2005). These factors combined have precipitated behavioral and physiological changes that have contributed to the recent rise in obesity and related chronic diseases.

Moderate increases in the percentage of calories from dietary fat intake, and consequently increases in the energy density of the diet, have contributed to the increase in the prevalence of obesity (Astrup et al., 2008; Goris and Westerterp, 2008; James, 2008). Americans consume diets with an average of about 34% of total energy from fat. When high-fat diets are fed to laboratory rodents, the majority become obese. Obesity appears to result both from an increased voluntary energy intake due to high-fat diets and from the body's ability to assimilate excess dietary fat more efficiently than excess dietary carbohydrate or protein (Horton et al., 1995). Furthermore, macronutrient distributions also influence the metabolism of energy intakes. High-protein diets have been explored as a means of promoting weight loss, in an attempt to moderate insulin action and capitalize on the energy cost of gluconeogenesis. Similarly, the consumption of refined sugars, especially fructose and sucrose, is controversially linked to an increased risk for obesity (Tappy and Lê, 2010).

While Americans are consuming more energy, they are also expending less energy through physical activity. In 2005, 39.6% of U.S. adults were inactive or reported no leisure-time physical activity (Figure 23-5) (Centers for Disease Control and Prevention [CDC], 2007). Physical activity levels were more likely to be inadequate in older adults, less educated people, and racial and ethnic minorities. Such trends in limited physical activity have ramifications on the development of obesity, but also numerous additional health outcomes. Much of the decline in physical activity can be attributed to modernization, which has made it easier to be sedentary both at work and at home. The increased availability of automobiles and labor-saving devices has substantially reduced the amount of time spent being physically active. An increase in the time spent in sedentary activities, including watching television and sitting at the computer, is thought to play a role in reducing physical activity in children. The highly attractive nature of these sedentary activities is an additional challenge to promoting more physically active behaviors (Physical Activity Guidelines Advisory Committee, 2008). During the period from 2001 to 2005, the proportion of U.S. adults meeting physical activity recommendations

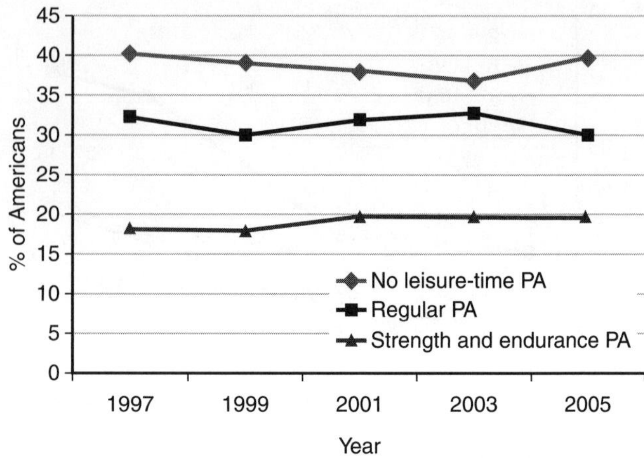

FIGURE 23-5 Changes in physical activity (PA) of U.S. adults between 1997 and 2005. (Based on data from CDC. [2010]. *DATA2010: The Healthy People 2010 Database.* Retrieved from http://wonder.cdc.gov/data2010)

(i.e., moderate intensity activity for at least 30 min/day, 5 or more days a week; or vigorous intensity activity for at least 20 min per day, 3 or more days per week) increased modestly from 45.3% to 48.8%, but the rates of obesity continued to rise.

Many other factors dictate the metabolic utilization of energy intakes. Alterations in the dietary habits of individuals in poverty as well as those suffering from food insecurity have been linked to increased rates of obesity (Drewnowski and Darmon, 2005; Dinour et al., 2007). A greater reliance on foods that are energy-dense, nutrient-poor, and inexpensive commonly leads to diets that are high in fat; these habits have precipitated poor health outcomes, including increased fat deposition and increased risk for several chronic diseases. Physiological responses to food components and contaminants have also been discovered. Changes in gut microflora due to dietary practices or consumption of chemical contaminants, such as bisphenol A in plastics, are two examples (Grün, 2010; Musso et al., 2010). There is even some evidence that infectious agents can influence obesity onset (Mitra and Clarke, 2010). Importantly, the varied rates of obesity within individuals exposed to the same potentially obesogenic environments suggest that many factors, including consumption of high-fat diets or physical inactivity, should not be viewed as known causes of obesity. Rather, these environmental factors increase the probability of an imbalance between energy intake and energy expenditure for individuals living in that environment. Much research has also indicated that the intrauterine growth environment during pregnancy can have an impact on physiology in childhood and adulthood, altering the propensity to develop obesity and chronic diseases (Varvarigou, 2010).

Interactions of Genes and Environment

Obesity is most likely to occur when a genetically susceptible individual encounters an environment conducive to obesity, sometimes referred to as an obesogenic environment. An example is provided by Pima Indians living in Arizona as compared to those in northern Mexico. These populations

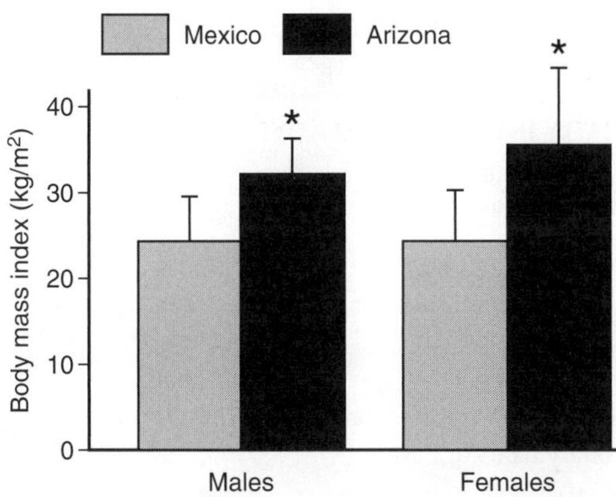

FIGURE 23-6 Mean body mass index (BMI) (± standard deviation) of Pima Indians living in either a traditional lifestyle in Maycoba, Mexico, or a modern lifestyle in Arizona. *In both sexes, BMI was significantly higher ($P \leq 0.0001$) in Pima Indians living in Arizona compared with BMI of Pima Indians living in Mexico. (Modified from Ravussin, E., & Tataranni, P. A. [1997]. Dietary fat and human obesity. *Journal of the American Dietetic Association, 97,* S42–S46. Copyright American Dietetic Association.)

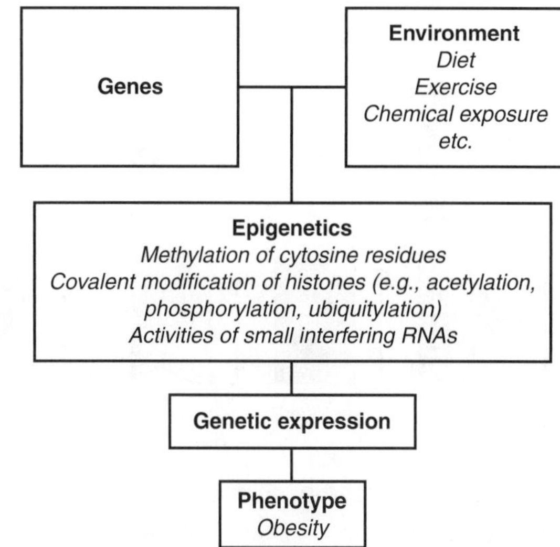

FIGURE 23-7 The role of epigenetics in the interaction of genes and the environment.

are genetically similar but have very different lifestyle patterns and rates of obesity. Pima Indians in Arizona show an extremely high prevalence of obesity and report low levels of physical activity combined with high intakes of energy-dense diets (Figure 23-6). In contrast, Mexican Pima Indians are farmers, consuming food that they grow and engaging in high levels of physical activity (Esparza et al., 2000). The Mexican Pima Indians are significantly less obese than the Arizona Pima Indians, demonstrating the importance of environmental factors on body weight. However, the mean BMI for the Mexican Pima Indians is still greater than would be expected for a highly active population consuming a low-fat diet, suggesting that Pima Indians, regardless of environment, have genes that favor high body weight. Interestingly, *FTO* gene variants appear to have some role in influencing BMI in the Pima Indian population (Rong et al., 2009).

Additional studies beyond those in Pima Indians provide further evidence of such an *FTO* gene–environment interaction. For specific *FTO* variants, BMI is greater in individuals who are sedentary, whereas this association is attenuated in those who are physically active (Andreasen et al., 2008; Ruiz et al., 2010). These results suggest that genetic susceptibility toward obesity induced by variation in at least *FTO* can be overcome to some degree by lifestyle modifications. It should be noted that no studies have yet shown a similar gene–environment interaction for *MC4R*, although data are limiting.

Epigenetics, or the heritable changes in gene function that occur without a change in the nucleotide sequence, is another means by which genes interact with the environment (Figure 23-7). Epigenetic changes often involve changes in DNA methylation or histone modification. Although this is an emerging field, there are several examples in which environmental exposure to nutrients can alter epigenetic factors (Campión et al., 2009). An example is the agouti gene from mouse studies. Increased agouti gene expression can result in obesity; expression of this gene is influenced by DNA methylation. Dietary intake of methyl donors, such as folic acid, can alter DNA methylation of this gene, which in turn controls expression of this obesity-inducing gene. How obesity susceptibility is influenced by epigenetic modifications in humans is being intensively studied.

As other gene variants are identified, more large-scale studies will be needed to identify additional gene–environment interactions. A better understanding of the interaction of lifestyle with genetics may hold important public health messages. They may identify environments most problematic for particular genetic variants and remove the fatalistic view of obesity susceptibility genes, because they may reveal that a healthy lifestyle can overcome genetics to some degree.

HEALTH CONSEQUENCES OF OBESITY

Obesity is associated with many physiological and psychosocial risks. Because of the underlying energy balance etiology of obesity, the synergistic impact of the contributing lifestyle behaviors and physiological changes resulting from obesity lead to an increased risk for numerous acute and chronic health conditions. Although obesity is considered a risk factor for many disease states, the causal mechanisms are not known for all associations.

Comorbidities

The data in Figure 23-8 illustrate the strong relationships between BMI and the risks of type 2 diabetes, coronary heart disease, high blood pressure, and metabolic syndrome (Nguyen et al., 2008). Significant associations were also found between BMI and the prevalence of hypercholesterolemia, asthma, and fair or poor general health. Box 23-1 lists the most frequently observed comorbidities associated with obesity. The risk of developing a comorbidity is influenced by the extent of obesity, the location of excess body fat, and the degree of weight gain over the adult years. In general, obesity-associated morbidity and mortality increase in direct proportion to increases in BMI. Furthermore,

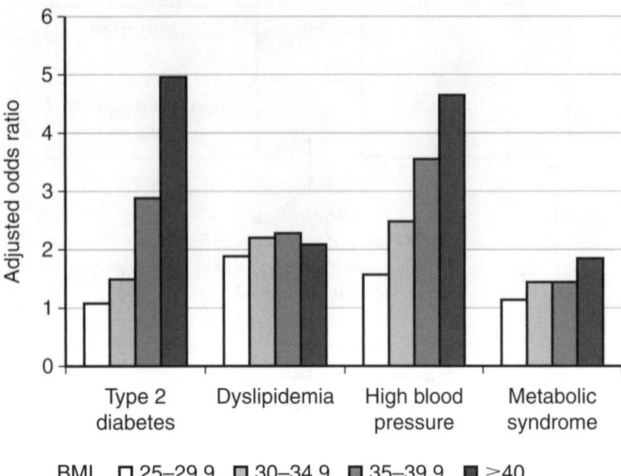

FIGURE 23-8 Adjusted odds ratios for risk of medical conditions by BMI for adults in the United States. The odds ratios shown are the prevalence of the given disease in adults who are overweight (BMI = 25–29.9 kg/m^2) or obese (BMI ≥30 kg/m^2) compared to the prevalence in those with a healthy BMI (18.5–24.9 kg/m^2). The prevalence of disease in adults with a healthy BMI is thus set at 1.0 (not shown), and increased prevalence is indicated by an odds ratio greater than 1.0. Data are from NHANES 1999–2004. Data were adjusted for age, gender, race/ethnicity, smoking, and physical activity. (Based on data reported by Nguyen, N. T., Magno, C. P., Lane, K. T., Hinojosa, M. W., & Lane, J. S. [2008]. Association of hypertension, diabetes, dyslipidemia, and metabolic syndrome with obesity: Findings from the National Health and Nutrition Examination Survey, 1999 to 2004. *Journal of the American College of Surgeons, 207*, 928–934.)

BOX 23-1 Comorbidities Frequently Associated With Obesity

GREATLY INCREASED (RELATIVE RISK >3)

Type 2 diabetes
Gallbladder disease
Dyslipidemia
Insulin resistance
Breathlessness
Sleep apnea

MODERATELY INCREASED (RELATIVE RISK ~2 TO 3)

Coronary heart disease
Hypertension
Osteoarthritis (knees)
Hyperuricemia and gout

SLIGHTLY INCREASED (RELATIVE RISK ~1 TO 2)

Cancer (breast cancer in postmenopausal women, endometrial cancer, colon cancer)
Reproductive hormone abnormalities
Polycystic ovary syndrome
Impaired fertility
Low back pain due to obesity
Increased anesthetic risk
Fetal defects associated with maternal obesity

Modified from World Health Organization. (1997). *Obesity: Preventing and managing the global epidemic: Report of a WHO Consultation on Obesity*. Geneva: WHO.

health care costs have been estimated to be approximately 22% higher in individuals presenting with central adiposity (Højgaard et al., 2008). The combination of increased BMI and the presence of central adiposity further increases the risk of comorbid conditions.

When all-cause mortality (risk of death from any cause) is plotted against BMI, an increased risk in mortality is evident with BMIs nearing 30 kg/m^2 and increases steeply as BMIs increase above 30 kg/m^2 (see Figure 23-2). Obesity has been linked to significantly increased risk of mortality from cardiovascular disease and obesity-related cancers, compared to risk in normal-weight adults (Flegal et al., 2007). A meta-analysis of prospective studies found that overweight participants had significantly increased incidence of type 2 diabetes; all cancers except esophageal (female subjects only), pancreatic, and prostate cancers; all cardiovascular diseases (except congestive heart failure); asthma; gallbladder disease; osteoarthritis; and chronic back pain (Guh et al., 2009). The greatest relative risk for chronic disease in obese men and women was seen for type 2 diabetes. The odds ratio (the ratio of the odds of the disease occurring in the obese group compared to the non-obese group) was 6.74 (95% confidence interval: 5.55–8.19) for obese men and 12.41 (95% confidence interval: 9.03–17.06) for obese women.

Metabolic Syndrome

Along with the increase in the prevalence of obesity during the last decades, a new heterogeneous clinical disorder strongly associated with central obesity and insulin resistance has been identified. This disorder has been called syndrome X and insulin-resistance syndrome, and it is now commonly known as metabolic syndrome (Moller and Kaufman, 2005). A joint conference of the American Heart Association (AHA), the National Heart, Lung, and Blood Institute (NHLBI), and the American Diabetes Association (ADA) identified the major components of the syndrome as central obesity, insulin resistance with or without glucose intolerance, atherogenic dyslipidemia, elevated blood pressure, a proinflammatory state, and a prothrombotic state (Grundy et al., 2004). Individuals with this metabolic syndrome are at increased risk for development of type 2 diabetes, atherosclerotic cardiovascular disease, and cardiovascular death. Individuals with metabolic syndrome also seem to be more susceptible to some other conditions, including polycystic ovary syndrome, fatty liver, cholesterol gallstones, asthma, sleep disturbances, and some forms of cancer.

In addition to the presence of central adiposity and insulin resistance, abnormal levels of various compounds that may serve as either markers or mediators of metabolic syndrome commonly aggregate in individuals with metabolic syndrome. These include altered levels of plasma lipids (elevated serum triacylglycerols, elevated apolipoprotein B, elevated small dense low-density lipoprotein particles, and depressed levels of high-density lipoprotein cholesterol); altered levels of coagulation factors (elevated levels of plasminogen activator inhibitor 1 and fibrinogen); elevated

TABLE 23-2 Criteria for Clinical Diagnosis of Metabolic Syndrome

CLINICAL MEASURE*	ATP III/NCEP†	WHO‡	AHA/NHLBI§	IDF¶¶
Waist circumference	≥102 cm in men ≥88 cm in women	Central obesity determined by waist to hip ratio	≥102 cm in men ≥88 cm in women	Specific to ethnicity
BMI		BMI >30 kg/m²		
Triacylglycerol level	≥150 mg/dL	≥150 mg/dL	≥150 mg/dL	≥150 mg/dL
HDL-C	<40 mg/dL in men <50 mg/dL in women	<5 mg/dL in men <39 mg/dL in women	<40 mg/dL in men <50 mg/dL in women	<40 mg/dL in men <50 mg/dL in women
Blood pressure	≥130/85 mm Hg	≥140/90 mm Hg	≥130/85 mm Hg	≥130/85 mm Hg
Glucose level	Fasting >110 mg/dL	IGT, IFG, T2D, or fasting >110 mg/dL	Fasting ≥100 mg/dL	Fasting ≥100 mg/dL or previous diagnosis of T2D

BMI, Body mass index; *HDL-C,* high-density lipoprotein cholesterol; *IFG,* impaired fasting glucose; *IGT,* impaired glucose tolerance; *T2D,* type 2 diabetes.

*Values are for levels prior to treatment to lower blood lipids or glucose levels or to reduce blood pressure.

†National Cholesterol Education Program. (2002). Third report of the National Cholesterol Education Program (NCEP) Expert Panel on Detection, Evaluation, and Treatment of High Blood Cholesterol in Adults (Adult Treatment Panel III) final report. *Circulation, 106,* 3143–3421.

‡Alberti, A. G., & Zimmet, P. Z. (1998). Definition, diagnosis and classification of diabetes mellitus and its complications. I: Diagnosis and classification of diabetes mellitus provisional report of a WHO consultation. *Diabetic Medicine, 15,* 539–553.

§Grundy, S. M., Cleeman, J. I., Daniels, S. R., Donato, K. A., Eckel, R. H., Franklin, B. A., … Costa, F.; American Heart Association; National Heart, Lung, and Blood Institute. (2005). Diagnosis and management of the metabolic syndrome: An American Heart Association/National Heart, Lung, and Blood Institute scientific statement. *Circulation, 112,* 2735–2752.

¶¶Alberti, K. G., Zimmet, P., & Shaw, J. (2006). Metabolic syndrome—A new world-wide definition. A Consensus Statement from the International Diabetes Federation. *Diabetic Medicine, 23*(5), 469–480.

levels of cytokines (tumor necrosis factor-α and interleukin 6); and elevated levels of acute phase proteins associated with inflammatory states (e.g., C-reactive protein).

Several diagnostic criteria have been developed by various organizations for the identification of metabolic syndrome. Table 23-2 presents the diagnostic criteria of Third Adult Treatment Panel (ATP III)/National Cholesterol Education Program (NCEP), WHO, AHA/NHLBI, and the International Diabetes Federation (IDF). The various definitions specify that a set number of disease features must be present for a diagnosis of metabolic syndrome to be made; however, the clinical values and superseding factors differ across the definitions. Therefore, despite an agreement about the underlying role of obesity in this cluster of metabolic abnormalities, the various groups charged with setting the diagnostic criteria do not always agree about the key elements of metabolic syndrome or the etiologies underlying metabolic syndrome.

The ATP III/NCEP and AHA/NHLBI criteria for a clinical diagnosis of metabolic syndrome require that any three or more of five criteria must be present for a diagnosis of metabolic syndrome (NCEP, 2002; Grundy et al., 2005). In contrast, WHO (Alberti and Zimmet, 1998) and IDF (Alberti et al., 2006) require the presence of what is seen as a central feature plus two additional criteria, for a total of three criteria. WHO requires that evidence of diabetes or insulin resistance be present along with two additional criteria. The base requirement for evidence of impaired glucose regulation or insulin resistance is met by the presence of type 2 diabetes mellitus, impaired fasting glycemia (>110 mg/dL), impaired glucose tolerance, or (for those with normal fasting glucose levels) glucose uptake below the lowest quartile under hyperinsulinemic euglycemic conditions. The IDF holds central adiposity as the driving force in the syndrome that must be present with two additional risk factors for diagnosis in adolescents and adults. The IDF recommends use of ethnicity-specific standards for threshold values for WC rather than a single threshold as their definition of central adiposity.

Prevalence of Metabolic Syndrome

Characteristics of metabolic syndrome occur in some children and adolescents, but the prevalence clearly increases with age so that the highest prevalence is observed in older persons. However, frequency rises rapidly in middle age and parallels, with some time lag, the development of obesity in the population. Using the criteria of the ATP III/NCEP, the overall prevalence of metabolic syndrome from 1988 to 1994 in U.S. adults was estimated to be approximately 24% (Ford et al., 2002). Data from 2003 to 2006 suggest that the prevalence had increased to an age-adjusted rate of 34% of adults (Ervin, 2009). For adults older than 60 years, the prevalence was much higher at approximately 42% in 1988–1994, increasing to 54% in 2003–2006. Obese men and women were 32 times and 17 times, respectively, more likely to present with metabolic syndrome than their underweight or normal-weight counterparts. Non-Hispanic white males were significantly more likely to present with metabolic syndrome than non-Hispanic black males; however, non-Hispanic white females were significantly less likely to present with metabolic syndrome than non-Hispanic black and Mexican American women.

Etiology of Metabolic Syndrome

There are differing viewpoints regarding the etiologies of the composite factors of metabolic syndrome. Furthermore, the defining cornerstone condition is also up for debate. Several camps contend that the clustering of cardiovascular disease and diabetes results from the increasing rates of obesity; however, others contend that an underlying insulin resistance syndrome produces the resultant hyperlipidemia, hyperglycemia, and hypertension. Whether anchored in obesity or insulin resistance, the risk of metabolic disease is further exacerbated by genetic factors and any additional metabolic imbalances that alter the function of insulin action. For example, individuals with a family history of type 2 diabetes are at increased risk for metabolic syndrome, and this risk is further increased in those who become overweight or obese and in those who adopt sedentary lifestyles. Also, women with a history of gestational diabetes or polycystic ovary syndrome have an increased risk of metabolic syndrome. The subset of clinical features exhibited by individuals may also be strongly influenced by underlying genetic predispositions; whether dyslipidemia, glucose intolerance, or visceral fat accumulation is the predominant phenotypic expression of metabolic syndrome may depend on an individual's genetic makeup.

Most persons with multiple metabolic risk factors for metabolic syndrome are insulin resistant. Insulin resistance is strongly associated with atherogenic dyslipidemia and a proinflammatory state, but it is less tightly associated with hypertension and the prothrombotic state. There is no doubt that insulin resistance leads to impaired glucose tolerance and type 2 diabetes, but a causal relationship between insulin resistance and the other risk factors of metabolic syndrome is less certain owing to the complex interactions between obesity and defects in insulin signaling. Therefore the mechanistic links between insulin resistance and most of the components of the metabolic syndrome remain unclear.

Most commonly, the metabolic syndrome is associated with central obesity. An excess of visceral fat may be particularly pathogenic, but abdominal subcutaneous adipose tissue likely contributes as well, as can total body fat. Visceral adipose tissue may be particularly active in producing a number of less favorable adipokines and secretory molecules. These include free (nonesterified) fatty acids, which can provoke peripheral insulin resistance and decreased peripheral glucose utilization; proinflammatory and atherogenic adipokines (tumor necrosis factor-α and interleukin 6); resistin, an adipokine that can induce insulin resistance; and plasminogen activator inhibitor 1, a protease inhibitor, which is also produced by the liver and endothelial cells, that acts to inhibit fibrinolysis (the breakdown of blood clots). Adiponectin and leptin are two other adipokines produced by white adipose tissue that play a role in metabolic syndrome. In obesity, adiponectin levels fall and leptin levels rise; leptin insensitivity also develops (Robinson and Graham, 2004). Although adipocyte-derived factors clearly appear to be involved in inducing insulin resistance and other features of the metabolic syndrome, the mechanism is likely very complex and largely unknown.

THERAPEUTIC APPROACHES TO THE TREATMENT OF OBESITY

Because of the interrelations of lifestyle behaviors and risk factors associated with obesity, chronic disease, and metabolic syndrome, therapeutic approaches should be established to prevent or reverse weight gain and combat comorbidities. Therapeutic lifestyle changes (TLC) is a term first used by the NCEP to describe the changes in diet, weight management, and physical activity that they recommend for lowering low-density lipoprotein (LDL) levels (NCEP, 2002). Following TLC can result in improvements in weight status, glycemic control (plasma insulin and blood glucose), blood lipid patterns (LDL, high-density lipoprotein, and triacylglycerol levels), and blood pressure (NCEP, 2002; Appel et al., 2005; Wister et al., 2007).

Prevention of weight gain should be the first goal in obesity management, with a progression toward the healthful promotion of weight loss. Weight loss of as little as 5 to 20 kg (11 to 12 lb) can facilitate substantial reductions in hypertension and cardiovascular disease risk (Hamman et al., 2006; Moore et al., 2005). One kilogram of weight loss has been shown to produce a 16% reduction in the risk of developing diabetes (Hamman et al., 2006).

Although weight loss can produce meaningful improvements in chronic disease risk and is useful in treatment of metabolic syndrome, many factors compete with the ability of individuals to implement and sustain the needed TLC to support weight loss. The physical and built environments impact the access to food and the types of food available for individuals. For example, the availability and accessibility of grocery stores or fast food restaurants may drive consumer behaviors and dietary habits. Similarly, the infrastructures of communities, such as access to recreational facilities or the presence of sidewalks and walking trails, can impact a person's level of physical activity. However, personal factors, such as knowledge, beliefs, attitudes, self-efficacy, and skills, play an equally strong role in driving personal lifestyle behavior choices. Significant drivers in individual food intake behaviors include taste, cost, convenience, perceived health benefit, time, food preparation skills, and cultural paradigms. Thus the process of weight loss counseling should involve a comprehensive assessment of personal, socioeconomic, psychological, and environmental factors involved in food intake behaviors.

The most successful weight loss programs involve modifications in dietary intake habits, promotion of regular moderate physical activity, and behavioral therapy. Dietary interventions should focus on the creation of energy deficits to promote weight loss. Several approaches to facilitate this change include altering meal frequency and patterns, controlling portion size, using meal replacements, and including nutrition education that focuses on healthy cooking and reading nutrition labels. Setting realistic goals will also facilitate greater adherence to treatment regimens to develop manageable, long-term solutions to weight issues. Paramount to facilitating an energy deficit is an accurate assessment of energy needs, either through indirect calorimetry or estimating equations.

For obese adults (BMI ≥30 kg/m^2) who are unable to lose weight or maintain weight loss after diet or exercise alone, alternative approaches to weight loss may be recommended. Drug therapy may also be appropriate in persons with BMIs greater than 27 kg/m^2 if they also have other significant conditions such as hypercholesterolemia. However, the choice of drugs for pharmacological treatment of obesity is very limited and safety of such products remains a concern. Amphetamines and amphetamine derivatives are no longer considered appropriate for use as appetite suppressants because they have a number of potentially dangerous side effects, including physical and psychological addiction, and can be used for only a few weeks. Sibutramine, an appetite suppressant, was taken off the market in the United States and Canada in 2010 due to evidence it increased the risk of cardiovascular events. Another appetite suppressant, rimonabant, was never approved in the United States and Canada, but was sold in Europe prior to 2008 when it was removed due to safety concerns. Phentermine is approved for short-term use in combination with exercise and diet.

The only antiobesity drug currently approved for use in the United States is orlistat. Orlistat is an over-the-counter lipase inhibitor that acts nonsystemically in the gut to inhibit pancreatic lipase, which is necessary for triacylglycerol digestion and absorption. In patients taking orlistat, approximately 25% of dietary fat passes through the bowel undigested and is excreted in the feces. Orlistat is sold as a prescription drug in many countries under the trade name Xenical, and in some including the United States as a nonprescription drug under the trade name Alli. Orlistat causes gastrointestinal side effects including steatorrhea, limiting its acceptability. Orlistat is intended to be used in adults in conjunction with a weight loss program (reduced calorie diet, increased exercise) and is expected to result in modest weight loss. Clinical trials suggest that patients given orlistat in addition to lifestyle modifications, such as diet and exercise, lose about 2 to 3 kg more than those not taking the drug over the course of 1 to 4 years (Torgerson et al., 2004). It also reduced the incidence of diabetes in the obese patient population.

Surgical treatment is an option for long-term weight control in the severely obese. Surgical treatment is considered appropriate only for those with BMIs greater than or equal to 40 kg/m^2, or for those with BMIs greater than or equal to 35 kg/m^2 who also have a life-threatening or disabling condition related to obesity, such as high blood pressure, cardiac illness, or type 2 diabetes. Gastrointestinal surgery (adjustable banded gastroplasty or Roux-en-Y gastric bypass) has produced losses of 50% or more of the excess weight in obese patients; weight loss was sustained for 5 or 10 years with significant improvement in comorbid conditions (Günther et al., 2006; Karlsson et al., 2007). Patients should not be considered for surgery unless they have first tried more conventional treatments and undergo careful examination by a multidisciplinary team with medical, surgical, psychiatric, and nutritional expertise. Lifelong TLC and medical surveillance after surgery are required. In bariatric surgery, the goals of treatment are to promote sustained weight loss and prevent common weight regain.

LIPODYSTROPHY

Obesity and lipodystrophy (lipoatrophy) represent extreme opposites in the adiposity spectrum yet share many common metabolic outcomes. Both disorders occur because of disturbances in adipose tissue mass. Although obesity has been studied extensively for a number of years, the more recent investigations of lipodystrophies have advanced our understanding of the physiological roles and importance of adipose tissue in energy balance and metabolism.

DEFINITION AND TYPES OF LIPODYSTROPHY

Lipodystrophies are a heterogeneous group of disorders characterized by loss of adipose tissue mass. Lipodystrophies can be secondary due to illness or drugs (acquired lipodystrophies) or inherited (congenital or familial lipodystrophies). The extent of fat loss may also vary from impacting adipose tissue in only parts of the body (partial or localized lipodystrophies) or more globally (generalized lipodystrophies). Acquired localized lipodystrophies are common at injection sites for specific drugs, such as steroids or insulin. An acquired, generalized form of lipodystrophy is associated with long-term HIV treatment with antiretroviral drugs, which results in adipose tissue loss from the face, arms, legs and buttocks along with an accumulation of fat on the neck and upper back.

Congenital and familial lipodystrophies are very rare disorders, which may be apparent at birth or later in life. Eight different genetic loci, including those containing the genes encoding 1-acylglycerol-3-phosphate *O*-acyltransferase 2 (AGPAT2), Berardinelli-Seip congenital lipodystrophy 2 (BSCL2), caveolin 1, lamin A/C, peroxisome proliferator-activated receptor gamma, Akt2, zinc metalloprotease, and lipase maturation factor 1, have been linked to different lipodystrophy syndromes (Simha and Garg, 2009). Some are severe, such as those caused by gene mutations in *AGPAT2* and *BSCL2*, and result in near total absence of adipose tissue mass from birth. How these genetic variants result in loss of adipose tissue mass is not always understood, but some, such as those of the *AGPAT2* gene that encodes an enzyme required for triacylglycerol and glycerophospholipid synthesis, appear to result in defects in the proliferation and differentiation of adipocytes or in their premature death.

METABOLIC CONSEQUENCES OF LIPODYSTROPHY

The metabolic consequences of lipodystrophy depend on the severity of the loss of adipose tissue mass. For localized forms, such as those caused at injection sites, the problem could be merely cosmetic. In general, the more severe the loss of adipose tissue mass, especially of subcutaneous fat mass, the more significant the metabolic disturbances.

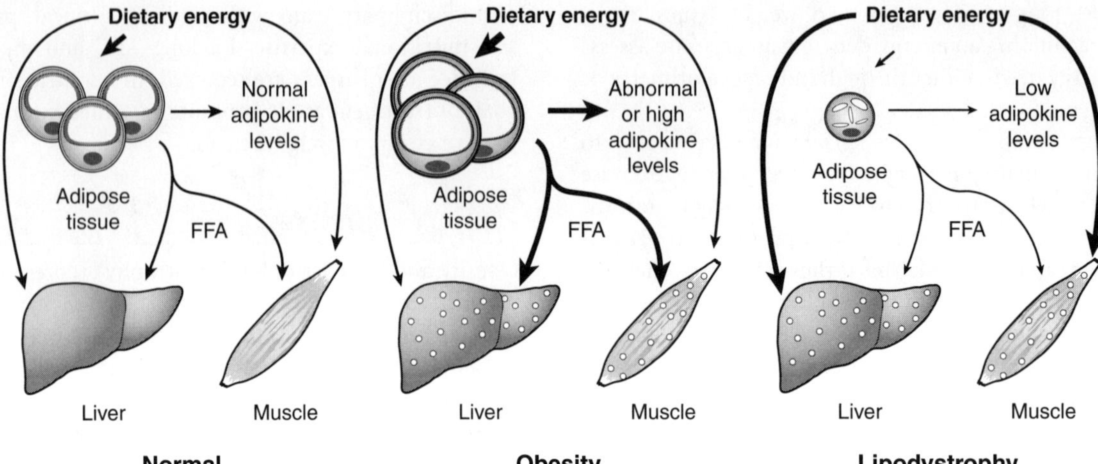

FIGURE 23-9 Schematic diagram comparing the role of adipose tissue in normal energy metabolism with its functions in states of obesity and lipodystrophy. Under normal conditions, adipose tissue is a major site to store excess energy, reducing the need to store excess fat energy in other tissues, such as the liver and muscle. Under obese states, many tissues become insulin resistant, and adipose tissue is enlarged and overwhelmed with the energy provided. With lipodystrophy, there is absolute or relative loss of adipose tissue mass, making this tissue incapable of storing the excess energy. In both lipodystrophy and obesity, the energy that cannot be stored in adipose tissue is redirected into nonadipose sites; in the illustration, ectopic storage of fat in liver and muscle is noted by white circles. The excess or lack of adipose tissue in individuals with obesity or lipodystrophy, respectively, also results in changes in adipokine secretions, which may also have broad impacts on overall energy balance. (Modified from Garg, A. [2006]. Adipose tissue dysfunction in obesity and lipodystrophy. *Clinical Cornerstone, 8*, S7–S13. Copyright [2006] Elsevier.)

Interestingly, obesity and lipodystrophy represent extreme opposites in adipose tissue mass, with obesity resulting from an excess and lipodystrophy from a lack of adipose tissue, yet they result in similar metabolic problems. Most notably, insulin resistance and hypertriglyceridemia are hallmarks of both conditions. How these two extremes can result in similar clinical outcomes remains unresolved, but overlapping mechanisms are implicated. The ability of adipose tissue to store excess fat appears to be important for insulin resistance. Inflammation and ectopic fat deposition (i.e., the spilling over of fat into other nonadipose tissues) appear to be common features of both extremes and likely contribute to the overlap of clinical outcomes (Figure 23-9). Interestingly, both conditions result in abnormal adipokine levels, but changes tend to be in opposite directions, with most adipokines being elevated in obesity and decreased in lipodystrophy in accordance with the adipose tissue mass. However, adiponectin, which is positively correlated with insulin sensitivity, is decreased in both conditions and so may contribute to their common metabolic disturbances.

STARVATION AND PROTEIN-ENERGY MALNUTRITION

Starvation and protein-energy malnutrition (PEM) occur when insufficient or no energy intake is supplied to balance energy expenditure. The reduced energy intake results in decreased body weight. The decreased body weight is usually due to a combined reduction of lean and fat mass. PEM is especially problematic in children in whom adequate nutrient intake is important for maintaining a satisfactory growth rate.

DEFINITIONS OF PEM

The term *PEM,* or *protein-energy malnutrition,* is applied to a group of related disorders. These include the clinical syndromes of marasmus, kwashiorkor, intermediate states of marasmic kwashiorkor, and milder forms of malnutrition (Table 23-3). While PEM specifically refers to a deficiency of all or some of the energy macronutrients, micronutrient deficiencies often accompany PEM and contribute to the various clinical manifestations of PEM. Starvation can be considered a severe form of PEM in which no nutrients are consumed.

Marasmus is caused by an insufficient energy intake, resulting in emaciation. The term *marasmus* is derived from the Greek *marasmos,* which means "withering or wasting." Children with marasmus appear emaciated with marked loss of subcutaneous fat and skeletal muscle. Marasmic children have retarded growth and feel hungry. In contrast, kwashiorkor generally results from an adequate energy intake but an inadequate amount or poor quality of dietary protein, leading to decreased protein synthesis. The term *kwashiorkor* is taken from the Ga language of Ghana and means "first child–second child." The term referred to the sickness observed in children who were weaned because of the birth of a second child, when breast milk was replaced by foods that are high in starch and low in protein (e.g., yam, cassava, sweet potato, or green banana). In addition to retarded growth, children with kwashiorkor typically have edema, a swollen abdomen, and a fatty liver, and often have characteristic skin changes and depigmentation of the hair. Children with intermediate forms of marasmic kwashiorkor typically have some edema and more body fat than those with marasmus.

TABLE 23-3 General Comparison of Marasmus and Kwashiorkor

	MARASMUS	KWASHIORKOR
Main deficiency*	Insufficient protein and calorie intake	Insufficient protein
Meaning	Greek for "withering or wasting"	Ga for "first child–second child"
Body weight	Significantly decreased	Slightly decreased
Adipose stores	Significantly decreased	Varies, typically normal amount or slightly decreased
Clinical symptoms	Extensive tissue and muscle wasting Normal liver function Dry, loose skin Dehydration Impaired immunity Anemia Lethargy	Edema Swollen abdomen and legs Fatty liver Skin changes Depigmentation of hair Impaired immunity Anemia Lethargy

*Typically accompanied by deficiencies in many micronutrients.

CAUSES OF PEM

PEM can be primary, caused by insufficient intake of protein or energy, or both, or it can be secondary, brought on by a drug or disorder that interferes with nutrient availability. PEM most frequently occurs in young children in developing countries and in institutionalized elderly people who have inadequate intake of nutrients. At times, severe food shortages in poor, underdeveloped countries have led to overwhelming famine and starvation. Ineffective weaning practices, economic factors, and maternal malnutrition may also play a role. Children are especially vulnerable because of their dependence on others for food and because of their high requirements for protein and energy per kilogram body weight due to their rapid growth. The clinical outcomes can be very severe and lifelong if PEM occurs in youth. When PEM occurs during the first 5 years of life, the damage to physical and cognitive development is usually irreversible. Further, malnourished people who survive childhood often have lifelong disabilities. Undernourished women are more likely to produce an underweight newborn baby; in some countries (e.g., India and Bangladesh) more than 30% of all children are born underweight (Food and Agriculture Organization [FAO], 2004). If intrauterine malnutrition is compounded after birth or after weaning by insufficient food to satisfy the infant's needs for catch-up growth, PEM often results. Interestingly, although low birth weight and undernutrition early in life are associated with an increased prevalence of PEM in environments with limited food resources, low birth weight and undernutrition early in life are associated with increased risk of obesity and diet-related diseases in adulthood in industrialized countries.

The origin of PEM can be secondary, when it is the result of other diseases that lead to low food ingestion, inadequate nutrient absorption or utilization, increased nutritional requirements, increased nutrient losses, or a combination of these. Common causes of secondary PEM include gastrointestinal disorders or infections, wasting disorders, and conditions that increase metabolic demand. Gastrointestinal infections are a very common cause because of associated diarrhea, anorexia, vomiting, increased metabolic needs, and decreased intestinal absorption. Diseases such as cystic fibrosis, chronic renal failure, childhood malignancies, congenital heart disease, and neuromuscular diseases also are commonly associated with secondary PEM. Those who intentionally alter eating patterns, such as individuals who practice fad diets or inappropriately manage food allergies, and those who have psychiatric diseases, such as anorexia nervosa or depression, can also develop severe PEM. In contrast to the prevalence of primary PEM in developing countries, malnutrition more commonly is secondary to another disorder in industrialized countries.

PREVALENCE OF PEM

Starvation affects many populations all over the world. Worldwide, primary PEM is the most common cause of malnutrition and the current statistics are alarming. PEM is the most important nutritional disease in developing countries because of its high prevalence and its relationship with child mortality rates, impaired physical growth, and inadequate social and economic development. The FAO (2009) estimates suggest that approximately 1.2 billion people worldwide were undernourished in 2009. The number of undernourished people in the world increased by 75 million during 2007 and by 40 million during 2008. This growth is largely attributed to the world's economic crisis during this time period. The distribution of those undernourished by region is shown in Figure 23-10. Importantly, one out of four children (146 million) in developing countries is underweight, and 6.5 million children under the age of 5 years die in developing countries each year from malnutrition and hunger-related causes.

Undernutrition also is present in many institutionalized and hospitalized patients (Hudson et al., 2000; Omran and Morley, 2000). These populations are susceptible to starvation because of an inability to eat (e.g., difficulty chewing and swallowing, nausea, lack of appetite) or to the substantial

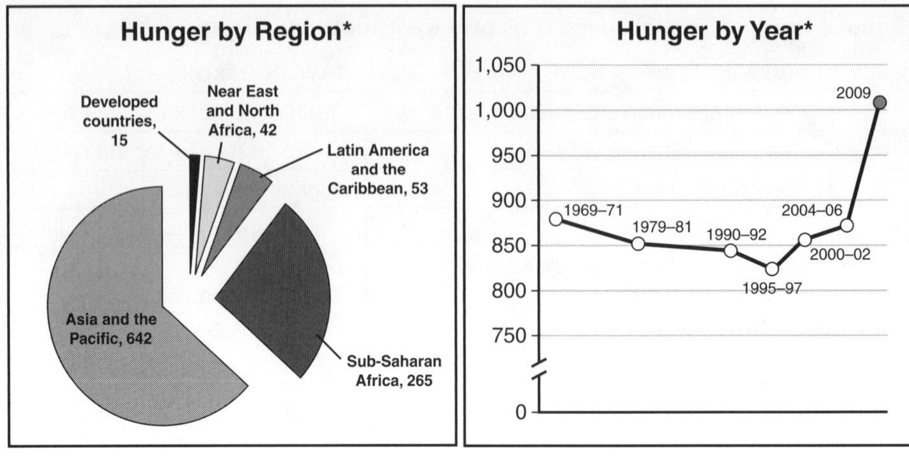

FIGURE 23-10 Statistics on hunger. (Redrawn from data of Food and Agriculture Organization. [2009]. *The state of food insecurity in the world 2009: Economic crises—Impacts and lessons learned.* Rome: FAO.) FAO measures hunger as "the number of people who do not consume the minimum daily energy requirement, which is the amount of calories needed for light activity and a minimum acceptable weight for attained height."

increase in energy expenditure that results from severe trauma or infection. The elderly are particularly susceptible to PEM because of functional declines, illness, poverty, and long-term residential care situations. Although data are lacking regarding prevalence, estimates usually suggest that 20% to 40% of all institutionalized elders are undernourished (Avery et al., 2010). Moderate PEM may lead to unintentional weight loss, weakened grip, and inability to perform high-energy tasks, whereas more severe PEM may lead to loss of more than 20% of body weight, the inability to eat normal-sized meals, a slow heart rate, low blood pressure, and low body temperature. Kwashiorkor-like PEM may occur in patients who have been severely burned, suffered trauma, or had sepsis or other life-threatening illness. In cases of sudden onset of severe PEM, body fat and muscle mass may be relatively normal.

COMORBIDITIES OF PEM

Primary or secondary PEM can subsequently alter risk for other conditions. The degree of risk depends on the age of the individual, the severity and length of the malnutrition, and the presence of any additional micronutrient deficiencies. For example, depletion of more than 10% of body protein is associated with an increased risk of morbidity and debility, a state that would be significantly more traumatic to an infant.

Regarding specific morbidities, PEM can notably alter immunity, making an individual much more susceptible to conditions related to immune function than an individual who is well nourished. In fact, malnutrition is considered by some to be the most common cause of immunodeficiency worldwide (Chandra, 2002). Impairments in immune function include processes related to cell-mediated immunity, phagocyte function, cytokine production, and the complement system. Specific defects in the immune system include depressed thymic function, atrophy of lymphoid organs, and profound T-lymphocyte deficiency. In addition, PEM weakens the body's natural barriers to infectious agents, such as mucous membranes and skin. Further, the hypothalamic–pituitary–adrenal axis is activated and increases glucocorticoid levels. The result is that PEM increases susceptibility to pathogens, reactivates viral infections, and promotes the development of opportunistic infections, such as those caused by parasites. Because PEM results in increased infection but reduced ability to fight the infection, the immune response is further weakened, leading to an even greater alteration in immune cell populations and a generalized increase in inflammatory mediators. Two groups that are already at a disadvantage in terms of immunity, young infants and the elderly, are especially prone to immune impairments with PEM.

Another consideration for individuals with PEM is that drug pharmacokinetics are altered (Oshikoya et al., 2010), making it more challenging to fight an infection or treat the underlying disease in the case of secondary PEM. PEM also alters cognitive performance and promotes dementia in the elderly (Morley, 2010).

METABOLIC ADAPTATION TO SHORT-TERM OR PROLONGED STARVATION

The response to starvation can best be understood as a protective mechanism in which the body attempts to maintain energy balance and avoid loss of body mass. When energy intake is low, the body relies on endogenous fuel sources, which are mainly adipose tissue triacylglycerols and skeletal muscle proteins. The primary metabolic signals triggering these events are a fall in the plasma level of insulin and increases in the concentrations of glucagon and glucocorticoids, caused by the limited intake of dietary carbohydrate and thus a low plasma glucose concentration. Hypoinsulinemia facilitates mobilization of free fatty acids, starvation ketosis, and net catabolism of skeletal muscle protein to provide substrates for visceral protein synthesis and for gluconeogenesis.

The essential features of the metabolic response to starvation are altered rates and patterns of fuel utilization and protein metabolism, aimed at minimizing fuel needs and limiting lean tissue loss. The nature of the starvation diet determines the pattern of hormone levels and fuel consumption. In total fasting, the liver glycogen stores are rapidly depleted and the body turns to gluconeogenesis, mainly from amino acid carbon skeletons, to maintain plasma glucose levels. Therefore starvation changes overall protein metabolism, resulting in an initial rapid loss of body protein; but this is followed by a prolonged period during which further protein losses are minimized to protect lean body mass; this is associated with a slower rate of synthesis and breakdown of body protein.

In prolonged starvation, fat oxidation becomes the dominant fuel (Owen et al., 1998). Hepatic ketogenesis from fatty acids provides an additional fuel for most tissues. The brain switches from using exclusively glucose to using predominantly ketone bodies. Ketone bodies provide an additional fuel to resting muscle during prolonged starvation, being oxidized along with fatty acids. The metabolic ketoacidosis of prolonged fasting induces a compensatory increase in renal production of ammonia to increase removal of hydrogen ions from the body as ammonium. This change is associated with augmented renal gluconeogenesis and a somewhat greater loss of body nitrogen than would occur without the acidosis. Loss of more than 40% of body weight is usually fatal, with death usually resulting from heart failure, electrolyte imbalance, or low body temperature. The survival of a nonobese fasting individual coincides roughly with the predicted time of depletion of fat, approximately 60 days. Obviously, obese individuals with their greater stores of fat have a survival advantage under starvation conditions. Obese individuals have a larger fat mass and also lose lean mass at a slower rate than do lean individuals (Elia et al., 1999). Nevertheless, the requirement of gluconeogenic substrates would still necessitate the catabolism of muscle protein during prolonged starvation in the obese individual, and death of a very obese individual during prolonged starvation would be expected to occur due to loss of essential lean body mass before the depletion of the enlarged fat stores.

TREATMENT OF PROTEIN-ENERGY MALNUTRITION

Treatment for PEM depends on the severity, duration, and causes. For severe PEM, the first steps are correcting fluid and electrolyte abnormalities and treating infections with antibiotics. The next step is oral feeding, which usually involves the introduction of a nutritious liquid formula, with the daily amount gradually increased over 1 to 3 weeks. Introduction of food may be delayed if diarrhea is severe. During refeeding, the shift from the fasting state to intake of a mixed diet can stimulate sodium and water retention, hypophosphatemia, and other electrolyte shifts, as well as deplete thiamin and other B vitamins. Electrolyte levels and edema should be carefully monitored. After several weeks, the formula can be replaced by solid foods. If PEM is secondary, the underlying cause of the condition should also be treated or managed.

THINKING CRITICALLY

1. Describe some of the metabolic consequences of obesity. Describe some of the metabolic consequences of protein-energy malnutrition. How do these imbalances act to increase disease risk?
2. Atrophy of adipose tissue (lipodystrophies) and accumulation of excess adipose tissue (obesity) result in many similar abnormalities. What does the similarity of metabolic changes associated with both obesity and lipodystrophy suggest about the mechanism by which either leads to metabolic syndrome?

REFERENCES

Alberti, K. G., & Zimmet, P. Z. (1998). Definition, diagnosis and classification of diabetes mellitus and its complications, I: Diagnosis and classification of diabetes mellitus provisional report of a WHO consultation. *Diabetic Medicine, 15*, 539–553.

Alberti, K. G., Zimmet, P., & Shaw, J. (2006). Metabolic syndrome—A new world-wide definition. A Consensus Statement from the International Diabetes Federation. *Diabetic Medicine, 23*, 469–480.

Andreasen, C. H., Stender-Petersen, K. L., Mogensen, M. S., Torekov, S. S., Wegner, L., Andersen, G., … Hansen, T. (2008). Low physical activity accentuates the effect of the FTO rs9939609 polymorphism on body fat accumulation. *Diabetes, 57*, 264–268.

Appel, L. J., Sacks, F. M., Carey, V. J., Obarzanek, E., Swain, J. F., Miller, E. R., 3rd, ... OmniHeart Collaborative Research Group. (2005). Effects of protein, monounsaturated fat, and carbohydrate intake on blood pressure and serum lipids: Results of the OmniHeart randomized trial. *The Journal of the American Medical Association, 294*, 2455–2464.

Astrup, A., Dyerberg, J., Selleck, M., & Stender, S. (2008). Nutrition transition and its relationship to the development of obesity and related chronic diseases. *Obesity Reviews, 9*(Suppl. 1), 48–52.

Avery, E., Kleppinger, A., Feinn, R., & Kenny, A. M. (2010). Determinants of living situation in a population of community-dwelling and assisted living–dwelling elders. *Journal of the American Medical Directors Association, 11*, 140–144.

Campión, J., Milagro, F. I., & Martínez, J. A. (2009). Individuality and epigenetics in obesity. *Obesity Reviews, 10*, 383–392.

Centers for Disease Control and Prevention. (2007). Prevalence of regular physical activity among adults—United States, 2001 and 2005. *Morbidity and Mortality Weekly Report, 56*, 1209–1212.

Chandra, R. K. (2002). Nutrition and the immune system from birth to old age. *European Journal of Clinical Nutrition, 56*(Suppl. 3), S73–S76.

Dinour, L. M., Bergen, D., & Yeh, M. C. (2007). The food insecurity-obesity paradox: A review of the literature and the role food stamps may play. *Journal of the American Dietetic Association, 107*, 1952–1961.

Drewnowski, A., & Darmon, N. (2005). Food choices and diet costs: An economic analysis. *The Journal of Nutrition, 135*, 900–904.

Drolet, R., Richard, C., Sniderman, A. D., Mailloux, J., Fortier, M., Huot, C., … Tchernof, A. (2008). Hypertrophy and hyperplasia of abdominal adipose tissues in women. *International Journal of Obesity (London), 32*, 283–291.

Elia, M., Stubbs, R. J., & Henry, C. J. K. (1999). Differences in fat, carbohydrate, and protein metabolism between lean and obese subjects undergoing total starvation. *Obesity Research, 7*, 597–604.

Ervin, R. B. (2009). *Prevalence of metabolic syndrome among adults 20 years of age and over, by sex, age, race and ethnicity, and body mass index: United States, 2003–2006. National Health Statistics Reports; no. 13*. Hyattsville, MD: National Center for Health Statistics.

Esparza, J., Fox, C., Harper, I. T., Bennett, P. H., Schulz, L. O., Valencia, M. E., & Ravussin, E. (2000). Daily energy expenditure in Mexican and USA Pima Indians: Low physical activity as a possible cause of obesity. *International Journal of Obesity and Related Metabolic Disorders, 24*, 55–59.

Fernandez, J. R., Redden, D., Pietrobelli, A., & Allison, D. B. (2004). Waist circumference percentiles in nationally representative samples of African-American, European-American, and Mexican-American children and adolescents. *The Journal of Pediatrics, 145*, 427–430.

Flegal, K. M., Carroll, M. D., Ogden, C. L., & Curtin, L. R. (2010). Prevalence and trends in obesity among US adults, 1999–2008. *The Journal of the American Medical Association, 303*, 235–241.

Flegal, K. M., Graubard, B. I., Williamson, D. F., & Gail, M. H. (2007). Cause-specific excess deaths associated with underweight, overweight, and obesity. *The Journal of the American Medical Association, 298*, 2028–2037.

Food and Agriculture Organization (2004). *The state of food insecurity in the world 2004: Monitoring progress towards the World Food Summit and Millennium*. Rome: FAO.

Food and Agriculture Organization (2009). *The state of food insecurity in the world 2009: Economic crises—Impacts and lessons learned*. Rome: FAO.

Ford, E., Giles, W., & Dietz, W. (2002). Prevalence of the metabolic syndrome among U.S. adults. Findings from the Third National Health and Nutrition Examination Survey. *The Journal of the American Medical Association, 287*, 356–359.

Frühbeck, G. (2008). Overview of adipose tissue and its role in obesity and metabolic disorders. *Methods in Molecular Biology, 456*, 1–22.

Galic, S., Oakhill, J. S., & Steinberg, G. R. (2010). Adipose tissue as an endocrine organ. *Molecular and Cellular Endocrinology, 316*, 129–139.

Goris, A. H., & Westerterp, K. R. (2008). Physical activity, fat intake and body fat. *Physiology & Behavior, 94*, 164–168.

Grün, F. (2010). Obesogens. *Current Opinion in Endocrinology, Diabetes, and Obesity, 17*, 453–459.

Grundy, S., Brewer, H. B., Jr., Cleeman, J. I., Smith, S. C., Jr., & Lenfant, C. (2004). AHA/NHLBI/ADA conference proceedings: Definition of metabolic syndrome. Report of the National Heart, Lung, and Blood Institute/American Heart Association conference on scientific issues related to definition. *Circulation, 109*, 433–438.

Grundy, S. M., Cleeman, J. I., Daniels, S. R., Donato, K. A., Eckel, R. H., Franklin, B. A., Gordon, D. J., Krauss, R. M., Savage, P. J., Smith, S. C., Jr., Spertus, J. A., Costa, F., American Heart Association, & National Heart, Lung, and Blood Institute. (2005). Diagnosis and management of the metabolic syndrome: An American Heart Association/National Heart, Lung, and Blood Institute Scientific Statement. *Circulation, 112*, 2735–2752.

Guh, D. P., Zhang, W., Bansback, N., Amarsi, Z., Birmingham, C. L., & Anis, A. H. (2009). The incidence of co-morbidities related to obesity and overweight: A systematic review and meta-analysis. *BMC Public Health, 9*, 88.

Günther, K., Vollmuth, J., Weissbach, R., Hohenberger, W., Husemann, B., & Horbach, T. (2006). Weight reduction after an early version of the open gastric bypass for morbid obesity: Results after 23 years. *Obesity Surgery, 16*, 288–296.

Hamman, R. F., Wing, R. R., Edelstein, S. L., Lachin, J. M., Bray, G. A., Delahanty, L., ... Wylie-Rosett, J. (2006). Effect of weight loss with lifestyle intervention on risk of diabetes. *Diabetes Care, 29*, 2102–2107.

Harman-Boehm, I., Blüher, M., Redel, H., Sion-Vardy, N., Ovadia, S., Avinoach, E., ... Rudich, A. (2007). Macrophage infiltration into omental versus subcutaneous fat across different populations: Effect of regional adiposity and the comorbidities of obesity. *The Journal of Clinical Endocrinology and Metabolism, 92*, 2240–2247.

Højgaard, B., Olsen, K. R., Søgaard, J., Sørensen, T. I., & Gyrd-Hansen, D. (2008). Economic costs of abdominal obesity. *Obesity Facts, 1*, 146–154.

Horton, T. J., Drougas, H., Brachey, A., Reed, G. W., Peters, J. C., & Hill, J. O. (1995). Fat and carbohydrate overfeeding in humans: Different effects on energy storage. *The American Journal of Clinical Nutrition, 62*, 19–29.

Hudson, H. M., Daubert, C. R., & Mills, R. H. (2000). The interdependency of protein-energy malnutrition, aging, and dysphagia. *Dysphagia, 15*, 31–38.

James, W. P. (2008). The fundamental drivers of the obesity epidemic. *Obesity Reviews, 9*(Suppl. 1), 6–13.

Karlsson, J., Taft, C., Rydén, A., Sjöström, L., & Sullivan, M. (2007). Ten-year trends in health-related quality of life after surgical and conventional treatment for severe obesity: The SOS intervention study. *International Journal of Obesity, 31*, 1248–1261.

Lee, M. J., Wu, Y., & Fried, S. K. (2010). Adipose tissue remodeling in pathophysiology of obesity. *Current Opinion in Clinical Nutrition and Metabolic Care, 13*, 371–376.

Mathieu, P., Lemieux, I., & Després, J. P. (2010). Obesity, inflammation, and cardiovascular risk. *Clinical Pharmacology and Therapeutics, 87*, 407–416.

McPherson, R. (2007). Genetic contributors to obesity. *The Canadian Journal of Cardiology, 23*(Suppl. A), 23A–27A.

Mitra, A. K., & Clarke, K. (2010). Viral obesity: Fact or fiction? *Obesity Reviews, 11*, 289–296.

Moller, D. E., & Kaufman, K. D. (2005). Metabolic syndrome: A clinical and molecular perspective. *Annual Review of Medicine, 56*, 45–62.

Moore, L. L., Visioni, A. J., Qureshi, M. M., Bradlee, M. L., Ellison, R. C., & D'Agostino, R. (2005). Weight loss in overweight adults and the long-term risk of hypertension: The Framingham Study. *Archives of Internal Medicine, 165*, 1298–1303.

Morley, J. E. (2010). Nutrition and the brain. *Clinics in Geriatric Medicine, 26*, 89–98.

Müller, H. P., Raudies, F., Unrath, A., Neumann, H., Ludolph, A. C., & Kassubek, J. (2011). Quantification of human body fat tissue percentage by MRI. *NMR in Biomedicine, 24*, 17–24.

Musso, G., Gambino, R., & Cassader, M. (2010). Obesity, diabetes, and gut microbiota: The hygiene hypothesis expanded? *Diabetes Care, 33*, 2277–2284.

National Cholesterol Education Program. (2002). Third Report of the National Cholesterol Education Program (NCEP) Expert Panel on Detection, Evaluation, and Treatment of High Blood Cholesterol in Adults (Adult Treatment Panel III) final report. *Circulation, 106*, 3143–3421.

National Institutes of Health. (1998). Clinical guidelines on the identification, evaluation, and treatment of overweight and obesity in adults—The evidence report. *Obesity Research, 6*(Suppl. 2), 51S–209S.

Nguyen, N. T., Magno, C. P., Lane, K. T., Hinojosa, M. W., & Lane, J. S. (2008). Association of hypertension, diabetes, dyslipidemia, and metabolic syndrome with obesity: Findings from the National Health and Nutrition Examination Survey, 1999 to 2004. *Journal of the American College of Surgeons, 207*, 928–934.

Ogden, O., & Carroll, M. (2010). *Prevalence of obesity among children and adolescents: United States, trends 1963–1965 through 2007–2008*. National Center for Health Statistics, Health E-Stats. Retrieved from www.cdc.gov/nchs/fastats/overwt.htm

Omran, M. L., & Morley, J. E. (2000). Assessment of protein energy malnutrition in older persons, Part I: History, examination, body composition, and screening tools. *Nutrition, 16*, 50–63.

Oshikoya, K. A., Sammons, H. M., & Choonara, I. (2010). A systematic review of pharmacokinetics studies in children with protein—Energy malnutrition. *European Journal of Clinical Pharmacology, 66*, 1025–1035.

Owen, O. E., Smalley, K. J., D'Alessio, D. A., Mozzoli, M. A., & Dawson, E. K. (1998). Protein, fat, and carbohydrate requirements during starvation: Anaplerosis and cataplerosis. *The American Journal of Clinical Nutrition, 68*, 12–34.

Physical Activity Guidelines Advisory Committee. (2008). *Physical Activity Guidelines Advisory Committee report, 2008*. Washington, DC: U.S. Department of Health and Human Services.

Pi-Sunyer, F. X. (1993). Medical hazards of obesity. *Annals of Internal Medicine, 119*, 655–660.

Pouliot, M.-C., Despres, J.-P., Lemieux, S., Moorjani, S., Bouchard, C., Tremblay, A., … Lupien, P. J. (1994). Waist circumference and abdominal sagittal diameter: Best simple anthropometric indexes of abdominal visceral adipose tissue accumulation and related cardiovascular risk in men and women. *The American Journal of Cardiology, 73*, 460–468.

Rankinen, T., Zuberi, A., Chagnon, Y. C., Weisnagel, S. J., Argyropoulos, G., Walts, B., … Bouchard, C. (2006). The human obesity gene map: The 2005 update. *Obesity, 14*, 529–644.

Robinson, L. E., & Graham, T. E. (2004). Metabolic syndrome, a cardiovascular disease risk factor: Role of adipocytokines and impacts of diet and physical activity. *Canadian Journal of Applied Physiology, 29*, 808–829.

Rong, R., Hanson, R. L., Ortiz, D., Wiedrich, C., Kobes, S., Knowler, W. C., … Baier, L. J. (2009). Association analysis of variation in/near FTO, CDKAL1, SLC30A8, HHEX, EXT2, IGF2BP2, LOC387761, and CDKN2B with type 2 diabetes and related quantitative traits in Pima Indians. *Diabetes, 58*, 478–488.

Ruiz, J. R., Labayen, I., Ortega, F. B., Legry, V., Moreno, L. A., Dallongeville, J., … Meirhaeghe, A. (2010). Attenuation of the effect of the FTO rs9939609 polymorphism on total and central body fat by physical activity in adolescents: The HELENA Study. *Archives of Pediatrics & Adolescent Medicine, 164*, 328–333.

Silventoinen, K., Rokholm, B., Kaprio, J., & Sørensen, T. I. (2010). The genetic and environmental influences on childhood obesity: A systematic review of twin and adoption studies. *International Journal of Obesity, 34*, 29–40.

Simha, V., & Garg, A. (2009). Inherited lipodystrophies and hypertriglyceridemia. *Current Opinion in Lipidology, 20*, 300–308.

Tan, S., Scherag, A., Janssen, O. E., Hahn, S., Lahner, H., Dietz, T., … Hinney, A. (2010). Large effects on body mass index and insulin resistance of fat mass and obesity associated gene (FTO) variants in patients with polycystic ovary syndrome (PCOS). *BMC Medical Genetics, 11*, 12.

Tao, Y. X. (2010). The melanocortin-4 receptor: Physiology, pharmacology, and pathophysiology. *Endocrine Reviews, 31*, 506–543.

Tappy, L., & Lê, K. A. (2010). Metabolic effects of fructose and the worldwide increase in obesity. *Physiological Reviews, 90*, 23–46.

Torgerson, J., Hauptman, J., Boldrin, M., & Sjöström, L. (2004). XENical in the prevention of diabetes in obese subjects (XENDOS) study: A randomized study of orlistat as an adjunct to lifestyle changes for the prevention of type 2 diabetes in obese patients. *Diabetes Care, 27*, 155–161.

Varvarigou, A. A. (2010). Intrauterine growth restriction as a potential risk factor for disease onset in adulthood. *Journal of Pediatric Endocrinology & Metabolism, 23*, 215–224.

Weisberg, S. P., McCann, D., Desai, M., Rosenbaum, M., Leibel, R. L., & Ferrante, A. W., Jr. (2003). Obesity is associated with macrophage accumulation in adipose tissue. *The Journal of Clinical Investigation, 112*, 1796–1808.

Wister, A. P., Loewen, N., Kennedy-Symonds, H. M., McGowan, B., McCoy, B., & Singer, J. P. (2007). One-year follow-up of a therapeutic lifestyle intervention targeting cardiovascular disease risk. *Canadian Medical Association Journal, 177*, 859–865.

World Health Organization. (1997). *Obesity: Preventing and managing the global epidemic*. Geneva: WHO.

World Health Organization. (2005). *The WHO global database on body mass index (BMI)*. Geneva: WHO.

RECOMMENDED READINGS

Frühbeck, G. (2008). Overview of adipose tissue and its role in obesity and metabolic disorders. *Methods in Molecular Biology, 456*, 1–22.

Galic, S., Oakhill, J. S., & Steinberg, G. R. (2010). Adipose tissue as an endocrine organ. *Molecular and Cellular Endocrinology, 316*, 129–139.

Institute of Medicine. (2002). *Dietary Reference Intakes: Energy, carbohydrate, fiber, fat, fatty acids, cholesterol, protein, and amino acids*. Washington, DC: The National Academies Press.

Lee, M. J., Wu, Y., & Fried, S. K. (2010). Adipose tissue remodeling in pathophysiology of obesity. *Current Opinion in Clinical Nutrition and Metabolic Care, 13*, 371–376.

Simha, V., & Garg, A. (2009). Inherited lipodystrophies and hypertriglyceridemia. *Current Opinion in Lipidology, 20*, 300–308.

RECOMMENDED WEBSITES

Detailed advice for weight reduction can be obtained from obesity guidelines at websites maintained by:

American Heart Association, www.heart.org/HEARTORG/

American Obesity Association (AOA), www.obesity.org

Centers for Disease Control and Prevention (CDC), National Center for Chronic Disease Prevention and Health Promotion, www.cdc.gov/obesity/index.html

National Heart, Lung and Blood Institute (NHLBI), www.nhlbi.nih.gov

Information about worldwide nutrition problems related to energy is available at websites maintained by:

Food and Agriculture Organization of the United Nations (FAO), www.fao.org

United Nations System Standing Committee on Nutrition (SCN), www.unscn.org

World Health Organization (WHO), www.who.int/en/

UNIT VI

The Vitamins

Vitamins are defined as organic compounds that are required in the diet in only small amounts to maintain fundamental functions of the body (growth, metabolism, and cellular integrity). This definition distinguishes vitamins from the organic macronutrients because vitamins are not catabolized to CO_2 and H_2O to satisfy part of the energy requirement and are not used for structural purposes; hence vitamins are required in much smaller amounts than are carbohydrates, proteins, and triacylglycerols. Vitamins are distinguished from the minerals (which also are required in relatively small amounts compared with nutrient sources of energy) by their organic rather than inorganic nature.

Well before the twentieth century, the curative effects of certain foods were recognized. An ancient Egyptian medical treatise recommended eating roast ox liver or black cock's liver to cure night blindness, and early reports indicate that writings as far back as 1500 BC stated that consumption of liver cured night blindness. It has been known for nearly three centuries that scurvy can be controlled by dietary means. In 1747 James Lind, a Scottish physician in the Royal Navy, hypothesized that various "acidic principles" might have antiscorbutic properties. Lind tested his theory by feeding a variety of acidic substances to sailors who had scurvy. The treatments included eating two oranges or one lemon per day, and these citrus fruits had miraculous curative powers. As early as 1855, beriberi, which was a common affliction among Japanese sailors, was found to be prevented or cured by adding meat, milk, and vegetables to the regular polished rice diet of Japanese seamen.

It was during the twentieth century, however, that the vitamins were isolated, identified, and chemically synthesized. The first of these essential dietary factors to be isolated and chemically identified was the antiberiberi substance, which was isolated from rice polishings by Casimir Funk, a Polish biochemist who was working at the Lister Institute in London. Funk called this factor *vitamine* based on evidence that it was an "amine" that was "vital" for life. In 1912 Funk extended the use of this term and the "vitamine theory" to include those other trace dietary essentials that were missing in individuals with rickets, scurvy, and pellagra as well as in those with beriberi. The name *vitamine* was changed to *vitamin* as the structures of additional essential organic factors were discovered and it became clear that most were not amines.

The first major subdivision of the vitamins stems from work that was done by Wilhelm Stepp in Germany, Elmer McCollum and Margaret Davis at the University of Wisconsin, and Thomas Osborne and Lafayette Mendel at Yale University. By using different solvents to extract growth factors from foods, these investigators found that one could separate "fat-soluble" and "water-soluble" factors. Around 1915 McCollum and Davis demonstrated that a fat-soluble factor "A" present in butterfat and egg yolk and a heat-labile, water-soluble factor "B" present in wheat germ were needed for growth in young rats. Ensuing efforts at a number of laboratories led to specific identification of the fat-soluble vitamins as belonging to groups now called A, D, E, and K.

In the search for factors that would prevent beriberi and pellagra, it became apparent that water-soluble factor B was not a single substance, as pointed out by Joseph Goldberger in the 1920s. The successive efforts of numerous investigators were required to unravel the "B complex." It took researchers about 25 years to identify all the B vitamins, beginning with the isolation of B_1 (thiamin) in 1926 and ending with the identification of the structure of vitamin B_{12} (cyanocobalamin) in 1955. The chemical synthesis of cyanocobalamin was not accomplished until 1970. Other workers investigating the effects of water-soluble vitamins realized that the factor shown by Axel Holst and Theodor Frolick in Oslo in 1907 to prevent a scurvylike condition in guinea pigs was the antiscorbutic activity associated with lemon juice. S. S. Zilva and others at the Lister Institute termed this factor vitamin C.

Over the course of the twentieth century, researchers identified 13 vitamins that are dietary essentials for humans. These include eight B vitamins (thiamin, niacin, riboflavin, folate, vitamin B_6, vitamin B_{12}, biotin, and pantothenic acid), vitamin C or ascorbic acid, and the fat-soluble vitamins A, D, E, and K. Choline, a micronutrient commonly grouped with the B vitamins, is an essential micronutrient for at least a subset of the population and has some of the characteristics of a vitamin and is thus included in this unit. As vitamins were further characterized, it was found that the activity of a particular vitamin was often found in several closely related compounds known as vitamers. For example, vitamin B_6 is used to refer not only to pyridoxine (pyridoxol), but also to pyridoxal and pyridoxamine; and vitamin A is used to refer to retinol, retinal, and retinoic acid.

In addition, as more has been learned about the vitamins, it has become clear that some of the vitamins are not strictly dietary essentials. Vitamin D is synthesized in the skin from an endogenous precursor (7-dehydrocholesterol) upon exposure to sunlight. Niacin-containing coenzymes, and subsequently niacin, are synthesized from the amino acid tryptophan.

Most vitamins are not related chemically, and they differ in their biochemical and physiological roles. The historical water-soluble and fat-soluble classification distinguishes vitamins by their physical solubility in solvents, and this classification also broadly separates the vitamins by some of the types of processes involved in their digestion, absorption, and transport, as well as by some aspects of their functions.

The most common function of vitamins is as essential components of coenzymes. All of the B vitamins, vitamin C, and reduced vitamin K are required as coenzymes or as components of coenzymes that are synthesized from the vitamins. Coenzymes are defined as small, organic molecules that are required by an enzyme and that participate in the chemistry of catalysis. Most coenzymes shuttle back and forth between two (or more) different forms. Coenzymes include ascorbic acid, reduced vitamin K, biotin (covalently bound to enzyme), nicotinamide adenine dinucleotide (NAD) and nicotinamide adenine dinucleotide phosphate (NADP) (niacin-containing), flavin adenine dinucleotide (FAD) and flavin mononucleotide (FMN) (riboflavin-containing), thiamin diphosphate, several folate coenzymes, methyl-B_{12} and deoxyadenosyl-B_{12}, pyridoxal phosphate and pyridoxamine phosphate (vitamin B_6 coenzymes), and coenzyme A and enzyme-bound 4′-phosphopantetheine (derivatives of pantothenic acid). These coenzymes may be covalently attached to the enzyme protein (biotin, FAD in a few cases, and 4′-phosphopantetheine), tightly associated with specific apoenzymes to form the active holoenzyme (FAD and FMN, B_{12} coenzymes, most folate coenzymes, and B_6 coenzymes), or only weakly associated with their apoenzymes such that the cofactors and substrates behave similarly (NAD and NADP, some folate coenzymes, coenzyme A, ascorbate, and reduced vitamin K). It should be noted that not all coenzymes are formed from vitamins; for example, coenzyme Q, lipoic acid, dolichol phosphate, and biopterin are synthesized in the body.

The other functions of vitamins are more varied. Two of the vitamins are required for synthesis of hormones: vitamin D is required for formation of 1,25-dihydroxyvitamin D, and vitamin A is required for formation of all-*trans*-retinoic acid. Vitamin A also acts as a visual pigment in the form of 11-*cis*-retinal. Vitamin E serves as a lipid-soluble antioxidant, and vitamin C also has antioxidant functions. The niacin-containing coenzyme NAD also serves as substrate for adenosine diphosphate (ADP)–ribosylation reactions.

In the following eight chapters, the vitamins are discussed. The details of coenzyme, hormone, and antioxidant function are discussed, because these biochemical and physiological functions are the bases of the requirements for these vitamins, and clinical signs of deficiency result from impairment of these functions. Some of the B vitamins have been grouped because they play major roles in particular areas of metabolism. Niacin, riboflavin, and thiamin are grouped together because these three vitamins play critical roles in the central pathways underlying energy-yielding nutrient metabolism. Folate, choline, vitamin B_{12}, and vitamin B_6 are grouped together because of their important roles as coenzymes and/or cosubstrates in the one-carbon (1-C) metabolic network. Biotin and pantothenic acid are covered in a single chapter because these two vitamins are intimately (but not exclusively) involved in lipid metabolism. Vitamin C, vitamin A, vitamin D, vitamin E, and vitamin K are covered in separate chapters because of their specialized functions in the body.

CHAPTER 24

Niacin, Riboflavin, and Thiamin

*W. Todd Penberthy, PhD**

COMMON ABBREVIATIONS

FAD	flavin adenine dinucleotide	**NaMN**	nicotinate (nicotinic acid) mononucleotide
FMN	flavin mononucleotide	**NE**	niacin equivalent
NAD	nicotinamide adenine dinucleotide	**NMN**	nicotinamide mononucleotide
NADP	nicotinamide adenine dinucleotide phosphate	**ThDP**	thiamin diphosphate

Vitamins B_3 (niacin), B_2 (riboflavin), and B_1 (thiamin or thiamine) are ultimately used by just over 400, 150, and 20 different proteins, respectively, and are thus intimately connected in essential bioenergetic, anabolic, and catabolic pathways. The thiamin and niacin deficiency diseases known as beriberi and pellagra, respectively, were the most devastating vitamin deficiency diseases in the history of the United States. These three vitamins are so important to human health that, together with folate, they are the only vitamins legally mandated for food enrichment by the government. Mandated enrichment is generally considered to have eliminated respective deficiency diseases; however, deficiency of these vitamins remains a primary concern in the modern developed world. This is due to poor food choices, adverse drug reactions, and infectious and autoimmune diseases, any of which can aggressively trigger pathways that actively deplete these vitamins. This chapter covers the history, physiological function, chemistry, and dietary requirements for each of these important vitamins.

NIACIN

Vitamin B_3 is the essential dietary precursor for endogenous formation of nicotinamide adenine dinucleotide (NAD). Ultimately NAD functions as either a cofactor in hundreds of oxidation–reduction (redox) reactions or as a substrate in enzyme-catalyzed reactions controlling DNA repair, transcriptional regulation, and other global genomic regulatory functions. NAD is involved in more reactions than any other known vitamin-derived molecule. Today, NAD research continues to expand because of the therapeutic benefit seen with NAD-mediated activation of sirtuins as well as the role of NAD-depleting poly (ADP-ribose) polymerase 1 (PARP1) enzyme in cancer.

NIACIN HISTORY

Niacin deficiency was first described in Europe by Casal in 1762 as a condition of melancholia, crusty skin, and extreme weakness. Casal coined the disease "pellagra," meaning angry skin. Pellagra became the most severe vitamin deficiency disease in U.S. history. Over 120,000 people died from pellagra epidemics during the first two decades of the twentieth century; pellagra was also the leading cause of death in mental hospitals in 1907.

By the 1950s medical doctors who witnessed pellagra noticed its similarities to schizophrenia. These doctors theorized that schizophrenics might have a genetic disorder that required far greater levels of dietary niacin. Experiments revealed that fixed administration of gram quantities of niacin to schizophrenic patients frequently resulted in therapeutic benefit with minimal or no adversity (Hoffer et al., 1957). However, this approach remains controversial and requires additional study. As a result of these initial experiments focused on schizophrenia, it was also determined that high-dose niacin (as nicotinic acid) is an effective treatment for dyslipidemia. Today high-dose niacin is a more effective elevator of high-density lipoprotein ("good" cholesterol) than any other pharmaceutical. This approach simultaneously lowers cholesterol, triacylglycerols, and very-low-density lipoprotein. Administration of high doses of various NAD precursors remains an active area of research, especially based on the many favorable results obtained in animal models of human diseases.

*This chapter is a revision of the chapter contributed by Donald B. McCormick, PhD, for the second edition.

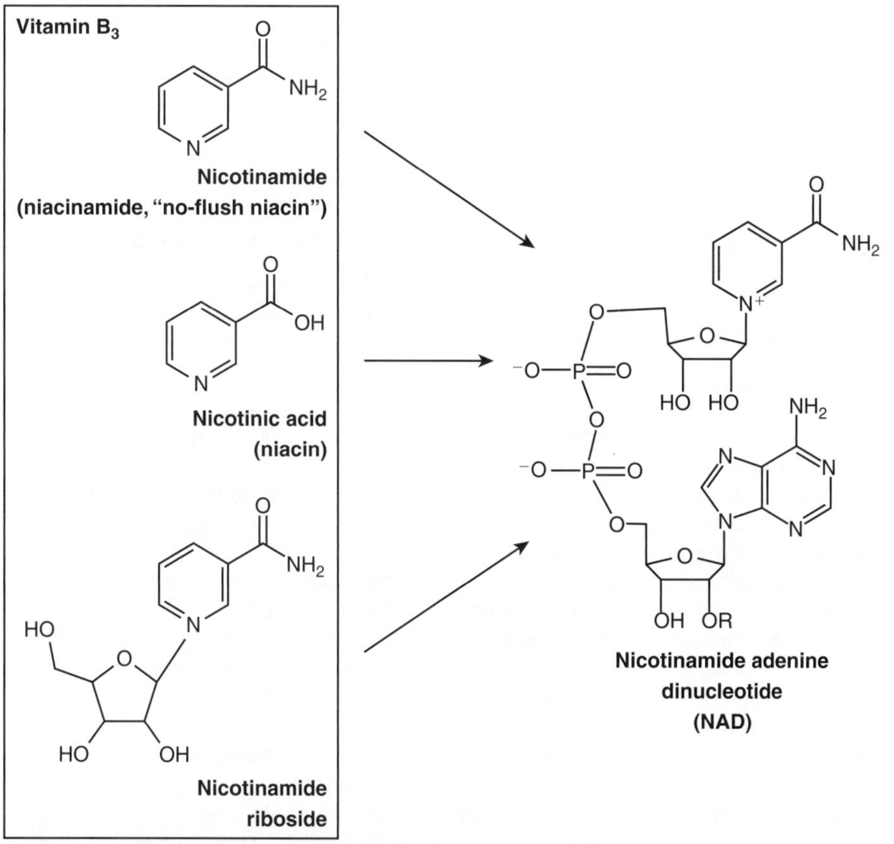

Vitamin B_3

Nicotinamide (niacinamide, "no-flush niacin")

Nicotinic acid (niacin)

Nicotinamide riboside

Nicotinamide adenine dinucleotide (NAD)

FIGURE 24-1 Three forms of vitamin B_3. Vitamin B_3 is a precursor to nicotinamide dinucleotide (NAD). The body converts the three forms of B_3 to NAD through two enzyme reactions, or three in the case of nicotinic acid. We must obtain nicotinic acid, nicotinamide, nicotinamide riboside, or tryptophan from our diet to ultimately synthesize the essential molecule NAD.

NIACIN NOMENCLATURE, STRUCTURE, AND BIOCHEMISTRY

Vitamin B_3 is defined as the precursor to NAD and potentially includes three different molecular forms: nicotinic acid, niacinamide, and nicotinamide riboside. Nicotinic acid or pyridine-3-carboxylic acid is sometimes referred to as "flushing" niacin, whereas niacinamide or pyridine-3-carboxamide is referred to as "flush-free" niacin. The third form of vitamin B_3, nicotinamide riboside, was recently discovered in 2004 and is not used clinically yet (Bieganowski and Brenner, 2004). Structures for the three molecules are shown in Figure 24-1.

NIACIN PHYSIOLOGICAL FUNCTION

Molecular biology uses the elimination of gene expression to determine protein function. We can consider similar loss-of-function analysis for determining nutrient function. However, nutrient loss-of-function analysis is much more practically useful because we can readily address the loss-of-function symptoms by administering the vitamin molecule. Experiments involving vitamin deficiencies cannot usually be performed on humans; however, we can still learn from the history of pellagra in human populations and through experimentally controllable animal models.

DIETARY DEFICIENCIES OF NIACIN

The first symptoms of niacin deficiency (i.e., pellagra) include weakness, lassitude, anorexia, and indigestion. These are followed by the classic "three D's": dermatitis, diarrhea, and dementia. Additional symptoms include (1) functional changes in the gastrointestinal tract manifested as an absence of normal response to histamine, diminished secretion of hydrochloric acid in the gastric juice, and impaired absorption of vitamin B_{12}, fat, glucose, and D-xylose; and (2) nonspecific lesions of the central nervous system. The dermatitis has a characteristic appearance on parts of the body exposed to sunlight, heat, or mild trauma, such as the face, neck, hands, feet, and elbows. These lesions are usually bilaterally symmetrical. Mental symptoms develop in untreated cases and include irritability, headaches, sleeplessness, loss of memory, and emotional instability. Pellagra-like symptoms are also seen in chronic alcoholism, in carcinoid syndrome, and in some patients who receive certain medications, such as the antituberculosis drug isoniazid or some chemotherapeutics.

NIACIN-RESPONSIVE GENETIC DISORDERS

Niacin-responsive genetic diseases such as aldehyde dehydrogenase and glucose-6-phosphate 1-dehydrogenase can be rescued with high doses of niacin (Table 24-1). High-dose vitamin therapies stimulate variant enzymes with decreased coenzyme binding affinity (increased K_m), thereby improving the metabolic dysfunction (Ames et al., 2002). Given that the number of proteins that require NAD is greater than that for any other cofactor, scores of unmapped genetic polymorphisms are predicted to be responsive to high doses of NAD precursors, many of which have yet to be examined.

PROTEINS THAT REQUIRE NIACIN

NAD participates in more reactions than any other known vitamin-derived molecule. Hundreds of redox reactions use NAD as a cofactor. Tens of reactions use NAD as a substrate and a few proteins use NAD as a ligand. At least 470 proteins use NAD or nicotinamide adenine dinucleotide phosphate (NADP[H]) in some capacity, and this number continually changes as more proteins are discovered. The function and importance of NAD concentrations remain active research areas.

REDOX REACTIONS

NAD(P[H]) is used as a cofactor in a highly diverse set of reactions including the conversion of alcohols (often sugars and polyols) to aldehydes or ketones, hemiacetals to lactones,

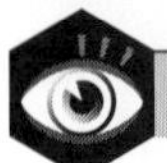

NUTRITION INSIGHT

Enrichment of Grain Products with B Vitamins

In the 1870s a technological development was made in mass grain milling. For the first time refined foods such as white flour and white rice became available to large segments of the population. Previously only wealthy individuals could have these. The milling of grains had the advantage of preventing spoilage; however, this processing depleted vitamins and minerals concentrated in the outer layers of the kernels (bran and aleurone) and germ. Wherever these refined foods were introduced, the diseases of pellagra and beriberi frequently appeared, depending on the variety of the diets.

Pellagra was particularly rampant in the southern United States, where diets frequently consisted simply of corn, molasses, and biscuits. For decades the search for the cause of pellagra centered on the association with corn-rich diets. Curiously, Native Americans did not suffer from pellagra, although corn was their main dietary staple. They treated corn with limewater, a process called nixtamalization, which released the NAD precursor tryptophan (and also inactivated mycotoxins), thus preventing pellagra.

Pellagra was finally understood in the 1930s thanks in large part to the initial work of the epidemiologist Dr. Joseph Goldberger. In 1926 he showed that a small amount of brewer's yeast could prevent pellagra. Initially Goldberger's hypothesis that pellagra was a deficiency disease was rejected in favor of hypotheses involving corn toxins or poor sanitation. In 1937 Dr. Conrad A. Elvjeham identified the pellagra-preventing factor as the molecule nicotinic acid. In these first experiments, dogs were fed deficient diets to cause tongue discoloration. The component of rice polishings that prevented tongue discoloration was subsequently isolated and named the pellagra-preventing factor.

Owing to the severity of the pellagra epidemics, the U.S. government established legally mandated standards of niacin enrichment of flour and other grain products. Beginning in the early 1940s these standards restored levels of thiamin, riboflavin, niacin, and iron to those found in whole-grain products. Enriched flour contains 2.9 mg thiamin, 1.8 mg riboflavin, 24.0 mg niacin, and 20 mg iron per pound of flour. Beginning as late as 1998, enriched-grain products have also been fortified with folate. Although products labeled "enriched" are responsible for eliminating pellagra epidemics, whole-grain products are still exceptional sources of nutrients because other vitamins and minerals lost in milling are not added as part of the enrichment program.

TABLE 24-1 Niacin-Responsive Genetic Disorders

DISEASE	SYMPTOMS	GENETIC MUTATION	NIACIN RESCUE
Hemolytic anemia	Anemia, jaundice, kernicterus, renal failure	*G6PD,* glucose-6-phosphate dehydrogenase (the single most common metabolic disorder; affects over 400 million people worldwide)	Unknown, but likely to help when K_m of G6PD is elevated
Hartnup disease	Psychological symptoms, ataxia, diplopia	*SLC6A19,* neutral amino acid transporter	Known relief of all symptoms
Ethanol-induced anginal attacks, increased incidence of esophageal cancer, alcohol-induced pancreatitis	Anginal attacks, esophageal cancer	*ALDH2,* aldehyde dehydrogenase 2 or acetaldehyde dehydrogenase	Potential reduction in anginal attacks, esophageal cancer, alcohol-induced pancreatitis
Dihydropteridine reductase (DHPR) deficiency (also known as atypical hyperphenylalaninemia)	Neurological symptoms	*DHPR,* dihydropteridine reductase	Potential reversal
Hydroxyacyl-coenzyme-A dehydrogenase (HADH) deficiency (also known as mitochondrial trifunctional protein deficiency)	Cardiomyopathy, hypoglycemia, fatty liver	*HADHA,* long-chain 3-hydroxyacyl-CoA dehydrogenase	Potential reversal

aldehydes to acids, and certain amino acids to keto acids. The common mechanism of operation for NAD(P[H]) cofactor redox reactions is generalized in Figure 24-2. Most dehydrogenases that use NAD or NADP function reversibly. Generally enzymes use NAD(H) in catabolic reactions, whereas NADP(H) is more commonly involved in anabolic (biosynthetic) reactions. For example, NADPH serves as an important reducing agent for the synthesis of fats and steroids (e.g., reactions catalyzed by 3-ketoacyl reductase, enoyl reductase, and 3-hydroxy-3-methylglutaryl-coenzyme A [HMG-CoA] reductase).

For pyridine nucleotide coenzymes to continue acting as catalysts, they must be recycled by coupling with other redox reactions. This may occur by coupling dehydrogenation reactions with hydrogenation reactions. For example, glyceraldehyde 3-phosphate dehydrogenase is coupled with lactate dehydrogenase in anaerobic glycolysis to produce NAD required for glycolysis. Similarly, NADPH produced by the pentose phosphate pathway is coupled to fatty acid synthesis. Alternatively dehydrogenation reactions are coupled with electron transport, as found in mitochondria.

Both NAD and NADP are part of the intracellular respiratory mechanism of all cells. They assist in the stepwise transfer of electrons or reducing equivalents from various energy substrates to the cytochromes. NADH usually donates its electrons to a flavin coenzyme in the mitochondrial electron transport chain responsible for ATP production. These reactions are outlined in Figure 24-3. A major source of NADH in the mitochondria is the β-oxidation of fatty acids. The main extramitochondrial source is NADH formed in glycolysis. Reducing equivalents are carried to the mitochondria by the malate–aspartate or the glycerol phosphate–dihydroxyacetone shuttles (see Chapter 12).

The approximately 57 different human cytochrome P450 monooxygenase systems use reducing equivalents of NADH and NADPH for a wide variety of functions, including synthesis and degradation of drugs, xenobiotics, prostaglandins, leukotrienes, retinoic acid, vitamin D, cholesterol, bile, and steroids (Nebert and Russell, 2002).

NONREDOX REACTIONS AND CONTROL OF NAD LEVELS

Four classes of enzymes play dominant roles in controlling NAD levels in response to DNA damage, immune activation, and other stimuli. These enzymes are poly(ADP-ribose) polymerase 1 (PARP1 through PARP18), the NAD-dependent deacetylases (sirtuin 1 through sirtuin 7), the ADP ribosyl-cyclases (CD38 and CD157), and indoleamine 2,3-dioxygenase (IDO). The first three of these enzymes produce nicotinamide as a side product that is recycled back to NAD via the salvage pathway as shown in Figure 24-4.

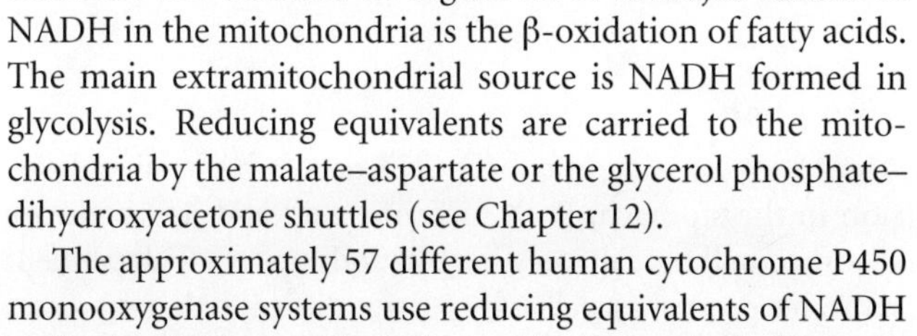

NAD-consuming activities are highly activated in response to any kind of DNA damage. PARP1 and PARP2 enzymes use NAD as a substrate to generate poly(ADP)ribose, an anionic polymer resembling DNA, to transfer ADP-ribose directly to histones and other proteins, including p53 and nuclear factor kappa B (NFκB). There are at least 18 different ADP-ribose transferring enzymes. PARP activation is directly proportional to the degree of DNA damage; it stops cell division and attempts DNA repair, a critical step in preventing cancer cells. More significantly, hyperactivation of PARP1 alone depletes intracellular NAD and ATP, which can lead to uncontrolled necrotic cell death.

Sirtuins can negatively regulate PARP activity by deacetylation. The sirtuins are NAD-dependent deacetylases that can target histones, p53, NFκB, and other important proteins. A tremendous amount of research has been devoted to sirtuins, owing to the general observation that increased NAD-mediated sirtuin activation affords health benefits. For example, sirtuin activators are useful for the treatment of diabetes and neurodegeneration in animal models.

We generally cannot change our genetics; however, we can change our epigenetics by altering NAD levels. Increased NAD activates sirtuin enzymes, which alters chromatin structure. For example, sirtuins are activated when calorie intake is reduced, and the resulting change in chromatin structure may be responsible for many of the therapeutically beneficial effects of calorie restriction. The other histone deacetylases are believed to possess constitutive activity that cannot be regulated. Thus NAD-dependent activation of sirtuin histone deacetylase activity is unique.

The ADP ribosyl-cyclase enzyme CD38 uses NAD as a substrate to generate the most potent known activators of intracellular calcium release, a mechanism required for chemotaxis of a variety of immune cells. The CD38-deficient mouse has persistent elevated NAD levels, increased energy expenditure, and does not become obese even when fed a high-fat diet. However, because CD38 is also required for chemotaxis of various immune cells, CD38-deficient mice are much more susceptible to infections. CD38 levels and activity are chiefly regulated at the transcriptional level, particularly by tumor necrosis factor-alpha (TNFα), which positively increases expression of CD38. CD157 is another NAD-dependent ADP ribosyl-cyclase that has important but less understood roles in neuron–glia cell interactions.

IDO plays major roles in controlling physiological NAD levels in humans by altering tryptophan concentrations within restricted cell types. Tryptophan is the essential substrate used for the de novo synthesis of NAD. IDO is highly activated within professional antigen-presenting immune cells (dendritic cells, macrophages, and B cells) during infections and in autoimmune disease. Unfortunately, persistent activation of IDO is pathogenic to neighboring cells because of this immune cell–specific consumption of tryptophan.

H2N C O R1 H C R2 X H N+ R NAD(P)+ ⇌ H2N C O HB HA N R NAD(P)H + C R2 X R1 + H+

FIGURE 24-2 Mechanism of substrate oxidation or reduction by pyridine nucleotide coenzymes. Typically, *X* is an electronegative atom (e.g., oxygen).

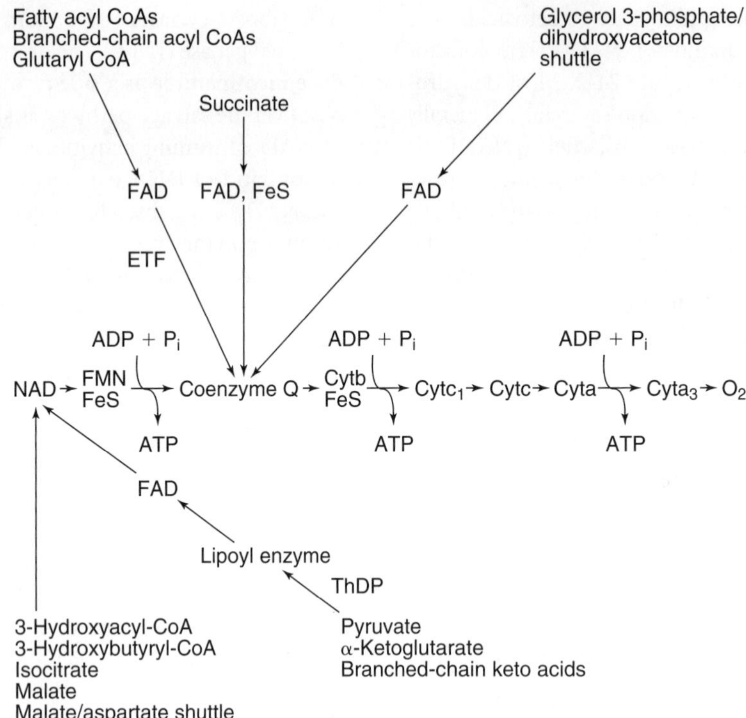

FIGURE 24-3 Pyridine nucleotides and flavocoenzymes funnel reducing equivalents to the mitochondrial respiratory chain. The main extramitochondrial source is NADH formed in glycolysis. These reducing equivalents are carried into the mitochondria by the malate–aspartate or the glycerol phosphate–dihydroxyacetone shuttles. NADH yields 3 ATPs, whereas $FADH_2$ yields 2 ATPs. *Cyt,* Cytochrome; *ETF,* electron transfer flavoprotein; *FAD,* flavin adenine dinucleotide; *FeS,* iron-sulfur protein domain; *FMN,* flavin mononucleotide; *ThDP,* thiamin diphosphate.

The IDO pathways are complicated, but they are an area of intense research for both autoimmune diseases and cancer.

NIACIN SOURCES, CHEMICAL STABILITY, AND ADMET

SOURCES

Nicotinic acid, nicotinamide, and nicotinamide riboside are widely distributed in foods of both plant and animal origin. Good sources of preformed NAD precursors include milk, beef, poultry, fish, legumes, peanuts, and some cereals. Enriched grain products and flours are good sources as well. In uncooked foods of animal origin, the major forms of niacin are the cellular pyridine nucleotides, NAD(H) and NADP(H).

CHEMICAL STABILITY

Niacin is relatively stable to heat but food preparation methods can affect the level of biologically available niacin. For example, roasting green coffee beans converts some of the trigonelline *N*-methylnicotinic acid betaine to nicotinic acid; also, pretreatment of corn with limewater, as in the traditional preparation of tortillas in Mexico and Central America, releases much of the bound NAD precursor, tryptophan.

ADMET

The physiological effect of any ingested molecule depends on absorption, distribution, metabolism, excretion, and toxicity, together abbreviated as ADMET.

Absorption

Absorption of some nicotinic acid occurs by passive diffusion in the stomach. Both nicotinic acid and its amide are absorbed in the small intestine by a sodium (Na^+)-dependent saturable process as well as by passive diffusion that increases at higher nonphysiological concentrations of the vitamin (Bechgaard and Jespersen, 1977).

Distribution and Metabolism

Coenzyme forms of niacin in the gastrointestinal tract are first rapidly hydrolyzed to nicotinamide mononucleotide (NMN) by nonspecific pyrophosphatases in the intestinal lumen (Gross and Henderson, 1983). Alkaline phosphatase catalyzes further cleavage to nicotinamide riboside, which is converted to NAD by a two-step pathway starting with a reaction catalyzed by nicotinamide riboside kinase (see Figure 24-4) (Bieganowski and Brenner, 2004). NAD glycohydrolases (NADases) within mucosal cells may contribute to the breakdown of the coenzymes to nicotinamide. Once in the plasma, niacin enters cells by active or passive diffusion followed by metabolic trapping. Active diffusion of niacin into erythrocytes involves an anion transporter protein. Both erythrocytes and liver rapidly remove and convert niacin to NAD.

Tryptophan is an essential amino acid and also a precursor to NAD. Deficiencies of tryptophan transport (Hartnup disease) are primarily rescued by administering nicotinamide or nicotinic acid. Tryptophan is required for endogenous synthesis of NAD via the de novo pathway, which begins as the kynurenine pathway. This pathway requires

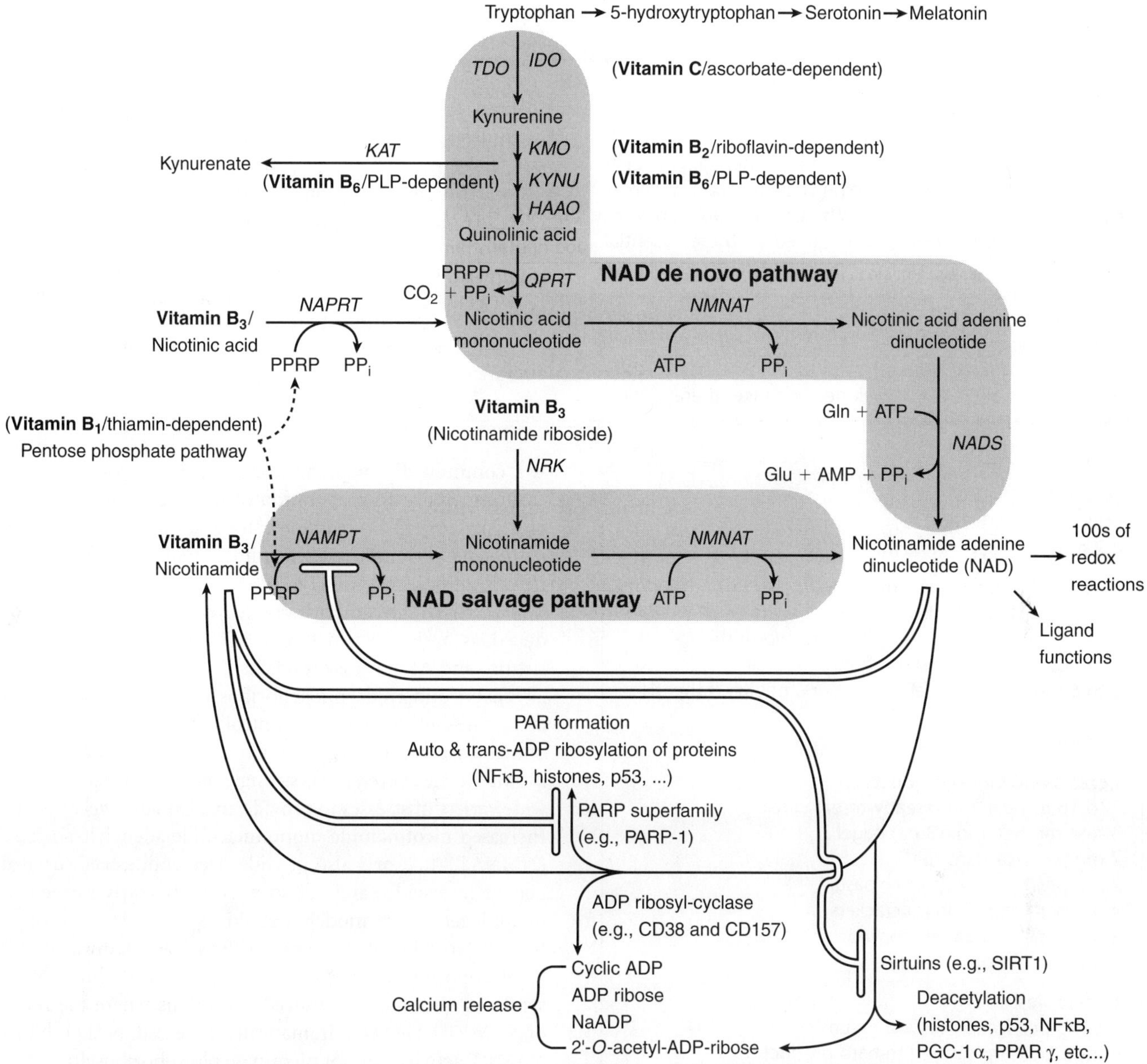

FIGURE 24-4 Pathways proceeding from vitamins or essential amino acid tryptophan to NAD synthesis and fates are shown. NAD is used by ADP ribosyl-cyclase and sirtuin to generate potent activators of intracellular calcium release. Additional vitamins required for completion of the de novo NAD synthesis pathway starting from tryptophan include vitamin B_2 (riboflavin), vitamin B_6 (pyridoxyl phosphate), and vitamin C (ascorbate). Otherwise, vitamin B_1 (thiamin) is required for synthesis of phosphoribosylpyrophosphate (PRPP) in the pentose phosphate pathway. Feedback inhibition loops are drawn with double lines. Nicotinic acid has distinguished capacity as a provider of NAD because nicotinate phosphoribosyltransferase (NAPRT) is not inhibited by NAD feedback inhibition (see text). By contrast when starting from nicotinamide, nicotinamide phosphoribosyltransferase (NAMPT) is inhibited by NAD. Nicotinic acid is converted to NAD via three reactions, whereas nicotinamide and nicotinamide riboside are converted to NAD via two reactions. The Preiss-Handler pathway begins with nicotinate combining with PRPP to make nicotinate mononucleotide (NaMN) in a reaction catalyzed by NAPRT. NaMN is then adenylated to form nicotinic acid adenine dinucleotide (NaAD) in an ATP-requiring reaction catalyzed by nicotinamide mononucleotide adenylyltransferase (NMNAT). NaAD is then converted to NAD by an ATP-requiring NAD synthetase (NADS) reaction, which transfers the amide from glutamine to NaMN to produce NAD. Nicotinamide and nicotinamide riboside are converted to NAD by just two reactions. Both are first converted to nicotinamide mononucleotide (NMN) followed by conversion to NAD in a reaction that requires ATP and is catalyzed by NMNAT. The NMNAT enzymes are used in NAD synthesis from all NAD precursors including tryptophan and nicotinic acid. *Gln,* Glutamine; *Glu,* glutamate; *HAAO,* 3-hydroxyanthranilate 3,4-dioxygenase; *IDO,* indoleamine 2,3-dioxygenase; *KAT,* kynurenine aminotransferase; *KMO,* kynurenine 3-monooxygenase; *KYNU,* kyureninase; *NRK,* nicotinamide riboside kinase; *PAR,* poly(ADP-ribose); *PARP,* PAR polymerase; *PPAR,* peroxisome proliferator-activated receptor, *QPRT,* quinolinate phosphoribosyltransferase; *TDO,* tryptophan 2,3-dioxygenase.

CLINICAL CORRELATION

Niacin and Cancer

Cancer cells require more NAD and ATP to survive than nontransformed healthy cells. The rate of glycolysis in a cancer cell is at least 30 times greater than that of a nontransformed cell, making it more susceptible to cell death when deprived of essential molecules. Essentially all cells starve to death after some point of deprivation, whereas cancer cells will starve to death sooner than nontransformed cells when both are deprived of these essential molecules. Inhibition of NAD pathways kills cancer cells with greater sensitivity than healthy cells. New chemotherapeutics are being developed to target inhibition of the NAD-synthesizing enzymes NAMPT and IDO, essentially using a metabolic approach to killing cancer. PARP1 inhibitors are also being developed as cancer therapeutics.

Thinking Critically

1. Given that cancer is a disease defined by genetic mutation and rapid cellular proliferation, should niacin intake be restricted during chemotherapy?
2. Caloric restriction also delays the onset of cancer. The body normally undergoes the process of cachexia during cancer. Given that cachexia resembles pellagra, which involves vitamin depletion, and that inhibition of NAD biosynthesis is more likely to kill rapidly growing cancer cells rather than healthy cells, is it possible that cachexia may be in part a desirable response of the body to attempt to control cancer?

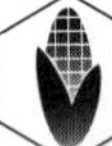

FOOD SOURCES OF PREFORMED NIACIN

Milk and Milk Products
0.2 mg per 1 cup whole milk

Meat and Meat Substitutes
14 mg per 3 oz beef liver
10 to 11 mg per 3 oz tuna, halibut, swordfish
7 mg per 3 oz rainbow trout
2 to 6 mg per 3 oz beef, lamb, pork, poultry, other fish
4 mg per 1 oz peanuts
0.05 mg per 1 egg

Cereals and Grain Products
2 to 10 mg per 1 cup ready-to-eat cereal
3 to 4 mg per 4-in. (3-oz) bagel
2 mg per 2-oz hard roll
2 mg per 1 cup noodles or pasta
4 mg per 1 cup graham crackers
3 mg per 1 cup barley, cooked
3 mg per 1 cup cooked rice

Vegetables
0.5 mg per 1 cup mustard greens
4 mg per 1 cup canned tomato product
3 mg per 1 cup mushrooms
2 mg per 1 cup corn
2 mg per 1 cup potatoes

Data from U.S. Department of Agriculture (USDA), Agricultural Research Service (ARS). (2010). *USDA National Nutrient Database for Standard Reference, Release 23.* Retrieved from www.ars.usda.gov/ba/bhnrc/ndl

riboflavin, pyridoxyl phosphate (vitamin B_6), and ascorbate (vitamin C) (see Figure 24-4). The de novo pathway is highly regulated by the immune system in specific cell types. Interferon gamma activates the rate-limiting enzyme, IDO, which is required for interferon gamma's biological activities. Many intermediates in this NAD synthetic pathway such as kynurenine and kynurenate have significant physiological roles. Persistent activation of IDO is seen in many autoimmune diseases and in cancer, where decreased serum tryptophan is a common diagnostic indicator of poor prognosis. The complementary administration of high doses of alternative NAD precursors has been repeatedly shown to rescue these pathogenic processes in both animal models and some clinical cases (Penberthy, 2007).

The NAD salvage pathway recycles nicotinamide produced as a side product of NAD-degradation by PARP, sirtuin, and ADP ribosyl-cyclases back to NAD (see Figure 24-4). Nicotinamide phosphoribosyltransferase (NAMPT) is the rate-limiting enzyme controlling the rate of recycling of nicotinamide to NAD (Revollo et al., 2004). Importantly, *NAMPT* gene expression is strongly induced in response to a wide variety of stresses to provide an adequate level of NAD. Increased nicotinamide mononucleotide adenylyltransferse (NMNAT)-1, 2, or 3 also provides tremendous cell survival benefit in a wide range of stresses, particularly as seen in neurodegenerative models (Sasaki et al., 2006). Although NAMPT may be rate limiting for the salvage pathway under basal conditions, the NMNAT enzymes may limit NAD synthesis under stress-induced conditions where the levels of NAMPT have been dramatically increased. NAD inhibits NAMPT activity but not nicotinate phosphoribosyltransferase (NAPRT). This is partially why nicotinic acid provides greater levels of intracellular NAD than nicotinamide for many cell types.

Excretion

Modest intake of niacin results in little excretion in the urine because both vitamers are actively reabsorbed from glomerular filtrates. Several *N*-methylnicotinate metabolites are formed enzymatically, primarily in the liver, and do appear in urine.

Toxicity

Over the past several decades, dyslipidemia has been commonly treated with 3 to 5 g of nicotinic acid daily without serious adverse events (Carlson, 2005; Guyton and Bays, 2007). However, the flush response can be exceedingly unpleasant. The upper tolerable intake level (UL) for adults is designated at 35 mg/day of niacin, limited to niacin

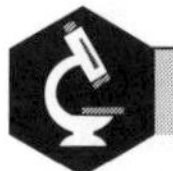

CLINICAL CORRELATION

Case Study of Pellagra in an Adult Woman

Oakley and Wallace (1994) reported a case involving a young woman in New Zealand who had a variety of neurological and dermal symptoms consistent with pellagra. However, she did not have diarrhea. Her symptoms were precipitated by prolonged lactation and increased activity. She had breast-fed her daughter for 3 years and had been particularly active while building her own home. Dietary intakes of niacin equivalents were within normal range. Her daily total excretion of urinary amino acids was abnormally high (77 mmol/L). Chromatography of urinary amino acids revealed elevated loss of tryptophan and other large neutral amino acids (alanine, serine, threonine, valine, methionine, isoleucine, tyrosine, and phenylalanine), whereas taurine, glycine, ornithine, lysine, arginine, and aspartate were present in normal amounts. Her symptoms were resolved after taking nicotinamide plus other B vitamins.

Thinking Critically

1. From the information given, what underlying metabolic abnormality was probably responsible for the development of pellagra in this woman with normal intake of niacin?
2. The first symptoms of pellagra secondary to inherited disorders usually occur in childhood. Why would periods of rapid growth or of prolonged lactation as in this case precipitate the appearance of pellagra? Why might increased activity precipitate the appearance of pellagra?

obtained from synthetic sources or fortified foods, based on the dose of nicotinic acid that can be associated with flushing effects. Although the flush can be uncomfortable, it is in fact linked to the beneficial effect of correcting dyslipidemia, because nicotinamide does not exert these therapeutically beneficial effects on lipid profiles.

BIOCHEMICAL ASSESSMENT OF NIACIN NUTRITURE, DIETARY REQUIREMENTS, AND HIGH-DOSE RESPONSES

BIOCHEMICAL ASSESSMENT OF NIACIN NUTRITURE

Biochemical assessment of niacin nutritional status is usually based on whole blood measures of NAD/NADP (Jacobson and Jacobson, 1997). Restricting niacin/tryptophan intake to 50% of the Recommended Dietary Allowance (RDA) decreases NAD by 70% within 5 weeks while NADP levels remain constant. A decrease in NAD levels precedes pellagra symptoms and are frequently seen in carcinoid syndrome patients.

DIETARY REQUIREMENTS

The RDA was first developed during World War II to set minimal standards for food relief during wartime. These standards are updated regularly. The Estimated Average Requirement (EAR) is a measure of the amount needed to satisfy the needs of 50% of the population, while the RDA is designed to satisfy the needs of 97% of the population. Because the amino acid tryptophan may also serve as a precursor for NAD synthesis, the term *niacin equivalent* (NE) is used to quantify niacin intakes and requirements.

For niacin the EAR is 12 mg and 11 mg of NEs per day for men and women, respectively. RDAs are calculated as 30% greater than the EAR (1 coefficient of variation = 15%). The RDA is relatively easy to meet, with typical intakes in the United States of 25 to 40 mg of NEs per day, but it should be recognized that tryptophan rather than niacin is the major source of NEs in typical diets.

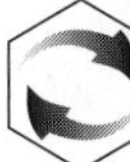

DRIs Across the Life Cycle: Niacin

	mg NE per Day	
Infants	RDA	UL*
0 through 6 mo	2 (AI)	ND
7 through 12 mo	4 (AI)	ND
Children		
1 through 3 yr	6	10
4 through 8 yr	8	15
9 through 13 yr	12	20
Males		
14 through 18 yr	16	30
≥19 yr	16	35
Females		
14 through 18 yr	14	30
≥19 yr	14	35
Pregnant		
<19 yr	18	30
≥19 yr	18	35
Lactating		
<19 yr	17	30
≥19 yr	17	35

Data from IOM. (1998). *Dietary Reference Intakes for thiamin, riboflavin, niacin, vitamin B_6, folate, vitamin B_{12}, pantothenic acid, biotin, and choline.* Washington, DC: National Academy Press.

AI, Adequate Intake; *DRI,* Dietary Reference Intake; *ND,* not determinable; *NE,* niacin equivalent; *RDA,* Recommended Dietary Allowance; *UL,* Tolerable Upper Intake Level.

*The niacin UL is in mg of preformed niacin and is not expressed in NEs. The UL applies to synthetic forms obtained from supplements, fortified foods, or a combination of the two.

The tryptophan content of proteins ranges from about 0.6% for corn to 1.5% for animal products. One should note that niacin values given in food composition tables usually do not take into account the bioavailability of niacin (e.g., from corn) and do not include an estimate of NEs available from tryptophan in the food. An estimated average conversion factor of 60 mg tryptophan to yield 1 mg niacin is used to calculate the NEs available from tryptophan. A diet in excess of 100 g protein per day can provide 16 mg NEs and meet the RDA without inclusion of preformed niacin.

Pregnancy, hormones, stress, and infections all affect tryptophan bioavailability. Steroid hormones (glucocorticoids and estrogens) elevate tryptophan dioxygenase and IDO. This decreases inflammation by reducing extracellular tryptophan while simultaneously increasing complementary NAD (Knox and Piras, 1967; Penberthy, 2009).

The upper tolerable intake level (UL) for adults is 35 mg/day of niacin, limited to preformed niacin obtained from synthetic sources or fortified foods, and is based on the dose of nicotinic acid that can be associated with flushing effects. The UL is not meant to apply to individuals who are receiving high-dose niacin for the treatment of dyslipidemia under medical supervision.

HIGH-DOSE NIACIN

Pharmacological doses of nicotinic acid (but not nicotinamide) exert lifesaving therapeutic benefits for heart disease by reducing serum cholesterol, triacylglycerol, and very-low-density lipoproteins (VLDLs) while increasing the concentration of high-density lipoproteins (HDLs) in plasma. All of these are therapeutically desirable changes for treating dyslipidemia. Ultimately high doses of niacin reduce mortality from heart disease even 10 years after discontinuation of the niacin (Canner et al., 1986).

The high-dose niacin effect on lipodystrophy occurs in part through activation of the high affinity nicotinic acid G protein–coupled receptors (GPCRs), GPR109a and GPR10b. Nicotinamide does not have appreciable affinity for these receptors and does not have the same beneficial effects on lipid profiles. Nicotinic acid–mediated activation of these receptors inhibits lipolysis in adipocytes, which ultimately exerts some beneficial effects on lipid parameters. Nicotinic acid GPCR signaling occurs via decreased intracellular cAMP (Tunaru et al., 2003). Prostaglandins are released from Langerhans cells followed by release from keratinocytes (Hanson et al., 2010). The prostaglandins PGE_2 and PGD_2 ultimately cause a strong vasodilation (flush) that can be very uncomfortable to some. The niacin flush is reduced in schizophrenics, so this is now used as a marker for schizophrenia (Messamore et al., 2003).

RIBOFLAVIN

Riboflavin (also known as vitamin B_2) serves a staggeringly wide range of vital functions and is similar to niacin in this respect. Riboflavin is required for fatty acid oxidation and mitochondrial electron transfer for ATP production. It is also required for essential human functions in vitamin B_6 coenzyme synthesis, DNA replication, DNA repair, protein disulfide formation, immune function, chromatin modification, cellular redox regulation, immunity, neurotransmitter clearance, regulation of blood pressure, amine catabolism, and circadian rhythm. The two physiological flavocoenzymes derived from the vitamin are riboflavin 5′-phosphate or flavin mononucleotide (FMN) and the more commonly used flavin adenine dinucleotide (FAD). There are approximately 170 proteins known to use FAD or FMN.

RIBOFLAVIN HISTORY

Riboflavin was originally isolated as a fluorescent fraction from milk by A. Wynter Blythe in 1879. However, it was not until 1933 that Kuhn, Gyorgy, and Wagner discovered physiological growth-promoting activities for the fluorescent component from thiamin-replete rice extracts in a rat model. Thiamin provided the heat-sensitive growth-promoting activity, whereas riboflavin provided the fluorescent heat-stable growth-promoting activity. One year later the independent laboratories of Kuhn and Karrer solved the structure of riboflavin.

Unlike pellagra and beriberi, no particular epidemic disease was historically ascribed to riboflavin deficiency or ariboflavinosis. Riboflavin has received the least biomedical research attention of the three B vitamins covered in this chapter, despite its essential roles described above. Today riboflavin deficiency continues to afflict populations of affluent societies and is endemic in some regions of the world.

RIBOFLAVIN NOMENCLATURE, STRUCTURE, AND BIOCHEMISTRY

Riboflavin is also known as 7,8-dimethyl-10-(1′-D-ribityl) isoalloxazine. "Ribo" refers to the ribityl side chain, and "flavin" is now synonymous with any substituted isoalloxazine. Riboflavin is also known as lactoflavin or vitamin G. The structure for this yellow, fluorescent, water-soluble compound is shown in Figure 24-5.

The isoalloxazone ring of FAD and FMN is considered the most chemically versatile redox cofactor in the cell. It is capable of one or two electron transfers in electron transport chains and in enzymes. This can lead to formation of double bonds, removal of double bonds or amine groups, and hydroxylation of aromatic molecules. Flavocoenzymes participate in oxidation–reduction reactions in numerous pathways and in energy production via the respiratory chain as shown in Figure 24-6.

Some flavoprotein-catalyzed dehydrogenations are pyridine nucleotide–dependent, whereas other dehydrogenations are independent reactions in which the pyridine nucleotides act as electron donors or acceptors. Other reactions involve sulfur-containing compounds, hydroxylations, oxidative decarboxylations, dioxygenations, and reduction of oxygen to hydrogen peroxide.

Most flavin coenzymes are noncovalently associated with the apoenzymic proteins, but a few flavins are covalently bound. Humans only possess a few known covalent flavoproteins. These are the mitochondrial 8α-*N*(3)-histidyl

Riboflavin (Vitamin B_2) **Flavin mononucleotide (FMN)** **Flavin adenine dinucleotide (FAD)**

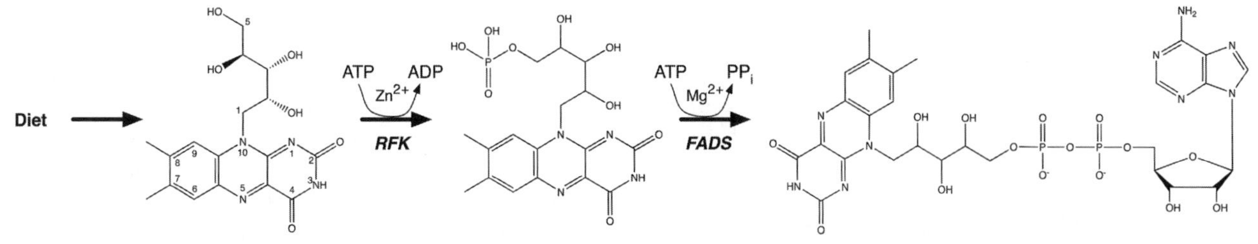

FIGURE 24-5 Riboflavin structure with numbering and pathway from vitamin to cofactor. We obtain vitamin B_2 from the plants or microbes that synthesize it. FAD is made by our bodies via reactions catalyzed by riboflavin kinase (RFK) and FAD synthetase (FADS, also known as FMN adenylyltransferase).

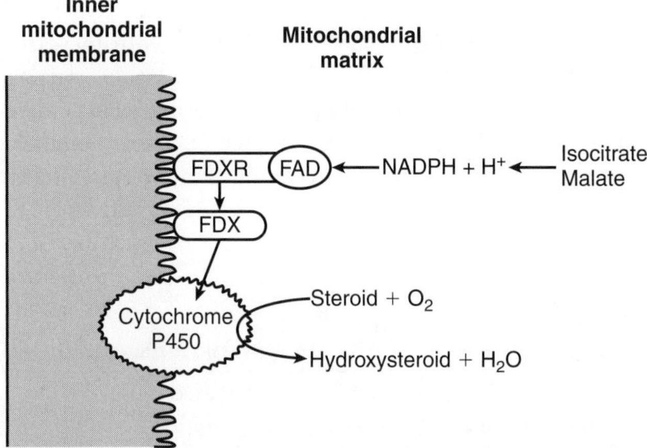

FIGURE 24-6 Obtaining reducing equivalents in the mitochondria for cytochrome P450. NADH and NADPH cannot be transported across the inner mitochondrial membrane, so reducing equivalents are obtained through malate or isocitrate, which enter via specific transporters. Electrons are transported via the flavin-dependent enzyme ferrodoxin reductase to cytochrome P450. Cytochrome P450 functions in the metabolism of cholesterol, xenobiotics, drugs, steroids, prostaglandins, and vitamins A and D. *FDXR,* Ferrodoxin reductase; *FDX,* ferrodoxin/adrenodoxin.

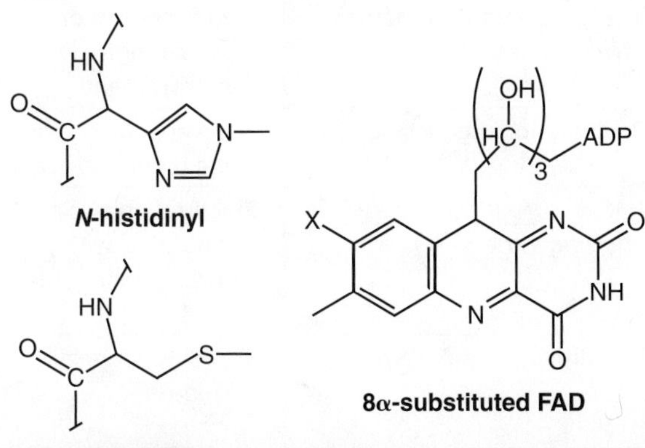

FIGURE 24-7 Representative covalent flavins in mammals where 8α-attachment is to such electronegative atoms as *N* or *S* within amino acid residues of enzymes.

(peptide)-FADs dehydrogenases (for succinate, sarcosine, and dimethylglycine), 8α-*S*-cysteinyl(peptide)-FAD of monoamine oxidase, and the nuclear lysine-specific demethylase. Structures for these mammalian covalent flavins are illustrated in Figure 24-7.

RIBOFLAVIN PHYSIOLOGICAL FUNCTION

Riboflavin ultimately serves a wide variety of physiological functions that have been identified in animal models and people with clinically important riboflavin deficiencies or riboflavin-responsive genetic disorders.

DIETARY DEFICIENCIES OF RIBOFLAVIN

The physiological responses to inadequate dietary intake of riboflavin are numerous and most strongly resemble both pellagra and vitamin B_6 deficiency. In people with ariboflavinosis, growth typically is stunted and a variety of skin lesions appear. Clinical features of ariboflavinosis include dermatitis, anemia, muscular weakness, soreness of the mouth and tongue, burning of the eyes, superficial vascularization of the cornea, and neuropathy.

Riboflavin serves essential roles early in development. Maternal ariboflavinosis can result in multiple acyl-CoA dehydrogenase deficiency (MADD) in the fetus (Chiong et al., 2007). A pregnancy-specific riboflavin binding protein is produced by the mother to insure that adequate riboflavin is delivered to the developing fetus. Experimental inactivation of pregnancy-specific riboflavin-binding protein leads to degeneration of the fetus due to absence of fetal FAD. This has been observed in monkeys, mice, and rats. Secretion of flavin into milk is an important source of riboflavin for the newborn (Roughead and McCormick, 1990). Riboflavin and its coenzyme derivatives are light sensitive. Newborn infants with hyperbilirubinemia treated with phototherapy commonly require additional riboflavin during treatment because of photoinactivation of riboflavin.

Enzyme activities are altered during ariboflavinosis. Riboflavin kinase is unstable in the absence of its riboflavin substrate, whereas FAD synthetase activity increases. Other proteins also become unstable. These changes may explain the relatively greater decrease in hepatic FMN than in FAD levels that occur in riboflavin deficiency. Marked decreases in the activities of FMN- and FAD-requiring enzymes, such as xanthine oxidase and glutathione reductase, also occur in tissues of riboflavin-deficient animals. Riboflavin deficiency in chicks further reveals nerve demyelination.

RIBOFLAVIN-RESPONSIVE GENETIC DISORDERS

The most common riboflavin-responsive genetic disorders are the multiple acyl-CoA dehydrogenase disorders (MADD), which arise from mutations in electron transfer flavoproteins (Table 24-2 [Er et al., 2010]). FAD-dependent acyl-CoA dehydrogenase enzymes catalyze the first step in the β-oxidation of lipids. Acyl-CoA dehydrogenase proteins transfer electrons from oxidized fatty acids to the electron transfer flavoprotein (ETF) complex—ETFα, ETFβ, and ETF dehydrogenase. Eventually these electrons are transferred to ubiquinone oxidoreductase in the respiratory chain. This pathway is a major source of energy for tissues including the heart, skeletal muscle, and liver. Mutation in any of these three ETFs results in MADD, some mutations of which are responsive to high-dose riboflavin administration. In MADD, these flavoproteins are less stable and have reduced half-life inside the cell.

Depending on the type of mutation, these diseases present phenotypes that range from neonatal cardiac defect with hepatic failure to adolescent myopathies. Null mutations are always associated with the severe phenotype, whereas missense mutations are sometimes responsive to riboflavin administration. Adult-onset MADD is strikingly responsive to riboflavin therapy, with plasma acylcarnitine and acid profiles returning to normal after administration of 100 mg/day of riboflavin in combination with carnitine (Liang et al., 2009). Administration of hundreds of milligrams of riboflavin also results in significant motor and cognitive improvement in patients with a mutation in another dehydrogenase encoding gene, the *L2HGDH* gene (Yilmaz, 2009), which converts L-2-hydroxyglutaric acid to α-ketoglutarate in a FAD-dependent fashion.

The methylenetetrahydrofolate reductase *(MTHFR)* genetic polymorphism C677T is correlated with increased incidence of cardiovascular disease, neural tube defects, Down syndrome, congenital cardiac malformations, dementia, and other conditions (see Chapter 25). This polymorphism is located in the FAD binding domain resulting in decreased FAD binding, decreased MTHFR activity, and

TABLE 24-2 Riboflavin-Responsive Genetic Disorders

DISEASE	SYMPTOMS	GENETIC MUTATION	RIBOFLAVIN RESCUE
Multiple acyl-CoA dehydrogenase deficiency, MADD (also known as glutaric aciduria type II)	Excessive excretion of glutaric, lactic, ethylmalonic, butyric, isobutyric, 2-methyl butyric, and isovaleric acids; symptoms range from fetal lethal hepatic failure to adult-onset myopathy	Electron transfer flavoprotein (ETF) A (alpha subunit) and B (beta subunit) and ETF dehydrogenase (ETFDH) resulting in glutaric aciduria IIA, IIB, and IIC respectively (the most common fatty acid metabolism error)	Increased muscle strength, correction of β-oxidation, reduced hydroxyglutarate
Very-long-chain acyl-CoA dehydrogenase (VLCAD) deficiency	Neonatal cardiomyopathy, infantile hepatic coma, or adult-onset myopathy	*VLCAD*	Unknown
Other acyl-CoA dehydrogenase deficiencies (unidentified at present)	Wide range	Unknown	Unknown
L-2-Hydroxyglutaric aciduria, LHGuria	Macrocephaly, cerebellar ataxia, central nervous system tumors, and mental retardation	*L2HGDH,* L-2-hydroxyglutarate dehydrogenase	Significant motor and cognitive improvement
Glutathione reductase	Lupus-like symptoms	*GSR,* glutathione reductase	Recovery of glutathione reductase activity
Succinate CoQ reductase deficiency (also known as defective mitochondrial complex II)	Progressive motor and mental deterioration	*SDHAF* or *SDHAF1,* succinate dehydrogenase	Stabilization of clinical conditions with cognitive impairment
Mitochondrially encoded tRNA leucine 1 (MTTL1) deficiency	Severe muscle weakness	*MTTL,* mitochondrial tRNA leucine	Improved muscle strength
Combined oxidative phosphorylation deficiency 6, COXPD6	Early onset neurodegeneration	*AIFM1,* apoptosis-inducing factor	Some improvement of movement ability

ultimately increased plasma homocysteine. Riboflavin supplementation of *MTHFR* C677T-containing lymphocytes increases the stability of this otherwise labile enzyme. Thus it makes sense to consider supplementing with riboflavin in these individuals (Ames et al., 2002).

PROTEINS THAT REQUIRE RIBOFLAVIN

One of the most exciting discoveries in riboflavin research has been elucidation of the role of FAD in TNF-mediated activation of NADPH oxidase (Yazdanpanah et al., 2009). FAD plays a central role in energy production as part of both β-oxidation and the electron transport system. However, flavins also participate in a wide range of enzyme functions besides mitochondrial bioenergetics, including:

- Detoxification (flavin monooxygenases)
- Redox status regulation (glutathione reductase, thioredoxin reductase, and quinone oxidoreductase)
- Basic protein disulfide maturation (Ero1-α)
- Detoxification (flavin monooxygenases)
- Neurotransmitter catabolism (monoamine oxidase)
- Cellular methylation (methylenetetrahydrofolate reductase)
- Circadian rhythm (cryptochromes)
- DNA repair (cryptochromes)
- Amine catabolism (spermine oxidase)
- DNA replication (methylenetetrahydrofolate reductase)
- Immune function (NADPH oxidases and nitric oxide synthases)
- Histone methylation-mediated transcriptional regulation (lysine-specific demethylase)

The functions of proteins that use FAD or FMN are overwhelming; however, the therapeutic potential of high-dose riboflavin is largely unexamined. There are over 150 different flavoproteins; several of the most significant ones are briefly covered here. The photoresponsive chromophore in the cryptochrome flavoproteins is involved in both photoreactive repair of UV-damaged DNA and in controlling light-responsive circadian rhythm. Absence of cryptochromes results in a mouse with no internal clock. Both glutathione reductase and thioredoxin reductase are flavoproteins that serve essential functions in controlling endogenous antioxidant levels in the cell. The sulfhydryl oxidase Ero1 (endoplasmic reticulum oxidoreductase 1) is rate limiting in controlling disulfide bond formation, an essential process

CLINICAL CORRELATION

Multiple Acyl-CoA Dehydrogenase Disorders and Riboflavin

Multiple acyl-CoA dehydrogenase disorders (MADD) (also known as glutaric acidemia type II) result in excretion of various organic acids and esters of fatty acids with glycine or carnitine in the urine. The omega-oxidation of fatty acids to dicarboxylic acids and the transesterification of acyl groups with carnitine and glycine are the result of alternative pathways of metabolism for substrates that accumulate because they cannot enter the normal catabolic pathways.

Cultured skin fibroblasts from patients with MADD have a severely reduced capacity for oxidation of a variety of organic acyl CoAs, including short-, medium-, and long-chain fatty acyl CoAs. Although the oxidation of these metabolites requires several different substrate-specific dehydrogenases, this group of dehydrogenases shares a common oxidation agent, an electron transfer flavoprotein (ETF) that contains tightly bound flavin adenine diphosphate (FAD). The ETF-$FADH_2$ complex is reoxidized by ETF dehydrogenase with reduction of coenzyme Q (ubiquinone) to connect the flow of electrons to the electron transfer chain and eventually oxygen, to form water and generate ATP. Multiple acyl-CoA dehydrogenase deficiencies are attributed to a defect of either ETF or ETF dehydrogenase.

Multiple acyl-CoA dehydrogenase disorders most commonly present in infancy with failure to thrive and repeated episodes of vomiting, lethargy, and coma with dicarboxylate aciduria and hypoglycemia. Mild or late-onset forms of multiple acyl-CoA dehydrogenase disorders are more rare and the clinical picture is variable.

Diagnosis of MADD was made for a 62-year-old man who was admitted to a hospital because of easy fatigue to his legs during walking (Araki et al., 1994). He had also experienced fatigue to his neck muscles from holding his head erect. Biopsied muscle samples showed excessive lipid accumulation. The muscle-free carnitine concentration was at the lower end of the normal range, and the ratio of acylcarnitine to free carnitine in skeletal muscle was elevated. The concentrations of lactate and pyruvate in the blood were within the normal range in the resting state but were markedly increased after a 7.5-minute walk. Riboflavin therapy resulted in a dramatic improvement in both clinical and biochemical parameters.

Thinking Critically

1. In this adult patient, how could you explain the excessive lipid storage in muscle? How would you explain muscle fatigue?
2. In this situation, a defect in FAD binding to ETF dehydrogenase was suspected. Why?
3. What dietary recommendations would you make for children with multiple acyl-CoA dehydrogenase deficiency in terms of fat, carbohydrate, and protein intake? Would energy production via aerobic oxidation of glucose be affected in these patients? Explain.
4. Secondary carnitine deficiency has been diagnosed in a number of cases, as in this adult patient. Plasma-free carnitine is typically lower or undetectable, but acylcarnitine is present in plasma. Marked improvements have been observed in patients following carnitine supplementation. What is the possible basis for the carnitine deficiency or the accumulation of acylcarnitine?

particularly crucial for maturation of secreted proteins. This includes riboflavin-binding protein itself, which requires formation of nine disulfide bonds. Lysine-specific demethylase uses covalently bound FAD to remove methyl groups from histones, to loosen chromatin structure, and to allow gene transcription. Both NADPH oxidase and nitric oxide synthase use FAD. NADPH oxidase catalyzes the first step in controlled endogenous free radical generation in the neutrophil oxidative burst. After riboflavin kinase binds both the NADPH oxidase enzyme and the TNFα-receptor, riboflavin kinase converts riboflavin to FMN (see Figure 24-5). Elimination of riboflavin kinase results in an embryonic lethal mouse phenotype. Significantly, administration of TNFα increases production of FAD starting from riboflavin, where FAD can substitute for TNFα in signaling for activation of the NADPH oxidase free radical generating pathway. This is consistent with the many previous examples revealing antiinfectious activities for riboflavin as described in the next section. Although the current RDA is enough under otherwise healthy conditions, these studies collectively indicate that higher doses of riboflavin may be needed to treat infectious disease.

NADPH oxidase functions in immune responses, angiogenesis, intracellular redox reactions, cell growth, and cross talk with the nitric oxide systems. Nitric oxide enzymes control blood flow, blood pressure, and immune response to infection. Kynurenine monooxygenase is needed for the essential production of NAD starting from the endogenous substrate tryptophan. NAD(P)H:quinone oxidoreductases (NQO) and quinone reductases (QR) prevent generation of semiquinones by directing two hydride reductions to hydroquinones. Otherwise, the semiquinone species react with oxygen to produce oxygen radicals. Thus, NQO serves important roles in detoxification of environmental quinones, as NQO expression is highly induced in response to various stressors. A similar protein, QR, is associated with the proteosome and controls protein degradation. The potential dependence of these physiological activities on riboflavin concentration is poorly understood. Whether FAD is actively depleted by activation of any particular enzymes is largely unknown. This stands in stark contrast to the well-established major NAD-consuming pathways described in the previous section.

RIBOFLAVIN SOURCES, CHEMICAL STABILITY, AND ADMET

SOURCES

Riboflavin is made only in plants and some bacteria, where riboflavin biosynthesis is regulated by a unique mechanism involving RNA that specifically recognizes riboflavin. Riboflavin in most foods is mainly in coenzymatic forms, with over two thirds typically as FAD. Milk and eggs, however, possess relatively large amounts of free riboflavin bound to specific binding proteins. The exceptionally high total riboflavin content in milk and eggs is indicative of the particularly important role of riboflavin in fetal development.

FOOD SOURCES OF RIBOFLAVIN

Milk and Milk Products
0.5 mg per 8 oz yogurt
0.45 mg per 1 cup milk
0.4 mg per 1 cup cottage cheese

Cereals and Grain Products
0.4 to 1.0 mg per 1 cup ready-to-eat cereal
0.3 mg per 4-in. (3-oz) bagel
0.2 mg per 1 cup graham crackers

Meat and Meat Substitutes
0.3 mg per 3 oz pork
0.25 mg per 1 egg

Vegetables
0.3 mg per 1 cup spinach
0.3 mg per 1 cup mushrooms
0.3 mg per 1 cup soybeans

Data from USDA, ARS. (2010). *USDA National Nutrient Database for Standard Reference, Release 23.* Retrieved from www.ars.usda.gov/ba/bhnrc/ndl

Approximately one third of the adult RDA for riboflavin is supplied in the American diet by milk and milk-based products (Block et al., 1985). Meats and green vegetables supply much of the rest. Although cereals are rather poor sources, enriched flour and breakfast cereals contribute significant amounts of riboflavin.

CHEMICAL STABILITY

Riboflavin and its phosphate, flavin mononucleotide (FMN), are relatively heat stable in slightly acidic and neutral conditions and become more labile in basic conditions. Cleavage of the ribityl side chain with loss of vitamin activity occurs when solutions that contain riboflavin are exposed to light, producing the photoproducts lumichrome and lumiflavin. The use of riboflavin for the inactivation of pathogens of the blood supply is under investigation. Riboflavin-induced photo-activation of pathogens in blood components that contain no nucleic acids (e.g., erythrocytes, thrombocytes, and plasma) is due to the ability of light-excited flavin to photooxidize bases, especially guanyl residues, in the nucleic acids of bacterial and viral pathogens (Goodrich, 2000).

ADMET

Absorption

After ingestion, gastric acidification and subsequent proteolysis releases flavocoenzymes from their noncovalent bonds to proteins. Nonspecific action by pyrophosphatases (nucleotidohydrolases) and phosphomonoesterase (alkaline phosphatase) on the flavin coenzymes occurs in the upper small intestine.

Riboflavin is absorbed by two different concentration-dependent mechanisms. At physiological concentrations (less than 12 nM), riboflavin is absorbed by a saturable active sodium-dependent transporter that brings the vitamin into the cell. Three high affinity riboflavin transporters (RFT1, RFT2, and RFT3) have been identified in humans (Yao et al., 2010; Yonezawa et al., 2008). These are most highly expressed in placenta (RFT1), testes (RFT2), and brain (RFT3); RFT1 and RFT2 are also highly expressed in small intestine. At higher pharmacological concentrations (greater than 12 nM), riboflavin can enter cells by diffusion, only limited by the low solubility of riboflavin. Intake and apparent absorption increase proportionately up to about 27 mg in a single dose with little further absorption observed at higher intakes (Zempleni et al., 1996).

Distribution

Riboflavin circulating in plasma is loosely associated with albumin, immunoglobulins, and other proteins (Innis et al., 1985). FAD concentrations vary in different tissues; for example, hepatocytes are more susceptible to riboflavin deficiency than lymphocytes. Ultimately this results in less hepatic secretion, greater oxidative damage, and fewer liver cells (Werner et al., 2005).

Metabolism

Flavocoenzymes are formed by a sequential pathway that involves two molecules of ATP, riboflavin kinase, and FAD synthetase, as shown in Figure 24-5. These cytosolic enzymes are widely distributed in tissues. Thyroid hormone increases riboflavin kinase activity by conversion of the enzyme from a less active to a more active form (Lee and McCormick, 1985). The FAD synthetase is inhibited by its product, FAD (Yamada et al., 1990). In the covalent attachment of FAD, the apoenzyme itself catalyzes the flavinylation (Decker, 1993). Phosphorylation of riboflavin by riboflavin kinase results in the metabolic trapping of riboflavin-5-phosphate inside the cell (Aw et al., 1983; Bowers-Komro and McCormick, 1987). Riboflavin catabolism in mammals varies, and many products reflect the action of microflora in the gut and the effects of photodegradation (Chastain, 1991).

Excretion

Most flavins are noncovalently bound to enzymes as FAD. However, unbound FAD is relatively labile in vivo, where it is rapidly hydrolyzed back to riboflavin, readily diffuses out of cells, and is excreted in the urine as riboflavin or 7-hydroxymethylriboflavin. Riboflavin is removed from both peripheral circulation and the brain via active sodium-dependent transporters expressed in renal tubular cells and the choroid plexus. Because there is little storage of riboflavin, the urinary excretion of flavins (0.3 mg/day in normal adults) reflects dietary intake. For normal adults eating varied diets, riboflavin accounts for 60% to 70% of urinary flavin. Negligible amounts of riboflavin are excreted in the urine of people with ariboflavinosis.

Toxicity

Riboflavin has low toxicity, with no reported cases in humans. This may be due to its low solubility or to the ready excretion of unbound riboflavin in the urine.

BIOCHEMICAL ASSESSMENT OF RIBOFLAVIN NUTRITURE AND DIETARY REQUIREMENTS

BIOCHEMICAL ASSESSMENT OF RIBOFLAVIN NUTRITURE

The most common method to assess riboflavin status is the augmentation of glutathione reductase activity in freshly lysed erythrocytes after incubation with FAD in vitro. Either a low absolute activity of erythrocyte glutathione reductase or an elevated fractional stimulation of that activity by addition of FAD is indicative of riboflavin deficiency. Urinary riboflavin excretion (24 hours) of less than 10% of that ingested also may reflect inadequate nutrition. The concentration of riboflavin in erythrocytes has also been used as an indicator of riboflavin status, with values less than 0.15 mg/L considered as low or deficient. The activity of pyridoxine 5'-phosphate oxidase (see Chapter 25), a FMN-dependent enzyme, is responsive to changes in riboflavin intake and is a potentially superior biomarker of riboflavin status for people with glucose-6-phosphate dehydrogenase deficiency (Mushtaq et al., 2009), the most common human enzyme defect.

DIETARY REQUIREMENTS

Riboflavin requirements have been related to protein allowances, lean body mass, metabolic body size, and energy intake. Urinary excretion of riboflavin rises as dietary riboflavin is increased from 0.5 to 0.75 mg/1,000 kcal. Based on intakes that prevent clinical and biochemical signs of deficiency, the Institute of Medicine (IOM, 1998) set the EAR for riboflavin at 1.1 mg/day for men and 0.9 mg/day for women. The RDA was set as the EAR +20% (IOM, 1998), with slightly higher increments for pregnant and lactating women. The IOM (1998) established Adequate Intake (AI) for infants from birth through 6 months of age based on the average intake of riboflavin by breast-fed infants (0.35 mg riboflavin/L milk × 0.78 L milk/day + 0.3 mg/day). The AI for older infants was extrapolated from values for younger infants and adults. EARs and RDAs for children were estimated by extrapolation from adult values on the basis of metabolic body weight plus an allowance for growth. Based on data from the National Health and Nutrition Examination Survey (NHANES) III, the median intake of riboflavin from food in the United States is 2.0 mg/day for men and 1.6 mg/day for women. The range of intakes (5th to 95th percentile levels) is 1.2 to 3.6 mg/day for men and 1.0 to 2.8 mg/day for women. Therefore intakes for nearly all adults in the United States exceed the RDA.

Riboflavin deficiencies have been associated with increased risk for anemia, cancer, cardiovascular disease, and neurodegeneration. Riboflavin deficiency is endemic in populations that do not consume milk and milk products. In the Western world, the populations at greatest risk for ariboflavinosis are the young, immunocompromised, and the elderly, most of whom are highly responsive to even minimal amounts (e.g., 1 mg) of riboflavin (Gariballa et al., 2009).

Riboflavin-deficient diets have been shown to cause corneal vascularization, opacity, and cataracts; however, clinical

NUTRITION INSIGHT

Riboflavin Status Biomarkers

Ideally, a biomarker for riboflavin should correlate with as many physiologically significant changes as possible while being detectable as early as possible. Given that over 150 unique proteins use riboflavin, it comes as no surprise that the biochemical assessment of riboflavin status continues to be an active area of research, and up to 14 different biomarkers have been considered (Hoey et al., 2009). For example, glutathione reductase is insensitive to poor riboflavin status in individuals with glucose-6-phosphate dehydrogenase (G6PD) deficiency. By contrast the FMN-dependent enzyme pyridoxamine phosphate oxidase (PPO) activity is detectably increased and responds to riboflavin in individuals with G6PD deficiency. Thus PPO is a more physiologically sensitive indicator of riboflavin status. This is likely because PPO itself serves immediately essential functions in the conversion of vitamin B_6 to its active form.

Thinking Critically

1. Given the wide array of symptoms connected with ariboflavinosis, what would be the most reliable physiological indicator?
2. Given the many functions of riboflavin, which physiological activity or pathogenic process would you predict to be most likely to cause a loss of riboflavin-associated coenzymes: intense physical exercise, DNA damaging agents, hyperexcitable tissues (e.g., seizures), accumulation of toxins such as polychlorobiphenols, bacterial infections, yeast infections, or compromised immune systems?
3. Vigorous exercise can deplete riboflavin. However, little difference in riboflavin status is observed in athletes compared to nonathletes. Why might this be and what are the implications?

studies are lacking. Riboflavin-responsive night blindness has also been observed, and there are well-characterized riboflavin-dependent photoreceptors and cryptochromes. These cryptochromes are known to play a role in dark adaptation.

Anemia, defined as a hemoglobin concentration less than 110g/L, has been observed in 48% of rural Chinese women in their third trimester. A systematic study of supplementations revealed that riboflavin increased the hemoglobin counts more than iron and folate alone (Ma et al., 2008).

There have been several studies examining riboflavin for treating migraines. Benefits have been reported for children and adolescents treated with 200 to 400 mg/day (Condo et al., 2009). No adverse events were seen. However, the current opinion in the field remains uncertain.

Several genetic diseases arising from mutations in the FAD-binding domain of proteins are known to result in an increased K_m for the coenzyme. These diseases are dramatically responsive to higher doses of riboflavin. MADD in newborns can also arise from nongenetic causes such as maternal riboflavin deficiency.

DRIs Across the Life Cycle: Riboflavin

	mg Riboflavin per Day*
Infants	RDA
0 through 6 mo	0.3 (AI)
7 through 12 mo	0.4 (AI)
Children	
1 through 3 yr	0.5
4 through 8 yr	0.6
9 through 13 yr	0.9
Males	
≥14 yr	1.3
Females	
14 through 18 yr	1.0
≥19 yr	1.1
Pregnant	1.4
Lactating	1.6

Data from IOM. (1998). *Dietary Reference Intakes for thiamin, riboflavin, niacin, vitamin B_6, folate, vitamin B_{12}, pantothenic acid, biotin, and choline.* Washington, DC: National Academy Press.
AI, Adequate Intake; *DRI*, Dietary Reference Intake; *RDA*, Recommended Dietary Allowance.
*Note: There is no established Tolerable Upper Intake Level (UL) for riboflavin.

THIAMIN

Thiamin is the first identified B vitamin. Although it is essential for all known forms of life for energy production and DNA synthesis, only bacteria, plants, and fungi are capable of synthesizing thiamin. Thiamin is also distinguished as the only vitamin covered in this chapter for which a toxin evolved in nature to specifically target its destruction.

THIAMIN HISTORY

Feeding chicks with a heat sensitive thiamin-containing factor present in rice polishings can reverse polyneuropathy in spastic chicks fed only white rice. Christiaan Eijkman was awarded the Nobel Prize in 1929 for this work performed in the 1890s with spastic chicks (Eijkman, 1990). Dr. Umetaro Suzuki made similar observations independently in Japan. All of this work led to the discovery that a component of rice hulls could reverse the thiamin deficiency disease beriberi.

It was not until 1933 that Dr. Roger J. Williams purified thiamin. When dogs were fed a thiamin-deficient diet of boiled meat and polished rice, they succumbed to beriberi within weeks; but the addition of thiamin rescued them. Eijkman, like Joseph Goldberg with the disease of pellagra, advanced research by reversing previous misunderstandings of these as infectious diseases, revealing the cause as dietary deficiency.

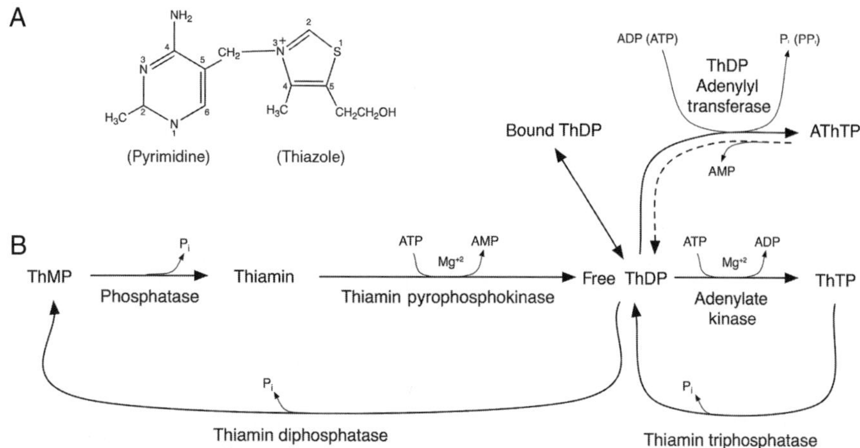

FIGURE 24-8 Thiamin structure (**A**) and phosphorylation (**B**). Thiamin has two functional aromatic rings, pyrimidine and thiazole. Two phosphates are attached to the hydroxyl group of thiamin to make thiamin diphosphate (ThDP; also known as thiamin pyrophosphate), the active form of cofactor. ThDP can be converted back to either thiamin triphosphate (ThTP) or thiamin monophosphate (ThMP). Little is known regarding the physiological significance of the adenosine thiamin triphosphate (AThTP). AThTP is present in muscle and brain, but the pathways are not entirely understood.

THIAMIN NOMENCLATURE, STRUCTURE, AND BIOCHEMISTRY

NOMENCLATURE AND STRUCTURE

Vitamin B_1 is a pyrimidyl-substituted thiazole (3-[2-methyl-4-aminopyrimidinyl]methyl-4-methyl-5-[β-hydroxyethyl] thiazole), as illustrated in Figure 24-8. The principal if not sole coenzyme form of thiamin is thiamin diphosphate (ThDP), which is also known as thiamin pyrophosphate. In eukaryotes, approximately 80% to 90% of thiamin is observed as ThDP, with approximately 10% as free thiamin. ThDP is also the precursor for thiamin monophosphate (ThMP; approximately less than 1% of cellular thiamin), thiamin triphosphate (ThTP; approximately 0.1% to 1% of cellular thiamin), and thiaminylated adenines (adenosine thiamin triphosphate [AThTP]; adenosine thiamine diphosphate [AThDP]). Very little is understood regarding the functions of ThMP, ThTP, AThTP, and AThDP.

BIOCHEMISTRY

The two major types of ThDP-dependent biochemical reactions are decarboxylations and the transfer of two carbon fragments from a ketose to an aldose. Decarboxylation of α-keto acids involves condensation of the thiazole with the α-carbonyl carbon on the acid, which leads to loss of CO_2 with production of a resonance-stabilized carbanion. These ThDP-dependent (and FAD- and NAD-dependent) α-keto acid dehydrogenase complexes are used to catalyze the oxidative decarboxylation of pyruvate to acetyl-CoA, α-ketoglutarate to succinyl-CoA, and the α-keto acids from branched-chain amino acids to their respective acyl-CoAs. ThDP is also used for transformation of α-ketols (ketose phosphates); these sugar rearrangements are essential for synthesis of ribose and oxidation of glucose by the pentose phosphate pathway. Another important role of ThDP is in the α-oxidation of 3-methyl-branched fatty acids, such as phytanic acid, which undergo shortening by one carbon in a process that includes activation, 2-hydroxylation, a ThDP-dependent cleavage, and aldehyde dehydrogenation. Failure of this system, mostly linked to the second enzyme of the sequence, phytanoyl-CoA hydroxylase, results in Refsum disease (Casteels et al., 2003). Metabolic pathways critically dependent upon ThDP are summarized in Figures 24-9 and 24-10.

THIAMIN PHYSIOLOGICAL FUNCTION

We can learn about thiamin function by considering the clinical symptoms of thiamin deficiency or the phenotype of thiamin-responsive genetic disorders. Thiamin is required for the synthesis of all nucleotides and is therefore required for production of ATP, ribose, and NAD, as well as DNA. Thiamin deficiency affects a wide range of cellular functions with diverse effects on the human body.

DIETARY DEFICIENCIES OF THIAMIN

Dietary thiamin deficiency results when milled unenriched grains such as rice and wheat make up the majority of the diet. Clinical signs of deficiency primarily involve the nervous and cardiovascular systems. In infants, symptoms appear suddenly and severely, often involving cardiac failure and cyanosis (bluish coloration of skin and mucous membranes due to deficient oxygenation of the blood). Adult symptoms most frequently observed are mental confusion, anorexia, muscular weakness, ataxia, eye paralysis, edema (wet beriberi), muscle wasting (dry beriberi), tachycardia, and an enlarged heart.

Commonly, the distinction between wet (cardiovascular) and dry (neuritic) manifestations of beriberi relate to duration and severity of the deficiency, the degree of physical exertion, and caloric intake. The wet or edematous condition results from severe physical exertion and high carbohydrate intake. The dry or polyneuritic form stems from

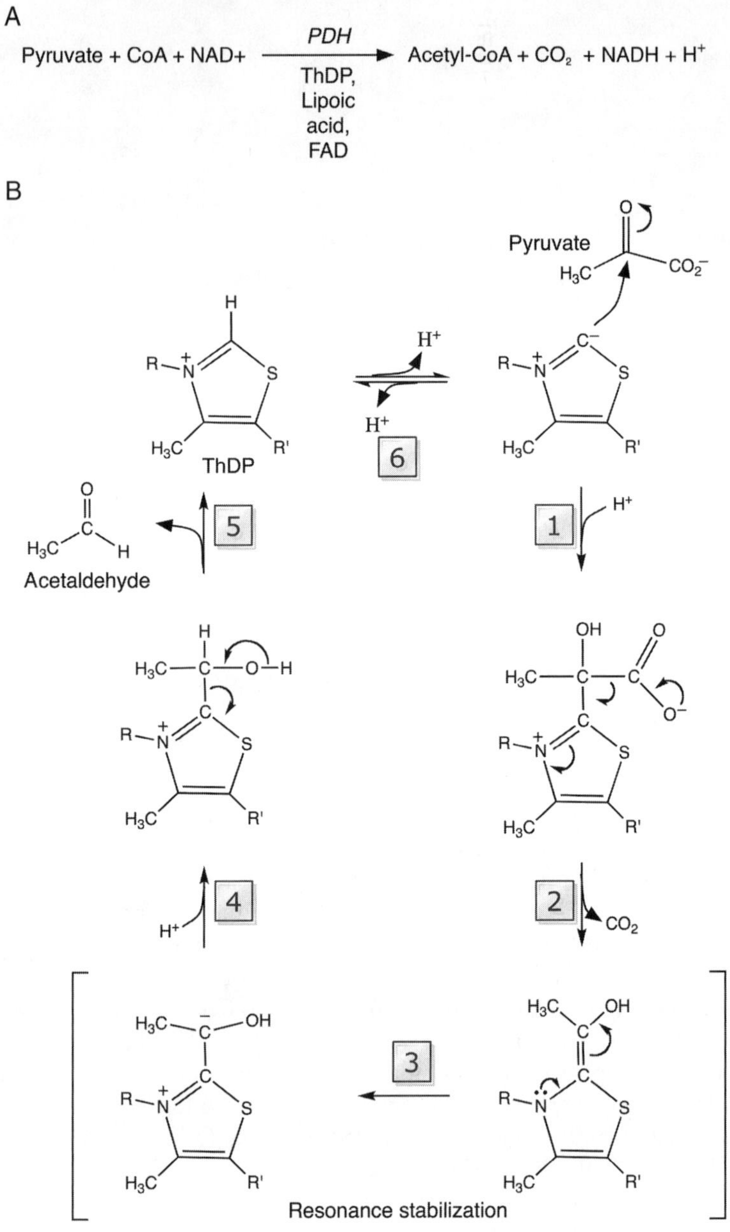

FIGURE 24-9 The role of thiamin disphosphate (ThDP) in pyruvate decarboxylase (E1, the first of three enzymes in the pyruvate dehydrogenase [PDH] complex) is shown. **A,** The *PDH* enzyme is above the reaction arrow, and cofactors are shown below the arrow. **B,** The enzyme mechanism involving ThDP and the E1 of the PDH complex is shown. Acetaldehyde is depicted here as a free molecule, but it actually is transferred to the lipoic acid moiety of the E2 (second enzyme) of the PDH complex.

relative inactivity with caloric restriction along with chronic thiamin deficiency. The three major physiological derangements that involve the cardiovascular system are peripheral vasodilation that leads to a high cardiac output state, myocardial failure, and water retention that leads to edema. Nervous system involvement includes peripheral neuropathy, Wernicke encephalopathy, and the amnesic psychosis of Korsakoff syndrome.

Thiamin deficiency can be caused by ingestion of agents that actively destroy endogenous thiamin, such as excessive alcohol, sulfites, thiaminase toxin, or certain drugs. Chronic alcoholism is a common contributor to deficiency in that there is not only a low intake of thiamin (and other B vitamins) but also impaired absorption and storage. Sulfites are used by the food and the wine industries to kill bacteria; however, they can degrade thiamin by breaking the methylene bridge to the thiazole nitrogen. Ingestion of sulfites can lead to sudden breathing difficulties or migraines within minutes. In rare cases, sulfite consumption has even resulted in death. In 1986 use of sulfites for preventing spoilage of raw fruits and vegetables was banned. Raw fish and ferns contain thiaminases, which are enzymes that hydrolytically destroy thiamin in the gastrointestinal tract. Others who are at risk of thiamin deficiency include patients undergoing long-term renal dialysis, treatment with loop diuretics (e.g., furosemide), and even those with chronic febrile infections.

THIAMIN-RESPONSIVE GENETIC DISORDERS

Thiamin-responsive genetic disorders commonly manifest as diabetes and anemia, indicating chief roles for thiamin in controlling glucose homeostasis and hematopoiesis. Thiamin-responsive inborn errors of metabolism are shown in Table 24-3.

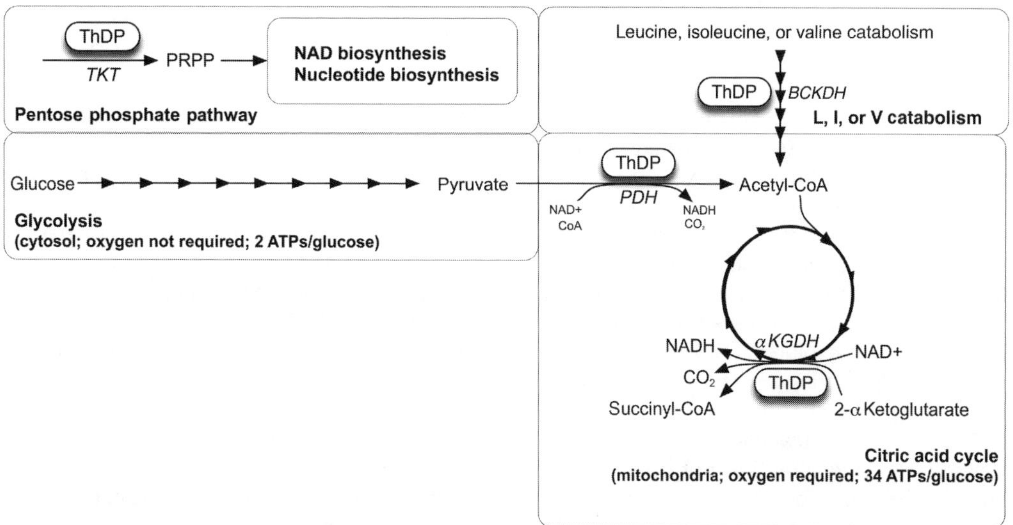

FIGURE 24-10 Thiamin diphosphate (ThDP) is required for biochemical synthesis of ATP, NAD, and nucleotides. Accordingly, thiamin is essential to life on multiple levels. ThDP-dependent reactions include the cytosolic transketolase (pentose phosphate pathway) and three mitochondrial enzyme complexes: pyruvate dehydrogenase (PDH) complex, α-ketoglutarate dehydrogenase (αKGDH) complex, and branched-chain α-ketoglutarate dehydrogenase (BCKDH) complex. *PRPP,* Phosphoribosylpyrophosphate; *TKT*, transketolase.

TABLE 24-3 Thiamin-Responsive Genetic Disorders

DISEASE	SYMPTOMS	GENETIC MUTATION	THIAMIN RESCUE
Pyruvate decarboxylase deficiency (also known as pyruvate dehydrogenase deficiency or as ataxia with lactic acidosis)	Ataxia, severe lactic acidosis usually leading to death in the newborn; lethargic, seizures, mental retardation	*PDHA1*, E1-α polypeptide of the pyruvate dehydrogenase complex	Improvement in lactic acid levels, pyruvate levels, and neurological symptoms
Wernicke-Korsakoff syndrome	Amnesia, ataxia, ocular abnormalities including nystagmus	Unknown	Nystagmus in minutes; ataxia recovery in days to weeks
Maple syrup urine disease, branched-chain α-keto acid dehydrogenase deficiency	Mental and physical retardation, block on oxidative phosphorylation	α-Ketoglutarate dehydrogenase complex-associated gene products: *BCKDHA* or *BCKDHB* or *DBT/BCATE2* or *DLD*	Hyperaminoaciduria corrected
Thiamin-responsive megaloblastic anemia syndrome, TRMA (also known as thiamin responsive with diabetes mellitus and sensorineural deafness, or as Roger syndrome)	Anemia, deafness, diabetes	*SLC19A2*, thiamin transporter	Potential recovery from all symptoms
Encephalopathy	Double vision, seizures, and white matter changes in the thalamus	*SLC25A2*, thiamin transporter	Seizures eliminated
Amish microcephaly	Microcephaly and anemia	*SLC25A2*, mitochondrial thiamin transporter	Never tested
Wolfram syndrome	Diabetes insipidus and mellitus with optic atrophy and deafness; DIDMOAD	*WFS1*, wolframin protein	Corrected hematological abnormalities and restored insulin sensitivity

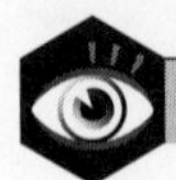

NUTRITION INSIGHT

Thiaminase Poisoning

Perhaps the most notorious case of thiaminase poisoning was that of Australian explorers Robert Burke and William Wills, who completed the first transcontinental crossing of Australia in the nineteenth century. Unfortunately, these explorers succumbed to beriberi within days after eating flour prepared from thiaminase-rich nonbracken nardoo ferns after depleting their previous source of thiamin, which was pork. Although they observed the Aborigines eating cooked nardoo, the explorers decided to eat raw nardoo fern rather than preparing it. Tragically, these non-bracken ferns possess up 100 times greater thiaminase than bracken ferns. They began complaining in their journals of increasing weakness and starvation, but not from want of food. Wills wrote, "I have a good appetite and relish the nardoo much but it seems to give us no nutriment." Thiamin and niacin are known to control appetite as well. They also complained of edema, wet beriberi, and an increased sensitivity to cold. Ultimately they would die.

Thiaminase poisoning occurs most commonly with livestock grazing in lush pastures with many ferns. Horses eating hay contaminated with at least 20% snake grass will show signs of thiamin deficiency within 2 to 5 weeks. Snake grass is an ancient plant that reproduces using spores, not seeds. This confirms the ancient nature of the thiaminase toxin. Fortunately, thiaminase-poisoned animals can readily recover once treated by injection of several hundred milligrams thiamin.

Interestingly, Native Americans had been eating corn as a staple for hundreds of years, but Europeans were first introduced to corn only upon their arrival to the New World. The European settlers unwittingly left the NAD precursor tryptophan biologically unavailable, because they did not treat corn with lye (a strongly alkaline solution). Native Americans did not experience pellagra, yet their diets were very similar to those of the European settlers. This unfortunate lack of communication regarding proper preparation of ferns and corn would tragically result in the settlers suffering from beriberi and pellagra, respectively.

Pyruvate decarboxylase deficiency disease is one of the most common causes of primary lactic acidosis in children and results from mutations in the E1 of the pyruvate dehydrogenase complex. The disease is characterized by chronic neurological dysfunction with neurodegeneration in the central nervous system, and it generally includes lactic acidosis. Symptoms include fevers preceding ataxia, with increased plasma levels of pyruvate and lactate. High doses of thiamin improve lactate, pyruvate, and many physical symptoms in most cases (Brunette et al., 1972; Lonsdale et al., 1969; Naito et al., 2002; Wick et al., 1977).

Mutation of the *WFS1* gene encoding the wolframin protein, a calcium channel, results in symptoms similar to that of Roger syndrome and includes diabetes insipidus, diabetes mellitus, optic atrophy, and deafness (DIDMOAD) as well as anemia. DIDMOAD patients are commonly legally blind and suffer from severe depression with psychosis. Treatment with thiamin may correct glucose abnormalities and hematological symptoms in the DIDMOAD patient (Borgna-Pignatti et al., 1989); however, neurological abnormalities are sometimes less responsive to thiamin supplementation.

Maple syrup urine disease (MSUD) is caused by mutations in one of the subunits of the branched-chain α-ketoglutarate dehydrogenase complex. This is characterized by sugary smelling urine and neurological disorders. There are five different types of MSUD, only one of which is responsive to thiamin (Duran et al., 1978; Scriver et al., 1971). Branched-chain α-keto acid dehydrogenase (BCKDH) activity is reduced by 30% to 40% because of a mutation that decreases the affinity for thiamin (Chuang et al., 1982). ThDP not only serves as cofactor in this reaction but also increases the stability and biological half-life of this membrane bound mitochondrial BCKDH (Elsas and Danner, 1982).

Thiamin-responsive megaloblastic anemia syndrome (TRMA, also known as Roger syndrome) arises from a mutation in the high-affinity thiamin transporter, SLC19A2 (for a review, see Neufeld et al., 2001). This disease is characterized by excessive, large, immature blood cells (megaloblastic anemia); diabetes mellitus; and sensorineural hearing loss. Patients respond well to pharmacological doses of thiamin (100 mg/day), which can diffuse into the cell at these high concentrations, independent of the presence of SLC19A2. The fact that genetic dysfunction of the thiamin transporter SLC19A2 leads to diabetes with neurodegeneration speaks volumes about the importance of thiamin in both glucose metabolism and neural function. In SLC19A2-deficient mice, insulin secretion is decreased, suggesting that thiamin may serve critical functions in controlling insulin secretion itself. Mutations in the mitochondrial ThDP transporter SLC25A19 results in Amish microencephaly followed by death, generally at approximately 6 months of age. This phenotype demonstrates the importance of mitochondrial thiamin.

Wilson disease is caused by a mutation in ATP7B, an ATPase copper-transporting protein. Loss of ATP7B leads to toxic accumulation of copper, which ultimately inhibits two thiamin-dependent enzymes, α-ketoglutarate dehydrogenase and pyruvate dehydrogenase. Administration of high doses of thiamin and lipoic acid to cells or mice is able to rescue the defects from loss of ATP7B function (Sheline and Choi, 2004), supporting the idea that high doses of thiamin can be used to successfully treat Wilson disease.

Clinical thiamin deficiency is most commonly recognized in the Western world because of its high association with alcoholics suffering from Wernicke-Korsakoff syndrome

(WKS), also known as Wernicke encephalopathy. Alcohol inhibits absorption of thiamin. WKS is characterized by an unsteady gate, confusion, and involuntary eye movement (nystagmus). There is a genetic susceptibility to WKS, but the gene(s) involved have not been determined. Acquired immunodeficiency syndrome (AIDS), chemotherapy, carcinoma, chronic vomiting, and other conditions can also bring on WKS. Encephalopathy is the first acute phase, and psychosis is the long-lasting, chronic stage characterized by an inability to learn. Consequently, it is most important to treat WKS early with intravenous thiamin (usually 500 mg for 3 days) to prevent permanent brain damage. The pill form of thiamin is insufficient. Relief from involuntary eye movements occurs within minutes after thiamin administration. Analysis of WKS patient pathology typically reveals damage to many brain regions, including the brainstem, cerebellum, cerebral cortex, diencephalon, and forebrain (Langlais et al., 1996).

UNKNOWN FUNCTIONS

There are several thiamin-derived isoforms present in the cell that most likely function as something other than cofactors. These are thiamin triphosphate (ThTP), thiamin monophosphate (ThMP), and adenosine thiamin triphosphate (AdThTP). These are still poorly understood, but research has revealed some aspects of their functions.

ThTP possesses two high-energy phosphoanhydride bonds resembling those of ATP, which has long been held to be the only molecule capable of phosphorylation of eukaryotic proteins. However, ThTP can also phosphorylate proteins in mammals (Makarchikov et al., 2003). ThTP synthesis in mammalian brain is coupled to the respiratory chain similar to ATP synthesis (Gangolf et al., 2010). ThTP can serve as a substrate instead of a cofactor in the phosphorylation of rapsyn, which is a protein that induces clustering of other proteins at neuromuscular synapses. High concentrations of thiamin phosphate esters are present at nerve terminals. Whether loss of mitochondrial ThTP in the mammalian brain is an important part of the neurodegeneration seen in beriberi remains to be determined. The nonmetabolic roles of thiamin in excitable tissues such as nerves remain a great medical mystery at the nexus of biochemistry and neurobiology.

PROTEINS THAT REQUIRE THIAMIN

There are approximately 21 unique human proteins that use ThDP, based on the presence of conserved distinguishable domains for binding pyrophosphate and pyrimidine (TEED: *www.teed.uni-stuttgart.de/*; Widmann et al., 2010). These can be sorted into four types of enzymes: decarboxylases, transketolases, oxidoreductases, and α-keto acid dehydrogenases. Although the total number of ThDP-dependent enzymes is approximately an order of magnitude less than that of NAD- or FAD-associated enzymes, thiamin is still the least stable of these three molecules and is particularly susceptible to degradation.

Transketolase directs glucose to either glycolysis or the pentose phosphate pathway; the latter uses glucose-derived carbons for synthesis of ribose, which is required for DNA synthesis, cell proliferation, and NAD synthesis (see PRPP in Figure 24-4). Cancer is a disease involving accelerated replication of cells. Transketolase is expressed at exceptionally high levels in pancreatic cancer (Liu et al., 2010a). For this reason, thiaminase is being examined as a potential therapeutic adjuvant to kill cancer cells (Liu et al., 2010b). Thiamin working through transketolase can redirect the glycolytic intermediate fructose-6-phosphate from glycolysis toward the pentose-phosphate pathway. This redirection removes toxic glucose-derived metabolites (Beltramo et al., 2008; Hammes et al., 2003), which is particularly important in diabetes. Diabetic nephropathy has been shown to be especially responsive to thiamin administration (Babaei-Jadidi et al., 2003; Rabbani et al., 2009). Genetic abnormalities described earlier as causes of diabetes, such as DIDMOAD and Roger syndrome, can also be treated with thiamin (see Table 24-3). Nonetheless, the potential therapeutic benefit of administering high doses of thiamin for treating diabetes remains largely unexamined.

THIAMIN SOURCES, CHEMICAL STABILITY, AND ADMET

SOURCES

Thiamin is essential to all life from prokaryotes to mammals, but only prokaryotes, plants, and fungi are capable of synthesizing it. Thiamin biosynthesis is regulated by a unique mechanism involving RNA structures that specifically recognize ThDP and negatively regulate expression of thiamin biosynthetic enzymes. Abundant food sources for thiamin are unrefined cereal germs, whole grains, meats (especially pork), nuts, and legumes. Enriched flours and grain products in the United States contain added thiamin (Gubler, 1991).

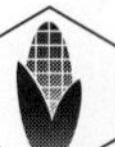

FOOD SOURCES OF THIAMIN

Meat and Meat Substitutes
0.4 to 1.0 mg per 3 oz pork or ham
0.4 mg per 1 cup black beans, green peas
0.3 mg per 1 cup lentils or beans (pinto, kidney, great northern, limas)

Cereals and Grain Products
0.3 to 0.9 mg per 1 cup ready-to-eat cereals
0.4 mg per 4-in. (3-oz) bagel
0.3 mg per 2-oz hard roll
0.3 mg per 1 cup noodles or pasta
0.2 mg per 1 cup cooked rice

Fruits
0.3 mg per 6 oz grapefruit juice
0.3 mg per 1 cup orange juice

Data from USDA, ARS. (2010). *USDA National Nutrient Database for Standard Reference, Release 23.* Retrieved from www.ars.usda.gov/ba/bhnrc/ndl

CHEMICAL STABILITY

Elevation of temperature, especially in aqueous media above neutral pH, leads to rapid loss of thiamin activity. Whether fever itself can cause thiamin breakdown is not known. Nonetheless, thiamin-responsive illnesses preceded by febrile attacks have been observed in the clinic (Adamolekun and Eniola, 1993). Rupture of the methylene bridge to the thiazole nitrogen also occurs readily when thiamin is exposed to sulfites, which are formed during food preservation with sulfur dioxide.

ADMET

Absorption

At normal physiological concentrations, active transport is required for cellular uptake of thiamin. At supraphysiological concentrations humans, thiamin can be absorbed by passive diffusion. Thiamin phosphate derivatives are first hydrolyzed by phosphatases present in the small intestine, after which the vitamin is readily absorbed by ubiquitous high-affinity thiamin transporters encoded by human genes *SLC19A2* and *SLC19A3* (Table 24-3). Both SLC19A2 and SLC19A3 transporters are localized to the plasma membrane. A third transporter, SLC19A1, is localized to the mitochondria. Folate is also transported by the SLC19 family of transporters. These transporters are inhibited by alcohol consumption or the drug pyrithiamine.

Distribution

Thiamin is carried by the portal circulation to the liver and then to the general circulation. There is a marked variation of transport capacity among tissues. Just 30 to 50 mg of thiamin is stored in the body. About half of thiamin stores are localized to skeletal muscle, with the rest present primarily in heart, liver, brain, and kidney. Free thiamin occurs in the plasma, whereas ThDP predominates in the cellular components because thiamin is phosphorylated immediately after cell entry. Most of the ThDP is transported intracellularly to the mitochondria, with some ThDP sent to peroxisomes.

Metabolism

The three main enzymes catalyzing conversions of thiamin and its phosphate esters are shown in Figure 24-8. A pyrophosphokinase catalyzes formation of the coenzyme ThDP. Some of this is routed to the monophosphates by thiamin diphosphatase and to triphosphates by ThDP adenylyl transferase. Approximately 80% of thiamin exists as the diphosphate, 10% as the triphosphate, and the rest as thiamin and its monophosphate.

Thiamin triphosphate concentrations vary widely depending on the species of animal and tissue analyzed. It is consistently detected in the human brain where it is restricted to mitochondria. Adenylated thiamins are detectable in human tissues at concentrations that are orders of magnitude less than other adenine nucleotides, such as AMP, ATP, or NAD. AThTP and ThTP have high phosphate energy potential and appear likely to be involved in phosphorylation reactions. The functional significance of AThDP is unknown.

Excretion

The half-life for thiamin in a healthy individual is 18 to 24 days but merely 6 days in a deficient individual. When thiamin is present at a concentration higher than a tissue needs, it is rapidly excreted in the urine. As with some urinary flavins, several of the numerous metabolites of thiamin arise from action of symbiotic microflora in the gut.

Toxicity

There are no well-established toxic effects from the consumption of excess thiamin in food or through long-term oral supplementation. Megadosing up to 1 g thiamin/day has been done without adverse events (Ames et al., 2002). No UL was set by the IOM (1998) because no adverse effects were reported from consuming excess thiamin in food and supplements. Supplements containing up to 100 mg/day are widely available.

Intravenous thiamin has been administered without significant reported adverse effects. The kidneys readily clear thiamin. Injection of doses up to 200 times the daily maintenance dose generally has not led to toxic effects, but some individuals appear to develop a hypersensitivity to thiamin. Although thiamin injection at high doses is generally considered safe, a small number of life-threatening anaphylactic reactions have been observed with large intravenous doses of thiamin.

BIOCHEMICAL ASSESSMENT OF THIAMIN NUTRITURE AND DIETARY REQUIREMENTS

BIOCHEMICAL ASSESSMENT OF THIAMIN NUTRITURE

Numerous methods have been used to assess the state of thiamin nutrition in humans (McCormick and Greene, 1999). The most common of these are the measurement of the activity of erythrocyte transketolase and the measurement of blood levels of pyruvate and α-ketoglutarate. The measurement of whole blood or erythrocyte transketolase activity (basal level) and the enhancement of basal enzymatic activity by the addition of ThDP are considered to be the most reliable methods and are used in a clinical setting. ThDP stimulation of greater than 16% indicates possible deficiency. Symptoms of beriberi (such as peripheral neuropathy and cardiac abnormalities) usually do not appear until the ThDP stimulation of erythrocyte transketolase activity is about 40%.

DIETARY REQUIREMENTS

Signs of inadequate thiamin levels are apparent first in the brain, within just 2 to 3 weeks of deficient intake. This is likely due to the brain's great dependency on glucose as an energy source. Ultimately, this can lead to irreversible neurodegeneration if it is not quickly treated. Based on intakes that prevent clinical and biochemical signs of deficiency, the IOM (1998) set the EAR for thiamin at 1.1 mg/day for men and 0.9 mg/day for women. The RDA was set as the EAR + 20% (IOM, 1998), with slightly higher increments for pregnant

CLINICAL CORRELATION

Infantile Thiamin Deficiency in Industrialized Nations

Kelsey Shields, BS, and Marie A. Caudill, PhD, RD

Thiamin deficiency in infants is extremely rare in industrialized nations. Nevertheless, in October and November 2003, approximately 20 Israeli infants were seriously affected after being fed thiamin-deficient soy-based formula (Fattal-Valevski et al., 2009). Upon admission to the hospital, the infants were experiencing a series of wet and dry beriberi-like symptoms in the form of Wernicke encephalopathy, apneic episodes, convulsions, and megaloblastic anemia (Abu-Kishk et al., 2009). These infants had high circulating concentrations of lactate and pyruvate along with elevated erythrocyte transketolase activities (Fattal-Valevski et al., 2005). The infants were treated with high-dose thiamin intravenously, and symptoms improved within hours of administration. However, 2 of the original 20 infants died of cardiomyopathy, and 10 exhibited residual neurological and developmental damage. Findings of a 5-year follow-up with seven of the affected infants showed an association of infantile thiamin deficiency with severe speech and motor retardation, dysfunction of the brainstem and basal ganglia, and seizure recurrence (Fattal-Valevski et al., 2009). Thus, despite treatment, certain pathologies remained.

Thinking Critically

1. Explain the relationship between the biochemical panel results (i.e., high lactate concentrations) and the diagnosis of thiamin deficiency.
2. Based on thiamin's role in carbohydrate oxidation, would it be safe to administer a glucose load to the affected infants? Why or why not?

and lactating women to cover the estimated requirements for growth in maternal and fetal compartments, secretion in the milk, and small increases in energy use. Recommendations for infants are based on the thiamin content of human breast milk and on caloric intake.

Thiamin dietary requirements are elevated in individuals who eat a high-carbohydrate diet, chronically consume excess alcohol, need dialysis, or have chronic febrile infections. Folate deficiency depresses thiamin absorption. The depression of thiamin absorption observed in alcoholics may be secondary to a folate deficiency. Individuals deplete body stores of thiamin rapidly during starvation or semistarvation. High-dose thiamin supplementation (100 mg/day) clearly increases serum thiamin levels and has been shown to decrease exercise-induced fatigue and blood glucose levels in human subjects post-exercise (Suzuki and Itokawa, 1996).

The median intake of thiamin by adults is about 1.7 mg/day for men and 1.4 mg/day for women based on NHANES III. Most individuals in the United States have intakes greater than the EAR. However, up to 10% of the elderly population is deficient in thiamin, partly because of a decreased ability to absorb thiamin. Intravenous administration of thiamin to the elderly has been able to correct some problems.

DRIs Across the Life Cycle: Thiamin

	mg Thiamin per Day*
Infant	RDA
0 through 6 mo	0.2 (AI)
7 through 12 mo	0.3 (AI)
Children	
1 through 3 yr	0.5
4 through 8 yr	0.6
9 through 13 yr	0.9
Males	
≥14 yr	1.2
Females	
14 through 18 yr	1.0
≥19 yr	1.1
Pregnant	1.4
Lactating	1.4

Data from IOM. (1998). *Dietary Reference Intakes for thiamin, riboflavin, niacin, vitamin B_6, folate, vitamin B_{12}, pantothenic acid, biotin, and choline.* Washington, DC: National Academy Press.

AI, Adequate Intake; *DRI*, Dietary Reference Intake; *RDA*, Recommended Dietary Allowance.

*Note: There is no established Tolerable Upper Intake Level (UL) for thiamin.

INTERDEPENDENCE OF B_3, B_2, AND B_1

Thiamin, riboflavin, and niacin are frequently dependent on each other to perform functions. All three are required for the human essential protein complexes pyruvate dehydrogenase (PDH) (Figure 24-11) and α-ketoglutarate dehydrogenase (αKGDH). Both of these also require lipoic acid and coenzyme-A, whereas PDH additionally uses pantothenate. Figure 24-11 shows the oxidative decarboxylation of pyruvate by the PDH complex. ThDP serves as the coenzyme for pyruvate decarboxylase (E1), whereas FAD and NAD are required for dihydrolipoyl dehydrogenase (E3) activity. Ultimately, all three vitamins are required for the metabolism of fuels to generate ATP, the universal energy equivalent.

NAD synthesis requires both riboflavin and thiamin. Going backward in the pathway, thiamin is required for synthesis of phosphoribosylpyrophosphate (PRPP). The ThDP-dependent enzyme transketolase converts six-carbon sugars to five- and seven-carbons sugars, where the five-carbon sugar ribose is subsequently converted to PRPP and used for synthesis of NAD. Starting from B vitamins niacin/nicotinic acid or niacinamide/nicotinamide, the PRPP is used to synthesize NAD in reactions catalyzed by NAMPT and NMNAT, as shown in Figure 24-4. Thus a deficiency of

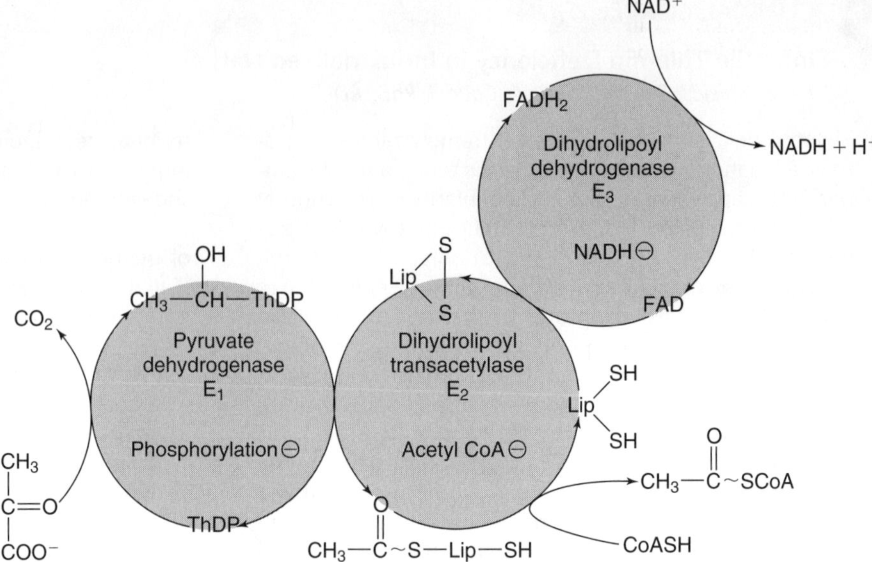

FIGURE 24-11 Oxidative decarboxylation of pyruvate by the pyruvate dehydrogenase complex. *FAD,* Flavin adenine dinucleotide; *Lip,* enzyme-bound lipoate; *NAD,* nicotinamide adenine dinucleotide; *ThDP,* thiamin diphosphate. Negative effectors of E_1, E_2, and E_3 enzymes are shown.

thiamin is likely to cause a deficiency of NAD. In fact, beriberi (thiamin deficiency) and pellagra (niacin deficiency) have very similar symptoms. Riboflavin is required not only for completion of the kynurenine pathway going from tryptophan to NAD, but also for synthesis of the active form of vitamin B_6, which itself is required for completion of the kynurenine pathway, as shown in Figure 24-4. Again, the symptoms of ariboflavinosis resemble pellagra. However, NAD precursors cannot rescue all of the effects of ariboflavinosis or beriberi.

One particularly exciting area of modern vitamin research involves the function of NAD and FAD as protein chaperones. These activities are responsible for proper protein folding. Alzheimer disease is generally considered irreversible and is specifically defined by the appearance of insoluble protein plaques in postmortem brains. Notably, overexpression of the NAD biosynthesis gene encoded by *NMNAT* prevents neurodegeneration under otherwise lethal conditions (Sasaki et al., 2006), and this effect has been determined to be due to chaperone activities in experiments with *Drosophila* (Zhai et al., 2008). FAD has also been shown to increase the half-life of several proteins, and it assists in the proper formation of disulfide bonds in proteins via the FAD-dependent enzyme Ero1. Absence of NAD causes dementia, whereas the most common cause of dementia today is Alzheimer disease, which is the result of improperly processed proteins.

THINKING CRITICALLY

1. Beriberi (vitamin B_1/thiamin deficiency) and pellagra (vitamin B_3/NAD deficiency) have many similar symptoms. This is in part because thiamin is needed for synthesis of NAD. During thiamin deficiency, can you still make NAD?
2. What are the vitamins needed to synthesize NAD starting from tryptophan?
3. What molecules and enzymes are required for biosynthesis of NAD when starting from nicotinic acid?
4. What molecules and enzymes are required for biosynthesis of NAD when starting from nicotinamide?

REFERENCES

Abu-Kishk, I., Rachmiel, M., Hoffmann, C., Lahat, E., & Eshel, G. (2009). Infantile encephalopathy due to vitamin deficiency in industrial countries. *Child's Nervous System, 25,* 1477–1480.

Adamolekun, B., & Eniola, A. (1993). Thiamine-responsive acute cerebellar ataxia following febrile illness. *The Central African Journal of Medicine, 39,* 40–41.

Ames, B. N., Elson-Schwab, I., & Silver, E. A. (2002). High-dose vitamin therapy stimulates variant enzymes with decreased coenzyme binding affinity (increased K(m)): Relevance to genetic disease and polymorphisms. *The American Journal of Clinical Nutrition, 75,* 616–658.

Araki, E., Kobayashi, T., Kohtake, N., Goto, I., & Hashimoto, T. (1994). A riboflavin-responsive lipid storage myopathy due to multiple acyl-CoA dehydrogenase deficiency: An adult case. *Journal of the Neurological Sciences, 126,* 202–205.

Aw, T. Y., Jones, D. P., & McCormick, D. B. (1983). Uptake of riboflavin by isolated rat liver cells. *The Journal of Nutrition, 113,* 1249–1254.

Babaei-Jadidi, R., Karachalias, N., Ahmed, N., Battah, S., & Thornalley, P. J. (2003). Prevention of incipient diabetic nephropathy by high-dose thiamine and benfotiamine. *Diabetes, 52,* 2110–2120.

Bechgaard, H., & Jespersen, S. (1977). GI absorption of niacin in humans. *Journal of Pharmaceutical Sciences, 66,* 871–872.

Beltramo, E., Berrone, E., Tarallo, S., & Porta, M. (2008). Effects of thiamine and benfotiamine on intracellular glucose metabolism and relevance in the prevention of diabetic complications. *Acta Diabetologica, 45,* 131–141.

Bieganowski, P., & Brenner, C. (2004). Discoveries of nicotinamide riboside as a nutrient and conserved NRK genes establish a Preiss-Handler independent route to NAD+ in fungi and humans. *Cell, 117*, 495–502.

Block, G., Dresser, C. M., Hartman, A. M., & Carroll, M. D. (1985). Nutrient sources in the American diet: Quantitative data from the NHANES II survey. I. Vitamins and minerals. *American Journal of Epidemiology, 122*, 13–26.

Borgna-Pignatti, C., Marradi, P., Pinelli, L., Monetti, N., & Patrini, C. (1989). Thiamine-responsive anemia in DIDMOAD syndrome. *The Journal of Pediatrics, 114*, 405–410.

Bowers-Komro, D. M., & McCormick, D. B. (Eds.). (1987). Riboflavin uptake by isolated rat kidney cells. In *Flavins and flavoproteins* (pp. 449–453). Berlin, Germany: Walter de Gruyter.

Brunette, M. G., Delvin, E., Hazel, B., & Scriver, C. R. (1972). Thiamine-responsive lactic acidosis in a patient with deficient low-KM pyruvate carboxylase activity in liver. *Pediatrics, 50*, 702–711.

Canner, P. L., Berge, K. G., Wenger, N. K., Stamler, J., Friedman, L., Prineas, R. J., & Friedewald, W. (1986). Fifteen year mortality in Coronary Drug Project patients: Long-term benefit with niacin. *Journal of the American College of Cardiology, 8*, 1245–1255.

Carlson, L. A. (2005). Nicotinic acid: The broad-spectrum lipid drug. A 50th anniversary review. *Journal of Internal Medicine, 258*, 94–114.

Casteels, M., Foulon, V., Mannaerts, G. P., & Van Veldhoven, P. P. (2003). Alpha-oxidation of 3-methyl-substituted fatty acids and its thiamine dependence. *European Journal of Biochemistry, 270*, 1619–1627.

Chastain, J. L. (1991). Flavin metabolites. In F. Muller (Ed.), *Chemistry and biochemistry of flavins* (Vol. I, pp. 195–200). Boca Raton, FL: CRC Press.

Chiong, M. A., Sim, K. G., Carpenter, K., Rhead, W., Ho, G., Olsen, R. K., & Christodoulou, J. (2007). Transient multiple acyl-CoA dehydrogenation deficiency in a newborn female caused by maternal riboflavin deficiency. *Molecular Genetics and Metabolism, 92*, 109–114.

Chuang, D. T., Ku, L. S., & Cox, R. P. (1982). Biochemical basis of thiamin-responsive maple syrup urine disease. *Transactions of the Association of American Physician, 95*, 196–204.

Condo, M., Posar, A., Arbizzani, A., & Parmeggiani, A. (2009). Riboflavin prophylaxis in pediatric and adolescent migraine. *The Journal of Headache and Pain, 10*, 361–365.

Decker, K. F. (1993). Biosynthesis and function of enzymes with covalently bound flavin. *Annual Review of Nutrition, 13*, 17–41.

Duran, M., Tielens, A. G., Wadman, S. K., Stigter, J. C., & Kleijer, W. J. (1978). Effects of thiamine in a patient with a variant form of branched-chian ketoaciduria. *Acta Paediatrica Scandinavica, 67*, 367–372.

Eijkman, C. (1990). Anti-neuritis vitamin and beriberi. Nobel prize paper. 1929. *Nederlands Tijdschrift voor Geneeskunde, 134*, 1654–1657.

Elsas, L. J., & Danner, D. J. (1982). The role of thiamin in maple syrup urine disease. *Annals of the New York Academy of Sciences, 378*, 404–421.

Er, T. K., Liang, W. C., Chang, J. G., & Jong, Y. J. (2010). High resolution melting analysis facilitates mutation screening of ETFDH gene: Applications in riboflavin-responsive multiple acyl-CoA dehydrogenase deficiency. *Clinica Chimica Acta, 411*, 690–699.

Fattal-Valevski, A., Bloch-Mimouni, A., Kivity, S., Heyman, E., Brezner, A., Strausberg, R., ... Goldberg-Stern, H. (2009). Epilepsy in children with infantile thiamine deficiency. *Neurology, 73*, 828–833.

Fattal-Valevski, A., Kesler, A., Sela, B., Nitzan-Kaluski, D., Rotstein, M., Mesterman, R., ... Eshel, G. (2005). Outbreak of life-threatening thiamine deficiency in infants in Israel caused by a defective soy-based formula. *Pediatrics, 115*, 233–238.

Gangolf, M., Wins, P., Thiry, M., El Moualij, B., & Bettendorff, L. (2010). Thiamine triphosphate synthesis in rat brain occurs in mitochondria and is coupled to the respiratory chain. *The Journal of Biological Chemistry, 285*, 583–594.

Gariballa, S., Forster, S., & Powers, H. (2009). Riboflavin status in acutely ill patients and response to dietary supplements. *Journal of Parenteral and Enteral Nutrition, 33*, 656–661.

Goodrich, R. P. (2000). The use of riboflavin for the inactivation of pathogens in blood products. *Vox Sanguinis, 78*(Suppl 2), 211–215.

Gross, C. J., & Henderson, L. M. (1983). Digestion and absorption of NAD by the small intestine of the rat. *The Journal of Nutrition, 113*, 412–420.

Gubler, C. J. (1991). Thiamin. In M. Dekker (Ed.), *Handbook of vitamins* (pp. 233–281). New York: MacMillan.

Guyton, J. R., & Bays, H. E. (2007). Safety considerations with niacin therapy. *The American Journal of Cardiology, 99*, 22C–31C.

Hammes, H. P., Du, X., Edelstein, D., Taguchi, T., Matsumura, T., Ju, Q., ... Brownlee, M. (2003). Benfotiamine blocks three major pathways of hyperglycemic damage and prevents experimental diabetic retinopathy. *Nature Medicine, 9*, 294–299.

Hanson, J., Gille, A., Zwykiel, S., Lukasova, M., Clausen, B. E., Ahmed, K., ... Offermanns, S. (2010). Nicotinic acid- and monomethyl fumarate-induced flushing involves GPR109A expressed by keratinocytes and COX-2-dependent prostanoid formation in mice. *The Journal of Clinical Investigation, 120*, 2910–2919.

Hoey, L., McNulty, H., & Strain, J. J. (2009). Studies of biomarker responses to intervention with riboflavin: A systematic review. *The American Journal of Clinical Nutrition, 89*, 1960S–1980S.

Hoffer, A., Osmond, H., Callbeck, M. J., & Kahan, I. (1957). Treatment of schizophrenia with nicotinic acid and nicotinamide. *Journal of Clinical and Experimental Psychopathology, 18*, 131–158.

Innis, W. S., McCormick, D. B., & Merrill, A. H. (1985). Variations in riboflavin binding by human plasma: Identification of immunoglobulins as the major proteins responsible. *Biochemical Medicine, 34*, 151–165.

Institute of Medicine. (1998). *Dietary reference intakes for thiamin, riboflavin, niacin, vitamin B_6, folate, vitamin B_{12}, pantothenic acid, biotin, and choline.* Washington, DC: National Academy Press.

Jacobson, E. L., & Jacobson, M. K. (1997). Tissue NAD as a biochemical measure of niacin status in humans. *Methods in Enzymology, 280*, 221–230.

Knox, W. E., & Piras, M. M. (1967). Tryptophan pyrrolase of liver. 3. Conjugation in vivo during cofactor induction by tryptophan analogues. *The Journal of Biological Chemistry, 242*, 2959–2965.

Langlais, P. J., Zhang, S. X., & Savage, L. M. (1996). Neuropathology of thiamine deficiency: An update on the comparative analysis of human disorders and experimental models. *Metabolic Brain Disease, 11*, 19–37.

Lee, S. S., & McCormick, D. B. (1985). Thyroid hormone regulation of flavocoenzyme biosynthesis. *Archives of Biochemistry and Biophysics, 237*, 197–201.

Liang, W. C., Ohkuma, A., Hayashi, Y. K., Lopez, L. C., Hirano, M., Nonaka, I., ... Nishino, I. (2009). ETFDH mutations, CoQ10 levels, and respiratory chain activities in patients with riboflavin-responsive multiple acyl-CoA dehydrogenase deficiency. *Neuromuscular Disorders, 19*, 212–216.

Liu, H., Huang, D., McArthur, D. L., Boros, L. G., Nissen, N., & Heaney, A. P. (2010a). Fructose induces transketolase flux to promote pancreatic cancer growth. *Cancer Research, 70*, 6368–6376.

Liu, S., Monks, N. R., Hanes, J. W., Begley, T. P., Yu, H., & Moscow, J. A. (2010b). Sensitivity of breast cancer cell lines to recombinant thiaminase I. *Cancer Chemotherapy and Pharmacology, 66*, 171–179.

Lonsdale, D., Faulkner, W. R., Price, W., & Smeby, R. R. (1969). Pyruvic acidemia with hyperalaninemia: Vitamin B1 dependency. *The Journal of Pediatrics 74*, 827–828.

Ma, A. G., Schouten, E. G., Zhang, F. Z., Kok, F. J., Yang, F., Jiang, D. C., … Han, X. X. (2008). Retinol and riboflavin supplementation decreases the prevalence of anemia in Chinese pregnant women taking iron and folic acid supplements. *The Journal of Nutrition, 138*, 1946–1950.

Makarchikov, A. F., Lakaye, B., Gulyai, I. E., Czerniecki, J., Coumans, B., Wins, P., … Bettendorff, L. (2003). Thiamine triphosphate and thiamine triphosphatase activities: From bacteria to mammals. *Cellular and Molecular Life Sciences, 60*, 1477–1488.

McCormick, D. B., & Greene, H. L. (1999). Vitamins. In C. A. Burtis & E. R. Ashwood (Eds.), *Textbook of clinical chemistry* (pp. 999–1029). Philadelphia: Saunders.

Messamore, E., Hoffman, W. F., & Janowsky, A. (2003). The niacin skin flush abnormality in schizophrenia: A quantitative dose-response study. *Schizophrenia Research, 62*, 251–258.

Mushtaq, S., Su, H., Hill, M. H., & Powers, H. J. (2009). Erythrocyte pyridoxamine phosphate oxidase activity: A potential biomarker of riboflavin status? *The American Journal of Clinical Nutrition, 90*, 1151–1159.

Naito, E., Ito, M., Yokota, I., Saijo, T., Matsuda, J., Ogawa, Y., … Kuroda, Y. (2002). Thiamine-responsive pyruvate dehydrogenase deficiency in two patients caused by a point mutation (F205L and L216F) within the thiamine pyrophosphate binding region. *Biochimica et Biophysica Acta, 1588*, 79–84.

Nebert, D. W., & Russell, D. W. (2002). Clinical importance of the cytochromes P450. *Lancet, 360*, 1155–1162.

Neufeld, E. J., Fleming, J. C., Tartaglini, E., & Steinkamp, M. P. (2001). Thiamine-responsive megaloblastic anemia syndrome: A disorder of high-affinity thiamine transport. *Blood Cells, Molecules & Disease, 27*, 135–138.

Oakley, A., & Wallace, J. (1994). Hartnup disease presenting in an adult. *Clinical and Experimental Dermatology, 19*, 407–408.

Penberthy, W. T. (2007). Pharmacological targeting of IDO-mediated tolerance for treating autoimmune disease. *Current Drug Metabolism, 8*, 245–266.

Penberthy, W. T. (2009). Nicotinic acid–mediated activation of both membrane and nuclear receptors towards therapeutic glucocorticoid mimetics for treating multiple sclerosis. *PPAR Research, 2009*, 853707.

Rabbani, N., Alam, S. S., Riaz, S., Larkin, J. R., Akhtar, M. W., Shafi, T., & Thornalley, P. J. (2009). High-dose thiamine therapy for patients with type 2 diabetes and microalbuminuria: A randomised, double-blind placebo-controlled pilot study. *Diabetologia, 52*, 208–212.

Revollo, J. R., Grimm, A. A., & Imai, S. (2004). The NAD biosynthesis pathway mediated by nicotinamide phosphoribosyltransferase regulates Sir2 activity in mammalian cells. *The Journal of Biological Chemistry, 279*, 50754–50763.

Roughead, Z. K., & McCormick, D. B. (1990). Flavin composition of human milk. *The American Journal of Clinical Nutrition, 52*, 854–857.

Sasaki, Y., Araki, T., & Milbrandt, J. (2006). Stimulation of nicotinamide adenine dinucleotide biosynthetic pathways delays axonal degeneration after axotomy. *The Journal of Neuroscience, 26*, 8484–8491.

Scriver, C. R., Mackenzie, S., Clow, C. L., & Delvin, E. (1971). Thiamine-responsive maple-syrup-urine disease. *Lancet, 1*, 310–312.

Sheline, C. T., & Choi, D. W. (2004). Cu^{2+} toxicity inhibition of mitochondrial dehydrogenases in vitro and in vivo. *Annals of Neurology, 55*, 645–653.

Suzuki, M., & Itokawa, Y. (1996). Effects of thiamine supplementation on exercise-induced fatigue. *Metabolic Brain Disease, 11*, 95–106.

Tunaru, S., Kero, J., Schaub, A., Wufka, C., Blaukat, A., Pfeffer, K., & Offermanns, S. (2003). PUMA-G and HM74 are receptors for nicotinic acid and mediate its anti-lipolytic effect. *Nature Medicine, 9*, 352–355.

Werner, R., Manthey, K. C., Griffin, J. B., & Zempleni, J. (2005). HepG2 cells develop signs of riboflavin deficiency within 4 days of culture in riboflavin-deficient medium. *The Journal of Nutritional Biochemistry, 16*, 617–624.

Wick, H., Schweizer, K., & Baumgartner, R. (1977). Thiamine dependency in a patient with congenital lacticacidaemia due to pyruvate dehydrogenase deficiency. *Agents and Actions, 7*, 405–410.

Widmann, M., Radloff, R., & Pleiss, J. (2010). The thiamine diphosphate dependent Enzyme Engineering Database: A tool for the systematic analysis of sequence and structure relations. *BMC Biochemistry, 11*, 9.

Yamada, Y., Merrill, A. H., Jr., & McCormick, D. B. (1990). Probable reaction mechanisms of flavokinase and FAD synthetase from rat liver. *Archives of Biochemistry and Biophysics, 278*, 125–130.

Yao, Y., Yonezawa, A., Yoshimatsu, H., Masuda, S., Katsura, T., & Inui, K. (2010). Identification and comparative functional characterization of a new human riboflavin transporter hRFT3 expressed in the brain. *The Journal of Nutrition, 140*, 1220–1226.

Yazdanpanah, B., Wiegmann, K., Tchikov, V., Krut, O., Pongratz, C., Schramm, M., … Krönke, M. (2009). Riboflavin kinase couples TNF receptor 1 to NADPH oxidase. *Nature, 460*, 1159–1163.

Yilmaz, K. (2009). Riboflavin treatment in a case with l-2-hydroxyglutaric aciduria. *European Journal of Paediatric Neurology, 13*, 57–60.

Yonezawa, A., Masuda, S., Katsura, T., & Inui, K. (2008). Identification and functional characterization of a novel human and rat riboflavin transporter, RFT1. *American Journal of Physiology. Cell Physiology, 295*, C632–C641.

Zempleni, J., Galloway, J. R., & McCormick, D. B. (1996). Pharmacokinetics of orally and intravenously administered riboflavin in healthy humans. *The American Journal of Clinical Nutrition, 63*, 54–66.

Zhai, R. G., Zhang, F., Hiesinger, P. R., Cao, Y., Haueter, C. M., & Bellen, H. J. (2008). NAD synthase NMNAT acts as a chaperone to protect against neurodegeneration. *Nature, 452*, 887–891.

RECOMMENDED READING

Ames, B. N., Elson-Schwab, I., & Silver, E. A. (2002). High-dose vitamin therapy stimulates variant enzymes with decreased coenzyme binding affinity (increased K(m)): Relevance to genetic disease and polymorphisms. *The American Journal of Clinical Nutrition, 75*(4), 616–658.

RECOMMENDED WEBSITES

OMIM—Online Mendelian Inheritance in Man. http://www.ncbi.nlm.nih.gov/sites/entrez?db=omim

Thiamine diphosphate dependent Enzyme Engineering Database, TEED. http://www.teed.uni-stuttgart.de/

CHAPTER 25

Folate, Choline, Vitamin B_{12}, and Vitamin B_6

Marie A. Caudill, PhD, RD; Joshua W. Miller, PhD; Jesse F. Gregory III, PhD; and Barry Shane, PhD

COMMON ABBREVIATIONS

AdoHcy	*S*-adenosylhomocysteine
AdoMet	*S*-adenosylmethionine
Cbl	cobalamin, vitamin B_{12}
DAG	diacylglycerol
DFE	dietary folate equivalent
MTHFR	5,10-methylenetetrahydrofolate reductase
NTD	neural tube defect
PEMT	phosphatidylethanolamine *N*-methyltransferase
PL	pyridoxal
PLP	pyridoxal 5′-phosphate
PM	pyridoxamine
PMP	pyridoxamine 5′-phosphate
PN	pyridoxine or pyridoxol
PNP	pyridoxine 5′-phosphate
PtdCho	phosphatidylcholine
TC	transcobalamin
THF	tetrahydrofolate

The grouping of the nutrients folate, choline, vitamin B_{12}, and vitamin B_6 arises from their important roles as coenzymes, cosubstrates, or both in the one-carbon (1-C) metabolic network. Folate polyglutamates function in the transfer of 1-C units and are required for nucleotide biosynthesis and methionine reformation from homocysteine. Vitamin B_6–dependent enzymes are intimately involved in the supply of 1-C units and in homocysteine catabolism. Vitamin B_{12} deficiency can cause a secondary deficiency of folate resulting in diminished nucleotide biosynthesis and cell division. Because choline serves as an alternative route to folate and vitamin B_{12}–dependent homocysteine remethylation, there is an added layer of nutrient intermingling.

FOLATE

Folate was initially investigated as a dietary factor that prevented megaloblastic anemia of pregnancy and as a growth factor present in green leafy vegetables (foliage), hence its name. As a donor and acceptor of 1-C moieties, folate participates in nucleotide biosynthesis and the remethylation of homocysteine to methionine. Because of the role of folate coenzymes in the synthesis of DNA precursors, folate antagonists have found widespread clinical use as anticancer and antimicrobial agents. Periconceptional supplementation with folic acid, a synthetic form of this vitamin, reduces the incidence of neural tube defects and has led to folic acid fortification programs in the United States, Canada, and approximately 50 other countries.

CHEMISTRY OF FOLATE

Folate is the generic name for this water-soluble B vitamin. Common structural features of folate derivatives include (1) a pteridine bicyclic ring system, (2) *p*-aminobenzoic acid, and (3) one or more glutamic acid residues (Figure 25-1). Folic acid is the synthetic, monoglutamate, fully oxidized, and most stable form of the vitamin (see Figure 25-1). Folate metabolism involves the reduction of the pyrazine ring of the pterin moiety to the coenzymatically active tetrahydrofolate (THF) form, the elongation of the glutamate chain by the addition of L-glutamate residues in an unusual γ-peptide linkage, and the acquisition and oxidation or reduction of 1-C units at the N5 and/or N10 positions (see Figure 25-1).

SOURCES OF FOLATE

Folates are synthesized by microorganisms and plants as the 7,8-dihydrofolate (DHF) form, and all naturally occurring folates are reduced THF derivatives. Good sources of naturally occurring food folate are shown in the box, "Food Sources of Folate and Folic Acid." Fully oxidized synthetic folic acid is found in the diet only when foodstuffs are fortified with folic acid or when dietary folates are oxidized. Fully oxidized folic acid is also the common form of folate found in vitamin supplements. Reduced folates are less stable than folic acid, and their stability varies depending on the 1-C substitution. Large losses of food

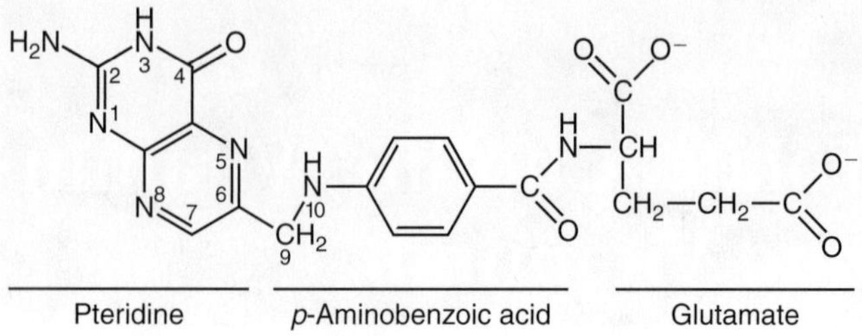

Pteridine | p-Aminobenzoic acid | Glutamate

Folic acid (oxidized, monoglutamate form)

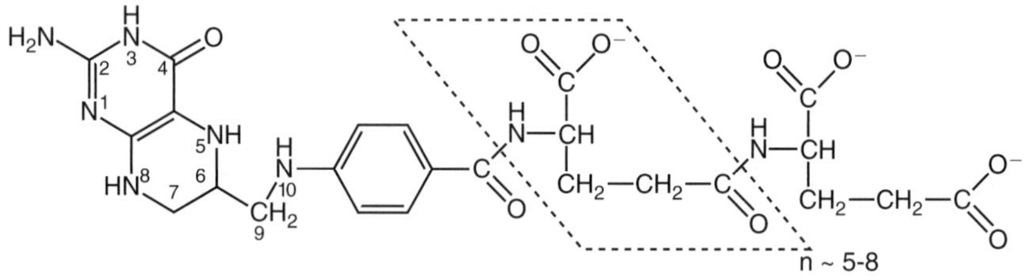

n ~ 5-8

Tetrahydrofolate (THF: reduced, polyglutamate form)

One-carbon substituent		Position	Oxidation state
Methyl	$—CH_3$	N5	Methanol
Methylene	$—CH_2—$	N5, N10	Formaldehyde
Methenyl	—CH=	N5, N10	Formate
Formyl	—CHO	N5 or N10	Formate
Formimino	HN=CH—	N5	Formate

FIGURE 25-1 Structure of folic acid and tetrahydrofolate (THF) poly-γ-glutamate. THF polyglutamates usually contain about 5-8 glutamates (n ~ 5-8). One-carbon substituents can be at the N-5 and/or N-10 positions of the reduced THF molecule.

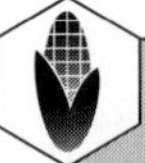

FOOD SOURCES OF FOLATE AND FOLIC ACID

Food Sources High in Naturally Occurring Folate

Legumes

180 μg DFE* per ½ cup lentils

110 to 150 μg DFE per ½ cup pinto, black, navy, kidney beans

60 to 80 μg DFE per ½ cup lima beans, kidney beans, split peas

Vegetables

120 to 130 μg DFE per ½ cup okra, spinach, asparagus

80 to 85 μg DFE per ½ cup broccoli, Brussels sprouts

50 to 70 μg DFE per ½ cup beets, corn, peas

Food Sources High in Folic Acid (Fortified and Enriched Foods)

Cereal and Grain Products

807 μg DFE per ¾ cup General Mills, Whole Grain Total

650 μg DFE per ½ cup Kellog's All-Bran cereal

150 to 400 μg DFE per 1 cup ready-to-eat cereal (e.g., Cheerios)

75 to 120 μg DFE per ½ cup cooked white enriched rice

140 μg DFE per 10 pretzels

200 μg DFE per 4-in. (3-oz) plain bagel

Data from U.S. Department of Agriculture (USDA), Agricultural Research Service (ARS). (2010). *USDA National Nutrient Database for Standard Reference, Release 23*. Retrieved from www.ars.usda.gov/ba/bhnrc/ndl

DFE, dietary folate equivalent.

*1 μg DFE = 1 μg of food folate = 0.6 μg of folic acid in fortified/enriched foods.

folate can occur during food processing or preparation, especially from heating under oxidative conditions. Additional losses can occur by the leaching of folate from food into the cooking water.

FOLATE ABSORPTION

Most naturally occurring dietary folates are polyglutamate derivatives and must be hydrolyzed by a brush border membrane γ-glutamylhydrolase (glutamate carboxypeptidase II, GCPII) in the small intestine to monoglutamate forms before absorption across the intestinal mucosa. As folic acid is a monoglutamate, hydrolysis of glutamates by GCPII is not required. Absorption of folate monoglutamate is via a saturable carrier-mediated process, but a diffusion-like process also occurs at high folate concentrations. The main intestinal transporter, proton-coupled folate transporter (PCFT) encoded by the *SLC46A1* gene, is a transmembrane protein that is highly expressed in enterocytes. PCFT belongs to the superfamily of solute carriers, functions optimally at low pH, and has a similar affinity for reduced folates and folic acid (Zhao et al., 2009a). Hereditary folate malabsorption is a consequence of loss-of-function mutations in the *SLC46A1* gene.

Metabolism of folate, primarily to 5-methyltetrahydrofolate (5-methyl-THF), occurs in the intestinal cell but is not required for transport. When pharmacological doses of various folates are given, most of the transported vitamin appears unchanged in portal and peripheral circulation.

FOLATE BIOAVAILABILITY

Bioavailability is a function of absorptive and metabolic processes that are influenced by many factors, including nutrient form, dietary intake, and individual genetic variation (McNulty and Pentieva, 2009; Caudill, 2010). In contrast to the high bioavailability of folic acid when given as a supplement or in fortified food, the bioavailability of naturally occurring food folate is variable and often incomplete. Several luminal factors can contribute to the lower bioavailability of food folate, including (1) entrapment of naturally occurring folates in the cellular structure or insoluble matrix of certain foods, (2) destruction of labile tetrahydrofolates during passage through the stomach, (3) inhibition of the intestinal deconjugation of polyglutamyl folates by food constituents, and (4) impairment of folate deconjugation by alteration of jejunal pH. Although pharmacological doses of folic acid are well absorbed, most of the vitamin is not retained in the body because tissues have a limited capacity to retain large amounts of folate.

TRANSPORT OF FOLATE

After folate absorption into the portal circulation (predominately 5-methyl-THF), much of this folate can be taken up by the liver via PCFT (Shane, 2009; Zhao et al., 2009a) (Figure 25-2). This folate–proton symporter is highly expressed on human liver basolateral membranes, which transport folates from the portal circulation. Liver and most, if not all, tissues also express the bidirectional reduced folate carrier (RFC), a product of the *SLC19A1* gene (Zhao et al., 2009a). RFC is a transmembrane protein whose specificity for various folates differs among tissues and between the apical and basolateral membranes of cells. Affinities of RFC for reduced folates are in the low micromolar range, whereas affinities for folic acid are lower in the mid-micromolar range.

Folate monoglutamates are exported from cells by RFC but also by select ATP-binding cassette (ABC) exporters such as the multidrug resistance (MDR)–associated proteins (Zhao et al., 2009a). 5-Methyl-THF is the predominate form of folate exported to plasma and is thus the circulatory form. Some folate is secreted in bile, but this can be reabsorbed in the intestine via an enterohepatic circulation.

Folate receptors (FRα, FRβ, and FRγ), also referred to as folate-binding proteins, are a distinct class of folate transporters that are expressed by several peripheral tissues and display a high affinity for folic acid (in the nanomolar range). There are at least three distinct genes that code for the receptors, and the encoded protein is usually attached to the plasma membrane of cells via a glycosylphosphatidylinositol anchor (Zhao et al., 2009a). Internalization of folate occurs via a receptor-mediated endocytotic process. In the internalized endosome, folate is released from the receptor and is exported from the endosome into the cytosol by a mechanism that appears to be mediated by PCFT (Zhao et al., 2009b). Folate receptors are highly expressed in the choroid plexus, kidney proximal tubes, erythropoietic cells, and placenta, and in a number of human tumors. The presence of this high affinity transporter in the choroid plexus is thought to protect the brain from the effects of folate deficiency, as folate levels in the cerebrospinal fluid are considerably higher than in the peripheral circulation. A soluble form of folate-binding protein is also present at low levels in plasma and at high levels in human milk.

TISSUE ACCUMULATION OF FOLATE

More than 95% of tissue folates are polyglutamate species, primarily with chain lengths between five and eight glutamates. With most folate-dependent enzymes, the polyglutamates usually exhibit greatly increased affinities for these enzymes and are more effective than monoglutamates as substrates. The polyanionic nature of the polyglutamate chain, coupled with binding of folate polyglutamates by intracellular proteins, allows tissues to retain and concentrate polyglutamate forms of the vitamin. Folate coenzymes are found primarily in the mitochondria and cytosol of the cell, and accumulation of folate in these compartments requires the conversion of folates to polyglutamates, which is catalyzed by the enzyme folylpolyglutamate synthetase (Shane, 2009):

$$\text{MgATP} + \text{THF(glu}_n) + \text{Glutamate} \rightarrow \text{MgADP} + \text{THF(glu}_{n+1}) + \text{P}_i$$

Folylpolyglutamate synthetase is encoded by a single human gene, and cytosolic and mitochondrial isozymes are generated by alternative transcription start sites for the gene and by alternative translational start sites for its messenger RNA (mRNA). THF and its polyglutamate forms are the preferred substrates for folylpolyglutamate synthetase, whereas 5-substituted folates such as 5-methyl-THF are poor substrates. Because 5-methyl-THF is the major folate transported into most tissues, the extent of folate accumulation depends on a tissue's ability to metabolize 5-methyl-THF to THF via the methionine synthase reaction. Unmetabolized 5-methyl-THF is rapidly effluxed from the tissue to plasma, as is folic acid, which appears in the circulation when the metabolic capacity of DHF reductase is exceeded.

The major hepatic mitochondrial folates are 10-formyl-tetrahydrofolate (10-formyl-THF) and THF, and much of the latter is bound to two folate enzymes, dimethylglycine dehydrogenase and sarcosine dehydrogenase. In the cytosol, a large proportion of the 5-methyl-THF is bound to glycine *N*-methyltransferase, whereas much of the cytosolic THF is bound to 10-formyl-THF dehydrogenase.

FOLATE TURNOVER

Tissues contain a soluble lysosomal γ-glutamylhydrolase activity, sometimes called folate conjugase, which is involved in the hydrolysis of polyglutamates with their subsequent release from the tissue in the monoglutamate form. However, the major route of folate turnover and catabolism appears to involve the degradation of folate coenzymes to pterin derivatives and aminobenzoylpolyglutamates via oxidative cleavage

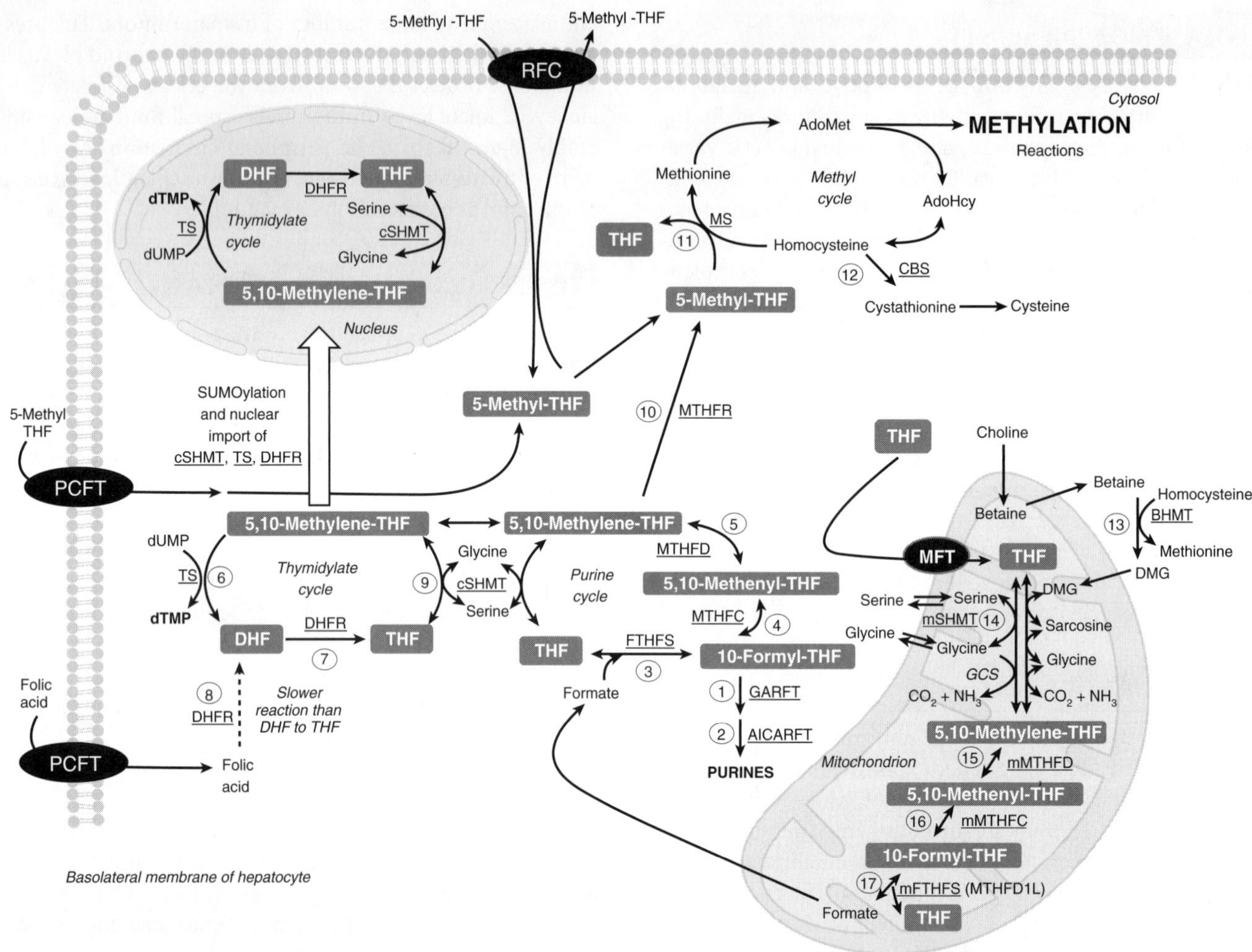

FIGURE 25-2 Proposed route of folate entry and metabolism in liver cells. The major metabolic cycles of folate-dependent one-carbon (1-C) metabolism occur in the cytosol and nucleus of cells. Provision of 1-C moieties for cytosolic 1-C metabolism in the form of formate occurs mainly in the mitochondrion through the catabolism of serine, glycine, and choline. Refer to Table 25-1 for a description of the reaction that corresponds to each number. *AdoHcy*, *S*-Adenosylhomocysteine; *AdoMet*, *S*-adenosylmethionine; *AICAR*, 5-amino-4-imidazolecarboxamide ribonucleotide; *AICARFT*, AICAR formyltransferase; *BHMT*, betaine homocysteine methyltransferase; *c*, cytosolic; *CBS*, cystathionine β synthase; *DHF*, dihydrofolate; *DHFR*, DHF reductase; *DMG*, dimethylglycine; *dTMP*, 2-deoxythymidine 5′-monophosphate; *dUMP*, 2-deoxyuridine 5′-monophosphate; *FTHFS*, formyltetrahydrofolate synthetase; *GARFT*, glycinamide ribonucleotide formyltransferase; *GCS*, glycine cleavage system; *m*, mitochondrial; *MFT*, mitochondrial folate transporter; *MS*, methionine synthase; *MTHFC*, methenyltetrahydrofolate cyclohydrolase; *MTHFD*, methylenetetrahydrofolate dehydrogenase; *MTHFR*, methylenetetrahydrofolate reductase; *PCFT*, proton-coupled folate transporter; *RFC*, reduced folate carrier; *SHMT*, serine hydroxymethyltransferase; *THF*, tetrahydrofolate; *TS*, thymidylate synthase.

at the C9, N10 bond (see Figure 25-1). Methenyl-THF synthetase, the normal enzymatic function of which is the conversion of 5-formyl-THF to 5,10-methenyl-THF, is responsible for some of this cleavage. The aminobenzoylpolyglutamates generated are hydrolyzed to aminobenzoylglutamate by lysosomal γ-glutamylhydrolase and are partly *N*-acetylated, at least in liver, and the *N*-acetyl-aminobenzoylglutamate is excreted in the urine. In human populations, only small amounts of intact folate are usually found in urine (except in populations exposed to folic acid fortification and/or consuming supplemental folate), and cleavage products represent the bulk of the excretion. Under normal conditions of dietary intake and status, whole-body folate stores turn over slowly with a half-life in excess of 100 days.

METABOLIC FUNCTIONS OF FOLATE

Folate coenzymes act as acceptors or donors of 1-C units in a variety of reactions involved in nucleotide biosynthesis and methyl metabolism in mammalian tissues. Methionine, thymidylate, and purine synthesis are the major pathways of 1-C metabolism and occur in the cytosol and nucleus (see Figure 25-2). These biosynthetic cycles are interconnected, and interconversion of the folate coenzymes is mediated by the trifunctional enzyme, C1-THF synthase. Consequently, folate metabolism and its regulation are interwoven, and factors that regulate any one cycle of 1-C metabolism will influence folate availability for the other cycles. Extensive folate metabolism also occurs in the mitochondria, where

TABLE 25-1 Major Metabolic Reactions for Folate*

REACTION	ENZYME	ABBREVIATION	REACTION CATALYZED
1	Glycinamide ribonucleotide (GAR) formyltransferase	GARFT	10-Formyl-THF + GAR → THF + Formyl-GAR
2	5-amino-4-imadazolecarboxamide ribonucleotide (AICAR) formyltransferase	AICARFT	10-Formyl-THF + AICAR → THF + Formyl-AICAR
3	10-Formyl-THF synthetase	FTHFS	Formate + MgATP + THF → 10-Formyl-THF + MgADP + P_i
4	5,10-Methenyl-THF cyclohydrolase	MTHFC	10-Formyl-THF + H^+ ↔ 5,10-Methenyl-THF + H_2O
5	5,10-Methylene-THF dehydrogenase	MTHFD	5,10-Methenyl-THF + NADPH + H^+ ↔ 5,10-Methylene-THF + $NADP^+$
6	Thymidylate synthase	TS	5,10-Methylene-THF + dUMP → Dihydrofolate + dTMP
7	Dihydrofolate reductase	DHFR	Dihydrofolate + NADPH + H^+ → THF + $NADP^+$
8	Dihydrofolate reductase	DHFR	Folic acid + NADPH + H^+ → DHF + $NADP^+$
9	Cytosolic serine hydroxymethyltransferase	cSHMT	Serine + THF ↔ 5,10-Methylene-THF + Glycine
10	Methylene-THF reductase	MTHFR	5,10-Methylene-THF + NADPH + H^+ → 5-Methyl-THF + $NADP^+$
11	Methionine synthase	MS	5-Methyl-THF + Homocysteine → THF + Methionine
12	Cystathionine β-synthase	CBS	Serine + Homocysteine → Cystathionine + H_2O
13	Betaine-homocysteine methyltransferase	BHMT	Betaine + Homocysteine → Methioinine + Dimethylglycine
14	Mitochondrial serine hydroxymethyltransferase	mSHMT	Serine + THF ↔ 5,10-Methylene-THF + Glycine
15	Mitochondrial 5,10-methylenene-THF dehydrogenase	mMTHFD	5,10-Methylene-THF + NAD^+ ↔ 5,10-Methenyl-THF + NADH + H^+
16	Mitochondrial 5,10-methenyl cyclohydrolase	mMTHFC	5,10-Methenyl-THF + H_2O ↔ 10-Formyl-THF + H^+
17	Mitochondrial 10-formyl-THF synthetase	mFTHFS	10-Formyl-THF + MgADP + P_i ↔ Formate + MgATP + THF

*As shown in Figure 25-2. Reactions 3, 4, and 5 represent activities of the cytosolic trifunctional enzyme, C1-THF synthase.

mitochondrial folate metabolism plays an important role in the provision of 1-C units for cytosolic 1-C metabolism.

NUCLEOTIDE SYNTHESIS

Purine Cycle

The C-8 and C-2 positions of the purine ring are derived from 10-formyl-THF in reactions catalyzed by glycinamide ribonucleotide formyltransferase (GARFT) (see reaction 1 in Figure 25-2 and Table 25-1) and 5-amino-4-imidazolecarboxamide ribonucleotide formyltransferase (AICARFT) (see reaction 2 in Figure 25-2 and Table 25-1). 10-Formyl-THF is formed by the formylation of THF in a reaction catalyzed by 10-formyl-THF synthetase (see reaction 3 in Figure 25-2 and Table 25-1), a step that represents the primary entry point of 1-C units for cytosolic folate-dependent biosynthetic reactions (Stover, 2009).

10-Formyl-THF synthetase activity resides on the C-terminal domain of the trifunctional enzyme, C1-THF synthase, which is encoded by the *MTHFD1* gene. The N-terminal domain of C1-THF synthase contains cyclohydrolase and dehydrogenase activities, which enable the reversible interconversions of 10-formyl-THF to 5,10-methenyl-THF (see reaction 4 in Figure 25-2 and Table 25-1) and 5,10-methenyl-THF to 5,10-methylene-THF (see reaction 5 in Figure 25-2 and Table 25-1). Because of the reversibility of these reactions, 10-formyl-THF can also be obtained by the oxidation of 5,10-methylene-THF. In vivo, however, this pathway is driven in the reductive direction (i.e., toward 5,10-methylene-THF) by the higher ratio of NADPH to $NADP^+$ in the cytosol of cells.

Thymidylate Cycle

Folate, as 5,10-methylene-THF, is required for the synthesis of the pyrimidine, thymidylate. Thymidylate synthase catalyzes the transfer of formaldehyde from folate to the 5-position of deoxyuridine monophosphate (dUMP) for the formation of deoxythymidine monophosphate (dTMP) (see reaction 6 in Figure 25-2 and Table 25-1). The THF of 5,10-methylene-THF provides the reducing component for reduction of the transferred methylene moiety to a methyl group of dTMP and is oxidized to DHF in the process. DHF is inactive as a coenzyme and has to be reduced back to THF, in a reaction catalyzed by DHF reductase, before it can play a further role in 1-C metabolism (see reaction 7 in Figure 25-2 and Table 25-1). The major role of DHF reductase is the reduction of DHF formed during thymidylate synthesis to THF. Dihydrofolate reductase also catalyzes the reduction of synthetic folic acid to DHF (see reaction 8 in Figure 25-2 and Table 25-1) and then THF; however, folic acid is a poorer substrate than DHF (Bailey and Ayling, 2009).

5,10-Methylene-THF is generated from 10-formyl-THF through the cyclohydrolase and dehydrogenase activities of the trifunctional protein, C1-THF synthase, as previously described. Alternatively, 5,10-methylene-THF is obtained by cytosolic serine hydroxymethyltransferase (cSHMT), a pyridoxal 5′-phosphate (PLP)-dependent enzyme that catalyzes the reversible transfer of formaldehyde from serine to THF to generate 5,10-methylene-THF and glycine (see reaction 9 in Figure 25-2 and Table 25-1). Mammalian cells have two genes that encode SHMT isozymes. These isozymes share 63% amino acid sequence identity and are encoded by *SHMT1* and *SHMT2* (Stover, 2009). *SHMT1* encodes the cytosolic isozyme, and *SHMT2* encodes the mitochondrial isozyme found in mature cells. However, *SHMT2* has recently been shown to encode two transcripts, one for *SHMT2* (mitochondrial) and one for *SHMT2α*. The transcript for *SHMT2α* lacks exon 1 and encodes a protein that is found in the cytosol and nucleus during the S (DNA synthesis) phase of the cell cycle (see next paragraph) (Anderson and Stover, 2009). The C3 of serine, a nonessential amino acid derived from glucose or the diet, is a major source of 1-C units for folate metabolism that mainly enter cytosolic folate-mediated 1-C metabolism as formate (Davis et al., 2004).

The three enzymes that constitute the de novo thymidylate synthesis pathway in mammals—cytosolic serine hydroxymethyltransferase (SHMT1 and SHMT2α), thymidylate synthase, and DHF reductase—undergo sumoylation and nuclear import during the S phase of the cell cycle (Anderson et al., 2007; Woeller et al., 2007). Thymidylate synthase activity is expressed only in replicating tissues, and expression of thymidylate synthase and DHF reductase mRNA is highest during the S phase of the cell cycle. Compartmentation of the thymidylate biosynthetic enzymes in the nucleus may allow for folate-dependent deoxythymidine triphosphate (dTTP) biosynthesis directly at the replication fork (Anderson and Stover, 2009).

METHYL METABOLISM

Methionine Cycle

A major cytosolic cycle of 1-C incorporation involves the reduction of 5,10-methylene-THF to 5-methyl-THF, followed by the transfer of the methyl group to homocysteine to form methionine and regenerate THF. 5,10-Methylene-THF reduction is catalyzed by the flavoprotein methylenetetrahydrofolate reductase (MTHFR) (see reaction 10 in Figure 25-2 and Table 25-1). The reaction is irreversible under in vivo conditions and is the committed step in the flux of 1-C units to the methionine resynthesis cycle. The next enzyme in this cycle, methionine synthase, is one of only two vitamin B_{12}–dependent mammalian enzymes, and it catalyzes the transfer of the methyl group from 5-methyl-THF to homocysteine (see reaction 11 in Figure 25-2 and Table 25-1). The methionine synthase reaction is the only reaction in which the methyl group of 5-methyl-THF can be metabolized in mammalian tissues. Although methionine is an essential amino acid, the methionine synthase reaction plays a major role in methyl group metabolism because it allows the reuse of the homocysteine backbone as a carrier of methyl groups derived primarily from the C3 of serine. The enzyme contains tightly bound cob(I)alamin, and the reaction proceeds via a methylcob(III)alamin intermediate as described in the vitamin B_{12} section of this chapter.

Homocysteine is not found in the diet but arises from hydrolysis of *S*-adenosylhomocysteine (AdoHcy), the product of *S*-adenosylmethionine (AdoMet)–dependent methylation reactions. Homocysteine can be metabolized to cysteine in reactions catalyzed by two PLP-dependent enzymes, cystathionine β-synthase (see reaction 12 in Figure 25-2 and Table 25-1) and cystathionine γ-lyase. Alternatively, homocysteine can be converted back to methionine via the folate-dependent methionine synthase reaction (see reaction 11 in Figure 25-2) or by betaine–homocysteine methyltransferase, which catalyzes the transfer of one of the methyl groups of betaine to homocysteine to generate methionine and dimethylglycine (see reaction 13 in Figure 25-2 and Table 25-1). The extent of homocysteine remethylation or transsulfuration is tissue-dependent, and many tissues export homocysteine and cystathionine into the circulation. Tissue levels of homocysteine are normally low; elevated homocysteine levels increase AdoHcy levels, an inhibitor of many methylation reactions. Kidney and liver are thought to be important organs for homocysteine remethylation and for transsulfuration.

Remethylation is also dependent on the methyl group status of the tissue. The major regulator of the folate-dependent methionine cycle is AdoMet, which is a potent allosteric inhibitor of MTHFR. Liver contains a high K_m AdoMet synthetase, and hepatic levels of AdoMet reflect methionine status. High levels of AdoMet inhibit MTHFR, reducing synthesis of 5-methyl-THF and hence remethylation of homocysteine. At the same time, the high levels of AdoMet activate cystathionine β-synthase, stimulating transsulfuration of homocysteine to cysteine. Conversely, when AdoMet is low, remethylation of homocysteine is favored and transsulfuration is inhibited. MTHFR activity is also modified by the well-described genetic variant, 677C→T within this gene, which reduces enzyme activity and modifies disease risk (Christensen and Rozen, 2009).

Liver and kidney also contain a major cytosolic protein, glycine *N*-methyltransferase, which acts as a sink for excess methyl groups. This enzyme catalyzes the AdoMet-dependent methylation of glycine to sarcosine. Although folate is not a substrate for glycine *N*-methyltransferase, 5-methyl-THF is a potent inhibitor and the protein is a major cytosolic folate-binding protein. When AdoMet levels are high, MTHFR is inhibited, reducing 5-methyl-THF formation and relieving inhibition of glycine *N*-methyltransferase, and consequently allowing removal of excess methyl groups. At low AdoMet concentrations, MTHFR is more active, 5-methyl-THF polyglutamates accumulate, and glycine *N*-methyltransferase is inhibited. Excess methionine, which can be toxic, results in an elevated level of sarcosine, some of which is excreted in urine.

SOURCES OF 1-C UNITS FOR BIOSYNTHETIC REACTIONS

Mitochondrial Generation of 1-C Units

Mitochondrial folate-mediated 1-C metabolism generates 1-C units in the form of formate through the catabolism of serine, glycine, and choline. Redox and equilibrium conditions support the flow of 1-C units through the mitochondria in the oxidative direction of 5,10-methylene-THF to 10-formyl-THF to formate (Tibbetts and Appling, 2010); however, many questions remain regarding the control of 1-C flux through the mitochondria, which may be tissue and species specific.

Reduced monoglutamate coenzyme forms, likely the monoglutamate of THF or 5-formyl-THF, are transported across the mitochondrial inner membrane by the mitochondrial folate transporter (MFT) (Tibbetts and Appling, 2010; Titus and Moran, 2000) and then undergo polyglutamation. Entry of serine, glycine, and other 1-C donors into the mitochondria occurs via carrier-mediated processes, although the proteins involved in these transport processes are not well defined.

Mitochondrial PLP-dependent serine hydroxymethyltransferase (mSHMT) catalyzes the reversible transfer of serine C3 to THF to form glycine and 5,10-methylene-THF (see reaction 14 in Figure 25-2 and Table 25-1). 5,10-Methylene-THF can also be produced by the transfer of 1-C units to THF from dimethylglycine, sarcosine, and glycine. The dehydrogenase and cyclohydrolase activities of the mitochondrial bifunctional C_1-THF synthase catalyze the reversible conversions of 5,10-methylene-THF to 5,10-methenyl-THF, and 5,10-methenyl-THF to 10-formyl-THF (see reactions 15 and 16, respectively, in Figure 25-2 and Table 25-1). The bifunctional C_1-THF synthase encoded by the *MTHFD2* gene is expressed in mammalian embryos (Christensen and Mackenzie, 2008), whereas the enzyme encoded by the putative *MTHFD2L* gene is expressed in mammalian adults (Tibbetts and Appling, 2010). It is hypothesized that *MTHFD2L* expression replaces *MTHFD2* as development progresses, thereby maintaining mitochondrial dehydrogenase/cyclohydrolase activities throughout development and adulthood (Tibbetts and Appling, 2010). A separate gene, *MTHFD1L*, encodes a monofunctional 10-formyl-THF synthetase for mitochondrial formate production and THF regeneration (see reaction 17 in Figure 25-2 and Table 25-1). Efflux of formate into the cytosol enables its use in cytosolic folate mediated 1-C metabolism. The 1-C units can also be disposed of by conversion to CO_2 in a reaction catalyzed by 10-formyl-THF dehydrogenase:

$$\text{10-Formyl-THF} + \text{NADP}^+ + H_2O \rightarrow \text{THF} + CO_2 + \text{NADPH} + H^+$$

Alternatively, the 1-C can be used for mitochondrial protein synthesis whereby the initiator methionyl-tRNA (Met-tRNA^{fMet}) is formylated to formylmethionyl-tRNA (fMet-tRNA^{fMet}) (Li et al., 2000) in a reaction catalyzed by methionyl-tRNA formyltransferase:

$$\text{10-Formyl-THF} + \text{Met-tRNA}^{fMet} + H_2O \rightarrow \text{THF} + \text{fMet-tRNA}^{fMet}$$

Cytosolic Generation of 1-C Units

In addition to 1-Cs derived from mitochondrial and cytosolic serine catabolism, 1-C units are also derived from histidine and purine degradation (Stover, 2009). 1-C units derived from histidine and purines enter cytosolic folate-mediated metabolism as 5,10-methenyl-THF, which exists in equilibrium with 10-formyl-THF. The C2 of the imidazole ring of histidine provides 1-C units at the oxidation level of formate. Cytosolic formiminoglutamate formiminotransferase catalyzes the transfer of a formimino group from formiminoglutamate, an intermediate in the histidine catabolism pathway, to THF:

$$\text{Formiminoglutamate} + \text{THF} \rightarrow \text{5-Formimino-THF} + \text{Glutamate}$$

The formimino moiety is converted to 5,10-methenyl-THF in a formiminotetrahydrofolate cyclodeaminase catalyzed reaction:

$$\text{5-Formimino-THF} + H^+ \rightarrow \text{5,10-Methenyl-THF} + NH_3$$

Formiminotransferase and cyclodeaminase activities reside on a single bifunctional protein. In folate deficiency, formiminoglutamate catabolism is impaired, and formiminoglutamate is excreted in elevated amounts in urine.

FOLATE DEFICIENCY: SYMPTOMS, METABOLIC BASES, AND DISEASE

Folate deficiency is usually caused by a dietary insufficiency, although it can arise from other causes such as malabsorption syndromes, genetic heterogeneity, or drug treatment. As might be expected from its metabolic roles, the clinical effects of deficiency are related to defects in DNA synthesis, particularly in fast-growing tissues, and in methyl group metabolism. The classic symptom is a megaloblastic anemia reflecting deranged DNA synthesis in erythropoietic cells. Folate deficiency is also associated with increased risk for vascular disease and an increased incidence of some cancers. Depression and polyneuropathy have also been reported, although the evidence linking folate deficiency to neurological disease is not conclusive. However, in frank genetic diseases involving rare cases of severe defects in various folate-dependent enzymes, neurological symptoms have been clearly documented, with many cases of mental retardation.

MEGALOBLASTIC ANEMIA

Megaloblastic anemia is characterized by enlarged red blood cells (RBCs) and hypersegmentation of the nuclei of circulating polymorphonuclear leukocytes with reduced cell number. Megaloblastic changes also occur in other tissues, but the condition is usually detected clinically by the anemia. The megaloblastic anemia of folate deficiency is identical to that observed in vitamin B_{12} deficiency. Megaloblastic cells have almost twofold the normal content of DNA, and the cells are arrested in the G2 phase of the cell cycle (i.e., in the gap between DNA synthesis and mitosis), preventing cell division. The DNA contains breaks suggesting a defect in DNA synthesis or repair. If cell division occurs, the cells undergo apoptosis (programmed cell death).

These defects are thought to be caused by defective thymidylate synthesis coupled with an enlarged deoxyuridine triphosphate (dUTP) pool that results in uracil misincorporation into DNA. Damaged reticulocytes and RBCs are normally removed by the spleen. Splenectomized individuals with low RBC folate concentrations have an increased uracil content and double-strand breaks in their DNA, and folate supplementation reverses these abnormal findings (Blount et al., 1997). Uracil in DNA normally arises from deamination of cytosine, which constantly occurs at a slow rate. Because uracil behaves exactly as thymine in DNA and base-pairs with adenine, cytosine deamination to uracil can lead to a mutagenic change from a cytosine-guanine (C-G) base pair to a uracil (thymine)-adenine [U(T)-A] base pair during replication. Normally, this potential damage is repaired by uracil–DNA glycosylase, which removes the uracil base. A few additional bases are removed on either side of the damage, and the DNA is repaired by complementary base pairing, with a C being reinserted opposite the G.

Tissues also contain a dUTPase, which hydrolyzes dUTP to deoxyuridine monophosphate (dUMP) and keeps dUTP levels very low. Uridine misincorporation in place of thymidine during DNA synthesis or repair is normally minimized by competition between the small dUTP pool and the larger dTTP pool. If U is misincorporated in place of T (opposite an A), the uracil–DNA glycosylase removes the U, and a T is then reinserted. In folate deficiency, dTTP pools are depressed and dUTP pools are increased, leading to increased incorporation of dUTP instead of dTTP. Increased repair by the glycosylase would lead to more transient single-strand breaks. In addition, repair of the damage by reinsertion of T is inefficient because of the smaller dTTP pools, which increases the probability of U being reinserted by mistake, which in turn leads to more single-strand breaks. If U is misincorporated on both DNA strands in proximity, a double-strand break, which cannot be repaired, can occur during the uracil–DNA glycosylase–mediated repair; unfortunately, an increase in double-strand breaks incurs a higher risk of cancer.

CANCER

Folate deficiency is associated with increased risk for certain types of cancer, including colon cancer, in epidemiological studies (Chen et al., 2009). The underlying mechanism has not been ascertained, but uracil misincorporation arising from defective thymidylate synthesis is hypothesized as one possibility. In many genes, transcription is turned off during development by methylation of cytosine residues (at the C5 position) in CpG islands located in promoter regions of some genes. (Designation of nucleotides separated by a single phosphate moiety [e.g., CpG] is used to distinguish linear sequences of nucleotides in a strand of DNA from base-pairs [e.g., C-G] between strands of DNA.) Epigenetic changes in DNA methylation play important roles in chromosome stability, X chromosome inactivation, and imprinting. Changes in gene expression and DNA methylation are early events in the progression of many human cancers, and both hypermethylation and hypomethylation have been implicated in the inappropriate regulation of proto-oncogenes and tumor suppressor genes (Ciappio and Mason, 2009). Although improved folate status may be beneficial in reducing cancer risk, it is also recognized that once foci of precancerous cells are established, increasing folate intake may increase cancer risk.

Because folate is required for cell division and proliferation, folate antagonists have been used extensively for the treatment of a variety of cancers. Methotrexate, a 4-aminofolic acid analog, is a potent inhibitor of DHF reductase and is used therapeutically for the treatment of cancers. Treatment of rapidly growing cells with this drug causes trapping of folate in the nonfunctional dihydrofolate form. Slowly growing tissues, which have negligible or low levels of thymidylate synthase activity, do not convert reduced folate to the dihydrofolate form as rapidly, so are less affected by a dihydrofolate reductase inhibitor. Clinical resistance to drugs such as methotrexate often develops. Mechanisms for resistance include a decrease in the level of, or a mutation in, the RFC, resulting in decreased methotrexate uptake; amplification of the dihydrofolate reductase gene resulting in an increase in the level of dihydrofolate reductase activity; and a decrease in folylpolyglutamate synthetase activity, which reduces accumulation of the drug by the tissue.

VASCULAR DISEASE

Chronic mild hyperhomocysteinemia is recognized as a risk factor for occlusive vascular disease. However, decreasing homocysteine levels through treatment with folic acid and other B vitamins (B_{12} and B_6) has not been shown to be effective in the prevention of a heart attack (Clarke et al., 2010; M. Lee et al., 2010; Mei et al., 2010; Miller et al., 2010). Efficacy of B vitamin supplementation in the reduction of stroke is also largely negative, although potential mild benefits in primary stroke prevention were shown (M. Lee et al., 2010). Thus although elevated plasma homocysteine concentrations

CLINICAL CORRELATION

Folate and Cancer Risk: A Complex Relationship

Joel B. Mason, MD

A large body of epidemiological evidence has emerged over the past two decades that indicates that those individuals who habitually consume an abundant quantity of folate in their diet have an approximately 20% to 50% reduced risk of developing certain cancers compared to those whose diets contain the lowest amounts of the vitamin. Additionally, the relationship generally remains robust even after other known risk factors for cancer are removed by statistical regression. Interestingly, the protective effect tends to be more pronounced among those who are moderate-to-heavy consumers of alcohol, a known inhibitor of folate metabolism. Although a few notable null studies exist, the overwhelming consensus of studies in this field is that adequate folate intake does exert a protective effect. The most compelling evidence in this regard pertains to colorectal cancer, although lesser degrees of evidence exist for other common cancers such as those of the breast, lung, and pancreas.

Evidence in support of a true causal relationship between folate intake and colorectal cancer risk is bolstered by several other types of scientific evidence. For instance, in several rodent models of colorectal cancer, the consumption of adequate amounts of folate conveys a cancer-protective effect compared to diets mildly inadequate in folate. Also, homozygosity for the common C677T polymorphism in the MTHFR gene is associated with a reduced risk of colorectal cancer, further implicating a true mechanistic role for folate metabolism in the determination of cancer risk. Moreover, a protective role for folate is eminently plausible from a biological perspective, because two of the major biochemical functions of folate in the cell—nucleotide synthesis (and by extension DNA synthesis and repair) and biological methylation—are each considered major pathways by which cancer may develop when these processes go awry.

However, more is not necessarily better when it comes to folate consumption. Several lines of evidence suggest that an excessive intake of folate may play a paradoxical, cancer-promoting role in select circumstances, especially when existing clones of precancerous or cancerous cells are present. Moreover, there is a genuine possibility that the lifestyle habits of many Americans, in conjunction with public health policy and the practices of the food industry, have inadvertently created these circumstances among certain segments of the population. Observations supporting this concept date back to two human trials conducted in subjects with acute leukemia in the 1940s. More rigorously conducted, contemporary studies—including two intervention trials—have recapitulated these early studies and underscore the point that relatively modest levels of folate supplementation can create this cancer-promoting effect (Cole et al., 2007; Ebbing et al., 2009; Figueiredo et al., 2009). Moreover, nationally representative colorectal cancer incidence in North America increased by about 5 cancer cases per 100,000 individuals in conjunction with the institution of mandatory folic acid fortification of enriched cereal grains in both the United States and Canada in the mid 1990s, which translates to 15,000 additional cases in the United States each year (Mason et al., 2007). Organs prone to contain indolent foci of precancerous tissue (so-called dysplasia) in the elderly, such as the colorectum and prostate, seem to be most vulnerable to this effect. This is of considerable concern in the United States, where 35% to 50% of adults over the age of 50 years harbor one or more colonic adenomas and the majority of men over the age of 70 contain foci of precancerous tissue in their prostate.

The quantity of folate consumed by many U.S. adults does seem to fall within a range that might produce this cancer-promoting effect. In addition to the folate obtained from natural sources in the diet, there are a plethora of foodstuffs that are fortified with folic acid either at the discretion of the food industry or because of federally mandated fortification of enriched flour. Moreover, 40% of U.S. adults over the age of 59 years consume a vitamin supplement at least five times per week; this appears to be the major source of excess folate consumption. By consuming a multivitamin and a bowl of fortified ready-to-eat cereal in the morning, federally mandated fortified flour in various foodstuffs during the course of the day, and a vitamin B-complex tablet at night, one can easily exceed 2,000 dietary folate equivalents (DFEs) in a day.

The cancer-promoting effect of folate is likely related to the fact that a neoplastic colonic epithelium has an exceptionally high rate of proliferation and therefore a heightened demand for nucleotides. Accelerated proliferation might therefore be induced by excess folate because the vitamin is an essential cofactor for de novo thymidine synthesis, a rate-limiting step for DNA synthesis. The fact that folic acid, which is not a naturally occurring form of the vitamin, is used by food and pharmaceutical industries for fortification and supplementation may also be important. Folic acid is usually converted to a natural biological form of the vitamin (i.e., 5-methyltetrahydrofolate) as it passes through the intestinal wall. However, oral doses of as little as 200 μg can saturate this conversion mechanism, resulting in circulating folic acid (Sweeney et al., 2007). There is some concern that this oxidized, nonsubstituted form of folate might be detrimental because it bypasses certain regulatory modes and enters folate metabolism in the form of tetrahydrofolate, which is converted directly to 5,10-methylene-THF, the essential cofactor for thymidine synthesis. More than 80% of individuals who are regular users of vitamin supplements have detectable levels of unmetabolized folic acid in their plasma.

This "dual effect of folate," as it pertains to cancer risk, is creating considerable consternation for those who are trying to establish guidelines for the healthful intake

CLINICAL CORRELATION—cont'd

Folate and Cancer Risk: A Complex Relationship

Joel B. Mason, MD

of folate, particularly because it underscores the point that the level of intake of a micronutrient that is safe and healthful for one person may be potentially harmful to another. The issue is particularly poignant at present, because many countries are debating whether to institute, or increase, mandatory folic acid fortification of grains, the latter being an effective means of preventing births complicated by a neural tube defect.

There is good evidence that folate may promote cancer development under certain experimental conditions. The challenge before us is to determine whether we have inadvertently enabled it to play this paradoxical role as a cancer-promoting agent throughout the population. The evidence to support such a contention is sparse, but it is not a possibility that we should cast aside without careful consideration.

are a marker of increased risk for cardiovascular disease, the routine use of folic acid and other B vitamins for cardiovascular prevention is not supported by the current available evidence.

BIRTH DEFECTS

Neural tube defects (NTDs) are congenital malformations of the brain and spinal cord caused by the failure of the neural tube to close during early embryogenesis. NTDs constitute the third largest congenital burden after congenital heart disease and Down syndrome. NTD risk is modified by numerous genetic and environmental factors including exposure to folic acid. The observation that periconceptual supplementation with folic acid reduced the incidence of these defects by 50% to 75% led to mandated folic acid fortification programs in the United States and approximately 50 other countries (Berry et al., 2009). As a result of these fortification programs, folate intake and status have increased dramatically (Berry et al., 2009). Notably, incidence of newborns with NTDs has decreased in several populations, in the range of 19% to 78% (Berry et al., 2009), with the greatest percent declines occurring in groups with the highest baseline rates.

Although folate status affects the risk for NTDs, this condition is not thought to result from folate deficiency per se. It appears to be a genetic disease, possibly multigenetic, with a phenotype that can be modified by increased folate in the subset of individuals who are folate-responsive. The mechanism by which improved maternal folate status affords protection is unknown. However, emerging data emphasize the importance of folate and the thymidylate biosynthesis pathway in proper neural tube closure (Beaudin and Stover, 2009). Neural crest cells, which participate in neural tube closure, have an especially high demand for folate to support cellular growth, diffentiation, and migration (Wallis et al., 2009). Disruptions in the normal methylation states of genes could also be a contributing factor (Beaudin and Stover, 2007, 2009).

There is some evidence that folic acid supplementation may reduce the risk of orofacial clefts (Wallis et al., 2009; Hobbs et al., 2009; Wehby and Murray, 2010) and congenital heart defects (Wallis et al., 2009), although results are mixed. Interestingly, neural crest cells are involved in the development of the craniofacial structure, the neural tube, and the heart and thus provide a link between these diverse anatomical structures (Wallis et al., 2009). Preliminary data also suggest that folic acid supplementation throughout pregnancy may reduce the risk of certain adverse pregnancy outcomes such as preterm birth (Czeizel et al., 2010; Tamura et al., 2009) but paradoxically increase the risk of others (i.e., asthma in children [Whitrow et al., 2009]).

FOLATE STATUS ASSESSMENT

Folate status is most commonly assessed by measurements of serum (or plasma) or RBC folate concentrations. Mature RBCs do not transport or accumulate folate; their folate stores are formed during erythropoiesis and are retained, probably because of binding to hemoglobin, through the 120-day life span of the human RBC. Thus RBC folate concentrations are often used as a measure of long-term folate status. Fasting serum folate concentrations also are an indicator of status but can be influenced by recent dietary intake. Serum folate concentrations of less than 3 ng/mL and RBC folate concentrations of less than 140 ng/mL are indicative of folate deficiency (Institute of Medicine [IOM], 1998). Plasma concentrations of total homocysteine, which increase when there is a deficiency of 5-methyl-THF, are used as a functional indicator of folate status. However, because homocysteine metabolism is affected by the availability of other B vitamins (i.e., vitamin B_{12}), it is not considered a specific marker. Various cutoff values of elevated plasma homocysteine have been reported and range from higher than 10 to higher than 16 μmol/L.

Since folic acid fortification of the U.S. food supply in 1998, the prevalence of low blood folate in the entire U.S. population has decreased substantially such that less than 1% and 6% have low serum folate and RBC folate concentrations, respectively (Pfeiffer et al., 2007). Similarly, the prevalence of elevated plasma homocysteine concentrations, defined as higher than 13 μmol/L, is 5% of the U.S. population (Pfeiffer et al., 2005). Thus in the era of folic acid fortification, an elevated fasting plasma homocysteine is more likely due to vitamin B_{12} than folate deficiency.

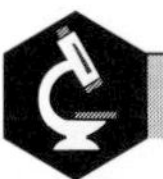

CLINICAL CORRELATION

Folic Acid and Neural Tube Defects: Are We Any Closer to Understanding Mechanisms?

Patrick J. Stover, PhD

Neural tube defects (NTDs) are a class of common birth defects that include anencephaly, exencephaly, and spina bifida. They arise from the failure to complete the closure of the neural tube during a critical developmental window which extends from the 23rd to 28th day following human conception. NTD etiology is heterogeneous and multifactorial. Over the past two decades numerous genetic, nutritional, and other environmental risk factors have been identified. However, 95% of NTD-affected pregnancies are born into families with no history of these disorders (American College of Obstetricians and Gynecologists, 2008). The strongest association to date is between the B-vitamin folate and NTD risk. Although the mechanisms resulting in failure of neural tube closure are unknown, up to 70% of NTDs can be prevented by maternal folic acid supplementation.

Closure of the neural tube during early embryonic development requires rapid cell proliferation, survival, differentiation, and migration of the neural epithelium. Therefore it is not surprising that hundreds of genes have been identified as causing neural tube closure defects when disrupted in mice. However, only a few of these NTD mouse models have been shown to be prevented by maternal folic acid supplementation, and none has been found to contribute significantly to the overall genetic risk for human NTDs.

The metabolic mechanisms underlying the association between folate and NTD pathogenesis have yet to be identified. Disruption of Folbp1, a folate receptor responsible for folate transport in the developing neural epithelium, results in folate responsive neural tube defects in mice (Piedrahita et al., 1999). This mouse model confirms the essential role of folate in neural tube closure defects. Although elevated plasma homocysteine, which occurs during folate deficiency, is a risk factor for NTDs, disruption of genes that encode enzymes involved in folate-dependent homocysteine remethylation do not cause NTDs, nor does disruption of genes involved in homocysteine metabolism through the transsulfuration pathway. These results indicate that the genetic contribution to NTDs is not associated with homocysteine metabolism or folate-dependent methionine biosynthesis. Disruption of *Shmt1*, an enzyme that supplies folate-activated 1-C units for de novo thymidylate biosynthesis, results in folate-responsive exencephaly in mice but not spina bifida (Beaudin et al., 2011). Additional investigation of mouse models of folate-dependent nucleotide biosynthesis may reveal the full range of metabolic disruptions that lead to NTDs and untangle the relative contributions of nutritional deficiency and genetic risk factors to NTD pathogenesis.

Determining the precise metabolic impairments that cause NTDs has the potential to design improved nutritional interventions that target both susceptible subgroups of the population and the metabolic pathway that causes neural tube closure defects.

FOLATE DIETARY RECOMMENDATIONS

DIETARY REFERENCE INTAKES

Because folic acid added to food is more bioavailable than food folate, folate recommendations are now stated as dietary folate equivalents (DFEs): 0.6 μg of folic acid is equivalent to 1 μg of folate from food:

$$\mu g \text{ of DFEs} = \mu g \text{ of Food folate} + (1.7 \times \mu g \text{ of Folic acid})$$

The Institute of Medicine (IOM, 1998) set the Estimated Average Requirement (EAR) for adults as 320 μg of DFEs per day, based mainly on controlled studies in which participants received a folate-depleted diet supplemented with various levels of folic acid. Assuming a 10% coefficient of variation, the Recommended Dietary Allowance (RDA) for adult men and women was set as the EAR + 20%. A higher intake is recommended for pregnant and lactating women to cover the accelerated demands placed on the supply of folate for DNA synthesis (and other 1-C transfer reactions) and the amount of folate secreted in milk, respectively. Recommendations for children were based on extrapolation from adult EARs on the basis of metabolic body weight ($kg^{0.75}$). Adequate Intakes (AIs) for infants were based on the folate content of milk of well-nourished mothers. The AI of folate for infants during the first 6 months after birth was based on a mean daily intake of 0.78 L of milk that contains 85 μg/L of folate. The AI for infants ages 7 through 12 months was extrapolated from the AI or EARs for other age groups. Increases in dietary intake of folate do not affect maternal milk folate levels. Because no information is available on the bioavailability of milk folate in infants compared to that of folic acid added to formula, DFEs are not used to calculate the level of folic acid to add to formula.

FOLATE INTAKE

The 2003-2006 data from the National Health and Nutrition Examination Survey (NHANES) showed that the median (50th percentile) intake of dietary folate in U.S. women ages 31 to 50 years is 437 μg DFE/day, with a range (5th to 95th percentile) from 215 to 834 μg DFE/day (Bailey et al., 2010a). Median dietary folate intake for men ages 19 to 50 years is 607 μg DFE/day, and dietary folate intake by U.S. men ranges from 339 to 1047 μg DFE/day. Compared to the EAR for folate, most of the adult U.S. population (more than 75%) is getting adequate dietary folate intake. When supplemental folic acid and dietary folate intake are combined, more than 85% are above the EAR.

DRIs Across the Life Cycle: Folate

	µg DFEs per Day	
Infants	RDA	UL*
0 through 6 mo	65 (AI)	ND
7 through 12 mo	80 (AI)	ND
Children		
1 through 3 yr	150	300
4 through 8 yr	200	400
9 through 13 yr	300	600
14 through 18 yr	400	800
Adults		
≥19 yr	400†	800
Pregnant women		
<19 yr	600	800
≥19 yr	600	1,000
Lactating women		
<19 yr	500	800
≥19 yr	500	1,000

Data from IOM. (1998). *Dietary Reference Intakes for thiamin, riboflavin, niacin, vitamin* B_6*, folate, vitamin* B_{12}*, pantothenic acid, biotin, and choline*. Washington, DC: National Academy Press.

1 µg DFE = 1 µg food folate = 0.5 µg of folic acid taken on an empty stomach = 0.6 µg of folic acid with meals.

AI, Adequate Intake; *DFEs*, dietary folate equivalents; *DRI;* Dietary Reference Intake; *ND*, not determinable; *RDA*, Recommended Dietary Allowance; *UL*, Tolerable Upper Intake Level.

*The UL for folate applies to synthetic folic acid obtained from supplements, fortified foods, or a combination of the two.

†To minimize the risk of neural tube defects, it is recommended that women capable of becoming pregnant consume 400 µg of folic acid per day (from supplements and/or fortified foods) in addition to normal food folate intake.

FOLIC ACID INTAKE RECOMMENDATION FOR NEURAL TUBE DEFECT RISK REDUCTION

The folate intervention trials that established the protective effect of folic acid, coupled with other surveys, led to recommendations by the U.S. Public Health Service (1992) and the IOM (1998) that women capable of becoming pregnant consume 400 µg of synthetic folic acid per day to reduce their risk of having a baby with a NTD. It is not known whether lower levels of supplementation would be as effective, nor is it known whether disease risk could be reduced by dietary folate alone. Food folate is less bioavailable than folic acid. Post–folic acid fortification NHANES data indicate that the majority of women in the United States are not consuming the recommended 400 µg synthetic folic acid per day for NTD risk reduction (U.S. Department of Agriculture, 2010) and that meeting this level of intake requires the use of supplements containing folic acid (Yang et al., 2010).

GENETIC POLYMORPHISMS

Genetic variation within genes encoding proteins involved in folate metabolism and transport alters the risk of developing diseases such as NTDs, cancer, cardiovascular disease, and dementia (Christensen and Rozen, 2009). The gene–disease relationship is often modified by folate status such that effects of the polymorphism are only observed under conditions of suboptimal folate status. Therefore ensuring an adequate folate intake in individuals harboring deleterious functional variants (i.e., those modulating gene expression or protein function) is an important consideration when establishing nutrient recommendations designed to improve human health.

Historically, this genetic heterogeneity has been accounted for when setting RDAs by adding two coefficients of variation (CV) to the EAR. For establishing the RDAs for folate, a CV of 10% was assumed based on variation in basal metabolic rate (IOM, 1998); thus the RDA for folate may not adequately capture the impact of genetic variation in folate-metabolizing genes on requirements.

The *MTHFR* 677C→T single nucleotide polymorphism is the most common genetic cause of mild hyperhomocysteinemia and is frequently associated with lower folate status (Christensen and Rozen, 2009). The 677C→T polymorphism causes a substitution of valine for alanine in the protein's catalytic domain and yields a thermolabile enzyme that is more likely to dissociate from its riboflavin-derived flavin adenine dinucleotide (FAD) cofactor (Yamada et al., 2001). The prevalence of the MTHFR 677TT (homozygous) genotype varies by ethnicity and geographic location but averages 11% in the United States (Yang et al., 2008). Research examining the adequacy of the current RDA of 400 µg DFE/day has shown it to be sufficient for women with the 677TT genotype (Guinotte et al., 2003; Shelnutt et al., 2003) yet insufficient for men with the 677TT genotype (Solis et al., 2008).

FOLATE TOXICITY

There is no evidence of adverse effects of high intakes of naturally occurring food folate. Large doses of folic acid, however, can produce a hematological response in people with megaloblastic anemia caused by vitamin B_{12} deficiency. When folate was first isolated, and before the isolation of vitamin B_{12}, many patients with pernicious anemia were treated with large quantities of folic acid. Folic acid does not correct the severe neurological symptoms of vitamin B_{12} deficiency, and some studies suggested that folic acid treatment of vitamin B_{12}–deficient subjects may have exacerbated the development of neurological defects. Because large doses of folic acid may mask the development and diagnosis of anemia in vitamin B_{12}–deficient people and thus increase the risk that vitamin B_{12} deficiency will be recognized only when irreversible neurological symptoms develop, the IOM (1998) set the Tolerable Upper Intake Level (UL) at 1 mg per day of folic acid from fortified food or supplements. Excessive folic acid intake may also promote the growth of established tumors.

NHANES 2003–2006 survey data showed that 2.7% of U.S. adults (Yang et al., 2010) and 5% of those older than 50 years (Bailey et al., 2010a) consumed more than the UL of folic acid. However, U.S. adults who do not consume supplements or who consume an average of 400 µg or less of folic acid per day from supplements are unlikely to exceed the UL at current fortification levels (Yang et al., 2010). In U.S. children aged 1 to 13 years, more than half (53%) of dietary supplement users exceeded the UL as compared with 5% of nonusers (Bailey et al., 2010b).

THINKING CRITICALLY

Folate

Genetic Variation

1. Describe the MTHFR 677C→T genetic variant.
2. What are the effects of homozygosity for this genetic variant on serum folate and homocysteine? Explain why these effects are observed.
3. In the era of folic acid fortification of the food supply, robust effects of the MTHFR 677TT genotype are not observed. Why?
4. What are the challenges, advantages, and limitations to establishing dietary recommendations based on genetic background? Should separate recommendations be established for various subgroups based on genotype?

Cancer

1. Identify the mechanisms by which folate deficiency can increase cancer risk.
2. Explain how excess folic acid might increase cancer progression.
3. Explain why folate-related proteins (i.e., enzymes and transporters) are therapeutic targets in the treatment of cancer.
4. Based on the dual role of folate in cancer, explain the title below.

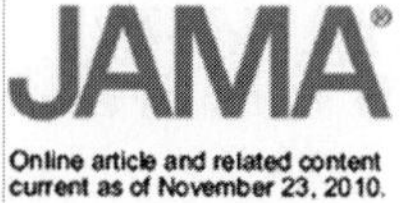
JAMA
Online article and related content current as of November 23, 2010.

Folate and Cancer—Timing Is Everything
Cornelia M. Ulrich; John D. Potter
JAMA. 2007;297(21):2408-2409 (doi:10.1001/jama.297.21.2408)
http://jama.ama-assn.org/cgi/content/full/297/21/2408

CHOLINE

Choline was first isolated from ox bile (the Greek word for bile is *chole*) by Andreas Strecker in 1862 and chemically synthesized in 1866. The nutritional importance of choline was recognized in the early 1930s by Best and Huntsman when it was demonstrated that dietary choline deficiency caused fatty liver in rodents. Over the next decade, a general consensus emerged on the dietary essentiality of choline for several mammalian species including the rat, dog, chicken, pig, rhesus monkey, and baboon. Dietary choline deprivation in these mammals resulted in serious physiological changes with rapid accumulation of triacylglycerol in the liver being the most common manifestation. Recognition that choline may also be an essential nutrient for humans was advanced by studies in men and women on parenteral nutrition (Buchman et al., 2001). A dietary requirement for choline was also demonstrated in healthy men participating in a choline depletion–repletion metabolic study (Zeisel et al., 1991), the results of which guided the establishment of choline adequate intake levels in 1998 (IOM, 1998).

CHOLINE CHEMISTRY

Choline (2-hydroxyethyl-trimethyl-ammonium) is a trimethylated, positively charged, quaternary, saturated amine (Figure 25-3) that serves as the precursor molecule of several metabolites and is commonly grouped with the water-soluble B vitamins. Betaine, dimethylglycine, and sarcosine are oxidized derivatives of choline, each possessing one or more labile methyl groups. Phosphatidylcholine (PtdCho), the main form of choline in food and in the body, is a phospholipid with choline as its polar head group. PtdCho can be made from choline by the cytidine diphosphate choline (CDP-choline) pathway (also known as the Kennedy pathway) or it can be synthesized by the sequential methylation of phosphatidylethanolamine via the phosphatidylethanolamine *N*-methyltransferase (PEMT) pathway (see Figure 25-3). The PEMT pathway forms a "new" choline moiety and is often referred to as the de novo pathway. Sphingomyelin, a sphingolipid, can be derived from PtdCho, whereas lysophosphatidylcholine and glycerophosphocholine are degradation products of PtdCho (see Figure 25-3).

FOOD SOURCES OF CHOLINE

Foods contain water-soluble forms of choline (i.e., free choline, phosphocholine, glycerophosphocholine) and lipid-soluble forms (i.e., sphingomyelin, lysophosphatidylcholine [lysoPtdCho], and PtdCho) (Zeisel et al., 2003). Approximately two thirds of choline in food is found in the lipid-soluble form, mainly as PtdCho. The remaining one third is present in water-soluble forms, mostly as free choline and glycerophosphocholine. Dietary choline intake is determined by summing all forms of choline, including PtdCho, sphingomyelin, lysoPtdCho, free choline, glycerophosphocholine, and phosphocholine. Betaine, although derived from choline, is not included in this summation because it cannot be converted back to choline. However, a high consumption of dietary betaine may have a choline-sparing effect (Dilger et al., 2007). Choline is widely distributed in the food supply, but animal products are generally a more concentrated source than plant materials. Choline is not usually found in vitamin and mineral supplements but it can be purchased as a choline salt, CDP-choline, or PtdCho (i.e., lecithin).

CHOLINE ABSORPTION

Digestion and absorption of choline metabolites varies depending upon the form. The majority of PtdCho is digested by the action of phospholipase A2, yielding a free fatty acid and lysoPtdCho, both of which are absorbed by enterocytes, as described in Chapter 10. Within the enterocyte, a portion of the lysoPtdCho is reacylated to PtdCho and incorporated into chylomicrons. The remainder is further hydrolyzed to glycerophosphocholine and subsequently glycerophosphate and free choline. Both the choline and the glycerophosphate can be

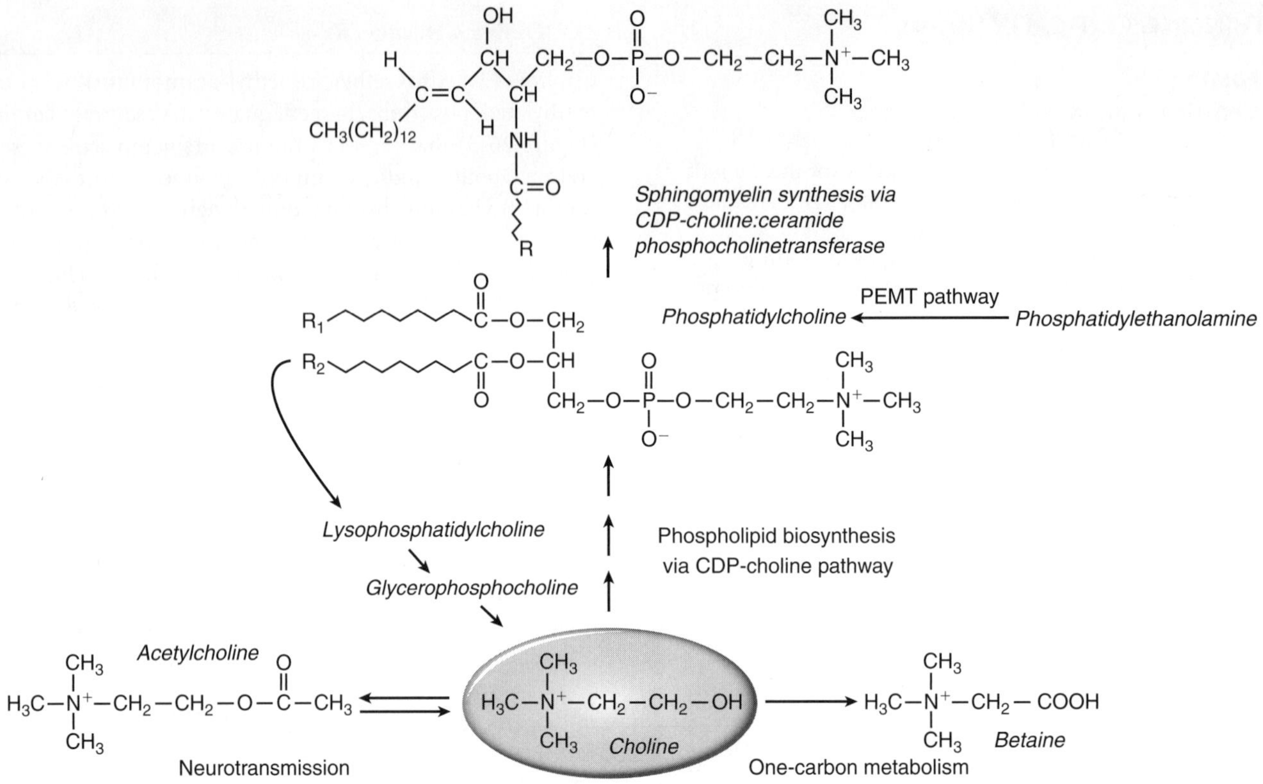

FIGURE 25-3 Choline: structure and aspects of its metabolism. *CDP*, Cytidine diphosphate; *PEMT*, phosphatidylethanolamine *N*-methyltransferase.

transported by the portal blood for use in the liver or other tissues.

Free choline is absorbed mainly in the jejunum and ileum via a sodium-independent carrier mediated transport system that is saturable and substrate-specific (Kamath et al., 2003). Passive diffusion also occurs at high choline concentrations. Within the enterocyte a portion of the absorbed free choline is oxidized to betaine. The osmotic properties of betaine may play an important role in the enterocyte. Dietary betaine is absorbed mainly in the duodenum via a carrier-mediated transport system that is distinct from that used for choline. Choline efflux across the basolateral membrane and entry into the hepatic portal venous system is less well characterized but may involve a proton antiport system.

Unabsorbed choline reaching the large intestine is metabolized in part to methylamines by gut bacteria (Zeisel et al., 1983). The methylamines, mainly trimethylamine and its oxide (trimethylamine *N*-oxide), are excreted in urine and feces. Excessive excretion of trimethylamine is responsible for the fishy body odor that occurs with large oral doses of free choline. Impaired oxidation of trimethylamine to its nonodorous counterpart, trimethylamine *N*-oxide, can also arise from genetic errors in the flavin-containing monooxygenase 3 gene, *FMO3*. Individuals harboring this genetic aberration require diets low in free choline to avoid trimethylamine excess and fishy body odor.

CHOLINE BIOAVAILABLITY

The bioavailability of free choline appears to be very high. Studies with CDP-choline (cytidine 5′-diphosphocholine) show virtually complete absorption of free choline (after its hydrolysis from cytidine in the small intestine) and its wide distribution in the body (Secades and Lorenzo, 2006). The bioavailability of PtdCho varies depending upon the food source. Chick growth bioassays show that soybean PtdCho is fully available, peanut and soybean meal PtdCho are 76% and 83% available, respectively, and canola meal PtdCho is 24% available (Emmert and Baker, 1997). Factors limiting PtdCho bioavailability are unclear. In rat and human studies, the fatty acid composition of the PtdCho molecule does not alter bioavailability. The total choline content of food is not changed by heat treatment (although interconversions between choline forms may occur).

Because of absorptive and transport differences between water and lipid-soluble choline metabolites (i.e., portal blood versus the lymphatic system, which bypasses the liver), differences in the distribution and metabolic fate of the choline moiety may exist. In a study in which ^{14}C-methyl-labeled choline, phosphocholine, glycerophosphocholine, and PtdCho were added to infant formula and fed to rat pups, uptake of label from choline and PtdCho was similar (Cheng et al., 1996). Label from the water-soluble metabolites (choline, phosphocholine, and glycerophosphocholine) appeared rapidly within blood and liver, reaching peak levels by 5 hours;

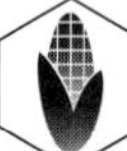

FOOD SOURCES OF CHOLINE

Meat and Meat Substitutes
365 mg per 3 oz beef liver
258 mg per 3 oz chicken giblets
87 to 106 mg per 3 oz beef
85 to 95 mg per 3 oz pork
65 to 70 mg per 3 oz crustacean meat (lobster, crab), tuna, trout, swordfish, halibut, cod
23 mg per ¼ block tofu
100 to 125 mg per 1 large egg scrambled, fried, poached

Milk and Milk Products
220 mg per 1 cup condensed, sweetened milk
58 mg per 1 cup soy milk
43 mg per 1 cup milk
40 mg per 1 cup cottage cheese
34 mg per 8 oz yogurt

Legumes
70 to 80 mg per 1 cup navy, garbanzo, kidney, lima beans
65 mg per 1 cup lentils, peas

Vegetables
100 mg per 1 cup tomato
60 mg per 1 cup Brussels sprout, broccoli, cauliflower, artichokes, collard greens

Grains
36 to 40 mg per 1 cup whole grain wheat flour, bulgur
34 mg per 1 cup buckwheat groats
30 mg per 1 cup oat bran
26 mg per 1 cup whole grain yellow cornmeal

USDA, ARS. (2010). *USDA National Nutrient Database for Standard Reference, Release 23*. Retrieved from *www.ars.usda.gov/ba/bhnrc/ndl*.

label in brain continued to increase for more than 24 hours. Label from the lipid-soluble metabolite, PtdCho, took longer to appear in blood and liver, consistent with its absorption via the slower lymphatic route versus the portal blood route, but remained elevated for more than 24 hours. Label from PtdCho in brain continued to increase for more than 24 hours but failed to achieve the concentrations attained by treatment with the water-soluble choline metabolites. These putative bioavailability inequities should be considered when selecting the form of choline to be used in the preparation of infant formula, supplements, and research studies.

TRANSPORT OF CHOLINE

Because choline is a charged hydrophilic cation, transport mechanisms are required for its entry into most cells (Lockman and Allen, 2002). There are two main groups of choline transporters: (1) the high-affinity (K_m of 20 μm or less), saturable, sodium-dependent choline transporters (CHTs) that provide choline for acetylcholine synthesis in the presynaptic nerve terminal; and (2) the low-affinity (K_m greater than 30 to 100 μm), sodium-independent choline transporters, which are ubiquitously expressed in plasma membranes and provide choline for phospholipid synthesis. Additional less common choline transport systems have been described including a high-affinity, sodium-dependent transport system residing in the blood brain–barrier.

METABOLISM OF CHOLINE

As the precursor of several metabolites, choline has many physiological functions throughout the body that depend on its available local supply. The main tissue involved in choline metabolism is the liver, where choline has two main fates: phospholipid biosynthesis (i.e., PtdCho and sphingomyelin) or conversion to the methyl donor betaine (Figure 25-4). Small amounts of free choline are also converted to acetylcholine in specific tissue types. In lung, PtdCho with palmitate esterified to the *sn*1 and *sn*2 positions of the glycerol backbone (i.e., dipalmitoylphosphatidylcholine) is the most active component of lung surfactant.

PHOSPHATIDYLCHOLINE

Phosphatidylcholine accounts for about 95% of the total choline pool in most tissues and is the predominate phospholipid in mammalian cells (Li and Vance, 2008). In the liver, PtdCho can be used for membrane biogenesis, formation of bile, secretion in very-low-density lipoprotein (VLDL), and production of sphingomyelin (see Figure 25-4). All mammalian cells with a nucleus can make PtdCho through the CDP-choline pathway. This pathway is critical to cell vitality and its impairment leads to programmed cell death (apoptosis). An alternate pathway involving methylation of phosphatidylethanolamine (a noncholine metabolite) also exists and is most active in liver. Catabolism of PtdCho by several phospholipases enables choline recycling as well as the generation of several cellular signaling molecules.

CDP-Choline Pathway

Upon entry into a cell, free choline is rapidly phosphorylated to phosphocholine by choline kinase, a cytosolic enzyme that catalyzes the initial and committed step of the CDP-choline pathway (see reaction 1 in Figure 25-4 and Table 25-2). Choline kinase is encoded by two genes, *CHKA* and *CKHB*. Disruption of the *CHKA* gene is lethal at an early stage of embryogenesis in mice (Wang et al., 2005).

In the second and rate-limiting step of the CDP-choline pathway, phosphocholine is activated to CDP-choline in a CTP-dependent reaction catalyzed by CTP:phosphocholine cytidylyltransferase (see reaction 2 in Figure 25-4 and Table 25-2). Two genes, *PCYT1A* and *PYCT1B*, encode the α and β isoforms of human CTP:phosphocholine cytidylyltransferase, respectively. The α isoform is ubiquitously expressed and contains an N-terminal nuclear localization signal that directs the enzyme to the nucleus in many cultured and primary cells (Gehrig et al., 2009). Nuclear localization of the α isoform may be important for coordinating PtdCho synthesis with the cycle cell as well as nuclear envelope architecture and proliferation (Lagace and Ridgway, 2005). The α isoform of CTP:phosphocholine cytidylyltransferase

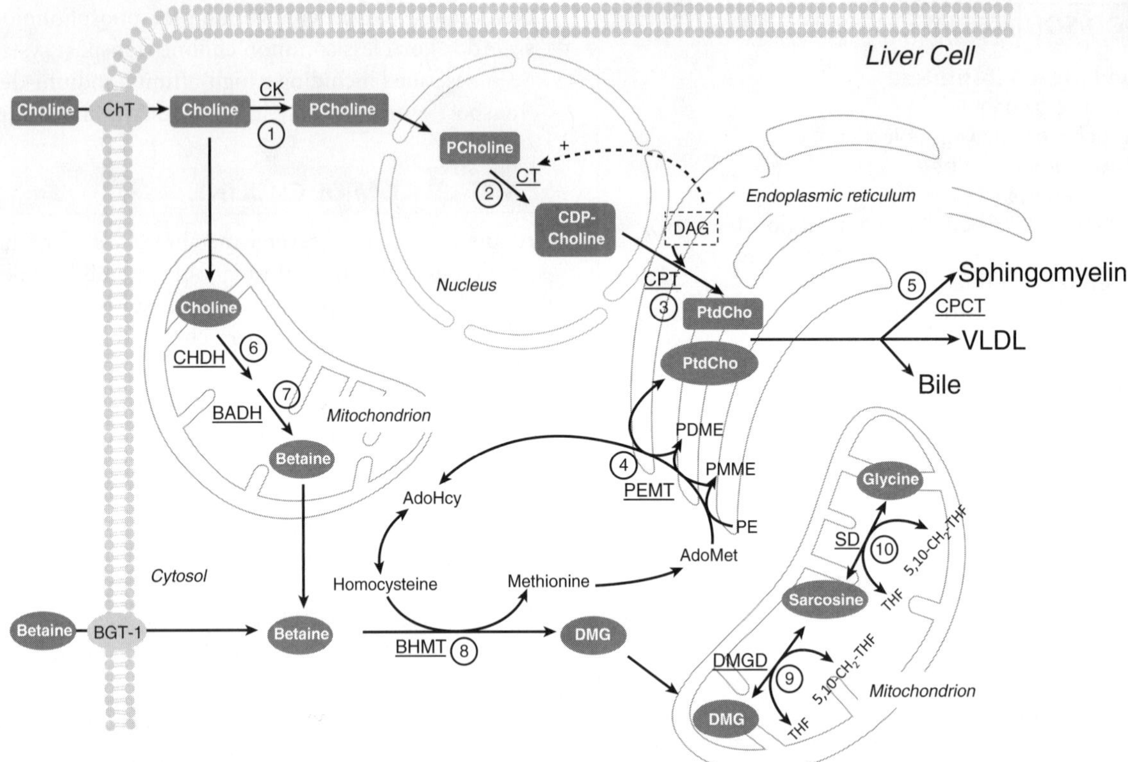

FIGURE 25-4 Hepatic choline metabolism. Entry of choline into hepatocytes is carrier mediated (CLT). Choline is preferentially directed toward the CDP-choline pathway for phosphatidylcholine (PtdCho) biosynthesis (metabolites with rectangular backgrounds). CTP-phosphocholine cytidylyltransferase is the rate-limiting enzyme of the CDP-choline pathway and is activated by diacylglycerol (DAG). As free choline levels rise within the cell, oxidation to betaine occurs. Betaine can also enter the hepatocyte via facilitated diffusion (BGT-1). Betaine participates in one-carbon metabolism (metabolites with circular backgrounds) and is used for the remethylation of homocysteine to methionine. Phosphatidylethnaolamine *N*-methyltransferase (PEMT), a main consumer of methyl groups, provides an alternative pathway for PtdCho biosynthesis. Once synthesized, PtdCho has several fates, including conversion to sphingomyelin; incorporation into very-low-density lipoproteins, bile, or biomembranes; and hydrolysis to free choline. Refer to Table 25-2 for a description of the reaction that corresponds to each number. *AdoHcy, S*-adenosylhomocysteine; *AdoMet, S*-adenosylmethionine; *BADH,* betaine aldehyde dehydrogenase; *BGT-1,* betaine/gamma amino butyric acid transporter; *BHMT,* betaine-homocysteine methyltransferase; *CDP,* cytidine diphosphate; *CHDH,* choline dehydrogenase; *CK,* choline kinase; *ChT,* choline transporter (low affinity); *CPCT,* phosphatidylcholine-ceramide-phosphocholine transferase; *CPT,* choline phosphotransferase; *CT,* cytidine triphosphate:phosphocholine cytidylyltransferase; *DMG,* dimethylglycine; *DMGD,* dimethylglycine dehydrogenase; *PCholine,* phosphocholine; *PDME,* phosphatidyldimethylethanolamine, *PE,* phosphatidylethanolamine; *PEMT,* phosphatidylethanolamine N-methyltransferase; *PMME,* phosphatidylmonomethylethanolamine; *PtdCho,* phosphatidylcholine; *SD,* sarcosine dehydrogenase; *THF,* tetrahydrofolate; *VLDL,* very-low-density lipoproteins.

translocates to the nuclear envelope and regulates its proliferation by mechanisms involving membrane binding and increased PtdCho synthesis. However, the α isoform of CTP:phosphocholine cytidylyltransferase is also found in the cytosol and in association with the endoplasmic reticulum (ER) and Golgi complex membranes in certain cell types. Nuclear export of the α isoform occurs in response to increased demand for PtdCho (Gehrig et al., 2009). Thus, depending on the cell type and demand for PtdCho, the α isoform of CDP-phosphocholine cytidylyltransferase can be found in nuclear, ER, and Golgi complex membranes. The β isoforms of CTP:phosphocholine cytidylyltransferase do not contain an N-terminal nuclear localization signal and are located in the cytosol and on the ER membrane, primarily in brain tissue (Ridsdale et al., 2001), where they are important in neurite outgrowth and branching (Carter et al., 2008).

CTP:phosphocholine cytidylyltransferase enzymes exist in an inactive soluble form and an active membrane insoluble form. Movement of the enzyme on and off the membrane is a major mode of regulation. The α isoform of CTP:phosphocholine cytidylyltransferase translocates to the nuclear membrane in response to numerous stimuli, including PtdCho degradation, fatty acids, and diacylglycerol. Activating lipids (i.e., diacylglycerol [DAG]) or PtdCho depletion increases membrane lateral packing stress, which is sensed by a long amphipathic α-helix portion of the CTP:phosphocholine cytidylyltransferase enzyme and results in its insertion into the membrane bilayer (Gehrig et al., 2009). Transcriptional regulation of CTP:phosphocholine cytidylyltransferase expression also occurs and is largely governed by transcription factors linked to the cell cycle, cell growth, and differentiation (Sugimoto et al., 2008).

TABLE 25-2 Major Metabolic Reactions for Choline*

REACTION	ENZYME	ABBREVIATION	REACTION CATALYZED
1	Choline kinase	CK	ATP + Choline → ADP + Phosphocholine
2	CTP-phosphocholine cytidylyltransferase	CT	CTP + Phosphocholine → Diphosphate + CDP-choline
3	Choline phosphotrans-ferase	CPT	CDP-choline + 1,2-Diacylglycerol → CMP + Phosphatidylcholine
4	Phosphatidylethanolamine *N*-methyltransferase	PEMT	3 AdoMet + Phosphatidylethanolamine → 3 AdoHcy + Phosphatidylcholine
5	Ceramide-phosphocholine transferase	CPCT	Phosphatidylcholine + Ceramide → Sphingomyelin + 1,2-Diacylglycerol
6	Choline dehydrogenase	CHDH	Choline + Acceptor → Betaine aldehyde + Reduced acceptor
7	Betaine aldehyde dehydrogenase	BADH	Betaine aldehyde + NAD^+ + H_2O → Betaine + NADH + 2 H^+
8	Betaine-homocysteine methyltransferase	BHMT	Betaine + Homocysteine → Dimethylglycine + Methionine
9	Dimethylglycine dehydrogenase	DMGD	Dimethylglycine + THF + H_2O ↔ Sarcosine + 5,10-Methylene-THF
10	Sarcosine dehydrogenase	SD	Sarcosine + THF + H_2O ↔ Glycine + 5,10-Methylene-THF

*As shown in Figure 25-4.

In the third and final step of the CDP-choline pathway, choline phosphotransferase catalyzes the transfer of phosphocholine from CDP-choline to DAG (see reaction 3 in Figure 25-4 and Table 25-2). Two human genes, *CEPT1* and *CPT1*, code the proteins that can convert CDP-choline to PtdCho. The protein encoded by *CEPT1* is localized to the nuclear and ER membranes and transfers a phosphobase from either CDP-choline or CDP-ethanolamine to DAG to synthesize PtdCho or phosphatidylethanolamine, respectively, along with release of CMP (Henneberry et al., 2002). In proliferating cells, the ER appears to be a major site of PtdCho synthesis. *CPT1* codes for a protein that localizes to the Golgi complex and uses DAG and CDP-choline for the exclusive synthesis of PtdCho. New PtdCho is distributed throughout the cell via membrane lateral diffusion, vesicular transport, or protein carriers.

PEMT Pathway

Phosphatidylethanolamine *N*-methyltransferase (PEMT) catalyzes the sequential methylation of phosphatidylethanolamine to phosphatidylmonomethylethanolamine, phosphatidyldimethylethanolamine, and finally PtdCho (see reaction 4 in Figure 25-4 and Table 25-2). In mammalian cells, all three steps in the PEMT pathway are catalyzed by PEMT, which is an integral membrane protein. Although PEMT has been detected in several tissues including brain and mammary epithelial cells, it is quantitatively significant only in the liver, where it accounts for about 30% of the PtdCho synthesized in rodents (Reo et al., 2002). The human *PEMT* gene generates three unique transcripts encoding two distinct isoforms, PEMT1 (most abundant) and PEMT2 (Shields et al., 2001). Both isoforms localize to the ER and a subfraction of ER membranes that cofractionate with mitochondria, known as mitochondria-associated membranes (Shields et al., 2003). Though PEMT1 activity is important in generating PtdCho for VLDL and bile biosynthesis, PEMT2 activity appears to inhibit hepatocyte cell growth, possibly by decreasing the expression of CTP:phosphocholine cytidylyltransferase and down-regulating the CDP-choline pathway.

The methyl donor for PEMT methylation reactions is AdoMet (*S*-adenosylmethionine), which binds to several residues of PEMT exposed on the cytosolic surface of the ER and Golgi complex membranes. PEMT is a main consumer of AdoMet and thus a main producer of AdoHcy (*S*-adenosylhomocysteine), the product of all AdoMet-dependent methylation reactions and the precursor of homocysteine. Deletion of the *PEMT* gene in mice results in a 50% reduction in circulating homocysteine compared to levels observed in wild-type mice (Jacobs et al., 2005), indicating that the PEMT reaction is a major source of circulating homocysteine.

Hepatic PEMT activity is increased under conditions of dietary choline deficiency. Other factors involved in the regulation of PEMT include concentrations of phosphatidylethanolamine and the ratio of AdoMet to *S*-adenosylhomocysteine. The PEMT gene also contains estrogen response elements such that expression and activity is induced by estrogen in human and mouse primary hepatocytes (Resseguie et al., 2007).

Molecular Distinctions Between Phosphatidylcholine Derived from the CDP-Choline Pathway versus the PEMT Pathway

Although PtdCho is the product of both the CDP-choline and the PEMT pathways, the fatty acid profiles of the PtdCho molecules differ. PEMT-derived PtdCho is enriched in long-chain polyunsaturated fatty acids, particularly docosahexaenoic acid (DHA, C22:6n-3) (DeLong et al., 1999; Pynn et al., 2011), whereas CDP-choline–derived PtdCho is enriched in linoleic acid (C18:2n-6). As newly synthesized PtdCho is incorporated into VLDL and exported from liver, PEMT plays a major role in providing DHA to extrahepatic tissues (Pynn et al., 2011).

SPHINGOMYELIN

Sphingomyelin is synthesized from PtdCho and ceramide at the luminal surface of the *cis*-medial Golgi complex. In a reaction catalyzed by phosphatidylcholine-ceramide-phosphocholine transferase, the phosphocholine head group is transferred to ceramide forming sphingomyelin and DAG (see reaction 5 in Figure 25-4 and Table 25-2). Removal of DAG, a potent second messenger, is believed to occur through its conversion to triacylglycerol. Ceramide is the hydrophobic precursor for all sphingolipids and is synthesized in the ER. Vesicular transport of newly synthesized sphingomyelin to other cell surfaces appears to be the major route of transport.

BETAINE

In mammals, betaine is an important source of methyl groups in liver and plays an essential role as an organic osmolyte in the kidney. Betaine is derived primarily from the oxidation of choline but it is also present preformed in food. The main transporter of betaine into cells is the betaine/gamma-amino butyric acid transporter (BGT-1), a sodium- and chloride-dependent transporter expressed in several tissues including kidney, brain, liver, heart, skeletal muscle, and to a lesser extent, placenta. Less specific transporters, including a sodium-dependent carnitine transporter in human placental cells, can also be used for cellular uptake of betaine. As intracellular concentrations of free choline rise, choline kinase, the first enzyme in the CDP-choline pathway, becomes saturated and the majority of choline then enters the mitochondria where it is converted to betaine in a two-step reaction. Choline oxidation may therefore serve as a "spillover" pathway under conditions of high dietary choline.

The first and rate-limiting step of choline oxidation to betaine produces betaine aldehyde and is catalyzed by an FAD-linked choline dehydrogenase situated on the inner side of the mitochondrial inner membrane (see reaction 6 in Figure 25-4 and Table 25-2). In rat liver, choline oxidation is controlled by a choline-specific transporter that enables choline passage through the inner membrane of the mitochondria (Kaplan et al., 1993). An NAD-linked betaine aldehyde dehydrogenase located in the mitochondrial matrix catalyzes the second step to form betaine (see reaction 7 in Figure 25-4 and Table 25-2). Once formed, betaine diffuses into the cytosol where it functions as a methyl donor in the formation of methionine from homocysteine. This reaction is carried out by betaine-homocysteine methyl transferase (BHMT) and provides a folate-independent route for homocysteine remethylation (see reaction 8 in Figure 25-4 and Table 25-2). However, unlike the ubiquitous expression of methionine synthase, the expression of BHMT is limited to the liver, kidney (proximal tubules of the cortex), and lens of eye. Dimethylglycine, the other product of BHMT reactions, enters the mitochondria where the two remaining labile methyl groups are donated to THF in reactions catalyzed by dimethylglycine dehydrogenase and sarcosine dehydrogenase (see reactions 9 and 10, respectively, in Figure 25-4 and Table 25-2). These reactions together result in the formation of two molecules of 5,10-methylene THF and one molecule of glycine per molecule of dimethylglycine. The 1-C units associated with folate are subsequently oxidized to formate, which enters the cytosol to partake in folate mediated 1-C metabolism (see Figure 25-2).

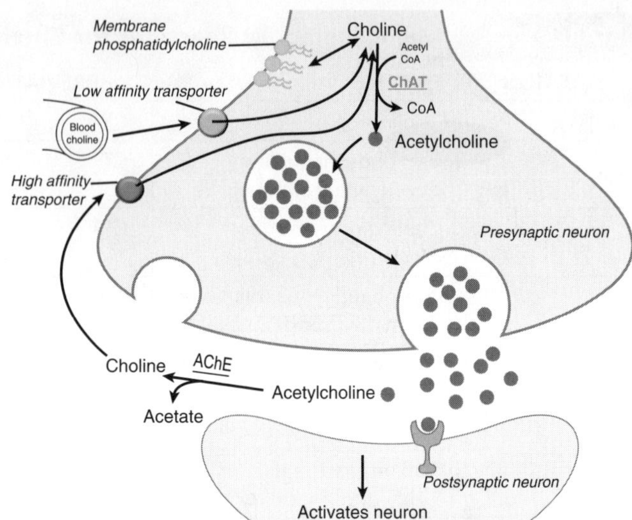

FIGURE 25-5 Acetylcholine biosynthesis and release from a presynaptic neuron. *AChE,* acetylcholine esterase; *ChAT,* choline acetyltransferase.

BHMT activity is regulated by the dietary intake of betaine, choline, and methionine. Choline deficiency dramatically curtails choline oxidation to betaine in mice (Li et al., 2005), whereas diets supplemented with choline and betaine increase BHMT activity. Low dietary methionine intake increases BHMT expression and activity, as do relatively high methionine intakes (Slow and Garrow, 2006). Like MTHFR, BHMT activity is also suppressed by high cellular AdoMet concentrations and enhanced by diminished AdoMet concentrations (Finkelstein, 2001).

ACETYLCHOLINE

Acetylcholine has widespread actions as a neurotransmitter in the central and peripheral nervous systems. Within the mammalian central nervous system, cholinergic neurons modulate diverse cognitive processes, including arousal, attention, and memory (Ferguson and Blakely, 2004). Acetylcholine also controls the output of many organs, including the heart, lungs, exocrine and endocrine glands, gut, and bladder. Choline acetyltransferase catalyzes the formation of acetylcholine from choline and acetyl CoA (Figure 25-5). The expression of choline acetyltransferase is largely confined to cholinergic neurons, although it is also expressed in several noncholinergic tissues including placenta (Bhuiyan et al., 2006).

Free choline that has traversed the blood brain barrier can enter presynaptic cholinergic neurons via the common lower affinity (but higher capacity) route that provides choline for PtdCho biosynthesis (see Figure 25-5). Once formed, membrane PtdCho can be hydrolyzed by phospholipase D to provide free choline for acetylcholine biosynthesis. Presynaptic cholinergic neurons also express a high-affinity, sodium-dependent choline transporter that is encoded by *SLC5A7* in humans. High-affinity choline transporters reside on plasma membranes of cholinergic presynaptic terminals, allowing them to efficiently take up choline. Once inside the neuron, choline is efficiently acetylated by choline acetyltransferase to generate acetylcholine (Ferguson and Blakely, 2004). Acetylcholine is packaged into synaptic vesicles by a second cholinergic neuron–specific transporter, vesicular acetylcholine transporter.

In response to potassium evoked depolarization of neuron membranes and/or elevated cytosolic Ca^{2+} concentrations, acetylcholine-containing vesicles fuse with the plasma membrane and acetylcholine is released into the synaptic cleft where it temporarily binds receptors (muscarinic and nicotinic receptors) on the postsynaptic neuron to transmit the signal (see Figure 25-5). Acetylcholinesterase terminates cholinergic signaling by hydrolyzing acetylcholine within the synaptic cleft to acetate and choline. The choline is recycled by high-affinity choline transporters, which enable choline uptake followed by its conversion to acetylcholine. Neurons undergoing sustained firing meet the increased demand for free choline by increasing the number of high-affinity choline transporters expressed in the plasma membranes of cholinergic presynaptic terminals (Ferguson and Blakely, 2004).

PHYSIOLOGICAL FUNCTIONS OF CHOLINE

The physiological functions of choline relate mainly to the role of choline-containing moieties in lipid biosynthesis and metabolism, membrane formation, neurotransmission, and 1-C metabolism.

BILE FORMATION

Biliary lipids protect hepatocytes and bile duct epithelia cells against the cytotoxicity of bile salts (Oude Elferink and Groen, 2000). The main biliary phospholipid comprising more than 95% of the total is PtdCho. Biliary PtdCho is molecularly distinct in that it contains predominately palmitic acid (C16:0) and linoleic acid (C18:0) esterified at the *sn*-1 and *sn*-2 positions on the glycerol backbone. Bile acids synthesized in liver from cholesterol are transported across the apical membrane of hepatocytes into the lumen of bile canaliculi as described in Chapter 7 (see Figure 7-9). Bile acid secretion into the canalicular space drives the secretion of PtdCho and cholesterol from liver cells into bile. The origin of the PtdCho destined for bile formation appears to be a preformed hepatic microsomal pool and circulating lipoproteins, mainly HDLs. Although newly synthesized PtdCho contributes only a small percentage of biliary PtdCho, both betaine-homocysteine methyltransferase and PEMT are localized to the canalicular membranes and thereby enable the synthesis of PtdCho close to its biliary excretion site (Sehayek et al., 2003). PtdCho is delivered to the canalicular membrane by a phospholipid transport protein and across the membrane by the ABCB4 (MDR3) transporter. MDR3, a PtdCho-specific phospholipid flippase, translocates PtdCho from the inner leaflet of the cell membrane to the outer leaflet. Exposure to bile salts in the canalicular space extracts the PtdCho into bile. Large amounts of bile acids, phospholipids, and cholesterol are secreted into bile at rates of 24, 11, and 1.2 grams per day, respectively. Approximately 95% of biliary PtdCho is reabsorbed by the intestine and mainly incorporated into chylomicrons. Only about 40% of this PtdCho is returned to the liver as the other 55% is used by extrahepatic tissues.

MEMBRANE STRUCTURE AND STABILITY

Phosphatidylcholine, the main constituent of membranes, is localized primarily to the outer leaflet of the lipid bilayer (as is sphingomyelin). PtdCho can be transferred from one population of membranes to another via a soluble intracellular protein. Intramembrane transport, which entails the transbilayer movement of the PtdCho molecule, also occurs. An adequate supply of PtdCho and other membrane substrates is critical for cellular division, and demand for this vital amine is increased during periods of rapid growth (i.e., gestation).

VLDL BIOSYNTHESIS AND SECRETION

Phosphatidylcholine, the major lipid on the surface monolayer of VLDL particles, is packaged with triacylglycerol mainly in the Golgi cisternae. Both the CDP-choline and the PEMT pathways contribute to the PtdCho destined for secretion in VLDL (Pynn et al., 2011). Newly synthesized PtdCho is a requisite for VLDL biosynthesis and thus export of fat from liver (Li and Vance, 2008).

SECRETORY PATHWAY

Vesicles budding from the *trans* Golgi apparatus require the release of DAG from PtdCho. DAG recruits specific proteins to the Golgi apparatus that function in vesicular transport (Baron and Malhotra, 2002) and is derived via degradation of PtdCho with phospholipase D followed by conversion of phosphatidic acid to DAG. The generated DAG is subsequently reincorporated into PtdCho by choline phosphotransferase located at the Golgi apparatus. The CDP-choline substrate required for this reaction is generated by CTP-phosphocholine cytidylyltransferase localized to the *trans* Golgi compartment. A recent study in stimulated macrophages derived from *PCYT1A*-null mice showed that the α isozyme of CTP-phosphocholine cytidylyltransferase (and PtdCho resynthesis) was necessary for cytokine secretion from the Golgi apparatus (Tian et al., 2008).

BRAIN DEVELOPMENT AND COGNITION

Choline is essential for numerous processes that comprise brain development (Zeisel, 2004). Studies in rodents have shown that choline availability in utero (and in the early postnatal period) produces lasting changes in neural systems that underlie learning and memory and exerts lifelong effects on cognitive functioning.

METHYL GROUP DONOR

As a source of labile methyl groups in liver and kidney (described in previous text), choline availability modulates the pool of AdoMet that is used by over 60 methyltransferases for the production and regulation of various molecules, including creatine phosphate, DNA and histones, neurotransmitters, phospholipids, and hormones. Alterations in promoter region DNA methylation and gene expression in the offspring of rodents exposed to varying amounts of choline during gestation is of particular interest (Davison et al., 2009; Kovacheva et al., 2009; Napoli et al., 2008), because it implies a role for choline in prenatal programming.

CELL SIGNALING

In the cell membrane, phospholipids are important precursors of second messengers that control a number of processes inside the cell (Zeisel and Blusztajn, 1994). Membrane PtdCho is a source of DAG following its hydrolysis by phospholipase C. DAG then is able to activate protein kinase C, which phosphorylates and affects the activity of numerous target proteins inside the cell. PtdCho is also a major source of arachidonic acid for the biosynthesis of eicosanoids after its release by phospholipase A2. Phosphatidate (diacylglycerol 3-phosphate), lysophosphatidate, lysoPtdCho, and platelet-activating factor are other potent signaling molecules derived from PtdCho hydrolysis. Signaling molecules derived from the degradation of sphingomyelin include sphingosylphosphorylcholine and ceramide.

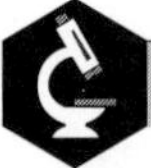

CLINICAL CORRELATION

Perinatal Choline Supplementation: A Therapy for Cognitive Dysfunction During Aging, Alzheimer Disease, and Down Syndrome?

Barbara J. Strupp, PhD

The nutritional requirements of the developing nervous system remain poorly understood. It is known that choline derivatives are essential for neuronal and glial progenitor cell division, axon and dendrite growth, synapse formation, and myelination (Cermak et al., 1998). However, the amount of choline that must be ingested by the mother during pregnancy to ensure optimal brain development of her child is unknown. In rats consuming a standard laboratory chow diet, pregnancy causes a pronounced depletion of choline pools (Zeisel et al., 1995), indicating that choline requirements during pregnancy are increased and that the need for this nutrient by the mother and the fetuses may commonly exceed the amount consumed by the mother. Consistent with this view, rodent studies have shown that supplementing the maternal diet with additional choline (approximately four times the amount of choline in normal chow) leads to a significant enhancement of memory and attentional abilities of the offspring when tested as adults (McCann et al., 2006; Meck and Williams, 2003). Moreover, supplementing the maternal diet with extra amounts of this single nutrient for as short a period as 5 days during a critical period of pregnancy substantially lessens aging-related memory decline of the offspring (Meck et al., 2008). Although the mechanism(s) by which increased choline availability produces these lifelong cognitive benefits are incompletely understood, organizational effects on brain development have been demonstrated, as have lasting increases in central cholinergic activity, hippocampal long-term potentiation, neurogenesis, and neurotrophins. These lasting effects may arise, at least in part, from changes in DNA methylation and gene expression patterns, secondary to choline's role as a methyl donor.

The benefits of increased maternal choline intake may even be more profound for fetuses with Down syndrome, the most common known cause of mental retardation, affecting approximately 1 in 800 live births. A recent study using the Ts65Dn mouse model of Down syndrome demonstrated that supplementing the maternal diet with excess choline during pregnancy and lactation substantially improved attentional function of the trisomic offspring, and partially normalized the heightened emotional responses exhibited by these mice (Moon et al., 2010). These findings offer the exciting possibility that increasing the choline intake of pregnant and lactating women might significantly lessen the cognitive and affective dysfunction in Down syndrome offspring. With the relatively recent realization that individuals with Down syndrome exhibit not only mental retardation but also early-onset Alzheimer disease, there is a growing need to identify effective interventions for this disorder. Although the mechanism(s) responsible for these lasting beneficial effects of increased maternal choline intake in this Down syndrome model are unknown, several lines of reasoning suggest that this early nutritional intervention may offer some protection to basal forebrain cholinergic neurons, which normally atrophy by 6 months of age in this mouse model. These changes in the mouse brain recapitulate the loss of neurons in Down syndrome humans coincident with the onset of neuropathology similar to Alzheimer disease. If this hypothesis proves to be correct, recommendations to increase maternal choline intake may offer protection against Alzheimer disease in the population at large.

In summary, these studies collectively raise the possibility that women may need to increase their intake of choline during pregnancy to ensure optimal cognitive functioning of their offspring, including successful aging. Definitive recommendations, however, await replication of these benefits in humans with randomized controlled clinical trials.

OSMOLYTE

Betaine and glycerophosphocholine are compatible (nonperturbing) organic osmolytes that protect against damage caused by hyperosmolality (most often in the form of salt and urea). Most notably osmolytes reduce osmotic potential and stabilize native protein structure (i.e., protect proteins from misfolding) (Burg and Ferraris, 2008). In mammals, betaine and glycerophosphocholine accumulate in renal medullary cells as these cells are exposed to extremely high concentrations of NaCl and urea because of their roles in concentrating urine. In these cells, betaine can be synthesized from choline or can be taken up from the extracellular fluid by the betaine transporter, BGT1. Hypertonicity increases the uptake of betaine by increasing the number of betaine transporters present in the basolateral membrane of the renal medullary cell (Burg and Ferraris, 2008). Glycerophosphocholine is derived from PtdCho via the action of phospholipase B. High NaCl and/or urea increase glycerophosphocholine synthesis; high NaCl also reduces its degradation. The cells of other tissues that experience milder forms of hyperosmolality also accumulate organic osmolytes.

CHOLINE DEFICIENCY

Choline deficiency has been described in a variety of animal species and manifests in growth, hepatic, pancreatic, lipoprotein, memory, and renal abnormalities in some species (Zeisel and Blusztajn, 1994). Fatty liver and liver dysfunction are the main clinical manifestations of choline deficiency in humans (Buchman, 2009; Zeisel et al., 1991). Triacylglycerol accumulation in liver is due to the requirement for PtdCho in the biosynthesis of VLDL. Liver damage/dysfunction is a consequence of disrupted membrane integrity, apoptosis, and decreased membrane fluidity (Li et al., 2006).

In choline deficiency, the plasma membrane ratio of PtdCho to phosphatidylethanolamine is diminished, which contributes to the leakage of the liver cytosolic enzymes, alanine aminotransferase and aspartate aminotransferase, into the blood. Diminished membrane integrity is not restricted to plasma membranes or to liver tissue. Choline deficiency can result in dysfunctional mitochondrial membranes such that free radicals, normally contained within the mitochondria, escape and contribute to the oxidative damage of DNA and proteins in other cellular compartments (Hensley et al., 2000). Leakage of creatine phosphokinase from muscle cells under conditions of choline deficiency has also been reported (da Costa et al., 2004).

CHOLINE AND DISEASE

DISEASE RISK

Epidemiological studies show associations between choline intake or status and certain diseases. However, it is important to remember that choline is not consumed in isolation of other nutrients, that diseases often alter nutrient metabolism, and that the causal role of choline in the development of these diseases remains unclear.

Birth Defects

Independent of folate intake, a higher maternal choline intake is associated with a 40% to 50% lower risk of having a baby with an NTD (Shaw et al., 2004) or cleft lip (Shaw et al., 2006) in a comparison of extreme quartiles. A strong inverse relationship between maternal serum total choline concentrations measured at midgestation, and NTD risk was also observed in a prospective study that included 180,000 pregnant women in the United States who were exposed to folic acid fortification (Shaw et al., 2009). That choline may modify NTD risk is supported by population-based studies demonstrating associations between genetic variants in choline-metabolizing genes and risk of NTDs (Enaw et al., 2006).

Cancer

In recent years several population-based studies have examined the relationship between dietary choline intake (and other 1-C metabolism nutrients) and breast cancer risk. Among premenopausal and postmenopausal women from the Nurses' Health Study cohort, a high dietary choline intake was not prospectively associated with reduced breast cancer risk (Cho et al., 2007, 2010). However, in a smaller case control study of premenopausal and postmenopausal women in the United States, a higher choline intake was associated with a 24% lower risk of breast cancer (Xu et al., 2009), and breast cancer risk was modified by genetic variation in choline-metabolizing enzymes (Xu et al., 2009).

Conversely, a higher dietary choline intake was linked to an increased risk of distal colorectal adenoma in women (Cho et al., 2007). No associations between colorectal cancer risk and dietary choline intake were detected in men (J. E. Lee et al., 2010). However, in a prospective investigation of seven circulating B vitamins and prostate cancer risk, a higher plasma choline concentration was associated with increased risk (Johansson et al., 2009).

DISEASE TREATMENT

Cognitive Deficits

Because Alzheimer disease is characterized by diminished acetylcholine synthesis and cholinergic dysfunction, the efficacy of supplemental choline in treating neurological deficits has been explored. Though choline salts and PtdCho are not effective therapies (Amenta and Tayebati, 2008), a meta-analysis of controlled clinical trials conducted in elderly subjects with neurological deficits indicated that CDP-choline supplementation improved memory and behavior (Fioravanti and Yanagi, 2005). CDP-choline may also reduce cognitive deficits following a stroke when administered within the first 24 hours of the cerebral event (Alvarez-Sabin and Roman, 2011; Davalos et al., 2002). CDP-choline's therapeutic action has been attributed to its role in stabilizing cell membranes, reducing the presence of free radicals, increasing the release of dopamine neurotransmitters in the brain, and activating the central cholinergic system.

Nonalcoholic Fatty Liver Disease

Nonalcoholic fatty liver disease (NAFLD) is a term that encompasses a disease spectrum ranging from triacylglycerol accumulation in hepatocytes (hepatic steatosis) to hepatic steatosis with inflammation (steatohepatitis), fibrosis, and cirrhosis. The efficacy of high-dose betaine in the treatment of NAFLD is an active area of scientific inquiry.

CHOLINE HOMEOSTASIS

Steady-state concentrations of choline metabolites are maintained in animals and humans through several adaptive mechanisms. During choline deficiency, rodents maintain their levels of choline-containing lipids (e.g., PtdCho) in liver and extrahepatic tissues by (1) increasing hepatic de novo biosynthesis through the PEMT pathway, (2) activating the CDP-choline pathway in liver to ensure efficient conversion of choline to PtdCho, (3) depressing hepatic oxidation of choline to betaine, (4) increasing cellular choline uptake, and (5) redistributing choline among tissues. Notably, during severe and prolonged choline deficiency, redistribution of choline among tissues allows the brain to maintain a stable level of total choline (Li et al., 2007). Conversely, studies in rodents demonstrated rapid removal of free choline from portal blood by the liver and enhanced hepatic oxidation to betaine following choline supplementation. Moreover, in cells manipulated to generate excess PtdCho, catabolism of PtdCho is markedly enhanced (Walkey et al., 1994), as is degradation of CPT1, the terminal enzyme in the CDP-choline pathway (Butler and Mallampalli, 2010).

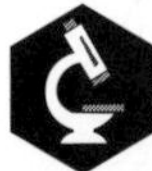

CLINICAL CORRELATION

Betaine and Nonalcoholic Fatty Liver Disease

Elango Kathirvel, PhD; Kengathevy Morgan, PhD; and Timothy R. Morgan, MD

Nonalcoholic fatty liver disease (NAFLD) refers to the accumulation of fat (triacylglycerols) in hepatocytes (the primary cells in the liver) in someone who does not drink excessive amounts of alcohol (i.e., less than two drinks per day for men or one drink per day for women) (Perlemuter et al., 2007). Recent studies suggest that up to 40% of adults in the United States have NAFLD (Williams et al., 2011). Patients with NAFLD are usually overweight but asymptomatic, and may have either normal liver blood tests or blood tests suggesting liver injury. Approximately 20% of patients with NAFLD have liver inflammation and fibrosis, which can progress to cirrhosis, liver failure, and hepatocellular carcinoma. Unfortunately, there is no safe and effective treatment for NAFLD.

Insulin resistance is the underlying pathophysiological abnormality in NAFLD (Perlemuter et al., 2007). NAFLD can be created in rodents by feeding a diet containing high sucrose or 20% or more of calories from fat (for comparison, standard rodent diets contain 10% of calories from fat) (Kathirvel et al., 2010; Song et al., 2007). After several months mice become overweight, have insulin resistance as shown by abnormal glucose tolerance test and elevated fasting insulin levels, and have fat in the liver (steatosis).

Betaine may play an important role in NAFLD. The betaine content in the liver is significantly reduced in mice with NAFLD (Kathirvel et al., 2010). Administration of betaine to mice with NAFLD reverses the betaine deficiency in the liver (indeed, it leads to supranormal levels of betaine in the liver). Betaine administration also reverses insulin resistance (i.e., restores a normal glucose tolerance test) and reduces fat in the liver but doesn't significantly reduce body weight.

The mechanisms by which betaine reverses insulin resistance and hepatic steatosis are incompletely understood. Using a dietary sucrose feeding model of NAFLD, Song and colleagues (2007) reported that betaine supplementation increased activation of hepatic AMP-activated protein kinase (AMPK), which would decrease gluconeogenesis and lipogenesis and increase fatty acid oxidation in the liver. Betaine supplementation also decreased nuclear localization of SREBP-1c and ChREBP, two transcription factors involved in regulating expression of lipogenic genes, as well as decreasing expression of genes for acetyl-CoA carboxylase and fatty acid synthase, two genes critical in fatty acid synthesis. Kathirvel and co-workers (2010), using a high-fat model of NAFLD in mice, found that betaine supplementation restored hepatic betaine concentration but did not restore hepatic choline level. Betaine supplementation might reduce fatty liver by increasing PtdCho synthesis via the PEMT pathway, permitting increased synthesis of VLDL and export of triacylglycerols from hepatocytes. In support of this hypothesis, betaine supplementation activated the PEMT pathway and reversed fatty liver in rats fed ethanol (Kharbanda et al., 2007).

Studies of betaine supplementation as a treatment of NAFLD in humans are limited and results are conflicting. An uncontrolled trial in patients with NAFLD suggested that betaine reduced liver injury (Abdelmalek et al., 2001), but a subsequent small, randomized, placebo-controlled trial found no benefit with betaine treatment (Abdelmalek et al., 2009).

In summary, hepatic betaine deficiency is present in animals with NAFLD. Betaine supplementation restores hepatic betaine level and reverses insulin resistance and liver steatosis. Betaine is available as a dietary supplement (i.e., over the counter) in the United States and appears to be safe. Further studies are needed to determine whether betaine might be a suitable treatment for humans with either insulin resistance or NAFLD.

In humans, a minimal concentration of plasma-free choline is maintained despite consumption of a diet devoid of choline and signs of organ dysfunction (da Costa et al., 2005). After oral administration of 2,200 mg choline per day (as choline chloride) to men for 12 weeks, fasting plasma choline concentration doubled from about 6 to 13 μmol/L (Veenema et al., 2008); however, this rise represented less than 5% of the administered dose, which is consistent with the liver's ability to act as a sink for choline (Zeisel et al., 1980). An insignificant amount of free choline is excreted in the urine by healthy individuals, rarely exceeding 2% of the administered dose.

STATUS ASSESSMENT OF CHOLINE

Sensitive and specific biomarkers of choline status are lacking. Plasma-free choline is a specific marker of choline status but appears to be tightly regulated and relatively unresponsive to changes in dietary choline intake (Abratte et al., 2009). Plasma-free choline concentrations range from about 6 to 13 μmol/L with a median of 8.6 μmol/L in healthy, nonfasted adults (Holm et al., 2007). In studies where choline intake is manipulated, several nonspecific biomarkers can be examined, including measurements of circulating liver and muscle enzyme concentrations; plasma PtdCho, which measures PtdCho in circulating concentrations of lipoproteins; plasma homocysteine, especially after a methionine load; and genomic endpoints, such as DNA damage and methylation of cytosine residues (Shin et al., 2010).

DIETARY RECOMMENDATIONS, FACTORS AFFECTING DIETARY REQUIREMENTS, AND DIETARY CHOLINE INTAKE

DIETARY RECOMMENDATIONS

In 1998 dietary recommendations for choline, in the form of Adequate Intake (AI) levels, were established for the first time (IOM, 1998). For men and women, the AI was based on a single study showing that 500 mg/day of choline (~7 mg/kg/day) was enough to prevent elevations in alanine aminotransferase (a marker of liver dysfunction) in healthy men. The AI was calculated as 7 mg/kg times the reference weight of a man (76 kg) or woman (61 kg), with rounding. Upward adjustments during pregnancy and lactation were made based on the amount of choline accretion by the fetus and placenta and the amount secreted in human milk, respectively. For infants of ages 0 through 6 months, the AI reflects the observed mean intake of choline by infants consuming human milk. For all other age groups, AIs were extrapolated from adult values.

The neonatal requirement for a dietary supply of choline was recognized by the American Academy of Pediatrics in 1985, when it recommended that infant formulas contain at least 7 mg of choline per 100 kcal. Choline chloride and choline bitartrate are the forms usually added to infant formulas and milk products.

FACTORS INFLUENCING CHOLINE REQUIREMENTS

Dietary Availability of Other Methyl Donors

Because other methyl donors (i.e, dietary betaine, folate, methionine, and vitamin B_{12}) influence the metabolic demand for choline and its biosynthesis, the requirement for choline will vary depending on the availability of these methyl donors. The intermingling of choline and folate, and the choline sparing effect of folate, was recognized approximately 70 years ago (reviewed in Caudill, 2009). More recently, human feeding studies (Abratte et al., 2008, 2009) have reported declines in plasma PtdCho with folate depletion, increases with folate repletion, or both.

Genetic Variation

Genetic deficiencies in choline or 1-C metabolizing enzymes also influence choline requirements (Zeisel, 2011; West and Caudill, 2010). For example, a guanine (G) to adenine (A) substitution at nucleotide 1958 in the *MTHFD1* gene (MTHFD1 1958G→A, rs2236225) prompts the substitution of a glutamine for arginine in the 10-formyl-THF synthetase domain of C1-THF synthase. In premenopausal women consuming a choline-deficient diet, one or two copies of the variant 1958A allele markedly increased the risk of exhibiting signs of choline deficiency (i.e., organ dysfunction) (Kohlmeier et al., 2005). Single nucleotide polymorphisms in the *PEMT* gene (e.g., −744G→C; rs12325817) have also been associated with increased risk of choline deficiency (da Costa et al., 2006; Fischer et al., 2010). The PEMT −744C risk allele is located in close proximity to a critical estrogen

DRIs Across the Life Cycle: Choline

	mg Choline per Day	
Infant	AI	UL
0 through 6 mo	125	ND
7 through 12 mo	150	ND
Children		
1 through 3 yr	200	1,000
4 through 8 yr	250	1,000
9 through 13 yr	375	2,000
Males		
≥14 yr	550	3,000
Females		
14 through 18 yr	400	3,000
≥19 yr	425	3,500
Pregnant		
<19 yr	450	3,000
≥19 yr	450	3,500
Lactating		
<19 yr	550	3,000
≥19 yr	550	3,500

Data from IOM. (1998). *Dietary Reference Intakes for thiamin, riboflavin, niacin, vitamin B_6, folate, vitamin B_{12}, pantothenic acid, biotin, and choline.* Washington, DC: National Academy Press.

AI, Adequate Intake; *DRI*, Dietary Reference Intake; *ND*, not determinable; *UL*, Tolerable Upper Intake Level.

response element and impairs hormone-inducible PEMT expression (Resseguie et al., 2011).

Males and postmenopausal women have a higher requirement for dietary choline than do premenopausal women (Fischer et al., 2007, 2010). The lower dietary choline requirement of premenopausal women is likely due to the presence of estrogen, which increases PEMT activity (Resseguie et al., 2007) and thus the endogenous production of the choline moiety.

Comorbidites

The requirement for choline is higher in certain disease states. In children with cystic fibrosis, PtdCho and lysoPtdCho fecal excretion is increased and is associated with choline depletion and perturbations in markers of 1-C metabolism (Chen et al., 2005).

DIETARY INTAKE

The majority of the U.S. population is not consuming sufficient choline to meet the current AI. Based on the 2007–2008 NHANES data, mean choline intakes in the U.S. are about 400 mg/day for men and 260 mg/day for women (U.S. Department of Agriculture, 2010). However, unlike an EAR, an AI cannot be used to estimate the prevalence of inadequacy.

CHOLINE TOXICITY

High doses of supplemental choline have been associated with fishy body odor, hypotension, vomiting, salivation, sweating, and gastrointestinal effects (IOM, 1998). In deriving a UL (Tolerable Upper Intake Level), hypotension was selected as the critical effect and fishy body odor was selected as the secondary consideration. A lowest-observed-adverse-effect level of 7.5 g/day choline was divided by an uncertainty factor of two to obtain a UL of 3.5 g/day for adults after rounding (IOM, 1998). The adult UL was adjusted for children and adolescents on the basis of relative body weight. No UL was established for infants due to insufficient data.

THINKING CRITICALLY

Choline

KL is in her third trimester of pregnancy and has developed fatty liver and liver dysfunction (e.g., elevated serum concentrations of alanine aminotransferase).

1. How might choline deficiency be contributing to the fatty liver and liver dysfunction? Propose two mechanisms based on the physiological functions of this nutrient.
2. Identify two genetic variants that may increase the dietary requirement for choline. Explain.
3. Would supplementing with folate be helpful in attenuating the fatty liver or liver dysfunction? Explain and propose a mechanism(s) based on the metabolic intermingling of folate and choline metabolism.

VITAMIN B_{12}

In the mid nineteenth century Thomas Addison described a megaloblastic anemia that appeared to be associated with degenerative disease of the stomach. It was called pernicious anemia because of its invariably fatal outcome. In the 1920s George Minot and William Murphy described the first effective treatment of this disease—1 pound of raw liver per day—for which they received a Nobel Prize. It soon became apparent that normal gastric juice contained a factor (intrinsic factor) that was required for the use of a dietary component (extrinsic factor or vitamin B_{12}) that was needed to prevent the anemia. Because of the identical anemia that arises from folate or B_{12} deficiency, it was originally thought that extrinsic factor was folic acid, and folic acid was used to treat pernicious anemia patients when it was isolated in the 1940s. With the isolation of B_{12} a few years later, it became clear that pernicious anemia was due to B_{12} deficiency.

CHEMISTRY OF VITAMIN B_{12}

The term *vitamin B_{12}* refers specifically to cyanocobalamin, the supplement form of the vitamin. But it also is used to refer generally to all cobalt-containing, bioactive members of the cobalamin family. Cobalamins consist of a central cobalt atom surrounded by a heme-like planar corrin ring (Figure 25-6), with four pyrrole nitrogens coordinated to the cobalt. Cobalamins also contain a phosphoribosyl-5,6-dimethylbenzimidazole side group, with one of the nitrogens linked to the cobalt by coordination at the "bottom" position. When bound to enzymes, this lower axial ligand is replaced by an active-site histidine residue. The upper axial position can be occupied by a number of different ligands, including hydroxyl (hydroxycobalamin or aquocobalamin), cyano (cyanocobalamin), methyl (methylcobalamin), and 5′-deoxyadenosyl (5′-deoxyadenosylcobalamin) moieties (Figure 25-7). Cyanocobalamin is rarely found naturally but arises as an artifact from extraction of trace amounts of cyanide during purification of the vitamin from natural sources. Cobalamins are complex molecules, and Nobel Prizes were awarded to Dorothy Hodgkin in 1964 for the determination of their structure by X-ray crystallography and to Robert Woodward in 1965 for their synthesis. Metal–carbon bonds are rare in nature, and the pyrrole structure is the only example of a cobalt–carbon bond.

In cobalamins, the oxidation state of the cobalt plays an important role in cofactor function. For biological activity in eukaryotic cells, both cyanocobalamin and hydroxycobalamin, in which the cobalt atom is trivalent Co^{3+} [cob(III) alamin], must be reduced to the Co^{1+} [cob(I)alamin] derivative. They must also be converted to methylcob(III)alamin or 5′-deoxyadenosylcob(III)alamin (also known as coenzyme B_{12}). These two cofactor forms of the vitamin are very sensitive to oxidation and photolysis.

Chemical analogs of vitamin B_{12}, called corrinoids, exist in nature and can be identified in blood and excreta of humans.

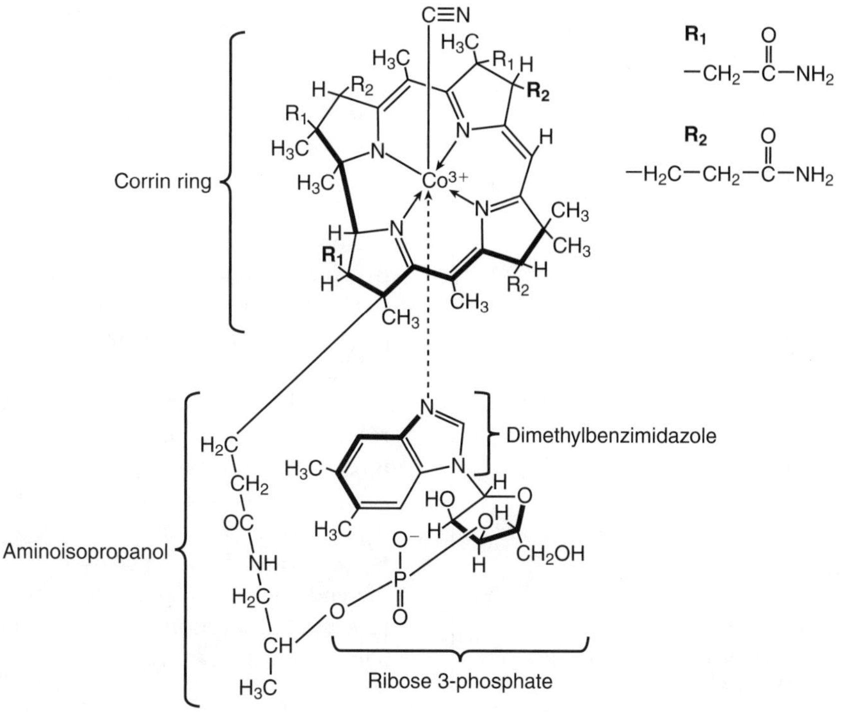

FIGURE 25-6 Structure of vitamin B_{12} (cyanocobalamin).

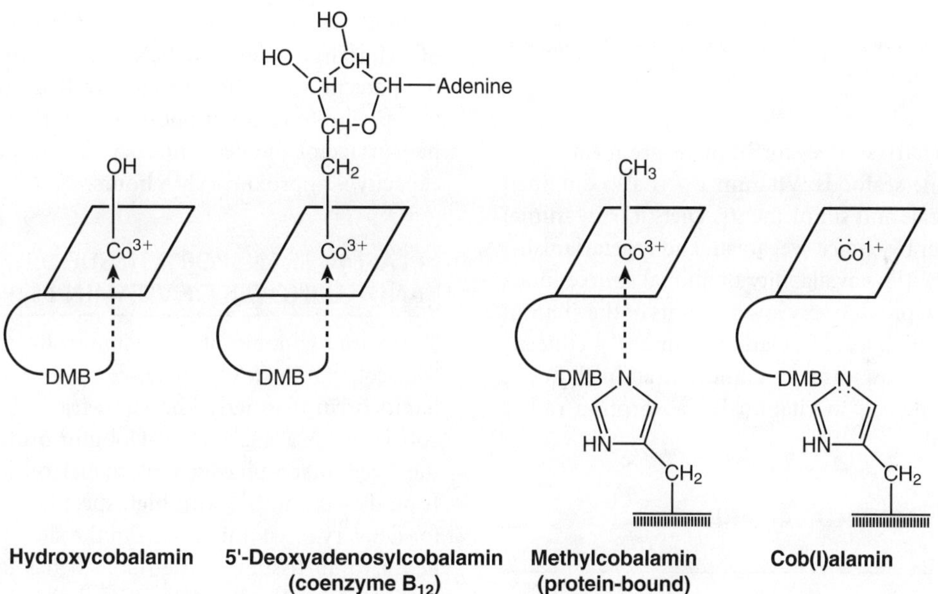

FIGURE 25-7 Intracellular forms of vitamin B_{12}. In vitamin B_{12}–dependent enzymes, the ligand to the lower axial position of the cobalt atom is an imidazole nitrogen of a histidyl residue within the protein instead of the dimethylbenzimidazolyl (DMB) side group of the vitamin B_{12} molecule. This is shown for methylcobalamin bound to methionine synthase. The nitrogen-cobalt ligand detaches (base-off form) in the cob(I)alamin-enzyme derivative.

These corrinoids are generally of two types: (1) cobamides, which have a chemically altered lower axial ligand; and (2) cobinamides, which lack the lower axial ligand. It is unclear if these analogs come from the diet, gut microflora, or endogenous breakdown of vitamin B_{12} within cells. Vitamin B_{12} analogs do not support cellular functions or growth in mammals, and it is unknown if they are inhibitors of vitamin B_{12}–dependent reactions.

SOURCES OF VITAMIN B_{12}

Vitamin B_{12} is synthesized solely by anaerobic microorganisms. Except for some algae, such as seaweed, plant sources do not contain vitamin B_{12}. Ruminant animals acquire vitamin B_{12} from gut microflora, whereas other animals acquire vitamin B_{12} through copraphagia, bacterial contamination of the diet, or by eating animal source foods containing vitamin

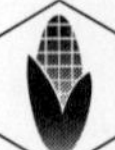

FOOD SOURCES HIGH IN VITAMIN B_{12}

Mollusks and Crustaceans
42 to 84 μg per 3 oz clams
13 μg per 3 oz oysters
9 μg per 3 oz crab
2.6 μg per 3 oz lobster
1 μg per 3 oz shrimp

Fish
8 μg per 3 oz sardines
5 μg per 3 oz canned salmon
1 to 2 μg per 3 oz flounder, sole, swordfish, roughy, catfish

Meats
1.4 to 2.5 μg per 3 oz beef
2 to 2.2 μg per 3 oz lamb
0.5 to 0.6 μg per 3 oz pork

Milk and Milk Products
1.0 to 1.3 μg per 1 cup milk
1.3 to 1.4 μg per 8 oz yogurt
0.6 to 0.8 μg per ½ cup cottage cheese
0.6 μg per 1 oz mozzarella cheese

Other
0.6 μg per 1 large egg
1.5 μg per ½ cup soy milk

USDA, ARS. (2010). *USDA National Nutrient Database for Standard Reference, Release 23*. Retrieved from www.ars.usda.gov/ba/bhnrc/ndl.

B_{12}. The major dietary sources for humans are meat, dairy products, and some seafoods. Vitamin B_{12} is also obtained from fortified cereals and supplements. Diets low in animal source foods, either by choice (veganism and vegetarianism) or by circumstance (low availability of animal source foods in the food supply), provide very low amounts of the vitamin and are associated with low circulating vitamin B_{12} concentrations. However, most cases of clinical vitamin B_{12} deficiency arise from defects in vitamin B_{12} absorption rather than deficient intake.

ABSORPTION AND BIOAVAILABILITY OF VITAMIN B_{12}

Vitamin B_{12} absorption occurs via complex mechanisms within discrete anatomical areas of the gastrointestinal tract (Figure 25-8). Dietary vitamin B_{12} is released from proteins by pepsin, a proteolytic enzyme produced by gastric chief cells, and by stomach acid produced by gastric parietal cells. The released vitamin B_{12} initially binds to salivary R-binder (a member of a family of vitamin B_{12}–binding proteins called haptocorrins), which has high affinity for vitamin B_{12} under acidic conditions. As the vitamin B_{12}–R-binder complex passes into the small intestine, the R-binder is hydrolyzed by pancreatic proteases, and the freed vitamin B_{12} binds to intrinsic factor (IF), a 45-kDa glycoprotein secreted by the gastric parietal cells. Sufficient IF is released following a meal to bind 2 to 4 μg of vitamin B_{12}.

Absorption of vitamin B_{12} occurs via two distinct mechanisms. The first mechanism is passive diffusion, which occurs throughout the gastrointestinal tract. It is estimated that 1% of any given dose of vitamin B_{12} is absorbed in this manner. The second mechanism is active or physiological absorption of vitamin B_{12}, which occurs via a 460-kDa receptor called "cubilin," located in the distal ileum at the end of the small intestine. Cubilin recognizes the IF–vitamin B_{12} complex but not unbound vitamin B_{12} or vitamin B_{12}–free IF. Cubilin interacts with a second protein, amnionless (AMN), which is required for the apical localization of cubilin in polarized cells. In the presence of Ca^{2+}, the IF–B_{12} complex binds to cubilin and the complex is internalized by receptor-mediated endocytosis. The cubilin-AMN receptor is recycled to the membrane, whereas the internalized IF-B_{12} complex remains in the late endosomes. The late endosomes then fuse with lysosomes, the IF is degraded, and the vitamin B_{12} is released into the cytosol. Vitamin B_{12} then traverses the endothelial cell and enters the portal circulation. This process of absorption across the gut epithelium takes about 3 to 4 hours.

The bioavailability of vitamin B_{12} is limited by the physiological absorption mechanism, which can become saturated with relatively small amounts of oral vitamin B_{12}. The maximal amount that can be absorbed from a given dose of B_{12} is about 1.5 μg. For doses of 3 μg or less, approximately 50% of a vitamin B_{12} dose will be absorbed. For doses above 3 μg, the percent absorption progressively decreases. The refractory period to restore unbound cubilin density on the luminal surface of the ileal enterocytes and maximal absorptive capacity is approximately 6 hours.

PLASMA TRANSPORT, TISSUE UPTAKE, AND TURNOVER OF VITAMIN B_{12}

There are two main plasma vitamin B_{12} transport proteins, transcobalamin (formerly known as transcobalamin II) and haptocorrin (formerly known as transcobalamin I). Transcobalamin is a 45.5-kDa β-globulin protein synthesized in the liver, macrophages, endothelial cells, and enterocytes. It binds vitamin B_{12} with high specificity and is responsible for delivery of vitamin B_{12} from the site of absorption in the ileum to all tissues of the body. It has long been thought that vitamin B_{12} enters the circulation bound to transcobalamin. Recent evidence, however, suggests that free vitamin B_{12} exits the enterocyte via the multidrug resistance protein 1 (MRP1/ABCC1) before being bound to transcobalamin in the blood (Beedholm-Ebsen et al., 2010). The plasma half-life of the transcobalamin–vitamin B_{12} complex is approximately 6 minutes. Because of this short half-life, transcobalamin is typically only 10% to 20% saturated and carries only about 20% to 30% of the total circulating vitamin B_{12} at any given time. The transcobalamin–vitamin B_{12} complex is taken up into tissues by receptor-mediated endocytosis. The transcobalamin–vitamin B_{12} receptor, which has recently been cloned, is a 58-kDa membrane glycoprotein (Quadros et al., 2009). In the kidney and the yolk sac,

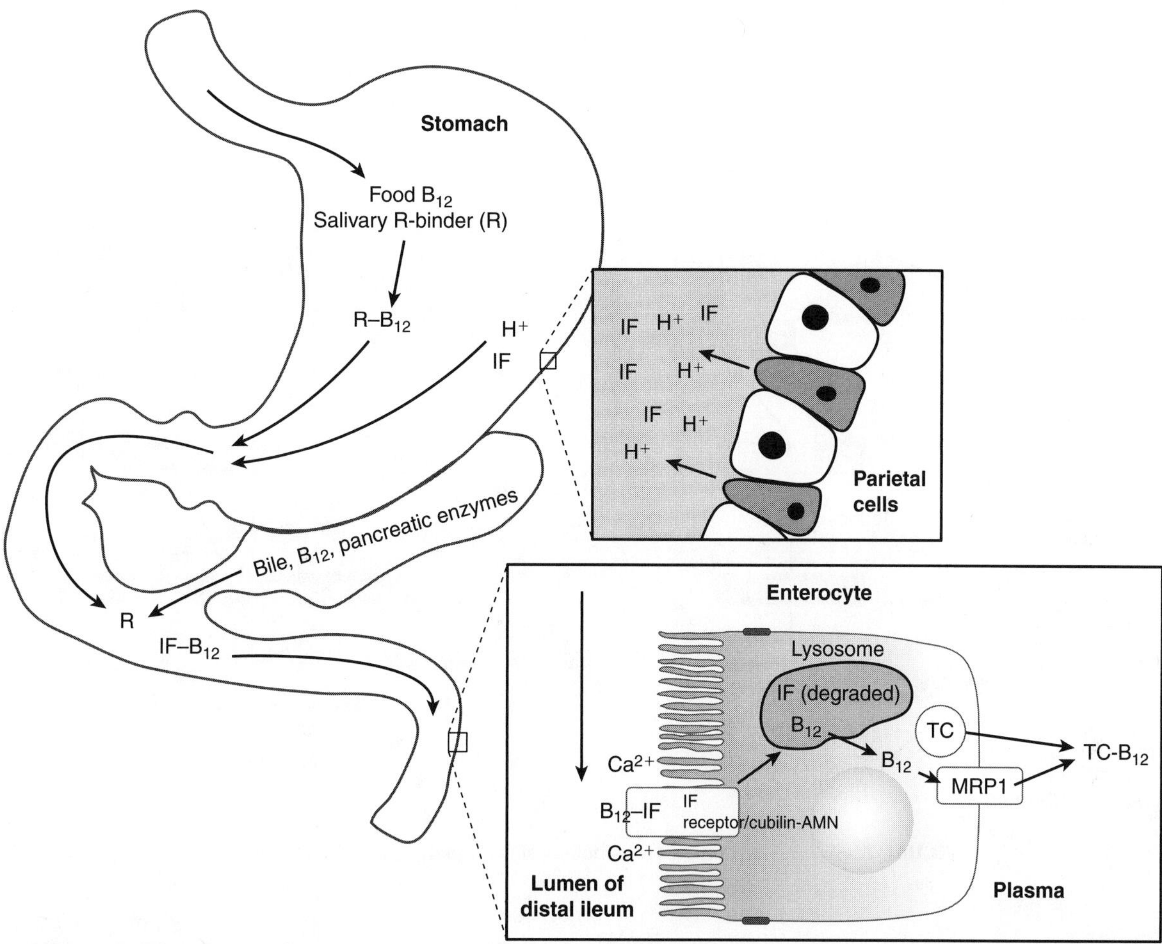

FIGURE 25-8 Absorption and processing of dietary vitamin B_{12}. *IF,* Intrinsic factor; *MRP1,* multidrug resistance protein 1; *TC,* transcobalamin.

tissue uptake of transcobalamin–vitamin B_{12} also occurs via a cubilin-mediated process.

Haptocorrin is an approximately 150,000-kDa glycoprotein derived primarily from neutrophil-specific granules. In contrast to transcobalamin, the plasma half-life of haptocorrin-B_{12} is long (~10 days). As a result, haptocorrin is typically 80% to 90% saturated and carries about 70% to 80% of circulating vitamin B_{12}. The physiological role of haptocorrin is not clearly understood. It does not appear to bind vitamin B_{12} after absorption across the enterocyte, and it is unknown how circulating vitamin B_{12} becomes bound to it. Moreover, the haptocorrin–vitamin B_{12} complex is not recognized by the transcobalamin–vitamin B_{12} receptor. Instead, it is recognized by asialoglycoprotein receptors in the liver. Unlike transcobalamin, haptocorrin not only binds vitamin B_{12} but also binds other corrinoids and cobinamides. This suggests a potential function of haptocorrin may be to transport corrinoids and cobinamides to the liver, from which these compounds are excreted in the bile into the upper small intestine. Because IF does not bind corrinoids and cobinamides, they are not reabsorbed and are excreted in the stool.

Most of the body store of vitamin B_{12}, estimated at about 2 to 3 mg, is in the liver. 5′-Deoxyadenosylcobalamin is the major form of the vitamin in liver, whereas methylcobalamin is the major form in plasma. The vitamin is excreted via the urine and via the bile. Normally, the enterohepatic circulation results in effective reuptake of biliary vitamin B_{12} via the IF-mediated process. Turnover rates of whole-body vitamin B_{12} have been estimated at approximately 0.1%/day (i.e., 2 to 3 μg/day in an adult).

INTRACELLULAR METABOLISM AND METABOLIC FUNCTIONS OF VITAMIN B_{12}

Mammals need vitamin B_{12} as a cofactor for two enzymes, cytosolic methionine synthase, which uses methylcobalamin as a cofactor, and mitochondrial methylmalonyl CoA mutase, which uses 5′-deoxyadenosylcobalamin as its cofactor. Upon endocytosis into cells, the transcobalamin–vitamin B_{12} complex is degraded in the lysosome and the free vitamin B_{12} is transported into the cytosol (Figure 25-9). Vitamin B_{12} is released into the cytosol of cells as hydroxycob(III)alamin, which is now available for coenzyme synthesis. In the cytosol, hydroxycob(III)alamin is reduced to the cob(I)alamin derivative. Cob(I)alamin is then methylated to the methylcob(III) alamin derivative after binding to methionine synthase. Alternatively, vitamin B_{12} can be transported into the mitochondria and reduced, and the 5′-deoxyadenosyl ligand added from ATP

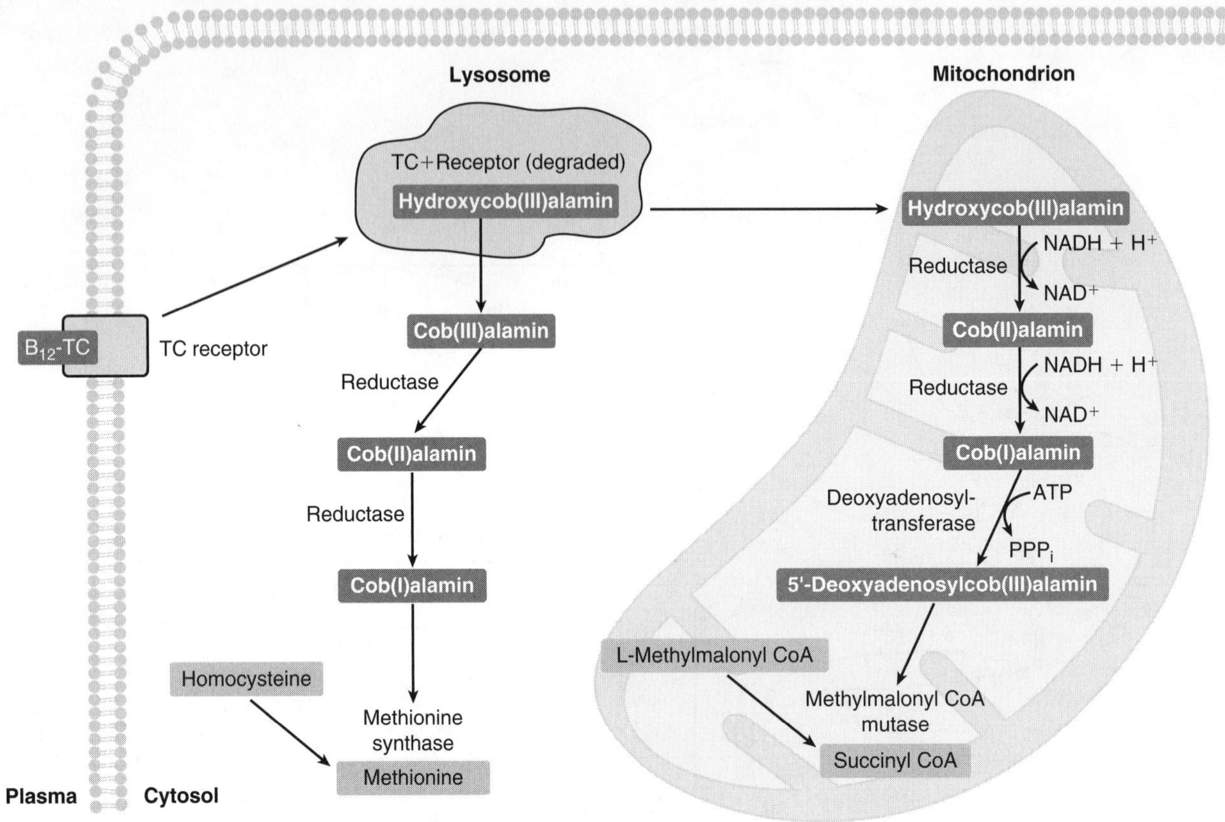

FIGURE 25-9 Tissue uptake and metabolism of vitamin B_{12}. *TC,* Transcobalamin.

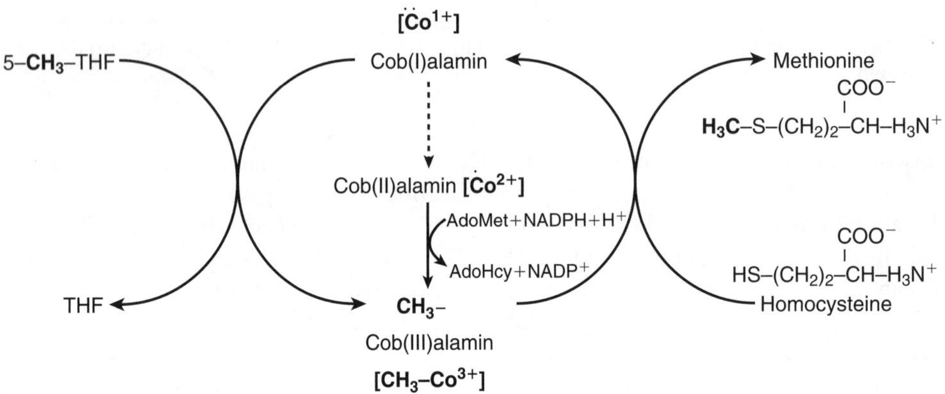

FIGURE 25-10 Remethylation of homocysteine via the methionine synthase reaction. Enzyme-bound cob(I)alamin is methylated by 5-methyl-THF to generate the methylcob(III)alamin intermediate, or it is oxidized to the nonfunctional cob(II) alamin form. Cob(II)alamin is reduced and methylated by methionine synthase reductase using *S*-adenosylmethionine (AdoMet) as the methyl donor.

in a reaction catalyzed by a deoxyadenosyltransferase. At least nine proteins are involved in the metabolism and trafficking of vitamin B_{12} within the cell. Rare human genetic defects in these proteins have been described that are associated with impaired vitamin B_{12} metabolism and function, often with severe clinical consequences depending on the nature of the defect.

METHIONINE SYNTHASE

Methylcobalamin is a cofactor for the previously described folate-dependent methionine synthase involved in homocysteine remethylation (Figure 25-10). Methionine synthase is a large, monomeric zinc metalloprotein (~140 kDa) consisting of three domains: a catalytic domain containing the binding sites for 5-methyl-THF and homocysteine, a vitamin B_{12} domain in which the vitamin B_{12} cofactor binds, and an accessory protein domain. Most of the methionine synthase in mammalian tissues is normally present as the holoenzyme form, containing a tightly bound vitamin B_{12} cofactor. The cob(I)alamin cofactor is methylated by 5-methyl-THF, generating enzyme-bound methylcob(III)alamin and releasing THF. The methylcob(III)alamin transfers its methyl group to homocysteine to generate methionine. Heterolytic cleavage of the cobalt-carbon bond regenerates the enzyme-bound cob(I)alamin derivative. The cofactor is occasionally oxidized to the nonfunctional cob(II)alamin derivative during catalysis. When this occurs, the enzyme is reactivated by methionine synthase reductase, an accessory protein that catalyzes the AdoMet- and NADPH-dependent reductive methylation of enzyme-bound cob(II)alamin to methylcob(III)alamin. Human mutations that result in loss of methionine synthase activity and early onset megaloblastic anemia fall into two complementation groups. The cblG complementation group results from mutations in the structural gene for methionine synthase *(MTR)*, whereas mutations in the methionine synthase reductase gene *(MTRR)* are responsible for the cblE complementation group.

Methionine synthase can also catalyze the reduction of the anesthetic gas nitrous oxide to nitrogen. During this process, a hydroxyl radical is formed, which can destroy the polypeptide backbone of the protein and inactivate the enzyme, as well as irreversibly oxidize the vitamin B_{12} cofactor. Chronic exposure to nitrous oxide will cause functional vitamin B_{12} deficiency. Nitrous oxide is sometimes used to inactivate methionine synthase in experimental animals to generate a model for the metabolic effects of vitamin B_{12} deficiency.

Many organisms do not use vitamin B_{12} cofactors and instead possess a vitamin B_{12}–independent methionine synthase that catalyzes the 5-methyl-THF–dependent methylation of homocysteine to methionine. This enzyme, which is not found in mammalian tissues, is absolutely specific for a folylpolyglutamate substrate. Many bacteria express the vitamin B_{12}–dependent enzyme when cultured in the presence of cobalamin, whereas the vitamin B_{12}–independent enzyme is induced in the absence of cobalamin. A question that arises is why some organisms, such as mammals, retained the vitamin B_{12}–dependent enzyme, which necessitates a very complex process for vitamin B_{12} transport and metabolism and makes the organism susceptible to defects in these processes, rather than simply using the vitamin B_{12}–independent methionine synthase expressed by other nonmammalian organisms. The answer is not obvious but may be related to the very poor catalytic activity of the vitamin B_{12}–independent enzyme. In organisms such as yeast, or bacteria cultured in the absence of cobalamin, the vitamin B_{12}–independent enzyme is induced to very high levels to compensate for its poor catalytic activity, becoming one of the major proteins expressed by these organisms. The more catalytically effective vitamin B_{12}–dependent enzyme is a low-abundance protein.

METHYLMALONYL-CoA MUTASE

Mitochondrial β-oxidation of odd-chain fatty acids produces both acetyl CoA and propionyl-CoA. Propionyl-CoA is converted to D-methylmalonyl-CoA in a reaction catalyzed by the biotin-dependent propionyl-CoA carboxylase. Propionyl-CoA and methylmalonyl-CoA can also arise during catabolism of isoleucine, valine, methionine, and threonine. A racemase converts D-methylmalonyl-CoA to L-methylmalonyl-CoA, and the 5′-deoxyadenosylcobalamin–dependent methylmalonyl-CoA mutase catalyzes the conversion of L-methylmalonyl CoA to succinyl-CoA (Figure 25-11). The mutase reaction involves the breakage and migration of a carbon–carbon bond. All these reactions occur in the mitochondria, and the succinyl-CoA that is formed has several potential fates, including entry into the citric acid cycle and heme biosynthesis. In liver, conversion of propionyl-CoA to succinyl-CoA allows the carbon skeletons of some amino acids, as well as propionyl-CoA from odd-chain fatty acid metabolism, to be used for gluconeogenesis.

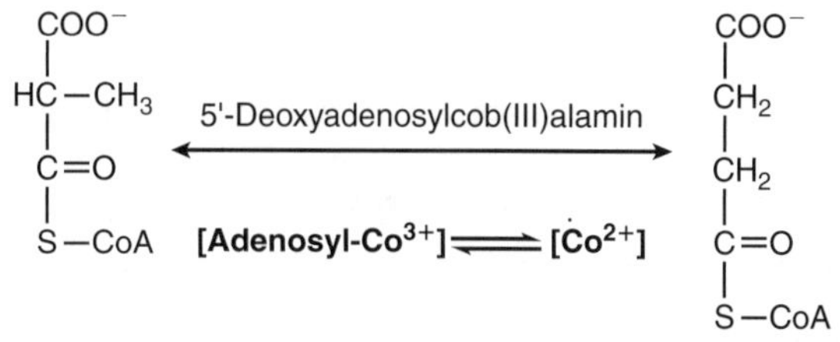

5'-Deoxyadenosylcob(III)alamin

[Adenosyl-Co^{3+}] ⇌ [Co^{2+}]

L-Methylmalonyl-CoA **Succinyl-CoA**

FIGURE 25-11 The methylmalonyl-CoA mutase reaction. The mutase catalyzes the hemolytic cleavage of coenzyme B_{12} (5′-deoxyadenosylcob(III)alamin) to generate an adenosyl radical, which interacts with the substrate, and a vitamin B_{12} cofactor radical.

VITAMIN B_{12} DEFICIENCY: SYMPTOMS AND METABOLIC BASES

Vitamin B_{12} deficiency can arise from both dietary insufficiency and malabsorption syndromes. Low dietary intake, once thought to be a relatively uncommon cause of vitamin B_{12} deficiency that was restricted to vegans and vegetarians, is now recognized as highly prevalent in developing countries in which the availability of animal source foods is limited. Severe clinical vitamin B_{12} deficiency, however, most commonly arises from a defect in vitamin B_{12} absorption. The primary manifestations of vitamin B_{12} deficiency are (1) megaloblastic anemia identical to that observed in folate deficiency, and (2) severe and often irreversible neurological disease affecting the spinal cord (subacute combined degeneration), the peripheral nerves (peripheral neuropathy), and the brain (memory loss, dementia, and depression). These neurological manifestations are the consequence of demyelination of neuronal axons and are likely related to metabolic disturbances in 1-C metabolism. Although the development of anemia often precedes the neurological disease and allows the detection and treatment of vitamin B_{12} deficiency before the development of neurological damage, this is not always the case. Some patients develop neurological disease in the absence of anemia. Neurological symptoms occur in 75% to 90% of patients with clinical vitamin B_{12} deficiency and may be the only symptom in 25%. The presentation of neurological symptoms in the absence of anemia may occur when excess folic acid from food or supplements is consumed and alleviates or prevents the anemia but does not affect the neurological deterioration. This "masking" of vitamin B_{12} deficiency by folic acid may prevent its early detection (i.e., by observation of megaloblastic anemia), thus allowing neurological deterioration to continue until clinical and often irreversible neurological damage occurs. In addition to this proposed masking effect, some observational data suggest that excess folic acid intake exacerbates vitamin B_{12} deficiency (Morris et al., 2007; Selhub et al., 2007; Miller et al., 2009), but firm evidence in support of this hypothesis is lacking.

VITAMIN B_{12} MALABSORPTION

The classical cause of vitamin B_{12} malabsorption is pernicious anemia, which is a lack of IF caused by autoimmune destruction of the gastric parietal cells. Pernicious anemia is primarily a disease of older adults, affecting an estimated 2% to 3% of those aged 65 years and older, though it is not restricted to any age group. Because body vitamin B_{12} stores are usually ample at the onset of the disease and the turnover of body stores is slow, it can take many years before deficiency symptoms become apparent. Whole-body turnover is increased, owing to an inability to reabsorb both biliary and dietary vitamin B_{12}. The destruction of the parietal cells decreases acid production, which also impairs release of dietary vitamin from proteins that bind vitamin B_{12}.

Malabsorption of vitamin B_{12} from food sources often occurs in individuals with atrophic gastritis, a condition of reduced stomach acid production and consequent reduced capacity to extract vitamin B_{12} from foods. Individuals with atrophic gastritis may efficiently absorb crystalline vitamin B_{12} from supplements, but not vitamin B_{12} from foods. The prevalence of atrophic gastritis increases with age, perhaps exceeding 30% in older adults (age 65 years and older), thus accounting for the majority of cases of vitamin B_{12} deficiency in older adults. Infection with *Helicobacter pylori* and bacterial overgrowth in the gut may contribute to atrophic gastritis or the inhibition of vitamin B_{12} absorption from food. Other less common causes of vitamin B_{12} malabsorption include pancreatic insufficiency, intestinal disorders such as Crohn disease and tropical sprue, infestation with fish tapeworm, and genetic defects affecting the physiological absorption process. Surgical gastric resection, a procedure that is sometimes used for the treatment of obesity, can also lead to decreased acid and IF production and consequent vitamin B_{12} malabsorption, as can chronic use of proton pump inhibitors used to treat acid reflux.

The Schilling test has been the gold standard for clinical diagnosis of pernicious anemia. The test consists of oral consumption of radioactively labeled vitamin B_{12} (typically labeled with ^{57}Co), followed by intramuscular injection of a large dose of unlabeled vitamin B_{12} up to 2 hours after the oral dose. The unlabeled vitamin B_{12} saturates all the plasma vitamin B_{12} proteins, thus causing any newly absorbed vitamin B_{12} to be flushed into the urine. High levels of radioactivity appearing in the urine over the 24 hours after the oral dose indicate an intact capacity to absorb the vitamin, whereas low levels indicate malabsorption. If malabsorption is suspected, the test is repeated with the radioactive vitamin B_{12} combined with an exogenous source of IF. If vitamin B_{12} absorption is restored by the addition of IF, then this is diagnostic for pernicious anemia. If absorption is not restored with IF, then other intestinal disorders may be responsible for the malabsorption syndrome. A variation of the Schilling test, called the food-bound or egg yolk vitamin B_{12} absorption test, uses radioactively labeled vitamin B_{12} bound to food proteins. This simulates endogenous vitamin B_{12} absorption from food sources. In recent years, the Schilling test has been rarely performed in the clinical setting because of issues of expense, radioactive waste disposal, and reduced availability of the test components. The test also requires normal renal function, which is often impaired in older adults. Diagnosis of pernicious anemia is now most often made based on low circulating vitamin B_{12} concentrations accompanied by anemia or neurological symptoms and a positive test for circulating autoantibodies for IF or the gastric parietal cells.

Standard treatment for pernicious anemia and other severe malabsorption syndromes is monthly intramuscular injections of 1 mg vitamin B_{12}. An alternative regimen is large daily oral doses of crystalline vitamin B_{12} (1 to 2 mg/day). This strategy exploits the fact that about 1% of a given dose of vitamin B_{12} is absorbed by passive diffusion. Malabsorption of vitamin B_{12} due to atrophic gastritis and other causes not affecting the IF-mediated absorption process may be treated with smaller daily oral doses of crystalline vitamin B_{12} (25 to 500 μg/day).

MEGALOBLASTIC ANEMIA

Megaloblastic anemia occurs in both folate and vitamin B_{12} deficiency. This is best explained by the methyl trap hypothesis. Folate, in the form of 5-methyl-THF, serves as substrate and vitamin B_{12}, in the form of methylcobalamin, serves as cofactor for methionine synthase. In patients with severe vitamin B_{12} deficiency, methionine synthase activity in bone marrow is reduced by more than 85%, and most of the protein is present in the apoenzyme form. This causes an accumulation of cellular folate as 5-methyl-THF because the methionine synthase reaction, which is severely impaired, is the only reaction capable of converting 5-methyl-THF back to free THF. The trapping of folate as 5-methyl-THF results in lack of folate for other reactions of 1-C metabolism, including thymidylate and purine synthesis. The lack of synthesis of thymidylate and purines is the underlying biochemical cause of megaloblastic anemia. Thus vitamin B_{12} deficiency causes a functional folate deficiency and has the same clinical outcome (i.e., megaloblastic anemia) as a folate deficiency.

Vitamin B_{12} deficiency also impairs the tissue accumulation of folates. 5-Methyl-THF enters cells in the monoglutamate form. Retention of folate in the cell requires conversion of the methylated monoglutamate to THF, which then serves as the substrate for polyglutamation. The polyglutamate forms of folate do not cross cell membranes and thus are retained in cells. A block in methionine synthase activity due to vitamin B_{12} deficiency prevents the conversion of 5-methyl-THF to THF and subsequent polyglutamation. This results in an inability of tissues to accumulate exogenous folate, such that most of the transported 5-methyl-THF is released back into the circulation. This reduction in the ability of tissues to accumulate folate, coupled with turnover of tissue folate pools, leads to a reduction in tissue folate levels, and an absolute tissue folate deficiency ensues on top of the functional deficiency caused by the methyl trap. In experimental animals placed on a vitamin B_{12}–deficient diet, or in animals treated with nitrous oxide to inhibit methionine synthase activity, plasma folate levels initially increase because tissues are unable to retain entering folate, but folate then eventually drops to low levels because the body is unable to retain it.

SUBACUTE COMBINED DEGENERATION

The mechanism underlying the neurological symptoms of vitamin B_{12} deficiency is not well understood. Most experimental animals do not develop neurological symptoms when placed on a vitamin B_{12}–deficient diet, in part because it is difficult to eliminate gut bacterial synthesis of vitamin B_{12} as a source of the vitamin. Although rarely used as a model, the South African fruit bat does display neurological abnormalities when made vitamin B_{12}–deficient, as do nonhuman primates.

Because mammals have only two vitamin B_{12}–dependent enzymes and methionine synthase is the locus of the defect causing anemia, attention has been focused on the role of methylmalonyl-CoA mutase in the etiology of the neurological defects. Vitamin B_{12} deficiency causes accumulation of methylmalonyl-CoA in the mitochondria, an elevation in circulating methylmalonic acid, acidosis, and elevated methylmalonic acid excretion. The accumulation of mitochondrial methylmalonyl-CoA depletes the CoA pool available for other mitochondrial enzymes and metabolites, resulting in increased concentrations of methylmalonic acid and propionic acid which can be used for cytosolic synthesis of long-chain fatty acids in place of acetyl-CoA or malonyl-CoA. A role for the accumulation of unusual fatty acids in myelin as a reason for the demyelination has been proposed, but evidence for this is not convincing. In any case, demyelination is not caused by a block in methylmalonyl-CoA mutase activity. Humans with severe genetic impairment of the *MUT* locus encoding the methylmalonyl-CoA mutase have a variety of severe clinical conditions and metabolic abnormalities but do not develop subacute combined degeneration of the spinal cord or megaloblastic anemia.

Monkeys treated with nitrous oxide develop neurological disease similar to that observed in humans, and these symptoms are prevented by methionine supplementation, suggesting that the neurological disease of vitamin B_{12} deficiency may result from inhibition of methionine synthase. In the few known cases of genetic defects in methionine synthase or in the enzymes responsible for methylcobalamin synthesis, the patients exhibit the expected megaloblastic anemia and some also exhibit demyelination. Similarly, some patients with defects in MTHFR (methylenetetrahydrofolate reductase) exhibit the same neurological symptoms as are observed in vitamin B_{12} deficiency. These patients do not exhibit megaloblastic anemia, because a defect in MTHFR prevents the formation of 5-methyl-THF and thus prevents trapping of THF and increases folate coenzyme availability for nucleotide synthesis. Although the mechanism responsible for the neurological disease of vitamin B_{12} deficiency is not understood, current evidence supports the hypothesis that it is related to defective methionine synthesis and that the locus of the defect is methionine synthase. A mouse knockout model for methionine synthase has been developed. The homozygous deletion is embryonically lethal, as might be predicted because of the expected derangement in DNA synthesis caused by the methyl trap. The heterozygote may prove to be a useful animal model for elucidating the development of neurological disease resulting from vitamin B_{12} deficiency.

A model for vitamin B_{12} deficiency in the rat, involving the totally gastrectomized animal, has been described (Scalabrino, 2009). Removal of the stomach induces severe vitamin B_{12} deficiency, and the rats develop neurological abnormalities similar to those observed in humans, including vacuolization, intramyelinic and interstitial edema of the white matter of the central nervous system, and astrogliosis. This is accompanied by overproduction of tumor necrosis factor-alpha (TNFα) and reduced synthesis of two neurotrophic agents, epidermal growth factor (EGF) and interleukin-6 (IL6) and has led to the hypothesis that dysregulation of these agents is induced by vitamin B_{12} deficiency and is responsible for subacute combined degeneration. It remains to be established how vitamin B_{12} deficiency affects TNFα and EGF levels and whether the dysregulation in these agents causes the subacute combined degeneration or results from it in this extreme animal model.

HYPERHOMOCYSTEINEMIA

The relationship of hyperhomocysteinemia to vascular disease risk is described earlier in this chapter. Plasma homocysteine is elevated in pernicious anemia because of the block in methionine synthase activity. In population studies, individuals with the lowest deciles of plasma vitamin B_{12} had the highest plasma homocysteine values. Although a slight correlation was observed between dietary vitamin B_{12} and homocysteine levels, it was weaker than that for plasma homocysteine and plasma vitamin B_{12}, indicating that defects in absorption rather than dietary content play a greater role in the development of impaired vitamin B_{12} status. As indicated previously, with the improvement of folate status of the U.S. population following food fortification, vitamin B_{12} status has become the major nutritional determinant of fasting homocysteine levels.

ASSAY AND DETECTION OF VITAMIN B_{12} DEFICIENCY

Assays for total plasma vitamin B_{12} have evolved over the last several decades. The first assays were microbiological, using *Lactobacillus leichmannii* and other vitamin B_{12}–dependent organisms. Some of the original microbiological assays measured both true vitamin B_{12} and its analogs. More recently, radioisotope dilution assays and nonradioactive enzyme-linked and chemiluminescence assays have been employed. The latter assays are often automated for use in high-throughput clinical laboratories. The most widely used test is a competitive radioassay procedure for plasma vitamin B_{12} that uses IF as the protein binder. IF will not bind vitamin B_{12} analogs and thus this test is specific for biologically active forms of the vitamin. A plasma level of less than 150 pmol/L (200 pg/mL) is typically considered indicative of deficiency. However, plasma levels greater than 150 pmol/L are often seen in subjects who, by other criteria such as elevated homocysteine and methylmalonic acid levels, are at risk of deficiency symptoms. Though plasma vitamin B_{12} level is a relatively good screening test for vitamin B_{12} status, it does suffer from fairly poor sensitivity. Other tests that are considered more sensitive and that have relatively high specificity include plasma and urinary methylmalonic acid and the amount of the total plasma vitamin B_{12} that is bound to transcobalamin (i.e., the amount of holotranscobalamin).

Because vitamin B_{12} deficiency induces a folate deficiency, many of the biochemical effects of vitamin B_{12} deficiency are identical to those seen in folate deficiency. Although plasma folate level is initially elevated, as the deficiency progresses plasma and RBC folate concentrations are reduced, plasma homocysteine is elevated, and urinary formiminoglutamate excretion is increased. By using these biochemical tests, it is not possible to distinguish whether an individual is deficient in folate, vitamin B_{12}, or both. A low plasma vitamin B_{12} level or elevated methylmalonic acid concentration would indicate vitamin B_{12} deficiency, whereas a normal plasma vitamin B_{12} coupled with low plasma or red cell folate would suggest folate deficiency.

A diagnosis of megaloblastic anemia can be confirmed by the appearance and size of blood cells. Because of the severe and sometimes irreversible nature of the neurological disease in untreated B_{12} deficiency, early detection of neurological impairment is critical. The use of a tuning fork to check for an absent vibration sensation is a simple neurological test that can detect early stages of neurological impairment.

DRIs Across the Life Cycle: Vitamin B_{12}

	μg Vitamin B_{12} per Day
Infants	RDA
0 through 6 mo	0.4 (AI)
7 through 12 mo	0.5 (AI)
Children	
1 through 3 yr	0.9
4 through 8 yr	1.2
9 through 13 yr	1.8
14 through 18 yr	2.4
Adults	
19 through 50 yr	2.4
≥51 yr	2.4*
Pregnant women	2.6
Lactating women	2.8

Data from IOM. (1998). *Dietary Reference Intakes for thiamin, riboflavin, niacin, vitamin B_6, folate, vitamin B_{12}, pantothenic acid, biotin, and choline*. Washington, DC: National Academy Press.

AI, Adequate Intake; *DRI*, Dietary Reference Intake; *RDA*, Recommended Dietary Allowance.

*Adults older than 50 years are advised to obtain most of the RDA for vitamin B_{12} from foods fortified with vitamin B_{12} or a vitamin B_{12}–containing supplement.

VITAMIN B_{12} REQUIREMENTS

The adult EAR for vitamin B_{12} is 2.0 μg/day. This is based on hematological evidence and plasma vitamin B_{12} values. The RDA is set at 20% above the EAR, or 2.4 μg/day. Intake of 2.6 μg/day is recommended for pregnant women to allow for fetal deposition of 0.1 to 0.2 μg/day, and intake of 2.8 μg/day is recommended for lactating women to allow for secretion of vitamin B_{12} in breastmilk. Because of the decreased absorption of vitamin B_{12} from food in older adults, it is recommended that individuals older than 50 years meet the RDA by ingesting foods fortified with vitamin B_{12} or by taking a supplement. EAR values for children were extrapolated from adult values based on body weight ($kg^{0.75}$), and the RDA values were set as 1.2 times the EAR. Adequate Intake (AI) for infants is based on the vitamin B_{12} content of breastmilk of well-nourished mothers (0.42 μg/L).

VITAMIN B_{12} DIETARY INTAKES

Based on the 2001–2002 NHANES data (Moshfegh et al., 2005), the median intake of vitamin B_{12} by women (19+ years) in the United States is 3.8 μg/day. Intake for women ranges (5th to 95th percentile) from 1.7 to 9.0 μg/day. For men (19+ years), the median intake is 5.7 μg/day, and intake ranges from 2.8 to 12.6 μg/day. Nearly all U.S. adults less than 50 years of age have vitamin B_{12} intakes above the EAR. For those aged 50 years and older, a comparison to the EAR was not made because up to about 30% of older people may inadequately absorb food-bound vitamin B and it is recommended they obtain vitamin B_{12} from supplements or fortified sources.

VITAMIN B_{12} TOXICITY

No toxicity associated with high doses of oral or intramuscular vitamin B_{12} has been reported, and milligram doses are used to treat pernicious anemia with no apparent side effects. Therefore no UL (Tolerable Upper Intake Level) has been established for vitamin B_{12}.

THINKING CRITICALLY

Vitamin B_{12}

During a diet history, you discover that your 73-year-old client has been taking 4 mg of folic acid daily for the past 5 years. In addition, he is a daily user of the antacid drug omeprazole (Prilosec).

1. In regard to vitamin B_{12}, what is the danger of taking such high doses of folic acid? Be specific and include an explanation of the "methyl trap."
2. Explain the significance of the daily use of omeprazole (Prilosec) in relation to vitamin B_{12} status.
3. What are the biochemical and clinical signs of vitamin B_{12} deficiency?
4. What assessment tests would you run on this patient to assess his vitamin B_{12} status? Explain.

VITAMIN B_6

Vitamin B_6 was originally isolated as an antidermatitis and antianemia factor for animals. The classical clinical symptoms of vitamin B_6 deficiency are a seborrheic dermatitis, microcytic anemia, epileptiform convulsions, depression, and confusion. Microcytic anemia is a reflection of decreased hemoglobin synthesis. More recently, several studies have reported that low vitamin B_6 status is a risk factor for cardiovascular disease and certain cancers, but the mechanisms responsible have not been determined.

CHEMISTRY OF VITAMIN B_6

Vitamin B_6 compounds are 4-substituted 2-methyl-3-hydroxy-5-hydroxymethylpyridine compounds (Figure 25-12). There are six major derivatives with vitamin activity: pyridoxal (PL), the 4-formyl derivative; pyridoxine (PN), the 4-hydroxymethyl derivative; pyridoxamine (PM), the 4-aminomethyl derivative; and their respective 5′-phosphate derivatives (PLP, PNP, and PMP). The major forms in animal tissues are the coenzyme species PLP and PMP. PN is usually the main form in plant foods, and a large proportion of the PN in plants can be present as a glucoside derivative. PN is the form of the vitamin normally present in supplements or fortified foods. The major excreted form of vitamin B_6 is the 4-carboxylate derivative known as 4-pyridoxic acid.

Vitamin B_6 compounds, and in particular PL and PLP, are light sensitive. Large losses of food vitamin B_6 can occur during heating and by leaching of the vitamin during food preparation.

SOURCES OF VITAMIN B_6

Cereals, meat, fish, poultry, and noncitrus fruits are the major contributors of vitamin B_6 in the American diet. Rich sources are highly fortified cereals, beef liver, and other organ meats.

ABSORPTION OF VITAMIN B_6

Vitamin B_6 is absorbed in the small intestine by a nonsaturable passive diffusion mechanism. The 5′-phosphate derivatives are hydrolyzed by a phosphatase before uptake. PN glucoside is normally deconjugated by a mucosal glucosidase. In humans, some PN glucoside is absorbed intact and can be hydrolyzed to PN in various tissues.

BIOAVAILABILITY OF VITAMIN B_6

The bioavailability of vitamin B_6 supplements is greater than 90%. Bioavailability of nonglucoside forms of the vitamin in foods is greater than 75%, whereas the bioavailability of PN

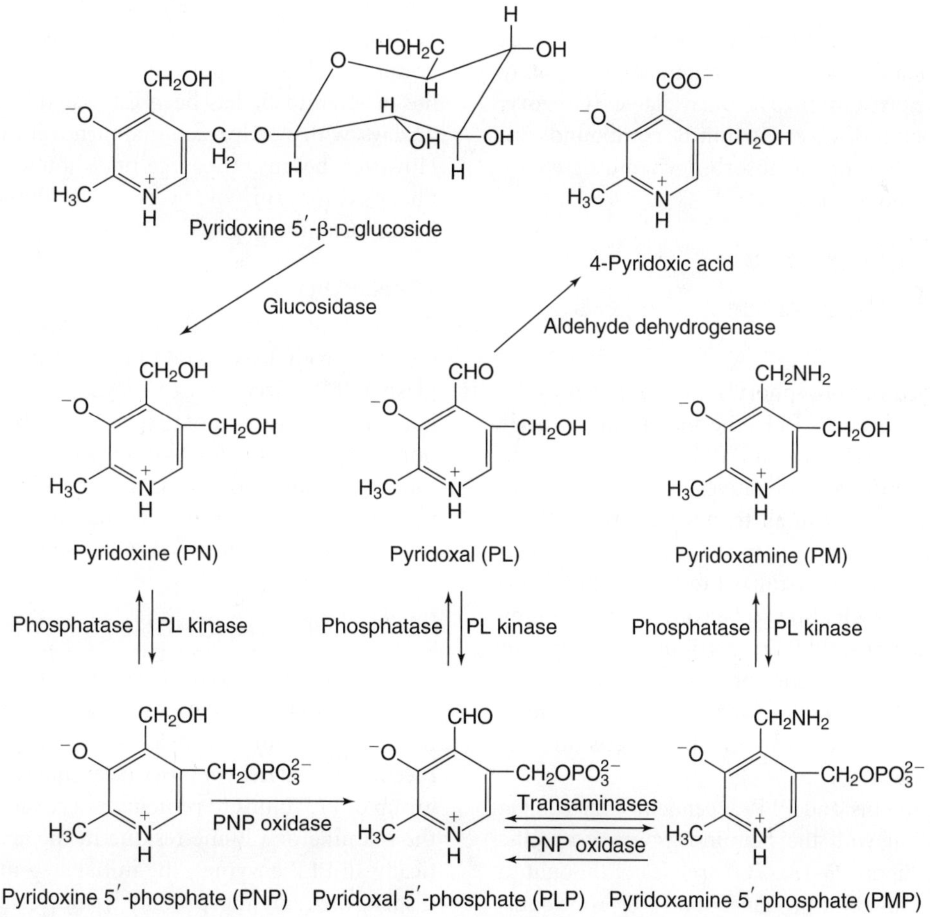

FIGURE 25-12 Vitamin B_6 compounds and their interconversion and metabolism.

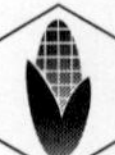

FOOD SOURCES HIGH IN VITAMIN B_6

Cereals and Grains
0.3 to 1.0 mg per 1 cup ready-to-eat cereal
0.3 mg per ½ cup cooked enriched rice
0.15 mg per ½ cup brown rice

Vegetables
0.15 to 0.2 mg per ½ cup pinto beans, lentils, lima beans
0.1 mg per ½ cup lima beans, kidney beans, chickpeas
0.15 to 0.2 mg per ½ cup Brussels sprouts, spinach, sweet red peppers, broccoli, sauerkraut, winter squash
0.25 mg per ½ cup carrot juice

Meat, Poultry, and Fish
0.4 mg per 3 oz turkey
0.3 to 0.4 mg per 3 oz pork
0.2 to 0.4 mg per 3 oz fish
0.25 to 0.5 mg per 3 oz beef

Other
0.3 mg per ½ cup prunes
0.2 mg per 1 cup orange juice
0.35 mg per 1 oz pistachio nuts
0.2 mg per 1 oz sunflower seeds

USDA, ARS. (2010). *USDA National Nutrient Database for Standard Reference, Release 23.* Retrieved from www.ars.usda.gov/ba/bhnrc/ndl.

glucoside in food is about half as much. Overall, vitamin B_6 in a mixed diet, which would typically contain approximately 15% PN glucoside, is about 75% bioavailable (Gregory, 1997). Pharmacological doses of vitamin B_6 compounds are well absorbed, but most of the absorbed vitamin is eliminated in the urine at high doses.

METABOLISM, TURNOVER, AND TRANSPORT OF VITAMIN B_6

METABOLISM

Most of the absorbed nonphosphorylated B_6 is taken up by the liver and metabolized to PLP, the major coenzymatic form (Figure 25-13). PN, PL, and PM are converted to their respective 5′-phosphate derivatives by the enzyme PL kinase. PL kinase is present in all tissues, including RBCs. PNP, which is normally found only at very low concentrations in tissues, and PMP are oxidized to PLP by the flavoprotein PNP oxidase. PMP also can be converted to PLP by transamination reactions. PLP is distributed throughout various subcellular compartments, but most is in the cytosol and mitochondria. Most of the PL kinase activity is found in the cytosol, and the mechanism by which PLP gets into the mitochondria is unclear.

PLP binds to proteins and PLP-dependent enzymes via Schiff base formation with the ε-amino group of specific lysine residues (see Figure 25-13). PLP itself is not thought to cross membranes. However, protein-bound PLP is in equilibrium with free PLP, and free PLP can be hydrolyzed to PL by various phosphatases and released by the tissue; protein binding protects PLP from the action of these phosphatases. Conditions of increased phosphatase activity, both in tissues and in plasma, can lead to increased hydrolysis of PLP. Tissue protein capacity for binding PLP limits tissue accumulation of vitamin B_6. At high intakes of vitamin B_6, tissue-binding capacity is exceeded and the free PLP is rapidly hydrolyzed to the nonphosphorylated PL, which is released by the liver and other tissues into the circulation. Product inhibition of the PNP oxidase by PLP makes the relationship between PN intake and PLP concentration in tissues and plasma very nonlinear. However, the high PLP-binding capacities of proteins in muscle (phosphorylase), plasma (albumin), and RBCs (hemoglobin) allow them to accumulate high levels of PLP even when other tissues are saturated.

TURNOVER

PL in liver can be oxidized to the inactive excretory metabolite pyridoxic acid by a flavoprotein aldehyde dehydrogenase. On normal diets, urinary pyridoxic acid excretion accounts for about half the vitamin B_6 compounds. With large doses of vitamin B_6, the proportion of unmetabolized vitamin B_6 excreted increases, and at very high doses of PN much of the dose is excreted unchanged in the urine Vitamin B_6 is also excreted in feces, but this may be due to biosynthesis in the lower gut.

Estimates of total body vitamin B_6 stores in healthy adults range from approximately 400 μmol to 1,000 μmol (60 to 170 mg), and 80% to 90% of this is in muscle, primarily bound to glycogen phosphorylase. The overall body half-life of vitamin B_6 has been estimated to be approximately 25 days, with a daily fractional turnover rate of less than 3%. However, because the large pool bound to glycogen phosphorylase may turn over very slowly, the actual half-life may be significantly longer.

TRANSPORT

Plasma PLP, a major form of the vitamin in plasma, is secreted from liver as a PLP–albumin complex. Because plasma PLP reflects liver PLP levels (and stores), plasma PLP is a sensitive indicator of tissue vitamin B_6 status. Circulating nonphosphorylated forms of the vitamin can be transported into tissues and blood cells. Plasma PLP is also a source of vitamin B_6 for tissue uptake, but it must dissociate from albumin and be hydrolyzed to PL before it is available.

METABOLIC FUNCTIONS OF VITAMIN B_6

PLP serves as a coenzyme for more than 100 enzymes, which include primarily enzymes involved in amino acid metabolism, such as aminotransferases, decarboxylases, aldolases, racemases, and dehydratases (see Chapter 14). The carbonyl group of PLP binds to proteins as a covalent Schiff base with the ε-amine of a lysine residue in the active site. For practically all PLP enzymes, the initial step in catalysis involves displacement of the protein lysine residue by the amino group of the entering amino acid, which forms a new Schiff

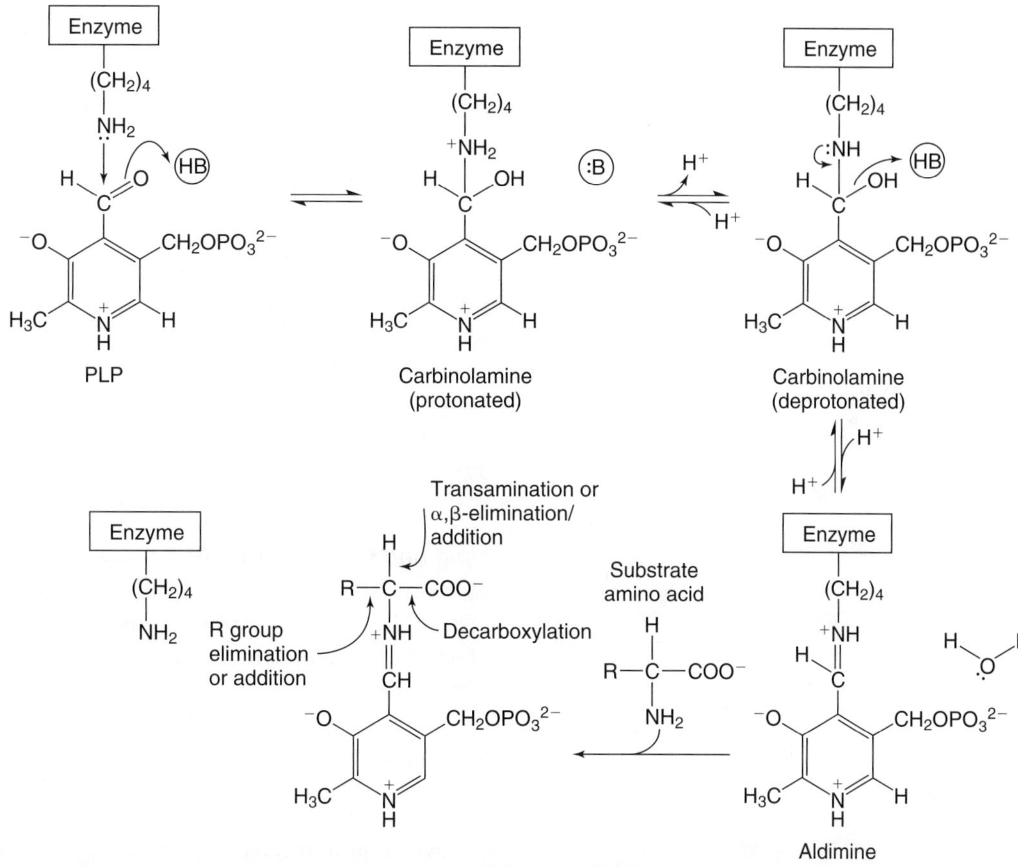

FIGURE 25-13 Schiff base formation between pyridoxal 5′-phosphate (PLP) and the ε-amino group of a lysine residue at the active site of an enzyme (HB, residue on the enzyme that acts as an acid–base catalyst). An entering amino acid substrate displaces the lysine residue and forms a Schiff base with the coenzyme. The coenzyme remains tightly bound to the protein via electrostatic interactions through its 5′-phosphate. Labilization of the various bonds around the α-carbon of the amino acid can result in elimination, addition, transamination, or decarboxylation reactions.

base with the coenzyme (see Figure 25-13). The coenzyme is no longer covalently attached to the enzyme but the aldimine derivative remains tightly bound. Electron movement and labilization of the different bonds around the α-carbon of the amino acid can lead to transamination, decarboxylation, racemization, α,β-elimination/addition, or R-group elimination/addition.

TRANSAMINATION

The catabolism of nearly all amino acids involves transfer of their amino groups to α-keto acids. The major amino group acceptors are α-ketoglutarate and pyruvate; transamination with these keto acids results in formation of glutamate and alanine, respectively, whereas the amino acid substrate is converted to its respective keto acid (see Chapter 14).

These transamination (aminotransferase) reactions initially generate the keto acid of the amino acid and PMP (Figure 25-14). Reversal of this reaction using α-ketoglutarate or pyruvate as the entering keto acid generates glutamate or alanine. Aminotransferase reactions normally result in the transfer of the α-amino group of an amino acid to a keto acid. However, the PMP that is formed in the first part of the reaction sometimes dissociates from the enzyme before the keto acid can interact, which yields a slow conversion of PLP to PMP. A PMP–enzyme intermediate is not formed in other PLP-enzyme–catalyzed reactions.

DECARBOXYLATION

Decarboxylases are involved in many areas of metabolism, including the formation of a number of hormones and neurotransmitters, such as epinephrine, serotonin, and dopamine. Elimination of CO_2 from a compound results in a large drop in free energy, and decarboxylase reactions are essentially irreversible. The mitochondrial glycine cleavage system, which is a glycine decarboxylase, serves an important role in regulating glycine concentration.

HEME SYNTHESIS

PLP is a cofactor for mitochondrial δ-aminolevulinate synthase, which catalyzes the first and rate-limiting step in heme biosynthesis in liver (Figure 25-15). Labilization of the R group of glycine and addition of succinate yields the transient intermediate α-amino-β-ketoadipate, which is rapidly decarboxylated to δ-aminolevulinate. Two molecules of aminolevulinate condense to form porphobilinogen, and further condensation and metabolism yields heme. The synthesis of D-aminolevulinate synthase is regulated by heme.

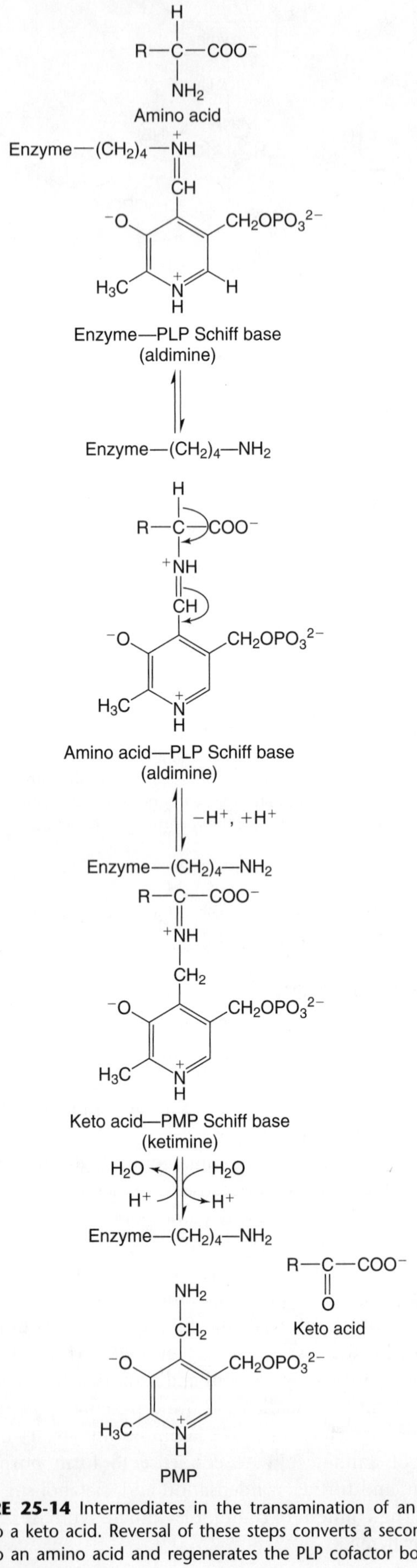

FIGURE 25-14 Intermediates in the transamination of an amino acid to a keto acid. Reversal of these steps converts a second keto acid to an amino acid and regenerates the PLP cofactor bound to the enzyme.

One-carbon Metabolism

PLP is a cofactor for serine hydroxymethyltransferase, which is involved in serine biosynthesis, and for cystathionine β-synthase and cystathionine γ-lyase, which catalyze the two steps in the transsulfuration pathway for homocysteine catabolism and cysteine synthesis (see Figure 25-2). PLP also serves as a cofactor for the glycine cleavage system, which is a three-protein complex in mitochondria that catalyzes the net catabolism of glycine to CO_2 and NH_3, along with the transfer of the glycine α-carbon to THF to form 5,10-methylene-THF. Recent studies have shown that this process is a major supplier of 1-C units in 1-C metabolism in humans (Lamers et al., 2009a). Probably at least a part of this substantial production of 5,10-methylene-THF by the glycine cleavage system is used in the conversion of glycine to serine for use in gluconeogenesis.

Lipid and Carbohydrate Metabolism

PLP enzymes are also involved in lipid and carbohydrate metabolism. PLP is a cofactor in the muscle glycogen phosphorylase reaction, but in this reaction the 5′-phosphate group, rather than the 4-carbonyl group, is directly involved in catalysis. Most of the PLP in the body is associated with muscle glycogen phosphorylase. PLP is a cofactor for serine palmitoyl transferase, an enzyme involved in sphingolipid synthesis.

Several studies have suggested that PLP modifies the properties of the glucocorticoid receptor, and it has been proposed that PLP may play a role in steroid hormone action. Similarly, PLP has been shown to affect the transcription rate of some genes. However, high levels of PLP were used in these in vitro studies, and it has not been established that these observations have physiological relevance.

VITAMIN B_6 DEFICIENCY: SYMPTOMS AND METABOLIC BASES

Vitamin B_6 deficiency can lead to seborrheic dermatitis, microcytic anemia, convulsions, depression, and confusion. Electroencephalographic abnormalities have also been reported in controlled studies of B_6 depletion. With the exception of the anemia, the exact mechanisms underlying these abnormalities and their clinical relevance at the more typical marginal to moderate levels of vitamin B_6 deficiency have not been established.

MICROCYTIC ANEMIA

Microcytic anemia is a reflection of decreased hemoglobin synthesis. Replication of the erythroid cell is regulated by its heme content, and reticulocyte cell division stops when the hemoglobin protein concentration reaches approximately 20%. Cells that are defective in heme biosynthesis continue to replicate; cell number can increase, but the cells are small (microcytic) and total blood concentration of hemoglobin is reduced (anemia). The role of PLP as a cofactor for δ-aminolevulinate synthase, the first enzyme in heme

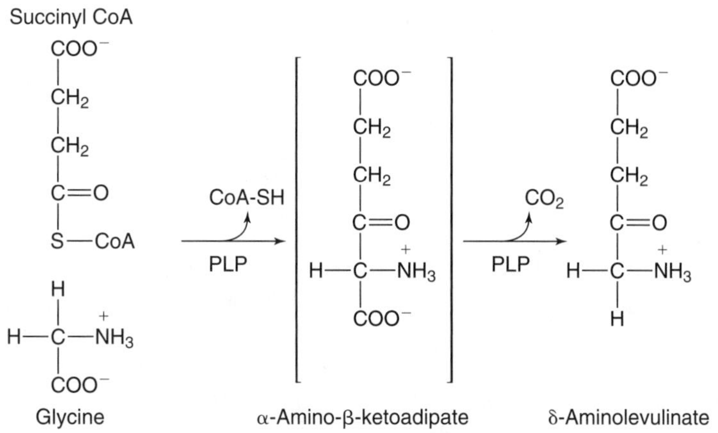

Succinyl CoA + Glycine → (CoA-SH, PLP) → [α-Amino-β-ketoadipate] → (CO_2, PLP) → δ-Aminolevulinate

FIGURE 25-15 The δ-aminolevulinate synthase reaction.

biosynthesis, can entirely explain this vitamin B_6–deficiency syndrome.

CONVULSIONS AND ELECTROENCEPHALOGRAPHIC ABNORMALITIES

PLP is a cofactor for decarboxylases that are involved in synthesis of neurotransmitters such as serotonin and dopamine, and vitamin B_6 status has been shown to influence biogenic amine levels in the brain. Reduced activity of some of these decarboxylases could reasonably explain the convulsions and electroencephalographic abnormalities, but the responsible biogenic amine has not been established. It has also been proposed that the convulsions are caused by abnormal tryptophan metabolites that accumulate in the brain in vitamin B_6 deficiency. An outbreak of convulsions occurred in the 1950s in infants who were fed a formula that contained very low vitamin B_6 content, and these convulsions did respond to PN administration. Although occasional cases of convulsions in breast-fed infants of mothers with poor vitamin B_6 status have been reported since then, these are quite rare, and the possibility that other factors were responsible for the convulsions has not been eliminated.

HYPERHOMOCYSTEINEMIA

The increase in plasma homocysteine following a methionine load or a meal is responsive to, and primarily affected by, vitamin B_6 status, reflecting the ability of PLP-dependent cystathionine β-synthase to catalyze the transsulfuration and removal of homocysteine (see Figure 25-2). Elevation of preprandial plasma homocysteine is more sensitive to insufficiency of folate and/or vitamin B_{12} than of vitamin B_6.

ALCOHOL

Low plasma PLP levels and a decreased vitamin B_6 status are associated with alcoholism but they are largely independent of poor diet and of defects in metabolism caused by liver damage. Acetaldehyde, the oxidation product of ethanol, decreases cellular PLP. Acetaldehyde is thought to displace PLP from proteins, making PLP more susceptible to hydrolysis by phosphatases.

VITAMIN B_6 AND DISEASE RISK

Many studies have shown relationships between low vitamin B_6 status and elevated risk of cardiovascular disease, but the mechanism responsible has not been determined. Low vitamin B_6 intake or low plasma PLP level, or both, are associated with greater risk of coronary artery disease, stroke, and venous thrombosis (Verhoef et al., 1996; Rimm et al., 1998; Dalery et al., 1995; Kelly et al., 2003). These associations are largely independent of folate status and plasma homocysteine concentration. Recent findings of inverse associations between inflammatory markers and plasma PLP concentration (Morris et al., 2010) suggest a possible role of inflammation. Whether low vitamin B_6 status is mechanistically involved or may be a correlate of inflammatory status affecting cardiovascular disease remains to be determined. Low vitamin B_6 status may impair the production of glutathione in a subset of individuals (Lamers et al., 2009b), which could indicate a connection between vitamin B_6 insufficiency, oxidant defense, and disease risk.

Several studies also have reported that low vitamin B_6 status is a risk factor for certain cancers, including colorectal and lung cancers (Larsson et al., 2010; Johansson et al., 2010). Again, the mechanisms responsible have not been determined.

DETECTION OF VITAMIN B_6 DEFICIENCY

A variety of biochemical indicators have been used to assess vitamin B_6 status. Plasma PLP is a reflection of liver PLP and thus tissue stores, and it generally correlates with other indices of B_6 status. Plasma PLP level is normally measured by an enzymatic assay using the apoenzyme form of tyrosine decarboxylase or by high performance liquid chromatograpy. A plasma PLP level of less than 20 nmol/L is considered to reflect inadequate vitamin status in the adult, although some support a threshold of 30 nmol/L for assessing sufficiency. Plasma PLP increases approximately 12 nmol/L for each 1 mg/day increase in vitamin B_6 intake (Morris et al., 2008). Clinical symptoms of vitamin B_6 deficiency and abnormal electroencephalographic patterns have been observed in some vitamin-depleted subjects when their plasma PLP levels fell to 10 nmol/L.

The stimulation of RBC aspartate aminotransferase or alanine aminotransferase activities by PLP has been used to evaluate vitamin B_6 status. These tests assess the amount of enzyme in the apoenzyme versus holoenzyme form, the proportion of which increases with vitamin B_6 depletion. The excretion of tryptophan catabolites following a loading dose of tryptophan also has been used to assess vitamin B_6 status. The urinary excretion of xanthurenate, which is normally a minor tryptophan catabolite, is increased in vitamin B_6 deficiency. Although tryptophan is catabolized primarily to CO_2 (see Chapter 14), a number of branch points in this pathway can lead to the synthesis of quantitatively minor metabolites such as NAD and xanthurenate. The activity of one of the enzymes in tryptophan catabolism, the PLP-dependent kynureninase, is reduced in vitamin B_6 deficiency, which diverts the metabolic flow into the xanthurenate synthesis pathway. Urinary excretion of xanthurenate can be a nonspecific test, however, because the first enzyme in the tryptophan catabolic pathway, tryptophan dioxygenase, may be induced by steroid hormones, and the level of kynureninase itself is decreased during pregnancy. Xanthurenate, as well as other tryptophan catabolites, is elevated in pregnant women and in high-dose oral contraceptive users in the absence of a vitamin B_6 deficiency.

An increase in plasma homocysteine levels following a methionine challenge dose is a fairly specific test of vitamin B_6 status. Recent studies have shown that plasma cystathionine concentration is a very sensitive biomarker for vitamin B_6 insufficiency because of the accumulation of cystathionine associated with reduced activity of cystathionine γ-lyase. An advantage of cystathionine as a biomarker is that it can be measured in a fasting blood sample and does not require the methionine challenge dose.

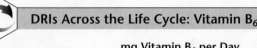

DRIs Across the Life Cycle: Vitamin B_6

	mg Vitamin B_6 per Day	
Infants	RDA	UL
0 through 6 mo	0.1 (AI)	ND
7 through 12 mo	0.3 (AI)	ND
Children		
1 through 3 yr	0.5	30
4 through 8 yr	0.6	40
9 through 13 yr	1.0	60
Males		
14 through 18 yr	1.3	80
19 through 50 yr	1.3	100
≥51 yr	1.7	100
Females		
14 through 18 yr	1.2	80
19 through 50 yr	1.3	100
≥51 yr	1.5	100
Pregnant		
<19 yr	1.9	80
≥19 yr	1.9	100
Lactating		
<19 yr	2.0	80
≥19 yr	2.0	100

Data from IOM. (1998). *Dietary Reference Intakes for thiamin, riboflavin, niacin, vitamin B_6, folate, vitamin B_{12}, pantothenic acid, biotin, and choline.* Washington, DC: National Academy Press.
AI, Adequate Intake; *DRI;* Dietary Reference Intake*; ND,* not determinable; *RDA,* Recommended Dietary Allowance; *UL,* Tolerable Upper Intake Level.

VITAMIN B_6 REQUIREMENTS

The primary criterion used in setting the EAR for vitamin B_6 was a plasma PLP value of at least 20 nmol/L (IOM, 1998). The EAR for vitamin B_6 is 1.1 mg/day for adults from 19 to 50 years, and the RDA is 1.3 mg/day or 20% more than the EAR to allow for variance in need. The estimated EARs were higher for adults older than 50 years, and higher for men than women in this older age group. Therefore the EARs for women and men older than 50 years are 1.3 and 1.4 mg/day, respectively, and the RDAs are 1.5 and 1.7 mg/day, respectively. Upward adjustments to the EAR for vitamin B_6 were also made to cover the higher requirement of this vitamin during pregnancy and lactation. AIs for infants are based on the vitamin B_6 content of milk of well-nourished mothers and the mean volume of milk consumed (0.13 mg/L × 0.78 L/day = 0.1 mg/day). Recommendations for older infants and children were estimated by extrapolation from adults.

Clinical symptoms of vitamin B_6 deficiency have never been observed in experimental subjects receiving intakes of 0.5 mg/day, although such studies have been relatively short-term. Metabolic effects of marginal vitamin B_6 status (e.g., elevated plasma glycine and cystathionine levels) often are observed in humans having plasma PLP concentrations in the 20 to 30 nmol/L range. Evidence such as this, along with epidemiological observations associating low vitamin B_6 status and disease risk, are considered by some investigators to suggest that a higher RDA may be prudent. Recent data from NHANES 2003–2004 suggest that a daily vitamin B_6 intake of 3.0 to 4.9 mg is generally adequate to maintain an acceptable plasma PLP concentration, but segments of the population do not maintain adequate vitamin B_6 status at that intake level (Morris et al., 2008). For example, low plasma PLP is common in women using modern formulations of oral contraceptives (Morris et al., 2008). Whether this association of oral contraceptive use with low plasma PLP reflects actual vitamin B_6 deficiency or a redistribution of PLP into tissues remains unclear.

VITAMIN B_6 INTAKE

NHANES 2001–2002 data (Moshfegh et al., 2005) showed that median (50th percentile) vitamin B_6 dietary intake of U.S. women (19 years or older) is 1.45 mg/day. Intake of women ranges (5th to 95th percentile) from 0.79 to 2.51 mg/day. For men (19 years or older), the median dietary vitamin B_6 intake is 2.11 mg/day, and daily intake ranges from 1.17 to 3.68 mg/day. Compared to the EAR for vitamin B_6,

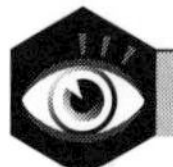

NUTRITION INSIGHT

Vitamin B_6 Status and Oral Contraceptive Usage

Evidence linking the usage of oral contraceptive agents (OCAs) to apparently low vitamin B_6 status has been discussed and debated since the early 1970s. At that time, the primary findings associating OCAs with low vitamin B_6 status was the tryptophan load test, in which the pattern of tryptophan metabolites is examined following an orally administered challenge dose of tryptophan. Because of the involvement of several PLP-dependent enzymes in tryptophan metabolism, changes in the profile of metabolites (particularly elevation in xanthurenic acid) occur in vitamin B_6 deficiency and indicate altered tryptophan metabolism. As stated earlier, however, tryptophan dioxygenase activity is influenced by other factors including estrogens, so its application in the context of OCAs yields ambiguous results. Studies in the 1970s provided little evidence of impaired vitamin B_6 status in OCA users. Good summaries of the issues and their interpretation have been published (Leklem, 1986; Miller, 1986).

Modern OCAs, termed third-generation OCAs, provide much lower estrogen doses, and most of the nutrition community assumed that any effect on vitamin B_6 metabolism, status, or function would be minimal. Morris and colleagues (2008) evaluated plasma PLP data from the National Health and Nutrition Evaluation Survey 2003–2004 and observed a surprisingly high incidence of very low plasma PLP values in the range considered to be indicative of vitamin B_6 deficiency among women who were oral contraceptive users. For example, these investigators observed a mean of 13 nmol/L, with 78% under the 20 nmol/L lower limit of the normal range, in women using OCAs (Morris et al., 2008). Although this observation from the nationally representative NHANES study has not yet been confirmed, similar findings were reported from an Italian study (Lusana et al., 2003). Whether these data indicate a true problem of frequent vitamin B_6 inadequacy associated with oral contraceptive use, or perhaps a suppression of plasma PLP while functional vitamin B_6 status remains adequate, remains to be determined.

most U.S. men are consuming adequate dietary vitamin B_6, whereas dietary intake in 28% of women is below the EAR.

VITAMIN B_6 TOXICITY

A severe sensory neuropathy has been described in subjects taking very large doses of PN (1 to 6 g/day) for the treatment of conditions such as carpal tunnel syndrome, premenstrual syndrome, asthma, and sickle cell disease. The reason for the sensory neuropathy is not known, but modification of proteins by PLP may be involved in the development of this condition. Although the efficacy of PN megadoses for treatment of these conditions has little scientific rationale, the toxic effects of megadoses have been clearly demonstrated. Because few studies have specifically looked for adverse effects of high doses of vitamin B_6, the highest safe dose is not known. Some evidence for toxicity has been reported for daily doses of 500 mg, whereas the absence of adverse effects has been rigorously documented in subjects taking daily doses of 100 mg or 300 mg of PN. A safe UL of 100 mg/day has been recommended by the IOM (1998); 100 mg of PN is approximately equal to body stores of total vitamin B_6 in healthy individuals. High doses of PN are used in certain forms of genetic disease such as homocysteinuria, but little evidence of toxicity has been reported.

THINKING CRITICALLY

Vitamin B_6

1. Describe three ways in which vitamin B_6 deficiency can adversely affect 1-C metabolism.
2. How would supplementing with amino acids impact the demand for vitamin B_6? In your answer, describe the metabolic reaction that may be affected by excess amino acid intake.
3. Contrast the anemia observed in vitamin B_6 deficiency to that observed in folate or vitamin B_{12} deficiency.

REFERENCES

Abdelmalek, M. F., Angulo, P., Jorgensen, R. A., Sylvestre, P. B., & Lindor, K. D. (2001). Betaine, a promising new agent for patients with nonalcoholic steatohepatitis: Results of a pilot study. *The American Journal of Gastroenterology, 96*, 2711–2717.

Abdelmalek, M. F., Sanderson, S. O., Angulo, P., Soldevila-Pico, C., Liu, C., Peter, J., … Lindor, K. D. (2009). Betaine for nonalcoholic fatty liver disease: Results of a randomized placebo-controlled trial. *Hepatology, 50*, 1818–1826.

Abratte, C. M., Wang, W., Li, R., Axume, J., Moriarty, D. J., & Caudill, M. A. (2009). Choline status is not a reliable indicator of moderate changes in dietary choline consumption in premenopausal women. *The Journal of Nutritional Biochemistry, 20*, 62–69.

Abratte, C. M., Wang, W., Li, R., Moriarty, D. J., & Caudill, M. A. (2008). Folate intake and the MTHFR C677T genotype influence choline status in young Mexican American women. *The Journal of Nutritional Biochemistry, 19*, 158–165.

Alvarez-Sabin, J., & Roman, G. C. (2011). Citicoline in vascular cognitive impairment and vascular dementia after stroke. *Stroke, 42*, S40–S43.

Amenta, F., & Tayebati, S. K. (2008). Pathways of acetylcholine synthesis, transport and release as targets for treatment of adult-onset cognitive dysfunction. *Current Medicinal Chemistry, 15*, 488–498.

American College of Obstetricians and Gynecologists. (2008). *Neural tube defects.* ACOG Practice Bulletin, number 44, July 2003 (reaffirmed 2008).

Anderson, D. D., & Stover, P. J. (2009). SHMT1 and SHMT2 are functionally redundant in nuclear de novo thymidylate biosynthesis. *PLoS One, 4,* e5839.

Anderson, D. D., Woeller, C. F., & Stover, P. J. (2007). Small ubiquitin-like modifier-1 (SUMO-1) modification of thymidylate synthase and dihydrofolate reductase. *Clinical Chemistry and Laboratory Medicine, 45,* 1760–1763.

Bailey, R. L., Dodd, K. W., Gahche, J. J., Dwyer, J. T., McDowell, M. A., Yetley, E. A., Sempos, C. A., Burt, V. L., Radimer, K. L., & Picciano, M. F. (2010a). Total folate and folic acid intake from foods and dietary supplements in the United States: 2003–2006. *The American Journal of Clinical Nutrition, 91,* 231–237.

Bailey, R. L., McDowell, M. A., Dodd, K. W., Gahche, J. J., Dwyer, J. T., & Picciano, M. F. (2010b). Total folate and folic acid intakes from foods and dietary supplements of US children aged 1–13 y. *The American Journal of Clinical Nutrition, 92,* 353–358.

Bailey, S. W., & Ayling, J. E. (2009). The extremely slow and variable activity of dihydrofolate reductase in human liver and its implications for high folic acid intake. *Proceedings of the National Academy of Sciences of the United States of America, 106,* 15424–15429.

Baron, C. L., & Malhotra, V. (2002). Role of diacylglycerol in PKD recruitment to the TGN and protein transport to the plasma membrane. *Science, 295,* 325–328.

Beaudin, A. E., Abarinov, E. V., Noden, D. M., Perry, C. A., Chu, S., Stabler, S. P., … Stover, P. J. (2011). Shmt1 and de novo thymidylate biosynthesis underlie folate-responsive neural tube defects in mice. *The American Journal of Clinical Nutrition, 93,* 1–10.

Beaudin, A. E., & Stover, P. J. (2007). Folate-mediated one-carbon metabolism and neural tube defects: Balancing genome synthesis and gene expression. Birth Defects Research. Part C. *Embryo Today: Reviews, 81,* 183–203.

Beaudin, A. E., & Stover, P. J. (2009). Insights into metabolic mechanisms underlying folate-responsive neural tube defects: A minireview. Birth Defects Research. Part A. *Clinical and Molecular Teratology, 85,* 274–284.

Beedholm-Ebsen, R., van de Wetering, K., Hardlei, T., Nexo, E., Borst, P., & Moestrup, S. K. (2010). Identification of multidrug resistance protein 1 (MRP1/ABCC1) as a molecular gate for cellular export of cobalamin. *Blood, 8,* 1632–1639.

Berry, R., Mullinare, J., & Hamner, H. C. (2009). Folic acid fortification: Neural tube defect risk reduction—A global perspective. In L. Bailey (Ed.), *Folate in health and disease* (2nd ed., pp. 179–204). Boca Raton, FL: CRC Press.

Bhuiyan, M. B., Murad, F., & Fant, M. E. (2006). The placental cholinergic system: Localization to the cytotrophoblast and modulation of nitric oxide. *Cell Communication and Signaling, 4,* 4.

Blount, B. C., Mack, M. M., Wehr, C. M., MacGregor, J. T., Hiatt, R. A., Wang, G., … Ames, B. N. (1997). Folate deficiency causes uracil misincorporation into human DNA and chromosomal breakage: Implications for cancer and neuronal damage. *Proceedings of the National Academy of Sciences of the United States of America, 94,* 3290–3295.

Buchman, A. L. (2009). The addition of choline to parenteral nutrition. *Gastroenterology, 137,* S119–S128.

Buchman, A. L., Ament, M. E., Sohel, M., Dubin, M., Jenden, D. J., Roch, M., … Ahn, C. (2001). Choline deficiency causes reversible hepatic abnormalities in patients receiving parenteral nutrition: Proof of a human choline requirement: A placebo-controlled trial. *Journal of Parenteral and Enteral Nutrition, 25,* 260–268.

Burg, M. B., & Ferraris, J. D. (2008). Intracellular organic osmolytes: Function and regulation. *The Journal of Biological Chemistry, 283,* 7309–7313.

Butler, P. L., & Mallampalli, R. K. (2010). Cross-talk between remodeling and de novo pathways maintains phospholipid balance through ubiquitination. *The Journal of Biological Chemistry, 285,* 6246–6258.

Carter, J. M., Demizieux, L., Campenot, R. B., Vance, D. E., & Vance, J. E. (2008). Phosphatidylcholine biosynthesis via CTP:phosphocholine cytidylyltransferase 2 facilitates neurite outgrowth and branching. *The Journal of Biological Chemistry, 283,* 202–212.

Caudill, M. (2009). Folate and choline interrelationships: Metabolic and potential health implications. In L. Bailey (Ed.), *Folate in health and disease* (pp. 449–465). Boca Raton, FL: CRC Press.

Caudill, M. A. (2010). Folate bioavailability: Implications for establishing dietary recommendations and optimizing status. *The American Journal of Clinical Nutrition, 91,* 1455S–1460S.

Cermak, J. M., Holler, T., Jackson, D. A., & Blusztajn, J. K. (1998). Prenatal availability of choline modifies development of the hippocampal cholinergic system. *The FASEB Journal, 12,* 349–357.

Chen, A. H., Innis, S. M., Davidson, A. G., & James, S. J. (2005). Phosphatidylcholine and lysophosphatidylcholine excretion is increased in children with cystic fibrosis and is associated with plasma homocysteine, *S*-adenosylhomocysteine, and *S*-adenosylmethionine. *The American Journal of Clinical Nutrition, 81,* 686–691.

Chen, J., Xu, X., Liu, A., & Ulrich, C. (2009). Folate and cancer: Epidemiological perspective. In L. Bailey (Ed.), *Folate in health and disease* (2nd ed., pp. 205–234). Boca Raton, FL: CRC Press.

Cheng, W. L., Holmes-McNary, M. Q., Mar, M. H., Lien, E. L., & Zeisel, S. H. (1996). Bioavailability of choline and choline esters from milk in rat pups. *The Journal of Nutritional Biochemistry, 7,* 457–464.

Cho, E., Holmes, M., Hankinson, S. E., & Willett, W. C. (2007). Nutrients involved in one-carbon metabolism and risk of breast cancer among premenopausal women. *Cancer Epidemiology, Biomarkers & Prevention, 16,* 2787–2790.

Cho, E., Holmes, M. D., Hankinson, S. E., & Willett, W. C. (2010). Choline and betaine intake and risk of breast cancer among post-menopausal women. *British Journal of Cancer, 102,* 489–494.

Christensen, K. E., & Mackenzie, R. E. (2008). Mitochondrial methylenetetrahydrofolate dehydrogenase, methenyltetrahydrofolate cyclohydrolase, and formyltetrahydrofolate synthetases. *Vitamins and Hormones, 79,* 393–410.

Christensen, K. E., & Rozen, R. (2009). Genetic variation: Effect on folate metabolism and health. In L. Bailey (Ed.), *Folate in health and disease* (2nd ed., pp. 75–110). Boca Raton, FL: CRC Press.

Ciappio, E., & Mason, J. B. (2009). Folate and carcinogenesis: Basic mechanisms. In L. Bailey (Ed.), *Folate in health and disease* (2nd ed., pp. 235–262). Boca Raton, FL: CRC Press.

Clarke, R., Halsey, J., Lewington, S., Lonn, E., Armitage, J., Manson, J. E., … Collins, R. (2010). Effects of lowering homocysteine levels with B vitamins on cardiovascular disease, cancer, and cause-specific mortality: Meta-analysis of 8 randomized trials involving 37485 individuals. *Archives of Internal Medicine, 170,* 1622–1631.

Cole, B. F., Baron, J. A., Sandler, R. S., Haile, R. W., Ahnen, D. J., Bresalier, R. S., … Greenberg, E. R.; Polyp Prevention Study Group. (2007). Folic acid for the prevention of colorectal adenomas. *The Journal of the American Medical Association, 297,* 2351–2359.

Czeizel, A. E., Puho, E. H., Langmar, Z., Acs, N., & Banhidy, F. (2010). Possible association of folic acid supplementation during pregnancy with reduction of preterm birth: A population-based study. *European Journal of Obstetrics, Gynecology, and Reproductive Biology, 148*, 135–140.

da Costa, K. A., Badea, M., Fischer, L. M., & Zeisel, S. H. (2004). Elevated serum creatine phosphokinase in choline-deficient humans: Mechanistic studies in C2C12 mouse myoblasts. *The American Journal of Clinical Nutrition, 80*, 163–170.

da Costa, K. A., Gaffney, C. E., Fischer, L. M., & Zeisel, S. H. (2005). Choline deficiency in mice and humans is associated with increased plasma homocysteine concentration after a methionine load. *The American Journal of Clinical Nutrition, 81*, 440–444.

da Costa, K. A., Kozyreva, O. G., Song, J., Galanko, J. A., Fischer, L. M., & Zeisel, S. H. (2006). Common genetic polymorphisms affect the human requirement for the nutrient choline. *The FASEB Journal, 20*, 1336–1344.

Dalery, K., Lussier-Cacan, S., Selhub, J., Davignon, J., Latour, Y., & Genest, J. (1995). Homocysteine and coronary artery disease in French Canadian subjects: Relation with vitamins B_{12}, B_6, pyridoxal phosphate, and folate. *The American Journal of Cardiology, 75*, 1107–1111.

Davalos, A., Castillo, J., Alvarez-Sabin, J., Secades, J. J., Mercadal, J., Lopez, S., … Lozano, R. (2002). Oral citicoline in acute ischemic stroke: An individual patient data pooling analysis of clinical trials. *Stroke, 33*, 2850–2857.

Davis, S. R., Stacpoole, P. W., Williamson, J., Kick, L. S., Quinlivan, E. P., Coats, B. S., … Gregory, J. F., 3rd. (2004). Tracer-derived total and folate-dependent homocysteine remethylation and synthesis rates in humans indicate that serine is the main one-carbon donor. *American Journal of Physiology. Endocrinology and Metabolism, 286*, E272–E279.

Davison, J. M., Mellott, T. J., Kovacheva, V. P., & Blusztajn, J. K. (2009). Gestational choline supply regulates methylation of histone H3, expression of histone methyltransferases G9a (Kmt1c) and Suv39h1 (Kmt1a), and DNA methylation of their genes in rat fetal liver and brain. *The Journal of Biological Chemistry, 284*, 1982–1989.

DeLong, C. J., Shen, Y. J., Thomas, M. J., & Cui, Z. (1999). Molecular distinction of phosphatidylcholine synthesis between the CDP-choline pathway and phosphatidylethanolamine methylation pathway. *The Journal of Biological Chemistry, 274*, 29683–29688.

Dilger, R. N., Garrow, T. A., & Baker, D. H. (2007). Betaine can partially spare choline in chicks but only when added to diets containing a minimal level of choline. *The Journal of Nutrition, 137*, 2224–2228.

Ebbing, M., Bonaa, K., Nygard, O., Arnesen, E., Ueland, P., Nordrehaug, J., … Vollset, S. (2009). Cancer incidence and mortality after treatment with folic acid and vitamin B_{12}. *The Journal of the American Medical Association, 302*, 2119–2126.

Emmert, J. L., & Baker, D. H. (1997). A chick bioassay approach for determining the bioavailable choline concentration in normal and overheated soybean meal, canola meal and peanut meal. *The Journal of Nutrition, 127*, 745–752.

Enaw, J. O., Zhu, H., Yang, W., Lu, W., Shaw, G. M., Lammer, E. J., & Finnell, R. H. (2006). CHKA and PCYT1A gene polymorphisms, choline intake and spina bifida risk in a California population. *BMC Medicine, 4*, 36.

Ferguson, S. M., & Blakely, R. D. (2004). The choline transporter resurfaces: New roles for synaptic vesicles? *Molecular Interventions, 4*, 22–37.

Figueiredo, J., Grau, M., Haile, R., Sandler, R., Summers, R., Bresalier, R., … Baron, J. (2009). Folic acid and risk of prostate cancer: Results from a randomized trial. *Journal of the National Cancer Institute, 101*, 432–435.

Finkelstein, J. D. (2001). Regulation of homocysteine metabolims. In R. J. D. Carmel (Ed.), *Homocysteine in health and disease* (pp. 92–99). Cambridge, MA: Cambridge University Press.

Fioravanti, M., & Yanagi, M. (2005). Cytidinediphosphocholine (CDP-choline) for cognitive and behavioural disturbances associated with chronic cerebral disorders in the elderly. *The Cochrane Database of Systematic Reviews* (2), CD000269.

Fischer, L. M., daCosta, K. A., Kwock, L., Galanko, J., & Zeisel, S. H. (2010). Dietary choline requirements of women: Effects of estrogen and genetic variation. *The American Journal of Clinical Nutrition, 92*, 1113–1119.

Fischer, L. M., daCosta, K. A., Kwock, L., Stewart, P. W., Lu, T. S., Stabler, S. P., … Zeisel, S. H. (2007). Sex and menopausal status influence human dietary requirements for the nutrient choline. *The American Journal of Clinical Nutrition, 85*, 1275–1285.

Gehrig, K., Morton, C. C., & Ridgway, N. D. (2009). Nuclear export of the rate-limiting enzyme in phosphatidylcholine synthesis is mediated by its membrane binding domain. *Journal of Lipid Research, 50*, 966–976.

Gregory, J. F., 3rd. (1997). Bioavailability of vitamin B-6. *European Journal of Clinical Nutrition, 51*, S43–S48.

Guinotte, C. L., Burns, M. G., Axume, J. A., Hata, H., Urrutia, T. F., Alamilla, A., … Caudill, M. A. (2003). Methylenetetrahydrofolate reductase 677C→T variant modulates folate status response to controlled folate intakes in young women. *The Journal of Nutrition, 133*, 1272–1280.

Henneberry, A. L., Wright, M. M., & McMaster, C. R. (2002). The major sites of cellular phospholipid synthesis and molecular determinants of fatty acid and lipid head group specificity. *Molecular Biology of the Cell, 13*, 3148–3161.

Hensley, K., Kotake, Y., Sang, H., Pye, Q. N., Wallis, G. L., Kolker, L. M., … Floyd, R. A. (2000). Dietary choline restriction causes complex I dysfunction and increased H(2)O(2) generation in liver mitochondria. *Carcinogenesis, 21*, 983–989.

Hobbs, C. A., Shaw, G. M., Werler, M. M., & Mosley, B. (2009). Folate status and birth defect risk. In L. Bailey (Ed.), *Folate in health and disease* (2nd ed., pp. 133–153). Boca Raton, FL: CRC Press.

Holm, P. I., Hustad, S., Ueland, P. M., Vollset, S. E., Grotmol, T., & Schneede, J. (2007). Modulation of the homocysteine-betaine relationship by methylenetetrahydrofolate reductase 677 C→T genotypes and B-vitamin status in a large-scale epidemiological study. *The Journal of Clinical Endocrinology and Metabolism, 92*, 1535–1541.

Institute of Medicine. (1998). *Dietary Reference Intakes for thiamin, riboflavin, niacin, vitamin B_6, folate, vitamin B_{12}, pantothenic acid, biotin, and choline*. Washington, DC: National Academy Press.

Jacobs, R. L., Stead, L. M., Devlin, C., Tabas, I., Brosnan, M. E., Brosnan, J. T., & Vance, D. E. (2005). Physiological regulation of phospholipid methylation alters plasma homocysteine in mice. *The Journal of Biological Chemistry, 280*, 28299–28305.

Johansson, M., Relton, C., Ueland, P. M., Vollset, S. E., Midttun, O., Nygard, O., … Brennan, P. (2010). Serum B vitamin levels and risk of lung cancer. *The Journal of the American Medical Association, 303*, 2377–2385.

Johansson, M., Van Guelpen, B., Vollset, S. E., Hultdin, J., Bergh, A., Key, T., … Stattin, P. (2009). One-carbon metabolism and prostate cancer risk: Prospective investigation of seven circulating B vitamins and metabolites. *Cancer Epidemiology, Biomarkers & Prevention, 18*, 1538–1543.

Kamath, A. V., Darling, I. M., & Morris, M. E. (2003). Choline uptake in human intestinal Caco-2 cells is carrier-mediated. *The Journal of Nutrition, 133*, 2607–2611.

Kaplan, C. P., Porter, R. K., & Brand, M. D. (1993). The choline transporter is the major site of control of choline oxidation in isolated rat liver mitochondria. *FEBS Letters, 321*, 24–26.

Kathirvel, E., Morgan, K., Nandgiri, G., Sandoval, B. C., Caudill, M. A., Bottiglieri, T., ... Morgan, T. R. (2010). Betaine improves nonalcoholic fatty liver and associated hepatic insulin resistance: A potential mechanism for hepatoprotection by betaine. *American Journal of Physiology. Gastrointestinal and Liver Physiology, 299*, G1068–G1077.

Kelly, P. J., Shih, V. E., Kistler, J. P., Barron, M., Lee, H., Mandell, R., & Furie, K. L. (2003). Low vitamin B_6 but not homocyst(e)ine is associated with increased risk of stroke and transient ischemic attack in the era of folic acid grain fortification. *Stroke, 34*, e51–e54.

Kharbanda, K. K., Mailliard, M. E., Baldwin, C. R., Beckenhauer, H. C., Sorrell, M. F., & Tuma, D. J. (2007). Betaine attenuates alcoholic steatosis by restoring phosphatidylcholine generation via the phosphatidylethanolamine methyltransferase pathway. *Journal of Hepatology, 46*, 314–321.

Kohlmeier, M., da Costa, K. A., Fischer, L. M., & Zeisel, S. H. (2005). Genetic variation of folate-mediated one-carbon transfer pathway predicts susceptibility to choline deficiency in humans. *Proceedings of the National Academy of Sciences of the United States of America, 102*, 16025–16030.

Kovacheva, V. P., Davison, J. M., Mellott, T. J., Rogers, A. E., Yang, S., O'Brien, M. J., & Blusztajn, J. K. (2009). Raising gestational choline intake alters gene expression in DMBA-evoked mammary tumors and prolongs survival. *The FASEB Journal, 23*, 1054–1063.

Lagace, T. A., & Ridgway, N. D. (2005). The rate-limiting enzyme in phosphatidylcholine synthesis regulates proliferation of the nucleoplasmic reticulum. *Molecular Biology of the Cell, 16*, 1120–1130.

Lamers, Y., Williamson, J., Theriaque, D. W., Shuster, J. J., Gilbert, L. R., Keeling, C., Stacpoole, P. W., & Gregory, J. F. (2009a). Production of 1-carbon units from glycine is extensive in healthy men and women. *The Journal of Nutrition, 139*, 666–671.

Lamers, Y., O'Rourke, B., Gilbert, L. R., Keeling, C., Matthews, D. E., Stacpoole, P. W., & Gregory, J. F. (2009b). Vitamin B-6 restriction tends to reduce red blood cell glutathione synthesis rate without affecting red blood cell or plasma glutathione concentrations in healthy men and women. *The American Journal of Clinical Nutrition, 90*, 336–343.

Larsson, S. C., Orsini, N., & Wolk, A. (2010). Vitamin B-6 and risk of colorectal cancer. A meta-analysis of prospective studies. *The Journal of the American Medical Association, 303*, 1077–1083.

Lee, J. E., Giovannucci, E., Fuchs, C. S., Willett, W. C., Zeisel, S. H., & Cho, E. (2010). Choline and betaine intake and the risk of colorectal cancer in men. *Cancer Epidemiology, Biomarkers & Prevention, 19*, 884–887.

Lee, M., Hong, K. S., Chang, S. C., & Saver, J. L. (2010). Efficacy of homocysteine-lowering therapy with folic acid in stroke prevention: A meta-analysis. *Stroke, 41*, 1205–1212.

Leklem, J. E. (1986). Vitamin B-6 requirement and oral contraceptive use—A concern? *The Journal of Nutrition, 116*, 475–477.

Li, Y., Holmes, W. B., Appling, D. R., & RajBhandary, U. L. (2000). Initiation of protein synthesis in *Saccharomyces cerevisiae* mitochondria without formylation of the initiator tRNA. *Journal of Bacteriology, 182*, 2886–2892.

Li, Z., Agellon, L., & Vance, D. E. (2005). Phosphatidylcholine homeostasis and liver failure. *The Journal of Biological Chemistry, 280*, 37798–37802.

Li, Z., Agellon, L. B., & Vance, D. E. (2007). Choline redistribution during adaptation to choline deprivation. *The Journal of Biological Chemistry, 282*, 10283–10289.

Li, Z., Agellon, L. B., Allen, T. M., Umeda, M., Jewell, L., Mason, A., & Vance, D. E. (2006). The ratio of phosphatidylcholine to phosphatidylethanolamine influences membrane integrity and steatohepatitis. *Cell Metabolism, 3*, 321–331.

Li, Z., & Vance, D. E. (2008). Phosphatidylcholine and choline homeostasis. *Journal of Lipid Research, 49*, 1187–1194.

Lockman, P. R., & Allen, D. D. (2002). The transport of choline. *Drug Development and Industrial Pharmacy, 28*, 749–771.

Lussana, F., Zighetti, M. L., Bucciarelli, P., Cugno, M., & Cattaneo, M. (2003). Blood levels of homocysteine, folate, vitamin B_6 and B_{12} in women using oral contraceptives compared to non-users. *Thrombosis Research, 112*, 37–41.

Mason, J. B., Dickstein, A., Jacques, P. F., Haggarty, P., Selhub, J., Dallal, G., & Rosenberg, I. H. (2007). A temporal association between folic acid fortification and an increase in colorectal cancer rates may be illuminating important biological principles: A hypothesis. *Cancer Epidemiology, Biomarkers & Prevention, 16*, 1325–1329.

McCann, J. C., Hudes, M., & Ames, B. N. (2006). An overview of evidence for a causal relationship between dietary availability of choline during development and cognitive function in offspring. *Neuroscience and Biobehavioral Reviews, 30*, 696–712.

McNulty, H., & Pentieva, K. (2009). Folate bioavailability. In L. Bailey (Ed.), *Folate in health and disease* (2nd ed., pp. 25–47). Boca Raton, FL: CRC Press.

Meck, W. H., & Williams, C. L. (2003). Metabolic imprinting of choline by its availability during gestation: Implications for memory and attentional processing across the lifespan. *Neuroscience and Biobehavioral Reviews, 27*, 385–399.

Meck, W. H., Williams, C. L., Cermak, J. M., & Blusztajn, J. K. (2008). Developmental periods of choline sensitivity provide an ontogenetic mechanism for regulating memory capacity and age-related dementia. *Frontiers in Integrative Neuroscience, 1*, 7.

Mei, W., Rong, Y., Jinming, L., Yongjun, L., & Hui, Z. (2010). Effect of homocysteine interventions on the risk of cardiocerebrovascular events: A meta-analysis of randomised controlled trials. *International Journal of Clinical Practice, 64*, 208–215.

Miller, E. R., 3rd, Juraschek, S., Pastor-Barriuso, R., Bazzano, L. A., Appel, L. J., & Guallar, E. (2010). Meta-analysis of folic acid supplementation trials on risk of cardiovascular disease and risk interaction with baseline homocysteine levels. *The American Journal of Cardiology, 106*, 517–527.

Miller, J. W., Garrod, M. G., Allen, L. H., Haan, M. N., & Green, R. (2009). Metabolic evidence of vitamin B_{12} deficiency, including high homocysteine and methylmalonic acid and low holotranscobalamin, is more pronounced in older adults with elevated plasma folate. *The American Journal of Clinical Nutrition, 6*, 1586–1592.

Miller, L. T. (1986). Do oral contraceptive agents affect nutrient requirements—Vitamin B-6? *The Journal of Nutrition, 116*, 1344–1345.

Moon, J., Chen, M., Gandhy, S. U., Strawderman, M., Levitsky, D. A., Maclean, K. N., & Strupp, B. J. (2010). Perinatal choline supplementation improves cognitive functioning and emotion regulation in the Ts65Dn mouse model of Down syndrome. *Behavioral Neuroscience, 124*, 346–361.

Morris, M. S., Jacques, P. F., Rosenberg, I. H., & Selhub, J. (2007). Folate and vitamin B-12 status in relation to anemia, macrocytosis, and cognitive impairment in older Americans in the age of folic acid fortification. *The American Journal of Clinical Nutrition, 1*, 193–200.

Morris, M. S., Picciano, M. F., Jacques, P. F., & Selhub, J. (2008). Plasma pyridoxal 5′-phosphate in the US population: The National Health and Nutrition Examination Survey, 2003–2004. *The American Journal of Clinical Nutrition, 87*, 1446–1454.

Morris, M. S., Sakakeeny, L., Jacques, P. F., Picciano, M. F., & Selhub, J. (2010). Vitamin B-6 intake is inversely related to, and the requirement is affected by, inflammation status. *The Journal of Nutrition, 140*, 103–110.

Mosfegh, A., Goldman, J., & Cleveland, L. (2005). *What we eat in America. NHANES 2001-2002. Usual nutrient intakes from food compared to Dietary Reference Intakes.* Washington, DC: U.S. Department of Agriculture, Agricultural Research Service.

Napoli, I., Blusztajn, J. K., & Mellott, T. J. (2008). Prenatal choline supplementation in rats increases the expression of IGF2 and its receptor IGF2R and enhances IGF2-induced acetylcholine release in hippocampus and frontal cortex. *Brain Research, 1237,* 124–135.

Oude Elferink, R. P., & Groen, A. K. (2000). Mechanisms of biliary lipid secretion and their role in lipid homeostasis. *Seminars in Liver Disease, 20,* 293–305.

Perlemuter, G., Bigorgne, A., Cassard-Doulcier, A. M., & Naveau, S. (2007). Nonalcoholic fatty liver disease: From pathogenesis to patient care. *Nature Clinical Practice. Endocrinology & Metabolism, 3,* 458–469.

Pfeiffer, C. M., Caudill, S. P., Gunter, E. W., Osterloh, J., & Sampson, E. J. (2005). Biochemical indicators of B vitamin status in the US population after folic acid fortification: Results from the National Health and Nutrition Examination Survey 1999–2000. *The American Journal of Clinical Nutrition, 82,* 442–450.

Pfeiffer, C. M., Johnson, C. L., Jain, R. B., Yetley, E. A., Picciano, M. F., Rader, J. I., Fisher, K. D., Mulinare, J., & Osterloh, J. D. (2007). Trends in blood folate and vitamin B-12 concentrations in the United States, 1988–2004. *The American Journal of Clinical Nutrition, 86,* 718–727.

Piedrahita, J. A., Oetama, B., Bennett, G. D., van Waes, J., Kamen, B. A., Richardson, J., … Finnell, R. H. (1999). Mice lacking the folic acid-binding protein Folbp1 are defective in early embryonic development. *Nature Genetics, 23,* 228–232.

Pynn, C. J., Henderson, N. G., Clark, H., Koster, G., Bernhard, W., & Postle, A. D. (2011). Specificity and rate of human and mouse liver and plasma phosphatidylcholine synthesis analyzed in vivo. *Journal of Lipid Research, 52,* 399–407.

Quadros, E. V., Nakayama, Y., & Sequeira, J. M. (2009). The protein and the gene encoding the receptor for the cellular uptake of transcobalamin-bound cobalamin. *Blood, 1,* 186–192.

Reo, N. V., Adinehzadeh, M., & Foy, B. D. (2002). Kinetic analyses of liver phosphatidylcholine and phosphatidylethanolamine biosynthesis using (13)C NMR spectroscopy. *Biochimica et Biophysica Acta, 1580,* 171–188.

Resseguie, M., Song, J., Niculescu, M. D., da Costa, K. A., Randall, T. A., & Zeisel, S. H. (2007). Phosphatidylethanolamine N-methyltransferase (PEMT) gene expression is induced by estrogen in human and mouse primary hepatocytes. *The FASEB Journal, 21,* 2622–2632.

Resseguie, M. E., da Costa, K. A., Galanko, J. A., Patel, M., Davis, I. J., & Zeisel, S. H. (2011). Aberrant estrogen regulation of PEMT results in choline deficiency-associated liver dysfunction. *The Journal of Biological Chemistry, 286,* 1649–1658.

Ridsdale, R., Tseu, I., Wang, J., & Post, M. (2001). CTP phosphocholine cytidylyltransferase alpha is a cytosolic protein in pulmonary epithelial cells and tissues. *The Journal of Biological Chemistry, 276,* 49148–49155.

Rimm, E. B., Willett, W. C., Hu, F. B., Sampson, L., Colditz, G. A., Manson, J. E., … Stampfer, M. J. (1998). Folate and vitamin B_6 from diet and supplements in relation to risk of coronary heart disease among women. *The Journal of the American Medical Association, 279,* 359–364.

Scalabrino, G. (2009). The multi-faceted basis of vitamin B_{12} (cobalamin) neurotrophism in adult central nervous system: Lessons learned from its deficiency. *Progress in Neurobiology, 3,* 203–220.

Secades, J. J., & Lorenzo, J. L. (2006). Citicoline: Pharmacological and clinical review, 2006 update. *Methods and Findings in Experimental and Clinical Pharmacology, 28,* 1–56.

Sehayek, E., Wang, R., Ono, J. G., Zinchuk, V. S., Duncan, E. M., Shefer, S., … Breslow, J. L. (2003). Localization of the PE methylation pathway and SR-BI to the canalicular membrane: Evidence for apical PC biosynthesis that may promote biliary excretion of phospholipid and cholesterol. *Journal of Lipid Research, 44,* 1605–1613.

Selhub, J., Morris, M. S., & Jacques, P. F. (2007). In vitamin B_{12} deficiency, higher serum folate is associated with increased total homocysteine and methylmalonic acid concentrations. *Proceedings of the National Academy of Sciences of the United States of America, 50,* 19995–20000.

Shane, B. (2009). Folate chemistry and metabolism. In L. Bailey (Ed.), *Folate in health and disease* (2nd ed., pp. 1–24). Boca Raton, FL: CRC Press.

Shaw, G. M., Carmichael, S. L., Laurent, C., & Rasmussen, S. A. (2006). Maternal nutrient intakes and risk of orofacial clefts. *Epidemiology, 17,* 285–291.

Shaw, G. M., Carmichael, S. L., Yang, W., Selvin, S., & Schaffer, D. M. (2004). Periconceptional dietary intake of choline and betaine and neural tube defects in offspring. *American Journal of Epidemiology, 160,* 102–109.

Shaw, G. M., Finnell, R. H., Blom, H. J., Carmichael, S. L., Vollset, S. E., Yang, W., & Ueland, P. M. (2009). Choline and risk of neural tube defects in a folate-fortified population. *Epidemiology, 20,* 714–719.

Shelnutt, K. P., Kauwell, G. P., Chapman, C. M., Gregory, J. F., 3rd, Maneval, D. R., Browdy, A. A., … Bailey, L. B.(2003). Folate status response to controlled folate intake is affected by the methylenetetrahydrofolate reductase 677C→T polymorphism in young women. *The Journal of Nutrition, 133,* 4107–4111.

Shields, D. J., Agellon, L. B., & Vance, D. E. (2001). Structure, expression profile and alternative processing of the human phosphatidylethanolamine N-methyltransferase (PEMT) gene. *Biochimica et Biophysica Acta, 1532,* 105–114.

Shields, D. J., Lehner, R., Agellon, L. B., & Vance, D. E. (2003). Membrane topography of human phosphatidylethanolamine N-methyltransferase. *The Journal of Biological Chemistry, 278,* 2956–2962.

Shin, W., Yan, J., Abratte, C. M., Vermeylen, F., & Caudill, M. A. (2010). Choline intake exceeding current dietary recommendations preserves markers of cellular methylation in a genetic subgroup of folate-compromised men. *The Journal of Nutrition, 140,* 975–980.

Slow, S., & Garrow, T. A. (2006). Liver choline dehydrogenase and kidney betaine-homocysteine methyltransferase expression are not affected by methionine or choline intake in growing rats. *The Journal of Nutrition, 136,* 2279–2283.

Solis, C., Veenema, K., Ivanov, A. A., Tran, S., Li, R., Wang, W., … Caudill, M. A. (2008). Folate intake at RDA levels is inadequate for Mexican American men with the methylenetetrahydrofolate reductase 677TT genotype. *The Journal of Nutrition, 138,* 67–72.

Song, Z., Deaciuc, I., Zhou, Z., Song, M., Chen, T., Hill, D., & McClain, C. J. (2007). Involvement of AMP-activated protein kinase in beneficial effects of betaine on high-sucrose diet-induced hepatic steatosis. *American Journal of Physiology. Gastrointestinal and Liver Physiology, 293,* G894–G902.

Stover, P. (2009). Folate biochemical pathways and their regulation. In L. Bailey (Ed.), *Folate in health and disease* (2nd ed., pp. 49–74). Boca Raton, FL: CRC Press.

Sugimoto, H., Banchio, C., & Vance, D. E. (2008). Transcriptional regulation of phosphatidylcholine biosynthesis. *Progress in Lipid Research, 47,* 204–220.

Sweeney, M. R., McPartlin, J., & Scott, J. (2007). Folic acid fortification and public health: Report on threshold doses above which unmetabolised folic acid appear in serum. *BMC Public Health, 7,* 41.

Tamura, T., Picciano, M. F., & McGuire, M. K. (2009). Folate in pregnancy and lactation. In L. Bailey (Ed.), *Folate in health and disease* (2nd ed., pp. 111–131). Boca Raton, FL: CRC Press.

Tian, Y., Pate, C., Andreolotti, A., Wang, L., Tuomanen, E., Boyd, K., … Jackowski, S. (2008). Cytokine secretion requires phosphatidylcholine synthesis. *The Journal of Cell Biology, 181*, 945–957.

Tibbetts, A. S., & Appling, D. R. (2010). Compartmentalization of mammalian folate-mediated one-carbon metabolism. *Annual Review of Nutrition, 30*, 57–81.

Titus, S. A., & Moran, R. G. (2000). Retrovirally mediated complementation of the glyB phenotype. Cloning of a human gene encoding the carrier for entry of folates into mitochondria. *The Journal of Biological Chemistry, 275*, 36811–36817.

U.S. Department of Agriculture, Agricultural Research Service. (2010). *What we eat in America. NHANES 2007–2008*. Washington, DC: Author.

Veenema, K., Solis, C., Li, R., Wang, W., Maletz, C. V., Abratte, C. M., & Caudill, M. A. (2008). Adequate intake levels of choline are sufficient for preventing elevations in serum markers of liver dysfunction in Mexican American men but are not optimal for minimizing plasma total homocysteine increases after a methionine load. *The American Journal of Clinical Nutrition, 88*, 685–692.

Verhoef, P., Stampfer, M. J., Buring, J. E., Gaziano, J. M., Allen, R. H., Stabler, S. P., … Willett, W. C. (1996). Homocysteine metabolism and risk of myocardial infarction: Relation with vitamins B_6, B_{12}, and folate. *American Journal of Epidemiology, 143*, 845–859.

Walkey, C. J., Kalmar, G. B., & Cornell, R. B. (1994). Overexpression of rat liver CTP:phosphocholine cytidylyltransferase accelerates phosphatidylcholine synthesis and degradation. *The Journal of Biological Chemistry, 269*, 5742–5749.

Wallis, D., Ballard, J. L., Shaw, G. M., Lammer, E. J., & Finnell, R. H. (2009). Folate-related birth defects: Embryonic consequences of abnormal folate transport and metabolism. In L. Bailey (Ed.), *Folate in health and disease* (2nd ed., pp. 155–178). Boca Raton, FL: CRC Press.

Wang, L., Magdaleno, S., Tabas, I., & Jackowski, S. (2005). Early embryonic lethality in mice with targeted deletion of the CTP:phosphocholine cytidylyltransferase alpha gene (Pcyt1a). *Molecular and Cellular Biology, 25*, 3357–3363.

Wehby, G. L., & Murray, J. C. (2010). Folic acid and orofacial clefts: A review of the evidence. *Oral Diseases, 16*, 11–19.

West, A. A., & Caudill, M. A. (2010). Genetic variation: Impact on folate (and choline) bioefficacy. *International Journal for Vitamin and Nutrition Research, 80*, 319–329.

Whitrow, M. J., Moore, V. M., Rumbold, A. R., & Davies, M. J. (2009). Effect of supplemental folic acid in pregnancy on childhood asthma: A prospective birth cohort study. *American Journal of Epidemiology, 170*, 1486–1493.

Williams, C. D., Stengel, J., Asike, M. I., Torres, D. M., Shaw, J., Contreras, M., … Harrison, S. A. (2011). Prevalence of nonalcoholic fatty liver disease and nonalcoholic steatohepatitis among a largely middle-aged population utilizing ultrasound and liver biopsy: A prospective study. *Gastroenterology, 140*, 124–131.

Woeller, C. F., Anderson, D. D., Szebenyi, D. M., & Stover, P. J. (2007). Evidence for small ubiquitin-like modifier-dependent nuclear import of the thymidylate biosynthesis pathway. *The Journal of Biological Chemistry, 282*, 17623–17631.

Xu, X., Gammon, M. D., Zeisel, S. H., Bradshaw, P. T., Wetmur, J. G., Teitelbaum, S. L., … Chen, J. (2009). High intakes of choline and betaine reduce breast cancer mortality in a population-based study. *The FASEB Journal, 23*, 4022–4028.

Yamada, K., Chen, Z., Rozen, R., & Matthews, R. G. (2001). Effects of common polymorphisms on the properties of recombinant human methylenetetrahydrofolate reductase. *Proceedings of the National Academy of Sciences of the United States of America, 98*, 14853–14858.

Yang, Q., Cogswell, M. E., Hamner, H. C., Carriquiry, A., Bailey, L. B., Pfeiffer, C. M., & Berry, R. J. (2010). Folic acid source, usual intake, and folate and vitamin B-12 status in US adults: National Health and Nutrition Examination Survey (NHANES) 2003–2006. *The American Journal of Clinical Nutrition, 91*, 64–72.

Yang, Q. H., Botto, L. D., Gallagher, M., Friedman, J. M., Sanders, C. L., Koontz, D., … Steinberg, K. (2008). Prevalence and effects of gene-gene and gene-nutrient interactions on serum folate and serum total homocysteine concentrations in the United States: Findings from the third National Health and Nutrition Examination Survey DNA Bank. *The American Journal of Clinical Nutrition, 88*, 232–246.

Zeisel, S. H. (2004). Nutritional importance of choline for brain development. *Journal of the American College of Nutrition, 23*, 621S–626S.

Zeisel, S. H. (2011). Nutritional genomics: Defining the dietary requirement and effects of choline. *The Journal of Nutrition, 140*, 1S–4S.

Zeisel, S. H., & Blusztajn, J. K. (1994). Choline and human nutrition. *Annual Review of Nutrition, 14*, 269–296.

Zeisel, S. H., Da Costa, K. A., Franklin, P. D., Alexander, E. A., Lamont, J. T., Sheard, N. F., & Beiser, A. (1991). Choline, an essential nutrient for humans. *The FASEB Journal, 5*, 2093–2098.

Zeisel, S. H., Growdon, J. H., Wurtman, R. J., Magil, S. G., & Logue, M. (1980). Normal plasma choline responses to ingested lecithin. *Neurology, 30*, 1226–1229.

Zeisel, S. H., Mar, M. H., Howe, J. C., & Holden, J. M. (2003). Concentrations of choline-containing compounds and betaine in common foods. *The Journal of Nutrition, 133*, 1302–1307.

Zeisel, S. H., Wishnok, J. S., & Blusztajn, J. K. (1983). Formation of methylamines from ingested choline and lecithin. *The Journal of Pharmacology and Experimental Therapeutics, 225*, 320–324.

Zeisel, S. H., Mar, M.-H., Zhou, Z.-W., & da Costa, K.-A. (1995). Pregnancy and lactation are associated with diminished concentrations of choline and its metabolites in rat liver. *The Journal of Nutrition, 125*, 3049–3054.

Zhao, R., Matherly, L. H., & Goldman, I. D. (2009a). Membrane transporters and folate homeostasis: Intestinal absorption and transport into systemic compartments and tissues. *Expert Reviews in Molecular Medicine, 11*, e4.

Zhao, R., Min, S. H., Wang, Y., Campanella, E., Low, P. S., & Goldman, I. D. (2009b). A role for the proton-coupled folate transporter (PCFT-SLC46A1) in folate receptor-mediated endocytosis. *The Journal of Biological Chemistry, 284*, 4267–4274.

RECOMMENDED READINGS

Bailey, L. B. (Ed.). (2009). *Folate in health and disease* (2nd ed.). Boca Raton, FL: CRC Press.

Caudill, M. A. (2010). Pre- and postnatal health: Evidence of increased choline needs. *Journal of the American Dietetic Association, 110*, 1198–1206.

Chanarin, I. (1979). *The megaloblastic anemias* (2nd ed.). Oxford: Blackwell Scientific Publications.

Folates and pterins. (1986). In R. L. Blakley & V. M. Whitehead (Eds.), *Nutritional, pharmacological, and physiological aspects* (Vol. 3). New York: Wiley.

Green, R., & Miller, J. W. (2007). Vitamin B_{12}. In J. Zempleni & R. B. Rucker (Eds.), *Handbook of vitamins* (4th ed., pp. 413–457). Boca Raton, FL: CRC Press.

Li, A., & Vance, D. E. (2008). Phosphatidylcholine and choline homeostasis. *Journal of Lipid Research, 49*, 1187–1194.

Scriver, C. R., Sly, S. S., Childs, B., Beaudet, A. L., Valle, D., Kinzler, K. W., & Vogelstein, B. (Eds.). (2001). *The metabolic and molecular bases of inherited disease* (8th ed.). New York: McGraw-Hill.

Zeisel, S. H. (2011). Nutritional genomics: Defining the dietary requirement and effects of choline. *The Journal of Nutrition, 141*, 531–534.

Zeisel, S. H., & da Costa, K. A. (2009). Choline: An essential nutrient for public health. *Nutrition Reviews, 67*, 615–623.

Zempleni, J., Rucker, R. B., Suttie, J., & McCormick, D. B. (Eds.), (2007). *Handbook of vitamins* (4th ed.). New York: CRC Press.

CHAPTER 26

Biotin and Pantothenic Acid

*Donald M. Mock, MD, PhD, and Nell I. Matthews, BA**

COMMON ABBREVIATIONS

ACC	acetyl-CoA carboxylase
ACP	acyl carrier protein
CoA	coenzyme A
CPT	carnitine palmitoyltransferase
HCS	holocarboxylase synthetase
MCC	methylcrotonyl-CoA carboxylase
PC	pyruvate carboxylase
PCC	propionyl-CoA carboxylase

This chapter discusses the molecular, biochemical, and physiological roles of two micronutrients that are essential to human nutrition: the water-soluble vitamins biotin (vitamin B_7) and pantothenic acid (vitamin B_5). Biotin serves as an essential cofactor for five enzymes that transfer carbon dioxide (use free bicarbonate) to substrates that are crucial to intermediary metabolism. Pantothenic acid is metabolized to two major enzyme cofactors: coenzyme A (CoA) and the acyl carrier protein (ACP) domain of fatty acid synthase. About 4% of all cellular enzymes use CoA thioesters, or CoA derivatives such as acetyl-CoA, as substrates.

BIOTIN

Biotin is a water-soluble vitamin and is generally classified in the vitamin B complex group. Biotin was discovered by accident in nutritional experiments investigating the protein requirements of rats. Boas (1927) observed that rats fed dried egg white developed scaly dermatitis, hair loss, and neurological signs and pursued this observation by demonstrating that a water-soluble factor in many foodstuffs is capable of curing these signs of deficiency. Egg white contains avidin, a glycoprotein that binds biotin very specifically and tightly. From an evolutionary standpoint, avidin probably serves as a bacteriostat in egg white. Consistent with this possibility is the observation that avidin is resistant to a broad range of bacterial proteases in both the free and the biotin-bound form. Because avidin is also resistant to pancreatic proteases, dietary avidin binds to dietary biotin (and probably any biotin from intestinal microbes) and prevents its absorption. Cooking denatures avidin, rendering this protein susceptible to digestion and unable to interfere with the absorption of biotin.

BIOTIN SYNTHESIS

Mammals (including humans) cannot synthesize biotin. Rather, mammals depend on dietary biotin synthesized by microbes and plants. Although biotin is synthesized by many microbes in the human intestine, the contribution of microbial biotin to absorbed biotin, if any, remains unknown.

Biotin contains two five-member rings made from a ureido group attached to a tetrahydrothiophene ring (Figure 26-1). A valeric acid side chain is attached to the tetrahydrothiophene ring. The pathway for biosynthesis of biotin was largely elaborated by M.A. Eisenberg and associates working with *Escherichia coli* (Eisenberg, 1973).

HOLOCARBOXYLASES AND HOLOCARBOXYLASE SYNTHETASE

In mammals, biotin serves as an essential cofactor for five enzymes that catalyze critical steps in intermediary metabolism. All are carboxylases that facilitate the incorporation of a carboxyl group into a substrate, and all employ a similar catalytic mechanism.

Biotin is attached to the inactive apocarboxylase protein by a condensation reaction catalyzed by holocarboxylase synthetase (HCS) (see Figure 26-1). An amide bond is formed between the carboxyl group of the valeric acid side chain of biotin and the ε-amino group of a specific lysine residue in each of the apocarboxylases. These regions of each apocarboxylase contain sequences of amino acids (e.g., Met-Lys-Met at the attachment site) that are highly conserved for the individual carboxylases, and both the N- and C-terminus in HCS are important for recognition of the apocarboxylases (Hassan et al., 2009).

*This chapter is a revision of the chapter contributed by Lawrence Sweetman, PhD, for the second edition.

BIOTIN-CONTAINING CARBOXYLASES

CARBOXYLASE MECHANISM

In the carboxylase reaction, the carboxyl moiety is first attached to the biotin cofactor (of the holocarboxylase enzyme) at the ureido nitrogen opposite the side chain (Figure 26-2). Dehydration of HCO_3^- (bicarbonate) to CO_2, forming carboxyphosphate, is driven by the hydrolysis of ATP to ADP (see Figure 26-2). The carboxyphosphate then carboxylates a specific nitrogen (N1) in the ureido containing ring of biotin to form N1 carboxybiotinyl-enzyme, and inorganic phosphate is released. These two steps allow HCO_3^-, which is present at a higher concentration in the cell fluid than is CO_2, to be used for formation of the bound, chemically reactive form of CO_2. The carboxyl group can then be transferred to a substrate yielding a carboxylated product. Because the valeric acid side chain of biotin is coupled to the side chain of lysine in each holocarboxylase, this CO_2 is at the end of a long, flexible chain, allowing the biotinyl coenzyme to be carboxylated at one site and used as a CO_2 donor at a second site.

Whether expression of the mammalian biotin-dependent carboxylases is influenced by biotin status remains to be elucidated. However, the interaction of biotin synthesis and production of holo-(acetyl-CoA carboxylase) in *E. coli* has been extensively studied. In the bacterial system, which synthesizes both biotin and apocarboxylase, the availability of the apocarboxylase protein and of biotin (as the intermediate biotinyl-AMP) act together to control the rate of biotin synthesis by direct interaction with promoter regions of the biotin operon, which in turn controls a cluster of genes that encode enzymes that catalyze the synthesis of biotin.

The five biotin-dependent mammalian carboxylases are acetyl-CoA carboxylase isoforms 1 and 2 (formerly known as ACCα and ACCβ), pyruvate carboxylase, methylcrotonyl-CoA carboxylase, and propionyl-CoA carboxylase. An overview of the roles of these biotin-dependent carboxylases in the cell is given in Figure 26-3.

ACETYL-CoA CARBOXYLASE

Acetyl-CoA carboxylase (ACC) catalyzes the incorporation of bicarbonate into acetyl-CoA to form malonyl-CoA (Figure 26-4) and exists in two isoforms. Isoform 1 of ACC (ACC1) is encoded by the *ACACA* gene and is located in the cytosol. The malonyl-CoA produced by ACC1 is rate-limiting in fatty acid synthesis (elongation). Isoform 2 of ACC (ACC2) is encoded by the *ACACB* gene and is located on the outer mitochondrial membrane. ACC2 controls fatty acid oxidation in mitochondria through the inhibition of carnitine palmitoyltransferase I by its product malonyl-CoA. Carnitine palmitoyltransferase I catalyzes the rate-limiting step in fatty acid uptake into mitochondria and thus regulates the availability of fatty acids for oxidation.

Thus ACC1 and ACC2 are thought to have different, but complementary, roles in cellular metabolism; ACC1 regulates fatty acid synthesis, and activation of ACC2 inhibits fatty acid oxidation. An inactive mitochondrial form of ACC may also serve as storage for biotin.

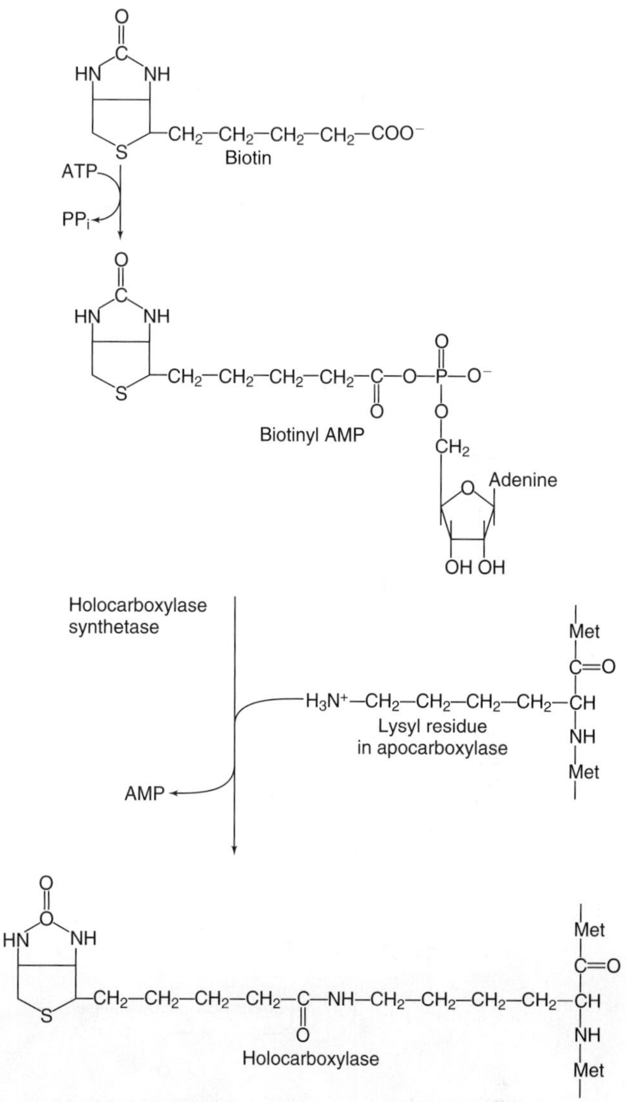

FIGURE 26-1 Holocarboxylase synthetase reaction. Each active holocarboxylase is formed in a reaction catalyzed in two sequential steps by holocarboxylase synthetase: (1) formation of biotinyl-AMP from biotin and ATP, and (2) formation of an amide bond between the carboxyl group of biotin and the ε-amino group on a specific lysine residue in each apocarboxylase, with the release of AMP.

Given that acetyl-CoA is the central compound of intermediary metabolism, it is not surprising that the regulation of ACC1 and ACC2 is complex. The active form of cytosolic ACC1 exists as a very large polymer with a molecular mass in the millions of daltons and is inactivated by dissociation into its protomer units. Citrate activates ACC1 by increasing polymerization. CoA itself activates ACC1 by lowering the K_m for acetyl-CoA. ACC1 is inhibited by the products of fatty acid synthesis, the long-chain acyl-CoAs, which also act to depolymerize the enzyme. In addition, ACC1 activity is regulated by covalent modification (phosphorylation) in response to the hormones insulin and glucagon. A high insulin-to-glucagon ratio typical of the immediate postprandial state (fed state with increased blood glucose level) favors dephosphorylation of ACC1 to an active form, whereas a low insulin-to-glucagon ratio (typical of a fasting state) favors

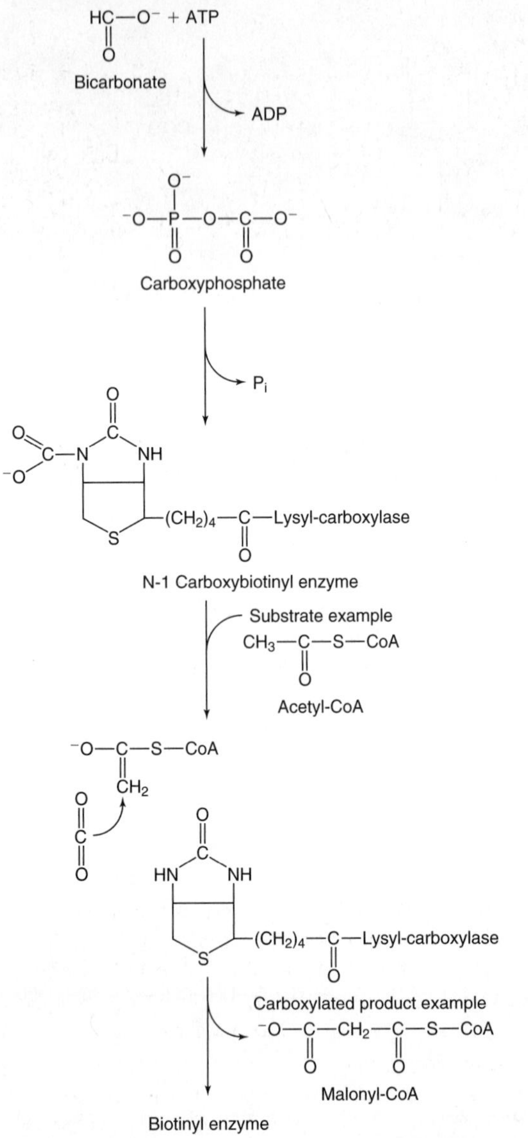

FIGURE 26-2 Mechanism of carboxylation by biotinyl enzymes. With energy provided by the hydrolysis of ATP, bicarbonate is attached to biotin to form N1 carboxybiotin. The carboxyl group is then transferred to the substrate to form the carboxylated product. The carboxylation of acetyl-CoA to malonyl-CoA is shown as an example.

phosphorylation to the inactive form. The amount of ACC1 protein also responds to changes in dietary and hormonal conditions. Regulation of ACC2 has not been as extensively studied but appears to operate through inactivation of ACC2 by phosphorylation catalyzed by AMP-activated protein kinase (Cho et al., 2009).

PYRUVATE CARBOXYLASE

The three remaining carboxylases are mitochondrial. Pyruvate carboxylase (PC) is encoded by the *PC* gene and catalyzes the incorporation of bicarbonate into pyruvate to form oxaloacetate, a central intermediate in carbohydrate, lipid, and amino acid metabolism (see Figure 26-4). The formation of oxaloacetate by PC serves an anaplerotic reaction, replenishing intermediates in the citric acid cycle. This supports synthesis of other intermediates such as α-ketoglutarate, a precursor of glutamate, and citrate, a precursor of cytosolic acetyl-CoA for fatty acid and cholesterol synthesis. Lack of sufficient oxaloacetate for citrate formation limits acetyl-CoA oxidation by the citric acid cycle, thus promoting formation of ketone bodies from acetyl-CoA in the liver. Oxaloacetate is also necessary for aspartate formation and the shuttling of amino acid nitrogen into the urea cycle. The PC reaction also plays a critical role in gluconeogenesis, allowing pyruvate to be converted back to phosphoenolpyruvate via intermediate formation of oxaloacetate. Deficiency of PC is probably the cause of lactic acidemia, central nervous system lactic acidosis, and abnormalities in glucose regulation which are commonly observed in biotin deficiency, genetic biotinidase deficiency, and holocarboxylase synthetase deficiency. Biotinidase is a biotin-amide hydrolase that hydrolyzes biocytin to biotin and lysine, playing a critical role in biotin recycling (see later). PC also plays a role in the formation of the protective myelin sheath that surrounds the axons of certain nerve cells and in the production of neurotransmitters, both of which may contribute to the phenotype of inherited PC deficiency.

In the "A" form of inherited PC deficiency, symptoms of affected infants in their first few months of life are mild or moderate lactic acidemia and psychomotor retardation. Lactic acidemia can lead to vomiting, abdominal pain, fatigue, muscle weakness, and difficulty breathing. Most children die within the first few years, and survivors have severe mental retardation.

In the more severe "B" form of PC deficiency, the initial presentation usually occurs shortly after birth with hypotonia, seizures, coma, severe lactic acidemia, and signs of liver failure such as elevated blood ammonia concentrations. Death usually occurs before 3 months of age.

PROPIONYL-CoA CARBOXYLASE

Propionyl-CoA carboxylase (PCC) catalyzes the incorporation of bicarbonate into propionyl-CoA to form methylmalonyl CoA (see Figure 26-4). Methylmalonyl-CoA then undergoes isomerization to succinyl-CoA, which enters the citric acid cycle; this isomerization is catalyzed by the vitamin B_{12}–dependent enzyme methylmalonyl-CoA mutase.

Sources of propionyl CoA include the propionyl-CoA formed from catabolism of the amino acids valine, isoleucine, threonine, and methionine; the propionyl-CoA formed in the final step in the β-oxidation of odd-numbered or branched-chain fatty acids; the propionyl-CoA released as a by-product of bile acid synthesis from cholesterol (i.e., shortening of the cholesterol side chain by 3 carbons); and a significant amount of propionate produced by the intestinal microflora. PCC is not rate limiting in the metabolism of propionyl-CoA, and the enzyme activity is not sensitively regulated by allosteric effectors or by dietary or hormonal changes. PCC is composed of two nonidentical subunits: a biotinylated α subunit encoded by the gene *PCCA* and a nonbiotinylated β subunit encoded by the gene *PCCB*.

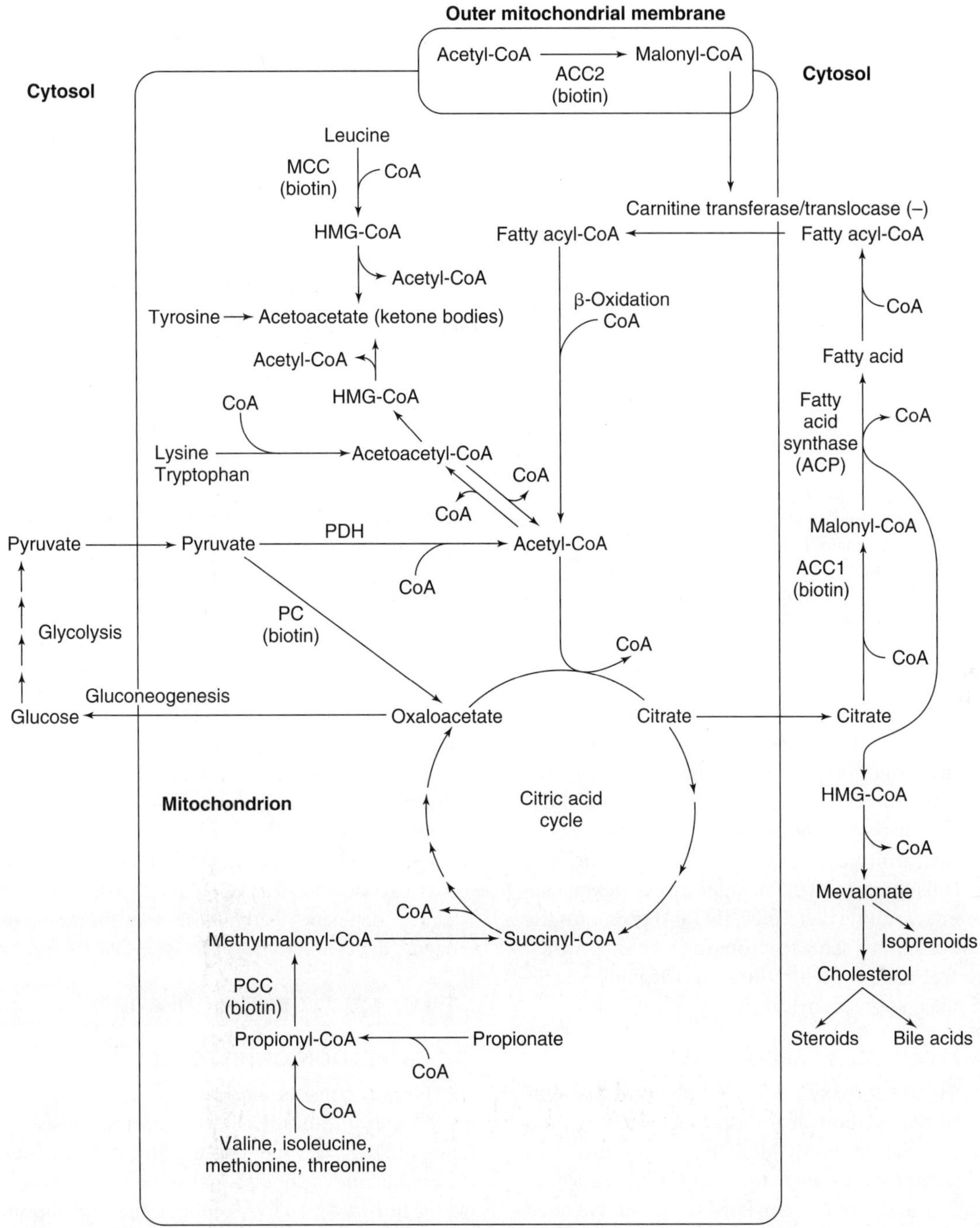

FIGURE 26-3 Roles of the five biotin-dependent carboxylases, of coenzyme A (CoA), and of acyl carrier protein (ACP) within the cell. Shown is an overview of the metabolic pathways of ACC1 (cytosolic) and ACC2 (outer mitochondrial membrane), and the three mitochondrial carboxylases, PCC, MCC, and PC. *ACC1* and *ACC2*, acetyl-CoA carboxylase 1 and 2; *HMG-CoA*, 3-hydroxy-3-methylglutaryl-CoA; *MCC*, methylcrotonyl-CoA carboxylase; *PC*, pyruvate carboxylase; *PCC*, propionyl-CoA carboxylase; *PDH*, pyruvate dehydrogenase.

Propionic acidemia is the disease caused by an inherited deficiency of PCC. Affected individuals have repeated, life-threatening episodes of severe ketosis and metabolic acidosis that often begin in infancy. Findings include vomiting, dehydration, and lethargy, which can progress to coma and death if not treated. Frequent neurological complications include developmental delay, seizures, and cerebral atrophy. The concentration of propionyl-CoA increases due to the metabolic block in propionate metabolism caused by decreased PCC activity, and a lack of PCC results in increased urinary excretion of a constellation of propionate metabolites that are diagnostic of propionic acidemia. These include 3-hydroxypropionate, propionylglycine, propionylcarnitine, and methylcitrate.

The most important treatment for propionic acidemia is restriction of dietary protein, thereby limiting the amino acid precursors of propionate. Use of special formulas that

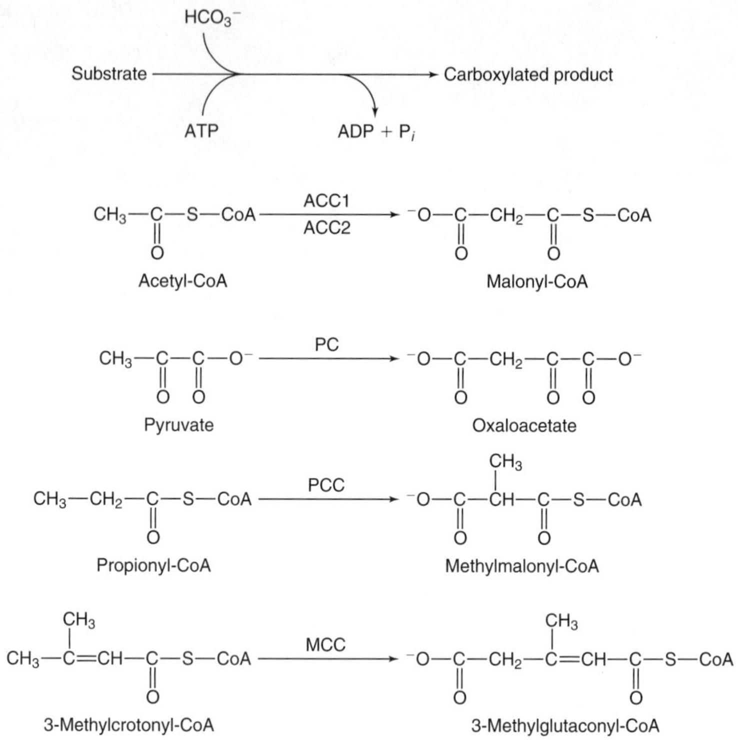

$$\text{Substrate} + HCO_3^- + \text{ATP} \longrightarrow \text{Carboxylated product} + \text{ADP} + P_i$$

$$\underset{\text{Acetyl-CoA}}{CH_3{-}C({=}O){-}S{-}CoA} \xrightarrow[\text{ACC2}]{\text{ACC1}} \underset{\text{Malonyl-CoA}}{{}^{-}O{-}C({=}O){-}CH_2{-}C({=}O){-}S{-}CoA}$$

$$\underset{\text{Pyruvate}}{CH_3{-}C({=}O){-}C({=}O){-}O^-} \xrightarrow{\text{PC}} \underset{\text{Oxaloacetate}}{{}^{-}O{-}C({=}O){-}CH_2{-}C({=}O){-}C({=}O){-}O^-}$$

$$\underset{\text{Propionyl-CoA}}{CH_3{-}CH_2{-}C({=}O){-}S{-}CoA} \xrightarrow{\text{PCC}} \underset{\text{Methylmalonyl-CoA}}{{}^{-}O{-}C({=}O){-}CH(CH_3){-}C({=}O){-}S{-}CoA}$$

$$\underset{\text{3-Methylcrotonyl-CoA}}{CH_3{-}C(CH_3){=}CH{-}C({=}O){-}S{-}CoA} \xrightarrow{\text{MCC}} \underset{\text{3-Methylglutaconyl-CoA}}{{}^{-}O{-}C({=}O){-}CH_2{-}C(CH_3){=}CH{-}C({=}O){-}S{-}CoA}$$

FIGURE 26-4 Carboxylase reactions. The substrates and products of the five mammalian biotin-containing carboxylases are shown. Bicarbonate is incorporated as a carboxyl moiety in the products, and the reaction is driven by energy released from the hydrolysis of ATP. *ACC1*, acetyl CoA carboxylase 1; *ACC2*, acetyl-CoA carboxylase 2; *MCC*, methylcrotonyl-CoA carboxylase; *PC*, pyruvate carboxylase; *PCC*, propionyl-CoA carboxylase.

have very low levels of isoleucine, valine, methionine, and threonine has the same goal. The minimum requirement for these essential amino acids is met by the addition of other proteins after calculation of the content of each amino acid. Loss of propionylcarnitine can lead to a secondary deficiency of carnitine. Thus therapy often includes supplemental carnitine to prevent carnitine deficiency; this also promotes the conversion of propionyl-CoA to propionylcarnitine, which helps restore free CoA concentrations and facilitates excretion of propionate as propionylcarnitine.

METHYLCROTONYL-CoA CARBOXYLASE

Methylcrotonyl-CoA carboxylase (MCC) catalyzes an essential step in the degradation of the branched-chain amino acid leucine (see Figure 26-4). MCC is composed of two nonidentical subunits: a biotinylated α subunit encoded by the gene *MCCC1* and a nonbiotinylated β subunit encoded by the gene *MCCC2*. MCC is not regulated by small molecules or by dietary or hormonal factors. Deficient activity of MCC leads to metabolism of 3-methylcrotonyl-CoA to 3-hydroxyisovaleric acid, 3-hydroxyisovalerylcarnitine, and 3-methylcrotonylglycine by an alternate pathway (Stratton et al., 2010). Thus increased urinary excretion of these abnormal metabolites reflects deficient activity of MCC.

The inherited deficiency of MCC characteristically presents with recurrent episodes of vomiting, diarrhea, lethargy, hypotonia, severe metabolic acidosis, hypoglycemia, and carnitine depletion. Moderate restriction of dietary protein to limit leucine intake and carnitine supplementation to correct or prevent carnitine deficiency generally result in normal development. Some cases respond to biotin supplementation. Newborn screening of acylcarnitines has identified a much higher incidence of asymptomatic MCC deficiency than expected from the number of patients ascertained by clinical symptoms; this observation suggests that many patients may have a benign clinical course. Of note, newborn screening has detected babies with elevated blood 3-hydroxyisovalerylcarnitine levels who do not have the enzyme deficiency but whose asymptomatic mothers are enzyme deficient.

BIOTIN AND GENE REGULATION

BIOTINYLATION OF HISTONES

Chromatin consists of repetitive nucleoprotein complexes called nucleosomes. Each nucleosome consists of 146 base pairs of DNA, wrapped around an octamer of core histones. These histones play essential roles not only in DNA packaging but also in DNA repair, gene replication, and gene regulation.

The core histones are designated H2A, H2B, H3, and H4; each nucleosome contains one H3/H3/H4/H4 tetramer and two H2A/H2B dimers. Mammals also express a fifth class of histones: histone H1, which serves as a linker between nucleosomes. Each core histone has a globular domain and a flexible *N*-terminal tail. The *N*-terminal tails of core histones protrude from the nucleosomal surface, and covalent modifications of these tails play critical roles in gene regulation (Camporeale et al., 2004; Chew et al., 2006; Kobza et al., 2008).

In 1995 Hymes and Wolf discovered that biotinidase can act as a biotinyl-transferase; biocytin serves as the source of biotin, and histones are specifically biotinylated (Hymes et al., 1995). Zempleni and co-workers reported that the abundance of biotinylated histones varies with the cell cycle and that biotinylated histones are increased approximately twofold in activated, dividing lymphocytes compared to quiescent lymphocytes (Stanley et al., 2002). These observations suggested that biotinylation of histones might play a role in regulating DNA transcription as an additional element in the "histone code." Based on this initial work, it was believed that biotinylation of histones was catalyzed by biotinidase (Hymes et al., 1995). Indeed, approximately 25% of total cellular biotinidase activity is located in the nucleus, and histones are biotinylated enzymatically in a process that is catalyzed in vitro by biotinidase.

However, subsequent studies provided evidence that HCS is substantially more important than biotinidase for biotinylation of histones in vivo (Chew et al., 2008; Gralla et al., 2008; Kobza et al., 2008). Fibroblasts from patients with inherited deficiency of HCS exhibit decreased biotinylation of histones. In contrast, biotin can be removed from histones by biotinidase, and debiotinylation of histones is decreased in samples from biotinidase-deficient patients. Current understanding is that HCS plays the predominant role in histone biotinylation and biotinidase plays the predominant role in histone debiotinylation.

Biotinylation of distinct lysine residues as a covalent modification of histones that affects DNA transcription has several supporting lines of investigation. Currently, about a dozen biotinylation sites have been identified in histones H2A, H3, and H4. HCS is present in both nuclear and cytoplasmic compartments; in the nucleus, HCS is associated with chromatin. Nevertheless, controversy exists as to whether biotin attachment to histones occurs in vivo (Healy et al., 2009).

Although the mechanisms remain to be elucidated, biotin status clearly affects gene expression. Cell culture studies suggest that cell proliferation generates an increased demand for biotin, perhaps stemming from increased synthesis of biotin-dependent carboxylases. Evidence is emerging that this demand is met by an upregulation of biotin transporter expression that is mediated by biotinylation of lysine 12 in histone H4 (H4K12bio) (Gralla et al., 2008). Another function of H4K12bio appears to be chromosomal stability (Camporeale et al., 2007; Chew et al., 2008; Gralla et al., 2008; Wijeratne et al., 2010). Low levels of histone biotinylation have been reported in biotin-deficient cells and model organisms (Chew et al., 2008); reduced histone biotinylation has been linked to increased frequency of retrotransposition events, consistent with a role for histone biotinylation in chromosomal stability.

Other roles for biotin in affecting gene expression have been observed. Pioneering studies by Dakshinamurti and co-workers reported a role for biotin in the regulation of the glucokinase gene (Dakshinamurti and Cheah-Tan, 1968). Solorzano-Vargas and colleagues (2002) reported that biotin deficiency reduces messenger RNA (mRNA) levels of HCS, ACC1, and PCC and postulated that a cyclic GMP–dependent signaling pathway is involved in the pathogenesis. Zempleni and co-workers have demonstrated involvement of nitric oxide in the cyclic GMP signaling pathway (Rodriguez-Melendez and Zempleni, 2009; Zempleni et al., 2009).

BIOTIN DIGESTION AND ABSORPTION

The content of free biotin and protein-bound biotin in foods is variable, but the majority of biotin in meats and cereals appears to be protein-bound via an amide bond between biotin and lysine. Upon digestion, the lysine and small lysine-containing peptides with covalently attached biotin are released. The released lysine with biotin covalently attached is called biocytin. Because the amide bond between biotin and lysine is not hydrolyzed by most pancreatic or cellular proteases, release is likely mediated by biotinidase. Biotinidase mRNA is present in the pancreas and, in lesser amounts, in intestinal mucosa.

At physiological pH, the carboxyl group of biotin is negatively charged. Thus biotin is at least modestly water-soluble and requires a transporter to cross cell membranes such as enterocytes for absorption (reviewed by Said, 2008). In intact intestinal preparations such as loops and everted gut sacks, biotin transport exhibits two components. One component is saturable at a K_m of approximately 10 μM biotin. The other is not saturable, even at very large concentrations of biotin, which is consistent with passive diffusion. Absorption of biocytin is inefficient relative to biotin, suggesting that biotinidase plays a critical role in generating free biotin from biocytin (and dietary protein) and making biotin available for absorption.

Human intestinal epithelial cells are highly specialized. Biotin transport must occur across two structurally and functionally different membrane domains: the brush border membrane that faces the intestinal lumen and the basolateral membrane that faces the interstitium, which is in contact with the blood that perfuses the intestine (Said, 2008).

In the brush border membrane, transport occurs via a Na^+-dependent, electroneutral, carrier-mediated mechanism that saturates at the micromolar range, accounting for the overall limitation in nondiffusion transport (Said, 2008). In the presence of a Na^+ gradient, biotin transport occurs against a concentration gradient. This biotin transporter can also transport pantothenic acid and lipoic acid and hence has been named SMVT (sodium-dependent multivitamin transporter). Human SMVT is the product of the *SLC5A6* gene, and is exclusively targeted to the apical (brush border) membrane.

Biotin transport across the basolateral membrane also occurs by a carrier-mediated mechanism. However, this carrier is Na^+-independent, electrogenic, and cannot accumulate biotin against a concentration gradient (Said, 2008).

Intestinal biotin transport is upregulated in response to biotin deficiency in both humans and animal models. The mechanism likely involves induction of SMVT mRNA synthesis and an increased number of SMVT transporters per cell. The increase in SMVT is likely mediated by an induction in the activity of P1, which is one of two promoter regions upstream from the *SMVT* gene (Said, 2008).

Although carrier-mediated transport of biotin is most active in the proximal small bowel of the rat, the absorption of biotin from the proximal colon is still significant, supporting the potential nutritional significance of biotin synthesized and released by enteric flora. However, the quantitative importance of the contribution of enteric biotin synthesis to absorbed biotin remains to be determined.

Based on a study in which biotin was administered orally in pharmacological amounts, bioavailability of free biotin is approximately 100%. Thus the pharmacological doses of biotin given to treat biotin-dependent inborn errors of metabolism are likely to be well absorbed. Moreover, the finding of high bioavailability of biotin at pharmacological doses provides at least some basis for predicting that bioavailability will also be high at the physiological doses at which the biotin transporter mediates uptake. Little is known about the bioavailability of protein-bound biotin.

BIOTIN UPTAKE AND TRANSPORT IN TISSUES

Biotin concentrations in plasma are low relative to other water-soluble vitamins. Most biotin in plasma is free and dissolved in the aqueous phase of plasma. However, approximately 7% is reversibly bound to plasma protein, and approximately 12% is covalently bound to plasma protein. Binding to plasma albumin likely accounts for the reversible binding. Biotinidase has been proposed as a biotin-binding protein or biotin-carrier protein for the transport of biotin into cells. A biotin-binding plasma glycoprotein has been observed in pregnant rats.

BIOTIN UPTAKE BY LIVER

SMVT is widely expressed in human tissues. Studies by Said and co-workers (Said, 2008) using RNA interference specific for SMVT provide strong evidence that biotin uptake by the liver (and likely many other somatic tissues) occurs via SMVT. Metabolic trapping (e.g., biotin bound covalently to intracellular proteins) is also important. After entering the hepatocyte, biotin diffuses into the mitochondria via a pH-dependent process suggesting that biotin enters the mitochondria in the neutral, protonated form and dissociates into the anionic form in the more alkaline mitochondrial environment, thereby becoming trapped by the charge. The pH of the mitochondrial matrix is about 7.5 compared to about 7.2 for cytosol. Based on a study in rats, biliary excretion of biotin is quantitatively negligible.

BIOTIN UPTAKE INTO CENTRAL NERVOUS SYSTEM

Using rats, Spector and Mock (1987) demonstrated that biotin is transported across the blood–brain barrier by a structurally specific, saturable system; the apparent K_m is several orders of magnitude greater than the concentration of free biotin in plasma. Additional animal studies indicated a specific transport system for biotin into the neurons after biotin crosses the blood–brain barrier.

A child with a very high biotin requirement and an observed defect in biotin transport by lymphocytes has been reported (Mardach et al., 2002). This 18-month-old boy presented with sudden onset of coma; both the neurological problems and a pattern of organic aciduria consistent with multiple carboxylase deficiency were responsive to pharmacological doses of biotin (i.e., 10 mg/d). Continued high-dose biotin supplementation was needed to prevent symptomatic relapse. As the *SMVT* gene sequence was normal, these investigators speculated that the lymphocyte biotin transporter is expressed in other tissues and mediates some critical aspect of biotin homeostasis. An additional biotin transporter has been proposed; Zempleni and co-workers provided evidence that monocarboxylate transporter 1 (MCT1) is a biotin transporter in human lymphocytes (Daberkow et al., 2003). MCT1 may also be responsible for biotin transport in other tissues (Grafe et al., 2003).

Ozand and collaborators recently described several patients in Saudi Arabia with biotin-responsive basal ganglia disease. Symptoms include confusion, lethargy, vomiting, seizures, dystonia, dysarthria, dysphagia, seventh nerve paralysis, quadriparesis, ataxia, hypertension, chorea, and coma. The signs and symptoms recurred if biotin was discontinued. A defect in the biotin transporter system across the blood–brain barrier was postulated. Additional work by Gusella and co-workers identified a genetic defect in *SLC19A3*, but Said and associates conclusively proved that *SLC19A3* codes for THTR2, the thiamine transporter located in the apical membrane of intestinal, renal tubule, and hepatic cells (Subramanian et al., 2006). THTR2 does not transport biotin, leaving the biotin responsiveness of these patients unexplained.

BIOTIN UPTAKE FROM RENAL FILTRATE

Because biotin is a small molecule (244 Da) and mainly not bound to protein in plasma, most of the biotin will appear in glomerular filtrate. Thus like many of the water-soluble vitamins, the specific system for the reabsorption of biotin from the glomerular filtrate is important to avoid substantial losses of biotin in urine. A biotin transport system was identified by Said and co-workers in brush border membrane vesicles from human kidney cortex and in human-derived proximal tubular epithelial HK-2 cells (Balamurugan et al., 2005). Uptake is electroneutral, structurally specific, and saturable. It occurs against a biotin concentration gradient and depends on an inwardly directed Na^+ gradient; it is inhibited by pantothenic acid, lipoate, and small interfering RNA specific for SMVT, providing conclusive proof that SMVT is the principal renal biotin reabsorption transporter. Biotin uptake by SMVT is adaptively regulated by biotin deficiency, consistent with previous studies demonstrating reduced biotin excretion in the early stages of experimentally induced biotin deficiency in human subjects.

PLACENTAL TRANSPORT OF BIOTIN

Biotin concentrations are 3 to 17 times greater in human fetal plasma than in maternal plasma, suggesting active placental transport. SMVT is expressed in normal human placenta and in fact was originally discovered in human chorionic carcinoma cells. However, in the isolated, perfused single cotyledon from placenta, transport of biotin across the placenta is relatively weak, potentially allowing greater fetal deficiency than maternal deficiency, as reported in mice (Mock, 2009).

TRANSPORT OF BIOTIN INTO HUMAN MILK

Greater than 95% of the biotin in human milk is free in the aqueous phase of the skim milk fraction. A steady increase in the biotin concentration is observed during the first 18 days postpartum in about half of women; after that, biotin concentrations vary substantially. In early and transitional human milk, bisnorbiotin (an inactive metabolite; see later) accounts for about half of the total biotin plus metabolites. With postpartum maturation, the proportion of the total due to biotin increases; however, bisnorbiotin still accounts for about 25% of the total at 5 weeks postpartum. The concentration of biotin in human milk is 10 to 100 times that in plasma, indicating that a system (or systems) exists for transporting biotin into milk. These have yet to be elucidated.

BIOTIN DEGRADATION

In the normal turnover of carboxylases and histones, the biotin released may be metabolized to inactive metabolites instead of incorporation back into these proteins. Biotin, possibly in the form of biotinyl-CoA, can be oxidized to bisnorbiotin and tetranorbiotin (metabolites with two and four fewer carbons, respectively, in the valeric acid side chain). The sulfur can be oxidized to sulfoxide (one oxygen on the sulfur) and possibly to sulfone (two oxygens on the sulfur). Biotin, bisnorbiotin, and biotin sulfoxide are present in mole ratios of about 3:2:1 in human urine and plasma. Biotin catabolism is accelerated during pregnancy, with cigarette smoking, and with antiepileptic therapy, leading to an increase in the ratio of biotin catabolites to biotin. This accelerated degradation may contribute to biotin depletion.

BIOTIN DEFICIENCY

CIRCUMSTANCES LEADING TO DEFICIENCY

The requirement for biotin by normal humans has been clearly documented in three situations: prolonged consumption of raw egg white, parenteral nutrition without biotin supplementation in patients with short-gut syndrome, and infant feeding with an elemental formula devoid of biotin. Because biotin could not legally be added as a supplement to infant formulas in Japan until 2003, all reports related to infant formula have come from Japan. Fujimoto and colleagues (2005) described the ninth such infant and provided an excellent summary of the other eight infants. Often, feeding of an elemental formula was required to treat intractable, chronic diarrhea. The infants typically developed both the classic cutaneous manifestations of biotin deficiency and the characteristic pattern of organic aciduria. Biotinidase deficiency and HCS deficiency were ruled out by the gradual weaning of biotin supplementation.

Biotin deficiency likely also occurs in children with severe protein-energy malnutrition as judged by decreased lymphocyte carboxylase activity and plasma biotin levels, and may contribute to the clinical syndrome of protein-energy malnutrition. Long-term antiepileptic therapy in adults can lead to biotin depletion. The depletion can be severe enough to interfere with leucine degradation and cause increased urinary excretion of 3-hydroxyisovaleric acid. The mechanism of biotin depletion during antiepileptic therapy is not known, but may involve accelerated biotin catabolism, impaired biotin absorption, impaired biotin transport in plasma, impaired renal reclamation biotin, or a combination of these.

Studies of biotin status during pregnancy provide evidence that a marginal degree of biotin deficiency develops in at least one third of women during normal pregnancy (Mock, 2009). Although the degree of biotin deficiency was not severe enough to produce overt manifestations of biotin deficiency, the deficiency was sufficiently severe to produce metabolic derangements. A similar marginal degree of biotin deficiency causes high rates of fetal malformations in some mammals. Takechi and colleagues have shown in human embryonic palatal mesenchymal cells that biotin deficiency reduces biotin-dependent carboxylases, biotinylated histones, and cell proliferation (Takechi et al., 2008). Moreover, a posthoc analysis of data from a large multivitamin supplementation study (Czeizel and Dudás, 1992) provided interesting, although indirect, evidence that the marginal degree of biotin deficiency that occurs spontaneously in normal human gestation may be teratogenic (Mock, 2009). Biotin deficiency has also been reported or inferred in several other clinical circumstances. These include Leiner disease, renal dialysis, and alcoholism.

CLINICAL FINDINGS OF OVERT BIOTIN DEFICIENCY

The clinical findings of overt biotin deficiency in adults and older children have been quite similar to those reported by Sydenstricker in his pioneering study of egg-white feeding (Sydenstricker et al., 1942). Clinical signs of overt biotin deficiency begin to appear gradually several weeks to months after the initiation of egg-white feeding or 6 months to 3 years after the initiation of long-term total parenteral nutrition without biotin. Thinning of hair, often with loss of hair color, was reported in most patients. A skin rash described as scaly (seborrheic) and red (eczematous) was present in the majority; in several, the rash was distributed around the eyes, nose, and mouth. Depression, lethargy, hallucinations, and paresthesias of the extremities were prominent neurological symptoms in the majority of adults.

In infants, the signs and symptoms of biotin deficiency developed within 3 to 6 months after initiation of long-term total parenteral nutrition or biotin-free formula. The rash typically appeared first around the eyes, nose, and mouth.

Ultimately, the ears and perineal orifices were involved. The appearance of the rash was similar to that of cutaneous *Candida* infection (i.e., an erythematous base and crusting exudates); typically, *Candida* could be cultured from the lesions. The rash of biotin deficiency is also similar but not identical to the rash of zinc deficiency. In infants, hair loss, including eyebrows and lashes, can occur after 6 to 9 months of parenteral nutrition. These cutaneous manifestations, in conjunction with an unusual distribution of facial fat, have been dubbed "biotin deficiency facies." The most striking neurological findings in biotin-deficient infants were hypotonia, lethargy, and developmental delay. A failure to interact with caregivers was observed and might reflect the same central nervous system dysfunction diagnosed as depression in the adults.

LABORATORY FINDINGS OF BIOTIN DEFICIENCY

Indicators of biotin deficiency have been validated mainly experimentally, by inducing progressive but asymptomatic biotin deficiency with a diet high in egg whites. The urinary excretion of biotin declines dramatically, reaching abnormal values in about 90% of subjects after 3 weeks. Urinary excretion of 3-hydroxyisovaleric acid and plasma and urinary 3-hydroxyisovalerylcarnitine increase to greater than the normal range in about 90% of subjects after 2 weeks of eating egg whites, providing evidence that biotin depletion decreases the activity of the biotin-dependent enzyme MCC (Horvath et al., 2010a, 2010b; Stratton et al., 2010). Serum concentrations of free biotin decrease to abnormal values in less than half of the subjects, confirming the impression of many investigators in this field that blood biotin concentration is not an early or sensitive indicator of impaired biotin status.

The best indicator of biotin status is activity of the biotin-dependent enzyme PCC in lymphocytes isolated from venous blood samples. The assay quantitates the catalysis by PCC of ^{14}C-bicarbonate incorporation into acid-precipitable material (i.e., methylmalonyl-CoA). Unfortunately, this assay is technically demanding, and the blood samples require special handling and storage.

INBORN ERRORS OF BIOTIN METABOLISM

HOLOCARBOXYLASE SYNTHETASE DEFICIENCY

Genetic deficiencies of HCS and biotinidase cause two types of multiple carboxylase deficiency which were previously designated the neonatal and juvenile forms. The inherited deficiency of HCS activity results in decreased activities of all five of the biotin-dependent carboxylases. In turn, these multiple carboxylase deficiencies result in clinical findings arising from the roles of all five carboxylases in metabolism. In patients with a severe HCS deficiency, illness often occurs in the neonatal period and includes severe ketoacidosis, seizures, and lethargy; if not recognized and treated, coma and death can ensue. In patients with a milder form of HCS deficiency, hair loss (alopecia) and an erythematous skin rash typical of biotin deficiency can appear at several months of age. Elevated urinary excretions of the metabolites characteristic of deficiency of several of the biotin-dependent carboxylase are seen. Treatment with large oral doses of biotin (e.g., 10 to 60 mg per day) usually results in dramatic improvement of the biochemical abnormalities, skin rash, alopecia, and neurological findings, provided irreversible neurological damage has not occurred.

A variety of mutations of the HCS gene have been reported. When studied, the concentration of biotin needed to attain half of the maximal reaction rate (the K_m) generally was found to be increased far above biotin levels found in normal cells. In contrast, the maximal enzyme activity (V_{max}) usually was greater than zero and approached normal at the higher levels of biotin. These observations explain why treatment with very large doses of biotin that increased tissue levels of biotin far above normal can result in enough activity of HCS to convert apocarboxylases to active holocarboxylases, correcting the multiple carboxylase deficiencies. A complete absence of HCS activity, which would mean no activity of any of the five carboxylases, would probably be fatal in utero.

BIOTINIDASE DEFICIENCY

In the normal turnover of cellular proteins, holocarboxylases are degraded to biocytin or biotin linked to an oligopeptide containing at most a few amino acid residues. Biotinidase likely plays a critical role by releasing biotin for recycling from intracellular proteins such as carboxylases and histones during protein turnover. Consistent with this global role, biotinidase is found in many tissues, including heart, brain, liver, lung, skeletal muscle, kidney, plasma, placenta, pancreas, and intestine.

The gene for human biotinidase has been identified, sequenced, and characterized. The biotinidase gene is a

DRIs Across the Life Cycle: Biotin

	μg Biotin per Day
Infant	AI
0 through 6 mo	5
7 through 12 mo	6
Children	
1 through 3 yr	8
4 through 8 yr	12
9 through 13 yr	20
14 through 18 yr	25
Males	
≥19 yr	30
Females	
≥19 yr	30
Pregnant	30
Lactating	35

Data from IOM. (2006). In J. J. Otten, J. P. Hellwig, & L. D. Meyers (Eds.), *Dietary Reference Intakes: The essential guide to nutrient requirements* (p. 196). Washington, DC: The National Academies Press.

AI, Adequate Intake; *DRI*, Dietary Reference Intake.

Note: There is no established Tolerable Upper Intake Level (UL) for biotin.

single copy gene of 1,629 bases encoding a 543–amino acid protein; the mRNA is present in multiple tissues, including heart, brain, placenta, liver, lung, skeletal muscle, kidney, and pancreas. Biotinidase activity is greatest in serum, liver, kidney, and adrenal gland. The liver is thought to be the source of plasma biotinidase.

Individuals with less than 10% of normal activity in plasma exhibit seizures, hypotonia, skin rash, and alopecia, usually presenting in infancy (reviewed by Barry Wolf [2010], the person who discovered biotinidase). Many children have ataxia, developmental delay, conjunctivitis, hearing loss, visual problems including optic atrophy, and a characteristic organic aciduria. If untreated, progression to coma or death can occur. Some children only manifest one or two features, or they develop motor limb weakness, spastic paresis, and eye problems, such as loss of visual acuity and scotomata, later in life. Once hearing loss, optic atrophy, and moderate or severe developmental delay appear, they are often irreversible despite treatment with biotin. If treatment is begun before onset of clinical findings, signs and symptoms appear to be preventable.

Thus the clinical findings and biochemical abnormalities of biotinidase deficiency resemble those of biotin deficiency (dermatitis, alopecia, conjunctivitis, ataxia, developmental delay), suggesting that they are caused by biotin deficiency. However, the signs and symptoms of biotin deficiency and biotinidase deficiency are not identical. Seizures, irreversible neurosensory hearing loss, and optic atrophy have been observed in biotinidase deficiency, but not in biotin deficiency. A knockout mouse model of biotinidase deficiency recapitulates many of the clinical findings observed in human biotinidase deficiency (Pindolia et al., 2010).

DIETARY SOURCES AND RECOMMENDED INTAKES

Because biotin cannot be synthesized by mammals, humans must derive biotin from other sources. The ultimate source of biotin appears to be de novo synthesis by bacteria; primitive eukaryotic organisms such as yeast, molds, and algae; and some plant species.

FOOD SOURCES OF BIOTIN

Most measurements of the biotin content of various foods have been made with bioassays and are likely to contain substantial errors. However, some worthwhile generalizations can still be made. Biotin is widely distributed in natural foodstuffs, but the absolute content of even the richest sources is low when compared with the content of most other water-soluble vitamins. Foods relatively rich in biotin include egg yolk, liver, nuts, legumes, and some vegetables. The average daily dietary biotin intake is about 35 to 70 μg based on microbial assay data.

RECOMMENDED INTAKES

Data providing an accurate estimate of the biotin requirement for infants, children, and adults are lacking; not surprisingly, recommendations often vary among countries. Because of these limitations, the Food and Nutrition Board of the Institute of Medicine (IOM, 1998) has offered only Adequate Intakes (AIs) for biotin. The AI for preterm infants is not different from that of the AI for infants through the first 6 months of life, which was based on average biotin intake of breast-fed infants and is 5 μg/day. The AIs for older infants (6 μg/day), children (8 to 12 μg/day), adolescents (25 μg/day), and adults (30 μg/day) were all extrapolated from the values for younger infants. No increment was added for pregnancy, but the AI for lactating women is 35 μg/day (30 μg/day plus 5 μg/day to cover biotin in the milk).

TOXICITY

No Tolerable Upper Intake Level (UL) for biotin has been established. Daily use of up to 100 mg orally or up to 20 mg intravenously for treatment of subjects with biotin-responsive inborn errors of metabolism has not produced any signs of toxicity.

THINKING CRITICALLY

Biotin

1. You suspect that pregnancy contributes to biotin deficiency. What measures of biotin status would you choose to determine whether biotin status of pregnant women is diminished? For each measure, specify the directions of change with deficiency, the mechanisms underlying the changes, and the appropriate controls for interpretation.
2. Based on the test results from your biotin status diagnostic workup ordered for question 1, you conclude that biotin status is reduced in the first trimester of pregnancy. Propose a mechanism that can lead to decreased biotin status and the design of a clinical study for testing the proposed mechanism. Confine your experimental design to studies that can be performed on human participants.
3. In your clinical study of biotin status in pregnancy, you find that impaired biotin status is associated with birth defects. Propose two different biochemical mechanisms for the teratogenesis. What could you measure in umbilical cord blood to confirm the mechanism?
4. You know that biotin transport in the intestine is upregulated in response to a diet that induces biotin deficiency. Describe a mechanism that could result in such upregulation and an experimental approach for testing your hypothesized mechanism.
5. The first cases of human biotin deficiency were described in two circumstances: (1) individuals consuming diets high in raw egg whites, and (2) individuals on long-term total intravenous nutrition without biotin supplementation. The patients requiring intravenous nutrition often had short gut syndrome and were receiving broad-spectrum antibiotics. In both of these circumstances, net biotin absorption may have been impaired by mechanisms affecting multiple sources of biotin, multiple mechanisms of absorption, or both. Describe these, and explain your thinking.

Several studies of plasma levels, pharmacokinetics, and bioavailability after acute or chronic oral, intramuscular, or intravenous administration of biotin in cattle, swine, fish, and humans have been conducted. High doses (e.g., 1200 μg) result in high biotin concentrations in blood and the urinary excretion of a large proportion as unchanged biotin. Increased blood concentrations of bisnorbiotin and biotin sulfoxide and increased urinary excretion of bisnorbiotin and biotin sulfoxide are also reported, providing evidence that these biotin metabolites originate from human tissues rather than enteric bacteria.

PANTOTHENIC ACID

Pantothenic acid (vitamin B_5) is classified with the water-soluble B vitamins. Pantothenic acid was isolated, identified, and named by Roger John Williams in 1933 (Williams et al., 1933). Williams named it from Greek roots, *panton* meaning "of all things," to reflect the ubiquitous presence of pantothenic acid in bacteria, algae, molds, plants, and animals.

Pantothenic acid (pantothenate, the ionized form) is a precursor to coenzyme A (CoA). About 4% of all cellular enzymes use CoA or its thioester derivatives as substrates (Zhyvoloup et al., 2002). Indeed, the CoA ester of acetic acid, acetyl-CoA, is considered to be a central common compound of mammalian intermediary metabolism. In addition, acyl carrier protein (ACP) is also formed from pantothenic acid and serves as an essential carrier of acyl groups during the synthesis of fatty acids (Byers and Gong, 2007).

PANTOTHENIC ACID SYNTHESIS

Synthesis of pantothenic acid is limited to plants, eubacteria, and archaea. The synthetic pathway is well established for *E. coli*, and a route has been proposed for its synthesis in plants (Smith et al., 2007). The final step in its synthesis involves the linkage of β-alanine and pantoic acid by a peptide (amide) linkage.

DIETARY SOURCES AND INTAKE

The dietary sources of pantothenic acid are CoA and ACP, which are obtained from both plants and animals. Rich sources include liver, kidney, egg yolk, broccoli, and yeast (IOM, 1998). Fish, shellfish, chicken, milk, yogurt, legumes, mushrooms, avocado, and sweet potatoes are also good sources. Whole grains are good sources of pantothenic acid; however, processing and refining of grains may result in a 35% to 75% loss. Freezing and canning of foods result in similar losses. Large national nutritional surveys were unable to estimate pantothenic acid intake because data on the pantothenic acid content of foods are scarce. Smaller studies estimate the average daily intake of pantothenic acid for adults to be 5 to 6 mg/day. For more information on the nutrient content of foods, search the U.S. Department of Agriculture nutrient database (*www.ars.usda.gov/nutrientdata*).

Vitamin B_5 is commercially available as D-pantothenic acid; calcium pantothenate, which is more stable and soluble as an oral supplement; as well as the D isomer of panthenol (dexpanthenol), which is biologically active but mainly used in cosmetics due to its moisturizing properties.

DIGESTION, ABSORPTION, AND TRANSPORT

Within the lumen of the intestine, pantothenic acid is formed by the hydrolysis of CoA and ACP to 4′-phosphopantetheine, which is then dephosphorylated to pantetheine. Pantetheinase, an intestinal enzyme, then hydrolyzes pantetheine into free pantothenic acid. Free pantothenic acid is taken up into the enterocyte by SMVT (the sodium-dependent multivitamin transporter) and released into the portal blood (Zempleni, 2005).

Free pantothenic acid is found in plasma. Uptake of pantothenic acid from plasma into heart, liver, muscle, and kidney occurs by active transport via the SMVT, whereas uptake by brain occurs by facilitated diffusion (Spector, 1986). High concentrations of total pantothenate are found within red blood cells (RBCs) because pantothenate diffuses into the RBC and is phosphorylated to 4′-phosphopantothenic acid (Annous and Song, 1995). Although phosphorylation is the first step of synthesis of CoA in most cells, the mature RBC no longer has an endoplasmic reticulum or nucleus; thus further metabolism to CoA cannot occur. Consequently, 4′-phosphopantothenic acid is trapped in the RBC because the phosphorylated pantothenic acid is unable to diffuse back through the membrane (Annous and Song, 1995). Active uptake via the SMVT occurs in heart, liver, muscle, and kidney; uptake by brain occurs by facilitated diffusion (Spector, 1986).

METABOLISM OF PANTOTHENIC ACID TO CoA AND ACP

Pantothenic acid combines with mercaptoethylamine (cysteamine), adenine, and ribose 3′-phosphate moieties to form CoA (Figure 26-5). The biosynthesis of CoA in mammalian cells utilizes pantothenate, ATP, and cysteine as substrates. There are five enzymatic steps in CoA biosynthesis (Figure 26-6). In the first step, which is the rate-limiting reaction, pantothenate is phosphorylated to 4′-phosphopantothenate by pantothenate kinase. As is often the case, the enzyme catalyzing the committed controlling step is inhibited by CoA, the end product of the pathway (classic negative feedback). Next, 4′-phosphopantothenate is condensed with cysteine to form 4′-phosphopantothenoylcysteine, which is then decarboxylated to 4′-phosphopantetheine. These two reactions are catalyzed by the 4′-phosphopantothenoylcysteine synthase and 4′-phosphopantothenoylcysteine decarboxylase. These two activities are due to two distinct domains of a single bifunctional enzyme in archaea (Zhyvoloup et al., 2002) and bacteria, but in eukaryotes these are two distinct

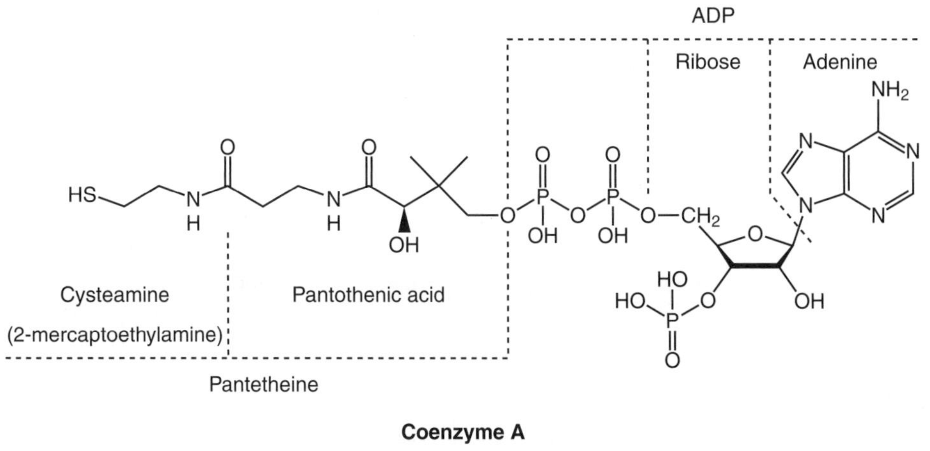

FIGURE 26-5 Pantothenic acid structure. Pantothenic acid combines with 2-mercaptoethylamine (cysteamine), adenine, and ribose 3′-phosphate moieties to form CoA.

proteins. 4′-Phosphopantetheine is subsequently converted to dephospho-CoA by phosphopantetheine adenylyltransferase and phosphorylated by dephospho-CoA kinase at the 3′-OH of the ribose to form CoA. These latter two enzymatic activities are catalyzed by two separate enzymes in prokaryotes and plants; however, in mammals the reactions are catalyzed by a single bifunctional enzyme, termed CoA synthase.

ACP is produced by addition of 4′-phosphopantothenic acid to a serine residue on the ACP domain of fatty acid synthase (Figure 26-7). In mammals, the ACP domain of fatty acid synthase is highly conserved. It functions as a separate domain within the large multidomain fatty acid synthase (Byers and Gong, 2007). The ACP domain is synthesized as an enzymatically inactive apoprotein, which is converted to the holo-ACP by the covalent attachment of 4′-phosphopantetheine from CoA. This step is catalyzed by 4′-phosphopantetheinyl transferase. ACP serves as a carrier of acyl intermediates during fatty acid syntheses.

FUNCTIONS OF CoA AND ACP

Both CoA and ACP are essential carriers of the de facto substrates for critical pathways in intermediary metabolism (see Figure 26-3). ACP is essential for synthesis of palmitate. CoA is essential to the entrance of acetyl-CoA into the citric acid cycle for complete oxidation of glucose or fatty acids and for other reactions involving citric acid cycle intermediates; synthesis of cholesterol, steroid hormones, and bile acids; fatty acid synthesis; and fatty acid oxidation. CoA serves this role by forming high-energy thioesters for many metabolic intermediates. CoA has additional important roles in oxidative metabolism of pyruvate via pyruvate dehydrogenase and in the metabolism of a wide variety of organic acids, including those formed in the catabolism of many amino acids. Ketone "bodies" (acetone, acetoacetate, and 3-hydroxybutyrate) are made in the hepatic mitochondria from acetyl-CoA, which in turn can arise from fatty acids from adipose tissue among others sources. Acetoacetate and 3-hydroxybutyrate are released from the liver to spare glucose consumption during prolonged starvation. In particular, the brain derives about 30% of its energy from ketone bodies after only 3 days of fasting. In such ketone body–consuming organs, the ketone bodies are converted back to acetyl-CoA and produce energy via the citric acid cycle (see Figure 26-3).

CoA AND CARNITINE

Long-chain fatty acids cannot cross from the cytosol into the mitochondria directly. Instead, the free long-chain fatty acids are activated to fatty acyl-CoA by acyl-CoA synthetases; ATP hydrolysis provides the energy for the formation of this high-energy thioester bond (see Figure 26-3). Then, on the outer mitochondrial membrane, the enzyme carnitine palmitoyltransferase 1 (CPT1) transesterifies the fatty acyl-CoA to a fatty acyl carnitine, releasing free CoA (see Chapter 16, Figure 16-10). A carnitine acylcarnitine translocase subsequently moves the acylcarnitine into the mitochondrial matrix while simultaneously moving a free carnitine out of the mitochondria. Finally, carnitine palmitoyltransferase 2, which is present on the inner mitochondrial membrane, regenerates the fatty acyl-CoA and releases free carnitine. The fatty acyl-CoA is now available for fatty acid oxidation within the mitochondrial matrix. Similar processes occur for short- and medium-chain fatty acids.

Free carnitine and carnitine esters act as a buffer to maintain a normal ratio of free CoA to acyl-CoA when specific CoA intermediates accumulate (such as might be seen in an inborn error in a particular enzymatic pathway; or in vitamin deficiency such as biotin deficiency that decreases activity of a biotin-dependent carboxylase). If acyl-CoAs accumulate, free CoA could be depleted below the levels needed for its essential roles in metabolism. The conversion of some acyl-CoAs to acylcarnitines frees up CoA and maintains a more normal ratio of free to esterified CoA. Large amounts of the acylcarnitines accumulate within the cell, enter the blood circulation, and are excreted in urine as a means of removing accumulated esters of CoA that may be toxic. Not surprisingly, secondary carnitine depletion has been observed in such situations, as previously discussed in the biotin section of this chapter.

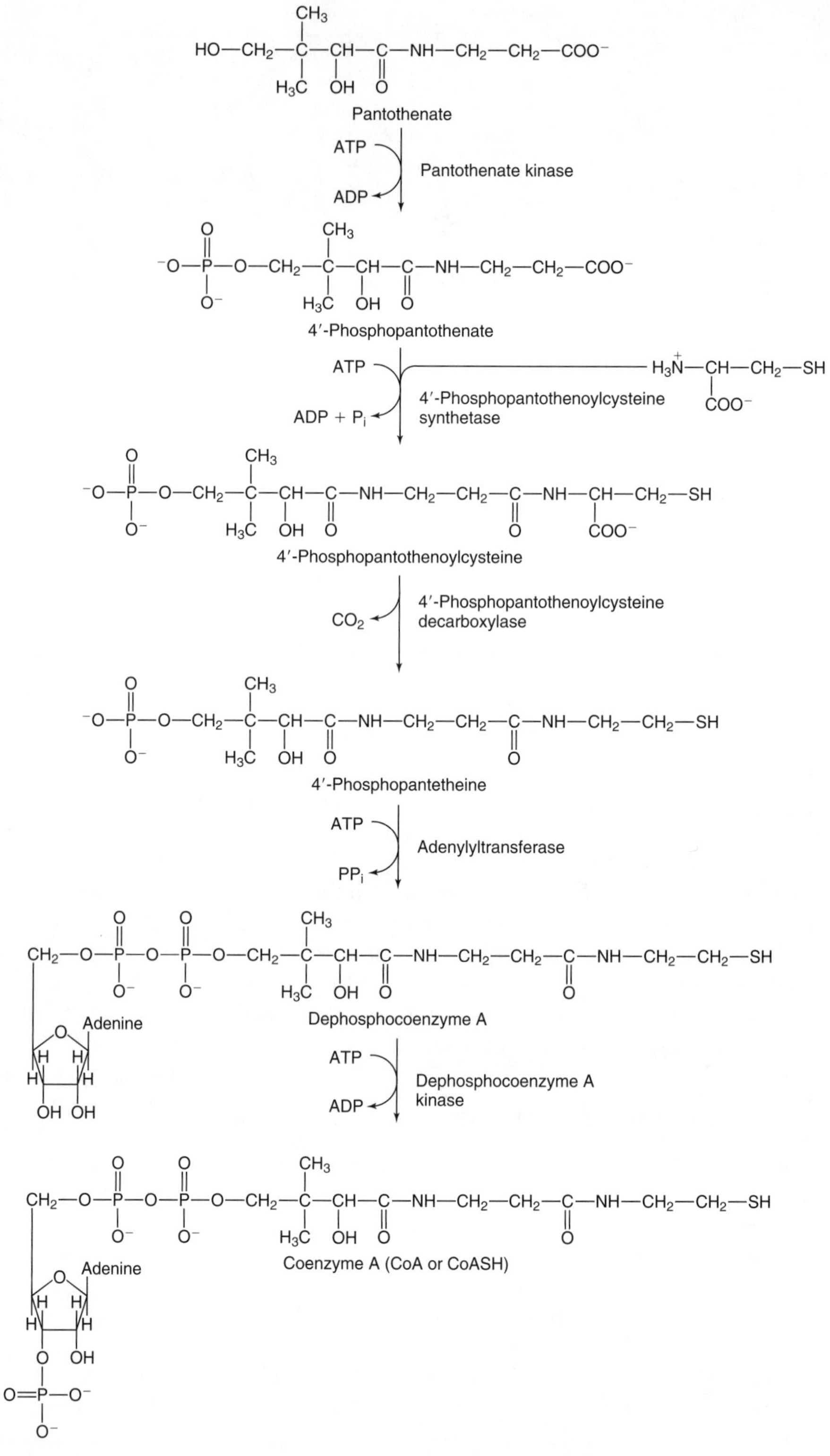

Pantothenate

ATP → ADP — Pantothenate kinase

4′-Phosphopantothenate

ATP → ADP + P_i (+ H_3N^+—CH(COO^-)—CH_2—SH) — 4′-Phosphopantothenoylcysteine synthetase

4′-Phosphopantothenoylcysteine

→ CO_2 — 4′-Phosphopantothenoylcysteine decarboxylase

4′-Phosphopantetheine

ATP → PP_i — Adenylyltransferase

Dephosphocoenzyme A

ATP → ADP — Dephosphocoenzyme A kinase

Coenzyme A (CoA or CoASH)

FIGURE 26-6 There are five enzymatic steps in CoA biosynthesis: (1) pantothenate is phosphorylated to 4′-phosphopantothenate by pantothenate kinase; (2) 4′-phosphopantothenate is condensed with cysteine to form 4′-phosphopantothenoylcysteine; (3) 4′-phosphopantothenoylcysteine is then decarboxylated to 4′-phosphopantetheine; (4) 4′-phosphopantetheine is subsequently converted to dephospho-CoA by phosphopantetheine adenylyltransferase; (5) dephospho-CoA is phosphorylated by dephospho-CoA kinase at the 3′-OH of the ribose to form CoA.

DIETARY REQUIREMENT

The Food and Nutrition Board of the IOM in 1998 felt the existing scientific evidence was insufficient to calculate a Recommended Dietary Allowance for pantothenic acid, but an Adequate Intake (AI) has been established. The AI for pantothenic acid is based on estimated dietary intakes in healthy populations (IOM, 1998).

PANTOTHENIC ACID DEFICIENCY

There are no reports of spontaneous pantothenic acid deficiency with associated disease states. Historical records of severe malnutrition in prisoners of war indicate that numbness, burning, and tingling of feet was relieved when prisoners were fed yeast extracts and other vitamins in an urgent repletion effort. The credit to pantothenic acid specifically

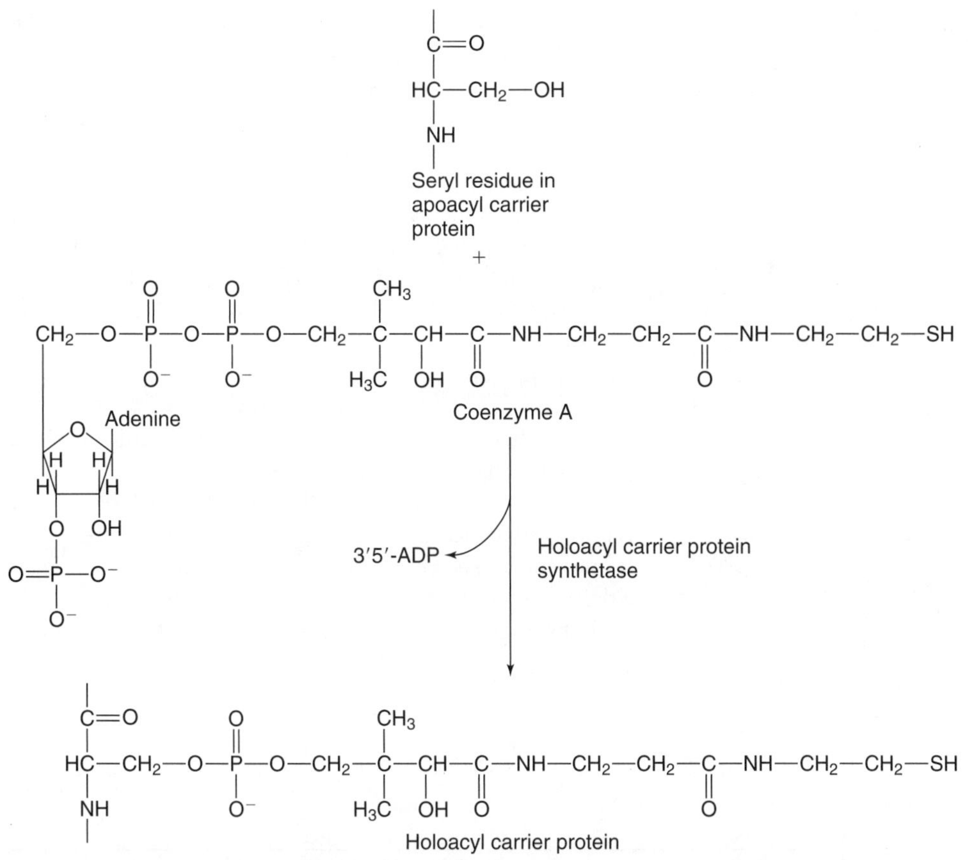

FIGURE 26-7 Acyl carrier protein (ACP) is the product of 4′-phosphopantothenic acid and serine. The ACP domain is synthesized as an enzymatically inactive apoprotein, which is converted to the holo-ACP by the covalent attachment of 4′-phosphopantetheine from CoA to a specific serine residue of the ACP. This step is catalyzed by 4′-phosphopantetheinyl transferase (holoacyl carrier protein synthetase).

for relieving these symptoms is probably a post hoc reflection based on the study of experimental pantothenic acid deficiency in human volunteers (Bean et al., 1955). Within 25 days of beginning a pantothenic acid–depleted diet that included the agonist ω-methylpantothenic acid, participants complained of numbness and tingling of the hands and feet; one subject had "an especially disagreeable burning sensation." Participants also experienced severe diarrhea and altered mental affect described as quarrelsome, sullen, and petulant. Further evidence of physical effects of deficiency was documented in weanling pigs receiving suboptimal amounts of pantothenate. Pigs developed diarrhea and hind limb weakness after 2 to 4 weeks of a pantothenic acid–depleted diet (Stothers et al., 1955). In other animal models of deficiency, pantothenic acid deficiency damaged the adrenal glands in rats, whereas monkeys developed anemia due to decreased synthesis of heme. Dogs with pantothenic acid deficiency developed low blood glucose levels, rapid breathing and heart rates, and convulsions. Chickens developed skin irritation, feather abnormalities, and spinal nerve damage associated with the degeneration of the myelin sheath. Pantothenic acid–deficient mice showed decreased exercise tolerance and diminished storage of glucose (in the form of glycogen) in muscle and liver. Mice also developed skin irritation and graying of the fur, which was reversed by giving pantothenic acid. This finding led to the idea of adding pantothenic acid to shampoo, although it has not been successful in restoring hair color in humans. In rats, pantothenic acid deficiency affected testicular function (Yamamoto et al., 2009).

PURPORTED THERAPEUTIC USES OF PANTOTHENIC ACID

The physical findings and symptoms that occurred in severe deficiency experimentally induced in animals have led to numerous claims for very large doses of pantothenic acid as treatment or cure for a host of conditions. The National Institutes of Health (NIH) website (*www.nlm.nih.gov/medlineplus/druginfo/natural/853.html*) includes a long list of conditions and diseases that oral pantothenic acid supplementation is supposed to benefit; these include acne, attention-deficit/hyperactivity disorder, dandruff, retarded growth, dizziness, shingles, and wound healing. This NIH site notes that there is not sufficient scientific evidence to determine effectiveness of treatment. For instance, treatment of acne with about 10 g pantothenic acid per day is recommended by several commercial sites, which offer their products. Evidence of effectiveness, when cited at all, is based on a publication by Lit-Hung Leung in 1995 in the journal *Medical Hypotheses* (Leung, 1995b). Leung published other articles, including on the use of pantothenic acid as a weight loss supplement (Leung, 1995a). No references to any placebo-controlled, blinded studies published in English were found.

DRIs Across the Life Cycle: Pantothenic Acid

	mg Pantothenic Acid per Day*
Infant	AI
0 through 6 mo	1.7
7 through 12 mo	1.8
Children	
1 through 3 yr	2
4 through 8 yr	3
9 through 13 yr	4
14 through 18 yr	5
Males	
≥19 yr	5
Females	
≥19 yr	5
Pregnant	6
Lactating	7

Data from IOM. (1998). *Dietary reference intakes for thiamin, riboflavin, niacin, vitamin B_6, folate, vitamin B_{12}, pantothenic acid, biotin, and choline.* Washington, DC: National Academy Press.
AI, Adequate Intake; *DRI*, Dietary Reference Intake.
*There is no established Tolerable Upper Intake Level (UL) for pantothenic acid.

There are two recent reports of use of dexpanthenol, the alcohol analog of pantothenic acid, to treat testicular torsion experimentally induced in rats (Etensel et al., 2007a, 2007b). The proposed mechanism is prevention of free radical oxygen injury in ischemia followed by reperfusion. Reduction of oxidation injury by pantothenic acid and dexpanthenol is proposed to involve an increase in free glutathione (Slyshenkov et al., 2004). Other reports of pantothenic acid or dexpanthenol for wound healing are not as well documented (Abdelatif et al., 2008; Ellinger and Stehle, 2009).

TOXICITY

As with other water-soluble vitamins, there is little evidence of toxicity from pantothenic acid taken for prolonged periods in amounts 1,000 times the AI. There are occasional reports of diarrhea and heartburn from prolonged use. There is one report of eosinophilic pleuropericardial effusion in an elderly woman taking biotin (10 mg/day) and pantothenic acid (300 mg/day) in combination for 2 months (Debordeau et al., 2001).

REFERENCES

Abdelatif, M., Yakoot, M., & Etmaan, M. (2008). Safety and efficacy of a new honey ointment on diabetic foot ulcers: A prospective pilot study. *Journal of Wound Care, 17*(3), 108–110.

Annous, K. F., & Song, W. O. (1995). Pantothenic acid uptake and metabolism by red blood cells of rats. *The Journal of Nutrition, 125*, 2586–2593.

Balamurugan, K., Vaziri, N. D., & Said, H. M. (2005). Biotin uptake by human proximal tubular epithelial cells: Cellular and molecular aspects. *American Journal of Physiology. Renal Physiology, 288*, F823–F831.

Bean, W. B., Hodges, R. E., & Daum, K. (1955). Pantothenic acid deficiency induced in human subjects. *The Journal of Clinical Investigation, 37*(7), 1073–1084.

Boas, M. A. (1927). The effect of desiccation upon the nutritive properties of egg-white. *The Biochemical Journal, 21*, 712–724.

Byers, D. M., & Gong, H. (2007). Acyl carrier protein: Structure–function relationships in a conserved multifunctional protein family. *Biochemistry and Cell Biology, 85*(6), 649–662.

Camporeale, G., Oommen, A. M., Griffin, J. B., Sarath, G., & Zempleni, J. (2007). K12-biotinylated histone H4 marks heterochromatin in human lymphoblastoma cells. *The Journal of Nutritional Biochemistry, 18*(11), 760–768.

Camporeale, G., Shubert, E. E., Sarath, G., Cerny, R., & Zempleni, J. (2004). K8 and K12 are biotinylated in human histone H4. *European Journal of Biochemistry, 271*(11), 2257–2263.

Chew, Y. C., Camporeale, G., Kothapalli, N., Sarath, G., & Zempleni, J. (2006). Lysine residues in N-terminal and C-terminal regions of human histone H2A are targets for biotinylation by biotinidase. *The Journal of Nutritional Biochemistry, 17*(4), 225–233.

Chew, Y. C., West, J. T., Kratzer, S. J., Ilvarsonn, A. M., Eissenberg, J. C., Dave, B. J., … Zempleni, J. (2008). Biotinylation of histones represses transposable elements in human and mouse cells and cell lines and in *Drosophila melanogaster*. *The Journal of Nutrition, 138*(12), 2316–2322.

Cho, Y. S., Lee, J. I., Shin, D., Kim, H. T., Jung, H. Y., Lee, T. G., … Heo, Y. S. (2009). Molecular mechanism for the regulation of human ACC2 through phosphorylation by AMPK. *Biochemical and Biophysical Research Communications, 391*(1), 187–192.

Czeizel, A. E., Dudas, I. (1992). Prevention of the first occurrence of neural-tube defects by periconceptional vitamin supplementation. *New England Journal of Medicine, 327*, 1832–1835.

Daberkow, R. L., White, B. R., Cederberg, R. A., Griffin, J. B., & Zempleni, J. (2003). Monocarboxylate transporter 1 mediates biotin uptake in human peripheral blood mononuclear cells. *The Journal of Nutrition, 133*, 2703–2706.

Dakshinamurti, K., & Cheah-Tan, C. (1968). Liver glucokinase of the biotin deficient rat. *Canadian Journal of Biochemistry, 46*, 75–80.

Debourdeau, P. M., Djezzar, S., Estival, J. L., Zammit, C. M., Richard, R. C., & Castot, A. C. (2001). Life-threatening eosinophilic pleuropericardial effusion related to vitamins B5 and H. *The Annals of Pharmacotherapy, 35*(4), 424–426.

Eisenberg, M. A. (1973). Biotin: Biogenesis, transport, and their regulation. *Advances in Enzymology & Related Areas of Molecular Biology, 38*, 317–372.

Ellinger, S., & Stehle, P. (2009). Efficacy of vitamin supplementation in situations with wound healing disorders: Results from clinical intervention studies. *Current Opinion in Clinical Nutrition and Metabolic Care, 12*(6), 588–595

Etensel, B., Ozkisacik, S., Ozkara, E., Karul, A., Oztan, O., Yazici, M., & Gursoy, H. (2007a). Dexpanthenol attenuates lipid peroxidation and testicular damage at experimental ischemia and reperfusion injury. *Pediatric Surgery International, 23*, 177–181.

Etensel, B., Ozkisacik, S., Ozkara, E., Serbest, L. A., Yazici, M., & Gursoy, H. (2007b). The protective effect of dexpanthenol on testicular atrophy at 60th day following experimental testicular torsion. *Pediatric Surgery International, 23*, 270–275.

Fujimoto, W., Inaoki, M., Fukui, T., Inoue, Y., & Kuhara, T. (2005). Biotin deficiency in an infant fed with amino acid formula. *The Journal of Dermatology, 32*(4), 256–261.

Grafe, F., Wohlrab, W., Neubert, R. H., & Brandsch, M. (2003). Transport of biotin in human keratinocytes. *The Journal of Investigative Dermatology*, *120*(3), 428–433.

Gralla, M., Camporeale, G., & Zempleni, J. (2008). Holocarboxylase synthetase regulates expression of biotin transporters by chromatin remodeling events at the SMVT locus. *The Journal of Nutritional Biochemistry*, *19*(6), 400–408.

Hassan, Y. I., Moriyama, H., Olsen, L. J., Bi, X., & Zempleni, J. (2009). N- and C-terminal domains in human holocarboxylase synthetase participate in substrate recognition. *Molecular Genetics and Metabolism*, *96*(4), 183–188.

Healy, S., Perez-Cadahia, B., Jia, D., McDonald, M. K., Davie, J. R., & Gravel, R. A. (2009). Biotin is not a natural histone modification. *Biochimica et Biophysica Acta*, *1989*(11–12), 719–733.

Horvath, T. D., Stratton, S. L., Bogusiewicz, A., Owen, S. O., Mock, D. M., & Moran, J. H. (2010a). Quantitative measurement of urinary excretion of 3-hydroxyisovaleryl carnitine by LC-MS/MS as an indicator of biotin status in humans. *Analytical Chemistry*, *82*(22), 9543–9548.

Horvath, T. D., Stratton, S. L., Bogusiewicz, A., Pack, L., Moran, J., & Mock, D. M. (2010b). Quantitative measurement of plasma 3-hydroxyisovaleryl carnitine by LC-MS/MS as a novel biomarker of biotin status in humans. *Analytical Chemistry*, *82*(10), 4140–4144.

Hymes, J., Fleischhauer, K., & Wolf, B. (1995). Biotinylation of biotinidase following incubation with biocytin. *Clinica Chimica Acta*, *233*, 39–45.

Institute of Medicine. (1998). *Dietary reference intakes for thiamin, riboflavin, niacin, vitamin B_6, folate, vitamin B_{12}, pantothenic acid, biotin, and choline*. Washington, DC: National Academy Press.

Kobza, K., Sarath, G., & Zempleni, J. (2008). Prokaryotic BirA ligase biotinylates K4, K9, K18 and K23 in histone H3. *BMB Reports*, *41*(4), 310–315.

Leung, L. H. (1995a). Pantothenic acid as a weight-reducing agent: Fasting without hunger, weakness and ketosis. *Medical Hypotheses*, *44*(5), 403–405.

Leung, L. H. (1995b). Pantothenic acid deficiency as the pathogenesis of acne vulgaris. *Medical Hypotheses*, *44*(6), 490–492.

Mardach, R., Zempleni, J., Wolf, B., Cress, S., Boylan, J., Roth, S., … Mock, D. (2002). Biotin dependency due to a defect in biotin transport. *The Journal of Clinical Investigation*, *109*(12), 1617–1623.

Mock, D. M. (2009). Marginal biotin deficiency is common in normal human pregnancy and is highly teratogenic in the mouse. *The Journal of Nutrition*, *139*(1), 154–157.

Pindolia, K., Jordan, M., Guo, C., Matthews, N., Mock, D. M., Strovel, E., … Wolf, B. (2010). Development and characterization of a mouse with profound biotinidase deficiency: A biotin-responsive neurocutaneous disorder. *Molecular Genetics and Metabolism*, *102*(2), 161–169.

Rodriguez-Melendez, R., & Zempleni, J. (2009). Nitric oxide signaling depends on biotin in Jurkat human lymphoma cells. *The Journal of Nutrition*, *139*, 429–433.

Said, H. (2008). Cell and molecular aspects of the human intestinal biotin absorption process. *The Journal of Nutrition*, *139*(1), 158–162.

Slyshenkov, V. S., Dymkowska, D., & Wojtczak, L. (2004). Pantothenic acid and pantothenol increase biosynthesis of glutathione by boosting cell energetics. *FEBS Letters*, *569*, 169–172.

Smith, A. G., Croft, M. T., Moulin, M., & Webb, M. E. (2007). Plants need their vitamins too. *Current Opinion in Plant Biology*, *10*(3), 266–275.

Solorzano-Vargas, R. S., Pacheco-Alvarez, D., & Leon-Del-Rio, A. (2002). Holocarboxylase synthetase is an obligate participant in biotin-mediated regulation of its own expression and of biotin-dependent carboxylases mRNA levels in human cells. *Proceedings of the National Academy of Sciences of the United States of America*, *99*(8), 5325–5330.

Spector, R. (1986). Pantothenic acid transport and metabolism in the central nervous system. *The American Journal of Physiology*, *250*, R292–R297.

Spector, R., & Mock, D. (1987). Biotin transport through the blood-brain barrier. *Journal of Neurochemistry*, *48*(2), 400–404.

Stanley, J. S., Mock, D. M., Griffin, J. B., & Zempleni, J. (2002). Biotin uptake into human peripheral blood mononuclear cells increases early in the cell cycle, increasing carboxylase activities. *The Journal of Nutrition*, *132*(7), 1854–1859.

Stothers, S. C., Schmidt, D. A., Johnston, R. L., Hoefer, J. A., & Luecke, R. W. (1955). The pantothenic acid requirement of the baby pig. *The Journal of Nutrition*, *57*, 47–53.

Stratton, S. L., Horvath, T. D., Bogusiewicz, A., Matthews, N. I., Henrich, C. L., Spencer, H. J., … Mock, D. M. (2010). Plasma concentration of 3-hydroxyisovaleryl carnitine is an early and sensitive indicator of marginal biotin deficiency in humans. *The American Journal of Clinical Nutrition*, *92*, 1399–1405.

Subramanian, V. S., Marchant, J. S., & Said, H. M. (2006). Biotin-responsive basal ganglia disease-linked mutations inhibit thiamine transport via hTHTR2: Biotin is not a substrate for hTHTR2. *American Journal of Physiology. Cell Physiology*, *291*(5), C851–C859.

Sydenstricker, V. P., Singal, S. A., Briggs, A. P., & DeVaughn, N. M. (1942). Preliminary observations on "Egg white injury" in man and its cure with a biotin concentrate. *Science*, *95*, 176–177.

Takechi, R., Taniguchi, A., Ebara, S., Fukui, T., & Watanabe, T. (2008). Biotin deficiency affects the proliferation of human embryonic palatal mesenchymal cells in culture. *The Journal of Nutrition*, *138*, 680–684.

Wijeratne, S. S., Camporeale, G., & Zempleni, J. (2010). K12-biotinylated histone H4 is enriched in telomeric repeats from human lung IMR-90 fibroblasts. *The Journal of Nutritional Biochemistry*, *21*(4), 310–316.

Williams, R. J., Lyman, C. M., Goodyear, G. H., Truesdail, J. H., & Holaday, D. (1933). Pantothenic acid, a growth determinant of universal biological occurrence. *Journal of the American Chemical Society*, *55*, 2912–2927.

Wolf, B. (2010). Clinical issues and frequent questions about biotinidase deficiency. *Molecular Genetics and Metabolism*, *100*(1), 6–13.

Yamamoto, T., Jaroenporn, S., Pan, L., Azumano, I., Onda, M., Nakamura, K., …Taya, K. (2009). Effects of pantothenic acid on testicular function in male rats. *The Journal of Veterinary Medical Science*, *71*(11), 1427–1432.

Zempleni, J. (2005). Uptake, localization, and noncarboxylase roles of biotin. *Annual Review of Nutrition*, *25*, 175–196.

Zempleni, J., Wijeratne, S. S., & Hassan, Y. I. (2009). Biotin. *BioFactors*, *35*(1), 36–46.

Zhyvoloup, A., Nemazanyy, I., Babich, A., Panasyuk, G., Pobigailo, N., Vudmaska, M., … Gout, I. T. (2002). Molecular cloning of CoA synthase: The missing link in CoA biosynthesis. *The Journal of Biological Chemistry*, *277*(25), 22107–22110.

CHAPTER 27

Vitamin C

*Alexander Michels, PhD, and Balz Frei, PhD**

COMMON ABBREVIATIONS

ER	endoplasmic reticulum
GLUT	glucose transporter
GSH	glutathione
GSSG	glutathione disulfide
SVCT	sodium-dependent vitamin C transporter

Vitamin C is an essential micronutrient in the human diet. The electron donating or reducing capacity of ascorbate, the ionized form of ascorbic acid, allows it to participate in various enzymatic and nonenzymatic reactions that encompass all of its known biological functions. These include, for example, several enzymatic hydroxylation reactions in the biosynthesis of collagen, carnitine, and norepinephrine, as well as various nonenzymatic reactions that may protect cells against damaging free radicals and reactive oxygen species. Although vitamin C, also known as ascorbic acid or ascorbate, was discovered early in the twentieth century, our knowledge of vitamin C transport and distribution in the human body and its metabolism and biological functions remains incomplete. Long known for its role in the prevention of the deficiency disease scurvy, emerging research suggests an important role for vitamin C in the prevention of chronic diseases, particularly cardiovascular diseases, and novel applications of vitamin C in the treatment of cancer. As our understanding of the role of vitamin C in biology evolves, dietary intake recommendations to promote human health will need to be reevaluated.

VITAMIN C NOMENCLATURE, STRUCTURE, AND CHEMICAL PROPERTIES

The reduced form of vitamin C, ascorbic acid, is a six-carbon lactone synthesized from glucose by many animals (Figure 27-1). Most mammals synthesize ascorbic acid in the liver, but in reptiles and some birds synthesis occurs in the kidneys (Chatterjee, 1973). Vitamin C synthesis is coupled to glycogenolysis, and thus is downregulated in animals on carbohydrate-restricted diets or when glycogen is depleted during fasting (Banhegyi et al., 1997). Several species are unable to synthesize ascorbic acid, including humans and other simian primates, guinea pigs, Indian fruit bats, capybaras, and various bird and fish species. Humans lack gulonolactone oxidase, the terminal enzyme in the biosynthetic pathway of ascorbic acid. The gene encoding the enzyme in these species has undergone substantial mutation so that no protein is produced (Nishikimi et al., 1994). Animals unable to synthesize ascorbic acid must ingest it to survive, so ascorbic acid is a vitamin for humans.

At neutral pH ascorbic acid exists primarily as the ascorbate monoanion (Figure 27-2), although a small amount of the dianion also exists. For this reason, the term ascorbate is used synonymously with ascorbic acid, although in many cases the ascorbate anions are the reacting molecules. The fully protonated molecule, ascorbic acid, only exists in low pH environments. Although the term *vitamin C* typically refers to the reduced forms of the molecule (ascorbic acid or ascorbate), it can also be understood as the combination of these reduced forms and oxidized forms (ascorbyl radical and dehydroascorbic acid).

ASCORBATE

Ascorbate acts as an electron donor (reducing agent), which accounts for all of its known biochemical and molecular functions. Two electrons of the 2-ene-2,3-diol (ene-diol) structural element of ascorbate are available for donation (see Figure 27-2). The full oxidation of ascorbic acid to dehydroascorbic acid reflects the ascorbate donation of both of these electrons to one or more acceptor molecules. However, the full oxidation of ascorbate in a single step is an unlikely occurrence because electrons are usually lost sequentially (Halliwell, 1996), with formation of the intermediate free radical called ascorbyl radical (sometimes also termed semidehydroascorbic acid, monodehydroascorbic acid, or ascorbate free radical). Because of resonance stabilization of the unpaired electron across the ene-diol and 1-oxo groups (see Figure 27-2), the ascorbyl radical reacts poorly with other molecules (Buettner and Jurkiewicz, 1996). The reactivity of ascorbate with many potentially harmful radical

*This chapter is a revision of the chapter contributed by Mark Levine, MD, for the second edition.

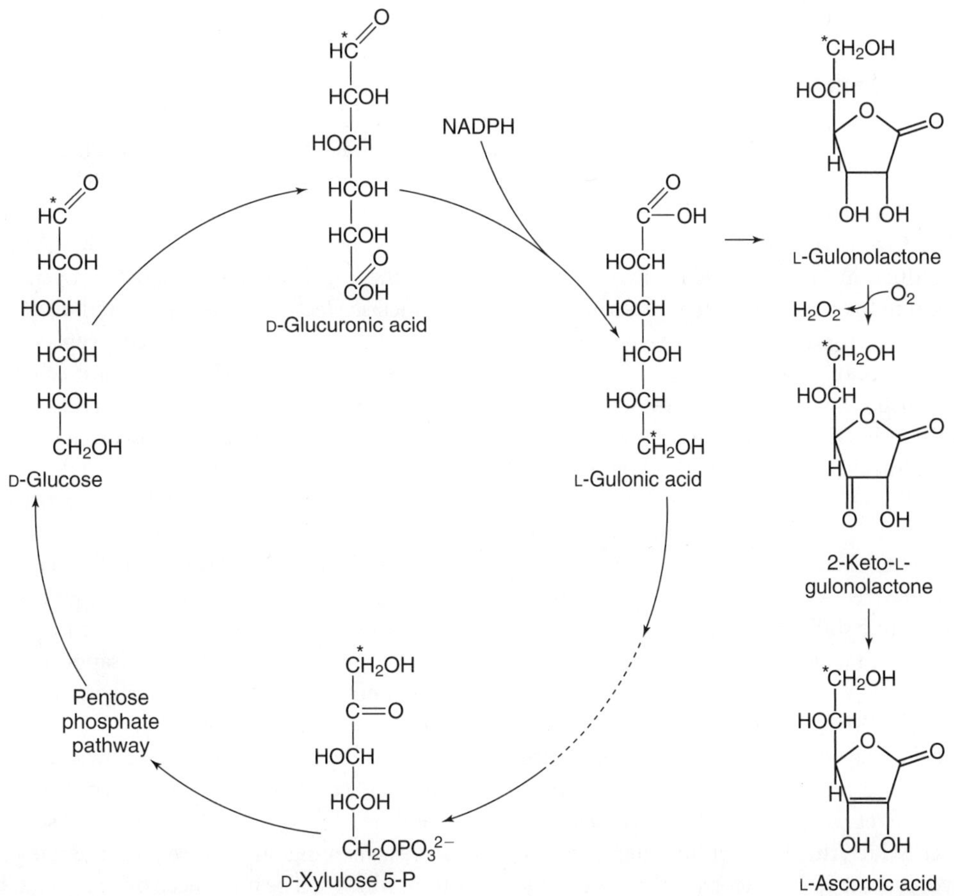

FIGURE 27-1 Pathway for the biosynthesis of ascorbic acid from glucose in mammals. Humans, primates, and some other species lack gulonolactone oxidase and cannot convert L-gulonolactone to 2-keto-L-gulonolactone. The conversion of 2-keto-L-gulonolactone to L-ascorbic acid is a spontaneous reaction that does not require an enzyme. The asterisk denotes the carbon in the C1 position of a glucose molecule that will eventually become the carbon in the C6 position of ascorbic acid.

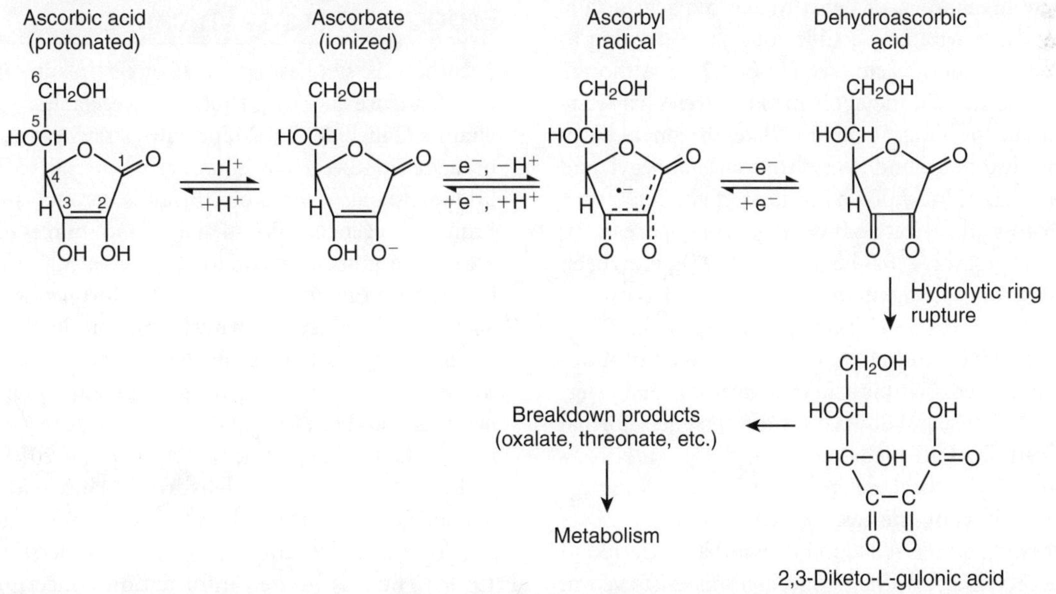

FIGURE 27-2 Ascorbic acid oxidation. Ascorbic acid at physiological pH is present predominantly as the ascorbate anion. Release of one electron ($e^{\bullet -}$) and one proton (H^+) (together a hydrogen atom) from ascorbate leads to formation of the ascorbyl radical. The single unpaired electron of the ascorbyl radical is highly delocalized, making it a relatively stable radical species. Release of another electron from the ascorbyl radical leads to formation of dehydroascorbic acid. Dehydroascorbic acid exists in more than one configuration, but only one is shown for simplicity. Formation of 2,3-diketo-L-gulonic acid by hydrolytic ring rupture is an irreversible step in ascorbate metabolism, leading to nonenzymatic formation of breakdown products that are further metabolized in the cell.

species and the relative stability of its free-radical form make ascorbate an ideal electron donor and strong antioxidant in biological systems. These roles of ascorbic acid are discussed later in this chapter.

ASCORBYL RADICAL

The ascorbyl radical, formed by partial oxidation of ascorbate, can be reduced to ascorbate, although the enzymes that catalyze this reduction have not been fully characterized. Ascorbyl radical reducing activities have been observed in membranes of mitochondria, endoplasmic reticulum (ER) and erythrocytes (May et al., 2001a), which may be a component of a transmembrane electron transfer system (see later section, Vitamin C Transport and Tissue Distribution). The ascorbyl radical can also be reduced by the cytosolic selenium-containing enzyme thioredoxin reductase (May et al., 1998). Furthermore, two molecules of ascorbyl radical react readily with each other in a nonenzymatic dismutation reaction that reduces one molecule of ascorbyl radical to ascorbate, while the other molecule is oxidized to dehydroascorbic acid (Bors and Buettner, 1997).

DEHYDROASCORBIC ACID

Dehydroascorbic acid may exist in one of several forms, and it is likely that the dominant form in vivo is the bicyclic hemiketal (Corpe et al., 2005). The term *dehydroascorbic acid* is used widely in the scientific literature; the designation "dehydroascorbate" is incorrect, because dehydroascorbic acid is not ionized under physiological conditions. Although dehydroascorbic acid is more stable than the ascorbyl radical, dehydroascorbic acid degradation at physiological pH occurs within minutes. At acidic pH, especially below pH 4, dehydroascorbic acid stability improves markedly. The breakdown of dehydroascorbic acid occurs through hydrolysis, with irreversible rupture of the ring to yield 2,3-diketo-L-gulonic acid (see Figure 27-2). Although 2,3-diketo-L-gulonic acid metabolism is not well characterized, its metabolic products include oxalate, threonate, threose, xylonate, lyxonate, and L-erythrulose (Banhegyi and Loewus, 2004). These breakdown products of vitamin C may enter the pentose phosphate pathway, gluconeogenesis, or other metabolic pathways (Banhegyi et al., 1997). It has been reported that carbons from vitamin C are released as carbon dioxide from cells or expired by animals (Baker et al., 1975). Additionally, murine and human erythrocytes can produce lactate when provided ascorbic acid (Braun et al., 1997), suggesting that ascorbate breakdown products can enter normal pathways of carbohydrate metabolism.

Like the ascorbyl radical, dehydroascorbic acid is rapidly reduced in vivo, either by one-electron reduction to the ascorbyl radical or two-electron reduction to ascorbate, referred to as "ascorbate recycling." Recycling mechanisms exist even in animals that synthesize ascorbic acid (Banhegyi et al., 1997), allowing them to recycle ascorbate that has been oxidized in the body or dehydroascorbic acid that has been ingested in the diet. Dehydroascorbic acid reduction in biological systems is accomplished through several pathways that ultimately require NADPH as the electron-donating agent (Arrigoni and De Tullio, 2002; Winkler et al., 1994). Dehydroascorbic acid can be reduced chemically by glutathione (GSH) or enzymatically by the GSH-dependent enzymes: glutaredoxin, protein disulfide isomerase, and dehydroascorbate [*sic*] reductase. Glutathione disulfide (GSSG) produced in these reactions is reduced back to GSH by the NADPH-dependent enzyme, glutathione disulfide reductase (Figure 27-3). In addition, dehydroascorbic acid can be reduced by the NADPH-dependent enzymes, 3α-hydroxysteroid dehydrogenase and thioredoxin reductase. Because depleting intracellular GSH leads to deficits in dehydroascorbic acid reduction capacity (May et al., 2001b; May et al., 1996), GSH-dependent mechanisms for ascorbate recycling appear to predominate in cells.

Nevertheless, recycling of ascorbate by reduction of dehydroascorbic acid and the ascorbyl radical in humans appears to be inefficient, because total body ascorbate is depleted over time on a vitamin C–free diet. Hence, nonsynthesizing species require vitamin C in the diet to make up for the deficit between recycling and destruction mechanisms. Currently there are no means to measure these rates separately in humans. What can be measured is ascorbate disappearance as a function of time and ascorbate dose, usually in plasma or blood cells. Such data show that when vitamin C ingestion ceases, healthy humans become vitamin C–deficient after approximately 30 days (Levine et al., 1996b; Levine et al., 2001). However, the time needed to reach a deficiency state depends on body stores when ingestion ceases and the rate of ascorbate oxidation, which can be influenced by many factors. Additionally, it is currently unknown if the rate of disappearance of vitamin C in plasma is indicative of the vitamin C status in all tissues. Some tissues, such as the brain, maintain higher vitamin C levels despite lower concentrations in other tissues.

FOOD SOURCES OF VITAMIN C

Ascorbate is synthesized in all green plants and is found in abundance in many fruits and vegetables. Fruits high in vitamin C include cantaloupe, kiwi, strawberries, lemons, and oranges. Good vegetable sources are broccoli, red pepper, cauliflower, spinach, tomatoes, Brussels sprouts, and asparagus. Fruit and vegetable juices that are good sources of the vitamin are orange, grapefruit, and tomato juices. Many foods, such as breakfast cereals and fruit drinks, are fortified with vitamin C. Vitamin C is present in many animal products, such as meat, poultry, and eggs, but is generally lost upon cooking or heating, making these foods unreliable sources of the vitamin. Unfortified grains and cereals and dairy products are generally low in vitamin C (U.S. Department of Agriculture, 2010).

Both ascorbate and dehydroascorbic acid are present in foods. Ascorbate predominates, accounting for 80% to 90% of the total vitamin C content (Vanderslice and Higgs, 1991). There is limited information concerning the relationship between food aging and progressive ascorbate oxidation and dehydroascorbic acid formation, but increased oxidation is expected during prolonged storage, which may be slowed by cooling or freezing (Vanderslice and Higgs, 1991). Food preparation also can have a significant effect on vitamin C content. Heating destroys vitamin C in foods,

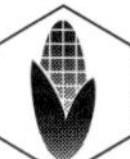

FOOD SOURCES OF VITAMIN C

Juices
60 to 90 mg per 6 fl oz orange juice
50 to 70 mg per 6 fl oz grapefruit juice
30 to 35 mg per 6 fl oz tomato juice
15 to 20 mg per 6 fl oz carrot or pineapple juice

Fruits
~180 mg per 1 papaya (304 g)
~70 mg per 1 kiwi fruit (76 g)
35 to 50 mg per ½ cup pineapple, papaya, oranges, or strawberries
15 to 35 mg per ½ cup raspberries, blackberries, grapefruit, or melon (honeydew or cantaloupe)

Vegetables
~90 to 150 mg per 1 sweet pepper, green or red (119 g)
~60 to 110 mg per 1 hot pepper, green or red (45 g)
35 to 50 mg per ½ cup broccoli, Brussels sprouts, kolhrabi, or edible pod peas
15 to 35 mg per ½ cup cauliflower, collards, kale, asparagus, cabbages, spinach, or soybeans

U.S. Department of Agriculture, Agricultural Research Service. (2010). *USDA National Nutrient Database for Standard Reference, Release 23.* Retrieved from www.ars.usda.gov/ba/bhnrc/ndl.

which is accelerated by the presence of metals like copper or iron, which may be released from the cooked food or from cooking receptacles. Foods cooked quickly will retain some vitamin C, and quick boiling or microwave steaming is usually recommended for preserving vitamin C in cooked vegetables (Miglio et al., 2008; Vanderslice and Higgs, 1991). Foods treated with heat before or during preservation (e.g., pasteurization) contain less vitamin C than the fresh food. Although vitamin C is relatively stable for extended periods of time in neutral or basic solutions, it is best preserved at acidic pH. Oxygen and light exposure also affect the vitamin C content of food.

Vitamin C is added to many food products to preserve freshness and enhance shelf life. Usually the amount of vitamin C added is minimal, and it may be oxidized during storage. The ascorbate epimer, erythorbic acid, also called D-isoascorbic acid and D-araboascorbic acid, is an antioxidant food additive used to preserve smoked or cured meats and some beverages. Although erythorbic acid has no vitamin C–like (antiscorbutic) activity, consumption of large amounts may result in false indications of ascorbate concentrations in blood or urine samples (Sauberlich et al., 1996).

VITAMIN C SUPPLEMENTS

L-Ascorbic acid can be synthesized inexpensively and is widely available as a dietary supplement. Natural and synthetic L-ascorbic acid are indistinguishable and readily bioavailable when taken in the diet or as a supplement. Vitamin C tablets are available in many forms, including as potassium, calcium, or magnesium salts or mixtures of ascorbic acid with other compounds purported to enhance vitamin C absorption. Mineral ascorbate formulations or other buffered preparations are beneficial for individuals with sensitivity to the acid content of vitamin C supplements. However, neither the mineral ascorbates nor alternative formulations of vitamin C have been demonstrated to have significantly increased bioavailability compared to free ascorbic acid or sodium ascorbate. There are no known factors that increase absorption of vitamin C into the body, but as research into vitamin C transporters continues, there is the possibility that dietary factors, or other coadministered supplements, that enhance vitamin C absorption will be discovered.

VITAMIN C TRANSPORT

VITAMIN C ABSORPTION AND BIOAVAILABILITY

Studies in guinea pigs have shown that ascorbic acid and dehydroascorbic acid are absorbed primarily in the jejunum of the small intestine (Rose, 1988). Ascorbate absorption is a sodium-dependent process, whereas absorption of dehydroascorbic acid is sodium-independent. Once absorbed, dehydroascorbic acid is reduced to ascorbate in enterocytes. Thus ingestion of either form of vitamin C results in ascorbate accumulation in the blood. In animals that are unable to synthesize vitamin C, ingested dehydroascorbic acid can prevent scurvy; but because there is extensive degradation of dehydroascorbic acid, much higher doses are needed compared to ascorbate (Ogiri et al., 2002). Dietary supplementation with dehydroascorbic acid should be avoided because of possible negative metabolic consequences of high intakes of dehydroascorbic acid (Arrigoni and De Tullio, 2002).

NUTRITION INSIGHT

What Is Bioavailability?

Bioavailability is a measure of the amount of substance absorbed into the bloodstream. To measure bioavailability, a substance is administered to a subject and the change in plasma concentration is measured by serial blood sampling over time. The data from the blood measurements are then displayed as a function of time. Differences between doses administered or the differences in absorption at a given dose in relation to route of delivery can be measured in this fashion. The *absolute bioavailability* is the difference between oral and intravenous administration of a substance at a given dose, measured by the difference in the area under the curve for the data collected. Thus absolute bioavailability is a measure of the amount of a vitamin or nutrient the subject absorbed through the gastrointestinal tract in relation to direct delivery into the bloodstream. Bioavailability is usually expressed as a percentage. One hundred percent bioavailability represents complete absorption. Many factors can affect bioavailability, including current status of the individual for a given nutrient, general health of the individual and delivery mechanisms that may increase or decrease absorption by the gut.

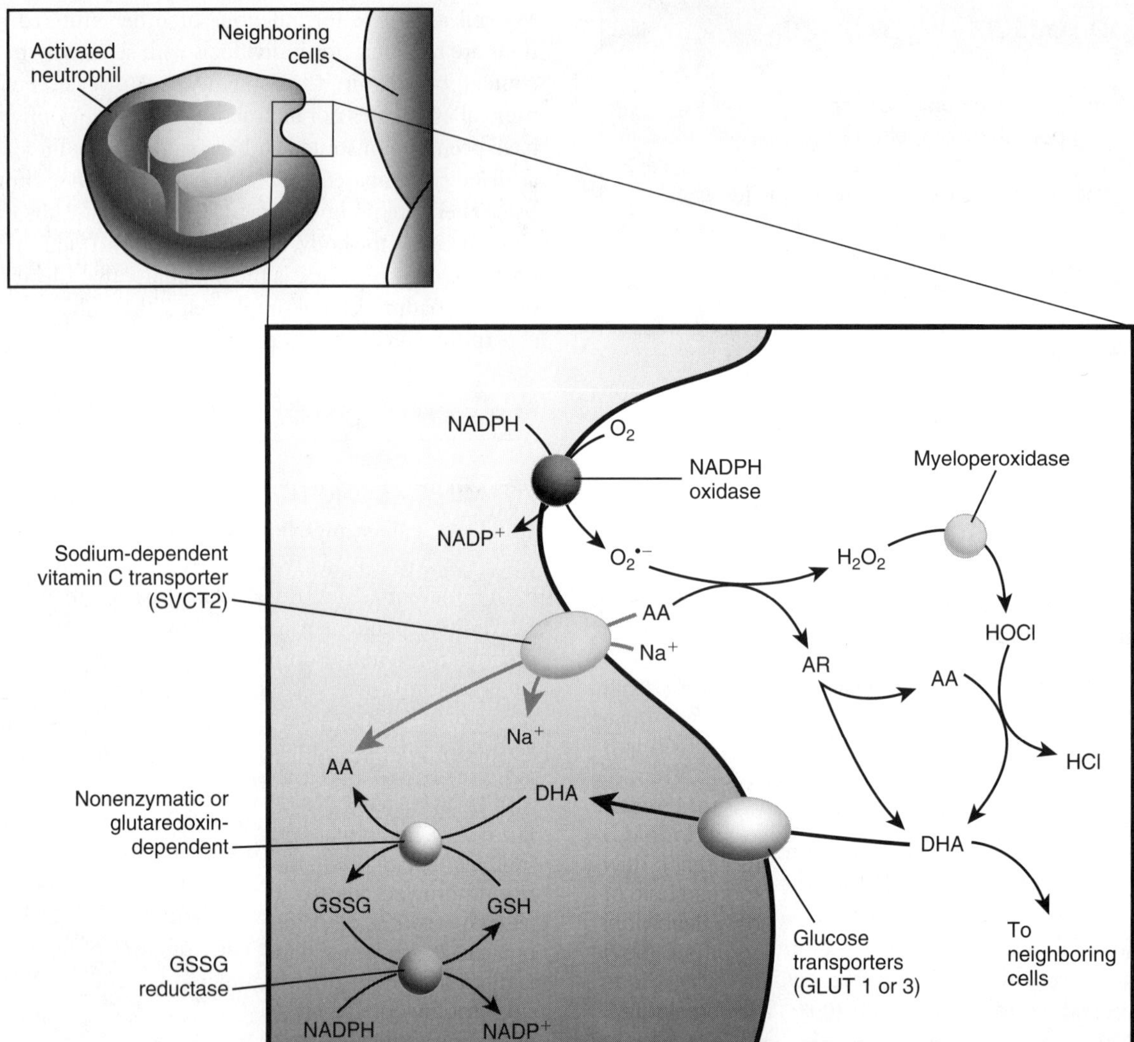

FIGURE 27-3 Mechanisms of vitamin C accumulation in human neutrophils. Vitamin C accumulation in neutrophils can occur by ascorbic acid (AA) uptake via the sodium-dependent vitamin C transporter 2 (SVCT2) or dehydroascorbic acid (DHA) transport and intracellular AA recycling. Activated neutrophils secrete superoxide radicals ($O_2^{\bullet-}$) from NADPH oxidase and release myeloperoxidase that produces hypochlorous acid (HOCl) from hydrogen peroxide (H_2O_2) and chloride. Both $O_2^{\bullet-}$ and HOCl may oxidize extracellular AA to ascorbyl radical (AR) and DHA. DHA is rapidly transported into neutrophils or nearby cells by glucose transporters (i.e., GLUT1 and GLUT3) and is immediately reduced intracellularly to AA by glutathione (GSH)-dependent reactions, either nonenzymatically or catalyzed by an enzyme such as glutaredoxin. GSH oxidized to glutathione disulfide (GSSG) during DHA reduction is regenerated by GSSG reductase and NADPH. NADPH is a product of glucose metabolism through the pentose phosphate pathway. Although the figure shows DHA uptake by GLUT1 and GLUT3, different cell types might use other glucose transporters.

The bioavailability and pharmacokinetics (or more appropriately, "micronutrient kinetics") of vitamin C have been determined in young, healthy individuals. These studies indicate that greater than 80% of a single vitamin C dose between 15 and 100 mg is absorbed (Graumlich et al., 1997; Levine et al., 1996b). Bioavailability declines for higher doses and is slightly less than 50% for a dose of 1,250 mg. Pharmacokinetic data for plasma and leukocyte vitamin C concentrations obtained from seven healthy young men previously depleted of vitamin C (Levine et al., 1996b) are shown in Figures 27-4 and 27-5, respectively. Similar results were obtained in women (Levine et al., 2001). At low doses of vitamin C (30 to 100 mg/day), there was a steep dose-dependent increase of plasma and cell ascorbate levels. Plasma ascorbate levels reached near-saturation at daily doses of 200 to 400 mg of vitamin C (see Figure 27-4), whereas cell ascorbate levels reached near-saturation at doses between 100 and 200 mg/day (see Figure 27-5). The shape of these curves for ascorbic acid bioavailability and pharmacokinetics is determined by the regulation of vitamin C transport mechanisms.

VITAMIN C TRANSPORT AND TISSUE DISTRIBUTION

After passing the small intestinal mucosa, vitamin C enters the mesenteric vein and hepatic portal venous system. Some of the vitamin C in the portal blood passes directly through the liver sinusoidal system into the hepatic vein, while a portion is retained by hepatocytes. Vitamin C distributes into the general circulation and extravascular space, where it

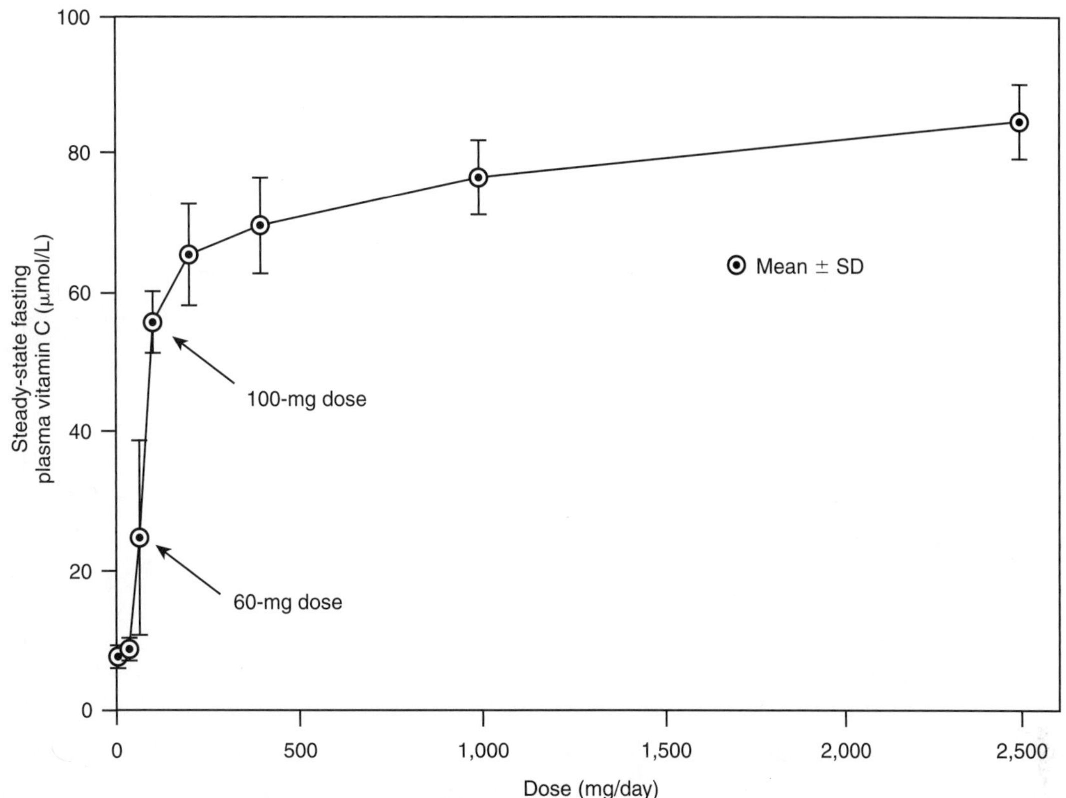

FIGURE 27-4 Steady-state fasting plasma vitamin C concentrations (mean ± SD) as a function of dose among seven healthy men previously depleted of vitamin C. Volunteers (ages 20 to 26 years) were studied as inpatients (study duration 146 ± 23 days, mean ± SD) and consumed a vitamin C–deficient diet throughout the depletion phase of the study, resulting in plasma and tissue vitamin C depletion before the start of the supplementation phase of the study. Vitamin C in solution was then administered by mouth at the doses shown until steady state was reached for each dose. Plasma vitamin C concentrations achieved by 60 mg/day and 100 mg/day oral vitamin C are indicated by the arrows in the figure. (Data from Levine, M., Conry-Cantilena, C., Wang, Y., Welch, R. W., Washko, P. W., Dhariwal, K. R., Park, J. B., Lazarev, A., Graumlich, J. F., King, J., & Cantilena, L. R. [1996]. Vitamin C pharmacokinetics in healthy volunteers: Evidence for a recommended dietary allowance. *Proceedings of the National Academy of Sciences of the United States of America, 93,* 3704-3709.)

can be taken up by peripheral tissues. When vitamin C in blood reaches the kidneys, it is freely filtered through the glomeruli and then reabsorbed in the proximal convoluted renal tubules and returned to the bloodstream. When tubular uptake of ascorbate is saturated because of high concentrations of ascorbate in the luminal fluid (i.e., the renal threshold of plasma ascorbate has been reached), any excess vitamin C that cannot be reabsorbed is excreted in the urine.

TRANSPORT OF ASCORBATE ACROSS CELL MEMBRANES

Ascorbate concentrations in plasma (usually 30 to 80 μmol/L) are lower than in tissues, most of which accumulate vitamin C in millimolar concentrations (Figure 27-6). Higher levels of ascorbate accumulate in extracellular fluids other than plasma, including air surface liquid of the respiratory tract (van der Vliet et al., 1999), gastric juices (Waring et al., 1996), cerebrospinal fluid (Bowman et al., 2010), seminal fluid (Fraga et al., 1991), and the aqueous humor of the eye (Taylor et al., 1991). It should be emphasized that the tissue concentrations of ascorbate shown in Figure 27-6 were obtained from limited literature sources, which are mostly compiled from older historical data (Hornig, 1975). The reported concentrations of ascorbate in most human tissues were not determined using modern techniques for preservation and analysis. More recent data, although limited, show that vitamin C levels in human tissues are higher than previously reported (Atanasova et al., 2005; Brubaker et al., 2000; Kathir et al., 2010; Kuiper et al., 2010; Waring et al., 1996) and similar to those measured in guinea pigs. Thus it is generally believed that adrenals, corneal epithelium, and pituitary glands have the highest concentrations of ascorbate in the human body. Other parts of the brain and eye, and spleen, pancreas, liver, and kidney also have high ascorbate levels, whereas most other tissues maintain relatively low millimolar levels ranging from 1 mg to 15 mg per 100 g of tissue (see Figure 27-6). In the blood, leukocytes maintain millimolar concentrations of ascorbate (Levine et al., 2001), whereas erythrocytes have the lowest cellular level because they do not concentrate vitamin C from the plasma (Evans et al., 1982).

RELATIONSHIP BETWEEN PLASMA AND TISSUE ASCORBATE LEVELS

It is often assumed that the relationship between vitamin C levels in plasma and tissues is the same regardless of the organ studied. However, data from vitamin C depletion studies in experimental animals suggest otherwise. Ascorbate levels do

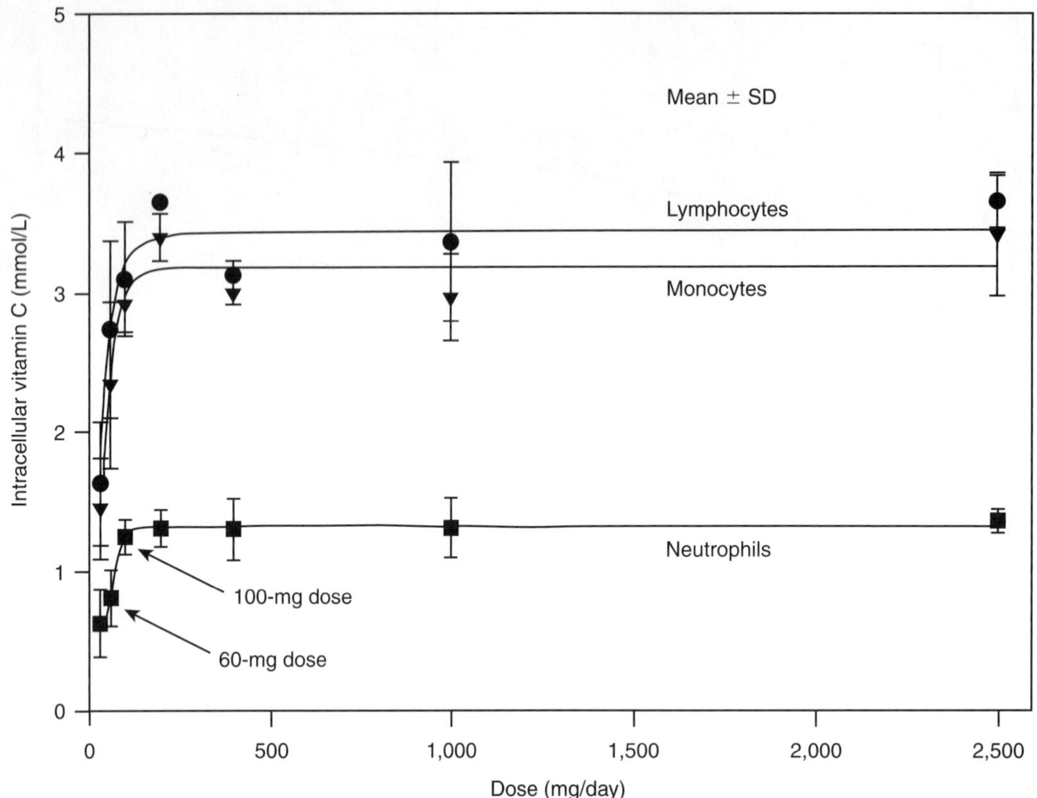

FIGURE 27-5 Intracellular vitamin C concentrations (mean ± SD) in circulating cells as a function of dose among seven healthy men previously depleted of vitamin C. Cells were isolated when steady state was achieved for each dose. Note that neutrophil vitamin C concentrations did not increase appreciably after the 100 mg/day dose. Eighty percent neutrophil saturation was achieved between 60 mg/day and 100 mg/day, and the neutrophil vitamin C concentrations at these doses are indicated in the figure. *Closed squares,* neutrophils; *closed triangles,* monocytes; *closed circles,* lymphocytes. (Data from Levine, M., Conry-Cantilena, C., Wang, Y., Welch, R. W., Washko, P. W., Dhariwal, K. R., Park, J. B., Lazarev, A., Graumlich, J. F., King, J., & Cantilena, L. R. [1996]. Vitamin C pharmacokinetics in healthy volunteers: Evidence for a recommended dietary allowance. *Proceedings of the National Academy of Sciences of the United States of America, 93,* 3704 -3709.)

not decline at the same rate in various tissues when plasma levels decrease. In particular, the brain and eye are less rapidly depleted than other organs of the body (Harrison et al., 2010b; Hill et al., 2003; Parsons et al., 2006; Tanaka et al., 1997). Upon Vitamin C-repletion, it is believed that ascorbate levels saturate in the brain before any other tissues, but the exact relationship with dietary vitamin C dose or plasma concentration is unknown. The organ-specific variation in vitamin C accumulation rates is considered an effect of the various vitamin C transporters in the body.

ACCUMULATION OF ASCORBATE IN TISSUES

Ascorbate is transported into cells by sodium-dependent vitamin C transporters (SVCTs) that exist in two different isoforms, SVCT1 and SVCT2 (Tsukaguchi et al., 1999). These two transporters belong to the nucleobase transporter superfamily (Hogue and Ling, 1999) but are otherwise dissimilar to other sodium-dependent transporters. Both transporters are highly specific for ascorbate and do not transport dehydroascorbic acid, glucose, or many other structurally related compounds (Rumsey et al., 1997; Tsukaguchi et al., 1999). However, some ascorbic acid derivatives with small structural changes are recognized by SVCTs (Corpe et al., 2005; Rumsey et al., 1999). SVCT1 and SVCT2 are also specific for transport of the sodium ion, cotransporting one or two sodium ions with each molecule of ascorbate into cells, although SVCT2 also requires calcium and magnesium for activity (Godoy et al., 2007). Removal of sodium from the extracellular fluid or inhibition of the Na^+/K^+-ATPase effectively halts all SVCT ascorbate-transport activity (Luo et al., 2008).

Primarily located on the apical side of polarized epithelial cells, SVCT1 is expressed in intestine, liver, kidney, lung, epididymis, ovary, prostate, placenta, pancreas, and skin (see Figure 27-6). SVCT1 has a K_m of approximately 60 to 200 μmol/L (Savini et al., 2008) and achieves a velocity approaching V_{max} at a concentration of about 1 mmol/L (Varma et al., 2008). SVCT1 is responsible for intestinal absorption of ascorbate by the enterocyte and renal reabsorption of ascorbate in the proximal tubules of the kidneys. SVCT1 knockout mice continuously excrete vitamin C in the urine and, as a result, have very low plasma vitamin C concentrations (Corpe et al., 2010).

SVCT2 is widely distributed in the body and expressed in every cell type except erythrocytes (May et al., 2007). SVCT2 has a reported K_m of approximately 5 to 60 μmol/L with a velocity approaching V_{max} at a concentration of about 60 to

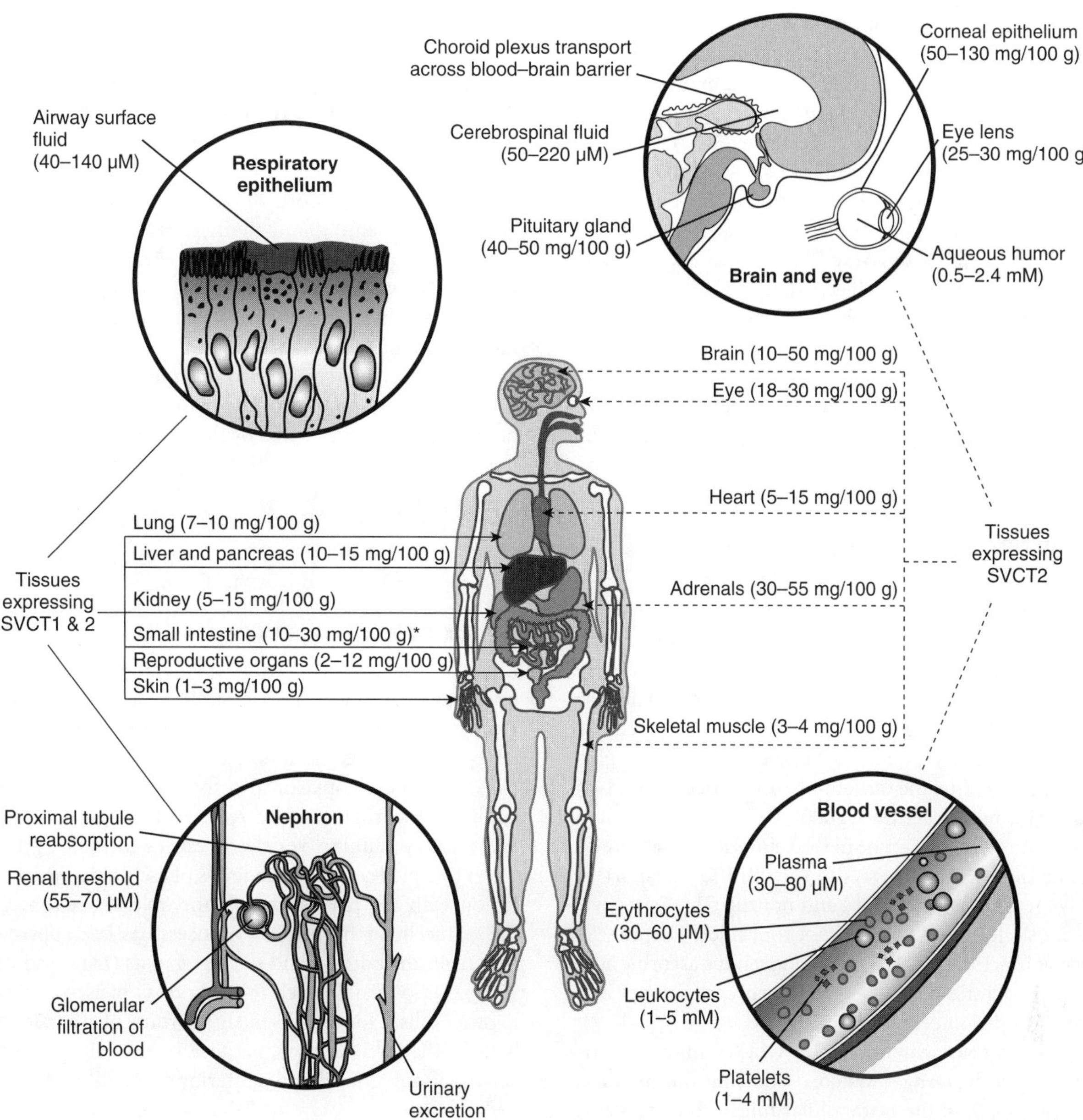

FIGURE 27-6 Tissue distribution of vitamin C and its transport proteins in the human body. Tissues in the body require the activity of sodium-dependent vitamin C transport proteins (SVCTs) to maintain physiological ascorbic acid levels. Tissues that primarily express SVCT2 have some of the highest vitamin C concentrations in the body, in particular, brain, eye, adrenal glands, leukocytes, and platelets. SVCT2 is also responsible for the maintenance of high ascorbic acid levels in cerebrospinal fluid and the aqueous humor of the eye. Tissues expressing SVCT1 also express SVCT2, and many of these tissues are also involved in the redistribution of vitamin C throughout the body (liver, kidney) or the interaction with the environment (lung, skin). SVCT1 helps maintain the plasma ascorbic acid concentration by controlling ascorbate reabsorption in the proximal tubules of the kidney, preventing loss of ascorbate in the urine. The ascorbate concentrations are from limited human data and are represented as mg/100 g wet weight for tissues and molarity (mM or μM) for intracellular and extracellular fluids. Asterisk indicates that the tissue concentrations of ascorbate in the small intestine are heavily dependent on recent dietary intake.

100 μmol/L (Savini et al., 2008). Hence, compared to SVCT1, which is responsible for bulk vitamin C transport, SVCT2 is a high-affinity, low-capacity vitamin C transporter. In epithelial cells that express both SVCTs, SVCT1 is found on the apical side and SVCT2 on the basolateral side (Boyer et al., 2005; Maulen et al., 2003; Subramanian et al., 2004). Thus, SVCT2 is responsible for the exit of ascorbate from enterocytes or renal proximal tubules so that it can enter the circulation. SVCT2 also is responsible for uptake of ascorbic acid into tissues from the extracellular fluid, and genetic deficiency of SVCT2 is associated with near-depletion of vitamin C in every tissue examined (Sotiriou et al., 2002). SVCT2 is required for the accumulation of vitamin C in tissues that display the highest concentrations (10 to 25 mmol/L) of the vitamin, such as brain and adrenals. SVCT2 knockout mice do not survive past birth, because they quickly develop cerebral hemorrhage

and are unable to breathe (Sotiriou et al., 2002), underscoring the need for vitamin C in normal prenatal development.

The regulatory mechanisms of SVCT gene expression and protein synthesis and activity are incompletely understood. In cell culture systems, SVCT2 messenger RNA (mRNA) levels increase in response to oxidative stress (Chi and May, 2009; May et al., 2010; Qiao et al., 2009; Savini et al., 2007) and factors that stimulate cell division (Fujita et al., 2001; Liang et al., 2002; Qiao and May, 2009; Wu et al., 2007). In general, these observations suggest that SVCT2 is a redox-sensitive vitamin C transporter. SVCT1 gene expression is regulated by the transcription factor, hepatocyte nuclear factor 1 (HNF1) (Michels and Hagen, 2009), but the exact mechanisms of this regulation are still under investigation. Both SVCT proteins may undergo posttranslational modification, influencing their activity and presentation on the surface of the plasma membrane (Savini et al., 2008).

CELLULAR UPTAKE OF DEHYDROASCORBIC ACID

As indicated earlier, SVCTs do not transport dehydroascorbic acid (Corpe et al., 2005; Daruwala et al., 1999; Takanaga et al., 2004). However, dehydroascorbic acid may be transported into cells by facilitated glucose transporters (Rumsey et al., 1997; Vera et al., 1993; Washko et al., 1993). Glucose transporters (GLUT) 1, 3, and 4 transport dehydroascorbic acid with high affinity, equal to or higher than that for glucose, which is due to the structural similarities of the two molecules (Rumsey et al., 1997, 2000). Dehydroascorbic acid is rapidly reduced to ascorbate in the cell, as described previously. The dominant pathways for vitamin C transport in the body seem to be the SVCTs and not the GLUTs, as evidenced most clearly by SVCT2 knockout mice. Despite the presence of functional GLUTs and endogenous ascorbic acid synthesis, these mice display severe ascorbate deficiency and die at birth (Sotiriou et al., 2002).

Dehydroascorbic acid uptake by GLUTs may be considered a rapid "scavenger system," allowing the oxidized form of vitamin C in the extracellular milieu to be recycled intracellularly. It has been proposed that erythrocytes, which contain GLUTs but no SVCTs in their plasma membrane, take up dehydroascorbic acid formed in plasma and reduce it intracellularly to ascorbate (May et al., 2001b). Heightened production and release of reactive oxygen species by activated phagocytes may result in oxidation of extracellular ascorbate to dehydroascorbic acid, followed by rapid, GLUT-mediated uptake of dehydroascorbic acid and intracellular ascorbate recycling (see Figure 27-3). This may occur by either the phagocytes themselves or other nearby cells, a process called the "bystander effect" (Nualart et al., 2003). Because of rapid scavenging mechanisms and the high rate of spontaneous decomposition (Retsky et al., 1993), dehydroascorbic acid cannot be reliably detected in plasma or tissues.

VITAMIN C UPTAKE BY CELLULAR ORGANELLES

Cellular organelles accumulate vitamin C, but neither the exact mechanism of ascorbate transport or steady-state levels of ascorbate in various cellular compartments have been determined. GLUTs have been implicated in the transport of dehydroascorbic acid across the membrane of the ER, where ascorbate transport is lacking (Banhegyi et al., 1998). Though not an ascorbate transport mechanism per se, single electrons from cytosolic ascorbate may be transferred via membrane-bound cytochrome b561 to the ER lumen, where they may be used to reduce ascorbyl radicals to ascorbate (Dhariwal et al., 1991; Fleming and Kent, 1991; Szarka et al., 2002). This process also provides reducing equivalents for enzymes that reside within the ER/Golgi/vesicular system such as dopamine β-hydroxylase (see later). The cytosolic ascorbyl radical produced by transfer of an electron from ascorbate to cytochrome b561 may then dismutate to form ascorbate and dehydroascorbic acid. By proximity, this dehydroascorbic acid may be transported by the GLUT transporters across the ER membrane. In the ER lumen, it can be recycled back to ascorbate thereby adding to its vitamin C content. A similar system has been described for electron transfer across the plasma membrane and is thought to occur primarily in erythrocytes (Lane and Lawen, 2009).

EFFLUX OF ASCORBATE FROM CELLS

Efflux of ascorbic acid from cells and tissues is not well understood but has been measured in several organs (Lane and Lawen, 2009). It has been proposed that general volume-sensitive organic anion channels may release ascorbate from the cytoplasm in response to osmotic stress. In addition, ascorbate can be released through exocytosis of ascorbate-containing vesicles. Vesicles formed by ER and Golgi complex contain high levels of ascorbate, which, upon fusion with the plasma membrane, release vitamin C into the extracellular milieu. This process has been observed in cells from the adrenal and salivary glands (Lane and Lawen, 2009). Although it is unclear if exocytosis of ascorbate occurs in other cells, exocytosis is likely the route of efflux for ascorbate synthesized de novo, because L-gulonolactone oxidase activity is only found in the interior of the ER of liver.

ENZYMATIC FUNCTIONS OF VITAMIN C

Vitamin C is known to participate as an electron donor required for maximum activity of several biosynthetic enzymes (Englard and Seifter, 1986; Levine, 1986). Three enzymes are found in fungi and are involved in reutilization pathways for pyrimidines or the deoxyribose moiety of deoxynucleosides. Because these enzymes are not known to be involved in reactions in mammals, they will not be discussed further. The known vitamin C–dependent mammalian enzymes participate in hydroxylation of procollagen and other proteins, amidation of peptide hormones tyrosine metabolism, and carnitine and norepinephrine biosynthesis. Additional enzymes using vitamin C as a reducing agent may exist, but the specificity of these enzyme reactions for ascorbate has not been experimentally established.

Enzymes that require ascorbate have either monooxygenase or dioxygenase activity. The monooxygenases, dopamine β-hydroxylase and peptidylglycine α-monooxygenase,

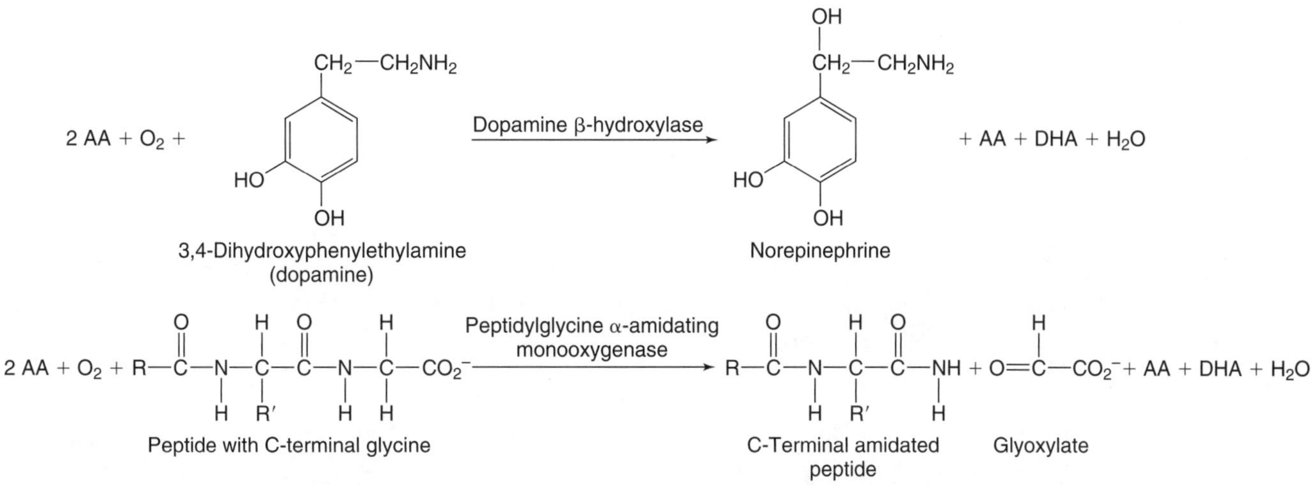

2 AA + O_2 + 3,4-Dihydroxyphenylethylamine (dopamine) —Dopamine β-hydroxylase→ Norepinephrine + AA + DHA + H_2O

2 AA + O_2 + Peptide with C-terminal glycine —Peptidylglycine α-amidating monooxygenase→ C-Terminal amidated peptide + Glyoxylate + AA + DHA + H_2O

FIGURE 27-7 The reactions of ascorbic acid–requiring monooxygenases. The action of dopamine β-hydroxylase is the addition of a single oxygen atom to the ethylamine side chain on dopamine, forming a hydroxyl group. The other atom of oxygen is incorporated into water. Peptidylglycine α-amidating monooxygenase catalyzes the hydroxylation of a peptide with a C-terminal glycine meeting certain target signal criteria, followed by the cleavage of glyoxylate. This results in a shorter peptide with an amide group. *AA,* Ascorbic acid; *DHA,* dehydroascorbic acid.

incorporate a single oxygen atom into a substrate, either dopamine or a peptide with a terminal glycine (Figure 27-7). Both monooxygenase enzymes require two copper atoms in their active site to be reduced by ascorbate, receiving one electron from each of two ascorbate molecules (Fleming and Kent, 1991; Stewart and Klinman, 1988). The ascorbyl radicals formed during this reaction dismutate, resulting in the full oxidation of one molecule of ascorbate per enzyme cycle.

The remaining enzymes are dioxygenases, which incorporate molecular oxygen (O_2), with each oxygen atom incorporated in a different way. Most of these dioxygenases require α-ketoglutarate as a cosubstrate and incorporate one oxygen atom into α-ketoglutarate (with decarboxylation and formation of succinate) and the other oxygen atom into the enzyme-specific substrate (Figure 27-8). One exception is 4-hydroxyphenylpyruvate dioxygenase, which incorporates both oxygen atoms into different locations of the same substrate (4-hydroxyphenylpyruvate). These dioxygenase enzymes can proceed along their normal biological reaction sequence in the absence of ascorbate as long as sufficient substrate is present, incorporating electrons from the α-keto acid cosubstrate into the specific substrate. If the substrate concentration becomes limiting, however, the enzyme performs an uncoupled reaction oxidizing its iron center so that the enzymatic reaction can no longer proceed. In this case, ascorbate donates its electrons to the resulting Fe(IV)=O/Fe(III)-$O^{\bullet-}$ complex, restoring the enzyme to an active state (see Figure 27-8). In this manner, ascorbate acts as a "pseudo-cofactor" for the reaction. However, uncoupled enzyme activity and formation of an oxidized iron complex have not been demonstrated unequivocally in vivo, leaving the exact role of ascorbate in dioxygenase function subject to further debate.

Although ascorbate is required for maximum activity of these enzymes, at least in vitro, other electron donors can take the place of ascorbate in vivo as well as in cultured cells devoid of ascorbate. Various molecules may serve in this role if ascorbate is limiting. However, the K_m for ascorbate of these monooxygenases and dioxygenases is relatively low (less than 1 mmol/L), below the ascorbate concentration in most cells, suggesting that small amounts of vitamin C in the diet may be sufficient to sustain full enzyme activity in vivo. Nevertheless, prolonged vitamin C deficiency results in impairments in the activities of these enzymes.

MONOOXYGENASES

Dopamine β-Hydroxylase

Dopamine β-hydroxylase is necessary for hydroxylation of dopamine during the synthesis of the catecholamine, norepinephrine, in peripheral neurons, central neurons, and the adrenal medulla. Because of its abundance, the enzyme from the adrenal medulla has been characterized in detail. The enzyme is a tetrameric glycoprotein, with subunits arranged as pairs of disulfide-linked monomeric species. There are both membrane-bound and soluble enzyme forms, which probably differ in subunit composition (Fleming and Kent, 1991). The enzyme contains two copper atoms per subunit. Dopamine β-hydroxylase is localized in neurosecretory vesicles of neurons and in secretory vesicles (chromaffin granules) of the adrenal medulla (Levine et al., 1991).

The enzyme uses molecular oxygen and dopamine as substrates and ascorbate as the preferred electron donor, as shown in Figure 27-7. The kinetics for ascorbate in norepinephrine biosynthesis were determined in situ, meaning in intact animal tissue (Levine et al., 1991). The K_m of dopamine β-hydroxylase for intravesicular ascorbate was found to be approximately 0.5 mmol/L, which is similar to that of the isolated enzyme (Kaufman, 1974). Intact secretory vesicles of the brain and adrenals contain 10 to 15 mmol/L of ascorbate, which is sufficient to saturate dopamine β-hydroxylase with ascorbate.

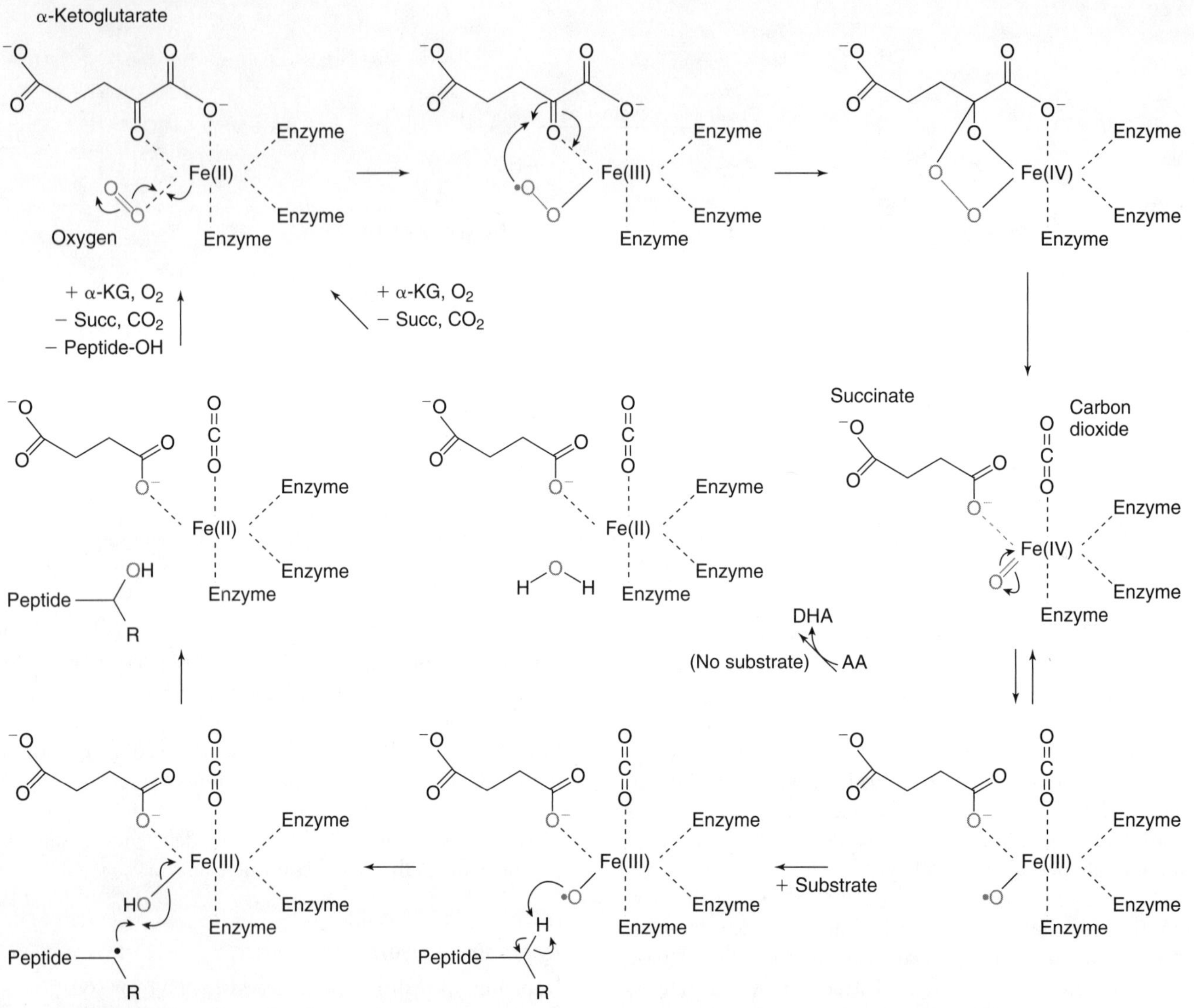

FIGURE 27-8 Reaction mechanisms of prolyl hydroxylase and lysyl hydroxylase. The order of binding of O_2 and the polypeptide substrate are uncertain, as is the order of release of the hydroxylated peptide and CO_2. The reaction may proceed in the absence of ascorbate if sufficient substrate polypeptides are available. If the polypeptide substrate polypeptide concentration becomes limiting, the enzyme catalyzes an uncoupled decarboxylation reaction of α-ketoglutarate cosubstrate that results in oxidation of the enzyme's iron center. After such an event, the enzyme cannot perform any catalytic reactions because the reactive iron–oxo complex is probably converted to an Fe(III)–$O^{\bullet-}$ complex. Ascorbate is needed to reactivate the enzyme by reducing Fe(III) to Fe(II). *AA,* Ascorbic acid; *α-KG,* α-ketoglutarate; *DHA,* dehydroascorbic acid; *Enzyme,* enzyme peptide residues linking the iron center; *Peptide-OH,* hydroxylated peptide; *Succ,* succinate.

Peptidylglycine α-Amidating Monooxygenase

Many biologically active peptides are synthesized from inactive precursors by posttranslational modification. To confer activity to many bioactive peptides, a carboxy-terminal α-amide group must be added by a process called α-amidation. α-Amidation is mediated by peptidylglycine α-amidating monooxygenase (PAM) (Eipper et al., 1993; Prigge et al., 2000). Amidated peptide hormones include thyrotropin-releasing hormone, gonadotropin-releasing hormone, oxytocin, vasopressin, cholecystokinin, gastrin, calcitonin, substance P, and neuropeptide Y.

PAM is a bifunctional enzyme that contains two distinct monofunctional domains connected by a linker region (Eipper et al., 1993; Prigge et al., 2000). The two domains are peptidylglycine α-hydroxylating monooxygenase (PHM) and peptidyl-α-hydroxyglycine α-amidating lyase (PAL). PAM is localized in secretory vesicles, where it is anchored to the vesicle membrane (Eipper et al., 1993; Prigge et al., 2000). Amidation is a two-step reaction, with each reaction mediated by one of the PAM domains. The initial, rate-limiting reaction is mediated by PHM and results in hydroxylation of the C-terminal glycine of the substrate peptide with formation of peptidylhydroxyglycine. In the second step, which is mediated by PAL, the peptidylhydroxyglycine moiety is cleaved into glyoxylate and the amidated peptide. The overall reaction is shown in Figure 27-7.

PHM is similar to dopamine β-hydroxylase in several respects. Both enzymes are monooxygenases. PHM and dopamine β-hydroxylase share significant amino acid sequence similarity, indicating that these enzymes are evolutionarily linked. The enzymes have 28% identity extending through a common catalytic domain of approximately 270 residues (Eipper et al., 1993; Prigge et al., 2000). Like dopamine β-hydroxylase, PHM requires ascorbate, oxygen, and copper. In addition, PAM uses intravesicular ascorbate maintained by transmembrane transfer, similar to dopamine β-hydroxylase (Eipper et al., 1993; Prigge et al., 2000).

DIOXYGENASES

Prolyl 4-Hydroxylase, Prolyl 3-Hydroxylase, and Lysyl Hydroxylase

A cardinal symptom of vitamin C deficiency is poor wound healing, which provided an early clue that vitamin C may be involved in collagen biosynthesis (Lind, 1753; Peterkofsky, 1991). The well-characterized enzymatic role of vitamin C in collagen biosynthesis is its participation in prolyl and lysyl hydroxylase reactions. Hydroxylation of the proline residues greatly increases the stability of collagen under physiological conditions, whereas some of the hydroxylysine residues undergo further modifications that aid collagen's function. Newly synthesized collagen precursor proteins, called procollagen, undergo modification in the ER before translocation to the Golgi apparatus (see Chapter 5). Hydroxylation of certain proline and lysine residues occurs along the length of procollagen polypeptides (Figure 27-9), which stimulates proper folding of the polypeptides and increases extracellular stability of mature collagen. Vitamin C acts with prolyl 3-hydroxylase, prolyl 4-hydroxylase, and lysyl hydroxylase for procollagen hydroxylation (Myllyharju, 2003; Peterkofsky, 1991).

Much of what is known about dioxygenase reactions and the role of ascorbate has been derived from the study of prolyl and lysyl hydroxylases. These dioxygenases have specific binding sites for ascorbate near the iron center (Majamaa et al., 1986), but it is not clear whether ascorbate binds to these sites during the normal catalytic cycle. If this were the case, ascorbate might help prevent the active-site iron from becoming oxidized, without ascorbate being oxidized itself. However, the only experimentally verified reaction of the enzyme with ascorbate is the reduction by ascorbate of the enzyme's oxidized iron center following an uncoupled reaction, as shown in Figure 27-8.

Vitamin C also appears to affect procollagen gene transcription and mRNA stability and the release of mature collagen from cells, but the underlying mechanisms are currently poorly understood (Peterkofsky, 1991).

Hypoxia Inducible Factor Hydroxylases

Hydroxylation of proline and asparagine residues has been described as a regulatory mechanism for the transcription factor, hypoxia inducible factor 1α (HIF-1α). HIF-1α is synthesized constitutively in cells, but under normal cellular oxygen concentrations (normoxia) key proline and asparagine residues are hydroxylated (see Figure 27-9), leading to HIF-1α proteosomal degradation (Figure 27-10). Hydroxylation of HIF-1α does not occur under some conditions, in particular, low oxygen concentrations (hypoxia). Without hydroxylation, HIF-1α binds with HIF-1β to form a stable dimer, which induces hypoxia-responsive genes that play a role in angiogenesis, erythropoiesis, and glycolysis (Bardos and Ashcroft, 2005; Marin-Hernandez et al., 2009; Pugh and Ratcliffe, 2003). HIF-1α is critical to initiating apoptosis in neutrophils, a normal process critical for the resolution of inflammation (Vissers and Wilkie, 2007). Elevated HIF-1α levels have been found in many solid tumors and are linked to poor prognosis in cancer patients (Rankin and Giaccia, 2008). It is not clear if the increase in HIF-1α in tumors is due to the hypoxia that normally occurs in large, poorly vascularized tumors, or if its expression is enhanced during cancer progression as a consequence of gene dysregulation. In either case, HIF-1α is considered a promising target for cancer therapy.

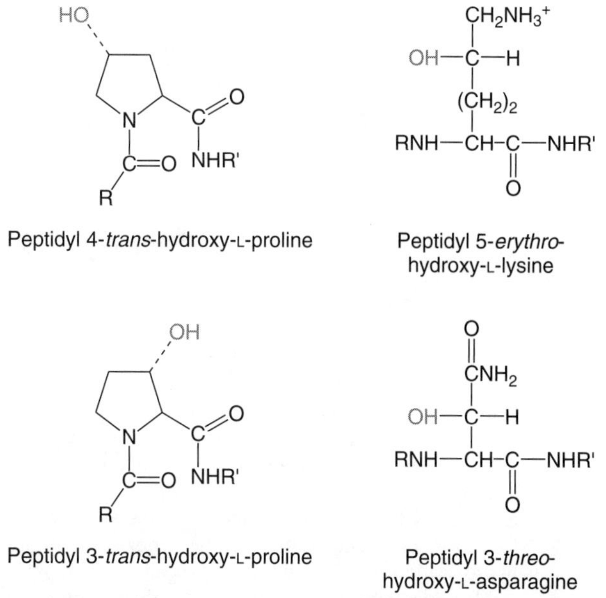

Peptidyl 4-*trans*-hydroxy-L-proline

Peptidyl 5-*erythro*-hydroxy-L-lysine

Peptidyl 3-*trans*-hydroxy-L-proline

Peptidyl 3-*threo*-hydroxy-L-asparagine

FIGURE 27-9 Reaction products of prolyl, lysyl, and asparaginyl hydroxylases. R and R′ represent the N- and C-terminal portions of the polypeptide containing the hydroxylated residue.

HIF-1α proline hydroxylation is accomplished by a distinct family of prolyl 4-hydroxylases (PH) termed PHD1, PHD2, and PHD3. In addition, a protein called factor inhibiting HIF (FIH) acts as the associated HIF-1α asparaginyl hydroxylase. These enzymes require ascorbate for full activity in a similar fashion to the collagen prolyl and lysyl hydroxylases (Bruick and McKnight, 2001; Myllyharju, 2003). Ascorbate deficiency is thought to lead to loss of hydroxylation and stabilization of HIF-1α under normoxic conditions (Bruick and McKnight, 2001; Myllyharju, 2003).

Currently, the effects of low tissue ascorbate levels are being investigated in cancer, anemia, and ischemic heart disease for HIF-1α hydroxylase involvement (Chen et al., 2009; Rankin and Giaccia, 2008).

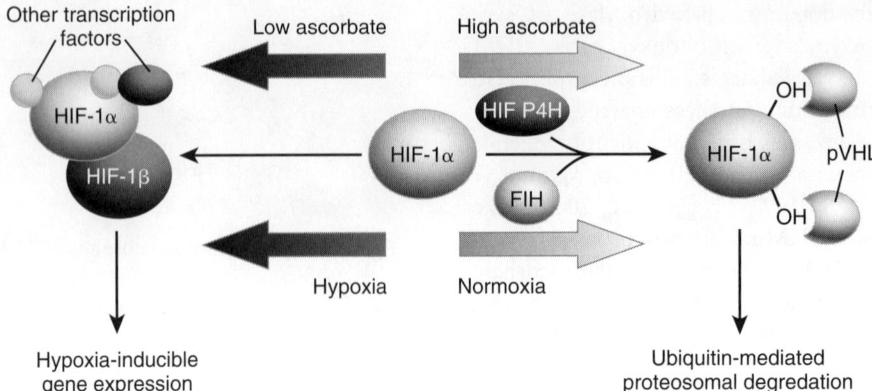

FIGURE 27-10 Regulation of the hypoxia-inducible transcription factor, HIF-1α, by oxygen- and ascorbate-dependent prolyl 4-hydroxylation. Under normoxia (*right-pointing arrows*), HIF-1α undergoes prolyl 4-hydroxylation by HIF prolyl 4-hydroxylase (HIF P4H) and asparaginyl hydroxylation by factor-inhibiting HIF-1 (FIH). The same reactions also occur when intracellular vitamin C concentrations are above the K_m for each of these enzymes (~150 to 300 μmol/L). Hydroxylation is necessary for subsequent binding of the von Hippel–Lindau (pVHL) E3 ubiquitin ligase complex, which targets HIF-1α for proteosomal degradation. Under hypoxia and/or ascorbate concentrations below the K_m of HIF P4H and FIH, no prolyl hydroxylation of HIF-1α occurs (*left-pointing arrows*). Under these conditions, HIF-1α is not degraded and instead forms a stable dimer with HIF-1β. This dimer is then translocated to the nucleus, where it binds to HIF-responsive elements in the promoter region of hypoxia-inducible genes, inducing their expression.

Trimethyllysine Hydroxylase and γ-Butyrobetaine Hydroxylase

One of the first clinical effects of vitamin C deprivation is fatigue (Levine et al., 1996b, 2001; Lind, 1753), a symptom that precedes scurvy (see later). L-Carnitine, a zwitterionic quaternary amino acid, is required to form acyl carnitine derivatives that transfer long-chain fatty acids into mitochondria for subsequent β-oxidation and ATP synthesis (see Chapter 16). Ascorbic acid participates in two hydroxylation reactions that are required for the synthesis of carnitine from its amino acid precursors, lysine and methionine.

In mammals, certain proteins containing lysine are methylated using *S*-adenosylmethionine to form ε-*N*-trimethyllysine residues, which are subsequently released by proteolytic cleavage. The free trimethyllysine may then undergo a four-step reaction sequence to form carnitine (Figure 27-11). The first reaction is hydroxylation of ε-*N*-trimethyllysine to β-hydroxy-ε-*N*-trimethyllysine catalyzed by trimethyllysine hydroxylase. In the second reaction, glycine is released to form γ-trimethylaminobutyraldehyde, which undergoes dehydrogenation in the third reaction to form γ-butyrobetaine. In the fourth reaction, γ-butyrobetaine is hydroxylated by γ-butyrobetaine hydroxylase, with carnitine as the product (Dunn et al., 1984; Englard and Seifter, 1986; Rebouche, 1991).

The two hydroxylation reactions in the carnitine synthesis pathway are catalyzed by dioxygenases that require iron, α-ketoglutarate, and ascorbate (Dunn et al., 1984). Although it has not been extensively studied, the mechanism of ascorbate action is probably similar to that in the prolyl and lysyl hydroxylase reactions, where ascorbate maintains iron in a reduced state, while the reducing equivalents for the hydroxylation reaction are obtained via the oxidative decarboxylation of cosubstrate α-ketoglutarate (Englard and Seifter, 1986).

Although these two enzymes for carnitine biosynthesis are most active with ascorbate as a reductant, carnitine

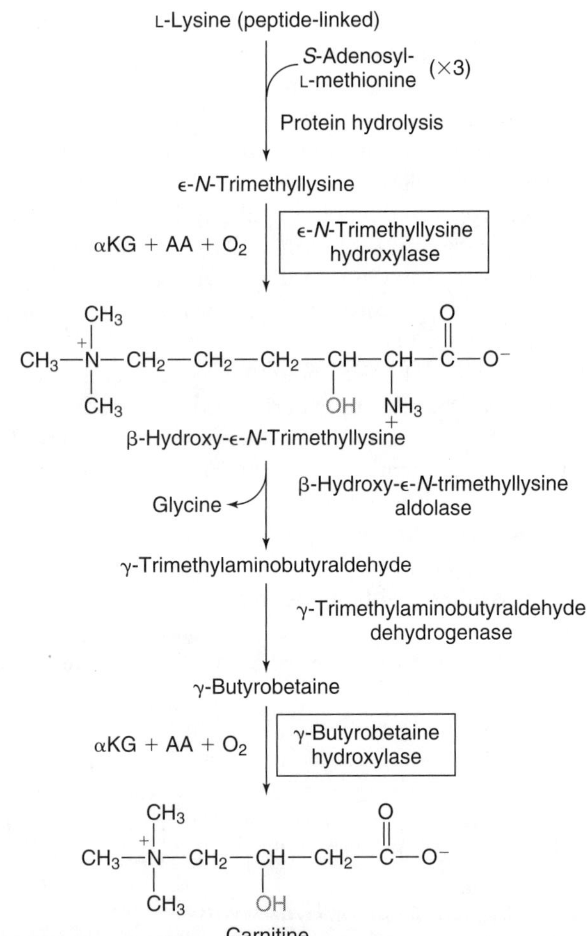

FIGURE 27-11 Pathway of carnitine biosynthesis in mammals. ε-*N*-trimethyllysine hydroxylase and γ-butyrobetaine hydroxylase are the enzymes that use ascorbic acid (AA). *αKG*, α-Ketoglutarate. (Redrawn from Rebouche, C. J. [1991]. Ascorbic acid and carnitine biosynthesis. *The American Journal of Clinical Nutrition, 54,* 1147S-1152S.)

biosynthesis is not strictly dependent on ascorbate. Vitamin C–deficient guinea pigs provided with excess substrate for these hydroxylation reactions, such as trimethyllysine or γ-butyrobetaine, showed nearly normal rates of carnitine biosynthesis, indicating that other reducing agents can replace ascorbate in vivo (Rebouche, 1995). Furthermore, recent data show that vitamin C–deficient gulonolactonase-knockout mice exhibit no changes in the capacity to synthesize carnitine (Furusawa et al., 2008), and lethargy in ascorbate-deficient SVCT1 knockout mice is not affected by carnitine supplementation (Corpe et al., 2010). Together, these findings suggest that carnitine biosynthesis is not strictly dependent on the availability of vitamin C, and conversely carnitine levels are not a sensitive indicator of vitamin C status.

4-Hydroxyphenylpyruvate Dioxygenase

As part of tyrosine catabolism, 4-hydroxyphenylpyruvate dioxygenase catalyzes the conversion of 4-hydroxyphenylpyruvate to homogentisate (Moran, 2005). The enzyme uses molecular oxygen to catalyze coupled oxidations. It appears to be a true dioxygenase and is similar to other keto acid–dependent dioxygenases, such as the α-ketoglutarate-dependent dioxygenases that are involved in prolyl and lysyl hydroxylation and carnitine synthesis. However, in the hydroxyphenylpyruvate reaction, the α-keto acid required for electron donation is part of the same molecule that is hydroxylated (Figure 27-12) (Englard and Seifter, 1986).

As for other dioxygenases, ascorbate is used by hydroxyphenylpyruvate dioxygenase as a pseudo-cofactor to reduce the iron center after an uncoupled enzyme reaction has occurred. Animal studies and clinical trials support a relationship between ascorbate deficiency and tyrosine metabolism (Englard and Seifter, 1986). Scorbutic guinea pigs have excess tyrosine in the circulation (tyrosinemia) and excrete 4-hydroxyphenylpyruvate in urine. Premature human infants display the same pattern. In both guinea pigs and premature infants, ascorbate administration eliminates tyrosinemia and hydroxyphenylpyruvate excretion. Nevertheless, it remains possible that the effect of ascorbate is indirect (Englard and Seifter, 1986).

OTHER ENZYMES

Ascorbate has been postulated to act as a reducing agent for a number of other hydroxylases and dioxygenases, but they are not considered canonical ascorbate-dependent enzymes because there is no conclusive supporting evidence. Good candidate enzymes for the influence of ascorbate on catalytic activity are cholesterol-7α-hydroxylase (Bjorkhem and Kallner, 1976; Holloway et al., 1981), indoleamine 2,3-dioxygenase (Littlejohn et al., 2000; Werner and Werner-Felmayer, 2007), and β-carotene-15,15′-dioxygenase (von Lintig and Vogt, 2000), which are involved in bile acid production, tryptophan metabolism, and retinoid formation, respectively. Additionally, many of the α-ketoglutarate–dependent dioxygenases have been presumed to require ascorbate as a pseudo-cofactor, although empirical data are lacking in support of these claims.

NONENZYMATIC FUNCTIONS OF VITAMIN C

Vitamin C has numerous nonenzymatic functions, some of which remain controversial, as the validity and physiological relevance of some of the experimental systems used to investigate these functions are unclear. Similar to its function in enzymatic reactions, ascorbate also acts as an electron donor in all of its nonenzymatic reactions. Though in some of these reactions ascorbate acts as an antioxidant, it can also function as a prooxidant. It is important to note that ascorbate does not function in either role alone but within a certain context involving other biological reactants. Interpreting the role of vitamin C in biological systems should be done with caution, because ascorbate can function simultaneously as an antioxidant and a prooxidant. It is also important to note that whereas ascorbate and the ascorbyl radical can act as electron donors, dehydroascorbic acid cannot. The functions of dehydroascorbic acid in biological systems are limited and may have little relevance in vivo.

VITAMIN C AS A BIOLOGICAL REDUCTANT

Iron Absorption

Vitamin C supplements are used clinically to increase nonheme iron absorption. In the small intestine, vitamin C strongly enhances iron absorption by reducing dietary ferric

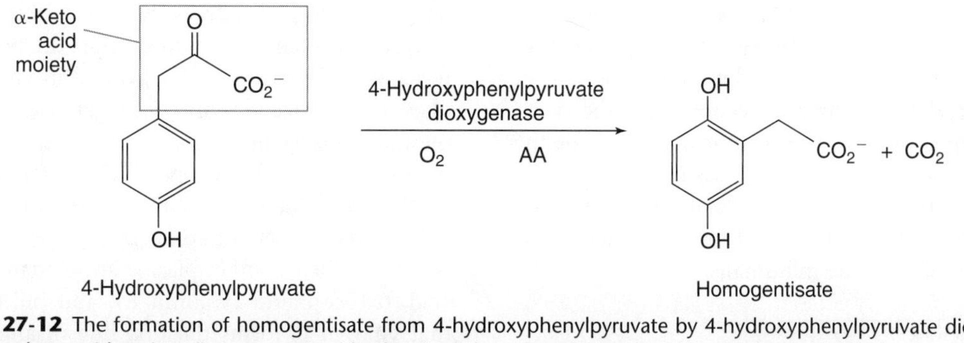

FIGURE 27-12 The formation of homogentisate from 4-hydroxyphenylpyruvate by 4-hydroxyphenylpyruvate dioxygenase. The α-keto acid moiety (i.e., pyruvate side-chain) of the substrate (enclosed in the rectangle) is the source of the electrons needed to complete the enzymatic reaction, resulting in the addition to a hydroxyl substituent on C4 of the hydroxyphenyl ring and the oxidative decarboxylation and rearrangement of the pyruvate side chain on the phenyl ring, called the NIH shift. *AA,* Ascorbic acid.

(Fe^{3+}) iron to ferrous (Fe^{2+}) iron and forming an absorbable iron–ascorbic acid complex. Soluble inorganic iron absorption is increased 1.5 to 10 times by vitamin C coingestion, depending on body iron status, vitamin C dose, and whether food is involved in the delivery. Amounts of vitamin C that enhance iron absorption are commonly found in foods that are good sources of the vitamin (Hallberg, 1995). The effect of vitamin C on iron absorption can result in a modest elevation of hemoglobin concentration in anemic patients, at least in the short term (Cook and Reddy, 2001).

Reactions with Dietary Nitrates

Vitamin C can readily react with nitrites and nitrates. Although nitrites and nitrates can be formed by reactions with nitric oxide, they are commonly found in the diet. Not only are nitrates found in vegetables, but they are used as preservatives and curing agents in many processed foods. These compounds have the potential for reacting with proteins in the digestive tract, producing *N*-nitroso compounds that have been linked to gastric cancer. Ascorbate, when present during the digestion of nitrites and nitrates, especially in the stomach, reduces them to less harmful products, including nitric oxide, thereby preventing protein damage and reducing cancer risk (Mirvish et al., 1998).

Ascorbylation

Although not a reduction reaction per se, ascorbate can act as a nucleophile and react with electrophiles, many of which are present in the diet or formed upon lipid peroxidation. The process of this ascorbic acid adduction has been called ascorbylation, and it may help detoxify these electrophilic compounds (Kesinger and Stevens, 2009; Miranda et al., 2009). As with the reactions with nitrate, ascorbylation is more likely to occur in the digestive tract, before absorption can occur, although some reactions may occur in plasma and tissues.

Recycling of Tetrahydrobiopterin

Ascorbate has been shown to maintain or increase tetrahydrobiopterin levels in cells, most likely by reduction of one of the oxidized forms of tetrahydrobiopterin, trihydrobiopterin. Tetrahydrobiopterin is a cofactor needed in several enzymes, some of which have hydroxylase activity. One of these enzymes, endothelial nitric oxide synthase (eNOS), produces nitric oxide, a gaseous substance that exerts a variety of effects in the vasculature, including vasodilation by smooth muscle relaxation and inhibition of platelet aggregation. Recycling of tetrahydrobiopterin, rather than scavenging of superoxide radicals, is now thought to be the mechanism by which vitamin C increases nitric oxide synthesis and biological activity in the vasculature (Heller et al., 2001), thereby improving endothelial function and potentially reducing blood pressure in humans.

VITAMIN C AS AN ANTIOXIDANT

The most important nonenzymatic function of vitamin C is to act as a biological antioxidant or "free radical scavenger." The standard one-electron reduction potential of ascorbic acid, which measures the ability of a molecule to donate an electron to another molecule, is approximately 0.28 volts, and that of the ascorbyl radical about −0.17 volts. The standard reduction potentials of various redox-active compounds are shown in Table 27-1. As suggested by their placement in the "pecking order" of electron donors and acceptors, ascorbate and the ascorbyl radical have the potential to reduce a variety of harmful biological oxidants, or "reactive oxygen species". If left unchecked, these reactive oxygen species can alter cell signaling pathways and enhance inflammatory gene transcription, impair cell function, and initiate apoptosis. They may also react with and oxidatively damage biological macromolecules, such as lipids, proteins, and DNA, which has been implicated in many human diseases (Halliwell and Gutterige, 2007).

In addition to its favorable one-electron reduction potential, another reason ascorbate is such an efficient antioxidant is that its one-electron oxidation product, the ascorbyl radical, is a highly delocalized, and thus relatively stable, radical species that does not cause oxidative damage. Instead, the ascorbyl radical can scavenge another free radical species or, more likely, readily undergo dismutation to ascorbate and dehydroascorbic acid, thereby regenerating one molecule of ascorbate available for another free-radical scavenging reaction (see Figure 27-2).

In biological systems, many different reactive oxygen and nitrogen species are formed that have the potential to cause oxidative and "nitrative" damage. For example, superoxide radicals, peroxynitrite, hydrogen peroxide, and hypochlorous acid (the active component in bleach) are all formed during the "oxidative burst" of neutrophils (see Figure 27-3), with the primary purpose of killing invading pathogens. However, these neutrophil-derived reactive species may also damage host tissues, especially under conditions of chronic inflammation. Whether ascorbate can effectively inactivate reactive oxygen and nitrogen species depends not only on their respective one-electron reduction potentials (see Table 27-1), but also on the rate constants of the reactions between these reactive species and ascorbate (Table 27-2). For example, ascorbate reacts rapidly with most oxygen radical species and hypochlorous acid as well as several reactive nitrogen species. Based on its one-electron reduction potential and high rate constants with many oxidants, vitamin C has been called "the terminal water-soluble small molecule antioxidant" in biological systems (Buettner, 1993).

Strong evidence exists to support the potent antioxidant functions of vitamin C in vitro and in vivo. When human plasma is oxidized in vitro, endogenous vitamin C protects plasma lipids against oxidative damage, as measured by the formation of lipid hydroperoxides (Frei, 1991; Frei et al., 1989; Frei et al., 1988) or F_2-isoprostanes, a validated biomarker of lipid peroxidation (Lynch et al., 1994). Vitamin C is oxidized before other plasma antioxidants, including uric acid, α-tocopherol (vitamin E), and bilirubin, suggesting that vitamin C forms the first line of antioxidant defense in extracellular fluids and is the only biological antioxidant in plasma capable of preventing detectable lipid peroxidation (Frei, 1991; Frei et al., 1988, 1989). Several studies have

TABLE 27-1 Standard Reduction Potential of Ascorbate Compared to Other Redox-Active Compounds

	OXIDIZED FORM/REDUCED FORM	STANDARD REDUCTION POTENTIAL (MV)
Highly reducing	$CO_2/CO_2^{\bullet -}$	–1800
↑	O_2, $H^+/HO_2^{\bullet}$	–460
	Fe^{3+}/Fe^{2+} (transferrin bound)	–400
	$O_2/O_2^{\bullet -}$	–330
	$NAD(P)^+$, H^+/NAD(P)H	–320
	Fe^{3+}/Fe^{2+} (ferritin bound)	–190
	FAD, $2H^+/FADH_2$	–180
	Dehydroascorbic acid/ascorbyl radical$^{\bullet -}$	**–174**
	CoQ, $H^+/CoQH^{\bullet}$ (coenzyme Q)	–40
	Fe^{3+}/Fe^{2+} (citrate bound)	10
	$CoQH^{\bullet}$, $H^+/CoQH_2$ (coenzyme Q)	20
	Fe^{3+}/Fe^{2+} (cytochrome *c* bound)	260
	Ascorbyl radical$^{\bullet -}$, H^+/ascorbate$^-$	**282**
	α-Toc$^{\bullet}$, H^+/α-Toc (α-tocopherol)	500
	$UH^{\bullet -}$, H^+/UH_2^- (urate)	590
	PUFA$^{\bullet}$, H^+/PUFA-H (polyunsaturated fatty acid)	600
	Cys$^{\bullet}$/Cys- (cysteine)	920
	$O_2^{\bullet -}$, $2H^+/H_2O_2$	940
	$RO_2^{\bullet}$, H^+/ROOH	770–1440
↓	$HO_2^{\bullet}$, H^+/H_2O_2	1060
Highly oxidizing	$^{\bullet}OH$, H^+/H_2O	2310

The standard reduction potential represents a measure of a compound's ability to accept an electron (i.e., become reduced). Higher (more positive) values represent more oxidizing compounds (i.e., compounds that will accept electrons from other compounds), whereas lower (more negative) values represent compounds more likely to donate electrons. Ascorbate lies near the center of these reduction potentials. The one-electron oxidation of ascorbate to the ascorbyl radical (the opposite of the reduction described above, producing a potential of –282 mV) has the capacity to reduce any compound with a more positive reduction potential, and thus may reduce many oxidizing species such as superoxide radicals ($O_2^{\bullet -}$), alkyl peroxyl radicals ($RO_2^{\bullet}$), and cysteine thiyl radicals (Cys$^{\bullet}$). Ascorbate may also reduce other antioxidant radicals, such as α-tocopherol radicals (α-Toc$^{\bullet}$) and urate radicals ($UH^{\bullet -}$). However, it must be noted that the reaction rate is dependent on several factors besides reduction potentials, including chemical structure, concentrations of reactants, and temperature. Although the ascorbyl radical has a more negative reduction potential than ascorbate, its most likely reaction is with itself (dismutation to ascorbate and dehydroascorbic acid) rather than reactive oxygen species. (Adapted from Buettner, G. R. [1993]. The pecking order of free radicals and antioxidants: Lipid peroxidation, alpha-tocopherol, and ascorbate. *Archives of Biochemistry and Biophysics, 300*, 535-543.)

shown that vitamin C also acts as an antioxidant in vivo. For example, SVCT2-deficient mice, which have low systemic concentrations of vitamin C, exhibit increased levels of oxidative damage (Harrison et al., 2010a). In humans, vitamin C supplementation has been shown to reduce elevated plasma levels of F_2-isoprostanes in smokers and in non-smokers exposed to environmental tobacco smoke (Dietrich et al., 2002, 2003; Reilly et al., 1996). Similarly, elevated levels of F_2-isoprostanes in patients with liver cirrhosis are reduced by vitamin C supplements (Meagher et al., 1999; Reilly et al., 1996). In addition, increased ascorbate levels in humans have been correlated with decreased protein carbonyls and protein aggregation (Carr and Frei, 1999a; Carty et al., 2000), both markers of oxidative damage to proteins.

Vitamin C also protects against oxidative damage associated with inflammation, which has been demonstrated in several systems in vivo, such as endotoxemia (Wilson, 2009) and vascular inflammation and atherosclerosis in experimental animals (Aguirre and May, 2008). In human study participants, vitamin C supplementation reduced elevated levels of C-reactive protein, a systemic marker of inflammation and independent risk factor for cardiovascular diseases (Block et al., 2009; Langlois et al., 2001). Conversely, many lifestyle factors and disease conditions that increase oxidant production have been shown to lower vitamin C levels in humans. Smoking, excessive alcohol consumption, metabolic syndrome, diabetes, and obesity are all associated with increased oxidative stress and decreased vitamin C status

TABLE 27-2 Reactive Species Scavenged by Ascorbate

CHEMICAL SPECIES	REACTION RATE CONSTANT (liter/mole•s)	SOURCES IN THE BODY
REACTIVE OXYGEN SPECIES		
Superoxide radical ($O_2^{\bullet-}$) Hydroperoxyl radical ($HO_2^\bullet$)	1×10^5	• Uncoupled electron transfer in mitochondria • NADPH oxidase activity • Reaction of O_2 with reduced free transition metal ions (Fe^{2+}, Cu^+)
Hypochlorous acid (HOCl)	6×10^6	• Myeloperoxidase activity in neutrophils (see Figure 27-3)
Peroxyl radicals ($RO_2^\bullet$)	1×10^6	• Reaction of hydroperoxyl radicals with lipids • Decomposition of lipid peroxides • Reaction of O_2 with carbon-centered radicals (formed by the reaction of hydroxyl radicals)
Alkoxyl radical ($RO^\bullet$)	1.6×10^9	• Decomposition of lipid peroxides
Hydroxyl radical ($^\bullet OH$)	1.1×10^{10}	• Fenton chemistry: Reaction of H_2O_2 with reduced free transition metal ions (Fe^{2+}, Cu^+) • Ultraviolet breakdown of H_2O_2 • Ionizing radiation of exposure • Reaction of HOCl with $O_2^{\bullet-}$
REACTIVE NITROGEN SPECIES		
Nitrogen dioxide ($^\bullet NO_2$)	1×10^7	• Reaction of O_2 with nitric oxide ($NO^\bullet$) produced by nitric oxide synthases (NOS)
Dinitrogen trioxide (N_2O_3) Dinitrogen tetroxide (N_2O_4)	1.2×10^9	• Reactions of $^\bullet NO_2$ with $NO^\bullet$
Peroxynitrite ($ONOO^-$)	235	• Reaction of $NO^\bullet$ with $O_2^{\bullet-}$
REACTIVE SULFUR SPECIES		
Thiyl radicals ($RS^\bullet$) Sulphonyl radicals ($RSO^\bullet$)	6×10^8	• Reaction of thiols with $OH^\bullet$, $RO_2^\bullet$, $RO^\bullet$, or carbon-centered radicals • Reactions with oxidized free transition metal ions (Fe^{3+}, Cu^{2+}) • UV reaction with protein disulphides
ANTIOXIDANT RADICALS		
α-Tocopherol radical (α-$Toc^\bullet$)	2×10^5	• Reaction of α-Toc with $RO^\bullet$ or RO_2
Urate radical ($UH^{\bullet-}$)	1×10^6	• Reaction of UH_2 with $RO_2^\bullet$ or $^\bullet OH$
Glutathione radical ($GS^\bullet$)	6×10^8	• See thiyl radicals, earlier in table

The actual reaction rate of ascorbate with any given compound listed in this table is dependent on specific reaction conditions, including temperature, pH, concentrations of reactants, and competing side reactions. (Data from Halliwell, B. G., & Gutterige, J. M. C. [2007]. *Free radicals in biology and medicine* (4th ed.). New York: Oxford University Press.)
UV, ultraviolet.

(Bingham et al., 2008; Carr and Frei, 1999b; Khaw et al., 2008; Sargeant et al., 2000).

Nevertheless, the role of vitamin C in the prevention of oxidative damage in vivo remains somewhat controversial, mainly because of technical challenges of measuring antioxidant activity in humans. Many of the pitfalls can be avoided by using validated oxidative stress biomarkers, such as F_2-isoprostanes; specific methodologies for sample collection, storage, and vitamin C analysis that avoid ex vivo oxidation artifacts; and proper study design (Carr and Frei, 1999a, 1999b; Lykkesfeldt and Poulsen, 2010).

THE ANTIOXIDANT NETWORK

Ascorbate has been shown to react with other biological antioxidants. This has given rise to the theory of an "antioxidant network" in the body, where ascorbate acts as a central

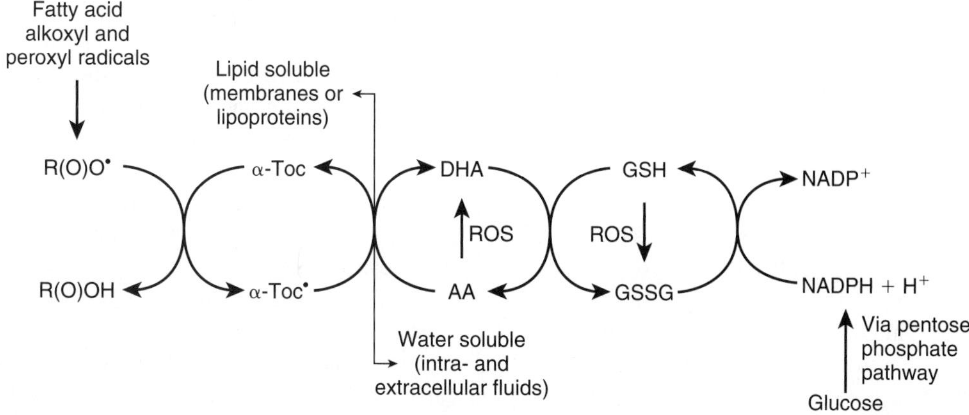

FIGURE 27-13 The antioxidant network. Fatty acid–derived alkoxyl and peroxyl radicals can be reduced by vitamin E (α-tocopherol; α-Toc), forming the α-tocopherol radical (α-Toc•), which can be reduced by vitamin C (ascorbic acid; AA). Dehydroascorbic acid (DHA) is reduced to AA by glutathione (GSH), which is oxidized to glutathione disulfide (GSSG). Finally, GSSG is reduced to GSH by GSSG reductase at the expense of NADPH. Although the full sequence of antioxidant interactions occurs in the cytosol and cellular membranes, portions of it may occur in organelles as well as in extracellular fluids and lipoproteins. Note that AA and GSH also directly react with, and are oxidized by, reactive oxygen species (ROS) in addition to acting as part of the antioxidant network.

reducing agent. Based on its one-electron reduction potential, ascorbate can reduce the radical species formed upon one-electron oxidation of urate and α-tocopherol (see Table 27-1), thereby regenerating these biological antioxidants after they have reacted with free radical species. The interaction of vitamin C at the water–lipid interface with vitamin E allows the reducing power of ascorbate to affect lipid-soluble radicals in membranes and lipoproteins, with which it could not otherwise react (see Chapter 29). The dehydroascorbic acid produced by these reactions can be reduced by GSH-dependent mechanisms (Figure 27-13). The role of GSH as an electron donor in the antioxidant network is beneficial in several ways: diet-derived antioxidants such as vitamins E and C and metabolic antioxidants such as urate can be regenerated and will not be lost; GSH can be synthesized by all cells; and GSSG is readily reduced by NADPH-dependent mechanisms. The interactions of vitamin E and GSH with vitamin C have been demonstrated in vivo (Bruno et al., 2006; Meister, 1994; Traber, 2007), supporting the important role of vitamin C as a biological reductant in the antioxidant network.

PROOXIDANT EFFECTS OF VITAMIN C

Although vitamin C at physiological concentrations did not appear to exert prooxidant effects in healthy human study participants (Carr and Frei, 1999a; Levine et al., 2001), it has the potential to behave as a prooxidant under certain conditions. Ascorbate may donate an electron to molecular oxygen to form superoxide radicals (Buettner and Jurkiewicz, 1996). However, this direct reaction of ascorbate with molecular oxygen is thermodynamically highly unfavored (see Table 27-1) and can be observed only at high, nonphysiological concentrations of both reactants. Furthermore, this reaction is more likely to occur with the ascorbate dianion, a molecular species that exists in very small quantities in biological fluids. A chemically more favored prooxidant action of vitamin C is mediated by redox-active transition metals, such as iron

$$AscH^- + Fe^{3+} \longrightarrow Asc^{\bullet -} + H^+ + Fe^{2+}$$
$$O_2 + Fe^{2+} \longrightarrow O_2^{\bullet -} + Fe^{3+}$$
$$2\,O_2^{\bullet -} + 2\,H^+ \longrightarrow H_2O_2 + O_2$$
$$H_2O_2 + Fe^{3+} \longrightarrow Fe^{3+} + OH^- + {}^{\bullet}OH$$

FIGURE 27-14 Reaction sequence for the iron-dependent prooxidant activity of vitamin C. *AscH⁻*, Ascorbate; *Asc•⁻*, ascorbyl radical; *H_2O_2*, hydrogen peroxide; *$O_2^{\bullet -}$*, superoxide radical; *•OH*, hydroxyl radical.

or copper (Figure 27-14). If these metals are present free in solution, they are readily reduced by ascorbate (as occurs in the active site of ascorbate-dependent enzymes). The reduced metal ions, Fe^{2+} or Cu^+, rapidly reduce molecular oxygen to superoxide radicals that subsequently may dismutate to molecular oxygen and hydrogen peroxide, which can produce highly damaging hydroxyl radicals in the presence of Fe^{2+} or Cu^+ (called the Fenton reaction). In this case, ascorbate is not directly donating electrons to oxygen but using metal ions as intermediaries. The removal of metal ions from solution prevents these reactions. In vitro this is often done by using chelators (metal-binding chemicals), and in vivo most of these metals are sequestered by binding to metal-binding proteins.

Interestingly, hydrogen peroxide formation has been detected in cell culture and extracellular fluids in vivo in the presence of millimolar concentrations of ascorbate, which can be achieved in humans by intravenous (but not oral) administration of vitamin C (Chen et al., 2005, 2007). The detection of ascorbyl radicals in fluids from human study participants receiving high-dose intravenous vitamin C has been used as evidence that vitamin C acts as a prooxidant in vivo under these conditions (Chen et al., 2007). Since ascorbate-generated hydrogen peroxide selectively kills cancer cells but not normal cells (Chen et al., 2005, 2008), intravenous administration of vitamin C is currently being studied for its potential use in cancer therapy.

IN VITRO EFFECTS OF VITAMIN C: INTERPRET CAREFULLY

Antioxidant or prooxidant effects of ascorbate observed in vitro do not automatically confer relevance in vivo, for several reasons (Halliwell, 2003). In cell culture, prooxidant effects of ascorbate are favored because of exposure to ambient oxygen and light as well as the presence of significant amounts of iron and other trace metals in culture media. All of these factors contribute to artificial ascorbate oxidation that would not occur under physiological conditions.

Standard culture media do not contain significant amounts of vitamin C either because it is not added or, if initially present, because it oxidizes within 24 hours because of the factors just mentioned. For this reason, cells in culture lack vitamin C unless they have been freshly isolated from tissue or the culture medium is regularly supplemented with vitamin C (Smith et al., 2002). Hence effects of extracellular or intracellular vitamin C on cell function are usually tested in cells devoid of the vitamin, which has little or no physiological relevance. As discussed earlier, in vivo intracellular ascorbate concentrations are in the millimolar range, and even in the presence of severe deficiency most cells still retain some vitamin C. Therefore it would be more appropriate if comparisons were made between cells that have either low or high intracellular concentrations of ascorbate to study the effects of vitamin C, but this is not usually done.

Similarly, in ex vivo studies using samples obtained from human study participants or animals, investigators must take special precautions to prevent artificial oxidation of ascorbate. Free metals in solutions, often present as contaminants, need to be controlled; light and oxygen exposure should be limited; and additional steps must be taken to stabilize ascorbate in biological fluids, cells, and tissues. This includes, but is not limited to, minimizing time of sample processing, keeping samples at low temperature and in the dark, and acidifying samples because ascorbate is more stable at low pH.

Thus data from in vitro studies must be interpreted carefully, which requires a good understanding of the chemistry of vitamin C. Furthermore, although vitamin C has been proposed to have many roles in vitro, such as effects on gene transcription and protein synthesis (Arrigoni and De Tullio, 2002), such findings will remain controversial until and unless they are confirmed in vivo.

VITAMIN C AND HUMAN HEALTH

VITAMIN C DEFICIENCY: SCURVY

Scurvy, which was not attributed to vitamin C deficiency until the twentieth century, was first described several thousand years ago. Although many treatments for scurvy have been described over the years, a specific cure was not found until 1753 when the Scottish physician James Lind noted that the disease could be prevented by ingesting lemon juice (Lind, 1753). The active protective compound, ascorbic acid, was isolated and characterized between 1928 and 1932 in the laboratories of Albert Szent-Györgyi and Charles King (King and Waugh, 1932; Svirbely and Szent-Györgyi, 1932). Once the vitamin was identified, its deficiency state was studied more systematically.

When vitamin C is absent from the diet, levels of vitamin C in the body decline because of the inefficiency of recycling mechanisms. Tissue levels of vitamin C during depletion depend on several factors, including initial body store and rate of ascorbate use in enzymatic reactions and nonenzymatic, primarily antioxidant, reactions. To some degree, nutritional status can determine the length of time until scurvy symptoms appear, because diets rich in other antioxidants can preserve some vitamin C in the body. However, on a diet specifically lacking vitamin C, plasma levels in human study participants with sufficient but not maximal vitamin C stores drop to near-scurvy levels in approximately 30 days (Levine et al., 1996b, 2001). Interestingly, in some animal species that are unable to synthesize ascorbic acid, vitamin C levels drop much more rapidly than in humans (Harrison et al., 2010b; Hill et al., 2003; Parsons et al., 2006; Tanaka et al., 1997), possibly due to higher metabolic rates. Based on animal studies, it appears that vitamin C levels do not decline in all tissues at the same rate; thus scurvy symptoms are usually progressive, with some symptoms developing earlier than others.

The signs of scurvy are considered to be an effect of a general lack of vitamin C for associated enzyme functions. Petechial hemorrhage (small areas of bleeding under the skin), coiled hair, bleeding gums, ecchymoses (larger areas of bleeding under the skin), hyperkeratosis (increased skin cells around hair follicles), arthralgias (joint pain), and joint effusions (abnormal amounts of fluid in joints) are commonly observed in scurvy (Hirschmann and Raugi, 1999; Hood et al., 1970) and are related to loss of prolyl and lysyl hydroxylase activity for collagen biosynthesis. Loss of catecholamine synthesis and neuroendocrine peptide maturation can occur with impaired activity of dopamine β-hydroxylase and peptidylglycine α-amidating monooxygenase, and this may be responsible for reports of hypochondriasis (excessive fear of having a serious disease) and depression in scorbutic patients (Baker et al., 1971; Hodges et al., 1971; Kinsman and Hood, 1971). Impaired carnitine biosynthesis, along with deficits in neurotransmitter and bioactive peptides, may contribute to fatigue—an important early symptom in vitamin C deficiency first mentioned in Lind's classic work (Lind, 1753). In vitamin C depletion–repletion studies conducted at the National Institutes of Health (NIH), healthy volunteers were made vitamin C–deficient but did not develop signs of scurvy. However, the majority of human study participants experienced fatigue (Levine et al., 1996b, 2001), which was reversed when plasma concentrations exceeded 20 μmol/L ascorbate.

Scurvy is rare in developed countries because it can be prevented by as little as 10 mg of vitamin C daily. It is often difficult for health professionals to recognize subclinical vitamin C deficiency because its only symptom, fatigue, is nonspecific and has many causes. Overt vitamin C deficiency in the United States today is seen in malnourished populations, including those with cancer cachexia, poor dietary habits, malabsorption (sometimes associated with gastric bypass surgery), alcoholism, or chemical dependency. Scurvy may also occur in children or the elderly, who are unwilling or unable to eat vitamin C–containing foods. Patients with end-stage renal disease are often treated using hemodialysis, which removes vitamin C, and many patients who receive this treatment have low plasma and tissue vitamin C concentrations and require supplementation.

VITAMIN C IN DISEASE PREVENTION

Because about one third of Americans have inadequate intakes of vitamin C from food, subclinical vitamin C deficiency is surprisingly common in the United States (Hampl et al., 2004). Although overt vitamin C deficiency causes scurvy, covert deficiency is believed to increase the risk of certain chronic diseases. Much of the available information on vitamin C and chronic disease risk is derived from prospective cohort studies in which vitamin C intake is assessed at baseline in a large number of people who are then followed over time to monitor morbidity and mortality from chronic disease. Prospective studies must be interpreted with a full understanding of their limitations. In prospective cohort studies, investigators do not usually measure vitamin C levels in study participants, but rely instead on voluntary reporting of dietary and supplemental intake, which is inherently inaccurate (Dehghan et al., 2007). In addition to dietary or supplemental vitamin C intake, numerous other factors determine vitamin C body status, including polymorphisms in the genes for SVCT1 and SVCT2 (Timpson et al., 2010) and numerous lifestyle factors, such as cigarette smoking and excessive alcohol consumption. These factors need to be controlled for in observational studies for proper interpretation, but since they are incompletely understood and other factors may exist that remain unknown, residual confounding is unavoidable. These limitations make data interpretation uncertain; highlighting the need for well-designed, well-executed, randomized controlled trials of vitamin C supplementation. Nevertheless, randomized controlled trials of micronutrients such as vitamin C have serious limitations and shortcomings that make their interpretation problematic (Blumberg et al., 2010; Frei, 2004; Lykkesfeldt and Poulsen, 2010).

One of the most compelling prospective cohort studies investigating the relationship between vitamin C and chronic disease outcome is the European Prospective Investigation into Cancer and Nutrition study of subjects recruited from the Norfolk area in the United Kingdom (EPIC-Norfolk). The strength of this study lies within its large population of over 30,000 men and women and its use of plasma vitamin C levels measured at baseline, rather than estimates of vitamin C intake from dietary records. Some of the major findings of this study include significant inverse associations between vitamin C status and risk of all-cause mortality and incidence of several diseases (Khaw et al., 2001; Myint et al., 2008). Specifically, those individuals with the highest plasma vitamin C levels had a 71% and 68% decreased risk of death from cardiovascular disease and ischemic heart disease, respectively, when compared to those individuals with the lowest vitamin C status. The study group also reported a 17% decrease in relative risk in incidence of stroke for every 20 μmol/L increase in plasma vitamin C levels. Furthermore, in men, a 20 μmol/L increase in plasma vitamin C levels was associated with a 15% decreased risk of death from all types of cancer.

CARDIOVASCULAR DISEASES

A meta-analysis of 14 prospective cohort studies published in 2008 concluded that higher dietary intakes of vitamin C were associated with a significantly reduced risk of coronary artery disease (CAD) (Ye and Song, 2008). However, the meta-analysis did not show an association of vitamin C supplement intake with CAD risk. Dietary vitamin C intake has also been associated with a significantly lower risk of death from stroke and incidence of ischemic stroke and intracerebral hemorrhage (Gale et al., 1995; Hirvonen et al., 2000; Voko et al., 2003). However, no relation was found between dietary vitamin C intake and cerebral infarction or subarachnoid hemorrhage. Both observational studies and randomized controlled trials have found inverse associations between vitamin C intake (either through supplement or diet) or plasma vitamin C levels and blood pressure (Frikke-Schmidt and Lykkesfeldt, 2009; Jacques, 1992) or plasma C-reactive protein level (Block et al., 2009; Boekholdt et al., 2006; Oliveira et al., 2009), and direct associations with serum high-density lipoprotein cholesterol (Boekholdt et al., 2006; Jacques, 1992). Overall, the protective effect of vitamin C in cardiovascular diseases may occur at daily intakes of about 100 to 200 mg of vitamin C, a range resulting in near-saturation of plasma and tissues, as discussed earlier (Carr and Frei, 1999b).

CANCER

Most case-control and prospective cohort studies have reported that dietary vitamin C intake is associated with a decreased risk of cancers of the digestive tract, including the oral cavity, esophagus, and stomach (Carr and Frei, 1999b). Evidence suggests that dietary vitamin C is not significantly associated with the development of cancers at other sites. Protective effects have generally been observed in study participants consuming at least 80 to 110 mg of vitamin C daily. Consumption of a diet high in vitamin C–rich fruits and

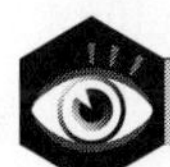

NUTRITION INSIGHT

The Common Cold

Linus Pauling popularized the idea that large doses of vitamin C may prevent or reduce the severity of the common cold. Since his publications, many controlled vitamin C trials have been conducted with a variety of doses and populations. In certain groups, such as those experiencing physical stress or chronic exposure to extreme environments, vitamin C may help reduce cold incidence (Douglas et al., 2007). Current evidence suggests that supplemental vitamin C has little impact as a prophylaxis against the common cold in the general population but may shorten the duration of the cold and lessen its severity.

vegetables has been associated with reduced mortality from cancer overall (Khaw et al., 2001; Pocobelli et al., 2009) but it is difficult to attribute these effects to vitamin C intake alone.

OTHER DISEASES

The relationship between plasma ascorbate levels or use of vitamin C supplements has been postulated to have a significant effect on eye-related diseases. Though there is no strong evidence that taking vitamin C supplements can prevent the development of cataracts (AREDS, 2001; Chasan-Taber et al., 1999; Rautiainen et al., 2010), several studies have found an inverse association between plasma vitamin C levels and cataract risk (Dherani et al., 2008; Simon and Hudes, 1999; Valero et al., 2002). On the other hand, no association has been found with risk of age-related macular degeneration and vitamin C consumption.

Vitamin C doses of up to 3 g/day have been reported to increase urinary excretion of uric acid, a condition known as hyperuricosuria. The effect of this supplementation is to lower uric acid in the blood and decrease the risk for uric acid crystallization, or gout. A few observational studies have examined the relationship between intake of vitamin C and gout, and the results are consistently positive, showing an inverse association of gout risk with increasing consumption of the vitamin (Choi et al., 2009; Gao et al., 2008; Huang et al., 2005).

VITAMIN C IN DISEASE TREATMENT

In addition to prevention of certain chronic diseases, vitamin C may be efficacious in treatment of established disease. Impaired vasodilation is becoming increasingly recognized as an independent risk factor for cardiovascular mortality, and vitamin C supplementation has been consistently shown to improve vasodilation in individuals with established CAD as well as in those with angina pectoris, congestive heart failure, diabetes mellitus, high serum cholesterol, and high blood pressure (Frikke-Schmidt and Lykkesfeldt, 2009; Gokce et al., 1999; Levine et al., 1996a; Versari et al., 2009). Studies in individuals with hypertension found that vitamin C supplementation significantly decreased systolic blood pressure (Duffy et al., 1999, 2001). Improved vasodilation and lowered blood pressure have been demonstrated at oral doses of about 500 mg of vitamin C daily.

The efficacy of vitamin C in cancer treatment is still under debate. Studies conducted by Linus Pauling and Ewan Cameron suggested that very large doses of vitamin C, given orally or administered intravenously, were helpful in increasing the survival time and improving the quality of life of terminal cancer patients (Cameron and Pauling, 1976). Although this was not replicated in later oral dosing studies at the Mayo Clinic (Creagan et al., 1979; Moertel et al., 1985), recent work at the NIH has suggested that intravenous doses of vitamin C have the potential to produce hydrogen peroxide (Chen et al., 2005, 2007, 2008), which is selectively toxic to cancer cells. Currently, several phase I and phase II clinical trials in cancer patients are being conducted with intravenous vitamin C (Hoffer et al., 2008).

POPULATIONS POTENTIALLY ADVERSELY AFFECTED BY EXCESS VITAMIN C

Although vitamin C—even in large gram doses—is safe in healthy people, in some individuals with chronic diseases or inherited conditions, adverse effects of vitamin C supplementation have been reported. It is generally accepted that dietary sources of vitamin C are safe in these individuals, and frequent consumption of vitamin C–rich foods is encouraged. The data suggesting adverse effects of vitamin C supplementation in these study participants are often inconclusive.

Vitamin C has been reported to increase kidney stone formation in those with renal disease by increasing oxalate levels in the blood (Chai et al., 2004; Massey et al., 2005; Taylor et al., 2004; Traxer et al., 2003). Individuals with renal disease or on hemodialysis are encouraged by physicians not to consume large amounts of supplemental vitamin C. However, in the Dietary Approaches to Stop Hypertension (DASH) study, kidney stone formers who ate a diet high in vitamin C and other micronutrients showed a decreased risk of stone formation (Taylor et al., 2009). Vitamin C acquired through diet or supplement did not augment stone formation risk. Although vitamin C can break down into oxalate, a component of kidney stones, it has been suggested that vitamin C supplementation may increase oxalate solubility, causing increased oxalate in the urine without increased stone formation. Furthermore, dialysis patients are particularly at risk for vitamin C deficiency due to loss of vitamin C through the dialysis procedure (Deicher et al., 2005; Singer et al., 2008; Tomson et al., 1989), suggesting the need for supplemental vitamin C. The optimum intake of vitamin C in these patients is unknown, but recent data show beneficial effects of ascorbic acid doses of at least 250 mg daily (Abdollahzad et al., 2009; Chao et al., 2002; Ferretti et al., 2008; Tarng et al., 2004), with few adverse side effects (Singer, 2010).

As described previously, vitamin C promotes iron absorption from the small intestine. In theory, vitamin C consumed with iron could increase the risk of iron overload in susceptible individuals (Gerster, 1999), such as patients with hemochromatosis, thalassemia major, sickle cell disease, or sideroblastic anemia, and those who require frequent blood transfusions. Patients with these conditions should not avoid eating fruits and vegetables (Barton et al., 1998), but instead should limit intake of iron. Whether vitamin C exacerbates iron overload in patients with these conditions remains unclear.

Glucose-6-phosphate dehydrogenase deficiency is an X-linked inherited disease that can cause hemolytic crises, sometimes precipitated as a consequence of oxidative stress. In study participants with glucose-6-phosphate dehydrogenase deficiency, hemolysis has been reported subsequent to vitamin C administration (Levine et al., 1999). However, this association has not been seen in all individuals with the disease.

Several harmful effects have been erroneously attributed to vitamin C supplementation, including hypoglycemia, rebound scurvy, DNA damage and mutagenesis, infertility, and destruction of vitamin B_{12}. None of these conditions is caused by either dietary or supplemental vitamin C.

DIETARY REFERENCE INTAKES FOR VITAMIN C

The earliest recommendation for vitamin C intake of 10 mg daily was based on studies conducted by the British Royal Air Force during World War II, which indicated that this amount of vitamin C was needed to prevent scurvy, with an added safety margin (Bartley et al., 1953). When it was recognized that the Royal Air Force data probably underestimated vitamin C intake, depletion–repletion studies were conducted using prisoners in Iowa (Baker et al., 1969, 1971; Hodges et al., 1971). Results of these studies were used to set the 1980 and 1989 Recommended Dietary Allowance (RDA) of vitamin C at 60 mg daily. At the time it was believed that 60 mg daily was adequate to protect against signs and symptoms of scurvy for at least 1 month if vitamin C ingestion suddenly stopped. It was also thought that this dose would provide sufficient vitamin C to compensate for metabolic losses while minimizing urinary excretion. Because these studies were done with male adults, recommendations were extrapolated for women and across age ranges of both sexes.

Nevertheless, there were a number of serious limitations in the Iowa studies. The vitamin C assay was imprecise, a narrow dose range was tested, and the number of participants was small (Baker et al., 1971; Hodges et al., 1971). In one of the depletion–repletion studies, study participants were fed a diet that was deficient in other nutrients besides vitamin C (Baker et al., 1969). In addition, the conclusion that 60 mg daily would compensate for metabolic losses was based on data obtained in deficient patients (Hodges et al., 1971). Because vitamin C metabolism changes as a function of depletion or repletion, use of data from deficient study participants to calculate metabolism for the general population is questionable. Perhaps more important, the 1980 and 1989 RDAs were based on the amount needed to prevent deficiency and not on a functional measure of vitamin C status or on the amount needed to maintain optimum health (Levine, 1986). Indeed, at that time, functional measures were not considered as a basis for establishing RDAs for any of the vitamins.

In setting the Dietary Reference Intakes (DRIs) for vitamin C in 2000, the Institute of Medicine (IOM) included consideration of functional data as well as newly published depletion–repletion data from studies conducted at the NIH. Data from healthy young men (Levine et al., 1996b) were used to determine the DRIs for vitamin C (IOM, 2000), and data from healthy women were published subsequently (Levine et al., 2001). Data from both men and women provided comprehensive concentration and pharmacokinetic data over a wide dose range of vitamin C (Graumlich et al., 1997; Levine et al., 1996b, 2001). Both male and female study participants consumed a diet only deficient in vitamin C, without any other nutrient deficiencies. Study participants consumed vitamin C–depleted diets for approximately 4 weeks and then were repleted stepwise with increasing doses of vitamin C. Steady-state fasting plasma concentrations were determined for each of seven doses, which ranged from 30 to 2,500 mg daily (see Figure 27-4). At steady-state for each dose, vitamin C concentrations were determined in circulating cells (see Figure 27-5), vitamin C excretion in urine was measured, and bioavailability was assessed.

The IOM based the Estimated Average Requirement (EAR) on neutrophil vitamin C concentrations in men (Levine et al., 1996b), putative vitamin C antioxidant action in neutrophils (Anderson and Lukey, 1987; Halliwell et al., 1987), and urinary vitamin C excretion in men (Levine et al., 1996b). Neutrophils accumulate vitamin C via SVCT2, and vitamin C accumulation is more avid in the presence of extracellular oxidants when it is also mediated by dehydroascorbic acid uptake via GLUT1 or GLUT3 and ascorbate recycling, as described earlier (see Figure 27-3). An EAR was selected to achieve near-maximal intracellular vitamin C concentration in activated neutrophils for self-protection against the oxidants they produce, as determined in studies conducted in vitro (Anderson and Lukey, 1987; Anderson et al., 1987), while also minimizing urinary loss of vitamin C in men (Levine et al., 1996b).

DRIs Across the Life Cycle: Vitamin C

	mg Vitamin C per Day*	
Infants	RDA	UL
0 through 6 mo	40 (AI)	ND
7 through 12 mo	50 (AI)	ND
Children		
1 through 3 yr	15	400
4 through 8 yr	25	650
9 through 13 yr	45	1,200
Males		
14 through 18 yr	75	1,800
≥19 yr	90	2,000
Females		
14 through 18 yr	65	1,800
≥19 yr	75	2,000
Pregnant		
<19 yr	80	1,800
≥19 yr	85	2,000
Lactating		
<19 yr	115	1,800
≥19 yr	120	2,000

Data from IOM. (2006). In J. J. Otten, J. P. Hellwig, & L. D. Meyers (Eds.), *Dietary Reference Intakes: The essential guide to nutrient requirements.* Washington, DC: The National Academies Press.

AI, Adequate Intake; *DRI*, Dietary Reference Intake; *ND*, not determinable; *RDA*, Recommended Dietary Allowance; *UL*, Tolerable Upper Intake Level.

*An additional intake of approximately 35 mg vitamin C per day is recommended for smokers.

As shown in Figure 27-4, at the 100-mg oral dose of vitamin C, mean neutrophil ascorbate concentrations were nearly at the saturation level of 1.25 ± 0.12 mmol/L (mean ± SD), and urinary loss of the vitamin C dose was approximately 25%. A dose that would achieve 80% neutrophil saturation was chosen by the IOM to provide antioxidant protection with minimal urinary loss. By regression analysis the dose corresponding to 80% saturation was found to be approximately 75 mg (IOM, 2000). This value was selected as the EAR for adult males aged 19 to 50 years, and EARs for other age and sex groups were derived by extrapolation from this value based on relative body weights. The EAR for pregnant women was increased by an estimate of that needed to ensure adequate transfer of vitamin C to the fetus, and the EAR for lactating women was increased by the average amount secreted in the milk. RDAs were set as the EAR + 20%, with rounding.

However, more recent data from depletion–repletion studies in 15 healthy young women (Levine et al., 2001) suggest that the current RDA for vitamin C set by the IOM in 2000 is too low. These studies concluded that the vitamin C dose required for saturation of plasma and circulating cells is 400 mg/day (Levine et al., 2001), suggesting that some revision in the EAR and RDA for vitamin C may be necessary in the future.

Like other nutrients, Adequate Intakes (AIs) of vitamin C were set for infants. The AI for infants through 6 months of age was calculated as the average intake of vitamin C from human milk during the first 6 months of life (50 mg of vitamin C per L milk × 0.78 L milk consumed per day). For infants from 7 through 12 months of age, the AI is based on intake from human milk plus complementary foods. For children, the recommendation is based on estimated body size in relation to the adult.

Based on lower plasma vitamin C levels measured in smokers, the RDA for men and women who smoke is 35 mg/day higher than for nonsmokers. No pharmacokinetic studies have been performed in older adults, a group thought to have decreased absorption and increased requirements for vitamin C (Brubacher et al., 2000).

In the studies used to calculate the EARs, vitamin C was given as pure vitamin C in a solution that was administered at half-dose twice daily in the fasting state. It is not known whether vitamin C in food consumed during several daily meals is bioavailable to the same extent as pure vitamin C given once during the fasting state. Therefore the intake of vitamin C from foods may need to be higher than the present DRIs if the bioavailability of vitamin C from foods is less than that from the pure solutions used in the depletion–repletion studies (Levine et al., 1996b, 2001). On the other hand, increasing the frequency of vitamin C consumption throughout the day, to reflect a normal eating pattern, may result in higher plasma and tissue ascorbate levels than discrete, large doses (Duconge et al., 2008).

Despite the prevalence of vitamin C in foods, dietary intake data from NHANES III, 1988 to 1994, showed that the median vitamin C intake from foods was about 100 mg/day for individuals in the United States; the 5th to 95th percentile range was 58 to 167 mg/day (IOM, 2000). When supplement use was included, median intake was estimated at 116 mg/day and the 5th to 95th percentile range was 61 to 430 mg/day. Although these data suggest that vitamin C intake in the U.S. population meets current recommendations, the true measure of vitamin C status in humans is plasma ascorbate concentration. The ascorbate level in the blood is determined not only by dietary intake but also, for example, by single nucleotide polymorphisms in the gene encoding SVCT1, smoking status, alcohol consumption, and age. When plasma vitamin C levels are measured instead of using dietary records, vitamin C consumption in many individuals appears far from adequate. In NHANES III, for example, 14% of men and 10% of women had plasma vitamin C concentrations less than 11 μmol/L, which is considered deficient. Other specific groups, including smokers, had significantly lower plasma vitamin C levels than the general population (Hampl et al., 2004).

The IOM set the Tolerable Upper Intake Level (UL) for oral vitamin C ingestion for adults at 2 g daily, based on gastrointestinal disturbances observed in some individuals at higher doses, although these effects are usually transient (Cameron and Pauling, 1974; IOM, 2000). No other adverse health effects in generally healthy people were found for vitamin C intake, even at doses much greater than the UL.

THINKING CRITICALLY

1. Vitamin C transport and metabolism maintain vitamin C levels in the plasma within a certain range. Describe the mechanisms by which "steady-state" plasma ascorbate concentrations are achieved at a given vitamin C dose. Consider the effects of the dietary asborption, urinary excretion, and tissue uptake.
2. Manifestations of scurvy include bleeding gums, fatigue, and depression. Provide a biochemical explanation for each of these manifestations based on the enzymatic functions of vitamin C.
3. Epidemiological studies suggest that high dietary intake of vitamin C is protective against several chronic diseases. Provide a mechanism by which vitamin C may be exerting its protective effects. What is an alternative explanation for this relationship? Describe the type of study that would enable a causal inference.
4. Although dehydroascorbic acid is not a reducing agent, it may have beneficial effects when present in the diet. Explain. Why is consuming dehydroascorbic acid not very effective?
5. Consuming iron and ascorbic acid is considered both beneficial and detrimental, depending on the conditions. Provide an example of a positive and adverse effect of vitamin C in the presence of iron. How does oxygen play a role?

REFERENCES

Abdollahzad, H., Eghtesadi, S., Nourmohammadi, I., Khadem-Ansari, M., Nejad-Gashti, H., & Esmaillzadeh, A. (2009). Effect of vitamin C supplementation on oxidative stress and lipid profiles in hemodialysis patients. *International Journal for Vitamin and Nutrition Research, 79*, 281–287.

Aguirre, R., & May, J. M. (2008). Inflammation in the vascular bed: Importance of vitamin C. *Pharmacology & Therapeutics, 119*, 96–103.

Anderson, R., & Lukey, P. T. (1987). A biological role for ascorbate in the selective neutralization of extracellular phagocyte-derived oxidants. *Annals of the New York Academy of Sciences, 498*, 229–247.

Anderson, R., Lukey, P. T., Theron, A. J., & Dippenaar, U. (1987). Ascorbate and cysteine-mediated selective neutralisation of extracellular oxidants during N-formyl peptide activation of human phagocytes. *Agents and Actions, 20*, 77–86.

AREDS. (2001). A randomized, placebo-controlled, clinical trial of high-dose supplementation with vitamins C and E and beta carotene for age-related cataract and vision loss: AREDS report no. 9. *Archives of Ophthalmology, 119*, 1439–1452.

Arrigoni, O., & De Tullio, M. C. (2002). Ascorbic acid: Much more than just an antioxidant. *Biochimica et Biophysica Acta, 1569*, 1–9.

Atanasova, B. D., Li, A. C., Bjarnason, I., Tzatchev, K. N., & Simpson, R. J. (2005). Duodenal ascorbate and ferric reductase in human iron deficiency. *The American Journal of Clinical Nutrition, 81*, 130–133.

Baker, E. M., Halver, J. E., Johnsen, D. O., Joyce, B. E., Knight, M. K., & Tolbert, B. M. (1975). Metabolism of ascorbic acid and ascorbic-2-sulfate in man and the subhuman primate. *Annals of the New York Academy of Sciences, 258*, 72–80.

Baker, E. M., Hodges, R. E., Hood, J., Sauberlich, H. E., & March, S. C. (1969). Metabolism of ascorbic-1-14C acid in experimental human scurvy. *The American Journal of Clinical Nutrition, 22*, 549–558.

Baker, E. M., Hodges, R. E., Hood, J., Sauberlich, H. E., March, S. C., & Canham, J. E. (1971). Metabolism of 14C- and 3H-labeled L-ascorbic acid in human scurvy. *The American Journal of Clinical Nutrition, 24*, 444–454.

Banhegyi, G., Braun, L., Csala, M., Puskas, F., & Mandl, J. (1997). Ascorbate metabolism and its regulation in animals. *Free Radical Biology & Medicine, 23*, 793–803.

Banhegyi, G., & Loewus, F. L. (2004). Ascorbic acid catabolism: Breakdown pathways in animals and plants. In H. Asard, J. M. May, & N. Smirnoff (Eds.), *Vitamin C: Functions and biochemistry in animals and plants* (pp. 31–48). London: BIOS Scientific Publishers.

Banhegyi, G., Marcolongo, P., Puskas, F., Fulceri, R., Mandl, J., & Benedetti, A. (1998). Dehydroascorbate and ascorbate transport in rat liver microsomal vesicles. *The Journal of Biological Chemistry, 273*, 2758–2762.

Bardos, J. I., & Ashcroft, M. (2005). Negative and positive regulation of HIF-1: A complex network. *Biochimica et Biophysica Acta, 1755*, 107–120.

Bartley, W., Krebs, H. A., & O'Brien, J. R. P. (1953). *Vitamin C requirements of human adults* (Vol. 280). London: Medical Research Council, H.M. Stationary Office.

Barton, J. C., McDonnell, S. M., Adams, P. C., Brissot, P., Powell, L. W., Edwards, C. Q., … Kowdley, K. V. (1998). Management of hemochromatosis. Hemochromatosis Management Working Group. *Annals of Internal Medicine, 129*, 932–939.

Bingham, S., Luben, R., Welch, A., Low, Y. L., Khaw, K. T., Wareham, N., & Day, N. (2008). Associations between dietary methods and biomarkers, and between fruits and vegetables and risk of ischaemic heart disease, in the EPIC Norfolk Cohort Study. *International Journal of Epidemiology, 37*, 978–987.

Bjorkhem, I., & Kallner, A. (1976). Hepatic 7alpha-hydroxylation of cholesterol in ascorbate-deficient and ascorbate-supplemented guinea pigs. *Journal of Lipid Research, 17*, 360–365.

Block, G., Jensen, C. D., Dalvi, T. B., Norkus, E. P., Hudes, M., Crawford, P. B., … Harmatz, P. (2009). Vitamin C treatment reduces elevated C-reactive protein. *Free Radical Biology & Medicine, 46*, 70–77.

Blumberg, J., Heaney, R. P., Huncharek, M., Scholl, T., Stampfer, M., Vieth, R., Weaver, C. M., & Zeisel, S. H. (2010). Evidence-based criteria in the nutritional context. *Nutrition Reviews, 68*, 478–484.

Boekholdt, S. M., Meuwese, M. C., Day, N. E., Luben, R., Welch, A., Wareham, N. J., & Khaw, K. T. (2006). Plasma concentrations of ascorbic acid and C-reactive protein, and risk of future coronary artery disease, in apparently healthy men and women: The EPIC-Norfolk prospective population study. *The British Journal of Nutrition, 96*, 516–522.

Bors, W., & Buettner, G. R. (1997). The vitamin C radical and its reactions. In L. Packer & J. Fuchs (Eds.), *Vitamin C in health and disease* (pp. 75–94). New York: Marcel Dekker, Inc.

Bowman, G. L., Shannon, J., Frei, B., Kaye, J. A., & Quinn, J. F. (2010). Uric acid as a CNS antioxidant. *Journal of Alzheimer's Disease, 19*, 1331–1336.

Boyer, J. C., Campbell, C. E., Sigurdson, W. J., & Kuo, S. M. (2005). Polarized localization of vitamin C transporters, SVCT1 and SVCT2, in epithelial cells. *Biochemical and Biophysical Research Communications, 334*, 150–156.

Braun, L., Puskas, F., Csala, M., Meszaros, G., Mandl, J., & Banhegyi, G. (1997). Ascorbate as a substrate for glycolysis or gluconeogenesis: Evidence for an interorgan ascorbate cycle. *Free Radical Biology & Medicine, 23*, 804–808.

Brubacher, D., Moser, U., & Jordan, P. (2000). Vitamin C concentrations in plasma as a function of intake: A meta-analysis. *International Journal for Vitamin and Nutrition Research, 70*, 226–237.

Brubaker, R. F., Bourne, W. M., Bachman, L. A., & McLaren, J. W. (2000). Ascorbic acid content of human corneal epithelium. *Investigative Ophthalmology & Visual Science, 41*, 1681–1683.

Bruick, R. K., & McKnight, S. L. (2001). A conserved family of prolyl-4-hydroxylases that modify HIF. *Science, 294*, 1337–1340.

Bruno, R. S., Leonard, S. W., Atkinson, J., Montine, T. J., Ramakrishnan, R., Bray, T. M., & Traber, M. G. (2006). Faster plasma vitamin E disappearance in smokers is normalized by vitamin C supplementation. *Free Radical Biology & Medicine, 40*, 689–697.

Buettner, G. R. (1993). The pecking order of free radicals and antioxidants: Lipid peroxidation, alpha-tocopherol, and ascorbate. *Archives of Biochemistry and Biophysics, 300*, 535–543.

Buettner, G. R., & Jurkiewicz, B. A. (1996). Catalytic metals, ascorbate and free radicals: Combinations to avoid. *Radiation Research, 145*, 532–541.

Cameron, E., & Pauling, L. (1974). The orthomolecular treatment of cancer. I. The role of ascorbic acid in host resistance. *Chemico-Biological Interactions, 9*, 273–283.

Cameron, E., & Pauling, L. (1976). Supplemental ascorbate in the supportive treatment of cancer: Prolongation of survival times in terminal human cancer. *Proceedings of the National Academy of Sciences of the United States of America, 73*, 3685–3689.

Carr, A., & Frei, B. (1999a). Does vitamin C act as a pro-oxidant under physiological conditions? *The FASEB Journal, 13*, 1007–1024.

Carr, A. C., & Frei, B. (1999b). Toward a new recommended dietary allowance for vitamin C based on antioxidant and health effects in humans. *The American Journal of Clinical Nutrition, 69*, 1086–1107.

Carty, J. L., Bevan, R., Waller, H., Mistry, N., Cooke, M., Lunec, J., & Griffiths, H. R. (2000). The effects of vitamin C supplementation on protein oxidation in healthy volunteers. *Biochemical and Biophysical Research Communications, 273*, 729–735.

Chai, W., Liebman, M., Kynast-Gales, S., & Massey, L. (2004). Oxalate absorption and endogenous oxalate synthesis from ascorbate in calcium oxalate stone formers and non-stone formers. *American Journal of Kidney Diseases, 44*, 1060–1069.

Chao, J. C., Yuan, M. D., Chen, P. Y., & Chien, S. W. (2002). Vitamin C and E supplements improve the impaired antioxidant status and decrease plasma lipid peroxides in hemodialysis patients small star, filled. *The Journal of Nutritional Biochemistry, 13*, 653–663.

Chasan-Taber, L., Willett, W. C., Seddon, J. M., Stampfer, M. J., Rosner, B., Colditz, G. A., & Hankinson, S. E. (1999). A prospective study of vitamin supplement intake and cataract extraction among U.S. women. *Epidemiology, 10*, 679–684.

Chatterjee, I. B. (1973). Evolution and the biosynthesis of ascorbic acid. *Science, 182*, 1271–1272.

Chen, L., Endler, A., & Shibasaki, F. (2009). Hypoxia and angiogenesis: Regulation of hypoxia-inducible factors via novel binding factors. *Experimental & Molecular Medicine, 41*, 849–857.

Chen, Q., Espey, M. G., Krishna, M. C., Mitchell, J. B., Corpe, C. P., Buettner, G. R., … Levine, M. (2005). Pharmacologic ascorbic acid concentrations selectively kill cancer cells: Action as a prodrug to deliver hydrogen peroxide to tissues. *Proceedings of the National Academy of Sciences of the United States of America, 102*, 13604–13609.

Chen, Q., Espey, M. G., Sun, A. Y., Lee, J. H., Krishna, M. C., Shacter, E., … Levine, M. (2007). Ascorbate in pharmacologic concentrations selectively generates ascorbate radical and hydrogen peroxide in extracellular fluid in vivo. *Proceedings of the National Academy of Sciences of the United States of America, 104*, 8749–8754.

Chen, Q., Espey, M. G., Sun, A. Y., Pooput, C., Kirk, K. L., Krishna, M. C., … Levine, M. (2008). Pharmacologic doses of ascorbate act as a prooxidant and decrease growth of aggressive tumor xenografts in mice. *Proceedings of the National Academy of Sciences of the United States of America, 105*, 11105–11109.

Chi, X., & May, J. M. (2009). Oxidized lipoprotein induces the macrophage ascorbate transporter (SVCT2): Protection by intracellular ascorbate against oxidant stress and apoptosis. *Archives of Biochemistry and Biophysics, 485*, 174–182.

Choi, H. K., Gao, X., & Curhan, G. (2009). Vitamin C intake and the risk of gout in men: A prospective study. *Archives of Internal Medicine, 169*, 502–507.

Cook, J. D., & Reddy, M. B. (2001). Effect of ascorbic acid intake on nonheme-iron absorption from a complete diet. *The American Journal of Clinical Nutrition, 73*, 93–98.

Corpe, C. P., Lee, J. H., Kwon, O., Eck, P., Narayanan, J., Kirk, K. L., & Levine, M. (2005). 6-Bromo-6-deoxy-L-ascorbic acid: An ascorbate analog specific for Na+-dependent vitamin C transporter but not glucose transporter pathways. *The Journal of Biological Chemistry, 280*, 5211–5220.

Corpe, C. P., Tu, H., Eck, P., Wang, J., Faulhaber-Walter, R., Schnermann, J., … Levine, M. (2010). Vitamin C transporter Slc23a1 links renal reabsorption, vitamin C tissue accumulation, and perinatal survival in mice. *The Journal of Clinical Investigation, 120*, 1069–1083.

Creagan, E. T., Moertel, C. G., O'Fallon, J. R., Schutt, A. J., O'Connell, M. J., Rubin, J., & Frytak, S. (1979). Failure of high-dose vitamin C (ascorbic acid) therapy to benefit patients with advanced cancer. A controlled trial. *New England Journal of Medicine, 301*, 687–690.

Daruwala, R., Song, J., Koh, W. S., Rumsey, S. C., & Levine, M. (1999). Cloning and functional characterization of the human sodium-dependent vitamin C transporters hSVCT1 and hSVCT2. *FEBS Letters, 460*, 480–484.

Dehghan, M., Akhtar-Danesh, N., McMillan, C. R., & Thabane, L. (2007). Is plasma vitamin C an appropriate biomarker of vitamin C intake? A systematic review and meta-analysis. *Nutrition Journal, 6*, 41.

Deicher, R., Ziai, F., Bieglmayer, C., Schillinger, M., & Horl, W. H. (2005). Low total vitamin C plasma level is a risk factor for cardiovascular morbidity and mortality in hemodialysis patients. *Journal of the American Society of Nephrology, 16*, 1811–1818.

Dhariwal, K. R., Shirvan, M., & Levine, M. (1991). Ascorbic acid regeneration in chromaffin granules. In situ kinetics. *The Journal of Biological Chemistry, 266*, 5384–5387.

Dherani, M., Murthy, G. V., Gupta, S. K., Young, I. S., Maraini, G., Camparini, M., … Fletcher, A. E. (2008). Blood levels of vitamin C, carotenoids and retinol are inversely associated with cataract in a North Indian population. *Investigative Ophthalmology & Visual Science, 49*, 3328–3335.

Dietrich, M., Block, G., Benowitz, N. L., Morrow, J. D., Hudes, M., Jacob, P., 3rd, … Packer, L. (2003). Vitamin C supplementation decreases oxidative stress biomarker f2-isoprostanes in plasma of nonsmokers exposed to environmental tobacco smoke. *Nutrition and Cancer, 45*, 176–184.

Dietrich, M., Block, G., Hudes, M., Morrow, J. D., Norkus, E. P., Traber, M. G., … Packer, L. (2002). Antioxidant supplementation decreases lipid peroxidation biomarker F(2)-isoprostanes in plasma of smokers. *Cancer Epidemiology, Biomarkers & Prevention, 11*, 7–13.

Douglas, R. M., Hemila, H., Chalker, E., & Treacy, B. (2007). Vitamin C for preventing and treating the common cold. *The Cochrane Database of Systematic Reviews*, (3), CD000980.

Duconge, J., Miranda-Massari, J. R., Gonzalez, M. J., Jackson, J. A., Warnock, W., & Riordan, N. H. (2008). Pharmacokinetics of vitamin C: Insights into the oral and intravenous administration of ascorbate. *Puerto Rico Health Sciences Journal, 27*, 7–19.

Duffy, S. J., Gokce, N., Holbrook, M., Huang, A., Frei, B., Keaney, J. F., Jr., & Vita, J. A. (1999). Treatment of hypertension with ascorbic acid. *Lancet, 354*, 2048–2049.

Duffy, S. J., Gokce, N., Holbrook, M., Hunter, L. M., Biegelsen, E. S., Huang, A., … Vita, J. A. (2001). Effect of ascorbic acid treatment on conduit vessel endothelial dysfunction in patients with hypertension. *American Journal of Physiology. Heart and Circulatory Physiology, 280*, H528–H534.

Dunn, W. A., Rettura, G., Seifter, E., & Englard, S. (1984). Carnitine biosynthesis from gamma-butyrobetaine and from exogenous protein-bound 6-N-trimethyl-L-lysine by the perfused guinea pig liver. Effect of ascorbate deficiency on the in situ activity of gamma-butyrobetaine hydroxylase. *The Journal of Biological Chemistry, 259*, 10764–10770.

Eipper, B. A., Bloomquist, B. T., Husten, E. J., Milgram, S. L., & Mains, R. E. (1993). Peptidylglycine alpha-amidating monooxygenase and other processing enzymes in the neurointermediate pituitary. *Annals of the New York Academy of Sciences, 680*, 147–160.

Englard, S., & Seifter, S. (1986). The biochemical functions of ascorbic acid. *Annual Review of Nutrition, 6*, 365–406.

Evans, R. M., Currie, L., & Campbell, A. (1982). The distribution of ascorbic acid between various cellular components of blood, in normal individuals, and its relation to the plasma concentration. *The British Journal of Nutrition, 47*, 473–482.

Ferretti, G., Bacchetti, T., Masciangelo, S., & Pallotta, G. (2008). Lipid peroxidation in hemodialysis patients: Effect of vitamin C supplementation. *Clinical Biochemistry, 41*, 381–386.

Fleming, P. J., & Kent, U. M. (1991). Cytochrome b561, ascorbic acid, and transmembrane electron transfer. *The American Journal of Clinical Nutrition, 54*, 1173S–1178S.

Fraga, C. G., Motchnik, P. A., Shigenaga, M. K., Helbock, H. J., Jacob, R. A., & Ames, B. N. (1991). Ascorbic acid protects against endogenous oxidative DNA damage in human sperm. *Proceedings of the National Academy of Sciences of the United States of America, 88*, 11003–11006.

Frei, B. (1991). Ascorbic acid protects lipids in human plasma and low-density lipoprotein against oxidative damage. *The American Journal of Clinical Nutrition, 54,* 1113S–1118S.

Frei, B. (2004). Efficacy of dietary antioxidants to prevent oxidative damage and inhibit chronic disease. *The Journal of Nutrition, 134,* 3196S–3198S.

Frei, B., England, L., & Ames, B. N. (1989). Ascorbate is an outstanding antioxidant in human blood plasma. *Proceedings of the National Academy of Sciences of the United States of America, 86,* 6377–6381.

Frei, B., Stocker, R., & Ames, B. N. (1988). Antioxidant defenses and lipid peroxidation in human blood plasma. *Proceedings of the National Academy of Sciences of the United States of America, 85,* 9748–9752.

Frikke-Schmidt, H., & Lykkesfeldt, J. (2009). Role of marginal vitamin C deficiency in atherogenesis: In vivo models and clinical studies. *Basic & Clinical Pharmacology & Toxicology, 104,* 419–433.

Fujita, I., Hirano, J., Itoh, N., Nakanishi, T., & Tanaka, K. (2001). Dexamethasone induces sodium-dependant vitamin C transporter in a mouse osteoblastic cell line MC3T3-E1. *The British Journal of Nutrition, 86,* 145–149.

Furusawa, H., Sato, Y., Tanaka, Y., Inai, Y., Amano, A., Iwama, M., … Ishigami, A. (2008). Vitamin C is not essential for carnitine biosynthesis in vivo: Verification in vitamin C–depleted senescence marker protein-30/gluconolactonase knockout mice. *Biological & Pharmaceutical Bulletin, 31,* 1673–1679.

Gale, C. R., Martyn, C. N., Winter, P. D., & Cooper, C. (1995). Vitamin C and risk of death from stroke and coronary heart disease in cohort of elderly people. *BMJ, 310,* 1563–1566.

Gao, X., Curhan, G., Forman, J. P., Ascherio, A., & Choi, H. K. (2008). Vitamin C intake and serum uric acid concentration in men. *The Journal of Rheumatology, 35,* 1853–1858.

Gerster, H. (1999). High-dose vitamin C: A risk for persons with high iron stores? *International Journal for Vitamin and Nutrition Research, 69,* 67–82.

Godoy, A., Ormazabal, V., Moraga-Cid, G., Zuniga, F. A., Sotomayor, P., Barra, V., … Vera, J. C. (2007). Mechanistic insights and functional determinants of the transport cycle of the ascorbic acid transporter SVCT2. Activation by sodium and absolute dependence on bivalent cations. *The Journal of Biological Chemistry, 282,* 615–624.

Gokce, N., Keaney, J. F., Jr., Frei, B., Holbrook, M., Olesiak, M., Zachariah, B. J., … Vita, J. A. (1999). Long-term ascorbic acid administration reverses endothelial vasomotor dysfunction in patients with coronary artery disease. *Circulation, 99,* 3234–3240.

Graumlich, J. F., Ludden, T. M., Conry-Cantilena, C., Cantilena, L. R., Jr., Wang, Y., & Levine, M. (1997). Pharmacokinetic model of ascorbic acid in healthy male volunteers during depletion and repletion. *Pharmaceutical Research, 14,* 1133–1139.

Hallberg, L. (1995). Iron and vitamins. *Bibliotheca Nutritio et Dieta, 52,* 20–29.

Halliwell, B. (1996). Vitamin C: Antioxidant or pro-oxidant in vivo? *Free Radical Research, 25,* 439–454.

Halliwell, B. (2003). Oxidative stress in cell culture: An under-appreciated problem? *FEBS Letters, 540,* 3–6.

Halliwell, B., Wasil, M., & Grootveld, M. (1987). Biologically significant scavenging of the myeloperoxidase-derived oxidant hypochlorous acid by ascorbic acid. Implications for antioxidant protection in the inflamed rheumatoid joint. *FEBS Letters, 213,* 15–17.

Halliwell, B. G., & Gutterige, J. M. C. (2007). *Free radicals in biology and medicine* (4th ed.). New York: Oxford University Press.

Hampl, J. S., Taylor, C. A., & Johnston, C. S. (2004). Vitamin C deficiency and depletion in the United States: The Third National Health and Nutrition Examination Survey, 1988 to 1994. *American Journal of Public Health, 94,* 870–875.

Harrison, F. E., Dawes, S. M., Meredith, M. E., Babaev, V. R., Li, L., & May, J. M. (2010a). Low vitamin C and increased oxidative stress and cell death in mice that lack the sodium-dependent vitamin C transporter SVCT2. *Free Radical Biology & Medicine, 49,* 821–829.

Harrison, F. E., Green, R. J., Dawes, S. M., & May, J. M. (2010b). Vitamin C distribution and retention in the mouse brain. *Brain Research, 1348C,* 181–186.

Heller, R., Unbehaun, A., Schellenberg, B., Mayer, B., Werner-Felmayer, G., & Werner, E. R. (2001). L-Ascorbic acid potentiates endothelial nitric oxide synthesis via a chemical stabilization of tetrahydrobiopterin. *The Journal of Biological Chemistry, 276,* 40–47.

Hill, K. E., Montine, T. J., Motley, A. K., Li, X., May, J. M., & Burk, R. F. (2003). Combined deficiency of vitamins E and C causes paralysis and death in guinea pigs. *The American Journal of Clinical Nutrition, 77,* 1484–1488.

Hirschmann, J. V., & Raugi, G. J. (1999). Adult scurvy. *Journal of the American Academy of Dermatology, 41,* 895-906; quiz 907–910.

Hirvonen, T., Virtamo, J., Korhonen, P., Albanes, D., & Pietinen, P. (2000). Intake of flavonoids, carotenoids, vitamins C and E, and risk of stroke in male smokers. *Stroke, 31,* 2301–2306.

Hodges, R. E., Hood, J., Canham, J. E., Sauberlich, H. E., & Baker, E. M. (1971). Clinical manifestations of ascorbic acid deficiency in man. *The American Journal of Clinical Nutrition, 24,* 432–443.

Hoffer, L. J., Levine, M., Assouline, S., Melnychuk, D., Padayatty, S. J., Rosadiuk, K., … Miller, W. H., Jr. (2008). Phase I clinical trial of i.v. ascorbic acid in advanced malignancy. *Annals of Oncology, 19,* 1969–1974.

Hogue, D. L., & Ling, V. (1999). A human nucleobase transporter-like cDNA (SLC23A1): Member of a transporter family conserved from bacteria to mammals. *Genomics, 59,* 18–23.

Holloway, D. E., Peterson, F. J., Prigge, W. F., & Gebhard, R. L. (1981). Influence of dietary ascorbic acid upon enzymes of sterol biosynthesis in the guinea pig. *Biochemical and Biophysical Research Communications, 102,* 1283–1289.

Hood, J., Burns, C. A., & Hodges, R. E. (1970). Sjogren's syndrome in scurvy. *New England Journal of Medicine, 282,* 1120–1124.

Hornig, D. (1975). Distribution of ascorbic acid, metabolites and analogues in man and animals. *Annals of the New York Academy of Sciences, 258,* 103–118.

Huang, H. Y., Appel, L. J., Choi, M. J., Gelber, A. C., Charleston, J., Norkus, E. P., & Miller, E. R. (2005). The effects of vitamin C supplementation on serum concentrations of uric acid: Results of a randomized controlled trial. *Arthritis and Rheumatism, 52,* 1843–1847.

Institute of Medicine. (2000). *Dietary reference intakes for vitamin C, vitamin E, selenium carotenoids.* Washington, DC: National Academy Press.

Jacques, P. F. (1992). Effects of vitamin C on high-density lipoprotein cholesterol and blood pressure. *Journal of the American College of Nutrition, 11,* 139–144.

Kathir, K., Dennis, J. M., Croft, K. D., Mori, T. A., Lau, A. K., Adams, M. R., & Stocker, R. (2010). Equivalent lipid oxidation profiles in advanced atherosclerotic lesions of carotid endarterectomy plaques obtained from symptomatic type 2 diabetic and nondiabetic subjects. *Free Radical Biology & Medicine, 49,* 481–486.

Kaufman, S. (1974). Dopamine-beta-hydroxylase. *Journal of Psychiatric Research, 11,* 303–316.

Kesinger, N. G., & Stevens, J. F. (2009). Covalent interaction of ascorbic acid with natural products. *Phytochemistry, 70,* 1930–1939.

Khaw, K. T., Bingham, S., Welch, A., Luben, R., Wareham, N., Oakes, S., & Day, N. (2001). Relation between plasma ascorbic acid and mortality in men and women in EPIC-Norfolk prospective study: A prospective population study. European Prospective Investigation into Cancer and Nutrition. *Lancet, 357,* 657–663.

Khaw, K. T., Wareham, N., Bingham, S., Welch, A., Luben, R., & Day, N. (2008). Combined impact of health behaviours and mortality in men and women: The EPIC-Norfolk prospective population study. *PLoS Medicine 5*, e12.

King, C. C., & Waugh, W. A. (1932). The chemical nature of vitamin C. *Science, 75*, 357–358.

Kinsman, R. A., & Hood, J. (1971). Some behavioral effects of ascorbic acid deficiency. *The American Journal of Clinical Nutrition, 24*, 455–464.

Kuiper, C., Molenaar, I. G., Dachs, G. U., Currie, M. J., Sykes, P. H., & Vissers, M. C. (2010). Low ascorbate levels are associated with increased hypoxia-inducible factor-1 activity and an aggressive tumor phenotype in endometrial cancer. *Cancer Research, 70*, 5749–5758.

Lane, D. J., & Lawen, A. (2009). Ascorbate and plasma membrane electron transport—Enzymes vs efflux. *Free Radical Biology & Medicine, 47*, 485–495.

Langlois, M., Duprez, D., Delanghe, J., De Buyzere, M., & Clement, D. L. (2001). Serum vitamin C concentration is low in peripheral arterial disease and is associated with inflammation and severity of atherosclerosis. *Circulation, 103*, 1863–1868.

Levine, G. N., Frei, B., Koulouris, S. N., Gerhard, M. D., Keaney, J. F., Jr., & Vita, J. A. (1996a). Ascorbic acid reverses endothelial vasomotor dysfunction in patients with coronary artery disease. *Circulation, 93*, 1107–1113.

Levine, M. (1986). New concepts in the biology and biochemistry of ascorbic acid. *New England Journal of Medicine, 314*, 892–902.

Levine, M., Conry-Cantilena, C., Wang, Y., Welch, R. W., Washko, P. W., Dhariwal, K. R., … Cantilena, L. R. (1996b). Vitamin C pharmacokinetics in healthy volunteers: Evidence for a recommended dietary allowance. *Proceedings of the National Academy of Sciences of the United States of America, 93*, 3704–3709.

Levine, M., Dhariwal, K. R., Washko, P. W., Butler, J. D., Welch, R. W., Wang, Y. H., & Bergsten, P. (1991). Ascorbic acid and in situ kinetics: A new approach to vitamin requirements. *The American Journal of Clinical Nutrition, 54*, 1157S–1162S.

Levine, M., Rumsey, S. C., Daruwala, R., Park, J. B., & Wang, Y. (1999). Criteria and recommendations for vitamin C intake. *The Journal of the American Medical Association, 281*, 1415–1423.

Levine, M., Wang, Y., Padayatty, S. J., & Morrow, J. (2001). A new recommended dietary allowance of vitamin C for healthy young women. *Proceedings of the National Academy of Sciences of the United States of America, 98*, 9842–9846.

Liang, W. J., Johnson, D., Ma, L. S., Jarvis, S. M., & Wei-Jun, L. (2002). Regulation of the human vitamin C transporters expressed in COS-1 cells by protein kinase C [corrected]. *American Journal of Physiology. Cell Physiology, 283*, C1696–C1704.

Lind, J. (1753). *A treatise on the scurvy*. London: A. Millar.

Littlejohn, T. K., Takikawa, O., Skylas, D., Jamie, J. F., Walker, M. J., & Truscott, R. J. (2000). Expression and purification of recombinant human indoleamine 2,3-dioxygenase. *Protein Expression and Purification, 19*, 22–29.

Luo, S., Wang, Z., Kansara, V., Pal, D., & Mitra, A. K. (2008). Activity of a sodium-dependent vitamin C transporter (SVCT) in MDCK-MDR1 cells and mechanism of ascorbate uptake. *International Journal of Pharmaceutics, 358*, 168–176.

Lykkesfeldt, J., & Poulsen, H. E. (2010). Is vitamin C supplementation beneficial? Lessons learned from randomised controlled trials. *The British Journal of Nutrition, 103*, 1251–1259.

Lynch, S. M., Morrow, J. D., Roberts, L. J., 2nd, & Frei, B. (1994). Formation of non-cyclooxygenase-derived prostanoids (F2-isoprostanes) in plasma and low density lipoprotein exposed to oxidative stress in vitro. *The Journal of Clinical Investigation, 93*, 998–1004.

Majamaa, K., Gunzler, V., Hanauske-Abel, H. M., Myllyla, R., & Kivirikko, K. I. (1986). Partial identity of the 2-oxoglutarate and ascorbate binding sites of prolyl 4-hydroxylase. *The Journal of Biological Chemistry, 261*, 7819–7823.

Marin-Hernandez, A., Gallardo-Perez, J. C., Ralph, S. J., Rodriguez-Enriquez, S., & Moreno-Sanchez, R. (2009). HIF-1alpha modulates energy metabolism in cancer cells by inducing over-expression of specific glycolytic isoforms. *Mini Reviews in Medicinal Chemistry, 9*, 1084–1101.

Massey, L. K., Liebman, M., & Kynast-Gales, S. A. (2005). Ascorbate increases human oxaluria and kidney stone risk. *The Journal of Nutrition, 135*, 1673–1677.

Maulen, N. P., Henriquez, E. A., Kempe, S., Carcamo, J. G., Schmid-Kotsas, A., Bachem, M., … Vera, J. C. (2003). Up-regulation and polarized expression of the sodium-ascorbic acid transporter SVCT1 in post-confluent differentiated CaCo-2 cells. *The Journal of Biological Chemistry, 278*, 9035–9041.

May, J. M., Cobb, C. E., Mendiratta, S., Hill, K. E., & Burk, R. F. (1998). Reduction of the ascorbyl free radical to ascorbate by thioredoxin reductase. *The Journal of Biological Chemistry, 273*, 23039–23045.

May, J. M., Li, L., & Qu, Z. C. (2010). Oxidized LDL up-regulates the ascorbic acid transporter SVCT2 in endothelial cells. *Molecular and Cellular Biochemistry, 343*, 217–222.

May, J. M., Qu, Z., & Cobb, C. E. (2001a). Recycling of the ascorbate free radical by human erythrocyte membranes. *Free Radical Biology & Medicine, 31*, 117–124.

May, J. M., Qu, Z., & Morrow, J. D. (2001b). Mechanisms of ascorbic acid recycling in human erythrocytes. *Biochimica et Biophysica Acta, 1528*, 159–166.

May, J. M., Qu, Z. C., Qiao, H., & Koury, M. J. (2007). Maturational loss of the vitamin C transporter in erythrocytes. *Biochemical and Biophysical Research Communications, 360*, 295–298.

May, J. M., Qu, Z. C., Whitesell, R. R., & Cobb, C. E. (1996). Ascorbate recycling in human erythrocytes: Role of GSH in reducing dehydroascorbate. *Free Radical Biology & Medicine, 20*, 543–551.

Meagher, E. A., Barry, O. P., Burke, A., Lucey, M. R., Lawson, J. A., Rokach, J., & FitzGerald, G. A. (1999). Alcohol-induced generation of lipid peroxidation products in humans. *The Journal of Clinical Investigation, 104*, 805–813.

Meister, A. (1994). Glutathione-ascorbic acid antioxidant system in animals. *The Journal of Biological Chemistry, 269*, 9397–9400.

Michels, A. J., & Hagen, T. M. (2009). Hepatocyte nuclear factor 1 is essential for transcription of sodium-dependent vitamin C transporter protein 1. *American Journal of Physiology. Cell Physiology, 297*, C1220–C1227.

Miglio, C., Chiavaro, E., Visconti, A., Fogliano, V., & Pellegrini, N. (2008). Effects of different cooking methods on nutritional and physicochemical characteristics of selected vegetables. *Journal of Agricultural and Food Chemistry, 56*, 139–147.

Miranda, C. L., Reed, R. L., Kuiper, H. C., Alber, S., & Stevens, J. F. (2009). Ascorbic acid promotes detoxification and elimination of 4-hydroxy-2(E)-nonenal in human monocytic THP-1 cells. *Chemical Research in Toxicology, 22*, 863–874.

Mirvish, S. S., Grandjean, A. C., Reimers, K. J., Connelly, B. J., Chen, S. C., Morris, C. R., … Lyden, E. R. (1998). Effect of ascorbic acid dose taken with a meal on nitrosoproline excretion in subjects ingesting nitrate and proline. *Nutrition and Cancer, 31*, 106–110.

Moertel, C. G., Fleming, T. R., Creagan, E. T., Rubin, J., O'Connell, M. J., & Ames, M. M. (1985). High-dose vitamin C versus placebo in the treatment of patients with advanced cancer who have had no prior chemotherapy. A randomized double-blind comparison. *New England Journal of Medicine, 312*, 137–141.

Moran, G. R. (2005). 4-Hydroxyphenylpyruvate dioxygenase. *Archives of Biochemistry and Biophysics, 433*, 117–128.

Myint, P. K., Luben, R. N., Welch, A. A., Bingham, S. A., Wareham, N. J., & Khaw, K. T. (2008). Plasma vitamin C concentrations predict risk of incident stroke over 10 y in 20 649 participants of the European Prospective Investigation into Cancer Norfolk prospective population study. *The American Journal of Clinical Nutrition, 87*, 64–69.

Myllyharju, J. (2003). Prolyl 4-hydroxylases, the key enzymes of collagen biosynthesis. *Matrix Biology, 22*, 15–24.

Nishikimi, M., Fukuyama, R., Minoshima, S., Shimizu, N., & Yagi, K. (1994). Cloning and chromosomal mapping of the human nonfunctional gene for l-gulono-gamma-lactone oxidase, the enzyme for L-ascorbic acid biosynthesis missing in man. *The Journal of Biological Chemistry, 269*, 13685–13688.

Nualart, F. J., Rivas, C. I., Montecinos, V. P., Godoy, A. S., Guaiquil, V. H., Golde, D. W., & Vera, J. C. (2003). Recycling of vitamin C by a bystander effect. *The Journal of Biological Chemistry, 278*, 10128–10133.

Ogiri, Y., Sun, F., Hayami, S., Fujimura, A., Yamamoto, K., Yaita, M., & Kojo, S. (2002). Very low vitamin C activity of orally administered L-dehydroascorbic acid. *Journal of Agricultural and Food Chemistry, 50*, 227–229.

Oliveira, A., Rodriguez-Artalejo, F., & Lopes, C. (2009). The association of fruits, vegetables, antioxidant vitamins and fibre intake with high-sensitivity C-reactive protein: Sex and body mass index interactions. *European Journal of Clinical Nutrition, 63*, 1345–1352.

Parsons, K. K., Maeda, N., Yamauchi, M., Banes, A. J., & Koller, B. H. (2006). Ascorbic acid-independent synthesis of collagen in mice. *American Journal of Physiology. Endocrinology and Metabolism, 290*, E1131–E1139.

Peterkofsky, B. (1991). Ascorbate requirement for hydroxylation and secretion of procollagen: Relationship to inhibition of collagen synthesis in scurvy. *The American Journal of Clinical Nutrition, 54*, 1135S–1140S.

Pocobelli, G., Peters, U., Kristal, A. R., & White, E. (2009). Use of supplements of multivitamins, vitamin C, and vitamin E in relation to mortality. *American Journal of Epidemiology, 170*, 472–483.

Prigge, S. T., Mains, R. E., Eipper, B. A., & Amzel, L. M. (2000). New insights into copper monooxygenases and peptide amidation: Structure, mechanism and function. *Cellular and Molecular Life Sciences, 57*, 1236–1259.

Pugh, C. W., & Ratcliffe, P. J. (2003). Regulation of angiogenesis by hypoxia: Role of the HIF system. *Nature Medicine, 9*, 677–684.

Qiao, H., Li, L., Qu, Z. C., & May, J. M. (2009). Cobalt-induced oxidant stress in cultured endothelial cells: Prevention by ascorbate in relation to HIF-1alpha. *Biofactors, 35*, 306–313.

Qiao, H., & May, J. M. (2009). Macrophage differentiation increases expression of the ascorbate transporter (SVCT2). *Free Radical Biology & Medicine, 46*, 1221–1232.

Rankin, E. B., & Giaccia, A. J. (2008). The role of hypoxia-inducible factors in tumorigenesis. *Cell Death and Differentiation, 15*, 678–685.

Rautiainen, S., Lindblad, B. E., Morgenstern, R., & Wolk, A. (2010). Vitamin C supplements and the risk of age-related cataract: A population-based prospective cohort study in women. *The American Journal of Clinical Nutrition, 91*, 487–493.

Rebouche, C. J. (1991). Ascorbic acid and carnitine biosynthesis. *The American Journal of Clinical Nutrition, 54*, 1147S–1152S.

Rebouche, C. J. (1995). Renal handling of carnitine in experimental vitamin C deficiency. *Metabolism, 44*, 1639–1643.

Reilly, M., Delanty, N., Lawson, J. A., & FitzGerald, G. A. (1996). Modulation of oxidant stress in vivo in chronic cigarette smokers. *Circulation, 94*, 19–25.

Retsky, K. L., Freeman, M. W., & Frei, B. (1993). Ascorbic acid oxidation product(s) protect human low density lipoprotein against atherogenic modification. Anti- rather than prooxidant activity of vitamin C in the presence of transition metal ions. *The Journal of Biological Chemistry, 268*, 1304–1309.

Rose, R. C. (1988). Transport of ascorbic acid and other water soluble vitamins. *Biochimica et Biophysica Acta, 947*, 35–366.

Rumsey, S. C., Daruwala, R., Al-Hasani, H., Zarnowski, M. J., Simpson, I. A., & Levine, M. (2000). Dehydroascorbic acid transport by GLUT4 in *Xenopus* oocytes and isolated rat adipocytes. *The Journal of Biological Chemistry, 275*, 28246–28253.

Rumsey, S. C., Kwon, O., Xu, G. W., Burant, C. F., Simpson, I., & Levine, M. (1997). Glucose transporter isoforms GLUT1 and GLUT3 transport dehydroascorbic acid. *The Journal of Biological Chemistry, 272*, 18982–18989.

Rumsey, S. C., Welch, R. W., Garraffo, H. M., Ge, P., Lu, S. F., Crossman, A. T., … Levine, M. (1999). Specificity of ascorbate analogs for ascorbate transport. Synthesis and detection of [(125)I]6-deoxy-6-iodo-L-ascorbic acid and characterization of its ascorbate-specific transport properties. *The Journal of Biological Chemistry, 274*, 23215–23222.

Sargeant, L. A., Wareham, N. J., Bingham, S., Day, N. E., Luben, R. N., Oakes, S., … Khaw, K. T. (2000). Vitamin C and hyperglycemia in the European Prospective Investigation into Cancer–Norfolk (EPIC-Norfolk) study: A population-based study. *Diabetes Care, 23*, 726–732.

Sauberlich, H. E., Tamura, T., Craig, C. B., Freeberg, L. E., & Liu, T. (1996). Effects of erythorbic acid on vitamin C metabolism in young women. *The American Journal of Clinical Nutrition, 64*, 336–346.

Savini, I., Rossi, A., Catani, M. V., Ceci, R., & Avigliano, L. (2007). Redox regulation of vitamin C transporter SVCT2 in C2C12 myotubes. *Biochemical and Biophysical Research Communications, 361*, 385–390.

Savini, I., Rossi, A., Pierro, C., Avigliano, L., & Catani, M. V. (2008). SVCT1 and SVCT2: Key proteins for vitamin C uptake. *Amino Acids, 34*, 347–355.

Simon, J. A., & Hudes, E. S. (1999). Serum ascorbic acid and other correlates of self-reported cataract among older Americans. *Journal of Clinical Epidemiology, 52*, 1207–1211.

Singer, R., Rhodes, H. C., Chin, G., Kulkarni, H., & Ferrari, P. (2008). High prevalence of ascorbate deficiency in an Australian peritoneal dialysis population. *Nephrology (Carlton), 13*, 17–22.

Singer, R. F. (2010). Vitamin C supplementation in kidney failure: Effect on uraemic symptoms. *Nephrology, Dialysis, Transplantation, 26*(2), 614–620.

Smith, A. R., Visioli, F., & Hagen, T. M. (2002). Vitamin C matters: Increased oxidative stress in cultured human aortic endothelial cells without supplemental ascorbic acid. *The FASEB Journal, 16*, 1102–1104.

Sotiriou, S., Gispert, S., Cheng, J., Wang, Y., Chen, A., Hoogstraten-Miller, S., … Nussbaum, R. L. (2002). Ascorbic-acid transporter Slc23a1 is essential for vitamin C transport into the brain and for perinatal survival. *Nature Medicine, 8*, 514–517.

Stewart, L. C., & Klinman, J. P. (1988). Dopamine beta-hydroxylase of adrenal chromaffin granules: Structure and function. *Annual Review of Biochemistry, 57*, 551–592.

Subramanian, V. S., Marchant, J. S., Boulware, M. J., & Said, H. M. (2004). A C-terminal region dictates the apical plasma membrane targeting of the human sodium-dependent vitamin C transporter-1 in polarized epithelia. *The Journal of Biological Chemistry, 279*, 27719–27728.

Svirbely, J. L., & Szent-Györgyi, A. (1932). The chemical nature of vitamin C. *The Biochemical Journal, 26*, 865–870.

Szarka, A., Stadler, K., Jenei, V., Margittai, E., Csala, M., Jakus, J., … Banhegyi, G. (2002). Ascorbyl free radical and dehydroascorbate formation in rat liver endoplasmic reticulum. *Journal of Bioenergetics and Biomembranes, 34*, 317–323.

Takanaga, H., Mackenzie, B., & Hediger, M. A. (2004). Sodium-dependent ascorbic acid transporter family SLC23. *Pflügers Archiv, 447*, 677–682.

Tanaka, K., Hashimoto, T., Tokumaru, S., Iguchi, H., & Kojo, S. (1997). Interactions between vitamin C and vitamin E are observed in tissues of inherently scorbutic rats. *The Journal of Nutrition, 127*, 2060–2064.

Tarng, D. C., Liu, T. Y., & Huang, T. P. (2004). Protective effect of vitamin C on 8-hydroxy-2′-deoxyguanosine level in peripheral blood lymphocytes of chronic hemodialysis patients. *Kidney International, 66*, 820–831.

Taylor, A., Jacques, P. F., Nadler, D., Morrow, F., Sulsky, S. I., & Shepard, D. (1991). Relationship in humans between ascorbic acid consumption and levels of total and reduced ascorbic acid in lens, aqueous humor, and plasma. *Current Eye Research, 10*, 751–759.

Taylor, E. N., Fung, T. T., & Curhan, G. C. (2009). DASH-style diet associates with reduced risk for kidney stones. *Journal of the American Society of Nephrology, 20*, 2253–2259.

Taylor, E. N., Stampfer, M. J., & Curhan, G. C. (2004). Dietary factors and the risk of incident kidney stones in men: New insights after 14 years of follow-up. *Journal of the American Society of Nephrology, 15*, 3225–3232.

Timpson, N. J., Forouhi, N. G., Brion, M. J., Harbord, R. M., Cook, D. G., Johnson, P., … Davey, S. G. (2010). Genetic variation at the SLC23A1 locus is associated with circulating concentrations of L-ascorbic acid (vitamin C): Evidence from 5 independent studies with >15,000 participants. *The American Journal of Clinical Nutrition, 92*, 375–382.

Tomson, C. R., Channon, S. M., Parkinson, I. S., McArdle, P., Qureshi, M., Ward, M. K., & Laker, M. F. (1989). Correction of subclinical ascorbate deficiency in patients receiving dialysis: Effects on plasma oxalate, serum cholesterol, and capillary fragility. *Clinica Chimica Acta, 180*, 255–264.

Traber, M. G. (2007). Vitamin E regulatory mechanisms. *Annual Review of Nutrition, 27*, 347–362.

Traxer, O., Huet, B., Poindexter, J., Pak, C. Y., & Pearle, M. S. (2003). Effect of ascorbic acid consumption on urinary stone risk factors. *Journal of Urology, 170*, 397–401.

Tsukaguchi, H., Tokui, T., Mackenzie, B., Berger, U. V., Chen, X. Z., Wang, Y., … Hediger, M. A. (1999). A family of mammalian Na+-dependent L-ascorbic acid transporters. *Nature, 399*, 70–75.

U.S. Department of Agriculture/Agricultural Research Service. (2010). *USDA National Nutrient Database for Standard Reference, Release 23.* Retrieved from www.ars.usda.gov/ba/bhnrc/ndl

Valero, M. P., Fletcher, A. E., De Stavola, B. L., Vioque, J., & Alepuz, V. C. (2002). Vitamin C is associated with reduced risk of cataract in a Mediterranean population. *The Journal of Nutrition, 132*, 1299–1306.

van der Vliet, A., O'Neill, C. A., Cross, C. E., Koostra, J. M., Volz, W. G., Halliwell, B., & Louie, S. (1999). Determination of low-molecular-mass antioxidant concentrations in human respiratory tract lining fluids. *The American Journal of Physiology, 276*, L289–L296.

Vanderslice, J. T., & Higgs, D. J. (1991). Vitamin C content of foods: Sample variability. *The American Journal of Clinical Nutrition, 54*, 1323S–1327S.

Varma, S., Campbell, C. E., & Kuo, S. M. (2008). Functional role of conserved transmembrane segment 1 residues in human sodium-dependent vitamin C transporters. *Biochemistry, 47*, 2952–2960.

Vera, J. C., Rivas, C. I., Fischbarg, J., & Golde, D. W. (1993). Mammalian facilitative hexose transporters mediate the transport of dehydroascorbic acid. *Nature, 364*, 79–82.

Versari, D., Daghini, E., Virdis, A., Ghiadoni, L., & Taddei, S. (2009). Endothelium-dependent contractions and endothelial dysfunction in human hypertension. *British Journal of Pharmacology, 157*, 527–536.

Vissers M. C., & Wilkie R. P. (2007). Ascorbate deficiency results in impaired neutrophil apoptosis and clearance and is associated with up-regulation of hypoxia-inducible factor 1alpha. *Journal of Leukocyte Biology 42*, 1236–1244.

Voko, Z., Hollander, M., Hofman, A., Koudstaal, P. J., & Breteler, M. M. (2003). Dietary antioxidants and the risk of ischemic stroke: The Rotterdam Study. *Neurology, 61*, 1273–1275.

von Lintig, J., & Vogt, K. (2000). Filling the gap in vitamin A research. Molecular identification of an enzyme cleaving beta-carotene to retinal. *The Journal of Biological Chemistry, 275*, 11915–11920.

Waring, A. J., Drake, I. M., Schorah, C. J., White, K. L., Lynch, D. A., Axon, A. T., & Dixon, M. F. (1996). Ascorbic acid and total vitamin C concentrations in plasma, gastric juice, and gastrointestinal mucosa: Effects of gastritis and oral supplementation. *Gut, 38*, 171–176.

Washko, P. W., Wang, Y., & Levine, M. (1993). Ascorbic acid recycling in human neutrophils. *The Journal of Biological Chemistry, 268*, 15531–15535.

Werner, E. R., & Werner-Felmayer, G. (2007). Substrate and cofactor requirements of indoleamine 2,3-dioxygenase in interferon-gamma-treated cells: Utilization of oxygen rather than superoxide. *Current Drug Metabolism, 8*, 201–203.

Wilson, J. X. (2009). Mechanism of action of vitamin C in sepsis: Ascorbate modulates redox signaling in endothelium. *Biofactors, 35*, 5–13.

Winkler, B. S., Orselli, S. M., & Rex, T. S. (1994). The redox couple between glutathione and ascorbic acid: A chemical and physiological perspective. *Free Radical Biology & Medicine, 17*, 333–349.

Wu, X., Zeng, L. H., Taniguchi, T., & Xie, Q. M. (2007). Activation of PKA and phosphorylation of sodium-dependent vitamin C transporter 2 by prostaglandin E2 promote osteoblast-like differentiation in MC3T3-E1 cells. *Cell Death and Differentiation, 14*, 1792–1801.

Ye, Z., & Song, H. (2008). Antioxidant vitamins intake and the risk of coronary heart disease: Meta-analysis of cohort studies. *European Journal of Cardiovascular Prevention and Rehabilitation, 15*, 26–34.

RECOMMENDED READINGS

Asard, H., May, J. M., & Smirnoff, N. (Eds.). (2004). *Vitamin C: Functions and biochemistry in animals and plants.* London, UK: BIOS Scientific Publishers.

Carr, A. C., & Frei, B. (1999). Toward a new recommended dietary allowance for vitamin C based on antioxidant and health effects in humans. *The American Journal of Clinical Nutrition, 69*, 1086–1107.

Drake, V. J., & Frei, B. (2011). Vitamin C in human disease prevention. In R. Obeid & W. Herrmann (Eds.), *Vitamins in the prevention of human diseases.* Berlin, Germany: Walter de Gruyter.

Englard, S., & Seifter, S. (1986). The biochemical functions of ascorbic acid. *Annual Review of Nutrition, 6*, 365–406.

Institute of Medicine. (2000). *Dietary reference intakes for vitamin C, vitamin E, selenium, and carotenoids.* Washington, DC: National Academy Press.

Levine, M., Katz, A., & Padayatty, S. J. (2005). Vitamin C. In M. E. Shils, M. Shike, A. C. Ross, B. Caballero, & R. J. Cousins (Eds.), *Modern nutrition in health and disease* (10th ed., pp. 507–524). Baltimore: Lippincott, Williams, and Wilkins.

CHAPTER 28

Vitamin K

Reidar Wallin, PhD

COMMON ABBREVIATIONS

ER	endoplasmic reticulum
Gla	γ-carboxyglutamic acid
Glu	glutamic acid
MK	menaquinone
KH_2	reduced vitamin K, or vitamin K hydroquinone
K>O	vitamin K 2,3-epoxide
VKOR	vitamin K 2,3-epoxide reductase

Vitamin K, a fat-soluble vitamin, was first identified as an antihemorrhagic factor in the late 1930s (Dam, 1934) and is so named because a lack of this vitamin causes a defect in blood *koagulation* (German word for coagulation). Vitamin K serves as a cofactor in a posttranslational modification reaction converting a specific set of glutamic acid (Glu) residues in precursors of vitamin K–dependent proteins to γ-carboxyglutamic acid (Gla) residues which can bind Ca^{2+}. The vitamin K–dependent modification system is located on the luminal side of the endoplasmic reticulum (ER) where newly synthesized proteins undergo folding and modifications (Stanton et al., 1991). The first proteins to be characterized as vitamin K–dependent proteins were those belonging to the blood coagulation system (Monroe et al., 2002). The independent discovery by Stenflo and colleagues (1974) and Nelsestuen and co-workers (1974) that the vitamin K–dependent modification was a postribosomal modification converting Glu residues to Ca^{2+}-binding Gla residues in newly synthesized vitamin K–dependent proteins yielded the clinically important understanding as to why Ca^{2+} is essential for hemostasis. Ca^{2+} binding by the clotting factors, prothrombin and factors VII, IX and X, is essential for assembly of coagulation complexes on phospholipids at the site of an injury in the vessel wall, where blood platelets are first to aggregate and provide the phospholipids.

Following the discovery of vitamin K–dependent proteins belonging to the coagulation system, several vitamin K–dependent proteins that do not belong to the coagulation system have been identified, including matrix Gla protein (MGP) involved in inhibition of pathological bone formation; osteocalcin, involved in bone metabolism; and Gas6, involved in cell survival (Booth, 2009). A role for vitamin K in regulation of calcification, energy metabolism, and inflammation has been suggested (Booth, 2009).

NOMENCLATURE OF VITAMIN K ACTIVE COMPOUNDS

Compounds with vitamin K activity are 2-methyl-1,4-naphthoquinones with an isoprenoid hydrophobic side chain at the 3 position (Figure 28-1). Phylloquinone, also known as vitamin K_1, is the form of vitamin K that is isolated from green plants. Phylloquinone has a phytyl group at the 3 position of the naphthoquinone ring. The vitamin K_2 forms of

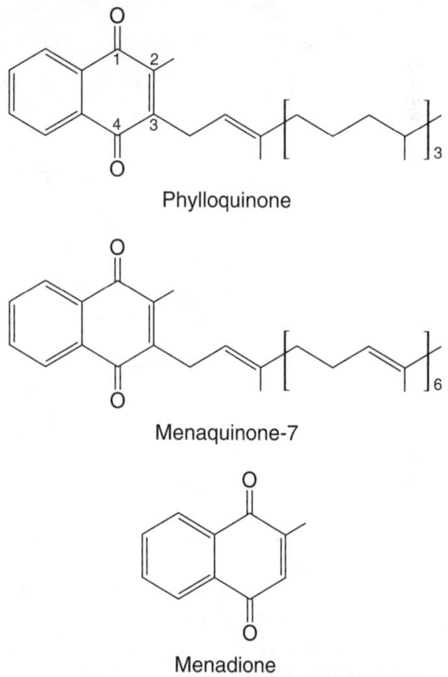

Phylloquinone

Menaquinone-7

Menadione

FIGURE 28-1 Structures of compounds with vitamin K activity. Phylloquinone synthesized in plants is the main dietary form of vitamin K. Menaquinone-7 is one of a series of menaquinones produced by intestinal bacteria, and menadione is a synthetic compound that can be converted to menaquinone-4 by animal tissues.

the vitamin that are synthesized by bacteria are now more properly designated as menaquinones. These forms of the vitamin have a side chain composed of unsaturated isoprene units at the 3 position (see Figure 28-1). Although a wide range of menaquinones (abbreviated as MK-n) are synthesized by bacteria, long-chain menaquinones with 6 to 10 isoprene groups in the side chain (MK-6 to MK-10) are the most common. The synthetic compound menadione (2-methyl-1,4-naphthoquinone) (see Figure 28-1) was shown very early to have vitamin K activity and commonly is used as a source of the vitamin in animal feeds. Menadione itself is not a substrate for the vitamin K–dependent carboxylase, but it is alkylated in mammalian tissues to an active form, MK-4, having a geranylgeranyl side chain in the 3 position.

MECHANISM OF ACTION OF VITAMIN K

DISCOVERY OF THE PHYSIOLOGICAL MECHANISM OF VITAMIN K ACTION

The discovery of vitamin K as an antihemorrhagic factor directed focus on the blood coagulation system as the physiological system targeted by the vitamin. The initial models of the system proposed by Macfarlane (1965) and Davie and Ratnof (1964) involve a cascade of activations of blood coagulation factors that result in conversion of the soluble plasma protein fibrinogen into fibrin, a protein that aids formation of blood clots. These early models have been modified extensively, and a simplified version of the current model of the blood coagulation system leading to fibrin clot formation is shown in Figure 28-2. The four vitamin K–dependent clotting factors (prothrombin and factors VII, IX, and X) involved in the intrinsic and extrinsic pathways of the cascade are circled in Figure 28-2. These proteins were shown to bind calcium ions (Ca^{2+}) and to bind to negatively charged phospholipid surfaces.

The intrinsic and the extrinsic pathways of blood clotting converge at the formation of active factor Xa (FXa) from its inactive proenzyme factor X (FX) form. Studies of prothrombin production became the key to determining the mechanism of action of vitamin K. Experiments with whole animals carried out in the mid-1960s strongly suggested that vitamin K was involved in converting an inactive hepatic precursor of plasma prothrombin to a biologically active prothrombin form found in plasma. This hypothesis was strengthened

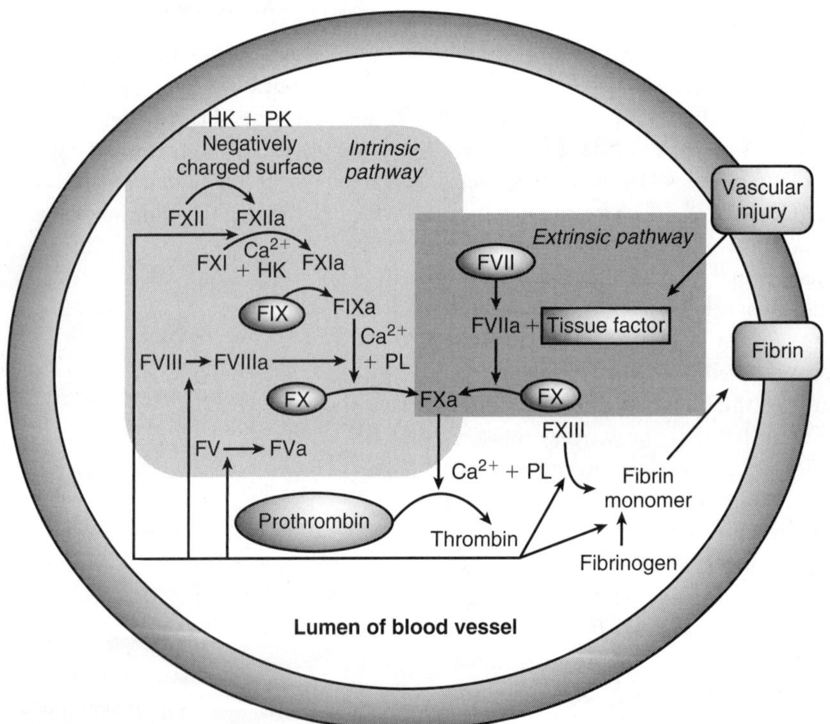

FIGURE 28-2 Vitamin K–dependent proteins involved in coagulation of blood. The figure shows a simplified version of the blood coagulation system, including an intrinsic and an extrinsic pathway. The extrinsic pathway is initiated when contact is made between blood and exposed negatively charged surfaces (e.g., upon vascular injury which leads to exposure of tissue factor, a subendothelial cell-surface glycoprotein that binds phospholipid [PL]).The intrinsic pathway is initiated when plasma prekallikrein (*PK*), plasma high-molecular weight kininogen (*HK*), factor (*F*) XII, and FXI bind to a negatively charged surface (e.g., phosphatidylserine on the surface of platelets). Each pathway consists of inactive proenzymes of coagulation factors that are converted to active proteases in a cascade of proteolytic reactions catalyzed by serine protease activities of many of the clotting factors. Both pathways converge at the point of conversion of the proenzyme factor X (*FX*) to the active protease factor Xa (*FXa*). Factor Xa activates the proenzyme prothrombin to thrombin, and thrombin converts the plasma protein fibrinogen to fibrin. Fibrin is an insoluble polymer involved in arrest of blood loss at the site of vessel injury. Thrombin also can activate FXI, FVIII, and FV, amplifying the cascade. Several proteins of the blood coagulation system undergo vitamin K–dependent posttranslational modification, converting these proteins into γ-carboxyglutamic acid (Gla)-containing proteins. These proteins are circled in the figure.

by clinical observations that an immunochemically similar, but biologically inactive, form of prothrombin was present in increased concentrations in the plasma of patients treated with anticoagulants that antagonized vitamin K action. The inactive proteins were called PIVKA factor (proteins induced in vitamin K absence) (Hemker and Reekers, 1974). Characterization of this "abnormal prothrombin" isolated from the plasma of cows fed the anticoagulant dicoumarol revealed that it lacked the specific Ca^{2+}-binding sites present in normal prothrombin, and it did not demonstrate a Ca^{2+}-dependent association with negatively charged phospholipid surfaces. These findings suggested that the function of vitamin K was to modify a liver precursor of this plasma protein to facilitate calcium binding. The action of the vitamin was therefore not at the level of gene transcription, but occurred after messenger RNA (mRNA) translation. By comparing peptides obtained from proteolytic digests of normal bovine prothrombin and abnormal prothrombin obtained from cows treated with dicumarol, Stenflo and colleagues (1974) identified the vitamin K modification as γ-carboxylation of Glu residues in newly formed vitamin K–dependent protein precursors. The structure of Gla, a previously unrecognized acidic amino acid (Nelsestuen et al., 1974; Stenflo et al., 1974), is shown in Figure 28-3. It was found that that all 10 of the Glu residues in the first 42 residues of bovine prothrombin were converted to Gla. The discovery of Gla in vitamin K–dependent coagulation factors revealed, for the first time, the role of Ca^{2+} in blood clotting. Calcium-binding by the Gla residues is essential for anchoring these coagulation factors to negatively charged lipids at the site of injury (Furie and Furie, 1992). The function of Gla residues in the vitamin K–dependent proteins that do not belong to the blood clotting system is less understood.

VITAMIN K: A SUBSTRATE FOR A γ-CARBOXYLASE

The discovery of Gla residues in prothrombin led to the demonstration (Esmon et al., 1975) that crude rat liver microsomal preparations (vesicles derived from the ER when cells are disrupted) contained an enzymatic activity that promoted a vitamin K–dependent incorporation of $^{14}CO_2$ into endogenous precursors of vitamin K–dependent proteins present in these preparations. Subsequent studies established that the $^{14}CO_2$ was present in Gla residues. Small peptides containing adjacent Glu-Glu residues such as Phe-Leu-Glu-Glu-Val were shown to be substrates for the enzyme present in detergent-solubilized microsomal preparations, and they were used to study the properties of this unique vitamin K–dependent γ-carboxylase. It is now well established that vitamin K–dependent γ-carboxylation of Glu residues in proteins is a posttranslational modification reaction that occurs on the luminal side of the rough ER. The majority of vitamin K–dependent proteins are secretory proteins that migrate through the ER and the Golgi apparatus before the proteins are secreted from the cells as mature proteins (Stanton et al., 1991). As shown in Figure 28-4, the vitamin K–dependent proteins are equipped with a signal peptide for penetration into the ER lumen. Upon entering the lumen, the N-terminal signal peptide is removed by signal peptidase. In addition, all precursors of vitamin K–dependent proteins are equipped with a unique propeptide that, in most of the proteins, constitutes the N-terminal part of the precursors after the signal peptide is removed. These propeptides are recognized by the γ-carboxylase in the ER membrane. They anchor the vitamin K–dependent protein precursors to the enzyme for γ-carboxylation of Glu residues in a reaction that requires reduced vitamin K (KH_2) as the active cofactor. Upon completion of γ-carboxylation, the vitamin K–dependent proteins are released from the γ-carboxylase and exit the ER in secretory vesicles for transport to the Golgi apparatus for additional modifications. The major modifications these proteins undergo in the Golgi apparatus are glycosylations. The proteins move through the *cis*-, *medial*-, and *trans*-Golgi compartments (see Figure 28-4).

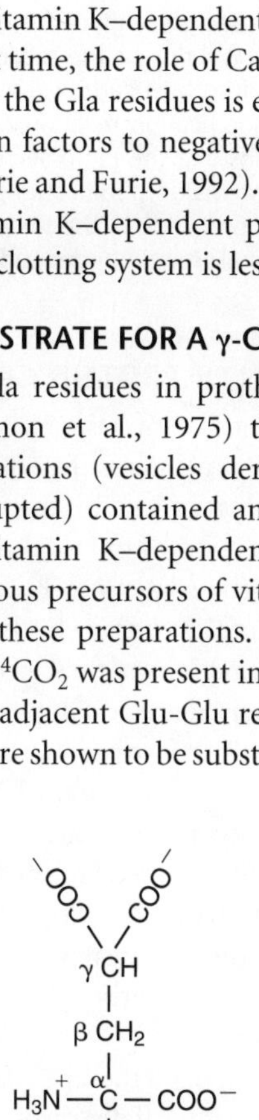

Because of the addition of sialic acid residues, the vitamin K–dependent proteins become more acidic in the Golgi apparatus. The propeptide stays attached to the protein during its migration through the Golgi apparatus but is proteolytically released from the protein in the *trans*-Golgi apparatus by the protease furin (Stanton et al., 1991). Release of the propeptide is essential for the coagulation factors to function as zymogens in the blood coagulation system. Bleeding disorders have been shown to result in the appearance of vitamin K–dependent coagulation factors in blood with the propeptide still attached (Diuguid et al., 1986).

THE VITAMIN K CYCLE AND THE VITAMIN K–DEPENDENT γ-CARBOXYLATION SYSTEM

As indicated in Figure 28-5, reduced vitamin K (KH_2 or vitamin K hydroquinone) is the γ-carboxylase cofactor. When one Glu residue is converted to one Gla residue, the cofactor KH_2 is converted to vitamin K 2,3-epoxide (K>O) (see Figure 28-5). The epoxide (K>O) is reduced back to the hydroquinone (KH_2) cofactor by the enzyme vitamin K 2,3-epoxide reductase (VKOR). VKOR is inhibited by warfarin, a derivative of the anticoagulant drug dicoumarol. The oxidation of vitamin KH_2 in the γ-carboxylation reaction and the reduction of K>O back to KH_2 by VKOR constitute the vitamin K cycle. DT-diaphorases, enzymes that are able to use either NADH or NADPH, can reduce vitamin K to KH_2 but cannot reduce K>O (see Figure 28-5). The warfarin-insensitive DT-diaphorase pathway for vitamin K reduction has a high K_m for vitamin K_1 and can only produce enough KH_2

FIGURE 28-3 Structure of γ-carboxyglutamic acid (Gla). Gla is a Ca^{2+}-binding amino acid.

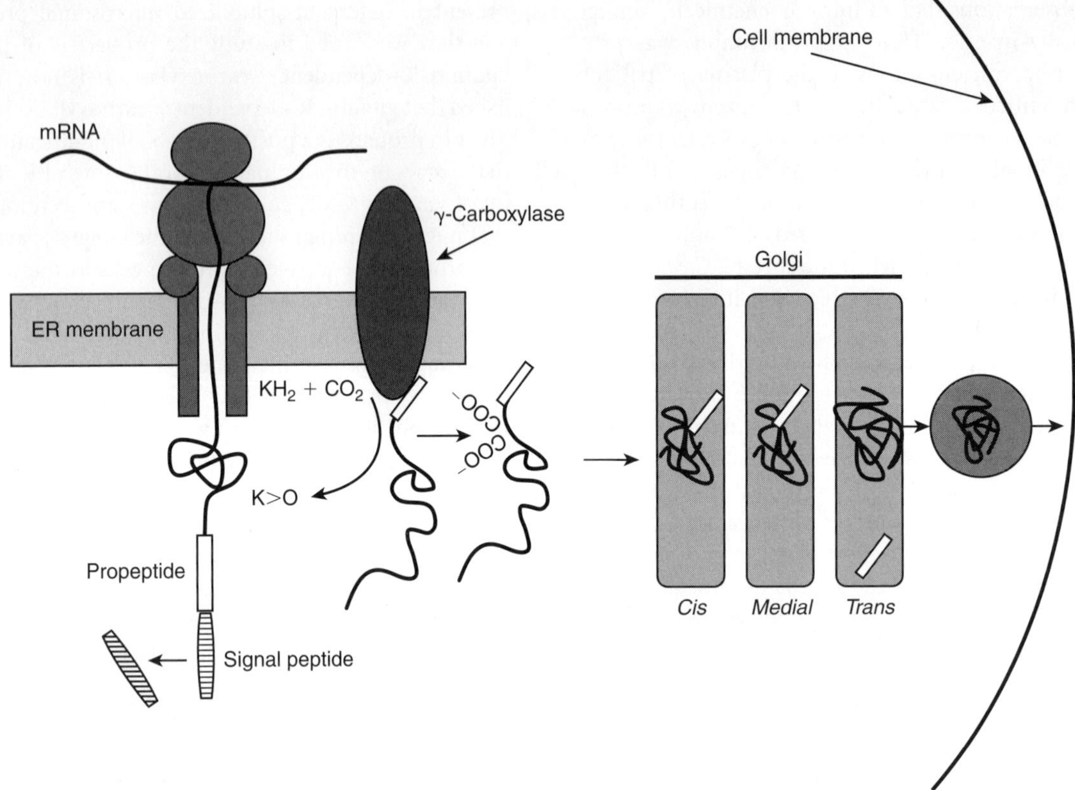

FIGURE 28-4 Posttranslational vitamin K–dependent modification of secretory vitamin K–dependent protein in the ER and transport through the secretory pathway of the cell. Vitamin K–dependent proteins are secretory glycoproteins. They are equipped with a signal peptide for translocation into the ER lumen and a propeptide that serves as the recognition signal that destines these proteins for vitamin K–dependent γ-carboxylation of glutamate residues by γ-carboxylase, which is an integral protein in the ER membrane. Reduced vitamin K (KH_2) is a cofactor for the modification reaction and vitamin K epoxide (K>O) is a product. γ-Carboxylated precursors of vitamin K–dependent proteins exit the ER in secretory vesicles and migrate through the *cis, medial, and trans* compartments of the Golgi apparatus. The major modifications the proteins undergo in the Golgi apparatus are glycosylations. The propeptide is released from the precursor in the trans-Golgi apparatus by the protease furin. Release of the propeptide is required for synthesis of functional vitamin K–dependent proteins.

cofactor for the γ-carboxylase to optimally produce fully γ-carboxylated proteins when high tissue concentrations of vitamin K are present (Wallin and Martin, 1987).

CHEMISTRY OF VITAMIN K ACTION

It has been a challenge over the years to determine how vitamin KH_2 can be the trigger for γ-carboxylation of specific Glu residues in vitamin K–dependent proteins. The first fundamental and critical role of vitamin KH_2 to initiate γ-carboxylation is its conversion into a strong base by removal of a H^+ from one of the OH groups on the napthoquinone ring system by a strong basic amino acid residue (B:) in the γ-carboxylase enzyme (Figure 28-6). The strong vitamin K base (K^-) thus formed then extracts a H^+ at the γ-carbon of the targeted Glu residue in the protein, and the resulting carbanion is then attacked by CO_2, resulting in addition of an extra COOH group to the γ-carbon on the Glu residue. Thus, a new Ca^{2+}-binding Gla residue forms in the protein sequence. For a more detailed understanding of the chemical reaction modeling, the reader is referred to papers by Dowd and co-workers (1995) and by Rishavy and associates (2006).

γ-CARBOXYLATION OF PROTEIN GLU RESIDUES

The physiological role of the vitamin K–dependent γ-carboxylase poses an interesting question in terms of enzyme–substrate recognition. This microsomal (ER) enzyme recognizes a small fraction of the total hepatic secretory protein pool and then carboxylates 9 to 12 Glu sites in the first 45 N-terminal residues of the vitamin K–dependent plasma proteins. The propeptide regions of these proteins show sequence homology. The propeptide region appears to be both a docking and a recognition site for the γ-carboxylase; it modulates the activity by decreasing the apparent K_m of the γ-carboxylase for the Glu-containing protein substrates. The propeptide domain is undoubtedly of major importance in directing the efficient γ-carboxylation of the multiple Glu sites in these substrates, but it is not known if the enzyme starts at one end of the Gla region and sequentially carboxylates all Glu sites or if the enzyme carboxylates randomly within this region. Reduction of KH_2 levels by anticoagulant therapy results in the production of a complex mixture of partially carboxylated forms of prothrombin, and the available data suggest that in the least carboxylated forms the potential Gla residue that is closest to the amino-terminal is preferentially carboxylated (Malhotra, 1972).

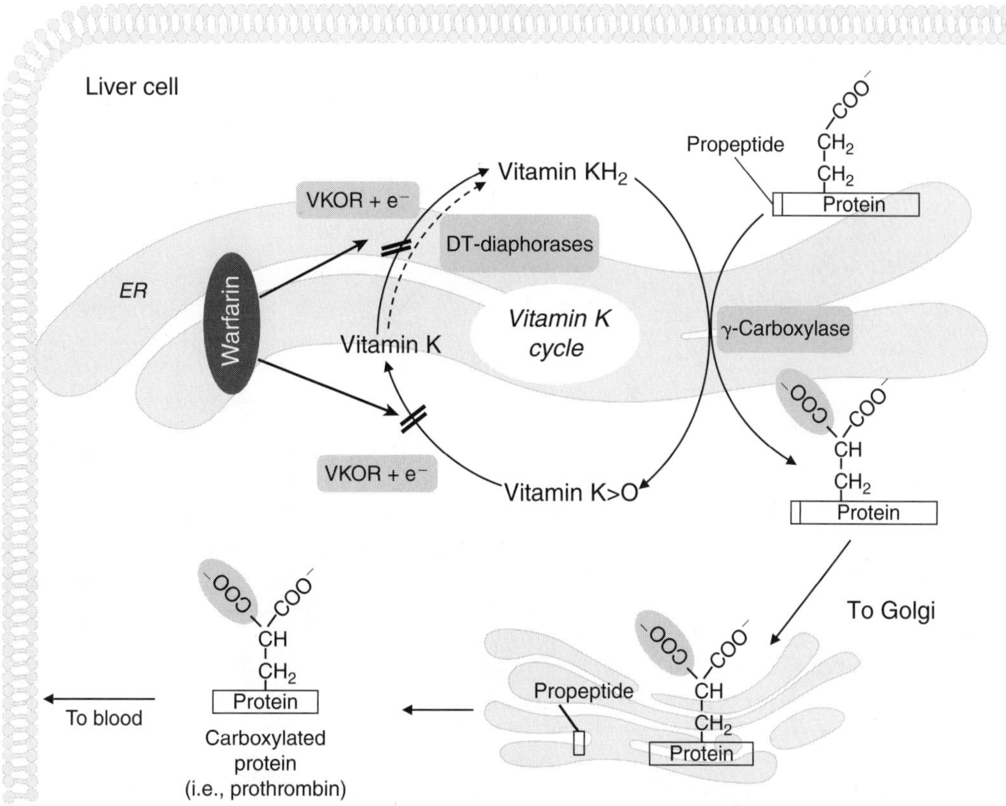

FIGURE 28-5 The vitamin K–dependent γ-carboxylation system in liver. Reduced vitamin K (vitamin KH_2) is a cofactor for γ-carboxylase. Concomitant with γ-carboxylation, vitamin KH_2 is converted to vitamin K 2,3-epoxide (vitamin K>O). Vitamin K>O is reduced back to the vitamin KH_2 cofactor by vitamin K 2,3-epoxide reductase (VKOR). These enzyme activities constitute the vitamin K cycle. VKOR is inhibited by warfarin and other coumarin anticoagulant drugs. DT-diaphorases are flavoproteins that can reduce vitamin K quinone (vitamin K) but not the vitamin K epoxide. The complete set of enzyme reactions shown in the figure constitutes the vitamin K–dependent γ-carboxylation system. After removal of the propeptide in the Golgi apparatus, the carboxylated protein is secreted into circulation.

The molecular mechanism resulting in the appearance in blood of vitamin K–dependent, under–γ-carboxylated coagulation factors (PIVKA factors), when the γ-carboxylation system is not functioning optimally, is unknown.

A model for Glu γ-carboxylation in the presence of sufficient KH_2 cofactor for the γ-carboxylase has been proposed by Stenina and colleagues (2001). Their data are consistent with a model of tethered processivity of γ-carboxylation. Finished Gla residues are bound to the active γ-carboxylation site on the γ-carboxylase that exposes a new targeted Glu residue for γ-carboxylation. This process will continue until the Gla region is completed. The finished vitamin K–modified protein then leaves the γ-carboxylase.

PURIFICATION AND CHARACTERIZATION OF γ-CARBOXYLASE

Early studies of γ-carboxylation were hampered by the lack of purified γ-carboxylase. By using an affinity approach, where the ligand was a large peptide containing the propeptide region and the Gla region of factor IX, Wu and colleagues (1991) purified a microsomal protein of molecular weight 94 kDa that exhibited γ-carboxylase activity and that required lipid for activity. Data from a topological study carried out by Tie and colleagues (2000) predict that γ-carboxylase spans the ER membrane at least five times. Therefore γ-carboxylase is considered a true integral protein of the ER membrane. For a more detailed description of γ-carboxylase, the reader should refer to the paper by Rishavy and co-workers (2006).

ANTAGONISM OF VITAMIN K ACTION BY CLINICALLY USED INHIBITORS

Dicoumarol was isolated from moldy sweet clover and identified in 1939 as the factor responsible for a hemorrhagic disease of cattle that was common in the midwestern United States in the early 1920s. This led to the use of dicoumarol (marketed in the United States as dicumarol) as the first anticoagulant drug to be used clinically. However, the toxicity of dicoumarol led to synthesis of many new versions of 4-hydroxycoumarins to find a clinically safe drug, and warfarin (Figure 28-7), synthesized under the leadership of Dr. Karl P. Link at the University of Wisconsin, became the most successful anticoagulant drug. Warfarin is an indirect vitamin K antagonist in that it does not inhibit the γ-carboxylase (Hildebrandt and Suttie, 1982) but rather inhibits VKOR and therefore the regeneration of vitamin KH_2 from K>O.

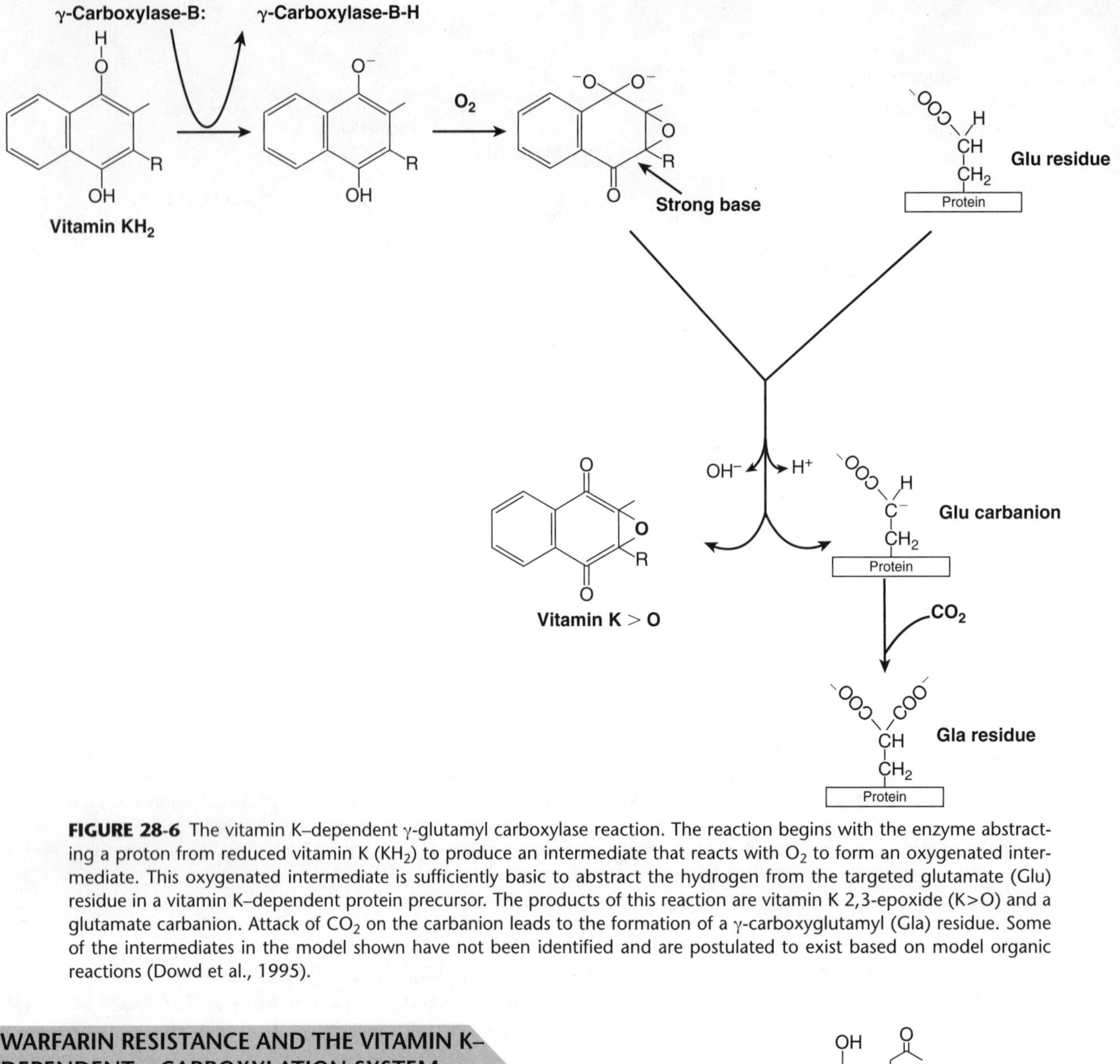

FIGURE 28-6 The vitamin K–dependent γ-glutamyl carboxylase reaction. The reaction begins with the enzyme abstracting a proton from reduced vitamin K (KH_2) to produce an intermediate that reacts with O_2 to form an oxygenated intermediate. This oxygenated intermediate is sufficiently basic to abstract the hydrogen from the targeted glutamate (Glu) residue in a vitamin K–dependent protein precursor. The products of this reaction are vitamin K 2,3-epoxide (K>O) and a glutamate carbanion. Attack of CO_2 on the carbanion leads to the formation of a γ-carboxyglutamyl (Gla) residue. Some of the intermediates in the model shown have not been identified and are postulated to exist based on model organic reactions (Dowd et al., 1995).

WARFARIN RESISTANCE AND THE VITAMIN K–DEPENDENT γ-CARBOXYLATION SYSTEM

As shown in Figure 28-5, the anticoagulant warfarin inhibits VKOR of the vitamin K cycle. Warfarin resistance is a problem in prophylactic medicine and also in rodent pest control. The problem can be pharmacological, nutritional, or genetic. Pharmacological resistance is associated with high turnover of the drug in the liver by the cytochrome P450 system where cytochrome P450-2C9 is the most active cytochrome involved in metabolism of warfarin (Hanatani et al., 2003). Nutritional resistance to warfarin results from high vitamin K intake (Suttie, 1978), and administration of vitamin K is the standard procedure used to treat warfarin intoxication in patients and animals.

The mechanism by which vitamin K works as an antidote to warfarin has been established (Wallin and Martin, 1987). When the liver concentration of vitamin K is elevated, vitamin K can be reduced by DT-diaphorases, enzymes that are able to use either NADH or NADPH for vitamin K reduction (Wallin and Martin, 1987; see Figure 28-5). Warfarin does not inhibit these enzymes. Therefore if the VKOR pathway for vitamin K reduction is blocked by warfarin, the alternative pathway can "drive" vitamin KH_2 cofactor production and maintain a normally functioning blood

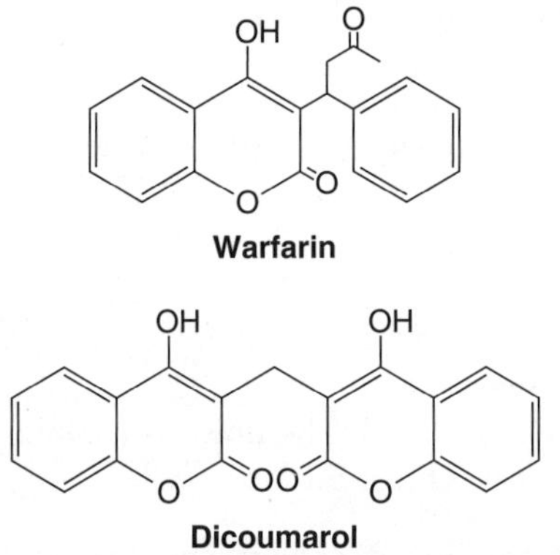

FIGURE 28-7 Clinically used 4-hydroxycoumarin anticoagulants. The 4-hydroxycoumarins, dicoumarol and warfarin, do not inhibit the carboxylase enzyme but prevent recycling of vitamin K–epoxide to the enzymatically active form of the vitamin.

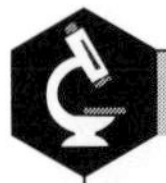

CLINICAL CORRELATION

Warfarin and Pharmacogenetics

Warfarin is the most used anticoagulant in the world to control unwanted clotting or thrombosis in patients. However, a variety of factors including genetics can influence a patient's response to warfarin, making it difficult to determine the correct dose for an individual. Two genes have been identified that account for most of the genetic variation in response to warfarin in the human population. These are *CYP2C9* and *VKORC1*.

CYP2C9 encodes a cytochrome P450 enzyme that is responsible for the metabolism of warfarin to inactive metabolites. Several single nucleotide polymorphisms in *CYP2C9* have been found, and several of these variant alleles encode proteins that have very low enzymatic activities. The most common of these polymorphisms are CYP2C9*2 and CYP2C9*3 (with CYP2C9*1 being the wild type); the haplotype frequencies for CYP2C9*1/*2 and CYP2C9*1/*3 are about 20% and 12%, respectively, in the Caucasian population. In contrast, these CYP2C9 polymorphisms are rare in Asian and African-American populations. Patients with these variant alleles are "warfarin sensitive" and require much lower doses of warfarin than patients with the wild-type allele. There is evidence of a gene-dose effect such that patients who are homozygous for the variant allele are more sensitive than those with one variant allele and one wild-type allele.

The second gene affecting an individual's response to warfarin, *VKORC1,* encodes the enzyme vitamin K epoxide reductase. VKORC1 polymorphisms have been identified that cause either warfarin sensitivity or warfarin resistance. For example, the -1639G>A promoter polymorphism results in less promoter activity for gene transcription. These patients have less VKORC and thus need less warfarin to achieve sufficient inhibition of vitamin K recycling.

The basis of warfarin resistance is less worked out than that for warfarin sensitivity. Several single-point mutations that result in amino acid substitutions have been associated with warfarin resistance. Among warfarin resistant patients in a Israeli Jewish population, Loebstein et al. (2007) identified a 5417G>T (Asp36Tyr) polymorphism in 7 of 15 resistant patients. This variant was significantly and consistently associated with the highest warfarin dose category. Analysis of ethnic groups within this population showed over-representation of the Asp36Tyr polymorphism in individuals of Ethiopian descent (15%) and Ashkenazi descent (4%).

Testing for the more common polymorphisms affecting warfarin response are now available. Consideration of genetic test results, along with other clinical information, is useful for recommending doses for patients starting warfarin therapy.

Thinking Critically

John, a 55-year-old male with a history of myocardial infarction, is prescribed warfarin. Prothrombin time measures reveal that the dose is ineffective. John is queried on his use of nutritional supplements (i.e., vitamin K) and blood is drawn for genotyping of the *VKORC1* gene (produces VKOR).

1. Describe the mechanism by which warfarin decreases blood clot formation.
2. What does prothrombin time reveal?
3. Why was John asked about his use of vitamin K supplements?
4. From the following choices, select the type of genetic variant in the *VKORC1* gene that may have contributed to John's decreased sensitivity to warfarin (may be more than one possible answer).
   a. Loss-of-function genetic variant (i.e., diminished production of VKOR)
   b. Gain-of-function genetic variant (i.e., greater production of VKOR)
   c. Genetic variant that diminishes warfarin binding

coagulation system as long as vitamin K levels are elevated. Because the DT-diaphorases cannot reduce K>O (vitamin K 2,3 epoxide), vitamin K cannot be effectively recycled for participation in a second carboxylation reaction.

Genetic warfarin resistance has been described in humans (Vermeer and Schurgers, 2000; Voora et al., 2009), and resistance to some of the second-generation anticoagulants has been seen in rodents. Members of two families with familial multiple coagulation factor deficiency (FMFD), a disease in which patients are deficient in all vitamin K–dependent coagulation factors, were investigated by Fregin and colleagues (2002), who mapped the disease to the 16p12-q21 region on chromosome 16. They noted that a linkage group of genes on 16p11 is orthologous to genes around warfarin resistance loci *Rw* in rats (Greaves and Ayres, 1967; Kohn et al., 2003) and *War* in mice (Wallace and MacSwiney, 1976). This homology led the investigators to propose that FMFD and warfarin resistance may be caused by allelic mutations in the same gene.

DNA sequencing of genes in the region resulted in identification of missense mutations in a gene of unknown function from all of the FMFD patients studied. The wild-type gene in unaffected individuals codes for an 18-kDa ER membrane protein, now known as VKOR complex subunit 1 (VKORC1); overexpression of this gene yielded a protein that exhibited warfarin-sensitive VKOR activity. Furthermore, it was shown that certain missense mutations in the gene resulted in significant warfarin resistance in the host (Rost et al., 2004). Using synthetic short interfering RNAs (siRNAs) to silence genes in the warfarin-resistant region on chromosome 16, Li and colleagues (2004) identified the same gene as that responsible for expression of warfarin-sensitive VKOR activity.

It has been proposed that additional forms of genetic warfarin resistance exist. One form has been shown to be associated with overexpression of the chaperone protein calumenin in rat liver (Wallin et al., 2001a). Calumenin belongs to the CREC (Cab45, reticulocalbin, ERC-45, calumenin) subfamily of Ca^{2+}-binding proteins (Honore, 2009; Honore and Vorum, 2000). The CREC proteins are found in the secretory pathways of cells, and most of the proteins have been shown to have chaperone functions. Despite being a hydrophilic, water-soluble, acidic protein, calumenin appears to be associated with ER membrane proteins. Data supporting this concept include immunocytochemical studies of the ER membrane (Honore and Vorum, 2000) and the demonstration that calumenin is strongly associated with lipid–detergent micelles, derived from the ER membrane, which also carry the VKOR enzyme complex (Wallin et al., 2001a).

Expression of calumenin in cell lines has been shown to inhibit VKOR activity and confer warfarin resistance to the VKOR enzyme complex. In addition, calumenin has been shown to be associated with the γ-carboxylase and to inhibit its activity (Wajih et al., 2004). Therefore calumenin appears to be a chaperone that regulates the capacity of the vitamin K–dependent γ-carboxylation system for production of functional vitamin K–dependent proteins. This regulatory role puts calumenin in a central position regarding maintenance of a normal blood coagulation system. In a recent human genetic study by Voora and co-workers (2009) calumenin was found to be a marker for warfarin resistance in African Americans and to have a role in the γ-carboxylation system, as suggested earlier by Wallin and colleagues (2001a).

SOURCES OF VITAMIN K

FOOD SOURCES

The major form of vitamin K in the diet is phylloquinone (vitamin K_1) of plant origin. Tables of vitamin K content of foods that were compiled before the mid-1990s were based on the chick bioassay and generally reported higher values for vitamin K than have been obtained with more modern methods involving lipid extraction followed by high-performance liquid chromatography (HPLC). Many foods and edible oils have been analyzed by these modern HPLC-methods, and good estimates of the phylloquinone content of a wide range of foods are now available in the U.S. Department of Agriculture (USDA) *National Nutrient Database for Standard Reference, Release 23* and other publications (Booth and Suttie, 1998; Dismore et al., 2003).

In general, green vegetables are the major source of phylloquinone in the diet, and foods such as kale, collards, spinach, parsley, broccoli, Brussels sprouts, cabbage, and lettuce are excellent sources of the vitamin. Green leafy vegetables can provide as much as 400 to 500 μg per ½-cup serving. Plant oils and margarine are the second major source of phylloquinone in the diet. The phylloquinone content of plant oils is variable, with soybean and canola oils containing greater than 100 μg phylloquinone per 100 g (7.4 tbsp), cottonseed oil and olive oil containing about 50 μg per 100 g, and corn oil containing less than 5 μg per 100 g. Fruits and nuts are not very important sources of vitamin K, but a few fruits (e.g., blueberries, blackberries, grapes, kiwi fruit, avocado, and prunes) provide on the order of 10 to 30 μg per ½-cup serving.

Hydrogenation of phylloquinone-rich vegetable oils results in some conversion of phylloquinone to 2′,3′-dihydrophylloquinone (Booth et al., 1996). These hydrogenated vegetable oils are widely used by the food industry, and dihydroquinone is found in margarines, infant formulas, and many prepared foods. The estimated intake of 2′,3′-dihydrophylloquinone is 12 to 24 μg/day for older children and adults (Booth et al., 1996). Administration of the dihydrophylloquinone to rats counteracted warfarin-induced prolonged blood coagulation and decreased the effects of warfarin on serum total osteocalcin levels (Sato et al., 2003). Dihydrophylloquinone was absorbed and detected in tissues of the rats, but it was not converted to MK-4 as is phylloquinone. In humans, dihydrophylloquinone was not absorbed as well and phylloquinone had no measurable biological effect on measures of bone formation and resorption (Booth et al., 2001). With trends in reducing commercially hydrogenated oils from the food supply, it is anticipated that there will be a concomitant decline in dihydrophylloquinone in the food supply.

Animal products are not rich sources of vitamin K. Limited amounts of MK-4 and higher menaquinones (i.e., MK-5 to MK-10) have been found in some animal products, including eggs, butter, various cheeses, beef and pork liver, and fermented soybean products (Koivu-Tikkanen et al., 2000). A high amount of MK-4 was found in chicken meat. Although the higher menaquinones were found to be essentially absent in the milk of several species, MK-4 has been measured in the milk of various species and in a range of infant formulas (Indyk and Woollard, 1997). The total vitamin K content calculated from the sum of phylloquinone, MK-4, and higher menaquinones in animal products was generally low in terms of total dietary phylloquinone content.

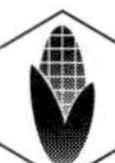

FOOD SOURCES OF PHYLLOQUINONE

Vegetables
400 to 500 μg per ½ cup kale, collards, spinach
75 to 150 μg per ½ cup Brussels sprouts, broccoli, asparagus
30 to 50 μg per ½ cup leaf lettuce, cabbage, rhubarb
5 to 20 μg per ½ cup green peas, tomato sauce, soybeans, carrots, cauliflower, green beans

Fruits
30 μg per 1 medium kiwi fruit
15 μg per ½ cup blueberries, blackberries
13 μg per ½ cup seedless grapes

Plant Oils
15 to 25 μg per 1 tbsp soybean, canola oil
5 to 20 μg per 1 tbsp (oil-based) salad dressings
5 to 15 μg per 1 tbsp margarine
7 μg per 1 tbsp olive oil

U.S. Department of Agriculture, Agricultural Research Service. (2010). *USDA National Nutrient Database for Standard Reference, Release 23.* Retrieved from www.ars.usda.gov/ba/bhnrc/ndl.

INTESTINAL BACTERIA

Intestinal anaerobes such as *Escherichia coli* and *Bacteroides fragilis* produce menaquinones, and the human gut contains large quantities of bacterially produced vitamin K. Early studies indicated that germ-free animals had an increased vitamin K requirement, but the nutritional significance of menaquinones produced in the large intestine is not yet clear. The extent or mechanism of menaquinone absorption from the large intestine has not been clearly established, although human liver does contain significant quantities of menaquinones. Cases of patients exhibiting a vitamin K–responsive hypoprothrombinemia after antibiotic administration have been reported. These episodes usually have been ascribed to an influence of the antibiotic on menaquinone synthesis in the large intestine, but the limited data available indicate that most antibiotics do not negatively influence menaquinone production. Many of the case reports may simply reflect very low dietary intakes of vitamin K due to limited food intake in severely ill patients or, perhaps, hematological responses to various underlying illnesses. An argument against the intestinal absorption of menaquinones produced by bacteria and their physiological use is the observation that one way to induce vitamin K deficiency and severe bleeding in rats untreated with antibiotics is to prevent them from eating their feces.

Nevertheless, the historical difficulty in producing vitamin K deficiency in human subjects suggests that menaquinones synthesized in the large intestine are of nutritional importance. The total hepatic pool of menaquinones in humans is approximately 10 times that of phylloquinone, and this source of vitamin K appears to be used at least to some extent. However, the high concentration in liver may reflect a slow turnover of this form of the vitamin. Limited data obtained from a rat model suggest that when a typical long-chain bacterial menaquinone (MK-9) is present in liver at concentrations similar to those of phylloquinone, it is not used as effectively as phylloquinone. Taken together, current data suggest that menaquinones provide only a minor portion of the vitamin K needed to satisfy the human requirement.

VITAMIN K_1 CONVERSION TO MK-4 IN EXTRAHEPATIC TISSUES

POTENTIAL CLINICAL SIGNIFICANCE

In studies with germ-free rats, Ronden and colleagues (1998) found that phylloquinone was converted into MK-4 in extrahepatic tissues. The exact enzymatic pathway leading to the conversion has not yet been established. A physiological function for extrahepatic MK-4 has been the motivation for several studies. The studies have elucidated new functions for vitamin K and the potential of MK-4 as a prophylactic agent in treatment of osteoporosis (Iwamoto et al., 2003; Cockayne et al., 2006), arterial calcification (Spronk et al., 2003), and liver cancer (Habu et al., 2004). MK-4 has also been found to be the major form of vitamin K in the brain, where it is concentrated in myelinated regions (Carrie et al., 2004). More than 93% of ingested vitamin K_1 is converted to MK-4 in the brain. Because dysregulation of myelin sulfatides is a risk factor for cognitive decline with age, Crivello and co-workers (2010) studied MK-4 in the brain and found significant positive correlations between sulfatides and MK-4 in the hippocampus. But it remains to be determined whether long-term supplementation with menadione and/or higher dietary vitamin K consumption would be sufficient to affect brain region-specific changes in the (1) number and/or metabolic activity of oligodendrocytes, (2) rate of myelin formation and loss, and (3) activity of genes responsible for the synthesis of myelin constituents. Other support of an important function for MK-4 in the brain comes from the observation that mothers who use warfarin during pregnancy have an increased risk of damage to the central nervous system of the fetus (Pati and Helmbrecht, 1994). Interestingly, Sundaram and Lev (1988) found that warfarin administration reduces synthesis of sulfatides and other sphingolipids in mouse brain.

MK-4 has also been shown to be a ligand for the steroid and xenobiotic receptor SXR (Ichikaw et al., 2006), which translocates to the nucleus and can affect gene expression of alkaline phosphatase, osteoprotegerin, osteopontin, and matrix Gla protein (Tabb et al., 2003). These proteins are involved in bone formation and regulation of bone formation (Wallin et al., 2001b). Additionally, Horie-Inoue and Inoue (2008) have identified MK-4 gene regulation of a small leucine-rich repeat proteoglycan, tsukushi, which contributes to collagen accumulation. The protein may interact with another MK-4–inducible SXR target, matrilin-2, a member of the matrilin family, which functions as a collagen adaptor. Besides functioning as a xenobiotic biosensor, their findings show that SXR is a MK-4 target and an important transcriptional factor that regulates homeostasis in bone cells. It is also possible that several new genes may be found to be transcriptionally regulated by MK-4.

More recent research has focused on the enzymes and pathways that are involved in conversion of vitamin K_1 to MK-4. Okano and colleagues (2008) have carried out an extensive study on identifying the enzymes involved in the conversion of administered vitamin K_1 to MK-4 in the rodent brain. They used deuterium-labeled vitamin K compounds with the radioactive label in the napthoquinone ring and the side chain, respectively. Their data clearly demonstrate that enzymatic cleavage of the side chain from vitamin K_1 and prenylation of the side chain–free napthoquinone ring system (menadione) of the vitamin is responsible for MK-4 generated in tissues from ingested vitamin K_1. An interesting observation by these authors is that labeled MK-4 was detected in the brain only when vitamin K was administered orally, suggesting an important role of the intestine in the release of menadione from phylloquinone. Menadione was effective whether administered enterally, parenterally, or intracerebroventricularly.

BIOAVAILABILITY

The bioavailability of phylloquinone to humans has not been studied extensively. Based on the appearance of vitamin K in plasma following a single meal, the absorption of food-bound phylloquinone appeared to be much slower than that of pure phylloquinone or food-bound menaquinones (Booth et al., 2002; Garber et al., 1999; Schurgers and Vermeer, 2002). However, in a longer-term metabolic study involving 36 participants and a crossover design, no difference in the relative bioavailability of phylloquinone from broccoli or fortified oil was observed. Supplementation of a mixed diet containing 100 μg of phylloquinone with an additional 400 μg of phylloquinone, from either broccoli or fortified oil, for 5 days yielded similar increases in the plasma phylloquinone concentration and similar decreases in the percentage of osteocalcin with reduced γ-carboxylation (Booth et al., 1999). In addition, the plasma level of deuterium labeled phylloquinone was extensively enriched after intake of broccoli or collards grown hydroponically with deuterium oxide in order to label vitamin K within the food matrix (Dolnikowski et al., 2002; Erkkila et al., 2004). Nevertheless, because of the uncertain bioavailability of food phylloquinone, the Institute of Medicine (IOM, 2002) recommends that phylloquinone from vegetable sources not be considered to be more than 20% as available as phylloquinone consumed as a supplement.

ABSORPTION, TRANSPORT, AND METABOLISM OF VITAMIN K

Dietary phylloquinone is absorbed from the gut into the lymphatic system, and any conditions that result in a general impairment of lipid absorption will also adversely influence vitamin K absorption. Following incorporation into chylomicrons in the mucosa of the duodenum and jejunum, the vitamin is secreted into the lymph and ultimately enters the liver in association with the chylomicron remnant particles. Circulating phylloquinone is found in the high-density (HDL), low-density (LDL), and very-low-density (VLDL) lipoprotein fractions, and its concentration is increased in hyperlipidemic patients. The apolipoprotein E (apo E) genotype is known to influence plasma lipoprotein clearance and has also been demonstrated to influence circulating phylloquinone concentrations.

Circulating phylloquinone concentrations are highly dependent on recent dietary intake, and even postabsorptive values cover a wide range. Plasma phylloquinone concentrations in the healthy population appear to be about 1 nmol/L, with a range from 0.3 to 2.5 nmol/L (0.15 to 1.15 μg/L) (Sadowski et al., 1989). The plasma phylloquinone concentration of the healthy newborn is only approximately 0.05 nmol/L. Early studies did not detect circulating menaquinones in plasma but, more recently, measurable concentrations of some of the long-chain menaquinones, mainly MK-7 and MK-8, have been reported (Suttie, 1995).

Measurements of human liver vitamin K content also are available. Values have been reported in the range of 2 to 20 ng of phylloquinone per gram of liver (Usui et al., 1990). A broad spectrum of bacterially produced long-chain menaquinones (MK-7 through MK-10) also is found in human liver, and the total concentration of menaquinones appears to be about ten times higher than that of phylloquinone (Suttie, 1995) and may reflect a slower turnover of long-chain menaquinones relative to phylloquinone. Both forms of the vitamin are rapidly concentrated in liver of experimental animals following ingestion. In contrast to the other fat-soluble vitamins, which have a significant tissue storage pool, phylloquinone has a very rapid turnover in liver.

Phylloquinone is excreted predominantly in feces via the bile, but significant amounts also are excreted in the urine (Shearer and Newman, 2008). Very little dietary phylloquinone is excreted unmetabolized, but the major metabolites are not well characterized. They appear to represent the stepwise oxidation of the side chain at the 3 position, followed by formation of conjugates with glucuronic acid. The 2,3-epoxide, which is formed as the result of the biochemical role of vitamin K as substrate for the liver microsomal γ-glutamyl carboxylase, appears to be subject to the same general pathways of oxidative degradation as is the parent vitamin. Very limited information suggests that the pathway of degradative metabolism of menaquinones is similar to that of phylloquinone.

PHYSIOLOGICAL ROLES OF VITAMIN K–DEPENDENT PROTEINS

The vitamin K–dependent formation of Gla is evolutionarily old, and some sea snails have Gla peptides that are used as potent neurotoxins (Bush et al., 1999). Vitamin K–dependent proteins are produced in a variety of tissues in the body. The most studied and best understood of these are the vitamin K–dependent plasma proteins involved in blood clotting, which are synthesized in the liver. These proteins include the coagulation cascade zymogens: prothrombin, factor VII, factor IX, and factor X (see Figure 28-2). Other vitamin K–dependent plasma proteins are involved in anticoagulation; these include protein C, protein S, and protein Z (Broze, 2001; Furie and Furie, 1992).

The first extrahepatic vitamin K–dependent protein to be discovered was isolated from bone and contained three Gla residues. It is the second most abundant protein in bone and is called osteocalcin or bone Gla protein (BGP). Osteocalcin is a small 8-kDa protein synthesized by the bone-forming cells (osteoblasts). A small amount of this bone protein circulates in plasma, and the degree of γ-carboxylation of plasma osteocalcin is sensitive to vitamin K nutritional status. Osteocalcin is believed to play a regulatory role in bone formation, and mice without functional osteocalcin characteristically acquire increased bone density, suggesting that osteocalcin is a negative regulator of bone formation (Ducy et al., 1996). However, the functional mechanism by which osteocalcin works is still not known. The plasma level of under-γ-carboxylated osteocalcin has been associated with the onset of osteoporosis in some studies, but administration of vitamin K_1 to prevent osteoporosis has yielded conflicting results (Tsugawa et al., 2008).

Matrix Gla protein (MGP) is a 14-kDa vitamin K–dependent protein synthesized by chondrocytes, osteoblasts, vascular smooth muscle cells, and other cell types (Loeser et al., 1993; Wallin et al., 2001b). MGP is unique among the members of the vitamin K–dependent protein family by retaining the propeptide as part of the mature protein sequence (Sweatt et al., 2003). MGP null mice show extensive calcification of the arterial wall and cartilage, and MGP is believed to be an important calcification inhibitor (Luo et al., 1997). One hypothesis for MGP's mechanism of action as a calcification inhibitor is its binding to bone morphogenetic protein-2 (BMP-2), a potent growth factor that transforms preosteoblastic cells into bone-forming cells (Abedin et al., 2004). It has been demonstrated that the Gla modification of MGP is essential for the protein to bind BMP-2. This finding leads to the prediction that vitamin K deficiency may trigger the pathology of arterial calcification. Reports supporting this hypothesis are emerging (Schori and Stungis, 2004). Murshed and co-workers (2004) showed that only the locally made MGP in the vessel wall can work as a calcification inhibitor of the wall; blood-borne MGP cannot.

The vitamin K–dependent protein Gas6 (growth arrest gene 6), a homolog of the anticoagulation factor protein S, is a ligand for the Axl receptor, which is a member of a family of cell adhesion molecule–related tyrosine kinase receptors (Stitt et al., 1995). Gas6 has been shown to induce Axl tyrosine phosphorylation and promote cell survival, migration, and growth (Fridell et al., 1998). Gas6 is expressed extensively in the brain (Prieto et al., 1999). γ-Carboxylation of Gas6 is a prerequisite for the protein to promote growth of Schwann cells and smooth muscle cells in the central nervous system, and insufficient γ-carboxylation of Gas6 has been proposed as a possible mechanism underlying the pathology of Alzheimer disease (Li et al., 1996). Four vitamin K–dependent putative membrane proteins—PRGP1, PRGP2, TmG3, and TmG4—some of which are located in the brain, have also been described, but the functions of these proteins are unknown (Kulman et al., 1997, 2001). The most recently discovered vitamin K–dependent proteins are the 10.2-kDa Gla-rich protein (GRP) discovered in sturgeon cartilage (Viagas et al., 2008) and the matrix cellular protein periostin (Hamilton, 2008).

VITAMIN K DEFICIENCY

Although a primary vitamin K deficiency is uncommon in the adult human population, a vitamin K–responsive hemorrhagic disease of the newborn is also a rare but long-recognized syndrome. Vitamin K stores of the newborn are low because of poor placental transfer of the vitamin, and the sterile gut precludes any possible production and use of menaquinones during early life. These conditions are complicated by a general hypoprothrombinemia in infants caused by the inability of immature liver to synthesize normal levels of clotting factors.

The breast-fed infant is at particular risk. The vitamin K content of breastmilk is less than that of cow's milk, and a low intake of phylloquinone by nursing infants has been shown to be a strong contributing factor in the development of vitamin K deficiency in the newborn. Plasma vitamin K concentrations in a group of exclusively breast-fed infants averaged 1.2 μg/L at 2 weeks of age and had decreased to 0.2 μg/L by 6 weeks of age (Greer, 2001; the lower limit of adult normal levels is 0.5 μg/L.) Commercial infant formulas are now routinely supplemented with vitamin K. Nursing mothers can increase vitamin K levels in their milk by taking phylloquinone supplements (Thijssen et al., 2002). The American and Canadian pediatric societies recommend intramuscular administration of phylloquinone at birth as routine prophylaxis, and the practice of oral or intramuscular administration of vitamin K to the newborn is almost universal in developed countries. Hemorrhagic disease remains a potential problem for breast-fed infants in some areas of the world where routine vitamin K administration to newborns is not performed.

The most common condition known to result in a vitamin K–responsive hemorrhagic event in the adult is a low dietary intake of vitamin K by a patient who also is receiving antibiotics. These cases are numerous, which suggests that patients with restricted food intake who also are receiving antibiotics should be closely monitored for signs of vitamin K deficiency. These episodes historically have been attributed to an interference of antibiotics with the microbial synthesis of menaquinones in the gut, but evidence to substantiate this effect is lacking, as discussed previously in this chapter.

Vitamin K deficiency also has been reported in patients subjected to long-term total parenteral nutrition, and supplementation of the vitamin is advised in these circumstances. Supplementation in the case of biliary obstruction also is advisable because the impairment of lipid absorption resulting from the lack of bile salts adversely affects vitamin K absorption. Depression of the plasma levels of vitamin K–dependent coagulation factors frequently has been found in patients with malabsorption syndromes and other gastrointestinal disorders (e.g., cystic fibrosis, sprue, celiac disease, ulcerative colitis, regional ileitis, ascaris infection, and short bowel syndrome), and patients usually respond to vitamin K administration with an increase in the level of plasma coagulation factors.

ASSESSMENT OF VITAMIN K STATUS

Although recent advances in methodology have made it possible to routinely measure the plasma or serum phylloquinone concentration, the factors influencing these concentrations and their relationships to dietary intake have not yet been clarified. Alteration of plasma phylloquinone by dietary restriction of the vitamin has been reported in a number of studies (Braam et al., 2004). However, because of the close relationship of plasma phylloquinone to recent dietary intake, these measurements lack utility for assessing vitamin K status. The clinical "prothrombin time," which is a measure of the rate of thrombin generation in plasma, historically has been used to assess the activities of the vitamin K–dependent clotting factors. However, prothrombin time is an insensitive indicator of vitamin K status as relatively large decreases in vitamin K–dependent clotting factor synthesis is needed to produce an apparent deficiency (as indicated by increases in prothrombin time).

More sensitive clotting assays and the ability to immunochemically detect circulating forms of prothrombin that lack some or all of the normal content of Gla residues now permit monitoring of much milder forms of vitamin K deficiency. The plasma concentration of under–γ-carboxylated prothrombin is a sensitive measure of vitamin K status, with low intakes of phylloquinone being associated with elevated concentrations. There are a number of reports that vitamin K status may be important in maintaining skeletal health, and the extent of insufficient γ-carboxylation of circulating osteocalcin has been considered as a possible criterion of vitamin K sufficiency. Although it is clear that vitamin K intake affects the degree of osteocalcin γ-carboxylation, technical problems with current assays, as well as the uncertain physiological significance of the measure, limit the current usefulness of the degree of γ-carboxylation of osteocalcin for assessment of vitamin K status.

DRIs Across the Life Cycle: Vitamin K

	μg Vitamin K per Day
Infant	AI*
0 through 6 mo	2.0
7 through 12 mo	2.5
Children	
1 through 3 yr	30
4 through 8 yr	55
9 through 13 yr	60
14 through 18 yr	75
Males	
≥19 yr	120
Females	
≥19 yr	90
Pregnant/Lactating	
<19 yr	75
≥19 yr	90

Data from IOM. (2006). In J. J. Otten, J. P. Hellwig, & L. D. Meyers (Eds.), Dietary *Reference Intakes: The essential guide to nutrient requirements.* Washington, DC: National Academies Press.
AI, Adequate Intake; *DRI,* Dietary Reference Intake.
*No Tolerable Upper Intake Level for vitamin K.

RECOMMENDATIONS FOR VITAMIN K INTAKE

When the IOM (2002) set the DRIs, it did not set a Recommended Dietary Allowance (RDA) for vitamin K because it lacked adequate data to estimate the average requirement. Adequate Intakes (AIs) were based on representative dietary intake data from healthy individuals (Booth, 2009). The AI for infants is based on the average intake of milk (0.78 L/day) and the average phylloquinone concentration in human milk (2.5 μg/L), which yields an AI of 2.0 μg/day after rounding for infants through 6 months of age. This AI determination assumes that infants receive the recommended 1 mg of prophylactic vitamin K at birth. Because infant formulas typically provide 50 to 100 μg/L of phylloquinone, formula-fed infants have much higher intakes. The AI for 7- through 12-month-old infants was set at 2.5 μg/day by extrapolating up from the AI for younger infants, because an intake of 2.5 μg/day has not been associated with adverse clinical outcomes. The AI would have been much higher if it had been extrapolated down from the typical intakes of older children, and the intake of the older infant will generally be much higher than the AI because of intake of complementary foods.

The AIs for children were determined from the median intake of each age group reported by the National Health and Nutrition Examination Survey (NHANES III, 1988-1994) and rounding up to the nearest 5 μg/day. The AIs for men and women of all ages were set according to the highest median intake value observed among the four adult age groupings used in NHANES III. These AIs are 120 μg/day for men and 90 μg/day for women. No additional intake was recommended for pregnant or lactating women. The AI values set by the IOM (2002) would be judged adequate by the criteria used previously to set the 1989 RDAs, which was 1 μg per kg body weight per day based on limited studies indicating that the daily vitamin K requirement of humans was in the range of 0.5 to 1.5 μg/kg.

No Tolerable Upper Intake Level (UL) was established because ingestion of high doses of phylloquinone, the natural form of the vitamin, has no toxic effect. Menadione, a synthetic form of the vitamin, was previously administered to infants but was shown to be associated with hemolytic anemia and liver toxicity and is no longer used.

REFERENCES

Abedin, M., Tintut, Y., & Demer, L. L. (2004). Vascular calcification: Mechanisms and clinical ramifications. *Arteriosclerosis, Thrombosis, and Vascular Biology, 24,* 1161–1170.

Booth, S. L. (2009). Roles of vitamin K beyond coagulation. *Annual Review of Nutrition, 29,* 89–110.

Booth, S. L., Lichtenstein, A. H., & Dallal, G. E. (2002). Phylloquinone absorption from phylloquinone-fortified oil is greater than from a vegetable in younger and older men and women. *The Journal of Nutrition, 132,* 2609–2612.

Booth, S. L., Lichtenstein, A. H., O'Brien-Morse, M., McKeown, N. M., Wood, R. J., Saltzman, E., & Gundberg, C. M. (2001). Effects of a hydrogenated form of vitamin K on bone formation and resorption. *The American Journal of Clinical Nutrition, 74,* 783–790.

Booth, S. L., O'Brien-Morse, M. E., Dallal, G. E., Davidson, K. W., & Gundberg, C. M. (1999). Response of vitamin K status to different intakes and sources of phylloquinone-rich foods: Comparison of younger and older adults. *The American Journal of Clinical Nutrition, 70,* 368–377.

Booth, S. L., Pennington, J. A., & Sadowski, J. A. (1996). Dihydro-vitamin K_1: Primary food sources and estimated intakes in the American diet. *Lipids, 31,* 715–720.

Booth, S. L., & Suttie, J. W. (1998). Dietary intake and adequacy of vitamin K. *The Journal of Nutrition, 128,* 785–788.

Braam, L., McKeown, N., Jacques, P., Lichtenstein, A., Vermeer, C., Wilson, P., & Booth, S. (2004). Dietary phylloquinone intake as a potential marker for a heart-healthy dietary pattern in the Framingham Offspring cohort. *Journal of the American Dietetic Association, 104,* 1410–1414.

Broze, G. J., Jr. (2001). Protein Z dependent regulation of coagulation. *Thrombosis and Haemostasis, 86*, 8–13.

Bush, K. A., Stenflo, J., Roth, D. A., Czerwiec, E., Harrist, A., Begley, G. S., … Furie, B. (1999). Hydrophobic amino acids define the carboxylation recognition site in the precursor of the gamma-carboxyglutamic-acid-containing conotoxin epsilon-TxIX from the marine cone snail *Conus textile*. *Biochemistry, 38*, 14660–14466.

Carrie, I., Portaulalian, J., Vicaaretti, R., Rochford, J., Potvin, S., & Ferland, G. (2004). Menaquinone-4 concentration is correlated with sphingolipid concentration in rat brain. *The Journal of Nutrition, 134*, 167–172.

Cockayne, S., Adamson, J., Lanham-New, S., Shearer, M. J., Gilbody, S., & Torgerson, D. J. (2006). Vitamin K and the prevention of fractures: Systematic review and meta-analysis of randomized controlled trials. *Archives of Internal Medicine, 166*, 1256–1261.

Crivello, N. A., Casseus, S. L., Peterson, J. W., Smith, D. E., & Booth, S. L. (2010). Age-and brain region-specific effects of dietary vitamin K on myelin sulfatides. *The Journal of Nutritional Biochemistry, 21*, 1083–1088.

Dam, H. (1934). Haemorrhages in chicks reared on artificial diets: A new deficiency disease. *Nature, 133*, 909–910.

Davie, E. W., & Ratnof, O. D. (1964). Waterfall sequence for intrinsic blood clotting. *Science, 145*, 1310–1311.

Dismore, M. L., Haytowitz, D. B., Gebhardt, S. E., Peterson, J. W., & Booth, S. L. (2003). Vitamin K content of nuts and fruits in the US diet. *Journal of the American Dietetic Association, 103*, 1650–1652.

Diuguid, D. L., Rabiet, M. J., Furie, B. C., Liebman, H. A., & Furie, B. (1986). Molecular basis of hemophilia B: Defective enzyme due to an unprocessed propeptide is caused by a point mutation in the factor IX precursor. *Proceedings of the National Academy of Sciences of the United States of America, 83*, 5803–5807.

Dolnikowski, G. G., Sun, Z., Grusak, M. A., Peterson, J. W., Booth, S. L. (2002). HPLC and GC/MS determination of deuterated vitamin K (phylloquinone) in human serum after ingestion of deuterium-labeled broccoli. *Journal of Nutritional Biochemistry 13*, 168–174.

Dowd, P., Hershline, R., Ham, S. W., & Naganathan, S. (1995). Vitamin K and energy transduction: A base strength amplification mechanism. *Science, 269*, 1684–1691.

Ducy, P., Desbois, C., Boyce, B., Pinero, G., Story, B., Dunstan, C., … Karsenty, G. (1996). Increased bone formation in osteocalcin-deficient mice. *Nature, 382*, 448–452.

Erkkila, A.T., Lichtenstein, A. H., Dolnikowski, G. G., Grusak, M. A., Jalbert, S. M., Aquino, K. A., … Booth, S. L. (2004). Plasma transport of vitamin K in men using deuterium-labeled collard greens. *Metabolism 53*, 215–221.

Esmon, C. T., Sadowski, J. A., & Suttie, J. W. (1975). A new carboxylation reaction: The vitamin K–dependent incorporation of H14CO3 into prothrombin. *The Journal of Biological Chemistry, 250*, 4744–4748.

Fregin, A., Rost, S., Wolz, W., Krebsova, A., Muller, C. R., & Oldenburg, J. (2002). Homozygosity mapping of a second gene locus for hereditary combined deficiency of vitamin K–dependent clotting factors to the centromeric region of chromosome 16. *Blood, 100*, 3229–3232.

Fridell, Y. W., Villa, J., Jr., Attar, E. C., & Liu, E. T. (1998). GAS6 induces Axl-mediated chemotaxis of vascular smooth muscle cells. *The Journal of Biological Chemistry, 273*, 7123–7126.

Furie, B., & Furie, B. (1992). Molecular and cellular biology of blood coagulation. *New England Journal of Medicine, 326*, 800–806.

Garber, A. K., Binkley, N. C., Krueger, D. C., & Suttie, J. W. (1999). Comparison of phylloquinone bioavailability from food sources or a supplement in human subjects. *The Journal of Nutrition, 129*, 1201–1203.

Greaves, J. H., & Ayres, P. (1967). Heritable resistance to warfarin in rats. *Nature, 215*, 877–878.

Greer, F. R. (2001). Are breast-fed infants vitamin K deficient? *Advances in Experimental Medicine and Biology, 501*, 391–395.

Habu, D., Shiomi, S., Tamori, A., Takeda, T., Tanaka, T., Kubo, S., & Nishiguchi, S. (2004). Role of vitamin K_2 in the development of hepatocellular carcinoma in women with viral cirrhosis of the liver. *The Journal of the American Medical Association, 292*, 358–361.

Hamilton, D. W. (2008). Functional role of periostin in development and wound repair: Implications for connective tissue disease. *Journal of Cell Communication and Signaling, 2*, 9–17.

Hanatani, T., Fukuda, T., Onishi, S., Funae, Y., & Azuma, J. (2003). No major difference in inhibitory susceptibility between CYP2C9.1 and CYP2C9.3. *European Journal of Clinical Pharmacology, 59*, 233–235.

Hemker, H. C., & Reekers, P. P. M. (1974). Isolation and purification of proteins induced by vitamin K absence. *Thrombosis et Diathesis Haemorrhagica. Supplementum, 57*, 83–85.

Hildebrandt, E. F., & Suttie, J. W. (1982). Mechanism of coumarin action: Sensitivity of vitamin K metabolizing enzymes of normal and warfarin-resistant rat liver. *Biochemistry, 21*, 2406–2411.

Honore, B. (2009). The rapidly expanding CREC protein family: Members, localization, function, and role in disease. *BioEssays, 31*, 262–277.

Honore, B., & Vorum, H. (2000). The CREC family, a novel family of multiple EF-hand, low-affinity Ca^{2+}-binding proteins localized to the secretory pathway of mammalian cells. *FEBS Letters, 466*, 11–18.

Horie-Inoue, K., & Inoue, S. (2008). Steroid and xenobiotic receptor mediates a novel vitamin K_2 signaling pathway in osteoblastic cells. *Journal of Bone and Mineral Metabolism, 26*, 9–12.

Ichikawa, T., Horie-Inoue, K., Ikeda, K., Blumberg, B., & Inoue, S. (2006). Steroid and xenobiotic receptor SXR mediates vitamin K_2-activated transcription of extracellular matrix-related genes and collagen accumulation in osteoblastic cells. *The Journal of Biological Chemistry, 281*, 16927–16934.

Indyk, H. E., & Woollard, D. C. (1997). Vitamin K in milk and infant formulas: Determination and distribution of phylloquinone and menaquinone-4. *The Analyst, 122*, 465–469.

Institute of Medicine. (2002). *Dietary reference intakes for vitamin A, vitamin K, arsenic, boron, chromium, copper, iodine, iron, manganese, molybdenum, nickel, silicon, vanadium and zinc.* Washington, DC: National Academies Press.

Iwamoto, J., Takeda, T., & Ichimura, S. (2003). Combined treatment with vitamin K_2 and bisphosphonate in postmenopausal woman with osteoporosis. *Yonsei Medical Journal, 44*, 751–756.

Kohn, M. H., Pelz, H. J., & Wayne, R. K. (2003). Locus-specific genetic differentiation at Rw among warfarin resistant rat *(Rattus norvegicus)* populations. *Genetics, 164*, 1055–1070.

Koivu-Tikkanen, T. J., Ollilainen, V., & Piironen, V. I. (2000). Determination of phylloquinone and menaquinones in animal products with fluorescence detection after postcolumn reduction with metallic zinc. *Journal of Agricultural and Food Chemistry, 48*, 6325–6333.

Kulman, J. D., Harris, J. E., Haldeman, B. A., & Davie, E. W. (1997). Primary structure and tissue distribution of two novel proline-rich γ-carboxyglutamic acid proteins. *Proceedings of the National Academy of Sciences of the United States of America, 94*, 9058–9062.

Kulman, J. D., Harris, J. E., Xie, L., & Davie, E. W. (2001). Identification of two novel transmembrane gamma-carboxyglutamic acid proteins expressed broadly in fetal and adult tissues. *Proceedings of the National Academy of Sciences of the United States of America, 98*, 1370–1375.

Li, R., Chen, J., Hammonds, G., Phillips, H., Armanini, M., Wood, P., … Mather, J. P. (1996). Identification of Gas6 as a growth factor for human Schwann cells. *The Journal of Neuroscience, 16*, 2012–2019.

Li, T., Chang, C. Y., Jin, D. Y., Lin, P. J., Khvorova, A., & Stafford, D. W. (2004). Identification of the gene for vitamin K epoxide reductase. *Nature, 437*, 541–544.

Loebstein, R., Dvoskin, I., Halkin, H., Vecsler, M., Lubetsky, A., Rechavi, G., … Gak, E. (2007). A coding VKORC1 Asp36-Tyr polymorphism predisposes to warfarin resistance. *Blood, 109*, 2477–2480.

Loeser, R. F., Wallin, R., & Sadowski, J. (1993). Vitamin K and vitamin K–dependent proteins in the elderly: Implications for bone and cartilage biology. In R. R. Watson (Ed.), *Handbook of nutrition in the aged* (2nd ed., pp. 263–280). Boca Raton, FL: CRC Press.

Luo, G., Ducy, P., McKee, M. D., Pinero, G. J., Loyer, E., Behringer, R. R., & Karsenty, G. (1997). Spontaneous calcification of arteries and cartilage in mice lacking matrix Gla protein. *Nature, 386*, 78–81.

Macfarlane, R. G. (1965). The basis of the cascade hypothesis of blood coagulation. *Thrombosis et Diathesis Haemorrhagica, 15*, 591–602.

Malhotra, O. P. (1972). Terminal amino acids of normal and dicumarol-treated prothrombin. *Life Sciences, 11*, 445–454.

Monroe, D. M., Hoffman, M., & Roberts, H. R. (2002). Platelet and thrombin generation. *Arteriosclerosis, Thrombosis, and Vascular Biology, 22*, 1381–1389.

Murshed, M., Schinke, T., McKee, M. D., & Karsenty, G. (2004). Extracellular matrix mineralization is regulated locally: Different roles of two Gla-containing proteins. *The Journal of Cell Biology, 165*, 625–630.

Nelsestuen, G. L., Zytkovicz, T. H., & Howard, J. B. (1974). The mode of action of vitamin K: Identification of γ-carboxyglutamic acid as a component of prothrombin. *The Journal of Biological Chemistry, 249*, 6347–6350.

Okano, T., Shimomura, Y., Yamane, M., Suhara, Y., Kamao, M., Sugiura, M., & Nakagawa, K. (2008). Conversion of phylloquinone (vitamin K_1) into menaquinone-4 (vitamin K_2) in mice: Two possible routes for menaquinone-4 accumulation in cerebra of mice. *The Journal of Biological Chemistry, 283*, 11270–11279.

Pati, S., & Helmbrecht, G. D. (1994). Congenital schizencephaly associated with in utero warfarin exposure. *Reproductive Toxicology, 8*, 115–120.

Prieto, A. L., Weber, J. L., Tracy, S., Heeb, M. J., & Lai, C. (1999). Gas6, a ligand for the receptor protein-tyrosine kinase Tyro-3, is widely expressed in the central nervous system. *Brain Research, 816*, 646–661.

Rishavy, M. A., Hallgren, K. W., Yaubenko, A. V., Sthofman, R. L., Runge, K. W., & Berkner, K. L. (2006). Bronsted analysis reveals Lys218 as the carboxylase active site base that deprotonates vitamin K hydroqunone to initiate vitamin K–dependent protein carboxylation. *Biochemistry, 45*, 13239–13248.

Ronden, J. E., Drittij-Reijnders, M. J., Vermeer, C., & Thijssen, H. H. (1998). Intestinal flora is not an intermediate in the phylloquinone-menaquinone-4 conversion in the rat. *Biochimica et Biophysica Acta, 1379*, 69–75.

Rost, S., Fregin, A., Ivaskevicius, V., Conzelmann, E., Hortnagel, K., Pelz, H. J., … Oldenburg, J. (2004). Mutations in VKORC1 cause warfarin resistance and multiple coagulation factor deficiency type 2. *Nature, 437*, 537–541.

Sadowski, J. A., Hood, S. J., Dallal, G. E., & Garry, P. J. (1989). Phylloquinone in plasma from elderly and young adults: Factors influencing its concentration. *The American Journal of Clinical Nutrition, 50*, 100–108.

Sato, T., Ozaki, R., Kamo, S., Hara, Y., Konishi, S., Isobe, Y., … Harada, H. (2003). The biological activity and tissue distribution of 2′,3′-dihydrophylloquinone in rats. *Biochimica et Biophysica Acta, 1622*, 145–150.

Schori, T. R., & Stungis, G. E. (2004). Long-term warfarin treatment may induce arterial calcification in humans: Case report. *Clinical and Investigative Medicine, 27*, 107–109.

Schurgers, L. J., & Vermeer, C. (2002). Differential lipoprotein transport pathways of K-vitamins in healthy subjects. *Biochimica et Biophysica Acta, 1570*, 27–32.

Shearer, M. J., & Newman, P. (2008). Metabolism and cell biology of vitamin K. *Thrombosis and Haemostasis, 100*, 530–547.

Spronk, H. M., Soute, B. A., Schurgers, L. J., Thijssen, H. H., De Mey, J. G., & Vermeer, C. (2003). Tissue-specific utilization of menaquinone-4 results in the prevention of arterial calcification in warfarin-treated rats. *Journal of Vascular Research, 40*, 531–537.

Stanton, C., Taylor, R., & Wallin, R. (1991). Processing of prothrombin in the secretory pathway. *The Biochemical Journal, 277*, 59–65.

Stenflo, J., Fernlund, P., Egan, W., & Roepstorff, P. (1974). Vitamin K dependent modifications of glutamic acid residues in prothrombin. *Proceedings of the Society for Experimental Biology and Medicine, 71*, 2730–2733.

Stenina, O., Pudota, B. N., McNally, B. A., Hommema, E. L., & Berkner, K. L. (2001). Tethered processivity of the Vitamin K–dependent carboxylase: Factor IX is efficiently modified in a mechanism which distinguishes Gla's from Glu's and which accounts for comprehensive carboxylation in vivo. *Biochemistry, 40*, 10301–10309.

Stitt, T. N., Conn, G., Gore, M., Lai, C., Bruno, J., Radziejewski, C., … Yancopoulos, G. D. (1995). The anticoagulation factor protein S and its relative, Gas6, are ligands for the Tyro 3/Axl family of receptor tyrosine kinases. *Cell, 24*, 661–670.

Sundaram, K. S., & Lev, M. (1988). Warfarin administration reduces synthesis of sulfatides and other sphingolipids in mouse brain. *Journal of Lipid Research, 29*, 1475–1479.

Suttie, J. W. (1978). Vitamin K. In H. F. Deluca (Ed.), *Handbook of lipid research* (pp. 211–277). New York: Plenum Press.

Suttie, J. W. (1995). The importance of menaquinones in human nutrition. *Annual Review of Nutrition, 15*, 399–417.

Sweatt, A., Sane, D. C., Hutson, S. M., & Wallin, R. (2003). Matrix Gla protein (MGP) and bone morphogenetic protein-2 in aortic calcified lesions of aging rats. *Journal of Thrombosis and Haemostasis, 1*, 178–185.

Tabb, M. M., Sun, A., Zhou, C., Grun, F., Errandi, J., Romero, K., … Blumberg, B. (2003). Vitamin K_2 regulation of bone homeostasis is mediated by the steroid and xenobiotic receptor SXR. *The Journal of Biological Chemistry, 278*, 43919–43927.

Thijssen, H. H., Drittij, M. J., Vermeer, C., & Schoffelen, E. (2002). Menaquinone-4 in breast milk is derived from dietary phylloquinone. *The British Journal of Nutrition, 87*, 219–226.

Tie, J., Wu, S. M., Jin, D., Nicchitta, C. F., & Stafford, D. W. (2000). A topological study of the human gamma-glutamyl carboxylase. *Blood, 96*, 973–978.

Tsugawa, N., Shiraki, M., Suhara, Y., Kamao, M., & Ozaki, R. (2008). Low plasma phylloquinone concentration is associated with high incidence of vertebral fracture in elderly woman. *Journal of Bone and Mineral Metabolism, 26*, 79–85.

Usui, Y., Tanimura, H., Nishimura, N., Kobayashi, N., Okanoue, T., & Ozawa, K. (1990). Vitamin K concentrations in the plasma and liver of surgical patients. *The American Journal of Clinical Nutrition, 51*, 846–852.

Vermeer, C., & Schurgers, L. J. (2000). A comprehensive review of vitamin K and vitamin K antagonists. *Hematology/Oncology Clinics of North America, 14*, 339–353.

Viagas, C. S., Simes, D. C., Laize, V., Williamson, M. K., Price, P. A., & Cancela, M. L. (2008). GLA-rich protein (GRP): A new vitamin K–dependent protein identified from sturgeon cartilage and highly conserved in vertebrates. *The Journal of Biological Chemistry, 283*, 36655–36664.

Voora, D., Kobolt, D. C., King, C. R., Lenzini, P. A., Porche-Sorbet, R., Deych, E., … Gage, B. F. (2009). A polymorphism in the VKORC1 regulator calumenin predicts higher warfarin dose requirements in African Americans. *Clinical Pharmacology and Therapeutics, 87*, 445–451.

Wajih, N., Sane, D. C., Hutson, S. M., & Wallin, R. (2004). The inhibitory effect of calumenin on the vitamin K–dependent γ-carboxylation system: Characterization of the system in normal and warfarin resistant rats. *The Journal of Biological Chemistry, 279*, 25276–25283.

Wallace, M. E., & MacSwiney, F. J. (1976). A major gene controlling warfarin-resistance in the house mouse. *The Journal of Hygiene, 76*, 173–181.

Wallin, R., Hutson, S. M., Cain, D., Sweatt, A., & Sane, D. C. (2001a). A molecular mechanism for genetic warfarin resistance in the rat. *The FASEB Journal, 15*, 2542–2544.

Wallin, R., & Martin, L. F. (1987). Warfarin poisoning and vitamin K antagonism in rat and human liver. Design of a system in vitro that mimics the system in vivo. *The Biochemical Journal, 241*, 389–396.

Wallin, R., Wajih, N., Greenwood, G. T., & Sane, D. C. (2001b). Arterial calcification: A review of mechanisms, animal models, and the prospects for therapy. *Medicinal Research Reviews, 21*, 274–301.

Wu, S.-M., Morris, D. P., & Stafford, D. W. (1991). Identification and purification to near homogeneity of the vitamin K–dependent carboxylase. *Proceedings of the National Academy of Sciences of the United States of America, 88*, 2236–2240.

RECOMMENDED READINGS

Booth, S. L. (2009). Roles of vitamin K beyond coagulation. *Annual Review of Nutrition, 29*, 89–110.

Dowd, P., Ham, S.-W., Naganathan, S., & Hershline, R. (1995). The mechanism of action of vitamin K. *Annual Review of Nutrition, 15*, 419–440.

Wallin, R., & Hutson, S. M. (2004). Warfarin and the vitamin K–dependent gamma-carboxylation system. *Trends in Molecular Medicine, 10*, 299–302.

CHAPTER 29

Vitamin E

Robert S. Parker, PhD

Vitamin E was discovered more than 80 years ago as a lipid-soluble substance necessary for the prevention of fetal death and resorption in rats that had been fed a rancid lard diet (Evans and Bishop, 1922). Today, it is known that vitamin E deficiency results in species-specific abnormalities, including large motor dysfunction in humans. Though the causal molecular aspects of these abnormalities remain largely unknown, all are thought to be associated with the single consensus function of vitamin E, the trapping of lipophilic free radicals.

NOMENCLATURE AND STRUCTURE OF VITAMIN E

Vitamin E is the collective term for all of the structurally related tocopherols and tocotrienols (collectively termed tocochromanols, or the "vitamers" of vitamin E) and their derivatives that qualitatively exhibit the biological activity of RRR-α-tocopherol in prevention of rat fetal resorption. Therefore the term *vitamin E* is not synonymous with α-tocopherol, a common form of vitamin E. Tocopherol is derived from the Greek words *tokos* (childbirth), *phero* (to bring forth), and *ol* (alcohol), and relates to the role of vitamin E in reproduction in animals.

Four tocopherols and four tocotrienols occur naturally. All consist of a chromanol head group and a phytyl side chain and differ in the number and position of methyl groups on the phenol ring of the chromanol head group (Figure 29-1). The structure of a tocotrienol is similar to that of a tocopherol, except that the hydrophobic phytyl side chain of the tocotrienols contains double bonds at the 3′, 7′, and 11′ positions. In addition to these eight naturally occurring vitamers, synthetic α-tocopherol, as either free or ester forms, is available commercially. The tocopherol molecule has three chiral centers in its phytyl tail, making a total of eight stereoisomeric forms possible. The naturally occurring isomer of α-tocopherol (formerly known as D-α-tocopherol) biosynthesized by plants is the 2R, 4′R, 8′R stereoisomer, whereas synthetic α-tocopherol consists of a mixture of all eight possible stereoisomers. The tetrahedral arrangement of substituents around each asymmetric chiral center is designated R (from the Latin *rectus,* meaning "right") or S (from the Latin *sinister,* meaning "left").

To distinguish the naturally occurring stereoisomer of α-tocopherol from the synthetic mixture, naturally occurring α-tocopherol is designated as RRR-α-tocopherol, and the synthetic mixture of α-tocopherol stereoisomers (previously known as DL-α-tocopherol) is designated as all-racemic (all-rac)-α-tocopherol. Naturally occurring tocopherols in foods exist as the free (unesterified) forms. Synthetic ester forms of α-tocopherol are produced by forming ester linkages between the 6-hydroxyl group of the phenolic ring of α-tocopherol and the carboxylate group of acetic acid (see Figure 29-1) or succinic acid. The acetate or succinate ester forms of α-tocopherol are more chemically stable and are therefore more suitable for food fortification or vitamin supplement formulations than unesterified α-tocopherol. In addition, "natural source" vitamin E preparations are produced by methylation of mixtures of tocopherols (e.g., from soybean oil), resulting in products that contain predominantly α-tocopherol.

ABSORPTION, TRANSPORT, AND METABOLISM OF VITAMIN E

The absorption and plasma transport of vitamin E follows to a large extent the paths of cholesterol absorption and transport. Vitamin E is absorbed with other lipids, incorporated into chylomicrons, and eventually transported by other circulating lipoproteins. The tocochromanols are metabolized to water-soluble metabolites that are excreted primarily via the urine.

ABSORPTION

The process of intestinal absorption of vitamin E is similar to that of other lipid components of the diet. Tocopheryl esters, when present, are hydrolyzed to free tocopherol by pancreatic esterases in the proximal lumen of the small intestine. Tocopherols and tocotrienols, as constituents of bile salt micelles, are taken up, apparently by passive diffusion, into enterocytes lining the small intestine. Within the enterocyte, tocochromanols are incorporated, along with other lipids, into nascent triacylglycerol-rich chylomicrons. The chylomicrons are secreted into the intercellular space, from which they enter the lymphatics and eventually the bloodstream. Estimates of the absorption efficiency of tocopherols vary widely, but it appears that roughly half of the tocopherols consumed in foods is absorbed, with the remainder excreted in the feces. There appear to be no major differences in the rates of intestinal absorption of the various forms of vitamin E (Kayden and Traber, 1993).

PLASMA TRANSPORT AND TISSUE UPTAKE

Because of its virtual insolubility in water, vitamin E requires special transport mechanisms in the aqueous milieu of the body. As described, dietary tocopherols taken up by the small intestine are incorporated into triacylglycerol-rich chylomicrons, secreted into the intestinal lymph, and eventually delivered to the liver in the chylomicron remnants. Newly absorbed vitamin E taken up by parenchymal cells of the liver is either incorporated into nascent very-low-density lipoproteins (VLDLs) and secreted back into the bloodstream or metabolized within the liver to water-soluble metabolites. Endogenous vitamin E in other tissues appears to be released to high-density lipoproteins (HDLs) and other plasma lipoproteins and recirculated to the liver or other tissues. Tocopherols undergo exchange between lipoproteins, facilitated by a phospholipid transfer protein found in plasma (Kostner et al., 1995). Therefore, in the fasting state, tocopherols are approximately equally distributed between low-density lipoproteins (LDLs) and HDLs.

Tocopherols circulating in lipoproteins can be taken up by tissues via various receptor-mediated processes. Chylomicron remnants are taken up by the parenchymal cells of the liver via an apolipoprotein E–mediated mechanism, and LDL particles are taken up by liver and other tissues via apolipoprotein B100–mediated processes. Other mechanisms of cell uptake may involve selective uptake from HDLs via scavenger receptors, as is the case with cholesterol. In addition, some of the vitamin E in association with chylomicrons and VLDLs may be transferred to peripheral cells during the lipolysis of these triacylglycerol-rich lipoproteins by lipoprotein lipase. Studies of vitamin E delivery to tissues in transgenic mice overexpressing human lipoprotein lipase in muscle demonstrated enhanced vitamin E uptake by skeletal muscle but not by adipose tissue or brain (Sattler et al., 1996). (See Chapter 17 for an overview of lipoprotein metabolism.)

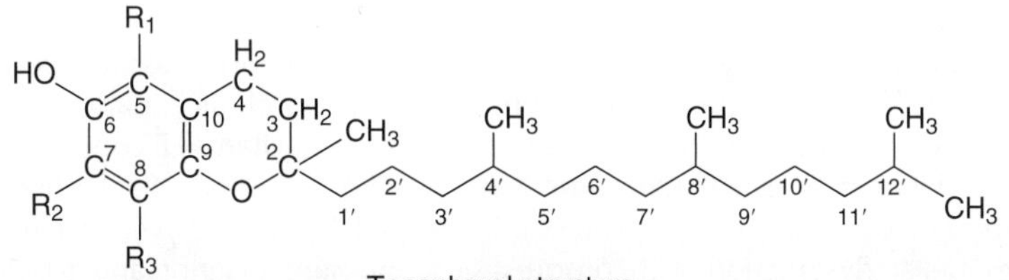

Tocopherol structure

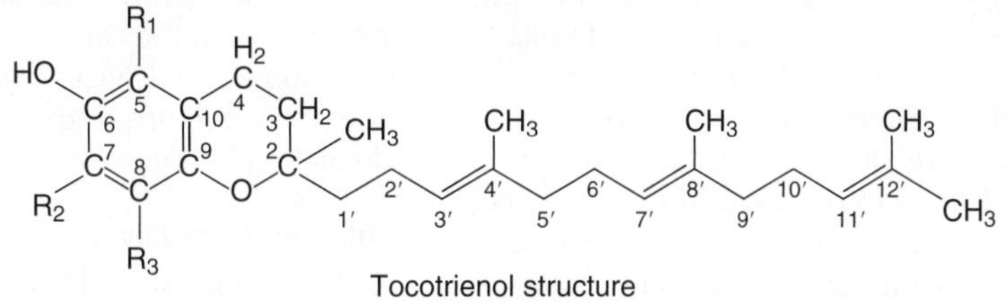

Tocotrienol structure

Position of methyls	Tocopherol structure	Tocotrienol structure
R_1,R_2,R_3	α-Tocopherol (α-T)	α-Tocotrienol (α-T-3)
R_1,R_3	β-Tocopherol (β-T)	β-Tocotrienol (β-T-3)
R_2,R_3	γ-Tocopherol (γ-T)	γ-Tocotrienol (γ-T-3)
R_3	δ-Tocopherol (δ-T)	δ-Tocotrienol (δ-T-3)

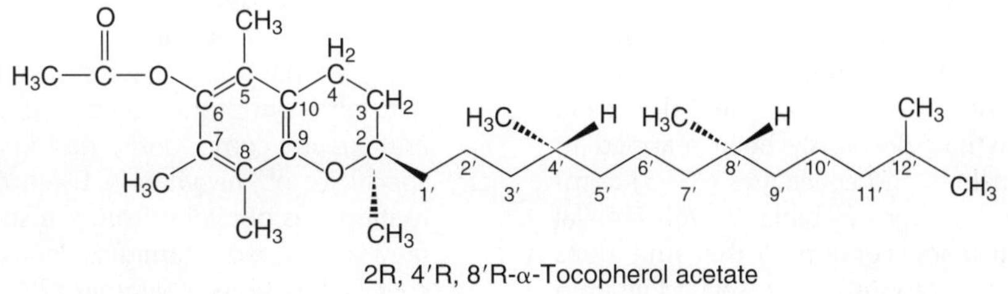

2R, 4′R, 8′R-α-Tocopherol acetate

FIGURE 29-1 Chemical structures of tocopherols, tocotrienols, and α-tocopheryl acetate.

Hepatic Secretion and the Role of α-Tocopherol Transfer Protein

The process of secretion of α-tocopherol from the liver via VLDLs is crucial to maintaining normal plasma vitamin E levels. A tocopherol-binding protein, called α-tocopherol transfer protein (α-TTP) plays an essential role in this process. This soluble protein is found predominantly in liver, and preferentially binds RRR-α-tocopherol relative to other forms of vitamin E (Manor and Morley, 2008). It is only one of two proteins known to bind vitamin E with high affinity; the other is cytochrome P450-4F2, as discussed later. α-TTP exhibits two unique properties: high affinity binding of α-tocopherol, and transfer of α-tocopherol from one membrane to another in a process involving direct membrane interaction (Morley et al., 2008). In the liver, α-TTP facilitates the secretion of α-tocopherol into the plasma lipoprotein pool (Traber et al., 1993) via a non–Golgi-dependent mechanism that has not been fully elucidated (Kaempf-Rotzoll et al., 2003). α-TTP has been reported to associate with lysosomes or late endosomes, where it presumably binds and transfers predominantly α-tocopherol to another vesicular compartment for translocation to the cell surface. The ATP-binding cassette transporter A1 (ABCA1), which lipidates apoA1 and lipid-poor HDL with phospholipid and cholesterol, has been reported to facilitate the secretion of vitamin E from cells (Oram et al., 2001; Qian et al., 2005), but a physical interaction between α-TTP and ABCA1 in the liver has yet to be demonstrated. This process contributes to the preferential enrichment of LDLs and HDLs with α-tocopherol compared with the other forms of vitamin E. A critical role for α-TTP in maintaining normal plasma tocopherol concentration has been demonstrated in patients with familial ataxia with isolated vitamin E deficiency, or AVED (Gotoda et al., 1995; Ouahchi et al., 1995; Kayden and Traber, 1993). These patients have clear signs of vitamin E deficiency (extremely

CLINICAL CORRELATION

α-Tocopherol Transfer Protein and Familial Isolated Vitamin E Deficiency

Secondary vitamin E deficiency occurs in patients with generalized fat malabsorption caused by disorders such as abetalipoproteinemia, cystic fibrosis, short bowel syndrome, and cholestatic liver disease. In these patients, prolonged deficiency of vitamin E eventually causes a decrease in the tocopherol content of nervous tissues and results in spinocerebellar dysfunction with progressive ataxia. In contrast, a number of patients have been documented as having specific inherited forms of vitamin E deficiency. These cases have been described as familial isolated vitamin E deficiency or ataxia with isolated vitamin E deficiency (AVED). Patients with this autosomal recessive neurodegenerative disease develop symptoms that resemble those of Friedreich ataxia. These patients have normal gastrointestinal absorption of dietary lipids and vitamin E (all forms), with normal intestinal secretion of lipids and vitamin E into chylomicrons. They have, however, an impaired ability to secrete α-tocopherol from the liver, a function that apparently allows healthy individuals to efficiently recirculate α-tocopherol obtained from lipoproteins back into the plasma lipoprotein pool. Therefore, in patients with familial isolated vitamin E deficiency, the absorption and postprandial transport of vitamin E to the liver are normal, but the hepatic secretion of vitamin E back into plasma is impaired; this results in a low or undetectable plasma vitamin E concentration and insufficient delivery of vitamin E to tissues.

The cDNA for α-TTP was isolated from rats and humans, and the human α-TPP gene was shown to be located at chromosome 8q13 (Arita et al., 1995). Familial vitamin E deficiency mutations had previously been mapped to this same location. Ouahchi and colleagues (1995) demonstrated α-TTP gene mutations in patients with familial isolated vitamin E deficiency, confirming that mutations of the gene for α-TTP are responsible for isolated vitamin E deficiency. Several mutations are now known. The type of mutation is associated with the degree of severity of the neurological damage and age of onset as well as with plasma vitamin E concentration. Interestingly, some mutations have no effect on α-tocopherol transfer activity of α-TTP in vitro, yet still result in vitamin E deficiency in humans (Manor and Morley, 2008). High doses of vitamin E can prevent or mitigate the neurological course of this disease. Serum vitamin E concentrations in patients increase when they are treated with large doses of vitamin E, presumably because of the direct transfer of tocopherol from chylomicrons or their remnants to tissues or to other circulating lipoproteins.

Thinking Critically

1. The affinity of α-TTP for various forms of vitamin E varies and is highest for RRR-α-tocopherol. There seems to be a linear relationship between the relative binding affinity (RRR-α-tocopherol, 100%; RRR-β-tocopherol, 38%; SRR-α-tocopherol, 11%; RRR-γ-tocopherol, 9%; and RRR-δ-tocopherol, 2%) and the known biological activity obtained from the rat resorption–gestation assay (Hosomi et al., 1977). How might α-TTP and the tocopherol-ω-oxidation pathway work together to determine the biological potency of the various forms of vitamin E? Explain. Do you think the type of tocopherol used as supplements for patients with familial isolated vitamin E deficiency would matter? Explain.
2. Many animal studies have shown that certain vitamin E deficiency symptoms can be partially reversed by other antioxidant compounds, raising questions about the specificity of the vitamin E requirement. What information was obtained from the studies of patients with familial isolated vitamin E deficiency with regard to specific functions of vitamin E?

low plasma vitamin E and neurological abnormalities) but have no fat malabsorption or lipoprotein abnormalities. Absence of functional α-TTP in these patients impairs secretion of α-tocopherol from liver into the bloodstream, resulting in very low concentrations of plasma vitamin E. Presumably the α-tocopherol not secreted into the bloodstream is secreted into the bile. The plasma vitamin E level of AVED patients can be normalized with high-dose vitamin E supplementation.

METABOLISM OF VITAMIN E AND THE ROLE OF CYTOCHROME P450-4F2

Tocopherols and tocotrienols other than α-tocopherol undergo extensive postabsorptive metabolism to water-soluble metabolites that are excreted primarily in the urine. This catabolic process involves severe truncation of the hydrophobic phytyl side chain, the moiety responsible for the fat-solubility of vitamin E. The metabolic pathway is depicted in Figure 29-2 and involves an initial hydroxylation of a terminal methyl group (ω-hydroxylation) of the phytyl side chain. In human beings, the enzyme cytochrome P450-4F2 (CYP4F2), an endoplasmic reticulum enzyme that requires NADPH and is expressed predominantly in the liver, has been implicated in this reaction (Sontag and Parker, 2002). The hydroxylated intermediate is further oxidized, apparently by an NAD-dependent dehydrogenase, to the corresponding ω-carboxychromanol. Truncation of the phytyl side chain subsequently occurs by sequential removal of two- or three-carbon units, ultimately yielding the 3′-carboxyethylhydroxychromanol (CEHC) (see Figure 29-2). Despite the relatively high water solubility of these short-chain metabolites, they appear to be largely conjugated with glucuronic acid by the action of uridine 5′-diphospho-glucuronosyltransferase, presumably at the phenolic hydroxyl group, to further facilitate their excretion in urine. α-Tocopherol is a relatively poor substrate for this catabolic pathway, whereas other tocopherols and the tocotrienols are good substrates (Sontag and Parker, 2007). Therefore the tocopherol-ω-oxidation pathway is considered to play a central role in the selective tissue deposition of α-tocopherol via the preferential elimination of the other forms of vitamin E, resulting in the "α-tocopherol phenotype." This phenotype is widely expressed in the animal kingdom. Though α-TTP also contributes to this phenotype (Figure 29-3), it does not appear

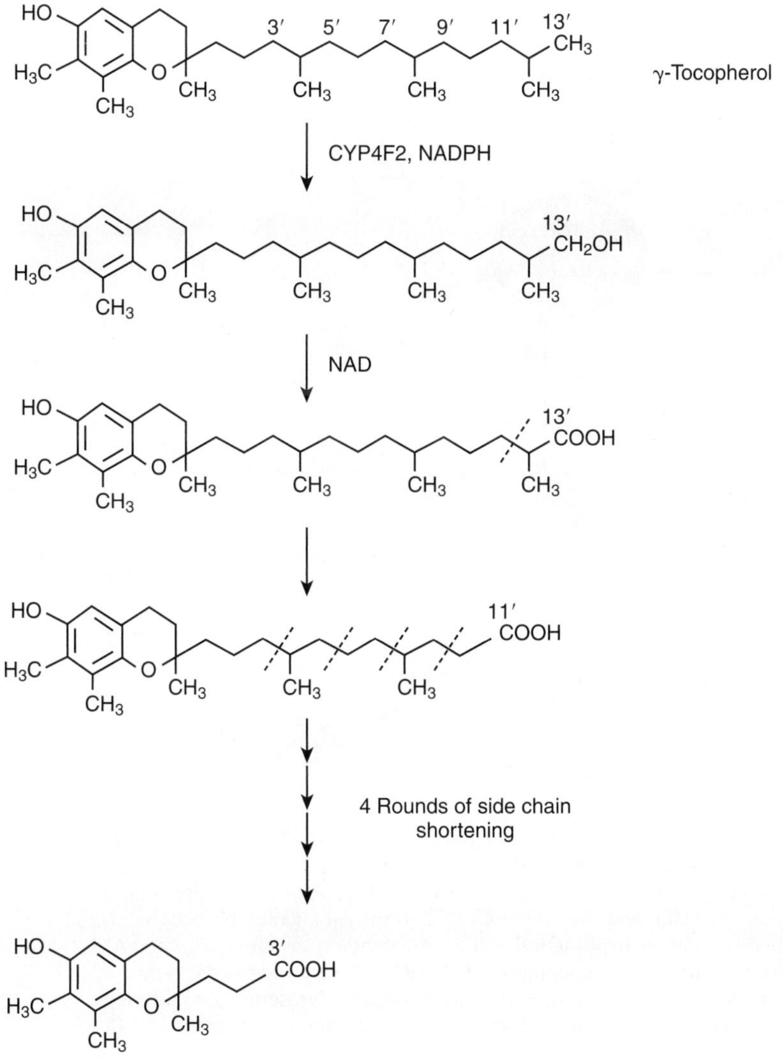

γ-Tocopherol

CYP4F2, NADPH

NAD

4 Rounds of side chain shortening

FIGURE 29-2 The ω-oxidation pathway of vitamin E metabolism. The pathway of ω-oxidation of the phytyl tail of tocopherols and tocotrienols, shown here with γ-tocopherol as substrate, involves an initial ω-hydroxylation at a terminal (13 or 13′) methyl group catalyzed by cytochrome P450-4F2 (CYP4F2). Subsequent reactions involve oxidation to the terminal carboxylic acid and sequential removal of 2- or 3-carbon moieties in a process analogous to the oxidation of fatty acids. The final products, 3′-carboxyethylhydroxychromanols (CEHC), are conjugated with glucuronic acid and excreted in the urine. Among the various forms of vitamin E, α-tocopherol is a poor substrate for CYP4F2. Therefore ω-oxidation contributes to the selective tissue enrichment with α-tocopherol via postabsorptive catabolism and elimination of the other forms of the vitamin.

to be essential, because the fruit fly, *Drosophila*, expresses the α-tocopherol phenotype and a cytochrome P450–mediated ω-oxidation pathway similar to that of mammals, yet does not express a protein with the hallmark activity of α-TTP (Parker and McCormick, 2005). To date ω-oxidation is the only known pathway of vitamin E metabolism.

PLASMA CONCENTRATION OF VITAMIN E AND RELATIONSHIP WITH DIETARY INTAKE

Usual plasma vitamin E concentrations in humans range from 20 to 30 μmol of α-tocopherol per liter or about 5 to 8 mmol α-tocopherol per mole of cholesterol. Plasma concentrations of γ-tocopherol are typically about one tenth those of α-tocopherol, and smaller amounts of δ-tocopherol are usually present. The relative proportions of tocopherols in plasma (and tissues) lie in stark contrast to those found in foods, as dietary intakes of γ-tocopherol, and occasionally even δ-tocopherol, exceed those of α-tocopherol. This difference, manifested as the "α-tocopherol phenotype," is brought about by the actions of α-TTP and the tocopherol-ω-oxidation pathway described in Figure 29-3.

With respect to α-tocopherol, plasma concentrations appear to be linearly related to intake over the range of intakes possible from foods (i.e., up to approximately 20 mg/day). At greater intakes (from supplements) plasma concentrations are nonlinearly related to intake such that only relatively small increases in plasma α-tocopherol are achieved even with a tenfold increase in intake over that from diet alone. A supplemental intake of α-tocopherol of roughly 400 mg/day is usually needed to achieve a doubling of the plasma α-tocopherol concentration, and the maximal plasma α-tocopherol concentration achievable is roughly 50 to 60 μmol/L (Princen et al., 1995). The reason for this nonlinearity at high intakes of α-tocopherol is not clear. A consequence of supplementation with α-tocopherol is suppression of the plasma concentrations of γ- and δ-tocopherols. The mechanism responsible for this suppression is not known. Supplementation with γ-tocopherol does not suppress concentrations of α-tocopherol.

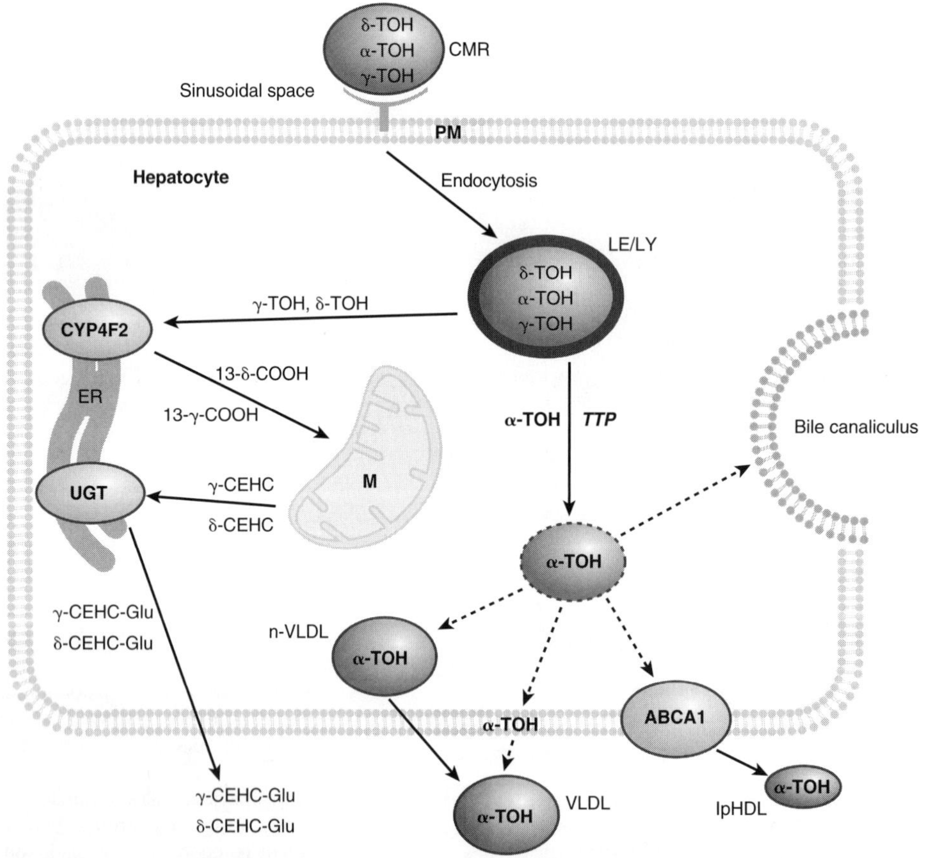

FIGURE 29-3 Functions of cytochrome P450-4F2 (CYP4F2) and α-tocopherol transfer protein (TTP) in the metabolism and secretion of vitamin E in hepatocytes, leading to the selective retention and tissue deposition of α-tocopherol. Illustrated is the role of TTP in the intracellular selection and secretion of α-tocopherol (α-TOH) to very-low-density lipoprotein (VLDL) and lipid-poor high-density lipoprotein (lpHDL), and the role of CYP4F2 in the ω-oxidation of tocopherols, particularly those other than α-tocopherol. Dashed features are hypothetical. *ABCA1,* ATP-binding cassette transporter A1; *CEHC,* carboxyethylhydroxychromanol; *CEHC-Glu,* glucuronide conjugate of CEHC; *CMR,* chylomicron remnant; 13-δ-COOH, 13-carboxy-delta tocopherol; *ER,* endoplasmic reticulum; *LE/LY,* late endosome–lysosome compartment; *M,* mitochondria; *PM,* plasma membrane; *TOH,* tocopherol; *UGT,* uridine 5′-diphospho-glucuronosyltransferase; *n-VLDL,* nascent very-low-density lipoprotein.

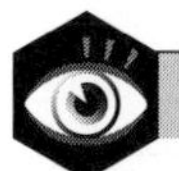

NUTRITION INSIGHT

The α-Tocopherol Phenotype: Are Non–α-Tocopherols Also Important for Health?

RRR-α-tocopherol is the predominant form of vitamin E in plasma and tissues of animals, despite the relative proportions of tocopherols and tocotrienols consumed. This "α-tocopherol phenotype" is one of the most striking aspects of vitamin E biology, but its biological significance remains unknown. RRR-γ-tocopherol is often the major form of vitamin E consumed in the diet, whereas the current dietary intake recommendations consider only RRR-α-tocopherol. Most supplements contain only α-tocopherol, and their use is associated with suppression of plasma levels of other tocopherols. RRR-α-tocopherol has traditionally been the focus of study because of its superior potency in bioassays for prevention of deficiency symptoms. However, results of several recent studies suggest that other forms of vitamin E may have beneficial biological effects, perhaps not involving antioxidant activity (Hensley et al., 2004; Jiang et al., 2001). Some have suggested that vitamin E supplements be composed of a mixture of tocopherols similar to that in a typical diet.

There are differences in the chemical reactivities of α-tocopherol and γ-tocopherol. In vitro, γ-tocopherol traps potentially mutagenic electrophiles, such as peroxynitrite and other reactive nitrogen oxide species. The 5 position of γ-tocopherol is highly nucleophilic and reactive toward electrophiles such as $NO^{\bullet}$ and $NO_2^{\bullet}$. In peroxynitrite-induced lipid peroxidation studies, α-tocopherol was converted to α-tocopherylquinone (a 2-electron oxidation product), whereas γ-tocopherol was converted to 5-NO_2-γ-tocopherol and its orthoquinone tocored (Christen et al., 1997). This ability is not shared by α-tocopherol, because it is methylated at C-5 on the phenol ring; α-tocopherol may trap the electrophile but is likely to remain chemically reactive. Supplementation with γ-tocopherol inhibited protein nitration and ascorbate oxidation in rats with inflammation (Jiang et al., 2002). Other studies in rats demonstrated that dietary supplementation with γ-tocopherol, but not α-tocopherol, reduced inflammation by suppressing the synthesis of various proinflammatory substances produced by cells of the immune system (Jiang and Ames, 2003). The 3′-carboxychromanol metabolite of γ-tocopherol has been shown to exhibit natriuretic activity in bioassays (Wechter et al., 1996), but its function in humans is currently uncertain.

Several human studies have reported an inverse association between serum or plasma concentrations of γ-tocopherol and risk for a variety of diseases. For example, in a Swedish study of male patients with coronary heart disease and healthy age-matched reference subjects, the serum α-tocopherol concentrations did not differ significantly between the groups (Ohrvall et al., 1996). However, the coronary heart disease group had a lower mean serum concentration of γ-tocopherol and a higher α- to γ-tocopherol ratio. The findings suggested that γ-tocopherol may be important, either itself or as a marker for another protective dietary factor. Another study found that men in the highest quartile of plasma γ-tocopherol concentration had a fivefold lower cancer incidence compared to men in the lowest quartile (Helzlsouer et al., 2000). Conversely, serum γ-tocopherol concentrations have been reported to be positively related to risk of cervical and oral and pharyngeal cancers (Zheng et al., 1993; Potischman et al., 1991).

Thinking Critically

1. Based on what is known or not known about the functions or effects of various forms of vitamin E, do you agree with the 2000 Dietary Reference Intake recommendation to consider only α-tocopherol as meeting nutrition needs?
2. Given that all forms of vitamin E are effective antioxidants and that antioxidation is the consensus function of vitamin E, how might the preferential accumulation of α-tocopherol (i.e., the α-tocopherol phenotype) be explained?

Because tocopherols are transported by plasma lipoproteins, individuals with higher plasma cholesterol levels typically have higher plasma tocopherol concentrations. In disorders causing lipid malabsorption (such as in individuals with cystic fibrosis or abetalipoproteinemia), plasma lipid, lipoprotein, and vitamin E concentrations frequently are all reduced concurrently (Machlin, 1991).

BIOLOGICAL FUNCTIONS OF VITAMIN E

The tocopherols and tocotrienols have long been recognized to be superior free radical antioxidants when tested in vitro, and it is this characteristic that is most often ascribed to their essentiality in vivo. Vitamin E (primarily α-tocopherol) is the major lipid-soluble, free radical chain-breaking antioxidant found in plasma, red blood cells, and tissues, and it plays an essential role in maintaining the integrity of biological membranes (Burton and Traber, 1990).

VITAMIN E AS A FREE RADICAL–SCAVENGING ANTIOXIDANT

Vitamin E is present in all cellular membranes, where it is thought to act to protect membrane lipids and perhaps proteins from free radical–induced oxidative damage. The reaction of α-tocopherol with polyunsaturated fatty acid peroxyl radicals to prevent uncontrolled lipid peroxidation is the best understood action of vitamin E. A variety of carbon- and oxygen-centered free radicals are generated during the course of normal metabolism in vivo. These include the superoxide, lipid alkoxyl, and peroxyl radicals. Among them, peroxyl radicals derived from polyunsaturated fatty acids have special significance because of their involvement in lipid peroxidation, which is the most common indicator of free radical production in living systems. (See Chapter 18 for more information on polyunsaturated fatty acids and lipid peroxidation.)

The process of lipid peroxidation (or autoxidation) can be divided into three phases: initiation, propagation, and termination. In the initiation phase (reaction I), carbon-centered lipid radicals (R•) can be produced by proton abstraction from a polyunsaturated fatty acid (RH) when a free radical initiator (I•) is present. Transition metal ions (Fe^{2+}, Cu^{2+}), ultraviolet light, and ionizing radiation have been implicated as initiators of lipid peroxidation. This lipid radical reacts readily with molecular oxygen to form a peroxyl radical (ROO•) (reaction II). In the propagation phase, the peroxyl radical formed can react with another polyunsaturated fatty acid (R′H) to form a fatty acid hydroperoxide (ROOH) and a new carbon-centered radical (reaction III). The propagative process can continue until all substrate fatty acids are oxidized or the chain reaction is broken (termination phase). Free radicals can be scavenged and the chain reaction terminated by self-quenching (reaction IV) or by the action of an antioxidant (AH) (reaction V), which generates an antioxidant free radical, A•. Of the free radical process inhibitors or antioxidants that are known, tocopherols are among the most effective chain-breakers.

$RH \xrightarrow{I^\bullet} R^\bullet$ (Reaction I)

$R^\bullet + O_2 \rightarrow ROO^\bullet$ (Reaction II)

$ROO^\bullet + R'H \rightarrow ROOH + R'^\bullet$ (Reaction III)

$R^\bullet (\text{or } ROO^\bullet) + R'^\bullet \rightarrow R\text{-}R' (\text{or } ROOR')$ (Reaction IV)

$R^\bullet (\text{or } ROO^\bullet) + AH \rightarrow RH (\text{or } ROOH) + A^\bullet$ (Reaction V)

The action of α-tocopherol in quenching lipid peroxyl radicals is shown in Figure 29-4; the 6-hydroxyl group of the chroman ring is the reactive portion of the tocochromanols. The phenolic hydrogen atom is donated to a free radical, resulting in the quenching of the free radical and the formation of the tocopheroxyl radical. Tocopherols react more rapidly with peroxyl radicals than do polyunsaturated fatty acids, and perhaps most importantly, the tocopherol radical is relatively unreactive. These two features conspire to render the tocopherols and tocotrienols extremely effective as free radical chain-breaking antioxidants. The tocopheroxyl radical has been shown in vitro to be reduced back to tocopherol by a variety of low-molecular-weight, water-soluble reducing substances such as ascorbic acid (Packer et al., 1995; Chow, 1991). The extent to which this regenerative process resulting from the interaction of these two vitamins occurs in vivo remains uncertain. Although the nature and extent of the vitamin E regenerative process in vivo remains speculative, it provides a working rationale for the observation that it is very difficult to deplete vitamin E in adult animals or humans. Although the oxidation of α-tocopherol to α-tocopheroxyl radical is reversible, further oxidation of the tocopheroxyl radical to α-tocopherylquinone is not reversible (see Figure 29-4).

Antioxidant activity of tocopherols is experimentally determined by their chemical reactivity with radicals or by their ability to inhibit autoxidation of fats and oils. The relative antioxidant activity of tocopherols varies considerably depending on the experimental conditions and the assessment method employed (Kamal-Eldin and Appelqvist, 1996). Efforts have also been made to compare the antioxidant efficacy of tocopherols and tocotrienols in living cells. In cells made selenium deficient, and therefore susceptible to adverse oxidation events (see Chapter 39 for discussion of the antioxidant function of selenium), tocopherols and tocotrienols exhibit different capacities to prevent cell death (Saito et al., 2003). However, the observed differences between the vitamers was mostly attributable to their ability to become associated with cell membranes, rather than to intrinsic differences in their chemical antioxidant activity. Tocopherol esters, which lack the critical free phenolic hydroxyl group, cannot function as antioxidants and must be hydrolyzed to free tocopherols in vivo before they can perform this function.

Vitamin E is not the only means by which cells are protected from oxidative damage. However, vitamin E occupies a unique position in the overall antioxidant picture owing to its localization in cell membranes and its efficacy at remarkably dilute concentrations. Cell membranes typically contain only one molecule of α-tocopherol per several hundred phospholipid molecules.

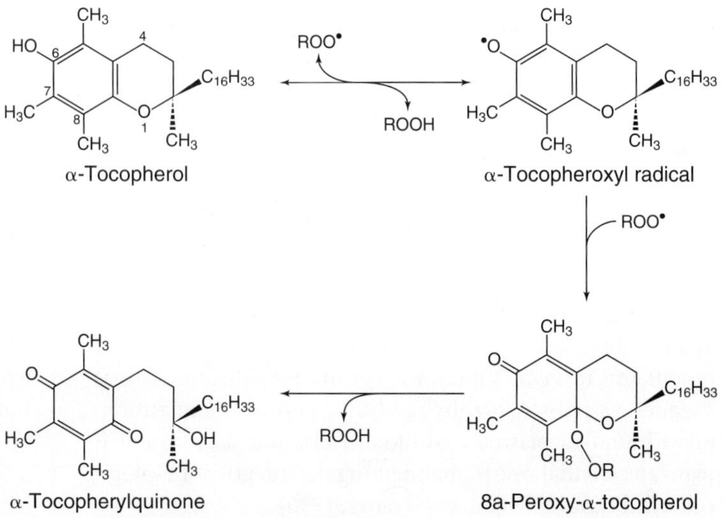

FIGURE 29-4 Reactions of α-tocopherol with peroxyl radicals. α-Tocopherol can scavenge two lipid peroxyl radicals (ROO•) as shown with the reaction of one peroxyl radical converting α-tocopherol to α-tocopheroxyl radical, which can react with a second peroxyl radical to form an adduct that is subsequently degraded to α-tocopherylquinone. Note the irreversibility of the latter steps.

OTHER FUNCTIONS OF VITAMIN E

Several nonantioxidant functions of vitamin E have been proposed. α-Tocopherol, for example, has been reported to influence protein kinase C activity and cell proliferation as well as synthesis of arachidonic acid metabolites involved in the immune response. Among these and other biological functions proposed for vitamin E, prevention of free radical–initiated lipid peroxidation and the resulting tissue damage is most widely accepted by investigators.

DEFICIENCY, HEALTH EFFECTS, AND BIOPOTENCY OF VITAMIN E

Much of what is known about the physiological consequences of vitamin E deficiency and toxicity has come from animal studies. Recent studies of patients with familial vitamin E deficiency have enhanced our understanding of the consequences of vitamin E deficiency in humans. Epidemiological studies and clinical intervention trials have provided new insights into the effect of vitamin E status on human health.

DEFICIENCY SYMPTOMS

A number of species-dependent, tissue-specific vitamin E deficiency symptoms have been reported. In some instances the development and severity of vitamin E deficiency symptoms are associated with the status of other nutrients, including selenium and sulfur-containing amino acids (Machlin, 1991). For example, the most common deficiency sign is necrotizing myopathy, which occurs in almost all species in the skeletal muscle and in some heart and smooth muscles. Myopathy primarily results from selenium deficiency in domestic animals, but rabbits and guinea pigs develop severe debilitating myopathy when fed a diet deficient in vitamin E but adequate in selenium. On the other hand, rats manifest a relatively benign myopathy when fed a vitamin E–deficient diet, and chickens do not develop myopathy unless the diet is depleted of both vitamin E and sulfur-containing amino acids. The reason for the species-dependent and tissue-specific vitamin E deficiency symptoms remains to be delineated.

In humans, lower plasma/serum levels of vitamin E (less than 12 μmol/L) are associated with a shorter lifespan of red blood cells and their increased susceptibility to hemolysis when exposed to an oxidizing agent. Vitamin E deficiency is rarely observed in adults. When it occurs, it is usually a result of lipoprotein or α-TPP deficiencies, or lipid malabsorption syndromes. Recent studies of children and adults with specific causes of fat/vitamin E malabsorption (such as abetalipoproteinemia, chronic cholestatic hepatobiliary disorder, and cystic fibrosis) have clearly shown that neurological abnormalities do occur in association with malabsorption syndromes of various etiologies (Kayden and Traber, 1993; Machlin, 1991). The similarity of the neurological abnormalities to those that occur in patients with familial isolated vitamin E deficiency suggests that the neurological symptoms are related specifically to the lack of adequate vitamin E in neural tissues.

Unlike the case of vitamin A, there is apparently no storage organ for vitamin E. Tocopherols accumulate in adipose tissue, but their mobilization from this tissue is slow and insufficient to prevent vitamin E deficiency in animals. The concentrations of tocopherols in fetal blood and tissues are considerably lower than those of the maternal system, apparently resulting from the low concentrations of lipoprotein carrier particles in fetal circulation. Infants born prematurely are susceptible to lung and ocular abnormalities that have been linked to insufficient antioxidant protection of these tissues.

HEALTH EFFECTS OF VITAMIN E

Increased intake of vitamin E has been associated with enhanced immune response and reduced risk of cardiovascular disease, certain cancers, and other degenerative diseases. Several indexes of immune response, including measures of delayed-type hypersensitivity, antibody production, lymphocyte proliferation and cytokine production are influenced by the status of essential nutrients, including vitamin E. Vitamin E supplementation is associated with enhanced production of the cytokine interleukin 2, enhanced lymphocyte proliferation, and decreased production of immunosuppressive prostaglandin E_2 (Meydani et al., 1990).

Several diet-related factors, including low vitamin E status, have been implicated in the increased incidence of coronary heart disease. Some, but not all, epidemiological studies have shown that a higher dietary intake or a higher plasma level of α-tocopherol is associated with decreased risk of cardiovascular diseases (Stampfer et al., 1993). The ability of vitamin E to prevent LDL oxidation, platelet adhesion, or both, may be responsible for the reduced risk of cardiovascular disease. Increased vitamin E intake from foods has been associated with reduced risk for a variety of cancers (Byers and Guerrero, 1995). Vitamin E may reduce disease risk by inactivating environmental mutagens/carcinogens, altering metabolic activation processes, enhancing the immune system, inhibiting cell proliferation, or other mechanisms that may or may not be related to its antioxidant activity. Paradoxically, clinical intervention trials using high doses of supplemental α-tocopherol have yielded inconsistent protective effects on prevention of cardiovascular diseases (Stocker, 1999; Vivekananthan et al., 2003). However, a recent meta-analysis has shown beneficial effects of vitamin E supplementation in diabetic individuals harboring a variant allele in the haptoglobin *(Hp)* gene (Blum et al., 2010).

BIOPOTENCY

The tocochromanols differ in their antioxidant and biological activities when examined in living organisms. α-Tocopherol is the most biologically active, owing to the retention function of α-TTP and the more extensive catabolism of other forms by CYP4F2. The comparative biological activity of tocopherols is assessed in bioassays by determining their relative ability to prevent deficiency symptoms such as fetal resorption or erythrocyte hemolysis in rats. The biological activity of various forms of vitamin

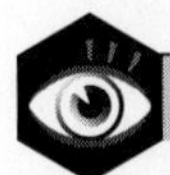

NUTRITION INSIGHT

Gene–Nutrient Interactions in Disease Risk

Sabrina Bardowell, RD

Vitamin E has been shown in cell culture and in cell-free systems to neutralize free radicals and prevent LDL oxidation and platelet adhesion, leading scientists to hypothesize that higher intake of vitamin E from food or supplements may reduce the risk of diseases such as cardiovascular disease and cancer. Along these lines, several observational studies have shown an association between higher dietary intakes of vitamin E or higher plasma levels of α-tocopherol and reduced risk of cardiovascular disease and a variety of cancers. However, large-scale randomized controlled clinical trials have yielded inconsistent findings, with the majority of the results indicating there is no protective effect of vitamin E supplementation against cardiovascular disease and cancer (Lippman et al., 2009; Lonn et al., 2005; Lee et al., 2005). The discrepancy between observational studies and clinical trials is likely to have many causes.

Recently, researchers are placing more emphasis on the interaction between genetics and nutrition in an effort to explain why clinical trials yield inconsistent results. A person's risk for disease can depend on their genetic makeup or the amounts of certain nutrients that the individual consumes. The interaction between these two factors, diet and genetics, can also affect a person's risk of disease. This is referred to as gene–nutrient interaction and may result in the protective effect of nutrients only for certain subgroups. In one circumstance (A), genetic polymorphisms can affect an individual's susceptibility to a disease process per se (e.g., expression of oncogenes in cancer), making supplementation with certain nutrients more or less effective. In another circumstance (B), genetic polymorphisms can alter the way some nutrients are metabolized in the body, making individuals with the polymorphism more or less responsive to supplementation with such nutrients. There are examples of both circumstances in the literature, demonstrating that the effectiveness of nutrient supplementation, including vitamin E, to prevent or treat disease may depend on the presence or absence of genetic polymorphisms.

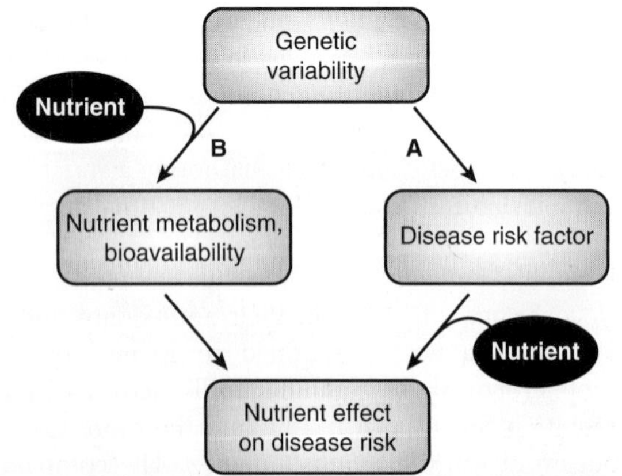

Circumstance A: In the Heart Outcomes Prevention Evaluation trial (HOPE), individuals with diabetes were given 400 IU α-tocopherol or placebo daily for an average of 7 years and were followed for the occurrence of major cardiovascular events. When examining the entire population studied, long-term supplementation with vitamin E did not prevent major cardiovascular events (Lonn et al., 2005). However, another research group recently reanalyzed the HOPE data according to haptoglobin (Hp) genotype and found that vitamin E supplementation selectively provided protection against cardiovascular disease in a subgroup of individuals with a polymorphism in the *Hp* gene (i.e., Hp 2-2 genotype) (Blum et al., 2010). *Hp* is a hemoglobin-binding protein that circulates in the plasma and functions as an antioxidant protein based on its ability to bind and clear hemoglobin molecules not contained within red blood cells. Hemoglobin molecules contain highly unstable heme iron that can cause oxidative damage via free radical mechanisms such as that depicted in Figure 29-4. There are two common allelic forms of the *Hp* gene in the human population, which are referred to as *Hp1* and *Hp2*. *Hp2* arose due to partial duplication of the *Hp1* gene, resulting in a mature Hp2 protein with a larger α-chain. The Hp2 protein has reduced ability to bind hemoglobin compared to the Hp1 protein, and thus individuals with diabetes and two *Hp2* alleles (Hp 2-2 genotype) are at increased risk for cardiovascular disease (Levy et al., 2002; Milman et al., 2008). The finding that vitamin E supplementation decreases cardiovascular events in a subgroup with increased oxidative stress has been replicated by additional prospective randomized clinical trials (Milman et al., 2008). This is one example in which large-scale intervention trials may miss beneficial effects of nutrients when only examining the population as a whole.

Circumstance B: It is also possible that subgroups of individuals may benefit from supplementation of a nutrient based on genetic polymorphisms that affect the metabolism of that nutrient. For example, data from the Alpha-Tocopherol, Beta-Carotene Cancer Prevention (ATBC) Study, in which subjects were given either 50 IU α-tocopherol per day or placebo for an average of 6 years, were reanalyzed based on polymorphisms in vitamin E transport genes. Supplementation with vitamin E reduced prostate cancer risk among men with common polymorphisms in vitamin E transport genes, including α-tocopherol transfer protein (Wright et al., 2009). Polymorphisms have also been identified in the gene encoding CYP4F2 (see Figure 29-2), which alter the metabolism of vitamin E (Bardowell et al., 2010). Researchers are now considering these gene–nutrient interactions when designing new studies or reanalyzing previous studies to identify genetic subgroups that may derive particular benefit from nutrient supplementation.

E has been expressed as units of activity in relation to that of all-rac-α-tocopheryl acetate, which is a common form of vitamin E used in vitamin supplements or for food fortification. The relative values in USP reference standard units (USP vitamin E unit) or international units (IUs) per milligram of compound assign 1 unit to 1.00 mg of all-rac-α-tocopheryl acetate. Vitamin E activity is also expressed as α-tocopherol equivalents (α-TE), and 1 α-TE is equivalent to 1.00 mg of RRR-α-tocopherol or 1.49 mg all-rac-α-tocopheryl acetate.

Forms of Vitamin E	Relative USP or IU Units per mg	α-Tocopherol Equivalents per mg
All-rac-α-tocopheryl acetate	1.00	0.67
All-rac-α-tocopherol	1.10	0.74
RRR-α-tocopheryl acetate	1.36	0.91
RRR-α-tocopherol	1.49	1.00

The relative activity of various tocopherols and tocotrienols based on bioassay methods is shown in Table 29-1.

TABLE 29-1 Relative Activity of Different Forms of Vitamin E

Form	Resorption–Gestation* (%)	Erythrocyte Hemolysis† (%)
RRR-α-tocopherol	100	100
RRR-β-tocopherol	25 to 50	15 to 27
RRR-γ-tocopherol	8 to 19	3 to 20
RRR-δ-tocopherol	0.1 to 3	0.3 to 2
RRR-α-tocotrienol	21 to 50	17 to 25
RRR-β-tocotrienol	4 to 5	1 to 5
RRR-α-tocopheryl acetate	91	—
All-rac-α-tocopherol‡	74	—
All-rac-α-tocopheryl acetate‡	67	—

Data from Machlin, L. J. (1991). In L. J. Machlin (Ed.), *Handbook of vitamins* (2nd ed., pp. 99 -114). New York: Marcel Dekker; Pryor, W. A. (1995). *Vitamin E and carotenoid abstracts.* La Grange, IL: VERIS, pp. vii -xi.

*Based on the fetal development and/or prevention of fetal loss in rats.

†Based on the prevention of hemoglobin release from red blood cells exposed to hydrogen peroxide.

‡A mixture of eight stereoisomers.

FOOD SOURCES AND INTAKE OF VITAMIN E

FOOD SOURCES

Tocopherols occur ubiquitously in plant and animal foods, but some foods are particularly rich sources. Oilseeds and their food products such as salad dressings, mayonnaise, margarines, and spreads are the best sources. The majority of the tocopherols consumed in the United States are not α-tocopherol. γ-Tocopherol, the predominant form of tocopherols present in soybean oil and corn oil, accounts for more than half of the estimated total tocopherol intake (Chow et al., 1967). Conversely, the major form in sunflower oil, safflower oil, and olive oil is α-tocopherol. Some foods and oils also contain β- and δ-tocopherols. Vitamin E–fortified breakfast cereals, peanut butter, eggs, potato chips, whole milk, and tomato products represent other major sources of vitamin E based on food consumption data. Tocotrienols are less widely distributed and are found in barley and rice brans and in palm oil.

DIETARY INTAKE OF VITAMIN E

Vitamin E intake is assessed by the combined use of food intake data and information on the tocopherol content of foods. These assessments are generally considered as rough estimates due to the inherent difficulty in obtaining accurate and complete food intake data coupled with incomplete food composition data. Some nutrient databases and nutrition labels do not distinguish among the various forms of tocopherols in foods. Estimates, based on the 1999–2000 data from the National Health and Nutrition Examination Survey (NHANES) place the median dietary intake of α-tocopherol alone at 7.6 mg/day for men and 5.8 mg/day for women aged 19 years or older (Moshfegh et al., 2005). The ranges of α-tocopherol intake

FOOD SOURCES OF VITAMIN E

	α-Tocopherol (mg)	Total tocopherols (mg)
Vegetable Oils (1 Tbsp, 14 g)		
Soybean oil	1	13
Olive oil	2	2
Corn, canola oils	2	6
Meats and Fish (3 oz, 85 g)		
Beef	0.3	0.3
Chicken (light or dark)	0.3	0.3
Salmon	0.7	0.7
Nuts (1/2 cup, 60 g)		
Walnuts	1	20
Pecans	1	14
Pistachios	1	15
Vegetables, Fruits, Legumes (½ cup)		
Red pepper, 75 g	2	3
Broccoli, 45 g	1	1
Spinach, 15 g	1	1
Tomato, 90 g	1	1
Apple, 55 g	0.1	0.1
Kidney beans, 125 g	0.2	2

Data from U.S. Department of Agriculture, Agricultural Research Service. (2010). *USDA National Nutrient Database for Standard Reference, Release 23.* Retrieved from www.ars.usda.gov/ba/bhnrc/ndl

(5th to 95th percentiles) are 4.1 to 14.2 mg/day for men and 3.1 to 11.0 mg/day for women. If supplement intake is included, median estimates of α-tocopherol intake are increased by approximately 0.4 mg/day.

RECOMMENDED INTAKE OF VITAMIN E AND ASSESSMENT OF VITAMIN E STATUS

The most recent U.S. recommendations were published in 2000 by the Institute of Medicine (IOM), National Institutes of Health. The 2000 Recommended Dietary Allowance (RDA) was based only on the α-tocopherol form of vitamin E and in this respect represents a change from the 1989 recommendations. Other forms of vitamin E (e.g., γ-tocopherol) were not considered to contribute to the RDA on the basis of poor in vitro binding to the α-TTP, despite their demonstrated value (albeit lower than α-tocopherol) in animal models of curative vitamin E deficiency. In addition, only the 2R stereoisomers of α-tocopherol are considered to satisfy the current RDA for vitamin E, based on their much higher affinity for α-TTP in comparison to the 2S stereoisomers found in synthetic preparations of α-tocopherol.

The nutritional status of vitamin E in humans is typically assessed on the basis of the concentration of α-tocopherol in serum (or plasma), usually normalized to plasma cholesterol. The only bioassay of vitamin E status conducted in humans is the susceptibility of red blood cells to hemolysis upon ex vivo exposure to hydrogen peroxide. The current RDA is based entirely on red blood cell hemolysis data obtained using erythrocytes from a small group of human subjects who were intentionally depleted of vitamin E and then repleted using varying levels of dietary α-tocopherol (Horwitt et al., 1963). In that study, erythrocytes isolated from subjects with plasma α-tocopherol concentrations less than 12 μmol/L exhibited increased hemolysis (breakdown of red blood cells leading to release of hemoglobin) when exposed to a particular concentration of hydrogen peroxide. Based on experimental data from these repletion studies with vitamin E–deficient subjects, the relationship between α-tocopherol intake and plasma α-tocopherol concentration was determined (Horwitt, 1960). The IOM (2000) used the intake needed to achieve a plasma concentration of 12 μmol/L as the basis for setting the Estimated Average Requirement (EAR) for adults of 12 mg RRR-α-tocopherol, or its equivalent, per day. The current RDA was set at two standard deviations (20%) greater than the EAR. No increment was added for pregnant women. For lactating women, the RDA was increased to 19 mg α-tocopherol per day to compensate for secretion in milk.

EARs and RDAs were set for children by extrapolation from adult values based on lean body mass and need for growth. Adequate Intakes (AIs) for infants from birth through 6 months of age were established based on α-tocopherol intake from human milk. Therefore the AI for infants during the first 6 months is 4 mg α-tocopherol/day (0.78 L milk/day with 4.9 mg α-tocopherol/L of milk). The AI for infants from 7 through 12 months of age is 5 mg/day and was extrapolated from that for younger infants.

Consequently, according to estimates of average daily intake of α-tocopherol of 6 to 8 mg, most individuals in the United States (89% to 97%) are not meeting the current recommendations (Maras et al., 2004; Moshfegh et al., 2005). Individuals consuming low-fat diets tend to have lower intakes of vitamin E, because the richest sources of vitamin E are vegetable oils and their products. However, the most recent data (NHANES 1999–2000) show that the arithmetic mean plasma α-tocopherol concentration of adults in the United States is approximately 30 μmol/L, only 2.5% exhibited concentrations less than 14 μmol/L, and nearly 80% were above 20 μmol/L (Ford et al., 2006). Serum γ-tocopherol concentrations averaged 5.7 μmol/L.

DRIs Across the Life Cycle: Vitamin E

mg α-Tocopherol per Day		
Infant	RDA	UL*
0 through 6 mo	4 (AI)	ND
7 through 12 mo	5 (AI)	ND
Children		
1 through 3 yr	6	200
4 through 8 yr	7	300
9 through 13 yr	11	600
14 through 18 yr	15	800
Males		
≥19 yr	15	1,000
Females		
≥19 yr	15	1,000
Pregnant		
<19 yr	15	800
≥19 yr	15	1,000
Lactating		
<19 yr	19	800
≥19 yr	19	1,000

Data from IOM. (2006). In J. J. Otten, J. P. Hellwig, & L. D. Meyers (Eds.), *Dietary Reference Intakes: The essential guide to nutrient requirements*. Washington, DC: The National Academies Press.
AI, Adequate Intake; *DRI*, Dietary Reference Intake; *ND*, not determinable; *RDA*, Recommended Dietary Allowance; *UL*, Tolerable Upper Intake Level.
*As α-tocopherol; applies to any form of synthetic α-tocopherol obtained from supplements, fortified foods, or a combination of the two. Little information exists on the adverse effects that might result from ingestion of other forms.

TOXICITY OF VITAMIN E

Vitamin E is a relatively nontoxic nutrient, probably due in part to the inability to accumulate concentrations more than about three times that resulting from usual intake from foods, as discussed in the preceding text. The most well-established symptom of high α-tocopherol intake is increased blood coagulation time and therefore increased risk of hemorrhage. The most recent vitamin E intake recommendations of the IOM established Tolerable Upper Intake Levels (ULs) for adults at 1,000 mg/day of any form of synthetic α-tocopherol based on the risk of hemorrhage (IOM, 2000).

REFERENCES

Arita, M., Sato, Y., Miyata, A., Tanabe, T., Takahashi, E., Kayden, H. J.,...Inoue, K. (1995). Human α-tocopherol transfer protein: cDNA cloning, expression and chromosomal localization. *The Biochemical Journal*, *306*, 437–443.

Bardowell, S. A., Stec, D. E., & Parker, R. S. (2010). Common variants of cytochrome P450 4F2 exhibit altered vitamin E-Ω-hydroxylase specific activity. *The Journal of Nutrition*, *140*(11), 1901–1906.

Blum, S., Vardi, M., Brown, J. B., Russell, A., Milman, U., Shapira, C.,...Levy, A. P. (2010). Vitamin E reduces cardiovascular disease in individuals with diabetes mellitus and the haptoglobin 2-2 genotype. *Pharmacogenomics*, *11*(5), 675–684.

Burton, G. W., & Traber, M. G. (1990). Vitamin E: Antioxidant activity, biokinetics, and bioavailability. *Annual Review of Nutrition*, *10*, 357–382.

Byers, T., & Guerrero, N. (1995). Epidemiologic evidence for vitamin C and vitamin E in cancer prevention. *The American Journal of Clinical Nutrition*, *62*, 1385S–1392S.

Chow, C. K. (1991). Vitamin E and oxidative stress. *Free Radical Biology & Medicine*, *11*, 215–232.

Chow, C. K., Draper, H. H., Csallany, A. S., & Chiu, M. (1967). The metabolism of C14-α-tocopheryl quinone and C14-α-tocopheryl hydroquinone. *Lipids*, *2*, 390–396.

Christen, S., Woodall, A. A., Shigenaga, M. K., Southwell-Keely, P. T., Duncan, M. W., & Ames, B. N. (1997). γ-Tocopherol traps mutagenic electrophiles such as NOx and complements α-tocopherol: Physiological implications. *Proceedings of the National Academy of Sciences of the United States of America*, *94*, 3217–3222.

Evans, H. M., & Bishop, K. S. (1922). On the existence of a hitherto unrecognized dietary factor essential for reproduction. *Science*, *56*, 650–651.

Ford, E. S., Schleicher, R. L., Mokdad, A. H., Ajani, U. A., & Liu, S. (2006). Distribution of serum concentrations of α-tocopherol and γ-tocopherol in the US population. *The American Journal of Clinical Nutrition*, *84*, 375–383.

Gotoda, T., Arita, M., Arai, H., Inoue, K., Yokota, T., Fukuo, Y.,... Yamada, N. (1995). Adult-onset spinocerebellar dysfunction caused by a mutation in the gene for the α-tocopherol-transfer protein. *New England Journal of Medicine*, *333*, 1313–1318.

Helzlsouer, K., Huang, H., Alberg, A., Hoffman, S., Burke, A., Norkus, E.,...Comstock, G. (2000). Association between alpha-tocopherol, gamma-tocopherol, selenium, and subsequent prostate cancer. *Journal of the National Cancer Institute*, *92*, 2018–2023.

Hensley, K., Benaksas, E., Bolli, R., Comp, P., Grammas, P., Hamdheydari, L.,...Floyd, R. (2004). New perspectives on vitamin E: γ-Tocopherol and carboxyethylhydroxychroman metabolites in biology and medicine. *Free Radical Biology & Medicine*, *36*, 1–15.

Hosomi, A., Arita, M., Sato, Y., Kiyose, C., Ueda, T., Igarashi, O.,... Inoue, K. (1977). Affinity for α-tocopherol transfer protein as a determinant of the biological activities of vitamin E analogs. *FEBS Letters*, *409*, 105–108.

Horwitt, M. (1960). Vitamin E and lipid metabolism in man. *The American Journal of Clinical Nutrition*, *8*, 451–461.

Horwitt, M., Century, B., & Zeman, A. (1963). Erythrocyte survival time and reticulocyte levels after tocopherol depletion in man. *The American Journal of Clinical Nutrition*, *12*, 99–106.

Institute of Medicine. (2000). *Dietary Reference Intakes for vitamin C, vitamin E, selenium and carotenoids*. Washington, DC: National Academy Press.

Jiang, Q., & Ames, B. (2003). Gamma-tocopherol, but not alpha-tocopherol, decreases proinflammatory eicosanoids and inflammation damage in rats. *The FASEB Journal*, *17*, 816–822.

Jiang, Q., Christen, S., Shigenaga, M., & Ames, B. (2001). γ-Tocopherol, the major form of vitamin E in the U.S. diet, deserves more attention. *The American Journal of Clinical Nutrition*, *74*, 714–722.

Jiang, Q., Lyddesfeld, J., Shigenaga, M., Shigeno, E., Christen, S., & Ames, B. (2002). Gamma-tocopherol supplementation inhibits protein nitration and ascorbate oxidation in rats with inflammation. *Free Radical Biology & Medicine*, *33*, 1534–1542.

Kaempf-Rotzoll, D., Traber, M., & Arai, H. (2003). Vitamin E and transfer proteins. *Current Opinion in Lipidology*, *14*, 249–254.

Kamal-Eldin, A., & Appelqvist, L. A. (1996). The chemistry and antioxidant properties of tocopherols and tocotrienols. *Lipids*, *31*, 671–701.

Kayden, H. J., & Traber, M. G. (1993). Absorption, lipoprotein transport, and regulation of plasma concentrations of vitamin E in humans. *Journal of Lipid Research*, *34*, 343–358.

Kostner, G. M., Oettl, K., Jauhiainen, M., Ehnholn, C., & Esterbauer, H. (1995). Human plasma phospholipid transfer protein accelerates exchange/transfer of α-tocopherol between lipoproteins and cells. *The Biochemical Journal*, *305*, 659–667.

Lee, I. M., Cook, N. R., Gaziano, J. M., Gordon, D., Ridker, P. M., Manson, J. E.,...Buring, J. E. (2005). Vitamin E in the primary prevention of cardiovascular disease and cancer: The Women's Health Study: A randomized controlled trial. *The Journal of the American Medical Association*, *294*(1), 56–65.

Levy, A. P., Hochberg, I., Jablonski, K., Resnick, H. E., Lee, E. T., Best, L., & Howard, B. V. (2002). Haptoglobin phenotype is an independent risk factor for cardiovascular disease in individuals with diabetes: The Strong Heart Study. *Journal of the American College of Cardiology*, *40*(11), 1984–1990.

Lippman, S. M., Klein, E. A., Goodman, P., Lucia, M. S., Thompson, I. M., Ford, L. G.,...Coltman, C. A., Jr. (2009). Effect of selenium and vitamin E on risk of prostate cancer and other cancers: The Selenium and Vitamin E Cancer Prevention Trial (SELECT). *The Journal of the American Medical Association*, *301*(1), 39–51.

Lonn, E., Bosch, J., Yusuf, S., Sheridan, P., Pogue, J., Arnold, J. M.,... Hope and HOPE-TOO Trial Investigators. (2005). Effects of long-term vitamin E supplementation on cardiovascular events and cancer: A randomized controlled trial. *The Journal of the American Medical Association*, *293*(11), 1338–1347.

Machlin, L. J. (1991). Vitamin E. In L. J. Machlin (Ed.), *Handbook of vitamins* (2nd ed., pp. 99–144). New York: Marcel Dekker.

Manor, D., & Morley, S. (2008). The α-tocopherol transfer protein. *Vitamins and Hormones*, *76*, 45–65.

Maras, J., Bermudez, O., Qiao, N., Bakun, P., Boody-Alter, E., & Tucker, K. (2004). Intake of α-tocopherol is limited among U.S. adults. *Journal of the American Dietetic Association*, *104*, 567–575.

Meydani, S. N., Barklund, M. P., Liu, S., Miller, R. A., Cannon, J. G., Morrow, F. D.,...Blumberg, J. B. (1990). Vitamin E supplementation enhances cell-mediated immunity in healthy elderly subjects. *The American Journal of Clinical Nutrition*, *52*, 557–563.

Milman, U., Blum, S., Shapira, C., Aronson, D., Miller-Lotan, R., Anbinder, Y.,...Levy, A. P. (2008). Vitamin E supplementation reduces cardiovascular events in a subgroup of middle-aged individuals with both type 2 diabetes mellitus and the haptoglobin 2-2 genotype: A prospective double-blinded clinical trial. *Arteriosclerosis, Thrombosis, and Vascular Biology*, *28*(2), 341–347.

Morley, S., Cecchini, M., Zhang, W., Virgulti, A., Noy, N., Atkinson, J., & Manor, D. (2008). Mechanism of ligand transfer by the hepatic tocopherol transfer protein. *The Journal of Biological Chemistry*, *283*, 17797–17804.

Moshfegh, A., Goldman, J., & Cleveland, L. (2005). *What we eat in America. NHANES 2001–2002. Usual nutrient intakes from food compared to dietary reference intakes.* Washington, DC: U.S. Department of Agriculture, Agricultural Research Service.

Ohrvall, M., Sundlof, G., & Vessby, B. (1996). Gamma, but not alpha, tocopherol levels in serum are reduced in coronary heart disease patients. *Journal of Internal Medicine, 239,* 111–117.

Oram, J., Vaughan, A., & Stocker, R. (2001). ATP-binding cassette transporter A1 mediates cellular secretion of α-tocopherol. *The Journal of Biological Chemistry, 276,* 39898–39902.

Ouahchi, K., Arita, M., Kayden, H., Hentati, F., Hamida, M. B., Sokol, R.,...Koenig, M. (1995). Ataxia with isolated vitamin E deficiency is caused by mutations in the α-tocopherol transfer protein. *Nature Genetics, 9,* 141–145.

Packer, L., Witt, E. H., & Trischler, H. J. (1995). Alpha-lipoic acid as a biological antioxidant. *Free Radical Biology & Medicine, 19,* 227–250.

Parker, R. S., & McCormick, C. C. (2005). Selective accumulation of alpha-tocopherol in Drosophila is associated with cytochrome P450 tocopherol-omega-hydroxylase activity but not alpha-tocopherol transfer protein. *Biochemical and Biophysical Research Communications, 338*(3), 1537–1541.

Potischman, N., Herrero, R., Brinton, A., Reeves, W., Stacewicz-Sapuntzakis, M., Jones, C.,...Gaitan, E. (1991). A case-control study of nutrient status and invasive cervical cancer. II. Serological indicators. *American Journal of Epidemiology, 134,* 1347–1355.

Princen, H., van Duyvenvoorde, W., Buytenhek, R., van der Laarse, A., van Poppel, G., Gevers Leuven, J., & van Hinsbergh, V. (1995). Supplementation with low doses of vitamin E protects LDL from lipid peroxidation in men and women. *Arteriosclerosis, Thrombosis, and Vascular Biology, 15,* 325–333.

Qian, J., Morley, S., Wilson, K., Nava, P., Atkinson, J., & Manor, D. (2005). Intracellular trafficking of vitamin E in hepatocytes: The role of tocopherol transfer protein. *Journal of Lipid Research, 46,* 2072–2082.

Saito, Y., Yoshida, Y., Adazawa, T., Takahashi, D., & Niki, E. (2003). Cell death caused by selenium deficiency and protective effect of antioxidants. *The Journal of Biological Chemistry, 278,* 39428–39434.

Sattler, W., Levak-Frank, S., Radner, H., Kostner, G. M., & Zechner, R. (1996). Muscle-specific overexpression of lipoprotein lipase in transgenic mice results in increased α-tocopherol levels in skeletal muscle. *The Biochemical Journal, 318,* 15–19.

Sontag, T. J., & Parker, R. S. (2002). Cytochrome P450 omega-hydroxylase pathway of tocopherol catabolism. Novel mechanism of regulation of vitamin E status. *The Journal of Biological Chemistry, 28,* 25290–25296.

Sontag, T. J., & Parker, R. S. (2007). Influence of major structural features of tocopherols and tocotrienols on their omega-oxidation by tocopherol-omega-hydroxylase. *Journal of Lipid Research, 48,* 1090–1098.

Stampfer, M. J., Henneckens, C. H., Ascherio, A., Giovannucci, E., Colditz, G. A., Rosner, B., & Willett, W. C. (1993). Vitamin E consumption and the risk of coronary disease in men. *New England Journal of Medicine, 328,* 1450–1456.

Stocker, R. (1999). The ambivalence of vitamin E in atherogenesis. *Trends in Biochemical Sciences, 24,* 219–223.

Traber, M. G., Sokol, R. J., Kohlschuetter, A., Yokota, T., Muller, D. P. R., Dufour, R., & Kayden, H. J. (1993). Impaired discrimination between stereoisomers of α-tocopherol in patients with familial isolated vitamin E deficiency. *Journal of Lipid Research, 34,* 201–210.

Vivekananthan, D., Penn, M., Sapp, S., Hsu, A., & Topol, E. (2003). Use of antioxidant vitamins for the prevention of cardiovascular disease: Meta-analysis of randomized trials. *Lancet, 361,* 2017–2023.

Wechter, W. J., Kantoci, D., Murray, E. D., Jr., D'Amico, D. C., Jung, M. E., & Wang W. H. (1996). A new endogenous natriuretic factor: LLU-alpha. *Proceedings of the National Academy of Sciences of the United States of America, 93,* 6002–6007.

Wright, M. E., Peters, U., Gunter, M. J., Moore, S. C., Lawson, K. A., Yeager, M.,...Albanes, D. (2009). Association of variants in two vitamin E transport genes with circulating vitamin E concentrations and prostate cancer risk. *Cancer Research, 69*(4), 1429–1438.

Zheng, W., Blot, W., Diamond, E., Norkus, E., Spate, V., Morris, J., & Comstock, G. (1993). Serum micronutrients and the subsequent risk of oral and pharyngeal cancer. *Cancer Research, 53,* 795–798.

RECOMMENDED READING

Institute of Medicine. (2000). *Dietary Reference Intakes for Vitamin C, vitamin E, selenium and carotenoids.* Washington, DC: National Academies Press. http://www.nap.edu/catalog.php?record_id=9810#toc

CHAPTER 30

Vitamin A

Noa Noy, PhD

COMMON ABBREVIATIONS

ARAT	acyl-CoA:retinol acyltransferase
CRABP	cellular retinoic acid–binding protein
CRALBP	cellular retinal-binding protein
CRBP	cellular retinol-binding protein
FABP	fatty acid binding protein
IPM	interphotoreceptor matrix
IRBP	interphotoreceptor retinoid-binding protein
LRAT	lecithin:retinol acyltransferase
PPAR	peroxisome proliferator-activated receptor
RA	retinoic acid
RAE	retinol activity equivalent
RAR	retinoic acid receptor
RBP	retinol-binding protein
RE	retinol equivalent
RPE	retinal pigment epithelium
RXR	retinoid X receptor

Vitamin A is essential during embryonic development and, in the adult, it is necessary for vision, immunity, proper regulation of metabolism, and cell proliferation, differentiation, and apoptosis. This chapter describes how vitamin A is obtained from the diet and processed in the body and it outlines available information on the mechanisms by which the vitamin exerts its diverse functions.

CHEMISTRY AND PHYSICAL PROPERTIES OF VITAMIN A AND CAROTENOIDS

Vitamin A was initially recognized as an essential growth factor present in foods of animal origin such as animal fats and fish oils, and this factor was called fat-soluble A (McCollum and Davis, 1913; Osborne and Mendel, 1919). It was also observed that some plants display an activity similar to this fat-soluble A factor. Subsequently, in the early 1930s it became clear that plant-derived compounds, known as carotenoids, are precursors for vitamin A and can be converted to retinol in animals.

NOMENCLATURE

Vitamin A nomenclature has undergone various changes since the discovery of this fat-soluble vitamin. Currently, the term *vitamin A* is used to generically describe compounds that exhibit the biological activity of retinol, the alcoholic form of vitamin A. The term can thus be applied to many naturally occurring and synthetic derivatives of retinol. Of the more than 600 carotenoids that are known to exist in nature, about 50 can serve as precursors for vitamin A. More recently, the term *retinoids* has been coined to describe compounds that share structural similarities with retinol regardless of their biological activity.

LABILITY AND LIMITED SOLUBILITY OF RETINOIDS IN WATER

The structures of some physiologically important retinoids as well as the most active provitamin A carotenoid, all-*trans*-β-carotene, are shown in Figure 30-1.

Retinoids are composed of three distinct structural domains: a β-ionone ring, a spacer of a polyunsaturated chain, and a polar end-group. The polar end-group of naturally occurring retinoids can exist at several oxidation states varying from the low oxidation state of retinol, to retinal, and to the even higher oxidation state in retinoic acid (RA). Vitamin A is stored in vivo in the form of retinyl esters in which the retinyl moiety is esterified with a long-chain fatty acid with concomitant loss of the polar end-group (see Figure 30-1). Retinol can also be converted in vivo to conjugated species with larger, more polar, end-groups (e.g., retinoyl β-glucuronide; see Figure 30-1).

In recent years a wide array of synthetic retinoid analogs have been developed. The β-ionone ring has been replaced systematically by multiple hydrophobic groups, the spacer chain has been derivatized to a variety of cyclic and aromatic rings, and the polar end-group has been converted into derivatives or precursors of active species. Active synthetic analogs, similar to naturally occurring retinoids, are amphipathic, typified by a hydrophobic moiety and a polar terminus.

The large hydrophobic moiety of retinoids results in a limited solubility of these compounds in water. In addition, the multiple double-bonds of the spacer chain render retinoids susceptible to photodegradation, isomerization, and oxidation. Therefore vitamin A and its analogs are stable in a crystalline form or when dissolved in organic solvents under nonoxidizing conditions, but they are labile when exposed to light or in aqueous solutions in the presence of oxygen.

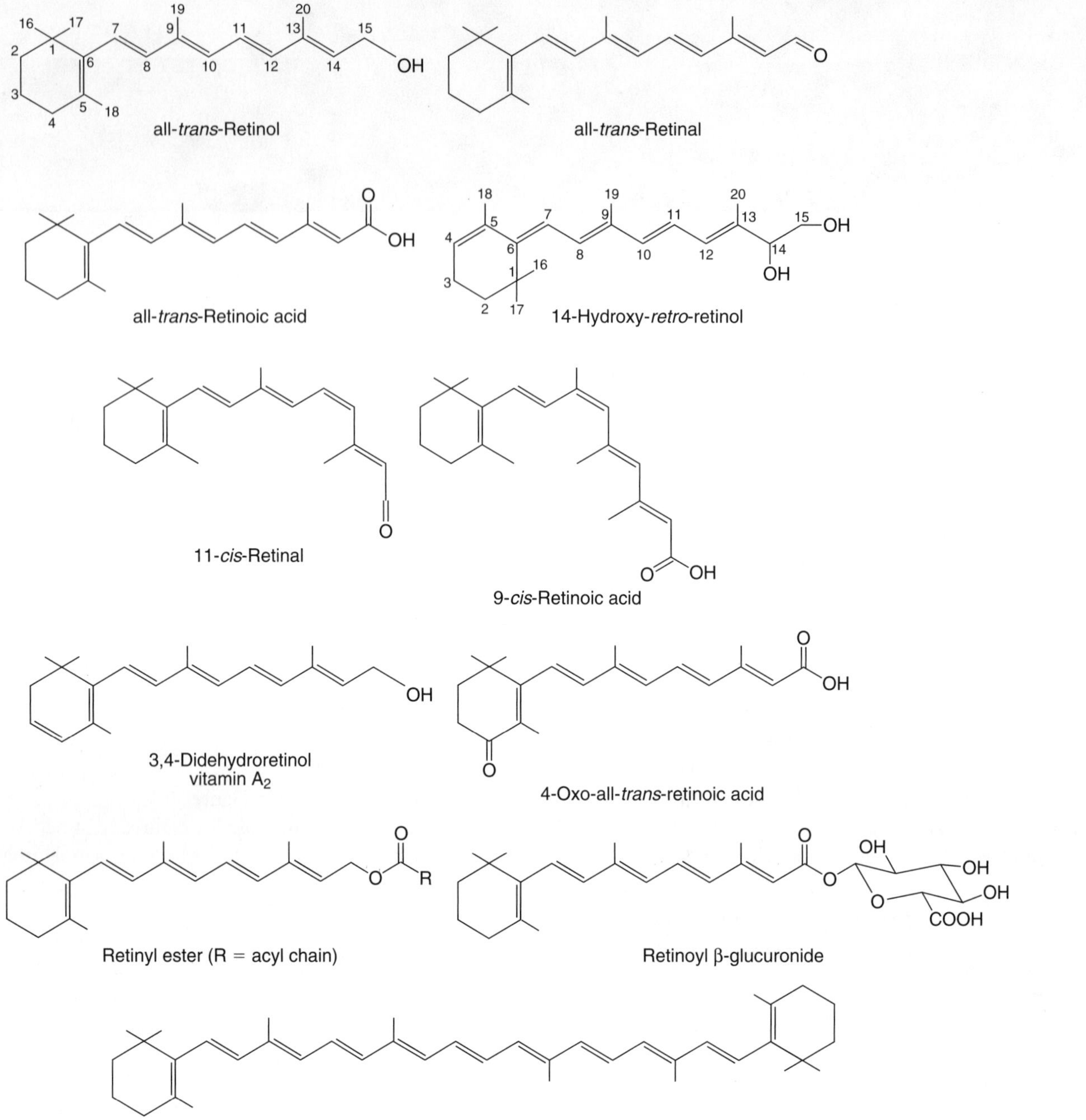

all-*trans*-Retinol

all-*trans*-Retinal

all-*trans*-Retinoic acid

14-Hydroxy-*retro*-retinol

11-*cis*-Retinal

9-*cis*-Retinoic acid

3,4-Didehydroretinol
vitamin A_2

4-Oxo-all-*trans*-retinoic acid

Retinyl ester (R = acyl chain)

Retinoyl β-glucuronide

all-*trans*-β-Carotene

FIGURE 30-1 Structures of vitamin A, β-carotene, and some of their biologically active derivatives.

The poor solubility and the lability of retinoids in aqueous phases raise important questions regarding their physiology: How do these insoluble compounds transfer across aqueous spaces between different organs, cells, and subcellular locations? How is their structural integrity retained in vivo when they traverse the aqueous phases of serum and cytosol?

OPTICAL PROPERTIES OF RETINOIDS AND CAROTENOIDS

Retinoids have absorption spectra with characteristic maxima in the 320- to 380-nm range. The absorption spectra of carotenoids center in the visible range at around 450 nm. Some retinoids, most notably retinols, are highly fluorescent and display fluorescence emission maxima in the range of 460 to 500 nm. In contrast, carotenoids do not significantly fluoresce at physiologically relevant temperatures. The optical properties of retinoids and, in particular, the environmental sensitivity of the fluorescence of retinols have been widely used to probe their interactions with cellular components such as membranes and specific binding proteins.

PHYSIOLOGICAL FUNCTIONS OF VITAMIN A

Vitamin A participates in a wide spectrum of biological functions. It is essential for vision, reproduction, immune function, and embryonic development, and it is involved in

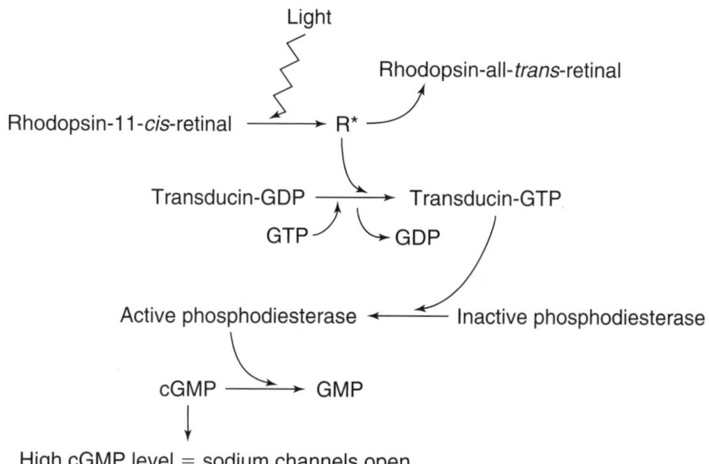

FIGURE 30-2 Early events in transduction of the visual signal. *c,* Cyclic; *GDP,* guanosine diphosphate; *GTP,* guanosine triphosphate; *R*,* metarhodopsin II.

regulation of cellular differentiation, proliferation, apoptosis, and metabolism. The diverse effects of the vitamin are exerted by several types of retinoids that function via different mechanisms. The 11-*cis*-isomer of retinal plays a critical role in visual transduction; RA and possibly other vitamin A metabolites regulate the transcription of multiple genes.

ROLE OF 11-*cis*-RETINAL IN VISION

Light is sensed in the vertebrate eye by rhodopsin, a membrane protein located in the outer segments of photoreceptor cells, which uses 11-*cis*-retinal as its chromophore. Two types of photoreceptor cells exist in the human retina: rods, which are stimulated by weak light of a broad range of wavelengths; and cones, which are responsible for color vision and function under bright light. Absorption of a photon by the 11-*cis*-retinal moiety of rhodopsin triggers a chain of events that culminates in hyperpolarization of the plasma membrane of the cell. Because photoreceptor cells form synapses with secondary neurons, the hyperpolarization is communicated further to transmit the visual signal to the brain.

The process of the visual signal transduction is a classical example of a G protein–mediated signaling cascade and is well characterized (Figure 30-2) (Wald, 1968; Travis et al., 2007; von Lintig et al., 2010). Absorption of a photon by rhodopsin-bound 11-*cis*-retinal results in isomerization of the chromophore to the all-*trans* form, a process that induces the protein to undergo several conformational changes through a series of short-lived intermediates. One of the protein intermediates (metarhodopsin II, R* in Figure 30-2) interacts with another membrane protein named transducin. Transducin is a G protein; its interaction with R* leads to an exchange of a transducin-bound guanosine diphosphate (GDP) for a guanosine triphosphate (GTP). In the GTP-bound (activated) state, transducin activates an enzyme called phosphodiesterase. Phosphodiesterase catalyzes the breakdown of cyclic guanosine monophosphate (cGMP), which keeps sodium channels in the plasma membranes of rod outer segments in the open state, to an inactive product, GMP. Because the level of cGMP

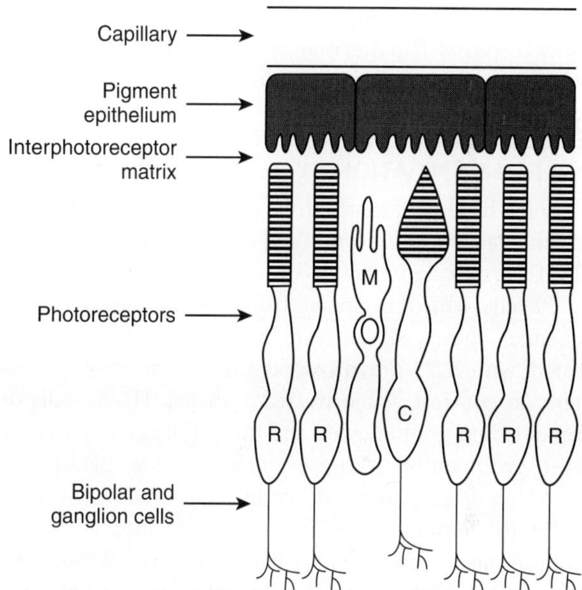

FIGURE 30-3 Schematic drawing of cells in the retina that are active in use and metabolism of retinoids. *C,* Cone; *M,* Müller cell; *R,* rod.

in rod outer segments in the dark is high (~0.07 mM), the sodium channels are open and the membranes of the cells are depolarized. Activation of phosphodiesterase following illumination results in lower levels of cGMP and leads to closing of the sodium channels and to hyperpolarization of the plasma membrane. The process of visual transduction is regulated further at several levels, including phosphorylation of rhodopsin intermediates, enzymatic hydrolysis of retinal from metarhodopsin II, and termination of the interaction between activated rhodopsin and transducin by the protein arrestin.

Bleached rhodopsin can be regenerated in the dark by 11-*cis*-retinal freshly supplied to the photoreceptors from the adjacent retinal pigment epithelium (RPE) cells (Figure 30-3), which take up vitamin A from blood and store it in the form of all-*trans*-retinyl esters. These storage species are enzymatically converted in RPE cells to 11-*cis*-retinal, which is then transported across the interphotoreceptor matrix to

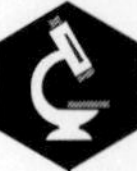

CLINICAL CORRELATION

Potential Therapeutic Uses of Ligands for Retinoid Nuclear Receptors

By virtue of their ability to modulate the rate of transcription of a variety of genes, retinoids can be potent therapeutic agents. Retinoic acid and synthetic ligands that activate retinoic acid receptor (RAR) are currently used in therapy and chemoprevention of several types of cancer, most notably promyelocytic leukemia. The ability of retinoid X receptor (RXR) to serve as a common partner for several nuclear receptors, such as RAR, vitamin D_3 receptor (VDR), thyroid hormone receptor (TR), liver X receptor (LXR), and peroxisome proliferator–activated receptor (PPAR), suggests that retinoid derivatives that are selective toward RXR might be useful in treating a variety of disorders. For example, it was reported that RXR-selective retinoids enhance sensitivity to insulin in mouse models of type 2 diabetes and obesity (Mukherjee et al., 1997). It was suggested that this antidiabetic activity is mediated by heterodimers of RXR with PPAR. It was also reported that retinoids increase the expression of apolipoproteins A-I and A-II in a human hepatoblastoma cell line, an activity that was ascribed to RXR-RAR heterodimers (Vu-Dac et al., 1996). Because apo-A–containing HDL is known to have a protective effect against coronary artery disease, these observations suggest that RXR ligands are potentially clinically useful in protecting against cardiovascular disease. It was recently reported that treatment of obese mice with all-*trans*-RA leads to weight loss and to enhanced insulin sensitivity (Berry and Noy, 2009). These effects were attributed to the ability of RA to activate both RAR and PPAR, which in turn enhance energy use and inhibit adipocyte differentiation.

photoreceptors. The metabolism and transport of retinoids in the eye are discussed later in this chapter.

REGULATION OF CELL PROLIFERATION AND DIFFERENTIATION BY RETINOIC ACIDS

Retinoids have profound effects on the differentiation and growth of a variety of normal and neoplastically transformed cells. One striking example is the differentiation pattern of HL-60 cells, which originated from a human promyelocytic leukemia. These cells differentiate into macrophages when treated with 1,25-dihydroxyvitamin D_3 or with phorbol esters. In contrast, when treated with RA, HL-60 cells differentiate into granulocytes, and this is followed by an arrest in cell proliferation. Other examples include the ability of RA to enhance neuronal differentiation or, in contrast, to inhibit the differentiation of fibroblasts into adipocytes. Retinoids also control the formation of particular patterns, such as digit development, during embryogenesis (Hoffman and Eichele, 1994). In addition, studies of isolated cells, animal models, and humans have demonstrated that retinoids can inhibit cancer development and, in some cases, induce transformed cells to revert to a normal phenotype. Indeed, RA is successfully used in treatment of human acute promyelocytic leukemia and other cancers (Soprano et al., 2004).

Many of the effects of retinoids on cells are due to the ability of the vitamin A metabolites all-*trans*-RA and 9-*cis*-RA to modulate the rate of transcription of genes, including those that encode growth factors, transcription factors, enzymes, extracellular matrix proteins, protooncogenes, and binding proteins. By regulating the expression of such proteins, RA controls a complex array of metabolic pathways and cellular behaviors.

ACTIVATION OF RETINOID NUCLEAR RECEPTORS

Retinoic acids regulate gene expression by activating specific transcription factors, termed retinoid receptors, which are members of a superfamily of the nuclear hormone receptor ligand-inducible transcription factors. Retinoid receptors bind to DNA recognition sequences (response elements) in regulatory regions of target genes, and upon binding of RA, facilitate the rate of transcription of these genes (Germain et al., 2006a, 2006b).

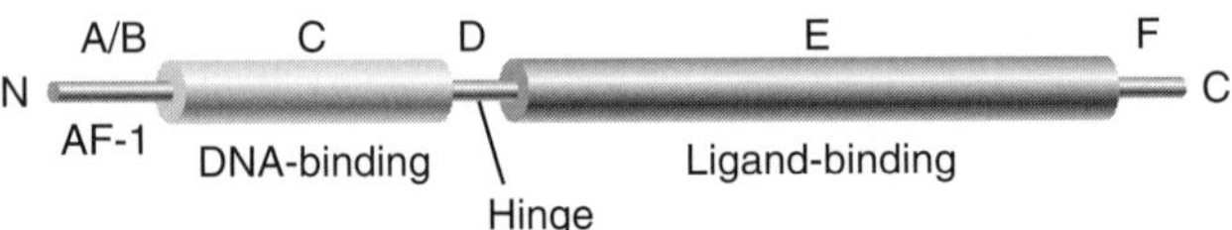

FIGURE 30-4 Structure of retinoid nuclear receptors. The receptors contain five domains. These include the N-terminal domain, A/B, which contains a basal transactivation function AF-1; domain C, which is the DNA-binding region and also participates in dimerization; domain D, which is a hinge region; and domain E, which contains the ligand-binding pocket and mediates interactions with accessory proteins. Domain E is important for ligand-dependent transcriptional activation and is also referred to as AF-2. The function of the carboxyl terminal domain F is not completely clear.

Structure of Retinoid Nuclear Receptors

Like other nuclear hormone receptors, retinoid receptors are composed of several functional domains (Figure 30-4). The N-terminal region of the receptors (A/B domain) which contains a basal, or ligand-independent, activation function termed AF-1. The DNA-binding domain (domain C) contains zinc-fingers responsible for the association of the receptor with DNA (see Chapter 37 for more information on the role of zinc finger motifs in DNA binding by proteins). Domain D is a hinge region that confers flexibility to the protein molecule. Domain E, termed the ligand binding domain, contains the ligand-binding pocket and is responsible for ligand-induced transcriptional activation by the receptors. The ligand-binding domain also contains regions that mediate the interactions of retinoid receptors with a variety of other proteins (see subsequent text). The C-terminal region, which is present in some but not all nuclear receptors, is termed the F domain, and its function is unknown at present.

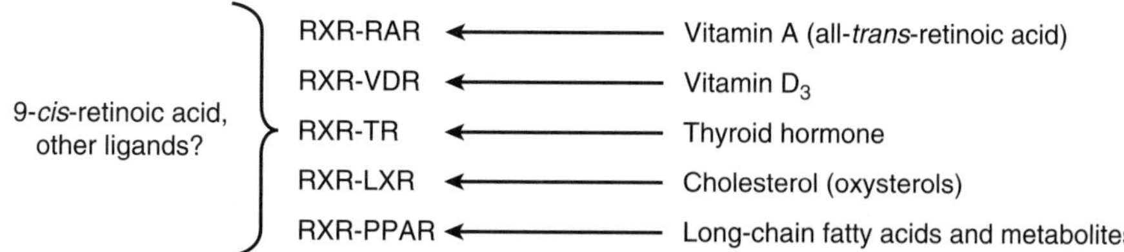

FIGURE 30-5 Heterodimerization partners of retinoid X receptor (RXR) and their respective ligands.

Types of Retinoid Receptors: RAR, PPARβ/δ), and RXR

All-*trans*-RA enhances the transcription of target genes by activating three RA receptors (RARα, RARβ, and RARγ) (Germain et al., 2006a) and a nuclear receptor termed peroxisome proliferator–activated receptor β/δ (PPARβ/δ) (Schug et al., 2007). The partitioning of the all-*trans*-RA hormone between these receptors is regulated by specific RA-binding proteins that selectively deliver it to particular receptors (see later). RARs and PPARβ/δ control the expression of a distinct array of target genes. As the binding proteins determine whether the hormone will be targeted to RAR or PPARβ/δ in a specific cell, cellular responses to RA vary depending on the relative expression levels of these proteins. A third type of retinoid receptors, termed the retinoid X receptors (RXRα, RXRβ, RXRγ), can be activated by the 9-*cis*-isomer of RA (9cRA). However, 9cRA is not found in all tissues that express RXR and it is uncertain whether this compound serves as the physiological ligand for this receptor (Calleja et al., 2006; Germain et al., 2006b).

RAR and PPARβ/δ Heterodimers

Like other nuclear hormone receptors, RAR, PPARβ/δ, and RXR bind to their DNA response elements as dimers. Dimerization, which is stabilized by strong interactions between the ligand-binding domains and by weaker interactions between the DNA-binding domains of the two monomers, serves to increase the specificity of binding of receptors to particular DNA sequences as well as the strength of their interactions with response elements. Mirroring dimer formation by the proteins, DNA response elements for retinoid receptors are usually arranged as two direct repeats of the same hexanucleotide sequence. RAR and PPARβ/δ homodimers do not readily form. Instead, these receptors associate with RXR with a high affinity to form heterodimers, and these RXR-RAR and RXR-PPAR heterodimers serve as the transcriptionally active species (Durand et al., 1992; Green and Wahli, 1994).

RXR Homo- and Heterodimers

In addition to heterodimerization with RAR and PPARβ/δ, RXRs can also interact with other members of the hormone receptor family. For example, they can form heterodimers with the vitamin D_3 receptor (VDR); the thyroid hormone receptor (TR); the peroxisome proliferator–activated receptors PPARα and PPARγ, which are activated by long-chain fatty acids and some of their metabolites; and with liver X receptor (LXR), which responds to cholesterol metabolites (Figure 30-5; also see Chapters 18 and 31 for more information on transcriptional control by fatty acids and vitamin D).

In addition, RXR can bind to DNA and regulate the transcription of target genes as a homodimer (RXR-RXR). RXR has also been reported to form active heterodimers with some orphan nuclear receptors (i.e., proteins that belong to the superfamily of nuclear receptors but for which the ligand is unknown). Heterodimers of RXR with other nuclear receptors can respond to the individual ligands of the two partners and consequently the transcriptional activities of RXR-heterodimers are regulated by more than one type of ligand. RXRs thus function as "master regulators" of several signaling nutrients and hormones as they converge at the genome to regulate gene expression (see Figure 30-5).

Role of Coregulatory Proteins

Modulation of gene transcription by nuclear receptors depends critically on binding of activating ligands, which controls the association of the receptors with coregulatory proteins (Hsia et al., 2010) (Figure 30-6). In the absence of ligands, nuclear receptors associate with proteins that function as transcriptional corepressors. These proteins display enzymatic activities that catalyze deacetylation of histones, resulting in a more compact chromatin structure that leads to repression of transcriptional rates. Upon ligand binding, nuclear receptors undergo a conformational change (Moras and Gronemeyer, 1998) that leads to dissociation of corepressors and recruitment of transcriptional coactivators. Some coactivators catalyze histone acetylation, thereby loosening the structure of the chromatin (Hsia et al., 2010), whereas others, such as components of the Mediator complex, interact with the general transcription machinery and stabilize the recruitment of RNA polymerase II to the target gene promoter (Ito and Roeder, 2001; Rachez and Freedman, 2001). Ligand-activated receptors thus facilitate the transcription of their target genes.

Unlike other receptors, including RAR and PPARβ/δ, the association of RXR with corepressors is weak, suggesting that ligand-dependent activation of this receptor might operate via a different mechanism. Indeed, it was demonstrated that RXR is unique in that, in the absence of its ligand, it exists as a transcriptionally silent homotetramer and that ligand binding results in rapid dissociation of RXR tetramers to the active dimeric species (Kersten et al., 1995, 1998; Gampe et al., 2000). Ligand-induced dissociation of RXR tetramers thus seems to be the first step in activation of this unusual receptor.

OTHER RETINOIDS AND THEIR FUNCTIONS

In addition to retinal and RA, other retinoids are endogenously present in a variety of tissues. The functions of these derivatives are not completely understood but some

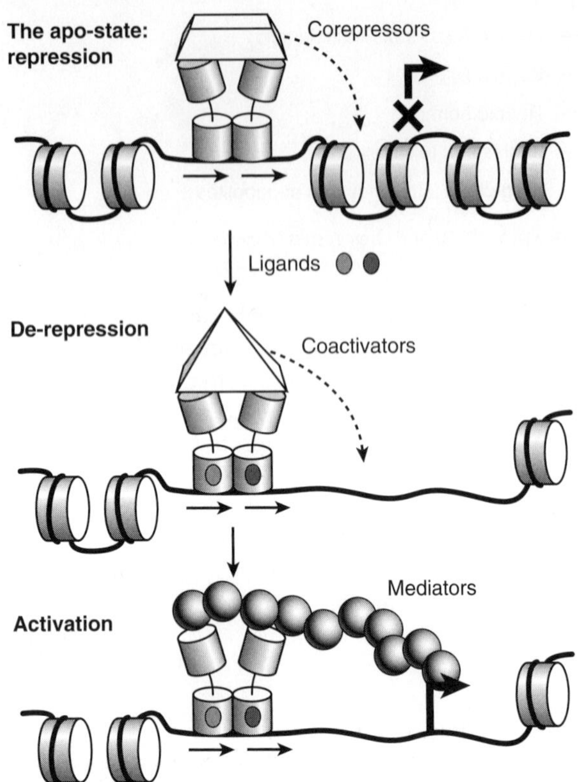

FIGURE 30-6 Transcriptional regulation by retinoid receptors. In the absence of ligand, the receptors associate with proteins that compact chromatin structure and repress transcription. Binding of ligands results in a conformational change that leads to an exchange of corepressors with coactivators. Coactivators modify chromatin to loosen up its structure. Subsequently, a different class of coactivators, termed the Mediator complex, bridge between the receptors and the general transcription machinery and enhance transcriptional rates.

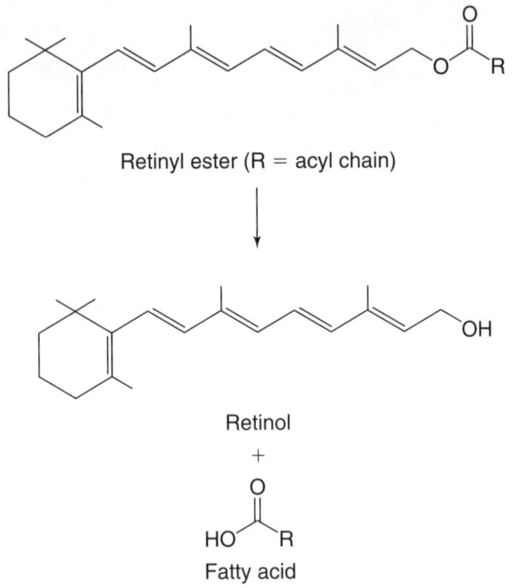

of them have been shown to be biologically active. For example, retinol itself as well as the metabolite 14-hydroxy-*retro*-retinol (see Figure 30-1), have been implicated in regulating lymphocyte physiology (Ross and Hammerling, 1994; Chiu et al., 2008). The mechanisms by which these compounds support lymphocyte growth are incompletely understood. They do not associate with any of the known nuclear retinoid receptors and may function by other signaling pathways.

Another biologically active retinoid is 3,4-didehydroretinol, also known as vitamin A_2. It is abundant in freshwater fish, where its metabolite 11-*cis*-dehydroretinal can serve as a ligand for visual pigments. In humans, 3,4-didehydroretinol was reported to accumulate in tissues of individuals with psoriasis and several other disorders of keratinization (Vahlquist and Torma, 1988). 3,4-Didehydroretinoic acid was found in chick limb buds, where it can affect development, presumably by activating retinoid nuclear receptors (Thaller and Eichele, 1990). It was reported that oxidized retinoid metabolites such as 4-oxo-RA avidly bind to RARβ and are important in determining the positions at which particular digits develop in early embryos (Pijnappel et al., 1993). In addition, it has been demonstrated that some proteins are modified by covalent retinoylation (Takahashi and Breitman, 1991). At present, the

Retinyl ester (R = acyl chain)

Retinol

\+

Fatty acid

FIGURE 30-7 Reaction catalyzed by retinyl ester hydrolase.

effects of retinoylation on the functions of proteins modified in this fashion are not known.

ABSORPTION, TRANSPORT, STORAGE, AND METABOLISM OF VITAMIN A AND CAROTENOIDS

ABSORPTION AND METABOLISM OF VITAMIN A IN THE INTESTINES

Two major forms of vitamin A are present in the diet: retinyl esters, which are derived from animal sources, and carotenoids, mainly β-carotene, which originate from plants (see Figure 30-1). Retinyl esters are hydrolyzed in the intestinal lumen to yield free retinol and the corresponding fatty acid (Figure 30-7). Retinyl ester hydrolysis requires the presence of bile salts that serve to solubilize the retinyl esters in mixed micelles and to activate the hydrolyzing enzymes. Several enzymes that are present in the intestinal lumen may be involved in the hydrolysis of dietary retinyl esters. Carboxylester lipase is secreted into the intestinal lumen from the pancreas and has been shown in vitro to display retinyl ester hydrolase activity. In addition, a retinyl ester hydrolase that is intrinsic to the brush border membrane of the small intestine has been characterized in rats and humans (Rigtrup and Ong, 1992). The different hydrolyzing enzymes are activated by different types of bile salts and have distinct substrate specificities. For example, whereas the pancreatic carboxylester lipase is selective for short-chain retinyl esters, the brush border membrane enzyme preferentially hydrolyzes retinyl esters containing a long-chain fatty acid such as palmitate or stearate. Following hydrolysis, retinol diffuses into the enterocytes in a concentration-dependent manner. In contrast, uptake of carotenoids is mediated by transporters (During and Harrison, 2007).

Absorbed β-carotene is centrally cleaved into two molecules of retinal by β-carotene 15,15′-monooxygenase (BCMO1)

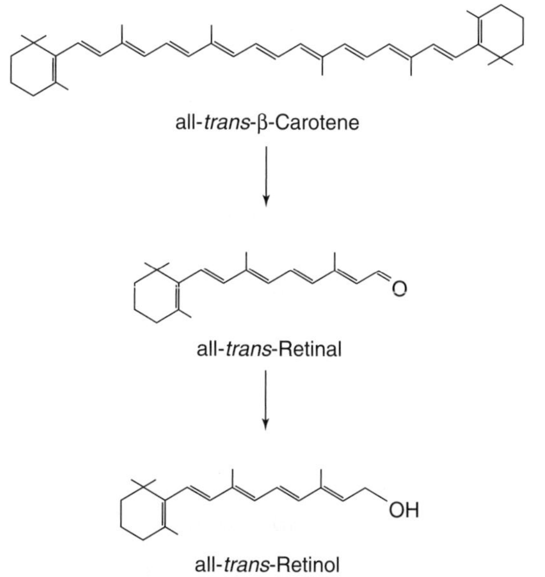

FIGURE 30-8 Cleavage of β-carotene.

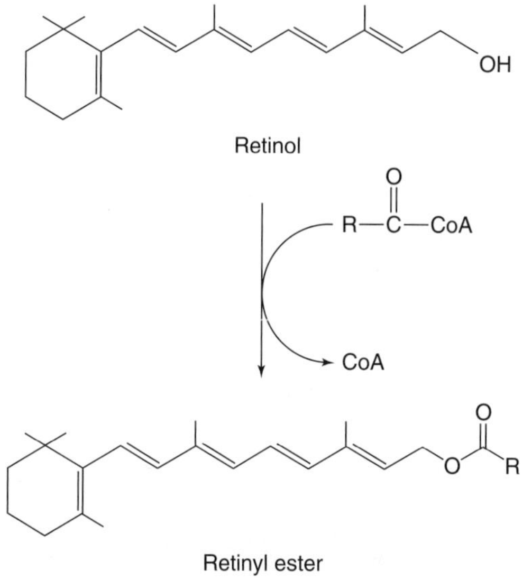

FIGURE 30-9 Reaction catalyzed by acyl CoA:retinol acyltransferase (ARAT).

(Figure 30-8). This enzyme is most highly expressed in the intestinal mucosa but is also found in liver, kidney, lungs, retina, and the brain. In addition, activities that catalyze eccentric cleavage have been reported. The amounts of carotenoids that can pass intact from intestinal cells into blood vary considerably between different species. In the rat, very limited amounts of carotenoids pass into the circulation. In humans, 60% to 70% of absorbed β-carotene is cleaved in the intestine, with the remainder transferred intact into blood and deposited in several tissues such as liver and adipose tissue. The serum level of carotenoids reflects dietary intake, suggesting that a significant fraction of newly absorbed carotenoids are exported from enterocytes into blood without being metabolically converted within these cells.

It has been suggested that carotenoids may have functions other than to serve as precursors for retinol. It should be noted, however, that there is no evidence to suggest that carotenoids are an essential nutrient.

ESTERIFICATION OF RETINOL BY ARAT AND LRAT

Vitamin A is transported in chylomicrons and stored in the liver in the form of retinyl esters in which retinol is esterified with a long-chain fatty acid. Esterification is accompanied by loss of the polar end-groups of both the retinyl and the fatty acyl moieties and results in exceedingly hydrophobic species, which accumulate within lipid droplets in storage cells. Two classes of enzymes that can catalyze the formation of retinyl esters have been identified (Blomhoff and Blomhoff, 2006; Moise et al., 2007). One of these uses activated fatty acids in the form of fatty acyl-CoAs and is termed acyl coenzyme A:retinol acyltransferase (ARAT) (Figure 30-9).

A second type of retinol-esterifying enzyme that functions independently of the presence of exogenous fatty acyl-CoAs is known as lecithin:retinol acyltransferase (LRAT) (Figure 30-10). This enzyme synthesizes retinyl esters by catalyzing the transesterification of a fatty acyl moiety from the *sn*-1 position of phosphatidylcholine to retinol.

Both ARAT and LRAT are integral membrane proteins and are associated with the microsomal (endoplasmic reticulum) fractions of cells of various tissues. Retinyl esters in plasma and in the liver mainly contain the fatty acyl moieties of palmitate and stearate, regardless of the composition of fatty acids in the diet. The composition of the acyl chains in retinyl esters thus corresponds to the primary species of fatty acids found in the *sn*-1 position of phosphatidylcholines, implicating LRAT as the predominant enzyme in esterification of retinol in the intestine and liver. LRAT messenger RNA (mRNA) is present in intestines, liver, testes, retina, and other tissues known for high activities of vitamin A processing. It is worth noting, however, that it has also been reported that retinol esterification in lactating mammary gland is catalyzed mainly by ARAT (Randolph et al., 1991). Hence the relative contributions of the two enzymes to retinyl ester synthesis may be tissue-specific.

ESTERIFICATION OF RETINOL IN THE INTESTINE

Formation of retinyl esters is the final step of vitamin A absorption in the intestine. Retinyl esters, along with other lipids, are then packaged in chylomicrons and secreted into the lymphatic system, which serves to deliver them to blood and subsequently to tissues for storage or use. Activities of both ARAT and LRAT have been noted in intestinal mucosa. The LRAT activity predominates, and ARAT activity contributes significantly to esterification only upon intake of large amounts of retinol.

Delivery of Retinyl Esters to the Liver

The major site of vitamin A storage in the body is the liver. It has been reported that retinyl esters in chylomicrons may be hydrolyzed by a lipoprotein lipase at the adipocyte surface, and it was suggested that this activity facilitates uptake

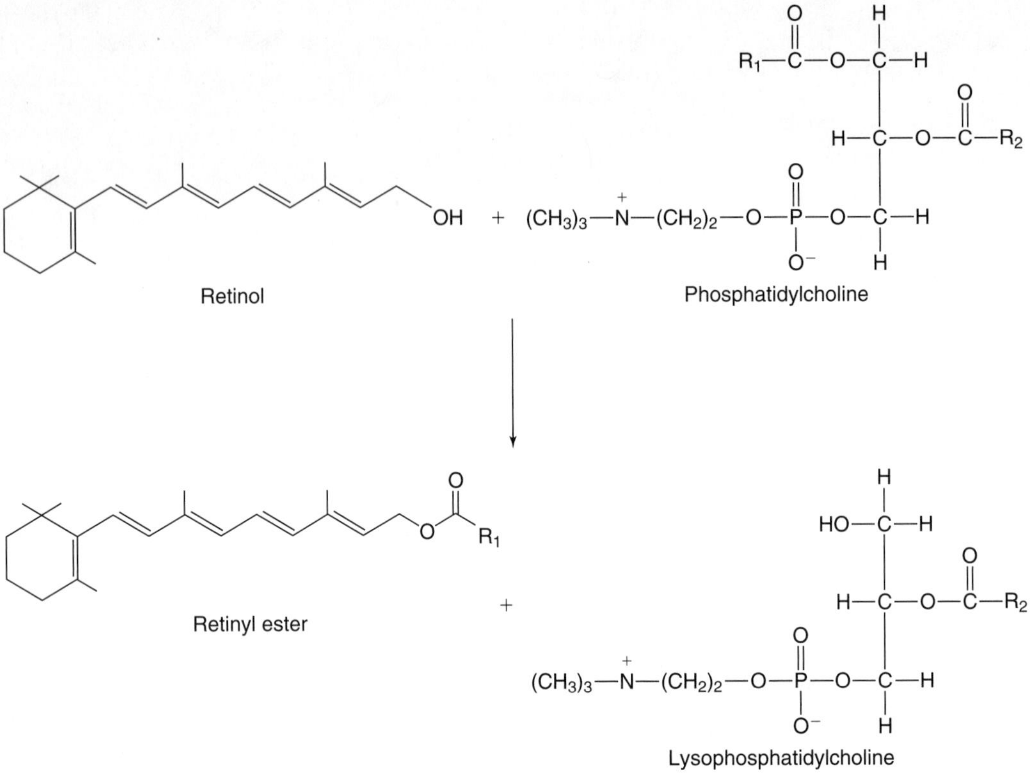

Retinol + Phosphatidylcholine → Retinyl ester + Lysophosphatidylcholine

FIGURE 30-10 Reaction catalyzed by lecithin:retinol acyltransferase (LRAT).

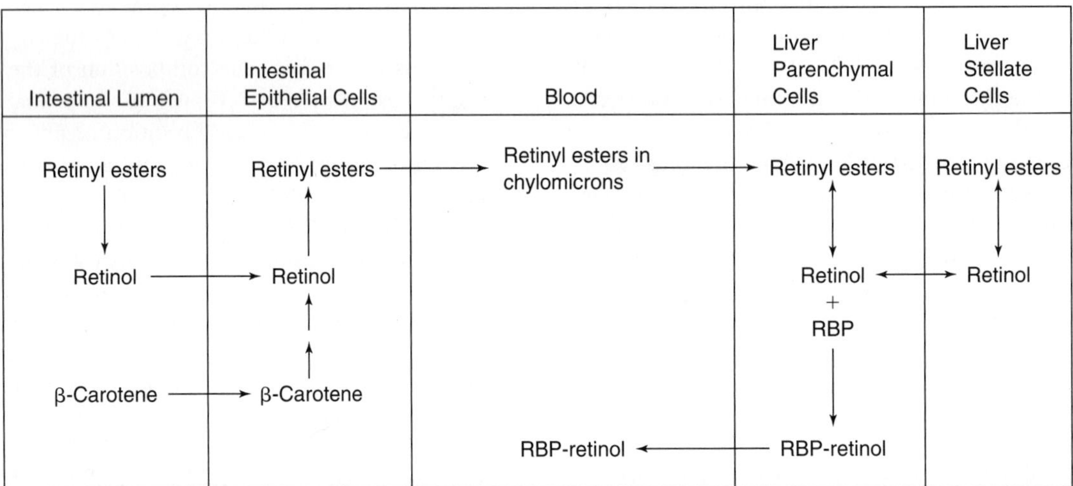

FIGURE 30-11 Movement of retinol between different organs and cells involves hydrolysis and formation of retinyl esters. *RBP*, Retinol binding protein.

of retinol by these cells (Blaner et al., 1994). However, a significant fraction of retinyl esters is retained in chylomicron remnants, and these are cleared from plasma into liver parenchymal cells by receptor-mediated endocytosis.

Hydrolysis and Re-formation of Retinyl Esters

Following uptake of retinyl esters from the circulation by hepatic parenchymal cells, vitamin A is transferred to hepatic stellate cells where it is stored. Although the mechanism by which vitamin A is transported between the two cell types is not completely understood, it has been shown that chylomicron retinyl esters are hydrolyzed in the parenchymal cells and that new retinyl esters are formed in the stellate cells. This suggests that vitamin A is transported between the two cell types in the form of free retinol (Blomhoff and Blomhoff, 2006).

Under normal dietary conditions, the main fraction of retinyl esters in the liver is found in the stellate cells where they accumulate in lipid droplets. In vitamin A–deficient animals, retinoids are mobilized from the stellate cells into parenchymal cells in a process that, again, seems to involve hydrolysis of retinyl esters. Therefore absorption and mobilization of vitamin A between different tissues and cells seems to require continuous hydrolysis and re-formation of retinyl esters (Figure 30-11).

Several distinct enzymatic activities catalyzing the hydrolysis of retinyl esters have been described in different membrane fractions of both parenchymal and stellate cells of the liver. Some retinyl ester hydrolases are activated by bile salts, but the activities of others are independent of bile salts. Reformation of retinyl esters is catalyzed in the liver by both LRAT and ARAT, with the former pathway predominating under physiological concentrations of retinol.

In addition to the liver, extrahepatic tissues play an important role in the overall metabolism and storage of vitamin A. Retinoids are found in extrahepatic organs including adipose depots, kidney, testis, lung, bone marrow, and the eye. These tissues contain significant amounts of retinol and retinyl esters and display esterification as well as retinyl ester hydrolase activities.

SYNTHESIS OF RETINAL AND RETINOIC ACID FROM RETINOL

Retinoic acid is produced from retinol by two sequential oxidation steps: retinol is converted to retinal, which is then oxidized into RA. These metabolic conversions are catalyzed, respectively, by retinol dehydrogenases and retinal dehydrogenases in reactions that entail the dehydrogenation of the substrates using the electron acceptors NAD^+ or $NADP^+$.

Retinol Dehydrogenases

Two classes of enzymes can function as retinol dehydrogenases in vitro: (1) cytosolic medium-chain alcohol dehydrogenases, and (2) members of the family of short-chain dehydrogenases/reductases (SDRs) that are associated with the membranes of the endoplasmic reticulum of various cells. In contrast to soluble alcohol dehydrogenases, it has been reported that some SDR-type retinol dehydrogenases are able to metabolize retinol when bound to the cellular retinol-binding protein (CRBP). Hence while the relative contributions of soluble versus microsomal activities to retinal synthesis in various tissues have not been completely established, it is currently believed that retinal formation in vivo occurs mainly by microsomal SDRs. The first such enzymes to be cloned were the hepatic all-*trans*-retinol dehydrogenase and the *cis*-retinol dehydrogenase that is highly expressed in the retinal pigment epithelium of the eye (Chai et al., 1995; Simon et al., 1996). Subsequently, multiple isozymes have been identified in various tissues. Some of these display a dual specificity toward *cis*- and all-*trans*-retinol, whereas others are more selective for particular isomeric configurations.

Retinal Dehydrogenases

Several mammalian cytosolic retinal dehydrogenases (RalDHs) that catalyze the NAD^+-dependent oxidation of all-*trans*-retinal to all-*trans*-RA have been identified. Recent studies using genetically manipulated mouse models indicated that these enzymes indeed play critical roles in RA synthesis in vivo. It was shown that genetic ablation of RalDH2 results in lethality on about embryonic day 9.5 because of severe trunk, hindbrain, and heart defects resembling those of vitamin A–deficient embryos (Niederreither et al., 1999). Homozygous RalDH1 knockout mice are viable and exhibit no gross malformations. However, it has been reported that RA synthesis in liver of these mice is greatly reduced, suggesting that RalDH1 participates in RA synthesis in vivo (Fan et al., 2003). Mice in which RalDH3 has been genetically knocked out display suppressed RA synthesis and ocular and nasal malformations similar to those observed in vitamin A–deficient fetuses (Dupe et al., 2003). These defects can be prevented by maternal treatment with RA, demonstrating the importance of the enzyme in RA synthesis. Less is known about the physiological function of RalDH4, which appears to display selectivity toward 9-*cis*-retinal, suggesting that it may play a role in synthesis of 9-*cis*-RA (Lin et al., 2003).

METABOLISM OF RETINOIC ACID

Retinoic acid is converted in vivo into several metabolites. The functional significance of these metabolites is incompletely understood.

Retinoic Acid Isomers

The most stable isomer of RA and the predominant species of this compound in vivo is the all-*trans* form. Another isomer, 13-*cis*-RA has been reported to be present in blood and in the small intestine. This isomer comprises a significant fraction of RA at equilibrium and may be present in vivo as a result of nonspecific isomerization. As discussed in the preceding text, another isomer, 9-*cis*-RA, binds to nuclear retinoid receptors with high affinity and is a powerful modulator of gene transcription.

Polar and Oxidized Metabolites of Retinoids

Several types of polar metabolites of retinoids are formed by the action of "detoxifying" enzymes, which catalyze the conjugation of polar groups onto hydrophobic substrates, thereby enhancing the solubility of the substrate and thus the ability of cells to secrete them. Retinoid β-glucuronides are synthesized from either RA or retinol in a variety of tissues including liver, kidney, and intestine, and are found in blood. Retinoid glucuronides are formed by microsomal UDP-glucuronyl transferases, which catalyze the conjugation of glucuronic acid to hydrophobic substrates. Retinoyl β-glucuronide can be hydrolyzed back to yield RA, a reaction that is catalyzed by the lysosomal β-glucuronidase.

Retinoic acid, retinol, and retinal are degraded by the microsomal cytochrome P450 system. Cytochrome P450 reactions, which require NADPH and molecular oxygen, convert these substrates to oxidized metabolites. Several isoforms of cytochrome P450-26, (Cyp26), that are highly specific toward RA have been identified (Haque and Anreola, 1998; Thatcher and Isoherranen, 2009). These enzymes catalyze the degradation of RA, thereby downregulating retinoid signaling. It may be worth noting, however, that some oxidized retinoids, such as 4-oxo-RA, can activate retinoid receptors and thus may be directly involved in affecting cellular physiology (Pijnappel et al., 1993; Nikawa et al., 1995).

RETINOID METABOLISM IN THE EYE

Synthesis of Retinyl Esters in Retinal Pigment Epithelium

The main vitamin A form that circulates in blood, all-*trans*-retinol, is taken up into the eye by the RPE (retinal pigment epithelium) (see Figure 30-3). RPE cells contain an unusually high level of enzymatic activity for conversion of retinol to retinyl esters. Esterification is catalyzed by an LRAT and results in formation of the vitamin A storage species all-*trans* retinyl esters. In turn, retinyl esters are precursors for the 11-*cis*-retinoids that participate in the visual cycle. LRAT of the RPE cells displays broad substrate specificity and, in the presence of 11-*cis*-retinol, can form 11-*cis*-retinyl esters. High levels of these esters have been shown to accumulate in RPE cells in the dark (Saari, 1999).

Formation of 11-cis-Retinoids

Conversion of all-*trans*-retinoids to the 11-*cis* configuration in the eye is a critical part of the visual cycle. This reaction is catalyzed in the RPE by a protein termed RPE65 (Travis et al., 2007; von Lintig et al., 2010). RPE cells of mice lacking functional RPE65 accumulate high levels of all-*trans*-retinyl esters but completely lack 11-*cis*-retinoids and thus are unable to generate visual pigments. Mutations in the *RPE65* gene in humans result in a severe recessive blinding disease called Leber congenital amaurosis. It has been suggested that isomerization of all-*trans*-retinoids to 11-*cis*-retinoids entails hydrolysis of all-*trans*-retinyl ester coupled with isomerization to produce 11-*cis*-retinol. This scenario suggests that the energy stored in the ester bond of the storage species is used to produce the 11-*cis* species (Deigner et al., 1989) (Figure 30-12). However, the exact mechanism by which RPE65 catalyzes retinol isomerization remains to be clarified.

11-*cis*-Retinol can also be produced in RPE cells by hydrolysis of 11-*cis*–retinyl esters, a reaction that is catalyzed by a microsomal retinyl ester hydrolase. This enzyme can also hydrolyze retinyl esters in the all-*trans* configuration but displays a significantly higher specific activity toward the *cis* substrates (Blaner et al., 1987).

11-*cis*-Retinol is oxidized to the retinoid that supports visual function, 11-*cis*-retinal, by a microsomal *cis*-retinol dehydrogenase. Several enzymes that function as *cis*-retinol dehydrogenases are expressed in the RPE (Parker and Crouch, 2010). This redundancy might suggest that loss-of-function mutations in any one of the genes that encode for these enzymes would result in only minor aberrations. Indeed, mutation of the 11-*cis*-retinol dehydrogenase RDH5 in humans leads to a nonprogressive night blindness without retinal dystrophy (Yamamoto et al., 1999). In contrast, it was reported that mutations in RDH12 are associated with a childhood-onset severe retinal dystrophy, suggesting that this isoform plays a more important role in the visual cycle (Janecke et al., 2004). Following its formation, 11-*cis*-retinal is exported from the RPE to photoreceptor cells where it serves to regenerate bleached rhodopsin.

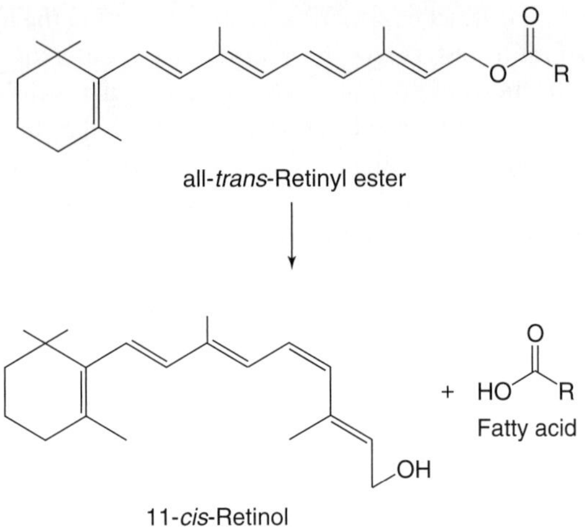

all-*trans*-Retinyl ester

11-*cis*-Retinol

+ Fatty acid

FIGURE 30-12 Reaction catalyzed by all-*trans*-retinyl ester isomerohydrolase.

It was suggested that, unlike rod photoreceptor cells that obtain 11-*cis*-retinal from the RPE, 11-*cis*-retinoids necessary for rhodopsin regeneration in cone cells originate in Müller cells (see Figure 30-3). Studies of retinas from animals that have mainly cones (chicken and ground squirrel) demonstrated an enzymatic activity in Müller cells that catalyzes direct isomerization of free (unesterified) all-*trans*-retinol (Mata et al., 2002). It was suggested that the resulting 11-*cis*-retinol is transported to cone cells where it is converted to 11-*cis*-retinal. It was further proposed that this alternative pathway for synthesis of 11-*cis*-retinal is significantly faster than that afforded by the RPE retinyl ester isomerohydrolase reaction and can support the higher rhodopsin turnover that characterizes bright-light vision mediated by cones.

Metabolism of Retinal in Photoreceptor Cells

Absorption of a photon by rhodopsin in photoreceptor cells leads to isomerization of rhodopsin-bound 11-*cis*-retinal to the all-*trans*-retinal. Photoisomerization initiates visual transduction and also results in the hydrolysis of the retinal–rhodopsin complex. Free all-*trans*-retinal is then converted by a retinol dehydrogenase to all-*trans*-retinol, which is transported to the RPE where it can be converted back to 11-*cis*-retinal. The major metabolic conversions of retinoids in photoreceptor and pigment epithelial cells are shown in Figure 30-13.

RETINOL-BINDING PROTEINS

Because of its amphipathic nature and its poor solubility in water, vitamin A can incorporate into the hydrophobic core of cellular membranes. However, the presence of excess vitamin A in membranes disrupts membrane structure and function. In addition, in order to reach their target cells and their sites of action inside cells, retinoids must move through the oxygen-rich aqueous spaces of plasma and cytosol. Therefore in considering retinoid biology it is important to understand how these poorly soluble and highly labile compounds

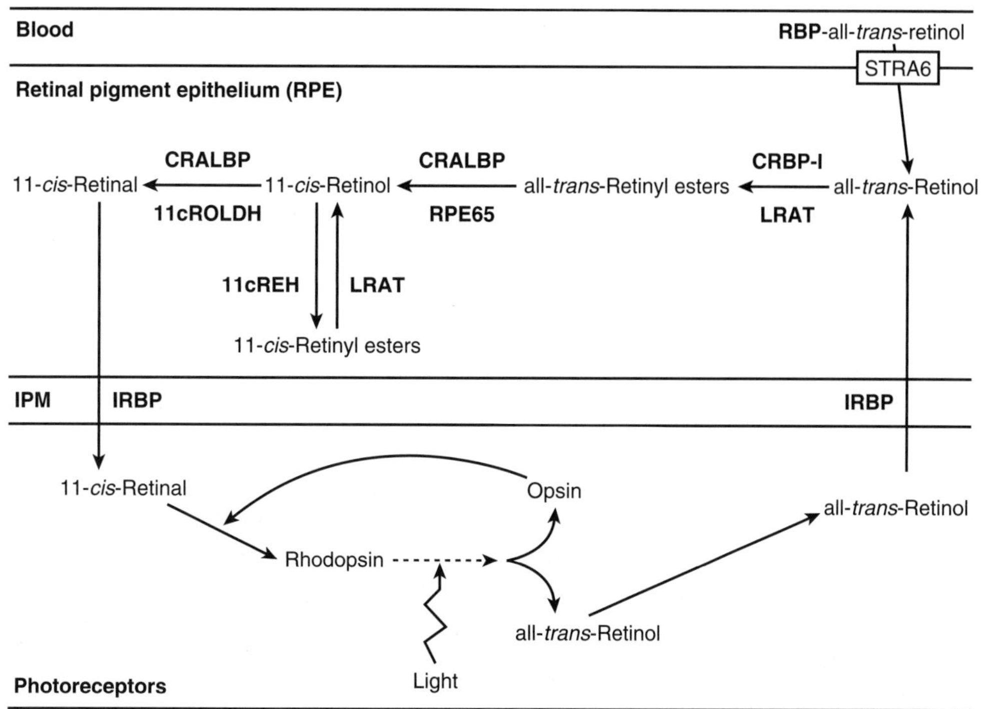

FIGURE 30-13 Major metabolic conversions of retinoids in the eye. Binding proteins and enzymes involved in retinoid metabolism in the eye are shown. *cREH, Cis*-retinyl ester hydrolase; *cROLDH, cis*-retinol dehydrogenase; *CRALP*, cellular retinal-binding protein; *CRBP*, cellular retinol-binding protein; *IPM*, interphotoreceptor matrix; *IRBP*, interphotoreceptor retinoid-binding protein; *LRAT*, lecithin:retinol acyltransferase; *RBP*, retinol-binding protein; *STRA6*, retinol transporter stimulated by RA-6.

TABLE 30-1 Retinoid-Binding Proteins

	M_r (kDa)	MAJOR LIGAND(S)	MAJOR LOCATION
Retinol-binding protein (RBP)	21.2	All-*trans*-retinol	Blood
Cellular retinol-binding protein (CRBP)	15.7	All-*trans*-retinol All-*trans*-retinal	Most tissues
Cellular retinol-binding protein II (CRBP-II)	15.6	All-*trans*-retinol All-*trans*-retinal	Small intestine, fetal liver
Cellular RA-binding protein I (CRABP-I)	15.5	All-*trans*-RA	Most tissues
Cellular RA-binding protein II (CRABP-II)	15.0	All-*trans*-RA	Skin, ovary, uterus, mammary
Cellular retinal-binding protein (CRALBP)	36.0	11-*cis*-retinal 11-*cis*-retinol	Retina
Interphotoreceptor retinoid-binding protein (IRBP)	136.0	11-*cis*-retinal All-*trans*-retinol	Interphotoreceptor matrix

M_r, Molecular mass; RA, retinoic acid.

traverse aqueous phases without loss of structural integrity, how their concentrations in cellular membranes are retained below membranolytic levels, and how they are directed to specific sites of metabolism and action. Answers to these questions were provided by the identification of multiple water-soluble proteins that specifically bind different vitamin A derivatives (Table 30-1). Retinol circulating in blood is bound to serum retinol-binding protein (RBP). In cells, there exist proteins that selectively bind retinol, retinal, and RA. In addition, the interphotoreceptor matrix (i.e., the extracellular space between the photoreceptors and RPE cells in the eye), contains a protein that displays a broad specificity for retinoids. Binding proteins for cellular retinol, retinal, and RA are highly conserved across species that use vitamin A, implying that they play critical roles in the biology of retinoids. The interactions of retinoids with these proteins retard their degradation, decrease their concentrations in membranes, and increase their concentrations in aqueous spaces. Importantly, in addition to these general roles, particular retinoid-binding proteins have critical and specific functions in regulating the metabolism and action of their respective ligands.

RETINOL-BINDING PROTEIN AND TRANSPORT OF RETINOL IN BLOOD

Retinol circulates in blood bound to a plasma protein named retinol-binding protein (RBP), which is a single polypeptide with a molecular weight of 21 kDa containing one binding site for retinol. The retinol-binding site of RBP is a hydrophobic β-barrel that encapsulates the retinol molecule with its β-ionone ring buried deep in the barrel, the isoprene chain stretched along the barrel axis, and the hydroxyl end-group lying almost at the surface of the protein (Newcomer et al., 1984).

The main site of synthesis and secretion of RBP is the liver, which is also the main storage site for vitamin A. Secretion of the protein from the liver is tightly regulated by the availability of retinol (Soprano and Blaner, 1994). During vitamin A deficiency, RBP secretion is inhibited and the protein accumulates in the ER. Upon an increase in retinol levels, RBP moves to the Golgi apparatus and is secreted into blood in the form of the holoprotein. Some extrahepatic tissues including adipose tissue, kidney, testis, brain, and the digestive tract also synthesize and secrete RBP. It was also reported that RBP is synthesized in extrahepatic tissues such as adipose tissue and RPE cells in the eye. RPE cells secrete the protein, not into the blood, but toward the retina into the interphotoreceptor matrix (Ong et al., 1994a). This suggests that RBP may serve as a carrier protein for retinol in compartments other than plasma.

In plasma, RBP is bound to another protein called transthyretin (TTR), a 56-kDa protein that, in addition to associating with RBP, functions as a carrier for thyroid hormones. It is believed that binding of RBP to TTR prevents the loss of the smaller protein from the circulation by filtration in the glomeruli. Although TTR is a tetrameric protein made up of four equivalent subunits, it is usually found bound to only one molecule of RBP. Therefore the protein complex responsible for the plasma transport of retinol contains TTR–RBP–retinol at a molar ratio of 1:1:1. The concentration of this complex in plasma is kept constant at 1 to 2 μmol/L, except in cases of vitamin A deficiency or in disease states. Interestingly, RBP levels in blood are elevated in obese rodents and humans and it has been shown that high serum levels of RBP contribute to insulin resistance (Yang et al., 2005; Graham et al., 2006). The mechanisms through which RBP induces insulin resistance and whether the effect stems from the function of the protein as a retinol carrier remain to be clarified.

Because most of the physiologically important retinoids differ from retinol only in the composition of their head groups, the structure of the RBP binding site suggests that it may bind other retinoids. Indeed, RBP displays a broad specificity for retinoids. However, in the presence of ligands with polar end-groups larger than a hydroxyl, such as the carboxyl group of RA, the interactions of RBP with TTR are hindered. Consequently, the only retinoid that is found to be associated with RBP in plasma is retinol. In contrast, RA circulates in plasma bound to serum albumin.

The tight interaction of retinol with the TTR–RBP complex allows this poorly soluble vitamin to circulate in the aqueous plasma. However, target tissues for vitamin A do not take up the protein complex. Hence to reach the interior of cells, retinol must dissociate from RBP before uptake. It was recently reported that uptake of retinol by target cells is mediated by a plasma membrane protein termed STRA6 (stimulated by RA 6), which functions as a retinol transporter to mobilize the vitamin from RBP in plasma RBP into the interior of cells (Kawaguchi et al., 2007). Mutations in STRA6 in humans lead to defects in embryonic development, resulting in multiple malformations collectively termed Matthew–Wood syndrome (Golzio et al., 2007; Pasutto et al., 2007). The basis for the critical need for STRA6 in embryonic development and whether such a need stems from the function of the protein as a retinol transporter are unknown at present.

CELLULAR BINDING PROTEINS FOR RETINOL AND RETINOIC ACID

Cells express several retinol- and RA-binding proteins. These proteins belong to the family of intracellular lipid binding proteins (iLBPs) and are characterized by a low molecular weight (~15 kDa) and by a shared β-clam structure composed of two five-stranded orthogonal β-sheets that form a ligand-binding pocket. A helix–loop–helix forms a "lid" over the entrance to the ligand-binding pocket of these proteins, raising the question of how respective ligands enter or exit the pocket (Kleywegt et al., 1994; Veerkamp and Maatman, 1995; Gutierrez-Gonzalez et al., 2002; Storch and Corsico, 2008). Although similar in their three-dimensional structures, iLBPs are less homologous in their primary sequences, and they bind lipophilic molecules with distinct selectivities. Several iLBPs are specifically involved in regulating retinoid metabolism and action.

Cellular Retinol-Binding Proteins

Four isotypes of cellular retinol-binding proteins (CRBP-I, II, III, and IV) have been identified to date, with the best characterized ones being CRBP-I and CRBP-II. CRBP-I is present in many tissues including liver, kidney, ovary, testis, lung, eye, spleen, and the small intestine. CRBP-II is found almost exclusively in the mucosal epithelium of the small intestine (Ong et al., 1994b). Although they are named for their interactions with retinol, both CRBP-I and CRBP-II also bind retinal. The affinity of CRBP-I for retinol was reported to be significantly stronger than that of CRBP-II. In contrast, the two proteins bind retinal with a similar affinity. The evolutionary conservation of the two proteins and their characteristic organ and cellular distribution suggest that they play important and distinct roles in the physiology of vitamin A.

CRBP-I and CRBP-II protect their ligands from the activity of some enzymes while allowing them to be metabolized by others. CRBP-II regulates such a selectivity in the intestine. In intestinal cells, free retinal is reduced efficiently to retinol by a soluble retinol dehydrogenase, but the reaction is inhibited when the substrate is bound to CRBP-II. In contrast, an intestinal microsomal dehydrogenase (associated with the ER) can reduce retinal both in the absence and the presence of the binding protein (Kakkad and Ong, 1988). Similarly, esterification of retinol by ARAT of the small intestine is inhibited in the presence of CRBP-II, but intestinal LRAT can metabolize both free and CRBP-II–bound retinol (Herr and Ong, 1992). Because most of the retinol in intestinal cells is bound to CRBP-II, these findings provide an explanation for the predominance of the LRAT-catalyzed reaction over the ARAT-catalyzed reaction in formation of retinyl esters in small intestine.

Similar to the ability of intestinal LRAT to access retinol when bound to CRBP-II, hepatic LRAT can metabolize retinol bound to CRBP-I. Interestingly, it was also reported that LRAT is inhibited by the addition of apo-CRBP-I (Herr and Ong, 1992) and that apo-CRBP-I activates liver retinyl ester hydrolase (Boerman and Napoli, 1991). The observations that apo-CRBP-I inhibits the LRAT reaction but activates the hydrolase suggest the following scenario. When the concentration of retinol, and thus the level of holo-CRBP-I, is high, retinyl ester formation will proceed at a fast rate. Conversely, when the availability of retinol decreases, apo-CRBP-I levels will increase, leading to lower rates of esterification and an enhanced retinyl ester hydrolysis. The notion that CRBP-I regulates the maintenance of vitamin A storage is supported by studies of mice in which the *CRBP-I* gene has been disrupted. This work revealed that *CRBP-I* deficiency is accompanied by a 50% reduction of retinyl ester pools in hepatic stellate cells, a reduction that appears to stem from decreased retinyl ester synthesis accompanied by an accelerated rate of clearance of hepatic retinyl esters (Ghyselinck et al., 1999).

The observation that retinol bound to CRBPs can serve as substrates for particular enzymes raises the question of how these enzymes access the ligand. This question is especially intriguing because retinol is bound to CRBP with the polar end-group buried deeply inside the binding pocket (Cowan et al., 1993). It is therefore difficult to envision how any enzyme could gain access to the ligand's end-group in such a location. One possibility is that protein–protein interactions between the binding protein and specific enzymes result in a conformational change in the CRBP region that covers the binding site, allowing for direct "channeling" of retinol from the binding protein into the enzyme's active site.

Cellular Retinoic Acid–Binding Proteins

In addition to binding to the nuclear hormone receptors RARs and PPARβ/δ, all-*trans*-RA associates in cells with three intracellular lipid-binding proteins: the cellular RA binding proteins CRABP-I and CRABP-II, and fatty acid binding protein 5 (FABP5). These proteins are highly conserved among species and they are expressed differentially across tissues and developmental stages. In the adult, CRABP-I and FABP5 are widely expressed, whereas CRABP-II displays a narrower tissue expression profile, which includes skin, ovary, uterus, mammary epithelium, and the choroid plexus of the brain.

It has been reported that increased expression of CRABP-I in cells enhances the rate of formation of polar metabolites of RA and decreases the transcriptional activity of the retinoid receptor RAR. It was also shown that the sensitivity of F9 teratocarcinoma cells to RA-induced differentiation is inversely correlated with the cellular level of CRABP-I (Boylan and Gudas, 1991, 1992). Although the molecular mechanism underlying these effects remains to be clarified, these observations suggest that CRABP-I dampens cellular response to RA, perhaps by facilitating its degradation.

In contrast to CRABP-I, CRABP-II and FABP5 enhance the sensitivity of cells to RA and they do so by cooperating with RA-activated nuclear receptors. Both CRABP-II and FABP5 are predominantly cytosolic in the absence of ligand, but they translocate to the nucleus upon binding of RA. In the nucleus, CRABP-II associates with RAR whereas FABP5 interacts with PPARβ/δ. Within the resulting CRABP-II/RAR and FABP5/PPARβ/δ complexes, RA is directly channeled from the binding pocket of the binding protein to the binding site of the respective receptor. Hence CRABP-II and FABP5 specifically deliver RA to RAR and to PPARβ/δ, respectively, thereby facilitating the ligation of the receptors and potentiating their ability to induce the expression of their target genes (Figure 30-14) (Dong et al., 1999; Tan et al., 2002; Donato et al., 2007; Schug et al., 2007). Consequently, RA activates RAR in cells in which the CRABP-II/FABP5 ratio is high but functions through PPARβ/δ in cells in which this ratio is low.

It is important to note that RAR and PPARβ/δ activate distinct sets of genes. For example, in various carcinoma cells RAR can induce the expression of genes involved in apoptosis, differentiation, and cell cycle control, and thus potently inhibits cell growth. In contrast, target genes for

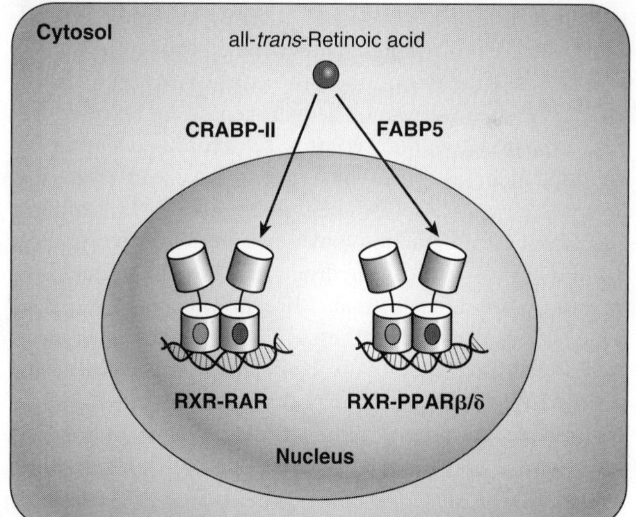

FIGURE 30-14 CRABP-II and FABP5 deliver retinoic acid to RAR and PPARβ/δ. In the absence of ligand, CRABP-II and FABP5 are present in the cytosol. Upon binding of retinoic acid, these proteins mobilize to the nucleus, where they associate with RAR and PPARβ/δ, respectively. Complex formation allows for direct channeling of RA from the binding pocket of the binding protein to the ligand-binding site of the receptor. Following ligand transfer, the complex dissociates and the binding protein returns to the cytosol. *CRABP*, Cellular retinoic acid binding protein; *FABP*, fatty acid binding protein; *PPAR*, peroxisome proliferator-activated protein; *RAR*, retinoic acid receptor; *RXR*, retinoic X receptor.

PPARβ/δ include genes that encode for growth factors and antiapoptotic proteins, and thus activation of this receptor often facilitates the growth and enhances the survival of cancer cells. Considering that the CRABP-II/FABP5 ratio in cells regulates the partitioning of RA between its two receptors, this ratio can determine the nature of cellular responses to RA. Indeed, it was reported that mammary tumor development in mouse models of breast cancer is accompanied by upregulation of FABP5 and a decrease in the expression of CRABP-II, resulting in a low CRABP-II/FABP5 ratio. It was shown further that as a result of the dysregulation of the expression of the binding proteins, RA treatment facilitates tumor growth in the mouse models (Budhu and Noy, 2002; Manor et al., 2003; Schug et al., 2008; for review, see Noy, 2010). FABP5 thus appears to function as an oncogene whereas CRABP-II is a tumor suppressor.

CELLULAR RETINAL-BINDING PROTEIN

The eye and the pineal gland contain a binding protein that is highly specific toward the 11-*cis* isomers of retinal and retinol. Cellular retinal-binding protein (CRALBP), a 36-kDa protein, is a member of the Sec14 lipid-binding/transfer protein family. This family encompasses approximately 20 members in mammals, including CRALBP and α-tocopherol transfer protein (see Chapter 29). The location of CRALBP in the retina and especially in RPE and the specificity of the protein toward 11-*cis*-retinoids suggest that it plays an important role in the homeostasis of the visual chromophore. Indeed, it has been shown that CRALBP is critical for the isomerization of all-*trans*–retinyl esters to 11-*cis*-retinol, a reaction catalyzed by RPE65. It is currently believed that CRALBP participates in the reaction by binding the product 11-*cis*-retinol, thereby preventing product inhibition and allowing the reaction to proceed. 11-*cis*-Retinol can be either oxidized by retinol dehydrogenase to 11-*cis*-retinal and exported to photoreceptor cells for regeneration of rhodopsin, or esterified by LRAT to form 11-*cis*–retinyl esters (see Figure 30-13). The presence of CRALBP inhibits the esterification reaction and stimulates the reaction catalyzed by 11-*cis*-retinol dehydrogenase, producing the visual chromophore 11-*cis*-retinal. Mice in which the *CRALBP* gene has been deleted synthesize 11-*cis*-retinal at a very slow rate and display a dramatically delayed recovery of visual sensitivity following light exposure (Saari et al., 2001). In accordance, mutations in the *CRALBP* gene in humans lead to progressive impairment of visual function (Burstedt et al., 2001).

INTERPHOTORECEPTOR RETINOID-BINDING PROTEIN

Regeneration of active visual pigments in the eye requires a continuous flux of retinoids between different cell types via the aqueous interphotoreceptor matrix space that separates them (see Figure 30-13). The low solubility of retinoids in water and the physiological requirement for their rapid transfer across an aqueous space raise questions regarding the mechanism by which the transport is accomplished.

The main soluble protein component of the interphotoreceptor matrix is a 136-kDa, highly glycosylated protein that binds retinoids and other hydrophobic ligands, such as long-chain fatty acids. It is believed that this protein, termed the interphotoreceptor retinoid-binding protein (IRBP), serves as a carrier for retinoids between the various cells that participate in the visual cycle (i.e., photoreceptors, RPE cells, and, perhaps, Müller cells). In contrast with other known retinoid-binding proteins, IRBP possesses three distinct sites for retinoids (Shaw and Noy, 2001). Participation of IRBP in shuttling of retinoids in the interphotoreceptor matrix is implied by the observations that the composition of retinoids associated with the protein in the interphotoreceptor matrix is modulated by light and that binding of retinoids to IRBP stabilizes them against degradation. It was also reported that IRBP can take up 11-*cis*-retinal from RPE and that it can efficiently deliver 11-*cis*-retinal to bleached-rod outer segments (Pepperberg et al., 1993; Saari, 1994). However, the exact role of IRBP in the transport process is not known. Theoretically, IRBP could serve simply as a storage compartment for retinoids in the interphotoreceptor matrix with the ability to bind and release these ligands according to their concentration gradients. Alternatively, IRBP could function to selectively target specific retinoids to particular locations in the eye by a yet unidentified mechanism. It has been reported that docosahexaenoic acid (DHA), which is a polyunsaturated fatty acid that is highly enriched in photoreceptor cells, specifically inhibits binding of the visual chromophore 11-*cis*-retinal to one of the IRBP retinoid binding sites. The following scenario was thus suggested. When IRBP is in the vicinity of the RPE, where the concentration of DHA is low, it will possess a high affinity for 11-*cis*-retinal and associate with it. Movement to the vicinity of photoreceptor cells will expose IRBP to high levels of DHA, resulting in rapid release of 11-*cis*-retinal from the regulated binding site (Chen et al., 1996).

NUTRITIONAL CONSIDERATIONS OF VITAMIN A

DIETARY REFERENCE INTAKES FOR VITAMIN A AND CAROTENOIDS

In establishing the Dietary Reference Intakes (DRIs), the Institute of Medicine (IOM, 2001) expresses vitamin A requirements as retinol activity equivalents (RAEs), which accounts for differences in bioconversion efficiencies. One μg RAE is equivalent to 1 μg of retinol, 12 μg of β-carotene, 24 μg of α-carotene, and 24 μg of β-cryptoxanthin. Thus a greater amount of provitamin A carotenoids (i.e., carotene-containing fruits and vegetables) is needed to meet the vitamin A requirement. The 1989 dietary recommendations were expressed as retinol equivalents (REs), where 1 μg RE is equivalent to 1 μg retinol, 6 μg β-carotene, and 12 μg of other dietary provitamin A carotenoids (National Research Council [NRC], 1989). The change in equivalency values from the NRC 1989 report to the IOM 2001 report was based in part on data showing that dietary carotenoids were less bioavailable than purified β-carotene in oil, which was used previously for establishing the REs (NRC, 1989).

Adequate Intakes (AIs) were set for infants based on their intake from human milk, and in the case of older infants, from complementary foods. These are 400 μg RAE (485 μg/L × 0.78 L milk/day) and 500 μg RAE (300 μg/day from milk + 200 μg/day from complementary food) per day for infants 0 through 6 months of age and 7 through 12 months of age, respectively. An adult Estimated Average Requirement (EAR) for vitamin A was based on the amount of dietary vitamin A required to maintain a given body pool size in well-nourished individuals (IOM, 2001). The EAR was set at 625 μg RAE/day for men and 500 μg RAE/day for women. The Recommended Dietary Allowances (RDAs) were set as the EAR + 40%, with rounding to the nearest 100 μg. DRIs for children were extrapolated from the adult EARs/RDAs, using metabolic weight ($kg^{0.75}$) as a basis for extrapolation. An increment of 50 μg RAE/day was added to the EAR for pregnant women age 19 or above, based on the accumulation of vitamin A in the liver of the fetus during gestation and an assumption that the liver contains approximately half of the fetus's vitamin A stores. An increment of 40 μg/day was added to the EAR for lactating women, based on the average secretion of vitamin A in human milk during the first 6 months of lactation. RDAs were set for pregnant and lactating women as the EAR + 40%.

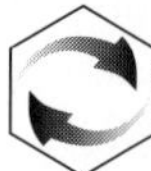

DRIs Across the Life Cycle: Vitamin A

	μg Retinol Activity Equivalents (RAE)* per Day	
Infants	RDA	UL†
0 through 6 mo	400 (AI)	600
7 through 12 mo	500 (AI)	600
Children		
1 through 3 yr	300	600
4 through 8 yr	400	900
9 through 13 yr	600	1,700
Males		
14 through 18 yr	900	2,800
≥19 yr	900	3,000
Females		
14 through 18 yr	700	1,700
≥19 yr	700	3,000
Pregnant		
<19 yr	750	2,800
≥19 yr	770	3,000
Lactating		
<19 yr	1,200	2,800
≥19 yr	1,300	3,000

Data from IOM. (2006). In J. J. Otten, J. P. Hellwig, & L. D. Meyers (Eds.), *Dietary Reference Intakes: The essential guide to nutrient requirements.* Washington, DC: National Academies Press.

AI, Adequate Intake; *DRI,* Dietary Reference Intake; *RDA,* Recommended Dietary Allowance; *UL,* Tolerable Upper Intake Level.

*1 μg RAE = 1 μg retinol, 12 μg β-carotene, 24 μg α-carotene, or 24 μg β-cryptoxanthin.

†The UL for vitamin A applies only to preformed vitamin A (e.g., retinol, the form of vitamin A found in animal foods, most fortified foods, and supplements). It does not apply to vitamin A derived from carotenoids.

The 2001–2002 data from the National Health and Nutrition Examination Survey (NHANES) showed that the median (50th percentile) intake of vitamin A for U.S. women (19 years and older) is 514 μg RAE/day, with a range (5th to 95th percentile) of 230 to 1064 μg RAE/day (Moshfegh et al., 2005). Dietary vitamin A intake for U.S. men (19 years and older) is 577 μg RAE/day, with a range of 238 to 1315 μg RAE/day. Compared to the EAR for vitamin A, many adults in the U.S. population (38% to 59%) do not have adequate dietary vitamin A intake.

Recommendations regarding daily intake of vitamin A have also been put forward by Expert Committees of the Food and Agriculture Organization and the World Health Organization (FAO/WHO, 2002). The FAO/WHO recommendations are given as REs and likely overestimate the vitamin A activity of plant carotenoids. The recommended safe intakes are 375 μg RE/day for infants from birth through 6 months of age, 400 μg RE/day for children from 7 months through 3 years of age, 450 μg RE/day for children 4 through 6 years of age, 500 μg RE/day for children 7 through 10 years of age, 600 μg RE/day for adolescents, 500 μg RE/day for female adults, 600 μg RE/day for male adults, 800 μg RE/day for pregnant women, and 850 μg/day for lactating women. The safe level of intake is defined as the average continuing intake of vitamin A required to permit adequate growth and other vitamin A–dependent

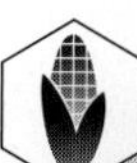

FOOD SOURCES OF RETINOL ACTIVITY EQUIVALENTS (RAE)*

Meat and Meat Substitutes

9000 μg per 3 oz turkey giblets
6500 μg per 3 oz beef liver
60 to 70 μg per 3 oz fish
80 to 90 μg per 1 egg

Vegetables and Fruits

300 to 900 μg per ½ cup pumpkin
200 to 270 μg per ½ cup winter squash
500 μg per ½ cup sweet potato
330 to 600 μg per ½ cup carrots
270 to 550 μg per ½ cup spinach, collards, kale
190 μg per ½ cup red pepper
190 μg per ½ cup cantaloupe
80 μg per ½ cup romaine lettuce

Milk and Milk Products/Fortified Products†

130 to 150 μg per ½ cup ricotta cheese
140 to 150 μg per 1 cup milk (vitamin A added)
120 μg per 1 tbsp margarine
110 to 160 μg per 1 cup ready-to-eat cereal

U.S. Department of Agriculture, Agricultural Research Service. (2011). *USDA National Nutrient Database for Standard Reference, Release 24.* Retrieved from www.ars.usda.gov/ba/bhnrc/ndl.

*1 μg RAE = 1 μg retinol, 12 μg β-carotene, 24 μg α-carotene, or 24 β-cryptoxanthin.

†Vitamin A in fortified foods and vitamin supplements is in the form of retinyl ester (e.g., retinyl acetate or retinyl palmitate).

functions and to maintain an acceptable total body reserve of the vitamin. These FAO/WHO safe levels of intake appear to be similar to the EARs established by the IOM (2001) for the U.S. and Canadian populations. However, the use of RE instead of RAE in fact yields average safe intakes that are substantially lower than those estimated by the IOM for the North American population. This factor needs further consideration, particularly because diets in most developing countries are low in preformed vitamin A and populations are dependent largely upon provitamin A carotenoids in plants as a source of REs.

VITAMIN A DEFICIENCY

Vitamin A deficiency is manifested by a number of symptoms, the most serious being ocular problems and a depressed immune function. In many developing countries in Southern and Southeastern Asia, Africa, and Central and South America, vitamin A deficiency is a serious nutritional problem that especially affects preschool-age children. Vitamin A deficiency is most common in populations consuming mainly plant-based diets with little dietary fat. Recent studies suggest that subclinical vitamin A deficiency is surprisingly common in developed countries and some extreme cases have been documented (Rodrigues and Dohlman, 2004).

Children younger than 6 years are particularly affected by vitamin A deficiency. It has been estimated that, worldwide, about 130 million preschoolers are vitamin A deficient, which contributes to blindness and poor immune function (West, 2003; Sommer, 2008). The initial signs of vitamin A deficiency are night blindness and impaired epidermal integrity manifested by hyperkeratosis. These conditions can be reversed upon supplementation of vitamin A. If left untreated, night blindness is followed by xerophthalmia, a disease associated with structural changes in the cornea. The first visible structural changes are drying of the conjunctiva and the cornea (xerosis) and the development of opaque areas called Bitot spots. This is followed by development of keratomalacia, which involves irreversible damage to the cornea and leads to blindness (Sommer, 2008).

In addition to keratinization of the cornea, deficiency of vitamin A results in keratinization of tracheal epithelium and in thinning of the intestinal epithelium. Xerophthalmia was reported to be accompanied by upper respiratory infection and diarrhea and to be exacerbated by protein-energy malnutrition. Vitamin A deficiency is also associated with a lower resistance to infections and with increased mortality in young children (Sommer, 1992). Mortality rates in children with night blindness or Bitot spots (white foamy patches on the conjunctiva) were reported to be threefold to eightfold greater when compared to children with no visible signs of vitamin A deficiency. Additionally, supplementation of vitamin A in children living in vitamin A–deficient areas was shown to significantly reduce the incidence of mortality (Sommer, 1992). The increased susceptibility to infection associated with vitamin A deficiency has been shown both by epidemiological evidence and by studies with laboratory animals to stem from compromised immune function.

It should be noted that although ocular symptoms are the most specific indicators of vitamin A deficiency, ocular manifestations occur only after other tissues have impaired functions that are less specific and less easily assessed. Low serum levels of retinol (less than 0.70 μmol/L) indicate subclinical vitamin A deficiency, but subclinical deficiency can be present with serum retinol levels as high as 1.05 μmol/L. Assessment of the response of persons to vitamin A supplementation can be used to identify individuals with critically depleted body stores.

VITAMIN A AND THE MAINTENANCE OF HEALTH

A diet rich in vitamin A and carotenoids can play a protective role against several physiological abnormalities. It was reported in early studies that epithelia of vitamin A–deficient organs are histologically similar to those of

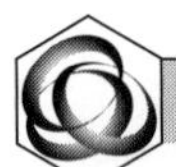

LIFE CYCLE CONSIDERATION

Vitamin A Supplements in Pregnancy

Studies in animals have shown that retinol can be teratogenic in early pregnancy and lead to fetal abnormalities including craniofacial, cardiac, thymic, and central nervous system malformations. In humans, the synthetic retinoid isotretinoin, which is used in treatment of severe acne, results in similar malformations. The period of sensitivity in humans is the second to the fifth week of pregnancy. The incidence of birth defects associated with cranial neural crest tissue in babies born to women who consumed more than 4,500 μg retinol per day was reported to be 3.5-fold higher than babies born to women whose daily consumption of vitamin A was 1,500 μg or less (Rothman et al., 1995). The increased incidence of defects was concentrated among babies born to women who consumed high levels of vitamin A before the seventh week of gestation. These observations suggest that intake of vitamin A at doses that are only several-fold higher than the RDA during early pregnancy is associated with a marked increase in the incidence of birth defects. Conversely, it was also reported that vitamin A supplements at a total dose exceeding 3,000 μg retinol did not result in a higher incidence of neural crest defects (Shaw et al., 1996; Werler et al., 1996). As pointed out by Gerster (1997), it seems prudent at the present time to follow the recommendations of the Teratology Society of the United States that the daily vitamin A dose for women should never exceed 3,000 μg RE (retinol equivalents) and that it is reasonable to replace part of the vitamin A supplement for pregnant women with β-carotene, which has never been shown to be teratogenic, either in animals or in humans.

neoplastic tissues (Wolbach and Howe, 1925), and a number of epidemiological studies have indicated that consumption of vitamin A and carotenoids is inversely correlated with development of several types of cancer. RA is clinically used for treatment of malignancies, such as promyelocytic leukemia, Kaposi sarcoma, and neuroblastoma, and premalignancies, such as leukoplakia, actinic keratosis, and xeroderma pigmentosum. However, cellular responses to RA vary and, in the context of some normal as well as carcinoma cells, this vitamin A metabolite fails to suppress growth or, paradoxically, actually enhances tumor growth. Hence use of RA in cancer therapy awaits better understanding of the basis for the resistance displayed by some tumors. Dietary vitamin A also plays an important role in enhancing immune responses. It has been reported that even mild vitamin A deficiency can lead to impaired immune response and lymphocyte function (Semba et al., 1992; Sommer and West, 1992; Sommer, 2008) and that vitamin A supplementation of children with no apparent deficiency results in significant reduction in disease mortality (Gerster, 1997). Vitamin A, via its metabolite RA, is also essential for embryogenesis. Vitamin A deficiency during gestation has been shown to induce fetal malformations in animals and is likely to have similar outcomes in humans. However, specific effects of vitamin A deficiency on fetal development in humans are difficult to discern because vitamin A deficiency is usually accompanied by general protein-energy malnutrition. Interestingly, the vitamin A–induced malformations that have been observed in animals with vitamin A deficiency are similar to those that are found in animals given excess vitamin A (Gerster, 1997).

VITAMIN A EXCESS

Acute vitamin A toxicity has been reported to occur following consumption of polar bear and seal liver by indigenous peoples of the Arctic and Arctic explorers. Chronic toxicity can occur following routine intake of smaller, but still large, doses of vitamin A over a period of several months and has been observed following daily ingestion exceeding 15,000 μg retinol. Higher sensitivity is observed in infants and young children in whom toxic manifestation can occur following daily ingestion of more than 6,000 μg retinol. Both acute and chronic forms of vitamin A toxicity are rare occurrences and are easily reversed following cessation of excessive intake. A third type of vitamin A toxicity can occur with ingestion of even lower doses of excess vitamin A during early pregnancy, where vitamin A can have teratogenic effects leading to fetal abnormalities. The teratogenic effects of vitamin A most likely stem from the high levels of RA formed upon excessive intake of vitamin A.

In establishing ULs (Tolerable Upper Intake Levels) for vitamin A intake, the IOM considered teratogenicity as the critical adverse effect on which to base a UL for women of childbearing age. Liver abnormalities (i.e., liver pathology characteristic of vitamin A intoxication) were considered as the critical adverse effect for setting ULs for other adults. Adverse effects have been observed due to intake of preformed vitamin A, so the ULs are stated in terms of vitamin A or retinol intake. The UL for adult men and women is 3,000 μg per day of preformed vitamin A. The UL, although based on different criteria, was the same for women 19 through 50 years of age and women 51 years of age or older.

THINKING CRITICALLY

1. Vitamin A transport and metabolism is linked to protein status.
   a. Consider the consequences of severe protein-energy malnutrition (PEM) on vitamin A status.
   b. Identify three biological consequences of PEM that relate to vitamin A function.
2. Which form of vitamin A accounts for most of its diverse biological functions? Explain.
3. What factors (environmental or genetic) may lead to apparent vitamin A deficiency? List a few examples.
4. Retinoic acid is a potent anticarcinogenic agent but its usage in oncology is limited by the development of retinoic acid resistance in tumors. What molecular mechanisms may underlie retinoic acid resistance?

REFERENCES

Berry, D. C., & Noy, N. (2009). All-*trans*-retinoic acid represses obesity and insulin resistance by activating both peroxisome proliferation-activated receptor beta/delta and retinoic acid receptor. *Molecular and Cellular Biology, 29,* 3286–3296.

Blaner, W. S., Das, S. R., Gouras, P., & Flood, M. T. (1987). Hydrolysis of 11-*cis*- and all-*trans*-retinyl palmitate by homogenates of human retinal epithelial cells. *The Journal of Biological Chemistry, 262,* 53–58.

Blaner, W. S., Obunike, J. C., Kurlandsky, S. B., al-Haideri, M., Piantedosi, R., Deckelbaum, R. J., & Goldberg, I. J. (1994). Lipoprotein lipase hydrolysis of retinyl ester. Possible implications for retinoid uptake by cells. *The Journal of Biological Chemistry, 269,* 16559–16565.

Blomhoff, R., & Blomhoff, H. K. (2006). Overview of retinoid metabolism and function. *Journal of Neurobiology, 66,* 606–630.

Boerman, M. H., & Napoli, J. L. (1991). Cholate-independent retinyl ester hydrolysis. Stimulation by Apo-cellular retinol-binding protein. *The Journal of Biological Chemistry, 266,* 22273–22278.

Boylan, J. F., & Gudas, L. J. (1991). Overexpression of the cellular retinoic acid binding protein-I (CRABP- I) results in a reduction in differentiation-specific gene expression in F9 teratocarcinoma cells. *The Journal of Cell Biology, 112,* 965–979.

Boylan, J. F., & Gudas, L. J. (1992). The level of CRABP-I expression influences the amounts and types of all-*trans*-retinoic acid metabolites in F9 teratocarcinoma stem cells. *The Journal of Biological Chemistry, 267,* 21486–21491.

Budhu, A. S., & Noy, N. (2002). Direct channeling of retinoic acid between cellular retinoic acid-binding protein II and retinoic acid receptor sensitizes mammary carcinoma cells to retinoic acid–induced growth arrest. *Molecular and Cellular Biology, 22,* 2632–2641.

Burstedt, M. S., Forsman-Semb, K., Golovleva, I., Janunger, T., Wachtmeister, L., & Sandgren, O. (2001). Ocular phenotype of bothnia dystrophy, an autosomal recessive retinitis pigmentosa associated with an R234W mutation in the RLBP1 gene. *Archives of Ophthalmology, 119*, 260–267.

Calleja, C., Messaddeq, N., Chapellier, B., Yang, H., Krezel, W., Li, M., … Chambon, P. (2006). Genetic and pharmacological evidence that a retinoic acid cannot be the RXR-activating ligand in mouse epidermis keratinocytes. *Genes & Development, 20*, 1525–1538.

Chai, X., Boerman, M. H., Zhai, Y., & Napoli, J. L. (1995). Cloning of a cDNA for liver microsomal retinol dehydrogenase: A tissue-specific, short-chain alcohol dehydrogenase. *The Journal of Biological Chemistry, 270*, 3900–3904.

Chen, Y., Houghton, L. A., Brenna, J. T., & Noy, N. (1996). Docosahexaenoic acid modulates the interactions of the interphotoreceptor retinoid-binding protein with 11-*cis*-retinal. *The Journal of Biological Chemistry, 271*, 20507–20515.

Chiu, H. J., Fischman, D. A., & Hammerling, U. (2008). Vitamin A depletion causes oxidative stress, mitochondrial dysfunction, and PARP-1-dependent energy deprivation. *The FASEB Journal, 22*, 3878–3887.

Cowan, S. W., Newcomer, M. E., & Jones, T. A. (1993). Crystallographic studies on a family of cellular lipophilic transport proteins. Refinement of P2 myelin protein and the structure determination and refinement of cellular retinol-binding protein in complex with all-*trans*-retinol. *Journal of Molecular Biology, 230*, 1225–1246.

Deigner, P. S., Law, W. C., Canada, F. J., & Rando, R. R. (1989). Membranes as the energy source in the endergonic transformation of vitamin A to 11-*cis*-retinol. *Science, 244*, 968–971.

Donato, L. J., Suh, J. H., & Noy, N. (2007). Suppression of mammary carcinoma cell growth by retinoic acid: The cell cycle control gene Btg2 is a direct target for retinoic acid receptor signaling. *Cancer Research, 67*, 609–615.

Dong, D., Ruuska, S. E., Levinthal, D. J., & Noy, N. (1999). Distinct roles for cellular retinoic acid-binding proteins I and II in regulating signaling by retinoic acid. *The Journal of Biological Chemistry, 274*, 23695–23698.

Dupe, V., Matt, N., Garnier, J. M., Chambon, P., Mark, M., & Ghyselinck, N. B. (2003). A newborn lethal defect due to inactivation of retinaldehyde dehydrogenase type 3 is prevented by maternal retinoic acid treatment. *Proceedings of the National Academy of Sciences of the United States of America, 100*, 14036–14041.

Durand, B., Saunders, M., Leroy, P., Leid, M., & Chambon, P. (1992). All-*trans* and 9-*cis* retinoic acid induction of CRABPII transcription is mediated by RAR-RXR heterodimers bound to DR1 and DR2 repeated motifs. *Cell, 71*, 73–85.

During, A., & Harrison, E. H. (2007). Mechanisms of provitamin A (carotenoid) and vitamin A (retinol) transport into and out of intestinal Caco-2 cells. *Journal of Lipid Research, 48*, 2283–2294.

Fan, X., Molotkov, A., Manabe, S., Donmoyer, C. M., Deltour, L., Foglio, M. H., … Duester, G. (2003). Targeted disruption of Aldh1a1 (Raldh1) provides evidence for a complex mechanism of retinoic acid synthesis in the developing retina. *Molecular and Cellular Biology, 23*, 4637–4648.

Food and Agriculture Organization/World Health Organization. (2002). Vitamin A. In *Human vitamin and mineral requirements. Report of a joint FAO/WHO expert consultation.* Rome: FAO/WHO.

Gampe, R. T., Jr., Montana, V. G., Lambert, M. H., Wisely, G. B., Milburn, M. V., & Xu, H. E. (2000). Structural basis for autorepression of retinoid X receptor by tetramer formation and the AF-2 helix. *Genes & Development, 14*, 2229–2241.

Germain, P., Chambon, P., Eichele, G., Evans, R. M., Lazar, M. A., Leid, M., … Gronemeyer, H. (2006a). International Union of Pharmacology. LX. Retinoic acid receptors. *Pharmacological Reviews, 58*, 712–725.

Germain, P., Chambon, P., Eichele, G., Evans, R. M., Lazar, M. A., Leid, M., … Gronemeyer, H. (2006b). International Union of Pharmacology. LXIII. Retinoid X receptors. *Pharmacological Reviews, 58*, 760–772.

Gerster, H. (1997). Vitamin A—Functions, dietary requirements and safety in humans. *International Journal for Vitamin and Nutrition Research, 67*, 71–90.

Ghyselinck, N. B., Bavik, C., Sapin, V., Mark, M., Bonnier, D., Hindelang, C., … Chambon, P. (1999). Cellular retinol-binding protein I is essential for vitamin A homeostasis. *The EMBO Journal, 18*, 4903–4914.

Golzio, C., Martinovic-Bouriel, J., Thomas, S., Mougou-Zrelli, S., Grattagliano-Bessieres, B., Bonniere, M., … Etchevers, H. C. (2007). Matthew-Wood syndrome is caused by truncating mutations in the retinol-binding protein receptor gene STRA6. *American Journal of Human Genetics, 80*, 1179–1187.

Graham, T. E., Yang, Q., Bluher, M., Hammarstedt, A., Ciaraldi, T. P., Henry, R. R., … Kahn, B. B. (2006). Retinol-binding protein 4 and insulin resistance in lean, obese, and diabetic subjects. *New England Journal of Medicine, 354*, 2552–2563.

Green, S., & Wahli, W. (1994). Peroxisome proliferator-activated receptors: Finding the orphan a home. *Molecular and Cellular Endocrinology, 100*, 149–153.

Gutierrez-Gonzalez, L. H., Ludwig, C., Hohoff, C., Rademacher, M., Hanhoff, T., Ruterjans, H., … Lucke, C. (2002). Solution structure and backbone dynamics of human epidermal-type fatty acid–binding protein (E-FABP). *The Biochemical Journal, 364*, 725–737.

Haque, M., & Anreola, F. (1998). The cloning and characterization of a novel cytochrome P450 family, CYP26, with specificity toward retinoic acid. *Nutrition Reviews, 56*, 84–85.

Herr, F. M., & Ong, D. E. (1992). Differential interaction of lecithin-retinol acyltransferase with cellular retinol binding proteins. *Biochemistry, 31*, 6748–6755.

Hoffman, C., & Eichele, G. (1994). Retinoids in development. In M. B.Sporn, A. B. Roberts, & D. S. Goodman (Eds.), *The retinoids, biology, chemistry and medicine* (pp. 387–441). New York: Raven Press.

Hsia, E. Y., Goodson, M. L., Zou, J. X., Privalsky, M. L., & Chen, H. W. (2010). Nuclear receptor coregulators as a new paradigm for therapeutic targeting. *Advanced Drug Delivery Reviews, 62*, 1227–1237.

Institute of Medicine. (2001). *Dietary reference intakes for vitamin A, vitamin K, arsenic, boron, chromium, copper, iodine, iron, manganese, molybendum, nickel, silicon, vanadium, and zinc.* Washington, DC: National Academy Press.

Ito, M., & Roeder, R. G. (2001). The TRAP/SMCC/Mediator complex and thyroid hormone receptor function. *Trends in Endocrinology and Metabolism, 12*, 127–134.

Janecke, A. R., Thompson, D. A., Utermann, G., Becker, C., Hubner, C. A., Schmid, E., … Gal, A. (2004). Mutations in RDH12 encoding a photoreceptor cell retinol dehydrogenase cause childhood-onset severe retinal dystrophy. *Nature Genetics, 36*, 850–854.

Kakkad, B. P., & Ong, D. E. (1988). Reduction of retinaldehyde bound to cellular retinol-binding protein (type II) by microsomes from rat small intestine. *The Journal of Biological Chemistry, 263*, 12916–12919.

Kawaguchi, R., Yu, J., Honda, J., Hu, J., Whitelegge, J., Ping, P., … Sun, H. (2007). A membrane receptor for retinol binding protein mediates cellular uptake of vitamin A. *Science, 315*, 820–825.

Kersten, S., Dong, D., Lee, W., Reczek, P. R., & Noy, N. (1998). Auto-silencing by the retinoid X receptor. *Journal of Molecular Biology, 284*, 21–32.

Kersten, S., Kelleher, D., Chambon, P., Gronemeyer, H., & Noy, N. (1995). Retinoid X receptor alpha forms tetramers in solution. *Proceedings of the National Academy of Sciences of the United States of America, 92*, 8645–8649.

Kleywegt, G. J., Bergfors, T., Senn, H., Le Motte, P., Gsell, B., Shudo, K., & Jones, T. A. (1994). Crystal structures of cellular retinoic acid binding proteins I and II in complex with all-*trans*-retinoic acid and a synthetic retinoid. *Structure, 2*, 1241–1258.

Lin, M., Zhang, M., Abraham, M., Smith, S. M., & Napoli, J. L. (2003). Mouse retinal dehydrogenase 4 (RALDH4), molecular cloning, cellular expression, and activity in 9-*cis*-retinoic acid biosynthesis in intact cells. *The Journal of Biological Chemistry, 278*, 9856–9861.

Manor, D., Shmidt, E. N., Budhu, A., Flesken-Nikitin, A., Zgola, M., Page, R., … Noy, N. (2003). Mammary carcinoma suppression by cellular retinoic acid binding protein-II. *Cancer Research, 63*, 4426–4433.

Mata, N. L., Radu, R. A., Clemmons, R. C., & Travis, G. H. (2002). Isomerization and oxidation of vitamin A in cone-dominant retinas: A novel pathway for visual-pigment regeneration in daylight. *Neuron, 36*, 69–80.

McCollum, E. V., & Davis, M. (1913). The necessity of certain lipins in the diet during growth. *The Journal of Biological Chemistry, 15*, 167–175.

Moise, A. R., Noy, N., Palczewski, K., & Blaner, W. S. (2007). Delivery of retinoid-based therapies to target tissues. *Biochemistry, 46*, 4449–4458.

Moras, D., & Gronemeyer, H. (1998). The nuclear receptor ligand-binding domain: Structure and function. *Current Opinion in Cell Biology, 10*, 384–391.

Moshfegh, A., Goldman, J., & Cleveland, L. (2005). *What we eat in America, NHANES 2001–2002: Usual nutrient intake from food compared to dietary reference intakes*. Washington, DC: U.S. Department of Agriculture, Agricultural Research Service.

Mukherjee, R., Davies, P. J., Crombie, D. L., Bischoff, E. D., Cesario, R. M., Jow, L., … Heyman, R. A. (1997). Sensitization of diabetic and obese mice to insulin by retinoid X receptor agonists. *Nature, 386*, 407–410.

National Research Council. (1989). *Recommended dietary allowances* (10th ed.). Washington, DC: National Academy Press.

Newcomer, M. E., Jones, T. A., Aqvist, J., Sundelin, J., Eriksson, U., Rask, L., & Peterson, P. A. (1984). The three-dimensional structure of retinol-binding protein. *The EMBO Journal, 3*, 1451–1454.

Niederreither, K., Subbarayan, V., Dolle, P., & Chambon, P. (1999). Embryonic retinoic acid synthesis is essential for early mouse post-implantation development. *Nature Genetics, 21*, 444–448.

Nikawa, T., Schulz, W. A., van den Brink, C. E., Hanusch, M., van der Saag, P., Stahl, W., & Sies, H. (1995). Efficacy of all-*trans*-beta-carotene, canthaxanthin, and all-*trans*-, 9-*cis*-, and 4-oxo-retinoic acids in inducing differentiation of an F9 embryonal carcinoma RAR beta-lacZ reporter cell line. *Archives of Biochemistry and Biophysics, 316*, 665–672.

Noy, N. (2010). Between death and survival: Retinoic acid in regulation of apoptosis. *Annual Review of Nutrition, 30*, 201–217.

Ong, D. E., Davis, J. T., O'Day, W. T., & Bok, D. (1994a). Synthesis and secretion of retinol-binding protein and transthyretin by cultured retinal pigment epithelium. *Biochemistry, 33*, 1835–1842.

Ong, D. E., Newcomer, M. E., & Chytil, F. (1994b). Cellular retinoid binding proteins. In M. B. Sporn, A. B. Roberts, & D. S. Goodman (Eds.), *The retinoids: Biology, chemistry, and medicine* (pp. 283–318). New York: Raven Press.

Osborne, T. B., & Mendel, L. B. (1919). The vitamins in green foods. *The Journal of Biological Chemistry, 37*, 187–200.

Parker, R. O., & Crouch, R. K. (2010). Retinol dehydrogenases (RDHs) in the visual cycle. *Experimental Eye Research, 91*, 788–792.

Pasutto, F., Sticht, H., Hammersen, G., Gillessen-Kaesbach, G., Fitzpatrick, D. R., Nurnberg, G., … Rauch, A. (2007). Mutations in STRA6 cause a broad spectrum of malformations including anophthalmia, congenital heart defects, diaphragmatic hernia, alveolar capillary dysplasia, lung hypoplasia, and mental retardation. *American Journal of Human Genetics, 80*, 550–560.

Pepperberg, D. R., Okajima, T. L., Wiggert, B., Ripps, H., Crouch, R. K., & Chader, G. J. (1993). Interphotoreceptor retinoid-binding protein (IRBP): Molecular biology and physiological role in the visual cycle of rhodopsin. *Molecular Neurobiology, 7*, 61–85.

Pijnappel, W. W., Hendriks, H. F., Folkers, G. E., van den Brink, C. E., Dekker, E. J., Edelenbosch, C., … Durston, A. J. (1993). The retinoid ligand 4-oxo-retinoic acid is a highly active modulator of positional specification. *Nature, 366*, 340–344.

Rachez, C., & Freedman, L. P. (2001). Mediator complexes and transcription. *Current Opinion in Cell Biology, 13*, 274–280.

Randolph, R. K., Winkler, K. E., & Ross, A. C. (1991). Fatty acyl CoA-dependent and -independent retinol esterification by rat liver and lactating mammary gland microsomes. *Archives of Biochemistry and Biophysics, 288*, 500–508.

Rigtrup, K. M., & Ong, D. E. (1992). A retinyl ester hydrolase activity intrinsic to the brush border membrane of rat small intestine. *Biochemistry, 31*, 2920–2926.

Rodrigues, M. I., & Dohlman, C. H. (2004). Blindness in an American boy caused by unrecognized vitamin A deficiency. *Archives of Ophthalmology, 122*, 1228–1229.

Ross, C. A., & Hammerling, U. G. (1994). Retinoids and the immune system. In M. B. Sporn, A. B. Roberts, & D. S. Goodman (Eds.), *The retinoids, biology, chemistry and medicine*. (pp. 521–544). New York: Raven Press.

Rothman, K. J., Moore, L. L., Singer, M. R., Nguyen, U. S., Mannino, S., & Milunsky, A. (1995). Teratogenicity of high vitamin A intake. *New England Journal of Medicine, 333*, 1369–1373.

Saari, J. C. (1994). Retinoids in photosensitive tissues. In M. B. Sporn, A. B. Roberts, & D. S.,Goodman (Eds.), *The retinoids, biology, chemistry and medicine* (pp. 351–386). New York: Raven Press.

Saari, J. C. (1999). Retinoids in mammalian vision. In H. Nau & W. S. Blaner (Eds.), *Retinoids: The biochemical and molecular basis of vitamin A and retinoid action* (pp. 563–588). Berlin: Springer-Verlag.

Saari, J. C., Nawrot, M., Kennedy, B. N., Garwin, G. G., Hurley, J. B., Huang, J., … Crabb, J. W. (2001). Visual cycle impairment in cellular retinaldehyde binding protein (CRALBP) knockout mice results in delayed dark adaptation. *Neuron, 29*, 739–748.

Schug, T. T., Berry, D. C., Shaw, N. S., Travis, S. N., & Noy, N. (2007). Opposing effects of retinoic acid on cell growth result from alternate activation of two different nuclear receptors. *Cell, 129*, 723–733.

Schug, T. T., Berry, D. C., Toshkov, I. A., Cheng, L., Nikitin, A. Y., & Noy, N. (2008). Overcoming retinoic acid-resistance of mammary carcinomas by diverting retinoic acid from PPAR-beta/delta to RAR. *Proceedings of the National Academy of Sciences of the United States of America, 105*, 7546–7551.

Semba, R. D., Muhilal, Scott, A. L., Natadisastra, G., Wirasasmita, S., Mele, L., … Sommer, A. (1992). Depressed immune response to tetanus in children with vitamin A deficiency. *The Journal of Nutrition, 122*, 101–107.

Shaw, G. M., Wasserman, C. R., Block, G., & Lammer, E. J. (1996). High maternal vitamin A intake and risk of anomalies of structures with a cranial neural crest cell contribution. *Lancet, 347*, 899–900.

Shaw, N. S., & Noy, N. (2001). Interphotoreceptor retinoid-binding protein contains three retinoid binding sites. *Experimental Eye Research, 72*, 183–190.

Simon, A., Lagercrantz, J., Bajalica-Lagercrantz, S., & Eriksson, U. (1996). Primary structure of human 11-*cis* retinol dehydrogenase and organization and chromosomal localization of the corresponding gene. *Genomics, 36*, 424–430.

Sommer, A. (1992). Vitamin A deficiency and childhood mortality. *Lancet, 340*, 488–489.

Sommer, A. (2008). Vitamin A deficiency and clinical disease: An historical overview. *The Journal of Nutrition, 138,* 1835–1839.

Sommer, A., & West, K. P., Jr. (1992). Vitamin A and childhood morbidity. *Lancet, 339,* 1302–1303.

Soprano, D. R., & Blaner, W. S. (1994). Plasma retinol-binding protein. In M. B. Sporn, A. B. Roberts, & D. S. Goodman (Eds.), *The retinoids, biology, chemistry, and medicine* (pp. 257–282). New York: Raven Press.

Soprano, D. R., Qin, P., & Soprano, K. J. (2004). Retinoic acid receptors and cancers. *Annual Review of Nutrition, 24,* 201–221.

Storch, J., & Corsico, B. (2008). The emerging functions and mechanisms of mammalian fatty acid–binding proteins. *Annual Review of Nutrition, 28,* 73–95.

Takahashi, N., & Breitman, T. R. (1991). Retinoylation of proteins in leukemia, embryonal carcinoma, and normal kidney cell lines: Differences associated with differential responses to retinoic acid. *Archives of Biochemistry and Biophysics, 285,* 105–110.

Tan, N. S., Shaw, N. S., Vinckenbosch, N., Liu, P., Yasmin, R., Desvergne, B., … Noy, N. (2002). Selective cooperation between fatty acid binding proteins and peroxisome proliferator-activated receptors in regulating transcription. *Molecular and Cellular Biology, 22,* 5114–5127.

Thaller, C., & Eichele, G. (1990). Isolation of 3,4-didehydroretinoic acid, a novel morphogenetic signal in the chick wing bud. *Nature, 345,* 815–819.

Thatcher, J. E., & Isoherranen, N. (2009). The role of CYP26 enzymes in retinoic acid clearance. *Expert Opinion on Drug Metabolism & Toxicology, 5,* 875–886.

Travis, G. H., Golczak, M., Moise, A. R., & Palczewski, K. (2007). Diseases caused by defects in the visual cycle: Retinoids as potential therapeutic agents. *Annual Review of Pharmacology and Toxicology, 47,* 469–512.

Vahlquist, A., & Torma, H. (1988). Retinoids and keratinization: Current concepts. *International Journal of Dermatology, 27,* 81–95.

Veerkamp, J. H., & Maatman, R. G. (1995). Cytoplasmic fatty acid–binding proteins: Their structure and genes. *Progress in Lipid Research, 34,* 17–52.

von Lintig, J., Kiser, P. D., Golczak, M., & Palczewski, K. (2010). The biochemical and structural basis for *trans*-to-*cis* isomerization of retinoids in the chemistry of vision. *Trends in Biochemical Sciences, 35,* 400–410.

Vu-Dac, N., Schoonjans, K., Kosykh, V., Dallongeville, J., Heyman, R. A., Staels, B., & Auwerx, J. (1996). Retinoids increase human apolipoprotein A-11 expression through activation of the retinoid X receptor but not the retinoic acid receptor. *Molecular and Cellular Biology, 16,* 3350–3360.

Wald, G. (1968). Molecular basis of visual excitation. *Science, 162,* 230–239.

Werler, M. M., Lammer, E. J., & Mitchell, A. A. (1996). Teratogenicity of high vitamin A intake. *New England Journal of Medicine, 334,* 1195–1196; author reply 1197.

West, K. P., Jr. (2003). Vitamin A deficiency disorders in children and women. *Food and Nutrition Bulletin, 24,* S78–S90.

Wolbach, S. B., & Howe, P. R. (1925). Tissue changes following deprivation of fat-soluble A vitamin.*The Journal of Experimental Medicine, 42* ,753–777.

Yamamoto, H., Simon, A., Eriksson, U., Harris, E., Berson, E. L., & Dryja, T. P. (1999). Mutations in the gene encoding 11-*cis* retinol dehydrogenase cause delayed dark adaptation and fundus albipunctatus. *Nature Genetics, 22,* 188–191.

Yang, Q., Graham, T. E., Mody, N., Preitner, F., Peroni, O. D., Zabolotny, J. M., … Kahn, B. B. (2005). Serum retinol binding protein 4 contributes to insulin resistance in obesity and type 2 diabetes. *Nature, 436,* 356–362.

RECOMMENDED READINGS

D'Ambrosio, D. N., Clugston, R. B., & Blaner, W. S. (2011). Vitamin A metabolism: An update. *Nutrients, 3, 63-103.*

Institute of Medicine. (2001). Vitamin A. In *Dietary reference intakes of vitamin A, vitamin K, arsenic, boron, chromium, copper, iodine, iron, manganese, molybdenum, nickel, silicon, vanadium, and zinc* (pp. 82–161). Washington, DC: National Academy Press.

Noy, N. (2010). Between death and survival: Retinoic acid in regulation of apoptosis. *Annual Review of Nutrition, 30,* 201–217.

Storch, J., & Thumser, A. E. (2010). Tissue-specific functions in the fatty acid–binding protein family. *The Journal of Biological Chemistry, 285,* 32679–32683.

CHAPTER 31

Vitamin D

Steven K. Clinton, MD, PhD*

COMMON ABBREVIATIONS

7-DHC	7-dehydrocholesterol
25OHD	25-hydroxyvitamin D; 25-hydroxycholecalciferol; calcidiol
$1,25(OH)_2D$	1,25-dihydroxyvitamin D; calcitriol
24-OH-ase	25-hydroxyvitamin D 24-hydroxylase
25-OH-ase	25-hydroxylase
1α-OH-ase	25-hydroxyvitamin D 1α-hydroxylase
D_2	vitamin D_2; ergocalciferol
D_3	vitamin D_3; cholecalciferol
PTH	parathyroid hormone
VDBP	vitamin D–binding protein
VDR	vitamin D receptor
VDRE	vitamin D response element

The discovery of vitamin D and its role in promoting bone health in the early decades of the twentieth century contributed to a dramatic decline in the incidence and prevalence of rickets that plagued children in the industrializing nations around the globe. In the years to come, many governments and medical organizations established public health guidelines for adequate intakes of vitamin D and calcium to promote bone health and prevent rickets and adult osteomalacia. In subsequent decades, the greater understanding of vitamin D biology coupled with the rapid growth of epidemiological and clinical studies examining relationships of vitamin D status to various diseases has stimulated an interest in the multifaceted and complex roles of this unique nutrient in an expanding array of human health outcomes. A distinctive aspect of vitamin D is that it can be synthesized by humans through the action of sunlight on exposed skin. Thus an understanding of vitamin D as both a hormone and nutrient presents challenges for the development of Dietary Reference Intake (DRI) values. The rapidly accumulating knowledge in recent years led to a revision of the DRIs for vitamin D and calcium (see Chapter 32) in 2011 by the Institute of Medicine (IOM) that will form the basis for efforts to promote health in the years to come.

Several key definitions are useful in the interpretation of this chapter and the published literature. Vitamin D levels in food and supplements are typically expressed in international units (IU) but may also be expressed as micrograms (μg). The biological activity of 1 μg of vitamin D_2 or D_3 is equivalent to 40 IU. Serum concentrations are expressed most commonly as nanomoles per liter (nmol/L) but can be converted into nanograms per milliliter (ng/mL) by multiplying by (384.6 ng/nmol) (L/1000mL).

*This chapter is a revision of the chapter contributed by Michael F. Holick, MD, PhD, for the second edition.

DIETARY AND ENDOGENOUS SOURCES OF VITAMIN D

The terms *vitamin D* and *calciferol* refer collectively to the two major nutritionally relevant chemical forms known as vitamin D_2 (ergocalciferol) and vitamin D_3 (cholecalciferol). Vitamin D_3 is the form produced in the skin of vertebrate animals when exposed to ultraviolet (UV) irradiation, whereas vitamin D_2 is produced from the precursor ergosterol by some phytoplankton, yeast, invertebrates, and fungi in response to UV irradiation. Vitamin D_2 is not synthesized by animals or land plants. Structural differences in the side chains (Figure 31-1) characterize the molecules, yet the biological activity of vitamin D_2 and D_3 are considered to be essentially equal in regards to correction of vitamin D deficiency. Vitamins D_2 and D_3 are both commercially synthesized and formulated into dietary supplements and may be added to fortify foods. Studies in animal models suggest that vitamin D_2 may have lower toxicity than vitamin D_3, but this has yet to be demonstrated in humans.

ENDOGENOUS SYNTHESIS AND METABOLISM OF VITAMIN D

Vitamin D can be synthesized by humans through an elegantly regulated multistep process that begins in the innermost strata of the skin, the stratum basal and stratum spinosum. 7-Dehydrocholesterol (7-DHC) is an immediate precursor of cholesterol synthesis and is abundantly synthesized by the differentiating cells of the epidermis and dermis. Following exposure to sunlight, 7-DHC in the skin absorbs ultraviolet B (UVB) photons with energies between

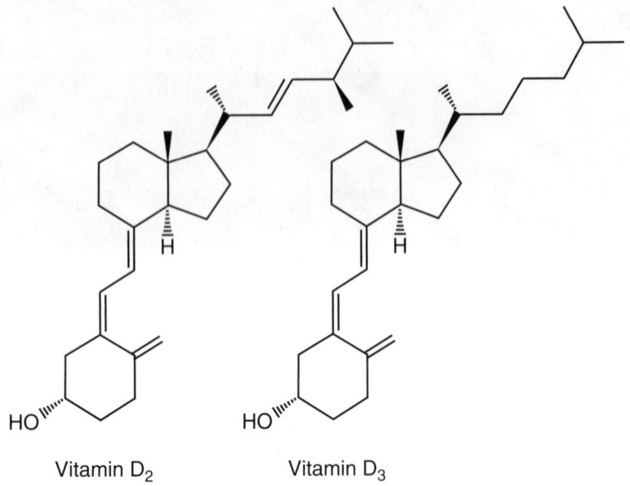

HO Vitamin D_2 HO Vitamin D_3

FIGURE 31-1 Comparison of vitamin D_2 and D_3 chemical structures.

290 and 320 nm. This process causes a transformation of 7-DHC to previtamin D_3 (Tian et al., 1994) (Figure 31-2). Although UV tanning lamps, including those in tanning beds, are dominated by light in the UVA spectrum, up to 10% of total UV exposure may be derived from UVB and impact vitamin D_3 synthesis. At normal body temperature, the previtamin D_3 undergoes a thermal isomerization of its double bonds to form vitamin D_3 (see Figure 31-2). As previtamin D_3 is converted to vitamin D_3, its three-dimensional structure changes, and this facilitates the translocation of vitamin D_3 from the skin cells to the bloodstream. In the circulation, the vitamin D_3 produced in the skin is bound to a specific α1-globulin known as vitamin D–binding protein (VDBP), the major plasma carrier of all vitamin D metabolites. VDBP may help sustain cutaneous synthesis by removing the end products and reducing negative feedback regulation.

The synthesis of vitamin D_3 is impacted by the availability of substrate, the intensity of irradiation reaching the dermis, and the length of exposure, ultimately reaching equilibrium between degradation and synthesis (Holick, 1995a). Indeed, toxic levels of vitamin D accumulating from skin synthesis are not known to occur. If vitamin D_3 does not exit from the skin into the circulation before being exposed to additional sunlight, it is degraded to many inactive forms, such as lumisterol and tachysterol (Holick, 1995a). In animals covered with fur or feathers, unique evolutionary adaptations allow vitamin D to be generated within the oily secretions deposited on the fur and feathers and ingested during grooming (Agarwal and Stout, 2004).

UPTAKE OF DIETARY VITAMIN D

Vitamin D can also be obtained from the diet as vitamin D_2 or vitamin D_3. Because vitamin D is fat-soluble, the vitamin is absorbed with other lipids in the intestine, a process facilitated by bile and pancreatic lipase (Holick, 1995b). Upon absorption, vitamin D appears in the chylomicrons that are released by the enterocytes and enters the lymphatic system, which drains into the venous bloodstream. Lipoprotein lipase, particularly in adipose tissue, acts upon chylomicron lipids and may result in a fraction of the vitamin D being taken up by fat cells. This observation suggests a mechanism whereby increased adiposity causes sequestering of vitamin D and is related to lower vitamin D status (IOM, 2011). Indeed, adipose tissue sequestration of vitamin D represents a nonspecific process, and these stores may not be actively used in periods of need (IOM, 2011). Thus obese individuals may require higher intakes of vitamin D to achieve serum concentrations of 25-hydroxyvitamin D (25OHD) comparable to those observed among lean individuals (IOM, 2011). Following depletion of triacylglycerols, the cholesterol-rich chylomicron remnants which still contain a significant fraction of the absorbed vitamin D are subsequently taken up by the liver.

METABOLISM OF VITAMIN D IN LIVER

Circulating vitamin D_2 or vitamin D_3 in chylomicron remnants, as well as VDBP-bound vitamin D_3 from endogenous synthesis, are taken up by the liver and hydroxylated by hepatic 25-hydroxylase (25-OH-ase), a mitochondrial and microsomal (endoplasmic reticulum) enzyme likely encoded by the gene *CYP2R1* (cytochrome P450 2R1) to form 25-hydroxycholecalciferol (25OHD) (see Figure 31-2). This enzyme is efficient and exhibits little or no feedback regulation. Like vitamin D, 25OHD circulates in plasma as a complex with VDBP. The plasma 25OHD level is currently considered to be the best measure of vitamin D status.

METABOLISM OF VITAMIN D IN KIDNEY

The subsequent metabolism of 25OHD to 1,25-dihydroxyvitamin D (1,25$[OH]_2$D) is the critical step in the endocrine regulatory process that is essential for maintaining homeostatic regulation of plasma calcium and phosphorus concentrations in ranges compatible with life and promotion of bone health. Delivery of 25OHD to the kidneys, and thus its conversion to 1,25$(OH)_2$D, depends upon the glomerular filtration of 25OHD–VDBP complexes from the plasma, followed by megalin-mediated endocytic uptake of 25OHD–VDBP from the glomerular filtrate into the proximal tubular cells of the kidney (Leheste et al., 2003). VDBP is a ligand of cubilin and megalin, which are two membrane-associated proteins that act in concert to mediate endocytic uptake of various small proteins and vitamin-carrier complexes across eptihelia. Therefore these endocytic receptors in the renal tubules are the major means by which 25OHD is targeted to the kidney (Nykjaer et al., 1999).

The enzymatic reaction producing 1,25$(OH)_2$D is highly regulated and is catalyzed by the action of mitochondrial 25-hydroxyvitamin D 1α-hydroxylase (1α-OH-ase), encoded by the *CYP27B1* (cytochrome P450 27B) gene. The expression of *CYP27B1* is stimulated by parathyroid hormone (PTH), whose main function is to respond to declining plasma calcium concentrations and act upon bone to stimulate calcium release, enhance active reabsorption of calcium from the kidney distal tubules, and stimulate production of 1,25$(OH)_2$D, which in turn will increase the

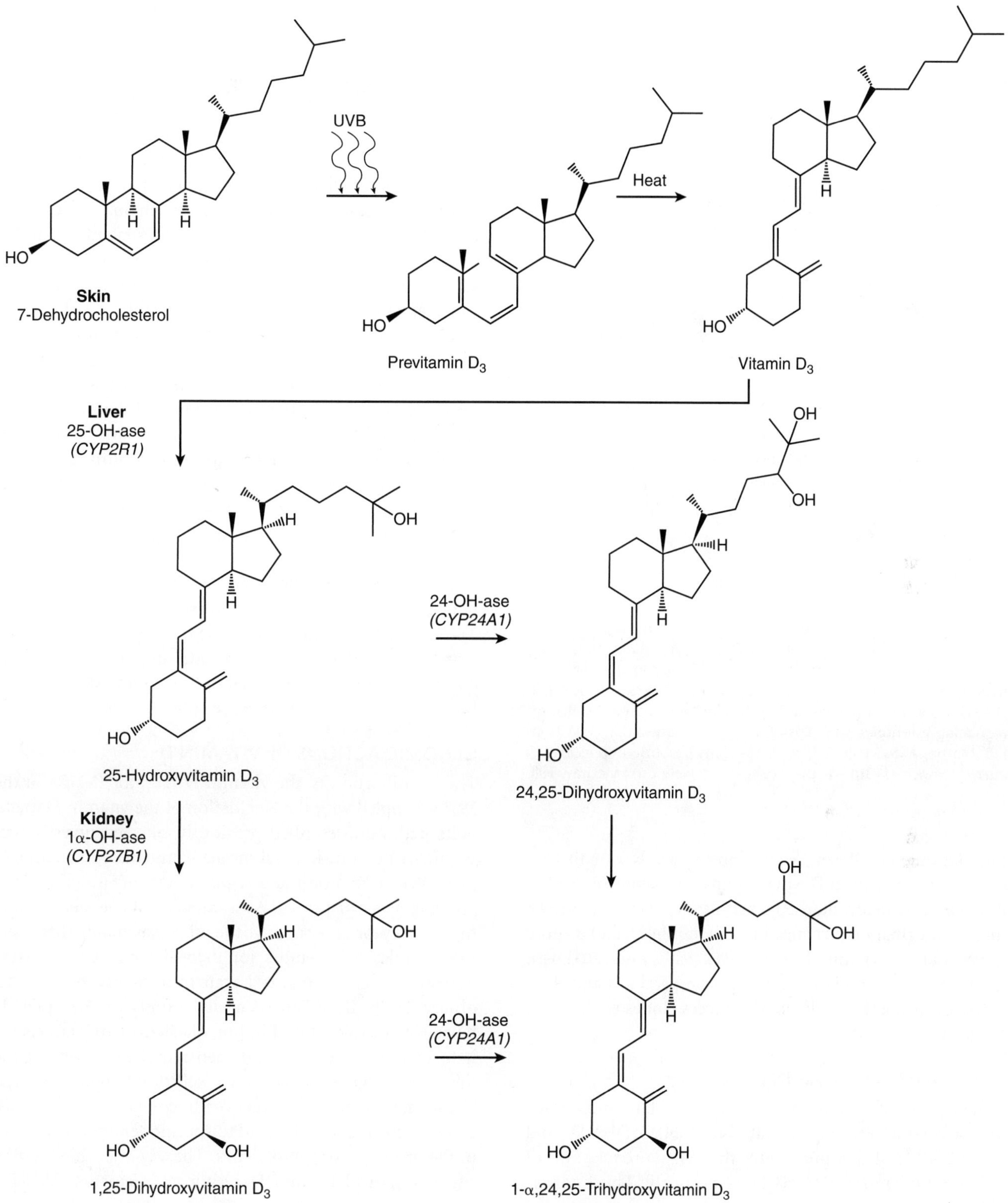

FIGURE 31-2 Vitamin D_3 synthesis and metabolism. The black triangular bonds indicate that the bond is coming toward you. The striped triangular bonds indicate that the bond is pointing away from you.

absorption of calcium by the intestine (Figure 31-3). As plasma concentrations of 1,25$(OH)_2$D increase, a negative feedback loop suppresses *CYP27B1* expression. Recently, the phosphaturic hormone, fibroblast-like growth factor-23, has been implicated as a counterregulatory hormone involved in suppressing *CYP27B1* expression (Galitzer et al., 2008; Bergwitz and Juppner, 2010; see Chapter 32, Figure 32-3).

1,25$(OH)_2$D is the high affinity ligand for the vitamin D receptor (VDR; see next section) and is transported from the kidney to target tissues via the VDBP. Studies in transgenic

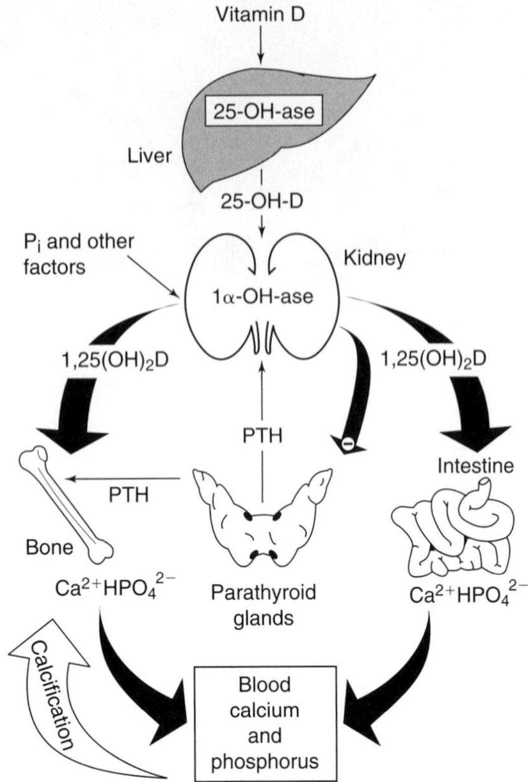

FIGURE 31-3 Metabolism of vitamin D and the biological actions of 1,25$(OH)_2$D. *25-OH-ase,* Vitamin D 25-hydroxylase; *1α-OH-ase,* 25-hydroxyvitamin D 1α-hydroxylase. Ca^{2+}, calcium ion, HPO_4^{2-}, hydrogen phophate ion. (From Holick, M. F., Krane, S., & Potts, J. T. [1994]. Calcium, phosphorus, and bone metabolism: Calcium-regulating hormones. In K. J. Isselbacher, E. Braunwald, J. D. Wilson, J. B. Martin, A. S. Fauci, & D. L. Kasper [Eds.], *Harrison's principles of internal medicine* [13th ed., pp. 2137–2151]. New York: McGraw-Hill.

mice lacking VDBP gene expression show only 10% to 15% of the plasma vitamin D when compared to controls. Other differences include a shortened half-life of plasma vitamin D, increased urinary concentrations of vitamin D, and a more rapid uptake of vitamin D by the liver that is associated with an increased catabolism to degradation products and their excretion primarily in the bile and feces (Jones et al., 1998; Berg, 1999).

CATABOLISM OF VITAMIN D

Catabolism of calciferol to more polar and readily excretable inactive metabolites, 24,25$(OH)_2$D and 1α,24,25$(OH)_2$D, begins with the 24-hydroxylation of either 25OHD or 1,25$(OH)_2$D, respectively. This hydroxylation reaction is catalyzed by the cytochrome P450 enzyme, 25-hydroxyvitamin D 24-hydroxylase (24-OH-ase), a protein encoded by the *CYP24A1* gene (Jones et al., 1998). Although *CYP24A1* is highly expressed in the kidney tubule, its tissue distribution is quite broad including the intestine, osteoblasts, placenta, keratinocytes, and prostate. The catabolic *CYP24A1* gene is potently induced by high plasma concentrations of 1,25$(OH)_2$D. Studies with mice lacking *CYP24A1* demonstrate an inability to clear plasma vitamin D, leading to a near 50% lethality at weaning (Masuda et al., 2005).

BIOLOGICAL ACTIONS OF VITAMIN D

1,25$(OH)_2$D is considered to be the biologically active hormonal form of vitamin D that is responsible for carrying out most, if not all, of the biological functions of vitamin D. A major function of 1,25$(OH)_2$D is to help maintain plasma concentrations of calcium within a normal range, which is achieved in part by increasing the efficiency of intestinal calcium absorption (Fleet and Schoch, 2010). 1,25$(OH)_2$D can dramatically impact the efficiency of intestinal calcium absorption from a basal level of 10% to 15% up to a level of 30% to 80%. 1,25$(OH)_2$D also increases the efficiency of intestinal phosphorus absorption. Other key tissues affected by 1,25$(OH)_2$D are the bones and kidneys. 1,25$(OH)_2$D along with PTH induces the formation and activation of osteoclasts, which function in the mobilization of calcium from bone (see Chapter 32, Figure 32-4). In addition, mature osteoblasts respond to 1,25$(OH)_2$D by increasing their expression of proteins involved in bone remodeling. 1,25$(OH)_2$D, together with PTH, also stimulates the renal distal tubule reabsorption of calcium. Thus overall, 1,25$(OH)_2$D acts on the intestines, bones, and kidneys to elevate plasma calcium (see Figure 31-3), which is required for mineralization of bone and for many other biological actions (see Chapter 32). Most of the effects of 1,25$(OH)_2$D on calcium homeostasis are mediated through alterations in gene expression.

GENOMIC ACTIONS OF VITAMIN D

The identification of the vitamin D receptor (VDR) in the 1970s, coupled with the elucidation of the vitamin D metabolic pathways described previously, allowed investigators to pursue the fundamental mechanisms whereby vitamin D promotes bone health and regulates various functions in a growing array of tissues. As a member of the steroid hormone receptor superfamily, the VDR has many characteristics similar to receptors for thyroid hormone, estrogen, testosterone, and retinoids. Localized primarily in the nuclei of target cells, the VDR has a high affinity for 1,25$(OH)_2$D hormone (or calcitriol). Binding of calcitriol to VDR causes it to be phosphorylated and then recruited by one of the three 9-*cis*-retinoid X receptors (RXRα, RXRβ, and RXRγ). These heterodimers interact with coregulatory proteins, allowing the complex to bind to specific genomic sequences in the promoter region of genes. The VDR-specific binding sites are named vitamin D–responsive elements (VDREs) (Figure 31-4).

The VDR and 1,25$(OH)_2$D ligand were found in the predicted target tissues of the intestine, bone, and kidney and strongly linked to the expected biological responses of increasing duodenal calcium absorption and enhanced bone mineralization. The best-characterized gene products that are induced by 1,25$(OH)_2$D in osteoblasts are osteocalcin, osteopontin, and alkaline phosphatase. Collectively, these proteins have a central role in the bone remodeling process. The major gene

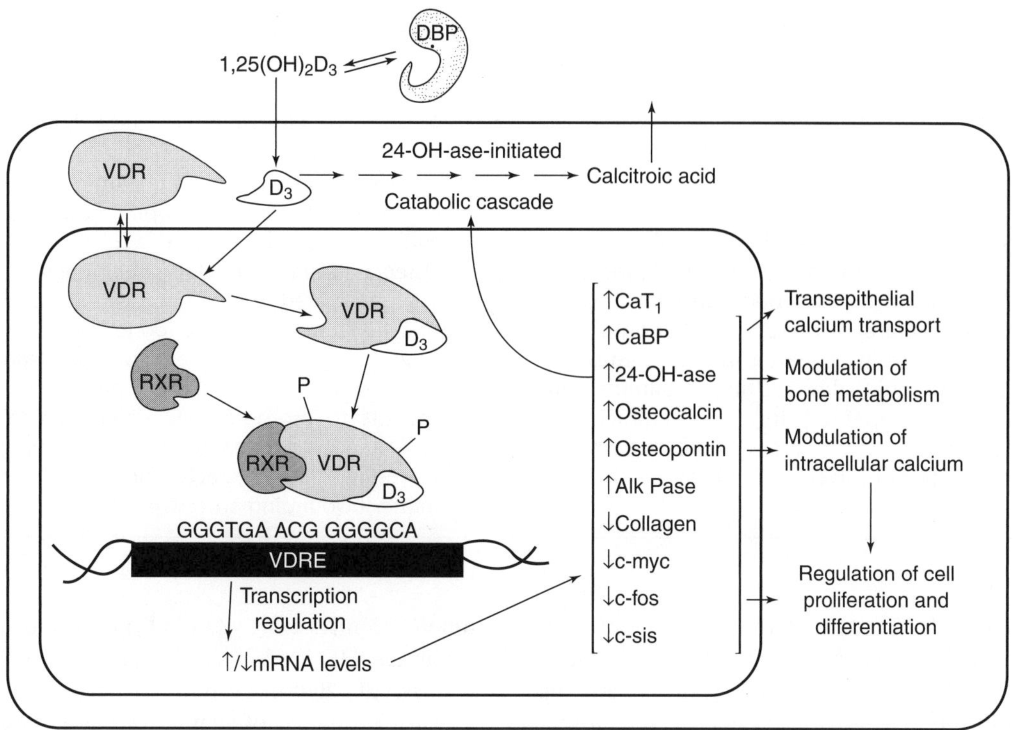

FIGURE 31-4 Cellular mechanisms of action. Proposed mechanism of action of $1,25(OH)_2D$ in target cells resulting in a variety of biological responses. The free form of $1,25(OH)_2D$ *(D_3)* enters the target cell and interacts with its nuclear vitamin D receptor *(VDR),* which is then phosphorylated *(P).* The $1,25(OH)_2D$–VDR complex combines with the retinoic acid X-receptor *(RXR)* to form a heterodimer, which in turn interacts with the vitamin D response element *(VDRE),* either enhancing or inhibiting transcription of vitamin D–responsive genes, such as for 25(OH)D-24-hydroxylase (24-OH-ase). (From Holick, M. F. [1996]. Vitamin D: Photobiology, metabolism, mechanism of action, and clinical applications. In M. J. Favus [Ed.], *Primer on the metabolic bone diseases and disorders of mineral metabolism* [3rd ed., pp. 74–81]. Philadelphia: Lippincott-Raven.) *Alk Pase,* alkaline phosphatase; *CaBP,* calcium binding protein; *CaT1,* epithelial calcium channel protein.

products induced in the small intestine by $1,25(OH)_2D$ are the epithelial calcium channel protein (CaT1) which directly affects the entry of calcium into the intestinal absorptive cell as well as several proteins that alter the flux of calcium across the intestinal absorptive cell (i.e., calcium binding protein [CaBP]) (see Figure 31-4). The translation of these laboratory findings to clinical application was rapid, with the demonstration that renal failure patients with poor synthesis of $1,25(OH)_2D$ responded to the pharmacological administration of the active hormone with enhanced calcium absorption and improved bone health (Brickman et al., 1972).

In recent decades, investigators have reported that the VDR is present in many tissues (Norman and Bouillon, 2010), most of which are not involved in calcium and phosphate homeostasis. The knowledge that the VDR acts as a transcription factor coupled with the presence of VDREs in the promoter regions of over 3% of genes in the human genome has greatly expanded research efforts to better elucidate the roles of vitamin D in the tissues and organs where the receptor is expressed. VDREs, considered the hallmark for vitamin D regulation of gene expression, are present in genes involved in a diverse range of processes, including the regulation of cell proliferation, differentiation, and apoptosis. In parallel, this knowledge also provides a molecular foundation for the study of an expanding array of disease processes that may theoretically be impacted by alterations in vitamin D status. Adding to the complexity of the vitamin D regulatory network, we now recognize that 1α-OH-ase is present in several tissues in addition to the kidney and that the local synthesis of the active hormone may have an autocrine or paracrine action to fine-tune tissue responses to vitamin D.

NONGENOMIC ACTIONS OF VITAMIN D

An emerging area of research focuses upon rapid steroid actions that mediate cellular effects occurring over seconds and minutes, as compared to the well-established genomic action of steroid hormones and receptor-mediated genomic actions that occur over hours or days and can be blocked by inhibitors of transcription (Mizwicki and Norman, 2009). Investigators have reported evidence for nongenomic actions of $1,25(OH)_2D$ that are independent of receptor-mediated transcription in a variety of cell types and tissues (Losel and Wehling, 2003; Norman, 2006; Mizwicki and Norman, 2009; Fleet and Schoch, 2010). Among the strongest examples for nongenomic actions of $1,25(OH)_2D$ is the induction of rapid intestinal absorption of calcium, called transcaltachia (Nemere et al., 1984; Huhtakangas et al., 2004; Fleet and Schoch, 2010), a process mediated by interactions with a membrane-associated, rapid response, steroid-binding protein (Nemere

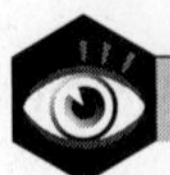

NUTRITION INSIGHT

Cells Involved in Bone Formation and Resorption

The major cells in bone that are concerned with bone formation and resorption are the osteoblasts, the osteocytes, and the osteoclasts. Osteoblasts are the bone-forming cells that secrete collagen, forming a matrix around themselves that then calcifies. Osteoblasts have VDRs and are responsive to changes in circulating concentrations of 1,25(OH)$_2$D. Osteoblasts arise from osteoprogenitor cells that are of mesenchymal origin. The osteoblasts seem to form at least a partial membrane that separates bone fluid (the fluid in most immediate contact with hydroxyapatites) from the extracellular fluid of the rest of the body. In this way, the calcium and phosphate concentrations in bone fluid can be carefully regulated.

As osteoblasts become surrounded by new bone (calcified matrix), they become osteocytes. Osteocytes remain in contact with one another and with osteoblasts via tight junctions between long protoplasmic processes that run through channels in the bone.

Osteoclasts are multinuclear cells that erode and resorb previously formed bone. Osteoclasts are derived from monocytic stem cells in the bone marrow as a result of stimulation of these cells by 1,25(OH)$_2$D–induced receptor activator of nuclear factor kappa B ligand (RANKL) on osteoblasts to promote their differentiation into osteoclasts. Osteoclasts appear to phagocytose and break down bone, resulting in a characteristic "chewed-out" edge on the bone surrounding an active osteoclast.

et al., 2004). Transcaltachia may lead to activation of multiple signaling cascades, such as phosphorylation of protein kinase C, the opening of cellular calcium channels resulting in an increase in intracellular calcium uptake, and further activation of the mitogen activiated protein kinase pathways. These cascades may enhance expression of the VDR, providing a basis for cross-talk and cooperation with the genomic pathway to induce biological responses.

EVALUATION OF VITAMIN D STATUS

Among scientists and the medical community, it is generally agreed that the serum concentration of 25OHD is the best surrogate biomarker of vitamin D status. Because the hepatic vitamin D 25-OH-ase is efficient and not tightly regulated, any increase in vitamin D intake or cutaneous production of vitamin D$_3$ leads to an increase in the circulating concentration of 25OHD. Hence, 25OHD is a valuable marker for determining an individual's vitamin D status at a specific time. Low or undetectable circulating concentrations of 25OHD (less than 10 ng/mL) are diagnostic of vitamin D deficiency. Currently, several different types of assays are employed, each with their own strengths and weaknesses (Carter et al., 2010). Antibody-based and liquid chromatography–based methods are currently used and are equivalent in terms of measuring total 25OHD. However, controversy remains over the performance of these assays in various clinical and research laboratories (IOM, 2011). For example, assay shift and drift must be considered in the evaluation of data from the NHANES (National Health and Nutrition Examination Survey) reports (IOM, 2011).

Serum vitamin D is not a biomarker for dietary intake as the relationship between dietary intake and circulating 25OHD is nonlinear. Many factors may impact the association between vitamin D intake and serum 25OHD; the most critical is endogenous synthesis (Cashman et al., 2008a, 2008b, 2009; Smith et al., 2009; IOM, 2011). Evidence suggests that increasing the serum level of 25OHD above 50 nmol/L requires more vitamin D intake than does increasing serum 25OHD levels when initial concentrations are lower (Aloia et al., 2008). A crude estimate is that for each additional 1,000 IU/day of vitamin D intake, the serum 25OHD concentration may increase by 10 to 20 nmol/L.

A key area of controversy relates to defining specific cutoff points of circulating 25OHD levels to define deficiency, marginal deficiency, normal ranges, and concentrations associated with toxicity. The recent National Academy of Sciences committee recognized the controversy regarding this issue, and many committee members suggested the need to develop a consensus that impacts the interpretation of clinical testing and the medical management of individuals, in addition to helping scientists and public health officials interpret human population-based studies (Ross et al., 2011). It is also important to consider the need for studies to define serum concentration standards in different age groups, from infants to the elderly, and to consider potential ethnic and gender differences. Finally, it is critical to develop studies to assess the combined and individual contributions of solar radiation and dietary intake to serum concentrations of 25OHD in healthy and diseased populations, in terms of mean values and the many genetic and environmental factors that may also impact vitamin D status.

In spite of the aforementioned limitations and concerns, a general strategy for interpretation of serum concentrations of 25OHD can be stated. Those with serum concentrations less than 5 ng/mL (12 nmol/L) are considered to be at risk of severe vitamin D deficiency (IOM, 2011). Individuals with a serum concentration in this range for 1 to 2 years may develop clinically relevant rickets or osteomalacia, particularly if dietary calcium intake is marginal (IOM, 2011). A serum concentration of 20 ng/mL (50 nmol/L) of 25OHD is considered adequate to satisfy the needs for bone health in the vast majority (97.5%) of healthy adults. The range of optimal serum 25OHD concentrations for other health outcomes related to vitamin D (such as cancer prevention or the prevention of frailty or falls in the elderly) is the subject of much debate. There is clearly a wide range of serum 25OHD concentrations where no clear evidence of toxicity has been reported. Many have assumed that the physiological production of vitamin D in humans with extensive exposure to the sun should provide information about levels of 25OHD that are not toxic. In studies of outdoor workers, such as lifeguards, mean serum concentrations of 25OHD of nearly 125 nmol/L (50 ng/mL) are observed (IOM, 2011). There are a few well-documented human studies of vitamin D toxicity in which serum 25OHD was measured (IOM, 2011). Based on these case-reports of vitamin D intoxication, serum concentrations above 100 to 150 ng/mL (250 to 375 nmol/L) raise concern for toxicity (IOM, 2011).

DIETARY SOURCES OF VITAMIN D

Total vitamin D intake includes both foods and dietary supplements. Foods naturally containing vitamin D are limited (U.S. Department of Agriculture [USDA], Agricultural Research Service [ARS], 2010). The richest sources of dietary vitamin D are fatty fish, such as salmon and sardines; liver oil extracts, such as cod liver oil; and egg yolks. In the United States, fluid milk is voluntarily fortified with 400 IU per quart (385 IU/L), and similar quantities are usually added to fortified plant-based milk substitutes. More recently, some cereals and breads have been fortified with vitamin D. Other milk-based products, including ice cream and cheeses, are not typically fortified with vitamin D, whereas some yogurts are fortified. In Canada, fortification of fluid milk (350 to 450 IU/L) and margarine (530 IU/g) is mandatory. Infant formulas are also fortified at levels consistent with those found in human milk and deemed to satisfy daily requirements (40 to 100 IU of vitamin D per 100 kcal in the United States and 40 to 80 IU per 100 kcal in Canada). Globally, many nations, particularly those in economically less developed areas, do not fortify with vitamin D, and the lack of reliable sources raises concerns for malnutrition in these populations.

The supplement industry is rapidly expanding and consumption of individual vitamin supplements is more prevalent today than in the past. Vitamin D is provided in supplements as either D_2 or D_3, with a trend toward vitamin D_3 being more common. In the United States, marketed supplements are increasingly being formulated at higher doses, often at 1,000 to 5,000 IU per dose, with some as high as 50,000 IU. In Canada, dosages of vitamin D above 1,000 IU are only available by prescription.

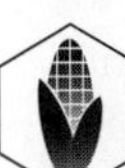

FOOD SOURCES OF VITAMIN D

- 815 IU per ½ fillet salmon (sockeye, cooked, dry heat)
- 706 IU per 1 piece swordfish (cooked, dry heat)
- 465 IU per 3 oz salmon (pink, canned, solids with bone and liquid)
- 367 IU per ½ fillet halibut (Atlantic and Pacific, cooked, dry heat)
- 154 IU per 3 oz tuna (light, canned in water, drained solids)
- 120 IU per 1 cup milk (fluid, 2% milk fat, with added vitamin A and D)
- 41 IU per 1 cup mushrooms, shiitake (cooked without salt)
- 40 to 100 IU per ¾ cup to 1⅓ cup various ready-to-eat cereals
- 36 IU per 1 medium egg (whole, raw, fresh)
- 21 IU per 3 oz pork (fresh, loin, center, bone-in, separable lean and fat, cooked, pan-fried)
- 9 IU per 1 tbsp butter, without salt
- 7 IU per 1 oz cheddar cheese
- 5 IU per 8 oz yogurt (plain, whole milk, 8 g protein per 8 oz)

Data from USDA, ARS. (2010). *USDA National Nutrient Database for Standard Reference, Release 23.* Retrieved from http://www.ars.usda.gov/ba/bhnrc/ndl.

SOLAR CONTRIBUTION TO VITAMIN D STATUS

Vitamin D synthesis in the skin occurs upon exposure to UVB radiation at wavelengths of 290 to 320 nm, and vitamin D synthesis in the skin can produce significant quantities of vitamin D. However, predicting vitamin D status based upon estimated sun exposure is difficult. The time of day, season, and latitude have dramatic effects on the amount of solar UVB radiation that reaches the earth's surface. In winter, vitamin-producing UVB photons pass through the ozone layer at an oblique angle, causing many to be absorbed by the ozone. More UVB photons penetrate the ozone layer in the spring, summer, and fall months because the sun is directly overhead. In general, reliable vitamin D synthesis to meet individual needs can be achieved at the equator and up to 40 degrees north and south. This leaves up to a third of the global population in areas where UVB is estimated to be marginal to provide adequate amounts of vitamin D.

Seasonal changes in vitamin D status are well documented and should be considered in the interpretation of epidemiological studies. In general, populations in temperate latitudes appear to experience increases in 25OHD serum concentrations in summer months as compared to winter (IOM, 2011). Yet latitude alone does not consistently correlate with average serum 25OHD concentrations of populations, and certainly not for individuals within a population (IOM, 2011); thus correlation of latitude with health or disease outcomes provides little insight into a mediating role of vitamin D.

Another key area of research concerns the synthesis of vitamin D in populations with differing skin pigmentation, (Armas et al., 2007; Snellman et al., 2009; Bogh et al., 2010). Skin color is mainly due to pigments called melanins, which are produced by melanocytes in the epidermis. Melanins can act as photoprotectants by absorbing UVB radiation. Loomis (1967) popularized the theory that melanin pigmentation in humans evolved to protect people who lived at or near the equator from producing excessive, toxic amounts of vitamin D_3. He further speculated that as populations migrated north and south of the equator, their skin pigmentation diminished to promote adequate vitamin D_3 synthesis in their skin, thus protecting their bones from rickets and osteomalacia. An individual with very dark skin pigmentation will require about ten times longer exposure to sunlight to produce the same amount of vitamin D_3 in his or her skin than a light-skinned person (Clemens et al., 1982). Indeed, NHANES data suggest that serum 25OHD concentrations are highest in whites, intermediate in Hispanics, and lowest in those of African descent living in the United States (Looker et al., 2008b). However, it must be noted that extensive variability exists among individuals within ethnic groups and that many other factors impact serum 25OHD concentrations (Aloia, 2008). In addition, fundamental differences in vitamin D metabolism and resultant bone health between ethnic groups are poorly understood (Talwar et al., 2007a, 2007b).

Similarly, extensive body covering with clothing may limit vitamin D synthesis (Diehl and Chiu, 2010). Populations such as bedouins, living in the Negev Desert in Israel, who are required to have most of the skin surface covered by clothing, are prone to developing vitamin D deficiency (Taha et al., 1984). Clothing absorbs most ultraviolet radiation; therefore covering the skin with most types of clothing will prevent or limit the cutaneous production of vitamin D_3 (Matsuoka et al., 1992).

Public health education has encouraged the use of sunscreens to reduce sun damage and skin cancer incidence. Interestingly, as sunscreens are evaluated in research settings and in free-living individuals where they are improperly or inadequately employed, the actual impact on vitamin D status is often difficult to quantify (Diehl and Chiu, 2010; Springbett et al., 2010). Less well studied are the effects of altitude, regular outdoor activities, and poorly understood genetic factors that influence the many steps in vitamin D metabolism and action. All of these issues must be taken into account when individuals are being evaluated for vitamin D–related medical conditions.

Declines in tissue and organ function are characteristics of aging. Therefore it is not surprising that aging reduces the capacity of human skin to synthesize vitamin D_3. Aging decreases the concentration of 7-DHC in the epidermis; the capacity of the skin to produce vitamin D_3 is reduced by approximately 75% by age 70 years compared to younger adults (Holick et al., 1989). It is recognized that elderly people may also exhibit a reduced ability to adapt to a low-calcium diet by increasing their efficiency of intestinal calcium absorption (Ireland and Fordtran, 1973). Additional evidence suggests that the ability of the kidneys to upregulate the production of $1,25(OH)_2D$ by PTH is less efficient with age (Riggs et al., 1981; Slovik et al., 1981). Furthermore, aging may also decrease the responsiveness of the intestinal VDR to $1,25(OH)_2D$ (Riggs et al., 1981; Ebeling et al., 1992). Thus multiple age-related changes in vitamin D metabolism support a greater need for dietary vitamin D intake to maintain optimal health.

Because UVB irradiation is not without risks, it is inappropriate to suggest that individuals choose sun exposure as an approach to satisfy vitamin D status in an era of readily available fortified foods and dietary supplements. Skin cancer, particularly the aggressive forms of malignant melanoma, are clearly related to UVB exposure, either from solar radiation or UV radiation from tanning beds.

VITAMIN D TOXICITY

It is difficult to achieve toxic levels of vitamin D from a combination of endogenous production and the consumption of typical supplements and fortified food sources. However, accidental toxic exposures that have significant impacts upon health can occur (IOM, 2011). Human vitamin D toxicity typically causes hypercalcemia. The pathogenesis is frequently due to excess vitamin D supplementation, leading to the production of high concentrations of 25OHD by the liver, a step that is efficient and lacks significant feedback regulation. Indeed, it is likely that manifestations of vitamin D toxicity in these cases may be mediated by the 25OHD rather than $1,25(OH)_2D$. Acute hypercalcemia in humans may present as loss of appetite, nausea, vomiting, dehydration, renal impairment, mental status changes, and coma, which if left untreated can be lethal. A more modest hypercalcemia with chronic duration may lead to ectopic tissue calcification and end-organ dysfunction, as has been clearly demonstrated in rodent models. Analysis of population studies suggested that risk of undesirable health outcomes, including pancreatic cancer, all cause mortality, cardiovascular disease, falls, and fractures, is elevated in people with serum 25OHD levels above 50 ng/mL (125 nmol/L) (IOM, 2011; Ross et al., 2011).

A subset of the population may be more sensitive to developing toxicity at serum 25OHD concentrations and vitamin D intakes within the normal range. For example, those with diseases that compromise the usual negative feedback on the renal 1α-OHase are at greater risk of toxicity. Those with chronic inflammatory diseases characterized by activation of monocytes and macrophages, such as sarcoidosis or tuberculosis, may have entopic activation of their 1α-OH-ase, which may result in excessive production of the active hormone leading to hypervitaminosis D. Patients may experience fatigue, weakness, and irritability, or memory and cognitive dysfunction; but because of compensatory suppression of PTH, frank hypercalcemia may not always occur. Interestingly, sarcoidosis can often be an undiagnosed indolent disease in a population, and its detection may be precipitated by vitamin D supplementation and hypercalcemia.

DIETARY REFERENCE INTAKES FOR VITAMIN D

The DRIs are public health recommendations and serve as a set of nutrient-based guidelines for good nutrition among healthy men and women over the life span as well as during uncomplicated pregnancy and lactation. The IOM in 2011 published new DRIs for calcium and vitamin D (IOM, 2011) following a two-year review of the current evidence-based literature. Reevaluation of the DRIs for calcium

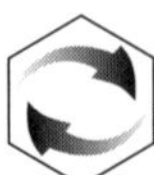

DRIs Across the Life Cycle: Vitamin D

	IU Vitamin D per Day	
Infants	RDA	UL
0 through 6 mo	400 (AI)	1,000
7 through 12 mo	400 (AI)	1,500
Children		
1 through 18 yr	600	2,500–4,000*
Adults		
19 through 50 yr	600	4,000
51 through 70 yr	600	4,000
≥71 yr	800	4,000
Pregnant	600	4,000
Lactating	600	4,000

Data from IOM. (2011). *Dietary Reference Intakes for calcium and vitamin D.* Washington, DC: The National Academies Press.
*UL is 2,500 IU for 1 through 3 years old, 3,000 IU for 4 through 8 years old, and 4,000 IU for 9 through 18 years old.
AI, Adequate Intake; *DRI,* Dietary Reference Intake; *IU,* international unit; *RDA,* Recommended Dietary Allowance; *UL,* Tolerable Upper Intake Level.

and Vitamin D was carried out because more information and higher quality studies had emerged since the previous evaluation in 1997.

The committee first examined the wealth of data related to health outcomes, including cancers, cardiovascular disease, hypertension, diabetes, metabolic syndrome, falls, immune system diseases, infectious disease, neuropsychological disease and functioning, diseases of pregnancy, and skeletal health. After a comprehensive review of published data, it was clear that bone health was the only area where conclusive evidence was available upon which DRIs could be established. In each of the other areas, studies often provided mixed or inconclusive results, particularly in regards to providing critical insight into dose–response relationships that are necessary to establish DRIs. Thus bone growth and maintenance served as the "indicator" health outcome for the 2011 DRIs.

The IOM committee recognized that seasonality of solar exposure, skin pigmentation, genetic factors, sunscreen use, latitude, outdoor activities, and religious and cultural habits related to body covering all contribute to heterogeneity in estimated endogenous vitamin D production. Therefore it would be impossible to define DRIs for varying levels of host vitamin D synthesis. Thus the DRIs are set with the assumption that dietary intake is the sole source of vitamin D.

The Estimated Average Requirement (EAR) corresponding to the median intake needs of the population was set at 400 IU/day across age groups, gender, and reproductive status, with the exception of infants for whom only an Adequate Intake based on typical intake was established. Recommended Dietary Allowances (RDAs), corresponding to two standard deviations above the EAR, was set at 600 IU/day for all individuals from 1 through 70 years of age, including pregnant and lactating women. However, because of inefficiencies in vitamin D absorption and metabolism that may impact bioavailability, the RDA was set at 800 IU/day for adults age 71 years and older. Recommended levels of intake are expected to provide serum concentrations of approximately 20 ng/mL (50 nmol/L) and to meet the needs for bone health in 97.5% of the healthy population (IOM, 2011).

The DRI process also includes defining an UL, the highest level of intake of a nutrient that is likely to pose no health risk. The starting point for defining the UL for vitamin D was 10,000 IU/day, a level of intake associated with hypercalcemia or acute toxicity. In addition, emerging data suggesting the potential for risk of certain cancers, all-cause mortality, and other outcomes to be increased at high levels of intake producing serum 25OHD levels above 50 ng/mL (125 nmol/L), provided a basis for defining the UL. The committee followed an approach to maximize public health protection and concluded that surpassing the 4,000 IU/day exposure leads to blood concentrations that begin to be associated with a greater risk of adverse health effects in some studies (IOM, 2011).

VITAMIN D AND HEALTH OUTCOMES

VITAMIN D IN BONE HEALTH

Vitamin D, along with calcium, plays a critical role in bone mineralization and bone disorders that may result from inadequate circulating levels of the biologically active metabolite of vitamin D. Vitamin D is a calciotropic hormone that acts to maintain blood calcium and phosphorus within the narrow physiological ranges for these ions. When the body's need for calcium to maintain metabolic functions is satisfied, calcium can be deposited into the skeleton. In periods of deficient vitamin D intake and resultant insufficient absorption of calcium, bone mineralization is compromised so that plasma calcium levels can be maintained within the normal range. Vitamin D deficiency reduces the efficiency of intestinal calcium absorption from an estimated 30% to 50% to no more than 10% to 15%, resulting in a decrease in plasma ionized calcium. The decreased plasma ionized calcium level is sensed by the parathyroid glands, which respond with an increase in PTH production and secretion. Release of PTH, in turn, leads to increased renal tubular calcium reabsorption and calcium conservation.

Rickets

Clinical vitamin D deficiency is commonly referred to as rickets in children and osteomalacia in adults. Rickets is characterized by a failure of the cartilage to mature and mineralize normally. The epiphyseal plates do not close until after puberty, so vitamin D deficiency in infants and children causes disorganization and hypertrophy of the chondrocytes at the mineralization front as well as a mineralization defect. The resultant characteristics of vitamin D–deficiency rickets (Figure 31-5) are short stature, a widening at the end of the long bones, rachitic rosary (i.e., enlargements of the costochondral junctions, which appear as a row of beadlike bumps that resemble rosary beads), and deformations in the skeleton. The bone deformities of the lower limbs are often

CLINICAL CORRELATION

Vitamin D–Dependent Rickets Type II

The vitamin D receptor (VDR) is a nuclear transcription factor that binds to the vitamin D response element (VDRE) of certain genes to regulate their expression. Vitamin D–dependent rickets type II (VDDRII) is a rare autosomal recessive disease that results from target organ resistance to the action of 1,25$(OH)_2$D. Mutations in the gene for VDR result in an inability of VDR to bind 1,25$(OH)_2$D or of the receptor-hormone complex to bind to VDRE in DNA. Affected patients usually present early in childhood with severe rickets, hypocalcemia, and growth retardation. Cultured fibroblasts obtained from these patients fail to respond to 1,25$(OH)_2$D by increasing synthesis of 25-hydroxyvitamin D 24-hydroxylase; this is used as a test for a defect in the 1,25$(OH)_2$D receptor–effector system. In patients with VDDRII, physiological doses of 1,25$(OH)_2$D have no therapeutic effect. In some patients, high-dose calcium therapy or pharmacological doses of vitamin D metabolites have resulted in biochemical and radiological improvement.

Thinking Critically

1. What effect would you expect a defect in the 1,25$(OH)_2$D receptor–effector system to have on calcium absorption? Why?
2. Would high-dose calcium therapy (intravenous or oral) potentially improve bone growth in patients with defects in the 1,25$(OH)_2$D receptor–effector system? Why?
3. For pharmacological doses of 1,25$(OH)_2$D to be effective, would some residual VDR need to be present? Why?

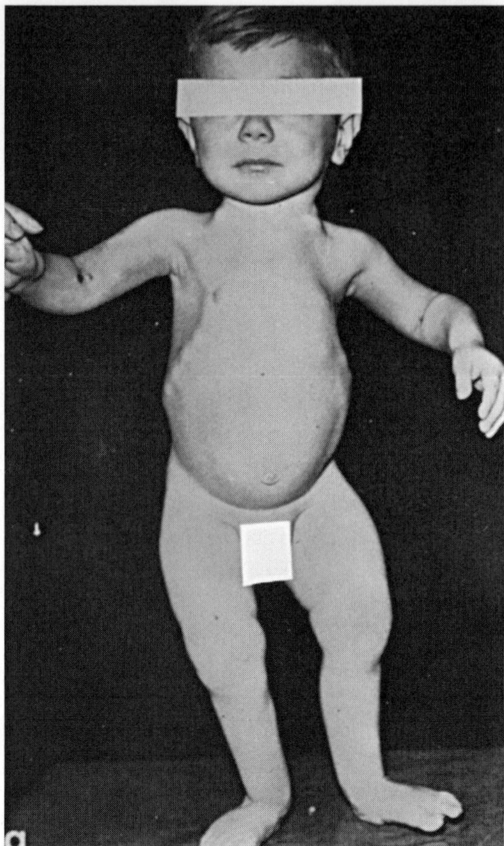

FIGURE 31-5 Child with rickets showing the characteristic bony deformities, including bowed legs and rachitic rosary of the rib cage. (From Fraser, D., & Scriver, C. R. [1994]. Disorders associated with hereditary or acquired abnormalities of vitamin D function: Hereditary disorders associated with vitamin D resistance or defective phosphate metabolism. In L. J. DeGroot [Ed.], *Endocrinology* [pp. 797–808]. New York: Grune and Stratton.)

referred to as "bowed legs" or "knocked knees." Remarkably, nutritional rickets continues to occur throughout the world, with reports documenting cases from over 60 nations in recent decades (Thacher et al., 2006).

The recent IOM report summarized the literature regarding serum 25OHD levels and the risk of rickets (IOM, 2011). The risk of rickets is higher in children who have serum 25OHD concentrations of 12 ng/mL (30 nmol/L) or below, but the risk is much less when the serum 25OHD is in the range of 12 to 20 ng/mL (30 to 50 nmol/L). The association of vitamin D status with incidence of rickets is dependent on adequate calcium intakes. For example, when calcium intakes are inadequate, vitamin D supplementation that increases serum concentration of 25OHD to 30 ng/mL (75 nmol/L) has no effect on development of rickets, illustrating the key role of calcium in this relationship. Importantly, the 25OHD concentration may only be marginally low in rickets if a simultaneous severe calcium deficiency is present (DeLucia et al., 2003).

Osteomalacia

In adults, the epiphyseal plates are closed, and hence adult vitamin D deficiency does not mimic the bony deformities observed in vitamin D–deficient children. Osteomalacia, characterized by poor mineralization of the collagen matrix of bone (i.e., the osteoid that forms before bone maturation), has emerged as a significant metabolic bone disease in our aging population (Bhan et al., 2010). Although osteomalacia does not cause dramatic bony deformities, it can cause severe osteopenia, which is reduced bone mineral density that can be observed as a reduced density of the skeleton as seen in radiographs. This mineralization defect contributes to an increased risk of skeletal fractures (Aaron et al., 1974a, 1974b). In some cases, osteomalacia can cause a localized or more generalized deep bone pain syndrome. This is thought to be due to the hydration of the unmineralized matrix in the bone, which exerts an outward pressure on the sensory fibers of the periosteum, resulting in throbbing bone pain (Holick, 2003; Bhan et al., 2010). The periosteum is a fibrous sheath covering bone that contains the blood vessels and nerves that provide nourishment and sensation to the bone. Laboratory testing of adults with osteomalacia may show hypocalcemia, hypophosphatemia, and increased serum bone alkaline phosphatase (Bhan et al., 2010). As vitamin D deficiency progresses, the associated PTH hypersecretion contributes to increased bone remodeling, bone resorption, and the cortical thinning noted on radographs.

Use of Bone Health Outcomes in Setting the DRIs

The IOM evaluated the relatonship between vitamin D status and bone health in establishing the current DRI for vitamin D (IOM, 2011). Unfortunately, many studies have not been conducted using a range of vitamin D doses. In addition, in many studies a combination of vitamin D and calcium have been administered, making interpretation very problematic, particularly for the purpose of establishing nutrient DRIs. Though some randomized controlled clinical studies suggested that serum 25OHD concentrations of 16 ng/mL (40 nmol/L) are sufficient to meet bone health requirements for the majority of healthy subjects, findings from other studies suggested that levels of 20 ng/mL (50 nmol/L) are consistent with optimal bone health. Observational studies (Cauley et al., 2008, 2009; Looker et al., 2008a; Ensrud et al., 2009; Melhus et al., 2010) have generally supported the findings of clinical investigations, suggesting a similar range of optimal serum 25OHD (IOM, 2011). A remarkable study by Priemel and associates (2010) was used by the recent DRI committee to support a serum 25OHD level of 20 ng/mL (50 nmol/L) as providing adequate vitamin D for at least 97.5% of the healthy population (IOM, 2011). The study examined bone biopsy specimens and serum 25OHD concentrations in a cohort of humans with unexpected deaths, for example from traumatic accidents. Evidence for loss of bone mineralization in individuals with with serum 25OHD levels above 20 ng/mL was not present. The data also indicated that even relatively low serum 25OHD levels were not associated with histological measures of osteomalacia in many individuals, a finding most likely related to the presence of adequate calcium intake. Furthermore, these data also indicated that in the setting of adequate calcium, vitamin D has less of an impact on bone health, whereas in periods of marginal calcium intake, vitamin D can play a more substantial role. The DRI committee employed this information to establish an EAR for young and middle-aged adults of 400 IU/day of vitamin D. This is consistent with a serum 25OHD concentration of 16 ng/mL (40 nmol/L) and a RDA of 600 IU/day providing a serum 25OH of 20 ng/mL (50 nmol/L) in healthy individuals.

For those over age 70 years, reduction in fracture risk was used by the IOM (2011) as a key outcome because of its greater prevalence and associated risk of significant morbidity and high subsequent mortality. Many but not all studies suggest that adequate vitamin D and calcium intake reduces the risk of falls and fractures (Jackson et al., 2006; Avenell et al., 2009; Bischoff-Ferrari et al., 2009a, 2009b; Sanders et al., 2010). Certainly, many factors contribute to the heterogeneity of this age group relative to obtaining adequate vitamin D and calcium, and aging is associated with inefficiencies in optimal metabolism of these nutrients. In addition, defining an independent effect of vitamin D or calcium with regard to bone events is difficult due to the design of many trials that incorporate both nutrients. Thus the DRI committee considered that a level of uncertainty should be included when defining the specifications of the RDA for vitamin D in people older than 70 years. With these considerations of uncertainty and heterogeneity, the RDA for the older population groups was established as 800 IU/day.

VITAMIN D AND EXTRASKELETAL HEALTH OUTCOMES

The discovery of VDRs (vitamin D receptors) and the presence of 1α-OH-ase activity in multiple tissues, including muscle cells, the immune system, vascular cells, many epithelial cell types, and the placenta, led to studies of possible autocrine and paracrine effects of vitamin D far beyond its role in skeletal health (Norman and Bouillon, 2010). Vitamin D may contribute to normal functions of nonskeletal tissues, whereas a deficiency—either systemically as defined by low circulating 25OHD or low active calcitriol in the blood, or within a tissue microenvironment because of aberrations in the local production of $1,25(OH)_2D$ or its signaling—may contribute to disease processes.

Mortality Rates

There is some evidence that overall mortality rates vary for populations differing in vitamin D status. For example, data from NHANES III suggested a risk of death (all-cause mortality) that was higher in those with 25OHD values of less than 10 ng/mL (25 nmol/L) compared to those with values higher than 20 ng/mL (50 nmol/L) (Ginde et al., 2009b). Confounding covariables may impact the interpretation of such studies. Although interesting, data such as these may reflect the fact that those with underlying illness, increased frailty, and reduced physical activity tend to have lower vitamin D levels secondary to poor nutrition and limited outdoor activity. For example, obesity is associated with many diseases that reduce longevity and is also associated with lower serum vitamin D concentrations. Thus vitamin D in this situation may not be the causative factor. A meta-analysis of 18 randomized controlled trials of vitamin supplementation with a mean follow-up time of 5.7 years in aging women reported a modest 7% lower risk of death in those with vitamin D supplementation between 300 and 2,000 IU/day (Autier and Gandini, 2007).

Cardiovascular Disease

Observational epidemiological studies suggest an enhanced risk of cardiovascular mortality and disease prevalence for those with lower vitamin D status, but the precise levels impacting risk, as well as mechanisms of action, remain undefined (Guallar et al., 2010; Pittas et al., 2010; Wang et al., 2010; IOM, 2011). For example, a reduced mortality was observed for those with 25OHD concentrations of 40 ng/mL (100 nmol/L) compared to those with values less than 10 ng/mL (25 nmol/L) (Ginde et al., 2009b). Another provocative cohort study examined patients undergoing angiography followed by serum 25OHD evaluations for 8 years. Those from the upper 25OHD quartile (median concentration of 28 ng/mL) had a lower mortality than those from the lowest quartile (median concentration of 8 ng/mL) (Dobnig et al., 2008). Vitamin D may also impact established risk factors for cardiovascular disease. The NHANES observational study of adolescents reported that 25OHD values below 15 ng/mL are associated with a doubled risk of hypertension compared to those with concentrations of 26 ng/mL or higher (Reis et al., 2009).

Similarly, adults with 25OHD concentrations less than 21 ng/mL show greater risks of hypertension, diabetes, obesity, and hyperlipidemia than those with concentrations greater than or equal to 37 ng/mL (Martins et al., 2007). However, a contrary hypothesis also suggests that under certain conditions vitamin D may accelerate vascular disease, perhaps by impacting vascular calcification. For example, a study of African Americans with type 2 diabetes mellitus reported that 25OHD status correlated with increased calcified plaques in the aorta and carotid arteries (Freedman et al., 2010).

Diabetes Mellitus

VDRs are present in pancreatic islet cells and addition of the vitamin D ligand may improve insulin secretory responses as well as insulin sensitivity of target cells. Yet the human literature regarding vitamin D status and risk of diabetes is particularly uninformative, because it does not fully address confounding variables and independent impacts of calcium and vitamin D (Pittas et al., 2007). For example, a meta-analysis of several observational studies of vitamin D supplementation versus no supplementation during childhood suggested a nearly 30% reduction in the risk of developing type 1 diabetes. Yet compliance, dosage, and impact of treatment on serum 25OHD data are not available in most of these reports included in the meta analysis (Zipitis and Akobeng, 2008). Similarly, the Harvard Nurses' Health Study reported that vitamin D and calcium supplementation were both related to a lower risk of developing type 2 diabetes (Pittas et al., 2006).

Neurological Disease

Multiple sclerosis is a relatively common disease and has received significant attention with regards to vitamin D status. The incidence of multiple sclerosis generally increases with higher latitudes, suggesting a hypothesis of limited UV exposure, reduced 25OHD status, and greater risk. One case-control study found that the risk of multiple sclerosis was lowest in those with higher 25OHD levels, yet this was limited to whites and was not observed in those of African descent (Munger et al., 2006). Anecdotal testimonials of the therapeutic benefits of vitamin D supplementation are common, yet therapeutic intervention trials have yielded unimpressive results (Ascherio et al., 2010). Various mental illnesses have also been associated with inadequate vitamin D status (McGrath et al., 2004). These are particularly difficult relationships to establish using cohort observational data, because the presence of disease may impact nutritional status or supplement usage patterns. Yet intriguing data from a randomized placebo-controlled study of overweight patients treated with high doses of vitamin D showed improvements in the depression survey scores (Jorde et al., 2008). At this time, data are limited and conclusions regarding a role for vitamin D in the etiology and therapy of neuropsychological disease are premature (IOM, 2011).

Immune Response and Infection

There is little doubt that vitamin D impacts immune cells and immune responses, with extensive supportive data from experimental studies in vitro and in vivo. Yet how these data can provide clear insight for testable hypotheses in human translational studies has been an elusive pursuit. Inconsistent and inconclusive data have resulted from studies of vitamin D and allergic diseases and autoimmune disorders (Wjst, 2007; Brehm et al., 2009; IOM, 2011). A role for vitamin D in the control of infectious diseases is particularly challenging because of the vast array of disease processes afflicting humans, and it is possible that a role for vitamin D may be unique to individual types of infections. For example, a meta-analysis of observational studies reported a lower risk of active tuberculosis in those with the highest values of 25OHD (Nnoaham and Clarke, 2008). Yet when tested in a randomized placebo-controlled trial of tuberculosis patients in West Africa, no impact of intervention with vitamin D on disease progression was noted (Wejse et al., 2009). The NHANES III study provided observational data indicating that those with serum 25OHD levels of less than 10 ng/mL (25 nmol/L) were more likely to report respiratory tract infections than those with higher concentrations, an effect that was strongest for those with asthma or chronic lung disease (Ginde et al., 2009a).

Cancers

The cancer literature in experimental models and in cell culture provide strong data supporting a hypothesis that vitamin D may impact risk of cancer or alter the course of the disease (Deeb et al., 2007; Fleet, 2007; Norman and Bouillon, 2010; IOM, 2011). Vitamin D plays a key role in the modulation of cellular growth, proliferation, differentiation, and survival, which are cellular processes that are disrupted in carcinogenesis. Unfortunately, human cancer is a complex process characterized by profound heterogeneity in etiology and response to therapy. The American Institute for Cancer Research (World Cancer Research Fund/American Institute for Cancer Research, 2007), the World Health Organization (International Agency for Research on Cancer, 2008), and the Agency for Healthcare Research and Quality (AHRQ) (Chung et al., 2009), which conducted a systematic review of the human literature, all conclude that a definitive causal role for vitamin D status in human cancer risk or prevention has not been established. The DRI committee conducted a thorough examination of past and recently published data and came to a similar conclusion (IOM, 2011).

CONTROVERSY OVER RECOMMENDATIONS FOR VITAMIN D INTAKE AND STATUS TESTING

Interestingly, many advocates for greater consumption of vitamin D selectively highlight data from the growing array of observational studies supporting positive health outcomes. Yet randomized controlled trials are few, and often do not confirm results of epidemiological studies that are best viewed as a basis for generating further hypotheses. In addition, many of the randomized trials included a very limited range of doses of vitamin D, leaving much speculation regarding an optimal level of intake.

The current recommendations by the DRI committee provide public health recommendations addressing the needs of a healthy North American population. Existing evidence indicates that the majority of healthy individuals are currently meeting their needs at the proposed RDAs for vitamin D and achieving a 25OHD serum concentration of at least 20 ng/mL (50 nmol/L). At this time, higher intake levels or greater achieved serum concentrations have not consistently conferred greater health benefits, a challenge to the concept that "more is better" (IOM, 2011; Ross et al., 2011).

The value of routine periodic vitamin D serum testing remains controversial for healthy individuals. The IOM committee found that the prevalence of vitamin D inadequacy in healthy North Americans has been frequently overestimated because the cutoff points used are not supported by scientific data and greatly exceed the levels identified as sufficient (20 ng/mL, or 50 nmol/L). Serum concentrations of 25OHD above 30 ng/mL (75 nmol/L) have not consistently been associated with health benefits, and some adverse risks have been suggested for various outcomes at 25OHD concentrations of 50 ng/mL (125 nmol/L) and higher.

Additional insights into the consequences of higher vitamin D intakes should come from a recently initiated study supported by the National Institutes of Health, which will compare placebo to 2000 IU/day of vitamin D and will involve 20,000 participants over a 5-year period. This study will examine many of the important health outcomes (Manson, 2010).

REFERENCES

Aaron, J. E., Gallagher, J. C., Anderson, J., Stasiak, L., Longton, E. B., Nordin, B. E., & Nicholson, M. (1974a). Frequency of osteomalacia and osteoporosis in fractures of the proximal femur. *Lancet, 1*, 229–233.

Aaron, J. E., Gallagher, J. C., & Nordin, B. E. (1974b). Seasonal variation of histological osteomalacia in femoral-neck fractures. *Lancet, 2*, 84–85.

Agarwal, S. C., & Stout, S. D. (2004). *Bone loss and osteoporosis: An anthropological perspective*. New York: Kluwer Academic/Plenum Publishers.

Aloia, J. F. (2008). African Americans, 25-hydroxyvitamin D, and osteoporosis: A paradox. *The American Journal of Clinical Nutrition, 88*, 545S–550S.

Aloia, J. F., Patel, M., Dimaano, R., Li-Ng, M., Talwar, S. A., Mikhail, M., ... Yeh, J. K. (2008). Vitamin D intake to attain a desired serum 25-hydroxyvitamin D concentration. *The American Journal of Clinical Nutrition, 87*, 1952–1958.

Armas, L. A., Dowell, S., Akhter, M., Duthuluru, S., Huerter, C., Hollis, B. W., ... Heaney, R. P. (2007). Ultraviolet-B radiation increases serum 25-hydroxyvitamin D levels: The effect of UVB dose and skin color. *Journal of the American Academy of Dermatology, 57*, 588–593.

Ascherio, A., Munger, K. L., & Simon, K. C. (2010). Vitamin D and multiple sclerosis. *Lancet Neurology, 9*, 599–612.

Autier, P., & Gandini, S. (2007). Vitamin D supplementation and total mortality: A meta-analysis of randomized controlled trials. *Archives of Internal Medicine, 167*, 1730–1737.

Avenell, A., Gillespie, W. J., Gillespie, L. D., & O'Connell, D. (2009). Vitamin D and vitamin D analogues for preventing fractures associated with involutional and post-menopausal osteoporosis. *The Cochrane Database of Systematic Reviews* (3), CD000227.

Berg, J. P. (1999). Vitamin D–binding protein prevents vitamin D deficiency and presents vitamin D for its renal activation. *European Journal of Endocrinology, 141*, 321–322.

Bergwitz, C., & Juppner, H. (2010). Regulation of phosphate homeostasis by PTH, vitamin D, and FGF23. *Annual Review of Medicine, 61*, 91–104.

Bhan, A., Rao, A. D., & Rao, D. S. (2010). Osteomalacia as a result of vitamin D deficiency. *Endocrinology and Metabolism Clinics of North America, 39*, 321–331.

Bischoff-Ferrari, H. A., Dawson-Hughes, B., Staehelin, H. B., Orav, J. E., Stuck, A. E., Theiler, R., ... Henschkowski, J. (2009a). Fall prevention with supplemental and active forms of vitamin D: A meta-analysis of randomised controlled trials. *BMJ, 339*, b3692.

Bischoff-Ferrari, H. A., Willett, W. C., Wong, J. B., Stuck, A. E., Staehelin, H. B., Orav, E. J., ... Henschkowski, J. (2009b). Prevention of nonvertebral fractures with oral vitamin D and dose dependency: A meta-analysis of randomized controlled trials. *Archives of Internal Medicine, 169*, 551–561.

Bogh, M. K., Schmedes, A. V., Philipsen, P. A., Thieden, E., & Wulf, H. C. (2010). Vitamin D production after UVB exposure depends on baseline vitamin D and total cholesterol but not on skin pigmentation. *The Journal of Investigative Dermatology, 130*, 546–553.

Brehm, J. M., Celedon, J. C., Soto-Quiros, M. E., Avila, L., Hunninghake, G. M., Forno, E., ... Litonjua, A. A. (2009). Serum vitamin D levels and markers of severity of childhood asthma in Costa Rica. *American Journal of Respiratory and Critical Care Medicine, 179*, 765–771.

Brickman, A. S., Coburn, J. W., & Norman, A. W. (1972). Action of 1,25-dihydroxycholecalciferol, a potent, kidney-produced metabolite of vitamin D, in uremic man. *New England Journal of Medicine, 287*, 891–895.

Carter, G. D., Berry, J. L., Gunter, E., Jones, G., Jones, J. C., Makin, H. L., ... Wheeler, M. J. (2010). Proficiency testing of 25-hydroxyvitamin D (25-OHD) assays. *The Journal of Steroid Biochemistry and Molecular Biology, 121*, 176–179.

Cashman, K. D., Hill, T. R., Cotter, A. A., Boreham, C. A., Dubitzky, W., Murray, L., ... Kiely, M. (2008a). Low vitamin D status adversely affects bone health parameters in adolescents. *The American Journal of Clinical Nutrition, 87*, 1039–1044.

Cashman, K. D., Hill, T. R., Lucey, A. J., Taylor, N., Seamans, K. M., Muldowney, S., ... Kiely, M. (2008b). Estimation of the dietary requirement for vitamin D in healthy adults. *The American Journal of Clinical Nutrition, 88*, 1535–1542.

Cashman, K. D., Wallace, J. M., Horigan, G., Hill, T. R., Barnes, M. S., Lucey, A. J., Bonham, M. P., Taylor, N., Duffy, E. M., Seamans, K., Muldowney, S., Fitzgerald, A. P., Flynn, A., Strain, J. J., & Kiely, M. (2009). Estimation of the dietary requirement for vitamin D in free-living adults ≥64 y of age. *The American Journal of Clinical Nutrition, 89*, 1366–1374.

Cauley, J. A., Lacroix, A. Z., Wu, L., Horwitz, M., Danielson, M. E., Bauer, D. C., ... Cummings, S. R. (2008). Serum 25-hydroxyvitamin D concentrations and risk for hip fractures. *Annals of Internal Medicine, 149*, 242–250.

Cauley, J. A., Parimi, N., Ensrud, K. E., Bauer, D. C., Cawthon, P. M., Cummings, S. R., ... Orwoll, E. (2009). Serum 25-hydroxyvitamin D and the risk of hip and nonspine fractures in older men. *Journal of Bone and Mineral Research, 25*, 545–553.

Chung, M., Balk, E. M., Brendel, M., Ip, S., Lau, J., Lee, J., … Trikalinos, T. A. (2009). *Vitamin D and calcium: A systematic review of health outcomes.* Evidence Report No. 183. In AHRQ Publication no. 09-E015. Rockville, MD: Prepared by the Tufts Evidence-based Practice Center.

Clemens, T. L., Adams, J. S., Henderson, S. L., & Holick, M. F. (1982). Increased skin pigment reduces the capacity of skin to synthesise vitamin D3. *Lancet, 1,* 74–76.

Deeb, K. K., Trump, D. L., & Johnson, C. S. (2007). Vitamin D signalling pathways in cancer: Potential for anticancer therapeutics. *Nature Reviews. Cancer, 7,* 684–700.

DeLucia, M. C., Mitnick, M. E., & Carpenter, T. O. (2003). Nutritional rickets with normal circulating 25-hydroxyvitamin D: A call for reexamining the role of dietary calcium intake in North American infants. *The Journal of Clinical Endocrinology and Metabolism, 88,* 3539–3545.

Diehl, J. W., & Chiu, M. W. (2010). Effects of ambient sunlight and photoprotection on vitamin D status. *Dermatologic Therapy, 23,* 48–60.

Dobnig, H., Pilz, S., Scharnagl, H., Renner, W., Seelhorst, U., Wellnitz, B., … Maerz, W. (2008). Independent association of low serum 25-hydroxyvitamin D and 1,25-dihydroxyvitamin D levels with all-cause and cardiovascular mortality. *Archives of Internal Medicine, 168,* 1340–1349.

Ebeling, P. R., Sandgren, M. E., DiMagno, E. P., Lane, A. W., DeLuca, H. F., & Riggs, B. L. (1992). Evidence of an age-related decrease in intestinal responsiveness to vitamin D: Relationship between serum 1,25-dihydroxyvitamin D3 and intestinal vitamin D receptor concentrations in normal women. *The Journal of Clinical Endocrinology and Metabolism, 75,* 176–182.

Ensrud, K. E., Taylor, B. C., Paudel, M. L., Cauley, J. A., Cawthon, P. M., Cummings, S. R., … Orwoll, E. S. (2009). Serum 25-hydroxyvitamin D levels and rate of hip bone loss in older men. *The Journal of Clinical Endocrinology and Metabolism, 94,* 2773–2780.

Fleet, J. C. (2007). What have genomic and proteomic approaches told us about vitamin D and cancer? *Nutrition Reviews, 65,* S127–S130.

Fleet, J. C., & Schoch, R. D. (2010). Molecular mechanisms for regulation of intestinal calcium absorption by vitamin D and other factors. *Critical Reviews in Clinical Laboratory Sciences, 47,* 181–195.

Freedman, B. I., Wagenknecht, L. E., Hairston, K. G., Bowden, D. W., Carr, J. J., Hightower, R. C., … Divers, J. (2010). Vitamin D, adiposity, and calcified atherosclerotic plaque in African-Americans. *The Journal of Clinical Endocrinology and Metabolism, 95,* 1076–1083.

Galitzer, H., Ben-Dov, I., Lavi-Moshayoff, V., Naveh-Many, T., & Silver, J. (2008). Fibroblast growth factor 23 acts on the parathyroid to decrease parathyroid hormone secretion. *Current Opinion in Nephrology and Hypertension, 17,* 363–367.

Ginde, A. A., Mansbach, J. M., & Camargo, C. A., Jr. (2009a). Association between serum 25-hydroxyvitamin D level and upper respiratory tract infection in the Third National Health and Nutrition Examination Survey. *Archives of Internal Medicine, 169,* 384–390.

Ginde, A. A., Scragg, R., Schwartz, R. S., & Camargo, C. A., Jr. (2009b). Prospective study of serum 25-hydroxyvitamin D level, cardiovascular disease mortality, and all-cause mortality in older U.S. adults. *Journal of the American Geriatric Society, 57,* 1595–1603.

Guallar, E., Miller, E. R., 3rd, Ordovas, J. M., & Stranges, S. (2010). Vitamin D supplementation in the age of lost innocence. *Annals of Internal Medicine, 152,* 327–329.

Holick, M. F. (1995a). Environmental factors that influence the cutaneous production of vitamin D. *The American Journal of Clinical Nutrition, 61,* 638S–645S.

Holick, M. F. (1995b). Vitamin D: Photobiology, metabolism, and clinical applications. In L. J. DeGroot, M. Besser, & H. G. Burgeret (Eds.), *Endocrinology* (3rd ed.). Philadelphia: Saunders.

Holick, M. F. (1996). Vitamin D: Photobiology, metabolism, mechanism of action, and clinical applications. In M. J. Favus (Ed.), *Primer on the metabolic bone diseases and disorders of mineral metabolism* (3rd ed., pp. 74–81). Philadelphia: Lippincott-Raven.

Holick, M. F. (2003). Vitamin D deficiency: What a pain it is. *Mayo Clinic Proceedings, 78,* 1457–1459.

Holick, M. F., Matsuoka, L. Y., & Wortsman, J. (1989). Age, vitamin D, and solar ultraviolet. *Lancet, 2,* 1104–1105.

Huhtakangas, J. A., Olivera, C. J., Bishop, J. E., Zanello, L. P., & Norman, A. W. (2004). The vitamin D receptor is present in caveolae-enriched plasma membranes and binds 1 alpha,25(OH)2-vitamin D3 in vivo and in vitro. *Molecular Endocrinology, 18,* 2660–2671.

Institute of Medicine. (2011). *Dietary Reference Intakes for calcium and vitamin D.* Washington, DC: The National Academies Press.

International Agency for Research on Cancer. (2008). Vitamin D and cancer. In P. Boyle & B. Levin (Eds.), *Reports IWG* (Vol. 5). Lyon, France: World Health Organization.

Ireland, P., & Fordtran, J. S. (1973). Effect of dietary calcium and age on jejunal calcium absorption in humans studied by intestinal perfusion. *The Journal of Clinical Investigation, 52,* 2672–2681.

Jackson, R. D., LaCroix, A. Z., Gass, M., Wallace, R. B., Robbins, J., Lewis, C. E., … Barad, D. (2006). Calcium plus vitamin D supplementation and the risk of fractures. *New England Journal of Medicine, 354,* 669–683.

Jones, G., Strugnell, S. A., & DeLuca, H. F. (1998). Current understanding of the molecular actions of vitamin D. *Physiological Reviews, 78,* 1193–1231.

Jorde, R., Sneve, M., Figenschau, Y., Svartberg, J., & Waterloo, K. (2008). Effects of vitamin D supplementation on symptoms of depression in overweight and obese subjects: Randomized double blind trial. *Journal of Internal Medicine, 264,* 599–609.

Leheste, J. R., Melsen, F., Wellner, M., Jansen, P., Schlichting, U., Renner-Muller, I., … Willnow, T. E. (2003). Hypocalcemia and osteopathy in mice with kidney-specific megalin gene defect. *The FASEB Journal, 17,* 247–249.

Looker, A. C., & Mussolino, M. E. (2008a). Serum 25-hydroxyvitamin D and hip fracture risk in older U.S. white adults. *Journal of Bone and Mineral Research, 23,* 143–150.

Looker, A. C., Pfeiffer, C. M., Lacher, D. A., Schleicher, R. L., Picciano, M. F., & Yetley, E. A. (2008b). Serum 25-hydroxyvitamin D status of the US population: 1988–1994 compared with 2000–2004. *The American Journal of Clinical Nutrition, 88,* 1519–1527.

Loomis, W. F. (1967). Skin-pigment regulation of vitamin-D biosynthesis in man. *Science, 157,* 501–506.

Losel, R., & Wehling, M. (2003). Nongenomic actions of steroid hormones. *Nature Reviews. Molecular Cell Biology, 4,* 46–56.

Manson, J. E. (2010). Vitamin D and the heart: Why we need large-scale clinical trials. *Cleveland Clinic Journal of Medicine, 77,* 903–910.

Martins, D., Wolf, M., Pan, D., Zadshir, A., Tareen, N., Thadhani, R., … Norris, K. (2007). Prevalence of cardiovascular risk factors and the serum levels of 25-hydroxyvitamin D in the United States: Data from the Third National Health and Nutrition Examination Survey. *Archives of Internal Medicine, 167,* 1159–1165.

Masuda, S., Byford, V., Arabian, A., Sakai, Y., Demay, M. B., St-Arnaud, R., & Jones, G. (2005). Altered pharmacokinetics of 1alpha,25-dihydroxyvitamin D3 and 25-hydroxyvitamin D3 in the blood and tissues of the 25-hydroxyvitamin D-24-hydroxylase (Cyp24a1) null mouse. *Endocrinology, 146,* 825–834.

Matsuoka, L. Y., Wortsman, J., Dannenberg, M. J., Hollis, B. W., Lu, Z., & Holick, M. F. (1992). Clothing prevents ultraviolet-B radiation-dependent photosynthesis of vitamin D3. *The Journal of Clinical Endocrinology and Metabolism, 75*, 1099–1103.

McGrath, J., Saari, K., Hakko, H., Jokelainen, J., Jones, P., Jarvelin, M. R., ... Isohanni, M. (2004). Vitamin D supplementation during the first year of life and risk of schizophrenia: A Finnish birth cohort study. *Schizophrenia Research, 67*, 237–245.

Melhus, H., Snellman, G., Gedeborg, R., Byberg, L., Berglund, L., Mallmin, H., ... Michaelsson, K. (2010). Plasma 25-hydroxyvitamin D levels and fracture risk in a community-based cohort of elderly men in Sweden. *The Journal of Clinical Endocrinology and Metabolism, 95*, 2637–2645.

Mizwicki, M. T., & Norman, A. W. (2009). The vitamin D sterol-vitamin D receptor ensemble model offers unique insights into both genomic and rapid-response signaling. *Science Signaling, 2*, re4.

Munger, K. L., Levin, L. I., Hollis, B. W., Howard, N. S., & Ascherio, A. (2006). Serum 25-hydroxyvitamin D levels and risk of multiple sclerosis. *The Journal of the American Medical Association, 296*, 2832–2838.

Nemere, I., Farach-Carson, M. C., Rohe, B., Sterling, T. M., Norman, A. W., Boyan, B. D., & Safford, S. E. (2004). Ribozyme knockdown functionally links a 1,25(OH)2D3 membrane binding protein (1,25D3-MARRS) and phosphate uptake in intestinal cells. *Proceedings of the National Academy of Sciences of the United States of America, 101*, 7392–7397.

Nemere, I., Yoshimoto, Y., & Norman, A. W. (1984). Calcium transport in perfused duodena from normal chicks: Enhancement within fourteen minutes of exposure to 1,25-dihydroxyvitamin D3. *Endocrinology, 115*, 1476–1483.

Nnoaham, K. E., & Clarke, A. (2008). Low serum vitamin D levels and tuberculosis: A systematic review and meta-analysis. *International Journal of Epidemiology, 37*, 113–119.

Norman, A. W. (2006). Minireview: Vitamin D receptor: New assignments for an already busy receptor. *Endocrinology, 147*, 5542–5548.

Norman, A. W., & Bouillon, R. (2010). Vitamin D nutritional policy needs a vision for the future. *Experimental Biology and Medicine, 235*, 1034–1045.

Nykjaer, A., Dragun, D., Walther, D., Vorum, H., Jacobsen, C., Herz, J., ... Willnow, T. E. (1999). An endocytic pathway essential for renal uptake and activation of the steroid 25-(OH) vitamin D3. *Cell, 96*, 507–515.

Pittas, A. G., Chung, M., Trikalinos, T., Mitri, J., Brendel, M., Patel, K., ... Balk, E. M. (2010). Systematic review: Vitamin D and cardiometabolic outcomes. *Annals of Internal Medicine, 152*, 307–314.

Pittas, A. G., Dawson-Hughes, B., Li, T., Van Dam, R. M., Willett, W. C., Manson, J. E., & Hu, F. B. (2006). Vitamin D and calcium intake in relation to type 2 diabetes in women. *Diabetes Care, 29*, 650–656.

Pittas, A. G., Lau, J., Hu, F. B., & Dawson-Hughes, B. (2007). The role of vitamin D and calcium in type 2 diabetes: A systematic review and meta-analysis. *The Journal of Clinical Endocrinology and Metabolism, 92*, 2017–2029.

Priemel, M., von Domarus, C., Klatte, T. O., Kessler, S., Schlie, J., Meier, S., ... Amling, M. (2010). Bone mineralization defects and vitamin D deficiency: Histomorphometric analysis of iliac crest bone biopsies and circulating 25-hydroxyvitamin D in 675 patients. *Journal of Bone and Mineral Research, 25*, 305–312.

Reis, J. P., von Muhlen, D., Miller, E. R., 3rd, Michos, E. D., & Appel, L. J. (2009). Vitamin D status and cardiometabolic risk factors in the United States adolescent population. *Pediatrics, 124*, e371–e379.

Riggs, B. L., Hamstra, A., & DeLuca, H. F. (1981). Assessment of 25-hydroxyvitamin D 1 alpha-hydroxylase reserve in postmenopausal osteoporosis by administration of parathyroid extract. *The Journal of Clinical Endocrinology and Metabolism, 53*, 833–835.

Ross, A. C., Manson, J. E., Abrams, S. A., Aloia, J. F., Brannon, P. M., Clinton, S. K., ... Shapses, S. A. (2011). The 2011 report on dietary reference intakes for calcium and vitamin D from the Institute of Medicine: What clinicians need to know. *The Journal of Clinical Endocrinology and Metabolism, 96*, 53–58.

Sanders, K. M., Stuart, A. L., Williamson, E. J., Simpson, J. A., Kotowicz, M. A., Young, D., & Nicholson, G. C. (2010). Annual high-dose oral vitamin D and falls and fractures in older women: A randomized controlled trial. *The Journal of the American Medical Association, 303*, 1815–1822.

Slovik, D. M., Adams, J. S., Neer, R. M., Holick, M. F., & Potts, J. T., Jr. (1981). Deficient production of 1,25-dihydroxyvitamin D in elderly osteoporotic patients. *New England Journal of Medicine, 305*, 372–374.

Smith, S. M., Gardner, K. K., Locke, J., & Zwart, S. R. (2009). Vitamin D supplementation during Antarctic winter. *The American Journal of Clinical Nutrition, 89*, 1092–1098.

Snellman, G., Melhus, H., Gedeborg, R., Olofsson, S., Wolk, A., Pedersen, N. L., & Michaelsson, K. (2009). Seasonal genetic influence on serum 25-hydroxyvitamin D levels: A twin study. *PLoS One, 4*, e7747.

Springbett, P., Buglass, S., & Young, A. R. (2010). Photoprotection and vitamin D status. *Journal of Photochemistry and Photobiology. B, Biology, 101*, 160–168.

Taha, S. A., Dost, S. M., & Sedrani, S. H. (1984). 25-Hydroxyvitamin D and total calcium: Extraordinarily low plasma concentrations in Saudi mothers and their neonates. *Pediatric Research, 18*, 739–741.

Talwar, S. A., Aloia, J. F., Pollack, S., & Yeh, J. K. (2007a). Dose response to vitamin D supplementation among postmenopausal African American women. *The American Journal of Clinical Nutrition, 86*, 1657–1662.

Talwar, S. A., Swedler, J., Yeh, J., Pollack, S., & Aloia, J. F. (2007b). Vitamin-D nutrition and bone mass in adolescent black girls. *Journal of the National Medical Association, 99*, 650–657.

Thacher, T. D., Fischer, P. R., Strand, M. A., & Pettifor, J. M. (2006). Nutritional rickets around the world: Causes and future directions. *Annals of Tropical Paediatrics, 26*, 1–16.

Tian, X. Q., Chen, T. C., Lu, Z., Shao, Q., & Holick, M. F. (1994). Characterization of the translocation process of vitamin D3 from the skin into the circulation. *Endocrinology, 135*, 655–661.

U.S. Department of Agriculture, Agricultural Research Service. (2010). *USDA National Nutrient Database for Standard Reference, Release 23*. Retrieved from http://www.ars.usda.gov/ba/bhnrc/ndl.

Wang, L., Manson, J. E., Song, Y., & Sesso, H. D. (2010). Systematic review: Vitamin D and calcium supplementation in prevention of cardiovascular events. *Annals of Internal Medicine, 152*, 315–323.

Wejse, C., Gomes, V. F., Rabna, P., Gustafson, P., Aaby, P., Lisse, I. M., ... Sodemann, M. (2009). Vitamin D as supplementary treatment for tuberculosis: A double-blind, randomized, placebo-controlled trial. *American Journal of Respiratory and Critical Care Medicine, 179*, 843–850.

Wjst, M. (2007). Public data mining shows extended linkage disequilibrium around ADAM33. *Allergy, 62*, 444–446.

World Cancer Research Fund/American Institute for Cancer Research. (2007). *Food, nutrition and the prevention of cancer: A global perspective*. Washington, DC: American Institute for Cancer Research.

Zipitis, C. S., & Akobeng, A. K. (2008). Vitamin D supplementation in early childhood and risk of type 1 diabetes: A systematic review and meta-analysis. *Archives of Disease in Childhood, 93*, 512–517.

UNIT VII

Minerals and Water

The organic components of the diet have been discussed in detail in the preceding chapters. In this unit, the biological roles of water and a number of essential elements that can be supplied in inorganic form are considered.

Water (H_2O) makes up the largest component of the body, accounting for about 73% of lean body mass in adults. As a percentage of total body weight, water content ranges from 75% of body weight in the neonate to 50% of body weight in older adults. Water serves as the principal fluid medium of the cell in which metabolic processes take place. The extracellular water bathing the cells serves as a medium for the transport of nutrients and oxygen to the cells and for removal of wastes from the body. In addition, water is necessary for organ formation and plays an important role in the regulation of body temperature.

From the 90 or so elements that occur naturally in the environment, a limited number (perhaps 22) are essential for human life. The organic nutrients—the carbohydrates, proteins, lipids, and vitamins—are made up almost entirely of six relatively small elements: hydrogen, carbon, nitrogen, oxygen, phosphorus, and sulfur. Two rather common features of the elements discussed in this unit, as opposed to those that make up the organic nutrients, are that these minerals are required in smaller amounts and for very specialized functions. In addition, although some of these elements (e.g., selenium and iodine) are also capable of forming covalent bonds, weaker types of bonds are much more common. In contrast to the strong covalent bonds found in organic molecules, in which each atom donates one electron to form a pair of outer orbital electrons that are shared, the ionic bonds (salt bridges) found in salts are formed by a single electron donated by one of the paired atoms. The coordinate covalent bonds found in metal chelates (e.g., heme and vitamin B_{12}) possess properties of both the covalent bond and the ionic bond: two electrons from one atom are donated to form the bond to another atom.

Minerals or inorganic nutrients are sometimes grouped by the amount of each element that is required by the human body. Essential elements include those classified as macroelements; calcium, phosphorus, magnesium, sodium, potassium, chloride, and sulfur are required at levels of greater than 100 mg/day by adults. Because the sulfur requirement is met by intake of sulfur amino acids, sulfur usually is not considered with the macroelements. The microelements may be considered in two groups: trace elements required in amounts ranging between 1 mg/day and 100 mg/day and ultratrace elements required in amounts in the microgram per day range (less than 1 mg/day). Trace elements include iron, zinc, manganese, copper, and fluorine. Ultratrace elements include selenium, molybdenum, iodine, chromium, boron, and cobalt. Some evidence of a benefit of arsenic, nickel, vanadium, and silicon comes from animal studies, but these four ultratrace elements have not been proved to be essential or beneficial for humans. Sulfate is not considered in detail in this unit because requirements for sulfate are thought to be met if the sulfur amino acid requirement is met as is discussed in Chapter 14. Similarly, cobalt is not considered in this unit because the only requirement humans have for cobalt is as part of preformed vitamin B_{12}, which is discussed in Chapter 25.

Minerals serve a diverse range of functions in the body, and many of these functions are discussed in the chapters in this unit. The deposition of calcium and phosphate as hydroxyapatite is essential for bone formation. Calcium is considered to be a second messenger molecule; binding of calcium to various proteins acts as a cellular signaling event. Sodium, potassium, chloride, calcium, magnesium, phosphate, and sulfate are all important inorganic electrolytes involved in ionic and osmotic balance and electrical gradients.

Many of the trace elements are found in association with enzymes and other proteins in which these metals serve structural, catalytic, or binding roles; examples include the role of zinc in the tertiary structure of various proteins, the catalytic role of copper or zinc at the active site of superoxide dismutase, and the role of iron in oxygen binding by hemoglobin. Some minerals are required solely for the synthesis of specialized organic compounds, as demonstrated by the incorporation of iodine into thyroid hormones, of selenium into selenocysteine for synthesis of selenoproteins, and of molybdenum into an organic cofactor required by several mammalian enzymes.

CHAPTER 32

Calcium and Phosphorus

*Sue A. Shapses, PhD**

COMMON ABBREVIATIONS

1,25(OH)$_2$D	1,25-dihydroxyvitamin D
25(OH)D	25-hydroxyvitamin D
FGF23	fibroblast growth factor 23
IP$_3$	inositol 1,4,5-triphosphate
P$_i$	inorganic phosphate, mainly HPO_4^{2-} and $H_2PO_4^-$ at physiological pH
PTH	parathyroid hormone
PTHrP	parathyroid hormone–related protein
TRPV	transient receptor potential (TRP) cation channel subfamily

The chemistry of calcium and phosphorus plays a unique biochemical role in living organisms. The important roles of these two elements are found in cell membrane function, cellular homeostasis, and the formation of the inorganic component of the skeleton. Several organs contribute to the intimate intertwining of calcium and phosphorus homeostasis by facilitating intestinal absorption, bone (re)modeling, and renal excretion and reabsorption and are the functional basis for discussing calcium and phosphate in a single chapter.

CHEMICAL PROPERTIES OF CALCIUM

The chemical characteristics of the calcium atom are important in the normal functions of this element in living organisms. Calcium belongs to the divalent metals in group IIA of the periodic table; this group of metals has two valence electrons that are lost when the metals ionize. Calcium gives up electrons readily and thus forms positive ions (Ca^{2+}) in solution. The double-positive charge on the Ca^{2+} nucleus pulls the outer electronic shells of the calcium ion into a tightly bound configuration. The relatively low ionic radius of calcium produces a high charge density or ionic potential. This electrostatic property of calcium has an important effect on the behavior of the ion in aqueous solution and on its participation in biological processes.

The biological activity and regulation of calcium is influenced by the concentration of the ionized or free Ca^{2+} in solution, the stability constant of Ca^{2+} with various ligands in solution, and the partition coefficient of Ca^{2+}, which defines the stability of Ca^{2+} binding in a nonaqueous phase such as cell membranes. The rate of movement of Ca^{2+} across cell membranes is limited by the permeability of the membrane to Ca^{2+}, as well as by the effect of Ca^{2+} itself on the membrane. The latter effect is due to an increase in rigidity and electrical resistance of the cell membrane when Ca^{2+} binds to membrane lipids. Moreover, binding of Ca^{2+} to the protein components of cell membranes can change the fluidity of the membrane by influencing the possibilities of cross-linking between proteins. These chemical properties of calcium selectively allow passage of ions; for example, the latter effect is important in determining the permeability of cells to sodium (Na^+) and potassium (K^+) ions. The flow of ions through channels in the membrane creates an electrical circuit that requires energy to drive the flow. The currents generated regulate many cellular functions.

Calmodulin is a highly conserved, ubiquitous calcium-binding protein in cells that modulates a wide variety of cellular reactions. Calmodulin contains four calcium-binding ("EF-hand") domains that contain a high proportion of glutamate and aspartate (acidic) residues. These calcium-binding domains are highly conserved and consist of approximately 30 to 40 amino acid residues in a helix-loop-helix structure known as an EF-hand (Figure 32-1). Calcium-binding domains usually occur in pairs and are also present in other cellular calcium-binding proteins, such as troponin C in muscle and calbindin-D9K in the intestine. Although many calcium-binding proteins contain calmodulin-like motifs, some other calcium-binding proteins, such as the vitamin K–dependent proteins that contain γ-carboxyglutamate (Gla) residues and the annexins, do not contain EF-hand domains.

In order for Ca^{2+} to function properly as a second messenger signaling molecule in mediating hormonal action, as a factor involved in motor nerve fiber function, and as a critical molecule in mineralization of bone tissue via the

*This chapter is a revision of the chapter contributed by Richard J. Wood, PhD, for the second edition.

formation of calcium phosphate complexes such as hydroxyapatite [$Ca_{10}(OH)_2(PO_4)_6$] crystals, the concentration of free Ca^{2+} in cells must be tightly regulated. The two important energy-requiring membrane pumps that eject calcium out of cells to help maintain calcium homeostasis are the Na^+,Ca^{2+}-exchange system in excitable cells and the magnesium (Mg^{2+})-dependent Ca^{2+}-ATPase enzyme system in nonexcitable cells. In addition, various other strategies are employed by the cell to control intracellular free Ca^{2+} concentrations, including the binding of Ca^{2+} to various cytosolic Ca^{2+}-binding proteins and small chelating ions, such as citrate, phosphate, ADP, and ATP, and the sequestering of Ca^{2+} within various subcellular compartments.

CHEMICAL PROPERTIES OF PHOSPHATE

In biological systems, phosphorus is present as free phosphate (or inorganic phosphate, P_i), phosphate anhydrides, or phosphate esters. The majority of the phosphorus in the body is found as phosphate (PO_4). The major forms of phosphate in aqueous environments are $H_2PO_4^-$ and HPO_4^{2-} ions. Phosphate is an important anion in the body and is involved in a variety of biochemical and physiological functions. Mg^{2+} and other cations, including Ca^{2+}, are found associated with phosphate compounds. In anhydrides and esters, phosphate is always negatively charged, and the terminal phosphate group is always partially protonated. Some anhydrides and esters of phosphate in the body include inositol 1,4,5-trisphosphate (IP_3), an important regulator of calcium release from intracellular stores; ATP, the major energy currency of the body; and phosphatidylcholine, a constituent of cell membranes. DNA and RNA are polymers based on phosphate ester monomers. A variety of enzymatic activities are controlled by alternate phosphorylation and dephosphorylation of proteins by cellular kinases and phosphatases. The metabolism of all major metabolic substrates depends on phosphate acting as a cofactor in a variety of enzymes and as the principal reservoir for metabolic energy in the form of ATP, creatine phosphate, and phosphoenolpyruvate.

Another important role of phosphate in the body is based on the fact that neutral molecules are soluble in lipid and will pass through membranes. Phosphorylation of molecules such as glucose causes the trapping of phosphorylated molecules within cells. The majority of phosphate in the body is found in bone where it combines with calcium to form hydroxyapatite, $Ca_{10}(OH)_2(PO_4)_6$, the principal inorganic compound found in the skeleton. Phosphate is also important in the control of acid–base balance in the body, including urinary excretion of phosphate as $H_2PO_4^-$.

PHYSIOLOGICAL AND METABOLIC FUNCTIONS OF CALCIUM AND PHOSPHATE

Both calcium and phosphate serve numerous roles in the body. These include roles as diverse as their structural role in formation of bone mineral, the regulation of enzyme activity by reversible phosphorylation of specific amino acid residues in the protein, the role of calcium as a second messenger in the cell, and the formation and hydrolysis of energy-rich phosphate bonds in ATP to fuel muscle contraction.

BIOLOGICAL FUNCTIONS OF CALCIUM

Calcium as a Second Messenger

Increased Cytosolic Ca^{2+}

Calcium acts as a second messenger by increasing cytosolic calcium, binding to Ca^{2+}-binding protein (i.e., calmodulin) to create a conformational change that alters cell activity, with subsequent removal of the Ca^{2+}. Almost all the calcium within cells is bound within organelles such as the endoplasmic reticulum (ER), the nucleus, and other membrane-bound compartments. Consequently, the free calcium in the cell cytosol is significantly lower than in the extracellular space, with a 10,000-fold chemical gradient for Ca^{2+} across cell membranes. Very small changes in the release of Ca^{2+} from intracellular sites or in its transport

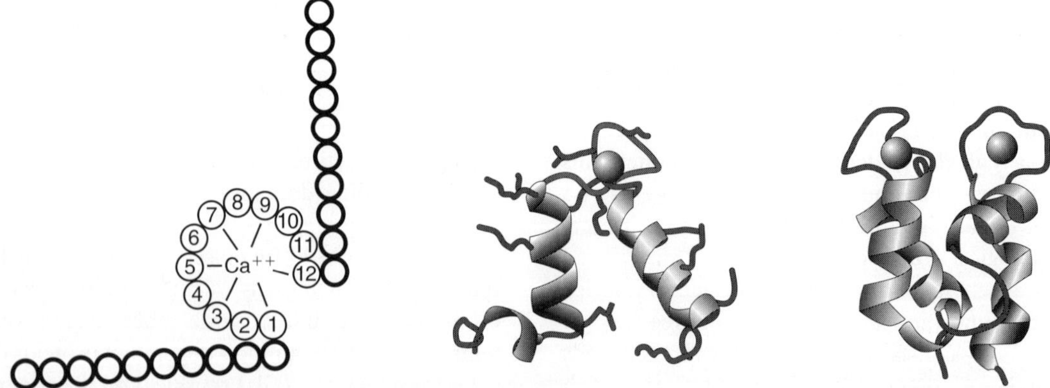

FIGURE 32-1 EF-hand calcium-binding motif. A commonly found calcium-binding motif in proteins is called the EF-hand structure. The EF-hand is composed of two perpendicular 10– to 12–amino acid alpha helices with a 12-residue calcium binding loop region (helix-loop-helix). Calcium ions bind within the calcium binding loop to oxygen ligands provided by amino acids 1, 3, 5, 7, 9, and 12. In most EF-hand proteins the residue at position 12 is a glutamate, which contributes both of its side-chain oxygens for calcium coordination. EF-hand elements usually occur in pairs and are found in a large number of calcium-binding proteins, such as calmodulin and calbindin D.

across the cell membrane will cause a large increase in cytosolic Ca^{2+} concentration. Changes in intracellular Ca^{2+} concentrations in response to cell-surface binding of peptide hormones or growth factors (first message) can act as a second messenger to elicit a variety of cellular activity, as summarized in Box 32-1.

Ligand binding to cell surface receptor proteins can result in the stimulation of the enzyme phospholipase C and in hydrolysis of phosphatidylinositol to diacylglycerol and IP_3 in the cell membrane. Increased cytosolic IP_3 causes the subsequent release of intracellular Ca^{2+} stores. Depolarization of excitable cells, such as heart muscle and nerve terminals, causes an opening of calcium-selective membrane channels and the release of Ca^{2+} from internal sources, mainly from the ER. The subsequent rise in free cytosolic Ca^{2+} concentration triggers muscle contraction or secretion of neurotransmitters.

BOX 32-1 Regulation of Selected Cellular Activities by Intracellular Calcium

- Locomotion and shape changes
  - Contraction/excitation of striated and smooth muscle
  - Movement of lymphocytes and other cells
- Movement of substances through cell membranes
- Permeability of cell membrane proteins
- Cell division and reproduction; cell–cell communication
- Exocrine and endocrine secretion of hormones
- Initiation of DNA synthesis, microtubule assembly, and chromosome movement
- Neurotransmitter release

Calcium-Dependent Trigger Proteins in Cells

Cytosolic Ca^{2+} can bind to cellular Ca^{2+}-binding proteins, including calmodulin, a ubiquitous cytosolic protein that can activate cellular kinases and other enzymes, and troponin C, a muscle protein that is bound to actinomycin contractile fibers. Binding of Ca^{2+} to calcium-dependent proteins such as calmodulin causes a conformational change in the protein that can then directly or indirectly alter cellular activity, as illustrated in Figure 32-2.

Removal of the Ca^{2+} Stimulus

Cell recovery involves removal of the stimulus to lower Ca^{2+} concentrations. This is done by a few methods, including (1) buffering free Ca^{2+} via molecular sequestration involving calcium-binding proteins, (2) compartmentalization of Ca^{2+} through uptake into cellular organelles, and (3) removal of excess Ca^{2+} from the cell via energy-dependent Ca^{2+} pumps found on the plasma membrane.

Role of Calcium in Activation of Other Proteins

Ca^{2+} binding to some proteins can affect cellular activity without first causing a conformational change in the Ca^{2+}-dependent protein. For example, cellular Ca^{2+} concentrations can control biological activity by facilitating the conversion of inactive proenzymes to active enzymes. This process is illustrated by considering some of the enzymes involved in digestion and blood clotting.

Phospholipase A2

Phospholipase A2 (PLA2) is an enzyme that releases fatty acids from the second carbon group of glycerol and has a strong, predetermined fold that generates a rather immobile cavity for Ca^{2+} binding. Ca^{2+} is needed to hold the phosphate

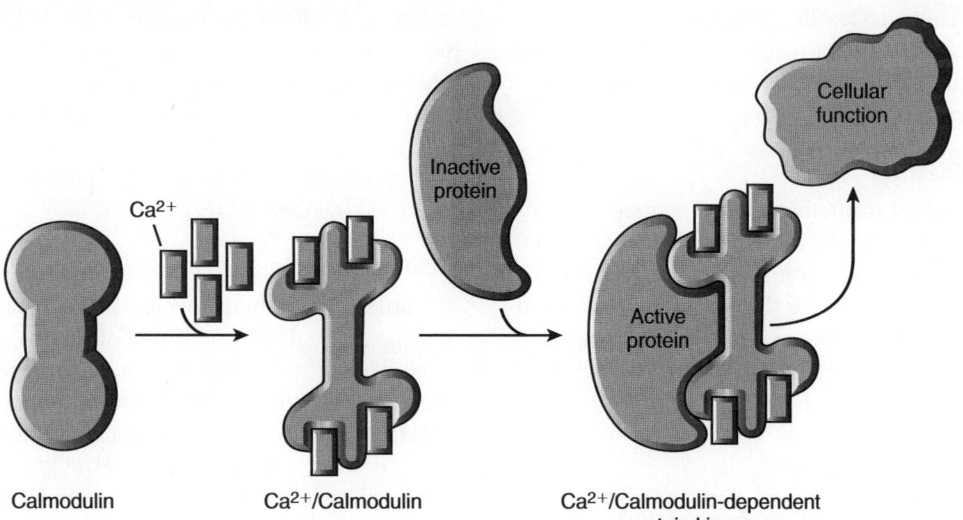

FIGURE 32-2 Calmodulin. Calcium ions (Ca^{2+}) bind to calmodulin, a ubiquitous cellular calcium-binding protein, resulting in a conformational change in this protein. The Ca^{2+}-dependent alteration of calmodulin structure exposes a region of the protein that can now bind to and activate a calmodulin-dependent target enzyme. The activation of the enzyme subsequently results directly or indirectly in a change in cellular function. The Ca^{2+} signal is turned off by lowering the cytosolic Ca^{2+} concentration, which can be achieved by sequestering free Ca^{2+} or pumping the Ca^{2+} out of the cell via plasma membrane Ca^{2+}-ATPase pumps. Also see Box 32-1 for cellular function of intracellular Ca^{2+}. (Modified from Cantley, L. [2009]. Signal transduction. In W. F. Boron & E. L. Boupaep (Eds.), *Medical physiology* [2nd ed., p. 62]. Philadelphia: Saunders.)

group of the phospholipid substrate in a suitable location for hydrolysis of the *sn*-2 ester linkage. Arachidonic acid is derived from membrane phospholipids by the action of PLA2 and is the rate-limiting step in prostaglandin synthesis, as described in Chapter 18. Phospholipases A2 include several protein families with common enzymatic activity with two Ca^{2+}-dependent families, the secreted and cytosolic PLA2. Two other families include Ca^{2+}-independent PLA2 (iPLA2) and lipoprotein-associated PLA2s (lp-PLA2), also known as platelet-activating factor acetylhydrolase (PAF-AH) (Burke and Dennis, 2009).

Calpains

Calpains are Ca^{2+}-dependent proteinases that contain calmodulin-like domains with EF-hand binding sites. Calpains are nonlysosomal, intracellular proteases present in both the cytoplasm and the nucleus and are active at neutral pH. Calpain proteinase complexes consist of an approximate catalytic and regulatory subunit. Progressive binding of Ca^{2+} to the calpain complex is linearly related to the dissociation of the two subunits, which reaches completion when all eight Ca^{2+}-binding sites of calpain (four per subunit) are occupied, whereas the activity of the catalytic subunit itself also is enhanced with greater physiological concentrations of Ca^{2+} (Reverter et al., 2001). There is increasing evidence that ubiquitous calpains participate in a variety of cellular processes including remodeling of cytoskeletal and membrane attachments, signal transduction pathways, and apoptosis. The activity of calpains is tightly controlled by the endogenous inhibitor calpastatin (Goll et al., 2003). In mammals and plants, calpain plays an essential role in development. Research suggests that calpains are involved in the cell degeneration processes that characterize numerous disease conditions linked to dysfunctions of cellular Ca^{2+} homeostasis, and especially in neurodegeneration. Atypical calpains may be associated with disease, such as calpain-10 that is linked to type 2 diabetes (Bertipaglia and Carafoli, 2007).

Blood-Clotting Enzymes

Two enzymes involved in the blood-clotting cascade, prothrombin and factor X, require calcium for their activation. Calcium binds to a protein site on prothrombin for its activation and to the phospholipid or the protein–phospholipid complex of factor X. In addition, calcium binding is essential for activation of protein S (Rezende et al., 2004), which is an important anticoagulant in the body.

Annexins

Annexins are a family of Ca^{2+}- and phospholipid-binding proteins present in all eukaryotes. Annexins are defined as being capable of binding negatively charged phospholipids in a Ca^{2+}-dependent reversible manner and must contain a 70–amino acid repeat sequence called an annexin repeat. Annexins are found both inside and outside of cells and act as membrane scaffold proteins involved in membrane–membrane and membrane–cytoskeleton interactions. They are involved in the mediation of Ca^{2+}-regulated processes including endocytosis, exocytosis, cytoskeletal regulation, and membrane conductance and organization (Fatimathas and Moss, 2010; Rescher and Gerke, 2004). Several pathological conditions may be modified by the annexins in the progression of cancer, diabetes, and the autoimmune disorder, antiphospholipid syndrome.

BIOLOGICAL FUNCTIONS OF PHOSPHATE

Inorganic phosphate has several important roles in many biological processes, including cell growth, cell signaling, nucleic acid synthesis, energy metabolism, membrane function, and bone mineralization. Phosphate also helps to maintain normal acid–base balance (pH) by acting as a buffer. Additionally, the phosphorus-containing molecule 2,3-diphosphoglycerate (2,3-DPG) binds to hemoglobin in red blood cells and influences oxygen delivery to the tissues of the body (Knochel, 2006). An acute decrease in plasma phosphate or a negative phosphate balance can lead to serious disease, including myopathy, cardiac dysfunction, abnormal neutrophil function, platelet dysfunction, and fragile red cell membrane. Chronically low phosphate balance will lead to impaired bone mineralization (rickets or osteomalacia). In contrast, elevated plasma phosphate will lead to secondary hyperparathyroidism, as is common in patients with chronic kidney disease.

Oxidative Phosphorylation to Form ATP

ATP serves as a common intermediate between cellular processes that generate free energy, such as glycolysis and respiration, and processes that consume free energy. Important cellular processes that require free energy (such as biosynthesis, contraction and motility, and active transport) depend largely on the energy released from splitting the energy-rich phosphate bond of ATP. Most catabolic pathways appear to be regulated by the energy state or the phosphorylation potential of the cell. AMP and ADP often serve as stimulatory regulators of catabolic reactions, whereas ATP often acts as an inhibitor of regulatory enzymes controlling the rate of catabolic pathways. Biosynthetic reactions are also regulated by AMP, ADP, and ATP.

Acid–Base Buffer System of HPO_4^{2-} and $H_2PO_4^-$

It is crucial for the body to maintain acid–base balance within narrow limits. Buffering is one of the major ways in which large changes in H^+ concentration are prevented. Phosphate is an effective buffer in the body to attenuate changes in the pH. If H^+ ions are added to the extracellular fluid, they will combine with HPO_4^{2-} to form $H_2PO_4^-$. Conversely, if H^+ ions are lost from the extracellular fluid, H^+ will be released from $H_2PO_4^-$.

DNA and RNA

Both DNA and RNA are linear polymers of nucleotides linked together by covalent phosphodiester linkages that join the 5′-carbon of one nucleotide to the 3′-carbon of the next nucleotide to form a sugar–phosphate backbone.

Phospholipids

Phospholipids are small molecules that resemble triacylglycerols because they are composed of fatty acids and glycerol. However, in phospholipids the glycerol is joined to only two fatty acids (a diacylglycerol), and the remaining site on glycerol is joined to a phosphate group. Additional charged groups such as choline are often attached to the phosphate (e.g., to form phosphatidylcholine); one exception to this rule is sphingomyelin, which is derived from sphingosine instead of glycerol. The fatty acid chains provide a hydrophobic tail for phospholipid molecules, whereas the phosphate-linked polar head group provides a hydrophilic head. The resulting structure is called a lipid bilayer. All biological membranes (except for those found in certain unusual bacteria) contain lipid bilayers as well as proteins, which provide membranes with stability and specialized biological functions.

Metabolic Trapping of Substrates

Neutral molecules can pass more readily across cell membranes than charged molecules. Phosphorylation of substrates can result in the metabolic trapping of the phosphorylated compounds within a cell and is considered a crucial event for intestinal absorption of riboflavin (Gastaldi et al., 2000) and vitamin B_6. Nonspecific phosphatases in the intestine hydrolyze the 5′-phosphate of each vitamin, allowing passage into the enterocyte via a nonsaturable, passive absorption process. After absorption, the vitamers (any chemical compound exhibiting vitamin-like activity) can be phosphorylated and thus retained.

Nucleotides, Creatine Phosphate, and Other Phosphoesters

Nucleotides consist of nucleosides (purine or pyrimidine bases attached to β-D-ribose or β-D-2-deoxyribose) that have one or more phosphate groups esterified to the sugar moiety (usually to the 5′-carbon). The most abundant nucleotide in cells is adenosine 5′-triphosphate (ATP). The major purine derivatives in cells are the adenosine and guanosine triphosphates and diphosphates, certain coenzymes or "activated" compounds that contain adenosine phosphate moieties, nucleotide derivatives such as guanosine diphosphate (GDP)-mannose, and, of course, DNA and RNA, which are polymers synthesized from nucleotide precursors including ATP and guanosine triphosphate (GTP). The major pyrimidine derivatives in cells are the uridine, cytidine, and thymidine triphosphates and diphosphates, nucleotide derivatives (such as uridine diphosphate [UDP]-glucose and cytidine diphosphate [CDP]-choline) that act as substrates for various reactions as well as building blocks for DNA and RNA.

Nucleotide triphosphates are required for synthesis of the active forms of a number of substrates and coenzymes for enzymatic reactions. Phosphate esters of sugars and their derivatives play major roles as intermediates in metabolism of glucose and other carbohydrates.

Coenzymes with catalytic functions in enzyme reactions transfer chemical groups to other molecules. Some coenzymes contain AMP moieties contributed by ATP in the coenzyme synthetic pathway, such as nicotinamide adenine dinucleotide (phosphate) [NAD(P)], whereas others are phosphate esters of vitamin precursors. Coenzymes are discussed in more detail in Chapters 24, 25, and 26.

Creatine phosphate is a high-energy phosphate ester that is stored in muscle to be used during exercise as a reservoir of available energy. Creatine phosphate is used to replenish ATP levels by transfer of the phosphate group from creatine phosphate to ADP in a reaction catalyzed by creatine kinase. (See Chapter 20 for more detail about the role of creatine phosphate in exercising muscle.)

Signaling Molecules: Cyclic AMP, Cyclic GMP, and Inositol Triphosphate

Another recognized function of nucleotides and their derivatives is their role as mediators of key metabolic processes. For example, 3′,5′-cyclic AMP (cAMP) functions as a second messenger in hormone-mediated control of glycogenolysis and glycogenesis. Cyclic 3′,5′-GMP (cGMP) also serves as an intracellular messenger by activating a specific protein kinase that phosphorylates target proteins in the cell.

IP_3 couples receptor activation at the plasma membrane to Ca^{2+} release from intracellular stores. Phosphatidylinositol (PtdIns) in the cell membrane is converted by a phosphorylation reaction (PtdIns kinase) into the polyphosphatidylinositols: phosphatidylinositol 4-phosphate (PIP) and phosphatidylinositol 4,5-bisphosphate (PI[4,5] P_2). Activation of a cell surface receptor activates a G protein in the cell membrane that in turn activates phospholipase C, which cleaves $PI(4,5)P_2$ to form IP_3 and diacylglycerol. Diacylglycerol can be further cleaved to yield arachidonic acid, which can be used to synthesize prostaglandins and other signaling molecules, or it can activate protein kinase C, which is a Ca^{2+}-dependent enzyme. (See Chapters 18 and 19 for more detail about these signaling processes.)

Reversible Covalent Modification of Proteins

Many protein molecules have two or more slightly different conformations that can alter their function. A common mechanism employed by the cell to control the shape of certain proteins involves covalent modification by transfer of a phosphate group from ATP to a serine, threonine, or tyrosine residue in the protein, forming a covalent linkage. The alternate phosphorylation and dephosphorylation of proteins via protein kinases and phosphatases is an important cellular control mechanism. (See Chapters 12 and 19 for more discussion of the role of phosphorylation in the regulation of enzyme activities). In addition, ATP-driven phosphorylation results in conformational changes in membrane-bound proteins that act as pumps to drive the influx or efflux of ions across the cell membrane (e.g., Na^+,K^+-ATPase pump) (see Chapter 34, Figure 34-2).

CALCIUM AND PHOSPHORUS AS COMPONENTS OF MINERALIZED TISSUE

The skeleton is an important reservoir for minerals in the body; it consists of 70% mineral, 20% collagen, 8% water, and 2% noncollagenous protein. Approximately 99% of the body's calcium, 85% of the phosphate, 70% of magnesium, and about 50% of sodium are found in bone (Driessens and Verbeeck, 1990). The mineral component of bone is largely calcium and phosphate. In the body, calcium is found mainly as the calcium phosphate compound hydroxyapatite. Forty-seven percent of skeletal weight is dry, fat-free bone, with 26% of the dry, fat-free bone weight contributed by calcium.

The skeleton is made up of two macroscopically recognizable types of bone tissue: cortical bone and trabecular bone. Approximately 80% of the skeleton is composed of dense cortical bone; the remainder is composed of sponge-like trabecular bone that is found mostly in the axial skeleton and in the ends of long bones. Trabecular bone is a frequent site of osteoporotic bone fracture and is particularly sensitive to calcium deficiency because of its relatively high rate of turnover. Compact bone consists mainly of extracellular substance or matrix; about 40% of the weight of the bone matrix is organic (nonmineral) components, primarily of type 1 collagen. Degradation products of type 1 collagen that are present in plasma or excreted in urine (e.g., deoxypyridinium or N-telopeptide or C-telopeptide regions of collagen) can be used as markers to estimate the rate of bone resorption (breakdown).

Teeth are the other mineralized tissue in the body. The hard outer layer of teeth is composed of enamel, which is 96% (by weight) inorganic matter, 3% water, and 1% organic matter. The inner dentine layer of the tooth is composed of 70% mineral, 20% organic matter, and 10% water. The major inorganic constituents of teeth are calcium and phosphate. The turnover of calcium in teeth is negligible.

Calcium-Binding Proteins in Bone

Osteonectin

Osteonectin is the most abundant noncollagenous protein in bone (Robey and Boskey, 2008). It accounts for approximately 20% to 25% of the total noncollagenous protein in compact bone and has a high affinity for binding calcium and hydroxyapatite. It is also called secreted protein acidic and rich in cysteine, sometimes abbreviated SPARC or basement membrane-40, BM-40. It is expressed in many mammalian tissues including muscle, brain, adipose, testes, kidney, skin, bone, and cartilage (Robey and Boskey, 2008). Osteonectin promotes osteoblast proliferation and survival and is critical for the maintenance of bone mass. It is also increased in wound healing, angiogenesis, tumor growth, and metastasis.

Gla Proteins

Vitamin K is a cofactor in the γ-glutamyl carboxylation pathway, a posttranslational conversion of specific glutamate residues into Gla residues (see Chapter 28). Three vitamin K–dependent proteins, osteocalcin, matrix Gla protein, and protein S, are found in the bone.

Osteocalcin is a highly conserved 5.7-kDa bone matrix protein found in bone, dentin, and exoskeleton and is synthesized by mature osteoblasts (Hauschka et al., 1989). Also called bone Gla protein, this molecule undergoes vitamin K–dependent γ carboxylation (Gla), which is necessary for conformational changes of the protein and binding capacity to hydroxyapatite. It regulates bone formation and activity of osteoclasts. Serum levels of osteocalcin are used as a biochemical marker of bone formation. However, mice lacking osteocalcin (knockout mouse) have an accelerated rate of bone formation (Ducy et al., 1996), suggesting a more complex role of osteocalcin. In addition, osteocalcin has been implicated as a hormone regulating energy metabolism (Lee et al., 2007) and has been shown to regulate beta cell proliferation and insulin secretion and sensitivity in animal models. Matrix Gla protein (MGP) is a 15-kDa, vitamin K–dependent noncollagenous protein originally isolated from bone, but is predominantly produced by vascular smooth muscle cell and chondrocytes. MGP is a potent inhibitor of vascular calcification, and MGP knockout (−/−) mice die within 6 to 8 weeks because of rupture of arteries (Luo et al., 1997). In humans, calcification is associated with decreased circulating MGP levels, because MGP has high affinity for hydroxyapatite. Protein S is a 70-kDa vitamin K–dependent anticoagulant Gla protein. Whereas protein S is synthesized by the osteoblast and a deficiency of protein S is associated with osteopenia (Maillard et al., 1992), the primary risk factor associated with protein S deficiency is thrombosis.

HORMONAL REGULATION OF CALCIUM AND PHOSPHATE METABOLISM

To maintain homeostasis and supply the mineral needs of the body, calcium and phosphate absorption by the intestine and reabsorption by the kidney, and bone turnover are coordinately regulated by the hormones $1,25(OH)_2D$ (also called calcitriol), parathyroid hormone (PTH), calcitonin and fibroblast growth factor 23 (FGF23) as summarized in Figure 32-3 and Box 32-2.

PARATHYROID HORMONE

PTH is a peptide hormone that is produced by the chief cells of the parathyroid gland and acts on certain cells through PTH receptors on the cell surface. The biologically active form of PTH is a single-chain polypeptide of 84 amino acids; however, only the first 31 amino acids of PTH are essential for biological activity. The parathyroid gland contains the extracellular calcium-sensing receptor (CaSR) that acts as a sensor of plasma ionized calcium levels (Thakker et al., 2010; dePaula and Rosen, 2010). Decreased ionized calcium in the blood is detected by the calcium sensor and leads to an increase in PTH secretion; conversely, secretion is inhibited by an increase in blood calcium. The rapid negative feedback regulation of PTH production is thus largely regulated by plasma calcium.

Bone and kidney are the primary target organs for PTH. The peptide hormone interacts with specific receptors on the plasma membrane of bone cells (osteoblasts) and tubular kidney cells to stimulate cAMP production. Cyclic AMP acts as a second messenger to activate certain enzymes, such as protein kinases, which trigger a cascade of biochemical events that ultimately result in expression of the physiological actions of PTH. Increased plasma PTH concentrations are detected by renal PTH receptors, causing the kidneys to rapidly increase the

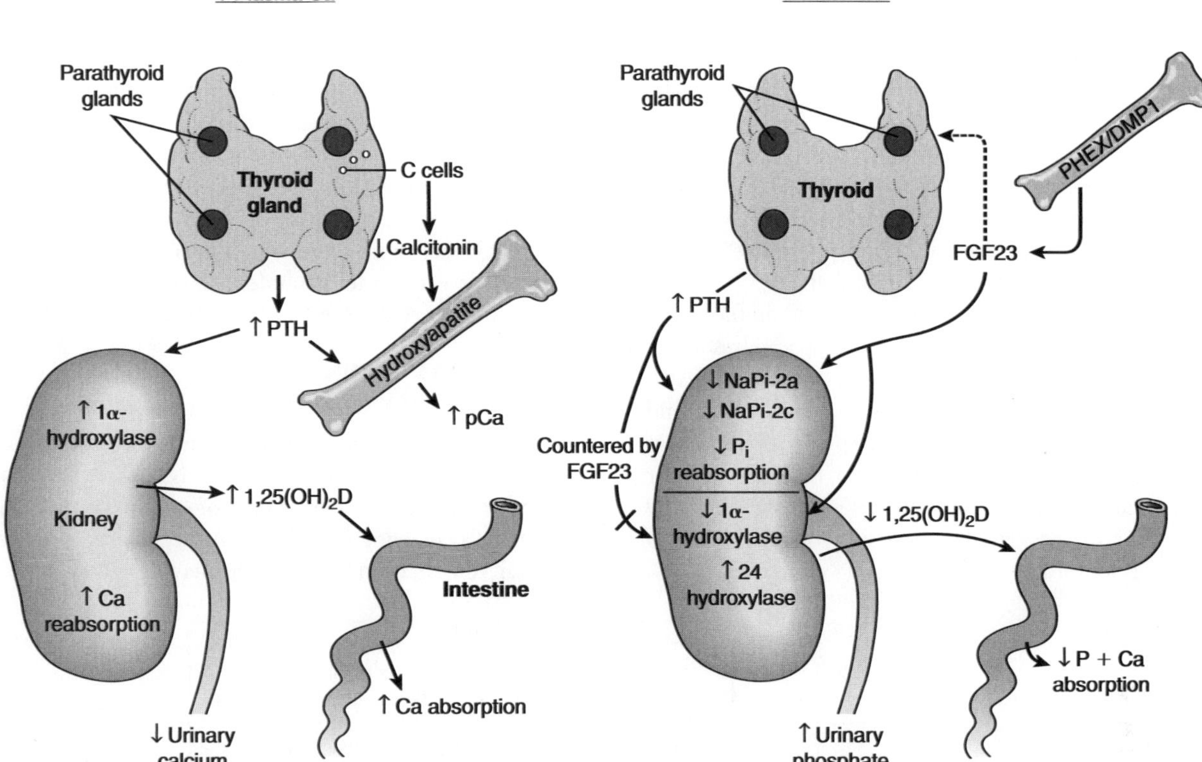

FIGURE 32-3 Hormonal control of calcium and phosphate metabolism. Calcium and phosphate homeostasis is maintained by the coordinated actions of the intestine, kidney, and bone. A fall in plasma ionic Ca^{2+} level is detected by a calcium-sensor protein in the parathyroid glands. This causes an increased secretion of parathyroid hormone (*PTH*) that then acts on receptors in the kidney and in bone osteoblasts. The renal effect of PTH results in an immediate increase in renal calcium reabsorption and a decrease in renal phosphate reabsorption. PTH also has a delayed effect on calcium and phosphate absorption by stimulating the activity of the renal 1α-hydroxylase that converts inactive 25-hydroxyvitamin D [*25(OH)D*] to the active vitamin D metabolite 1,25-dihydroxyvitamin D [*1,25(OH)$_2$D*]. In addition, 1,25(OH)$_2$D can also promote bone resorption by stimulating the production of osteoclasts. Fibroblast growth factor 23 (*FGF23*) is the most important regulator of phosphate renal reabsorption and acts to suppress sodium–phosphate cotransporter type-2a (NaPi-2a) and NaPi-2c and either alone or in conjunction with PTH acts to increase urinary phosphate excretion. In addition, FGF23 acts to lower plasma phosphorus by countering the actions of PTH on 1α-hydroxylase and 1,25(OH)$_2$D production and increasing the activity of 24 hydroxylase, which ultimately leads to lower intestinal phosphorus absorption. *DMP1*, Dentin matrix protein 1; *pCa*, plasma calcium; *PHEX*, phosphate-regulating gene with homologies to endopeptidases on the X chromosome.

BOX 32-2 Summary Points for Endocrine Regulation of Calcium and Phosphate

- The important regulators of calcium homeostasis are PTH, calcitonin, and 1,25(OH)$_2$D, and for phosphate they are FGF23, PTH, and 1,25(OH)$_2$D.
- PTH is upregulated by low plasma calcium and increased plasma phosphate concentrations. It is downregulated by increased plasma calcium and 1,25(OH)$_2$D levels and possibly increased plasma FGF23. PTH acts through PTH receptors to increase osteoblast activity (indirect action on osteoclast) with subsequent increases in plasma calcium. It acts on the kidney to increase calcium reabsorption (and plasma calcium levels) and decreases renal phosphate reabsorption to decrease plasma phosphate levels.
- Calcitonin acts in opposition to PTH and lowers blood calcium levels.
- 1,25(OH)$_2$D acts on the intestine to increase calcium and phosphate absorption with a net effect to increase plasma calcium and phosphate levels. FGF23 and PTH have opposite effects on the synthesis of 1,25(OH)$_2$D by decreasing and increasing it, respectively.
- FGF23 is a bone-derived growth factor from osteocytes that binds a Klotho–FGF receptor complex located in the distal tubule and inhibits renal phosphate reabsorption, suppresses expression of 1α- hydroxylase, and increases 24-hydroxylase activity in the kidney. FGF23 may also decrease PTH secretion by acting on the parathyroid glands. The primary effect is to reduce plasma phosphate.

rate of renal calcium reabsorption (which decreases urinary calcium loss) and decrease the rate of phosphate reabsorption (which increases urinary phosphate loss). PTH also increases the activity of the renal 25-hydroxyvitamin D 1α-hydroxylase that converts the biologically inactive 25-hydroxyvitamin D [25(OH)D] into the active hormonal form of vitamin D, $1,25(OH)_2D$. There are no PTH receptors in the intestine, but the PTH-mediated increase in circulating $1,25(OH)_2D$ leads to an increase in intestinal calcium and phosphate absorption. Also, despite the fact that PTH plays an important role in bone resorption, no PTH receptors are found on the osteoclasts (Gardella et al., 2010). PTH produces a bone-resorbing effect by stimulating expression of RANKL (receptor activator of nuclear factor kappa B [RANK] ligand) by osteoblasts and decreasing osteoprotegerin production by preosteoblast cells in bone (Figure 32-4). These factors work with RANK, a receptor for RANKL that is present on osteoclasts. Receptor activation by RANKL promotes osteoclast differentiation and activation into mature active bone-resorbing osteoclasts (Kearns et al., 2008). These three distinct but coordinated actions of PTH maintain calcium homeostasis by increasing calcium release from bone, reducing the renal clearance of calcium, and increasing absorption in the intestine. Hyperphosphatemia, which would result from the accompanying increased intestinal absorption and skeletal release of phosphorus, is prevented by the phosphaturic effect of PTH on the kidneys. In contrast to chronic high PTH that acts to resorb bone, lower dose intermittent PTH that is used in the treatment of osteoporosis and contains amino acids 1 to 34 (teriparatide) will stimulate bone formation (Dempster et al., 1993).

25-HYDROXYVITAMIN D AND 1,25-DIHYDROXYVITAMIN D

Vitamin D can enter the circulation after synthesis in the skin or absorption from the diet. Vitamin D is transported through the body via a vitamin D–binding protein. This complex binds to liver cells, allowing vitamin D to enter the hepatocytes. In the liver, the vitamin D molecule may be either stored or

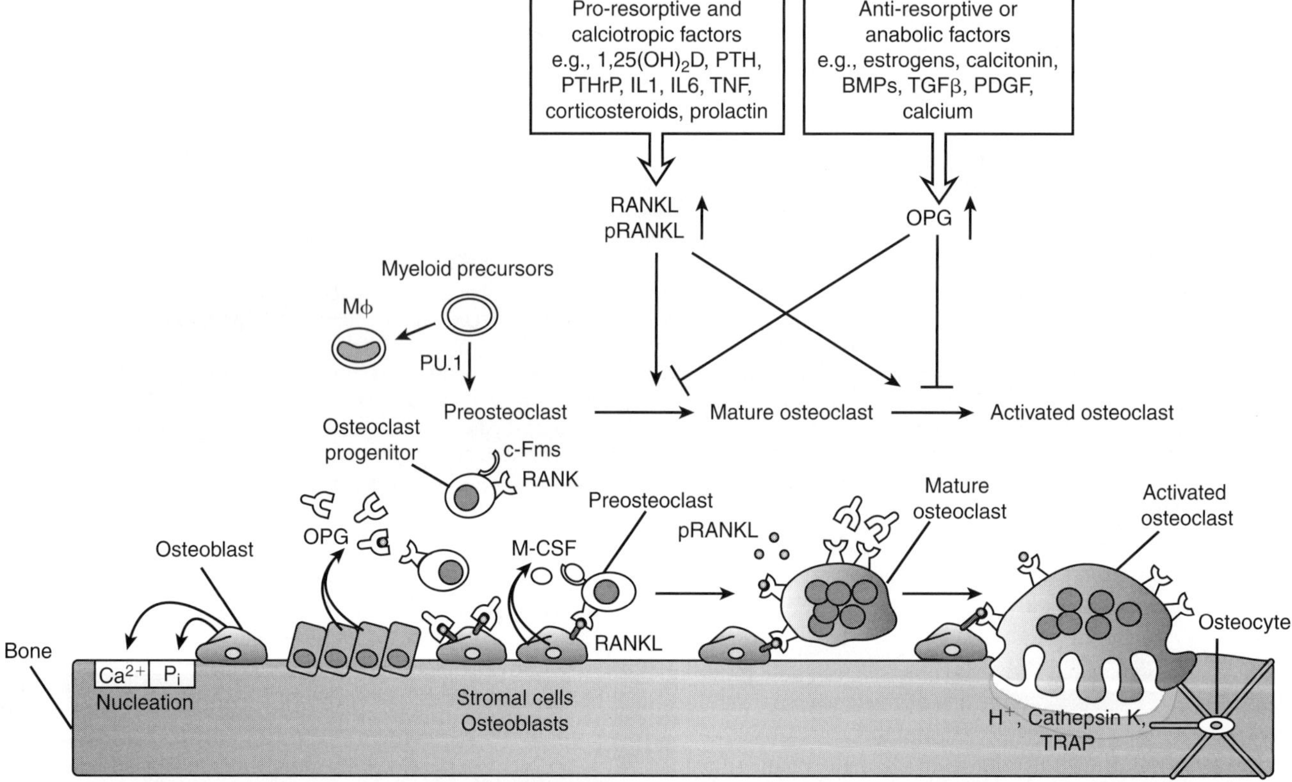

FIGURE 32-4 Osteoclastogenesis via osteoblast-mediated regulation. Transcription factor PU.1 is required for development of the osteoclast and macrophage (*M*) lineages from a common myeloid precursor. Macrophage-colony stimulating factor (*M-CSF*) produced by osteoblast cells acts upon the receptor c-Fms and the osteoclast progenitor is converted to a preosteoclast. Signaling through the membrane-bound receptor activator of nuclear factor-κB (*RANK*) promotes further differentiation of preosteoclasts to mature osteoclasts that secrete protons (H^+, acid) and proteolytic enzymes to resorb bone such as tartrate-resistant acid phosphatase (*TRAP*) and cathepsin K. RANK signaling is induced by receptor activator of nuclear factor-κB ligand (*RANKL*), present on osteoblasts, bone marrow stromal cells, lymphocytes, and possibly in a soluble form in plasma (*pRANKL*). The antagonist osteoprotegerin (*OPG*) competes with RANK for RANKL binding, thereby functioning as a negative regulator of osteoclast differentiation, activation, and survival. RANKL expression is induced by proresorptive factors (e.g., cytokines TNFα and IL1, PTH, and $1,25(OH)_2D$) that stimulate osteoclastogenesis. Conversely, osteoprotegerin is induced by factors that block bone catabolism and promote anabolic effects (e.g., bone morphogenic protein, BMP; transforming growth factor-β, TGFβ; platelet-derived growth factor, PDGF) to regulate bone resorption. *PTHrP*, Parathyroid hormone–related protein. (Modified from Maes, C., & Kronenberg, H. M. [2010]. Bone development and remodeling. In J. L. Jameson & L. J. De Groot [Eds.], *Endocrinology* [p. 1118]. Philadelphia: Saunders.)

hydroxylated at C25. The 25(OH)D that is formed by hydroxylation leaves the liver and is bound again in the blood by the vitamin D–binding protein. 25(OH)D can then be taken up by the kidney, where it can be further hydroxylated at the C1 position to form $1,25(OH)_2D$, the active hormone form of vitamin D. The renal conversion of 25(OH)D to $1,25(OH)_2D$ is regulated primarily by PTH, as described previously.

$1,25(OH)_2D$ likely plays many roles in the body and classically acts on cells through an intracellular receptor protein called the vitamin D receptor (VDR) that is found in many different tissues. In addition, a $1,25(OH)_2D$–membrane-associated rapid response to steroid-binding protein ($1,25D_3$-MARRS) has been found on plasma membranes, and it appears to regulate the rapid nongenomic aspects of $1,25(OH)_2D$ action (Nemere et al., 2004). However, the physiological importance of these rapid vitamin D–mediated effects on cells has yet to be determined. When activated by $1,25(OH)_2D$, the nuclear VDR interacts with specific gene promoter regions in DNA and affects transcription of these vitamin D–specific genes, such as increasing expression of the enterocyte membrane calcium channel (TRPV6, also called CaT1) (Wood et al., 2001) and calbindin-D_{9K}, a 9-kDa intracellular Ca^{2+}-binding protein that facilitates the absorption of calcium (Bronner, 2009). $1,25(OH)_2D$ also increases expression of a number of other proteins that are involved with other functions of vitamin D, such its immunological or antiproliferative effects (Wood et al., 2004). In addition, $1,25(OH)_2D$ increases the apical membrane Na^+-dependent phosphate transporter that facilitates phosphate absorption in the brush border membrane of the enterocyte.

Osteoblasts also have vitamin D receptors, and the effect of $1,25(OH)_2D$ on bone is to increase expression of RANKL by osteoblastic cells (see Figure 32-4). Receptor activation by RANKL leads to osteoclast differentiation, activation and survival, thereby promoting differentiation into osteoclasts and bone resorption (Maes and Kronenberg, 2010). However, this effect of $1,25(OH)_2D$ has only been shown with supraphysiological levels, and at physiological doses it suppresses PTH-induced RANKL expression and bone resorption (Suda et al., 2003) (see Chapter 31 for additional information on $1,25(OH)_2D$).

CALCITONIN

Calcitonin, synthesized by the C cells (previously termed the parafollicular cells) of the thyroid gland, is a polypeptide containing 32 amino acids, almost all of which are needed for biological activity. A rise in plasma Ca^{2+} is the strongest calcitonin secretagogue. When blood Ca^{2+} increases acutely, there is a parallel increase in calcitonin secretion, whereas an acute drop in plasma Ca^{2+} causes a decrease in calcitonin secretion. Calcitonin acts in opposition to PTH and lowers blood calcium levels. The best studied action of calcitonin, which appears to occur generally throughout all mammalian species, is to inhibit osteoclast activity (de Paula and Rosen, 2010). The plasma membrane of osteoclasts has calcitonin receptors that respond to calcitonin by increasing cAMP production, which in turn mediates the actions of calcitonin, including inhibition of the movement of osteoclasts. Inactivation of calcitonin occurs primarily in the kidney. Aside from the osteoclast calcitonin receptor, these receptors are found in other cells, such as monocytes, kidney, brain, pituitary, placenta, prostate, testis, lung, and lymphocytes (Martin et al., 2010). Calcitonin is used as a drug to treat diseases associated with high rates of bone resorption and hypercalcemia (Table 32-1), such as Paget disease and osteoporosis, to reduce vertebral fracture. Calcitonin also has been shown to reduce cartilage degradation in osteoarthritic patients (Karsdal et al., 2010) and has analgesic properties to inhibit bone pain (Knopp et al., 2005).

TABLE 32-1 Causes and Clinical Consequences of Hypocalcemia and Hypercalcemia

HYPOCALCEMIA

Causes

- Hypoparathyroidism due to primary or secondary causes, mutations, postradiation, infiltrative process (iron overload hemochromatosis, Wilson disease, tumor, Mg^{2+} excess or deficiency)
- Inadequate vitamin D production due to deficiency from poor nutrition, insufficient sunlight, malabsorption, chronic kidney disease, or end-stage liver disease
- PTH resistance (pseudohypoparathyroidism, Mg^{2+} deficiency)
- Vitamin D resistance (vitamin D–dependent rickets type 1 or 2)
- Miscellaneous causes: hyperphosphatemia, rapid transfusions, acute critical illness, osteoblastic metastasis, acute pancreatitis, rhabdomyolysis; drugs (foscarnet, IV bisphosphonate)

Clinical Consequences

- Asymptomatic, fatigue
- Neuromuscular irritability: tetany, carpopedal spasms, muscle twitching and cramping, circumoral tingling, abdominal cramps (Chvostek or Trousseau signs of neuromuscular irritability in the face or hand)
- Laryngospasm, bronchospasm
- Altered central nervous system function (seizures, altered mental status, depression, coma)
- Cardiomyopathy (prolonged QTc interval on electrocardiogram)

HYPERCALCEMIA

Causes

- Hyperabsorption of Ca (high PTH due to hyperparathyroidism or hypophosphatemia)
- Decreased urinary excretion (renal reabsorption defect)
- Increased bone resorption due to elevated PTH, $1,25(OH)_2D$, or skeletal metastasis
- Severe dehydration
- Idiopathic hypercalcemia and hypercalciuria (possibly related to TRPV5/6 mutations)

Clinical Consequences

- Fatigue, electrocardiogram abnormalities, nausea, vomiting, constipation, anorexia, abdominal pain, and hypercalciuria that may lead to kidney stones

FIBROBLAST GROWTH FACTOR 23

A major advance in understanding phosphate homeostasis was accomplished with the identification of FGF23 as a novel hormone that lowers blood phosphate levels (Kuro-o, 2010). When phosphate is in excess, FGF23 is secreted from osteocytes in bone, a process that is regulated by two bone proteins: phosphate-regulating gene with homology to endopeptidases on the X chromosome (PHEX) and dentin matrix protein 1 (DMP1) (see Figure 32-3). FGF23 acts on the kidney to suppress expression of the sodium-phosphate cotransporters (NaPi-2a, NaPi-2c) which facilitate the active reabsorption of phosphorus. Diminished expression of NaPi-2a and NaPi-2c occurs either directly or indirectly through stimulation of PTH activity, which increases urinary phosphate excretion (Bergwitz and Jüppner, 2010). In addition, FGF23 reduces plasma 1,25$(OH)_2$D levels by suppressing synthesis of 1α-hydroxylase and increasing catabolism by increasing 24-hydroxylase activity. The reduction in 1,25$(OH)_2$D levels results in a reduced phosphate intestinal absorption (and calcium absorption), thereby inducing a negative phosphate balance. FGF23 requires Klotho, a transmembrane protein, as a co-receptor for high affinity binding to FGF receptors. More specifically, FGF23 binds the Klotho–FGF receptor complex with much higher affinity than the FGF receptor alone.

There are hereditary disorders or tumor-induced osteomalacia that exhibit inappropriately high plasma FGF23 levels (and low 1,25$(OH)_2$D) and are characterized by phosphate wasting and impaired bone mineralization (Table 32-2). In contrast, defects in either FGF23 or Klotho are associated with phosphate retention and a premature aging syndrome. The causes and outcomes of hyperphosphatemia are outlined in Table 32-2. Several other phosphaturic peptides, such as secreted frizzled-related protein 4 (sFRP4), matrix extracellular phosphoglycoprotein, and fibroblast growth factor 7 (FGF7), have been shown to inhibit renal phosphate reabsorption and have a pathogenic role in several hypophosphatemic disorders. FGF23 and sFRP4 may be regulated by dietary phosphorus intake. Determination of levels of FGF23 and other phosphaturic peptides (phosphatonins) may improve the diagnosis and prognosis of various diseases association with abnormal mineral metabolism including chronic kidney disease.

TABLE 32-2 Causes and Clinical Consequences of Hypophosphatemia and Hyperphosphatemia

HYPOPHOSPHATEMIA

Causes

- Vitamin D deficiency or resistance (nutrition related, liver diseases, renal diseases, catabolism, anticonvulsants)
- Increased urinary loss due to autosomal dominant hypophosphatemic rickets and other related diseases with mutations that activate FGF23 or Klotho excess; renal phosphate wasting syndromes; hyperparathyroidism; osmotic diuresis; diabetic ketoacidosis; or medications, including calcitonin, diuretics, glucocorticoids, and bicarbonate
- Intracellular shifts (increased insulin, sepsis, tumors, acute respiratory alkalosis)

Clinical Consequences

- Central nervous system (irritability, seizures, delirium, coma)
- Hematopoietic system to decrease oxygen affinity, and affects leukocytes and platelets
- Muscle myopathy, bone resorption, decreased glomerular filtration rate , metabolic acidosis
- Electrolyte imbalances (glycosuria, hypercalciuria, hypermagnesiuria, hypophosphaturia)
- Metabolic abnormalities (insulin resistance, decreased gluconeogenesis, low PTH, high 1,25$(OH)_2$D)

HYPERPHOSPHATEMIA

Causes

- Decreased urinary excretion (renal insufficiency, hypoparathyroidism, acromegaly, bisphosphonates, tumoral calcinosis associated with FGF23 or Klotho inactivating mutations)
- Acute phosphate load
- Altered extracellular space (acidosis, hemolytic anemia, increased bone resorption, catabolic states)
- Pseudohyperphosphatemia (hyperglobulinemia, hyperlipidemia, hemolysis, hyperbilirubinemia)

Clinical Consequences

- Hypocalcemia and tetany, mild symptoms (intestinal distress or mild diarrhea), soft tissue calcification
- If secondary to renal diseases: hyperparathyroidism and renal osteodystrophy

OTHER HORMONES AFFECTING CALCIUM AND PHOSPHATE METABOLISM

Although PTH, 1,25$(OH)_2$D, FGF23, and calcitonin are the major calcium- and phosphate-regulating hormones, several other hormones, including parathyroid hormone–related protein (PTHrP), glucocorticoids, thyroid hormone, growth hormone, insulin, and estrogen, can also affect bone turnover and mineral metabolism.

PTHrP is closely related to PTH, and both of their amino-terminal portions activate the PTH receptor. Although the PTH receptor is present in a variety of tissues, it is found primarily in the kidney and bone, where it mediates mineral ion homeostasis. There may be other receptors for PTH and PTHrP for the C-terminal region, but their biological role is not well defined (Gardella et al., 2010). The common use of the PTH receptor allows PTHrP to act as a hormone mimicking the actions of PTH and has been shown to cause hypercalcemia in patients with certain cancers.

The main effect of glucocorticoids on bone is an inhibition of osteoblastic activity, although osteoclastic activity is also impaired. There is a reduced incorporation of sulfate into cartilage and of amino acids into collagen. Glucocorticoid treatment can reduce intestinal calcium absorption. An excess of glucocorticoids can lead to hypocalcemia and PTH stimulation, which reduces renal phosphate reabsorption and increases urinary phosphate losses. In patients who

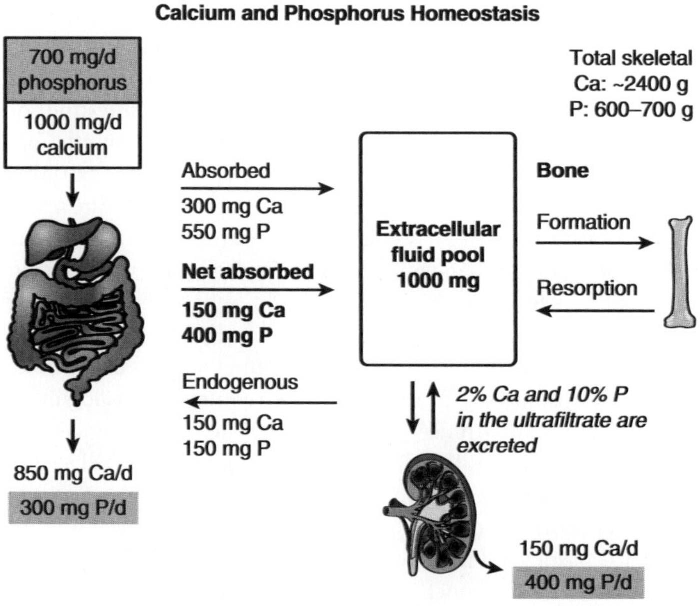

FIGURE 32-5 Calcium (Ca) and phosphorus (P) balance in normal physiology. Total absorption of dietary calcium and phosphorus is about 25% to 30% and 60% to 70%, respectively, for healthy adults. Yet some is secreted back into the intestine, so net absorption is always lower than total absorption at about 150 mg calcium/day and 400 mg phosphorus/day. In adults the exit from the exchangeable mineral pool into the skeleton, representing bone formation, is roughly equivalent to the entry into the exchangeable pool due to bone resorption (breakdown). The skeletal storage depot for calcium and phosphorus is 99% and 85%, respectively, of the total body pools (not shown). Most of the renal calcium and phosphorus is reabsorbed, so that only 2% calcium and 10% phosphorus that is filtered is then excreted in the urine.

have Cushing syndrome or who have arthritis that has been treated with cortisol, glucocorticoid excess can lead to bone loss, especially of trabecular bone, and result in osteoporosis. In children, excess glucocorticoid frequently causes delayed growth and skeletal maturation.

Thyroid hormone stimulates bone resorption, and both compact and trabecular bone are lost in hyperthyroidism. Increased urinary phosphate is observed in hyperthyroid patients in association with increased plasma phosphate. In hypothyroidism, the bone-mobilizing effect of PTH is impaired, leading to secondary hyperparathyroidism.

Growth hormone can stimulate the growth of cartilage and bone through the trophic action of insulin-like growth factor (IGF). Growth hormone can also stimulate the 1α-hydroxylase enzyme in the kidney, which increases plasma $1,25(OH)_2D$ levels. Levels of growth hormone and IGF decline with age. In senescent rats, growth hormone administration can increase calcium and phosphate absorption independent of changes in plasma $1,25(OH)_2D$ (Fleet et al., 1994).

Insulin, a pancreatic hormone involved primarily with regulating glucose metabolism, also stimulates the osteoblastic production of collagen. In addition, insulin can reduce the renal reabsorption of calcium and sodium and decrease urinary phosphate losses.

Estrogen receptors have been identified in bone, and gonadal hormones are important in the regulation of bone mass. Estrogen prevents bone resorption by inducing osteoclast apoptosis. Estrogen deficiency, which occurs in women after menopause, causes loss of bone and contributes to the development of osteoporosis. Estrogen or hormone replacement therapy in postmenopausal women reduces the rate of bone loss but increases the risk for venous thromboembolic events, cardiovascular disease, and breast cancer, which limits its use in the prevention of osteoporosis. Hypogonadism in adult men is a risk factor for osteoporosis, which may be related to the effects of testosterone on bone resorption.

CALCIUM AND PHOSPHATE HOMEOSTASIS

Mineral balance represents the equilibrium condition in which the amount of a mineral absorbed from the diet equals the sum of all the daily losses of the mineral from the body. Because 99% of calcium and 85% of the phosphorus in the body is found in the skeleton, changes in calcium balance are reflected in changes in bone mass. During growth, a positive calcium and phosphate balance must be maintained to supply sufficient amounts of these minerals for bone growth. In contrast, during periods of bone loss, as occur with immobilization and commonly during aging, loss of bone calcium causes a negative calcium balance. Coordination of calcium and phosphate fluxes across the intestine, kidney, and bone maintains calcium and phosphate homeostasis (Figure 32-5). This is needed to face marked changes in daily intakes of these minerals and longer-term metabolic changes associated with growth, aging, and disease.

INTESTINAL ABSORPTION

The unidirectional absorption of calcium or phosphate from the diet is called "true" absorption. However, there is also some obligatory mineral loss into the gastrointestinal tract, as part of digestive secretions and sloughed intestinal cells. Loss of endogenous calcium is referred to as endogenous fecal loss. The difference between true intestinal absorption and endogenous fecal loss is called "net" absorption, which is thus always lower than true absorption. Net absorption of calcium and phosphate is the nutritionally important absorbed amount that is available to build new bone, to maintain steady state plasma levels of these minerals, and to replace any skeletal and renal losses.

The rate of intestinal calcium absorption is regulated primarily by the circulating level of $1,25(OH)_2D$. The efficiency of true calcium absorption varies in response to the dietary calcium intake and throughout the life span as a function of metabolic need. Fractional calcium absorption is highest in infancy (~60%) and decreases to about 25% to 30% in young adults, except for rises during early puberty and during the last two trimesters of pregnancy (Institute of Medicine [IOM], 2011). Aging is associated with a gradual decline in intestinal calcium absorption (Avioli et al., 1965; Heaney et al., 1989), which may reflect both a decline in the plasma $1,25(OH)_2D$ concentration and an intestinal resistance to the action of the active hormone (Pattanaungkul et al., 2000; Wood et al., 1998). However, a more recent report suggests that there may be no decline in calcium balance up to 70 years of age (Hunt and Johnson, 2007). Calcium absorption also varies with estrogen status (Heaney et al., 1989), height (Bärger-Lux and Heaney, 2005), and obesity. It is higher in premenopausal than postmenopausal women and in severely obese compared to overweight individuals (Cifuentes et al., 2004; Riedt et al., 2006, 2007). Greater calcium absorption with excess adiposity may be related to higher estrogen levels in obese subjects (Shapses and Riedt, 2006), as intestinal calcium transport is enhanced by estrogen binding to the estrogen receptor in the intestine.

In general, a large increase in calcium intake is associated with lower absorption. Calcium absorption efficiency varies with calcium status (habitual calcium intake), so that individuals with low calcium intake will have higher calcium absorption. For example, middle-aged individuals with a high calcium intake (2,000 mg/day) only absorb 15%; but in those who consume only 200 mg/day, absorption is 45% (Heaney et al., 1989; Eastell et al., 1991). Though calcium absorption efficiency decreases with increasing intake, the total calcium absorbed increases with the total calcium load. This adaptation is helpful to increase the total calcium absorbed but cannot compensate for a very low calcium intake. Hence when calcium intake is low, bone accretion will be compromised in children and bone loss will occur in adults.

MECHANISM OF CALCIUM TRANSPORT

Kinetic studies of calcium transport suggest that there are two distinct pathways for calcium absorption in the intestine (Bronner, 2009). One pathway represents an active, energy-dependent, transcellular pathway with limited capacity that is under hormonal regulation of vitamin D. The second absorption pathway is a nonsaturable, energy-independent, concentration-dependent, paracellular transport pathway that is not regulated by vitamin D. Transcellular and paracellular transport is active during low and high calcium intakes, respectively.

Transcellular Ca^{2+} transport can be described as a three-step process consisting of passive entry of Ca^{2+} across the apical membrane, the transcellular movement of Ca^{2+} from the point of entry to the basolateral membrane, and its extrusion into the circulatory system. The active, saturable, transcellular transport pathway is found mainly in the duodenum and proximal jejunum. It is regulated by $1,25(OH)_2D$, the membrane channel protein transient receptor potential vanilloid (TRP) TRPV6/CaT1, the cytosolic calcium-binding protein calbindin D, and the basolateral Ca^{2+}-ATPase (Figure 32-6). For general transport across epithelial membranes (intestine or kidney), Ca^{2+} enters the cell at the luminal membrane via the epithelial Ca^{2+} channel TRPV6 (intestine) or TRPV5 (kidney) and is sequestered by calbindin-D_{9K} (intestine) or calbindin-D_{28K} (kidney). Next, the calbindin-bound Ca^{2+} diffuses to the basolateral side of the cell where it is extruded into the blood compartment. The plasma membrane Ca^{2+}-ATPase (PMCA1) is the primary pump in intestine; the Na^+/Ca^{2+} exchanger-1 (NCX1) is the main extruder in kidney, but it is also responsible for approximately 20% of Ca^{2+} extrusion in intestine (Dong et al., 2005; Perez et al., 2008; Schoeber et al., 2007). This final step in the process of transport out of the enterocyte requires that calcium be transported "uphill" against a 10,000-fold Ca^{2+} concentration gradient. Intracellular Ca^{2+} levels are maintained at 10^{-7} mol/L, whereas extracellular Ca^{2+} is 10^{-3} mol/L, and Ca^{2+} transport therefore requires an energy-dependent pump on the basolateral membrane.

Studies in knockout mice that cannot express calbindin or the vitamin D–sensitive TRPV6 calcium channel still seem capable of increasing calcium absorption in response to $1,25(OH)_2D$ (Christakos et al., 2007, 2010). Therefore other mechanisms of calcium transport may serve as a backup to the standard model but require future clarification. The downregulation of TRPV5 and TRPV6 is likely involved in the impaired calcium (re)absorption during aging and disease states (van Abel et al., 2005). In addition, estrogen affects transcription of both TRPV6 and VDR and may explain the lower levels of TRPV6 and VDR found in duodenal mucosal biopsies from postmenopausal women and their lower rates of calcium absorption compared to younger women (Walters et al., 2007). Calbindin D is believed to act as an intracellular calcium "ferry" that facilitates the diffusion of calcium across the aqueous cytosol to the basolateral membrane for extrusion out of the cell. There are two major subclasses of the calcium binding protein, calbindin D. There is calbindin-D_{9k} (9,000 Mr that is present in mammalian intestine and bovine, mouse, and neonatal rat kidney) and calbindin-D_{28K} (28,000 Mr, present in avian intestine, mammalian and avian kidney and pancreas, mammalian osteoblastic cells, and mammalian and molluskan brain) (Christakos et al., 2007).

Quantitatively, the most important site of calcium absorption in the intestine is the ileum, due to the relatively long sojourn of calcium in this segment of the intestine. It has been shown in humans that removal of the ileum has a more devastating effect on calcium absorption than removal of the jejunum. This can explain why calcium absorption remains at about 24% even after gastric bypass surgery for weight loss (Riedt et al., 2006), where the ileum remains intact and typically about half of the jejunum remains. Although calcium can also be absorbed by the colon, this segment of the intestine apparently plays a minor role in the overall economy of calcium absorption in humans. However, in rats the cecum has a high rate of vitamin D–dependent calcium absorption (Nellans and Goldsmith, 1983) and hence differs from humans. It is possible that vitamin D–dependent changes in membrane lipid composition and membrane fluidity are

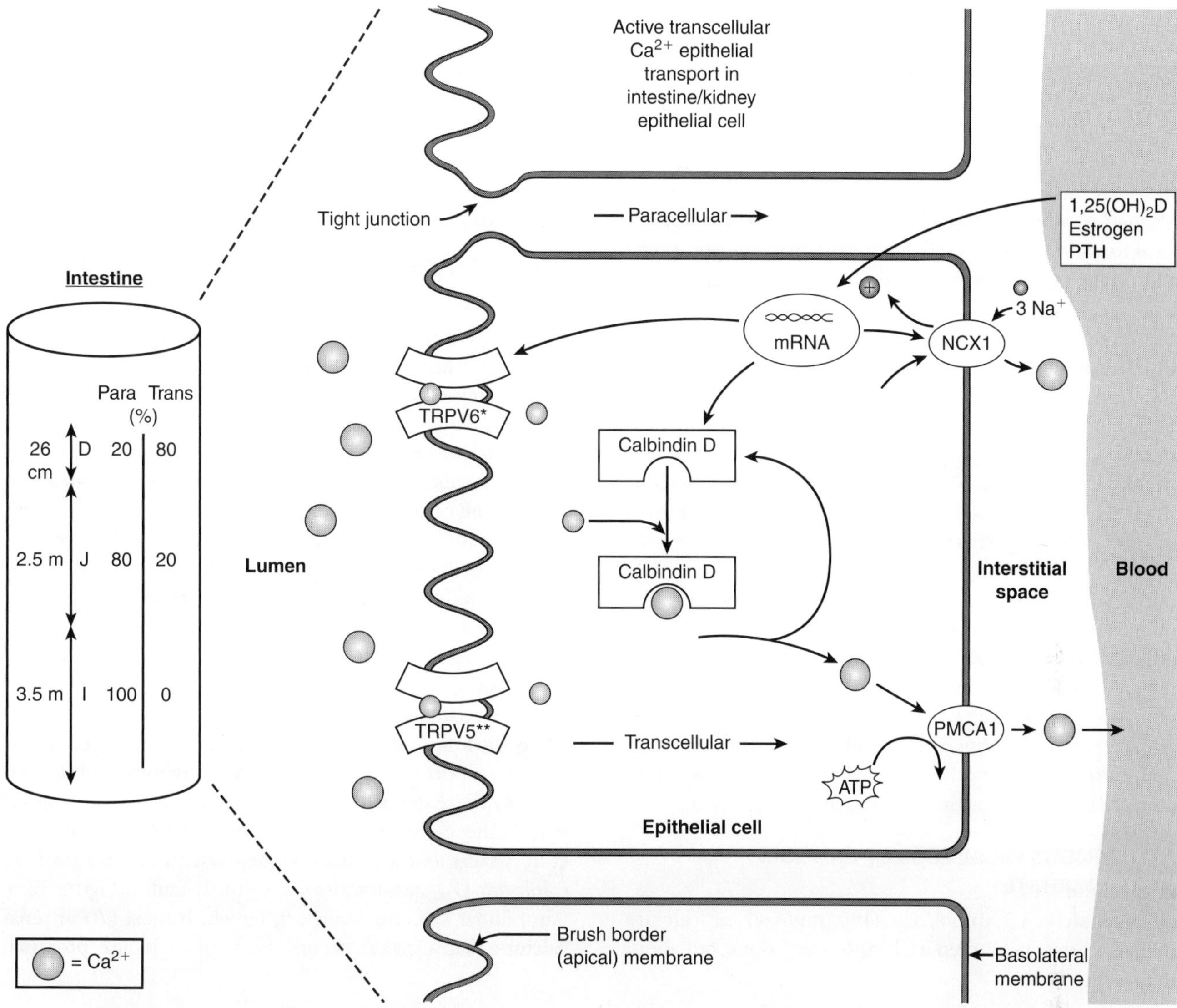

FIGURE 32-6 Model of paracellular (*para*) and transcellular (*trans*) Ca^{2+} transport (%) for a given location in the intestine and a detailed model of calcium transport across membranes (intestine and kidney). Calcium crosses the intestine by two routes. One pathway is the paracellular transport pathway, which is characterized by nonsaturable, energy-independent, concentration-dependent calcium transport. The calcium transcellular transport pathway is regulated primarily by $1,25(OH)_2D$ via a genomic mechanism that regulates the production of the brush border (apical) membrane calcium channels, the cytosolic mobile calcium buffer calbindin D, and the basolateral membrane exporter pumps. More specifically, Ca^{2+} enters the cell at the luminal membrane via the epithelial Ca^{2+} channel TRPV6 (intestine and kidney) or TRPV5 (kidney) and is sequestered by calbindin-D_{9K} (intestine and kidney) or calbindin-D_{28K} (primarily in kidney). Bound Ca^{2+} leaves these membranes by diffusing to the basolateral cell surface. There it is extruded into the blood compartment via the plasma membrane Ca^{2+}-ATPase (PMCA1, primary pump in intestine) and Na^+/Ca^{2+} exchanger-1 (NCX1, primary pump in kidney but also responsible for 20% of Ca^{2+} extrusion in intestine). The coordinated vitamin D–regulated actions efficiently increase calcium intestinal absorption or renal reabsorption to help maintain plasma calcium concentrations in the face of low dietary intake or increased calcium need. *D,* Duodenum; *I,* ileum; *J,* jejenum; measurements refer to length of each section of the small intestine.

partially responsible for altering the rate of calcium transport across the membrane (Fontaine et al., 1981). The multiple endocrine factors influencing calcium absorption are shown in Figure 32-3.

Calcium is absorbed in its ionized form; therefore it must be released from the insoluble salts in which it usually comes in food and dietary supplements. Even though most calcium salts are dissolved in the acidic pH of the stomach, absorption is not guaranteed. Calcium may form insoluble complexes with other dietary components, such as phytates, within the more alkaline pH found in the small intestine, limiting its bioavailability. Magnesium and calcium compete for intestinal absorption when an excess of either is present in the intestinal tract. In contrast, increased dietary protein has been shown to increase fractional calcium absorption (Kerstetter et al., 2005) that is partially due to greater transcellular calcium absorption (Gaffney-Stromberg et al., 2010).

INTESTINAL ABSORPTION OF PHOSPHATE

Phosphate absorption in humans has been shown to be linearly related to phosphate intake over a wide range of phosphate intakes. Approximately 60% to 70% of phosphate is absorbed from a typical mixed diet, making phosphate absorption about twice as efficient as calcium absorption. Phosphate absorption is influenced by vitamin D status, although to a less marked degree than calcium absorption. Administration of 1,25$(OH)_2$D directly increases phosphate absorption in all segments of the small intestine, but the major effect is in the jejunum (Renkema et al., 2008; Berndt and Kumar, 2009). Like calcium, phosphate is absorbed by both a saturable and a nonsaturable transport pathway.

Little is known about the molecular details of intestinal phosphate absorption. The preferred transport form is HPO_4^{2-}. The kinetics of phosphate uptake in vitro by isolated intestinal brush border vesicle preparations suggests that it crosses the apical membrane of the enterocyte by a carrier-mediated mechanism. Transport of phosphate into the intestinal cell is generally believed to be by an active, Na^+-dependent pathway mediated by the apical membrane phosphate transporter protein, but newer evidence with isotope studies shows that at high concentrations of phosphate, active Na^+-mediated transport is absent and passive diffusion occurs (Williams and DeLuca, 2007). In addition, intestinal adaptation to a low-phosphorus diet in VDR knockout mice indicate that absorption of phosphate is independent of the action of 1,25$(OH)_2$D on the nuclear VDR (Segawa et al., 2004).

ENDOGENOUS FECAL LOSS OF CALCIUM AND PHOSPHATE

Approximately 3.5 mmol/day (140 mg/day) of calcium enters the intestinal lumen in digestive secretions, but about 29% of this is reabsorbed, so that endogenous fecal calcium is usually 2.5 mmol/day (100 to 140 mg/day) (Heaney and Recker, 1994). Reports of endogenous fecal losses of phosphate have been variable but are usually lower than those observed for endogenous fecal calcium. Therefore endogenous loss of calcium and phosphate is about 15% of total fecal loss. Total loss is about 800 mg/day of calcium and 250 mg/day of phosphate (see Figure 32-5).

URINARY EXCRETION

Urinary Calcium

Because of the binding of plasma calcium to albumin, a significant portion of plasma calcium cannot enter the renal filtrate. Nevertheless, approximately 240 mmol (10,000 mg/day) of calcium is filtered by the kidneys. Urinary calcium excretion is usually only 2.5 to 6 mmol/day (100 to 240 mg/day) for normal individuals; this represents only about 1% to 2.5% of the calcium filtered by the kidney (see Figure 32-5). Approximately 50% of excreted calcium is in the free Ca^{2+} form, and the remainder is complexed with small anions such as sulfate, phosphate, citrate, and oxalate. Patients with renal stones (nephrolithiasis) frequently have hypercalciuria (urinary calcium greater than 250 mg/day) and kidney stones composed of calcium oxalate crystals.

Mechanisms of renal tubular calcium transport are similar to those found in the intestinal epithelium. Active calcium transport is found in the distal convoluted tubule and possibly the distal proximal tubule, and it involves an apical membrane calcium channel protein (TRPV5) (Nijenhuis et al., 2005) and a vitamin D–dependent, 28-kDa protein, calbindin-D_{28K}, as described previously and in Figure 32-6. Paracellular calcium transport, by which most (70%) renal calcium reabsorption occurs, takes place in the proximal

CLINICAL CORRELATION

Dietary Calcium, Protein, and Sodium Intake and Renal Stones

As many as 10% of men and 3% of women have a kidney stone during their adult lives. About 80% of all stones are composed of calcium oxalate, alone or with a nucleus of calcium phosphate apatite. A primary risk factor for calcium kidney stones (nephrolithiasis) is idiopathic (unknown cause) hypercalciuria and urinary supersaturation. In addition, a renal phosphate leak causing hypophosphatemia may predispose the individual to calcium stone formation by increasing the plasma calcitriol level, calcium excretion, and urinary saturation (Prié et al., 2001). Many people that develop renal stones exhibit a lower bone mineral content that may be due to consumption of a low-calcium diet (400 mg calcium/day) that had been previously recommended to patients with renal stones. A determining study by Borghi and colleagues (2002) showed that recurrent calcium oxalate stones and hypercalciuria can be prevented with a diet that has normal calcium (1,200 mg/day) and is low in animal protein (<60 g/day) and sodium (1.2 g/day). There is also epidemiological evidence showing that low-calcium diets are associated with an increased risk of nephrolithiasis, probably due to a greater degree of oxalate absorption from the intestine when diets are low in calcium (Curhan et al., 1993). Although use of calcium supplements also has been shown to be associated with increased risk of stone formation in the large Women's Health Initiative study (Jackson et al., 2006), intake was high at about 2,150 mg/day of calcium (and 765 IU/day of vitamin D) compared to the recommended calcium intake of 1,200 mg/day. There are few or no studies showing increased stone risk with calcium intake at recommended levels (Heaney, 2008). Overall, a diet with the recommended calcium intake of 1 to 1.2 g/day and adequate water intake (2 to 3 L/day) are important in the prevention of renal stones. In addition, reducing animal protein and consuming a low-sodium diet (1.2 g/day) will further prevent reoccurrence of stones in individuals with recurrent calcium oxalate stones and hypercalciuria.

tubule, the thick ascending limb of the loop of Henle, and the connecting and collecting ducts. Urinary calcium and urinary sodium losses are frequently found to be positively associated because these two minerals share a common mechanism that parallels water movement.

There are large diurnal fluctuations in the rate of urinary calcium excretion, due mainly to the calciuretic effect of various food components. Dietary calcium intake has a positive but weak relationship with urinary calcium excretion. In contrast, elevations in plasma phosphate reduce urinary calcium. This occurs because high plasma phosphate decreases ionic calcium and thereby causes an increase in PTH synthesis, which in turn increases calcium reabsorption in the kidney. Dietary intake of simple sugars and protein can increase urinary calcium losses. For example, it has been calculated that for each 50-g increment in daily protein intake, an additional 1.5 mmol (60 mg) of calcium is lost in the urine (Kerstetter and Allen, 1990). The mechanism of protein-induced hypercalciuria involves a reduction of renal calcium reabsorption mediated in part by the sulfur amino acid content of the protein. The metabolism of these amino acids generates an acid (fixed anion, SO_2^-) load, which can inhibit renal calcium reabsorption. Despite this higher urinary calcium excretion, dietary protein does not result in negative calcium balance because it is also associated with higher calcium absorption (Kerstetter et al., 2005) and possibly lower fecal calcium loss (Whiting and Draper, 1981). In addition, the anticalciuretic effect of phosphate has practical implications, because the high phosphate content of meat causes a considerable blunting of the usual hypercalciuric effect of consuming a high-protein diet (Hegsted et al., 1981).

Urinary Phosphate

The kidney can efficiently regulate plasma phosphate levels, and the fractional excretion of filtered phosphate by the kidneys varies from 0.1% to 20%. Approximately 40% of the total phosphate reabsorption in the kidney occurs within the first few convolutions of the proximal tubule, and 60% to 70% has occurred by the time the ultrafiltrate reaches the last segment of the cortical superficial nephrons. The transport of phosphate in the renal tubules occurs by two processes: one depends on sodium and the other does not. There is passive transport only at the basolateral membranes. In the proximal tubule, phosphate is reabsorbed by an active, sodium–phosphate cotransporter type-2a (NaPi-2a) on the brush border (Bergwitz and Jüppner, 2010). FGF23 acts on the kidney to suppress expression of NaPi-2a and NaPi-2c, and either alone or with PTH, it acts to increase urinary phosphate excretion (Renkema et al., 2008). Plasma PTH promotes urinary excretion of phosphate by inhibiting reabsorption by both the Na^+-dependent and the Na^+-independent phosphate transport pathways. Overall, factors that increase phosphate reabsorption and reduce excretion include phosphate depletion, parathyroidectomy, and presence of $1{,}25OH_2D$. Urinary excretion of phosphate is enhanced by PTH, FGF23, and high circulating levels of phosphate or calcium.

BONE RESORPTION AND FORMATION

Bone is composed of collagen fibers, noncollagenous proteins, and deposited minerals, primarily as hydroxyapatite. Crystals of hydroxyapatite are found in and on the collagen fibers and in the ground substance (glycoproteins and proteoglycans) of bone. Longitudinal bone growth occurs in children until closure of the epiphyses during adolescence. However, bone mineral density is attained at about 18 and 20 years of age in females and males, respectively; yet bone mass (the amount of bone tissue in the skeleton) continues to increase until about the age of 30 years (Recker et al., 1992) and then is continually remodeled throughout life. Bone turnover occurs over several weeks by clusters of osteoclasts and osteoblasts arranged within temporary anatomical structures known as basic multicellular units (BMUs). This remodeling process occurs at localized sites in both cortical and trabecular bone. Although the entire bone calcium pool turns over on average every 5 to 6 years, a given local bone surface on trabecular bone may undergo complete remodeling once every 2 years. However, the rate of remodeling varies greatly among specific bones, with the most rapid turnover seen in lumbar vertebrae. In bone, the osteoblasts and osteoclasts are specialized cells for bone formation and resorption, respectively. Osteocytes are mature osteoblasts and respond to the mechanical environment; they are associated with bone microdamage that arise from cracks or fractures (Raggot and Partridge, 2010).

Bone Formation

The activity of osteoblasts in bone determines the rate of bone matrix (collagen and ground substance) deposition. Osteoblasts descend from pluripotent mesenchymal stem cells. Mesenchymal cells can differentiate into a variety of cell types, including muscle cells (myoblasts), fat cells (adipocytes), chondrocytes, and osteoblasts. Canonical Wnt signaling has been shown to play a significant role in the control of osteoblastogenesis and bone formation. Mouse models provide compelling evidence that β-catenin is a crucial transcription factor determining the osteoblast lineage commitment by inducing osteoblastic and suppressing chondrocytic differentiation (Maes and Kronenberg, 2010). Osteoblasts are also controlled by master transcription factor, runt-related transcription factor 2 (Runx2), and to a lesser extent by osterix, another transcription factor involved in osteoblast differentiation. Osteoblasts, which have cellular receptors for PTH, estrogen, and $1{,}25(OH)_2D$, regulate the flux of calcium and phosphate in bone and presumably mediate the deposition of hydroxyapatite in bone tissue. Osteoblasts are usually found in clusters along the bone surface and lay down bone matrix that is initially unmineralized (Maes and Kronenberg, 2010). During bone formation and mineralization, most of the osteoblasts differentiate into flattened cells that line or cover the bone surface. Some osteoblasts become trapped within the mineralized matrix and differentiate into osteocytes that are connected with each other and with the bone lining cells on the surface by cytoplasmic processes. Because the plasma membrane of the osteoblast is rich in the enzyme alkaline phosphatase, biochemical measures of bone-specific serum alkaline phosphatase are used as a convenient marker of bone formation rates.

Bone Resorption

The activity of osteoclasts in bone determines the rate of bone breakdown. The osteoclast has a monocytic–phagocytic cell lineage and is characterized histologically as a giant multinucleated cell that is usually found in contact with a calcified bone surface within a lacuna (hole) that is the result of its own resorptive activity (Maes and Kronenberg, 2010) (see Figure 32-2). Usually, only one to five osteoclasts are associated with one of these resorptive cavities. The contact zone of the osteoclast with the bone is characterized by the presence of a ruffled border on the osteoclast. The ruffled border portion of the osteoclast plasma membrane is surrounded by a ring of contractile proteins, which attach the cell to the bone surface and seal off the subosteoclastic bone-resorbing compartment.

The attachment of the cell to the bone matrix is performed by integrin receptors that bind to specific sequences in matrix proteins (Raggot and Partridge, 2010). Lysosomal enzymes are actively secreted via the ruffled border of the osteoclast into the sealed-off extracellular bone-resorbing compartment. The osteoclast secretes collagenase as well as protons to acidify the bone-resorbing compartment. The acid environment dissolves the hydroxyapatite crystals, and the secreted enzymes break down the bone matrix. The dissolution of bone helps maintain calcium and phosphate concentrations in the plasma. End products of bone matrix breakdown, such as hydroxyproline and amino-terminal collagen peptides, are excreted in the urine and can be used as convenient biochemical measures of bone resorption rates.

The mode of regulation of osteoclast activity is complex. Osteoclasts have receptors for calcitonin, and their activity is decreased by calcitonin. However, osteoclasts also respond to other regulatory signals, such as PTH, 1,25(OH)$_2$D, and prostaglandin E_2, via osteoblast mediation. Figure 32-4 illustrates the role of the osteoprotegerin/RANKL/RANK system in the process of osteoclastogenesis (Maes and Kronenberg, 2010). In brief, various proresorptive cytokines (e.g., tumor necrosis factor-alpha [TNFα] and interleukin 1 [IL1]) stimulate the production of macrophage colony-stimulating factor (M-CSF) by preosteoblastic/stromal cells. M-CSF binds to its receptor (c-Fms) on osteoclast precursor cells, leading to an expansion of these precursor cells. M-CSF also directly increases the production of soluble and membrane-bound RANKL (RANK ligand) by osteoblasts. RANKL binds to its receptor (RANK) on osteoclasts; ligand binding stimulates the differentiation, fusion into multinucleated cells, activation, and survival of osteoclasts. Osteoprotegerin is a soluble factor produced by preosteoblasts that acts as a receptor decoy and binds RANKL, thereby slowing osteoclastogenesis. Hormones, such as PTH, 1,25(OH)$_2$D, glucocorticoids, TGFα, and estrogen, regulate RANKL and osteoprotegerin to affect bone resorption activity.

Bone Remodeling Cycle: "Coupled" Bone Formation and Bone Resorption

After the osteoclasts have finished removing a certain amount of bone, they are replaced by bone-forming osteoblasts that then proceed to replace the excavated bone material. The total resorptive period at a given bone site takes approximately 40 days to complete. About 1 week after the resorptive phase, the formation activity of osteoblasts begins and continues for about 145 days (Melsen and Mosekilde, 1988) in a recurring cycle involving the coordinated activities of osteoblasts and osteoclasts. This process of bone remodeling can be divided into five phases: activation, resorption, reversal, formation, and termination or resting. Activation is the process by which osteoclast precursor cells are transformed into osteoclasts. Prostaglandins or lymphokines produced by cells at the bone site probably attract osteoclasts to the specific area of bone to be resorbed. The reversal phase involves cells that may receive or produce coupling signals that allow transition from bone resorption to formation within the bone modeling unit (Raggot and Partridge, 2010). Bone resorption and formation are mediated by the activity of osteoclasts and osteoblasts. During the process of remodeling, a coupling is somehow established between bone resorption and bone formation, and this linkage ensures the overall integrity of the skeleton despite the ongoing bone remodeling. Factors leading to the uncoupling of bone formation and bone resorption are important in the development of osteoporosis.

Because the process of bone remodeling is relatively long, clinical trials evaluating potential therapeutic agents (such as calcium supplementation) on bone mass need to continue for at least 2 to 3 years. Otherwise, simple transient effects on bone remodeling caused by the intervention and due to the temporary disruption of the normal remodeling process would not be distinguished from changes that would have a sustained long-term benefit on the skeleton (Heaney and Recker, 1994).

DIETARY SOURCES, BIOAVAILABILITY, AND RECOMMENDED INTAKES FOR CALCIUM AND PHOSPHORUS

DIETARY SOURCES OF CALCIUM AND PHOSPHATE

The great majority of calcium in American diets is supplied by milk and milk products. If milk-based products are excluded from the diet or used in limited amounts, then the relatively low calcium content of many foods makes it difficult to ingest recommended amounts of calcium. Some relatively rich vegetarian sources of calcium include calcium-set tofu and certain green vegetables. In addition, during the past decade, new calcium-fortified foods such as orange juice and certain cereals are available to address inadequate intakes.

Phosphate is widely distributed in foodstuffs. In general, food sources high in protein (meats, milk, eggs, and cereals) are also high in phosphate. Dairy products, meat, fish, poultry, and eggs supply about 70% of typical phosphate intakes in the United States (U.S. Department of Agriculture [USDA],

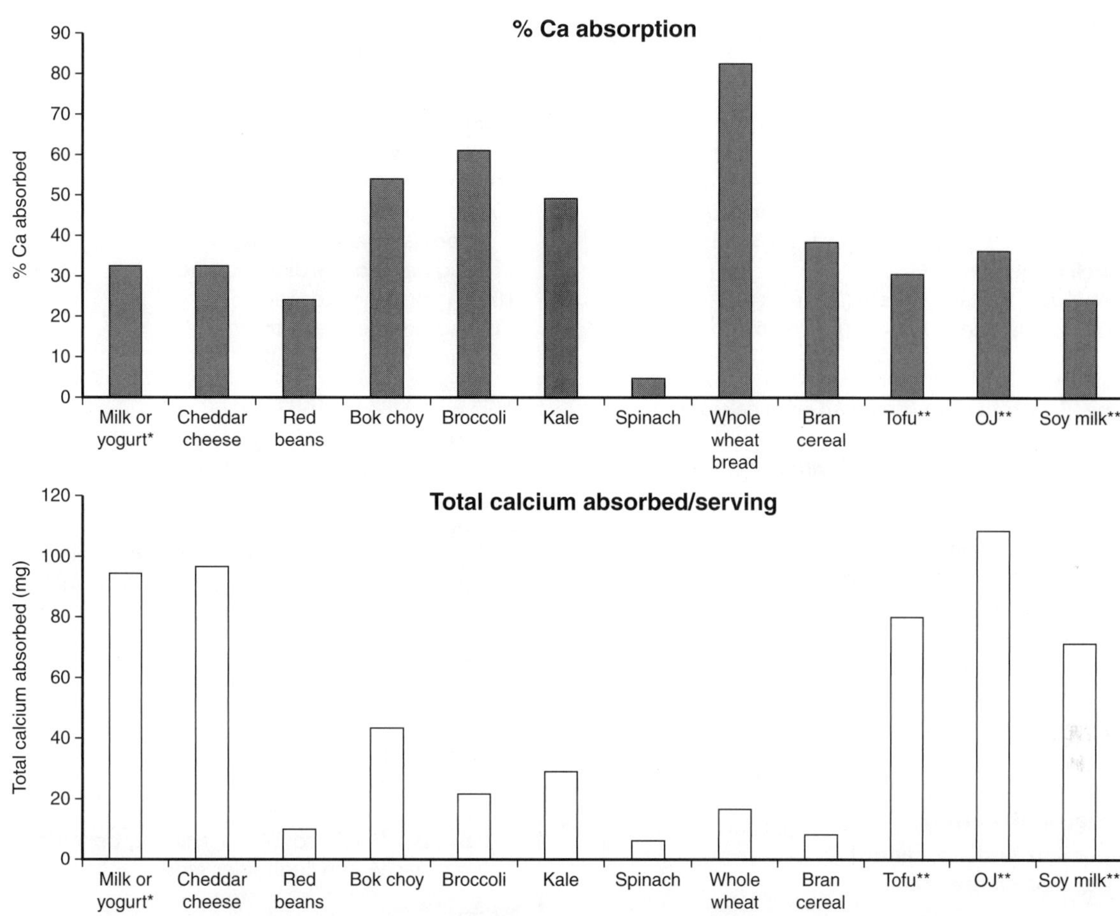

FIGURE 32-7 Percentage of calcium absorbed and total calcium absorbed from various food sources. The top bar graph is the percentage of calcium that is absorbed for each food source. Beneath is the total amount of calcium that would be absorbed (Percent absorption x Calcium content of food) for standard servings of a given food source. Serving size = 1 cup (240 g) of milk, yogurt, orange juice (OJ), or soy milk; 85 g of bok choy, kale, or spinach; 70 g of broccoli; 42 g of cheese; and 28 g of bread or cereal. *Nonfat, plain **Calcium-fortified. (Data from Weaver, C. M., & Heaney, R. P. [2005]. *Calcium in human health.* Totowa, NJ: Humana Press.)

2009, 2010). Processed foods and soda contains phosphorus as additives and can increase intake considerably.

CALCIUM AND PHOSPHATE BIOAVAILABILITY

Bioavailability refers to the fraction of a nutrient in food that is absorbed and metabolically available. For example, dietary factors that alter calcium absorption from food include dietary fiber, phytate, oxalate, and dietary protein, as discussed earlier. Ideally, an evaluation of dietary calcium and phosphate adequacy should consider not only the quantitative aspects of consumption but also the relative bioavailability of these minerals from food.

Milk has long been considered to be the best dietary source of calcium. However, large segments of the population are lactose-intolerant (see Chapter 8) and may avoid milk or consume only limited quantities. Investigators have used intrinsically incorporated stable isotopes of calcium to study the bioavailability of calcium from various foodstuffs and have compared the absorbability of calcium from several foods (Figure 32-7). Some low-oxalate green leafy vegetables have been shown to be sources of highly bioavailable calcium (Heaney and Weaver, 2005), but milk-based products, and fortified tofu and orange juice, are the richest sources of highly absorbable calcium per serving (see Figure 32-7).

Phosphate from meat is well absorbed (greater than 70%) by humans. Phosphate in grains is mostly in the form of phytate (*myo*-inositol hexaphosphate), an organophosphate compound used by plants to store phosphate. For example, more than 80% of the total phosphate in wheat, rice, seeds, legumes, and maize is found as phytate, which makes it less bioavailable because of its limited absorption. Inorganic phosphate is more readily absorbed by intestine; it is present in hidden ingredients such as additives in processed preserved foods or soft drinks. Therefore there has been concern about excessive phosphorus intake due to the greater bioavailability and intake of soft drinks and food additives as compared with natural sources (animal and vegetable) of food proteins. Overall, the type of dietary phosphorus (organic versus inorganic), source (animal versus plant derived), and ratio to protein intake can potentially influence phosphorus status and health (Kalantar-Zadeh et al., 2010).

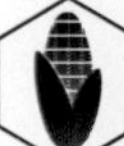

FOOD SOURCES OF CALCIUM

Milk and Milk Products

275 mg per 1 cup milk, whole
305 mg per 1 cup milk, skim
415 mg per 8-oz container yogurt, skim milk, plain
275 mg per 8-oz container yogurt, whole milk, plain
200 to 225 mg per 1 oz cheese (Swiss, provolone, mozzarella, cheddar)
70 mg per ½ cup cottage cheese (1% milk fat)
335 mg per ½ cup ricotta cheese (part-skim)

Tofu

170 mg per 3 oz tofu (firm, prepared with calcium sulfate)
95 mg per 3 oz tofu (soft, prepared with calcium sulfate)

Vegetables

160 mg per ½ cup collards, cooked
140 mg per ½ cup spinach, cooked
90 mg per ½ cup kale, cooked
75 mg per ½ cup baked beans
60 mg per ½ cup beans (navy, great northern)
175 mg per ½ cup rhubarb, cooked

Leavening Agents

340 mg per 1 tsp baking powder, double-acting

Fish (canned with bones)

325 mg per 3 oz sardines, canned
180 mg per 3 oz salmon, canned

Grains

120 to 150 mg per 1 cup Kix or Cheerios
30 mg per 1 cup Raisin Bran

Fortified Foods

1000 mg per 1 cup Total cereal
350 mg per 1 cup fortified orange juice

FOOD SOURCES OF PHOSPHORUS

Meat and Meat Substitutes

200 to 220 mg per 3 oz pork, fresh, cooked
170 to 200 mg per 3 oz beef, lean, cooked
200 mg per 3 oz chicken breast, cooked
200 to 285 mg per 3 oz fish (halibut, haddock, swordfish, salmon, tuna), cooked
415 mg per 3 oz sardines, canned
100 mg per egg, cooked
110 mg per piece soft tofu
130 mg per cup soy milk

Milk and Milk Products

200 to 225 mg per ½ cup cheese, ricotta
140 to 170 mg per ½ cup cheese, cottage
245 mg per 1 cup milk, skim
220 mg per 1 cup milk, whole
355 mg per 8-oz container yogurt, skim milk, plain
215 mg per 8-oz container yogurt, whole milk, plain

Legumes and Seeds

180 mg per ½ cup lentils, cooked
168 mg per ½ cup chickpeas, cooked
110 to 147 mg per ½ cup beans (pinto, kidney, black, white), cooked
151 mg per 1 oz cashews
132 mg per 1 oz peanuts
210 mg per ½ cup soybeans, mature, boiled
370 mg per ¼ cup sunflower seeds

Grains

205 mg per ½ cup wheat flour, whole grain
145 mg per ½ cup cornmeal, whole grain
125 mg per ½ cup white rice, dry
100 mg per 1 cup Total cereal
130 mg per 1 cup Cheerios
45 mg per 1 cup Kix
100–220 mg per 1 cup Raisin Bran

Data from U.S. Department of Agriculture, Agricultural Research Service. (2010). *USDA National Nutrient Database for Standard Reference, Release 23*. Retrieved from www.ars.usda.gov/ba/bhnrc/ndl

DIETARY REFERENCE INTAKES FOR CALCIUM AND PHOSPHORUS

Many people in the United States do not consume the recommended levels of dietary calcium (Bailey et al., 2010; IOM, 2011), although phosphate intakes are usually adequate. Recommended dietary intakes throughout the life cycle for the American and Canadian populations were updated in 1997 for phosphorus and more recently for calcium and vitamin D in 2011 (IOM, 1997, 2011). The DRIs Across the Life Cycle box shows the Recommended Dietary Allowance (RDA) and the Tolerable Upper Intake Level (UL) for calcium and phosphorus.

Calcium

The median (50th percentile) for dietary calcium intake in the United States ranges from 706 to 755 mg/day in women (19 years or older) and total calcium intake (with dietary supplements) ranges from 863 to 1,044 mg/day. Dietary calcium intake for men (19 years or older) in the United States is 833 to 1,127 mg/day. This level of intake is similar to many other countries such as Canada and those in Europe. The Estimated Average Requirement (EAR) for calcium ranges from 800 to 1,000 mg/day for adults of both genders, so many individuals are getting adequate calcium intake. However, the RDA (which meets or exceeds the requirement for 97.5% of the population) is not met by adult women of any age, or adult men after 70 years of age. The median intake for adolescent girls 14 through 18 years of age is 826 mg/day, which is much lower than the RDA of 1,300 mg/day for adolescents. More than 80% of all girls (ages 9 through 18 years) are below the adequate intake for calcium, whereas approximately 60% of adult women (any age) and men (older than 70 years) are below the EAR for calcium.

The calcium EARs and RDAs rely primarily upon calcium balance studies for persons 1 through 50 years of age. The effect of menopause on bone resulted in specifying different

CLINICAL CORRELATION

Phosphorus in the Diet and Complications in Disease

Although phosphate is important to numerous basic functions in the body, high blood levels are a problem for patients with chronic kidney disease (CKD). The goal in these patients is to reduce circulating phosphorus levels to lower the risk of vascular calcification. In CKD patients, the presence and extent of arterial calcification is independently predictive of cardiovascular disease and mortality. In animal models, phosphate binders that lower phosphate levels (reduction of 28% to 42%) demonstrate a consistent decrease in aortic calcium content when compared to untreated CKD (using knockout models of both *LDLr–/–* and *ApoE–/–*) (Shobeiri et al., 2010). It has been suggested that because protein and phosphorus intakes are closely correlated, the phosphorus/protein ratio in foods may be important to consider when advising patients depending on the stage of disease (Kalantar-Zadeh et al., 2010). High phosphorus intake can also negatively affect other diseases, such as in sarcoidosis, which is a chronic granulomatous disorder of unknown etiology that can affect multiple organ systems. Hypercalcemia and excessive endogenous $1,25(OH)_2D$ production are well-described complications. Chronic hypercalcemia and hypercalciuria associated with sarcoidosis include nephrocalcinosis, nephrolithiasis, nephrogenic diabetes insipidus, and soft tissue calcification. The hypercalcemia associated with sarcoidosis is more common in white than black individuals (even though the disease is more common in blacks), especially in the summer months when plasma vitamin D levels are increased. Demetriou and associates (2010) describe a case of sarcoidosis in a black patient who was experiencing diffuse soft tissue calcifications and acute kidney injury owing to sarcoidosis-induced hypercalcemia. His condition was believed to be exacerbated by sun exposure and increased phosphate consumption in the form of cola soft drinks, because reducing sun exposure and eliminating cola drinks resolved the soft tissue calcifications and kidney function improved. In addition, the treatment for this patient included hydration and glucocorticoid therapy. Therefore it is important to reduce phosphorus levels in these disease states to prevent hypercalcemia-induced soft tissue calcification. Excessive calcium intake and high vitamin D levels, through either the diet or sun exposure, should also be avoided. It is not known whether a high phosphorus diet in healthy individuals increases the risk of soft-tissue calcification, yet excessive phosphorus consumption should be avoided because it is theoretically possible.

EARs and RDAs for women and men 51 through 70 years of age. Hence women ages 51 through 70 years require greater calcium intake at 1,200 mg/day compared to men with 1,000 mg/day. After the age of 70 years, the effects of aging on bone loss are considered similar in men and women, so the EARs and RDAs are the same for men and women at 1,200 mg/day. The Adequate Intakes (AIs) for infants are based on the calcium content of human milk (0 through 6 months of age) or on the calcium content of human milk plus that obtained from infant foods (7 through 12 months of age). Children have an RDA that is not specific for males or females, and a higher calcium intake (1,300 mg/day) is recommended from 9 through 18 years of age. There is no evidence that calcium requirements are different for pregnant and lactating females compared with their nonpregnant or nonlactating counterparts.

A UL for calcium intake was set at 2,500 mg/day for children (less than 9 years) and adults below 51 years. It was set slightly higher during peak periods of growth (9 through 18 years) at 3,000 mg/day. A feeding study using high calcium levels provided evidence that among infants there is no elevation in calcium excretion (Sargent et al., 1999); the data allowed derivation of a UL for infants at 1,000 mg/day through 6 months of age and 1,500 mg/day from 6 through 12 months of age (IOM, 2011). Very high intakes of calcium (greater than 4,000 mg/day) have been associated with hypercalcemia and, consequently, calcium deposition in tissues and kidney failure. More recently, and in older women, total intake of calcium higher than 2,000 mg/day has been associated with an increased risk of kidney stones (Jackson et al., 2006) and possibly some cardiovascular-related risks (Bolland et al., 2010; Sanders et al., 2010) (see later discussion of excess intakes). Hence the new upper limit for calcium is set at 2,000 mg/day for older adults. High calcium intakes may also increase the risk of depletion of other minerals in vulnerable populations due to adverse effects of calcium on iron and zinc bioavailability. The UL for calcium is a conservative estimate and provides protection to adverse effects of high calcium intakes, such as calcium renal stones or hyperabsorptive hypercalciuria.

Phosphorus

Dietary phosphorus intake is 1,120 and 1,550 mg/day for women and men, respectively. The higher intake in men for both nutrients is simply a function of greater size and caloric intake of approximately 2,500 kcal/day in men compared to 1,800 kcal/day for women. In contrast to calcium intakes, only 5% of the adult population is below the EAR for phosphorus (USDA, 2009).

An EAR for phosphorus for children ages 1 through 18 years for each age group was based on a factorial approach (a summation of requirements for maintenance plus growth and correction for absorption efficiency). In contrast to the factorial methodology used to derive an EAR for growing children, the EAR for adults (19 years or older) was established on the basis of the amount of ingested phosphorus needed to maintain serum phosphate at the lower limit of the normal range (0.87 mmol/L) (IOM, 1997). The RDA for phosphorus for adults was set as the EAR + 20%, or 700 mg/day

DRIs Across the Life Cycle: Calcium and Phosphorus

	mg Calcium per Day		mg Phosphorus per Day	
Infant	RDA	UL	RDA	UL
0 through 6 mo	200 (AI)	1,000	100 (AI)	ND
7 through 12 mo	260 (AI)	1,500	275 (AI)	ND
Children				
1 through 3 yr	700	2,500	460	3,000
4 through 8 yr	1,000	2,500	500	3,000
9 through 13 yr	1,300	3,000	1,250	4,000
14 through 18 yr	1,300	3,000	1,250	4,000
Males				
19 through 70 yr	1,000	2,500	700	4,000
≥71 yr	1,200	2,000	700	3,000
Females				
19 through 50 yr	1,000	2,500	700	4,000
51 through 70 yr	1,200	2,000	700	4,000
≥71 yr	1,200	2,000	700	3,000
Pregnant/Lactating				
<19 yr	1,300	3,000	1,250	3,500/ 4,000
19 through 50 yr	1,000	2,500	700	3,500/ 4,000

Data from IOM. (1997). *Dietary Reference Intakes for calcium, phosphorus, magnesium, vitamin D, and fluoride.* Washington, DC: National Academy Press; IOM. (2011). *Dietary Reference Intakes for calcium and vitamin D.* Washington, DC: The National Academies Press.
AI, Adequate Intake; *DRI*, Dietary Reference Intake; *ND*, not determinable; *RDA*, Recommended Dietary Allowance; *UL*, Tolerable Upper Intake Level.

(22.6 mmol/day). Serum phosphate levels were used as the criterion of adequacy because it can be assumed that dietary phosphorus intakes are adequate to meet cellular and skeletal needs when serum phosphate levels are in the normal range. Conversely, phosphorus balance is not a good criterion of adequate intake because phosphate balance can be zero at an intake that is inadequate to maintain serum phosphate within a normal range. No increase in the RDA for phosphorus was recommended for pregnant or lactating women because there is increased intestinal absorption during pregnancy, and increased bone resorption and decreased urinary excretion of phosphorus during lactation needed for milk production (~100 mg/day). The AIs for infants were based on the phosphorus content of human milk (0 through 6 months of age) or the phosphorus content of human milk plus that obtained from infant foods (7 through 12 months of age).

There is no evidence for serious adverse effects of high dietary phosphorus intakes in healthy humans, but a conservative estimate of the UL was made based on phosphorus intakes associated with the upper boundary of adult normal values for serum phosphate. The basis for setting lower ULs for older adults and pregnant women was an increased prevalence of impaired renal function in older adults and the increased absorption efficiency for phosphorus during pregnancy.

CALCIUM AND PHOSPHATE DEFICIENCY, EXCESS, AND ASSESSMENT OF STATUS

Calcium deficiency is difficult to assess, and many possible indicators of calcium deficiency are also indicators of vitamin D status, bone diseases, and hormonal imbalances. In experimental animals that are severely restricted in dietary calcium (and develop hypocalcemia), increased serum levels of PTH and $1,25(OH)_2D$, higher fractional intestinal absorption of calcium and phosphate, and lower calcium but higher phosphate levels in urine are consistently observed. Bone resorption and turnover are also stimulated, and net loss of bone ensues.

Normal serum calcium concentrations range from 8.8 to 10.4 mg/dL (2.20 to 2.60 mmol/L) in adults and are tightly regulated by the concerted actions of intestinal calcium absorption, renal calcium reabsorption, and exchange of Ca^{2+} to and from bone. Total serum calcium consists of about 40% bound to plasma proteins (primarily albumin). The remaining 60% includes ionized calcium plus calcium complexed with phosphate and citrate. Most laboratories measure total calcium (i.e., protein-bound, complexed, and ionized) even though ionized or free calcium is the physiologically active form of calcium in plasma. Ionized calcium is difficult to measure, but in general neither serum total nor ionized calcium level reflects calcium status because the plasma calcium level is tightly controlled. Therefore poor dietary calcium intake does not necessarily reduce serum calcium levels. Low total serum calcium levels may be explainable by low levels of serum albumin rather than by a calcium deficiency. Hypocalcemia is total serum calcium concentration less than 8.8 mg/dL in the presence of normal plasma protein concentrations or a serum ionized calcium concentration less than 4.7 mg/dL (less than 1.17 mmol/L). Causes of hypocalcemia include hypoparathyroidism, vitamin D deficiency, and renal disease (Lewis et al., 2011) (see Table 32-1). Symptoms include paresthesias and tetany; when deficiency is severe, seizures, encephalopathy, and heart failure (Shoback, 2008) may occur. Chronic low intake of calcium will ultimately lead to lower peak bone density and/or increased loss after maturity (Boot et al., 2010).

Excess Calcium Intake

A large study from the Women's Health Initiative trial (Jackson et al., 2006) showed that supplementation with both calcium and vitamin D in 36,000 postmenopausal women results in a 17% greater risk of kidney stones (nephrolithiasis) compared to a placebo group. However, total calcium intake was significantly higher than recommended at about 2,100 mg/day, whereas the vitamin D intakes were not excessively high (about 800 IU/day). Calcification of vascular tissues has been reported with high calcium intake in patients with chronic kidney disease. In addition, high

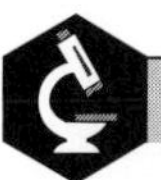

CLINICAL CORRELATION

Calcium and Osteoporosis

Osteoporosis is a multifactorial disease that is clinically characterized by low bone mass, bone pain, and an increased risk of bone fracture. The prevalence of osteoporosis is defined as a bone mineral density that is more than 2.5 standard deviations below the mean for young adults, which increases the risk of fracture, with hip fracture being the most serious outcome. In the United States and Europe, beginning at age 50 years, the lifetime risk of hip fracture is approximately 17% and 6% in white women and men, respectively. There is less variability and a lower risk of hip fracture in Asian and African heritages (Cummings and Melton, 2002). The prevalence of osteoporotic fracture is dramatically increased in elderly people, and estimates have recently been updated (Ettinger et al., 2010) using a relatively new and widely used fracture risk assessment tool, called FRAX (Kanis et al., 2007). The age-associated increase in the occurrence of osteoporosis has enormous public health significance because of the increasing proportion of elderly individuals in the U.S. population; the fastest growing segment of the population is those older than 85 years.

Several factors may be involved in the pathogenesis of postmenopausal osteoporosis, including reduced intestinal calcium absorption and increased urinary calcium loss. Some of the bone loss that is seen in elderly people can be ameliorated by calcium supplementation (Aloia et al., 1994; Reid et al., 1993; Dawson-Hughes et al., 1990). However, the role of dietary calcium in the causation and treatment of osteoporosis is still the focus of intense debate. Among the reasons for this debate is the complex nature of osteoporosis. Certainly the rather abrupt changes in bone and calcium metabolism that accompany menopause in women cannot be attributed solely to an abrupt decrease in calcium intake or absorption. Despite the fact that a number of investigators have noted a lack of association between current calcium intake and bone mineral density, the majority of studies show that both calcium and vitamin D supplementation can reduce the risk of fracture (Tang et al., 2007). Childhood is potentially an important time to intervene, because modeling suggests that a 10% increase in peak bone mass will delay the onset of osteoporosis by 13 years (Bonjour et al., 2009). Although twin studies show that most of this is genetically determined, peak bone mass can be positively influenced by environmental factors, including calcium and protein intakes and physical activity (Bonjour et al., 2009; Boot et al., 2010); prepubertal years may be the optimal for intervention. In addition, low bone mineral density in childhood is a risk factor for childhood fractures, so optimizing bone mass could also have a more immediate preventive effect on fracture rates in children. Another consideration is that optimal calcium intake may relate to nonskeletal endpoints (Heaney and Weaver, 2005). For example, a higher calcium intake reduces hypertension, particularly in the black population, and can attenuate blood lead levels that may be a concern for at-risk inner-city populations or developing countries. Both the skeletal and the nonskeletal outcome variables for calcium intake have been reviewed recently (IOM, 2011).

total calcium intake (~2,000 mg/day) may also contribute to increased vascular calcification and the risk of heart attack (Bolland et al., 2010). However, others claim no association between high calcium intake (~2,000 mg/day) and vascular calcification or disease (Lewis et al., 2011; Manson et al., 2010). Overall, there remains no evidence that consuming the recommended calcium intake in adults (total of 1,000 to 1,200 mg/day from supplements and diet) has any detrimental effect on cardiovascular events. In addition, increased calcium intake through dietary sources (not supplements) has never been associated with increased cardiovascular risks.

ASSESSMENT OF CALCIUM STATUS

Calcium balance data provide useful information on calcium status and whether calcium absorption is sufficient to replace calcium lost in urine, sweat, and feces. Because 99% of the body's calcium store is found in bone, a consistent negative calcium balance will result in bone loss. During growth, provision of sufficient dietary calcium in humans is necessary to achieve maximum levels of bone mineral density, but a positive calcium balance does not imply optimal bone mineralization (Bonjour et al., 1997, 2009). Precise bone densitometric techniques can be used to monitor the response of bone mineral density to dietary intervention. These sensitive techniques in the past decade have demonstrated the need for high calcium intakes to maximize bone growth in children and to retard bone loss in the elderly (Heaney and Weaver, 2005). New techniques to understand bone quality are currently being used, including magnetic resonance imaging and quantitative computed tomography.

PHOSPHATE DEFICIENCY, EXCESS, AND STATUS

Phosphorus deficiency is rare because of the high phosphorus content of the diet, efficient intestinal absorption, and the ability of the kidneys to produce an essentially phosphorus-free urine in response to hypophosphatemia. An exception to this general rule is the premature infant who is fed human milk, which has a much lower phosphorus content than cow's milk. Because the preterm infant has a high phosphorus deposition per unit of body size than full-term infants, they are vulnerable to hypophosphatemia, inadequate bone mineralization, and rickets despite an adequate vitamin D status.

Plasma phosphate depletion can also occur from excessive ingestion of aluminum hydroxide antacids, which can inhibit phosphorus absorption by binding dietary phosphorus in the gut. Abnormalities of phosphate homeostasis and depletion can also occur in association with various disease states. The symptoms of phosphate depletion include a diminished concentration of intracellular organic phosphoric acid esters, such as 2,3-diphosphoglycerate (in erythrocytes) and ATP (in muscle and other cell types). In the red blood cell, 2,3-diphosphoglycerate interacts with hemoglobin to promote the release of oxygen from oxyhemoglobin. Tissue oxygen levels can be lowered as a consequence of depleted 2,3-diphosphoglycerate levels because of a shift in the equilibrium for oxyhemoglobin dissociation so that less oxygen is liberated. Additional symptoms of severe phosphate depletion include hemolysis of red blood cells, diminished phagocytic function of granulocytes, severe muscle weakness, and hypercalciuria (see Table 32-2).

EXCESS PHOSPHORUS INTAKE

High intake of phosphorus can result in hyperphosphatemia and symptoms such as hypocalcemia and tetany, soft tissue calcification, and intestinal distress or mild diarrhea. In patients with chronic kidney disease, a high phosphorus burden will lead to hyperparathyroidism and renal osteodystrophy (see Table 32-2). Excess phosphorus is a particular concern because of its presence in additives and soft drinks and its greater bioavailability than natural sources, especially in certain disease states. Nevertheless, hyperphosphatemia due to excessive dietary intake is not a concern for most healthy individuals, except for the elderly who may have declining renal function.

ASSESSMENT OF PHOSPHATE STATUS

Use of plasma phosphate as an indicator of phosphate status may not be accurate since only 1% of total body phosphate is in the extracellular fluid. Plasma phosphate is determined by the tubular reabsorptive capacity of the kidney, which in turn is regulated by the level of PTH, growth hormone, and other factors. The level of phosphate in the plasma can be elevated because of muscle and bone catabolism, or it may be acutely decreased because of rapid shifts of phosphate into the intracellular compartment. Nevertheless, the plasma phosphate level is directly related to absorbed phosphorus and was used as a functional criterion to establish the EARs (and RDAs) for phosphorus for the adult population (IOM, 1997). Other approaches to assessing phosphate status are available. Intracellular phosphate levels in red blood cells, leukocytes, and platelets have been investigated as possible indicators of phosphate status and were found to correlate with circulating phosphate. Urinary phosphate levels reflect dietary phosphorus intake under normal conditions. Hypophosphaturia and hypercalciuria occur with phosphate depletion. Likewise, serum alkaline phosphatase and $1,25(OH)_2D$ may be elevated in phosphate deficiency, but these biochemical changes are not specific enough to predict body phosphate stores accurately.

CLINICAL DISORDERS INVOLVING ALTERED CALCIUM AND PHOSPHATE LEVELS

Several clinical disorders are associated with altered calcium and phosphate homeostasis (see Tables 32-1 and 32-2). Changes in calcium and phosphate stores may be caused by an increase or a decrease in intestinal absorption or renal reabsorption. In addition, rapid shifts in plasma phosphate levels occur in response to several conditions that stimulate movement of phosphate into or out of intracellular compartments. Intestinal disorders, such as Crohn's disease, celiac disease, and intestinal resection or bypass can result in poor mineral and vitamin D absorption owing in part to fat malabsorption. In chronic liver disease, poor mineral absorption can occur secondary to vitamin D deficiency caused by impaired hydroxylation of vitamin D. In chronic renal failure, impairment of calcium and phosphate homeostasis is associated with the reduced renal synthesis of $1,25(OH)_2D$ and the development of secondary hyperparathyroidism.

Excessive intestinal absorption of calcium occurs in sarcoidosis, a chronic granulomatous disease, because of enhanced extrarenal $1,25(OH)_2D$ production. Elevated $1,25(OH)_2D$ also explains hyperabsorption of calcium in primary hyperparathyroidism and the hyperabsorption of calcium found in many patients with renal calcium stones (nephrolithiasis). Hypercalcemia can be found in some cancer patients with tumors of the parathyroid glands, pancreatic islet cells, and anterior pituitary (Thakker et al., 2010).

Phosphate imbalance can occur in various disease states for several reasons (Bergwitz and Jüppner, 2010; Berndt and Kumar, 2009; Ruppe and Jan de Beur, 2008). In starvation, despite underlying phosphate depletion, normal plasma phosphate levels may be maintained because of increased muscle catabolism. Excessive amounts of phosphate can be lost in the urine of diabetics with poorly regulated glucose levels, owing to polyuria and the development of metabolic acidosis. However, plasma phosphate level can be normal or slightly elevated in ketotic patients because large amounts of phosphate may be released from intracellular sites. Recovering burn patients are at risk of hypophosphatemia due to massive diuresis. Likewise, excessive urinary phosphate losses are also seen in patients with dysfunctions of the proximal renal tubule, such as that seen in Fanconi syndrome. In alcoholism, phosphate depletion can occur because of low dietary phosphorus, intestinal malabsorption, increased urinary losses, secondary hyperparathyroidism, hypomagnesemia, and hypokalemia.

The clinical sequel of chronic hyperphosphatemia can result in soft tissue calcification. In chronic renal failure, reduced renal function may cause hyperphosphatemia, which may also be seen with severe hemolysis and various endocrine dysfunctions, such as hypoparathyroidism, acromegaly, and severe hyperthyroidism. Chronic hyperphosphatemia can be managed in these patients by limiting dietary phosphorus intake when possible and by administering oral phosphate binders containing aluminum, calcium, or magnesium salts.

MEDICATIONS THAT MAY INTERFERE WITH CALCIUM OR PHOSPHATE HOMEOSTASIS

There are many drugs that may deplete body stores of calcium that affect a wide range of patients. For example, corticosteroids, antibiotics, sulfonamides, mineral oil, and bile acid sequestrants will all cause malabsorption of calcium, whereas loop diuretics, aminoglycosides, corticosteroids, anticonvulsants, isoniazid, and thyroid hormones will deplete calcium stores and increase the risk of osteoporosis (Shapses et al., 2010). The beneficial effects of estrogens and thiazides on maintaining calcium balance should be considered when recommending these drugs to patients. Whether long-term proton pump inhibitor therapy increases the risk of fracture due to a reduction in calcium absorption remains controversial (Yang et al., 2006). Phosphate is affected by fewer drugs, but blood levels may be lowered by antacids, anticonvulsants, bile acid sequestrants, corticosteroids, diuretics, and insulin. The number of patients at risk of an imbalance of these minerals due to drug interactions is significant, and some supplementation of calcium or phosphorus may be necessary if dietary intake is inadequate.

REFERENCES

Aloia, J. F., Vaswani, A., Yeh, J. K., Ross, P. L., Flaster, E., & Dilmanian, F. A. (1994). Calcium supplementation with and without hormone replacement therapy to prevent postmenopausal bone loss. *Annals of Internal Medicine, 120*, 97–103.

Avioli, L. V., McDonald, J. E., & Lee, S. E. (1965). Influence of aging on the intestinal absorption of 47Ca in women and its relation to 47Ca absorption in postmenopausal osteoporosis. *The Journal of Clinical Investigation, 44*, 1960–1967.

Bailey, R. L., Dodd, K. W., Goldman, J. A., Gahche, J. J., Dwyer, J. T., Moshfegh, A. J., ... Picciano, M. F. (2010). Estimation of total usual calcium and vitamin D intakes in the United States. *The Journal of Nutrition, 140*, 817–822.

Barger-Lux, M. J., & Heaney, R. P. (2005). Calcium absorptive efficiency is positively related to body size. *The Journal of Clinical Endocrinology and Metabolism, 90*, 5118–5120.

Bergwitz, C., & Jüppner, H. (2010). Regulation of phosphate homeostasis by PTH, vitamin D, and FGF23. *Annual Review of Medicine, 61*, 91–104.

Berndt, T., & Kumar, R. (2009). Novel mechanisms in the regulation of phosphorus homeostasis. *Physiology (Bethesda), 24*, 17–25.

Bertipaglia, I., & Carafoli, E. (2007). Calpains and human disease. *Sub-cellular Biochemistry, 45*, 29–53.

Bolland, M. J., Avenell, A., Baron, J. A., Grey, A., MacLennan, G. S., Gamble, G. D., & Reid, I. R. (2010). Effect of calcium supplements on risk of myocardial infarction and cardiovascular events: Meta-analysis. *BMJ, 341*, c3691.

Bonjour, J. P., Carrie, A.-L., Ferrari, S., Clavien, H., Slosman, D., Theintz, G., & Rizzoli, R. (1997). Calcium-enriched foods and bone mass growth in prepubertal girls: A randomized, double-blind, placebo-controlled trial. *The Journal of Clinical Investigation, 99*, 1287–1294.

Bonjour, J. P., Chevalley, T., Ferrari, S., & Rizzoli, R. (2009). The importance and relevance of peak bone mass in the prevalence of osteoporosis. *Salud Pública de México, 51*(Suppl. 1), S5–S17.

Boot, A. M., de Ridder, M. A., van der Sluis, I. M., van Slobbe, I., Krenning, E. P., & Keizer-Schrama, S. M. (2010). Peak bone mineral density, lean body mass and fractures. *Bone, 46*, 336–341.

Borghi, L., Schianchi, T., Meschi, T., Guerra, A., Allegri, F., Maggiore, U., & Novarini, A. (2002). Comparison of two diets for the prevention of recurrent stones in idiopathic hypercalciuria. *New England Journal of Medicine, 346*, 77–84.

Bronner, F. (2009). Recent developments in intestinal calcium absorption. *Nutrition Reviews, 67*, 109–113.

Burke, J. E., & Dennis, E. A. (2009). Phospholipase A2 structure/function, mechanism, and signaling. *Journal of Lipid Research* (Suppl. 50), S237–S242.

Christakos, S., Dhawan, P., Ajibade, D., Benn, B. S., Feng, J., & Joshi, S. S. (2010). Mechanisms involved in vitamin D mediated intestinal calcium absorption and in non-classical actions of vitamin D. *The Journal of Steroid Biochemistry and Molecular Biology, 121*, 183–187.

Christakos, S., Dhawan, P., Benn, B., Porta, A., Hediger, M., Oh, G. T., ... Joshi, S. (2007). Vitamin D: Molecular mechanism of action. *Annals of the New York Academy of Sciences, 1116*, 340–348.

Cifuentes, M., Riedt, C. S., Field, M. P., Sherrell, R. M., Brolin, R. E., & Shapses, S. A. (2004). Weight loss and calcium intake influence calcium absorption in overweight postmenopausal women. *The American Journal of Clinical Nutrition, 80*, 123–130.

Cummings, S. R., & Melton, L. J. (2002). Epidemiology and outcomes of osteoporotic fractures. *Lancet, 359*, 1761–1767.

Curhan, G. C., Willett, W. C., Rimm, E. B., & Stampfer, M. J. (1993). A prospective study of dietary calcium and other nutrients and the risk of symptomatic kidney stones. *New England Journal of Medicine, 328*, 833–838.

Dawson-Hughes, B., Dallal, G., Krall, E. A., Sadowski, L., Sahyoun, N., & Tannenbaum, S. (1990). A controlled trial of the effect of calcium supplementation on bone density in postmenopausal women. *New England Journal of Medicine, 323*, 878–883.

Demetriou, E. T., Pietras, S. M., & Holick, M. F. (2010). Hypercalcemia and soft tissue calcification owing to sarcoidosis: The sunlight-cola connection. *Journal of Bone and Mineral Research, 25*, 1695–1699.

Dempster, D. W., Cosman, F., Parisien, M., & Shen, V. (1993). Anabolic actions of parathyroid hormone on bone. *Endocrine Reviews, 14*, 690–709.

de Paula, F. J., & Rosen, C. J. (2010). Back to the future: Revisiting parathyroid hormone and calcitonin control of bone remodeling. *Hormone and Metabolic Research, 42*, 299–306.

Dong, H., Sellers, Z. M., Smith, A., Chow, J. Y., & Barrett, K. E. (2005). Na(+)/Ca(2+) exchange regulates Ca(2+)-dependent duodenal mucosal ion transport and HCO(3)(−) secretion in mice. *American Journal of Physiology. Gastrointestinal and Liver Physiology, 288*, G457–G465.

Driessens, F. C. M., & Verbeeck, R. M. H. (1990). *Biominerals*. Boca Raton, FL: CRC Press.

Ducy, P., Desbois, C., Boyce, B., Pinero, G., Story, B., Dunstan, C., ... Karsenty, G. (1996). Increased bone formation in osteocalcin-deficient mice. *Nature, 382*, 448–452.

Eastell, R., Yergey, A. L., Vieira, N. E., Cedel, S. L., Kumar, R., & Riggs, B. L. (1991). Interrelationship among vitamin D metabolism, true calcium absorption, parathyroid function, and age in women: Evidence of an age-related intestinal resistance to 1,25-dihydroxyvitamin D action. *Journal of Bone and Mineral Research, 6*, 125–132.

Ettinger, B., Black, D. M., Dawson-Hughes, B., Pressman, A. R., & Melton, L. J., 3rd (2010). Updated fracture incidence rates for the US version of FRAX. *Osteoporosis International, 21*, 25–33.

Fatimathas, L., & Moss, S. E. (2010). Annexins as disease modifiers. *Histology and Histopathology, 25*, 527–532.

Fleet, J. C., Bruns, M. E., Hock, J. M., & Wood, R. J. (1994). Growth hormone and parathyroid hormone stimulate intestinal calcium absorption in aged female rats. *Endocrinology, 134*, 1755–1760.

Fontaine, O., Matsumoto, T., Goodman, D. B. P., & Rasmussen, H. (1981). Liponomic control of Ca^{2+} transport: Relationship to mechanism of 1,25-dihydroxyvitamin D3. *Proceedings of the National Academy of Sciences of the United States of America, 78*, 1751–1754.

Gaffney-Stomberg, E., Sun, B. H., Cucchi, C. E., Simpson, C. A., Gundberg, C., Kerstetter, J. E., & Insogna, K. L. (2010). The effect of dietary protein on intestinal calcium absorption in rats. *Endocrinology, 151*, 1071–1078.

Gardella, R. J., Jüppner, H., Brown, E. M., Kronenberg, H. M., & Potts, J. T., Jr. (2010). Parathyroid hormone and parathyroid hormone–related peptide in the regulation of calcium homeostasis and bone development. In J. L. Jameson & L. J. De Groot (Eds.), *Endocrinology* (pp. 1040–1073). New York: Saunders.

Gastaldi, G., Ferrari, G., Verri, A., Casirola, D., Orsenigo, M. N., & Laforenza, U. (2000). Riboflavin phosphorylation is the crucial event in riboflavin transport by isolated rat enterocytes. *The Journal of Nutrition, 130*, 2556–2561.

Goll, D. E., Thompson, V. F., Li, H., Wei, W., & Cong, J. (2003). The calpain system. *Physiological Reviews, 83*, 731–801.

Hauschka, P. V., Lian, J. B., Cole, D. E., & Gundberg, C. M. (1989). Osteocalcin and matrix Gla protein: Vitamin K–dependent proteins in bone. *Physiological Reviews, 69*, 990–1047.

Heaney, R. P. (2008). Calcium supplementation and incident kidney stone risk: A systematic review. *Journal of the American College of Nutrition, 27*, 519–527.

Heaney, R. P., & Recker, R. R. (1994). Determinants of endogenous fecal calcium in healthy women. *Journal of Bone and Mineral Research, 9*, 1621–1627.

Heaney, R. P., Recker, R. R., Stegman, M. R., & Moy, A. J. (1989). Calcium absorption in women: Relationships to calcium intake, estrogen status, and age. *Journal of Bone and Mineral Research, 4*, 469–475.

Heaney, R. P., & Weaver, C. M. (2005). Requirements for what endpoint? In C. M. Weaver & R. P. Heaney (Eds.), *Calcium in human health* (pp. 97–105). Totowa, NJ: Humana Press.

Hegsted, M., Schuette, S. A., Zemel, M. B., & Linkswiler, H. M. (1981). Urinary calcium and calcium balance in young men as affected by level of protein and phosphorus intake. *The Journal of Nutrition, 111*, 553–562.

Hunt, C. D., & Johnson, L. K. (2007). Calcium requirements: New estimations for men and women by cross-sectional statistical analyses of calcium balance data from metabolic studies. *The American Journal of Clinical Nutrition, 86*, 1054–1063.

Institute of Medicine. (1997). *Dietary Reference Intakes for calcium, phosphorus, magnesium, vitamin D, and fluoride*. Washington, DC: National Academy Press.

Institute of Medicine. (2011). *Dietary Reference Intakes for calcium and vitamin D*. Washington, DC: The National Academies Press.

Jackson, R. D., LaCroix, A. Z., Gass, M., Wallace, R. B., Robbins, J., Lewis, C. E., ... Women's Health Initiative Investigators. (2006). Calcium plus vitamin D supplementation and the risk of fractures. *New England Journal of Medicine, 354*, 669–683.

Kalantar-Zadeh, K., Gutekunst, L., Mehrotra, R., Kovesdy, C. P., Bross, R., Shinaberger, C. S., ... Kopple, J. D. (2010). Understanding sources of dietary phosphorus in the treatment of patients with chronic kidney disease. *Clinical Journal of the American Society of Nephrology, 5*, 519–530.

Kanis, J. A., Oden, A., Johnell, O., Johansson, H., De Laet, C., Brown, J., ... Yoshimura, N. (2007). The use of clinical risk factors enhances the performance of BMD in the prediction of hip and osteoporotic fractures in men and women. *Osteoporosis International, 18*, 1033–1046.

Karsdal, M. A., Byrjalsen, I., Henriksen, K., Riis, B. J., Lau, E. M., Arnold, M., & Christiansen, C. (2010). The effect of oral salmon calcitonin delivered with 5-CNAC on bone and cartilage degradation in osteoarthritic patients: A 14-day randomized study. *Osteoarthritis Cartilage, 18*, 150–159.

Kearns, A. E., Khosla, S., & Kostenuik, P. J. (2008). Receptor activator of nuclear factor kappaB ligand and osteoprotegerin regulation of bone remodeling in health and disease. *Endocrine Reviews, 29*, 155–192.

Kerstetter, J. E., & Allen, L. H. (1990). Dietary protein increases urinary calcium. *The Journal of Nutrition, 120*, 134–136.

Kerstetter, J. E., O'Brien, K. O., Caseria, D. M., Wall, D. E., & Insogna, K. L. (2005). The impact of dietary protein on calcium absorption and kinetic measures of bone turnover in women. *The Journal of Clinical Endocrinology and Metabolism, 90*, 26–31.

Knochel, J. P. (2006). Phosphorus. In M. E. Shils, M. Shike, A. C. Ross, B. Caballero, & R. J. Cousins (Eds.), *Modern nutrition in health and disease* (10th ed, pp. 211–222). Baltimore: Lippincott Williams & Wilkins.

Knopp, J. A., Diner, B. M., Blitz, M., Lyritis, G. P., & Rowe, B. H. (2005). Calcitonin for treating acute pain of osteoporotic vertebral compression fractures: A systematic review of randomized, controlled trials. *Osteoporosis International, 16*, 1281–1290.

Kuro-o, M. (2010). Overview of the FGF23-Klotho axis. *Pediatric Nephrology, 25*, 583–590.

Lee, N. K., Sowa, H., Hinoi, E., Ferron, M., Ahn, J. D., Confavreux, C., ... Karsenty, G. (2007). Endocrine regulation of energy metabolism by the skeleton. *Cell, 130*, 456–469.

Lewis, J. R., Calver, J., Zhu, K., Flicker, L., & Prince, R. L. (2011). Calcium supplementation and the risks of atherosclerotic vascular disease in older women: Results of a 5-year RCT and a 4.5-year follow-up. *Journal of Bone and Mineral Research, 26*, 35–41.

Luo, G., Ducy, P., McKee, M. D., Pinero, G. J., Loyer, E., Behringer, R. R., & Karsenty, G. (1997). Spontaneous calcification of arteries and cartilage in mice lacking matrix GLA protein. *Nature, 386*, 78–81.

Maes, C., & Kronenberg, H. M. (2010). Bone development and remodeling. In J. L. Jameson & L. J. De Groot (Eds.), *Endocrinology* (pp. 1111–1135). New York: Saunders.

Maillard, C., Berruyer, M., Serre, C. M., Dechavanne, M., & Delmas, P. D. (1992). Protein-S, a vitamin K-dependent protein, is a bone matrix component synthesized and secreted by osteoblasts. *Endocrinology, 130*, 1599–1604.

Manson, J. E., Allison, M. A., Carr, J. J., Langer, R. D., Cochrane, B. B., Hendrix, S. L., ... Women's Health Initiative—Coronary Artery Calcium Study Investigators. (2010). Calcium/vitamin D supplementation and coronary artery calcification in the Women's Health Initiative. *Menopause, 17*, 683–691.

Martin, T. J., Findlay, D. M., & Sexton, P. M. (2010). Calcitonin. In J. L. Jameson & L. J. De Groot (Eds.), *Endocrinology* (pp. 1074–1088). New York: Saunders.

Melsen, F., & Mosekilde, L. (1988). Calcified tissues: Cellular dynamics. In B. Nordin (Ed.), *Calcium in human biology* (pp. 187–208). London: Springer-Verlag.

Nellans, H. N., & Goldsmith, R. S. (1983). Mucosal calcium uptake by rat cecum: Identity with transcellular calcium absorption. *The American Journal of Physiology, 244*, G618–G622.

Nemere, I., Farach-Carson, M. C., Rohe, B., Sterling, T. M., Norman, A. W., Boyan, B. D., & Safford, S. E. (2004). Ribozyme knockdown functionally links a 1,25(OH)2D3 membrane binding protein (1,25D3-MARRS) and phosphate uptake in intestinal cells. *Proceedings of the National Academy of Sciences of the United States of America, 101*, 7392–7397.

Nijenhuis, T., Hoenderop, J. G., & Bindels, R. J. (2005). TRPV5 and TRPV6 in Ca(2+)(re)absorption: Regulating Ca(2+) entry at the gate. *Pflügers Archiv: European Journal of Physiology, 451*, 181–192.

Pattanaungkul, S., Riggs, B. L., Yergey, A. L., Vieira, N. E., O'Fallon, W. M., & Khosla, S. (2000). Relationship of intestinal calcium absorption to 1,25-dihydroxyvitamin D [1,25(OH)2D] levels in young versus elderly women: Evidence for age-related intestinal resistance to 1,25(OH)2D action. *The Journal of Clinical Endocrinology and Metabolism, 85*, 4023–4027.

Pérez, A. V., Picotto, G., Carpentieri, A. R., Rivoira, M. A., Peralta López, M. E., & Tolosa deTalamoni, N. G. (2008). Minireview on regulation of intestinal calcium absorption: Emphasis on molecular mechanisms of transcellular pathway. *Digestion, 77*, 22–34.

Prié, D., Ravery, V., Boccon-Gibod, L., & Friedlander, G. (2001). Frequency of renal phosphate leak among patients with calcium nephrolithiasis. *Kidney International, 60*, 272–276.

Raggot, L. J., & Partridge, N. C. (2010). Cellular and molecular mechanisms of bone remodeling. *The Journal of Biological Chemistry, 285*, 25103–25108.

Recker, R. R., Davies, K. M., Hinders, S. M., Heaney, R. P., Stegman, M. R., & Kimmel, D. B. (1992). Bone gain in young adult women. *The Journal of the American Medical Association, 268*, 2403–2408.

Reid, I. R., Ames, R. W., Evans, M. C., Gamble, G. D., & Sharpe, S. J. (1993). Effect of calcium supplementation on bone loss in postmenopausal women. *New England Journal of Medicine, 328*, 460–464.

Renkema, K. Y., Alexander, R. T., Bindels, R. J., & Hoenderop, J. G. (2008). Calcium and phosphate homeostasis: Concerted interplay of new regulators. *Annals of Medicine, 40*, 82–91.

Rescher, U., & Gerke, V. (2004). Annexins—Unique membrane binding proteins with diverse functions. *Journal of Cell Science, 117*, 2631–2639.

Reverter, D., Strobl, S., Fernandez-Catalan, C., Sorimachi, H., Suzuki, K., & Bode, W. (2001). Structural basis for possible calcium-induced activation mechanisms of calpains. *Biological Chemistry, 382*, 753–766.

Rezende, S. M., Simmonds, R. E., & Lane, D. A. (2004). Coagulation, inflammation, and apoptosis: Different roles for protein S and the protein S-C4b binding protein complex. *Blood, 103*, 1192–1201.

Riedt, C. S., Brolin, R. E., Sherrell, R. M., Field, M. P., & Shapses, S. A. (2006). True fractional calcium absorption is decreased after Rouxen-Y grastric bypass. *Obesity, 14*, 1940–1948.

Riedt, C. S., Schlussel, Y., von Thun, N., Ambia-Sobhan, H., Stahl, T., Field, M. P., ... Shapses, S. A. (2007). Premenopausal overweight women do not lose bone during moderate weight loss with adequate or higher calcium intake. *The American Journal of Clinical Nutrition, 85*, 972–980.

Robey, P. G., & Boskey, A. L. (2008). The composition of bone. In C. J. Rosen (Ed.), *Primer on the metabolic bone diseases and disorders of mineral metabolism* (pp. 32–38). Washington, DC: ASBMR Press.

Ruppe, M. D., & Jan de Beur, S. M. (2008). Disorders of phosphate homeostasis. In C. J. Rosen (Ed.), *Primer on the metabolic bone diseases and disorders of mineral metabolism* (pp. 317–324). Washington, DC: ASBMR Press.

Sanders, K. M., Stuart, A. L., Williamson, E. J., Simpson, J. A., Kotowicz, M. A., Young, D., & Nicholson, G. C. (2010). Annual high-dose oral vitamin D and falls and fractures in older women: A randomized controlled trial. *The Journal of the American Medical Association, 303*, 1815–1822. Erratum: *The Journal of the American Medical Association, 303,* 2357.

Sargent, J. D., Dalton, M. A., O'Connor, G. T., Olmstead, E. M., & Klein, R. Z. (1999). Randomized trial of calcium glycerophosphate-supplemented infant formula to prevent lead absorption. *American Journal of Clinical Nutrition, 69*(6), 1224–1230.

Schoeber, J. P., Hoenderop, J. G., & Bindels, R. J. (2007). Concerted action of associated proteins in the regulation of TRPV5 and TRPV6. *Biochemical Society Transactions, 35*, 115–119.

Segawa, H., Kaneko, I., Yamanaka, S., Ito, M., Kuwahata, M., Inoue, Y., ... Miyamoto, K. (2004). Intestinal Na-P(i) cotransporter adaptation to dietary P(i) content in vitamin D receptor null mice. *American Journal of Physiology. Renal Physiology, 287*, F39–F47.

Shapses, S. A., & Riedt, C. S. (2006). Bone, body weight, and weight reduction: What are the concerns? *The Journal of Nutrition, 136*, 1453–1456.

Shapses, S. A., Schlussel, Y., & Cifuentes, M. (2010). Drug-nutrient interactions that impact on mineral status. In J. I. Boullata & V. T. Armenti (Eds.), *Handbook of drug-nutrient interactions* (pp. 537–571). New York: Humana Press.

Shoback, D. (2008). Hypocalcemia: Definition, etiology, pathogenesis, diagnosis and management. In C. J. Rosen (Ed.), *Primer on the metabolic bone diseases and disorders of mineral metabolism* (pp. 313–317). Washington, DC: ASBMR Press.

Shobeiri, N., Adams, M. A., & Holden, R. M. (2010). Vascular calcification in animal models of CKD: A review. *American Journal of Nephrology, 31*, 471–481.

Suda, T., Ueno, Y., Fujii, K., & Shinki, T. (2003). Vitamin D and bone. *Journal of Cellular Biochemistry, 88*, 259–266.

Tang, B. M., Eslick, G. D., Nowson, C., Smith, C., & Bensoussan, A. (2007). Use of calcium or calcium in combination with vitamin D supplementation to prevent fractures and bone loss in people aged 50 years and older: A meta-analysis. *Lancet, 370*, 657–666.

Thakker, R. V., Bringhurst, R., & Jüppner, H. (2010). Calcium regulation, calcium homeostasis, and genetic disordersof calcium metabolism. In J. L. Jameson & L. J. De Groot (Eds.), *Endocrinology* (pp. 1136–1159). New York: Saunders.

U.S. Department of Agriculture, Agricultural Research Service. (2009). What we eat in America. NHANES 2005–2006, pp 1–24. Retrieved from www.ars.usda.gov/SP2UserFiles/Place/12355000/pdf/0506/usual_nutrient_intake_vitD_ca_phos_mg_2005-06.pdf

U.S. Department of Agriculture, Agricultural Research Service. (2010). *USDA National Nutrient Database for Standard Reference, Release 23.* Retrieved from www.ars.usda.gov/nutrientdata

van Abel, M., Hoenderop, J. G., & Bindels, R. J. (2005). The epithelial calcium channels TRPV5 and TRPV6: Regulation and implications for disease. *Naunyn-Schmiedeberg's Archives of Pharmacolog, 371*, 295–306.

Walters, J. R., Balesaria, S., Khair, U., Sangha, S., Banks, L., & Berry, J. L. (2007). The effects of vitamin D metabolites on expression of genes for calcium transporters in human duodenum. *The Journal of Steroid Biochemistry and Molecular Biology, 103*, 509–512.

Whiting, S. J., & Draper, H. H. (1981). Effect of chronic high protein feeding on bone composition in the adult rat. *The Journal of Nutrition, 111*, 178–183.

Williams, K. B., & DeLuca, H. F. (2007). Characterization of intestinal phosphate absorption using a novel in vivo method. *American Journal of Physiology. Endocrinology and Metabolism, 292*, E1917–E1921.

Wood, R. J., Fleet, J. C., Cashman, K., Bruns, M. E., & Deluca, H. F. (1998). Intestinal calcium absorption in the aged rat: Evidence of intestinal resistance to 1,25-dihydroxyvitamin D. *Endocrinology, 139*, 3843–3848.

Wood, R. J., Tchack, L., Angelo, G., Pratt, R. E., & Sonna, L. A. (2004). DNA microarray analysis of vitamin D–induced gene expression in a human colon carcinoma cell line. Physiological Genomics, 17, 122–129.

Wood, R. J., Tchack, L., & Taparia, S. (2001). 1,25-Dihydroxyvitamin D3 increases the expression of the CaT1 epithelial calcium channel in the Caco-2 human intestinal cell line. *BMC Physiology, 1*, 11.

Yang, Y. X., Lewis, J. D., Epstein, S., & Metz, D. C. (2006). Long-term proton pump inhibitor therapy and risk of hip fracture. *The Journal of the American Medical Association, 296*, 2947–2953.

RECOMMENDED READINGS

Anderson, J. B., Garner, S. C., & Klemmer, P. J. (Eds.). (2011). *Diet, nutrients, and bone health.* Boca Raton, FL: CRC Press, Taylor & Francis.

Bronner, F. (2009). Recent developments in intestinal calcium absorption. *Nutrition Reviews, 67,* 109–113.

Burckhardt, P., Dawson Hughes, B., & Weaver, C. M. (Eds.). (2010). *Nutritional aspects of osteoporosis.* London: Springer.

Holick, M. F., & Dawson-Hughes, B. (Eds.). (2004). *Nutrition and bone health.* Totawa, NJ: Humana Press.

Rosen, C. J. (Ed.). (2012). *Primer on the metabolic bone diseases and disorders of mineral metabolism* (9th ed). Washington, DC: American Society of Bone and Mineral Research.

Weaver, C. M., & Heaney, R. P. (Eds.). (2005). *Calcium in human health.* Totowa, NJ: Humana Press.

CHAPTER 33

Magnesium

*Jürgen Vormann, Dr. rer. nat.**

Magnesium (Mg^{2+}) plays an important role in numerous physiological processes. It is a cofactor for various enzymes that are involved in muscle contraction, neurotransmitter release, and the regulation of ion channels. The essential role of Mg^{2+} in fundamental cellular functions is mainly based on several properties of Mg^{2+}:

- Its action as an enzyme cofactor
- Its ability to chelate anionic ligands, especially adenosine triphosphate (ATP)
- Its ability to compete with calcium (Ca^{2+}) for binding sites, which modulates intracellular and extracellular free Ca^{2+} concentrations
- Its ability to cross-link negatively charged membrane constituents, which stabilizes them
- Its interaction with cell adhesion molecules

CHEMISTRY OF MAGNESIUM

Mg^{2+} is a divalent metal ion with an atomic number of 12 and a molecular weight of 24 g/mol. It is one of the most abundant elements in the earth's crust and is therefore also prevalent in seawater. In vertebrates, it is the fourth most abundant cation in the body and the second most abundant inside cells. Throughout evolution, Mg^{2+} has come to be involved in numerous biological processes.

ABSORPTION, BIOAVAILABILITY, AND EXCRETION OF MAGNESIUM

Mg^{2+} homeostasis in the body is obtained by balancing the intestinal absorption of Mg^{2+} with renal excretion.

INTESTINAL ABSORPTION

Intestinal Mg^{2+} absorption is inversely proportional to the amount ingested. Under normal dietary conditions in healthy individuals, approximately 30% to 50% of ingested Mg^{2+} is absorbed (Fine et al., 1991). Mg^{2+} is absorbed along the entire intestinal tract, but the sites of maximal Mg^{2+} absorption appear to be the distal jejunum and the ileum. The colon absorbs only small amounts of Mg^{2+}, which may be important in the context of dietary restriction or compromised Mg^{2+} absorption in the small intestine. When dietary intake is restricted, fractional absorption of Mg^{2+} may increase up to 80%. Conversely, it may be reduced to 20% with a diet high in Mg^{2+}. There is evidence that intestinal Mg^{2+} absorption is through paracellular and transcellular pathways (Quamme, 2008) (Figure 33-1). About 90% of normal Mg^{2+} absorption occurs passively through the paracellular pathway between the enterocytes, involving barrier proteins of the claudin family (claudin-16, claudin-19). The rate of Mg^{2+} absorption across the intestinal epithelium is dependent on the transepithelial electrical voltage (which is normally about +5 mV, lumen positive with respect to blood) and the transepithelial concentration gradient. The luminal Mg^{2+} concentration may be about 1.0 to 5.0 mM, depending on the dietary Mg^{2+} content and the presence of anionic chelators. Only the free Mg^{2+} moves through the paracellular pathway so that bound Mg^{2+} does not contribute to the transepithelial gradient. Plasma Mg^{2+} concentration is 0.5 to 0.7 mM, so there is normally a concentration gradient between the lumen and the blood. Various poorly understood hormonal and nonhormonal factors acting through a variety of intracellular signals might influence the passive transport.

At a low intraluminal Mg^{2+} concentration, however, absorption occurs primarily via the active transcellular route. Transcellular Mg^{2+} absorption is an active system where the Mg^{2+} entry is mainly mediated by the TRPM6 (transient receptor potential melastatin) channel kinase (see Figure 33-1). TRPM6 protein is localized to the apical membrane of the intestine, thus forming the entry pathway into the enterocyte. Low Mg^{2+} intake induces an increased expression of TRPM6, facilitating Mg^{2+} absorption (Groenestege et al., 2006). The basolateral exit of Mg^{2+} is less well understood. Most probably it consists of a Na^+/Mg^{2+} antiport system. In addition to these transporters, several other Mg^{2+}-sensitive genes have been described that are expressed in intestine and are probably involved in Mg^{2+} transport (Quamme, 2008).

*This chapter is a revision of the chapter contributed by Martin Konrad, MD, and Karl-Peter Schlingmann, MD, for the second edition.

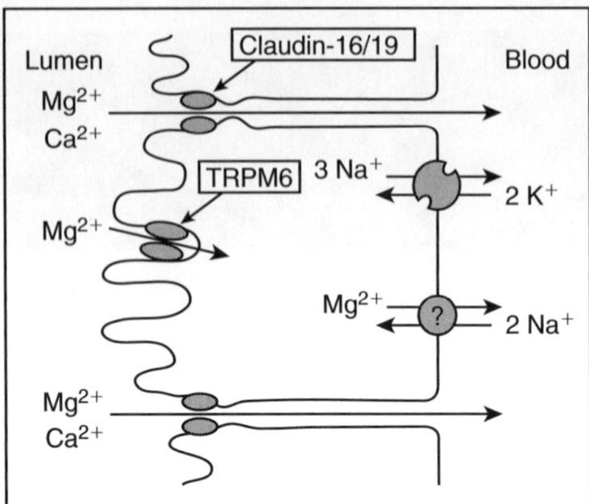

FIGURE 33-1 Proposed model of intestinal Mg^{2+} absorption by two independent pathways: passive paracellular absorption involving claudin-16 and claudin-19 and active transcellular transport involving TRPM6.

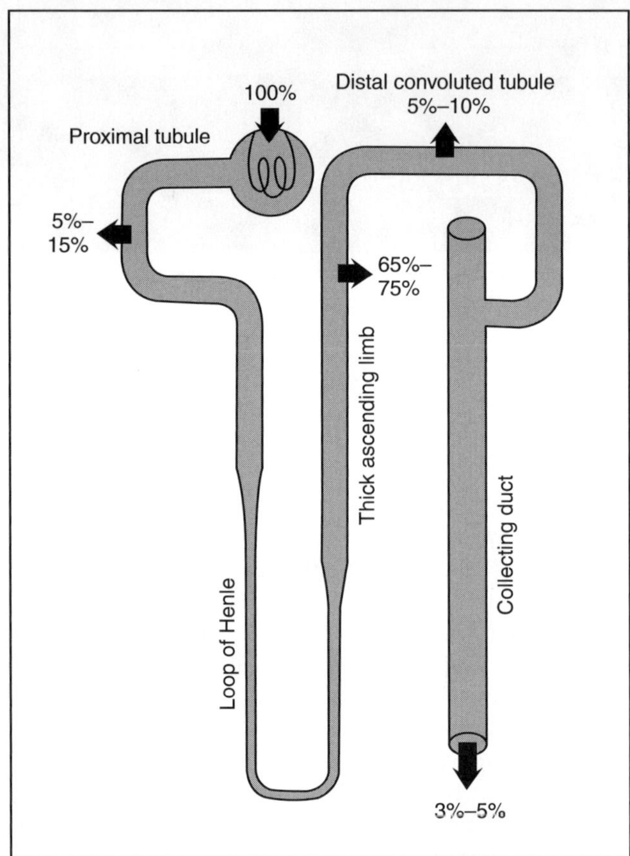

FIGURE 33-2 Summary of the tubular handling of Mg^{2+}. The 100% represents the total filtered load and the other percentage values represent the fraction of the filtered load absorbed at each tubular site.

BIOAVAILABILITY

Intestinal Mg^{2+} absorption can be affected by the presence of other nutrients and dietary constituents. High levels of dietary fiber from fruits, vegetables, and grains decrease fractional Mg^{2+} absorption (Siener and Hesse, 1995). However, diets high in vegetables are Mg^{2+}-rich, and the high Mg^{2+} content of these diets offsets decreased fractional absorption associated with the higher fiber intake. Many foods high in fiber also contain phytate, which may decrease intestinal Mg^{2+} absorption because Mg^{2+} binds to the phosphate groups on phytic acid. The ability of phosphate to bind Mg^{2+} may explain decreases in intestinal Mg^{2+} absorption in individuals on high-phosphate diets (Franz, 1989). Although dietary calcium has been reported to both decrease and increase Mg^{2+} absorption, human studies have shown no effect (Fine et al., 1991). It is likely that interactions between Ca^{2+} and Mg^{2+} occur at high local concentrations achieved with Mg^{2+} or Ca^{2+} supplements but not with usual dietary supply.

RENAL MAGNESIUM HANDLING

The kidney is the principal organ involved in Mg^{2+} homeostasis (Dimke et al., 2009). Under normal conditions, approximately 80% of the total plasma Mg^{2+} is filtered through the glomerulus, and most of this is reabsorbed (greater than 95%) as the filtrate passes through the nephrons (Figure 33-2). Therefore each day, only about 100 mg Mg^{2+} is excreted in the urine, whereas about 2,500 mg of Mg^{2+} is filtered by the glomeruli.

The major site of Mg^{2+} reabsorption is the cortical segment of the thick ascending limb of the loop of Henle, which accounts for 65% to 75% of renal Mg^{2+} reabsorption. This Mg^{2+} transport is passive and involves claudin-16, with movement from the tubular lumen to the interstitium driven by the lumen-positive transepithelial voltage (Figure 33-3, *A*). The transepithelial voltage is determined by Na^+, K^+, and Cl^- cotransport and active Na^+ reabsorption. Therefore any changes in these transport mechanisms consequently influence Mg^{2+} (and Ca^{2+}) reabsorption. Mg^{2+} reabsorption in the cortical thick ascending limb of the loop of Henle is regulated by a variety of hormones that act mainly by increasing the reabsorption rate. These hormonal responses are mediated by changes in both transepithelial voltage and paracellular permeability. It has been shown that 1,25-dihydroxyvitamin D influences Mg^{2+} transport in the cortical thick ascending limb by downregulating *claudin-16* expression at the transcriptional level (Efrati et al., 2005). The amount of reabsorbed Mg^{2+} is mediated by the extracellular Ca^{2+}/Mg^{2+}-sensing receptor (CaSR), which is expressed in the basolateral membrane. Activation of CaSR by increased blood concentrations of Ca^{2+} or Mg^{2+} leads to inhibition of salt reabsorption and paracellular Ca^{2+} and Mg^{2+} transport in the thick ascending limb, thereby increasing divalent cation excretion. Loop diuretics such as furosemide, which act to inhibit the Cl^- pump and subsequently block Na^+ reabsorption, may lead to hypomagnesemia, as these drugs have a large effect on transepithelial voltage.

Mg^{2+} reabsorption in the distal convoluted tubule is about 5% to 10% and is of crucial importance for regulating the final amount of excreted Mg^{2+}, because there is no evidence of Mg^{2+} reabsorption beyond this point. Reabsorption is mediated by an active transcellular transport mechanism, as shown

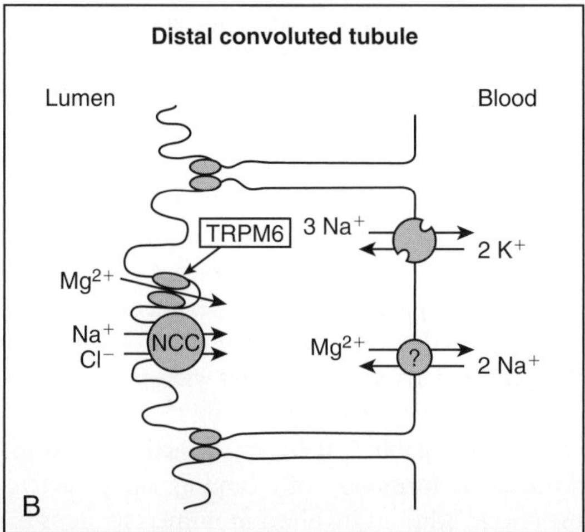

FIGURE 33-3 **A**, Mg^{2+} reabsorption in the thick ascending limb of Henle loop. Mg^{2+} transport is passive and involves claudin-16, with movement from the tubular lumen to the interstitium driven by the lumen-positive transepithelial voltage. **B**, Mg^{2+} reabsorption in the distal convoluted tubule. Reabsorption is mediated by an active transcellular transport mechanism and the TRPM6 channel. *NCC*, Sodium chloride cotransporter.

in Figure 33-3, *B*. Mg^{2+} enters the cell across the apical membrane through the TRPM6 channel. Uptake of Mg^{2+} is driven by the lumen-negative potential difference in this region of the tubule. Extrusion into the interstitium probably occurs by a Na^+-dependent exchange mechanism. Mutations in *TRPM6* were identified in patients with primary hypomagnesemia and with secondary hypocalcemia (Schlingmann et al., 2002; Walder et al., 2002). Mg^{2+} transport rates in the distal convoluted tubule change rapidly upon a decrease in Mg^{2+} availability, which allows efficient Mg^{2+} conservation. Conversely, during hypermagnesemia (or hypercalcemia), fractional excretion rates for Mg^{2+} are increased via activation of the CaSR, which results in inhibition of Mg^{2+} (or Ca^{2+}) reabsorption.

The epidermal growth factor (EGF) was identified as a magnesiotropic hormone. EGF stimulates the trafficking of TRPM6 channels to the luminal membrane, increasing the reabsorption of Mg^{2+} through TRPM6 (Thebault et al., 2009). Patients suffering from metastatic colorectal cancer are often treated with antibodies raised against the EGF receptor, such as cetuximab. Anti–EGF receptor monoclonal antibody therapy has been shown to result in hypomagnesemia in a significant number of patients (Tejpar et al., 2007). In addition, changes in acid–base balance significantly influence Mg^{2+} status, because production of TRPM6 is reduced in acidosis (Nijenhuis et al., 2006). In human volunteers a higher dietary acid load increased urinary Mg^{2+} losses (Rylander et al., 2006).

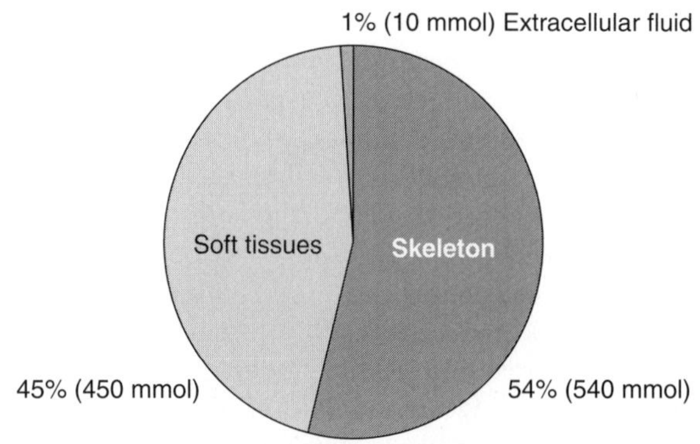

FIGURE 33-4 Distribution of Mg^{2+} in the body.

BODY MAGNESIUM CONTENT

The normal adult total body Mg^{2+} content is approximately 24 g, or 1,000 mmol, and 50% to 60% of this total resides in bone (Figure 33-4). Part of this Mg^{2+} is on the surface of bone and is in equilibrium with the extracellular Mg^{2+}. At reduced plasma concentrations Mg^{2+} can be rapidly released from the bone surface, and at increased plasma concentrations Mg^{2+} is bound to the surface (Elin, 1994). Based on investigations with the stable isotopes $^{25}Mg^{2+}$ and $^{26}Mg^{2+}$ in a kinetic model of Mg^{2+} metabolism in healthy men, 24% of the human total Mg^{2+} exchanges rapidly; of this, 79% turns over in 115 hours, representing probably the bone surface pool. The remaining part, which may represent plasma and easily accessible extracellular space, turns over in less than 9 hours (Sabatier et al., 2003). Therefore magnesium in bone represents a reservoir that buffers extracellular magnesium concentration. In humans this magnesium-buffering capacity is reduced with increasing age, because nearly half of the magnesium content of bone is lost over a lifetime (Vormann and Anke, 2002).

Extracellular Mg^{2+} accounts for only about 1% of total body Mg^{2+}. The normal serum Mg^{2+} concentration is 0.75 to 1.0 mmol/L (Weisinger and Bellorin-Font, 1998). Most of the plasma Mg^{2+}, approximately 60% to 65%, is ionized or free Mg^{2+}. Of the remaining 35% to 40%, 5% to 10% is complexed to anions such as phosphate, citrate, and sulfate, and 30% is bound to proteins (chiefly albumin).

Soft tissue contains about one half of the total body Mg^{2+}, approximately 470 mmol. The Mg^{2+} content of soft tissues varies between 2.5 and 9 mmol/kg wet tissue weight. In general, the higher the metabolic activity of the cell, the higher the Mg^{2+} content. Within the cell, significant amounts of Mg^{2+} are in the nucleus, mitochondria, and endoplasmic (or sarcoplasmic) reticulum as well as in the cytosol (Birch, 1993). Most of the Mg^{2+} is bound to proteins and other negatively charged molecules such as nucleoside triphosphates and diphosphates (e.g., ATP and ADP) and nucleic acids (e.g., RNA and DNA). In the cytoplasm, about 80% of the Mg^{2+} is complexed with ATP (Frausto da Silva and Williams, 1991). Only 1% to 5% of the total intracellular pool is free ionized Mg^{2+} (Romani et al., 1993). The concentration of free Mg^{2+} in the cytosol of mammalian cells has been reported to range from 0.2 to 1.0 mmol/L, but values vary with cell type and means of measurement. The free Mg^{2+} in the cell cytosol is maintained at a relatively constant level, even when the Mg^{2+} concentration in the extracellular fluid is experimentally varied above or below the physiological range (Romani, 2007).

The relative constancy of the free Mg^{2+} concentration in the intracellular milieu is attributed to the limited permeability of the plasma membrane to Mg^{2+} and to the operation of specific Mg^{2+} transport systems that regulate the rates at which Mg^{2+} enters or leaves cells. Cellular Mg^{2+} transport has been studied intensively, and it is mediated by a variety of Mg^{2+} transport proteins in different human tissues (Quamme, 2010). In most tissues, Mg^{2+} influx is dependent on TRPM7. This channel is ubiquitously expressed, whereas TRPM6 is only found along the intestine, kidney nephron, lung, and testis. However, total intracellular Mg^{2+} content is determined by a balance of Mg^{2+} influx and Mg^{2+} efflux. Whereas Mg^{2+} influx systems are quite well characterized, much less is known about the mechanisms underlying Mg^{2+} transport out of the cell. Mg^{2+} mainly leaves the cell through a Na^+/Mg^{2+} exchange mechanism, which depends on Na^+,K^+-ATPase activity (Wolf et al., 2008). Various other Mg^{2+} transport systems have been discovered in recent years; however, it is not known how they contribute to intracellular Mg^{2+} homeostasis (Quamme, 2010). It is also not known if polymorphisms of Mg^{2+} transporters influence Mg^{2+} status and affect Mg^{2+}-sensitive diseases.

PHYSIOLOGICAL ROLES OF MAGNESIUM

ENZYME AND ATP COFACTOR

The main biological role of Mg^{2+} in mammalian cells is anion charge neutralization (Romani, 2007; Cowan, 2002). Mg^{2+} is particularly found in association with organic polyphosphates such as nucleotide triphosphates and nucleotide diphosphates (e.g., ATP^{4-} and ADP^{3-}). Mg^{2+} is also found with other highly anionic species, including multisubstituted phosphates of sugars such as inositol triphosphate, nucleic acids (RNA and DNA), and some carboxylates (e.g., isocitrate-Mg^{2+} as substrate for isocitrate lyase; carboxylate groups on proteins).

Mg^{2+} is normally bound between the β- and γ-phosphates of nucleotide triphosphates, such as ATP, and between the α- and β-phosphates of nucleotide diphosphates, such as ADP (Figure 33-5). This arrangement neutralizes the negative charge density on the ATP or other nucleotide triphosphates or diphosphates, and it facilitates binding of the nucleotide phosphate to the enzymes that use them as substrates. In most reactions in which Mg^{2+} is involved, it is present as a complex with a nucleotide triphosphate or diphosphate, which serves as the substrate. The Mg^{2+} in these complexes does not interact directly with the enzyme in most cases, but it is linked by the substrate in an enzyme–substrate–metal type of substrate-bridged complex. Hence Mg^{2+} plays a dominant role in all enzymatic reactions that require nucleotide triphosphates or diphosphates. This reaction type is widespread in metabolism. Mg^{2+} also is required for binding to some enzymes or other proteins to stabilize them in the active conformation or to induce the formation of a binding site or active site. By these effects, Mg^{2+} is involved in numerous steps in central pathways of carbohydrate, lipid, and protein metabolism and in mitochondrial ATP synthesis. In addition, Mg^{2+} associates with nucleic acids, in which the phosphate groups in the nucleotide chains render the polymers negatively charged overall. Mg^{2+} stabilizes bending of RNA or DNA into particular curved or folded structures. This presumably occurs because of the cross-linking of the oxyanion centers of the phosphate residues by the divalent cation.

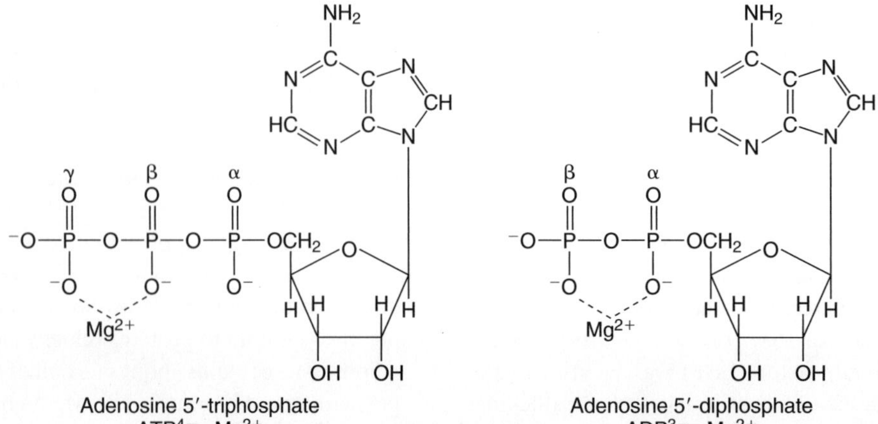

FIGURE 33-5 Physiological forms of Mg^{2+}-ATP and Mg^{2+}-ADP.

The transcription, translation, and replication of nucleic acids (RNA and DNA) require enzymes that catalyze the hydrolysis and formation of phosphodiester bonds. Almost all these enzymes require Mg^{2+} for optimal activity.

Replicating cells must be able to synthesize new protein, and all cells must continually replace protein that is degraded. Protein synthesis has been reported to be highly sensitive to Mg^{2+} depletion because it is required for virtually every step of protein biosynthesis. Formation of the aminoacyl–transfer RNA species (which requires Mg^{2+}-ATP), maintenance of its conformation (which is required for recognition by messenger RNA), and maintenance of the ribosomes all require Mg^{2+}. It is also required for structure and activity of elongation factor–guanosine triphosphate (GTP) complexes that allow protein synthesis to begin and for the GTPase activities that occur during elongation and termination of protein biosynthesis.

SECOND MESSENGER SYSTEMS

Many hormones, neurotransmitters, and other cellular effectors regulate cellular activity via the adenylate cyclase system. As is the case for other ATP-utilizing enzymes, the actual substrate for adenylate cyclase is Mg^{2+}-ATP (Figure 33-6). There is also evidence for a Mg^{2+} binding site on adenylate cyclase, through which Mg^{2+} directly increases enzyme activity.

Another group of hormones and neurotransmitters exert their effects by raising the ionized calcium (Ca^{2+}) concentration in the cytosol of their target cells through the activation of the phosphoinositol cycle (see Figure 33-6). One of the principal mechanisms by which this is thought to occur is by receptor-mediated activation of phospholipase C, which hydrolyzes a specific phospholipid in the plasma membrane, PIP_2 (phosphatidylinositol 4,5-bisphosphate), to yield two biologically active products, diacylglycerol and inositol 1,4,5-triphosphate (IP_3). Diacylglycerol activates protein kinase C, and IP_3 triggers calcium release from the endoplasmic reticulum. The IP_3 is rapidly inactivated by dephosphorylation. It appears that Mg^{2+} is essential for the normal functioning of this phosphoinositol cycle because the kinase that forms the PIP_2 and also the enzymes that inactivate IP_3 require Mg^{2+} at physiological concentrations (Volpe et al., 1990). In contrast, higher Mg^{2+} concentrations may decrease intracellular Ca^{2+} by two mechanisms: (1) noncompetitive inhibition of IP_3 binding to its receptor, and (2) inhibition of the release of Ca^{2+} via IP_3-gated channels (Volpe et al., 1990).

Ca^{2+} CHANNELS

Mg^{2+} has been called "nature's physiological calcium channel blocker" (Iseri and French, 1984). During Mg^{2+} depletion, intracellular Ca^{2+} rises. This may be caused by both uptake from extracellular Ca^{2+} and release from intracellular Ca^{2+} stores. Mg^{2+} has been demonstrated to decrease the inward Ca^{2+} flux through slow Ca^{2+} channels (O'Rourke, 1993; White and Hartzell, 1989). In addition, Mg^{2+} will decrease the transport of Ca^{2+} out of the endoplasmic reticulum into the cell cytosol. Consequently, because Ca^{2+} plays an important role in skeletal and smooth muscle contraction, a state of Mg^{2+} depletion may result in muscle cramps, hypertension, and coronary and cerebral vasospasm (Altura and Altura, 1995).

FOOD SOURCES, RECOMMENDED INTAKES, AND DIETARY INTAKES OF MAGNESIUM

FOOD SOURCES

Mg^{2+} is almost ubiquitous in foods. The primary dietary sources are whole grain cereals, legumes, nuts, and chocolate. Vegetables, fruits, meats, and fish have an intermediate

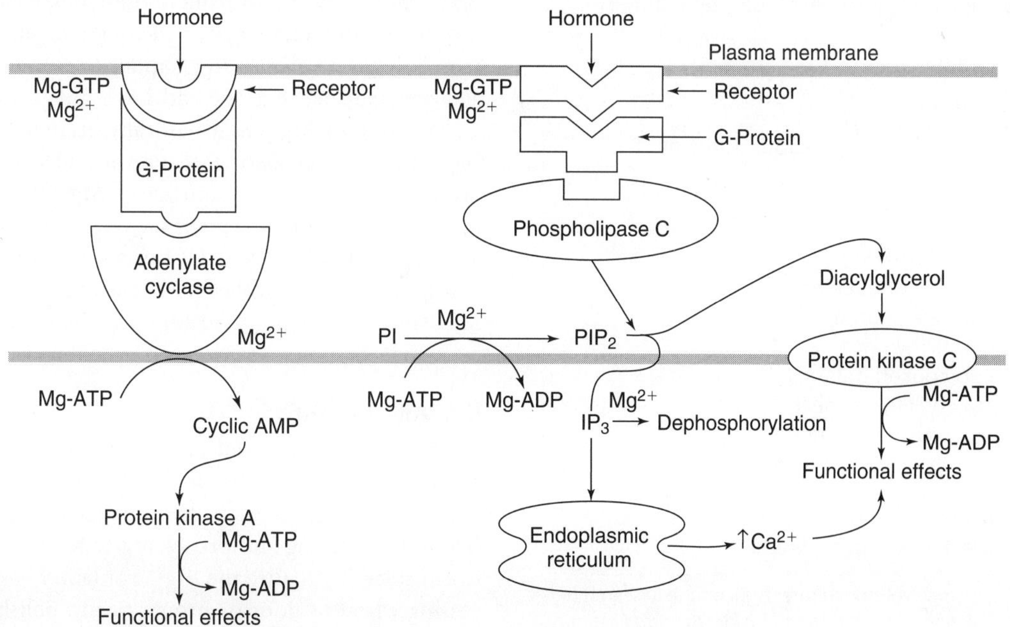

FIGURE 33-6 Schematic representation of the role of Mg^{2+} in two second messenger systems, adenylate cyclase and phosphatidylinositol. *GTP*, Guanosine triphosphate; *G-protein*, guanine nucleotide regulatory protein; *IP_3*, inositol 1,4,5-triphosphate; *PI*, phosphatidylinositol; *PIP_2*, phosphatidylinositol 4,5-bisphosphate.

CLINICAL CORRELATION

Magnesium Depletion in Patients with Diabetes Mellitus

Cardiovascular disease is a common cause of morbidity and mortality in patients with diabetes mellitus. This is in part due to hyperlipidemia and hypertension leading to coronary heart disease. Mg^{2+} deficiency has been linked to hypertension, perhaps by altering Ca^{2+} channels, resulting in increased Ca^{2+} in the vascular smooth muscle and causing vasoconstriction. Patients with diabetes mellitus are at risk for Mg^{2+} depletion. Renal Mg^{2+} loss has been correlated with high blood glucose and high urine glucose excretion. It is thought that the osmotic diuresis due to the glucose causes the kidney to waste Mg^{2+}. Medications may also contribute to Mg^{2+} loss. Patients with high blood pressure and heart disease frequently receive diuretics such as furosemide, which blocks the reabsorption of Mg^{2+} in the thick ascending limb of the loop of Henle. Because this is the major site of renal Mg^{2+} reabsorption, it causes marked urinary Mg^{2+} loss.

Thinking Critically

1. Why might individuals with diabetes mellitus be at risk of magnesium depletion?
2. How does magnesium depletion increase risk for cardiovascular disease?
3. Does magnesium deficiency contribute to heart dysrhythmias? How? (See Cardiovascular Manifestations.)

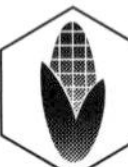

FOOD SOURCES OF MAGNESIUM

Legumes

60 to 75 mg per ½ cup soybeans, or white or black beans (cooked)
35 to 50 mg per ½ cup navy, lima, or kidney beans; chickpeas; split peas; or lentils (cooked)
60 mg per 1 cup soy milk

Nuts

100 mg per 1 oz Brazil nuts
80 mg per 1 oz almonds or cashews
70 mg per 1 oz pine nuts
45 mg per 1 oz hazelnuts or walnuts

Vegetables and Fruits

80 mg per ½ cup cooked spinach
40 mg per ½ cup cooked okra
30 mg per ½ cup sweet potato
20 mg per ½ cup edible pod peas, corn, or summer squash
20 mg per ½ cup bananas

Fish

40 to 90 mg per 3 oz serving (halibut, tuna, or haddock)
55 mg per 3 oz crab meat

Cereals and Grain Products

110 mg per ½ cup all bran cereal
40 mg per ¾ cup wheat bran flakes
40 mg per ½ cup brown rice
30 mg per ½ cup cooked bulgur
55 mg per 1 cup cooked oatmeal
25 to 30 mg per ½ cup white rice

Other

40 mg per 8 oz plain yogurt
40 mg per 1 tbsp blackstrap molasses

Data from U.S. Department of Agriculture, Agricultural Research Service. (2010). *USDA National Nutrient Database for Standard Reference, Release 23*. Retrieved from www.ars.usda.gov/ba/bhnrc/ndl

Mg^{2+} content, whereas milk-based products and beverages have a low Mg^{2+} content (Elin, 1994).

RECOMMENDED INTAKES

In the United States the Estimated Average Requirement (EAR) was set at 330 mg/day for men and 255 mg/day for women ages 19 through 30 years (Institute of Medicine [IOM], 1997). For adults older than 30 years, the EAR was set slightly higher at 350 and 265 mg/day for men and women, respectively. The Recommended Dietary Allowances (RDAs) for adults were set as the EAR + 20%. An incremental intake of an additional 40 mg/day was added to obtain RDAs for pregnant women. No increment was added for lactation. The magnesium requirements of children and adolescents were estimated from available balance study data or extrapolated from data of older children, and RDAs were set as the EAR + 20%. For infants, Adequate Intakes (AIs) were set based on the average intake from human milk during the first 6 months of life, or from human milk plus complementary foods for infants aged 7 through 12 months. Recommendations for dietary Mg^{2+} intake in other countries are also generally between 300 and 400 mg/day for adults.

Ingestion of Mg^{2+} as a naturally occurring substance in foods has not been associated with any adverse effects. However, because nonfood sources of Mg^{2+} (such as various Mg^{2+} salts) are used for pharmacological purposes, a Tolerable Upper Intake Level (UL) was set by the IOM (1997). Diarrhea was used as the most sensitive indicator of excess Mg^{2+} intake from nonfood sources. The UL for adolescents and adults is 350 mg/day of supplementary Mg^{2+}.

DIETARY INTAKES

A number of reports indicate that an increasing proportion of the general population does not consume adequate Mg^{2+} and consequently develops hypomagnesemia. This is largely due to the refining and processing of food, which is known to considerably reduce the Mg^{2+} content. For example, processing wheat to flour or brown rice to polished white rice reduces the Mg^{2+} content by approximately 80%.

The National Health and Nutrition Examination Survey 2005–2006 data (Moshfegh et al., 2009) showed that 53%

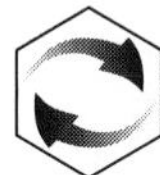

DRIs Across the Life Cycle: Magnesium

	mg Magnesium per day	
Infants	RDA	UL*
0 through 6 mo	30 (AI)	ND
7 through 12 mo	75 (AI)	ND
Children		
1 through 3 yr	80	65
4 through 8 yr	130	110
9 through 13 yr	240	350
Males		
14 through 18 yr	410	350
19 through 30 yr	400	350
≥31 yr	420	350
Females		
14 through 18 yr	360	350
19 through 30 yr	310	350
≥31 yr	320	350
Pregnant		
<19 yr	400	350
19 through 30 yr	350	350
≥31 yr	360	350
Lactating		
<19 yr	360	350
19 through 30 yr	310	350
≥31 yr	320	350

Data from IOM. (2006). In J. J. Otten, J. P. Hellwig, & L. D. Meyers (Eds.), *Dietary Reference Intakes: The essential guide to nutrient requirements.* Washington, DC: The National Academies Press.

AI, Adequate Intake; *DRI,* Dietary Reference Intake; *ND,* not determinable; *RDA,* Recommended Dietary Allowance; *UL,* Tolerable Upper Intake Level.

*The ULs for magnesium represent intake from pharmacological agents only and do not include intake from food and water.

of males (19 years or older) and 56% of females (19 years or older) consumed Mg^{2+} intakes below the EAR. Similar trends of low dietary Mg^{2+} intake were found in the United Kingdom (Henderson et al., 2003) and Germany (Nationale Verzehrs Studie II, 2008).

MAGNESIUM DEPLETION

CAUSES

Mg^{2+} may be lost via the gastrointestinal tract, either by excessive loss of secreted fluids or by impaired absorption (Box 33-1). The Mg^{2+} content of upper intestinal tract fluids is approximately 0.5 mmol/L, and vomiting or nasogastric suction may contribute to Mg^{2+} depletion from loss of these fluids. The Mg^{2+} content of diarrheal fluids and fistulous drainage is much higher (up to 7.5 mmol/L), and consequently Mg^{2+} depletion is common in patients with acute or chronic diarrhea, regional enteritis, ulcerative colitis, or an intestinal or biliary fistula. Malabsorption syndromes such as celiac sprue may result in Mg^{2+} deficiency. Steatorrhea and resection or bypass of the small bowel, particularly the ileum, often result in intestinal Mg^{2+} malabsorption and loss from the body. Lastly, acute severe pancreatitis may be associated with hypomagnesemia; this could be due to the clinical problem causing the pancreatitis (e.g., alcoholism) or to Mg^{2+} binding to necrotic fat surrounding the pancreas. A representative study showed that a high percentage of hospitalized patients (acute 26.1% and chronic 3.5%) are diagnosed with hypomagnesemia (Lum, 1992).

Excessive excretion of Mg^{2+} into the urine is another cause of Mg^{2+} depletion (see Box 33-1). Renal Mg^{2+} excretion is proportional to tubular fluid flow as well as to Na^+ and Ca^{2+} excretion. Therefore Mg^{2+} depletion may result from both chronic intravenous fluid therapy with Na^+-containing fluids and disorders such as primary aldosteronism in which there is extracellular volume expansion. Hypercalcemia and hypercalciuria have been shown to decrease renal Mg^{2+} reabsorption; these conditions are probably the cause of the excessive renal Mg^{2+} excretion and the hypomagnesemia observed in many hypercalcemic states. An osmotic diuresis will result in increased renal Mg^{2+} excretion due to excessive urinary volume. Osmotic diuresis caused by glucosuria can thus result in Mg^{2+} depletion, and diabetes mellitus is probably the most common clinical disorder associated with Mg^{2+} depletion. The degree of Mg^{2+} depletion in patients with diabetes mellitus has been related to the amount of glucose excreted into the urine and hence with the degree of osmotic diuresis.

A number of drugs can cause renal Mg^{2+} wasting and Mg^{2+} depletion. These include furosemide, aminoglycosides, amphotericin B, cisplatin, cyclosporine, pentamidine (Shah and Kirschenbaum, 1991), and also monoclonal antibodies against the EGF receptor (cetuximab), which are used in cancer therapy (Glaudemans et al., 2010). Proton pump inhibitors like omeprazole might induce severe Mg^{2+} deficits because gastric acid is needed to release bound Mg^{2+} in foodstuff (Hoorn et al., 2010). An elevated blood alcohol level has been associated with hypermagnesuria, and increased urinary excretion of Mg^{2+} is one factor contributing to Mg^{2+} depletion in chronic alcoholism. Metabolic acidosis also impairs renal conservation of Mg^{2+} (see earlier). Lastly, a number of rare inherited renal disorders are associated with Mg^{2+} wasting because of impaired renal reabsorption of Mg^{2+} (Naderi and Reilly, 2008).

MANIFESTATIONS

The biochemical and physiological manifestations of severe Mg^{2+} depletion are summarized in Box 33-2.

Hypokalemia

A common feature of Mg^{2+} depletion is hypokalemia (Whang et al., 1994). During Mg^{2+} depletion there is loss of K^+ from the cell, which is enhanced because the kidney is unable to conserve K^+. Attempts to replace this deficit with K^+ therapy alone are not successful without simultaneous Mg^{2+} therapy.

Hypocalcemia

Hypocalcemia is also a common manifestation of moderate to severe Mg^{2+} depletion (Rude et al., 2009). The hypocalcemia may be a major contributing factor to the increased neuromuscular excitability often present in Mg^{2+}-depleted patients. The pathogenesis of hypocalcemia

BOX 33-1 Causes of Magnesium Deficiency

GASTROINTESTINAL DISORDERS

Prolonged nasogastric suction/vomiting
Acute and chronic diarrhea
Malabsorption syndromes (e.g., celiac sprue)
Extensive bowel resection
Intestinal and biliary fistulas
Acute hemorrhagic pancreatitis

RENAL LOSS

Chronic parenteral fluid therapy
Osmotic diuresis (e.g., due to presence of glucose in diabetes mellitus)
Hypercalcemia
Alcohol
Metabolic acidosis (e.g., starvation, diabetic ketoacidosis, and alcoholism)
Renal diseases
- Chronic pyelonephritis, interstitial nephritis, and glomerulonephritis
- Diuretic phase of acute tubular necrosis
- Postobstructive nephropathy
- Renal tubular acidosis
- Postrenal transplantation

Endocrine disorders
- Hyperparathyroidism
- Hyperthyreosis
- Hyperaldosteronism
- Syndrome of inappropriate secretion of antidiuretic hormone (SIADH)

Drugs
- Diuretics (e.g., furosemide, hydrochlorothiazide)
- Aminoglycosides
- Calcineurin inhibitors (cyclosporin A, tacrolimus)
- Amphotericin B
- Pentamidine
- Cisplatin
- Beta-mimetics
- Catecholamines
- Anti–EGF receptor antibodies (cetuximab)
- Proton pump inhibitors (e.g., omeprazole)

Inherited defects of Mg^{2+} transporters

is multifactorial. Impaired parathyroid hormone (PTH) secretion appears to be a major factor in hypomagnesemia-induced hypocalcemia. Serum PTH concentrations are usually low in these patients, and Mg^{2+} administration will immediately stimulate PTH secretion. Patients with hypocalcemia due to Mg^{2+} depletion also exhibit both renal and skeletal resistance to exogenously administered PTH, as manifested by subnormal urinary cyclic AMP and phosphate excretion and a diminished calcemic response. All these effects are reversed following several days of Mg^{2+} therapy. Vitamin D metabolism and action may also be abnormal in hypocalcemic Mg^{2+}-deficient patients. Resistance to vitamin D therapy has been reported in such cases.

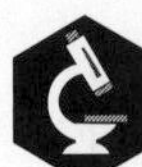

CLINICAL CORRELATION

Mg^{2+} Deficiency in Chronic Alcohol Abuse

Chronic alcoholics are prone to Mg^{2+} depletion for several reasons. First, as blood alcohol levels rise, the kidney is less efficient at reabsorbing Mg^{2+} from the tubular fluid. Alcoholics also have frequent episodes of diarrhea, which result in loss of large amounts of Mg^{2+}. Lastly, these individuals are usually poorly nourished and have a low Mg^{2+} intake. Alcohol and refined foods have very low Mg^{2+} content. Mg^{2+} is not included in routine blood tests, but other measurements may provide clues that suggest a Mg^{2+} deficiency. Low blood calcium is one such clue.

Thinking Critically

1. What is the effect of Mg^{2+} deficiency on calcium metabolism?
2. Would high-dose calcium correct the adverse effects of Mg^{2+} deficiency on calcium homeostasis? Why?
3. What would be the correct therapy? Why?

Neuromuscular Manifestations

Neuromuscular hyperexcitability may be the presenting complaint of patients with Mg^{2+} deficiency, and tetany and muscle cramps may be present. Generalized seizures (convulsions) may also occur. Other neuromuscular signs include dizziness, disequilibrium, muscular tremor, wasting, and weakness (Whang et al., 1994). Although hypocalcemia often contributes to the neurological signs, hypomagnesemia alone results in neuromuscular hyperexcitability.

Cardiovascular Manifestations

Mg^{2+} depletion may also result in electrocardiographic abnormalities and cardiac dysrhythmias, which may be manifested by a rapid heart rate (tachycardia), skipped heart beats (premature beats), or a totally irregular cardiac rhythm (fibrillation). Cardiac dysrhythmias are also known to occur during K^+ depletion; therefore the effect of Mg^{2+} deficiency on K^+ loss from the body may be the cause of the dysrhythmias (White and Hartzell, 1989; Whang et al., 1994). Several mechanisms may contribute to the K^+ loss. Mg^{2+} is necessary for the active transport of K^+ out of cells by the Na^+,K^+-ATPase pump. Mg^{2+}-depleted animals and humans have been found to have a reduction in the concentration of Na^+,K^+-ATPase pumps in skeletal muscle, and this reduction in number of transport systems may contribute to the decrease in cellular K^+ (Dorup, 1994). In addition, activity of the Na^+,K^+-ATPase pump is dependent on Mg^{2+}, as has been observed in heart, so Na^+ and K^+ transport activity may also be impaired during Mg^{2+} deficiency because of decreased activity of the Na^+,K^+-ATPase pump (Ryan, 1991).

Another mechanism for K^+ loss is an increased efflux of K^+ from cells via other Mg^{2+}-sensitive K^+ channels, as has been seen in skeletal muscle (Dorup, 1994). Mg^{2+} is also involved in regulating a number of K^+ channels in

BOX 33-2 Major Manifestations of Magnesium Depletion

BIOCHEMICAL

Hypokalemia
Excessive renal K^+ excretion
Decreased intracellular K^+
Hypocalcemia
Impaired parathyroid hormone (PTH) secretion
Renal and skeletal resistance to PTH
Resistance to vitamin D

NEUROMUSCULAR

Positive Chvostek and Trousseau signs
Spontaneous carpopedal spasm
Seizures
Vertigo, ataxia, nystagmus, athetoid and choreiform movements
Muscular weakness, tremor, fasciculation, and wasting
Headache

PSYCHIATRIC

Depression
Psychosis
Migraine

CARDIOVASCULAR

Electrocardiographic abnormalities
Prolonged PR and QT intervals
U waves
Cardiac dysrhythmias
Atrial tachycardia, fibrillations, torsades de pointes

GASTROINTESTINAL

Nausea, vomiting
Anorexia

heart muscle (Matsuda, 1991; White and Hartzell, 1989). Inwardly rectifying K^+ channels normally allow K^+ to pass more readily inward than outward, and intracellular Mg^{2+} appears to block the outward movement of K^+ through these channels in myocardial cells. In the absence of Mg^{2+}, K^+ is transported equally well in both directions, and a deficiency in Mg^{2+} may lead to a reduced amount of intracellular K^+. Because the resting membrane potential of heart muscle cells is determined in part by the intracellular K^+ concentration, a decreased concentration will result, by a complex mechanism, in partial depolarization (i.e., a less negative resting membrane potential) of electrical tissues at rest. In a study that provided only 101 mg Mg^{2+}/2,000 kcal a day to volunteers for up to 78 days, one third of the volunteers developed severe cardiac arrhythmias and required Mg^{2+} replacement therapy (Nielsen et al., 2007).

DIAGNOSIS OF MAGNESIUM DEFICIENCY

Routinely, only plasma Mg^{2+} concentrations are determined, because there is still no simple, rapid, and accurate laboratory test to determine total body Mg^{2+} status in humans (Arnaud, 2008). Plasma Mg^{2+} concentrations also exhibit a circadian rhythm, with higher values in the evening and lower values in the morning (Wilimzig et al., 1996). In addition, stress, physical performance, and acidosis might influence plasma Mg^{2+} level by Mg^{2+} release from the intracellular compartment. This release of Mg^{2+} from the intracellular compartment may yield artificially high plasma Mg^{2+} concentrations that obscure an existing Mg^{2+} deficit. A plasma concentration below the reference value therefore is indicative of a Mg^{2+} deficit, but a normal plasma Mg^{2+} concentration does not rule out Mg^{2+} deficiency (Ismail et al., 2010). New studies point to the possibility of measuring the expression of Mg^{2+}-sensitive genes in leukocytes to diagnose latent intracellular deficits (Vormann et al., 2009).

In patients who are at risk for Mg^{2+} deficiency but have normal serum Mg^{2+} levels, Mg^{2+} status can be further evaluated by determining the amount excreted in the urine following an intravenous infusion of Mg^{2+} (Arnaud, 2008). Healthy subjects excrete at least 80% of an intravenous Mg^{2+} load within 24 hours, whereas patients with Mg^{2+} deficiency excrete much less. The Mg^{2+} load test, however, requires normal renal handling of Mg^{2+}. If excess Mg^{2+} is being excreted by the kidneys through diuresis, the Mg^{2+} load test may yield an inappropriate negative result. Conversely, if renal function is impaired and less blood is being filtered, this test could give a false-positive result.

MAGNESIUM TOXICITY

Mg^{2+} intoxication is a rarely encountered clinical problem. Symptomatic hypermagnesemia is almost always caused by excessive intake or administration of Mg^{2+} salts in patients with renal failure or after Mg^{2+} infusion (Mordes, 1978). In persons without kidney failure, oral Mg^{2+} supplementation cannot lead to serum Mg^{2+} concentrations that could pose any harm.

MAGNESIUM AND DISEASE RISK

OSTEOPOROSIS

There is increasing awareness of the importance of Mg^{2+} for the skeleton. As most of the Mg^{2+} is located in bone, which is used as a buffer in times when Mg^{2+} level is low, reduced intake might contribute to osteoporosis (Rude et al., 2009). Supplementation studies with Mg^{2+} resulted in improved bone parameters, mineral content, and density (Stendig-Lindbergh et al., 1993; Dimai et al., 1998; Carpenter et al., 2006).

CARDIOVASCULAR DISORDERS

Several epidemiological studies suggested a protective effect of the cardiovascular system with high plasma Mg^{2+} concentration or high dietary Mg^{2+} intake. The Atherosclerosis Risk in Communities (ARIC) Study included more than 13,000 healthy subjects without coronary artery disease (CAD) on admission. After a 4- to 7-year follow-up, the data suggested that the highest risk for CAD occurred in subjects with the lowest serum Mg^{2+} and vice versa, even after controlling for the traditional CAD risk factors (Liao et al., 1998). The National Health and Nutrition Examination Survey Epidemiologic Follow-up Study (Ford, 1999) demonstrated an inverse association of serum Mg^{2+} and mortality from CAD and all causes. In a 30-year follow-up, low Mg^{2+} in the diet was found to increase the incidence of CAD by 2.1 times compared to high Mg^{2+} concentration, even after controlling for traditional CAD risk factors in the Honolulu heart program (Abbott et al., 2003). The health professional's follow-up study also showed a reduced incidence of CAD with high Mg^{2+} intake (Al-Delaimy et al., 2004). This epidemiological evidence is supported by several studies where Mg^{2+} supplementation proved to be effective in patients with cardiovascular disorders (Shechter, 2010). In addition, Mg^{2+} also has a mild antihypertensive effect (Jee et al., 2002).

TYPE 2 DIABETES MELLITUS

High Mg^{2+} intake is connected with a reduced risk to develop type 2 diabetes mellitus. Epidemiological studies with more than 300,000 participants demonstrated an increased risk for type 2 diabetes and also metabolic syndrome with reduced Mg^{2+} content of the diet. A meta-analysis showed a 15% reduced risk for diabetes per 100 mg/day additional dietary Mg^{2+} (Larsson and Wolk, 2007). A further investigation showed a close inverse correlation between serum Mg^{2+} concentration and development of type 2 diabetes in a 10-year follow-up (Guerrero-Romero et al., 2008). Intracellular Mg^{2+} plays a key role in regulating insulin action, insulin-mediated glucose uptake, and vascular tone. Reduced intracellular Mg^{2+} concentrations result in a defective tyrosine kinase activity, postreceptoral impairment in insulin action, and worsening of insulin resistance in diabetic patients (Barbagallo et al., 2007). Various studies demonstrated an improved insulin action in diabetics with Mg^{2+} supplementation (Song et al., 2006). Mg^{2+} status in diabetics is compromised because dietary intake is often low and urinary Mg^{2+} losses are high from polyuria and acidosis.

Hypomagnesemia is also correlated with increased concentrations of the inflammatory marker C-reactive protein (CRP) (Chacko et al., 2010), especially in patients with poor glycemic control (Guerrero-Romero and Rodriguez-Morán, 2006). In patients with heart failure and diabetes, Mg^{2+} supplementation significantly reduced CRP values (Almoznino-Sarafian et al., 2007). In sum, attention should be given to a sufficient Mg^{2+} supply, especially among individuals with diabetes mellitus.

CONCLUSION

Mg^{2+} has been called the "forgotten ion." During recent years, knowledge of Mg^{2+} homeostasis, requirements, connection to disease risks, and therapeutic use has increased tremendously. Because the usual dietary intake of Mg^{2+} is often low, individuals at risk of Mg^{2+} depletion should be advised to increase their dietary intake of Mg^{2+}-rich foods. An increased intake through Mg^{2+} supplements might be useful in patients with various diseases and especially in those taking medications that influence the Mg^{2+}-regulating systems in the kidneys.

REFERENCES

Abbott, R. D., Ando, F., Masaki, K. H., Tung, K. H., Rodriguez, B. L., Petrovitch, H., … Curb, J. D. (2003). Dietary magnesium intake and the future risk of coronary heart disease (The Honolulu Heart Program). *The American Journal of Cardiology, 92*, 665–669.

Al-Delaimy, W. K., Rimm, E. B., Willett, W. C., Stampfer, M. J., & Hu, F. B. (2004). Magnesium intake and risk of coronary heart disease among men. *Journal of the American College of Nutrition, 23*, 63–70.

Almoznino-Sarafian, D., Berman, S., Mor, A., Shteinshnaider, M., Gorelik, O., Tzur, I., … Cohen, N. (2007). Magnesium and C-reactive protein in heart failure: An anti-inflammatory effect of magnesium administration? *European Journal of Nutrition, 46*, 230–237.

Altura, B. M., & Altura, B. T. (1995). Role of magnesium in the pathogenesis of hypertension updated: Relationship to its actions on cardiac, vascular smooth muscle, and endothelial cells. In H. Laragh & B. M. Brenner (Eds.), *Hypertension: Pathophysiology, diagnosis, and management* (2nd ed., pp. 1214–1242). New York: Raven Press.

Arnaud, M. J. (2008). Update on the assessment of magnesium status. *The British Journal of Nutrition, 99*(Suppl. 3), S24–S36.

Barbagallo, M., Dominguez, L. J., & Resnick, L. M. (2007). Magnesium metabolism in hypertension and type 2 diabetes mellitus. *American Journal of Therapeutics, 14*, 375–385.

Birch, N. J. (1993). *Magnesium and the cell*. New York: Academic Press.

Carpenter, T. O., DeLucia, M. C., Zhang, J. H., Bejnerowicz, G., Tartamella, L., Dziura, J., … Cohen, D. (2006). A randomized controlled study of effects of dietary magnesium oxide supplementation on bone mineral content in healthy girls. *The Journal of Clinical Endocrinology and Metabolism, 91*, 4866–4872.

Chacko, S. A., Song, Y., Nathan, L., Tinker, L., de Boer, I. H., Tylavsky, F., Wallace, R., & Liu, S. (2010). Relations of dietary magnesium intake to biomarkers of inflammation and endothelial dysfunction in an ethnically diverse cohort of postmenopausal women. *Diabetes Care, 33*, 304–310.

Cowan, J. A. (2002). Structural and catalytic chemistry of magnesium-dependent enzymes. *Biometals, 15*, 225–235.

Dimai, H. P., Porta, S., Wirnsberger, G., Lindschinger, M., Pamperl, I., Dobnig, H., … Lau, K. H. (1998). Daily oral magnesium supplementation suppresses bone turnover in young adult males. *The Journal of Clinical Endocrinology and Metabolism, 83*, 2742–2748.

Dimke, H., Hoenderop, J. G., & Bindels, R. J. (2009). Hereditary tubular transport disorders: Implications for renal handling of Ca2+ and Mg2+. *Clinical Science, 118*, 1–18.

Dorup, I. (1994). Magnesium and potassium deficiency: Its diagnosis, occurrence and treatment in diuretic therapy and its consequences for growth, protein synthesis, and growth factors. *Acta Physiologica Scandinavica, 150*(Suppl. 618), 7–46.

Efrati, E., Arsentiev-Rozenfeld, J., & Zelikovic, I. (2005). The human paracellin-1 gene (hPCLN-1): Renal epithelial cell-specific expression and regulation. *American Journal of Physiology. Renal Physiology, 288,* F272–F283.

Elin, R. J. (1994). Magnesium: The fifth but forgotten electrolyte. *American Journal of Clinical Pathology, 102,* 616–622.

Fine, K. D., Santa Ana, C. A., Porter, J. L., & Fordtran, J. S. (1991). Intestinal absorption of magnesium from food and supplements. *The Journal of Clinical Investigation, 88,* 396–402.

Ford, E. S. (1999). Serum magnesium and ischemic heart disease: Findings from national sample of US adults. *International Journal of Epidemiology, 28,* 645–651.

Franz, K. B. (1989). Influence of phosphorus on intestinal absorption of calcium and magnesium. In Y. Itokawa & J. Durlach (Eds.), *Magnesium in health and disease* (pp. 71–78). London: John Libbey & Co.

Frausto da Silva, J. J. R., & Williams, R. J. P. (1991). The biological chemistry of magnesium: Phosphate metabolism. In *The biological chemistry of the elements* (pp. 241–267). Oxford: Oxford University Press.

Glaudemans, B., Knoers, N. V., Hoenderop, J. G., & Bindels, R. J. (2010). New molecular players facilitating Mg^{2+} reabsorption in the distal convoluted tubule. *Kidney International, 77,* 17–22.

Groenestege, W. M., Hoenderop, J. G., van den Heuvel, L., Knoers, N., & Bindels, R. J. (2006). The epithelial Mg2+ channel transient receptor potential melastatin 6 is regulated by dietary Mg2+ content and estrogens. *Journal of the American Society of Nephrology, 17,* 1035–1043.

Guerrero-Romero, F., Rascón-Pacheco, R. A., Rodríguez-Morán, M., de la Peña, J. E., & Wacher, N. (2008). Hypomagnesaemia and risk for metabolic glucose disorders: A 10-year follow-up study. *European Journal of Clinical Investigation, 38,* 389–396.

Guerrero-Romero, F., & Rodríguez-Morán, M. (2006). Hypomagnesemia, oxidative stress, inflammation, and metabolic syndrome. *Diabetes/Metabolism Research and Review, 22,* 471–476.

Henderson, L., Irving, K., Gregory, J., Bates, C. J., Prentice, A., Perks, J., … Farron, M. (2003). *The National Diet and Nutrition Survey: Adults aged 19 to 64 years. Volume 3: Vitamin and mineral intake and urinary analytes.* London: TSO.

Hoorn, E. J., van der Hoek, J., de Man, R. A., Kuipers, E. J., Bolwerk, C., & Zietse, R. (2010). A case series of proton pump inhibitor-induced hypomagnesemia. *American Journal of Kidney Diseases, 56,* 112–116.

Institute of Medicine. (1997). *Dietary Reference Intakes for calcium, phosphorus, magnesium, vitamin D, and fluoride.* Washington, DC: National Academy Press.

Iseri, L. T., & French, J. H. (1984). Magnesium: Nature's physiologic calcium blocker. *American Heart Journal, 108,* 188–193.

Ismail, Y., Ismail, A. A., & Ismail, A. A. (2010). The underestimated problem of using serum magnesium measurements to exclude magnesium deficiency in adults: A health warning is needed for "normal" results. *Clinical Chemistry and Laboratory Medicine, 48,* 323–327.

Jee, S. H., Miller, E. R., 3rd, Guallar, E., Singh, V. K., Appel, L. J., & Klag, M. J. (2002). The effect of magnesium supplementation on blood pressure: A meta-analysis of randomized clinical trials. *American Journal of Hypertension, 15,* 691–696.

Larsson, S. C., & Wolk, A. (2007). Magnesium intake and risk of type 2 diabetes: A meta-analysis. *Journal of Internal Medicine, 262,* 208–214.

Liao, F., Folsom, A. R., & Brancati, F. L. (1998). Is low magnesium concentration a risk factor for coronary heart disease? The Atherosclerosis Risk in Communities (ARIC) Study. *American Heart Journal, 136,* 480–490.

Lum, G. (1992). Hypomagnesemia in acute and chronic care patient populations. *American Journal of Clinical Pathology, 97,* 827–830.

Matsuda, H. (1991). Magnesium gating of the inwardly rectifying K^+ channel. *Annual Review of Physiology, 53,* 289–298.

Mordes, J. P. (1978). Excess magnesium. *Pharmacological Reviews, 29,* 273–300.

Mosfegh, A., Goldman, J., Ahuja, J., & Rhodes, D. (2009). *What we eat in America. NHANES 2005-2006. Usual nutrient intakes from food and water compared to Dietary Reference Intakes for Vitamin D, Calcium, Phosphorus, and Magnesium.* Washington, DC: U.S. Department of Agriculture, Agricultural Research Service.

Naderi, A. S., & Reilly, R. F., Jr. (2008). Hereditary etiologies of hypomagnesemia. *Nature Clinical Practice. Nephrology, 4,* 80–89.

Nationale Verzehrs Studie II. (2008). Max Rubner Institut, BFEL.

Nielsen, F. H., Milne, D. B., Klevay, L. M., Gallagher, S., & Johnson, L. (2007). Dietary magnesium deficiency induces heart rhythm changes, impairs glucose tolerance, and decreases serum cholesterol in post menopausal women. *Journal of the American College of Nutrition, 26,* 121–132.

Nijenhuis, T., Renkema, K. Y., Hoenderop, J. G., & Bindels, R. J. (2006). Acid-base status determines the renal expression of Ca^{2+} and Mg^{2+} transport proteins. *Journal of the American Society of Nephrology, 17,* 617–626.

O'Rourke, B. (1993). Ion channels as sensors of cellular energy: Mechanism for modulation by magnesium and nucleotides. *Biochemical Pharmacology, 46,* 1103–1112.

Peikert, A., Wilimzig, C., & Kohne-Volland, R. (1996). Prophylaxis of migraine with oral magnesium: Results from a prospective, multi-center, placebo-controlled and double-blind randomized study. *Cephalalgia, 16,* 257–263.

Quamme, G. A. (2008). Recent developments in intestinal magnesium absorption. *Current Opinion in Gastroenterology, 24,* 230–235.

Quamme, G. A. (2010). Molecular identification of ancient and modern mammalian magnesium transporters. *American Journal of Physiology. Cell Physiology, 298,* C407–C429.

Romani, A. (2007). Regulation of magnesium homeostasis and transport in mammalian cells. *Archives of Biochemistry and Biophysics, 458,* 90–102.

Romani, A., Marfella, C., & Scarpa, A. (1993). Cell magnesium transport and homeostasis: Role of intracellular compartments. *Mineral and Electrolyte Metabolism, 19,* 282–289.

Rude, R. K., Singer, F. R., & Gruber, H. E. (2009). Skeletal and hormonal effects of magnesium deficiency. *Journal of the American College of Nutrition, 28,* 131–141.

Ryan, M. F. (1991). The role of magnesium in clinical biochemistry: An overview. *Annals of Clinical Biochemistry, 28,* 19–26.

Rylander, R., Remer, T., Berkemeyer, S., & Vormann, J. (2006). Acid-base status affects renal magnesium losses in healthy, elderly persons. *The Journal of Nutrition, 136,* 2374–2377.

Sabatier, M., Pont, F., Arnaud, M. J., & Turnlund, J. R. (2003). A compartmental model of magnesium metabolism in healthy men based on two stable isotope tracers. *American Journal of Physiology. Regulatory, Integrative and Comparative Physiology, 285,* R656–R663.

Schlingmann, K. P., Weber, S., Peters, M., Niemann Nejsum, L., Vitzthum, H., Klingel, K., … Konrad, M. (2002). Hypomagnesemia with secondary hypocalcemia is caused by mutations in TRPM6, a new member of the TRPM gene family. *Nature Genetics, 31,* 166–170.

Shah, G. M., & Kirschenbaum, M. A. (1991). Renal magnesium wasting associated with therapeutic agents. *Mineral and Electrolyte Metabolism, 17,* 58–64.

Shechter, M. (2010). Magnesium and cardiovascular system. *Magnesium Research, 23,* 1–13.

Siener, R., & Hesse, A. (1995). Influence of a mixed and a vegetarian diet on urinary magnesium excretion and concentration. *The British Journal of Nutrition, 73,* 783–790.

Song, Y., He, K., Levitan, E. B., Manson, J. E., & Liu, S. (2006). Effects of oral magnesium supplementation on glycaemic control in type 2 diabetes: A meta-analysis of randomized double-blind controlled trials. *Diabetic Medicine, 23*, 1050–1056.

Stendig-Lindberg, G., Tepper, R., & Leichter, I. (1993). Trabecular bone density in a two year controlled trial of peroral magnesium in osteoporosis. *Magnesium Research, 6*, 155–163.

Tejpar, S., Piessevaux, H., Claes, K., Piront, P., Hoenderop, J. G., Verslype, C., & Van Cutsem, E. (2007). Magnesium wasting associated with epidermal-growth-factor receptor-targeting antibodies in colorectal cancer: A prospective study. *The Lancet Oncology, 8*, 387–394.

Thebault, S., Alexander, R. T., Tiel Groenestege, W. M., Hoenderop, J. G., & Bindels, R. J. (2009). EGF increases TRPM6 activity and surface expression. *Journal of the American Society of Nephrology, 20*, 78–85.

Volpe, P., Alderson-Lang, B. H., & Nickols, G. A. (1990). Regulation of inositol 1,4,5-trisphosphate-induced Ca^{2+} release. I. Effect of Mg^{2+}. *The American Journal of Physiology, 258*, C1077–C1085.

Vormann, J., & Anke, M. (2002). Dietary magnesium: Supply, requirements and recommendations—Results from duplicate and balance studies in man. *Journal of Clinical and Basic Cardiology, 5*, 49–53.

Vormann, J., Bednarik, R., Wolf, K., & Kolisek, M. (2009). New test for intracellular Mg^{2+} status by determining expression levels of Mg-sensitive marker genes. *Magnesium Research, 22*, 201.

Walder, R. Y., Landau, D., Meyer, P., Shalev, H., Tsolia, M., Borochowitz, Z., … Sheffield, V. C. (2002). Mutation of TRPM6 causes familial hypomagnesemia with secondary hypocalcemia. *Nature Genetics, 31*, 171–174.

Weisinger, J. R., & Bellorin-Font, E. (1998). Magnesium and phosphorus. *Lancet, 352*, 391–396.

Whang, R., Hampton, E. M., & Whang, D. D. (1994). Magnesium homeostasis and clinical disorders of magnesium deficiency. *The Annals of Pharmacotherapy, 28*, 220–226.

White, R. E., & Hartzell, H. C. (1989). Magnesium ions in cardiac function: Regulator of ion channels and second messengers. *Biochemical Pharmacology, 38*, 859–867.

Wilimzig, C., Latz, R., Vierling, W., Mutschler, E., Trnovec, T., & Nyulassy, S. (1996). Increase in magnesium plasma level after orally administered trimagnesium dicitrate. *European Journal of Clinical Pharmacology, 49*, 317–323.

Wolf, F. I., Trapani, V., & Cittadini, A. (2008). Magnesium and the control of cell proliferation: Looking for a needle in a haystack. *Magnesium Research, 21*, 83–91.

RECOMMENDED READINGS

Birch, N. J. (1993). *Magnesium and the cell*. New York: Academic Press.

Cittadini, A., & Wolf, F. I. (Eds.). (2003). Magnesium: From biochemistry and cell physiology to clinical implications. *Molecular Aspects of Medicine, 24*, 1–146.

Durlach, J. (1988). *Magnesium in clinical practice*. London: John Libbey & Co.

Seelig, M. S., & Rosanoff, A. (2003). *The magnesium factor*. New York: Avery.

CHAPTER 34

Sodium, Chloride, and Potassium

Hwai-Ping Sheng, PhD

COMMON ABBREVIATIONS

ANP atrial natriuretic peptide

AVP arginine vasopressin, also known as antidiuretic hormone (ADH)

FUNCTIONS AND DISTRIBUTION OF SODIUM, CHLORIDE, AND POTASSIUM

Sodium, chloride, and potassium are essential to the physiological well-being of human beings. They are the principal electrolytes of body fluids and exist largely as free hydrated ions that bind only weakly to organic molecules. These ions have complex physiological and biochemical functions because they are essential in maintaining the ionic and osmotic balance between the extracellular and intracellular fluids, stabilizing macroions such as proteins, and activating a small number of enzymes.

DISTRIBUTION IN THE BODY

A 70-kg adult has about 100 g of sodium, 95 g of chloride, and 140 g of potassium in the body (Forbes, 1987). Distribution of these electrolytes within the various fluid compartments and body tissues is highly variable in terms of concentration and content. Sodium and chloride are the major electrolytes found predominantly in extracellular fluid, whereas potassium is retained inside the cells (Figure 34-1). The concentration of sodium ions (Na^+) in the extracellular fluid, and thus in the plasma, is maintained within narrow limits at approximately 145 mmol/L. Its concentration in the intracellular fluid is low, about 12 mmol/L. Distribution of chloride ions (Cl^-) generally follows that of Na^+, with an extracellular concentration of about 110 mmol/L and an intracellular concentration of about 2 mmol/L. About one third of the body's sodium is sequestered as part of the integral structure of skeleton and therefore is not available for exchange with the fluid compartments. The concentration of potassium ions (K^+) is 150 mmol/L inside the cells and 4 to 5 mmol/L in the extracellular fluid. The largest fraction of body potassium, about 60% to 70% of the total, is located in the skeletal muscles, which make up about 40% of body weight.

PROPERTIES OF PLASMA MEMBRANES

Plasma membranes surrounding cells separate the body fluid compartment into an extracellular and an intracellular component. Movement of ions across cell membranes can occur by passive diffusion along a concentration or electrical gradient through ion channels or by an energy-yielding process of active transport of ions against these gradients. The selective permeability of the cell membranes prevents the movement of proteins and phosphates out of the cells. High concentrations of these intracellular organic anions require neutralization of the excess negative charges by cations, of which K^+ is the most important (see Figure 34-1). The intracellular accumulation of K^+ in exchange for Na^+, against their concentration gradients, is achieved by the Na^+,K^+-pump of the plasma membrane.

Sodium–Potassium Pump

This magnesium ion–dependent, Na^+- and K^+-activated ATPase (Na^+,K^+-ATPase) is the molecular basis of the Na^+,K^+-pump. The Na^+,K^+-ATPase belongs to the P-type ATPases, which are characterized by the transient phosphorylation of the ATPase protein during the transport cycle. Structurally, the functional unit of this enzyme is a heterodimer of two subunit proteins, the α-subunit and a smaller β-subunit. Other smaller membrane peptides, such as the γ-subunit, have been found to be closely associated with Na^+,K^+-ATPase, but their presence does not seem to affect the expression of the functional enzyme (Horisberger and Doucet, 2007). Several isoforms of both the α- and β-subunits have been identified in a variety of tissues; the relative proportion of each subunit isoform varies among tissues, and the isoforms are tissue-specific. At present, four different genes of α-subunits and three of β-subunits have been identified in mammalian Na^+,K^+-ATPases. Aside from their kinetic characteristics and tissue distribution, little is known regarding their differential physiological importance.

The larger α-subunit (~120 kDa) spans the membrane and has two large cytoplasmic domains. It binds ATP and both Na^+ and K^+ and contains the phosphorylation site. It is responsible for transport of Na^+ and K^+. The smaller β-subunit (~50 kDa), with a large extracellular domain,

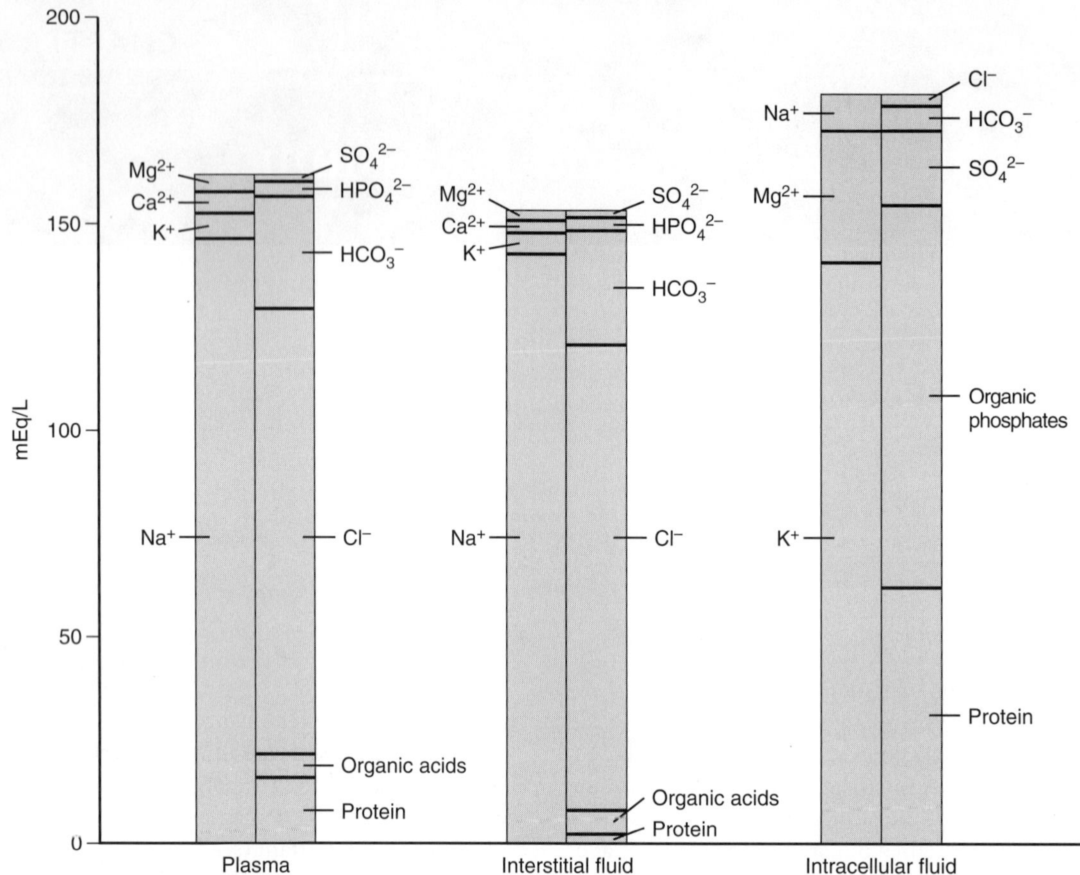

FIGURE 34-1 Ionic composition of plasma, interstitial, and intracellular compartments. Concentrations are expressed in milliequivalents (mEq) per liter (L).

is a glycoprotein that also spans the membrane. It is an essential component of the functional Na^+,K^+-ATPase. Affinity of the α-subunit for Na^+ and K^+ appears to be influenced by the particular β-subunit. As illustrated in Figure 34-2, the α-subunit binds ATP and three Na^+ from the cytoplasm. ATP activates the catalytic site of the transporter, which then cleaves the ATP and phosphorylates the aspartate residue on the α-subunit. A conformational change in the transport protein exposes the three Na^+ to the outside. The three Na^+ dissociate from the enzyme and are released into the extracellular fluid. The transporter is now available for binding two extracellular K^+. Binding of K^+ results in dephosphorylation of the α-subunit. The transport protein returns to its original conformation, and two K^+ are released into the cytosol in the process. The transport protein is ready for another cycle of transport.

The overall stoichiometry of the Na^+,K^+-ATPase reaction is that, with the hydrolysis of one molecule of ATP, three Na^+ and two K^+ are translocated in opposite directions across the cell membrane to maintain or restore the normally high K^+ and low Na^+ concentrations inside the cells. Because its activity results in a net movement of cations out of the cell and a negative charge is created in the cell relative to the outside, the Na^+,K^+-pump is an electrogenic pump.

Importance of the Sodium–Potassium Pump

The establishment of a differential electrical and chemical gradient for Na^+ and K^+ across cell membranes by the Na^+,K^+-pump generates and maintains a negative resting membrane potential of all cells, and this is the basis for excitability in nerve and muscle cells. Transport of three Na^+ in exchange for two K^+ also helps to maintain ionic homeostasis of the cells and to regulate cell volume. Furthermore, active transport of Na^+ out of the cells provides a driving force for the transport of other solutes, such as ions, sugars, amino acids, and neurotransmitters, across cell membranes through various Na^+-coupled cotransport systems.

IMPORTANCE OF SODIUM

A Major Determinant of Osmolarity and Extracellular Fluid Volume

The concentrations of the three major ions in body fluids are controlled within narrow limits in order for the body to function properly. The volume of the extracellular fluid compartment (interstitial fluid and plasma) is determined primarily by the total amount of osmotic particles present. Because of its high concentration, Na^+, together with its accompanying anions Cl^- and HCO_3^-, is the major determinant of osmolarity of plasma and extracellular fluid. The osmolarity of plasma and body fluids, at 290 mmol/L, can be estimated by doubling its Na^+ concentration of 145 mmol/L.

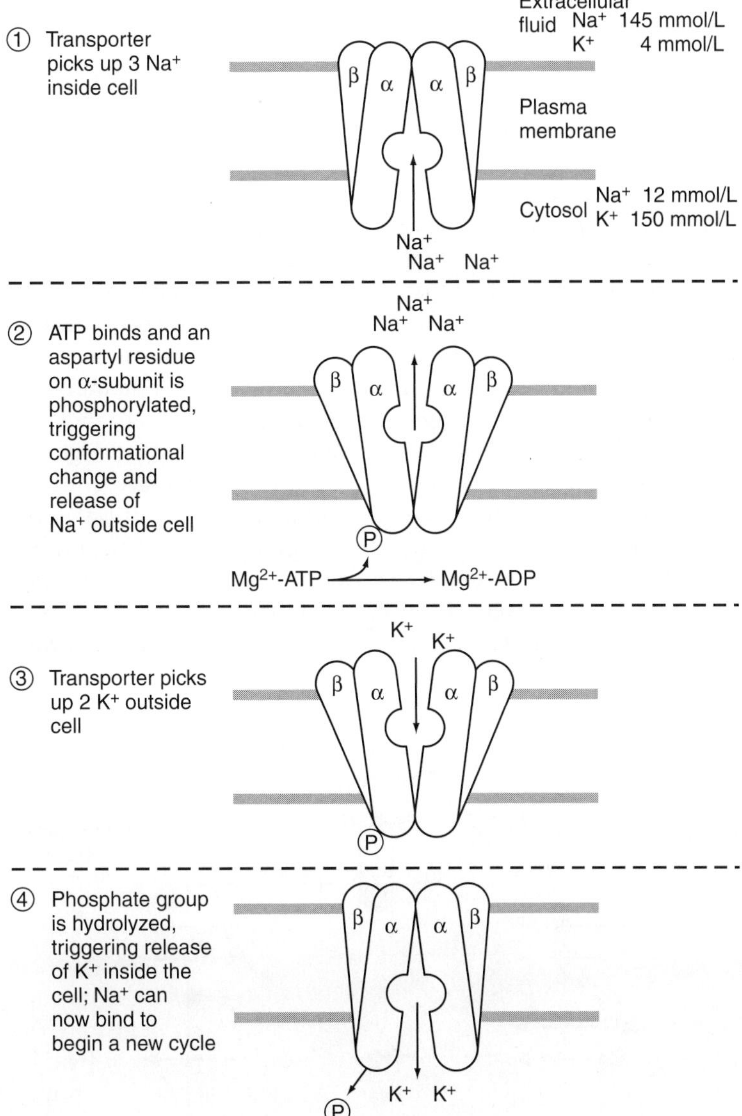
Extracellular fluid Na^+ 145 mmol/L
K^+ 4 mmol/L
Plasma membrane
Cytosol Na^+ 12 mmol/L
K^+ 150 mmol/L
① Transporter picks up 3 Na^+ inside cell
β α α β
Na^+ Na^+ Na^+
② ATP binds and an aspartyl residue on α-subunit is phosphorylated, triggering conformational change and release of Na^+ outside cell
P
Mg^{2+}-ATP
Mg^{2+}-ADP
③ Transporter picks up 2 K^+ outside cell
K^+ K^+
④ Phosphate group is hydrolyzed, triggering release of K^+ inside the cell; Na^+ can now bind to begin a new cycle

FIGURE 34-2 Schematic representation of the enzyme Na^+,K^+-ATPase, which is responsible for primary active transport of Na^+ and K^+ in opposite directions across plasma membranes. The enzyme consists of two types of subunits (α and β) and is thought to have the subunit composition $(\alpha\beta)_2$ and to have one set of cation-binding sites. The α-subunit contains the K^+ and Na^+ binding sites; it also contains a site for binding ATP and a phosphorylation site in the intracellular portion. Binding of Na^+ and ATP intracellularly activates the Na^+,K^+-ATPase, which cleaves one molecule of ATP to ADP and phosphorylates an aspartate residue on a subunit. Phosphorylation causes a conformational change in the carrier protein molecule, thereby extruding Na^+ on the extracellular surface and allowing extracellular K^+ to bind. K^+ binding activates intracellular hydrolysis of the bound phosphate group, resulting in a conformational change and release of K^+ inside the cell. The transporter is now ready to bind Na^+ for another transport cycle. For each ATP hydrolyzed, 3 Na^+ ions are moved out of the cell and 2 K^+ ions are moved into it. This accounts for the low intracellular Na^+ and high intracellular K^+ concentrations.

Any change in plasma Na^+ concentration will alter plasma osmolarity, or tonicity, and trigger physiological regulatory mechanisms to adjust water intake and water excretion to restore the osmolarity toward normal. Because the volume of extracellular fluid depends on the amount of Na^+ present in the extracellular space, regulation of plasma volume and extracellular fluid volume involves the regulation of ingestion and excretion of sodium (Hall, 2011d). Therefore, in the control of body fluid balance, sodium and water are the two primary variables, and balance can be achieved by adjustments of their ingestion and excretion.

Role of the Electrochemical Sodium Gradient in Nutrient Transport Processes

Absorption of dietary sodium in the small intestine and reabsorption of filtered sodium from the glomerular filtrate in the kidneys back into the circulation is important in many nutrient transport processes, for example, the absorption of chloride, amino acids, glucose, galactose, and water. Transepithelial transport of Na^+ involves movement across two membranes: the apical membrane facing the lumen of the intestine or the renal tubules, and the basolateral membrane, which faces the interstitial space. These two membranes have different transport properties. The apical membrane contains very few if any Na^+,K^+-ATPase transporters, whereas the basolateral membrane contains a large amount of Na^+,K^+-ATPase. Active extrusion of Na^+ across the basolateral membrane by the Na^+,K^+-ATPase reduces the concentration of intracellular Na^+ and provides an electrochemical potential gradient for the movement of Na^+ from the lumen into the cytosol to replace the Na^+ that is extruded. This transepithelial transport of Na^+ creates an electrochemical potential difference for Na^+ across the epithelial cells so that the epithelial cells are polarized, with the lumen slightly electronegative with respect to the interstitial fluid on the basal side of the epithelial cells (Hall, 2011e).

Entry of Na^+ down an electrical gradient across the apical membrane is either through the voltage-dependent Na^+ channels or by carrier-mediated transport (facilitated diffusion) in which other solutes are cotransported in the same direction or countertransported in the opposite direction. Absorption of Na^+ causes either the entry of an equimolar amount of Cl^- in the same direction as Na^+ movement or the secretion of an equimolar amount of K^+ or H^+ in the opposite direction in exchange for Na^+ (Figure 34-3). The absorption of Cl^- is either through the paracellular spaces (junctions between the apical borders of adjacent epithelial cells) or across the epithelial cells via the apical and basal membranes. Uptake of Na^+ and Cl^- across epithelial cells increases the intracellular concentrations of these two ions and provides an osmotic gradient for the absorption of water. A large proportion of water uptake occurs by the paracellular route, and only a small proportion of water flux is through the epithelial cells.

Some of the carrier proteins in the apical membrane, such as the sodium/glucose cotransporter 1 (SGLT1) and a number of the amino acid transport systems, have receptor sites for binding both Na^+ and a monosaccharide, or both Na^+ and an amino acid (see Figure 34-3). Because Na^+ is coupled to either a monosaccharide or an amino acid on the carrier protein, entry of Na^+ across the apical membrane also brings in a monosaccharide or an amino acid. This process of cotransport of these organic solutes is frequently referred to as secondary active transport because the energy used to establish the Na^+ gradient allows cotransport of these

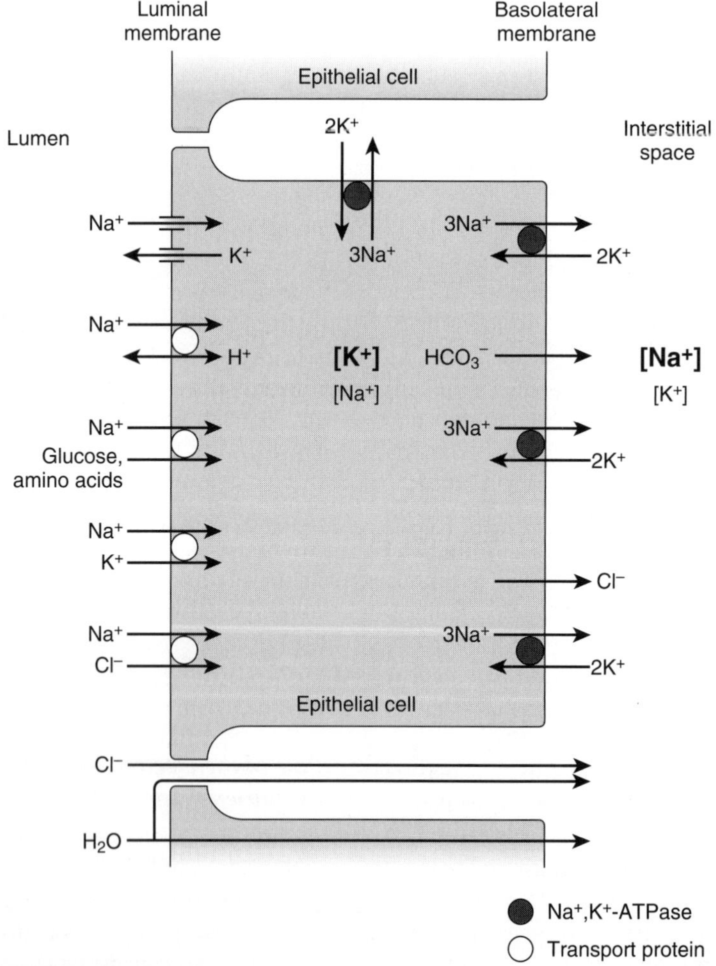

FIGURE 34-3 Schematic representation of how active extrusion of Na^+ via the enzyme Na^+,K^+-ATPase across the basolateral membrane of an epithelial cell creates an electrochemical gradient for the entry of Na^+ across the luminal membrane. Entry of Na^+ is by diffusion through ion channels or carrier-mediated transport (facilitated diffusion), which uses the electrochemical gradient created by the Na^+,K^+-ATPase as a driving force for cotransport or countertransport of other solutes. Only the most common types of transport are shown.

solutes to occur against their concentration gradients. The increase in concentrations of these organic solutes inside the epithelial cells then allows the diffusion, usually facilitated by another carrier, of these nutrients across the basolateral membrane into the interstitial fluid.

IMPORTANCE OF POTASSIUM

The high concentration gradient of K^+ between the intracellular and extracellular fluid is important for maintaining the normal resting membrane potential across cell membranes and for excitability of nerves and muscles. It plays a crucial role in the triggering of action potentials that initiate nerve impulse transmission and muscle contraction. Changes in the concentration of K^+ in the plasma alter this gradient and will adversely affect the aforementioned functions (Rodriguez-Soriano, 1995). For instance, in hyperkalemia, when the concentration of K^+ in the plasma exceeds 5.5 mmol/L, the membrane depolarizes, causing muscle weakness, flaccid paralysis, and cardiac dysrhythmias. Cardiac dysrhythmias associated with hyperkalemia range from sinus bradycardia to ventricular tachycardia, ventricular fibrillation, and ultimately cardiac arrest (asystole) when a plasma concentration of 8 mmol/L is reached. Because of the adverse effects of hyperkalemia on the heart, hyperkalemia constitutes a medical emergency. In contrast, in hypokalemia, when the concentration of K^+ in the plasma is less than 3.5 mmol/L, the membrane hyperpolarizes, and this can interfere with the normal functioning of nerves and muscles, resulting in muscle weakness and decreased smooth muscle contractility. Hypokalemia is also a risk factor for atrial and ventricular dysrhythmias (He and MacGregor, 2008). Severe hypokalemia can lead to paralysis, metabolic alkalosis, and death. Therefore physiological regulatory mechanisms are present to regulate the concentration of K^+ in the plasma within narrow limits.

OTHER FUNCTIONS OF ELECTROLYTES

Interactions with Macroions

Many macromolecules present in the extracellular and intracellular compartments contain multiple ionizing groups on their surfaces and are classified as macroions. Their behavior in solution depends on their surface charges, which either repel each other so that they remain separated in solution or attract each other so that they associate. Examples of macroions are proteins, nucleic acids, and a group of polysaccharides called the glycosaminoglycans. Proteins are polyampholytes that carry both acidic and basic groups on their surfaces. Depending on the pH of the solution, proteins may carry substantial net positive or net negative charges. At a plasma pH of 7.4, most plasma and intracellular proteins have net negative charges, but a few have net positive charges. The glycosaminoglycans carry carboxylate and sulfate groups and are of major structural importance. Chondroitin sulfates and keratan sulfates of connective tissue and dermatan sulfates of skin form matrices to hold together the protein components of connective tissue and skin. A very highly sulfated glycosaminoglycan is heparin, a natural anticoagulant produced by the mast cells that line the arterial walls. Heparan sulfate, which is less highly sulfated than heparin, is linked to many cell surface proteins and matrix proteoglycans.

Macroion surfaces are modified by a counterion atmosphere enriched in oppositely charged small ions, mainly Na^+, K^+, and Cl^-. The counterion atmosphere is greatly affected by the ionic strength of the solution. At low ionic strength, the counterion atmosphere is diffuse and there is minimal interference to interactions of macroions. At high ionic strength, the counterion atmosphere is concentrated about the macroions and effectively reduces their interactions. This explains the observation that increasing salt concentration of a solution containing protein increases the solubility of the protein.

Activation of Enzymes

Activators of enzyme-catalyzed reactions are frequently metal ions such as magnesium (Mg^{2+}), zinc (Zn^{2+}), manganese (Mn^{2+}), and calcium (Ca^{2+}); only a limited number of enzymes require the presence of Na^+, K^+, or Cl^-. The most common and most widely distributed enzyme in the cell membrane is the Na^+,K^+-ATPase, the activation of which requires the presence of Na^+ and K^+. Enzymes that require the presence of Cl^- for activation include the angiotensin-converting enzyme (ACE) that catalyzes the conversion of angiotensin 1 to angiotensin 2 (Bunning and Riordan, 1987). Although the presence of Mg^{2+} is required for activation of a number of enzymes by K^+ in mammalian tissues, K^+ by itself is important for the activity of pyruvate kinase (Larsen et al., 1994).

SODIUM, CHLORIDE, AND POTASSIUM BALANCE

A stable content of sodium, potassium, and chloride in the body is regulated by the neuroendocrine control systems. To maintain body balance, the amount consumed must equal the amount lost, which is mainly through renal excretion. In the growing child, a positive balance for these elements is important because of the accretion for tissue formation.

LOSS OF SODIUM, CHLORIDE, AND POTASSIUM

Obligatory loss of fluids through skin, feces, and urine inevitably causes loss of sodium and chloride (see Chapter 35). Minimum obligatory loss of sodium in the absence of profuse sweating and gastrointestinal and renal diseases has been estimated to be approximately 0.04 to 0.185 g/day, which consists of 0.005 to 0.035 g/day in urine, 0.01 to 0.125 g/day in feces, and dermal losses of 0.025 g/day (Dahl, 1958). Studies over a 12-day period have shown that sweat and fecal excretion accounted for only 2% to 5% of total sodium excretion in adults who consume an average intake of salt; the remainder of the salt consumed was excreted in the urine (Sanchez-Castillo et al., 1987b). However, loss of sodium can increase greatly under certain circumstances, such as diarrhea, diabetes, and profuse sweating during strenuous physical activity in hot weather. Under most but not all circumstances, loss of sodium is accompanied by a similar molar loss of chloride.

As with sodium and chloride, obligatory loss of fluid also causes loss of potassium. In a healthy adult, potassium loss via these routes is less than 0.8 g/day, with less than 0.4 g via fecal loss, 0.2 to 0.4 g via urinary loss, and negligible amounts from sweat (National Research Council, 1989).

INTAKE OF SODIUM AND CHLORIDE

Dietary Intake

Dietary sodium is consumed mainly as sodium chloride, with small amounts as sodium bicarbonate, sodium glutamate, and sodium citrate. These sodium salts are low in fresh vegetables and fresh fruits but high in cured meat products, processed foods, and canned vegetables. Studies in a British population found that only 10% of sodium intake came from natural foods, 15% from table salt added during cooking and at the table, and 75% from salts added during manufacturing and processing (Sanchez-Castillo et al., 1987a). The amount of chloride consumed parallels the amount of sodium, as dietary chloride is consumed almost exclusively as a salt of sodium.

Daily salt consumption has been estimated by assessing salt intake or measuring urinary sodium excretion. Usually consumption far exceeds the needs of an individual, although it varies widely between individuals and cultures. Americans consume between 1.8 and 5 g/day of sodium or between 4.8 and 13 g/day of sodium chloride (National Research Council, 1989). This wide range of reported intakes is due to the different methods of assessment and to the large variability of discretionary salt intake. Individuals consuming a diet high in processed foods have high salt intakes. In Japan, where consumption of salt-preserved fish and the use of salt for seasoning are customary, salt intake is high, ranging from 14 to 20 g/day (Kono et al., 1983). Conversely, salt consumption estimated from urinary sodium excretion of the Yanomami Indians in Brazil is very low, 0.053 g/day of sodium chloride (Mancilha-Carvalho and Souza e Silva, 2003). Vegetarians typically consume an average of 0.8 g/day of sodium chloride. Individuals with low or very low sodium intakes do not normally exhibit chronic deficiencies because of the efficiency of the body's mechanism of salt conservation.

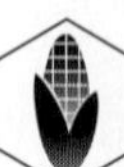

FOOD SOURCES HIGH IN SODIUM

Soups

2.5 g per 1 cup miso soup
0.7 to 1.1 g per 1 cup canned soup

Condiments and Leavening Agents

2.3 g per 1 tsp table salt
0.9 g per 1 tbsp soy sauce
0.8 g per 1 dill pickle (2 oz)
0.36 g per 1 tsp baking powder

Cured Meats

0.9 to 1.1 g per 3 oz ham
0.5 to 0.6 g per 1.7 oz hotdog
0.4 g per 3 medium slices cooked bacon
0.4 g per 2 slices (~2 oz) bologna

Cheese

0.4 g per ½ cup cottage cheese
0.4 g per 1 oz processed cheese
0.4 g per 1 oz blue cheese

Canned Vegetables and Tomato Sauce

0.8 g per ½ cup sauerkraut
0.6 g per ½ cup marinara/spaghetti sauce
0.2 g per ½ cup canned green peas

Data from U.S. Department of Agriculture [USDA], Agricultural Research Service. (2011). *USDA National Nutrient Database for Standard Reference, Release 24.* Retrieved from www.ars.usda.gov/ba/bhnrc/ndl

Recommended Intake

Daily minimum requirements of sodium and chloride in the adult can be estimated from the amount needed to replace obligatory losses. This amounts to not more than 0.18 g/day of sodium when substantial sweating does not occur (Institute of Medicine [IOM], 2004). The IOM does not establish an Estimated Average Requirement (EAR), and hence Recommended Dietary Allowance (RDA), for sodium because of inadequate data from dose–response studies. Instead Adequate Intakes (AIs) through the life span are provided.

The AIs were set based on a level that would meet the sodium needs and also allow intake of foods found in a Western type of diet and provide sufficient levels of other important nutrients. The AI for adult women and men who are 19 through 50 years of age is 1.5 g/day of sodium. The AI for chloride, at 2.3 g/day, is equimolar to that for sodium. These AIs are equivalent to the intake of 3.8 g of sodium chloride (table salt) per day. The AIs for sodium and chloride are intended to be sufficient for excess sodium chloride loss in sweat by unacclimatized persons who are exposed to high temperatures or who are moderately physically active. It will not be appropriate for individuals engaged in extreme endurance activity or prolonged exposure to heat, which will increase greatly the loss of sodium chloride through sweating. It should be noted that, based on NHANES 2001–2002 data, the estimated median intake of sodium from foods (not including salt added at the table) is 2.3 g for women and 4 g for men in the United States. This intake exceeds the AI for adults.

The AIs for older adults and for children were extrapolated from those for adults ages 19 through 50 years based on the mean energy intakes for various age–sex groups. The AIs for sodium and chloride are lower for older adults and the elderly because of their lower energy needs: 1.3 g/day of sodium and 2.0 g/day of chloride for adults from 51 through 70 years of age; and 1.2 g of sodium and 1.8 g of chloride for adults older than 70 years. These AIs are equivalent to the intake of 3.3 g and 3.0 g of sodium chloride per day. No increase in sodium or chloride intake is deemed necessary during pregnancy or lactation.

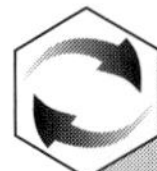

DRIs Across the Life Cycle: Sodium and Chloride

	g Sodium and Chloride per Day			
	Sodium		Chloride	
Infants	AI	UL	AI	UL
0 through 6 mo	0.12	ND	0.18	ND
7 through 12 mo	0.37	ND	0.57	ND
Children				
1 through 3 yr	1.0	1.5	1.5	2.3
4 through 8 yr	1.2	1.9	1.9	2.9
9 through 13 yr	1.5	2.2	2.3	3.4
14 through 18 yr	1.5	2.3	2.3	3.6
Adults				
19 through 50 yr	1.5	2.3	2.3	3.6
51 through 70 yr	1.3	2.3	2.0	3.6
≥71 yr	1.2	2.3	1.8	3.6
Pregnant	1.5	2.3	2.3	3.6
Lactating	1.5	2.3	2.3	3.6

Data from IOM. (2006). In J. J. Otten, J. P. Hellwig, & L. D. Meyers (Eds.), *Dietary Reference Intakes: The essential guide to nutrient requirements*. Washington, DC: The National Academies Press.
AI, Adequate Intake; *ND*, not determinable; *UL*, Tolerable Upper Intake Level.

The AIs for infants are based on typical intake from human milk (0.78 L/day and 0.16 g sodium/L of milk) and complementary foods. They are 0.12 g/day of sodium and 0.18 g/day of chloride for infants from birth through 6 months of age. For older infants between 7 and 12 months of age, the AI for sodium is 0.37 g/day, which is calculated as 0.08 g from human milk and 0.29 g from complementary foods. The AI for chloride is 0.57 g/day. The AIs for children 1 through 3 years of age are 1.0 g/day for sodium and 1.5 g/day for chloride, and for children 4 through 8 years of age are 1.2 g/day of sodium and 1.9 g/day of chloride. The AIs for boys and girls from 9 through 18 years of age are the same as those for young adults.

Development of hypertension appears to be associated with salt intake. Several trials have demonstrated that dietary sodium intake close to the AI (e.g., 1.2 g/day) was associated with lower blood pressure, compared to higher intakes (e.g., 2.3 g/day) (Johnson et al., 2001; Sacks et al., 2001; MacGregor et al., 1989). Based on these studies, the IOM (2004) has set a Tolerable Upper Intake Level (UL) for adults of 2.3 g (100 mmol)/day of sodium and 3.6 g (100 mmol)/day of chloride. The ULs for young children are somewhat lower.

INTAKE OF POTASSIUM

Dietary Intake

Potassium is widely distributed in foods, especially in vegetables and fruits. Intakes of potassium vary widely, depending on dietary habits. Based on the NHANES III data, the median intake of potassium in the United States is about 3.3 g/day for men and 2.2 g/day for women (IOM, 2004). These values do not include the use of salt substitutes or reduced-sodium salts. Salt substitutes contain from 0.4 to 2.8 g potassium per teaspoon as potassium chloride. Because of the growing evidence of the beneficial effects of potassium in protecting against cardiovascular diseases and reducing cardiovascular disease mortality, concern of possible underconsumption of potassium has led to recommendations for increased intake of dietary fruits and vegetables (He and MacGregor, 2008).

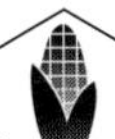

FOOD SOURCES HIGH IN POTASSIUM

Vegetables

0.3 to 0.4 g per ½ cup beans (soybean, pinto, kidney, navy, or lima)
0.35 g per ½ cup lentils
0.69 g per 1 cup carrot juice
0.55 g per 1 cup tomato juice
0.47 g per ½ cup marinara (spaghetti) sauce
0.4 to 0.5 g per ½ cup winter squash, sweet potato, or spinach
0.25 to 0.35 g per ½ cup cabbage, spinach, or pumpkin

Fruits

0.44 to 0.50 g per 1 cup orange juice
0.27 g per ¼ cup raisins
0.21 g per ½ cup melon
0.40 g per ½ cup plums
0.36 g per ½ cup plantains
0.27 g per ½ cup bananas

Fish

0.4 to 0.5 g per 3-oz serving (halibut, tuna, cod, or flounder)

Milk and Milk Products

0.39 g per 1 cup milk
0.55 g per 1 cup plain yogurt

Leavening Agents

0.495 g per 1 tsp cream of tartar

Data from USDA, Agricultural Research Service. (2011). *USDA National Nutrient Database for Standard Reference, Release 24*. Retrieved from www.ars.usda.gov/ba/bhnrc/ndl

Recommended Intake

To replace the obligatory loss of potassium, an adult should consume not less than 0.8 g/day of potassium. The IOM (2004) did not set an EAR or RDA for potassium because of insufficient dose–response data to establish an EAR. The adult AI for potassium was set at 4.7 g/day based upon the dietary level that would blunt the severe salt sensitivity prevalent in black men (Morris et al., 1999). This level of AI for potassium intake is also associated with a lower blood pressure, lower risk of kidney stones, and decreased bone loss. No increment was added to the AI for pregnant women, but the AI for lactating women was increased to 5.1 g/day to allow for the potassium content in human milk secreted during the first 6 months of lactation. Based on the NHANES III data, the percentage of adults who consume

DRIs Across the Life Cycle: Potassium

	g Potassium per Day
Infants	AI
0 through 6 mo	0.4
7 through 12 mo	0.7
Children	
1 through 3 yr	3.0
4 through 8 yr	3.8
9 through 13 yr	4.5
14 through 70 yr	4.7
≥71 yr	4.7
Pregnant	4.7
Lactating	5.1

Data from IOM. (2006). In J. J. Otten, J. P. Hellwig, & L. D. Meyers (Eds.), *Dietary Reference Intakes: The essential guide to nutrient requirements.* Washington, DC: The National Academies Press.
AI, Adequate Intake.

an amount of potassium that is equal to or greater than the AI is only 10% for men and less than 1% for women in the United States (IOM, 2004). A diet rich in fruits and vegetables is necessary to obtain the AI for potassium from natural foods.

The AIs for infants were based on typical intakes from human milk and complementary foods; they are 0.4 g/day of potassium for infants from birth through 6 months of age and 0.7 g/day for infants from 7 through 12 months of age. AIs for children over 1 year old were extrapolated from the adult AI on the basis of median energy intake levels.

There is no evidence that a high level of potassium from foods has adverse effects, so a UL for potassium was not set by the IOM (2004). However, in individuals with impaired urinary excretion of potassium, chronic consumption of a high level of potassium can result in hyperkalemia. Supplemental potassium should be used only under medical supervision in this case.

REGULATION OF SODIUM, CHLORIDE, AND POTASSIUM BALANCE

Sodium, chloride, and potassium normally are consumed in excess of their dietary requirements, and the excess has to be excreted. Excretion of these elements is under the control of various homeostatic regulatory mechanisms that effectively maintain a balance of these elements in the body despite a wide range of intakes and occasional large losses via the skin or the gastrointestinal tract. The kidneys are the main site of regulation of these balance; the intestines play only a relatively minor role. The kidneys respond to a deficiency of these elements in the diet by decreasing their excretion, and they respond to an excess by increasing their excretion in the urine. The amounts excreted by the kidneys can be adjusted either by changing the amount filtered at the glomerulus, which is accomplished by changing the glomerular filtration rate, or by changing the amount reabsorbed or secreted by tubular cells. For long-term regulation, controlling the filtration rate of these elements plays a relatively minor role. The amount excreted depends on the tubular functions of the kidneys. Excretion of Na^+ is controlled by varying the rate of Na^+ reabsorbed from the filtrate by the tubular cells, whereas excretion of K^+ is controlled by varying the rate of secretion of K^+ into the lumen by the distal tubules.

RENAL EXCRETION OF SODIUM, CHLORIDE, AND POTASSIUM

These electrolytes are filtered freely from the glomerular capillaries across the glomerular membrane into the Bowman's space of the nephrons (functional units of the kidneys) so that their concentrations in the glomerular filtrate are similar to those in the plasma. As the filtrate flows along the renal tubules, reabsorption of Na^+, Cl^-, and K^+ and secretion of K^+ by renal tubular cells alter the concentrations of these electrolytes in the urine. Figure 34-4 illustrates the basic renal processing of Na^+, Cl^-, and K^+. Normally 95% to 98% of the filtered load of these ions and water are reabsorbed by the proximal tubules, the thick ascending limbs of the loop of Henle, and the distal convoluted tubules, irrespective of intakes. Reabsorption of the remaining 2% to 5% of the filtered Na^+, Cl^-, and water, and the secretion of K^+ in the cortical collecting tubules are variable and depend greatly on the needs of the individual.

When intake of sodium is high, reabsorption of Na^+ from the cortical collecting tubule is low so that the excess Na^+ is excreted in the urine. However, when there is a sodium deficit due to low intake or excessive loss via the skin or the gastrointestinal tract, much of the Na^+ in the filtrate is reabsorbed, resulting in very low Na^+ concentration in the urine. In contrast to Na^+, K^+ is secreted by the tubular cells of the cortical collecting tubules (Rodriguez-Soriano, 1995). In the absence of disease, changes in K^+ excretion are not due to changes in reabsorption of K^+ in the proximal tubules but to changes in K^+ secretion by the cortical collecting tubules. During potassium depletion, most of the filtered K^+ is reabsorbed, and virtually no K^+ is excreted. The small amount of K^+ excreted comes from the filtered K^+ that escaped reabsorption. However, when potassium intake is high, secretion of K^+ is increased, thereby eliminating the excess potassium. A normal Western diet contains about 2 to 3 g/day of potassium and requires secretion of K^+ in order to maintain potassium balance.

Control of Renal Excretion of Sodium and Chloride

No important receptors capable of detecting the amount of sodium in the body have been identified. However, because Na^+ is the main determinant of extracellular fluid volume, physiological mechanisms that control the volume of extracellular fluid effectively maintain a balance for sodium and chloride (Hall, 2011c). Changes in extracellular fluid volume lead to corresponding changes in the effective circulating volume and affect the "fullness" or "pressure" in the circulation. This changes cardiac filling pressure, cardiac output, and arterial pressure. Volume or pressure

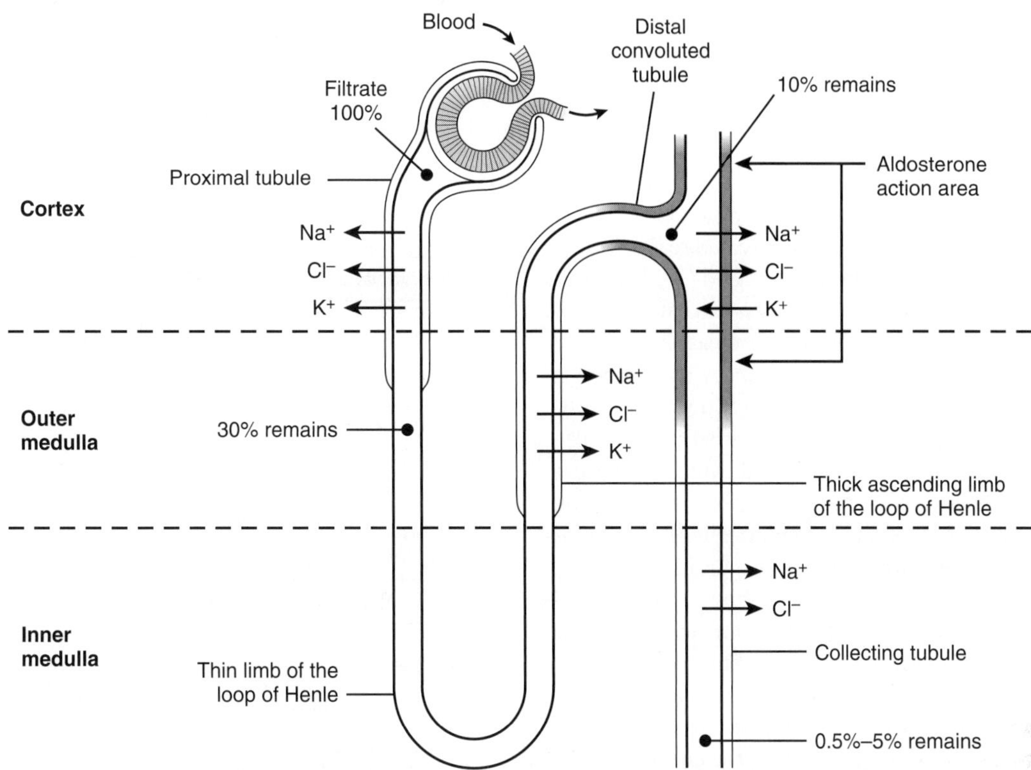

FIGURE 34-4 Reabsorption of Na^+, K^+, and Cl^- and secretion of K^+ at different parts of the nephron. The nephron is the functional unit of the kidney; there are approximately 1 million nephrons in each human kidney.

sensors (baroreceptors) that detect these changes are located throughout the vascular system. These baroreceptors send either excitatory or inhibitory signals to the central nervous system and the endocrine glands to effect appropriate responses by the kidneys to match the amount of sodium ingested. Three major mechanisms participate in the regulation of sodium balance: (1) vascular pressure receptors and their efferent renal sympathetic and arginine vasopressin (AVP) pathways, (2) the renin–angiotensin–aldosterone system, and (3) natriuretic peptides. Two of these mechanisms, vascular pressure receptors and their corresponding efferent pathways, and the renin–angiotensin–aldosterone system, respond effectively to hypovolemia by conservation of body sodium and water, whereas the natriuretic peptides are effective in hypervolemia when excess sodium and water are excreted in the urine (Hall, 2011b, 2011c, 2011d).

Vascular Pressure Receptors, Renal Sympathetic and Arginine Vasopressin Pathways

This reflex mechanism involves vascular pressure receptors (baroreceptors) that sense changes in circulating volume, afferent nerve fibers from these baroreceptors to the central nervous system, and the central efferent pathways to the kidneys. Secretion of a hormone, AVP (also called antidiuretic hormone), and changes in the renal sympathetic nerve activity modify renal excretion of sodium and water, thus minimizing the changes in circulating volume.

Baroreceptors and Afferent Pathways. Baroreceptors present in several sites within the vascular bed sense changes in a physical parameter, such as stretch or tension. There are essentially two kinds of vascular baroreceptors, low-pressure receptors and high-pressure receptors. The low-pressure receptors located in the central venous portion of the circulation respond primarily to changes in blood volume, which distends the walls of the cardiac atria and the pulmonary vein. The high-pressure receptors located in the arterial side of the vascular tree respond primarily to changes in blood pressure in the walls of the aortic arch and the carotid sinus. These baroreceptors send impulses to the hypothalamic and medullary regions of the central nervous system by way of the vagus and the glossopharyngeal nerves.

Efferent Pathways and Renal Effector Organ. Stimulation of baroreceptors in hypervolemia inhibits secretion of AVP from the posterior pituitary, which decreases plasma AVP level. Conversely, plasma AVP level is increased in hypovolemia. Arginine vasopressin increases the permeability of collecting ducts of the kidneys to water so that water is reabsorbed from the tubular lumen into the hyperosmotic medullary interstitium. It also enhances reabsorption of Na^+ and Cl^- by the thick ascending limb of the loops of Henle and, to a lesser degree, by the collecting ducts to decrease Na^+ and water excretion (Canessa et al., 1994). Thus in hypovolemia, conservation of body sodium and water occurs.

The renal sympathetic adrenergic nerves innervate all segments of the renal vasculature and tubules. Under normal arterial pressure, there is minimal sympathetic nerve activity to the kidneys. As part of a reflex response to a fall in systemic arterial pressure, the renal sympathetic nerves are activated to bring about a decrease in renal excretion of Na^+ and Cl^- (Hall, 2011b). Three major mechanisms are involved.

First, the α_1-adrenergic receptors of the afferent and efferent arterioles of the glomerulus are stimulated, and the overall renal vascular resistance is increased. The resultant decrease in renal blood flow and the glomerular filtration rate leads to an overall reduction in the filtered load of Na^+. Second, stimulation of Na^+,K^+-ATPase activity in the basolateral membrane and Na^+/H^+ exchanger in the apical membrane of the proximal tubular cells leads to an increased reabsorption, and thus decreased renal excretion of Na^+ and Cl^-. The stimulatory effect on Na^+,K^+-ATPase activity is mediated by activation of the α_1-adrenergic receptors, whereas that of Na^+/H^+ exchanger is mediated by stimulation of α_2-adrenergic receptors. Third, in addition to their effects on renal hemodynamics and reabsorption of Na^+, sympathetic nerves also stimulate the α_1-adrenergic receptors on the juxtaglomerular cells of the afferent and efferent arterioles to release renin. Renin subsequently increases the circulating levels of angiotensin 2 and aldosterone, which are important in stimulating reabsorption of Na^+. Studies in rats have shown that the basal level of the sympathetic nerve activity is sufficient to exert a tonic stimulation on renin release and tubular Na^+ and Cl^- reabsorption, whereas renal hemodynamics are affected only when sympathetic nerve activity is increased above the basal level. All these adaptive responses restore the effective circulating volume and blood pressure toward their normal values.

In summary, the regulation of volume by the two efferent pathways of the vascular pressure receptors, AVP and sympathetic nerves, is effective during hypovolemia. Activation of these pathways in low effective circulating volume increases the retention of Na^+, Cl^-, and water (Quail et al., 1987). Sympathetic nerve activity has smaller effects on renal excretion of Na^+ and Cl^- in hypervolemia because the sympathetic nerve activity to the kidneys is minimal in euvolemia and hence is not decreased substantially by hypervolemia.

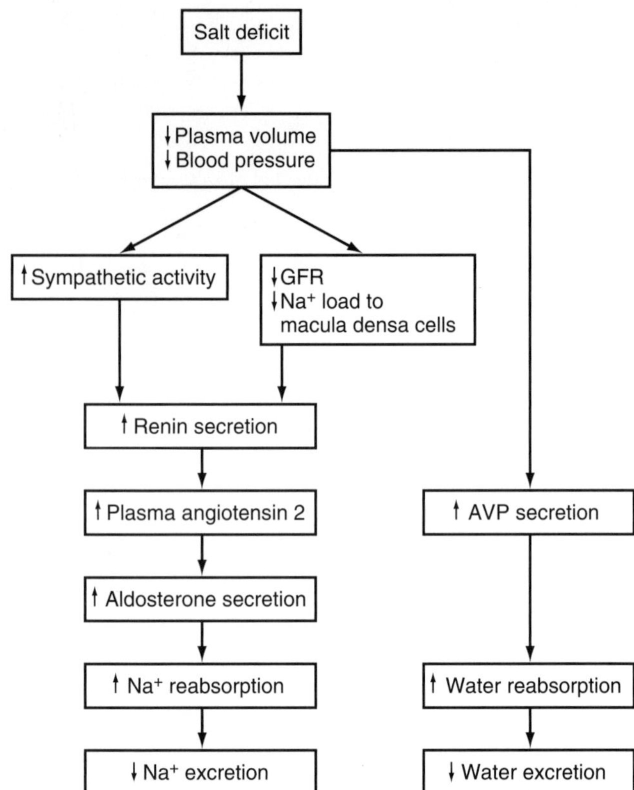

FIGURE 34-5 Schematic representation of the control of renal excretion of sodium and water during salt deficit. *AVP,* Arginine vasopressin; *GFR,* glomerular filtration rate.

Renin–Angiotensin–Aldosterone System

The renin–angiotensin–aldosterone system also plays an important role during hypovolemia to retain body sodium and water. This system is stimulated physiologically by baroreceptors, renal sympathetic nerves, and locally produced prostaglandins. Two distinct groups of sensors are located in the juxtaglomerular apparatus in the kidneys: the high-pressure baroreceptors located in the afferent arterioles of the glomerulus, and the chemoreceptors located in the macula densa area of the thick ascending limb of the renal tubules. The baroreceptors sense changes in perfusion pressure, whereas the chemoreceptors sense changes in the Na^+ load in the tubular fluid. These sensors respond to changes, especially in hypovolemia, by influencing the renin–angiotensin–aldosterone system, which has an important role in the regulation of renal hemodynamics and Na^+ transport (Figure 34-5) (Hall, 2011b).

Renin. Renin, a proteolytic enzyme, is synthesized and stored in an inactive form called prorenin in the juxtaglomerular cells of the afferent arterioles in the kidneys. A decrease in effective circulating volume increases the renal sympathetic nerves activity and also stimulates the intrarenal reflex mechanism of the juxtaglomerular apparatus to increase the secretion of renin. In the circulation, renin acts as an enzyme to split off a 10–amino acid peptide, angiotensin 1, from angiotensinogen. Angiotensinogen is an α_2-globulin produced by the liver and released into the circulation. Angiotensin 1 is biologically inactive and undergoes further cleavage to form angiotensin 2, an octapeptide. This reaction is catalyzed by angiotensin-converting enzyme (ACE), which is present in large amounts on the luminal surface of the endothelium of blood vessels in the lungs and other organs, including the liver and kidneys.

Angiotensin 2. Angiotensin 2 has significant physiological functions (Hall, 2011b). It is an important circulating vasoactive hormone, which causes arteriolar constriction, thereby raising peripheral resistance and maintaining blood pressure in response to a decrease in blood volume. Its central effects include stimulating secretion of AVP, increasing thirst sensation, and increasing the desire for salt. Furthermore, it conserves body sodium indirectly via stimulation of aldosterone secretion by the adrenal gland and directly by influencing renal hemodynamics and tubular epithelial Na^+ reabsorption and K^+ secretion. In its intrarenal effects, angiotensin 2 decreases renal plasma flow by its prominent vasoconstrictor effect on the efferent arterioles. The increase in arteriolar resistance causes a drop in hydrostatic pressure in the peritubular capillaries. This leads to an increase in Na^+ and fluid reabsorption in the proximal tubules in accordance with the Starling forces (see Chapter 35). In addition, angiotensin 2 acts directly on the tubular transport system in both the proximal and the distal tubules. In the proximal tubules, it increases the reabsorption of Na^+, Cl^-, and HCO_3^- by stimulating the Na^+,K^+-ATPase and the Na^+-HCO_3^- symporter in the basolateral membrane and the Na^+/H^+ exchanger in the apical membrane. In the distal tubules, angiotensin 2 stimulates the Na^+/H^+ exchanger in the apical membrane, and it also directly stimulates the Na^+ channel activity. The overall effect is an increase in reabsorption of NaCl and $NaHCO_3$ in the kidney.

Aldosterone. Aldosterone is a steroid hormone produced and secreted by the zona glomerulosa cells of the adrenal cortex. Its secretion is stimulated by a low plasma Na^+ concentration, a high plasma K^+ concentration, and angiotensin 2. In the kidneys, aldosterone stimulates reabsorption of Na^+ and secretion of K^+ by cells of the cortical collecting tubules, and to a lesser extent the distal convoluted and medullary collecting tubules. Aldosterone activates the electrogenic Na^+ and K^+ channels in the apical membrane, increases synthesis of these electrogenic ion channels, and increases synthesis of Na^+,K^+-ATPase in the basolateral membrane (Hall, 2011c). These changes increase the rate of reabsorption of Na^+ by increasing the active transport of Na^+ out of the cells across the basolateral membrane and the passive influx of Na^+ across the apical membrane. At the same time, the rate of movement of K^+ in the opposite direction is increased. The increased reabsorption of Na^+ also increases the potential difference across the tubular epithelial cells (the lumen becomes more negative), so that more K^+ is secreted into the lumen along the established electrical gradient.

Natriuretic Peptides

Natriuretic peptides, a group of peptides produced by the heart, vasculature, and brain, are composed of three structurally similar but genetically distinct groups: A-type natriuretic peptide (ANP), B-type natriuretic peptide (BNP), and C-type natriuretic peptide (CNP). These peptides are involved in the homeostatic control of body fluid and blood pressure. As opposed to the physiological effects of the renin–angiotensin–aldosterone system, which is effective in salt deficit, hypovolemia, and hypotension, the natriuretic peptides have potent natriuretic (excretion of large amount of sodium in the urine), diuretic, and vasodilating effects and are secreted during hypervolemia (Levin et al., 1998). Because of these effects, activation of the natriuretic peptides in left ventricular dysfunction improves the loading conditions of the heart.

A-type natriuretic peptide was first discovered as membrane-bound secretory granules in the myocytes of the cardiac atria. Both BNP and CNP were first isolated from porcine brain, but BNP was later found to be secreted predominantly from the heart, especially the cardiac ventricles. Both ANP and BNP are secreted into the circulation and act as hormones to induce natriuresis and diuresis. The major stimulus to ANP and BNP secretion from the cardiac atria and ventricles is atrial and ventricular distention induced by hypervolemia. Neurohumoral factors, such as AVP and angiotensin 2, and sympathetic stimulation can also modulate ANP and BNP release into the circulation (Vesely, 2007). These natriuretic peptides eliminate the excess fluid from the body indirectly by inhibiting the secretion of aldosterone from the adrenal cortex and directly by their action in the kidneys to increase Na^+ and water excretion by altering the renal hemodynamics. They increase the glomerular filtration rate and filtered load of Na^+ by their vasodilating action on the afferent arterioles at the glomerulus and also act directly on the cells in the medullary portion of the collecting duct to inhibit reabsorption of Na^+ and Cl^-. They also increase the excretion of water by inhibiting the secretion of AVP from the posterior pituitary. Taking all these effects together, the natriuretic peptides increase renal excretion of Na^+, Cl^-, and water in hypervolemia. Because expression of the natriuretic peptides are only upregulated in response to hypervolemia, there is no convincing evidence to indicate that circulating levels of ANP play an important role in hypovolemia.

C-type natriuretic peptide is expressed in the brain, blood vessel endothelium, heart, and kidneys. Its physiological effects differ from that of ANP and BNP. It has autocrine and paracrine effects in that it exerts its actions locally and does not have direct natriuretic effects (Barr et al., 1996). Abundant expression of CNP and its receptors in the hypothalamic and brainstem areas that are involved in blood pressure and volume regulation suggest its role as a neuromodulator in the brain to control intake and excretion of salt and water to maintain body fluid homeostasis (Antunes-Rodrigues et al., 2004). In the vascular endothelium, CNP functions in the local regulation of the vascular renin–angioiotensin system and inhibits the vasoconstrictor effect of angiotensin 1 causing vasodilation. It also controls local vasodilation in the kidneys.

Control of Plasma Concentration of Potassium

Regulation of plasma K^+ concentration involves cellular distribution and renal excretion, unlike Na^+ whose plasma concentration is regulated by renal excretion. Since more than 95% of body potassium is intracellular, physiological mechanisms to promote rapid entry of potassium into skeletal and hepatic cells immediately following a meal are important in minimizing the postprandial rise in plasma concentration. For example, if the potassium absorbed during a meal (about 1 g, or 25 mmol, which is approximately one third of median daily intake for males) were to remain in the extracellular fluid compartment, the concentration of K^+ in the plasma would increase to about 6 mmol/L. However, because of the increase in insulin and catecholamine release after meals, the rise in plasma K^+ is attenuated because both insulin and catecholamines cause rapid cellular uptake of K^+. This is essential in preventing the adverse effects of hyperkalemia, which can be life-threatening. However, to maintain longer lasting potassium balance, the excess potassium from the diet must be excreted by the kidneys.

Transmembrane Distribution of Potassium

As mentioned previously, changes in the concentration gradient of K^+ between the intracellular fluid and plasma adversely affect the normal resting membrane potential and excitability of nerves and muscles. Insulin, catecholamines, pH, and osmolarity all influence the transcellular distribution of K^+ to effect either an immediate rapid release of K^+ from the cells or an uptake of K^+ into the cells to maintain within narrow limits the concentration of K^+ in the plasma (Greenlee et al., 2009). Although aldosterone enhances secretion of K^+ by the tubular cells of the distal nephrons, its effects on transmembrane distribution of K^+ are controversial.

Insulin. Insulin is a major regulator of potassium homeostasis. During a meal, the high concentrations of glucose, amino acids, gastrointestinal hormones, and K^+ in the plasma cause insulin to be released from the beta cells of the pancreas. Insulin promotes uptake of K^+ by the liver, skeletal muscles, cardiac muscles, and adipocytes, thereby attenuating the rapid postprandial rise in plasma K^+ concentration (Greenlee et al., 2009). This reflex regulatory feedback mechanism helps to maintain the concentration of K^+ in plasma and the concentration gradient between plasma and intracellular fluid. The mechanism of insulin-mediated uptake of K^+ by cells is independent of its effects on uptake of glucose. Insulin stimulates tissue uptake of K^+ by stimulating Na^+,K^+-ATPase activity in plasma membranes. Other electroneutral transport pathways, such as Na^+/H^+ exchange and $Na^+/K^+/2Cl^-$ cotransporter in peripheral tissues, are also activated, but the roles of these in K^+ homeostasis is less clear.

Catecholamines. Both adrenergic sympathetic activity and circulating catecholamines can influence cellular uptake and release of K^+. Their dual effects on the movement of K^+ across cell membranes are due to activation of both the α-adrenergic and β-adrenergic receptors on cell membranes (Moratinos and Reverte, 1993). Stimulation of α_1- and α_2-adrenergic receptors increases plasma K^+ levels because of the activation of the hepatic Ca^{2+}-dependent K^+ channels, which release K^+ from the liver into the circulation. In contrast, stimulation of β_2-adrenergic receptors promotes cellular uptake of K^+ in the liver, muscles, and myocardium through stimulation of Na^+,K^+-ATPase and decreases plasma K^+ levels. The opposing effects of α- and β-adrenergic fibers have important physiological consequences. During exercise the sympathetic nervous system is activated; norepinephrine from the sympathetic nerve endings and epinephrine from the adrenal medulla are released. The released epinephrine potentially causes an initial rise in plasma K^+ concentration, owing to its action on the α-adrenergic receptors in the liver to release K^+, followed by sustained hypokalemia owing to its action on the β-adrenergic receptors in the muscles to promote cellular K^+ uptake. However, norepinephrine released by the sympathetic nerve endings during exercise also stimulates release of K^+ from the liver, and the dual effects of the two catecholamines ensure that hypokalemia does not occur during exercise.

Plasma pH. The effect of plasma pH on transmembrane distribution of K^+ is complex and depends on the presence of other physiological factors that affect distribution of K^+. In general, acute metabolic acidosis caused by accumulation of nonmetabolizable acids causes K^+ to leave cells in exchange for H^+ entry. The consequence is an increase in plasma K^+ concentration. Acute metabolic alkalosis generally induces the opposite response. Plasma K^+ concentration decreases because of movement of K^+ into the cells (Rodriguez-Soriano, 1995).

Renal Excretion of Potassium

Renal potassium excretion depends on glomerular filtration, reabsorption, and a highly regulated secretory process in the distal and collecting tubules of the kidneys. Normally, approximately 67% of filtered K^+ is reabsorbed from the proximal tubule and a further 20% is reabsorbed from the loop of Henle. Further reabsorption of K^+ occurs in the distal tubules when dietary intake is low. However, when K^+ intake is high, the excess K^+ is secreted in the distal and collecting tubules of the kidneys. The two most important homeostatic regulatory mechanisms for K^+ secretion are aldosterone and plasma K^+ concentration. In addition, other factors such as acid–base balance also influence K^+ secretion (Hall, 2011d).

Aldosterone. Aldosterone is the most important hormone regulating secretion of K^+. As mentioned above, either a high plasma K^+ or a low plasma Na^+ concentration will trigger its release from the adrenal cortex, thus providing a relatively large tolerance to changes in dietary potassium. Lack of aldosterone, for example in Addison disease, causes a marked depletion of body Na^+ and retention of K^+ (Nerup, 1974). Conversely, excess aldosterone, for example in Conn syndrome, is associated with depletion of K^+ and retention of Na^+ (Ganguly and Donohue, 1983).

Plasma Concentrations of Potassium and Hydrogen. Other factors that can directly affect secretion of K^+ by the distal nephrons are concentrations of plasma K^+ and H^+ (Hall, 2011d). Under normal circumstances, the concentration of K^+ in tubular cells reflects that of the plasma. This is because an increase in plasma K^+ concentration directly stimulates the Na^+,K^+-ATPase at the basolateral membrane of the distal nephrons. In addition, the resultant increased secretion of aldosterone from the high plasma K^+ further increases the uptake of K^+ by these cells. Increase in intracellular K^+ concentration increases the concentration gradient for K^+ across the apical membrane, promoting diffusion of K^+ into the lumen and increasing the excretion of K^+ in the urine. A decrease in the concentration of intracellular K^+ decreases the concentration gradient across the luminal membrane, and reduces the secretion of K^+.

Secretion of K^+ by the tubular cells in response to changes in acid–base balance is more complex. In general, acute acidosis decreases secretion of K^+, causing retention of potassium, whereas acute alkalosis increases secretion and loss of potassium from the body (Adrogue and Madias, 1981). In acute acidosis, the high plasma H^+ concentration inhibits the Na^+,K^+-ATPase activity at the basolateral membrane so that the intracellular K^+ concentration in the tubular cells is decreased, resulting in a decrease in secretion of K^+ by the tubular cells. However, with chronic acid–base disorders, the response of the kidney is varied. Secretion of K^+ depends on the etiology of the disorders and the presence of other processes that may be altered by changes in pH. Metabolic acidosis may be associated with an increase in K^+ secretion and mild K^+ depletion, which may be explained by an acidosis-induced increase in secretion of aldosterone. Metabolic alkalosis, however, is almost always accompanied by depletion of K^+.

CONTROL OF INTESTINAL ABSORPTION AND EXCRETION OF SODIUM, CHLORIDE, AND POTASSIUM

Under normal circumstances, about 99% of dietary Na^+, Cl^-, and K^+ is absorbed, and the remaining 1% is excreted in the feces. Analogies may be drawn between the excretion of these ions in the kidneys and the intestines. Absorption of Na^+ and Cl^- occurs along the entire length of the intestines; 90% to 95% is absorbed in the small intestine and the rest in the colon. Absorption of K^+ occurs in the small intestine, but normally there is net secretion of K^+ in the colon. In the colon, net absorption occurs during K^+ deficit, and net secretion occurs in K^+ excess. Intestinal absorption and secretion of Na^+, K^+, and Cl^- are subject to regulation by the nervous system, hormones, and paracrine agonists released from neurons in the enteric nervous system in the wall of the intestines. The most important of these factors is aldosterone, which stimulates absorption of Na^+ and secretion of K^+, mainly by the colon and, to a lesser extent, by the ileum. The mechanism of aldosterone action is similar to that in the renal tubules.

ACTIVATION OF SALT APPETITE

In the absence of excessive loss, our intake of sodium and water normally exceeds the amount needed for maintaining fluid balance. Any excess intake is excreted in the urine. However, prolonged sodium or salt (NaCl) deficiency and hypovolemia have been shown to motivate the search for and ingestion of sodium-containing foods and fluids. The presence of salt-seeking behavior in animals, for example in ruminants, is to ensure that there is an adequate intake of salt to protect the body from excessive loss of NaCl and water due to sweating, diarrhea, pregnancy, or lactation. This salt appetite or salt cravings behavioral drive to ingest salt is also present in salt-deficient humans. In adrenal-deficient patients, depletion of body sodium causes a strong desire for salty food because of taste alterations (Geerling and Loewy, 2008).

The exact mechanism responsible for salt cravings is incompletely understood. Both central and peripheral neural and hormonal systems have been implicated in the control of salt appetite. Behavioral studies in animals have shown the role of the gustatory neuraxis (which involves the facial nerves from the tongue to the brain) in their adaptive regulation of salt intake. Deprivation of this relay of sodium taste information to the brain abolishes the expression of sodium preferences and the ability of the animal to modify its behavior for sodium intake (Daniels and Fluharty, 2004). Hypovolemia and hypotension, which activate baroreceptors, are also implicated in the activation of salt appetite. Production of various hormones, such as aldosterone, AVP, oxytocin, and especially the renin–angiotensin system, is markedly elevated by prolonged sodium deprivation (Geerling and Loewy, 2008). These hormones promote renal conservation of sodium and water. In addition, these hormones also act centrally to stimulate salt appetite and thirst mechanism. Aldosterone-sensitive neurons are found in the brainstem and their activation is associated with a gradual increase in sodium appetite. All components of the renin–angiotensin system (renin, angiotensinogen, angiotensin-converting enzyme, and angiotensin receptors) are present in the neuronal centers in several brain regions known to have roles in the regulation of body fluid and electrolyte balance and the cardiovascular system. Centrally administered angiotensin receptor antagonists are found to disrupt sodium appetite and water drinking, sodium excretion, and AVP secretion. Evidence exists also that peripherally derived angiotensin 2 stimulates salt appetite in rats by its direct action on the brain.

INTERACTIONS AMONG SYSTEMS IN VOLUME REGULATION

The body employs a multifactorial system of feedback loops with their reinforcing and modulating pathways to effectively regulate circulating volume and blood pressure. The highly integrated pathways of the sympathetic nervous system, the renin–angiotensin–aldosterone system, AVP, and ANP when acting together provide multiple backup systems that permit the body to regulate the vasomotor tone and sodium and water balance in response to changes in volume, even when one of the regulatory systems fails. This regulatory feedback mechanism can be examined best by the following examples of changes in dietary NaCl.

To maintain a normal effective circulating volume, termed euvolemia, a precise balance of excretion of Na^+ and Cl^- to match their consumption is required. In euvolemic individuals, daily excretion of Na^+ and Cl^- equals the daily consumption. Excretion of Na^+ and Cl^- in the urine can vary over a wide range, from a very low level to as much as 23 g/day, depending on the diet.

In the case of positive salt balance, retention of sodium and chloride increases the volume of extracellular fluid and, hence, body weight. It is mainly this expansion of fluid volume that triggers the homeostatic regulatory mechanisms to increase the excretion of Na^+ and Cl^- via the following mechanisms: (1) stimulation of the low-pressure and high-pressure baroreceptors which suppresses the sympathetic nervous discharge to the kidneys by reflex pathways, (2) suppression of the renin–angiotensin–aldosterone system, (3) suppression of the AVP system, and (4) stimulation of the secretion of ANP from the cardiac atria. The loss of Na^+, Cl^-, and water from the body returns the volume of extracellular fluid and body weight to their original levels.

The opposite occurs in negative salt balance, in which acute depletion of Na^+ and Cl^- decreases the volume of extracellular fluid. The various control systems act together to conserve body Na^+ and Cl^- during depletion by stimulating the salt appetite and decreasing urinary excretion of Na^+ and Cl^-. Urinary excretion of Na^+ and Cl^- is decreased by reflex increase in sympathetic nervous discharge to the kidneys, stimulation of the renin–angiotensin–aldosterone system, and stimulation of the AVP system (see Figure 34-5).

SODIUM AND CHLORIDE IMBALANCE AND ITS CONSEQUENCES

In general, sodium retention results in proportionate water retention, and sodium loss results in proportionate water loss due to osmoregulation involving AVP. Various situations can cause an isotonic expansion or contraction of the extracellular volume. Physiological regulatory mechanisms for conservation of sodium seem to be better developed in humans than are mechanisms for excretion of sodium, possibly because of an evolutionary history during which salt deficit was more common than salt excess. Because of the well-developed capacity for retention of sodium, pathological states characterized by inappropriate retention of sodium are much more common than salt-losing conditions.

SODIUM CHLORIDE RETENTION

Retention of Na^+ occurs when Na^+ intake exceeds renal Na^+ excretory capacity. This situation can occur with rapid ingestion of large amounts of salt (e.g., ingestion of seawater) or during too-rapid saline infusion. Hypernatremia and hypervolemia resulting in acute hypertension usually occur in these situations (Table 34-1).The hypervolemia will initiate the Na^+ regulatory mechanisms to excrete the excess sodium and water. Hypervolemia can occur also in pathological conditions, such as congestive heart failure, renal failure, or when there is excessive production of aldosterone in Conn syndrome. In congestive heart failure, the kidneys often respond to circulatory insufficiency to retain Na^+. In these pathological states, despite the hypervolemia, the kidneys respond inappropriately by retaining more Na^+ instead of excreting the excess. This Na^+ retention, together with secondary water retention, causes accumulation of fluid in the vascular and interstitial spaces. Accumulation of fluid in the interstitial space is perceived as edema. In renal diseases and hyperaldosteronism, retention of sodium and water by the kidneys also causes hypervolemia and edema. In renal diseases, because retention of fluid is primarily due to failure of the kidneys, the retained fluid is less readily excreted. Therefore hypervolemia persists even though there is a sustained release of ANP. Edema and ultimately heart failure are signs of excess Na^+ and Cl^- that exceed the upper limits of tolerance or regulation (Hall, 2011a).

TABLE 34-1 Sodium Excess and Deficiency: Some Causes and Effects

	CAUSES	EFFECTS
Sodium excess	Excessive ingestion of salt Too-rapid infusion of saline Congestive heart failure Conn syndrome Renal failure	Hypernatremia, hypervolemia Hypertension Cardiovascular disease Edema and ultimately heart failure
Sodium deficit	Insufficient intake Profuse sweating Prolonged diarrhea and vomiting Addison disease Diabetes mellitus Diuretic therapy Renal diseases	Hypovolemia, dehydration, hypotension Increased pulse rate Dizziness and syncope Muscle weakness and cramps Circulatory shock

SODIUM CHLORIDE DEFICIENCY

Loss of sodium can occur through either renal or nonrenal routes. Hypovolemia and hyponatremia may occur through increased renal loss of Na^+ owing to decreased reabsorption (Hall, 2011a). In Addison disease where there is a deficiency in aldosterone, excretion of Na^+ is greatly enhanced. Loss of Na^+ and water also occur with the administration of diuretics, which inhibit NaCl reabsorption. In diabetes mellitus, the presence of glucose in excess of renal reabsorptive capacity causes diuresis and loss of Na^+. Transient increases in loss of Na^+ also occur in tubular necrosis and in certain toxic nephropathies. Chronic renal diseases that increase the permeability of the glomerular membranes or damage to tubular cells that decreases tubular capacity for reabsorption of Na^+ will result in Na^+ loss. The pathogenesis of increased Na^+ loss in chronic kidney diseases is a result of the increased filtered load of solutes and filtrate to the remaining functional nephrons.

The most common route for nonrenal loss of Na^+ is through the gastrointestinal tract from vomiting and diarrhea (Field et al., 1989). Severe and prolonged diarrhea causes hyponatremia, hypokalemia, and dehydration (see Table 34-1). Diseases causing diarrhea are among the leading sources of infant mortality and are a major world health problem. In an acute diarrheal episode in which an infant loses 5% of body weight, the infant is at risk for shock. A more gradual depletion of body fluid may not result in shock until the body weight has been reduced by about 10%. Although diarrhea causes losses of K^+, HCO_3^-, and Na^+, the immediate concern in treating severe diarrhea is to replace Na^+ and water to restore the circulatory volume. Dehydration in diarrhea can be reversed by oral or, in emergencies, intravenous rehydration therapy.

Substantial losses of water, sodium, chloride, and potassium can occur in the form of sweating during prolonged and strenuous exercise and manual work in a hot environment (see Table 34-1). Therefore there is a need to ensure adequate replacement of water and these ions. Manifestations of hypovolemia are a result of diminished regional tissue perfusion and they vary with the degree of volume contraction. The loss of Na^+ and hypovolemia produce symptoms that include orthostatic hypotension and increased pulse rate. Orthostatic hypotension occurs when a person moves suddenly, either from a reclining to an upright position or from a sitting to a standing position. Vasoconstriction and

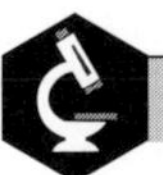

CLINICAL CORRELATION

Diarrhea

Each day, approximately 8 to 10 L of fluid passes through the gastrointestinal tract. About 2 L of these fluids are from the consumption of liquids and solid foods, and 6 to 8 L comprise secretions from the various parts of the gastrointestinal tract. The intestines absorb most of these fluids so that only 100 to 200 mL of fluid are lost daily in the stool of an adult. The average electrolyte contents of the stool are 35 to 50 mmol/L for Na^+, 75 to 90 mmol/L for K^+, 16 mmol/L for Cl^-, and 30 to 40 mmol/L for HCO_3^-.

Diarrhea is defined as an increase in stool liquidity and a fecal fluid volume of more than 200 mL/day in adults. Depending on the severity, several liters of fluid can be lost, leading to profound fluid and electrolyte imbalance. Although there are many causes of diarrhea, generally causes can be classified pathogenically into (1) osmotic, (2) secretory, (3) structural, and (4) primary motility disorders. Clinically the most common and important causes of diarrhea are osmotic and secretory.

Osmotic diarrhea can be caused either by ingestion of poorly absorbable solutes, such as magnesium sulfate, sorbitol, and lactulose, or by malabsorption or maldigestion of specific solutes because of enzyme deficiencies (e.g., lactase deficiency). The presence of these solutes (and their fermentation products in the large intestine) increases the intestinal luminal osmolarity. This creates an osmotic gradient across the mucosal cells of the intestines, resulting in a diffusion of water from the interstitial fluid compartment into the lumen of the intestines. In addition, the water that would normally be absorbed or reabsorbed along with the solutes remains in the lumen. Osmotic diarrhea ceases once the aggravating factor is passed out of the lumen.

Secretory diarrhea is characterized by either increased intestinal secretions or failure of distal reabsorption of normal secretions. Viral enteritis and bacterial infections are the most common causes of secretory diarrhea. Bacteria such as *Vibrio cholerae* and *Escherichia coli* release toxins that activate intestinal adenylate cyclase, resulting in increased secretion of sodium chloride and water, whereas enteroinvasive bacteria such as shigellae and salmonellae invade intestinal mucosa, producing ulceroinflammatory lesions.

The degree of dehydration due to diarrhea can range from mild to severe. This can be assessed clinically by examining the patient for skin turgor, mental status, blood pressure, urine output, and sunken eyeballs. Fluid replacement is of utmost importance to prevent circulatory collapse, especially in cases of severe dehydration, such as those seen in patients with cholera. Diarrhea also causes electrolyte and acid–base imbalances, including hypokalemia, hyperchloremia, and metabolic acidosis.

The World Health Organization (WHO) recommended the use of oral rehydration therapy for treatment of mild to moderate cases of diarrhea, especially in developing countries. Because of the high cost of intravenous fluid therapy and the distance of some areas from medical facilities, the program has been very successful in reducing mortality from diarrheal diseases, particularly in infants. Oral rehydration fluid contains 3.5 g of NaCl, 2.5 g of $NaHCO_3$, 1.5 g of KCl, and 20 g of glucose in 1 L of water. An alternative household remedy is to mix three "finger pinches" of salt and a "fistful of sugar" with about 1 quart of water to make the solution.

Thinking Critically

Diarrhea is characterized by dehydration, electrolyte imbalance, and acid–base imbalance. Discuss why hypokalemia, hyperchloremia, and metabolic acidosis occur.

decreased muscle perfusion during hypovolemia may also lead to muscular weakness and cramps. As hypovolemia becomes more severe, dizziness and syncope (fainting) may accompany the orthostatic hypotension. In severe forms of hypovolemia, the circulatory volume can be greatly compromised and circulatory shock may ensue. In hypovolemic individuals, mechanisms to conserve sodium are activated. If the loss is not of renal origin, the normal response is an immediate decrease in renal excretion of Na^+ to a very low level. In chronic sodium deficiency, the urine is virtually free of Na^+.

POTASSIUM IMBALANCE AND ITS CONSEQUENCES

HYPERKALEMIA

Retention of K^+ causing hyperkalemia occurs when potassium consumption exceeds the capacity of the kidneys to excrete K^+. Hyperkalemia is diagnosed when the plasma K^+ concentration exceeds 5.5 mmol/L (Evans and Greenberg, 2005). This rarely happens when the kidneys are functioning normally because their capacity to excrete K^+ is substantial. A reduced capacity occurs when there is a defect in the secretory process in the distal nephrons, a lack of aldosterone secretion, or a lack of responsiveness of the renal tubules to aldosterone.

Hyperkalemia can occur also in the absence of K^+ retention. A shift of intracellular K^+ into the plasma to cause hyperkalemia can occur in metabolic acidosis or from tissue damage, as in hemolysis, burns, major trauma, or lysis of tumor cells (Table 34-2). In the treatment of hyperkalemia, consumption of K^+ is restricted, but most importantly the underlying causes of hyperkalemia must be treated.

An important clinical manifestation of hyperkalemia is cardiac dysrhythmia, which ranges from sinus bradycardia to ventricular tachycardia, ventricular fibrillation, and ultimately cardiac arrest (asystole) when a plasma concentration of 8 mmol/L is reached. Because of the adverse effects of hyperkalemia on the heart, hyperkalemia constitutes a medical emergency. Other symptoms include paresthesia (an abnormal sensation of the skin), muscle weakness, and eventually flaccid paralysis (see Table 34-2) (Evans and Greenberg, 2005).

TABLE 34-2 Potassium Excess and Deficiency: Some Causes and Effects

	CAUSES	EFFECTS
Potassium excess	Lack of aldosterone secretion Metabolic acidosis Tissue damage Renal diseases	Hyperkalemia Cardiac dysrhythmias and ultimately cardiac arrest
Potassium deficit	Insufficient intake Prolonged vomiting and diarrhea Hyperaldosteronism Metabolic alkalosis Diuretic therapy	Hypokalemia Impaired muscle function such as muscle weakness, fatigue, and cramps Insulin resistance and glucose intolerance Cardiac dysrhythmias, paralysis

HYPOKALEMIA

Hypokalemia is diagnosed when the plasma K^+ concentration is less than 3.5 mmol/L. Because changes in plasma K^+ concentration usually parallel changes in intracellular K^+ concentration, it is usually associated with depletion of body potassium (Hall, 2011d). However, a low plasma K^+ concentration does not necessarily imply a depletion of body potassium or low intracellular concentration, because other factors may be present that shift K^+ from the extracellular to the intracellular compartment. This can occur in acute alkalosis or hyperinsulinemia.

Depletion of potassium can occur when intake is less than loss (see Table 34-2). Normally, potassium depletion rarely arises from insufficient consumption because the normal amount consumed usually exceeds that required for the replacement of obligatory losses and maintenance of tissues. It occurs only when intake is inadequate during prolonged fasting or when dietary potassium is severely restricted. In most cases, depletion of potassium and hypokalemia can occur through either renal or nonrenal routes. Renal K^+ loss can occur in endocrine and metabolic disorders such as hyperaldosteronism, metabolic alkalosis, and diuretic therapy. As with sodium depletion, the most common route for nonrenal loss is vomiting and diarrhea (see Table 34-2). In these situations, the normal reflex response (increased renal and colon K^+ absorption) is prevented because of the hypovolemia that accompanies the vomiting and diarrhea. Hypovolemia initiates regulatory reflex responses to retain Na^+ and water by the kidneys. The enhanced reabsorption of Na^+ from the cortical collecting tubules under the influence of aldosterone further exacerbates the loss of K^+.

Hypokalemia can result in muscle weakness, cardiac arrhythmias, insulin resistance, and glucose intolerance (see Table 34-2) (Greenlee et al., 2009). Manifestations of K^+ deficiency in cardiac and skeletal muscles are due to alterations of cellular metabolism and hyperpolarization of cellular membranes. Symptoms include depressed neuromuscular functions such as muscle weakness and cramps; in more severe hypokalemia, patients may experience cardiac dysrhythmias, paralysis, metabolic alkalosis, and death.

NUTRITIONAL CONSIDERATIONS

Both epidemiological and experimental studies have indicated that dietary factors play a major role in the prevalence of hypertension and cardiovascular diseases. Habitual high dietary salt intake has been implicated in the development of hypertension, hypertension-related cardiovascular diseases, renal diseases unrelated to blood pressure, gastric mucosal damage, gastric cancer, and bone demineralization with the consequence of osteoporosis (IOM, 2004; Ritz et al., 2009; Tsugane and Sasazuki, 2007). Hypertensive individuals who follow a salt-restricted diet usually experience a decrease in blood pressure and fewer additional complications (Jones, 2004). On the other hand, a diet rich in fruits and vegetables reduces the risk of the development and the progression of cardiovascular diseases, gastric cancer, and bone demineralization. Potassium, among the many nutrients and phytochemicals, is one of the nutrients that may be responsible for these protective actions (He and MacGregor, 2008; Tsugane and Sasazuki, 2007; Heaney, 2006).

No adverse effects of low sodium intakes between 1.1 g/day and 3.4 g/day have been found, although it has been reported in short-term clinical studies that a very low salt diet (0.46 to 0.69 g/day of sodium) increases risk factors for cardiovascular diseases (Fliser et al., 1993; Egan and Lackland, 2000). For example, some serum lipid fractions such as total cholesterol and low-density lipoprotein (LDL)-cholesterol concentrations, plasma levels of norepinephrine and insulin, and glucose-to-insulin ratio are increased in both normotensive and hypertensive people consuming severely restricted amounts of sodium. However, no obvious disorders of the serum lipid profile or carbohydrate metabolism are seen in cross-cultural studies where very low salt intake is associated with a low prevalence of hypertension (Stamler, 1997).

A low potassium intake that results in hypokalemia will show clinical manifestations of altered cellular metabolism and membrane potentials. Furthermore, because of the numerous protective actions of potassium, a deficit may increase the risks of hypertension, cardiovascular diseases, gastric mucosal damage, and osteoporosis.

HYPERTENSION AND CARDIOVASCULAR DISEASES

Hypertension, or high blood pressure, affects about one third of the adult population in the United States, and its incidence is rising. It is a major risk factor for cardiovascular disease, stroke, and renal failure in industrialized societies, and it is one of the leading causes of death. Genetic factors, organ disorders (primarily of kidney origin), and environmental factors, such as excessive salt intake and inadequate potassium intake, predispose an individual to hypertension. Both epidemiological and experimental studies implicate a primary role for dietary factors in their contribution to high blood pressure, and consequently hypertension-related cardiovascular diseases. Consumption of a high-fat, high-sodium, low-potassium, low-calcium, or low-magnesium diet may contribute to the development of hypertension (Reusser and McCarron, 1994). Therefore lifestyle modifications, including weight loss, increased physical activity, moderation of alcohol consumption, and an overall healthy dietary pattern such as the DASH (Dietary Approaches to Stop Hypertension) diet, have been recommended to help reduce blood pressure (Sacks et al., 2001). Recently the IOM (2010) recommended that the Food and Drug Administration (FDA) set mandatory national standards for the sodium content in foods—not banning the addition of salt to foods but beginning the process of reducing excess sodium in processed foods and menu items to a safer level. The goal of this recommendation is to reduce the prevalence of hypertension and ultimately decrease the mortality and morbidity due to cardiovascular diseases.

Association of High Salt Consumption with Hypertension

Although habitual high salt consumption and hypertension have been linked for more than a century, the mechanisms by which salt influences blood pressure and the relationship between sodium intake and cardiovascular morbidity and mortality are still controversial. This is not surprising, because individual differences are influenced by various dynamic variables, such as genetic susceptibility, body mass, cardiovascular factors, regulatory mechanisms mediated through the neural and hormonal systems, and the kidneys.

Implications of high salt intake in hypertension come from observations that the highest incidence of hypertension occurs in northern Japan, where salt intake may be as high as 20 g/day (Kono et al., 1983). In the United States, where salt intake averages between 5 and 13 g/day, results from the NHANES III collected over a period of 3 years (1988–1991) on 9,901 participants from age 18 through 74 years indicated that 24% of the adult population had hypertension. This number did not include normotensive individuals who were being treated for hypertension (Burt et al., 1995). Conversely, societies with low salt intake, such as the Yanomami Indians, have a low incidence of hypertension (Oliver et al., 1975).

The most comprehensive population-based study on the relationship between dietary salt and blood pressure was carried out by The INTERSALT Cooperative Research Group (Rose et al., 1998; Stamler, 1997). This group studied the association between blood pressure and 24-hour urinary excretion of Na^+ and K^+ in more than 10,000 men and women whose ages ranged from 20 to 59 years. Participants were from 52 geographically separate centers in 32 countries in Africa, the Americas, Asia, and Europe. Salt intake of the population in these diverse regions varies greatly. Highly standardized procedures were used in this international collaborative study so that comparisons could be made between centers. The variables measured include age, sex, body mass index, alcohol consumption, arterial blood pressure, and 24-hour urine collection for the analysis of urinary Na^+ and K^+ excretion. Median daily urinary excretion of sodium ranged between 4.6 mg and 5.6 g, but the distribution within this range was uneven. Four centers had mean values of less than 1.3 g/day, none had values between 1.3 and 2.4 g/day, four had values between 2.4 g and 3.2 g/day, and 44 had values between 3.2 g and 5.6 g/day. Therefore the bulk of the data on the association between blood pressure and excretion of sodium was for populations with high mean excretion of sodium (3.2 to 5.6 g/day).

Cross-center analyses of all 52 centers showed that median systolic blood pressure, but not diastolic pressure, was positively associated with median values of sodium excretion after adjustments for age, sex, body mass index, and consumption of alcohol. However, when the four centers with very low median values of sodium excretion were excluded from the analyses, the correlation between systolic blood pressure and excretion of sodium was not significant. The INTERSALT study also showed that populations in the four centers with median values for sodium excretion that were less than 1.3 g/day had low blood pressure, rare or absent hypertension, and no age-related rise in blood pressure, as occurred in populations in other centers. In centers where the average excretion of sodium was more than 2.4 g/day, median values for sodium excretion were related significantly to the age-related rise in blood pressure (Rodriguez et al., 1994). Although it was recognized that the association of blood pressure or prevalence of hypertension with median values for sodium excretion was relatively weak, the evidence supports the general contention that habitual intake of salt is an important factor in the occurrence of hypertension.

There may be direct association between sodium intake and incidence of cardiovascular disease, especially stroke and left ventricular hypertrophy independent of blood pressure (IOM, 2004). A recent meta-analysis of prospective studies showed greater risk of stroke and cardiovascular disease with higher salt intake (Strazzullo et al., 2009).

Genetic Factors

Although much is known about how lifestyle and diet affect blood pressure, the roles of genetic factors that predispose an individual to hypertension are just beginning to be understood. Numerous studies involving genome-wide scans using polymorphism markers have identified regions of chromosomes relating to salt sensitivity in salt-sensitive rodents and in hypertensive humans. Meta-analysis of data available from animal models of essential hypertension has identified numerous genes that associate with the onset of hypertension and with established hypertension in different organs (Marques et al., 2010). Perturbations in genes that regulate sodium and chloride reabsorption by the kidneys may be especially important determinants of salt sensitivity.

Abnormalities in membrane transport of sodium chloride in the distal tubules of the kidney have been identified. There is an association between hypertension and the T481S genotype in the chloride channel ClC-Kb, which is expressed in the basolateral membrane of the distal tubule and participates in renal Na^+ and Cl^- reabsorption (Jeck et al., 2004). In the white population studied, carriers of the variant 481S allele had significantly higher plasma Na^+ levels, higher systolic and diastolic blood pressures, and a significantly higher prevalence of hypertension. Thus 481S appears to be a gain-of-function genetic variant that results in higher ClC-Kb chloride channel activity and may lead to increased renal salt retention and consequently higher blood pressure. Patients with Bartter syndrome type 3 who lack this channel show characteristics of salt-wasting and hypotension (Simon et al., 1997). This inherited susceptibility is expressed in the presence of other predisposing factors, such as obesity, consumption of alcohol, unbalanced diet, and stress (Folkow, 1982). Polymorphisms in the *SPAK* gene that regulate the thiazide-sensitive Na^+-Cl^- cotransporter in the distal tubule have been implicated in a rare familial form of hypertension (Glover et al., 2011).

Dietary Salt Restriction

Questions still remain on whether moderate dietary sodium restriction should be recommended to all individuals to reduce blood pressure and also decrease the incidence of stroke and ischemic heart disease. Intervention studies of dietary salt restrictions to lower blood pressure have produced mixed results in both normotensive subjects and hypertensive patients. This may be explained by the fact that not all hypertensive patients are salt-sensitive, and many cases of hypertension are due to other causes. Nevertheless, results of the Trials of Hypertension Prevention (TOHP) (Cook et al., 1998) and the DASH-Sodium trial (Sacks et al., 2001) have demonstrated a lowering of blood pressure in response to dietary sodium reduction, thereby confirming the conclusions of the INTERSALT study (Jones, 2004). The response of blood pressure to salt restriction depended on age, the degree of restriction, and the initial blood pressure (Reusser and McCarron, 1994). Older patients seemed to have a greater response to salt restriction. The highest rate of success in reducing hypertension was obtained in nonoverweight, mildly hypertensive patients. Meta-analysis of clinical trials of modest sodium reduction lasting over 4 weeks involving both normotensive subjects and hypertensive patients have also shown a lowering of systolic and diastolic blood pressure with reduced salt intake. The reduction in blood pressure in normotensive patients is less pronounced than that in hypertensive patients (He and MacGregor, 2003).

Even in the absence of continued salt intervention, the beneficial effects of short-term sodium reduction on blood pressure and cardiovascular diseases are long term. Newborn infants randomly assigned to a low-sodium formula during their first 6 months have lower blood pressure at the end of the study period compared to those fed normal formula. This lower trend of blood pressure was maintained when they reach adolescence (Geleijnse et al., 1997). Long-term follow-up of adult participants in TOHP showed also that those who reduced their salt intake moderately for 18 months (TOHP I) and 36 to 48 months (TOHP II) have lower blood pressure, lower incidence of hypertension, and a reduction in the risk of cardiovascular diseases. including myocardial infarctions and strokes, even 7 years later (He et al., 2000, Cook et al., 2007). Thus reduced salt intake not only lowers blood pressure and reduces the incidence of hypertension and risks of cardiovascular diseases in the short term, but also has long-term beneficial effects.

Most recently, prospective data from the Third National Health and Examination Survey showed that a higher sodium intake was associated with increased all-cause mortality among U.S. adults (Yang et al., 2011). The study also found a significant positive correlation between the dietary ratio of sodium-to-potassium and risk of both cardiovascular disease and all-cause mortality (Yang et al., 2011). The later finding is consistent with previous work reporting a significant positive trend across quartiles of urinary sodium-to-potassium excretion ratio and cardiovascular disease risk (Cook et al., 2009). These findings collectively support public health recommendations that emphasize simultaneous reduction in sodium intake and elevation in potassium intake for reducing the risk of cardiovascular disease (see subsequent text).

Protective Action of Dietary Potassium Against Cardiovascular Diseases

The beneficial effects of K^+ on health have been of interest over the last few decades. Epidemiological studies and clinical intervention trials have shown that a potassium-rich diet protects against hypertension and cardiovascular diseases (Houston & Harper, 2008). Populations that ingest diets rich in potassium exhibit lower rates of hypertension and have a lower incidence of cardiovascular diseases, whereas those with diets habitually low in potassium (mainly industrialized cultures) appear to have an increased incidence of cardiovascular diseases (Young et al., 1995). The beneficial effects of high potassium intake on reduction of blood pressure and incidence of stroke and cardiovascular diseases are seen also in patients where no correlation has been found between blood pressure and intake of sodium. These results were substantiated by the INTERSALT study, which also showed that the inverse relationship between blood pressure and potassium intake is independent of sodium intake (Stamler, 1997).

The effects of high potassium intake independent of its effect on blood pressure is also seen in its prevention of heart failure and left ventricular hypertrophy, reduction of ventricular arrhythmias in patients with ischemic heart disease, reduction in the risk of stroke, and the prevention of renal vascular, glomerular, and tubular damage (He and MacGregor, 2001, 2008). Increasing intake of fruits and vegetables has been found to be associated with a 27% reduction in the risk of stroke, independent of blood pressure; although in this case, other nutrients and antioxidants found in fruits and vegetables may contribute to the effect (Bazzano et al., 2002).

Despite evidence supporting the cardiovascular protective action of potassium, its mechanism of action is still unknown. It has been proposed that increased potassium consumption increases plasma K^+ concentration, which in turn inhibits free radical formation in vascular endothelial cells, vascular smooth muscle cell proliferation, and platelet aggregation such that the rate of formation of atherosclerotic lesions is decreased (Young et al., 1995). A high-potassium diet and increases in serum potassium, even within the physiological range, may also promote vasodilatation of vascular endothelial and smooth muscle cells (Adrogué et al., 2007).

Dietary potassium intake can also modulate the expression of salt-sensitive blood pressure. Increasing potassium intake has been shown to reduce the frequency of salt sensitivity in men (Morris et al., 1999, Schmidlin et al., 1999). Animal models of both salt-sensitive and non–salt-sensitive rats have shown that supplementation with potassium protects against hypertension, stroke, cardiac hypertrophy, and renal glomerular lesions.

Data from studies on the usefulness of potassium supplementation to reduce blood pressure in hypertensive patients are mixed, because a number of studies did not document the amount of dietary potassium. Hence the total intake of potassium is unknown. Further, as with the studies of dietary sodium restriction in the treatment of hypertension, the success of potassium supplementation depends on the presence of other variables associated with hypertension (Krishna, 1994). In some clinical trials, supplementation with potassium or an increase in dietary potassium from natural foods reduced blood pressure and the incidence of stroke mortality (Young et al., 1995). In other trials, the beneficial effects of potassium were short-lived or nonexistent (Houston and Harper, 2008).

GASTRIC MUCOSAL DAMAGE

Association of High Salt Consumption

Diet, especially high salt intake, is thought to be important in the etiology of stomach cancer. Based on evidence from case-control and epidemiological studies, among the various risk factors that may contribute to atrophic gastritis and the development of gastric cancer are high intakes of salt; some traditionally preserved salted, pickled, or smoked foods; and dried meat and fish; whereas high intakes of fruits and vegetables decrease the risk (Krejs, 2010). Salt acts as an irritant that damages the stomach mucosa and makes the mucosal cells more susceptible to the carcinogenic polycyclic aromatic hydrocarbons and nitrosamines contained in most salted, smoked meat and fish products to induce glandular stomach tumors (Capoferro and Torgersen, 1974). *N*-Nitroso compounds are produced from nitrites present in preserved and smoked food by nitrosating bacteria present in the stomach. A high intragastric *N*-nitrosation of *N*-nitrosamines is related to intragastric lesions, and formation of intragastric *N*-nitrosamine is inhibited by fruit juices, which therefore decrease the risk of gastric cancer (Xu et al., 1993). Salt also enhances colonization of *Helicobacter pylori*, a gastric carcinogen, in the stomach (Fox et al., 1999). A positive association between consumption of salty foods and increased *H. pylori* infection has been reported in a cross-sectional study of Japanese men (Tsugane et al., 1994). Therefore a diet high in salt appears to enhance the initiation of cancer by damaging the gastric mucosal barrier, thereby facilitating the action of *H. pylori* and chemical carcinogens present in the diet, whereas high intake of fruits and vegetables protects the mucosal barrier and decreases the risk for gastric cancer.

THINKING CRITICALLY

J.S., a 45-year-old male, has been gaining weight slowly over the last few years, and lately he has been feeling excessively tired. He is a smoker and has a family history of high blood pressure. After much persuasion from his friends, he decides to go for a medical checkup. His blood pressure is 140/90 mm Hg. Two subsequent measurements yield the same result. His electrocardiogram, kidney function test, fasting blood glucose, and cholesterol levels are within the normal range.

His physician prescribes a thiazide diuretic. He is also encouraged to stop smoking, lose weight, exercise regularly, and follow a healthier diet. His recommended diet is low in sodium, rich in fruits and vegetables, and has reduced total and saturated fat intakes.

1. Why is a thiazide diuretic proposed as a medication for the treatment of J.S.'s high blood pressure?
2. How will these lifestyle changes lower his blood pressure?
3. What is likely to be the main source of sodium in J.S.'s diet? What strategies would you offer J.S. to reduce his sodium intake? Would these dietary strategies modulate his potassium intake? Explain.
4. What would be the best way to assess J.S.'s compliance with a low-sodium diet?

REFERENCES

Adrogué, H. J., & Madias, N. E. (1981). Changes in plasma potassium concentration during acid-base disturbances. *The American Journal of Medicine, 71*, 456–467.

Adrogué, H. J., & Madias, N. E. (2007). Sodium and potassium in the pathogenesis of hypertension. *The New England Journal of Medicine, 356*, 1966–1978.

Antunes-Rodrigues, J., De Castro, M., Elias, L. L. D., Valenca, M. M., & McCann, S. M. (2004). Neuroendocrine control of body fluid metabolism. *Physiological Reviews, 84*, 169–208.

Barr, C. S., Rhodes, P., & Struthers, A. D. (1996). C-type natriuretic peptide. *Peptides, 17*, 1243–1251.

Bazzano, L. A., He, J., Ogden, L. G., Loria, C. M., Vupputuri, S., Myers, L., & Whelton, P. K. (2002). Fruit and vegetable intake and risk of cardiovascular disease in US adults: The first National Health and Nutrition Examination Survey Epidemiologic Follow-up Study. *The American Journal of Clinical Nutrition, 76*, 93–99.

Bunning, P., & Riordan, J. F. (1987). Sulfate potentiation of the chloride activation of angiotensin-converting enzyme. *Biochemistry, 26*, 3374–3377.

Burt, V. L., Whelton, P., Rocella, E. J., Brown, C., Cutler, J. A., Higgins, M., Horan, M. J., & Labarthe, D. (1995). Prevalence of hypertension in the US adult population: Results from the Third National Health and Nutrition Examination Survey, 1988–1991. *Hypertension, 25*, 305–313.

Canessa, C. M., Schild, L., Buell, G., Thorens, B., Gautschi, I., Horisberger, J. D., & Rossier, B. C. (1994). Amiloride-sensitive epithelial Na^+ channel is made of three homologous subunits. *Nature, 367*, 463–467.

Capoferro, R., & Torgersen, O. (1974). The effect of hypertonic saline on the uptake of tritiated 7,12-dimethylbenz[a]anthracene by gastric mucosa. *Scandinavian Journal of Gastroenterology, 9*, 343–349.

Cook, N. R., Cutler, J. A., Obarzanek, E., Buring, J. E., Rexrode, K. M., Kumanyika, S. K., ... Whelton, P. K. (2007). Long term effects of dietary sodium reduction on cardiovascular disease outcomes: Observational follow-up of the trials of hypertension prevention (TOPH). *British Medical Journal, 334*, 885–888.

Cook, N. R., Kumanyika, S. K., & Cutler, J. A. (1998). Effect of change in sodium excretion on change in blood pressure corrected for measurement error. The Trials of Hypertension Prevention, Phase I. *American Journal of Epidemiology, 148*, 431–444.

Cook, N. R., Obarzanek, E., Cutler, J. A., Buring, J. E., Rexrode, K. M., Kumanyika, S. K., ... Whelton, P. K. (2009). Joint effects of sodium and potassium intake on subsequent cardiovascular disease: The trials of hypertension prevention follow-up study. *Archives of Internal Medicine, 169*, 32–40.

Dahl, L. K. (1958). Salt intake and salt need. *New England Journal of Medicine, 258*, 1152–1156.

Daniels, D., & Fluharty, S. J. (2004). Salt appetite: A neurohormonal viewpoint. *Physiology & Behavior, 81*, 319–337.

Egan, B. M., & Lackland, D. T. (2000). Biochemical and metabolic effects of very-low-salt diets. *The American Journal of the Medical Sciences, 320*, 233–239.

Evans, K. J., & Greenberg, A. (2005). Hyperkalemia: A review. *Journal of Intensive Care Medicine, 20*, 272–290.

Field, M., Rao, M. C., & Chang, E. B. (1989). Intestinal electrolyte transport and diarrheal disease. *New England Journal of Medicine, 321*, 800–806.

Fliser, D., Nowack, R., Allendorf-Ostwald, N., Kohl, B., Hubinger, A., & Ritz, E. (1993). Serum lipid changes on low salt diet: Effects of $\alpha 1$-adrenergic blockade. *American Journal of Hypertension, 6*, 320–324.

Folkow, B. (1982). Physiological aspects of primary hypertension. *Physiological Reviews, 62*, 347–504.

Forbes, G. B. (1987). *Human body composition: Growth, aging, nutrition, and activity* (pp. 169–195). New York: Springer-Verlag.

Fox, J. G., Dangler, C. A., Taylor, N. S., King, A., Koh, T. J., & Wang, T. C. (1999). High-salt diet induces gastric epithelial hyperplasia and parietal cell loss, and enhances *Helicobacter pylori* colonization in C57BL/6 mice. *Cancer Research, 59*, 4823–4828.

Ganguly, A., & Donohue, J. P. (1983). Primary aldosteronism: Pathophysiology, diagnosis and treatment. *Journal of Urology, 129*, 241–247.

Geerling, J. C., & Loewy, A. D. (2008). Central regulation of sodium appetite. *Experimental Physiology, 93*, 177–209.

Geleijnse, J. M., Hofman, A., Witteman, J. C., Hazebroek, A. A., Valkenburg, H. A., & Grobbee, D. E. (1997). Long-term effect of neonatal sodium restriction on blood pressure. *Hypertension, 29*, 913–917.

Glover, M., Zuber, A. M., & O'Shaughnessy, K. M. (2011). Hypertension, dietary salt intake, and the role of the thiazide-sensitive sodium chloride transporter NCCT. *Cardiovascular Therapeutics, 29*(1), 68–76.

Greenlee, M., Wingo, C. S., McDonough, A. A., Youn, J. H., & Kone, B. C. (2009). Narrative review: Evolving concepts in potassium homeostasis and hypokalemia. *Annals of Internal Medicine, 150*, 619–625.

Hall, J. E. (2011a). The body fluid compartments: Extracellular and intracellular fluids: Edema. In *Guyton and Hall textbook of medical physiology* (12th ed., pp. 285–301). Philadelphia: Saunders Elsevier.

Hall, J. E. (2011b). Urine formation by the kidneys: I. Glomerular filtration, renal blood flow, and their control. In *Guyton and Hall textbook of medical physiology* (12th ed., pp. 303–322). Philadelphia: Saunders Elsevier.

Hall, J. E. (2011c). Urine concentration and dilution: Regulation of extracellular fluid osmolarity and sodium concentration. In *Guyton and Hall textbook of medical physiology* (12th ed., pp. 345–360). Philadelphia: Saunders Elsevier.

Hall, J. E. (2011d). Renal regulation of potassium, calcium, phosphate, and magnesium: Integration of renal mechanisms for control of blood volume and extracellular fluid volume. In *Guyton and Hall textbook of medical physiology* (12th ed., pp. 361–378). Philadelphia: Saunders Elsevier.

Hall, J. E. (2011e). Digestion and absorption in the gastrointestinal tract. In *Guyton and Hall textbook of medical physiology* (12th ed., pp. 389–398). Philadelphia: Saunders Elsevier.

He, F. J., & MacGregor, G. A. (2001). Beneficial effects of potassium. *BMJ, 323*, 497–501.

He, F. J., & MacGregor, G. A. (2003). How far should salt intake be reduced? *Hypertension, 42*, 1093–1099.

He, F. J., & MacGregor, G. A. (2008). Beneficial effects of potassium on human health. *Physiologia Plantarum, 133*, 725–735.

He, J., Whelton, P. K., Appel, L. J., Charleston, J., & Klag, M. J. (2000). Long-term effects of weight loss and dietary sodium reduction on incidence of hypertension. *Hypertension, 35*, 544–549.

Heaney, R. P. (2006). Role of dietary sodium in osteoporosis. *Journal of the American College of Nutrition, 25*, S271–S276.

Horisberger, J.-D., & Doucet, A. (2007). Renal ion-translocating ATPases: The P-type family. In R. J. Alpern & S. C. Herbert (Eds.), *Seldin and Giebisch's the kidney: Physiology and pathophysiology* (4th ed., pp. 57–90). Oxford: Academic Press.

Houston, M. C., & Harper, K. J. (2008). Potassium, magnesium, and calcium: Their role in both the cause and treatment of hypertension. *Journal of Clinical Hypertension, 10*, 3–11.

Institute of Medicine. (2004). *Dietary Reference Intakes for water, potassium, sodium, chloride, and sulfate*. Washington, DC: The National Academies Press.

Institute of Medicine. (2010). *A population-based policy and systems change approach to prevent and control hypertension: Report brief.* Retrieved from http://www.iom.edu/Reports/2010/A-Population-Based-Policy-and-Systems-Change-Approach-to-Prevent-and-Control-Hypertension.aspx

Jeck, N., Waldegger, P., Doroszewicz, J., Seyberth, H., & Waldegger, S. (2004). A common sequence variation of the CLCNKB gene strongly activates CIC-Kb chloride channel activity. *Kidney International, 65*, 190–197.

Johnson, A. G., Nguyen, T. V., & Davis, D. (2001). Blood pressure is linked to salt intake and modulated by the angiotensinogen gene in normotensive and hypertensive elderly subjects. *Journal of Hypertension, 19*, 1053–1060.

Jones, D. W. (2004). Dietary sodium and blood pressure. *Hypertension, 43*, 932–935.

Kono, S., Ikeda, M., & Ogata, M. (1983). Salt and geographical mortality of gastric cancer and stroke in Japan. *Journal of Epidemiology and Community Health, 37*, 43–46.

Krejs, G. J. (2010). Gastric cancer: Epidemiology and risk factors. *Digestive Diseases, 28*, 600–603.

Krishna, G. G. (1994). Role of potassium in the pathogenesis of hypertension. *The American Journal of the Medical Sciences, 307*(Suppl. 1), S21–S25.

Larsen, T. M., Laughlin, L. T., Holden, H. M., Rayment, I., & Reed, G. H. (1994). Structure of rabbit muscle pyruvate kinase complexed with Mn^{2+}, K^+, and pyruvate. *Biochemistry, 33*, 6301–6309.

Levin, E. R., Gardner, D. G., & Samson, W. K. (1998). Natriuretic peptides. *New England Journal of Medicine, 339*, 321–328.

MacGregor, G. A., Markandu, N. D., Sagnella, G. A., Singer, D. R. D. J., & Cappuccio, F. P. (1989). Double-blind study of three sodium intakes and long-term effects of sodium restriction in essential hypertension. *Lancet, 2*, 1244–1247.

Mancilha-Carvalho, J. J., & Souza e Silva, N. A. (2003). The Yanomami Indians in the INTERSALT study. *Arquivos Brasileiros de Cardiologia, 80*, 289–300.

Marques, F. Z., Campain, A. E., Yang, Y. H. J., & Morris, B. J. (2010). Meta-analysis of genome-wide gene expression differences in onset and maintenance phases of genetic hypertension. *Hypertension, 56*, 319–324.

Moratinos, J., & Reverte, M. (1993). Effects of catecholamines on plasma potassium: The role of α- and β-adrenoceptors. *Fundamental & Clinical Pharmacology, 7*, 143–153.

Morris, R. C., Jr., Sebastian, A., Forman, A., Tanaka, M., & Schmidlin, O. (1999). Normotensive salt-sensitivity: Effects of race and dietary potassium. *Hypertension, 33*, 18–23.

National Research Council. (1989). *Recommended Dietary Allowances* (10th ed., pp. 247–261). Washington, DC: National Academy Press.

Nerup, J. (1974). Addison's disease—clinical studies: A report of 108 cases. *Acta Endocrinologica, 76*, 127–141.

Oliver, W. J., Cohen, E. L., & Neel, J. V. (1975). Blood pressure, sodium intake and sodium-related hormones in the Yanomamo Indians, a "no-salt" culture. *Circulation, 52*, 146–151.

Quail, A. W., Woods, R., & Korner, P. I. (1987). Cardiac and arterial baroreceptor influences in release of vasopressin and renin during hemorrhage. *The American Journal of Physiology, 252*, H1120–H1126.

Reusser, M. E., & McCarron, D. A. (1994). Micronutrient effects on blood pressure regulation. *Nutrition Reviews, 52*, 367–375.

Ritz, E., Koleganova, N., & Piecha, G. (2009). Role of sodium intake in the progression of chronic kidney disease. *Journal of Renal Nutrition, 19*, 61–62.

Rodriguez, B. L., Labarthe, D. R., Huang, B., & Lopez-Gomez, J. (1994). Rise of blood pressure with age: New evidence of population differences. *Hypertension, 24*, 779–785.

Rodriguez-Soriano, J. (1995). Potassium homeostasis and its disturbance in children. *Pediatric Nephrology, 9*, 364–374.

Rose, G., Stamler, J., Stamler, R., Elliott, P., Marmot, M., Pyorala, K., Kesteloot, H., Joossens, J., Hansson, L., Mancia, G., Dyer, A., Kromhout, D., Laaser, U., & Sans, S. (1998). Intersalt: An international study of electrolyte excretion and blood pressure. Results for 24 hour urinary sodium and potassium excretion. *British Medical Journal, 297*, 319–328.

Sacks, F. M., Svetkey, L. P., Vollmer, W. M., Appel, L. J., Bray, G. A., Harsha, D., … Lin, P. H. (2001). Effects of blood pressure of reduced dietary sodium and the Dietary Approaches to Stop Hypertension (DASH) diet. *New England Journal of Medicine, 344*, 3–10.

Sanchez-Castillo, C. P., Branch, W. J., & James, W. P. (1987a). A test of the validity of the lithium-marker technique for monitoring dietary sources of salt in men. *Clinical Science, 72*, 87–94.

Sanchez-Castillo, C. P., Warrender, S., Whitehead, T. P., & James, W. P. (1987b). An assessment of the sources of dietary salt in a British population. *Clinical Science, 72*, 95–102.

Schmidlin, O., Forman, A., Tanaka, M., Sebastian, A., & Morris, R. C. (1999). NaCl-induced renal vasoconstriction in salt-sensitive African-Americans: Antipressor and hemodynamic effects of potassium bicarbonate. *Hypertension, 22*, 633–639.

Simon, D. B., Bindra, R. S., Mansfield, T. A., Nelson-Williams, C., Mendonca, E., Stone, R., … Lifton, R. P. (1997). Mutations in the chloride channel gene, CLCNKB, cause Bartter's syndrome type III. *Nature Genetics, 17*, 171–178.

Stamler, J. (1997). The INTERSALT Study: Background, methods, findings, and implications. *The American Journal of Clinical Nutrition, 65*(Suppl.), S626–S642.

Strazzullo, P., D'Elia, L., Kandala, N. B., & Cappuccio, F. P. (2009). Salt intake, stroke, and cardiovascular disease: Meta-analysis of prospective studies. *BMJ 2009, 339*, b4567.

Tsugane, S., & Sasazuki, S. (2007). Diet and the risk of gastric cancer: Review of epidemiological evidence. *Gastric Cancer, 10*, 75–83.

Tsugane, S., Tei, Y., Takahashi, T., Watanabe, S., & Sugano, K. (1994). Salty food intake and risk of *Helicobacter pylori* infection. *Japanese Journal of Cancer Research, 85*, 474–478.

Vesely, D. L. (2007). Natriuretic hormones. In R. J. Alpern & S. C. Herbert (Eds.), *Seldin and Giebisch's the kidney: Physiology and pathophysiology* (4th ed., pp. 947–977). Oxford: Academic Press.

Xu, G. P., So, P. J., & Reed, P. I. (1993). Hypothesis on the relationship between gastric cancer and intragastric nitrosation: *N*-Nitrosamines in gastric juice of subjects from a high-risk area for gastric cancer and the inhibition of *N*-nitrosamine formation by fruit juices. *European Journal of Cancer Prevention, 2*, 25–36.

Yang, Q., Liu, T., Kuklina, E. A., Flanders, D., Hong, Y., Gillespie, C., … Hyu, F. B. (2011). Sodium and potassium intake and mortality among US adults: Prospective data from the Third National Health and Nutrition Examination Survey. *Archives of Internal Medicine, 171*(13), 1183–1191.

Young, D. B., Lin, H., & McCabe, R. D. (1995). Potassium's cardiovascular protective mechanisms. *The American Journal of Physiology, 268*, R825–R837.

RECOMMENDED READINGS

Adrogué, H. J., & Madias, N. E. (2007). Sodium and potassium in the pathogenesis of hypertension. *The New England Journal of Medicine, 356*, 1966–1978.

Bazzano, L. A., He, J., Ogden, L. G., Loria, C. M., Vupputuri, S., Myers, L., & Whelton, P. K. (2002). Fruit and vegetable intake and risk of cardiovascular disease in US adults: The first National Health and Nutrition Examination Survey Epidemiologic Follow-up Study. *The American Journal of Clinical Nutrition, 76*, 93–99.

Cook, N. R., Cutler, J. A., Obarzanek, E., Buring, J. E., Rexrode, K. M., Kumanyika, S. K., Appel, L. J., & Whelton, P. K. (2007). Long term effects of dietary sodium reduction on cardiovascular disease outcomes: Observational follow-up of the trials of hypertension prevention (TOPH). *British Medical Journal, 334*, 885–888.

Evans, K. J., & Greenberg, A. (2005). Hyperkalemia: A review. *Journal of Intensive Care Medicine, 20*, 272–290.

Greenlee, M., Wingo, C. S., McDonough, A. A., Youn, J. H., & Kone, B. C. (2009). Narrative review: Evolving concepts in potassium homeostasis and hypokalemia. *Annals of Internal Medicine, 150*, 619–625.

Hall, J. E. (2011). The body fluids and kidneys. In *Guyton and Hall textbook of medical physiology* (12th ed., pp. 285–398). Philadelphia: Saunders Elsevier.

Institute of Medicine. (2004). *Dietary Reference Intakes for water, potassium, sodium, chloride, and sulfate.* Washington, DC: The National Academies Press.

Jones, D. W. (2004). Dietary sodium and blood pressure. *Hypertension, 43*, 932–935.

Krejs, G. J. (2010). Gastric cancer: Epidemiology and risk factors. *Digestive Diseases*, *28*, 600–603.

National Research Council. (1989). *Recommended Dietary Allowances* (10th ed., pp. 247–261). Washington, DC: National Academy Press.

Stamler, J. (1997). The INTERSALT Study: Background, methods, findings, and implications. *The American Journal of Clinical Nutrition*, *65*(Suppl.), S626–S642.

Vesely, D. L. (2007). Natriuretic hormones. In R. J. Alpern, & S. C. Herbert (Eds.), *Seldin & Giebisch's the kidney: Physiology and pathophysiology* (4th ed., pp. 947–977). Oxford: Academic Press.

CHAPTER 35

Body Fluids and Water Balance

Hwai-Ping Sheng, PhD

COMMON ABBREVIATIONS

AVP arginine vasopressin, also known as antidiuretic hormone (ADH)
AQP aquaporin
C_{osm} osmolar clearance
C_{water} free-water clearance
Osm osmoles

PHYSIOLOGICAL FUNCTIONS OF WATER

Water is an essential nutrient vital to the existence of both animals and plants. In the body, water is present inside and around the cells and within all blood vessels. It lubricates joints and moistens tissues such as those in the eyes, nose, and mouth. The volume of the intracellular fluid provides turgor to the tissues, which is important for the tissue or organ form and ultimately the body form. Water performs several functions that are essential to life. It is the principal fluid medium in which nutrients, minerals, gases, and enzymes are dissolved. The extracellular water bathing the cells serves as a medium for the transport of nutrients and oxygen to the cells and for removing wastes from the cells, which will be eliminated by the liver and kidneys. The intracellular water establishes the physicochemical medium that allows various metabolic processes to take place. Another important physiological function of water is its role in the regulation of body temperature. This is achieved by removing excess heat from the body by evaporative water loss from the skin.

BODY WATER COMPARTMENTS

BODY WATER CONTENT

Water makes up the largest component of the body; its content in the body varies with age, sex, and adiposity of the individual. In the neonate, water makes up approximately 75% of body weight, decreasing progressively to about 60% in the young adult, and continuing to decline to approximately 50% at about 50 years of age. The higher proportion of water in the neonate is for the most part the result of a larger fraction of its body mass as extracellular fluid space. A combination of factors causes the proportion of extracellular fluid space to decrease gradually with an increase in age. These factors include an increase in the amount of cellular tissues, such as muscles, at the expense of extracellular space and an increase in the proportion of body mass made up of adipose tissues and the supporting structures of skeleton, cartilage, and connective tissues, all of which contain a relatively low water content.

Adult women have lower water content when compared with men of comparable age, and obese individuals have lower water content than their leaner counterparts. These variations can be attributed to differences in the proportion of adipose tissue relative to lean tissue in the body. Fat cells have a relatively low content of water, about 10%, whereas other cellular tissues such as muscles contain an average of 70% water. Therefore water content in the body varies inversely with the relative proportion of adipose tissue, and this can explain the lower water content both in women and in obese individuals. However, when body water is calculated on a lean body weight basis, it constitutes a relatively constant proportion, 73.2% for adults and 82% for neonates.

DISTRIBUTION OF BODY WATER

Water in the body is distributed throughout the various body fluid compartments. The simplest subdivision is into an intracellular and an extracellular compartment, with the two compartments separated by the cell membrane (Figure 35-1). On average, a 70-kg adult has 42 L of water, of which two thirds (28 L) is intracellular and one third (14 L) is extracellular. The extracellular fluid is made up of the interstitial fluid (11 L), which bathes the cells and includes the lymph, the plasma (3 L), and the cavity or transcellular fluids, of which the largest volume is secretory fluids in the lumen of the gastrointestinal tract.

The distribution of water in the various compartments determines the size of the compartments and is governed by solute particles and physical forces that maintain equilibrium across membranes separating these compartments. Osmotic forces and hydrostatic pressures are the prime determinants of water distribution in the body.

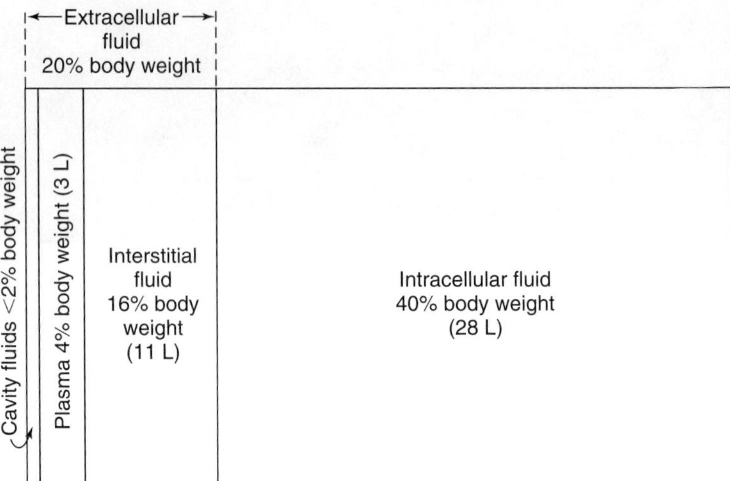

FIGURE 35-1 Major body fluid compartments of an adult. Intraluminal gastrointestinal water constitutes the largest fraction of the cavity fluids. In general, water moves freely between adjacent compartments along an osmotic gradient.

FLUID DISTRIBUTION BETWEEN EXTRACELLULAR AND INTRACELLULAR FLUID COMPARTMENTS

Osmosis and Osmotic Pressure

Osmotic forces across a semipermeable membrane (impermeable to solutes but permeable to water) separating two compartments govern the distribution and direction of water movement between these compartments. This concept is explained simply in Figure 35-2. The two compartments, A and B, which contain the same volume of fluid but different numbers of solute particles are separated by a semipermeable membrane. Water diffuses across the membrane in both directions, but more water molecules diffuse from compartment A, a region of higher water concentration (lower solute concentration), to compartment B, which is a region of lower water concentration (higher solute concentration). This process of net movement of water caused by a concentration difference of water or solutes is called osmosis. Osmosis of water results in the expansion of compartment B at the expense of compartment A. No further net diffusion of water occurs when the solute concentrations in both compartments are equal, that is, when osmotic equilibrium is established. To reach this state of equilibrium, the volume of compartment B has increased at the expense of compartment A. This situation can occur only when the two compartments are flexible volumetrically so that the net flow of water from one compartment to another does not create a pressure difference across the membrane. However, if the walls of compartment B do not expand, the increase in hydrostatic pressure in compartment B due to influx of water will oppose further inflow of water. The amount of pressure to be applied in order to prevent the inflow of water through the membrane into compartment B is called osmotic pressure (Rose and Post, 2001). The osmotic pressure of a solution therefore reflects the concentration of osmotically active particles in that solution.

The process of osmosis also explains the movement of water across cell membranes. Most cell membranes are semipermeable, that is, relatively impermeable to most solutes but highly permeable to water. Although water is a polar molecule, it is able to penetrate the nonpolar lipid region of membranes through a group of transmembrane channel proteins called aquaporins (AQPs), which form channels through which water can readily diffuse. The number of AQPs, also known as water channels, differs in membranes of different tissues. In some cells, the number of AQPs, and thus the permeability to water, can be altered in response to hormones. In the steady state, the volume of water that diffuses across the membrane in either direction is balanced precisely so that no net diffusion of water occurs and the volume of the cell remains unchanged. However, under certain conditions, when a concentration difference for water develops across the cell membrane by active transport of solutes, osmotic forces will develop across the cell membrane and water will move rapidly between these two compartments until an osmotic equilibrium is achieved. When this happens, net influx of water causes the cell to expand, whereas net efflux of water causes the cell to contract. Therefore at equilibrium the osmolar concentration (osmolarity) of the intracellular and interstitial fluid compartments remain similar, at approximately 290 mOsm/L.

Osmolality and Osmolarity

As noted, a difference in the solute concentrations of two fluid compartments separated by a semipermeable membrane causes osmotic movement of water. Therefore it is useful to have a concentration term that refers to the total concentration of solute particles that causes osmotic movement of water. Because it is the number and not the size or type of solute particles that causes water movement and hence contributes to the osmotic pressure of a solution, the term *osmole* (Osm, or osmol) is used to describe the number of osmotically active solute particles, regardless of their mass. One osmole is equal to 1 mole of an undissociated solute. One mole of a pure substance has a mass in grams equal to its molecular weight. A solution containing either 1 mole of glucose (180 g) or 1 mole of albumin (70,000 g) in 1 kg of water has a concentration of 1 Osm/kg of water, because

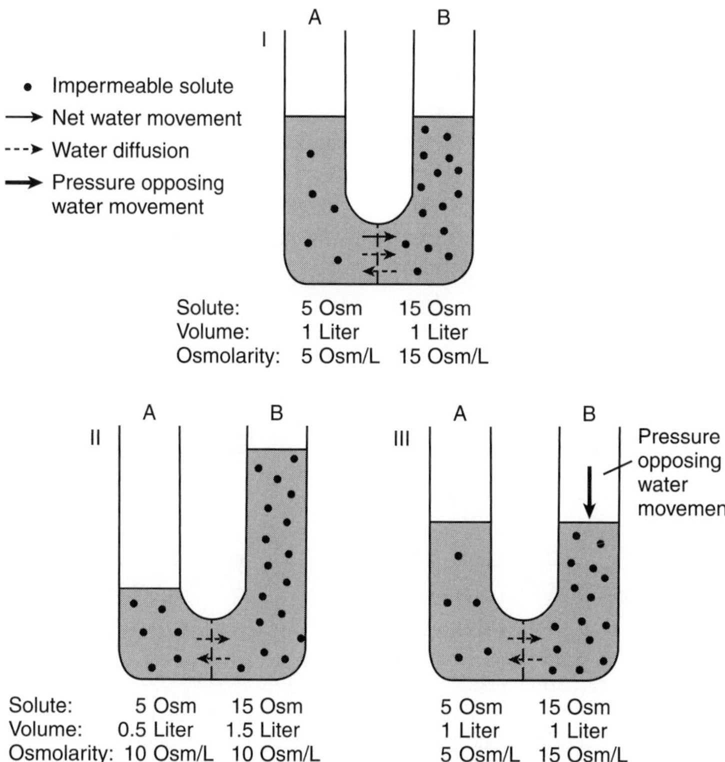

FIGURE 35-2 Osmosis and osmotic pressure can be illustrated by two compartments separated by a semipermeable membrane, permeable to water but not to solutes (circles). In diagram I, compartments A and B are shown filled with equal volumes of solution, but the solution in compartment A is hypo-osmotic with reference to the solution in compartment B. There is net movement of water from A to B until the solutions in the two compartments are iso-osmotic, as shown in diagram II. The movement of water across the semipermeable membrane leads to a change in the initial volumes at equilibrium. In this example, the volume of compartment B increased, whereas the volume of compartment A decreased. Because the volume of compartment B increased, there were no significant changes in hydrostatic pressure in the compartments. As shown in diagram III, application of a pressure can prevent osmotic movement of water across the semipermeable membrane. This pressure is called the osmotic pressure.

neither glucose nor albumin dissociates in solution. If the solute dissociates into 2 ions in solution, then 1 mole of the solute will contain 2 Osm. For example, 1 mole of sodium chloride (NaCl) dissociates to yield 1 mole each of sodium and chloride ions; therefore 1 mole of NaCl in 1 kg of water will have an osmolal concentration of 2 Osm/kg of water. Likewise, 1 mole of a solute that dissociates into 3 ions in solution (for example, $CaCl_2$) has an osmolal concentration of 3 Osm/kg.

Strictly speaking, ions in solutions exert interionic attraction to or repulsion from each other and can therefore change the actual number of osmotically active particles in the solution. Any deviations can be corrected for, if the osmotic coefficient for the molecule is known. For example, the osmotic coefficient for NaCl is 0.93. Therefore 1 mole of NaCl in 1 kg of water has an osmolal concentration of 1.86 rather than 2 mOsm/kg. In practice, the osmotic coefficients of different solutes are often disregarded when determining the osmolal concentrations of physiological solutions.

The concentration of body fluids can be expressed as Osm/kg water (osmolality) or Osm/L fluid (osmolarity). Therefore osmolarity is affected by the volume of solutes present in the body fluid, but osmolality is not. The normal osmolarity of plasma is approximately 290 mOsm/L. Solutes, mainly proteins, occupy about 5% of plasma volume. Therefore the osmolality of plasma is about 5% higher, at approximately 305 mOsm/kg of water. Because body fluids are dilute solutions, differences between osmolality and osmolarity are small and the two terms are often used synonymously. In practice, it is easier to express solute concentrations of plasma in mOsm/L than in mOsm/kg.

Iso-osmotic, Hypo-osmotic, and Hyperosmotic Solutions

The terms *iso-osmotic, hypo-osmotic,* and *hyperosmotic* are used to describe the relation of osmolar concentrations between different solutions. When two solutions are of equal osmolarity, they are iso-osmotic. A solution is hypo-osmotic when its osmolarity is lower than that of the reference solution and hyperosmotic when its osmolarity is higher. When cells are suspended in a hypo-osmotic solution, water enters the cells, causing them to expand. Conversely, when cells are suspended in a hyperosmotic solution, water diffuses out of the cells, causing them to contract. One would expect that, when cells are suspended in an iso-osmotic solution, no net flux of water would occur and cell size would remain the same. This is true only if cells are suspended in an iso-osmotic solution in which no net movement of solutes occurs across cell membranes. If cells are suspended in an iso-osmotic solution containing a highly permeant solute, such as urea, it diffuses into cells along its concentration gradient, causing an osmotic flow of water into cells, and the cells expand (Figure 35-3). Thus another term, *tonicity,* is used to describe the physiological osmolar concentration of a solution.

Isotonic, Hypotonic, and Hypertonic Solutions

Tonicity refers not only to the osmolarity of a solution relative to plasma but also to whether the solution will affect cell volume. An isotonic solution has an osmolarity of 290 mOsm/L, and when cells are placed in this solution, no net flux of water occurs. Solutions in which suspended cells shrink are hypertonic, and solutions in which suspended cells expand are hypotonic. Sodium chloride solution at

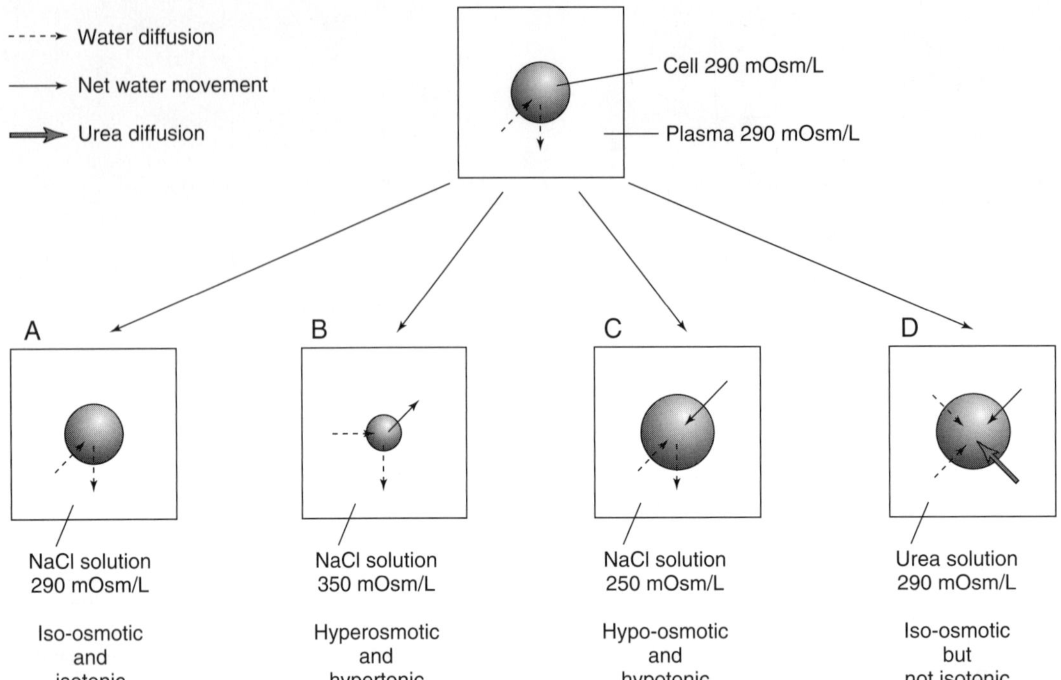

FIGURE 35-3 The concepts of osmolarity and tonicity can be illustrated by a red blood cell suspended in various media. In the body, red blood cells are suspended in plasma; because plasma is iso-osmotic and isotonic, the rate of water diffusion out of the cell is equal to that into the cell. No net movement of water occurs, and the cell volume remains the same. When a red blood cell is suspended in a 290 mOsm/L NaCl solution, no net movement of water occurs (**A**). The solution is iso-osmotic and isotonic. When a red blood cell is suspended in a 350 mOsm/L NaCl solution, there is a net movement of water out of the cell along an osmotic gradient (**B**). The cell will shrink. The solution is hyperosmotic and hypertonic. When a red blood cell is suspended in a 250 mOsm/L NaCl solution, there is a net movement of water into the cell, causing cell expansion and hemolysis (**C**). The solution is hypo-osmotic and hypotonic. When a red blood cell is suspended in a 290 mOsm/L urea solution, urea diffuses into the cell along its concentration gradient and water follows, resulting in net entry of water, which causes the cell to hemolyze (**D**). (The increased volume of water and solute in the cell causes the cell membrane to rupture.) The solution is iso-osmotic but not isotonic.

a concentration of 290 mOsm/L is an isotonic solution because sodium is kept out of cells by active transport processes. Conversely, a solution of urea at a concentration of 290 mOsm/L is iso-osmotic to plasma but not isotonic. Red blood cells suspended in an iso-osmotic solution of urea will expand and hemolyze because of influx of water. Urea diffuses readily into cells along its concentration gradient causing a progressive decrease in the osmolarity of the suspension fluid and causing water to move into the cells to maintain iso-osmolarity. It is important, therefore, to understand the difference between osmolarity and tonicity, especially in intravenous fluid therapy. A physiological saline solution contains 0.9% NaCl (290 mOsm/L), is isotonic with plasma, and is used commonly as replacement fluid during the postoperative period.

Osmolarity and Volume of Extracellular and Intracellular Fluid Compartments

In contrast to movement of water across cell membranes, movement of solutes is more variable and depends on the permeability characteristics of cell membranes as well as the presence of specific membrane transporters. Whereas cell membranes are relatively impermeable to proteins and organic phosphates, they selectively extrude sodium out of the cell in exchange for potassium. Therefore sodium and its accompanying anions, mainly chloride, are the major solutes in the extracellular fluid. Inside the cells, the major cations are potassium and magnesium, and the major anions are proteins and organic phosphates. Water will distribute passively between the intracellular and extracellular compartments according to the osmolar concentrations, which are determined by the quantity of diffusible and nondiffusible solutes present in each of these compartments. Consequently, the volume of each of these compartments depends on the amount of solutes present and the total volume of body water. Whenever an inequality of osmolar concentration occurs across the cell membrane, water diffuses rapidly from the compartment of lower osmolarity to one of higher osmolarity so that any differences in osmolarity are corrected within a few minutes. In the steady state, the osmolarity of extracellular and intracellular fluids are equal.

FLUID DISTRIBUTION BETWEEN PLASMA AND INTERSTITIAL FLUID COMPARTMENTS

Plasma circulates throughout the body and provides a medium for transporting water, solutes, and gases from one part of the body to another. As the blood flows through the capillaries, interstitial fluid is delivered continuously to tissues by ultrafiltration near the arterial ends and returned to the circulation near the venous ends by forces across the capillary endothelium. In this way, the absorbed solutes and water from the gastrointestinal tract and dissolved oxygen from the lungs are carried to the tissues by plasma and by interstitial fluid. Similarly, metabolic waste products, including dissolved carbon dioxide from tissues, are carried by the same route but in the opposite direction, to the kidneys, liver, and lungs to be eliminated. Therefore, as first described by Claude Bernard (1813–1879) as the milieu intérieur, the interstitial fluid constitutes the immediate environment of the body cells.

The interstitial fluid protects the cells in the body from direct contact with the external environment and acts as a buffer for the cells from sudden changes in solute and water content caused by ingestion or loss from the body. The body possesses various physiological control systems that regulate the elimination of solutes and water from the body, so that the composition and volume of the plasma and, indirectly, the composition and volume of the interstitial and intracellular fluids are maintained relatively constant.

A small fraction of interstitial fluid is continuously drained away through lymphatic channels. This fluid, called lymph, drains into the thoracic duct and returns to the circulation via the right subclavian vein. The total volume of lymph is small, about 1 to 2 L. Transcellular, or cavity, fluids are generally considered to be specialized secretory fluids produced by active transport processes occurring across epithelial cells. These fluids differ from interstitial fluid in that they are not simple ultrafiltrates of plasma; their compositions differ markedly from that of plasma and are adapted specifically to the function of a particular organ. Examples of transcellular fluids are fluids in the lumen of the gastrointestinal tract, the cerebrospinal fluid, and fluids in the intraocular, pleural, peritoneal, and synovial spaces. Of these, intraluminal gastrointestinal fluid constitutes the largest fraction. The total volume occupied by these fluids is small, about 1 to 2 L.

Movement of Fluid Across Capillary Endothelium

The fenestrations (20- to 100-nm diameter pores) of the capillary endothelium are highly permeable to almost all solutes in the plasma except proteins, so that interstitial fluid and plasma have a similar composition except for the higher concentration of proteins in the plasma. Except in the brain, diffusion and bulk flow of protein-free plasma constitute the most important means by which net movement of nutrients, gases, metabolic end products, and fluid occur across the capillary walls. Two factors, the Gibbs–Donnan equilibrium and the Starling forces, affect the distribution of solutes and flow of protein-free plasma through these fenestrations.

Gibbs–Donnan Equilibrium

On average, the concentration of proteins in the interstitial fluid is less than 10 g/L, compared with 73 g/L in the plasma. The differential concentration of protein affects the distribution of diffusible ions and osmotic pressures across the capillary endothelium. When two fluid compartments, A and B, are separated by a semipermeable membrane, the concentrations of any diffusible cation or anion are equal across the membrane so that no differences in concentration exist for any of the ions. On the basis of thermodynamic principles, Gibbs and Donnan showed that at equilibrium, the product of the concentrations of diffusible cations and anions in the two compartments are equal and electrical neutrality is maintained:

$$[\text{Cation}]_A \times [\text{Anion}]_A = [\text{Cation}]_B \times [\text{Anion}]_B$$

When a nondiffusible cation or anion is added to one of the compartments, the diffusible ions will redistribute themselves so that the concentration of each ion will no longer be equal across the cell membrane.

At normal plasma pH of 7.4, the majority of plasma proteins behave as negatively charged particles. Because proteins are confined to the vascular compartment, electrical neutrality in the plasma can be maintained only by an unequal distribution of the smaller diffusible ions, resulting in lower concentrations of each of the diffusible anions and higher concentrations of each of the diffusible cations in the plasma than in the interstitial fluid. At a normal concentration of plasma protein (73 g/L) this effect is small, with the concentration of monovalent anions (for example, chloride) about 5% lower and that of monovalent cations (for example, sodium and potassium) approximately 5% higher in the plasma than in the interstitial fluid. For all practical purposes, the concentrations of ions in the plasma and interstitial fluid can be considered to be about equal.

Starling's Law

The concentration difference of proteins across capillary endothelium not only affects the distribution of diffusible ions, but also causes an osmotic gradient across the capillary endothelium. This osmotic gradient exerts a pressure that is called the colloid osmotic pressure or oncotic pressure. Colloid osmotic pressure together with hydrostatic pressure are of physiological importance in determining net water movement across the capillary endothelium.

Starling first proposed the concept that the two opposing forces governing water movement across the capillary endothelium are created by the difference in hydrostatic pressure and the difference in colloid osmotic pressure across the capillary wall (Taylor, 1981). Therefore four variables determine the movement of fluid: hydrostatic pressures and protein concentrations in the plasma and the interstitial fluid. The following equations describe the forces responsible for net water movement across an idealized capillary endothelium:

$$\text{Net driving pressure} = (P_c - P_{if}) - (\pi_c - \pi_{if})$$

$$\text{Net volume of water flow} = K_f[(P_c - P_{if}) - (\pi_c - \pi_{if})]$$

where K_f is the permeability coefficient (product of water permeability and filtration surface area) of the capillary endothelium, P_c is the capillary hydrostatic pressure, P_{if} is the interstitial fluid hydrostatic pressure, π_c is the capillary colloid osmotic pressure, and π_{if} is the interstitial fluid colloid osmotic pressure.

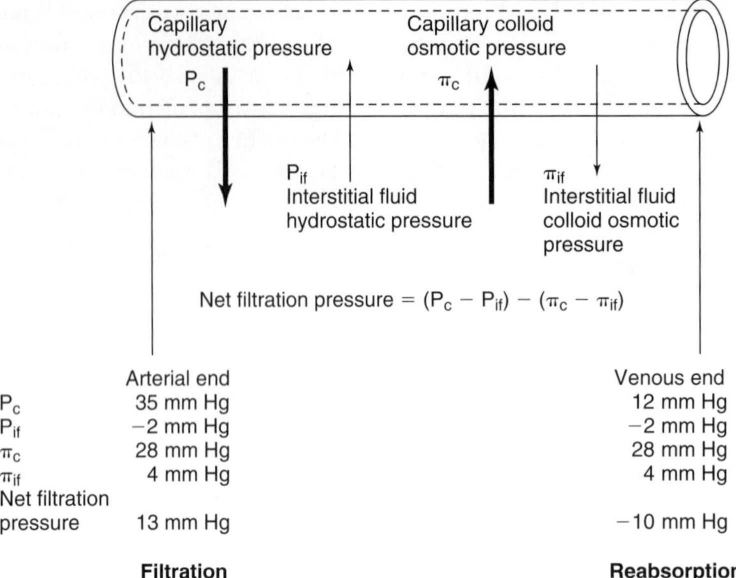

FIGURE 35-4 Illustration of the Starling forces across the capillary endothelium.

As blood flows along the capillary, the balance of these forces is a net pressure gradient favoring the movement of a small amount of fluid from the arterial end of the capillary into the interstitium. This causes hydrostatic pressure to decrease along the length of the capillary so that much of the fluid reenters the capillary at the venous end (Figure 35-4). The small amount of fluid that remains in the interstitium is returned to the circulation by the lymphatic vessels, which empty into the subclavian vein via the thoracic duct (Taylor, 1981).

Under normal circumstances, the difference in hydrostatic pressure between capillary blood and interstitial fluid favors filtration out of the capillary, and the difference in colloid osmotic pressure favors absorption of interstitial fluid into the capillary. An imbalance in any of these forces affects net movement of water across the capillary endothelium and ultimately will affect distribution of fluid between the plasma and interstitial compartments. For example, a decrease in plasma protein concentration in disease states, such as liver and kidney diseases, results in an accumulation of fluid in the interstitial spaces, causing edema.

Other factors that may affect the distribution of fluid across capillary endothelium include the integrity of the endothelium and the lymphatic drainage system. An increase in capillary permeability allows plasma albumin to enter the interstitium to an abnormal extent, thereby reducing the difference in colloid osmotic pressure (i.e., $\pi_c - \pi_{if}$ in Starling's equation). This increase in permeability occurs in sepsis, venom shock, drug overdose, and anaphylactic reactions, and it can cause large volumes of fluid to leak from the vascular to the interstitial space. The lymphatic system can reduce the volume of edema fluid by returning it to the intravascular system via the thoracic duct. Blockage of lymphatic drainage causes accumulation of fluid in the interstitial fluid compartment.

TABLE 35-1 Daily Water Balance in a 65-kg Man Calculated to Illustrate Minimal Required Drinking Water Intake

Water Intake		Water Loss	
SOURCE	LITERS	ROUTE	LITERS
Preformed water	0.85	Insensible—lungs	0.30
Metabolic water	0.37	Insensible—skin	0.40
Drinking—minimum	0.22	Feces	0.10
		Urine	0.64
Total	1.44	Total	1.44

WATER BALANCE

For an individual to maintain water balance, the amount of water consumed must equal the amount lost from the body. This is illustrated in Table 35-1 for a 65-kg man in a temperate environment who consumes a balanced diet that is adequate for his energy requirements. Even with the excretion of a maximally concentrated urine, water normally contained in the food (preformed water) and water produced by oxidation of food (metabolic water, or water of oxidation) are inadequate to compensate for losses of water from the respiratory tract, skin, gastrointestinal tract, and kidneys. Therefore an individual must ingest free water to maintain water balance. The body possesses several homeostatic regulatory mechanisms capable of maintaining balance of water over a wide range of water intakes so that health remains unimpaired. An inequality between intake and loss of water ultimately alters the composition and osmolarity of body fluids.

LOSS OF WATER

Water is lost from the body by essentially four different routes: respiratory tract, skin, gastrointestinal tract, and kidneys. Of these four, water loss from the kidneys is the most important and is regulated by various neuroendocrine pathways to maintain a constant osmolarity of the body fluids.

Water Loss through Respiratory Tract and Skin

Insensible Water Loss

Water is lost continuously from the body by two passive evaporative routes: from the upper respiratory tract during respiration and from the skin. These passive evaporative losses are termed "insensible losses" or "insensible perspiration" because they occur continuously and without our awareness. The amount of evaporative water loss from the respiratory tract depends on the ventilatory volume and water pressure gradient. A water pressure gradient occurs because expired air is saturated with moisture to a vapor pressure of about 47 mm Hg, whereas the vapor pressure of inspired air is usually less than 47 mm Hg. An individual loses an average of between 0.14 and 0.47 L daily by this route; the amount of the loss depends on body size, the degree of physical activity, and ambient temperature and humidity. It is to be expected that evaporative water loss from the lungs is increased in physical activity and when the atmospheric vapor pressure decreases (i.e., in cold, dry climates). Insensible water loss from the skin, which occurs independent of sweating, averages between 0.3 and 0.5 L daily for an individual living in a temperate environment and doing minimal physical activity (Geigy Scientific Tables, 1981).

On average, an individual will lose a total of 0.4 to 0.9 L of water daily from insensible loss through both the respiratory tract and skin. When body temperature rises higher than 39° C, evaporative loss from the respiratory tract increases because of a significant increase in the respiratory minute volume (Reithner, 1981). The increase in water loss by the respiratory route can be as much as an additional 0.1 L daily at elevated body temperatures. Dermal losses can increase much more due to sweating.

Sweat

Dermal losses due to sweating at high body temperatures can be substantial. Cutaneous water loss due mainly to sweating can increase by as much as 6 to 8 times the basal level when rectal temperature is above 39.5° C (Lamke et al., 1980).

The volume of water lost as sweat is highly variable, depending on the environment and the physical activity of the individual. In hot weather and during strenuous activity, evaporation of sweat from the skin is an effective means of dissipating the excess heat from the skin thus cooling the body and defending the core temperature of the body. For every gram of water that evaporates from the skin, 0.58 kcal of heat is lost from the body. Daily water losses as sweat are determined by the body's need for evaporative heat loss and are influenced by the environment and the metabolic rate. Water loss as sweat is substantially less in an environment of moderate temperature and humidity than in a warm, humid environment where loss through perspiration can be considerable.

Normally the volume of sweat in a 65-kg adult doing light work at an ambient temperature of 29° C (84.2° F) amounts to about 2 to 3 L daily, but it can increase to a maximum of about 2 to 4 L per hour for a short time in an unacclimatized individual who is performing heavy physical activity in a hot and humid environment. This levels off to about 0.5 L per hour over a 24-hour period as the duration of perspiration increases (Geigy Scientific Tables, 1981). Even at maximal sweating, the rate of heat loss may not be rapid enough to dissipate the heat from the body. When the body temperature rises to a critical level, higher than 40.5° C (105° F), the individual is likely to develop heatstroke. However, after acclimatization to hot weather for a few weeks, an individual will have greater tolerance of the hot and humid environment and can as much as double his or her sweating rate. Evaporation of this large volume of sweat effectively removes the excess heat from the body. Acclimatization also involves a decrease in the concentration of sodium chloride in the sweat, allowing for better conservation of sodium chloride (Takamata et al., 2001). The loss of several liters of sweat a day in a hot climate results in serious losses of both sodium chloride and water, which need to be replaced.

Water Loss by the Gastrointestinal Tract

The volume of water loss in feces is small, about 0.1 L a day, and does not cause problems with water balance unless excessive loss occurs during diarrhea. The volume of fluid ingested varies among individuals but averages about 1.7 L daily. Added to this ingested volume, the small intestine receives an additional 7 L of secretory fluids, which are made up of salivary, gastric, biliary, pancreatic, and intestinal secretions. Normally approximately 90% to 95% of these fluids is absorbed by the small intestine, and the remainder by the colon, leaving only approximately 0.1 L of water to be excreted in the feces. Absorption of water in the intestine is passive, along an osmotic gradient created by the absorption of nutrients from the lumen of the intestine into the plasma. In diseases of the gastrointestinal tract, large volumes of water can be lost in the feces, causing diarrhea. This occurs in gastroenteritis due to bacterial or viral infection or in any situation in which absorption of nutrients is compromised. Certain bacterial toxins, such as cholera toxin, can increase the secretion of sodium chloride from the crypt cells of the small intestinal mucosa into the lumen of the small intestine. The lumen becomes hyperosmotic, and water diffuses from the plasma into the lumen, causing diarrhea. Several liters of fluid, up to 10 to 20 L, can be lost, resulting in dehydration (Hall, 2011b).

Water Loss by the Kidneys

Renal water loss varies depending on solutes and water load. However, there is a minimal volume of water that has to be excreted because of the limit on how much the kidneys can concentrate urine. For a 65-kg reference man, the minimal urine volume that an adult must produce, assuming consumption of an average North American diet and normal

CLINICAL CORRELATION

Heat Acclimatization

Humans have relatively efficient heat dissipation mechanisms, but the thermoregulatory mechanism may be overwhelmed in a number of conditions, resulting in the development of hyperthermia. The risk of hyperthermia occurs when individuals move from a cool temperate climate to a tropical climate and perform physical exertion, or when athletes perform in tropical conditions without prior conditioning to the hot, and particularly hot and humid, ambient conditions. The inability to adequately dissipate body heat leads to a steady rise in body core temperature with the consequence of heat-related illness, which ranges from heat cramps to heatstroke. Prompt transfer to a cooler environment with adequate ventilation to accelerate body heat dissipation, adequate fluid replacement, and cessation of physical activity is essential for treatment of an individual with heat-related illness.

Conditioning the body to the hot environment by repeated bouts of exercise will improve the physiological responses of a healthy individual. This improvement of the individual's thermoregulatory responses to heat stress is known as heat acclimatization. The adaptation process is obtained several days after exposure and is usually fully achieved after 14 days, although it has been found that, in well-trained athletes, the heat-induced impairment of physiological responses and performances is still evident after 14 days (Voltaire et al., 2002). During acclimatization, a number of physiological adaptations to improve the individual's thermoregulatory ability occur. Typical physiological changes include heightened sweating response, reduced sodium concentration in the sweat, expanded plasma volume, and greater stability in cardiovascular function during exercise in the heat. Not only is sweating more profuse, it begins sooner and at a lower body temperature to improve dissipation of body heat. Water evaporation from the sweat provides the primary avenue of heat loss in order to defend the body's core temperature. Evaporation of 1 g of water from sweat at 30° C dissipates 0.58 kcal (2.43 kJ) of heat from the body (Geigy Scientific Tables, 1981). In addition, after adaptation, the greatly reduced sodium concentration in the sweat due to increased secretion of aldosterone is important, because it helps to conserve body sodium by minimizing sodium loss from the body. The resulting higher plasma osmolarity at a given sweat output will improve the thermoregulatory responses to heat stress (Takamata et al., 2001).

Heat stress, especially in competitive athletes, causes a spectrum of symptoms ranging from heat cramps to heatstroke (Squire, 1990). Heat cramps are an acute disorder of skeletal muscle characterized by brief, intermittent, and excruciating muscle cramps. Heat cramps often occur in people who are acclimatized to perform in hot climates and who consume a large amount of water to replace water losses without accompanying salt replacement. Although acclimatization is associated with diminished sodium concentration in the sweat, the loss of sodium in sweat can be considerable as the rate of sweat secretion increases. This condition can be prevented by adequate salt intake together with water replacement.

Heat exhaustion is caused by profuse sweating in a hot environment when the volume of water lost is not replaced by voluntary drinking and the plasma volume becomes depleted. There is dilation of blood vessels in the skin in an attempt to dissipate body heat. The resultant decrease in peripheral resistance together with depletion of plasma volume causes weakness and fainting. Body temperature in this individual is only moderately raised. The weakness and fainting is a safety mechanism, which, by the cessation of physical exertion in a hot and humid environment, prevents further rise in body temperature, thereby ensuring that the heat loss mechanism is not overextended. Treatment by external cooling and adequate hydration should be instituted in heat exhaustion. Prolonged untreated heat exhaustion can lead to heatstroke, in which body temperature increases steadily because of a complete breakdown in heat regulation. When this happens, the individual fails to sweat even in the face of a rapidly rising body temperature. When the elevated body temperature reaches a critical level, collapse, delirium, seizures, or coma occurs.

Thinking Critically

Exercise in the heat places the athlete at risk for heat illness. Children are at even greater risk for heat illness because their thermoregulatory mechanism is less efficient. Therefore it is important for the sports medicine team to be familiar with preventing and treating heat-related illness, especially in children and adolescents.

1. How does one prevent heat illness in athletes?
2. How does one treat heat illness when it occurs during sports competition?

renal function, is approximately 0.64 L a day (see Table 35-1). Metabolism of 70 g dietary protein results in the production of about 21 g of urea, which cannot be used by the body and has to be excreted in the urine. This 21 g of urea contributes 350 mOsm to the total osmotic load of substances presented to the kidneys. Added to this osmotic load is an additional 420 mOsm from phosphates, sulfates, other waste products, and ions (especially sodium chloride and potassium salts). Therefore the total load of osmotically active solutes requiring excretion by the kidneys is approximately 770 mOsm/day. Because the human kidneys can maximally concentrate urine to an osmolar concentration of 1,200 mOsm/L, the minimal volume of urine at maximal attainable osmolarity for this individual is 0.64 L a day. This volume of urine is known as the obligatory water loss.

INTAKE OF WATER

The minimal amount of water required daily to replace obligatory water losses from the respiratory tract, skin, feces, and urine is about 1.44 L (see Table 35-1). Water

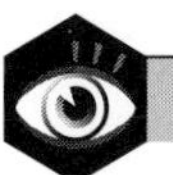

NUTRITION INSIGHT

Does Fluid Intake Reduce Energy Intake?

Humans habitually drink some form of beverage, be it milk, fruit juices, sugar-sweetened or nonnutritive sweetened beverages, or water. On average, the proportion of fluid consumed daily as water has diminished as people have shifted to other beverages. Whether such a trend will impact human health is unknown.

Two questions of interest have been raised. First, does drinking cold water burn calories and help a person lose weight? If a person were to drink a cup of ice-cold water at about 4° C, energy will be expended by the body to warm up the cold water until it reaches body temperature, or 37° C. One calorie (kilocalorie) is expended to raise 1 kg of water by 1° C. Therefore to raise the temperature of 1 cup (about 240 g) of ice-cold water to 35° C, an expenditure of 7.9 kilocalories (33 kcal × 0.24 kg water) is required. This amount of energy expended to warm up the cold water is insignificant in terms of the daily energy expenditure of an adult. An adult lying quietly expends about 1.3 kcal per minute.

Second, does water consumption with meals reduce energy intake of that meal and help a person lose weight? A recent systematic review of epidemiologic studies, relevant clinical trials, and intervention studies was conducted to address this question as well as whether drinking different beverages (i.e., milk and fruit juices) with meals will change the energy intake of the test meal (Daniels and Popkin, 2010). It was found that drinking water with meals does not change the total energy intake of the meal in nonobese, young to middle-aged adults, although removal of premeal water causes a small increase in the meal calories in both nonobese and overweight seniors. However, it has also emerged from these studies that different types of beverages consumed with a meal will affect the total energy intake of that meal. In preschool children, drinking milk with meals decreases the meal intake, but the total calorie intake of the meal is increased significantly. However, when preschoolers drink a fruit drink with a snack, their snack intake decreases because they reduced their snack calories to offset their beverage calories. Notably, if these preschoolers were to drink a diet fruit drink, they consumed fewer snack calories if the drink was served 30 minutes before the snack, but not if there was no delay or a 60-minute delay. Adults respond differently to milk, juices, or cola with meals. Their total meal energy intake increased with milk and juices but not with diet beverages. An increase in total meal energy intake was seen only at day 2.

Although these studies show that total meal energy intake increased with milk and juice consumption with meals, the data were collected from a single meal or from two or more meals during a 1- or 2-day period. This energy intake data should not be extrapolated to total daily energy intake because physiological regulatory mechanism for energy homeostasis to compensate for this increase may influence subsequent intake.

The benefit of drinking water as a weight loss intervention has also been reviewed. In a yearlong study involving German school children, schools that had educational and environmental interventions to increase water intake had a 31% reduced risk of overweight children compared to schools that did not introduce this intervention. The students at the intervention schools increased their water intake by an overall of 220 mL/day. Two 12-week clinical studies on weight loss intervention showed that older adults who drink water before meals and combine it with weight loss training lost 5.4 kg compared to 3.3 kg in the group that did not drink water before meals.

Although "water has a potentially important role to play in reducing energy intake, and consequently in obesity prevention" (Daniels and Popkin, 2010), there are many unanswered questions on the relationship between water consumption, energy metabolism, and weight status.

consumed by an individual comes from beverages, preformed water in food, and water produced by oxidation of food. If the composition of the ingested food is known, the yield of metabolic water can be calculated. Oxidation of 1 g each of carbohydrate, fat, and protein will yield approximately 0.6 g, 1.0 g, and 0.4 g of water, respectively. Assuming that the daily consumption of this 65-kg reference man is 400 g of carbohydrate, 100 g of fat, and 70 g of protein, the total yield of metabolic water from the food eaten amounts to 0.37 kg. Preformed water in food can be calculated from the difference between wet and dry weights of food; however, usually it is assumed that water makes up 60% of the wet weight. Therefore the weight of preformed water in the sample diet is about 0.85 kg, and the total volume of water (preformed plus metabolic) derived from ingested food is about 1.22 kg/day (1.22 L/day). Since the obligatory loss of water is 1.44 L/day, to remain in water balance the individual has to drink a minimum of 0.22 L of additional water. The ingested volume of water and other beverages varies greatly among individuals and depends on habit, custom, physical activity, and environment. On average, humans habitually drink between 1 and 2 L or more of water and beverages a day. The excess water is excreted by the kidneys to produce a less concentrated urine.

A reasonable allowance for water intake based on recommended energy intake is 1 mL/kcal expended, or about 35 mL/kg for adults and 1.5 mL/kcal or 150 mL/kg for infants (Institute of Medicine [IOM], 2004). Infants require more water on a body weight basis because of their relatively larger body surface area and metabolic rate, and the relatively limited capacity of their kidneys to handle the renal solute load. This is especially important for infants on formula, because most formula has a higher solute load than does human milk. Water loss can increase greatly in individuals doing heavy work, in athletes undergoing severe training in a hot climate, and in individuals with fever, vomiting, diabetes, or diarrhea. Under these circumstances, water needs are increased substantially.

RENAL EXCRETION OF WATER

As discussed in Chapter 34, the kidneys contribute significantly to homeostasis by stabilizing the volume and osmolarity of the body fluids. In their regulatory function, the kidneys process blood by removing substances that are in excess and conserving substances that are in deficit as these substances pass through the kidneys. Drinking large volumes of fluid causes a positive water balance so that the excess water will have to be excreted as dilute urine (hypo-osmotic with respect to plasma). Conversely, in water deficit, when there is a need to conserve body water, a smaller volume of concentrated (hyperosmotic) urine is excreted. Excretion of dilute urine involves the reabsorption of filtered solutes in excess of water, whereas the excretion of concentrated urine entails the reabsorption of water in excess of solutes (Hall, 2011a).

To understand how the kidneys produce either a dilute or concentrated urine, the following have to be considered:

- The transport and permeability characteristics of the various segments of the nephron
- The establishment of a hyperosmolar medullary gradient in the interstitium by the countercurrent multiplier system of the loops of Henle
- The final reabsorption of solutes and water from the renal tubules without affecting the hyperosmolar medullary gradient by the countercurrent exchanger system of the vasa recta
- The change in water permeability of the collecting tubules from a diuretic to an antidiuretic state under the influence of arginine vasopressin (AVP), which is also known as antidiuretic hormone (ADH).

TRANSPORT AND PERMEABILITY CHARACTERISTICS OF VARIOUS SEGMENTS OF THE NEPHRONS

The ultrafiltrate formed from filtration of plasma across the glomerular membrane into the Bowman space of the nephron is protein-free, and its ionic composition is similar to that of plasma except for the 5% difference due to the Gibbs-Donnan effect. As the filtrate flows along the nephrons, its composition and volume are altered by the permeability characteristics and the various transport processes that occur at the various nephron segments.

Proximal Tubules

Active reabsorption of sodium ions and the accompanying anions, and secondary active transport of organic nutrients in the proximal tubule create an osmotic gradient along which water is reabsorbed passively across the tubular cells. The rates of reabsorption of solutes and water are equal so that the osmolarity of the tubular fluid leaving the proximal tubule is similar to that of plasma, at 290 mOsm/L. This iso-osmotic reabsorption of 65% of the filtrate applies regardless of whether a dilute or concentrated urine is produced.

Tubular Cells Distal to the Proximal Tubules

Tubules distal to the proximal tubules are responsible for producing either a dilute or concentrated urine. This is achieved by the differences in permeability and transport characteristics of tubular cells in the different segments to sodium chloride, urea, and water. These differences establish a concentration and osmotic gradient across tubular cells, causing water to move passively along the osmotic gradient created. The establishment of this osmotic gradient in the medullary region of the kidneys is especially important because it allows the kidneys to excrete a concentrated urine. The final reabsorption of solutes (especially sodium chloride and urea) and water in the distal convoluted and collecting tubules is highly variable; it depends on the needs of the body and is influenced by hormones (Hall, 2011a).

Loops of Henle

The thin descending and ascending limbs are relatively permeable to sodium chloride and urea, thereby permitting these solutes to diffuse passively along their concentration gradient between the tubular and interstitial fluids. The thick ascending limb selectively transports sodium out of the fluid and it is relatively impermeable to urea. The thin descending limb is highly permeable to water, whereas the thin and thick ascending limbs are relatively impermeable to water.

Distal Nephrons

Active transport of sodium chloride out of the tubular fluid occurs along the distal convoluted tubules and throughout the length of the collecting tubules. The distal convoluted tubules and the cortical and outer medullary collecting tubules are relatively impermeable to urea. Conversely, the inner medullary collecting tubule is very permeable to urea because specialized urea transporters are present in the apical and basolateral plasma membranes (Knepper and Star, 1990). In the presence of AVP, the permeability to urea rises to a very high level; this response is mediated by the intracellular production of cyclic AMP (cAMP), which activates the apical urea transporter.

The first part of the distal convoluted tubules is relatively impermeable to water. The latter part of the distal convoluted tubule and the cortical and medullary collecting tubules are impermeable to water in the absence of AVP, but their permeability to water is increased in the presence of AVP. Thus final production of a concentrated or dilute urine is attributed to the water permeability of the latter part of the distal convoluted tubules and the cortical and medullary collecting tubules of the kidneys. In water deprivation, an increase in the secretion of AVP increases the water permeability of the collecting tubules and water diffuses out of the tubular lumen into the hyperosmotic interstitium, resulting in the excretion of a concentrated urine. This process

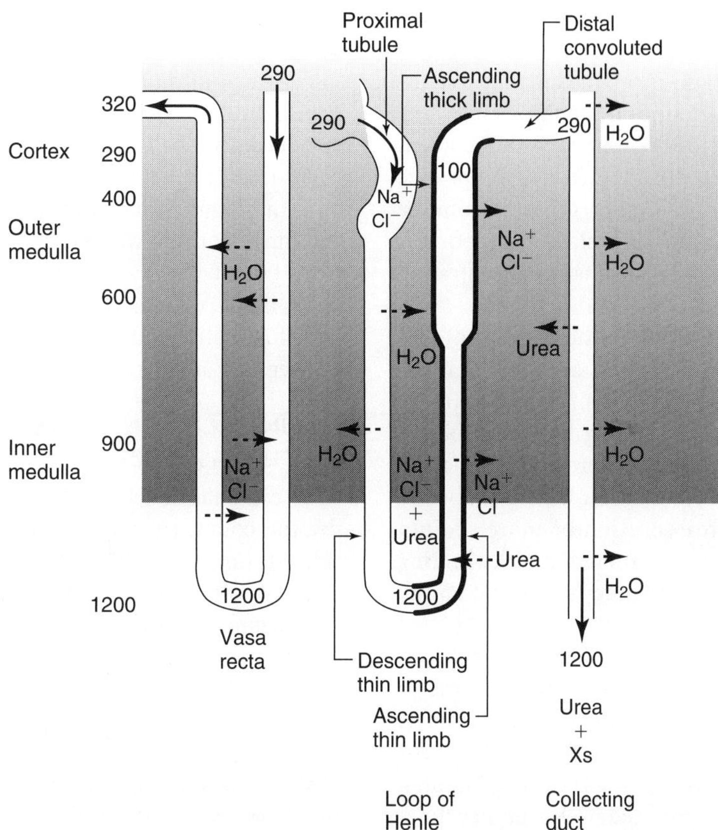

FIGURE 35-5 Establishment of an osmotic gradient in the medullary region of the kidney by the countercurrent multiplier system of the loop of Henle. Each human kidney contains approximately 1 million nephrons. The structures of only a single nephron with a long loop of Henle that penetrates into the inner medulla and of a single blood capillary are shown. Transport of NaCl out of the tubular fluid in the ascending limb and diffusion of water out of the tubular fluid in the descending limb create a small osmotic gradient that is multiplied by the counterflow of the tubular fluid. Tubular fluid is hypo-osmotic by the time it reaches the distal convoluted tubule. In the presence of arginine vasopressin (AVP), the late distal convoluted tubule and the collecting tubule are permeable to water. The tubular fluid equilibrates with the hypertonic interstitium, and concentrated urine is formed as shown. In the absence of AVP, the tubular fluid in the collecting tubule remains hypo-osmotic, and dilute urine is formed (see text for explanation). *Xs,* Solutes other than urea.

is important for water conservation in conditions of water deprivation. In the absence of AVP, the water permeability of the collecting tubules is low; water remains in the tubular lumen and a large volume of dilute urine is excreted. This is termed water diuresis.

COUNTERCURRENT MULTIPLIER SYSTEM OF THE LOOP OF HENLE

Establishment of an Osmotic Gradient

The establishment of an osmotic gradient from iso-osmotic in the corticomedullary region to hyperosmotic in the inner medullary region is made possible by the anatomical arrangements and the functional characteristics of the various segments of the distal tubules (Figure 35-5). Anatomically, loops of Henle in mammalian kidneys have different lengths, so they penetrate the medullary region to varying depths. The loops of Henle act as a countercurrent multiplier system, and the medullary blood vessels (i.e., the vasa recta) act as a countercurrent diffusion system. This arrangement, together with the different transport and permeability characteristics of the various segments of the distal tubules to sodium chloride, urea, and water, enable the kidney to establish an osmotic gradient in the medulla from 290 mOsm/L in the corticomedullary region to about 1,200 mOsm/L in the inner medullary region near the papillary tip of the kidneys. This osmotic gradient is made up of concentration gradients of mainly sodium chloride and urea and is essential for urine concentration in the collecting ducts.

Each loop of Henle consists of two parallel limbs of small diameter, with the tubular fluid flowing in opposite directions (countercurrent flow) and in close proximity. The hairpin conformation of the loop of Henle is such that fluid flows from the corticomedullary region to the medullary region in the thin descending limb and in the opposite direction in the thin and thick ascending limbs. Because of the counterflow and permeability characteristics, the loops of Henle operate as a countercurrent multiplier system and establish and maintain an osmotic gradient between the fluids in the corticomedullary region and the inner medullary region (Hall, 2011a).

Movement of Sodium Chloride, Urea, and Water

Active transport of sodium chloride out of the thick ascending limb is fundamental to the development of the osmotic gradient between the cortex and inner medulla. The highest levels of Na,K-ATPase are found in the thick ascending limbs, consistent with their role in powering countercurrent multiplication in the outer medulla. However, the passive movement of urea down its concentration gradient from the tubular fluid into the interstitium also plays an important role, especially when the kidney is maximally concentrating urine.

The mechanisms that contribute to the buildup of solutes, especially of sodium chloride and urea in the medullary region, are as follows: (1) active reabsorption of sodium chloride by the thick ascending limb produces a hypo-osmotic tubular fluid but a hyperosmotic interstitial fluid, because the thin and thick ascending limbs are impermeable to water; (2) reabsorption of more sodium chloride by the early distal convoluted and collecting tubules contribute further to the kidney's diluting ability (see Figure 35-5).

In water diuresis, when circulating AVP levels are low, the hypo-osmolarity is maintained and dilute urine is excreted. In antidiuresis, under the influence of AVP, water is removed from the late distal convoluted and the cortical and outer medullary portions of the collecting tubules, and in the process urea is concentrated in the tubular fluid. Because the inner medullary portion of the collecting tubule is permeable to urea and the permeability increases in the presence of AVP, urea moves from a concentrated tubular fluid down its concentration gradient into the interstitium, thereby increasing the osmolarity in the inner medullary region to a high level. Some of the urea in the interstitium diffuses passively into the lumen of both the thin descending and the ascending limbs along its concentration gradient.

The thin descending limb is very permeable to water but less so to sodium chloride and urea so that water moves out of the tubule and the osmolarity of the fluid flowing into this segment equilibrates with the surrounding hyperosmotic interstitial fluid. The fluid that enters the ascending limb has a higher concentration of sodium chloride because of the removal of water from the descending limb. Sodium chloride then moves passively from the tubular fluid in the thin ascending limb down its concentration gradient into the interstitium and adds further to the hyperosmolarity of the inner medullary region. There is more passive efflux of sodium chloride than passive influx of urea because the thin ascending limb is more permeable to sodium than urea, so there is a net efflux of osmotically active solutes. Because of the low water permeability, luminal fluid in the ascending limb is hypo-osmotic relative to its surrounding interstitium. Therefore both passive and active transport of sodium chloride out of the tubular fluid of the ascending limbs results in the formation of tubular fluid that is hypo-osmotic when it enters the distal convoluted tubule.

The countercurrent multiplier system in the kidneys is an energy efficient process. The establishment of a small osmotic gradient between the tubular fluid in the thin descending and ascending limbs of the loop of Henle with each pass of fluid can be multiplied by the continuous counterflow of fluid. By its operation, a considerable osmotic gradient (~900 mOsm/L) is generated between the plasma (290 mOsm/L) and the tubular fluids in the inner medullary region (1,200 mOsm/L) during antidiuresis. The energy cost associated with the establishment of this large osmotic gradient of 900 mOsm/L represents only the energy expended in generating small osmotic gradients between adjacent segments of the descending and ascending limbs of the loops of Henle.

COUNTERCURRENT EXCHANGER OF THE VASA RECTA

It is essential that the osmotic gradient that is established by the countercurrent multiplier system in the medullary interstitium be maintained and not dissipated by the blood supply. This goal is achieved by the specialized anatomical arrangement of the medullary blood vessels, the vasa recta. The descending vasa recta receive blood from the efferent arterioles of the nephrons and supply blood to the capillary plexuses at each level of the medulla. Blood from the capillary plexuses drains into the ascending vasa recta (Hall, 2011a). As the ascending vasa recta pass from the inner medulla toward the cortical region, they travel close to the descending vasa recta at the outer medullary region, which is a counterflow arrangement similar to that of the loops of Henle (see Figure 35-5).

Because the capillary endothelium is permeable to both solutes and water, the osmolarity of plasma in the vasa recta equilibrates with that of the medullary interstitial fluid at each level. The osmolarity of the descending vasa recta increases progressively from 290 mOsm/L at the corticomedullary region to 1,200 mOsm/L at the inner medullary area as they penetrate deeper into the medulla, gain solutes, and lose water. The reverse occurs at the ascending vasa recta as they leave the inner medulla. The plasma becomes progressively less hyperosmotic by passive loss of solutes and uptake of water as it flows from a region of higher to lower osmolarity. By the time the ascending vasa recta leave the medulla, the osmolarity of the plasma is only slightly higher than that of systemic plasma. This arrangement allows removal of the excess solutes and water that are reabsorbed by the various nephron segments in the medulla while at the same time providing a means of perfusion and maintaining the osmotic gradient in the medullary interstitium.

EXCRETION OF DILUTE AND CONCENTRATED URINE

Human kidneys can dilute urine to one sixth the osmolarity of plasma or concentrate it up to four times that of plasma; that is, humans can excrete urine of osmolarity between 50 and 1,200 mOsm/L. This is made possible by the countercurrent multiplier of the loop of Henle, which provides the mechanism for excretion of either dilute or concentrated urine, and the collecting duct, which harvests the work done by the loop of Henle. The collecting tubules run parallel and in close vicinity to the loops of Henle through an area of high osmolarity to drain into the ureter (see Figure 35-5).

Fluid leaving the thick ascending limb of the loop of Henle is hypo-osmotic, about 100 mOsm/L. When the circulating level of plasma AVP is low as in the condition of water excess, water permeability in the more distal portion of the distal convoluted tubule and in the collecting tubule is low. Further reabsorption of solutes, especially sodium chloride, by the tubular cells of the distal nephron dilutes the tubular fluid to an osmolarity of 50 mOsm/L. A dilute urine is excreted.

The production of a concentrated urine occurs when the circulating AVP levels are high, as occurs during dehydrated states. The permeability to water is increased in the more distal portions of the distal convoluted tubules and collecting tubules, and the permeability to urea is increased in the inner medullary collecting tubule. As the collecting tubule passes from the corticomedullary to inner medullary region, the tubular fluid equilibrates with the hyperosmotic interstitial fluid and water is removed. Removal of water concentrates the urea in the collecting tubule. The high permeability of the inner medullary tubule to urea under the influence of AVP causes urea to move from the tubular fluid into the interstitium, thereby further increasing the osmolarity in the interstitium. In antidiuresis, concentrated urine of an osmolarity as high as 1,200 mOsm/L is excreted.

CONCEPT OF FREE-WATER CLEARANCE

The excretion of a dilute urine entails removal of more water relative to solutes from the body in water excess. Relatively more solute is excreted in concentrated urine when an individual is dehydrated. Therefore dilute urine has an osmolar concentration less than that of plasma (about 290 mOsm/L), and the osmolar concentration of concentrated urine is more than 290 mOsm/L. Thus the fundamental process in the production of a dilute or concentrated urine can be viewed simply as the excretion of water and solutes separately by the kidneys. The relative proportion of excreted water and solutes changes with the hydration state of the individual.

In the excretion of a dilute urine, the volume of plasma that is cleared of this excess solute-free water per unit time by the kidney is called free-water clearance (C_{water}) and has the unit of volume/unit time, or liters/day (L/day). Similarly, in the excretion of a concentrated urine, the volume of plasma that is cleared of the excess solutes per unit time is called osmolar clearance (C_{osm}) and can be defined as the volume of water necessary for the excretion of the excess osmotic load in the urine so that urine is iso-osmotic with plasma. The C_{osm} can be calculated and also has the unit of L/day.

$$C_{osm} = (U_{osm} / P_{osm}) \times V$$

where U_{osm} is the osmolarity of urine (mOsm/L), V is the rate of urine flow (L/day), and P_{osm} is plasma osmolarity (mOsm/L).

Since the rate of urine flow (V in L/day) is the sum of solute-free water and solute clearance, that is sum of C_{water} and C_{osm},

$$V = C_{water} + C_{osm}$$

rearranging gives

$$C_{water} = V - C_{osm}$$

or

$$C_{water} = V - [(U_{osm} / P_{osm}) \times V]$$

Therefore when the rate of urine flow is greater than C_{osm} (i.e., when C_{water} is positive), relatively more water than solute is excreted in the urine; dilute or hypo-osmotic urine is excreted. Conversely, when the rate of urine flow is smaller than C_{osm} (i.e., when C_{water} is negative) relatively more solute is excreted in the urine, and urine is hyperosmotic.

Using the example of the reference man in Table 35-1, excretion of the daily solute load of 770 mOsm presented to the kidneys can be accomplished by producing a urine that is either iso-osmotic ($U_{osm}/P_{osm} = 1$), hyperosmotic ($U_{osm}/P_{osm} > 1$), or hypo-osmotic ($U_{osm}/P_{osm} < 1$) with respect to plasma. To produce a maximally concentrated urine of 1,200 mOsm/L, the minimal volume of water needed to excrete this 770 mOsm of solute load is 0.64 L/day. The C_{osm} can be calculated as follows:

$$C_{osm} = (1{,}200 \text{ mOsm/L}/290 \text{ mOsm/L}) \times 0.64 \text{ L/day} = 2.64 \text{ L/day}$$

and

$$C_{water} = V - C_{osm} = 0.64 \text{ L/day} - 2.64 \text{ L/day} = -2.0 \text{ L/day}$$

This negative C_{water} expresses the renal conservation of water in which solutes in excess of water are removed from the plasma and a concentrated urine is excreted. To excrete an iso-osmotic urine, the 770 mOsm of solutes would need to be excreted in 2.64 L/day of urine, or about four times the minimum obligatory urine volume. In this case of iso-osmotic urine excretion, C_{osm} equals urinary flow rate, C_{water} is equal to zero, and no excretion of solute-free water occurs. The production of a dilute urine requires a flow rate of more than 2.64 L/day; in this case, solute-free water is excreted by the kidneys and C_{water} is positive.

The determination of C_{water} provides important information on the functions of the segments of the nephron involved in the production of a dilute or concentrated urine. For the kidneys to excrete a maximal volume of solute-free water, AVP must be absent so that water reabsorption by the collecting tubules does not occur. Conversely, for the kidneys to excrete a concentrated urine, solute-free water is reabsorbed by the collecting tubules. This occurs only in the presence of AVP.

REGULATION OF WATER BALANCE

For an individual to maintain a constant osmolarity of the body fluids at 290 mOsm/L, the ratio of sodium chloride to total body water has to be regulated within narrow limits.

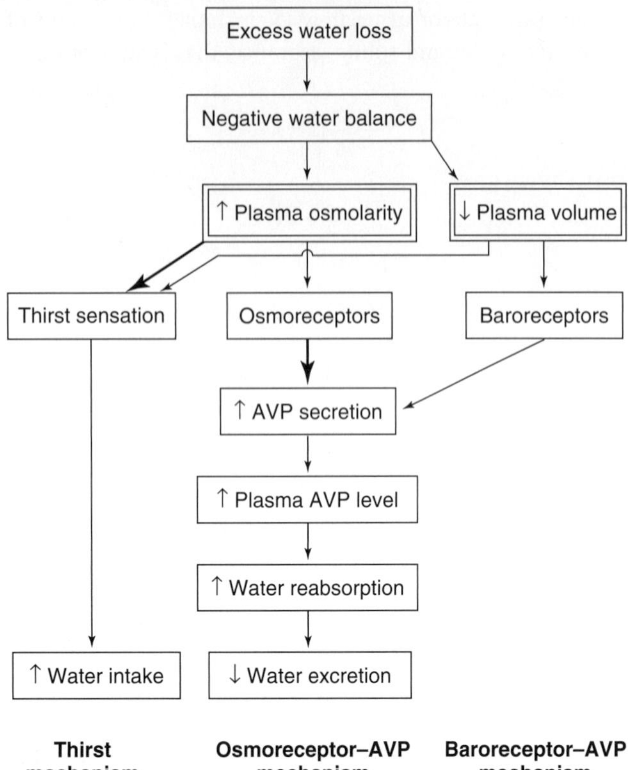

FIGURE 35-6 Integration of the osmoreceptor–AVP, baroreceptor–AVP, and thirst mechanisms in the regulation of water balance in water deficit.

Water excess or water deficit will invariably affect this ratio, thereby changing the plasma osmolarity, whereas disturbances in sodium balance will affect the volumes of body fluids. To maintain water balance, physiological feedback mechanisms are present to modify either water loss or water intake to bring plasma osmolarity back toward normal. These feedback mechanisms include the osmotic control pathways and baroreceptor pathways (Figure 35-6).

CENTRAL OSMORECEPTORS

A group of neurons that are sensitive to changes in the osmolarity of the extracellular fluid bathing them contributes to the regulation of water and sodium homeostasis. These osmoresponsive neurons are located in three loci associated with the lamina terminalis near the anterior part of the hypothalamus: the subfornical organ, the median preoptic nucleus, and the organum vasculosum lamina terminalis. These neurons effectively regulate intake of water and sodium by the sensation of thirst, which drives an individual to drink, and an appetite for salt. These osmoreceptors also regulate renal diuresis and natriuresis via their stimulation or inhibition of secretion of AVP and natriuretic peptides (Bourque and Oliet, 1997).

CONTROL OF RENAL EXCRETION OF WATER

The ability to excrete either concentrated or dilute urine depends on the circulating level of plasma AVP. In antidiuresis, when there is a need to conserve water, the circulating level of AVP is high and a concentrated urine is excreted. In water diuresis, the circulating level of AVP is low and a large volume of solute-free water is excreted.

Arginine Vasopressin

Synthesis of AVP

Arginine vasopressin, the principal hormonal regulator of body water balance, is a small peptide, nine amino acids in length. It is synthesized by the magnocellular neurons located within the supraoptic and paraventricular nuclei of the hypothalamus. Quantitatively, synthesis in the supraoptic nuclei is more important (Baylis and Thompson, 1988). The synthesized hormone is packaged as granules in vesicles in the neurons; transported in combination with a carrier protein, neurophysin, down the axons of these neurons; and stored as secretory granules in the nerve endings located in the neurohypophysis (posterior pituitary gland) until released.

Secretion of AVP

Stimulation of the magnocellular neurons transmits nerve impulses along the hypothalamic–hypophyseal tract to the nerve endings at the neurohypophysis to release the stored granules by exocytosis. After release, the neurophysin and AVP separate, and the AVP enters the circulation. Although AVP causes vessel constriction in the systemic circulation, its vasopressor effect is less potent than its antidiuretic effect in the kidneys. Some AVP is released into the brain where it may act centrally as a neuromodulator in the control of body fluid homeostasis (Kato et al., 2009).

Effects of AVP in the Kidney

Effects on Aquaporins. Reabsorption of water along an osmotic gradient across tubular epithelium can occur only if the epithelium is permeable to water. Water permeability depends largely on the presence of transporter proteins, called aquaporins, which function as water channels. To date, at least seven aquaporins (AQPs) have been shown to be expressed in discrete segments along the nephrons (Nielsen et al., 2002). Of these, AQP-2 is the predominant AQP responsive to AVP, and is therefore responsible for the majority of regulation of water reabsorption in the collecting tubule. AQP-2 is expressed in abundance in the apical plasma membrane and in intracellular vesicles of the collecting tubular cells. When AVP binds to receptors located on the basolateral membrane of the tubular cell, adenylate cyclase is activated and the intracellular level of cyclic AMP increases. This second messenger activates the AQP-2 proteins so that they "shuttle" from intracellular vesicles to be inserted into the apical plasma membrane and allow water reabsorption to take place (Figure 35-7). The time course for these reactions is rapid, within 40 seconds. This process temporarily provides channels that allow free diffusion of water from the tubular fluid into the cells along an osmotic gradient. When AVP is removed, these AQP-2 proteins are reinternalized in the cell, and the luminal membrane becomes impermeable to water. The downregulation of

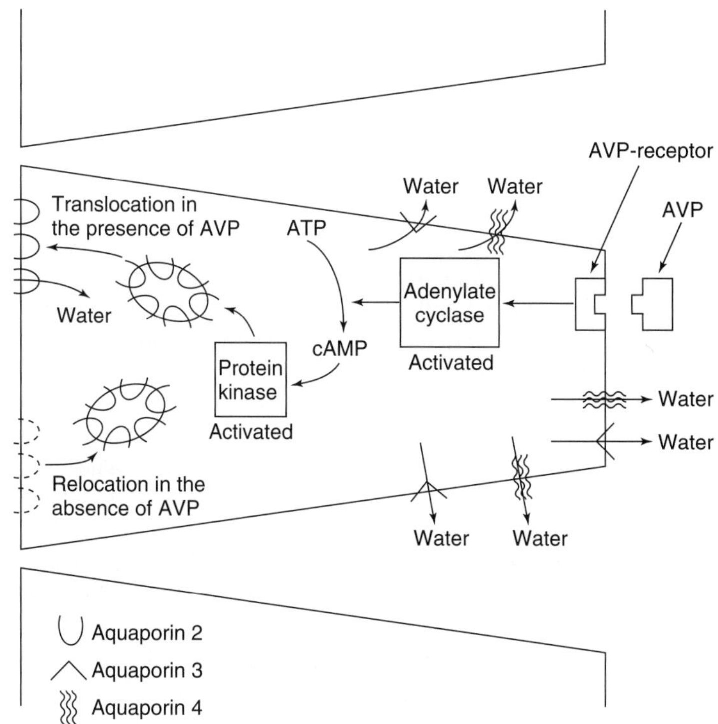

FIGURE 35-7 Proposed mechanism of some major events that result from the action of arginine vasopressin (*AVP*) on the collecting tubule to increase its water permeability.

AQP-2 in the apical membrane is rapid, occurring within minutes. Thus the insertion and removal of membrane vesicles containing water channels provide a rapid mechanism for controlling the permeability of the luminal membrane to water.

Other AQPs also have specific roles in water transport. Large numbers of AQP-3 proteins are located mainly in the lateral membrane, and AQP-4 proteins are located in both the basal and the lateral membranes of the tubular cells in the collecting tubule. AQP-3, but not AQP-4, is affected by AVP. The presence of AQP-3 and AQP-4 acts as exit channels for the water that is absorbed into the cells. By this route, a large volume of water can move from the lumen of the collecting tubules to the hyperosmotic interstitium of the medullary region. The presence of AQP-2 in the basolateral plasma membrane of the inner medullary collecting tubule further increases the permeability to water in the inner medullary region so that concentrated urine is excreted. In conditions of water excess, the collecting tubules are impermeable to water as a consequence of the absence of AVP, and a large volume of solute-free water is excreted.

Since AQPs are widely distributed and fulfill different functions in different tissues in the body, any dysfunction in AQPs may contribute to different disease states. In the kidneys, impairment of their function can result in disorders of body water homeostasis and nephrogenic diabetes. Results of a case-control study showed that reduced renal concentration and diluting capacity in moderately severe chronic kidney disease is partly due to an abnormally decreased response in the AVP–cAMP–AQPs axis (Pedersen et al., 2010).

Control of AVP Secretion

Secretion of AVP is influenced by many different stimuli, but the primary physiological factors are changes in plasma osmolarity and changes in effective circulating volume and pressure of the vascular system (Menninger, 1985) (see Figure 35-6). Other factors, such as stimuli to the central nervous system, neurotransmitters, various hormones, and drugs, can influence the secretion of AVP; the most prominent stimulus is activation of emetic centers in the brainstem by nausea-producing agents such as morphine, nicotine, and cholecystokinin (Verbalis et al., 1987; Miaskiewicz et al., 2011). Secretion of AVP is also stimulated by angiotensin 2 (Reis et al., 2010) and inhibited by glucocorticoid, ethanol, and central adiponectin (Bahr et al., 2006; Carney et al., 1995; Iwama et al., 2009).

Osmotic Control of AVP Secretion

Sodium chloride, the major contributor to the osmolar concentration in the plasma, is the most potent solute in stimulating the secretion of AVP. Administration of a hypertonic sodium chloride solution into the artery supplying the hypothalamus causes the release of AVP from the posterior pituitary. Conversely, injection of a hypotonic sodium chloride solution into the same artery inhibits AVP secretion (Zerbe and Robertson, 1983).

The magnocellular neurons that synthesize AVP in the supraoptic and paraventricular nuclei of the hypothalamus are intrinsically osmosensitive and respond to changes in osmolarity of the surrounding fluid. Their firing rate is modulated greatly by the osmosensitive neurons in the organum vasculosum lamina terminalis near the anterior pituitary (Bourque and Oliet, 1997). Increases in the firing rate of the magnocellular neurons increases the secretion of AVP from their nerve endings. Normally, the plasma osmolarity is "set" at 290 mOsm/L. A small increase of as little as 0.5% in the plasma osmolarity is sufficient to stimulate AVP secretion (Thompson et al., 1986). However, the sensitivity of this osmoregulatory system can be modified by various physiological and pathological states (Robertson, 1987).

Stimulatory potency of solutes depends on the permeability of the osmoreceptor to the solutes involved. For example, the plasma membrane of these osmometer cells is not permeable to sodium, and an osmotic gradient can be set up when plasma concentration of sodium changes. In contrast, urea, which penetrates cell membranes easily, is not an effective solute for changing AVP secretion. Because the half-life of the released AVP is short, less than 20 minutes, the circulating levels of AVP can decrease or increase rapidly within minutes in response to changes in the osmolarity of the plasma.

Baroreceptor Control of AVP Secretion

A decrease in effective circulating volume or arterial pressure stimulates secretion of AVP from the neurohypophysis (see Figure 35-6). However, the sensitivity of this system is less than that of the osmoreceptors. It requires a decrease of about 5% to 10% in blood volume or blood pressure before AVP secretion is stimulated, as compared to the 0.5% change in plasma osmolarity (Menninger, 1985).

Both the high-pressure or arterial baroreceptors (located in the aortic arch and carotid sinus) and the low-pressure or atrial receptors (located in the right atrium and pulmonary vein) are involved in the reflex control of AVP secretion (Thrasher, 1994). Under normal conditions, impulses from the afferent fibers of these baroreceptors tonically inhibit the secretion of AVP. In hypervolemia, stimulation of the baroreceptors sends signals to the brainstem (solitary tract nucleus of the medulla oblongata), which is part of the center that regulates heart rate and blood pressure. Signals are then relayed from the brainstem to hypothalamus to inhibit AVP secretion. Conversely, in hypovolemia these baroreceptors are not stimulated, and the secretion of AVP is increased.

THIRST MECHANISM IN CONTROL OF WATER INTAKE

Numerous physiological responses to an increase in plasma osmolarity or a decrease in blood volume or arterial pressure are involved in altering the desire for drinking water. This subjective feeling of thirst, which leads to increase in fluid intake necessary to counterbalance fluid loss, helps maintain a relatively constant plasma osmolarity. In addition to the feeling of thirst, an individual's habit also influences drinking.

Osmotic and Hypovolemic Stimulation of Thirst

Many stimuli alter the perception of thirst, but the most important stimulus is dehydration when the plasma osmolarity is increased. In humans, the osmoreceptors in the paraventricular nucleus that control osmotically stimulated AVP secretion are also involved in the perception of thirst (Bourque and Oliet, 1997). The osmotic threshold for thirst and AVP secretion is very similar. Above an osmotic threshold, the relationship between the increase in plasma osmolarity and increase in thirst and AVP is linear (Figaro and Mack, 1997). In addition, other peripheral osmoreceptors are present in the oropharyngeal area that are sensitive to a change in plasma osmolarity. In dehydration, dryness of the mucosa of the mouth and esophagus stimulates the oropharyngeal receptors, and afferent signals from these receptors contribute to the sensation of dry mouth and also increase AVP secretion.

A secondary stimulus to thirst sensation is a reduced effective circulating volume or arterial pressure (Thornton, 2010). The threshold for stimulating thirst by hypovolemia is significantly higher than that by osmotic stimulation. An increase of only 2% to 3% above basal level in plasma osmolarity produces a strong desire to drink, whereas a decrease of about 5% to 10% in blood volume or blood pressure is required before a similar thirst response is produced (IOM, 2004). Very little is known about the pathways involved in the response of thirst to decreased blood volume or arterial pressure, but it is believed that both the baroreceptor–AVP pathway and the renin–angiotensin–aldosterone system are involved. Angiotensin 2 increases blood pressure, and aldosterone retains body sodium and thus water, which increases blood volume. These effects indirectly reduce the thirst intensity. Angiotensin 2 may stimulate thirst by a direct effect on the brain.

Cessation of Thirst Sensation

The sensation of thirst is abolished when the osmolarity returns toward its set-point and plasma volume increases. However, an individual can find relief from thirst just by the act of drinking, even before water is absorbed from the gastrointestinal tract to have an effect on the plasma osmolarity. Receptors in the oropharynx, the gastrointestinal tract, and the liver–portal system probably are involved in this modulation of thirst (Figaro and Mack, 1997). Ingestion of water stimulates the oropharyngeal receptors, which reflexively diminishes the thirst drive and inhibits AVP secretion by sending signals to the magnocellular neurons. This inhibition of AVP secretion appears even before a substantive decrease in plasma osmolarity, indicating that the initial inhibition of AVP is via oropharyngeal stimulation by ingestion of water. This mechanism provides relief of thirst only temporarily. The increase in plasma osmolarity has to be corrected before the desire to drink is satisfied.

INTEGRATION OF OSMORECEPTOR–AVP, BARORECEPTOR–AVP, AND THIRST MECHANISMS

The osmoreceptor–AVP, baroreceptor–AVP, and thirst systems work in concert to regulate the osmolarity of body fluids and maintain water balance (see Figure 35-6). Under normal physiological conditions, the plasma osmolarity is maintained within narrow limits by the very sensitive osmoregulatory system for AVP secretion, which adjusts renal water excretion to small changes in osmolarity. In water deficit, plasma osmolarity increases and blood volume contracts. This stimulates the release of AVP to increase water reabsorption from the kidneys. However, the volume of water reabsorbed may be insufficient to correct fully for the water deficit. Stimulation of the thirst sensation to promote drinking leads to water intake, and the plasma osmolarity and blood volume are returned to normal. Conversely, when the plasma osmolarity is decreased and blood volume is increased in water excess, thirst sensation is suppressed, AVP is not secreted, and any unregulated water intake in excess of body need is excreted in the urine.

WATER IMBALANCE AND ITS CONSEQUENCES

Disturbances of water balance consist of either excess or depletion of water and are manifested by alterations in the body fluid osmolarity. Because the major determinant of plasma osmolarity is sodium ions, these disorders alter the plasma concentration of sodium ions. To understand the disturbances in volume, osmolarity, and distribution of body fluids, the following two fundamental physiological facts must be kept in mind:

1. Fluid compartments are in osmotic equilibrium because water permeates the cell membrane and diffuses freely between the extracellular and intracellular fluid compartments.
2. When the extracellular fluid becomes hypertonic, water diffuses out of cells until the osmolarities of the extracellular and intracellular fluids are equal; the reverse is true when extracellular fluid becomes hypotonic.

Changes in the osmolarity of the extracellular compartment will invariably affect the volume of the intracellular compartment. Water deficit is usually associated with hypernatremia (high plasma sodium concentration), and water excess is usually associated with hyponatremia (low plasma sodium concentration). Under normal circumstances, if the disturbances are not of renal origin, the kidneys compensate for the deficit or excess by appropriately adjusting urine volume and composition, thereby ensuring that the osmolarity of the body fluids is stabilized within narrow limits.

NEGATIVE WATER BALANCE AND HYPERNATREMIA

Dehydration, or excessive loss of body fluid, of 2% or more of body weight can lead to symptoms such as extreme thirst, decreased urine output, secretion of a concentrated urine, headaches, fatigue, muscle cramps, hypotension, and fever. It also adversely influences cognitive function and aerobic and endurance-type exercise performance (IOM, 2004). The effects of body water loss on exercise performance are to alter the functions of the central nervous system, thermoregulatory system, cardiovascular system, and metabolic functions.

In general, water is never lost without ions, nor ions without water; although the relative proportions of ions and water lost vary in different circumstances. Because of this relative loss of ions and water, there are three types of dehydration: isotonic (isonatremic), hypotonic (hyponatremic), and hypertonic (hypernatremic). In isotonic dehydration, there is equal loss of sodium and water; this is also known as hypovolemia and is the most common type of dehydration seen in humans. In situations where proportionately more sodium than water is lost from the body, hypotonic (or hyponatremic) dehydration results. When loss of water exceeds loss of sodium, hypertonic (hypernatremic) dehydration occurs.

When loss of water exceeds loss of sodium, the osmolarity of the extracellular fluid increases. Water diffuses out of the cells until the osmolarities across the cell membrane are equal. The volumes of both compartments will decrease and their osmolarities will increase. This can occur during heavy physical exertion in a hot and humid climate, leading to hypernatremia and hypovolemia (Randall, 1976). The thirst mechanism is stimulated, and AVP secretion occurs. Although the kidneys will conserve both electrolytes and water during dehydration by excreting a concentrated urine low in sodium, fluid loss ultimately has to be replaced by fluid intake.

POSITIVE WATER BALANCE AND HYPONATREMIA

Ingestion of an overly excessive amount of water does not normally occur in a healthy individual. It may occur in social situations such as drinking contests, in intensive exercise in a hot environment during which a large volume of fluid is consumed without proper replenishment of electrolytes, or in psychogenic polydipsia. This will increase total body water, diluting all the body fluid compartments where the volumes of both the intracellular and the extracellular compartments increase and their osmolarities decrease (hyponatremia and hypervolemia). Hyponatremia is defined by a plasma concentration of less than 135 mEq/L of sodium. The excess water will distribute throughout the body in proportion to the initial volumes of the intracellular and extracellular compartments.

Acute water intoxication caused by too rapid parenteral fluid replacement that greatly exceeded the kidney's maximal rate of excretion will cause expansion of brain cells. This swelling increases intracranial pressure, which leads to the observable symptoms of water intoxication such as headache, behavioral changes, confusion, and drowsiness. These are followed by nausea, vomiting, muscle twitching, convulsion, brain damage, coma, and finally death (IOM, 2004).

In a healthy individual, there are usually no adverse effects associated with overconsumption of water because the resultant hyponatremia inhibits secretion of AVP and the excess water is excreted to reestablish water balance. However, in conditions in which the low plasma osmolarity fails to inhibit secretion of AVP (such as in severe low-output congestive heart failure; Uretsky et al., 1985), cell expansion, hypervolemia, and hyponatremia occur.

Accumulation of Excess Fluid in Tissues: Edema

In edema, there is an accumulation of excess fluid in body tissues. Edema occurs when there is an imbalance of forces governing the diffusion of water across either the cell membrane or the capillary endothelium; it may also occur when the permeability of these membranes is increased. The most common edema occurs in the interstitial fluid compartment, but intracellular edema is also possible.

Edema commonly involves expansion of the interstitial space. Edema formation may be a result of an increase in filtration of plasma into the interstitial space or a failure of the lymphatics to return the filtered fluid to the circulation. An increase in filtration of plasma can result from an imbalance in any of the factors that affect net movement of water across the capillary endothelium. One example is an increase in permeability of the capillary endothelium that results from endothelial cell contraction elicited by chemical mediators of inflammation, such as histamine and bradykinin. Edema may also arise from the decrease in plasma oncotic pressure that results from a decrease in plasma protein concentration in individuals with liver cirrhosis, kidney diseases, or protein malnutrition. An increase in filtration pressure due to venous congestion secondary to congestive heart failure is another common cause of edema (Klabunde, 2005).

Intracellular edema can also occur when the permeability of the cell membrane to solutes is increased, when the concentration of a permeable solute in the plasma is increased, or when blood sodium level is low (hyponatremia). Both the increase in membrane permeability and the increase in plasma concentration of a permeable solute cause an influx of solutes into the cells. Water diffuses passively along the osmotic gradient into the cells, and the cells expand. In tissue inflammation, permeability of the cell membrane increases, and this causes an influx of sodium and other ions and, subsequently, water into the cells. In hyponatremia, water enters the cells along the osmotic gradient, causing the cells to expand.

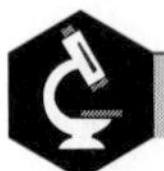

CLINICAL CORRELATION

Edema Formation

Edema, formerly known as hydropsy or dropsy, is the accumulation of an abnormal amount of fluid in the interstitial space. The extent of edema depends on the pathological states that affect lymphatic drainage or changes in any of the variables in Starling's equation, such as a decrease in plasma oncotic pressure, an increase in hydrostatic pressure in the capillaries, or an increase in capillary wall permeability. This will increase filtration across the capillary wall faster than the rate at which the lymphatics can drain.

LOCALIZED EDEMA

Edema can be localized or generalized. Localized edemas are restricted to a discrete vascular area or tissue, such as the swelling that accompanies injury or inflammation. Chemicals, such as bradykinin, histamine, and prostaglandins, are released locally in response to injury and they cause vasodilation and thus elevate capillary pressure and filtration. In addition, these chemicals increase permeability of capillary endothelial cells to proteins leading to the leakage of plasma proteins into the interstitial spaces in the injured tissues. This increases the oncotic pressure in the interstitial fluid, which then adds to the force for filtration, with the consequence of edema. Examples of edema in specific tissues are cerebral edema (extracellular fluid accumulation in the brain) and pulmonary edema (in left ventricular failure).

GENERALIZED EDEMA

Generalized edema exists when an abnormally large amount of fluid accumulates in the interstitial spaces throughout the body. Some common causes of generalized edema are congestive heart failure, nephrotic syndrome, liver disease, and nutritional or "hunger" edema.

A decrease in plasma oncotic pressure due to an abnormally low plasma protein concentration increases net capillary filtration pressure. Plasma protein concentration can be reduced when protein production is decreased in liver disease or when there is a loss of protein in urine. In healthy individuals, very little protein is filtered across the glomerular membrane. In individuals with membranous glomerulonephritis and focal segmental glomerulosclerosis, there is an increase in glomerular capillary wall permeability, so that large quantities of protein are filtered and excreted in the urine. This syndrome, nephrotic syndrome, is characterized by massive proteinuria, hypoalbuminemia, generalized edema, hyperlipidemia, and lipiduria. The shift of fluid from the intravascular to extravascular compartment causes a compensatory increase in the secretion of aldosterone, which further aggravates the condition by increasing reabsorption of filtered sodium from the renal tubules. Therapies consist of treatment of the underlying cause, sodium restriction, and judicious use of diuretics.

In congestive heart failure, impaired cardiac emptying results in a rise in ventricular end-diastolic pressure with the consequence of elevated venous pressure and elevated capillary hydrostatic pressure. This will promote transudation of fluids out of the vascular channel into the interstitial spaces, essentially diminishing the effective blood volume. The kidneys respond by retaining salt and water in an effort to increase intravascular fluid volume. However, because the cardiac output remains low, this leads to a vicious cycle that is self-perpetuating unless treatment to increase cardiac output is instituted. Treatment consists of reducing sodium and fluid retention through use of diuretics, improving cardiac output with inotropic agents such as digitalis, and reducing vascular resistance through use of vasodilating drugs. Edema can occur in either the pulmonary or the systemic capillary beds.

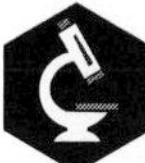

CLINICAL CORRELATION—cont'd

The systemic edema due to congestive heart failure is usually most prominent in the lower extremities when the patient is standing or sitting, and the edema shifts to the sacral area when the patient is lying down. Because gravity influences the distribution of the edema, it is termed dependent edema. If pressure is applied to the swollen area by depressing the skin with a finger or thumb, an indentation occurs and persists for some time after the release of the pressure. This is referred to as peripheral pitting edema.

Edema due to renal dysfunction tends to be massive and more equally distributed than edema of cardiac origin. Generalized massive edema is termed anasarca. When finger pressure is applied to the edematous area, temporary displacement of fluid leaves a pitted depression, hence the term pitting edema.

Another cause of edema is impaired lymphatic drainage. In filariasis, a parasitic worm infestation of the lymphatic system, lymphatic flow is obstructed. Obstruction to lymphatic flow is also seen following radical surgery for breast cancer in which axillary lymph nodes are removed. This edema is usually located distal to the point of obstruction.

Thinking Critically

Children with kwashiorkor, a form of protein-energy malnutrition, often present with signs of inanition and edema. Kwashiorkor is usually characterized by a diet poor in protein and relatively more adequate in total energy.

1. Why does edema develop in these children?
2. Discuss the occurrence of edema with regard to the Starling forces that determine fluid movement into and out of the vascular and interstitial spaces.

REFERENCES

Bahr, V., Franzen, N., Oelkers, W., Pfeiffer, A. F., & Diederich, S. (2006). Effect of exogenous glucocorticoid on osmotically stimulated antidiuretic hormone secretion and on water reabsorption in man. *European Journal of Endocrinology, 155*, 845–848.

Baylis, P. H., & Thompson, C. J. (1988). Osmoregulation of vasopressin secretion and thirst in health and disease. *Clinical Endocrinology, 29*, 549–576.

Bourque, C. W., & Oliet, S. H. R. (1997). Osmoreceptors in the central nervous system. *Annual Review of Physiology, 59*, 601–619.

Carney, S. L., Gillies, A. H., & Ray, C. D. (1995). Acute effect of ethanol on renal electrolyte transport in the rat. *Clinical and Experimental Pharmacology & Physiology, 22*, 629–634.

Daniels, M. C., & Popkin, B. M. (2010). Impact of water intake on energy intake and weight status: A systematic review. *Nutrition Reviews, 68*, 505–521.

Figaro, M. K., & Mack, G. W. (1997). Regulation of fluid intake in dehydrated humans: Role of oropharyngeal stimulation. *The American Journal of Physiology, 272*, R1740–R1746.

Geigy Scientific Tables. (1981). In C. Lintner (Ed.), *Geigy scientific tables* (8th ed., Vol. 1, p. 108). Basel, Switzerland: Ciba-Geigy Limited.

Hall, J. E. (2011a). Urine concentration and dilution: Regulation of extracellular fluid osmolarity and sodium concentration. In *Guyton and Hall textbook of medical physiology* (12th ed., pp. 345–360). Philadelphia: Saunders Elsevier.

Hall, J. E. (2011b). Digestion and absorption in the gastrointestinal tract. In *Guyton and Hall textbook of medical physiology* (12th ed., pp. 789–798). Philadelphia: Saunders Elsevier.

Institute of Medicine. (2004). Water. In *Dietary Reference Intakes for water, potassium, sodium, chloride, and sulfate* (pp. 73–185). Washington, DC: The National Academies Press.

Iwama, S., Sugimura, Y., Murase, T., Hiroi, M., Goto, M., Hayashi, M., … Oiso, Y. (2009). Central adiponectin functions to inhibit arginine vasopressin release in conscious rats. *Journal of Neuroendocrinology, 21*, 753–759.

Kato, K., Kannan, H., Ohta, H., Kemuriyama, T., Maruyama, S., Tandai-Hiruma, M., … Nishida, Y. (2009). Central endogenous vasopressin induced by central salt-loading participates in body fluid homeostasis through modulatory effects on neurones of the paraventricular nucleus in conscious rats. *Journal of Neuroendocrinology, 21*, 921–934.

Klabunde, R. E. (2005). Exchange function of the microcirculation. In *Cardiovascular physiology concepts* (pp. 171–184). Philadelphia: Lippincott Williams & Wilkins.

Knepper, M. A., & Star, R. A. (1990). The vasopressin-regulated urea transporter in renal inner medullary collecting duct. *The American Journal of Physiology, 259*, F393–F410.

Lamke, L. O., Nilsson, G., & Reithner, L. (1980). The influence of elevated body temperature on skin perspiration. *Acta Chirurgica Scandinavica, 146*, 81–84.

Menninger, R. P. (1985). Current concepts of volume receptor regulation of vasopressin release. *Federation Proceedings, 44*, 55–58.

Miaskiewicz, S. L., Stricker, E. M., & Verbalis, J. G. (2011). Neurohypophyseal secretion in response to cholecystokinin but not meal-induced gastric distention in humans. *The Journal of Clinical Endocrinology and Metabolism, 68*, 837–843.

Nielsen, S., Frøkaer, J., Marples, D., Kwon, T.-H., Agre, P., & Knepper, M. A. (2002). Aquaporins in the kidney: From molecules to medicine. *Physiological Reviews, 82*, 205–244.

Pedersen, E. B., Thomsen, I. M., & Lauridsen, T. G. (2010). Abnormal function of the vasopressin-cyclic-AMP-aquaporin2 axis during urine concentrating and diluting in patients with reduced renal function. A case control study. *BMC Nephrology, 11*, 26.

Randall, H. T. (1976). Fluid, electrolyte, and acid-balance. *The Surgical Clinics of North America, 56*, 1019–1058.

Reis, W. L., Saad, W. A., Camargo, L. A., Elias, L. L., & Antunes-Rodrigues, J. (2010). Central nitrergic system regulation of neuroendocrine secretion, fluid intake and blood pressure induced by antiotensin-II. *Behavioral and Brain Functions, 6*, 64.

Reithner, L. (1981). Insensible water loss from the respiratory tract in patients with fever. *Acta Chirurgica Scandinavica, 147*, 163–167.

Robertson, G. L. (1987). Physiology of ADH secretion. *Kidney International, 21*(Suppl.), S20–S26.

Rose, B. D., & Post, T. W. (2001). The total body water and the plasma sodium concentration. In *Clinical physiology of acid-base and electrolyte disorders* (5th ed., pp. 241–257). New York: McGraw-Hill.

Squire, D. L. (1990). Heat illness. Fluid and electrolyte issues for pediatric and adolescent athletes. *Pediatric Clinics of North America, 37*, 1085–1109.

Takamata, A., Yoshida, T., Nishida, N., & Morimoto, T. (2001). Relationship of osmotic inhibition in thermoregulatory responses and sweat sodium concentration in humans. *American Journal of Physiology. Regulatory, Integrative and Comparative Physiology, 280,* R623–R629.

Taylor, A. E. (1981). Capillary fluid filtration: Starling forces and lymph flow. *Circulation Research, 49,* 557–575.

Thompson, C. J., Bland, J., Burd, J., & Baylis, P. H. (1986). The osmotic thresholds for thirst and vasopressin release are similar in healthy man. *Clinical Science, 71,* 651–656.

Thornton, S. N. (2010). Thirst and hydration: Physiology and consequences of dysfunction. *Physiology & Behavior, 100,* 15–21.

Thrasher, T. N. (1994). Baroreceptor regulation of vasopressin and renin secretion: Low-pressure versus high-pressure receptors. *Frontiers in Neuroendocrinology, 15,* 157–196.

Uretsky, B. F., Verbalis, J. G., Generalovich, T., Valdes, A., & Reddy, P. S. (1985). Plasma vasopressin response to osmotic and hemodynamic stimuli in heart failure. *The American Journal of Physiology, 248,* H395–H402.

Verbalis, J. G., Richardson, D. W., & Stricker, E. M. (1987). Vasopressin release in response to nausea-producing agents and cholecystokinin in monkeys. *The American Journal of Physiology, 252,* R1138–R1142.

Voltaire, B., Galy, O., Coste, O., Recinais, S., Callis, A., Blonc, S., … Hue, O. (2002). Effect of fourteen days of acclimatization on athletic performance in tropical climate. *Canadian Journal of Applied Physiology, 27,* 551–562.

Zerbe, R. L., & Robertson, G. L. (1983). Osmoregulation of thirst and vasopressin secretion in human subjects: Effect of various solutes. *The American Journal of Physiology, 244,* E607–E614.

RECOMMENDED READINGS

Bourque, C. W., & Oliet, S. H. R. (1997). Osmoreceptors in the central nervous system. *Annual Review of Physiology, 59,* 601–619.

Daniels, M. C., & Popkin, B. M. (2010). Impact of water intake on energy intake and weight status: A systematic review. *Nutrition Reviews, 68,* 505–521.

Institute of Medicine. (2004). Water. In *Dietary Reference Intakes for water, potassium, sodium, chloride, and sulfate* (pp. 73–185). Washington, DC: The National Academies Press.

Thornton, S. N. (2010). Thirst and hydration: Physiology and consequences of dysfunction. *Physiology & Behavior, 100,* 15–21.

CHAPTER 36

Iron

Robert R. Crichton, PhD, FRSC

COMMON ABBREVIATIONS

BMP bone morphogenetic protein
DcytB duodenal cytochrome b
DMT1 divalent cation transporter1
HFE hereditary hemochromatosis genes
IrRE iron regulatory element (also abbreviated as IRE in the literature)
IrRP iron regulatory protein (also abbreviated as IRP in the literature)

Iron is an almost ubiquitous requirement for life in any form, and for humankind it is quite simply indispensable. Iron-related disorders leading to either exhaustion or overloading of iron stores are extremely common in all parts of the world. Iron deficiency as a cause of anemia has been known for centuries. Iron overload, whether due to failure to prevent unneeded dietary iron entering the circulation (genetic hemochromatosis) or as a long-term consequence of repeated blood transfusions, is also a well-established clinical condition. This unusual susceptibility of humans to iron-related disorders is due to their severely limited capacity both to excrete iron and to absorb dietary iron when compared to other mammals. It follows therefore that, as was originally suggested by McCance and Widdowson (1937), iron balance is primarily determined by iron absorption.

BIOLOGICAL FUNCTIONS OF IRON

It is doubtful that life on earth would be possible in the absence of iron. Iron is a transition element that is redox active, is a good Lewis acid, and is capable of forming bonds with electronegative elements (oxygen, nitrogen, and sulfur). The biological importance of iron resides to a great extent in its capacity to exist in several oxidation states, the principal ones being ferrous [Fe^{2+} or Fe(II)] and ferric [Fe^{3+} or Fe(III)], although higher valent forms, Fe^{4+} or Fe^{5+}, are generated during the catalytic cycle of a number of enzymes such as catalases, peroxidases, and cytochrome P450s.

Iron is a constituent of numerous proteins, particularly those involved in the transport and metabolism of oxygen, as can be seen from the examples in Box 36-1. Iron proteins can be classified according to the coordination chemistry of their iron: heme proteins, iron-sulfur (Fe-S) proteins, and non-heme, non–iron-sulfur proteins. This latter group includes proteins that contain single Fe atoms and diiron μ-oxygen-bridged centers as well as proteins involved in iron transport and storage. Iron most often has a coordination number of six, which gives octahedral stereochemistry; however, tetracoordinate iron (e.g., Fe-S clusters) and five-coordinate complexes are also occasionally found (Crichton, 2008, 2009).

HEME PROTEINS

The iron in heme proteins is present within a porphyrin, which consists of four pyrrole rings linked by methene bridges; in most hemoproteins the porphyrin is protoporphyrin IX, with four methyl, two vinyl, and two propionyl substituents as shown in Figure 36-1. Heme Fe is always coordinated to the four nitrogen atoms of the tetrapyrrole structure; the fifth, and in some cases the sixth, coordination position is occupied by amino acid residues of the protein. Heme itself is Fe^{2+}–protoporphyrin IX, whereas the corresponding Fe^{3+}–protoporphyrin IX complex is defined as hemin. In some heme proteins, such as cytochrome c, the porphyrin is covalently linked to amino acid residues of the protein.

Heme proteins are involved in a great number of functions (see Box 36-1). The heme proteins include the oxygen carriers hemoglobin and myoglobin and many heme-containing enzymes such as cytochrome oxidase, peroxidases, catalases, and cytochrome P450s, which are involved in the activation of O_2 or in the metabolism of peroxides (ROOHs). The iron atoms of these heme proteins possess an unoccupied sixth coordination site. This sixth site serves as the binding site for O_2, other inorganic ligands (e.g., nitric oxide [NO]), or organic ligands (e.g., through carbon–iron bonds in cytochrome P450s) (Crichton, 2009). Examples of such heme-containing enzymes are listed in Box 36-1 and include monooxygenases (hydroxylases), dioxygenases, and peroxidases. In contrast, in most of the electron transporting cytochromes, the sixth coordinate position of the Fe^{2+} of the heme is occupied by an amino acid residue of the protein (often a histidine or methionine residue). In contrast to cytochrome a_3 and cytochrome P450, which both bind oxygen and transfer electrons, most cytochromes only transfer electrons, with the iron in the heme alternating between the Fe^{2+} and Fe^{3+} states.

BOX 36-1 Types and Examples of Iron-Containing Proteins

I. Heme proteins
   A. O_2 carriers: hemoglobin, myoglobin
   B. Electron transport cytochromes: cytochromes a, b, and c of the mitochondrial electron transport chain
   C. Activators of molecular oxygen: monooxygenases, dioxygenases, and oxidases, such as cytochrome P450s, nitric oxide synthases, cytochrome c oxidase, peroxidases, and catalases

II. Iron-sulfur cluster proteins
   A. Components of electron transport chain enzymes such as mitochondrial aconitase and ferrochelatase

III. Mononuclear nonheme iron proteins
   A. Aromatic amino acid hydroxylases (monooxygenases) that require tetrahydrobiopterin as a cofactor; hydroxylation of aromatic amino acids
   B. Dioxygenases that require a keto acid cosubstrate (usually α-ketoglutarate) and a reducing agent (ascorbic acid), such as prolyl and lysyl hydroxylases
   C. Dioxygenases that add O_2 to a single substrate, for example, lipoxygenases

IV. Dinuclear nonheme iron proteins
   A. Proteins that react with dioxygen and that contain a four helical bundle protein fold surrounding a (μ-carboxylato) diiron core; examples are ribonucleotide reductase, fatty acyl-CoA desaturases, and H-chain ferritins

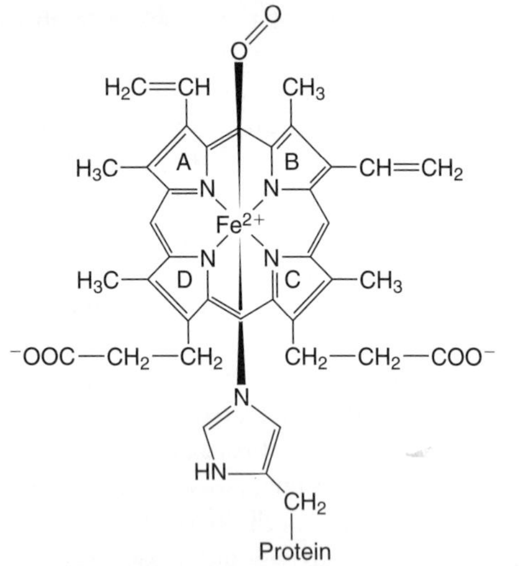

FIGURE 36-1 A detailed picture of the heme group (Fe^{2+}-protoporphyrin IX). The ferrous heme iron is shown bound to a histidine residue of the protein, and the sixth coordination site is occupied by oxygen as in oxygenated hemoglobin or myoglobin. In deoxyhemoglobin or deoxymyoglobin, the ferrous atom is five-coordinate.

IRON-SULFUR CLUSTER PROTEINS

The most common types of iron-sulfur centers are 2Fe-2S and 4Fe-4S clusters, which consist of equal numbers of iron and sulfide ions; the iron atoms of each cluster are also coordinated to the sulfur atoms of four cysteine residues in the protein, as shown in Figure 36-2. When both the sulfide atoms and the cysteine residues are considered, one can see that each Fe atom is tetrahedrally coordinated by four sulfur atoms. Most Fe-S cluster proteins are involved in electron transfer reactions. These include proteins of the mitochondrial electron transport chain as well as various mini–electron transport systems, such as the adrenodoxin (i.e., ferredoxin 1) component of mitochondrial cytochrome P450 systems. However, a number of Fe-S proteins have functions other than electron transfer, including catalysis and acting as biological sensors. The mitochondrial enzyme aconitase contains a 4Fe-4S center that acts as a Lewis acid in the dehydration reaction in which citrate is converted to isocitrate. As discussed later in this chapter, there is also a cytosolic aconitase, which is known as iron regulatory protein 1 (IrRP1) that acts as a biosensor for iron levels within the cell.

MONONUCLEAR NONHEME IRON PROTEINS

A number of enzymes contain a single Fe atom, which is coordinately bound to imidazole (histidine) or carboxylate (glutamate and aspartate) ligands on the protein; these enzymes are involved in reactions that use O_2 as substrate. The aromatic amino acid hydroxylases, which require tetrahydrobiopterin as a cofactor, constitute the first subgroup. A second subgroup requires a keto acid substrate (usually α-ketoglutarate) and a reducing agent (ascorbate). In these reactions, one of the oxygen atoms from O_2 is transferred to the substrate, which is hydroxylated, and the other oxygen atom is transferred to the keto acid cosubstrate, which undergoes oxidative decarboxylation. (See Chapter 27 for examples and an explanation of the role of ascorbic acid in these reactions.) Finally there are some other mononuclear iron-containing enzymes, which add both oxygen atoms from O_2 to a single substrate; these dioxygenases include the 15-lipoxygenase involved in eicosanoid synthesis and cysteine dioxygenase involved in cysteine catabolism and taurine synthesis (see Chapters 14 and 18).

DINUCLEAR NONHEME IRON PROTEINS

A family of proteins containing carboxylate-bridged dinuclear iron sites is involved in functions as diverse as the oxidation of Fe^{2+} to Fe^{3+} (e.g., the H-chain of ferritin), the catalysis of hydroxylation, epoxidation, and desaturation reactions; and the conversion of ribonucleotides into deoxyribonucleotides (e.g., ribonucleotide reductase) (Nordlund and Eklund, 1995; Sazinsky and Lippard, 2006). The common link in all of these dinuclear iron proteins is that they all contain a four helical bundle protein fold, which surrounds a (μ-carboxylato) diiron core with the two iron atoms separated by 0.4 nm or less, and that these iron atoms react with dioxygen (O_2). An example of this class of proteins is ribonucleotide reductase; ribonucleotide reductase catalyzes the reduction of the four common ribonucleotides to their corresponding deoxyribonucleotides, which is essential for deoxyribonucleic acid (DNA) synthesis. The structure of the diiron binding site is represented in Figure 36-3 (Nordlund and Eklund, 1995): each Fe^{2+} ion is octahedrally coordinated

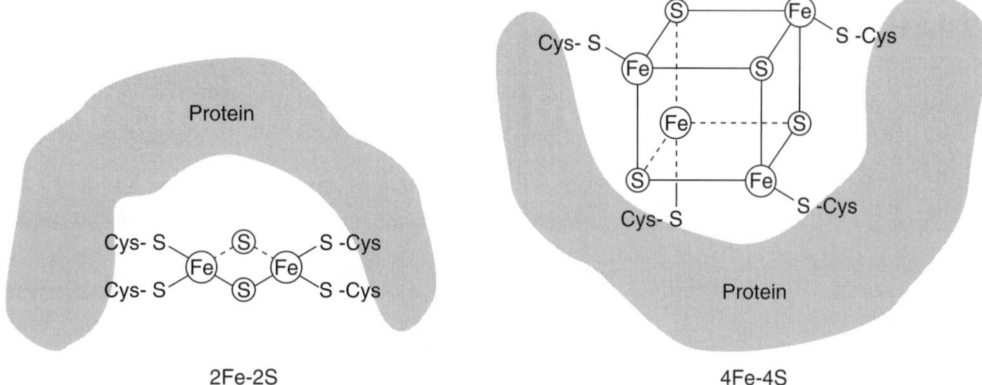

FIGURE 36-2 The two most common types of iron-sulfur clusters, namely 2Fe-2S and 4Fe-4S, consisting of equal numbers of iron and sulfide ions coordinated to four cysteinyl sulfhydryl groups of the protein.

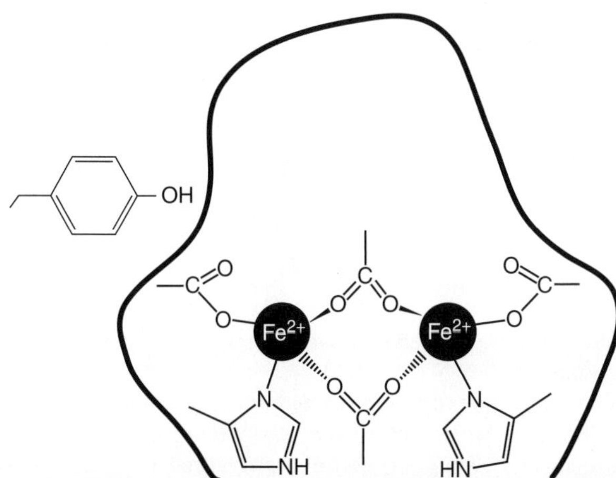

FIGURE 36-3 The active site of ribonucleotide reductase in the non–oxygen bound state. In the diiron site, the Fe^{2+} ions are indicated by solid circles. The tyrosine residue that is converted to a stable free radical during the reaction mechanism is indicated in the top left-hand corner of the figure. In the ribonucleotide reductase reaction, an oxygen atom binds to bridge the two iron atoms, displacing the glutamate carboxyl groups, and the tyrosine residue at the active site donates a proton to become a free radical. (Modified from Nordlund, P., & Eklund, H. [1995]. Diiron-carboxylate proteins. *Current Opinion in Structural Biology, 5*,758–766. Copyright 1995, Elsevier.)

by four carboxylate or imidazole groups of the protein. The reaction of the apoenzyme with O_2 results in formation of an Fe^{3+}–O–Fe^{3+} bridge and generation of a tyrosyl free radical in the protein, which plays an essential role in catalysis.

PROTEINS OF IRON TRANSPORT, STORAGE, AND RECYCLING

Given the many essential functions of iron in oxygen-requiring processes, electron transport, and deoxyribonucleotide synthesis, it is not surprising that efficient mechanisms have developed for iron assimilation and storage. The properties of iron that are so essential for cellular metabolism also make it possible for iron to participate in the generation of highly cytotoxic free radicals, notably the hydroxyl radical. In the aerobic extracellular environment, ferrous ions are readily oxidized to ferric ions, which can rapidly form complexes with hydroxide ions or water to form relatively insoluble polyhydroxides. If these polyhydroxides form in body fluids, the iron becomes unavailable for cellular uptake, and precipitation of these iron aggregates in tissues could have pathological consequences. Consequently, the mechanisms of iron exchange, transport, and storage must maintain an extremely low free iron concentration. Examples of some of the proteins involved in iron transport, storage, and recycling are given in Box 36-2. In addition to the major transport (transferrin and transferrin receptors) and storage (ferritins and hemosiderins) proteins, there are a number of other proteins involved in iron recycling.

PROTEINS OF IRON TRANSPORT

Transferrin

The major plasma protein involved in the transport of iron is transferrin (Crichton, 2009; Sargent et al., 2005; Wessling-Resnick, 2000). Transferrin, a glycoprotein synthesized principally in the liver, is composed of a single polypeptide chain of about 680 amino acids with two iron-binding sites. The closely related lactoferrin is found in human milk as well as in secretions such as tears and saliva, and is secreted by neutrophils; its principal function is as an iron scavenger preventing the proliferation of invading microorganisms. The transferrins have a characteristic bilobal structure, as shown for the diferric form of human lactoferrin in Figure 36-4, *A*. The similar amino- and carboxy-terminal lobes of transferrin are organized into two distinct domains, and each lobe contains one iron-binding site. The hexadentate iron binding site (Figure 36-4, *C*), consists of four protein ligands (an aspartate, a histidine, and two tyrosine residues) plus two oxygen atoms from the synergistically bound carbonate anion (CO_3^{2-}). Together they form a nearly ideal metal coordination sphere, with tight Fe^{3+} binding ($K_d = 10^{-19}$ to 10^{-20} M^{-1}). Neither Fe^{3+} nor CO_3^{2-} is bound significantly in the absence of the other. The multicopper oxidase ceruloplasmin and its enterocytic homolog hephaestin oxidize Fe^{2+} to Fe^{3+} before iron is incorporated into apotransferrin (the iron-free form of transferrin). Iron release from transferrin is described later.

Binding of iron by transferrin results in striking conformational changes in each of the two lobes (Figure 36-4, *B*). In the absence of bound Fe^{3+}, the apotransferrin molecule

BOX 36-2 Proteins Involved in Iron Transport, Storage, and Recycling

Protein	Function
IRON TRANSPORT/STORAGE PROTEINS	
Transferrin (Fe^{3+})	Transports iron in the circulation, supplies iron to cells
Lactoferrin (Fe^{3+})	Binds and removes iron from the circulation in infection
Divalent metal transporter 1 (DMT1) (Fe^{2+})	Transports Fe^{2+} across the apical membrane of enterocytes of the duodenum, and transports Fe^{2+} released from the transferrin–transferrin receptor complex, after its reduction by STEAP, out of endosomes; in both cases this symporter also transports H^+
Ferroportin (Fe^{2+})	Exports Fe^{2+} across the basolateral membrane of duodenal enterocytes and exports Fe^{2+} from macrophages and hepatocytes; acts with the multicopper oxidases ceruloplasmin and hephaestin to load apotransferrin with Fe^{3+}
Ferritins (Fe^{3+})	Stores iron in the cytosol of many cells; synthesis is subject to regulation by iron regulatory protein/iron regulatory element
Hemosiderin (Fe^{3+})	Stores iron within lysosomes in conditions of iron loading
TRANSFERRIN-BINDING PROTEINS	
Transferrin receptor 1	Principal protein for transferrin iron uptake, subject to regulation by iron regulatory proteins/iron regulatory elements
Transferrin receptor 2	Secondary protein for transferrin iron uptake, not subject to regulation by iron regulatory proteins/iron regulatory elements; involved in regulation of hepcidin transcription
PROTEINS OF IRON RECYCLING	
Ceruloplasmin	Multicopper oxidase that oxidizes Fe^{2+} to Fe^{3+} before its incorporation into apotransferrin
Hephaestin	Multicopper oxidase that oxidizes Fe^{2+} to Fe^{3+} before its incorporation into apotransferrin
Duodenal cytochrome b (DcytB)	Metalloreductase that reduces Fe^{3+} to Fe^{2+} before transport by DMT1 at the apical membrane of duodenal enterocytes
STEAP (six transmembrane epithelial antigen of the prostate)	Metalloreductase localized within endosomes that reduces Fe^{3+} to Fe^{2+} before transport by DMT1
Ferrochelatase	Inserts Fe^{2+} into protoporphyrin IX in last step of heme biosynthesis
Mitoferrin (Mfrn)	Transports iron into the mitochondria
Hemopexin	Binds heme with very strong affinity; undergoes endocytosis by target cells and is recycled, like transferrin, for reuse
Haptoglobins	Binds hemoglobin; undergoes endocytosis by target cells, but is not recycled
Heme oxygenase	Responsible for heme degradation and Fe^{2+} release in splenic macrophages

is flexible, with the two domains of each lobe free to swing apart and adopt an open conformation (Figure 36-4, *B*, left). In the presence of Fe^{3+} and CO_3^{2-} they take up a pincerlike closed position around the iron atom, bringing all six ligands involved in iron binding together (Baker et al., 2003).

In healthy individuals, transferrin is present in the plasma at a concentration of 25 to 50 μM but is only approximately 30% saturated with iron. The distribution of the plasma transferrin forms pool is 27% diferric, 34% monoferric (23% with iron bound to the N-lobe and 11% with iron bound to the C-lobe), and 39% apotransferrin. Thus plasma has significant excess iron-binding capacity. Transferrin is distributed throughout most of the extracellular fluids of the body.

Transferrin Receptors

Transferrin receptors are involved in the cellular uptake of iron from the circulation, and they have highest affinity for diferric transferrin. Transferrin receptor 1, is a transmembrane glycoprotein composed of two identical 95-kDa monomers linked by a pair of disulfide bridges. Each monomer consists of 760 amino acid residues organized into an amino-terminal cytoplasmic domain, required for intracellular trafficking of the transferrin–transferrin receptor complex, a short membrane-spanning segment, and a large extracellular domain. The three-dimensional structure of the human transferrin receptor 1-binding extracellular domain has been determined (Lawrence et al., 1999) as has that of the human diferric transferrin–transferrin receptor 1 complex (Cheng et al., 2004), shown in Figure 36-5. Each receptor dimer can bind two transferrin molecules, one to each subunit. The receptor is fundamental to the cellular binding and uptake of iron-bearing transferrin. A second transferrin receptor, transferrin receptor 2, has been identified, which binds transferrin with lower affinity than transferrin receptor 1. It appears to play an important role in the regulation of systemic iron homeostasis.

Other Transport Proteins

A number of other proteins present in plasma may play a role in iron transport. This is particularly likely in iron overload, hemolytic anemia, and conditions of ineffective erythropoiesis during which free hemoglobin or heme may be present in the plasma compartment. These transport proteins include haptoglobin, hemopexin, ferritin, lactoferrin, and albumin.

Haptoglobin binds free hemoglobin, and both hemopexin and albumin bind free heme and hemin. All three proteins are synthesized and secreted by the liver. The haptoglobin-hemoglobin complex is cleared from the plasma by the reticuloendothelial cells, mainly in the spleen. Hemopexin binds

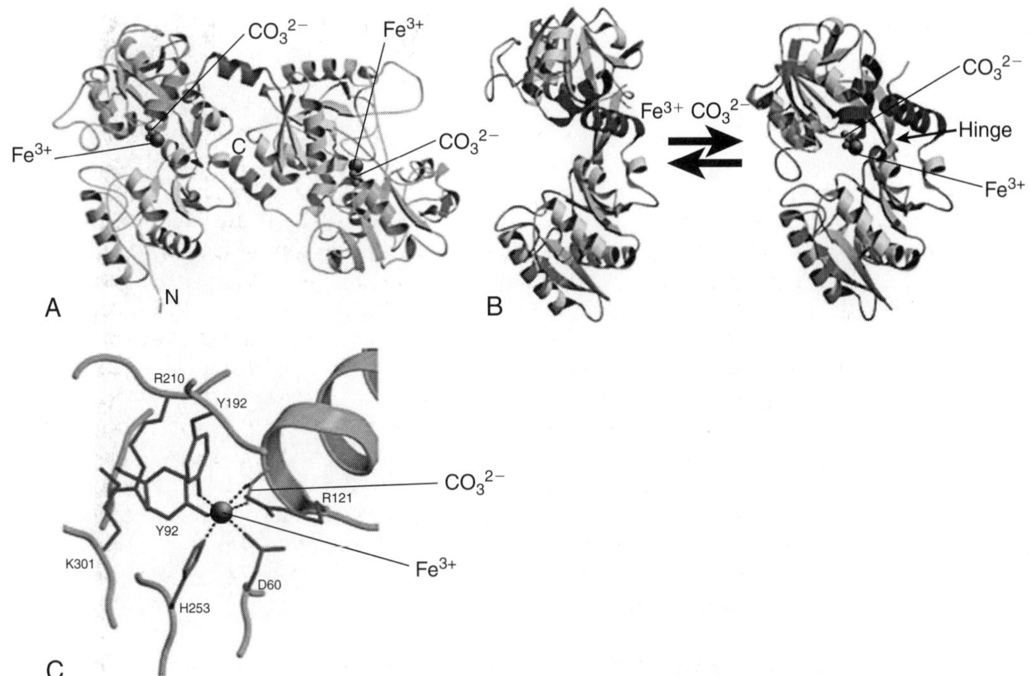

FIGURE 36-4 Ribbon diagram showing the characteristic bilobal structure of transferrins. **A,** Shown here is the iron-bound form of human lactoferrin, with the N-lobe on the left and the C-lobe on the right; the Fe^{3+} ion and CO_3^{2-} are bound in the interdomain cleft of each lobe. **B,** The conformational change that accompanies iron binding, shown here for the N-lobe of human transferrin. **C,** The canonical iron binding site of transferrins, shown here for the N-lobe of human lactoferrin, involves two tyrosine (Y), one aspartate (D), and one histidine (H) as ligands for the Fe^{3+} and a bidentate CO_3^{2-} ion pocket formed by an arginine (R) side chain and the N-terminus of an α-helix. (From Baker, H. M., Anderson, B. F., & Baker, E. N. [2003]. Dealing with iron: Common structural principles in proteins that transport iron and heme. *Proceedings of the National Academy of Sciences of the United States of America. 100*, 3579–3583. Copyright 2003, National Academy of Sciences, USA.)

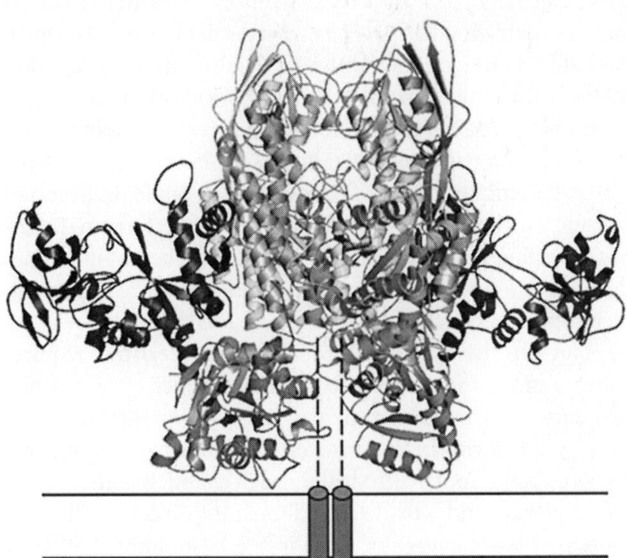

FIGURE 36-5 Structural model of two molecules of iron-free human transferrin bound to the ectodomain of the transferrin receptor dimer. The ribbon diagram of the ectodomain of the transferrin receptor is shown at top center with the stalks of the transferrin receptor, which links it to the membrane, shown as dotted lines and the transmembrane domains shown as cylinders. The transferrin molecules are shown bound on either side of the transferrin receptor ectodomain. (With kind permission from Springer Science+Business Media: Wally, J., & Buchanan, S. K. [2007]. A structural comparison of human serum transferrin and human lactoferrin. *Biometals. 20*, 249–262.)

heme with high affinity, and the hemopexin-heme complex is internalized mainly by liver cells. By removing hemoglobin and heme from the plasma, haptoglobin and hemopexin protect the body from the oxidative damage that can be caused by heme iron. In hemolytic anemias, plasma haptoglobin and hemopexin levels are low due to their function in scavenging hemoglobin and heme and their consequent endocytosis and removal from the plasma. Albumin is the most abundant plasma protein, and albumin binds heme and a number of other ligands with relatively high affinity. Albumin becomes the major scavenger of heme in patients with severe hematologic diseases characterized by excessive intravascular hemolysis. Albumin has a plasma half-life of 15 to 20 days and is cleared at a rate of about 15 g/day by the liver, kidney proximal tubular cells, and some other tissues via endocytotic mechanisms.

Lactoferrin is an iron-binding protein structurally similar to transferrin; it is found predominantly in neutrophils, secretory epithelium, and secretions, including milk. Amounts on the order of 2 to 3 mg/L (25 to 40 nmol/L) have been reported in human plasma. This concentration is several orders of magnitude lower than that of transferrin (30 μmol/L). Lactoferrin binds iron much more tightly than transferrin, particularly at acidic pH. The role of lactoferrin in iron transport is probably negligible. Its functional significance appears to relate to its antibacterial properties, due to its ability to sequester iron and thus reduce iron availability in infectious conditions. Ferritin is the intracellular storage form of iron, and very small levels

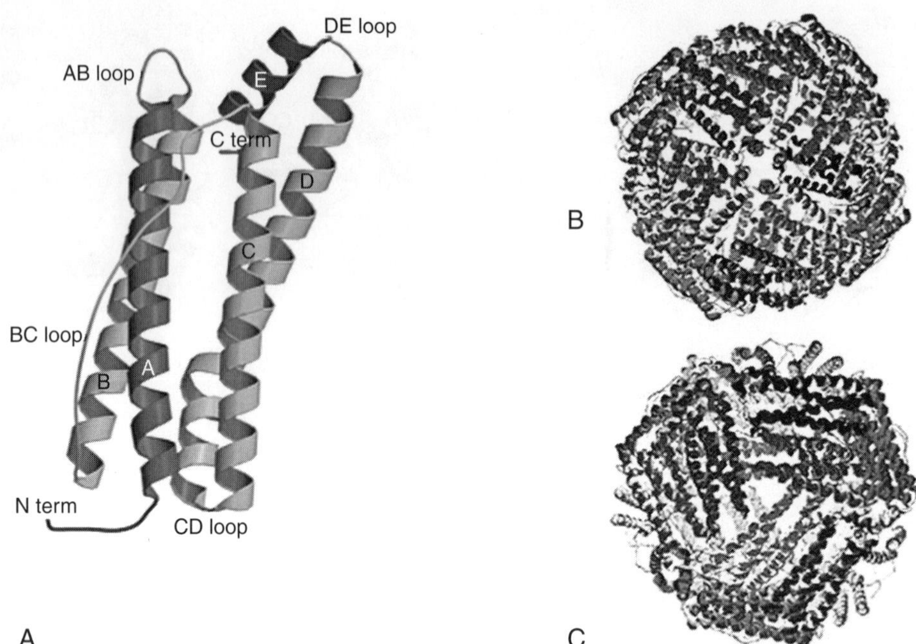

FIGURE 36-6 Ferritin structure. **A,** A ribbon diagram of the α-carbon backbone of the recombinant horse L-chain apoferritin subunit. **B, C,** Views of a ferritin molecule down the threefold and fourfold axes of symmetry, respectively. (From Crichton, R. R., & Declercq, J. P. [2010]. X-ray structures of ferritins and related proteins. *Biochimica et Biophysica Acta, 1800,* 706–718. Copyright [2010] Elsevier.)

are found circulating in the plasma. Whether plasma ferritin has a specific function is not known.

PROTEINS OF IRON STORAGE

Ferritin and Hemosiderin

To prevent the unwanted effects of iron-catalyzed free radical generation or iron oxidation and its subsequent precipitation, it is imperative that the cell stores excess iron safely. The iron-storage proteins ferritin and hemosiderin fulfill this cellular "housekeeping" function in all cells; in addition they serve as an iron reservoir in specialized cells (macrophages of the reticuloendothelial system and parenchymal cells of the liver) from which body iron pools can be replenished as iron is used or lost (Liu and Theil, 2005; Crichton, 2009; Arosio and Levi, 2010). The major storage sites of ferritin in normal subjects are liver, spleen, and skeletal muscle. Hemosiderin, which is thought to be the lysosomal degradation product of ferritin, represents a very small fraction of normal body iron stores, and is present mostly in macrophages. It can increase dramatically in iron overload.

The iron-free apoferritin molecule is composed of 24 subunits with molecular weights around 20 kDa each and has a total molecular mass of approximately 500 kDa. The apoferritin subunits form a hollow protein shell with an external diameter of 12 to 13 nm, delimiting a cavity of diameter 7 to 8 nm, within which iron can be stored in a nontoxic, water-soluble, yet bioavailable form. In mammalian ferritins, the iron core resembles the mineral known as ferrihydrite. The ferritin subunits (Figure 36-6, *A*) are roughly cylindrical, 5 nm long and 2.5 nm wide, with approximately 80% of the amino acid sequence present in five α-helices. Ferritin with its 24 subunits has a high degree of symmetry, and Figure 36-6, *B* and *C*, show a ferritin molecule viewed down the fourfold and threefold axes of symmetry, respectively (Crichton and Declercq, 2010).

Human ferritins are made up of two subunits of distinct amino acid sequence, known as H and L. The H subunits are characterized by a (μ-carboxylato) diiron core with ferroxidase activity, oxidizing Fe^{2+} to Fe^{3+}, whereas the L subunits, which lack this center, are thought to be involved in the nucleation of the iron core of ferritin. With two types of subunits, 25 "isoferritins" can be built. Variations in the proportions of the two subunits in ferritins of different tissues exist and reflect the tissue-specific functions of ferritin. For example, in liver and spleen, which play a major role in iron storage, ferritins have a much higher proportion of the L subunit, whereas in human heart and brain, where iron detoxification is more important, heteropolymers rich in H subunits are predominant.

The effective storage of iron in human ferritins requires contributions from both subunit types, which play complementary roles in storing, detoxifying, and maintaining Fe^{3+} in a soluble form. In the first step of iron incorporation, Fe^{2+} penetrates the apoferritin shell through channels at the surface of the protein and is oxidized at dinuclear iron centers (known as ferroxidase centers) localized in the H subunits. Fe^{3+} then migrates to nucleation centers within L subunits, in the interior of the protein shell. Once a nucleus of iron core has formed at the nucleation sites, deposition of iron on this inorganic core accomplishes the further incorporation of iron. The maximum storage capacity of each ferritin molecule is approximately 4,500 iron atoms. The mechanism of iron release from ferritin is not at all well understood, although its mobilization appears to require degradation of the ferritin molecule, within both the proteasome and the lysosome (De Domenico et al., 2006).

Hemosiderin is a lysosomal storage form of iron, which is found particularly in conditions of iron overload, such as hereditary hemochromatosis and transfusion-dependent hemoglobinopathies such as the thalassemias. The hemosiderins are thought to be the product of lysosomal degradation of ferritin (Crichton, 2009) The iron cores in hemosiderins isolated from iron-loaded animals and humans are ferrihydrite-like, similar to those in ferritin, but are less available to chelation than are those in ferritins (Ward et al., 2000).

BODY IRON COMPARTMENTS AND DAILY IRON EXCHANGE

Total body iron (approximately 40 mg/kg in women and 50 mg/kg in men) is made up of two major and one minor compartment—namely functional, storage, and transport iron—as summarized in Table 36-1. Functional iron is composed predominantly of the iron in hemoglobin of red blood cells and erythroid tissues, iron in myoglobin in the muscle, and iron-containing enzymes present in all cells of the body. The storage iron compartment is intrinsically more variable, accounting for between 0 and 20 mg of iron per kg of body weight. This iron is stored in ferritin, which is located predominantly in parenchymal cells of the liver and skeletal muscle, and in hemosiderin, which is stored mainly in macrophages of the reticuloendothelial system. These storage proteins serve as a repository for dietary iron absorbed in excess of that needed to replace losses from the functional compartment; this provides a mechanism to prevent accumulation of free iron ions, which would be toxic, and to provide an emergency reserve supply from which sudden deficits in the functional compartment may be replenished. Storage iron is usually present in roughly equal amounts in the macrophages of the mononuclear phagocytic cells, in hepatocytes, and in skeletal muscle. A very small amount of ferritin is found in plasma, and the serum ferritin level is used to assess iron stores, but the physiological function of plasma ferritin and its source are not yet clearly defined.

The much smaller transport compartment represents the interface between the storage and functional compartments, consisting essentially of transferrin-bound iron. It accounts for approximately 0.04 mg of iron per kg body weight. The total amount of plasma transferrin-bound iron in a 70-kg adult is only about 50 μmol, i.e., 2.8 mg in 2.5 L of plasma. Although the amount of iron bound to transferrin at any given time is quantitatively small, the flux of iron through this compartment is relatively large on a daily basis. The flux of iron through transferrin–iron pool is approximately 700 μmol/day in an adult (40 mg of Fe per day, or approximately 0.6 mg/kg per day) as determined by ferrokinetic evaluation. The transferrin molecule is significantly reused; it undergoes more than 100 cycles of iron delivery before it is finally removed from the circulation. Measurements of the transport compartment provide important, clinically useful information for defining the state of iron deficiency or excess.

Iron uptake from the diet amounts to release of about 1 to 2 mg of iron per day from enterocytes into the circulation, and this is balanced by iron losses from the body through various routes. In contrast to this "external" iron exchange, about 22 mg of iron from senescent or damaged erythrocytes is internally recycled each day. Thus, iron metabolism in the body is dominated by "internal" iron flux. Internal iron flux in other tissues also occurs due to movement of iron in and out of stores and to turnover of iron-containing proteins.

TABLE 36-1 Typical Iron Distribution in Adults

	mg Iron/kg Body Weight	
	MEN	WOMEN
Functional iron		
Hemoglobin	32	28
Myoglobin	5	4
Iron-containing enzymes	1–2	1–2
Storage iron		
Ferritin (and hemosiderin)	~11	~6
Transport iron		
Transferrin	0.04	0.04

INTERNAL IRON EXCHANGE AND CELLULAR IRON METABOLISM

The major pathways of internal iron exchange between different body compartments are dominated by heme synthesis for erythropoiesis and the turnover of senescent red blood cells (Figure 36-7). Transferrin transports iron between different cellular compartments, with about four fifths of the daily exchange cycling through the erythroid marrow and the mononuclear phagocytic system (i.e., monocytes and macrophages including those in the spleen and lymph nodes).

USE OF IRON FOR ERYTHROPOIESIS

Erythroblasts (nucleated, developing red blood cells) are generated by the bone marrow from stem cells. An erythroblast eventually loses its nucleus to become a reticulocyte and ultimately a mature red blood cell called an erythrocyte, by which stage hemoglobin synthesis has ceased. Transferrin-bound iron is taken up by erythroblasts and transported into the mitochondria, where it is incorporated into protoporphyrin IX by the mitochondrial enzyme ferrochelatase to form heme. Each day in the normal adult approximately 2×10^{11} red blood cells are produced, and this requires more than 2×10^{20} atoms, or almost 24 mg, of iron. The majority of this (~17 mg) is incorporated into hemoglobin.

RECYCLING OF IRON FROM SENESCENT OR DAMAGED RED BLOOD CELLS

Once released from the bone marrow, mature erythrocytes (red blood cells) circulate for approximately 120 days, and thereafter are recycled by cells of the mononuclear phagocytic system. As the erythrocytes circulate in the blood, a number of physicochemical changes occur. After senescent

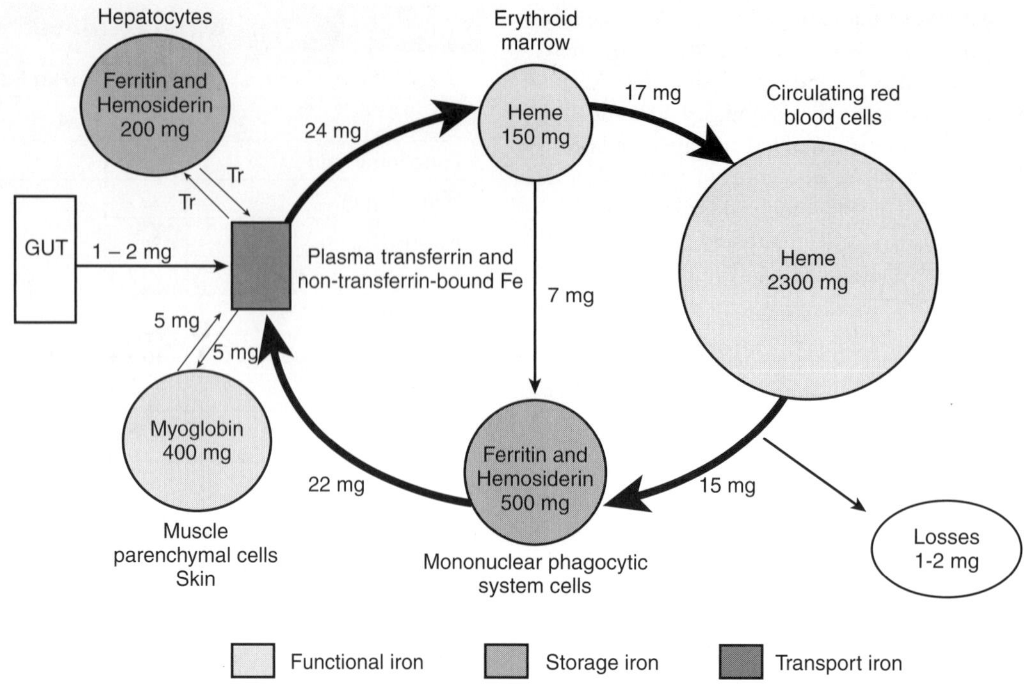

FIGURE 36-7 Body iron stores and daily iron exchange in humans. Iron content of various iron pools are shown inside circles, and daily exchange among pools is shown as values by the arrows. Endogenous iron losses occur mainly by shedding of cells from the skin and the lining of the intestines, urinary tract, and airways and essentially offset iron absorption from the diet. *Tr*, Trace.

erythrocytes are taken up and lysed within the lysosomes of mononuclear phagocytic cells (macrophages), the heme is broken down by heme oxygenase and the iron released from heme breakdown is exported from the lysosomes into the cytosol via NRAMP1 (natural resistance-associated macrophages protein 1, a divalent metal transporter homologous to DMT1). Export of iron from the macrophages occurs via ferroportin in conjunction with iron reduction by plasma ceruloplasmin and its loading onto plasma transferrin.

As iron is used for erythropoiesis and recovered from senescent erythrocytes by the mononuclear phagocytic system, a small amount of iron also moves in and out of iron storage forms, ferritin and hemosiderin, in these cells. In addition, a fraction of the newly formed erythrocytes are destroyed within the bone marrow itself (ineffective erythropoiesis) and their iron is released for reuse.

CENTRAL ROLE OF TRANSFERRIN IN IRON TRANSPORT AND CELLULAR UPTAKE

As mentioned earlier, transferrin has two iron-binding sites and transports iron between the erythroid marrow and the mononuclear phagocytic cells, as well as other tissues. The overall saturation of plasma transferrin with iron is normally about one third; so apotransferrin, the two monoferric transferrins, and diferric transferrin are all normally found in plasma.

Transferrin-dependent Cellular Iron Uptake

Transferrin-bound iron uptake by cells is mediated by expression of transferrin receptors on their plasma membranes. At physiological pH, the affinity of transferrin for its receptor correlates directly with the degree of iron occupancy. Apotransferrin has negligible affinity for the transferrin receptor at pH 7.4, whereas diferric transferrin has the highest affinity. Iron is delivered to cells via the transferrin-mediated cell cycle, as summarized in the upper left-hand corner of Figure 36-8. The diferric transferrin binds to its receptor and the complex is invaginated into clathrin-coated pits to form vesicles that fuse with endosomes. This delivers the vesicle contents into the interior of the endosome, where the pH is reduced to around 5 to 6 by the action of an ATP-dependent proton pump. Iron release from diferric transferrin is facilitated at acidic pH by protonation of the bound carbonate, thereby weakening the coordination of the iron, and by triggering conformational changes in both transferrin and the transferrin receptor, which stabilize the transferrin molecule in its apo-transferrin conformation. The Fe^{3+} is then reduced to Fe^{2+} by members of the six-transmembrane epithelial antigen of the prostate (STEAP) family of metalloreductases (Ohgami et al., 2005, 2006) for transport of Fe^{2+} out of the late endosome/lysosome into the cytosol via the divalent cation transporter, DMT1.

The apo-transferrin has an extremely high affinity for the transferrin receptor in the more acidic environment of the endosome. By remaining bound to the receptor, apo-transferrin largely escapes degradation by the lysosomal enzymes, and the majority of the apo-transferrin–transferrin receptor complexes are returned to the cell surface after iron is released. At the cell surface, the slightly alkaline pH allows the apo-transferrin to dissociate, leaving the transferrin receptor attached to the plasma membrane. Then the apo-transferrin is returned to the circulation where it is once again able to bind iron and participate in further cycles of iron delivery via the transferrin cycle, which ensures iron uptake by most cells.

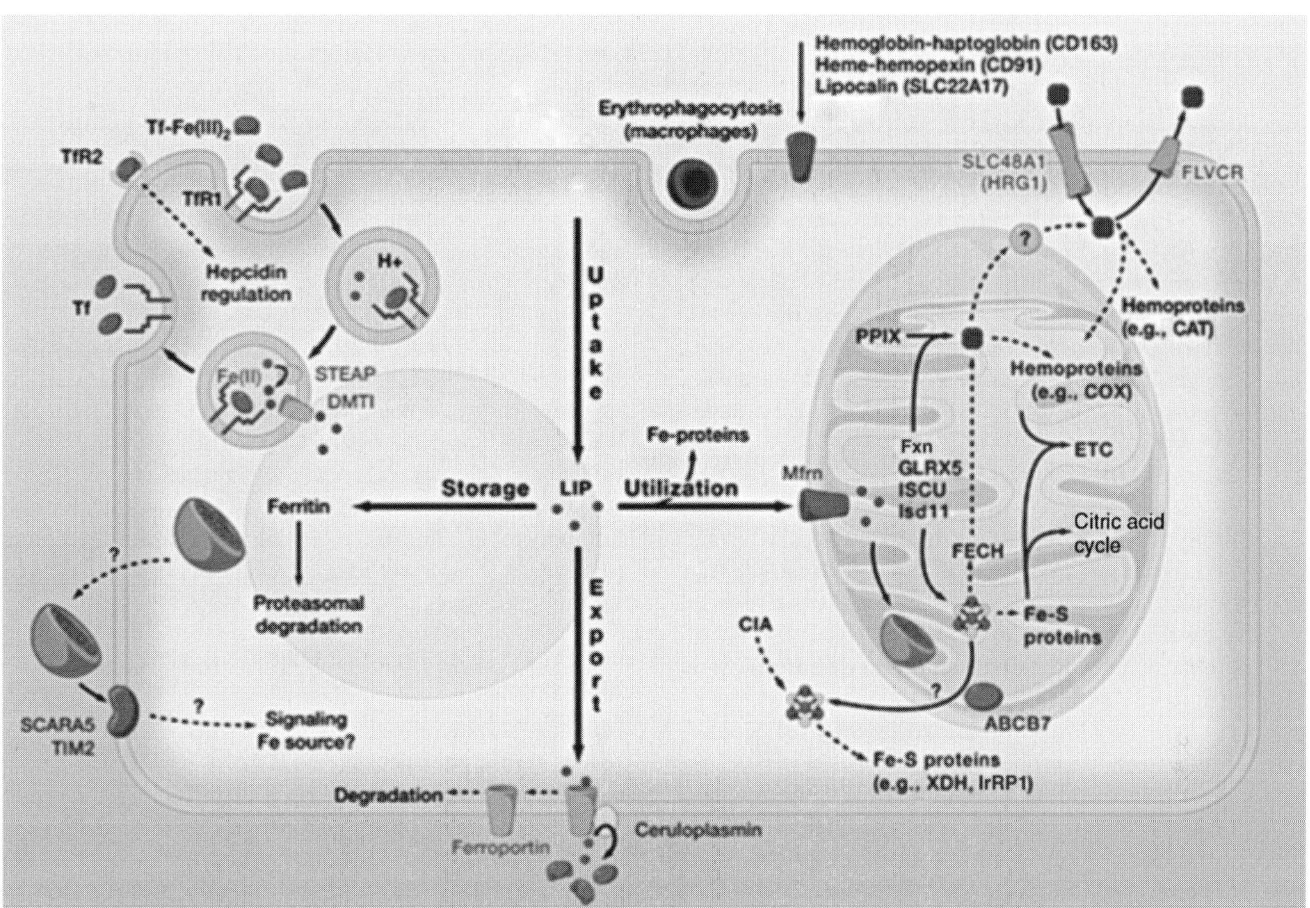

FIGURE 36-8 Cell biology of iron metabolism. A generic cell is indicated. Most cells acquire plasma iron via transferrin receptor 1 (TfR1)-mediated endocytosis of diferric transferrin, Tf-Fe(III)$_2$. In endosomes, iron is freed from transferrin and reduced to Fe(II) by STEAP metalloreductases prior to its release into the cytosol via divalent metal transporter 1 (DMT1); transferrin (Tf) and TfR1 return to the plasma membrane to be used for further cycles. (DMT1 also functions in the apical absorption of dietary iron after reduction by DcytB and possibly other ferrireductases in polarized epithelial cells such as enterocytes [not shown].) Other iron acquisition pathways are symbolized (e.g., acquisition of heme iron from red blood cells by macrophages). Iron uptake systems feed the so-called labile iron pool (LIP). The LIP is utilized for direct incorporation into iron proteins or iron transport to mitochondria via mitoferrin (Mfrn), where the metal is inserted into heme or Fe-S cluster prosthetic groups. The fraction of the LIP that is not utilized for metalation reactions can be exported via ferroportin, which works together with ferroxidases for iron loading onto transferrin, or stored in a nontoxic form in ferritin shells. The size of the LIP is determined by the rate of iron uptake, utilization, storage, and export; these processes must be coordinately regulated to avoid detrimental iron deficiency and prevent iron excess. Refer to the text for additional information. *ABCB7,* ATP binding cassette transporter 7; *CAT,* catalase; *CIA,* cytosolic iron-sulfur protein assembly; *COX,* cytochrome c oxidase; *ETC,* electron transport chain; *Fe,* iron; *Fe-S,* iron-sulfur; *FECH,* ferrochelatase; *FLVCR,* feline leukemia virus, subgroup C receptor; *Fxn,* frataxin; *GLRX5,* glutaredoxin 5; *ISCU,* iron-sulfur cluster scaffold homolog; *IrRP,* iron regulatory protein; *Isd11,* iron regulated surface determinant 11; *PPIX,* protoporphyrin IX; *SCARA5,* scavenger receptor class A, member 5; *TIM-2,* T-cell immunoglobulin and mucin domain containing 2; *XDH,* xanthine dehydrogenase.. (From Hentze, M. W., Muckenthaler, M. U., Galy, B., & Camaschella, C. [2010]. Two to tango: Regulation of mammalian iron metabolism. *Cell, 142,* 24–38. Copyright [2010] Elsevier.)

TRANSFERRIN AND FERROPORTIN-DEPENDENT IRON EXPORT

Export of ferrous iron from cells occurs via ferroportin, which works together with ferroxidases for iron loading onto plasma transferrin. Ferroportin levels are regulated by hepcidin, which is a central regulatory molecule of systemic iron homeostasis.

Ferroportin, the Cellular Iron Exporter

One of the most significant discoveries of the last decade has undoubtedly been the recognition of the key role of ferroportin, the only known cellular iron exporter, in systemic iron homeostasis. Ferroportin, the product of the *SLC40A1* gene, was independently identified by three laboratories in 2000 and shown to play a key role in the export of iron from a number of different cell types (McKie et al., 2000; Donovan et al., 2000; Abboud and Haile, 2000). Ferroportin is a transmembrane protein with 10 potential membrane-spanning regions. In polarized epithelial cells, it localizes to the basolateral membrane. It is expressed in many cells that play a critical role in mammalian iron metabolism, including placental syncytiotrophoblasts, duodenal enterocytes, hepatocytes, and reticuloendothelial macrophages. Targeted disruption of the mouse *SLC40A1* gene clearly established the unique and nonredundant functions of ferroportin in iron release from cells (Donovan et al., 2005). As illustrated in Figure 36-8 (lower center), ferroportin transports Fe^{2+} out of the cell, in concert with the ferroxidases (hephaestin in enterocytes and ceruloplasmin in other cell types). The ferroxidases facilitate the extraction of iron from the ferroportin channel and the subsequent loading of Fe^{3+} onto apotransferrin (De Domenico et al., 2007). Ferroportin expression is regulated by hepcidin, which triggers its degradation. Ferroportin mRNA translation is regulated by the IrRE/IrRP system in macrophages but not in erythroblasts.

Hepcidin

Since its serendipitous discovery in 2000 (Nicolas et al., 2001; Pigeon et al., 2001), the role of hepcidin as the key regulatory molecule of systemic iron homeostasis has become abundantly clear. It is a member of the defensin family of antimicrobial peptides, although, unlike the defensins whose purpose is to kill bacteria, hepcidin has only weak bactericidal activity. Hepcidin is synthesized by the liver hepatocytes as an 84-residue propeptide, which is cleaved by the protease furin in the Golgi apparatus to yield the mature, bioactive 25-residue peptide that is secreted. Hepcidin, like defensins, forms an amphipathic beta sheet and has four disulfide bonds.

Hepcidin is secreted into the bloodstream by the liver, and it acts systemically to downregulate ferroportin (Nemeth et al., 2004). Hepcidin binds to an amino acid sequence in the exterior segment of the transmembrane protein ferroportin, and this triggers ferroportin degradation (De Domenico et al., 2008). Subsequent to hepcidin binding, Janus kinase 2 (Jak 2) binds and phosphorylates ferroportin, resulting in its internalization, ubiquitination, and lysosomal degradation (De Domenico et al., 2009). Upregulation of hepcidin thus decreases iron efflux from the cell as well as its subsequent uptake into transferrin.

Hepatic hepcidin expression is regulated at the transcriptional level in response to multiple and in part opposing signals, including systemic iron availability, erythropoietic signals, hypoxia, and inflammatory and stress signals (Zhang and Enns, 2009; Hentze et al., 2010). Iron sensing appears to include mechanisms that respond to transferrin saturation and hepatic iron stores. The inflammatory cytokines interleukin 1 and interleukin 6 are both potent inducers of hepcidin expression. The inflammatory and iron stores regulators appear to operate independently, with integration occurring at the hepcidin gene promoter. Because an increase in hepcidin limits the recycling of heme iron needed to sustain erythropoiesis, upregulation of hepcidin secretion is an important contributor to the anemia of chronic disease.

HEMOGLOBIN AND HEME UPTAKE AND EFFLUX

Iron can also be taken up by transferrin-independent pathways. Hemoglobin and heme resulting from intravascular hemolysis are cleared by specific receptor-mediated scavenger systems (see Figure 36-8, upper right). Both the haptoglobin–hemoglobin and the hemopexin–heme complexes are internalized by receptor-mediated endocytosis and degraded. Lipocalin alpha(1)-microglobulin has been proposed to mediate heme uptake.

The presence of excess free heme in cells is highly toxic, and there is some evidence that heme efflux pathways exist, notably involving the feline leukemia virus, subgroup C receptor.

FERRITIN TRANSPORT

Although the physiological significance of ferritin transport is unknown, some proteins have been suggested to serve a role in ferritin uptake. Ferritin can enter cells via the Scara5 (scavenger receptor class A, member 5) and TIM-2 (T-cell immunoglobulin and mucin domain containing 2) receptors (see Figure 36-8, lower left). Mechanisms of ferritin efflux are unidentified.

INTRACELLULAR IRON TRAFFICKING, UTILIZATION, AND STORAGE

Iron uptake systems feed into the poorly characterized intracellular transit pool, usually referred to as the labile iron pool (see Figure 36-8), which has been described as "somewhat like the Loch Ness monster—only to disappear from view before its presence, or indeed its nature, can be confirmed" (Crichton, 1984). The labile iron pool represents iron in transit between storage, transport, functional, or recycled forms. Although the exact chemical nature of labile iron remains uncertain, it is thought to represent approximately micromolar concentrations of iron (Breuer et al., 2008). This pool reflects the readily available iron within the cell and is believed to be the key regulator of internal and external iron exchange.

The labile iron pool can be utilized (see Figure 36-8) for direct incorporation into iron proteins within the cytosol, or iron can be transported into the mitochondria by the inner mitochondrial membrane protein mitoferrin (see Figure 36-8, right of center). The majority of iron for cellular utilization is channeled through mitochondria-localized pathways that are involved in the insertion of iron into heme and Fe-S cluster prosthetic groups. Mitochondria represent the major subcellular site of iron utilization, so it is not surprising that they play a central role in the control of cellular iron metabolism (Sheftel and Lill, 2009). However, iron management within mitochondria remains poorly understood.

Heme Synthesis

In the mitochondria, Fe^{2+} is inserted into protoporphyrin IX by ferrochelatase to form heme. Heme is then incorporated into mitochondrial cytochromes such as cytochrome c oxidase; it can also be exported from the mitochondria via an undefined mechanism and incorporated into hemoproteins found in various parts of the cell (e.g., catalase in peroxisomes).

Iron-sulfur Cluster Synthesis

Iron-sulfur cluster (ISC) assembly begins in the mitochondria (Figure 36-9) with the assembly of a transiently bound Fe-S cluster on the scaffold protein ISCU. A cysteine desulfurase, Nfs1-Isd11, releases the sulfur required for Fe-S cluster formation from cysteine, generating a persulfide on a cysteine residue of Nsf1 and releasing the remainder of the substrate cysteine as alanine. Iron enters the mitochondria via mitoferin (Mfrn) and is donated to ISCU in a process that involves frataxin (Fxn). The electrons required for the reduction of S^0 (in cysteine) to sulfide (S^{2-}, present in Fe-S clusters) are supplied from NADH via ferredoxin (Fdx)/ferredoxin reductase (FdxR). The transfer of the Fe-S cluster from ISCU and its incorporation into recipient apoproteins (Apo) to generate the Fe-S–containing holoproteins requires a number of chaperones and the monothiol glutaredoxin (GLRX5).

Extramitochondrial Fe-S protein biogenesis requires the core ISC assembly machinery together with components of the ISC export machinery. The ATP-binding cassette (ABC) transporter B7 (ABCB7) exports an unknown component (X) to the cytosol for Fe-S protein assembly. Export may involve a sulfhydryl oxidase (ALR) and glutathione (GSH). In the cytosol, the cytosolic Fe-S protein assembly (CIA machinery) catalyzes Fe-S protein maturation. The Fe-S clusters are first assembled on Cfd1 and Nbp35 (P-loop NTPases), then transferred to the iron-only hydrogenase-like cytosolic factors (IOP1 and CIAO1), and finally incorporated into cytosolic and nuclear target apoproteins. (Lill and Mühlenhoff, 2008; Sheftel and Lill, 2009).

The importance of Fe-S proteins and Fe-S protein biogenesis in human health is underlined by the number of mutations in mitochondrial iron-sulfur cluster assembly

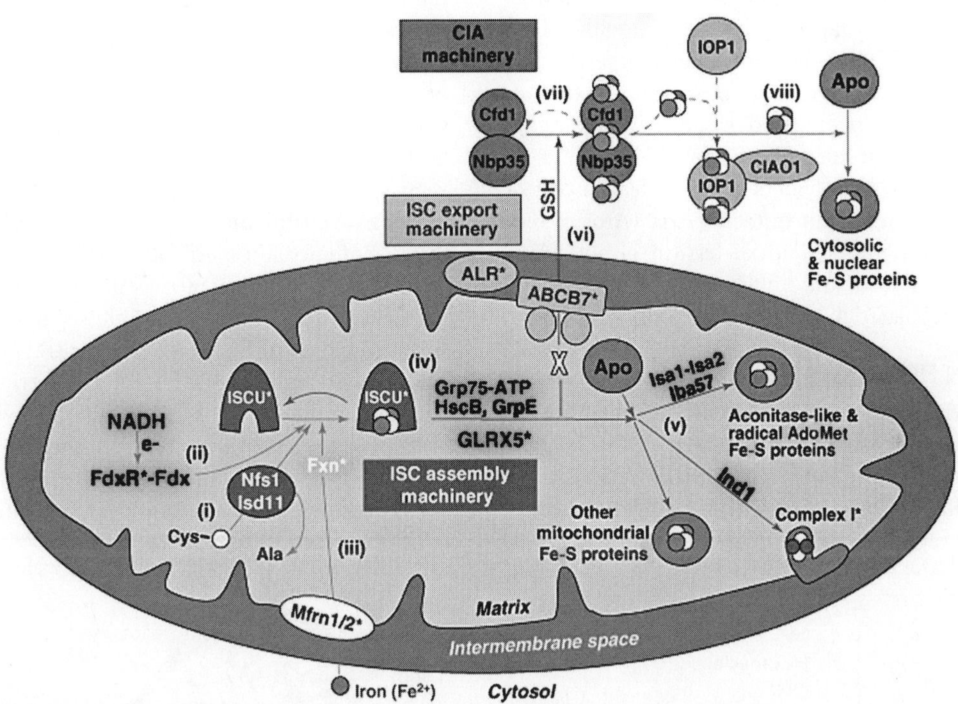

FIGURE 36-9 A current working model for Fe-S protein biogenesis in eukaryotes. The figure depicts the names used for human components. Components directly involved in human disease are marked with an asterisk. (i) A sulfur atom (white circle) is derived from cysteine (Cys) via the cysteine desulfurase Nfs1 in complex with iron-regulated surface determinant 11 (Isd11). (ii) The sulfur atom is transiently bound to Nfs1 as a persulfide, transferred to the iron sulfur cluster assembly scaffold protein (ISCU), and reduced to sulfide by electrons (e-) that presumably originate from NADH and pass through ferredoxin reductase (FdxR) and ferredoxin (Fdx). (iii) Iron (gray circle) enters the mitochondria through the carrier protein mitoferrin (Mfrn) and, by a process involving frataxin (Fxn), is combined with sulfide on the mitochondrial Fe-S scaffold ISCU. (iv) The Fe-S cluster transiently bound to ISCU is transferred to mitochondrial apoproteins (Apo) in an ATP-dependent process requiring an Hsp70-type chaperone system (potentially comprising the Hsp70 chaperone Grp75, HscB and GrpE) and glutaredoxin X5 (GLRX5). (v) Isa1, Isa2, and Iba57 play specific roles in delivering Fe-S clusters to a subset of Fe-S proteins that includes aconitase-like and S-adenosylmethionine (AdoMet) radical enzymes, whereas Ind1 is involved in the assembly of Fe-S clusters on respiratory complex I. An unknown intermediate (X) is synthesized in an iron-sulfur cluster (ISC) assembly machinery-dependent manner; and (vi) transported out of the mitochondria by the inner membrane ATP binding cassette transporter B7 (ABCB7) to assist the formation of cytosolic and nuclear Fe-S proteins. This process presumably involves the sulfhydryl oxidase ALR and glutathione (GSH). (vii) In the cytosol, a transiently bound iron-sulfur (Fe-S) cluster is formed on a scaffold complex consisting of the P-loop NTPases Cfd1 and Nbp35. (viii) The Fe-S clusters are then transferred and inserted into extramitochondrial apoproteins (Apo) in a reaction involving iron-only hydrogenase-like protein 1 (IOP1) and cytosolic iron-sulfur protein assembly protein 1 (CIAO1). (From Sheftel, A., Stehling, O., & Lill, R. [2010]. Iron-sulfur proteins in health and disease. *Trends in Endocrinology and Metabolism, 21*(5), 302–314. Copyright [2009] Elsevier.)

and the cytosolic Fe-S protein assembly components, which have been linked to hematological and neurological disorders (Sheftel et al., 2009). The first known examples were frataxin and ABC transporter B7. Depletion of frataxin in human cells by more than 70% causes the neurodegenerative disorder Friedreich's ataxia, the most common autosomal recessive ataxia. Friedreich's ataxia appears to be due mainly to the lack of Fe-S protein synthesis. Mutations in the human *ABCB7* gene cause a relatively rare form of X-linked sideroblastic anemia (so-named because the erythroblasts contain granules of ferritin) with cerebellar ataxia. The identification of other phenotypes associated with a lack of proteins involved in Fe-S protein biogenesis, such as a sideroblastic anemia associated with a lack of glutaredoxin 5, underlines the interplay between pathways of mitochondrial iron utilization and human health.

Storage of Iron as Ferritin

Iron from the cytosolic labile iron pool which is not required for exportation or for utilization, can be stored within ferritin (Arosio and Levi, 2010). The importance of ferritin in storing excess iron in a form that is not only nontoxic but potentially bioavailable is highlighted by the early lethality of H-chain ferritin knockout mice (Ferreira et al., 2000).

In some tissues, homopolymers of a nuclear-encoded H-chain ferritin are present in mitochondria (Arosio and Levi, 2010). However, mitochondrial ferritin is not present in gut, liver, or spleen, and unlike cytosolic ferritin, its expression is not regulated by the iron regulatory proteins.

CELLULAR IRON HOMEOSTASIS

Ferritin, transferrin receptor, and certain other proteins involved in iron homeostasis are regulated at the mRNA level by iron regulatory proteins (IrRPs) that bind to stem–loop structures in iron-responsive elements (IrREs) in the mRNAs. The regulatory mechanisms are best understood for ferritin and transferrin receptor expression.

Iron-Responsive Elements

Ferritin biosynthesis is regulated in response to changes in cellular iron content. This regulation involves a sequence of approximately 30 nucleotides in the 5′-untranslated region (5′-UTR) of the ferritin messenger RNA (mRNA), which is highly conserved through all ferritin genes (except mitochondrial ferritin). Biosynthesis of the transferrin receptor is also regulated posttranscriptionally, but in this case the regulation involves several nucleotide sequences in the 3′-untranslated region (3′-UTR) of the transferrin receptor mRNA. These sequences all show significant homology and have been termed iron-responsive elements (IrREs) (Muckenthaler et al., 2008).

A canonical IrRE can be defined by both its RNA sequence and its three-dimensional structure. An IrRE consists of a stem–loop secondary structure on the mRNA. The stem of the stem–loop structure contains an unpaired cytosine, which causes a bulge in the stem structure, and the loop consists of the unpaired nucleotide sequence, CAGUGN (where N = U, C, or A). The stem of the IrRE consists of five complementary base pairs above the unpaired cytosine plus a lower stem of variable length (Muckenthaler et al., 2008) (Figure 36-10). Based on the x-ray structure of an iron regulatory protein (IrRP) bound to the IrRE of ferritin mRNA (Walden et al., 2006), it appears that the high affinity and specificity of IrRP/IrRE interactions arise from two spatially distant sites that establish multiple RNA–protein contacts. These sites are clustered around the terminal loop and around the C-bulge of the IrRE.

As illustrated in Figure 36-11, transferrin receptor mRNA contains multiple IrREs in the 3′-UTR, whereas L and H chain mRNAs have a single IrRE in their 5′-UTRs. The binding of IrRPs to the 5′- and 3′-flanking IrREs results in different effects on translation, as is discussed later in this section.

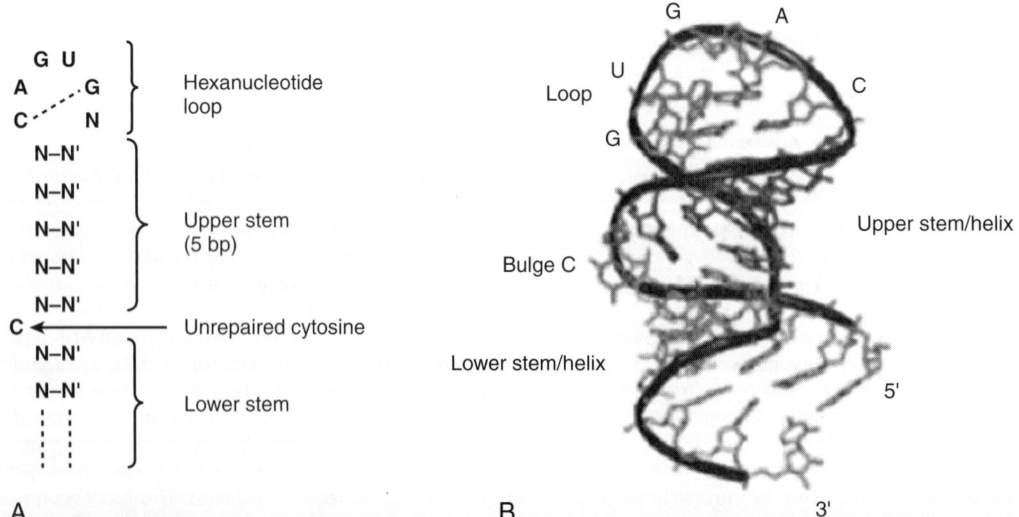

FIGURE 36-10 Structure of an iron regulatory element (IrRE). **A** Consensus sequence of an iron-responsive element (IrRE). The hexanucleotide loop has the sequence CAGUGN where N represents any nucleotide except G. The upper and lower stems are made up of base pairs (bp) of variable sequence (N-N′) which are separated by an unpaired C. **B** NMR structure of a consensus IrRE.

In addition to ferritin H and L chains and transferrin receptor mRNAs, the mRNAs for several other proteins have been found to contain IrREs or similar sequences. The mRNAs for the erythroid form of δ-aminolevulinic acid synthase 2, the first enzyme in the heme biosynthetic pathway; the mitochondrial form of aconitase; the iron export protein, ferroportin; and the hypoxia-inducible factor 2α also contain a single IrRE in the 5′-UTR. The divalent cation transporter protein DMT1 has a single IrRE in the 3′-UTR of its mRNA. Single IrRE-like structures have been found in the 3′-UTRs of several other mRNAs, such as CDC14A (cell division cycle 14 homologue A), but their functional roles remain unclear.

Iron Regulatory Proteins

Two cytosolic proteins interact directly with the IrREs to modulate mRNA translation; these proteins are designated iron regulatory proteins (IrRPs) or iron-responsive element binding proteins. IrRP1 and IrRP2 have a molecular weight of approximately 90 kDa and 105 kDa, respectively; the two proteins show significant sequence similarity but IrRP-2 has a 73-residue addition near its N-terminus.

In iron-replete cells, IrRP1 exists in a 4Fe-4S form, has aconitase activity, and lacks IrRE-binding activity. When the cellular iron concentration is low, the protein no longer has an Fe-S cluster. This apoprotein form of IrRP1 no longer has aconitase activity, but it now has IrRE-binding activity. Although the cysteine residues that coordinate the iron-sulfur cluster in IrRP1 are conserved in IrRP2, the latter has no detectable aconitase activity and does not appear to exist as an Fe-S protein.

IrRP2 is less abundant than IrRP1 in most cells, with greatest expression in intestine and brain. In iron-replete cells, IrRP2 is ubiquitinated and subjected to proteosomal degradation. This process involves the interaction of IrRP2 with the FBXL5 (F-box and leucine-rich repeat protein 5) adaptor protein, which recruits a SCF (SKP1-CUL1-F-box) E3 ligase complex, promoting ubiquitination and subsequent degradation by the proteosome (Salahudeen et al.,

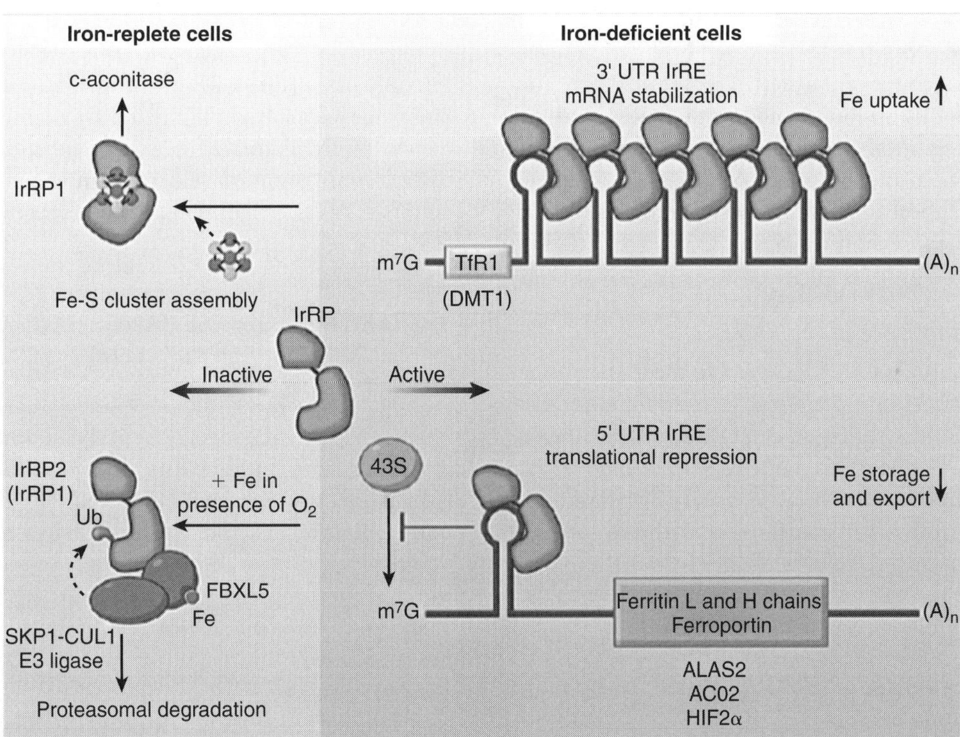

FIGURE 36-11 Regulation of cellular iron metabolism. In iron-deficient cells (right), iron regulatory protein 1 (IrRP1) or IrRP2 bind to *cis*-regulatory hairpin structures called iron regulatory elements (IrREs) that are present in the untranslated regions (UTRs) of mRNAs encoding proteins involved in iron transport and storage. The binding of IrRPs to single IrREs in the 5′ UTRs of target mRNAs (ferritin L chain, ferritin H chain, ferroportin) inhibits their translation, whereas IrRP interaction with multiple 3′ UTR IrREs in the *transferrin receptor 1* (*TfR1*) transcript increases its stability. As a consequence, TfR1-mediated iron uptake increases whereas iron storage in ferritin and export via ferroportin decrease, thereby increasing the labile iron pool. In iron-replete cells (left), FBXL5 iron-sensing F-box protein interacts with IrRP1 and IrRP2 and recruits the SKP1-CUL1 E3 ligase complex that promotes IrRP ubiquitination and degradation by the proteasome; IrRP1 is primarily subject to regulation via the assembly of a cubane Fe-S cluster that triggers a conformational switch precluding IrRE-binding and conferring aconitase activity to the holoprotein. In addition to ferritin H and L chains, ferroportin, and transferrin receptor mRNAs, the mRNAs for several other proteins have been found to contain IrREs or similar sequences. The mRNAs for the erythroid form of delta-aminolevulinic acid synthase 2 (ALAS2), the mitochondrial form of aconitase (ACO2), and the hypoxia-inducible factor 2α (HIF2α) also contain a single IrRE in the 5′-UTR. The divalent cation transporter protein (DMT1) has a single IrRE in the 3′-UTR of its mRNA. (From Hentze, M. W., Muckenthaler, M. U., Galy, B., & Camaschella, C. [2010]. Two to tango: Regulation of mammalian iron metabolism. *Cell, 142*, 24–38. Copyright [2010] Elsevier.)

2009; Vashisht et al., 2009) (see Figure 36-11). The FBXL5 protein contains a hemerythrin-like domain, which acts as an iron sensor. Direct binding of iron to this domain stabilizes FBXL5, and results in IrRP degradation; otherwise FBXL5 is degraded. The hemerythrin domain of FBXL5 also senses oxygen, and a lack of oxygen in the presence of sufficient iron also results in IrRP2 degradation. IrRP1 may also undergo regulated degradation by the ubiquitin-proteasome system, but the major mode of regulation of its IrRE-binding activity is the loss of the Fe-S cluster.

IrRP–IrRE Interactions

The specific mechanisms by which IrRE–IrRP interactions modulate protein biosynthesis in response to iron status are clearly different for IrREs located in the 5′- or 3′-UTRs.

Binding of IrRPs to IrREs in the 3′-UTR

When active IrRPs bind to the stem–loop structures on the 3′-end of the transferrin receptor mRNA, the transferrin receptor mRNA is stabilized against degradation, as illustrated in Figure 36-11. Consequently, when cytosolic iron levels are low, transferrin receptor mRNA concentrations increase and more transferrin receptor is synthesized, increasing the abundance of transferrin receptor. When iron is in excess, the IrRPs no longer bind to the IrREs, and the transferrin receptor mRNA, which is no longer protected by the IrRPs, is degraded and less transferrin receptor is synthesized. IrRPs also appear to positively regulate the expression of DMT1 mRNA expression via its single 3′-UTR IrRE, but the molecular mechanism is unclear.

Binding of IrRPs to IrREs in the 5′-UTR

When the iron supply is low, IrRPs bind to the 5′ stem–loop IrREs of the ferritin H or L chain mRNAs and inhibit translation of these mRNAs (see Figure 36-11). Conversely, when iron is abundant, the IrRPs are inactive, do not bind to the IrRE, and allow protein synthesis to occur. Translation of the iron export protein, ferroportin; the erythroid form of δ-aminolevulinic acid synthase (ALAS2); the mitochondrial form of aconitase (ACO2); and the hypoxia-inducible factor 2α (HIF2α) are similarly regulated.

Physiological Responses of IrRP-IrRE System to Iron and Non-iron Signals

When iron supplies are limiting, transferrin receptors are expressed, which allows the cell to take up more iron, but the synthesis of ferritin is blocked, consistent with the absence of a need to store excess iron. When the cellular levels of iron are adequate, ferritin is synthesized and the storage of potentially toxic iron in ferritin is thus facilitated, whereas the transferrin receptor mRNA is destroyed by ribonucleases so that iron uptake via transferrin receptor is decreased. Ferroportin mRNA translation by macrophages is also regulated by IrRP binding, whereas the ferroportin mRNA in erythroblasts lacks the 5′-IrRE. Thus, the capacity of certain cells to efflux iron via ferroportin is decreased in the iron-deficient state. Heme synthesis in erythroid cells is regulated in response to iron status through the interaction of IrRPs with the 5′-UTR of the mRNA for ALAS2, the first enzyme of protoporphyrin IX synthesis. Synthesis of ALAS2 and hence of heme is repressed in iron-deficient erythroid cells.

Although the major determinant of IrRP activity is the cytosolic content of exchangeable iron, the IrRPs also respond to noniron signals. IrRP2 is stabilized by hypoxia because oxygen, as well as iron, is required for stabilization of FBXL5 leading to IrRP2 degradation. In contrast, hypoxic conditions inactivate IrRP1 by favoring the holo-form of IrRP (with the 4Fe-4S cluster) (Meyron-Holz et al., 2004a). Reactive oxygen species selectively activate IrRP1 by causing disassembly of Fe-S clusters; nitric oxide, generated from L-arginine by nitric oxide synthase, is also able to modulate iron removal from iron-sulfur proteins (Muckenthaler et al., 2008). Clearly this could also result in modulation of the IrRE-binding activity of IrRP1 and might be one of the factors involved in posttranscriptional regulation of proteins of iron metabolism in situations of inflammation and stimulated cytokine production.

Genetic ablation of both IrRPs causes embryonic lethality (Smith et al., 2006; Galy et al., 2008), whereas animals lacking only one of the IrRPs are both viable and fertile. IrRP2 knockout mice have mild microcytic anemia and have a tendency toward increased neurodegeneration and abnormal body iron distribution (Cooperman et al., 2005; Galy et al., 2005). IrRP1 knockout mice are asymptomatic (Meyron-Holz et al., 2004b).

EXTERNAL IRON EXCHANGE, IRON ABSORPTION, AND SYSTEMIC IRON HOMEOSTASIS

External iron exchange is concerned with the processes by which iron is either lost from or added to the body. Normally only approximately 0.05% (2 to 2.5 mg) of body iron is lost each day. This iron loss must be replaced by absorption of a similar amount of iron from dietary sources. Net negative balance results when losses exceed absorption; this ultimately results in a depletion of the functional iron compartment and iron deficiency. When absorption exceeds losses, positive balance occurs; if this is sustained in an adult, it may ultimately lead to iron overload. Iron deficiency and iron overload are discussed separately later in this chapter.

IRON LOSSES AND REQUIREMENTS FOR ABSORBED IRON

In the basal state, iron is lost passively in cells that are shed from the skin surface or the epithelial lining of internal organs (intestines, urinary tract, and airways). Small amounts of red blood cells are also lost via the gastrointestinal tract. The normal amount of iron lost each day in men is about 14 μg/kg. These basal losses average 0.98 mg/day in a 70-kg man and 0.77 mg/day in a nonmenstruating 55-kg woman. In iron deficiency losses may be reduced by 50%, whereas in iron overload they are slightly increased. Menstruation increases the amount of iron loss, and absorption of 1.36 mg of iron is the median requirement for maintenance of iron balance in normal menstruating women. To maintain balance in 95% of women, absorption of 2.8 mg/day of iron is required.

The other physiological cause of increased iron loss is pregnancy. Although a pregnant woman should be in positive iron balance during the course of the pregnancy, it is not unusual for the course of pregnancy and parturition to result in a net loss of iron from the mother's body. The iron requirements specific to pregnancy over the 9-month gestational period, for a 55-kg woman, are calculated to be 830 mg (basal losses, 320 mg; products of conception, 360 mg [fetus, 270 mg; placenta and umbilical cord, 90 mg]; and peripartum blood loss, 150 mg). However, it should not be forgotten that during pregnancy, iron absorption will be upregulated. An additional 450 mg of iron is required for expanded maternal red cell mass; however, this iron will not be lost with parturition but will be returned to the mother during postpartum contraction of red cell mass. The greatest increases in total requirements (up to 6 mg of iron per day) are for fetal growth and erythroid expansion during the second and third trimesters, which are only slightly offset by the diminished loss of iron as a result of the amenorrhea of pregnancy. Lactation results in a further iron loss of 0.3 to 0.6 mg/day postpartum due to secretion in the milk, but this additional loss is largely balanced by the accompanying amenorrhea.

Growth markedly increases iron requirements for formation of both erythroid and nonerythroid tissues. In the first year of life the infant must absorb 0.3 mg of iron per day to maintain iron homeostasis. In the second year of life, growth causes this figure to rise to 0.4 mg/day. Slow growth from this time until puberty results in a gradual increase in requirements to 0.5 to 0.8 mg/day. Puberty and adolescent growth spurts increase iron requirements to 1.6 mg/day in boys and to 2.4 mg/day in girls (reflecting concomitant menarche).

Iron loss may be increased in situations of pathological and nonpathological blood loss. Pathological losses occur in situations such as bleeding from the urinary, genital, and gastrointestinal tracts. The gastrointestinal tract is the most common site of pathological bleeding, secondary to conditions such as esophagitis, gastritis, varices, peptic ulcers, neoplasms, diverticulosis, angiodysplasia, and inflammatory bowel disease. In developing regions of the world, infection with parasites such as hookworm may increase iron loss. Heavy infestation may cause bleeding of sufficient magnitude to increase requirements of iron by as much as 3 to 5 mg/day. Nonpathological increases in blood loss may be secondary to the effects of aspirin or nonsteroidal antiinflammatory drugs, which may cause gastric bleeding, or to voluntary blood donation.

Iron requirements are further increased by stimulation of erythropoiesis by administration of erythropoietin, which is used to treat disease states such as renal failure, or by endogenous erythropoietin, which is elevated in hemolytic states related to abnormalities in hemoglobin formation (e.g., thalassemia or sickle cell disease).

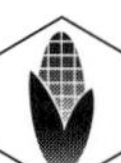

FOOD SOURCES OF IRON

Meat and Meat Substitutes
12 to 24 mg per 3 oz clams
6 mg per 3 oz oysters
5 mg per 3 oz beef liver
2 to 3 mg per 3 oz beef chuck or round
2 mg per 3 oz turkey
2 mg per 3 oz lamb

Legumes
4.5 mg per ½ cup soybeans
3 mg per ½ cup lentils
2.5 mg per ½ cup kidney or garbanzo beans
2 mg per ½ cup lima, navy, great northern, or black beans

Other Vegetables and Fruits
2 to 3 mg per ½ cup spinach
2 mg per ½ cup pumpkin
1 to 2 mg per ½ cup tomatoes
1.5 mg per ½ cup sour cherries
1.8 mg per ½ cup raisins
1 mg per ½ cup green peas
1 mg per ½ cup sweet potatoes

Cereal and Grain Products (Whole Grain, Enriched, or Fortified)
4 to 18 mg per 1 cup ready-to-eat cereals
3 to 3.5 mg per 3 oz bagel
3 mg per 3 oz graham crackers
2.5 mg per 10 pretzels (2 oz)
1 mg per ½ cup egg noodles
1 mg per ½ cup rice
1 mg per ½ cup couscous

Miscellaneous
2.6 mg per 3 oz semisweet chocolate
3.5 mg per 1 tbsp blackstrap molasses

Data from U.S. Department of Agriculture, Agricultural Research Service. (2011). *USDA National Nutrient Database for Standard Reference, Release 24*. Retrieved from http://www.ars.usda.gov/ba/bhnrc/ndl

IRON ABSORPTION

Intestinal iron absorption reflects a composite of three determinants: the iron content of the diet, the bioavailability of the dietary iron, and the capacity of the enterocytes to absorb the iron.

Iron Content of Diet

In terms of the iron content of the diet, western diets have remarkably consistent iron contents, averaging 5 to 6 mg/1,000 kcal. Iron in western diets tends to be highly bioavailable, with an estimated availability in the range of 14% to 17%. Therefore a 2,000-kcal diet should provide between 1.4 and 2 mg of absorbed iron/day.

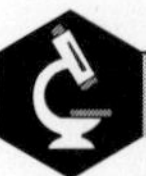

CLINICAL CORRELATION

Iron Deficiency and Low Iron Stores in Infants, Children, and Women of Child-Bearing Age

Iron deficiency affects a large number of infants, children, and women of child-bearing age in both developed nations and the developing world. Estimates of the prevalence of iron deficiency among women and children in developing countries are as high as 60%. Data from the third National Health and Nutrition Examination Survey (NHANES III), which was conducted during 1988 to 1994, indicated a low rate of iron deficiency in the United States (Centers for Disease Control and Prevention, 1998). Approximately 3% of children ages 12 to 36 months in the United States had iron deficiency anemia, and an additional 6% had low iron stores (based on elevated erythrocyte protoporphyrin concentration, low serum ferritin concentration, and low transferrin saturation). The NHANES III results indicated that 11% of nonpregnant women ages 16 to 49 years in the United States had low iron stores, and 3% to 5% also had iron deficiency anemia. The NHANES III data also indicated that the prevalence of iron deficiency is higher among children and women living at or below the poverty level than among those living above the poverty level.

Iron deficiency is of nutritional concern during infancy and childhood, especially among children less than 24 months of age. The iron stores of full-term infants are estimated to be adequate to meet iron requirements for 4 to 6 months, whereas those of preterm infants are smaller and may be depleted sooner. A rapid rate of growth, along with frequently inadequate intake of dietary iron, places young children at particular risk. Breast milk provides iron in a highly available form and is sufficient to meet an infant's needs through the first 6 months of life, but other sources of iron are recommended after 6 months. Iron-fortified formula and iron-fortified cereals are important sources of iron for infants in the first year of life. Risk for iron deficiency drops after 24 months of age because of the slower rate of growth and a more diversified diet.

Adolescent girls and women of child-bearing age (12 to 49 years) are also at some risk of iron deficiency. Most women in this age-group have high iron requirements due to menstrual blood losses and do not meet their needs for iron from dietary intake, partly because of relatively low energy expenditure and consequently low food intake. During pregnancy, iron requirement is high because there is an increase in blood volume and fetal and maternal tissues are growing. The requirement for absorbed iron during pregnancy (4.5 mg/day) is three times higher than during nonpregnancy (1.5 mg/day) and is only partially compensated for by increased iron absorption and decreased menstrual loss throughout pregnancy. Because most women enter pregnancy with low iron stores, routine iron supplementation during pregnancy has been the standard practice in many countries to prevent the development of iron deficiency anemia during the later part of pregnancy.

Consequences of iron deficiency include adverse developmental outcomes and greater risk of lead poisoning in children, reduced work capacity in adults, and possibly an increased risk of poor pregnancy outcomes, such as preterm delivery and higher maternal mortality.

Factors that Affect Iron Bioavailability

After dietary iron enters the common luminal pool in the gastrointestinal tract, it is subject to interactions with a number of ligands contained in the food and other food constituents that affect its absorption. The major ligands in foods that enhance nonheme iron absorption appear to be organic acids, such as ascorbic, citric, malic, and lactic acids, which are found particularly in citrus and deciduous fruits. Nonetheless, studies of the chronic ingestion of high doses of vitamin C or multivitamin supplements failed to show any effects of ascorbic acid on long-term iron status in subjects consuming mixed diets.

The major inhibitory ligands found in ingested foods include phytates, polyphenols, calcium, and fiber. Phytates are widely distributed in various grains and vegetables. Polyphenols are also widely distributed in various vegetables and are also found in beverages such as tea and coffee. Calcium and certain components of dietary fiber may also inhibit nonheme iron absorption.

Animal protein is a rich source of highly absorbable heme iron and has a marked enhancing effect on nonheme iron absorption.

Iron Absorption in the Duodenum

Iron absorption is most active in the proximal small intestine, near its junction with the stomach. The absorptive duodenal enterocytes originate by cellular division within the crypts of Lieberkühn. At this stage the crypt cells require iron for both cell development and differentiation and must obtain their iron from the plasma because they lack absorptive capacity. However, during the 48 hours of their migration from crypt to villous apex, they acquire capacity to absorb iron across their apical membranes from the lumen of the intestinal tract. The response of enterocytes to iron status appears to occur while these cells are in the crypts of the intestinal villus, because a delay of approximately 48 hours is required before any change in body iron requirements is reflected in altered absorption by the enterocytes.

MOLECULAR MECHANISMS OF IRON ABSORPTION

The two main pathways by which dietary iron is absorbed from the gastrointestinal tract are outlined in Figure 36-12.

Uptake of Luminal Inorganic Iron into Enterocytes: DMT1 and DcytB

Inorganic dietary iron is absorbed from the gastrointestinal tract by DMT1. Since dietary inorganic iron is thought to be mostly in the oxidized form, the Fe^{3+} must first be reduced to Fe^{2+} by an apical membrane–bound ferrireductase, duodenal cytochrome b (DcytB), before the Fe^{2+} is transported

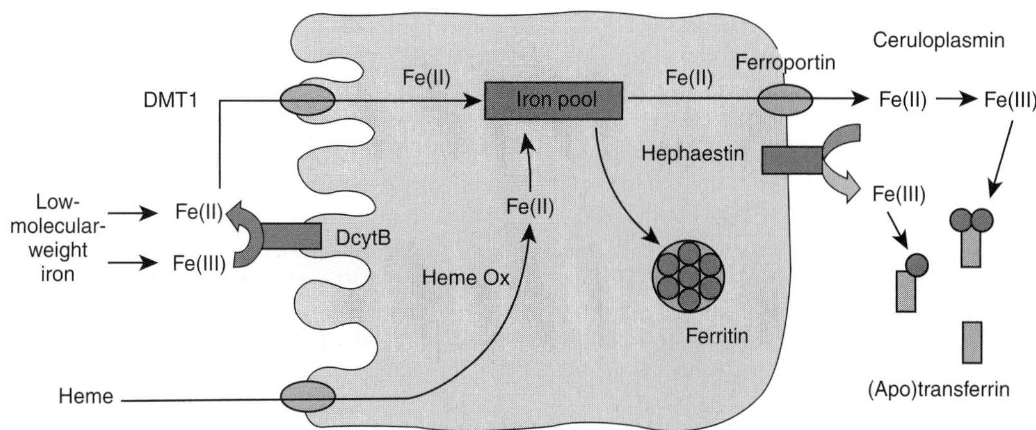

FIGURE 36-12 Schematic representation of iron absorption into an enterocyte. Iron is taken up from the gastrointestinal tract either as heme or nonheme iron. The former is degraded to release Fe(II) by heme oxygenase, whereas the latter is reduced by duodenal cytochrome b (DcytB) and transported across the apical membrane by divalent metal transporter 1 (DMT1). Within the enterocyte the iron pool can equilibrate with the intracellular storage protein ferritin. At the basolateral membrane, iron is transported out of the cell by ferroportin; its incorporation into apotransferrin requires the ferroxidase activity of hephaestin and/or ceruloplasmin.

by DMT1 into the enterocyte. Heme iron is thought to be taken up at the apical membrane of duodenal enterocytes by a specific heme transporter, and the Fe^{2+} is released intracellularly after the heme is degraded by heme oxygenase.

DMT1 was discovered in mk mice that have an autosomal recessive inherited defect in intestinal iron transport that results in microcytic anemia (Fleming et al., 1997). At around the same time, DMT1 was identified in the rat (Gunshin et al., 1997). The symporter DMT1 transports Fe^{2+} and other divalent metal ions, including Co^{2+}, Cu^{2+}, Mn^{2+}, Ni^{2+}, and Zn^{2+} (Gunshin et al., 1997), together with a proton. The DMT1 protein has 12 putative membrane-spanning domains, is expressed at the highest levels in the proximal duodenum, and is upregulated by dietary iron deficiency (Gunshin et al., 1997). The Belgrade rat, which has an autosomal recessively inherited anemia associated with both abnormal reticulocyte iron uptake and abnormal gastrointestinal iron absorption, has the same missense mutation in the *DMT1* gene as the mk mouse (Fleming et al., 1998). Due to mRNA processing in the nucleus, several variants of DMT1 mRNA exist in cells. Only the variant with an IrRE in its 3′-UTR is upregulated in the proximal duodenum during dietary iron starvation (Canonne-Hergaux et al., 1999). DMT1 is also called Nramp2, DCT1, and SLC11A2.

DcytB is a plasma membrane diheme protein (McKie et al., 2001) that is highly expressed in the apical membrane of duodenal enterocytes. It has around 50% sequence similarity to the cytochrome b_{561} family of plasma membrane reductases. Whether this is the only ferrireductase in the enterocyte apical membrane remains uncertain because DcytB knockout mice appear to have normal iron metabolism (Gunshin et al., 2005), although this has been challenged (McKie, 2008).

Uptake of Luminal Heme Iron into Enterocytes

The search for the mechanism of heme uptake, which in humans is a much more bioavailable source of iron than nonheme iron, seemed to have reached its conclusion when the putative heme transporter, designated heme carrier protein 1, was identified (Shayeghi et al., 2005). However, subsequent studies showed that the transporter had a 150-fold higher affinity for the B vitamin, folate (Qiu et al., 2006). Although the mechanism of heme uptake remains uncertain, the subsequent fate of heme iron is clear. It is degraded by heme oxygenase, mainly by the substrate-inducible heme oxygenase 1 enzyme located in the endoplasmic reticulum and perhaps other membrane fractions of cells (Ferris et al., 1999). Heme oxygenase catalyzes the cleavage of the α-methene bridge that joins the two pyrrole residues containing the vinyl substituents in the protoporphyrin. This results in release of Fe^{2+} and carbon monoxide (CO) from the tetrapyrrole structure as well as the conversion of the tetrapyrrole structure to biliverdin. Biliverdin is subsequently converted into bilirubin by biliverdin reductase.

Fate of Iron in Enterocytes: Storage as Ferritin or Export into Circulation via Ferroportin and Hephaestin

Within the intestinal cell, the Fe^{2+} derived from both heme and nonheme Fe^{2+} enters a low-molecular-weight pool. This iron can either be stored in ferritin in the mucosal cell or be transported across the basolateral membrane by the transmembrane transporter protein, ferroportin, to reach the interstitial fluid and plasma. The incorporation of iron into plasma apotransferrin is then facilitated by the oxidation of Fe^{2+} to Fe^{3+} by the multicopper oxidase hephaestin.

There appears to be little release of iron from ferritin within the enterocyte; the majority of enterocyte ferritin is apparently destined for excretion via the process of shedding of mucosal cells. Intestinal epithelial cells have a lifetime of about 3 to 4 days. Shedding of enterocytes represents an important mechanism for regulation of dietary iron uptake.

Transport of iron into the circulation at the basolateral membrane involves the iron exporter ferroportin which is localized in the basolateral membranes of enterocyes (McKie et al., 2000; Donovan et al., 2000; Abboud and Haile, 2000). Both ferroportin mRNA and protein levels are increased in enterocytes under conditions of increased iron absorption. Although the 5′-UTR of ferroportin mRNA in most cells contains a functional IrRE, which facilitates its translational repression in response to low iron status, a novel form of ferroportin lacking an IrRE was recently identified in enterocytes (Zhang et al., 2009). This alternative transcript may allow intestinal cells to express ferroportin and export iron into the circulation under low iron conditions.

Iron export from the enterocytes requires hephaestin, a multicopper oxidase homologous to ceruloplasmin, which oxidizes Fe^{2+} to Fe^{3+} for loading onto transferrin. Hephaestin was discovered in sex-linked anemia (*sla*) mice, which have a genetically inherited block in intestinal iron transport and develop a severe anemia; iron uptake from the intestinal lumen is normal in these mice, but they fail to transfer it to the circulation. Hence, iron accumulates in the enterocytes and is lost during the subsequent turnover of the intestinal epithelium. The mutant gene in *sla* mice (*HEPH*) encodes hephaestin. Hephaestin is highly expressed in intestine (Vulpe et al., 1999) and is inserted into the basolateral membrane of enterocytes by a glycosylphosphatidylinositol anchor.

REGULATION OF IRON ABSORPTION

Intestinal iron absorption is tightly controlled and depends on the iron requirements of the body. The process appears from recent studies to be regulated via a number of different pathways that modulate the expression of DMT1, DcytB, and ferroportin.

Induction of DMT1 and DcyB by Hypoxia

Because O_2 delivery to tissues depends on heme-proteins, oxygen and iron status are interrelated. A lack of adequate iron results in hypoxia in the tissues. Thus, it is not surprising that hypoxia-inducible factor (HIF)-mediated signaling plays a crucial role in regulating iron absorption. Hypoxia has been known for over 100 years to stimulate red blood cell production, and it was the interest in the physiological and molecular basis of the erythropoietic response that led to the discovery of erythropoietin. The search for the transcription factor that mediates the hypoxic induction of erythropoietin led to the discovery of HIF as a key mediator of cellular adaptation to low oxygen. Recent evidence suggests that HIF promotes erythropoiesis through coordinated hypoxia responses, which include increased erythropoietin production in the kidney and liver and enhanced iron uptake and utilization.

HIF is a heterodimeric nuclear transcription factor consisting of an oxygen-sensitive alpha subunit (HIF1α or HIF2α), and a ubiquitously expressed beta subunit, HIF1β. Under normal oxygen tension, the HIFα-subunits are modified by iron-dependent prolyl hydroxylases. The modified HIF interacts with von Hippel–Lindau factor and is subsequently targeted for proteasomal degradation through the ubiquitin–proteasome pathway. Under hypoxia, or following iron chelation, the prolyl hydroxylase activity is inhibited, resulting in the accumulation and translocation of HIF into the nucleus. Two recent studies show that acute iron deficiency induces HIF signaling via HIF2α in the duodenum, which upregulates the expression of DcytB and DMT1 resulting in increased iron absorption (Shah et al., 2009; Mastrogiannaki et al., 2009). Conditional knockout of intestinal HIF2α in mice abolished this response.

IrRPs Increase DMT1 and Decrease Ferroportin Translation

IrRPs are essential for iron absorption. One isoform of DMT1 has an IrRE in the 3′-UTR of its mRNA, and this isoform of DMT1 mRNA is stabilized by binding IrRP. On the other hand, ferroportin mRNA, except for a novel form in enterocytes, has an IrRE in the 5′-UTR, and IrRP binding inhibits its translation. Specific intestinal depletion of IrRP1 and IrRP2 in mice decreased DMT1 and increased ferroportin levels (Galy et al., 2008). The mice developed intestinal malabsorption and dehydration postnatally and died within 4 weeks of birth. These results demonstrate the critical role of IrRPs in the control of DMT1 and ferroportin expression. The expression of ferroportin mRNA with no IrRE in enterocytes may allow iron uptake across the basolateral membranes of enterocytes under conditions of low iron status. HIF2α mRNA also has an IrRE within its 5′-UTR (Sanchez et al., 2007), so in conditions of cellular hypoxia, translation of the HIF2α message is maintained through inhibition of IrRP1–dependent repression (Zimmer et al., 2008). This would facilitate the upregulation of duodenal expression of DMT1 as well as of DcytB.

Downregulation of Ferroportin by Hepcidin

The ferroportin protein is negatively regulated by hepcidin, the key iron regulatory hormone (Fleming and Sly, 2001) that is secreted predominantly by liver hepatocytes in response to high iron status. Hepcidin binds to ferroportin and triggers its internalization and degradation (De Domenico et al., 2009). Upregulation of hepcidin thus decreases iron efflux from the enterocyte via ferroportin and hence its subsequent uptake into transferrin.

DIETARY REFERENCE INTAKES FOR IRON

The Institute of Medicine (IOM, 2001) established Estimated Average Requirements (EARs), Recommended Dietary Allowances (RDAs) or Adequate Intakes (AIs), and Tolerable Upper Intake Levels (ULs) for iron in 2001. Except for infants during the first 6 months of life, the EARs and RDAs for iron are based on factorial modeling of iron needs. The main components of iron requirements considered by the IOM included basal iron losses, menstrual losses, and iron accretion during pregnancy and growth. An AI was set for infants from 0 through 6 months of age; this was calculated as the average iron concentration of human milk (0.35 mg/L) times the average daily intake of breast milk (0.78 L) and is 0.27 mg/day of iron.

The EAR for infants from 7 through 12 months of age, 6.9 mg/day, was based on the sum of the average requirements for absorbed iron for iron deposition (0.43 mg/day) and for replacement of basal iron losses (0.26 mg/day) corrected for a moderate bioavailability of 10%. The RDA was similarly calculated but based on the requirement of the 97.5th percentile group and is 11 mg/day of iron for infants 6 through 12 months. EARs and RDAs were similarly calculated for growing

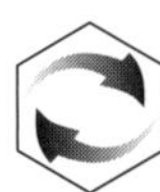

DRIs Across the Life Cycle: Iron

Iron

	mg Iron per Day	
Infants	RDA	UL
0 through 6 mo	0.27 (AI)	40
7 through 12 mo	11	40
Children		
1 through 3 yr	7	40
4 through 8 yr	10	40
9 through 13 yr	8	40
Males		
14 through 18 yr	11	45
≥19 yr	8	45
Females		
14 through 18 yr	15	45
19 through 50 yr	18	45
≥51 yr	8	45
Pregnant	27	45
Lactating		
<19 yr	10	45
≥19 yr	9	45

Data from IOM. (2006). In J. J. Otten, J. P. Hellwig, & L. D. Meyers (Eds.), *Dietary Reference Intakes: The essential guide to nutrient requirements* (p. 328). Washington, DC: The National Academies Press.
AI, Adequate Intake; *DRI*, Dietary Reference Intake; *RDA*, Recommended Dietary Allowance; *UL*, Tolerable Upper Intake Level.

children and adolescents except that a bioavailability of 18% was applied to convert the need for absorbed iron to the need for dietary iron. Replacement of menstrual iron losses was also considered for adolescent girls aged 14 through 18 years. The EARs range from 3.0 mg/day for children 1 through 3 years of age to 7.9 mg/day for girls aged 14 through 18 years; the RDAs range from 7 mg/day to 15 mg/day, respectively.

For adult men and postmenopausal women, the daily basal loss (0.014 mg/kg) was the only component used to estimate total needs for absorbed iron, and the need for absorbed iron was modeled at the 50th percentile for the EAR and at the 97.5th percentile for the RDA. A bioavailability of 18% was assumed. This approach yielded EARs of 6 mg/day for men of all ages and 5 mg/day of iron for women over 50 years of age. The RDA was set at 8 mg/day of iron for men and postmenopausal women. For women aged 19 through 50 years, menstrual losses were calculated to average 0.51 mg/day over a 28-day cycle. The need for iron to replace menstrual losses was added to the basal loss to yield an EAR and RDA of 8.1 mg/day and 18 mg/day, respectively, for women of childbearing age.

For pregnant women, the basal need is reduced because their are no menstrual losses of iron, but additional iron is needed to allow for iron deposition in the fetus and related tissues and for expansion of hemoglobin mass. Iron deposition in the fetus and related tissues is about 2.0 mg/day and the iron needed for expansion of hemoglobin mass is about 2.7 mg/day during pregnancy. The EAR and RDA for pregnant women (aged 19 through 50 years) are 22 mg/day and 27 mg/day, respectively. Similarly, for lactating women, an additional allowance was added to cover the replacement of the iron secreted in human milk (0.27 mg/day). However, the baseline requirement of lactating women was reduced due to assumed amenorrhea of lactation (e.g., 1.2 mg/day for woman aged 19 through 50 years). Using a bioavailability of 18%, the EAR and RDA for lactating women (aged 19 through 50 years) are 6.5 mg/day and 9 mg/day, respectively.

The toxicity of iron is related to the amount of elemental iron absorbed and can range from gastrointestinal irritation to systemic toxicity. For adults, based on gastrointestinal symptoms, a lowest observed adverse effect level of 70 mg/day was set according to the safe levels evaluated in the supplemental study of Frykman and colleagues (1994). Division of this value by an uncertainty factor of 1.5 led to an upper level of intake of 45 mg/day. This upper limit is above the 90th percentile intakes of any life stage and gender group except for pregnant and lactating women who usually are taking supplements as part of supervised pre- and postnatal care. In general, individuals are not likely to routinely ingest excess iron because of the gastrointestinal symptoms. For infants and young children an upper limit of 40 mg/day was set, based on potential adverse growth effects (Dewey et al., 2002).

According to the third National Health and Nutrition Examination Survey (NHANES III) (1988–1994), the median intake of iron from food is about 17.5 mg/day for adult men (aged 19 to 70 years) and 12.1 mg/day for adult women in the United States; the 5th to 95th percentile range of intakes was 10 to 31 mg/day for men and 7 to 21 mg/day for women (IOM, 2001). When iron intake from both food and supplements is considered, median intake is 18.4 mg/day for men and 13 mg/day for women.

Recommendations for iron intake deserve careful consideration, because iron deficiency severe enough to result in anemia is associated with significant morbidity, whereas uncontrolled iron absorption, as in hemochromatosis, causes multiorgan failure.

LABORATORY EVALUATION OF IRON STATUS

Changes in iron storage and distribution in the presence of different body iron contents are indicated in Figure 36-13, together with clinically available indicators of iron status. The single best measure to assess stores noninvasively is the ferritin concentration in serum. In the range of 20 to 200 μg/L, it bears a quantitative relationship to iron stores: 1 μg/L serum ferritin is indicative of 8 mg of storage iron. Careful phlebotomy studies have shown that plasma ferritin concentrations decrease until stores are exhausted, which is indicated by a serum ferritin of 12 μg/L. It should be noted, however, that alcohol consumption, infection, inflammation, neoplasia, and hepatic dysfunction may all spuriously raise the plasma ferritin concentration relative to stores and therefore result in a misleadingly high serum ferritin concentration. The size of stores also can be assessed invasively by measuring the iron content of bone marrow or liver biopsies, but these methods are unsuitable for routine use.

Measurements of serum total iron, transferrin, and particularly transferrin saturation reflect the balance between iron flowing into and out of the plasma iron pool. Once transferrin saturation drops below 15%, iron deficient erythropoiesis is already present.

The evaluation of hemoglobin concentration, hematocrit, mean red blood cell volume, and the red blood cell free erythrocyte protoporphyrin can be useful, but they usually become abnormal relatively late in the development of functional iron depletion because red blood cells survive in the circulation for a relatively long period (~120 days). In iron deficiency the numbers of transferrin receptors on the cell surface increase significantly. Because some of the transferrin receptors on the cell surface undergo proteolytic cleavage, releasing a soluble fragment of the transferrin receptor into the circulation (Baynes et al., 1994), the plasma concentration of soluble transferrin receptor fragment is a valuable marker of transferrin receptor levels. The soluble form of transferrin receptor is a good measure of truly functional iron depletion (Baynes et al., 1994), particularly in patients with infection, inflammation, or malignancy; serum ferritin is not a good indicator of iron deficiency in these patients.

Iron excess is best evaluated noninvasively; both an elevated serum ferritin concentration and a percent transferrin saturation in excess of normal indicate iron excess. When percent saturation exceeds 62%, the risk of non–protein-bound iron being present in the circulation and contributing to parenchymal tissue injury becomes very high. In iron overload, magnetic resonance imaging allows noninvasive evaluation of the progressive depletion of liver iron stores in the course of treatment (Tziomalos and Perifanis, 2010).

In individual patients, the results of a combination of measures of iron status can accurately define the precise stage of iron nutrition. Diagnosis of iron deficiency mandates a search for the underlying cause, because serious pathology might be present. There are concerns about relationships between iron level and heart disease and cancer (Reddy and Clark, 2004), so iron supplements should be used only when there is a definitive iron deficiency.

Early diagnosis of iron excess and early intervention are also important outcomes of iron status evaluation. If iron excess is not diagnosed and treated in its early stages, serious long-term organ damage may occur.

IRON DEFICIENCY

Iron deficiency is the most common and widespread nutritional disorder in the world. The World Health Organization (WHO) estimates that some 2 billion people (~ 30% of the world's population) are anemic, when defined as hemoglobin concentrations that are below recommended thresholds (WHO, 2007). Although not all anemia is due to iron deficiency, iron deficiency is the major cause of anemia; iron deficiency is exacerbated by infectious diseases such as malaria, hookworm infections, and schistosomiasis, HIV, and tuberculosis. Because anemia reflects the endpoint of functional iron deficiency, many additional people must be afflicted by depleted iron stores or lesser degrees of iron depletion. Anemia is also caused by deficiencies of other key micronutrients, including folate, vitamin B_{12}, and vitamin A, and by inherited conditions such as thalassemia that affect red blood cells.

In the developed world, only about 8% of the population is anemic. Conversely, in underdeveloped and developing regions of the world, approximately 36% of the population is anemic. Consequently, the iron nutritional imperatives are clearly different between developed and developing regions. The preliminary data from NHANES III suggest that iron deficiency anemia is currently an unusual finding in the United States (Centers for Disease Control and Prevention, 1998).

CONSEQUENCES OF IRON DEFICIENCY

The consequences of iron deficiency correlate with functional iron depletion; depletion of storage iron has no immediate functional consequence. A major concern arises from

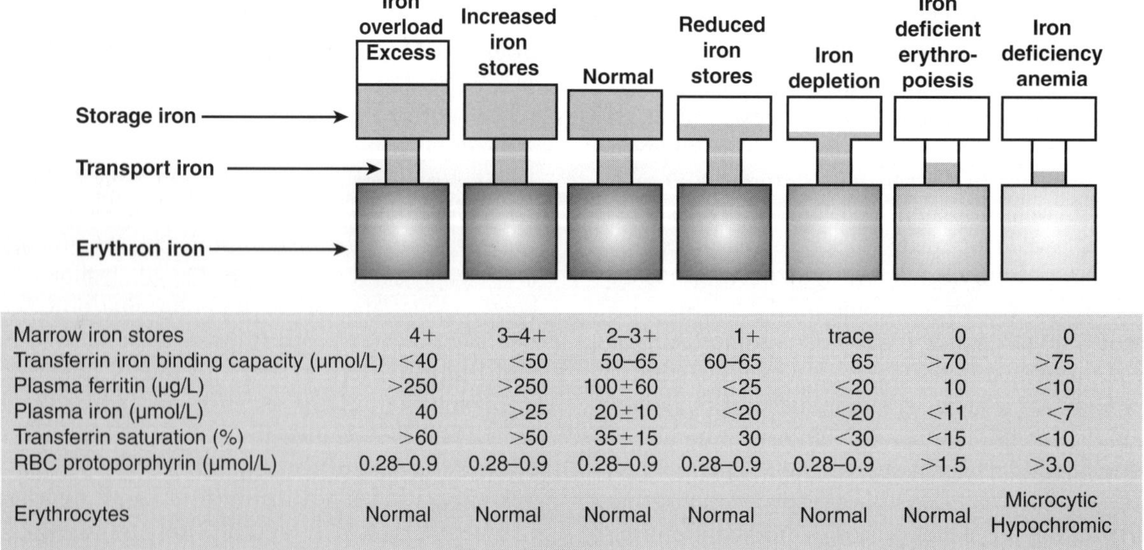

	Iron overload	Increased iron stores	Normal	Reduced iron stores	Iron depletion	Iron deficient erythropoiesis	Iron deficiency anemia
Marrow iron stores	4+	3–4+	2–3+	1+	trace	0	0
Transferrin iron binding capacity (μmol/L)	<40	<50	50–65	60–65	65	>70	>75
Plasma ferritin (μg/L)	>250	>250	100±60	<25	<20	10	<10
Plasma iron (μmol/L)	40	>25	20±10	<20	<20	<11	<7
Transferrin saturation (%)	>60	>50	35±15	30	<30	<15	<10
RBC protoporphyrin (μmol/L)	0.28–0.9	0.28–0.9	0.28–0.9	0.28–0.9	0.28–0.9	>1.5	>3.0
Erythrocytes	Normal	Normal	Normal	Normal	Normal	Normal	Microcytic Hypochromic

FIGURE 36-13 Sequential compartment depletions, stages of iron depletion, and the accompanying changes in iron-related measurements. (Modified from Bothwell, T. H., Charlton, R. W., Cook, J. D., & Finch, C. A. [1979]. *Iron metabolism in man* [p. 45]. Oxford, UK: Blackwell Scientific Publications.)

the demonstration that iron deficiency in infants appears to result in abnormal psychomotor development, which may be reversible only to a limited extent. Iron plays a key role in neurocognitive and neurobehavioral development (Beard, 2008). Iron requirements are expected to exceed iron intake during the first 6 to 18 months of postnatal life, which is a time of rapid neural development, when morphological, biochemical, and bioenergetic alterations may influence the way in which the brain functions in later life. Iron deficiency either in utero or in early postnatal life can result in abnormal cerebral development, because iron is essential for proper neurogenesis and differentiation of certain brain cells and brain regions.

That reductions in work performance, effort tolerance, and peak effort output result from iron deficiency is well documented. Where people depend upon manual labor for their livelihood, these impairments clearly translate into significant economic disadvantage. It also appears that iron deficiency contributes to adverse pregnancy outcomes, with higher rates of premature delivery and perinatal mortality in iron-deficient populations.

TREATMENT AND PREVENTION

Treatment of the individual subject with iron deficiency is obviously appropriate, but a search for the cause of the iron deficiency should also be undertaken. In populations with a low incidence of iron deficiency, identification and treatment of individuals are most appropriate. In most cases, the problem of iron deficiency is correctable with orally administered ferrous iron salts. Side effects of iron supplement ingestion frequently limit compliance, but they may be dramatically reduced by a formulation of iron that allows for its slow release over a number of hours within the stomach. Parenteral iron therapy is indicated in patients with poor absorption of iron, intolerance to iron with poor compliance, or where a rapid effect is required (Crichton et al., 2008).

In populations with a very high prevalence of iron deficiency, an appropriate prevention strategy would involve a pilot unscreened therapeutic supplementation trial. If the program is shown to be successful, then it should be rapidly translated into a regional or national program. In regions of intermediate prevalence, either a pilot fortification trial or a pilot prophylactic supplementation program would be appropriate. If successful, these should be extended regionally. The population's iron status should be surveyed to guard against the production of excessive positive iron balance.

In populations in which the prevalence of iron deficiency is low, a public health initiative aimed at improving overall iron nutrition is inappropriate. The only appropriate activity is the screening of high-risk groups, such as infants and pregnant women, and therapeutic supplementation of individuals who are identified as being iron-deficient. Indeed, if it appears that population iron status is increasing to levels higher than putative normal values, consideration should be given to reducing the levels of iron fortification and supplementation.

IRON EXCESS

The very limited ability of the human body to excrete iron led to the conclusion (McCance and Widdowson, 1937) that iron balance in humans is essentially determined by iron absorption. The consequence is that if we absorb a little more iron than we excrete, or if we receive a parenteral iron burden in the form of blood transfusions, we can become "iron-loaded." The excessive accumulation of iron results in tissue damage caused by iron-generated production of reactive free radicals, and ultimately in organ failure. There are a number of well-recognized situations of iron overload, which are presented in Box 36-3.

PRIMARY IRON OVERLOAD, HEREDITARY HEMOCHROMATOSIS

The common denominator in terms of pathophysiology in almost all forms of hereditary hemochromatosis is an inappropriately low level of hepcidin secretion. This results in elevated levels of the iron export protein ferroportin at the basolateral membrane of duodenal enterocytes, thereby increasing dietary iron absorption, and excess levels of ferroportin in cells of the mononuclear phagocytic system, thereby increasing iron recycling from these cells back into the circulation. The excess release of iron into the circulation from the enterocytes and from the mononuclear phagocytic cells results in high plasma transferrin saturation, an increase in non–transferrin-bound iron in the plasma, and increased iron deposition in tissues. Hereditary hemochromatosis is characterized by four common features (Pietrangelo, 2006): (1) its hereditary nature (usually autosomal recessive, although HFE-4 is autosomal dominant); (2) early and progressive rise of serum transferrin saturation, accompanied by highly toxic non–transferrin-bound iron in the plasma which is rapidly cleared from the plasma to the liver; (3)

BOX 36-3 Classification of Iron-Loading Disorders

PRIMARY IRON OVERLOAD, HEREDITARY HEMOCHROMATOSIS

Classic congenital hemochromatosis, mutations in HFE (HFE-1)
Juvenile hemochromatosis (HFE-2), mutations in hemojuvelin (HFE-2A) or in hepcidin (HFE-2B)
Transferrin receptor-2 mutations (HFE-3)
Ferroportin mutations (HFE-4)

SECONDARY IRON OVERLOAD*

Thalassemias
Pyruvate kinase deficiency
Dyserythropoietic anemia
Glucose 6-phosphate dehydrogenase deficiency
Hereditary spherocytosis
Sideroblastic anemia (deficiency of δ-aminolevulinic acid synthase)
Other anemias treated by multiple blood transfusions

*Usually associated with treatment of anemia with blood transfusions.

progressive parenchymal iron deposits (endocrine glands, heart, articulations, liver) with increasing probability of tissue damage; and (4) no impairment of erythropoiesis and a satisfactory response to therapeutic phlebotomy.

Regulation of Hepcidin Expression and Secretion by the Liver

Although the signaling mechanisms involved in iron sensing and regulation of hepcidin secretion by the liver are complex and not entirely understood, important insights into the regulation of hepcidin secretion have come from the various identified causes of hereditary hemochromatosis (Ganz and Nemeth, 2011).

Under normal conditions, the synthesis of hepcidin is regulated in response to iron status predominantly through regulation of transcription of the hepcidin (*HAMP*) gene. Hepcidin release is increased in response to increased iron concentrations and leads to downregulation of ferroportin levels and, hence, the sequestering of iron in enterocytes and the mononuclear phagocytic cells, which limits iron absorption and retains iron in intracellular ferritin. Bone morphogenetic protein receptor (BMPR) and its SMAD signaling pathway regulate hepcidin transcription. The signaling pathway is initiated by binding of bone morphogenetic protein 6 (BMP6), an iron-regulated ligand, to BMPR. Membrane-anchored hemojuvelin is a BMPR coreceptor that is also involved in regulation of hepcidin expression. Levels of hemojuvelin are possibly modulated in an iron-regulated manner. BMP signaling and hepcidin expression are also affected by two potential sensors of holo-transferrin concentrations, transferrin receptors 1 and 2, and their interacting partner, transmembrane protein HFE (high Fe). Increasing concentrations of holo-transferrin act to shift the interaction of HFE from transferrin receptor 1 to transferrin receptor 2, promoting stabilization of the transferrin receptor 2 protein and enhancing SMAD and Erk (extracellular signal-regulated kinase) signaling.

The regulation of hepcidin expression is complex and not fully understood. Evidence suggests the existence of a hepcidin-regulation signal that originates in erythroid

CLINICAL CORRELATION

Iron Overload

Iron overload can impair organ structure and function from the excessive deposition of iron in parenchymal cells of the organ. Hereditary hemochromatosis most frequently results from homozygosity for a mutant disease-causing *HFE* allelle and is limited largely to people of European origin. Homozygote frequencies are estimated to be between 1 in 100 and 1 in 1,000, with about 5% to 20% of the population being heterozygous for the *HFE* iron-loading gene. This abnormality leads to absorption of more iron than is required (a greater rate of iron absorption than is appropriate, given the body stores); the amount of iron absorbed in excess of requirements is only a few milligrams per day, but over a number of years this can result in an increase in iron stores to 20 to 50 times the normal levels, representing the accumulation of 20 to 40 g of surplus iron.

Because of interactions of genetics with iron supply and needs, phenotypic expression of this disorder is rare in populations where iron deficiency is prevalent (because of a lack of bioavailable iron in the diet), is encountered about 10 times more frequently in men than in women (owing to greater iron losses by women due to menstruation and the increased demands during pregnancy), and is typically diagnosed after the age of 40 years, with age at onset being younger in men than in women.

The earliest biochemical signs of iron overload are elevations in the plasma iron concentration, a high plasma transferrin saturation, and an elevated plasma ferritin concentration. As iron stores enlarge, hemosiderin deposits become more prominent in the liver; examination of liver biopsy specimens from patients with hereditary hemochromatosis reveals that the hepatocytes (parenchymal cells) are loaded with hemosiderin, whereas the Kupffer cells are relatively free of stored iron. Organ damage occurs only after the concentrations of stored iron are grossly elevated, but this damage is largely irreversible. Early diagnosis and treatment are essential to avoid tissue damage. Repeated phlebotomy to remove the excess iron (e.g., the removal of 500 mL of blood, which contains 200 to 250 mg of iron, each week over a period of 2 to 3 years), followed by less frequent removal of blood to prevent reaccumulation, is the usual treatment.

A picture resembling hemochromatosis may also be caused by iron-loading anemias. These iron-loading anemias include thalassemia major and certain other hereditary anemias in which erythropoiesis is ineffective. Thalassemia major occurs in patients who are homozygous for mutations that lead to a decrease in β-globin synthesis, which in turn leads to deficient hemoglobin synthesis and the accumulation of α-globin chains in the bone marrow. Iron overload occurs in these patients as a consequence of enhanced absorption of iron and of essential treatment of the anemia with multiple blood transfusions. In these chronic hyperplastic anemias, the iron deposition occurs in both reticuloendothelial and parenchymal cells, and organ damage tends to develop as parenchymal cell loading proceeds. Treatment of iron overload in these patients is by chelation therapy.

Thinking Critically

1. What effect would blood removal or chelation therapy over an extended period (~1 year) have on plasma iron concentration, transferrin saturation, total iron-binding capacity, and plasma ferritin levels?
2. Would you expect the prevalence of symptomatic hemochromatosis to increase or decrease with introduction of an iron fortification program or an increase in the intake of bioavailable iron? Why?

precursor cells in the bone marrow. This factor (or factors) suppresses hepcidin in proportion to the erythropoietic activity of the bone marrow; suppression of hepcidin allows for greater availability of iron for erythropoiesis. Erythroid factors might include the erythroid hormone erythropoietin, GDF15 (growth differentiation factor 15), or TWSG1 (twisted gastrulation homolog 1) that are secreted mainly by immature erythroid precursors. Hypoxia, via HIF, can suppress hepatic hepcidin expression independently of body iron status. In the nucleus, HIF binds to the hepcidin promotor, leading to suppression of hepcidin transcription, and to the furin promoter, leading to decreased processing of hemojuvelin, thereby increasing iron absorption and release from mononuclear phagocytic cells to meet the demands of increased erythropoiesis. Inflammation or infection, on the other hand, generates signals (e.g., interleukin 6 and other cytokines and microbial products) that increase hepcidin synthesis and secretion, resulting in less iron absorption and less iron recycling from macrophages for erythropoiesis and, consequently, the so-called anemia of inflammation or anemia of chronic disease in which plasma iron levels are low but cellular ferritin stores are high.

Major Forms and Causes of Hemochromatosis

The best defined and most prevalent form of hereditary hemochromatosis (called HFE-1) is due to mutations in the *HFE* gene, which account for more than 80% of the cases of hemochromatosis. The *HFE1* gene encodes a major histocompatibility complex class I–like molecule, called HFE (Feder et al., 1996). As mentioned above, HFE binds to both transferrin receptor 1 and 2 and is involved in hepcidin regulation by systemic iron availability (Goswami and Andrews, 2006). The most common mutation in the HFE protein, C282Y, is tenfold more prevalent than the mutation that causes most cases of cystic fibrosis. Were it not for the fact that the phenotype penetrance of the polymorphism is low (Beutler, 2007), HFE-related hemochromatosis would be the most frequently inherited metabolic disorder among white individuals. The prevalence of C282Y homozygosity among white subjects is 1:200 to 1:300; it is much less common in Hispanic, Asian American, Pacific Islander, and black populations. Approximately 80% of patients with hemochromatosis who are of northern European ancestry are homozygous for 282Y. The polymorphism probably arose from a mutation in a single Celtic or Viking ancestor who inhabited northwestern Europe centuries ago (Distante et al., 2004). A second mutation in HFE, H63D, has a higher prevalence in the general population, but only a small proportion or perhaps no individuals with this mutation exhibit clinical symptoms (i.e., very low penetrance).

Juvenile, or type 2, hemochromatosis (HFE-2) is rare, transmitted as a recessive trait, and characterized by early onset of iron overload and severe organ damage before 30 years of age. The disease is usually characterized by mutations in the hemojuvelin (*HFE2*) gene (Papanikolaou et al., 2004). An even rarer form of juvenile hematochromatosis is due to mutations in the gene (*HAMP*) for hepcidin (Roetto et al., 2003). Patients with juvenile hemochromatosis associated with mutations in either the *HFE2* or *HAMP* gene have low or absent urinary hepcidin levels, underlining the role of hemojuvelin in the regulation of hepatic hepcidin expression and the role of hepcidin itself.

In addition to HFE-1 and HFE-2, two other forms of hemochromatosis, HFE-3 and HFE-4, result from mutations in transferrin receptor 2 and ferroportin, respectively. HFE-3 is associated with mutations in the transferrin receptor 2 (*TRF2*) gene (Camaschella et al., 2000), causing a rare form of hereditary hemochromatosis with similar severity to HFE-1, consistent with HFE and transferrin receptor 2 being part of the same signaling pathway in hepcidin regulation by systemic iron availability (Goswami and Andrews, 2006).

An autosomal dominant form of iron storage disease, HFE-4, is caused by mutations in the ferroportin gene (*SLC40A1*), which is the target of hepcidin action (reviewed in Pietrangelo, 2004). The clinical features of HFE-4 are quite characteristic, with an early increase in serum ferritin despite low-normal transferrin saturation, progressive iron accumulation that is predominantly in reticuloendothelial macrophages, marginal anemia, and often low tolerance to phlebotomy. Mutations in ferroportin are widespread in the population, and it has been shown that a common polymorphism (Q248H) in ferroportin associates with a tendency to low hemoglobin and high ferritin in African and African American populations (Gordeuk et al., 2003).

NONHEMOCHROMATOTIC PRIMARY IRON OVERLOAD

Several other rare conditions have been described that result in iron loading. The importance of ceruloplasmin together with ferroportin in mobilizing cellular iron is underlined by mutations in the ceruloplasmin gene (aceruloplasminemia), which result in iron accumulation in brain and liver (Miyajima et al., 2003). Mutations in the transferrin gene result in severe iron deficiency and parenchymal iron overload (Beutler et al., 2000). Mutations in a number of other genes, including *DMT1*, lead to microcytic anemia and hepatic iron loading (Iolascon et al., 2009). Deficiency of the mitochondrial iron chaperone protein frataxin leads to massive iron accumulation in mitochondria in Friedreich ataxia, and iron chelation therapy seems to be an effective therapeutic strategy (Boddaert et al., 2007). And, of course, iron overload due to the custom of drinking a traditional fermented beverage with a high iron content has long been recognized in rural sub-Saharan African populations (Gordeuk, 2002).

TREATMENT AND PREVENTION OF IRON OVERLOAD

The first step in the treatment of iron overload involves diagnosis, which can be done noninvasively due to advances in imaging technology. Molecular genetics, which allows identification of the mutations involved, greatly facilitates the clinician's task when faced with the suspicion of excess tissue iron. Once iron overload has been established, therapeutic phlebotomy, in which one unit of blood (corresponding to 200 to 250 mg of iron) is removed weekly until serum ferritin is less than 30 μg/L and transferrin saturation drops below 30%, is the safest, most economical, and most effective treatment for hemochromatosis (Pietrangelo, 2006). Maintenance therapy (2 to 4 units/year) must be continued for the rest of the patient's life to keep transferrin saturation and serum ferritin normal.

SECONDARY IRON OVERLOAD

Secondary iron overload is most commonly encountered in the context of hematological diseases in which iron overload is a long-term consequence of repeated blood transfusions or enhanced dietary iron absorption on account of the underlying anemia, or both. In contrast to primary iron overload (hereditary hemochromatosis), iron deposition in secondary iron overload primarily affects cells of the mononuclear phagocytic system, with parenchymal loading only occurring at later stages of the disease.

Iron overload with cardiac and endocrine toxicity is well recognized in patients with transfusion-dependent anemias (see Box 36-3) such as β-thalassemia major (reviewed in Porter, 2009). The blood transfusions, along with the increased iron absorption observed in these conditions, lead to a massive increase in body iron content, the presence of non–transferrin-bound iron in the circulation, and ultimately extensive tissue damage. Tissue iron levels can be estimated by determination of serum ferritin levels (as long as there is no inflammatory-associated condition). However, more recently, magnetic resonance imaging (MRI) has proven effective in detecting and quantifying iron in both the heart and the liver (reviewed in Wood and Ghugre, 2008).

TREATMENT AND PREVENTION

The ravages of secondary iron overload can be reversed by hematopoietic stem cell transplantation (Smiers et al., 2010). This is the only curative option currently available and results in patients with hemoglobinopathy are excellent and still improving. However, secondary iron overload is usually treated by iron chelation therapy, which has as its primary aim the removal of iron from the body at a rate that is either greater than transfusional iron input (reduction therapy) or equal to transfusional iron input (maintenance therapy).

Three chelators are currently approved for clinical use (Figure 36-14). Desferrioxamine B (Desferal, Novartis AG, Basel, Switzerland) is a hexadentate chelator, one molecule binding one atom of iron. However, despite its impressive safety record, because it is not active by oral administration and is rapidly eliminated from the circulation, effective therapy usually requires subcutaneous or intravenous administration by a portable infusion pump for 9 to 10 hours, 5 to 6 days per week. This cumbersome and unpleasant regimen for administration increases the cost of treatment and poses serious problems of patient compliance.

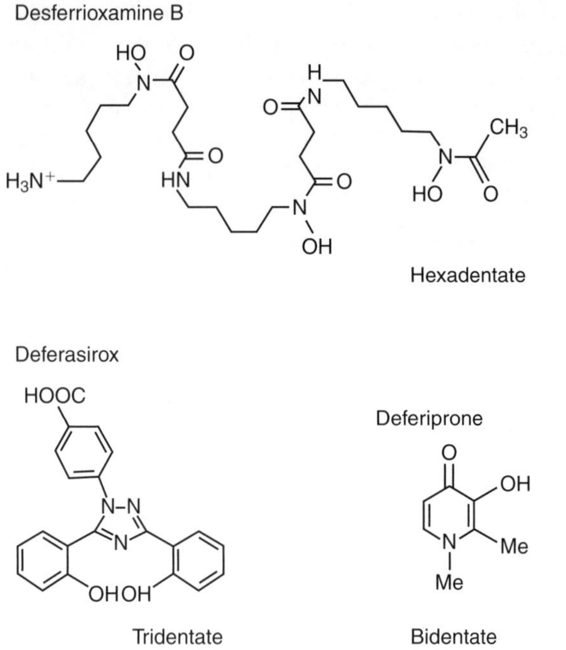

FIGURE 36-14 The structures of the iron chelators desferrioxamine B, deferasirox, and deferiprone.

The orally active bidentate chelator (forming a 3:1 chelator/iron complex) deferiprone (Ferriprox, Apotex, Toronto, Canada) is administered at 75 mg/day in three doses. Since its half-time is 3 to 4 hours, like desferrioxamine B it cannot give 24-hour chelation cover, and highly toxic labile plasma iron levels rebound between doses (Cabantchik et al., 2005). Deferiprone causes the serious problem of agranulocytosis in approximately 1% of patients. However, because of its ability to cross cellular membranes, it appears to have superior cardioprotective properties, and it may yield better cardioprotective results when used in tandem with desferrioxamine B (Beutler et al., 2003; Hershko, 2006).

Deferasirox (Exjade, ICL670, Novartis AG, Basel, Switzerland) is a new tridentate iron chelator (forming a 2:1 chelator/iron complex), which is not only orally active but also provides 24-hour chelation with a single dose per day. It has been shown in preclinical studies to be excreted predominantly by the fecal route, and large-scale prospective trials show efficacy with an acceptable safety profile in adults and children with up to 5 years follow-up (Porter, 2009; Cappellini and Pattoneri, 2009). The arrival of this orally active chelator, which can ensure 24-hour chelation coverage, means that patients with any form of secondary iron overload now have several therapeutic options, allowing treatment to be adjusted to the individual patient (Hershko, 2006).

REFERENCES

Abboud, S., & Haile, D. J. (2000). A novel mammalian iron-regulated protein involved in intracellular iron metabolism. *The Journal of Biological Chemistry, 275*, 19906–19912.

Arosio, P., & Levi, S. (2010). Cytosolic and mitochondrial ferritins in the regulation of cellular iron homeostasis and oxidative damage. *Biochimica et Biophysica Acta, 1800*, 783–792.

Baker, H. M., Anderson, B. F., & Baker, E. N. (2003). Dealing with iron: Common structural principles in proteins that transport iron and heme. *Proceedings of the National Academy of Sciences of the United States of America, 100*, 3579–3583.

Baynes, R. D., Skikne, B. S., & Cook, J. D. (1994). Circulating transferrin receptors and assessment of iron status. *The Journal of Nutritional Biochemistry, 5*, 322–330.

Beard, J. L. (2008). Why iron deficiency is important in infant development. *The Journal of Nutrition, 138*, 2534–2536.

Beutler, E. (2007). Iron storage disease: Facts, fiction and progress. *Blood Cells, Molecules & Diseases, 39*, 140–147.

Beutler, E., Gelbart, T., Lee, P., Trevino, R., Fernandez, M. A., & Fairbanks, V. F. (2000). Molecular characterization of a case of atransferrinemia. *Blood, 96*, 4071–4074.

Beutler, E., Hoffbrand, A. V., & Cook, J. D. (2003). Iron deficiency and overload. *Hematology/The Education Program of the American Society of Hematology, 2003*, 40–61.

Boddaert, N., Le Quan Sang, K. H., Rötig, A., Leroy-Willig, A., Gallet, S., Brunelle, F., … Cabantchik, Z. I. (2007). Selective iron chelation in Friedreich ataxia: Biologic and clinical implications. *Blood, 110*, 401–408.

Breuer, W., Shvartsman, M., & Cabantchik, Z. I. (2008). Intracellular labile iron. *The International Journal of Biochemistry & Cell Biology, 40*, 350–354.

Cabantchik, Z. I., Breuer, W., Zanninelli, G., & Cianciulli, P. (2005). LPI-labile plasma iron in iron overload. *Best Practice & Research. Clinical Haematology, 18*, 277–287.

Camaschella, C., Roetto, A., Cali, A., De Gobbi, M., Garozzo, G., Carella, M., … Gasparini, P. (2000). The gene TFR2 is mutated in a new type of haemochromatosis mapping to 7q22. *Nature Genetics, 25*, 14–15.

Canonne-Hergaux, F., Gruenheid, S., Ponka, P., & Gros, P. (1999). Cellular and subcellular localization of the Nramp2 iron transporter in the intestinal brush border and regulation by dietary iron. *Blood, 93*, 4406–4417.

Cappellini, M. D., & Pattoneri, P. (2009). Oral iron chelators. *Annual Review of Medicine, 60*, 25–38.

Centers for Disease Control and Prevention. (1998). Recommendations to prevent and control iron deficiency in the United States. *Morbidity and Mortality Weekly Report. Recommendations and Reports, 47*, 1–29.

Cheng, Y., Zak, O., Aisen, P., Harrison, S. C., & Walz, T. (2004). Structure of the human transferrin receptor-transferrin complex. *Cell, 116*(4), 565–567.

Cooperman, S. S., Meyron-Holtz, E. G., Olivierre-Wilson, H., Ghosh, M. C., McConnell, J. P., & Rouault, T. A. (2005). Microcytic anemia, erythropoietic protoporphyria, and neurodegeneration in mice with targeted deletion of iron-regulatory protein 2. *Blood, 106*, 1084–1091.

Crichton, R. R. (1984). Iron uptake and utilization by mammalian cells II. Intracellular iron utilization. *Trends in Biochemical Sciences, 9*, 283–286.

Crichton, R. R. (2008). *Biological inorganic chemistry: An introduction.* Amsterdam: Elsevier.

Crichton, R. R. (2009). *Inorganic biochemistry of iron metabolism: From molecular mechanisms to clinical consequences* (3rd ed.). New York: John Wiley and Sons.

Crichton, R. R., Danielson, B. G., & Geisser, P. (2008). *Iron therapy with special emphasis on intravenous administration* (4th ed.). Bremen, Germany: UNI-Med Verlag.

Crichton, R. R., & Declercq, J. P. (2010). X-ray structures of ferritins and related proteins. *Biochimica et Biophysica Acta, 1800*, 706–718.

De Domenico, I., Lo, E., Ward, D. M., & Kaplan, J. (2009). Hepcidin-induced internalization of ferroportin requires binding and cooperative interaction with Jak2. *Proceedings of the National Academy of Sciences of the United States of America, 106*, 3800–3805.

De Domenico, I., Nemeth, E., Nelson, J. M., Phillips, J. D., Ajioka, R. S., Kay, M. S., Kushner, J. P., Ganz, T., Ward, D. M., & Kaplan, J. (2008). The hepcidin-binding site on ferroportin is evolutionarily conserved. *Cell Metabolism, 8*, 146–156.

De Domenico, I., Vaughn, M. B., Li, L., Bagley, D., Musci, G., Ward, D. M., & Kaplan, J. (2006). Ferroportin-mediated mobilization of ferritin iron precedes ferritin degradation by the proteasome. *The EMBO Journal, 25*, 5396–5404.

De Domenico, I., Ward, D. M., di Patti, M. C., Jeong, S. Y., David, S., Musci, G., & Kaplan, J. (2007). Ferroxidase activity is required for the stability of cell surface ferroportin in cells expressing GPI-ceruloplasmin. *The EMBO Journal, 26*, 2823–2831.

Dewey, K. G., Domellöf, M., Cohen, R. J., Landa Rivera, L., Hernell, O., & Lönnerdal, B. (2002). Iron supplementation affects growth and morbidity of breast-fed infants: Results of a randomized trial in Sweden and Honduras. *The Journal of Nutrition, 132*, 3249–3255.

Distante, S., Robson, K. J., Graham-Campbell, J., Arnaiz-Villena, A., Brissot, P., & Worwood, M. (2004). The origin and spread of the HFE-C282Y haemochromatosis mutation. *Human Genetics, 115*, 269–279.

Donovan, A., Brownlie, A., Zhou, Y., Shepard, J., Pratt, S. J., Moynihan, J., … Zon, L. I. (2000). Positional cloning of zebrafish ferroportin1 identifies a conserved vertebrate iron exporter. *Nature, 403*, 776–781.

Donovan, A., Lima, C. A., Pinkus, J. L., Pinkus, G. S., Zon, L. I., Robine, S., & Andrews, N. C. (2005). The iron exporter ferroportin/Slc40a1 is essential for iron homeostasis. *Cell Metabolism, 1*, 191–200.

Feder, J. N., Gnirke, A., Thomas, W., Tsuchihashi, Z., Ruddy, D. A., Basava, A., … Wolff, R. K. (1996). A novel MHC class I-like gene is mutated in patients with hereditary hemochromatosis. *Nature Genetics, 13*, 399–408.

Ferreira, C., Bucchini, D., Martin, M. E., Levi, S., Arosio, P., Grandchamp, B., & Beaumont, C. (2000). Early embryonic lethality of H ferritin gene deletion in mice. *The Journal of Biological Chemistry, 275*, 3021–3024.

Ferris, C. D., Jaffrey, S. R., Sawa, A., Takahashi, M., Brady, S. D., Barrow, R. K., … Snyder, S. H. (1999). Haem oxygenase-1 prevents cell death by regulating cellular iron. *Nature Cell Biology, 1*, 152–157.

Fleming, M. D., Romano, M. A., Su, M. A., Garrick, L. M., Garrick, M. D., & Fleming, N. C. (1998). Nramp2 is mutated in the anemic Belgrade (b) rat: Evidence of a role for Nramp2 in endosomal iron transport. *Proceedings of the National Academy of Sciences of the United States of America, 95*, 1148–1153.

Fleming, M. D., Trenor, C. C. I., Su, M. A., Foernzler, D., Beier, D. R., Dietrich, W. F., & Andrews, N. C. (1997). Microcytic anemia mice have a mutation in Nramp2, a candidate iron transporter. *Nature Genetics, 16*, 383–386.

Fleming, R. E., & Sly, W. S. (2001). Hepcidin: A putative iron-regulatory hormone relevant to hereditary hemochromatosis and the anemia of chronic disease. *Proceedings of the National Academy of Sciences of the United States of America, 98*, 8160–8162.

Frykman, E., Bystrom, M., Jansson, U., Edberg, A., & Hansen, T. (1994). Side effects of iron supplements in blood donors: Superior tolerance of heme iron. *The Journal of Laboratory and Clinical Medicine, 123*, 561–564.

Galy, B., Ferring, D., Minana, B., Bell, O., Janser, H. G., Muckenthaler, M., … Hentze, M. W. (2005). Altered body iron distribution and microcytosis in mice deficient in iron regulatory protein 2 (IRP2). *Blood, 106*, 2580–2589.

Galy, B., Ferring-Appel, D., Kaden, S., Gröne, H. J., & Hentze, M. W. (2008). Iron regulatory proteins are essential for intestinal function and control key iron absorption molecules in the duodenum. *Cell Metabolism, 7*, 79–85.

Ganz, T., Nemeth, E. (2011). The hepcidin-ferroportin system as a therapeutic target in anemias and iron overload disorders. *Hematology American Society Hematology Education Program.* 2011:538–542.

Gordeuk, V. R. (2002). African iron overload. *Seminars in Hematology, 39*, 263–269.

Gordeuk, V. R., Caleffi, A., Corradini, E., Ferrara, F., Jones, R. A., Castro, O., … Pietrangelo, A. (2003). Iron overload in Africans and African-Americans and a common mutation in the SCL40A1 (ferroportin 1) gene. *Blood Cells, Molecules & Diseases, 31*, 299–304.

Goswami, T., & Andrews, N. C. (2006). Hereditary hemochromatosis protein, HFE, interaction with transferrin receptor 2 suggests a molecular mechanism for mammalian iron sensing. *The Journal of Biological Chemistry, 281*, 28494–28498.

Gunshin, H., Mackenzie, B., Berger, U. V., Gunshin, Y., Romero, M. F., Boron, W. F., … Hediger, M. A. (1997). Cloning and characterization of a mammalian proton-coupled metal-ion transporter. *Nature, 388*, 482–488.

Gunshin, H., Starr, C. N., Direnzo, C., Fleming, M. D., Jin, J., Greer, E. L., Sellers, V. M., Galica, S. M., & Andrews, N. C. (2005). Cybrd1 (duodenal cytochrome b) is not necessary for dietary iron absorption in mice. *Blood, 106*, 2879–2883.

Hentze, M. W., Muckenthaler, M. U., Galy, B., & Camaschella, C. (2010). Two to tango: Regulation of mammalian iron metabolism. *Cell, 142*, 24–38.

Hershko, C. (2006). Oral iron chelators: New opportunities and new dilemmas. *Haematologica, 91*, 1307–1312.

Institute of Medicine. (2001). *Dietary Reference Intakes for vitamin A, vitamin K, arsenic, boron, chromium, copper, iodine, iron, manganese, molybdenum, nickel, silicon, vanadium, and zinc.* Washington, DC: National Academy Press.

Iolascon, A., De Falco, L., & Beaumont, C. (2009). Molecular basis of inherited microcytic anemia due to defects in iron acquisition or heme synthesis. *Haematologica, 94*, 395–408.

Lawrence, C. M., Ray, S., Babyonyshev, M., Galluser, R., Borhani, D. W., & Harrison, S. C. (1999). Crystal structure of the ectodomain of human transferrin receptor. *Science, 286*, 779–782.

Lill, R., & Mühlenhoff, U. (2008). Maturation of iron-sulfur proteins in eukaryotes: Mechanisms, connected processes, and diseases. *Annual Review of Biochemistry, 77*, 669–700.

Liu, X., & Theil, E. C. (2005). Ferritins: Dynamic management of biological iron and oxygen chemistry. *Accounts of Chemical Research, 38*, 167–175.

Mastrogiannaki, M., Matak, P., Keith, B., Simon, M. C., Vaulont, S., & Peyssonnaux, C. (2009). HIF-2alpha, but not HIF-1alpha, promotes iron absorption in mice. *The Journal of Clinical Investigation, 119*, 1159–1166.

McCance, R. A., & Widdowson, E. M. (1937). Absorption and excretion of iron. *Lancet, 230*, 680–684.

McKie, A. T. (2008). The role of Dcytb in iron metabolism: An update. *Biochemical Society Transactions, 36*, 1239–1241.

McKie, A. T., Barrow, D., Latunde-Dada, G. O., Rolfs, A., Sager, G., Mudaly, E., … Simpson, R. J. (2001). An iron-regulated ferric reductase associated with the absorption of dietary iron. *Science, 291*, 1755–1759.

McKie, A. T., Marciani, P., Rolfs, A., Brennan, K., Wehr, K., Barrow, D., … Simpson, R. J. (2000). A novel duodenal iron-regulated transporter, IREG1, implicated in the basolateral transfer of iron to the circulation. *Molecular Cell, 5*, 299–309.

Meyron-Holz, E. G., Ghosh, M. C., & Rouault, T. A. (2004a). Mammalian tissue oxygen levels modulate iron-regulatory protein activities in vivo. *Science, 306*, 2087–2209.

Meyron-Holtz, E. G., Ghosh, M. C., Iwai, K., LaVaute, T., Brazzolotto, X., Berger, U. V., … Rouault, T. A. (2004b). Genetic ablations of iron regulatory proteins 1 and 2 reveal why iron regulatory protein 2 dominates iron homeostasis. *The EMBO Journal, 23*, 386–395.

Miyajima, H., Takahashi, Y., & Kono, S. (2003). Aceruloplasminemia, an inherited disorder of iron metabolism. *Biometals, 16*, 205–213.

Muckenthaler, M. U., Galy, B., & Hentze, M. W. (2008). Systemic iron homeostasis and the iron-responsive element/iron-regulatory protein (IRE/IRP) regulatory network. *Annual Review of Nutrition, 28*, 197–213.

Nemeth, E., Tuttle, M. S., Powelson, J., Vaughn, M. B., Donovan, A., Ward, D. M., … Kaplan, J. (2004). Hepcidin regulates cellular iron efflux by binding to ferroportin and inducing its internalization. *Science, 306*, 2090–2093.

Nicolas, G., Bennoun, M., Devaux, I., Beaumont, C., Grandchamp, B., Kahn, A., & Vaulont, S. (2001). Lack of hepcidin gene expression and severe tissue iron overload in upstream stimulatory factor 2 (USF2) knockout mice. *Proceedings of the National Academy of Sciences of the United States of America, 98*, 8780–8785.

Nordlund, P., & Eklund, H. (1995). Di-iron-carboxylate proteins. *Current Opinion in Structural Biology, 5*, 758–766.

Ohgami, R. S., Campagna, D. R., Greer, E. L., Antiochos, B., McDonald, A., Chen, J., Sharp, J. J., Fujiwara, Y., Barker, J. E., & Fleming, M. D. (2005). Identification of a ferrireductase required for efficient transferrin-dependent iron uptake in erythroid cells. *Nature Genetics, 37*, 1264–1269.

Ohgami, R. S., Campagna, D. R., McDonald, A., & Fleming, M. D. (2006). The STEAP proteins are metalloreductases. *Blood, 108*, 1388–1394.

Papanikolaou, G., Samuels, M. E., Ludwig, E. H., MacDonald, M. L., Franchini, P. L., Dube, M. P., … Goldberg, Y. P. (2004). Mutations in HFE2 cause iron overload in chromosome 1q-linked juvenile hemochromatosis. *Nature Genetics, 36*, 77–82.

Pietrangelo, A. (2004). The ferroportin disease. *Blood Cells, Molecules & Diseases, 32*, 131–138.

Pietrangelo, A. (2006). Hereditary hemochromatosis. *Annual Review of Nutrition, 26*, 251–270.

Pigeon, C., Ilyin, G., Courselaud, B., Leroyer, P., Turlin, B., Brissot, P., & Loreal, O. (2001). A new mouse liver-specific gene, encoding a protein homologous to human antimicrobial peptide hepcidin, is overexpressed during iron overload. *The Journal of Biological Chemistry, 276*, 7811–7819.

Porter, J. P. (2009). Pathophysiology of transfusional iron overload: Contrasting patterns in thalassemia major and sickle cell disease. *Hemoglobin, 33*, S37–S45.

Qiu, A., Jansen, M., Sakaris, A., Min, S. H., Chattopadhyay, S., Tsai, E., … Goldman, I. D. (2006). Identification of an intestinal folate transporter and the molecular basis for hereditary folate malabsorption. *Cell, 127*, 917–928.

Reddy, M. B., & Clark, L. (2004). Iron, oxidative stress, and disease risk. *Nutrition Reviews, 62*(8), 120–124.

Roetto, A., Papanikolaou, G., Politou, M., Alberti, F., Girelli, D., Christakis, J., … Camaschella, C. (2003). Mutant antimicrobial peptide hepcidin is associated with severe juvenile hemochromatosis. *Nature Genetics, 33*, 21–22.

Salahudeen, A. A., Thompson, J. W., Ruiz, J. C., Ma, H. W., Kinch, L. N., Li, Q., … Bruick, R. K. (2009). An E3 ligase possessing an iron-responsive hemerythrin domain is a regulator of iron homeostasis. *Science, 326*, 722–726.

Sanchez, M., Galy, B., Muckenthaler, M. U., & Hentze, M. W. (2007). Iron-regulatory proteins limit hypoxia-inducible factor-2alpha expression in iron deficiency. *Nature Structural & Molecular Biology, 14*, 420–426.

Sargent, P. J., Farnaud, S., & Evans, R. W. (2005). Structure/function overview of proteins involved in iron storage and transport. *Current Medicinal Chemistry, 12,* 2683–2693.

Sazinsky, M. H., & Lippard, S. J. (2006). Correlating structure with function in bacterial multicomponent monooxygenases and related diiron proteins. *Accounts of Chemical Research, 39,* 558–566.

Shah, Y. M., Matsubara, T., Ito, S., Yim, S. H., & Gonzalez, F. J. (2009). Intestinal hypoxia-inducible transcription factors are essential for iron absorption following iron deficiency. *Cell Metabolism, 9,* 152–164.

Shayeghi, M., Latunde-Dada, G. O., Oakhill, J. S., Laftah, A. H., Takeuchi, K., Halliday, N., … McKie, A. T. (2005). Identification of an intestinal heme transporter. *Cell, 122,* 789–801.

Sheftel, A. D., & Lill, R. (2009). The power plant of the cell is also a smithy: The emerging role of mitochondria in cellular iron homeostasis. *Annals of Medicine, 41,* 82–99.

Sheftel, A., Stehling, O., & Lill, R. (2009). Iron-sulfur proteins in health and disease. *Trends in Endocrinology and Metabolism 2010 May, 21*(5), 302–314.

Smiers, F. J., Krishnamurti, L., & Lucarelli, G. (2010). Hematopoietic stem cell transplantation for hemoglobinopathies: Current practice and emerging trends. *Pediatric Clinics of North America, 57,* 181–205.

Smith, S. R., Ghosh, M. C., Ollivierre-Wilson, H., Hang Tong, W., & Rouault, T. A. (2006). Complete loss of iron regulatory proteins 1 and 2 prevents viability of murine zygotes beyond the blastocyst stage of embryonic development. *Blood Cells, Molecules & Diseases, 36,* 283–287.

Tziomalos, K., & Perifanis, V. (2010). Liver iron content determination by magnetic resonance imaging. *World Journal of Gastroenterology, 16,* 1587–1597.

Vashisht, A. A., Zumbrennen, K. B., Huang, X., Powers, D. N., Durazo, A., Sun, D., … Wohlschlegel, J. A. (2009). Control of iron homeostasis by an iron-regulated ubiquitin ligase. *Science, 326,* 718–721.

Vulpe, C. D., Kuo, Y. M., Murphy, T. L., Cowley, L., Askwith, C., Libina, N., … Anderson, G. J. (1999). Hephaestin, a ceruloplasmin homologue implicated in intestinal iron transport, is defective in the sla mouse. *Nature Genetics, 21,* 195–199.

Walden, W. E., Selezneva, A. I., Dupuy, J., Volbeda, A., Fontecilla-Camps, J. C., Theil, E. C., & Volz, K. (2006). Structure of dual function iron regulatory protein 1 complexed with ferrtin IRE-RNA. *Science, 314,* 877–880.

Ward, R. J., Legssyer, R., Henry, C., & Crichton, R. R. (2000). Does the haemosiderin iron core determine its potential for chelation and the development of iron-induced tissue damage? *Journal of Inorganic Biochemistry, 79,* 311–317.

Wessling-Resnick, M. (2000). Iron transport. *Annual Review of Nutrition, 20,* 129–151.

Wood, J. C., & Ghugre, N. (2008). Magnetic resonance imaging assessment of excess iron in thalassemia, sickle cell disease and other iron overload diseases. *Hemoglobin, 32,* 85–96.

World Health Organization, Centers for Disease Control and Prevention. (2007). *Assessing the iron status of populations: A report of a joint World Health Organization/Centers for Disease Control technical consultation on the assessment of iron status at the population level.* Geneva, Switzerland. Available at http://whqlibdoc.who.int/publications/2004/9241593156_eng.pdf

Zhang, D. L., Hughes, R. M., Ollivierre-Wilson, H., Ghosh, M. C., & Rouault, T. A. (2009). A ferroportin transcript that lacks an iron-responsive element enables duodenal and erythroid precursor cells to evade translational repression. *Cell Metabolism, 9,* 461–473.

Zimmer, M., Ebert, B. L., Neil, C., Brenner, K., Papaioannou, I., Melas, A., … Iliopoulos, O. (2008). Small-molecule inhibitors of HIF-2a translation link its 5′UTR iron-responsive element to oxygen sensing. *Molecular Cell, 32,* 838–848.

RECOMMENDED READINGS

Beutler, E., Hoffbrand, A. V., & Cook, J. D. (2003). Iron deficiency and overload. *Hematology/The Education Program of the American Society of Hematology,* 40–61.

Crichton, R. R. (2009). *Inorganic biochemistry of iron metabolism: From molecular mechanisms to clinical consequences* (3rd ed.). New York: John Wiley and Sons.

Ganz, T., Nemeth, E. (2011). The hepcidin-ferroportin system as a therapeutic target in anemias and iron overload disorders. *Hematology American Society Hematology Education Program.* 2011:538–542.

CHAPTER 37

Zinc, Copper, and Manganese

Arthur Grider, PhD

COMMON ABBREVIATIONS

AE acrodermatitis enteropathica
CDF cation diffusion family; also known as zinc transporter (ZnT) family
DMT1 divalent metal transporter 1
IGF1 insulin-like growth factor 1
MD Menkes disease
MTF1 metal response element–binding transcription factor 1
SOD superoxide dismutase

Trace elements function in the body as components of enzymes and proteins involved in various biochemical pathways. Manganese is essential for certain enzymes involved in urea formation, carbohydrate metabolism, cartilage formation, and protection from reactive oxygen species. Copper is associated with numerous enzyme systems, such as those involved in collagen formation, neuropeptide and neurotransmitter synthesis, oxidative phosphorylation, iron metabolism, and protection from reactive oxygen species. Zinc is necessary for the activity of a number of enzymes, including those involved in alcohol metabolism, DNA metabolism, protein metabolism, glycolysis, bone formation, protection from reactive oxygen species, and signal transduction. Clearly, these trace elements, though present in relatively small concentrations, play a major role in maintaining our health and well-being.

ZINC, COPPER, AND MANGANESE IN ENZYME SYSTEMS

Zinc (Zn), copper (Cu), and manganese (Mn) are found within the periodic table as transition metals, defined as those elements containing *d* or *f* orbitals that are progressively filled with electrons. Manganese and copper contain partially filled *d* orbitals, whereas the *d* orbitals of zinc are completely filled. Zinc, copper, and manganese function as electron-pair acceptors (Lewis acids). In biological systems, the electron-pair donors (Lewis bases) are amino acids or water (Figure 37-1). A partial list of enzymes dependent on these minerals is contained in Table 37-1. Because more than 200 zinc-containing metalloenzymes with at least 20 distinct biological functions have been identified in various species, the metalloenzyme function is particularly associated with zinc. However, the metalloenzyme function is central to our understanding of the biology of copper, manganese, and zinc, and the loss of specific metalloenzyme function may account for the symptoms associated with deficiencies of these three metals.

There are four biological roles in which metals function: signaling, structural, catalytic, and regulatory. The last three roles relate directly to the functions of metals in proteins and enzyme systems. What makes zinc, copper, and manganese so useful in enzyme systems? Some general guidelines that can be followed to assess the likelihood that a mineral will fit a particular biological role include (1) the charge of the ion (determines the stability and reactivity of the metal in an enzyme), (2) the size of the atom (limits the sites a metal can fit), and (3) the natural abundance of a metal and its location within a cell (e.g., cytosolic versus extracellular will define the likelihood of incorporation into specific enzymes) (Glusker, 1991).

When the chemical features of zinc are examined, it becomes apparent why this metal is so prevalent in proteins and enzyme systems. First, with the exception of potassium (K^+) and magnesium (Mg^{2+}), zinc is the most common intracellular metal ion. It is found in the cytosol, in vesicles and organelles, and in the nucleus. Therefore it is in the correct proximity to be incorporated into many cellular enzymes. Next, zinc's flexible coordination geometry makes it ideal for the active site of enzymes. One hypothesis regarding metalloenzymes is that the active site of metalloenzymes is "poised for catalysis," a condition called the entatic state (Vallee and Galdes, 1984).

Researchers have defined the entatic state as the condition in which the geometry of the metal binding site in an enzyme is distorted and asymmetrical (Figure 37-2). When this strain is released by allowing the metal binding site to return to a less distorted form, the energy released may lower the energy of activation of the enzymatic reaction. Theoretically this permits a faster, more efficient

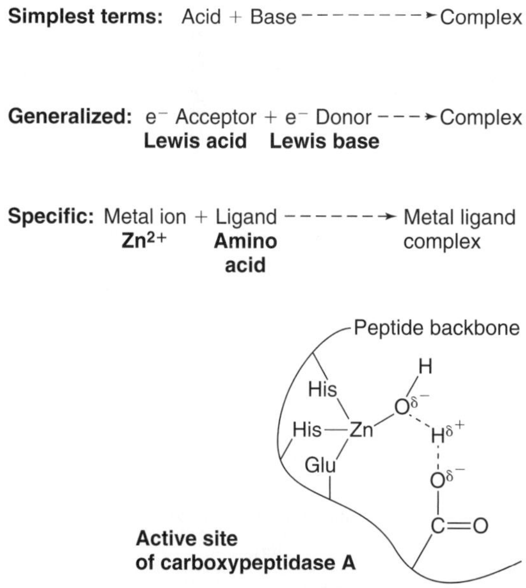

Simplest terms: Acid + Base ⟶ Complex

Generalized: e⁻ Acceptor + e⁻ Donor ⟶ Complex
Lewis acid **Lewis base**

Specific: Metal ion + Ligand ⟶ Metal ligand complex
Zn^{2+} **Amino acid**

Peptide backbone
His
His—Zn
Glu
H
$O^{\delta-}$
$H^{\delta+}$
$O^{\delta-}$
C=O
Active site of carboxypeptidase A

FIGURE 37-1 Metal–ligand complex formation. The biological roles of minerals like copper, zinc, or manganese frequently depend on their interaction with biological ligands such as amino acids in proteins. These interactions are defined by the chemistry of the mineral. This is illustrated in the figure using the general chemical principles of Lewis acid–base theory.

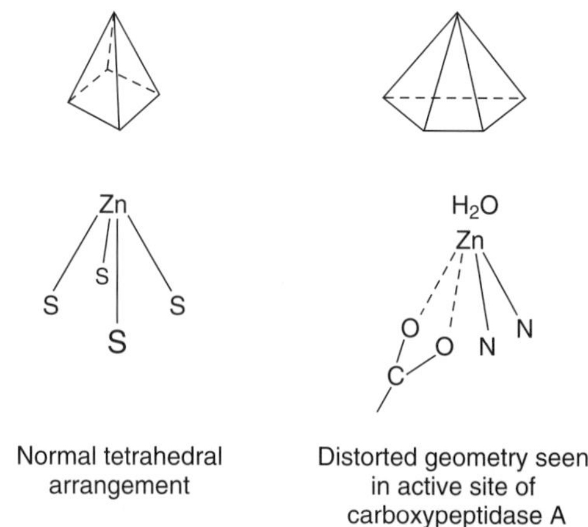

FIGURE 37-2 Distorted geometry of ligand binding is associated with the entatic state seen in the active site of enzymes. Zinc is shown bound to the enzyme via ligands to the sulfhydryl group of cysteine residues (*S*), the imidazole nitrogen of histidine residues (*N*), or the carboxylate group of glutamate residues (*COO⁻*).

enzymatic reaction. Zinc can sit in this entatic state because it has several possible coordination geometries, and because the coordination geometry is easily distorted. In addition, zinc is a strong Lewis acid (only copper is better), and its presence at an active site can supply a hydroxyl group (OH^-), which is important for many enzymatic reactions (see Figure 37-1). In this instance zinc uses water as a fourth ligand (the other three being amino acid residues in the enzyme). The hydroxyl group results when the water molecule forms a partial dipole that is loosely associated with zinc and with a negatively charged group in the enzyme (e.g., a carboxyl group from an aspartate residue).

Like zinc, manganese and copper can supply the hard base, OH^-, for enzymatic reactions when they are present in the active sites of enzymes. However, they have the advantage over zinc when redox reactions are required. Whereas manganese (Mn^{2+}, Mn^{3+}, and Mn^{7+}) and copper (Cu^{1+} and Cu^{2+}) have multiple valence states and can cycle between them as part of an enzymatic reaction, zinc has only one common valence state (Zn^{2+}) and cannot function in these situations. For example, Zn^{2+} serves a structural role in cytosolic and extracellular Cu/Zn superoxide dismutase (SOD), whereas the catalytic reaction of SOD in detoxifying superoxide involves a redox reaction that utilizes either copper (cytosolic and extracellular Cu/Zn-SODs) or manganese (mitochondrial Mn-SOD).

Understanding the central roles of zinc, copper, and manganese in association with proteins and enzymes also serves as a framework to explain how researchers have tried to develop functional status assessment tools that can be used in defining optimal dietary requirements.

ABSORPTION, TRANSPORT, STORAGE, AND EXCRETION OF ZINC, COPPER, AND MANGANESE

Humans or animals must effectively obtain and retain zinc, copper, and manganese so that these minerals may be utilized for their primary roles in enzyme systems or in other interactions with proteins and biological ligands. Though gaps remain in our knowledge of their metabolism, recent advances have increased our knowledge of the mechanisms for their cellular influx, efflux, and compartmentalization. Of the three metals, the least is known about the metabolism of manganese.

ABSORPTION

Zinc, copper, and manganese are each absorbed throughout the length of the small intestine but mainly in the jejunum. Copper may also be absorbed in the stomach. Absorption is regulated at the intestinal level for copper and zinc; despite limited evidence, this is also likely to be true for manganese. Absorption can be separated into a saturable, regulated portion and a nonregulated, diffusional component. Because of the existence of both carrier-mediated and nonregulated diffusional absorption of these minerals, the efficiency of absorption falls (i.e., lower fractional absorption), although the total amount of mineral entering the body increases as the dietary level of the mineral increases. Specific zinc and copper transporters have been identified as subsequently described. Intestinal manganese absorption may occur through the divalent metal transporter 1 (DMT1/SLC11A2), which transports iron, manganese, nickle, zinc, and the toxic metals cadmium and lead. Rats expressing a functionally impaired DMT1 exhibit reduced intestinal uptake of manganese (Bressler et al., 2007). (See Chapter 36 for a discussion of iron absorption.)

Zinc Absorption

Transcellular and paracellular transport are the two mechanisms for the intestinal transport of minerals from the lumen

TABLE 37-1 Vertebrate Enzymes Containing or Activated by Copper, Zinc, or Manganese

ENZYME	FUNCTION	ROLE OF METAL
COPPER		
Lysyl oxidase	Collagen synthesis	Catalytic
Peptidylglycine α-amidating monooxygenase	Neuropeptide synthesis	Catalytic
Superoxide dismutase (cytosolic and extracellular)	$O_2^{\cdot-}$ to H_2O_2	Catalytic
"Ferroxidase"/ceruloplasmin	Release of stored iron	Catalytic
Cytochrome c oxidase	Oxidative phosphorylation	Catalytic
Dopamine β-hydroxylase	Neurotransmitter synthesis	Catalytic
Tyrosine oxidase	Melanin synthesis	Catalytic
ZINC		
Alcohol dehydrogenase	Alcohol metabolism	Catalytic, noncatalytic
Superoxide dismutase (cytosolic)	$O_2^{\cdot-}$ to H_2O_2	Noncatalytic
Superoxide dismutase (extracellular)	$O_2^{\cdot-}$ to H_2O_2	Noncatalytic
Terminal deoxynucleotide transferase	Add deoxynucleotide triphosphates to 3′ end of DNA	?
Alkaline phosphatase	Bone formation	Catalytic, noncatalytic
5′-Nucleotidase	Hydrolysis of 5′-nucleotides	?
Fructose 1,6-bisphosphatase	Glycolysis	Regulatory
Aminopeptidase	Protein digestion	Catalytic, regulatory
Angiotensin-converting enzyme	Angiotensin I to II	Catalytic
Carboxypeptidases A and B	Protein digestion	Catalytic
Neutral protease	Protein digestion	Catalytic
Collagenase	Collagen breakdown	Catalytic
Carbonic anhydrase	$CO_2 \rightarrow HCO_3^-$	Catalytic
δ-Aminolevulinic acid dehydratase	Heme biosynthesis	Catalytic
MANGANESE		
Arginase	Urea formation	Catalytic
Pyruvate carboxylase	Gluconeogensis	Catalytic
Superoxide dismutase (mitochondrial)	$O_2^{\cdot-}$ to H_2O_2	Catalytic
Farnesyl pyrophosphate synthetase	Cholesterol synthesis	Catalytic
Glycosyltransferases	Cartilage formation	Regulatory
Phosphoenolpyruvate carboxylase	Gluconeogenesis	Regulatory
Xylosyltransferase	Cartilage formation	Regulatory

of the intestine to the portal circulation. Transcellular transport, the movement of zinc across the apical membrane through the cell and exiting at the basolateral membrane, is a carrier-mediated process. Paracellular transport occurs by simple diffusion as the concentration of zinc in the lumen exceeds the ability of the transcellular mechanism to transport zinc into the intestinal cell at its apical surface; zinc diffuses through the tight junctions between intestinal cells. The model for intestinal zinc absorption is shown in Figure 37-3.

Two zinc transporters that facilitate carrier-mediated zinc uptake into the intestinal cell have been identified, ZIP (Zrt/Irt-like protein 4; SLC39A4) and ZnT5 (zinc transporter 5; SLC30A5). Molecular studies of patients with the genetic disease acrodermatitis enteropathica (AE) have revealed that the *ZIP4/SLC394A4* gene is mutated in these individuals (Dufner-Beattie et al., 2003). This transporter protein is located at the apical surface of intestinal cells, and its presence is responsive to dietary zinc, increased with zinc deficiency,

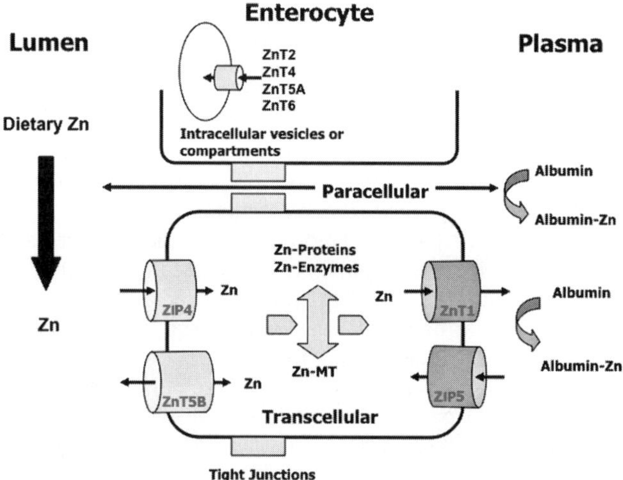

FIGURE 37-3 A proposed model for intestinal zinc absorption. Intraluminal zinc from dietary and endogenous sources can be transported across the intestinal epithelium in two ways, paracellular transport (diffusion) and transcellular transport (saturable). ZIP4 (defective in acrodermatitis enteropathica) and ZnT5B zinc transporters are located at the brush border membrane, whereas ZnT1 and ZIP5 zinc transporters are located at the basolateral membrane, of the enterocyte. The arrows indicate the direction of zinc transport. Inside the cell, zinc can be bound by metallothionein (*MT*) and be incorporated into other zinc-binding proteins and zinc-dependent enzymes involved in the biochemical and physiological functioning of the cell. Zinc can also be transported from the cytosol into various intracellular membrane vesicles and compartments, such as the Golgi apparatus and the endoplasmic reticulum, via zinc transporters ZnT2, ZnT4, ZnT5A, and ZnT6. Zinc that is transported out of the enterocyte by ZnT1 into the portal circulation will bind to albumin for transport to the liver. Zinc is transported both from the lumen to the portal circulation (ZIP4 → ZnT1) and from the portal circulation to the lumen (ZIP5 → ZnT5B).

and decreased during zinc sufficiency (Kim et al., 2004). The B splice variant of ZnT5 was found to be present at the apical surface of the Caco-2 intestinal cell line and the brush border membrane of human intestinal biopsies. Its messenger RNA (mRNA) expression was increased in these cells with 100 μM zinc supplementation, and it was shown to function as a zinc uptake transporter (Cragg et al., 2002). However, ZnT5 mRNA levels decreased when the cultured cells were grown in 200 μM zinc compared to 100 μM zinc (Cragg et al., 2005). Similarly, subjects consuming 25 mg zinc for 14 days exhibited reduced ZnT5 mRNA and ZnT5 protein in their intestinal biopsies (Cragg et al., 2005). Although ZnT5 is a member of the cation diffusion facilitator family, it may function as both an influx and an efflux zinc transporter in the intestinal cell (Valentine et al., 2007).

The control for intestinal zinc transport is not fully understood. The mechanism is likely to be complex, as recent cellular studies suggest. Elegant cell culture studies using cells transfected with the mouse *SLC39A4* gene showed that, under normal zinc levels, the ZIP4 transporter recycled rapidly via endocytosis between the plasma membrane and an endosomal vesicular compartment (Kim et al., 2004). Under zinc-deficient culture conditions, more of the ZIP4 transporter remained at the plasma membrane, whereas less was observed within the intracellular vesicular compartment. Conversely, when the cultured cells were exposed to an increasing concentration of zinc in the culture medium, less of the transporter was located at the plasma membrane, with a corresponding increase in the transporter within intracellular endosomal vesicles. Furthermore, the increased presence of the transporter at the plasma membrane corresponded with increased zinc uptake, with the converse also being true. Therefore these current studies with ZIP4 agree with whole animal and small intestine cell culture studies performed earlier, showing that zinc deficiency increases intestinal zinc transport and absorption. However, the zinc-dependent trigger for the translocation of the ZIP4 zinc transporter between the intracellular vesicles and the plasma membrane is not known at this time.

The mechanism of the intracellular transport of zinc from the apical to the basolateral intracellular surface for transport to the portal circulation is not known at this time. The transport of zinc from the enterocyte cytosol to the serosa across the basolateral membrane occurs via ZnT1 (SLC30A1), of the cation diffusion family of zinc transporters (McMahon and Cousins, 1998; Palmiter and Findley, 1995; Lichten and Cousins, 2009).

AE (acrodermatitis enteropathica) is caused by an autosomal recessive mutation and is characterized by symptoms normally associated with severe zinc deficiency. Symptoms include dermatitis, alopecia, poor growth, immune deficiencies, hypogonadism, night blindness, impaired taste, and diarrhea. Studies have shown that a primary defect in AE patients is reduced intestinal zinc absorption. Other studies have shown that cellular zinc uptake is reduced in intestinal biopsies and in cultured fibroblasts of patients with AE (Grider and Young, 1996). The AE mutation has been mapped to chromosomal region 8q24.3. Several mutations within the AE gene (*SLC39A4,* which encodes ZIP4) have been identified. The mutations, found in genomic DNA from patients with AE, include missense mutations and a premature termination codon. Several of the missense mutations have been studied thus far using transfected cell culture models; the mutations affect either the translocation of ZIP4 to the plasma membrane or its endocytosis from the plasma membrane (Wang et al., 2004). The posttranslational regulation of trafficking between membrane compartments has also been shown for the copper transporting P-type ATPases ATP7A and ATP7B.

Copper Absorption

As with zinc, manganese, and other trace elements, intestinal copper transport requires the following three steps:

1. Uptake from the intestinal lumen across the brush border membrane
2. Intracellular transport to the basolateral membrane
3. Transport across the plasma membrane to the portal circulation

CLINICAL CORRELATION

Copper versus Zinc Transporters: Lethal versus Nonlethal Mutations

Individuals diagnosed with Menkes disease (MD) are unable to absorb intestinal copper. Similarly, those afflicted with acrodermatitis enteropathica (AE) exhibit defective intestinal zinc transport. In both instances the affected transport proteins and their genes have been identified; MD involves the ATP7A copper transporter and AE involves the ZIP4 zinc transporter. MD causes the accumulation of copper in the intestinal cells, along with reduced serum copper and ceruloplasmin. In contrast, AE causes a reduction in the amount of zinc in intestinal cells along with a reduction in serum zinc. Furthermore, individuals afflicted with AE are successfully treated by the consumption of zinc supplements, whereas those afflicted with MD die despite attempts at copper supplementation.

Thinking Critically

1. Where do these transporters reside within the intestinal cell and how does their position within the cell affect the transport of their respective metal?
2. Why would an accumulation of intracellular copper be observed in the intestinal cells of MD patients but an accumulation of zinc not be observed in AE patients?
3. MD is lethal despite dietary copper supplementation because these patients die from copper deficiency but AE is treatable with dietary zinc supplementation. Why do the MD patients die while the AE patients thrive with the dietary supplementation of their respective metals?

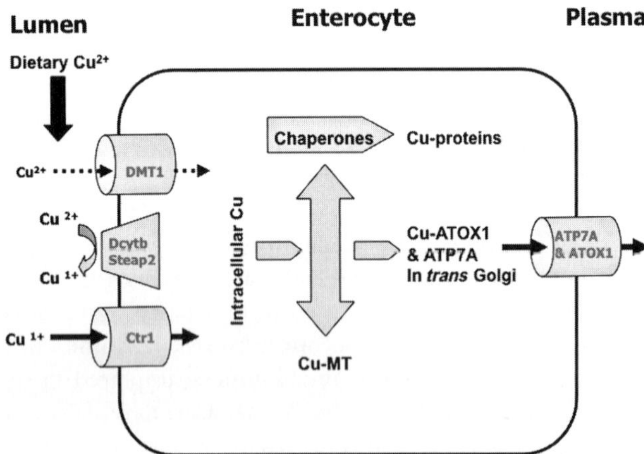

FIGURE 37-4 A proposed model for intestinal copper absorption. The primary transport mechanism is through the Ctr1 copper transporter following reduction to its cuprous form (Cu^{2+}) by duodenal cytochrome b (Dcytb) or six-transmembrane epithelial antigen of the prostate 2 (Steap2). Both Dcytb and Steap2 are reductases that reduce Fe^{3+}. Other reductants present in the luminal contents such as ascorbate may also be involved in reducing copper before its transport by Ctr1. The minor transport mechanism involves the Fe^{2+} transporter DMT1. Inside the cell, copper will bind to copper chaperones or metallothionein (*MT*); the chaperones will carry copper to various copper-dependent proteins such as superoxide dismutase. ATOX1 is the chaperone for the copper transporter ATP7A located in the *trans*-Golgi compartment. As a complex, ATOX1 and ATP7A translocate to the basolateral membrane, and copper is transported across the membrane to the portal circulation where it binds to albumin for transport to the liver.

The model for intestinal copper absorption is shown in Figure 37-4. Two potential apical membrane copper transporters have been identified in intestinal absorptive cells: (1) the Ctr1 (SLC31A1) copper transporter, and (2) the divalent metal transporter 1 (DMT1/SLC11A2; also called Nramp2). Ctr1 transports monovalent copper (Cu^{1+}) (Lee et al., 2002a, 2002b). DMT1 transports divalent iron but can also transport divalent copper (Cu^{2+}) (Gunshin et al., 2009). Most of the dietary copper is in its cupric state (Cu^{2+}). Luminal reduction of Cu^{2+} to Cu^{1+} may occur at the brush border membrane via duodenal cytochrome b (Dcytb/CYBRD1) or six-transmembrane epithelial antigen of the prostate 2 (Steap2), both serving as Fe^{3+} reductases that may also reduce Cu^{2+} (Prohaska, 2008).

Once inside the cell, copper is bound by chaperones that carry copper to various copper-binding proteins, cuproenzymes, or ATP7A, a membrane-associated copper transporting ATPase that is defective in Menkes syndrome (Figure 37-5). ATP7A is also called Menkes protein or MNKP. ATOX1 is a cytosolic copper chaperone that delivers copper from Ctr1 to ATP7A located at the *trans*-Golgi network. The copper is then exported from the intestinal cell at its basolateral side by this copper transporting ATPase. Menkes syndrome is an X-linked recessive genetic disorder caused by a mutation in the gene encoding for ATP7A that results in a lethal reduction in copper absorption (Tumer et al., 2003) (see subsequent text).

Inhibition of Intestinal Zinc and Copper Absorption by Metallothionein

At low zinc status, transcellular zinc absorption is at its most efficient; at high zinc status, zinc absorption is inhibited. Research suggests that this downregulation of zinc absorption is due to the production of metallothionein, a zinc-binding protein. Metallothionein is a low-molecular-weight protein (6.1 kDa) found in the cell cytosol, and it is produced in response to high levels of dietary zinc or copper, as well as toxic heavy metals such as cadmium (Cd^{2+}) and mercury (Hg^{2+}) (Cousins, 1985). It has been proposed that high levels of metallothionein in enterocytes act as a mucosal block by binding zinc and preventing its movement through the cell, thereby limiting absorption. The "blocked" metal is later lost from the body as the enterocyte is sloughed off into the intestine. Similarly, the induced production of metallothionein by copper may downregulate copper absorption by this same mechanism. Functions for metallothionein in tissues other than the intestine have also been proposed (discussed in subsequent text).

Some studies have shown that high levels of zinc can inhibit intestinal copper absorption; this observation has

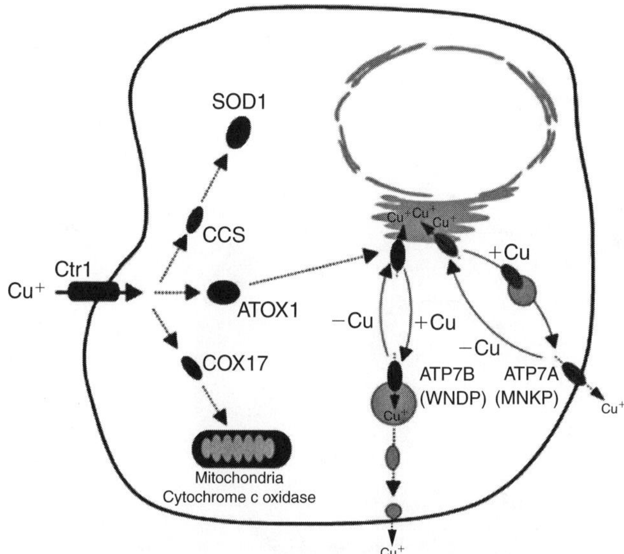

FIGURE 37-5 Schematic illustration depicting copper distribution in a generalized human cell. Copper uptake via human copper transporter 1 (Ctr1) provides copper to the copper chaperones ATOX1, CCS (copper chaperone for SOD), and COX17 (cytochrome c oxidase copper chaperone) for the transfer of copper to the ATPase Cu^{+2} transporting proteins ATP7A (which is also known as Menkes protein, MNKP), ATP7B (which is also known as Wilson disease protein, WNDP), Cu/Zn superoxide dismutase (SOD), and cytochrome c oxidase. ATP7A and ATP7B are shown in the *trans*-Golgi network (TGN), and the copper-induced recycling pathways are denoted by arrows. ATP7A and ATP7B in the *trans*-Golgi network provide copper to secreted cuproenzymes, such as tyrosinase and ceruloplasmin. Under excessive copper conditions, ATP7A and ATP7B are sorted to post-Golgi vesicles for exocytic trafficking. ATP7B traffics to a cytoplasmic vesicle compartment where it sequesters excess copper for subsequent excretion via a mechanism that presumably does not require ATP7B to be located at the plasma membrane. Elevated copper induces the trafficking of ATP7A to the plasma membrane of cells. As cytosolic copper concentrations decrease, ATP7A and ATP7B resume a steady state *trans*-Golgi location. (With kind permission from Springer Science+Business Media: Lutsenko, S., & Petris, M. J. [2002]. Function and regulation of the mammalian copper-transporting ATPases: Insights from biochemical and cell biological approaches. *Journal of Membrane Biology, 191*, 1–12, Figure 3.)

been used to reduce copper absorption and help minimize the copper toxicity that is characteristic of Wilson disease. This rare autosomal recessive genetic disorder is due to mutations in ATP7B (referred to as Wilson Disease Protein, WNDP), which encodes an ATPase similar to ATP7A in its copper transporting functions (see subsequent text). The high-zinc diet stimulates the production of metallothionein, which then reduces copper absorption by blocking transcellular transport. In contrast, high levels of dietary copper do not reduce zinc absorption. One explanation for this latter observation is that a high copper level is handled differently than a high zinc level. Zinc is a much stronger inducer of intestinal metallothionein than copper (Leone et al., 1985). In addition, copper may not reach the metal-regulatory element of the metallothionein gene as rapidly as zinc, when copper intake is excessive, because of its shuttling to various copper-binding protein compartments via chaperones.

Bioavailability

Just as the biological roles of copper, zinc, and manganese are defined by their chemical interactions with ligands, so are the interactions of these metals with dietary components. These interactions can influence how well copper, zinc, or manganese is absorbed from the diet, but the luminal interactions leading to increased or decreased absorption are less well characterized than those for ligand interactions of copper, zinc, and manganese with enzymes (Lonnerdal and Sandstrom, 1995).

Chemical similarities with other nutrients may result in competition for common binding sites between related minerals. This could explain the inhibition of manganese absorption caused by high dietary iron or the zinc–copper antagonism discussed previously. Binding of minerals to organic components of the diet in the lumen of the gastrointestinal tract can alter absorption. The classic example of this is the inhibitory effect that the phosphate-rich plant compound phytate (*myo*-inositol pentaphosphates and hexaphosphates) has on the absorption of zinc and many other minerals (e.g., copper and iron) from the diet (Torre et al., 1992). The presence of calcium and phytate together in the same meal enhances the inhibitory effect on mineral absorption because calcium stabilizes phytate. Others have suggested that binding of zinc or copper to low-molecular-weight ligands such as amino acids (e.g., histidine) may enhance intestinal absorption, but it is not clear how this enhancement would occur. Although ascorbate enhances iron absorption, it inhibits copper absorption. The chemical effects of ascorbate on iron and copper are the same; ascorbate promotes the reduction of both metals (to Fe^{2+} and Cu^{1+}). Dietary components can also influence other points of zinc or copper utilization. For example, high dietary molybdenum has been shown to increase urinary copper losses, and high dietary calcium increases exogenous zinc losses in the intestine.

TRANSPORT IN PLASMA AND TISSUE UPTAKE

Once absorbed, both copper and zinc are bound primarily to albumin in the plasma and transported to the liver.

Cellular Zinc Transporters

After reaching the liver, zinc is repackaged and released into the circulation bound to α_2-macroglobulin. At any given time, the relative distribution of zinc in the circulation is approximately 57% bound to albumin, 40% to α_2-macroglobulin, and 3% to low-molecular-weight ligands such as amino acids. There is evidence that the uptake of zinc into cells is regulated (note the discussion in the preceding text concerning the ZIP4 zinc transporter). Close to 200 zinc transporters, belonging either to the *SLC30* or *SLC39* gene families, have been identified, and are found in fungi, plants, insects, nematodes, and mammals (Liuzzi and Cousins, 2004; Lichten and Cousins, 2009). A total of 24 mammalian zinc transporters belonging to the *SLC30* (10 members; cation diffusion family, or CDF/ZnT family) and *SLC39* (14 members; zinc-responsive transport/iron responsive transport protein family, or ZIP family) gene families have been

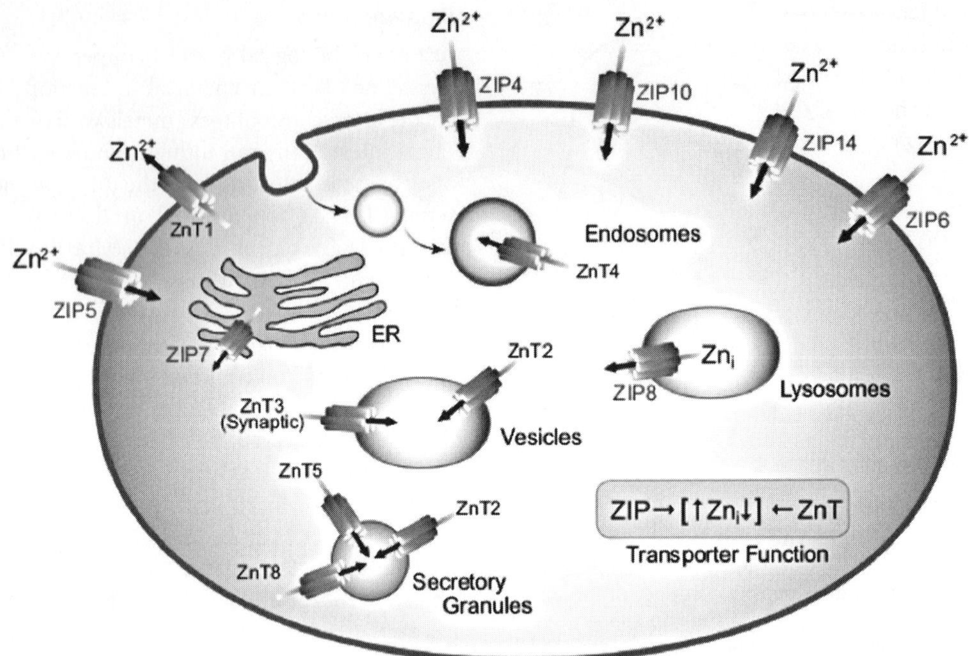

FIGURE 37-6 Generalized cell showing locations of some key zinc transporter proteins. The six and eight transmembrane domains for the majority of ZnT and ZIP proteins, respectively, are shown. Restricted localization to the plasma membrane on specific intracellular organelles has yet to be established for members of both protein families. As shown, the function of the ZnT and ZIP transporter families is to reduce and increase the cytoplasmic zinc concentrations, respectively. Such diverse distribution of these proteins suggests individual roles in executing the catalytic, structural, and regulatory roles of zinc. *ER*, Endoplasmic reticulum. (Used with permission of Annual Reviews, Inc. From Lichten, L. A., & Cousins, R. J. [2009]. Mammalian zinc transporters: Nutritional and physiologic regulation. *Annual Review of Nutrition, 29*, 153–176. Permission conveyed through Copyright Clearance Center.)

identified to date (reviewed in Kambe et al., 2004 and Lichten and Cousins, 2009). Figure 37-6 shows the membrane compartments containing these transporters and the direction of zinc transport. None of these transporters appears to require energy for its function. In endothelial cells, albumin is taken up by endocytosis as a part of transcytosis (Frank et al., 2009). This mechanism may provide for the majority of the internalization of zinc by cells because most zinc in the circulation is bound to albumin. A portion of this endocytosis occurs through non–clathrin-coated pits and may involve caveolae or lipid rafts, or both. These caveolae are specialized plasma membrane compartments that contain an unusually high amount of cholesterol and sphingolipids. They are involved in numerous signal transduction pathways and may be involved in some aspect of zinc uptake (Doherty and McMahon, 2009). After endocytosis the albumin likely releases the zinc, allowing it to be transported across the endosomal membrane and into the cytosol. Once in the cytosol it binds to proteins within the zinc-binding protein pool, including metallothionein.

The two types of transporters differ in several ways. The ZIP transporters that have been characterized thus far transport zinc into the cytosol, either into the cell from the extracellular milieu or into the cytosol from within intracellular membrane compartments. The ZnT transporters exhibit the opposite function, facilitating zinc efflux from the cytosol to the outside of the cell or into intracellular membrane compartments. Both transporter families are transmembrane proteins. The ZIP family contains proteins exhibiting seven or eight transmembrane domains, with extracellular amino and carboxyl ends. The ZnT family is made up mostly of proteins containing six transmembrane regions. Their amino and carboxyl ends are located intracellularly. The zinc transport/binding site for both families is an intracellular histidine-rich loop. However, this loop is located between transmembrane regions three and four in the ZIP family and between transmembrane regions four and five in the ZnT family. One of the members of the ZnT family, ZnT5, does not fit the general description of the other members of the ZnT family. It has 12 transmembrane regions and has been implicated in intestinal cell zinc influx and efflux at the brush border membrane (Cragg et al., 2002; Valentine et al., 2007). These transporter families are intimately involved in zinc acquisition from the environment as well as control of intracellular zinc influx and efflux within organelles (see Figure 37-6). The proliferation of these transporter families is indicative of the importance of zinc in cellular metabolism.

Copper and Ceruloplasmin

Once copper reaches the liver, it is incorporated into ceruloplasmin within the *trans*-Golgi network facilitated by ATP7B, a membrane-associated copper-transporting ATPase that is defective in Wilson disease. Then the copper–ceruloplasmin complex is released into the circulation for delivery to peripheral tissues. Scientists have traditionally thought that ceruloplasmin is a critical protein in the metabolism and function of copper (Vulpe and Packman, 1995). It is a large glycoprotein of 132 kDa, which contains 6% to 7% carbohydrate and which can bind six atoms of copper; 90% to 95% of serum copper is bound to ceruloplasmin. Ceruloplasmin is produced in the liver, and its synthesis is regulated by copper as well as inflammatory mediators such as interleukin 1 (IL1) and glucocorticoids. These and other factors associated with the acute-phase response are presumably responsible for the increase in serum copper and ceruloplasmin that occurs following acute inflammation or infection.

In cell culture studies, the mechanism of copper uptake into cells occurred through the binding of ceruloplasmin–copper to a cell-surface receptor (Percival and Harris, 1990). Whereas the circulating transferrin–iron complex is internalized after it binds to the transferrin receptor on the cell surface, copper is reduced and released from ceruloplasmin, at which point the copper can be taken up by the cell as the free metal through the Ctr1 copper transporter. Paradoxically, individuals who have a genetic mutation in the ceruloplasmin gene, leading to a total lack of ceruloplasmin in the serum (i.e., aceruloplasminemia), do not have overt symptoms of copper deficiency as one might predict from the cell culture studies (Harris et al., 1995). Instead, these individuals have altered iron metabolism. This raises questions regarding the biological role of ceruloplasmin in serum copper transport.

Other proteins are also involved in copper movement. Most if not all copper ions in cells are bound to SOD or other proteins. Studies in animals and cells have shown that a copper chaperone for SOD (CCS) is necessary for the insertion of copper into SOD. Rats fed copper-deficient diets displayed a dose-dependent increase in CCS expression in liver and erythrocytes (Bertinato et al., 2003).

Manganese Plasma Transport and Tissue Uptake

Manganese is handled slightly differently than are copper and zinc. Following absorption, manganese is thought to bind to α_2-macroglobulin for delivery to the liver. Because manganese can be oxidized to the Mn^{3+} state, it can bind to transferrin for subsequent delivery to other tissues. It is not clear, however, whether this system was intended to accommodate manganese or whether the binding is simply opportunistic. Regardless, this binding behavior suggests that manganese uptake into cells occurs by the same mechanism as iron uptake, by receptor-mediated endocytosis of the metal–transferrin complex.

STORAGE

When animals are fed experimental diets lacking copper, zinc, or manganese, their status rapidly declines. This suggests that there is not a storage pool of these minerals to be used during times of low intake or increased need (i.e., for the production of new metal-containing proteins and enzymes). For example, zinc can be localized in the bones under conditions of

CLINICAL CORRELATION

Role of Ceruloplasmin in Iron Metabolism

Subsequent to the identification of the mutated gene responsible for Wilson disease, it became possible to screen adult patients with neurological degeneration and low serum ceruloplasmin concentrations for molecular diagnosis of Wilson disease. Wilson disease is caused by defective coding for a putative copper-transporting ATPase located in hepatic membranes; this transport protein is required for copper trafficking into a common pool for biliary excretion and holoceruloplasmin biosynthesis. Failure to incorporate copper during ceruloplasmin biosynthesis results in unstable ceruloplasmin that lacks oxidase activity.

As patients were referred for molecular diagnosis, it became clear that some of the patients with low or absent ceruloplasmin did not have Wilson disease. Further molecular genetic analysis of patients with non–Wilson disease aceruloplasminemia revealed mutations in the ceruloplasmin gene that resulted in truncation of the open reading frame. Harris and colleagues (1995) described one of two sisters with undetectable ceruloplasmin. This patient was homozygous for a mutation in exon 7 of the ceruloplasmin gene. She had developed degeneration of the retina and basal ganglia during the fifth decade of life. Liver biopsy revealed a normal hepatic copper concentration but elevated iron stores. Indirect evidence for iron deposition in the basal ganglia of the brain was also obtained. The association of defects in ceruloplasmin synthesis with abnormalities in iron metabolism in this and other patients confirms an essential role of ceruloplasmin in human iron metabolism and supports a role of ceruloplasmin as a ferroxidase (Harris et al., 1995). However, the major problem in patients with aceruloplasminemia seems to be excessive iron deposition or storage, with much milder problems related to iron delivery or utilization. How a plasma protein can be involved in release of iron from tissue ferritin is not yet clear.

Thinking Critically

1. Explain how a lack of ceruloplasmin could result in iron overload in liver and other tissues.
2. A low serum iron concentration and an elevated serum ferritin concentration are found in patients with defects in the ceruloplasmin gene. Anemia is seen in some but not all patients with defects in the ceruloplasmin gene. (a) Explain how each of these clinical/biochemical manifestations could result from a defect in ferroxidase activity. (b) Are these changes in measures of iron status similar to or different from the changes that would occur in iron deficiency anemia? (See Chapter 36 for more information about iron metabolism.)
3. Copper metabolism and transport seem to be relatively normal in patients with defects in ceruloplasmin synthesis. What might this tell us about the role of ceruloplasmin in copper transport in the body?

high zinc intake, but this zinc cannot be specifically mobilized to serve the needs of the organism when intake is low. Mechanisms for the intracellular compartmentalization of excess intracellular zinc are complex and include metallothionein as well as zinc-containing vesicles called zincosomes.

Metallothionein

The only serious candidate for a zinc storage protein is metallothionein. Since its discovery in 1960, experiments on the biological role of this protein have been a central feature of zinc research. Metallothionein is a low-molecular-weight protein comprising 61 amino acids, of which 20 residues are cysteine residues (Cousins, 1985). It is surprising that there are no disulfide bridges in metallothionein; all the thiol groups are involved in metal binding. Seven atoms of zinc or the related transition elements (cadmium, mercury, copper, and silver) have been found to bind to metallothionein in vitro. The metals are normally bound in two clusters, with one cluster binding four metal ions and the other binding three. Under normal physiological conditions, zinc is the primary metal bound to metallothionein. It is unlikely that a significant amount of metal-free metallothionein exists. There are multiple isoforms of metallothionein in mammalian tissues; 4 isoforms have been identified in mice, and at least 12 metallothionein genes have been identified in humans.

Multiple functions of metallothionein have been identified. This protein is rapidly induced in liver, kidney, pancreas, and intestine by exposure to high levels of heavy metals, particularly zinc and cadmium; binding of these metals will control their intracellular concentrations. Hepatic levels of metallothionein are also directly induced by glucocorticoids and the cytokine interleukin 6 (IL6). This accounts for the redistribution of zinc from the plasma to the liver during the acute-phase response that occurs following bacterial infection or as a result of inflammatory conditions, such as rheumatoid arthritis and intense exercise. Hepatic metallothionein levels are also elevated in newborns and may serve as a short-term depot for zinc during the initial days of life. Metallothionein, because of its abundance of sulfhydryl groups, detoxifies reactive oxygen species. Furthermore, it is a marker for cell cycle progression.

Analysis of the promoter region of metallothionein reveals the factors involved in its expression and gives insight into its roles in cellular metabolism (Kimura and Itoh, 2008). Zinc promotes metallothionein gene transcription through metal response element–binding transcription factor 1 (MTF1; Palmiter, 1994). Under low zinc conditions, MTF1 is normally bound to a zinc-sensitive inhibitor (MTI). MTI dissociates from MTF1 in the presence of zinc, thereby allowing MTF1 to interact with the metal response elements in the metallothionein promoter to activate transcription of the metallothionein gene. MTF1 contains six zinc finger motifs (Figure 37-7) and is likely to function as an intracellular sensor of free zinc concentrations (Andrews, 2000). The actual site for transcriptional regulation by zinc or cadmium appears to be a cysteine-rich region that is outside of the zinc finger regions of this protein (Chen et al., 2004). The metallothionein promoter contains IL6 and glucocorticoid response elements as well. Transcription of the metallothionein is induced by cadmium and hydrogen peroxide, and involves interactions between the upstream stimulatory factor and an antioxidant response element (Andrews, 2000). Zinc binding to zinc finger transcription factors is modulated by metallothionein, suggesting a role for this protein in gene transcription (Laukens et al., 2009). Consequently the biological

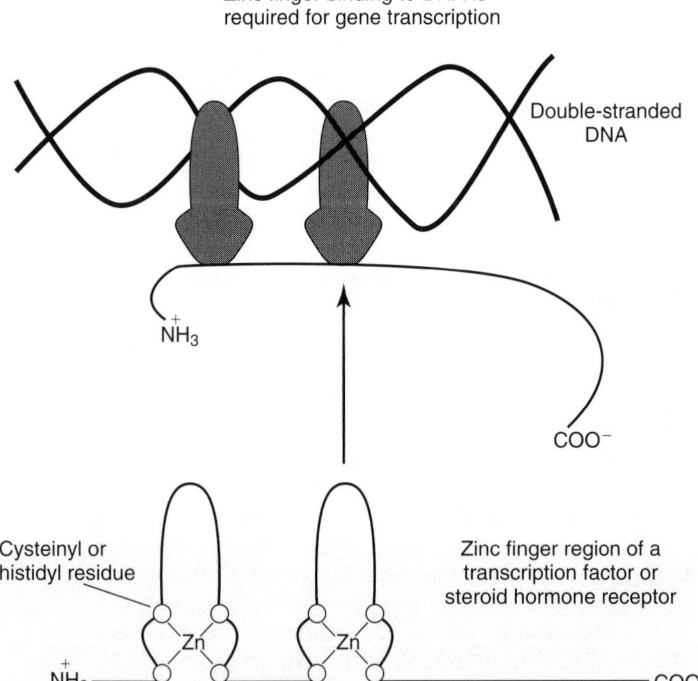

FIGURE 37-7 Zinc finger proteins are important for binding of transcription factors to DNA. By binding to histidine and cysteine residues in transcription factors and nuclear hormone receptors, zinc introduces a fingerlike secondary structure to the proteins. This structure allows the transcription factors to interact properly with response elements in the promoters of genes.

roles for metallothionein extend beyond metal binding, as was initially proposed. Metallothionein also functions as an antioxidant, is involved in the inflammatory response, and functions in the cell cycle.

Transgenic mice have been developed as a tool for understanding the role of metallothionein in normal zinc homeostasis. Mice that overexpress metallothionein I (the predominant form of the protein in mice) appear to resist dietary zinc deficiency compared with normal mice, which suggests that metallothionein functions as a repository for zinc (Dalton et al., 1996). In contrast, mice lacking the genes for metallothionein I and II (the forms found in intestine, liver, kidney, and most other cells except the brain) are born healthy and do not show any obvious symptoms of zinc deficiency when their mothers are fed a diet that contains adequate zinc (Kelly et al., 1996). However, kidney abnormalities are seen in newborn pups lacking metallothionein if their mothers are fed zinc-deficient diets while the pups are nursing. This suggests there may be a developmental role for metallothionein as a storage protein that protects the offspring when maternal zinc status is low.

Preliminary studies suggest that animals lacking metallothionein in the intestine do not reduce intestinal zinc absorption in response to high zinc status (Davis et al., 1996). This supports the proposed role of intestinal metallothionein in limiting the amount of zinc that leaves the enterocyte and enters the portal circulation. Finally, metallothionein knockout mice are excessively sensitive to cadmium toxicity, which supports the role of metallothionein as a heavy metal detoxification protein.

Mechanisms for Intracellular Zinc Homeostasis

Intracellular zinc homeostasis is also maintained by the transport of zinc into and out of cells and their intracellular vesicular compartments. One such mechanism involves coordinated transcription of metallothionein and ZnT1 via MTF1. The promoter regions of both of these genes contain metal response elements. As the intracellular zinc concentration increases, transcription of metallothionein and ZnT1 increases, resulting in increased cytosolic zinc binding and increased efflux of zinc across the plasma membrane (Heuchel et al., 1994; Langmade et al., 2000).

Zinc-containing vesicles, or zincosomes, were first identified by zinc-specific fluorescent probes that bound intracellular and intravesicular zinc (Zalewski et al., 1993; Coyle et al., 1994). It is proposed that transport of zinc between the cytosol and vesicles is mediated via certain *SLC30A* (ZnT) and *SLC39A* (ZIP) gene products (Lichten and Cousins, 2009). Using cultured cells as an experimental model, the binding characteristics of intravesicular zinc have been studied using x-ray absorption spectroscopy and micro x-ray fluorescence analysis. The results indicate that zinc within the zincosomes is bound in a manner similar to catalytic zinc sites within metalloenzymes (Wellenreuther et al., 2009). The binding characteristics support the potential for reversible zinc binding within the zincosomes, allowing for its subsequent release and transport to the cytosol via SLC39A zinc transporters. Furthermore, the binding characteristic permits the accumulation of zinc within zincosomes against a concentration gradient (Wellenreuther et al., 2009).

Menkes Syndrome and Wilson Disease: Copper Transporting P-Type ATPases

Both Menkes syndrome and Wilson disease are genetic disturbances in copper metabolism (DiDonato and Sarkar, 1997; Danks, 1995). Menkes syndrome is an X-linked recessive disorder that occurs at a rate greater than 1 in 300,000 live births and is usually fatal within 3 years after birth. It is characterized by low serum copper and ceruloplasmin levels and low copper levels in the liver and brain but markedly elevated cellular copper levels in the intestinal mucosa, muscle, spleen, and kidney. Other symptoms include abnormal ("steely") hair and progressive cerebral degeneration.

Wilson disease has autosomal recessive inheritance and occurs with an incidence greater than 1 in 100,000 live births. The onset of Wilson disease is much slower than that of Menkes syndrome, and it is usually diagnosed during or after the third decade of life. As in Menkes syndrome, serum ceruloplasmin levels are low in patients with Wilson disease, but in contrast to Menkes syndrome, copper accumulates in the liver and brain. Patients with Wilson disease appear to have a defect in the ability to excrete copper via the bile. Neurological damage and hepatic cirrhosis are end-stage effects of uncontrolled Wilson disease. If diagnosed early, patients can be treated by reducing copper intake, undergoing chelation therapy (with D-penicillamine), and taking oral zinc supplements (which will increase intestinal metallothionein and reduce copper absorption).

These diseases are caused by mutations in the genes encoding two P-type ATPases, ATP7A (Menkes syndrome) and ATP7B (Wilson disease) (Lutsenko and Petris, 2002). The P-type ATPases are a family of cation-transporting proteins found in all organisms and consists of over 200 members. Copper transport by ATP7A and ATP7B requires the catalytic hydrolysis of ATP. ATP7A and ATP7B are related but are two different proteins, exhibiting about 60% homology. The tissue distribution of these two transport proteins is different. ATP7A mRNA is found in all tissues except the liver, whereas ATP7B mRNA is highest in the liver, followed by the kidney, brain, placenta, heart, and lungs (Cox and Moore, 2002). Normally, increasing copper levels stimulates ATP7A, the Menkes protein, to translocate from the *trans*-Golgi network to the plasma membrane. ATP7B, however, travels from the *trans*-Golgi network to intracellular vesicles and liver bile canaliculi with increasing copper levels (see Figure 37-5). Therefore their movement between compartments is posttranslationally regulated in response to copper, as has been shown for the ZIP4 zinc transporter. The various genetic mutations underlying Menkes and Wilson diseases may result in the presence of mutant ATP7A or ATP7B proteins that display different patterns of copper-dependent trafficking between the *trans*-Golgi and their functional compartments.

EXCRETION

Under normal circumstances very little zinc, copper, or manganese is lost through the urine or through cutaneous losses; most is lost through the feces. Of the endogenous fecal loss, some is from the sloughing off of intestinal cells into the intestinal lumen and is considered nonspecific. However, when dietary zinc or copper intake is high and metallothionein levels are induced, this loss can be significant. The specific loss of copper and manganese through the gastrointestinal tract is via their secretion in the bile. The incorporation of manganese into bile is thought to be very rapid. When manganese is transported into the liver, it either rapidly enters the mitochondria (where it is incorporated into mitochondrial SOD) or is sequestered into lysosomes. Lysosomal manganese is then actively transported into the bile, and it is concentrated in the gallbladder to 150 times greater than that seen in the plasma. Almost all copper excretion is via the bile. Copper is transported to the *trans*-Golgi network via ATP7B. Copper-containing vesicles fuse with the bile canaliculi for excretion. Copper metabolism MURR1 domain (COMMD1), defective in Bedlington terriers afflicted with liver toxicosis, is essential for normal copper excretion. COMMD1 interacts with ATP7B as well as with X-linked inhibitor of apoptosis (XIAP), which is involved with COMMD1 degradation (Prohaska, 2008). Research efforts continue to further define the mechanism for copper excretion and identify the proteins involved.

Zinc excretion in urine varies with zinc intake, but urinary zinc generally amounts to less than 10% of total excretion. Approximately 90% of zinc excretion is through the feces; the actual level of excretion via the intestinal route varies with dietary intake and with the zinc status of the individual. As a result, the fine-tuning of zinc balance is mainly through intestinal secretion and fecal excretion. Although bile and gastroduodenal secretions contribute to endogenous zinc excretion, pancreatic secretions are the major contributor to endogenous zinc losses. The zinc-containing fraction of pancreatic secretions is made up of zinc-dependent enzymes, including carboxypeptidases A and B. These enzymes can be digested, and most of the zinc from them can be reabsorbed.

SELECTED FUNCTIONS OF ZINC, COPPER, AND MANGANESE

The following sections detail a few of the interesting biological functions of copper, zinc, and manganese for which mechanisms have been proposed.

ZINC FINGER PROTEINS AS GENE TRANSCRIPTION FACTORS

Zinc is involved in gene regulation through its binding to specific sequences within transcription factors. Klug coined the term *zinc finger* to describe the folding pattern of amino acids around zinc that he observed in the transcription factor TFIIIA (Rhodes and Klug, 1993). It is estimated that 10% of the human proteome are zinc-binding proteins; 27% of the zinc-binding proteins are zinc finger proteins with the same type of zinc-binding domain, Cys_2His_2 (Andrieni et al., 2006). The result of binding is formation of a loop, or "finger," in the protein that permits the folded region to bind DNA sequences in the promoter region of genes (see Figure 37-7). The transcription factor does not bind DNA in the absence of zinc. Other zinc-binding motifs have been identified, such as Cys_8 (steroid receptor), $Cys_3HisCys_4$, and $Cys_2HisCys_5$ (RING finger and LIM domain, respectively; also involved in protein–protein interactions) (Berg and Shi, 1996). The hypothesis that zinc is necessary for zinc finger function was supported by a study involving the estrogen receptor, apothionein (metallothionein without zinc), and metallothionein. Cano-Gauci and Sarkar (1996) found that the binding of the estrogen receptor to its response element was inhibited following incubation with apothionein and restored following incubation with metallothionein. These results indicate another role for metallothionein: a zinc buffer for activation and deactivation of transcription factors during gene expression.

ZINC REGULATION OF GROWTH

A primary feature of severe zinc deficiency in young animals and in children is slow growth. The classic observation, made over 30 years ago, was that low-zinc, high-phytate, plant-based diets stunted growth of Iranian adolescents (Reinhold, 1971). More recently, researchers have shown that low-income Hispanic children who fall in the lower growth percentiles and infants with a nutritional pattern of failure to thrive respond to zinc supplementation by growing. This suggests that mild zinc deficiency is one of the etiological factors contributing to these conditions. Numerous studies in humans and experimental animals report teratogenic effects and skeletal defects associated with zinc deficiency. Zinc has been shown to stimulate bone mineralization and protein synthesis in vitro (Yamaguchi, 1998).

Zinc deficiency appears to retard growth by disrupting the function of insulin-like growth factor 1 (IGF1), the factor that mediates the cellular effects of growth hormone. Studies have shown that serum IGF1 levels are reduced in zinc-deficient animals (Roth and Kirchgessner, 1994). However, normalizing serum levels of IGF1 by infusing zinc-deficient rats with IGF1 did not increase either food intake or growth, which suggests that additional points of growth regulation are also impaired (Browning et al., 1998). One possible mechanism is that zinc deficiency causes a reduction in the cellular levels of the IGF1 receptor (Williamson et al., 1997). Although this observation is preliminary, it is consistent with the observation that the promoter for the IGF1 receptor can be activated by a promoter-specific transcription factor (Sp1) that contains a zinc finger DNA–binding region. Based on studies defining the role of zinc in the signaling pathways of immune cells, it is no surprise that zinc is involved in similar pathways in other cells including osteoblasts and osteoclasts (Yamaguchi, 1998; Haase and Rink, 2009).

Recent studies have also linked one of the zinc transporters, ZIP13/SLC39A13, to connective tissue development.

This zinc transporter is located in the Golgi apparatus and normally functions to transport zinc from the Golgi to the cytoplasm; a defect causes the accumulation of zinc in the Golgi apparatus. ZIP13 knockout mice have been produced and their connective tissue development has been studied (Fukada et al., 2008). These mice exhibited defective chondrocytes and osteoblasts as well as impaired transforming growth factor-β and bone morphogenic protein signaling pathways. These mice exhibit a phenotype similar to humans afflicted with the spondylocheiro dysplastic form of Ehlers–Danlos syndrome, a disease affecting connective tissue (Giunta et al., 2008; Fukada et al., 2008). The homozygous mutation in *SLC39A13/ZIP13* causes the underhydroxylation of lysyl and prolyl residues of collagen despite normal hydroxylase activity. It is postulated that the accumulation of Zn^{2+} in the Golgi apparatus and endoplasmic reticulum competes with Fe^{2+}, which is required for proline and lysine hydroxylation (Giunta et al., 2008).

ZINC AND DIABETES

That insulin requires zinc for its crystallization (Scott, 1934) has been known since a decade after its discovery by Banting and Best. The specific role for zinc in insulin metabolism was reviewed in Emdin and associates (1980). Following the synthesis of proinsulin, zinc promotes the formation of proinsulin hexamers and increases its solubility before conversion to insulin. It is estimated that proinsulin binds 30 zinc ions, of which 2 to 4 are coordinated within the molecule. These zinc ions appear to be important for the solubility of the proinsulin hexamers. With the removal of the C-peptide from each proinsulin monomer, the resulting insulin increases its coordination of zinc to up to six ions per hexamer, which decreases its solubility and increases its crystallization within the secretory vesicle. The insulin, stored as a crystalline hexamer, is resistant from proteolytic attack within the vesicles (Emdin et al., 1980). Upon release of insulin into the bloodstream, the zinc is also released (Qian and Kennedy, 2001) and the insulin becomes soluble in the bloodstream (Emdin et al., 1980).

ZnT8/SLC30A8 is responsible for transporting zinc into secretory vesicles (Lichten and Cousins, 2009). Polymorphisms in the *SLC30A8/ZnT8* gene are associated with increased risk for types 1 and 2 diabetes (Boesgaard et al., 2008; Mocchegiani et al., 2008; Ingelsson et al., 2010). Antibodies against ZnT8 have been found in patients with type 1 diabetes (Jansen et al., 2009). Zinc is also involved with the insulin signaling pathway (Jansen et al., 2009), providing further evidence of the regulatory role of zinc in biochemical and physiological pathways.

IMMUNOREGULATION BY ZINC AND COPPER

Both zinc and copper deficiency impair immune function. Most of the work in this area has been conducted using mouse models. Studies in humans are more difficult because of the rarity of severe zinc or copper deficiency and the practical difficulties related to the identification of people with marginal zinc or copper deficiency. Nevertheless, in both animals and humans, zinc deficiency appears to reduce immune function because of an overall loss in the total numbers of lymphocytes (B and T cells) of the peripheral immune system (Walsh et al., 1994), whereas copper deficiency results in neutropenia (a lack of circulating neutrophil granulocytes) (Percival, 1995) and a lower number of T lymphocytes (Failla and Hopkins, 1997).

Zinc affects immunity in a multitude of ways and is involved in both innate and adaptive immunity. A number of signaling pathways in immune cells are sensitive to changes in intracellular zinc levels. In monocytes, zinc is required for activation of NF-κB (nuclear factor kappa B) and mitogen-activated protein kinase, leading to the secretion of proinflammatory cytokines. In macrophages, NF-κB and mitogen-activated protein kinase activation results in their maturation and antigen presentation (Haase and Rink, 2009). The effects of changes in intracellular zinc levels on lymphopoiesis mentioned previously are likely due to its actions on signaling pathways of the T-cell receptor and on pre–B cell development (Haase and Rink, 2009). The effects that zinc deficiency has on the lymphocytes may result partially from atrophy of the thymus, an organ that controls the development of T lymphocytes, and the loss of the zinc-dependent hormone thymulin that is secreted by the thymus gland. In zinc deficiency, the proportion of T lymphocytes and B lymphocytes (and subsets of these cell types) and the functional capacity of the lymphocytes present in zinc-deficient animals appear to be normal. Addition of copper to cultures of HL-60 cells (a promyelocytic cell line) promotes differentiation of these cells toward the granulocyte–neutrophil phenotype by enhancing the progression of the cells from promyelocytes to myelocytes. Therefore although both copper and zinc are important for optimal development of the immune system, their effects appear to be on different aspects of marrow stem cell differentiation (Figure 37-8).

Copper deficiency inhibits the proliferation of T cells (particularly helper T or $CD4^+$ cells) in response to mitogens. More detailed studies show that the T cell precursors can be activated and become competent during copper deficiency. Interleukin 2 (IL2) mediates T cell proliferation in response to mitogens, but copper-deficient cells do not make as much IL2 as do cells from copper-adequate animals. It is not clear how copper deficiency alters the production of IL2.

COPPER AND IRON METABOLISM

In addition to its proposed role as a plasma copper transport protein, ceruloplasmin has an enzymatic function as a ferroxidase, oxidizing Fe^{2+} released from iron stores to Fe^{3+}, which can then bind to transferrin and be delivered to cells for use in processes such as heme synthesis (Figure 37-9; see also Chapter 36). It also is possible that this ferroxidase function could be important in the plasma to help control the level of free Fe^{3+} and prevent it from initiating free radical damage. Copper is proposed to function in the catalytic site of ceruloplasmin/ferroxidase, where it exchanges electrons with iron. This ferroxidase role of ceruloplasmin was first proposed following observations of anemia in severely copper-deficient animals, which was characterized by

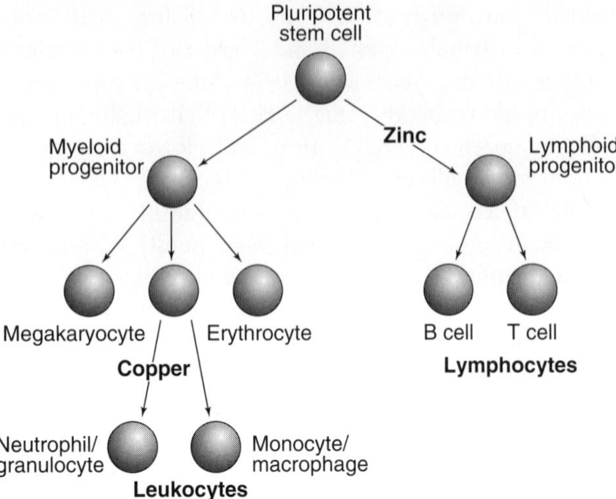

FIGURE 37-8 The putative sites of action for copper and zinc in immune cell differentiation. Severe copper deficiency results in reduced numbers of neutrophils, whereas severe zinc deficiency results in reduced numbers of T and B lymphocytes. This is partly due to impaired differentiation of these terminally differentiated cells from their precursors. The proposed points of action of copper and zinc on immune cell differentiation are shown in the figure.

normal hepatic iron stores (Owen, 1973). The anemia could be reversed by dietary copper but not iron. Other data are inconsistent with the proposed ferroxidase function of ceruloplasmin. However, individuals have been identified who genetically lack the ability to produce ceruloplasmin and are thus aceruloplasminemic, and these persons also show signs of irregular iron metabolism with tissue deposition of iron and mild anemia, providing additional support for a role for ceruloplasmin in iron metabolism (Harris et al., 1995).

COPPER IN BONE AND VASCULAR FUNCTION

Copper deficiency results in abnormal bone metabolism and in skeletal abnormalities in most species. This is not due to abnormal calcium metabolism or mineralization of bone but occurs because the collagen matrix of bone is incompletely formed. The root cause of this defect is reduced activity of the copper-containing enzyme lysyl oxidase (Rucker et al., 1996). Lysyl oxidase is required for the removal of the ε-amino group of lysyl and hydroxylysyl residues with oxidation of the ε-carbon to an aldehyde, which results in the production of a variety of cross-linkages with amino acid residues in collagen. A loss of lysyl oxidase activity results in lower strength and stability of bone collagen.

The lack of this cross-linking by lysyl oxidase also affects elastin. Elastin is a protein that normally gives the aorta its needed flexibility. During copper deficiency the aorta is weakened and aortic rupture may occur. Additional cardiac abnormalities have been observed in association with copper deficiency; these include cardiac hypertrophy, altered electrocardiograms, abnormal mitochondrial structure, and reduced levels of ATP and phosphocreatine. It is not clear what aspect of copper deficiency causes these latter effects, but they are not thought to be attributable to reduced lysyl oxidase activity.

SUPEROXIDE DISMUTASE AND FREE RADICAL PROTECTION

Superoxide dismutases are part of the body's natural defense against reactive oxygen species. Reactive oxygen species are free radicals that, if left uncontrolled, can damage DNA, proteins, and lipids within cells and can alter or inhibit cellular function (Noor et al., 2002; Halliwell, 1994). SODs catalyze the reaction by which superoxide is removed: $2O_2^{\cdot-} + 2H^+ \rightarrow H_2O_2 + O_2$. The hydrogen peroxide generated is further metabolized by either catalase (an iron-containing enzyme) or glutathione peroxidase (a selenium-containing enzyme). Cytosolic Cu/Zn-SOD is made up of two identical subunits, each of which contains one copper and one zinc. Extracellular Cu/Zn-SOD is a secreted tetrameric glycoprotein that is related but not identical to the cytosolic form of Cu/Zn-SOD. The manganese-containing SOD catalyzes the same reaction as the Cu/Zn-SOD, but Mn-SOD is located in the mitochondria as opposed to the cytosol or extracellular fluids. In the active site of the enzymes, copper or manganese is alternately reduced and oxidized by superoxide to produce hydrogen peroxide. Therefore the enzyme activity is completely inhibited in the absence of these minerals. In contrast, some Cu/Zn-SOD activity is retained when zinc is removed or replaced with other chemically similar metals (e.g., cadmium, mercury, or copper). Zinc may serve two functions: it may stabilize the native structure of the enzyme, and a zinc–histidyl–copper triad may act as a proton donor during the oxidation cycle of the enzyme.

The genetic overexpression of cytosolic Cu/Zn-SOD or Fe-dependent catalase in the fruit fly, an insect model of aging, prolongs life, presumably due to improved protection from free radical damage (Orr and Sohal, 1994). These types of studies have provided strong support for the free radical theory of aging. Experimental evidence shows that a reduction in cytosolic or extracellular Cu/Zn-SOD can also occur in animals fed zinc- or copper-deficient diets. This may have physiological consequences. For example, erythrocytes from

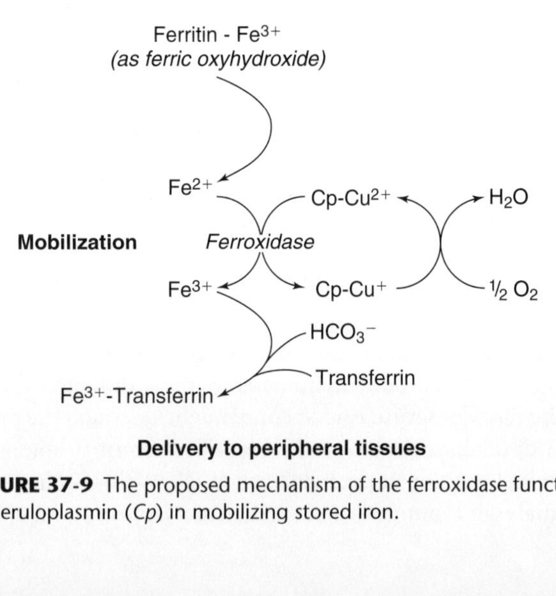

Stored iron in liver
Ferritin - Fe^{3+}
(as ferric oxyhydroxide)
Fe^{2+}
Cp-Cu^{2+}
H_2O
Mobilization
Ferroxidase
Fe^{3+}
Cp-Cu^{+}
½ O_2
HCO_3^-
Transferrin
Fe^{3+}-Transferrin
Delivery to peripheral tissues

FIGURE 37-9 The proposed mechanism of the ferroxidase function of ceruloplasmin (*Cp*) in mobilizing stored iron.

copper-deficient animals with low cytosolic Cu/Zn-SOD levels are more susceptible to lipid peroxidation and hemolysis in vitro (Rock et al., 1995). In addition, young rats fed a copper-deficient diet have lower Cu/Zn-SOD activity in the lung and liver and have shorter survival times when exposed to high-oxygen conditions. Collectively, these data suggest that dietary deficiencies of copper and zinc can have functional consequences related to reduced free radical defenses.

The mitochondria are the site of oxidative phosphorylation and are therefore a tremendous source of potentially hazardous reactive oxygen species and free radicals. Thus deficiency of manganese becomes a condition of superoxide radical poisoning, owing to the loss of Mn-SOD activity. This can have several identifiable consequences. First, researchers have identified abnormalities in cell function and ultrastructural abnormalities in mitochondria in manganese deficiency. The mitochondrial changes (elongation and reorientation of cristae, presence of vacuoles in the matrix, and separation of inner and outer mitochondrial membranes) are likely the result of observed increases in mitochondrial lipid peroxidation. Disruption of mitochondrial integrity may result in disturbed energy metabolism through disruption of oxidative phosphorylation. Manganese deficiency alters carbohydrate metabolism through the destruction of pancreatic beta cells. This could account for the decreased glucose utilization, reduced pancreatic insulin, and lower insulin output from perfused pancreas observed in manganese-deficient animals. Although it is not clear how manganese contributes to pancreatic beta cell abnormalities, researchers have proposed that free radical damage resulting from the lack of Mn-SOD activity is a factor.

MANGANESE IN CARTILAGE FORMATION

As with copper deficiency, skeletal abnormalities that are unrelated to impaired mineralization of bone are a characteristic of manganese deficiency. For example, in growing animals manganese deficiency results in an inhibition of endochondral osteogenesis at the growth plates and epiphyseal cartilages. This is caused by a reduction in the synthesis of proteoglycans such as chondroitin sulfate (the proteoglycan affected most by manganese deficiency) (Liu et al., 1994). Proteoglycans (glycosaminoglycan–protein complexes) are essential structural components of cartilage, which explains the sensitivity of the growth plate to manganese deficiency. Chondroitin sulfate synthesis is regulated by manganese at two sites. The polymerase responsible for the polymerization of uridine diphosphate-*N*-acetylgalactosamine to uridine diphosphate-glucuronic acid to form the glycosaminoglycan chain requires manganese. Galactotransferase, an enzyme that catalyzes the incorporation of galactose into a galactose–galactose–xylose trisaccharide, which is required for the linkage of the polysaccharide chain to the protein associated with it, is also a manganese-requiring enzyme. Other glycosyltransferases are also activated by manganese.

In the least severe stage of manganese deficiency, animals will give birth to viable offspring, but some of the young will exhibit ataxia and loss of equilibrium. This condition is the result of a structural defect in the development of the inner ear that impairs vestibular function. As with the bone defects noted earlier, these inner ear structural defects are also the result of impaired cartilage development associated with reduced proteoglycan formation.

ASSESSMENT OF ZINC, COPPER, AND MANGANESE STATUS AND DEFICIENCY SYMPTOMS

STATUS ASSESSMENT

The "Holy Grail" of status assessment is the availability of a functional parameter that changes with the dietary deficiency of a required nutrient. Unfortunately, there are no reliable functional assessment tools for zinc, copper, or manganese. Researchers have examined a number of metal-dependent enzymes for their ability to serve as sensitive indicators of zinc (e.g., alkaline phosphatase, Cu/Zn-SOD, 5′ nucleotidase) and copper (e.g., Cu/Zn-SOD) status (Delves, 1985). Recently, mice consuming a zinc-deficient diet exhibited changes in two zinc transport proteins located within their erythrocyte membranes (Ryu et al., 2008). ZIP10/SLC39A10 was upregulated and ZnT1 was downregulated following consumption of the zinc deficient diet. Whether these results will be replicated in humans remains to be determined. Although some of these assays show promise, none has to date been proved useful. The remaining option is static assessment tools, such as mineral levels in serum, hair, and red or white blood cells.

In healthy people, the plasma concentration of zinc does not appear to change except under conditions of extreme deficiency. Therefore plasma or serum zinc concentration is an inadequate measure for assessment of more subtle changes in status. The plasma zinc level does fall significantly during pregnancy, but this decrease is associated with a fall in plasma albumin concentration and an expansion of maternal blood volume. These changes may be important to the development of the fetus and the viability of the pregnancy, and it is not clear that this decline in plasma zinc indicates inadequate zinc intake during pregnancy (Swanson and King, 1983). Serum copper and ceruloplasmin have shown some utility as indicators of copper status, but these measures (as well as serum zinc) are very sensitive to acute inflammation. During acute inflammation, serum zinc levels fall and serum copper and ceruloplasmin levels increase, giving the false impression that zinc status is low and copper status is high. Although serum or plasma zinc lacks the sensitivity to determine the zinc status of individuals, there is a growing consensus among zinc researchers that serum zinc is useful for determining the risk of zinc deficiency within a population. Furthermore, if zinc supplementation of the population is deemed necessary, then serum zinc levels are considered to effectively determine the efficacy of the supplementation regimen (de Benoist, 2007; Hess et al., 2007; Hotz, 2007).

Hair mineral levels can be a useful crude measure of long-term mineral status, but hair mineral content is sensitive to contamination from the environment (e.g., shampoos and emissions). Erythrocyte or serum metallothionein levels have been evaluated as a measure of zinc status. Although extremes of zinc status can be assessed by this method, there is no indication that metallothionein concentration is useful for assessment of marginal zinc status. Lymphocyte zinc content has been shown to be more sensitive to marginal zinc intake in small, well-controlled studies. However, the association of lymphocyte zinc concentration with zinc intake has not been verified in larger groups, and the difficulty in isolating these white blood cells reduces the utility of this measure for assessing zinc status in the population. Finally, urinary excretion poorly reflects changes in intakes of zinc, copper, and manganese. Clearly, the development of reliable functional assessment tools is essential for establishing the true requirements for zinc, copper, and manganese and for defining the true health risks of inadequate intake of these minerals.

DEFICIENCY SYMPTOMS

Zinc

The symptoms of zinc deficiency have been observed in human populations consuming diets high in phytate and low in meat (e.g., the classic studies of zinc deficiency in Iranian children), as well as among individuals with acrodermatitis enteropathica (AE). As a result of its occurrence in humans, zinc deficiency has been studied extensively. Many symptoms of zinc deficiency have been characterized (Box 37-1), but the underlying biochemical defects responsible for most of them have not been found. For example, loss of appetite is one of the first signs associated with specific dietary zinc inadequacy. Although this clearly contributes to the growth depression seen in zinc-deficient children, the reason for the loss of appetite is not known. This is also true for the classic symptoms of zinc deficiency, such as loss of normal taste sensation, alopecia, hyperkeratinization of skin, and reproductive abnormalities. Because of the vast array of zinc-dependent enzymes, as well as the proposed importance of the zinc finger structure in modulating the interaction between transcription factors and DNA, it is unlikely that a single cause will be determined for many of these conditions.

Copper

Experimental copper deficiency has helped us understand the role of copper in iron metabolism, immune function, and cartilage production. The symptoms listed for copper deficiency in Box 37-1 are all associated with either severe dietary copper deficiency or copper deficiency associated with the genetic condition called Wilson disease. These conditions are rare in humans. In contrast, researchers have noted several symptoms (e.g., irregular heartbeat and impaired glucose utilization) that occur before the onset of severe deficiency and that may have more general relevance to human health. The degree of copper deficiency or low intake that leads to these milder symptoms is not clearly defined, but epidemiological evidence linking low serum copper levels to an elevated risk of cardiovascular disease suggests that marginal copper status may be of practical concern.

BOX 37-1 Characteristics of Zinc, Copper, and Manganese Deficiency in Animals and Humans

Zinc	Copper	Manganese
Loss of appetite	Anemia	Poor growth
Poor growth	Skeletal defects	Abnormal bone
Alopecia	Cardiac enlargement	Impaired glucose tolerance
Immune dysfunction	Altered pigmentation	Poor reproduction
Hypogonadism	Reproductive failure	Malformations in offspring
Poor wound healing	Lower aortic elasticity	
Impaired taste acuity	Neutropenia	

Manganese

Reduced growth is a general feature of manganese deficiency. Although food consumption does fall in manganese-deficient animals, it is not a prominent feature of the deficiency. As discussed earlier, some of the deficiency signs that have been observed for manganese can be linked to the loss of specific enzyme functions. In contrast, the cause of the disrupted reproductive ability (lower conception, increased spontaneous abortion, stillbirths, lower birth weights, defective ovulation, and testicular degeneration) observed in manganese-deficient animals is unknown. Similarly, although animal studies reveal a greater susceptibility to convulsions and electroencephalogram readings reminiscent of those for epileptics, the underlying basis for these phenomena is not clearly understood (see Box 37-1).

DIETARY REFERENCE INTAKES AND FOOD SOURCES OF ZINC, COPPER, AND MANGANESE

DIETARY REFERENCE INTAKES

The Institute of Medicine (IOM) published the Dietary Reference Intakes (DRIs) for zinc, copper, and manganese in 2001 (IOM, 2001). These DRIs replaced the Recommended Dietary Allowance (RDA) for zinc and the estimated safe and adequate daily dietary intakes for copper and manganese that had been set as part of the 1989 recommended dietary allowances.

Zinc

The Adequate Intake (AI) of zinc for infants from birth through 6 months of age was set as 2 mg/day. This value was based on the zinc intake of breast-fed infants, which declined from approximately 2.3 mg/day at 2 weeks to 1 mg/day at 6 months. The decline in intake with age is due to an unusually rapid physiological decline in the zinc concentration of

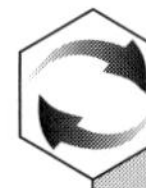

DRIs Across the Life Cycle: Zinc, Copper and Manganese

	mg Zinc per Day	mg Copper per Day	mg Manganese per Day
Infants	RDA	RDA	AI
0 through 6 mo	2.0 (AI)	0.20 (AI)	0.003
7 through 12 mo	3.0	0.22 (AI)	0.6
Children			
1 through 3 yr	3.0	0.34	1.2
4 through 8 yr	5.0	0.44	1.5
Males			
9 through 13 yr	8.0	0.70	1.9
14 through 18 yr	11.0	0.89	2.2
≥19 yr	11.0	0.90	2.3
Females			
9 through 13 yr	8.0	0.70	1.6
14 through 18 yr	9.0	0.89	1.6
≥19 yr	8.0	0.90	1.8
Pregnant	11.0	1.00	2.0
Lactating	12.0	1.30	2.6

Data from IOM. (2006). In J. J. Otten, J. P. Hellwig, & L. D. Meyers (Eds.), *Dietary Reference Intakes: The essential guide to nutrient requirements.* Washington, DC: The National Academies Press.

AI, Adequate Intake; *DRI,* Dietary Reference Intake; *RDA,* Recommended Dietary Allowance.

human milk from approximately 4 mg/L at 2 weeks postpartum to 1.2 mg/L at 6 months postpartum. Factorial estimates of zinc requirements based on fractional absorption of dietary zinc and endogenous losses yielded a similar range of estimates for the zinc requirement—2.1 mg/day at 1 month and 1.54 mg/day at 5 months—as did measurements of intake. There is some evidence that the zinc content of human milk is growth-limiting for some infants after 4 months of age, so the AI was set near the upper end of the range.

Human milk alone is an inadequate source of zinc after the first 6 months. For older infants and children, a factorial approach was used to arrive at the need for dietary zinc to replace losses and to support growth. In most cases, zinc losses were extrapolated from measurements made in adults, and requirements for growth were based on an average zinc content of 20 μg/g wet weight of tissue. For infants 7 through 12 months of age, total zinc losses were estimated as 64 μg/kg/day and the requirement for growth as 260 μg/day based on accretion of 13 g new tissue per day. For children ages 1 through 3 years, total losses were estimated as 48 μg/kg/day, and the requirement for growth was estimated as 20 μg/g × 6 g/day. For children ages 4 through 8 years, total losses were estimated as 48 μg/kg/day and the requirement for growth as 20 μg/g × 7 g/day. For children 9 through 13 years of age, total losses were estimated as 48 μg/kg/day and the requirement for growth as 20 μg/g × 10 g/day. Using an estimated fractional absorption of zinc of 0.3 and reference weights for each of the groups, the Estimated Average Requirements (EARs) were set as 2.5 mg/day for infants ages 7 through 12 months and for children aged 1 through 3 years, as 4 mg/day for children aged 4 through 8 years, as 7 mg/day for boys aged 9 through 13 years, and as 8 mg/day for girls aged 9 through 13 years. In the absence of information about the standard deviation of the requirement, the RDA was set as equal to the EAR plus 20%.

A similar factorial approach was also used in setting the DRIs for adolescents, ages 14 through 18 years, but with addition of an estimate to allow for semen or menstrual losses of zinc and using a fractional absorption estimate of 0.4 derived from studies with men. The EAR for adolescent boys and girls is 8.5 and 7.3 mg zinc/day, respectively.

The EAR of zinc for adults was also determined by factorial analysis. The average endogenous loss of zinc via all routes other than the intestine was calculated to be 1.27 mg/day for men and 1.0 mg/day for women. The minimum amount of absorbed zinc required to match endogenous zinc losses from the intestine was estimated as 2.57 mg/day for men and 2.3 mg/day for women. With fractional absorptions of 0.41 for men and 0.48 for women, the EARs were set as the amount of zinc required to replace the total calculated loss of zinc by men and women:

$$\text{Men: } (1.27 + 2.57)/0.41 = 9.3 \text{ mg/day}$$

$$\text{Women: } (1.0 + 2.3)/0.48 = 6.8 \text{ mg/day}$$

The RDA was set as the EAR + 20%: 11 mg/day for men and 8 mg/day for women.

The 2001–2002 data from the National Health and Nutrition Examination Survey (NHANES) (Moshfegh et al., 2005) showed that the median (50th percentile) dietary intake of zinc by U.S. men (≥19 years) is 13.6 mg/day, with a range (5th to 95th percentile) of 8.2 to 22.3 mg/day. For U.S. women (≥19 years), the median dietary intake of zinc is 9.2 mg/day, with a range of 5.4 to 15.7 mg/day. Compared to the EAR for zinc, most of the adult U.S. population (more than 80%) is consuming an adequate dietary intake.

Additional zinc intake is recommended for pregnant and lactating women. The EAR was increased by 2.7 mg/day for pregnant women, based on accumulation of absorbed zinc by maternal and fetal tissues during the fourth quarter of pregnancy, and by 3.6 mg/day for lactating adult women, based on the net additional loss of absorbed zinc during lactation.

Copper

The recommended intakes of copper for infants reflect the mean copper intake of infants principally fed human milk. The AI for infants from 0 through 6 months of age is 0.20 mg/day (0.25 mg copper/L milk × 0.78 L/day). For infants aged 7 through 12 months, the AI was based on copper intake from human milk (0.20 mg Cu/L milk × 0.6 L/day) plus an intake of 0.10 mg Cu/day from complementary foods, to yield a total of 0.22 mg/day. Because no data were available on which to base EARs for copper for children or adolescents, the EARs were estimated by extrapolating from the adult EAR (see subsequent text) using metabolic weight ($kg^{0.75}$) as the basis for the extrapolation.

The adult EAR for copper was established based on several studies of adult copper requirements that used biochemical indicators of copper status. The indicators included the concentrations of plasma and platelet copper, serum ceruloplasmin concentration, and erythrocyte SOD activity. The EAR for copper in men and women is 0.7 mg/day. Factorial analysis, used to determine the minimum amount of dietary copper intake to replace obligatory losses, yielded an estimate similar to that of the EAR for copper, which supported the EAR based on the indicators for copper status. The RDA for copper is defined as the EAR + 30%.

NHANES 2001–2002 survey data (Moshfegh et al., 2005) show that the median dietary intake of copper by U.S. men (≥19 years) is 1.44 mg/day, with a range (5th to 95th percentile) of 0.88 to 2.52 mg/day. For U.S. women (≥19 years), the median dietary intake of copper is 1.05 mg/day, with a range of 0.61 to 1.82 mg/day. Compared to the EAR for copper, most of the adult U.S. population (more than 90%) is consuming an adequate dietary intake.

An increase in the EAR by 0.10 mg copper/day was recommended for pregnant women based on the amount of copper accumulated by the maternal and fetal tissues adjusted by an estimate of copper absorption. An increase in the EAR by 0.30 mg/day was recommended for lactating women based on the amount of copper secreted in human milk adjusted by an estimate of copper absorption. Copper bioavailability was considered to be 65% to 70%.

Manganese

To date, no functional criteria for manganese status have been established. Therefore recommended intakes of manganese are set as AIs for all age and sex groups. For infants, the AIs are based on the manganese intake of breast-fed infants from human milk and from complementary foods during the second 6 months of life. Mean manganese concentration of human milk is approximately 4 μg/L at 1 month and 1.9 μg/L by 3 months postpartum. The AI for infants in the first 6 months of life is set as: 3.5 μg Mn/L × 0.78 L/day = 3 μg/day. This amount of manganese would be inadequate if complementary foods were not introduced into the diet of the infant. Based on average manganese intake by older infants of approximately 567 μg/day from complementary foods, the AI for infants that are 7 through 12 months of age is set as 600 μg/day or 0.6 mg/day. The AIs for children were set based on median manganese intake by children in the various age groups. These AIs range from 1.2 mg/day for children who are 1 through 3 years of age up to 2.2 mg/day for boys who are 14 through 18 years of age.

In adults, manganese balance has been observed to occur for a wide range of manganese intakes. Median intake of manganese in the United States is 2.25 mg/day for men and 1.74 mg/day for women (ages 19 to 70 years), based on the Total Diet Study (1991–1997). The AI was set at 2.3 mg/day for men and 1.8 mg/day for women. An increment of 0.2 mg/day was added for pregnant women, based on a gain of 16 kg body weight, to give an AI of 2 mg/day. The AI for lactating women was set at 2.6 mg/day based on the higher median intake of manganese by lactating women.

FOOD SOURCES

Zinc

Red meats, organ meats (e.g., liver), and shellfish (e.g., oysters) are generally the best dietary sources for zinc. Whole grain cereals are rich sources of zinc, but refined grain products are poor sources because the zinc is found primarily in the bran and germ. Many breakfast cereals made from refined grain products are supplemented with zinc and other nutrients during production and therefore may be good sources of zinc. Nuts and legumes are also relatively good plant sources of zinc. In contrast, fruits and

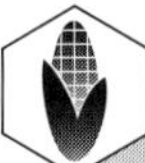

FOOD SOURCES OF ZINC, COPPER, AND MANGANESE

Zinc
- 2.5 to 6.5 mg per 3 oz crab
- 3 to 8 mg per 3 oz beef or lamb
- 1.7 to 4 mg per 3 oz pork, chicken, or turkey
- 0.9 to 4.6 mg per 1 cup ready-to-eat cereal (unfortified)
- 15 to 23 mg per 1 cup fortified cereal
- 0.7 to 1.5 mg per ½ cup legumes, mature seeds (chickpeas, lentils, soybeans, limas, or kidney), cooked
- 1.2 to 1.8 mg per 1 oz nuts, dry (pine nuts, cashews, or pecans)
- 2 mg per 8-oz container yogurt, plain
- 1.6 mg per ½ cup ricotta cheese, part skim

Copper
- 3.7 mg per 3 oz oysters
- 1.6 mg per 3 oz lobster
- 0.3 to 0.6 mg per 3 oz clams or crab
- 0.3 to 0.6 mg per 1 oz nuts (cashew, hazelnuts, walnuts)
- 0.1 to 0.4 mg per ½ cup legumes, mature seeds (soybeans, lentils, kidney, or limas)
- 0.1 to 0.2 mg per ½ cup green leafy vegetables (spinach, turnip greens, or kale), cooked
- 0.15 mg per ½ cup tomatoes (stewed)
- 0.13 mg per ½ cup potatoes, sweet potatoes, pumpkin
- 0.13 mg per ½ cup raspberries, blackberries, raw

Manganese
- 0.7 to 1.7 mg per 1 oz nuts (hazelnuts, pecans, or walnuts)
- 0.6 mg per 1 oz peanuts, roasted
- 0.3 to 0.9 mg per ½ cup legumes (chickpeas, limas, soybeans, or lentils)
- 0.9 mg per ½ cup brown rice, cooked
- 0.7 mg per ½ cup oatmeal, cooked
- 0.3 to 2.7 mg per 1 cup ready-to-eat cereal
- 0.3 to 0.5 mg per 6 oz tea
- 0.4 to 0.8 mg per ½ cup leafy green vegetables (spinach, collards, or turnip greens)
- 0.3 to 0.5 mg per ½ cup berries (raspberries, strawberries, or blueberries)

Data from U.S. Department of Agriculture, Agricultural Research Service. (2010). *USDA National Nutrient Database for Standard Reference, Release 23*. Retrieved from www.ars.usda.gov/ba/bhnrc/ndl

vegetables are generally low in zinc. Excessive intake of phytate-rich foods (e.g., some grains) is known to inhibit zinc bioavailability. Infant formulas are often supplemented with zinc, but this is up to the discretion of the producer.

Copper

Shellfish, nuts, legumes, the bran and germ portions of grains, and liver are rich sources of copper (greater than 0.3 mg of copper per 100 g). Most meats, mushrooms, tomatoes, dried fruits, bananas, potatoes, and grapes have moderate amounts of copper (0.1 to 0.3 mg/100 g). Poor sources of copper are cow's milk and dairy products, chicken, and many species of fish, fruits, and vegetables.

Manganese

Manganese can be found in unrefined cereals, nuts, tea, and leafy vegetables, but refined grains, meats, seafood, and dairy products are poor sources.

TOXICITY OF ZINC, COPPER, AND MANGANESE

As a general rule, zinc, copper, and manganese are relatively nontoxic when consumed in the diet. Toxic exposure is most likely to result from accidental exposure, from environmental contamination, or from overconsumption of dietary supplements.

ZINC

Manifestations of overt toxicity will occur with long-term exposure to as little as 100 to 300 mg of zinc per day. The symptoms of zinc toxicity include induced copper deficiency (characterized by anemia and neutropenia), impaired immune function, and reduction of high-density lipoprotein (HDL) cholesterol levels in some individuals. Extremely high zinc intake will cause vomiting, epigastric pain, lethargy, and fatigue. The most consistent adverse effect associated with excess zinc intake was reduced copper status, as measured by reduced erythrocyte Cu/Zn-SOD activity (IOM, 2001).

Because zinc intake in pharmacological amounts decreases copper absorption, the adverse effects of zinc supplements on copper metabolism (copper status) was used for establishing the Tolerable Upper Intake Level (UL) for zinc (IOM, 2001). The UL for zinc intake by adults was determined as that resulting in a reduction in erythrocyte Cu/Zn-SOD activity, a sensitive measure of copper status. The UL for zinc intake by adults is 40 mg/day, which includes zinc from foods, water, and supplements.

In 1996 Mossad and colleagues reported that taking zinc gluconate lozenges within 24 hours of the onset of cold symptoms reduced the duration of symptoms of the common cold. Although this is a potentially exciting finding, misuse of this product could result in zinc toxicity. To get the benefit of this product, users must take a lozenge containing 13.3 mg of zinc every 2 waking hours until the symptoms have been eliminated (4 to 7 days). This dose (greater than 150 mg/day) may have toxic effects, particularly if people attempt to use the lozenges prophylactically by consuming them throughout the cold and flu season (Mossad et al., 1996).

COPPER

Copper toxicity in humans has not been studied extensively. Wilson disease is a hereditary disease that causes copper accumulation in the liver and other organs and is an example of the damage excessive copper can cause. However, liver damage is rare for individuals with normal mechanisms for copper homeostasis when consuming up to 10 mg copper per day for 12 weeks (Pratt et al., 1985). There is a report of acute liver failure occurring in an individual consuming supplements containing 30 mg copper per day for 2 years, followed by the consumption of 60 mg of copper per day for 1 year (O'Donohue et al., 1993). Under conditions of chronic overconsumption of copper, toxicity occurs only when the capacity of the liver to bind and sequester copper is exceeded. The amount of dietary copper required to cause toxicity is not well established, but gastrointestinal discomfort has been seen with intakes of as little as 5 mg of copper per day. The consequences of copper toxicity are weakness, listlessness, and anorexia in the early stages, which can progress to coma, hepatic necrosis, vascular collapse, and death.

The IOM used liver damage as the critical endpoint for copper toxicity in setting the UL for copper at 10 mg/day (IOM, 2001). The UL was based on a no-observed-adverse-effect level of 10 mg/day, from a study of adults who consumed this level of copper for 12 weeks. Consumption of higher levels of copper resulted in acute liver failure.

MANGANESE

Manganese is considered one of the least toxic minerals. Oral toxicity is extremely rare. However, airborne manganese from industrial and automobile emissions can have serious toxic effects if exposure is sufficiently high. Symptoms associated with manganese toxicity include pancreatitis and neurological disorders that are similar to those observed in patients with schizophrenia and Parkinson disease. Manganese toxicity has been observed in children receiving long-term parenteral nutrition. In addition, the use of methylcyclopentadienyl manganese tricarbonyl as a gasoline additive in the United States has raised concerns that environmental exposure to manganese may increase in the future.

The UL for manganese intake from all sources was set at 11 mg/day (IOM, 2001). Available data indicate that individuals eating vegetarian and Western diets consume up to 11 mg/day of manganese. No adverse effects have been observed with the consumption of this level of manganese from the diet (Greger, 1999). Conversely, data from another study indicated that consumption of 15 mg/day of manganese for 25 days caused a significant increase in serum manganese concentration and, after 90 days, an increase in lymphocyte Mn-SOD activity (Davis and Greger, 1992). The latter may have been associated with an increase in the formation of reactive oxygen species. Therefore the lowest-observed-adverse-effect level was established at 15 mg of manganese per day.

REFERENCES

Andreini, C., Banci, L., Bertini, I., & Rosato, A. (2006). Counting the zinc-proteins encoded in the human genome. *Journal of Proteome Research, 5*, 196–201.

Andrews, G. K. (2000). Regulation of metallothionein gene expression by oxidative stress and metal ions. *Biochemical Pharmacology, 59*, 95–104.

Berg, J. M., & Shi, Y. (1996). The galvanization of biology: A growing appreciation for the roles of zinc. *Science, 271*, 1081–1085.

Bertinato, J., Iskandar, M., & L'Abbe, M. R. (2003). Copper deficiency induces the upregulation of the copper chaperone for Cu/Zn superoxide dismutase in weanling rats. *The Journal of Nutrition, 133*, 28–31.

Boesgaard, T. W., Zilinskaite, J., Vanttinen, M., Laakso, M., Jansson, P.-A., Hammarstedt, A., … Hansen, T. (2008). The common SLC30A8 Arg325Trp variant is associated with reduced first-phase insulin release in 846 non-diabetic offspring of type 2 diabetes patients—The EUGENE2 study. *Diabetologia, 51*, 816–820.

Bressler, J. P., Olivi, L., Cheong, J. H., Kim, Y., Maerten, A., & Bannon, D. (2007). Metal transporters in intestine and brain: Their involvement in metal-associated neurotoxicities. *Human & Experimental Toxicology, 26*, 221–229.

Browning, J. D., MacDonald, R. S., Thornton, W. H., & O'Dell, B. L. (1998). Reduced food intake in zinc deficient rats is normalized by megestrol acetate but not by insulin-like growth factor-I. *The Journal of Nutrition, 128*, 136–142.

Cano-Gauci, D. F., & Sarkar, B. (1996). Reversible zinc exchange between metallothionein and the estrogen receptor zinc finger. *FEBS Letters, 386*, 1–4.

Chen, X., Zhang, B., Harmon, P. M., Schaffner, W., Peterson, D. O., & Giedroc, D. P. (2004). A novel cysteine cluster in human metal-responsive transcription factor 1 is required for heavy metal-induced transcriptional activation in vivo. *The Journal of Biological Chemistry, 279*, 4515–4522.

Cousins, R. J. (1985). Absorption, transport, and hepatic metabolism of copper and zinc: Special reference to metallothionein and ceruloplasmin. *Physiological Reviews, 65*, 238–309.

Cox, D. W., & Moore, S. D. P. (2002). Copper transporting P-type ATPases and human disease. *Journal of Bioenergetics and Biomembranes, 34*, 333–338.

Coyle, P., Zalewski, P. D., Philcox, J. C., Forbes, I. J., Ward, A. D., Lincoln, S. F., … Rofe, A. M. (1994). Measurement of zinc in hepatocytes by using a fluorescent probe, zinquin: Relationship to metallothionein and intracellular zinc. *The Biochemical Journal, 303*, 781–786.

Cragg, R. A., Christie, G. R., Phillips, S. R., Russ, R. M., Kury, S., Mathers, J. C., … Ford, D. (2002). A novel zinc-regulated human zinc transporter, hZTL1, is localized to the enterocyte apical membrane. *The Journal of Biological Chemistry, 277*, 22789–22797.

Cragg, R. A., Phillips, S. R., Piper, J. M., Varma, J. S., Campbell, F. C., Mathers, J. C., & Ford, D. (2005). Homeostatic regulation of zinc transporters in the human small intestine by dietary zinc supplementation. *Gut, 54*, 469–478.

Dalton, T., Fu, K., Palmiter, R. D., & Andrews, G. K. (1996). Transgenic mice that overexpress metallothionein-I resist dietary zinc deficiency. *The Journal of Nutrition, 126*, 825–833.

Danks, D. M. (1995). Disorders of copper transport. In D. R. Scriver, A. L. Beaudet, W. S. Sly, & D. Valle (Eds.), *The metabolic and molecular bases of inherited disease* (7th ed., Vol. 2, pp. 2211–2235). New York: McGraw-Hill.

Davis, C. D., & Greger, J. L. (1992). Longitudinal changes of manganese-dependent superoxide dismutase and other indexes of manganese and iron status in women. *The American Journal of Clinical Nutrition, 55*, 747–752.

Davis, W., Chowrimootoo, G. F., & Seymour, C. A. (1996). Defective biliary copper excretion in Wilson's disease: The role of caeruloplasmin. *European Journal of Clinical Investigation, 26*, 893–901.

de Benoist, B., Darnton-Hill, I., Davidsson, L., Fontaine, O., & Hotz, C. (2007). Conclusions of the joint WHO/UNICEF/IAEA/IZiNCG interagency meeting on zinc status indicators. *Food and Nutrition Bulletin, 28*, S480–S484.

Delves, H. T. (1985). Assessment of trace element status. *Clinics in Endocrinology and Metabolism, 14*, 725–760.

DiDonato, M., & Sarkar, B. (1997). Copper transport and its alterations in Menkes and Wilson diseases. *Biochimica et Biophysica Acta, 1360*, 3–16.

Doherty, G. J., & McMahon, H. T. (2009). Mechanisms of endocytosis. *Annual Review of Biochemistry, 78*, 857–902.

Dufner-Beattie, J., Wang, F., Kuo, Y. M., Gitschier, J., Eide, D., & Andrews, G. K. (2003). The acrodermatitis enteropathica gene ZIP4 encodes a tissue-specific zinc-regulated zinc transporter in mice. *The Journal of Biological Chemistry, 278*, 33474–33481.

Emdin, S. O., Dodson, G. G., Cutfield, J. M., & Cutfield, S. M. (1980). Role of zinc in insulin biosynthesis. *Diabetologia, 19*, 174–182.

Failla, M. L., & Hopkins, R. G. (1997). Copper and immunocompetence. In R. W. F. Fischer, M. R. L'Abbe, K. A. Cockell, & R. S. Gibson (Eds.), *Trace elements in man and animals—9: Proceedings of the Ninth International Symposium on Trace Elements in Man and Animals* (pp. 425–428). Ottawa, Canada: NRC Research Press.

Frank, P. G., Pavlides, S., & Lisanti, M. P. (2009). Caveolae and transcytosis in endothelial cells: Role in atherosclerosis. *Cell & Tissue Research, 335*, 41–47.

Fukada, T., Civic, N., Furuichi, T., Shimoda, S., Mishima, K., et al. (2008). The zinc transporter SLC39A13/ZIP13 is required for connective tissue development; its involvement in BMP/TGF-β signaling pathways. *PLoS One, 3*(11), e3642.

Giunta, C., Elcioglu, N. U., Albrecht, B., Eich, G., Chambaz, C., Janecke, A. R., … Steinmann, B. (2008). Spondylocheiro dysplastic form of the Ehlers-Danlos syndrome—An autosomal-recessive entity caused by mutations in the zinc transporter gene SLC39A13. *American Journal of Human Genetics, 82*, 1290–1305.

Glusker, J. P. (1991). Structural aspects of metal liganding to functional groups in proteins. *Advances in Protein Chemistry, 42*, 1–76.

Greger, J. L. (1999). Nutrition versus toxicology of manganese in humans: Evaluation of potential biomarkers. *Neurotoxicology, 20*, 205–212.

Grider, A., & Young, E. M. (1996). The acrodermatitis enteropathica mutation transiently affects zinc metabolism in human fibroblasts. *The Journal of Nutrition, 126*, 219–224.

Gunshin, H., Mackenzie, B., Berger, U. V., Gunshin, Y., Romero, M. F., Boron, W. F., … Rink, L. (2009). Functional significance of zinc-related signaling pathways in immune cells. *Annual Review of Nutrition, 29*, 133–152.

Haase, H., & Rink, L. (2009). Functional significance of zinc-related signaling pathways in immune cells. *Annual Review of Nutrition, 29*, 133–152.

Halliwell, B. (1994). Free radicals and antioxidants: A personal view. *Nutrition Reviews, 52*, 253–265.

Harris, Z. L., Takahashi, Y., Miyajima, H., Serizawa, M., MacGillivray, R. T., & Gitlin, J. D. (1995). Aceruloplasminemia: Molecular characterization of this disorder of iron metabolism. *Proceedings of the National Academy of Sciences of the United States of America, 92*, 2539–2543.

Hess, S. Y., Peerson, J. M., King, J. C., & Brown, K. H. (2007). Use of serum zinc concentrations as an indicator of population zinc status. *Food and Nutrition Bulletin, 28*, S403–S429.

Heuchel, R., Radtke, F., Georgiev, O., Stark, G., Aguet, M., & Schaffner, W. (1994). The transcription factor MTF-1 is essential for basal and heavy metal-induced metallothionein gene-expression. *The EMBO Journal, 13*, 2870–2875.

Hotz, C. (2007). Dietary indicators for assessing the adequacy of population zinc intakes. *Food and Nutrition Bulletin, 28*, S430–S453.

Ingelsson, E., Langenberg, C., Hivert, M.-F., Prokopenko, I., Lyssenko, V., Dupuis, J., … MAGIC investigators. (2010). Detailed physiologic characterization reveals diverse mechanisms for novel genetic loci regulating glucose and insulin metabolism in humans. *Diabetes, 59*, 1266–1275.

Institute of Medicine. (2001). *Dietary Reference Intakes for vitamin A, vitamin K, arsenic, boron, chromium, copper, iodine, iron, manganese, molybdenum, nickel, silicon, vanadium, and zinc.* Washington, DC: National Academy Press.

Jansen, J., Karges, W., & Rink, L. (2009). Zinc and diabetes—Clinical links and molecular mechanisms. *The Journal of Nutritional Biochemistry, 20*, 399–417.

Kambe, T., Yamaguchi-Iwai, Y., Sasaki, R., & Nagao, M. (2004). Overview of mammalian zinc transporters. *Cellular and Molecular Life Sciences, 61*, 49–68.

Kelly, E. J., Quaife, C. J., Froelick, G. J., & Palmiter, R. D. (1996). Metallothionein I and II protect against zinc deficiency and zinc toxicity in mice. *The Journal of Nutrition, 126*, 1782–1790.

Kim, B. E., Wang, F., Dufner-Beattie, J., Andrews, G. K., Eide, D. J., & Petris, M. J. (2004). Zn^{2+}-stimulated endocytosis of the mZIP4 zinc transporter regulates its location at the plasma membrane. *The Journal of Biological Chemistry, 279*, 4523–4530.

Kimura, T., & Itoh, N. (2008). Function of metallothionein in gene expression and signal transduction: Newly found protective role of metallothionein. *Journal of Health Science, 54*, 251–260.

Langmade, S. J., Ravindra, R., Daniels, P. J., & Andrews, G. K. (2000). The transcription factor MTF-1 mediates metal regulation of the mouse ZnT1 gene. *The Journal of Biological Chemistry, 275*, 34803–34809.

Laukens, D., Waeytens, A., de Bleser, P., Cuvelier, C., & de Vos, M. (2009). Human metallothionein expression under normal and pathological conditions: Mechanisms of gene regulation based on in silico promoter analysis. *Critical Reviews in Eukaryotic Gene Expression, 19*, 301–317.

Lee, J., Pena, M. M. O., Nose, Y., & Thiele, D. J. (2002a). Biochemical characterization of the human copper transporter Ctr1. *The Journal of Biological Chemistry, 277*, 4380–4387.

Lee, J., Petris, M. J., & Thiele, D. J. (2002b). Characterization of mouse embryonic cells deficient in the Ctr1 high affinity copper transporter. *The Journal of Biological Chemistry, 277*, 40253–40259.

Leone, A., Pavlakis, G. N., & Hamer, D. H. (1985). Menkes' disease: Abnormal metallothionein gene regulation in response to copper. *Cell, 40*, 301–309.

Lichten, L. A., & Cousins, R. J. (2009). Mammalian zinc transporters: Nutritional and physiologic regulation. *Annual Review of Nutrition, 29*, 153–176.

Liu, A. C., Heinrichs, B. S., & Leach, R. M. (1994). Influence of manganese deficiency on the characteristics of proteoglycans of avian epiphyseal growth plate cartilage. *Poultry Science, 73*, 663–669.

Liuzzi, J. P., & Cousins, R. J. (2004). Mammalian zinc transporters. *Annual Review of Nutrition, 24*, 151–172.

Lonnerdal, B., & Sandstrom, B. (1995). Factors influencing the uptake of metal ions from the digestive tract. In G. Berthon (Ed.), *Handbook of metal-ligand interactions in biological fluids* (Vol. 1, pp. 331–337). New York: Marcel Dekker.

Lutsenko, S., & Petris, M. J. (2002). Function and regulation of the mammalian copper-transporting ATPases: Insights from biochemical and cell biological approaches. *The Journal of Membrane Biology, 191*, 1–12.

McMahon, R. J., & Cousins, R. J. (1998). Regulation of the zinc transporter ZnT-1 by dietary zinc. *Proceedings of the National Academy of Sciences of the United States of America, 95*, 4841–4846.

Mocchegiani, E., Giacconi, R., & Malavolta, M. (2008). Zinc signalling and subcellular distribution: Emerging targets in type 2 diabetes. *Trends in Molecular Medicine, 14*, 419–428.

Moshfegh, A., Goldman, J., & Cleveland, L. (2005). *What we eat in America, NHANES 2001–2002: Usual nutrient intakes from food compared to Dietary Reference Intakes.* Washington, DC: U.S. Department of Agriculture, Agricultural Research Service.

Mossad, S. B., Macknin, M. L., Medendorp, S. V., & Mason, P. (1996). Zinc gluconate lozenges for treating the common cold. A randomized, double-blind, placebo-controlled study. *Annals of Internal Medicine, 125*, 81–88.

Noor, R., Mittal, S., & Iqbal, J. (2002). Superoxide dismutase—Applications and relevance to human diseases. *Medical Science Monitor, 8*, RA210–RA215.

O'Donohue, J., Reid, M. A., Varghese, A., Portmann, B., & Williams, R. (1993). Micronodular cirrhosis and acute liver failure due to chronic copper self-intoxication. *European Journal of Gastroenterology & Hepatology, 5*, 561–562.

Orr, W. C., & Sohal, R. S. (1994). Extension of life-span by overexpression of superoxide dismutase and catalase in *Drosophila melanogaster*. *Science, 263*, 1128–1130.

Owen, C. A. (1973). Effects of iron on copper metabolism and copper on iron metabolism in rats. *The American Journal of Physiology, 224*, 514–518.

Palmiter, R. D. (1994). Regulation of metallothionein genes by heavy metals appears to be mediated by a zinc-sensitive inhibitor that interacts with a constitutively active transcription factor, MTF-1. *Proceedings of the National Academy of Sciences of the United States of America, 91*, 1219–1223.

Palmiter, R. D., & Findley, S. D. (1995). Cloning and functional characterization of a mammalian zinc transporter that confers resistance to zinc. *The EMBO Journal, 14*, 639–649.

Percival, S. S. (1995). Neutropenia caused by copper deficiency: Possible mechanisms of action. *Nutrition Reviews, 53*, 59–66.

Percival, S. S., & Harris, E. D. (1990). Copper transport from ceruloplasmin: Characterization of the cellular uptake mechanism. *The American Journal of Physiology, 258*, C140–C146.

Pratt, W. B., Omdahl, J. L., & Sorenson, J. R. (1985). Lack of effects of copper gluconate supplementation. *The American Journal of Clinical Nutrition, 42*, 681–682.

Prohaska, J. R. (2008). Role of copper transporters in copper homeostasis. *The American Journal of Clinical Nutrition, 88*, 826S–829S.

Qian, W.-J., & Kennedy, R. T. (2001). Spatial organization of Ca21 entry and exocytosis in mouse pancreatic β-cells. *Biochemical and Biophysical Research Communications, 286*, 315–332.

Reinhold, J. G. (1971). High phytate content of rural Iranian bread: A possible cause of human zinc deficiency. *The American Journal of Clinical Nutrition, 24*, 1204–1206.

Rhodes, D., & Klug, A. (1993). Zinc fingers. *Scientific American*, February, 56–65.

Rock, E., Gueux, E., Mazur, A., Motta, C., & Rayssiguier, Y. (1995). Anemia in copper-deficient rats: Role of alterations in erythrocyte membrane fluidity and oxidative damage. *The American Journal of Physiology, 269*, C1245–C1249.

Roth, H. P., & Kirchgessner, M. (1994). Influence of alimentary zinc deficiency on the concentration of growth hormone (GH), insulin-like growth factor I (IGF-I) and insulin in the serum of force-fed rats. *Hormone and Metabolic Research, 26*, 404–408.

Rucker, R. B., Romero-Chapman, N., Wong, T., Lee, J., Steinberg, F. M., McGee, C., … Keen, C. L. (1996). Modulation of lysyl oxidase by dietary copper in rats. *The Journal of Nutrition, 126,* 51–60.

Ryu, M.-S., Lichten, L. A., & Cousins, R. J. (2008). Zinc transporters ZnT1 (Slc30a1), Zip8 (Slc39a8), and Zip10 (Slc39a10) in mouse red blood cells are differentially regulated during erythroid development and by dietary zinc deficiency. *The Journal of Nutrition, 138,* 2076–2083.

Scott, D. A. (1934). Crystalline insulin. *The Biochemical Journal, 28,* 1592–1603.

Swanson, C. A., & King, J. C. (1983). Reduced serum zinc concentrations during pregnancy. *Obstetrics and Gynecology, 62,* 313–318.

Torre, M., Rodriguez, A. R., & Saura-Calixto, F. (1992). Effects of dietary fiber and phytic acid on mineral availability. *Critical Reviews in Food Science and Nutrition, 30,* 1–22.

Tumer, Z., Moller, L. B., & Horn, N. (2003). Screening of 383 unrelated patients affected with Menkes disease and finding of 57 gross deletions in ATP7A. *Human Mutation, 22,* 457–464.

Valentine, R. A., Jackson, K. A., Christie, G. R., Mathers, J. C., Taylor, P. M., & Ford, D. (2007). ZnT5 variant B is a bidirectional zinc transporter and mediates zinc uptake in human intestinal Caco-2 cells. *The Journal of Biological Chemistry, 282,* 14389–14393.

Vallee, B. L., & Galdes, A. (1984). The metallobiochemistry of zinc enzymes. *Advances in Enzymology and Related Areas of Molecular Biology, 56,* 283–430.

Vulpe, C. D., & Packman, S. (1995). Cellular copper transport. *Annual Review of Nutrition, 15,* 293–322.

Walsh, C. T., Sandstead, H. H., Prasad, A. S., Newbern, P. M., & Fraker, P. J. (1994). Zinc: Health effects and research priorities for the 1990s. *Environmental Health Perspectives, 102,* 5–46.

Wang, F., Kim, B. E., Dufner-Beattie, J., Petris, M. J., Andrews, G., & Eide, D. J. (2004). Acrodermatitis enteropathica mutations affect transport activity, localization and zinc-responsive trafficking of the mouse ZIP4 zinc transporter. *Human Molecular Genetics, 13,* 563–571.

Wellenreuther, G., Cianci, M., Tucoulou, R., Meyer-Klaucke, W., & Haase, H. (2009). The ligand environment of zinc stored in vesicles. *Biochemical and Biophysical Research Communications, 380,* 198–203.

Williamson, P. S., Brown, E. C., Browning, J. D., Wollard, L. C., Thornton, W. H., O'Dell, B. L., & MacDonald, R. S. (1997). Decreased insulin-like growth factor-I (IGF-I) receptor concentration and IGF-I binding in small intestine of zinc-deficient rats. *The FASEB Journal, 11,* A194.

Yamaguchi, M. (1998). Role of zinc in bone formation and bone resorption. *The Journal of Trace Elements in Experimental Medicine, 11,* 119–135.

Zalewski, P. D., Forbes, I. J., & Betts, W. H. (1993). Correlation of apoptosis with change in intracellular labile Zn(II) using zinquin[(2-methyl-8-p-toluenesulphonamido-6-quinolyloxy) acetic acid], a new specific fluorescent probe for Zn(II). *The Biochemical Journal, 296,* 403–408.

RECOMMENDED READINGS

Andreini, C., Banci, L., Bertini, I., & Rosato, A. (2006). Counting the zinc-proteins encoded in the human genome. *Journal of Proteome Research, 5,* 196–201.

Bressler, J. P., Olivi, L., Cheong, J. H., Kim, Y., Maerten, A., & Bannon, D. (2007). Metal transporters in intestine and brain: Their involvement in metal-associated neurotoxicities. *Human & Experimental Toxicology, 26,* 221–229.

Cox, D. W., & Moore, S. D. P. (2002). Copper transporting P-type ATPases and human disease. *Journal of Bioenergetics and Biomembranes, 34,* 333–338.

Haase, H., & Rink, L. (2009). Functional significance of zinc-related signaling pathways in immune cells. *Annual Review of Nutrition, 29,* 133–152.

Hess, S. Y., Peerson, J. M., King, J. C., & Brown, K. H. (2007). Use of serum zinc concentrations as an indicator of population zinc status. *Food and Nutrition Bulletin, 28,* S403–S429.

Hotz, C. (2007). Dietary indicators for assessing the adequacy of population zinc intakes. *Food and Nutrition Bulletin, 28,* S430–S453.

Institute of Medicine. (2001). *Dietary Reference Intakes for vitamin A, vitamin K, arsenic, boron, chromium, copper, iodine, iron, manganese, molybdenum, nickel, silicon, vanadium, and zinc.* Washington, DC: National Academy Press.

Jansen, J., Karges, W., & Rink, L. (2009). Zinc and diabetes—Clinical links and molecular mechanisms. *The Journal of Nutritional Biochemistry, 20,* 399–417.

Kimura, T., & Itoh, N. (2008). Function of metallothionein in gene expression and signal transduction: Newly found protective role of metallothionein. *Journal of Health Science, 54,* 251–260.

Laukens, D., Waeytens, A., de Bleser, P., Cuvelier, C., & de Vos, M. (2009). Human metallothionein expression under normal and pathological conditions: Mechanisms of gene regulation based on in silico promoter analysis. *Critical Reviews in Eukaryotic Gene Expression, 19,* 301–317.

Lichten, L. A., & Cousins, R. J. (2009). Mammalian zinc transporters: Nutritional and physiologic regulation. *Annual Review of Nutrition, 29,* 153–176.

Mocchegiani, E., Giacconi, R., & Malavolta, M. (2008). Zinc signalling and subcellular distribution: Emerging targets in type 2 diabetes. *Trends in Molecular Medicine, 14,* 419–428.

Prohaska, J. R. (2008). Role of copper transporters in copper homeostasis. *The American Journal of Clinical Nutrition, 88,* 826S–829S.

CHAPTER 38

Iodine

Elizabeth N. Pearce, MD, MSc, and Hedley C. Freake, PhD

COMMON ABBREVIATIONS

IDD	iodine deficiency disorder
NIS	sodium/iodide symporter
rT_3	reverse T_3
RXR	retinoid X receptor
T_3	3,5,3′-triiodothyronine
T_4	thyroxine
TR	thyroid hormone receptor
TRE	thyroid hormone response element
TRH	thyrotropin-releasing hormone
TSH	thyroid-stimulating hormone, thyrotropin

Iodine is responsible for just a single function in the body: the synthesis of thyroid hormones. However, the multiple actions of thyroid hormones mean that iodine has an impact on a wide range of metabolic and developmental functions. Deficiency of iodine is common, and the consequences of that deficiency are so profound, particularly in the fetal and neonatal period, that it represents one of the largest public health problems in the world today (World Health Organization [WHO], 2007). Yet eradicating iodine deficiency is relatively simple and in many parts of the world has resulted in dramatic improvements in human well-being.

PRODUCTION AND METABOLISM OF THYROID HORMONES

USE OF IODINE: THYROID HORMONES

Inorganic iodine occurs predominantly in nature in the form of the anion iodide. Its sole function in humans and other mammals is the synthesis of thyroid hormones. These iodinated derivatives of the amino acid tyrosine, shown in Figure 38-1, are thyroxine, or 3,5,3′,5′-tetraiodothyronine (T_4), and 3,5,3′-triiodothyronine (T_3). Because they are derived from amino acids, thyroid hormones are in the L-form. D-Isomers can be synthesized but have lower biological activity.

DIETARY SOURCES OF IODINE

Iodine is a reasonably abundant element, but its solubility leads to wide regional variations in its availability. The iodine content of soils is diminished by exposure to rain, snow, and glaciation, which leach out the mineral and deposit it in the oceans. Although iodine is volatilized from the sea and returns to land through rainwater, this does not make up for the long-term loss of iodine from older exposed soils. Iodine-deficient areas include mountainous regions, such as the Himalayas, Andes, and Alps, and also river deltas, such as the Ganges and the Yellow River, where frequent flooding has leached out the mineral (Zimmermann, 2009).

The iodine content of most food sources is low. The iodine content of plants averages 1 mg/kg dry weight, but it may be only 1% of that amount in plants grown in iodine-deficient areas. Its content in animal foods, including milk, reflects the amount found in the feeds supplied to the animals. Foods arising from the sea, such as fish and seaweed, provide a rich source. Foods of marine origin have greater amounts of iodine because marine animals can concentrate iodine from seawater. In more developed parts of the world, the food available to a particular community is usually drawn from a variety of geographical locations and thus, in aggregate, is less likely to be deficient in iodine. However, supplementation, particularly in the form of iodized salt as has been used in the United States and many other parts of the world, is the only reliable way to ensure an

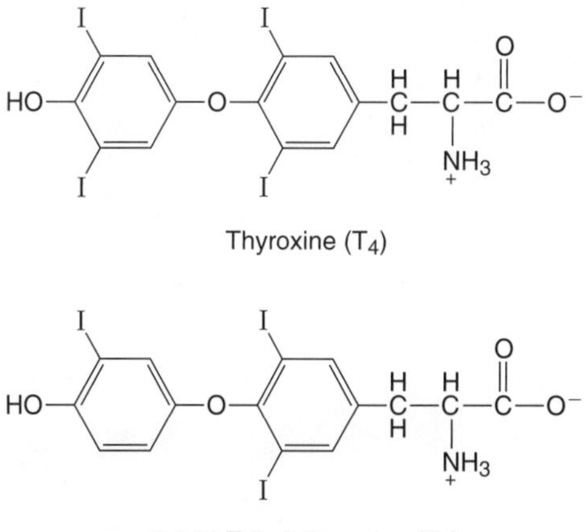

Thyroxine (T_4)

3,5,3′-Triiodothyronine (T_3)

FIGURE 38-1 Chemical structures of the thyroid hormones.

adequate dietary supply in low-iodine areas. This relatively simple public health program has reaped enormous benefits. Iodine intakes may also be increased by the use of iodine-containing products at various points in the food production process. For example, iodates are used in bread making, and iodine-containing antiseptics are used in dairy facilities (Pearce et al., 2004). Thus processed foods may contain enhanced levels of iodine from the addition of iodized salt or other additives.

FOOD SOURCES OF IODINE

Seafood (Fish, Shellfish, or Seaweed)
30 μg per 3 oz shrimp
100 to 140 μg per 3 oz haddock or cod
17 μg per 3 oz canned tuna

Vegetables, Meats, Eggs
60 μg per 1 medium baked potato
8 μg per ½ cup lima beans
24 μg per 1 large egg
99 μg per 3 oz baked cod

Iodized Salt
71 μg per 1.5 g (approximately ¼ tsp) salt

Bread (Iodates as Dough Improvers)
45 μg per 2 slices enriched white bread

Milk Products (Iodine-Based Antiseptics and Iodine in Cattle Feed)
56 μg per 8 oz milk
75 μg per 1 cup plain low-fat yogurt
12 μg per 1 oz cheddar cheese

Data from National Institute of Health Office of Dietary Supplements. Retrieved from *http://ods.od.nih.gov/factsheets/Iodine-Health Professional/*

ABSORPTION, STORAGE, AND EXCRETION OF IODINE

Iodine may be found in different forms in foods, including iodide (I^-) and iodate (IO^{3-}), the compound added to bread. Dietary iodine is reduced to iodide and absorbed efficiently along the length of the gastrointestinal tract, especially in the upper portion. The adult human body normally contains 15 to 20 mg of iodine, and about three fourths of this is found in the thyroid gland. The thyroid actively takes up iodide via the sodium/iodide symporter (NIS), which can be inhibited by environmental contaminants. Concentration of iodine in the gland is 40 times that in plasma under normal circumstances and can become still higher in iodine deficiency. Iodine accumulates to a much lesser extent in other tissues such as the salivary glands, stomach, ovaries, and testes. The kidneys are the other principal site for iodine removal from the circulation. They are incapable of conserving the mineral, and hence the kidneys represent the main route for excretion. The amount of iodine found in urine is proportional to the plasma concentration and can be used as a convenient index of iodine status in populations. Iodide is actively secreted into breast milk via NIS in lactating women. Small amounts of iodine are also lost in feces and sweat. Figure 38-2 provides a summary of the routes of iodine in the body from ingestion to excretion.

SYNTHESIS OF THYROID HORMONES

The process of thyroid hormone synthesis is illustrated in Figure 38-3. Iodide is actively transported across the basolateral membrane into the thyroid follicular cell cytoplasm by the NIS. It traverses the thyroid cells and is passively

HISTORICAL TIDBIT

The Goiter Belt

Until the 1920s endemic iodine deficiency disorders were prevalent in the Great Lakes, Appalachian, and Northwestern regions of the United States because of low soil iodine content. In the early 1900s goiter was present in up to 26% to 70% of schoolchildren living in this "goiter belt." The magnitude of the problem was noted at the time of World War I, when more military recruits from northern Michigan were determined to be unfit for duty because of goiter than for any other medical reason (Markel, 1987). In 1916 David Marine performed studies in schoolchildren that demonstrated that goiter could be eradicated by iodine supplementation (Marine and Kimball, 1917). Based primarily on his work, voluntary salt iodization was initiated in the United States in 1924, resulting in the elimination of the goiter belt.

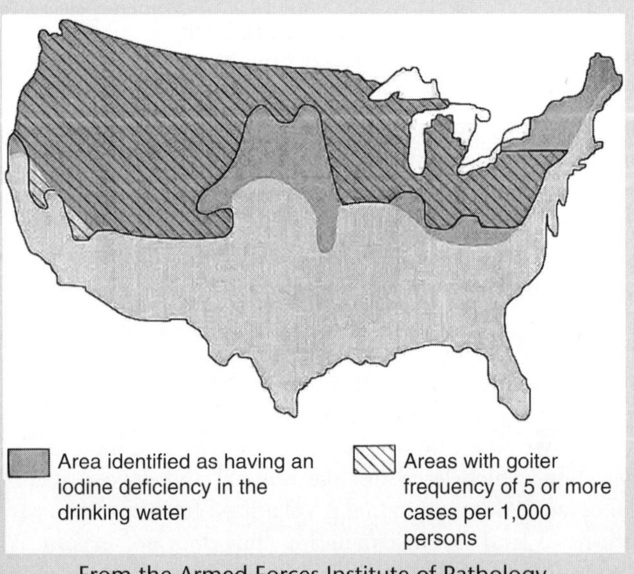

From the Armed Forces Institute of Pathology.

translocated into the follicular lumen by pendrin. Cloned in 1997, pendrin is a highly hydrophobic glycoprotein containing 780 amino acids. It is composed of 12 transmembrane domains and a carboxy-terminus inside the cytosol (Royaux et al., 2000). Pendrin is expressed not only in thyrocytes but also in kidney and inner ear cells. The apical iodide transporter (AIT), the cystic fibrosis transmembrane conductance regulator (CFTR), SLC5A8 (a member of the solute carrier 5A family), and the chloride channel 5 (ClCn5) are other putative transport proteins involved in iodide efflux across the apical membrane into the follicular lumen that have yet to be fully characterized.

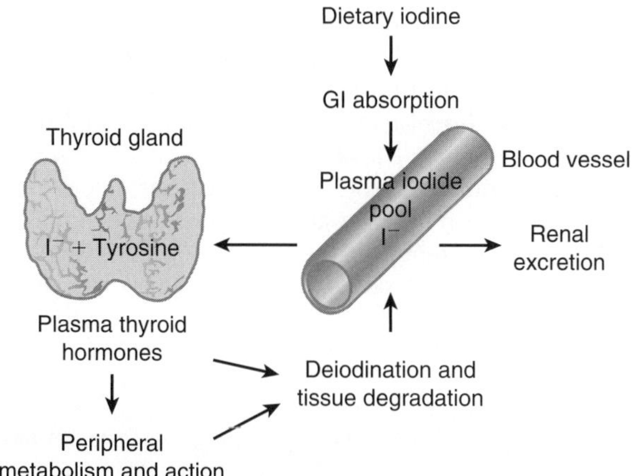

FIGURE 38-2 Routes of iodine in the body from ingestion to excretion. Iodine (as iodide, I^-) is readily absorbed along the gastrointestinal (*GI*) tract, and taken up by the thyroid from the plasma iodide (I^-) pool. Iodide is used to make thyroid hormone. Following deiodination of thyroid hormone, iodide may be taken up again by the thyroid or excreted in urine. Approximately 90% of ingested iodine is ultimately excreted by the kidneys, with additional losses in sweat, feces, and, in lactating women, breast milk.

The iodide is then oxidized by thyroid peroxidase, using hydrogen peroxide as a cosubstrate, and the reactive intermediate is coupled to tyrosyl residues in the protein thyroglobulin (a complex process referred to as organification). These then become monoiodotyrosyl or diiodotyrosyl residues, depending on whether one or two iodide molecules are incorporated. Thyroglobulin is a very large glycoprotein and may constitute up to one half the protein in the thyroid gland. Only selected tyrosyl residues in this protein become iodinated. Monoiodotyrosyl or diiodotyrosyl residues within thyroglobulin are coupled to form T_4 or T_3 residues. This reaction is also catalyzed by thyroid peroxidase. When the iodophenolic ring of one iodotyrosyl residue is coupled with another, the rest of the donor residue is left in the thyroglobulin chain in the form of a serine residue. Thyroid hormones are stored in the colloid space, still as a part of thyroglobulin.

For release of thyroid hormones, portions of colloid that contain iodinated thyroglobulin are taken into the thyroid follicular cells by pinocytosis. These endocytic vesicles then fuse with lysosomes within the cells, and the thyroglobulin within them is broken down by proteolytic enzymes. This results in the release of free thyroid hormones, which are able to diffuse into the circulation. T_4 is the predominant form released (approximately 80% of total hormone secreted), but T_3 is also secreted. The proportion of T_3 released appears to be increased under hypothyroid conditions due to increased intrathyroidal deiodination of T_4.

Hypothyroidism can result not only from insufficient dietary iodine but also from the ingestion of goitrogens. These are present in some foods, notably the cruciferous family of vegetables (e.g., broccoli and cabbage) and also cassava and millet. Cassava and millet may be more important, because they are dietary staples eaten in large quantities by some populations. Cruciferous vegetables themselves are not

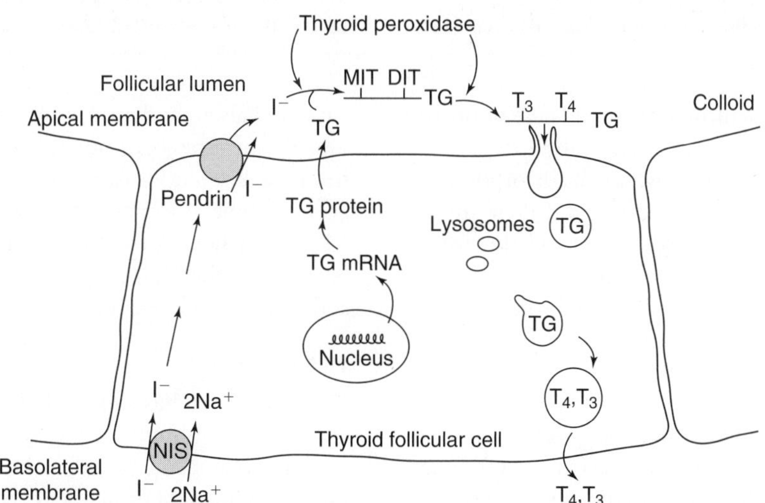

FIGURE 38-3 Synthesis of thyroid hormones in the thyroid follicular cells. Iodide is pumped into the follicular cells of the thyroid gland via the sodium/iodide symporter (NIS). It diffuses across the cells and enters the follicular lumen via pendrin where it is incorporated into thyroglobulin (*TG*) leading to the synthesis of MITs and DITs (monoiodotyrosines and diiodotyrosines), which then condense to form thyroid hormones. The hormones, still within thyroglobulin, are stored in the colloid space. When stimulated by thyroid-stimulating hormone (TSH), the secretion pathway begins with the uptake of a droplet of colloid via macropinocytosis and the fusion of the endocytic vesicle with a lysosome. The lysosomal enzymes degrade the thyroglobulin, leading to the release of the thyroid hormones and their secretion from the cell.

NUTRITION INSIGHT

Environmental Exposure to Perchlorate, a NIS Inhibitor

Perchlorate is a competitive inhibitor of the sodium/iodide symporter (NIS). When present in sufficiently high concentrations, perchlorate will decrease the active transport of iodide into the thyroid and decrease thyroid hormone synthesis. High doses of perchlorate were used in the 1950s as a treatment for hyperthyroidism. Perchlorate salts are used in the United States as oxidizers in solid propellants for rockets and missiles; in fireworks, road flares, and matches; and in air bag inflation systems. Perchlorate is also present in large concentrations in some fertilizers. In addition, low levels of perchlorate may be found in the environment as a product of natural processes. Perchlorate has been detected in the drinking water of communities around the United States, in foods such as lettuce and wheat, in cows' milk, and in multivitamins. There has been recent concern that low levels of perchlorate might pose a health hazard by inducing or aggravating underlying thyroid dysfunction.

Perchlorate exposure appears to be ubiquitous in the U.S. population. Detectable levels were found in all spot urine specimens analyzed for perchlorate in a random subsample (2,820 individuals) from the 2001–2002 National Health and Nutrition Examination Survey (NHANES). Children had higher levels than did adolescents and adults. Although exposure to perchlorate is widespread in the United States, estimated perchlorate exposures were all below the reference dose estimated by the Environmental Protection Agency to be without appreciable risk of adverse effects during a lifetime of exposure (Blount et al., 2007). Among women with urinary iodine values less than 100 μg/L in this data set, there was a significant positive correlation between urinary perchlorate concentrations and serum TSH and an inverse correlation between urinary perchlorate concentrations and serum T_4 values. However, no effect of perchlorate exposure on first-trimester thyroid function was seen in a recent cohort of iodine-deficient pregnant European women (Pearce et al., 2010).

The Environmental Protection Agency has determined that perchlorate may have an adverse effect on human health and is currently in the process of establishing a final drinking water standard for the U.S. public drinking water supplies.

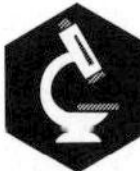

CLINICAL CORRELATION

Pendred Syndrome: Effects of Impaired Iodide Efflux

The most common genetic cause of deafness, accounting for 4% to 10% of all children with hereditary hearing loss, is Pendred syndrome, a disorder named after Waughan Pendred, the physician who first described it. The pendrin gene (*SLC26A4* or *PDS*) was identified in 1997 and is located on chromosome 7q22-31.1. Mutations of the pendrin gene, of which at least 150 have been described, account for the clinical manifestations in this autosomal recessive disorder, including sensorineural hearing loss, goiter, and defects in iodide organification (Kopp et al., 2008). The appearance of goiter is usually detected during childhood, although this may be noted earlier in states of iodine deficiency or later if masked by chronic high iodine intake. The extrathyroidal actions of pendrin include its role in maintaining the ionic composition of endolymph in the inner ear. Mutations in pendrin function result in an increased endolymph volume, and loss of inner ear sensory cells can be detected as early as infancy.

likely to be eaten in sufficient quantities to cause concern. Goitrogens work either by competitively inhibiting iodide uptake by the thyroid gland or by blocking its incorporation into the tyrosyl residues of thyroglobulin and their subsequent condensation. Antithyroid drugs, such as propylthiouracil and methimazole, work by the latter mechanism and are used clinically in the treatment of hyperthyroidism.

CIRCULATION

Thyroid hormones are carried in the blood by three proteins: thyroid-binding globulin, thyroid-binding prealbumin, and albumin. Prealbumin is also known as transthyretin and functions with retinol-binding protein in retinol transport (see Chapter 30). More than 99% of both T_4 and T_3 circulate bound to these proteins, but T_4 is bound 10 times more tightly than T_3. It appears likely that only the small free fraction is available for tissue uptake, either to exert biological activity or for further metabolism. This tight binding means that thyroid hormones, particularly T_4, have relatively long plasma half-lives (6 to 8 days) and also that there is a large plasma pool of thyroid hormones, which can become available to tissues after dissociation from the binding proteins. The T_4 plasma concentration in normal humans is approximately 100 nmol/L, which is 50- to 100-fold higher than that for T_3. The relative abundance of T_4 reflects both that T_4 is the primary product of the thyroid gland and that it has a longer plasma half-life than does T_3 (1 day).

TRANSPORT

Recent research has shown that thyroid hormone transport across cell membranes is energy dependent and mediated by specific organic anion and amino acid transporters, including the sodium taurocholate cotransporting polypeptide (NTCP), various sodium-independent organic anion transporting polypeptides, L-type amino acid transporters (LAT1 and LAT2), the fatty acid translocase (FAT, CD36), and the monocarboxylate transporters (MCT) 8 and 10. Congenital defects in MCT result in severe neurological and cognitive impairments (Heuer and Visser, 2009).

ACTIVATION

T_4, the predominant circulating thyroid hormone, is really a prohormone that requires deiodination at the 5′ position in the outer ring to generate the biologically active T_3. Deiodination serves not only to activate thyroid hormones but also to deactivate them (Figure 38-4). Removal of iodine from the inner ring of T_4 will result in the production of reverse T_3 (rT_3; 3,3′,5′-triiodothyronine), and similar processing of T_3 produces 3,3′-diiodothyronine, both of which are inactive metabolites.

A family of microsomal enzymes is responsible for deiodination (Bianco et al., 2002). The type 1 deiodinase is found in liver, kidney, and thyroid gland. It is associated with the plasma membrane and is thought to contribute significantly to circulating T_3 concentrations. It can perform inner ring as well as outer ring deiodinations, and its preferred substrate is rT_3. Type 1 deiodinase activity is increased in hyperthyroidism and decreased in the hypothyroid state. The type 2 deiodinase, located in brain, pituitary, and brown adipose tissue, operates solely on the outer ring. It is located in the endoplasmic reticulum and specifically functions to convert T_4 to T_3 for local use within these tissues. However, it is now appreciated that type 2 deiodinase can also contribute significantly to circulating levels of T_3 in plasma. In tissues containing the type 2 enzyme, thyroid hormone status will depend primarily on plasma levels of T_4 rather than T_3. The activity of this enzyme is increased in the hypothyroid state, which means that these tissues may be partially protected from the effects of hypothyroidism by this local production.

Type 3 deiodinase operates exclusively on the inner ring and therefore inactivates thyroid hormones. It has been found in brain and placenta, and its activity is increased with elevation of thyroid hormone status.

Genes encoding all three enzymes have now been cloned in multiple species and this has allowed many insights into the functioning and regulation of this enzyme family (Bianco et al., 2002). Of particular interest is the discovery that all three enzymes contain the unusual amino acid selenocysteine at their active site. This amino acid is similar to cysteine, except that the sulfur is substituted by selenium (see Chapter 39). The nucleotide triplet UGA encodes this substitution, which is critical for the catalytic properties of the enzyme. Under most circumstances this triplet is read as a stop codon but other sequences within the deiodinase messenger RNAs (mRNAs) override this coding and dictate the incorporation of selenocysteine. This linkage between thyroid hormone deiodination and selenium explains earlier work in rats, which showed that selenium deficiency reduced plasma T_3 and thereby impaired thyroid hormone status.

FURTHER METABOLISM AND EXCRETION

Removal of iodine from the inner ring is an irreversible degradative step. There are additional pathways of thyroid hormone metabolism. The phenolic hydroxyl group of the outer ring can be conjugated with glucuronate or sulfate. This occurs primarily in the liver, with glucuronidation being favored for T_4 and sulfation for T_3. These conjugates are then secreted into the bile and may be lost in the feces. However, a significant amount is likely to be hydrolyzed in the intestine, followed by reabsorption of the free thyroid hormones. Deamination or decarboxylation also occurs, resulting in carboxylate or amine analogs of the thyroid hormones, respectively. Although metabolic activity has been suggested for some of these analogs, this seems unlikely because their further degradation is very rapid. Any iodide produced by the extrathyroidal metabolism of thyroid hormones will be either taken up by the thyroid gland and used for further synthesis or excreted in the urine.

REGULATION OF THYROID HORMONE STATUS

From the preceding discussion it is apparent that thyroid hormone status can be modified at a number of different levels. The primary site may be output from the thyroid gland, but the rate of conversion of the prohormone to active T_3 is also important. Under normal circumstances, circulating thyroid hormone levels are tightly regulated because of a negative feedback loop controlling their production (Figure 38-5). Thyrotroph cells in the anterior pituitary produce thyrotropin, or thyroid-stimulating hormone (TSH), a glycoprotein that is a heterodimer of two subunits encoded by separate

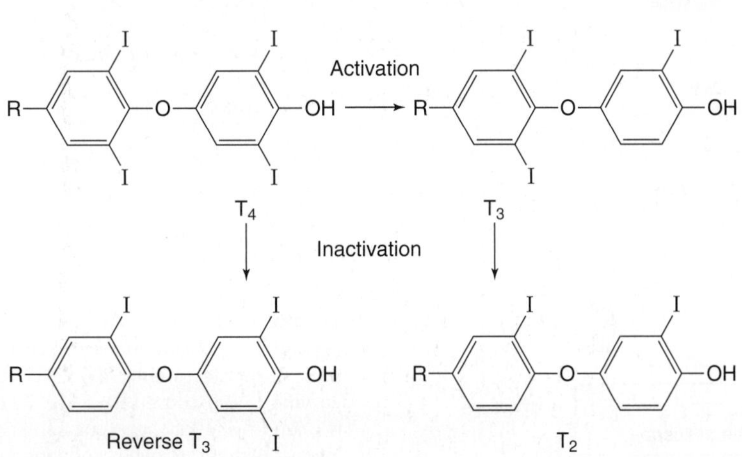

FIGURE 38-4 Deiodination pathways for thyroid hormones. The parent compound thyroxine (*T_4*) is activated by monodeiodination of the outer ring to form 3,5,3′-triiodothyronine (*T_3*). Either one of these may be inactivated by inner ring deiodination to form reverse T_3 or diiodothyronine (*T_2*).

genes. The α-subunit of TSH is similar to that of the gonadotropic pituitary hormones (luteinizing hormone and follicle-stimulating hormone), whereas the β-subunit is unique. TSH acts on the thyroid gland, primarily by a cyclic AMP–mediated mechanism, to stimulate iodide uptake and organification and release of thyroid hormones. T_4 travels back to the pituitary, where it is deiodinated by the type 2 enzyme. The T_3 that is produced operates at a transcriptional level to inhibit the production of TSH, thereby completing the cycle. TSH is also under the control of the hypothalamic tripeptide thyrotropin-releasing hormone (TRH), which is responsible for basal production of TSH by the pituitary. It provides a mechanism by which thyroid hormone status can be modulated at a central level, either positively (e.g., in response to cold) or negatively (e.g., in response to stress or illness). T_3 has also been shown to inhibit transcription of the *TRH* gene, meaning that the negative feedback loop extends up to the hypothalamus.

This hypothalamic–pituitary–thyroid axis is responsible for producing the appropriate amounts of thyroid hormones, but thyroid hormone status can also be regulated by altering the rate of T_4 to T_3 conversion. The deiodinase enzymes can be differentially regulated. This allows the possibility that tissues may differ in thyroid hormone status, according to whether they depend on the type 1 or type 2 deiodinase for supply of T_3. For example, plasma T_3 is reduced by fasting and increased by carbohydrate feeding in humans and these effects are achieved by altering the activity of the type 1 deiodinase. This response to decreased food availability helps conserve fuel by reducing metabolic rate. In particular, protein catabolism is minimized by a reduction in its T_3-stimulated turnover rate. However, because the type 2 enzyme is not affected by fasting, generation of T_3 in the brain and pituitary, and therefore T_3-dependent functions in those tissues, is maintained.

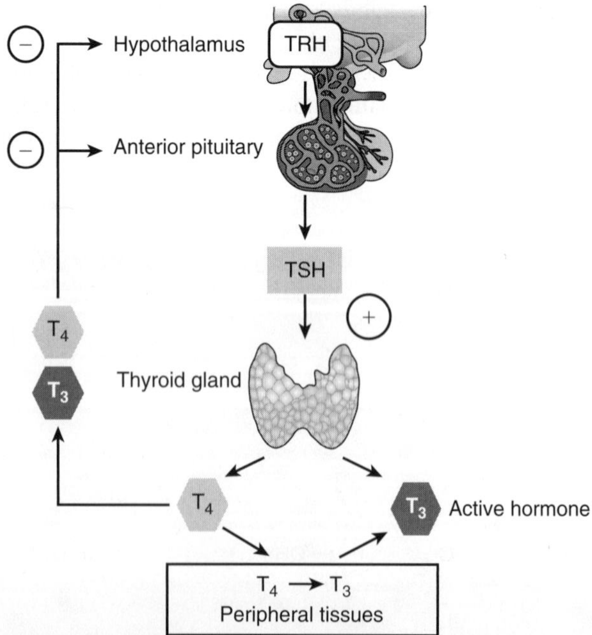

FIGURE 38-5 Feedback regulation of thyroid hormone status. *TRH*, Thyrotropin-releasing hormone; *TSH*, thyroid-stimulating hormone; *T_4*, thyroxine; *T_3*, 3,5,3′-triiodothyronine.

Measurement of serum TSH is widely used clinically as a sensitive indicator of thyroid hormone status. Elevated levels indicate hypothyroidism, whereas levels are low in hyperthyroidism. Circulating levels of T_3 may be maintained, even in the face of inadequate thyroid hormone production, both by increasing the proportion of T_3 produced by the thyroid gland and by stimulating peripheral conversion. Therefore plasma T_3 values may be within the normal range until late in the process of thyroid failure, despite reduced levels of T_4. This compensation may occur at the expense of the brain, because brain derives T_3 from plasma T_4 by the type 2 deiodinase-catalyzed reaction. Plasma TSH or T_4 concentrations are used to confirm normal thyroid hormone status in newborn infants.

MECHANISM OF ACTION OF THYROID HORMONES

Most and perhaps all actions of thyroid hormones are mediated by effects within the nucleus. This mechanism is outlined in Figure 38-6. Following dissociation from plasma proteins, T_4 and T_3 enter the cell. The T_4 is deiodinated and T_3 enters the nucleus. There it is bound by specific nuclear receptor proteins, which are associated with a set of target genes (Box 38-1). Hormone binding to these receptors alters these associations in a manner that leads to a change in the rate of transcription of the target genes. Changes in gene transcription in turn lead to changed amounts of mRNA, which are translated to correspondingly different amounts of protein. Thereby the physiological state is altered.

NUCLEAR RECEPTORS

Enormous progress has been made in the last 20 years in understanding the mechanism of action of thyroid hormone on a molecular level (Cheng et al., 2010). An important starting point for these advances was the cloning in 1986 of

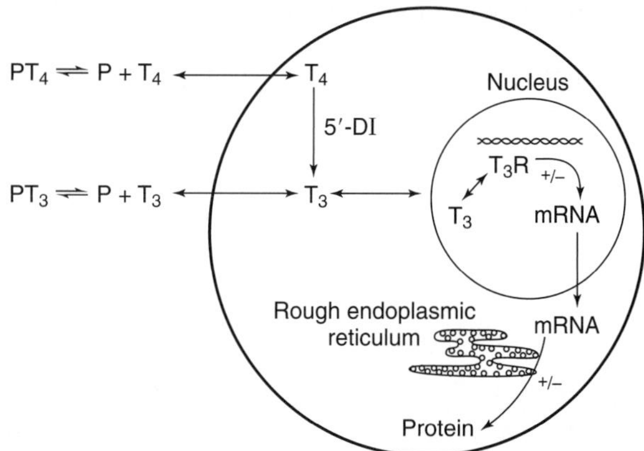

FIGURE 38-6 Outline of thyroid hormone action. Thyroid hormones (T_3 and T_4) circulate bound to plasma proteins (*P*), from which they must dissociate to enter the cell. Tissues containing the deiodinase enzyme (*5′-DI*) convert T_4 to T_3. T_3 travels to the nucleus, where it is bound by specific receptor transcription factors (*R*). Together they interact with target genes, resulting in a change in gene transcription rate. This results in altered mRNA levels, leading to different rates of protein synthesis and therefore different amounts of the protein products of the target genes, which ultimately produce the biological effect.

complementary DNAs (cDNAs) encoding thyroid hormone receptors (TRs) in two independent laboratories (Sap et al., 1986; Weinberger et al., 1986).

Functional Regions of Receptors

The realization that TRs are part of a family of nuclear acting proteins has facilitated progress in understanding their mechanism of action, because analogies can be drawn with other members of the class (Aranda and Pascual, 2001). This family includes receptors not only for steroid hormones but also for retinoic acid, 1,25-dihydroxyvitamin D, fatty acids, steroids, and a host of other lesser known or uncharacterized ligands. These receptors have a modular structure (Figure 38-7). They all have a carboxy-terminal region that binds to the ligand, and this region provides each receptor with its hormone ligand specificity. The area that is most highly conserved across the family is the DNA-binding region, through which the receptors recognize and bind to their target genes. This region contains conserved cysteine residues that coordinate two atoms of zinc. These stabilize a conformation required for binding to target genes. Regions that appear to be required for nuclear localization of the protein, that facilitate dimerization between receptors, or that are required for communicating the signal for altered transcription have also been described.

BOX 38-1 Selected Target Genes for Thyroid Hormones

METABOLIC
Fatty acid synthase
Malic enzyme
Pyruvate kinase
Spot 14
Phosphoenolpyruvate carboxykinase

CARDIAC
Myosin heavy chain
Calcium ATPase

ENDOCRINE
Growth hormone
Thyroid-stimulating hormone (TSH)
Thyroid hormone receptors (TR, α and β)

MITOCHONDRIAL
Cytochrome c

ION TRANSPORT
Na^+,K^+-ATPase

Multiple Thyroid Hormone Receptors

Two thyroid hormone receptors were identified in 1986, and although they were derived from different species, they appeared to be generated from independent genes. The existence of two human TR genes (α on chromosome 17 and β on chromosome 3) has subsequently been confirmed. In addition, these two genes result in multiple protein products. There are two thyroid hormone β receptors; β1 has a broad tissue distribution, including liver, muscle, brown fat, and kidney, and β2 is restricted to the pituitary and certain areas of the brain. Multiple products derived from the α gene have also been described; although only one of them, α1, retains an intact hormone-binding region and therefore appears capable of performing a receptor function. TRα1 is highly expressed in the brain, heart, and bone. Other α forms may play important roles, however, and it has been suggested that they may antagonize T_3 action. In particular, the non–hormone-binding variant α2 is expressed at high levels in the brain and in the testis, and it has been suggested that this could explain the metabolic nonresponsiveness of these tissues to T_3 in the adult (Lazar, 1993).

Response Elements in Target Genes

The TR must be capable of selecting the genes that it specifically regulates from among the background of the entire genome. This specificity is achieved by DNA sequences in the control regions of target genes, known as thyroid hormone response elements (TREs). A TRE consists of a hexanucleotide with the sequence AGGTCA, although some substitutions within that sequence are permissible. The TREs are usually found in pairs, although sometimes three or even more copies of this sequence are present. The same recognition motif is used by some other members of the nuclear receptor family, notably receptors for retinoic acid and vitamin D, which indicates that not only the recognition sequences but also their arrangement within the

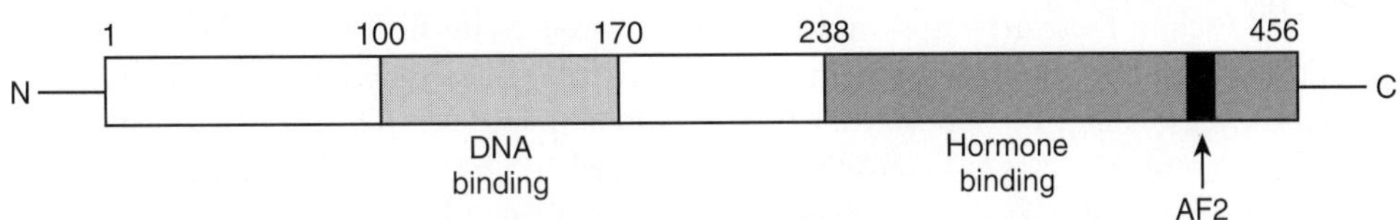

FIGURE 38-7 The modular structure of thyroid hormone receptors (TRs). In common with other members of the nuclear receptor family, the TRs have defined regions for DNA and hormone binding, separated by a hinge region. Sequences required for dimer formation have been described within both the DNA- and hormone-binding domains. The amino-terminal region does not appear to be required for function of TRs, although in other nuclear receptors this region contains an activation domain. The activation function-2 (*AF2*) domain is required for interaction with coactivating proteins. Sites required for interaction with corepressors have been located elsewhere in the ligand-binding domain as well as in the hinge region. The numbers shown represent amino acids in the human TRβ1 sequence.

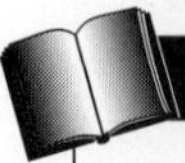

HISTORICAL TIDBIT

Accidental Cloning of Thyroid Hormone Receptors

Sap and colleagues (1986) and Weinberger and associates (1986), the groups that cloned the thyroid hormone receptors, were not thyroid hormone experts and were not deliberately seeking to clone the thyroid hormone receptor. Rather, they were following up on the observation that the glucocorticoid receptor and the estrogen receptor, which had both recently been cloned and sequenced, had a high degree of sequence homology to each other and also to a viral oncogene encoding the avian erythroblastosis virus *(erbA)*. Since oncogenes are derived from normal eukaryotic genes, they reasoned that mammalian and avian genomes would contain a homolog of *erbA* that would serve an important function. They identified complementary DNA (cDNA) generated by reverse transcription of the tissue mRNA that had sequences very similar to *erbA* from chick and human libraries and, because of their homology to the glucocorticoid and estrogen receptors, reasoned that these too would encode hormone receptors. When they expressed the encoded proteins, they found that they bound specifically to just one hormone, the thyroid hormone T_3. When they analyzed their data, they also realized they had cloned two different thyroid hormone receptors, although until that time it had been assumed there was only one. In the following years many other nuclear receptors, including those for vitamins A and D, were identifed using similar approaches.

promoter are important for determining target gene specificity. It has therefore been suggested that a TRE consists of two repeats of the sequence AGGTCA with a four-nucleotide separation. Although such a sequence certainly is able to respond to the thyroid hormone–receptor complex, the sequences actually found within target genes frequently deviate from this. Therefore, despite considerable attention to this question, the exact requirements for a DNA sequence to confer responsiveness to thyroid hormone remain to be established.

Heterodimerization of Receptors

The fact that recognition motifs for TRs, as well as for other members of the nuclear receptor family, are found in pairs suggests that the receptors might bind to the response elements as dimers. This has proved to be the case, although for thyroid hormone heterodimers rather than homodimers appear to be the favored form. Retinoic acid has a naturally occurring isomer, 9-*cis*-retinoic acid, which has its own nuclear receptor, termed the RXR, or retinoid X receptor. This is distinct from the receptor for all-*trans*-retinoic acid, the RAR. These retinoid receptors are discussed in detail in Chapter 30. Studies with in vitro systems have shown that, in the presence of T_3, TR–RXR heterodimers bind more tightly to TREs and confer a more robust transcriptional response than do TR–TR homodimers (Cheng et al., 2010). RXRs heterodimerize in a similarly effective way with both RARs and vitamin D receptors. Three distinct RXR genes have been discovered, and each of these generates multiple isoforms of the receptor. Given the multiple isoforms of TRs and RXRs, it appears reasonable to suppose that the combination of different receptor isoforms as heterodimerization partners would give a host of possibilities for achieving gene- and tissue-specific responses to thyroid hormone. The fact that a range of receptor heterodimers is available may also help explain why variations are observed in the response elements of target genes. The particular organization of a response element may favor a specific pair of TR/RXR isoforms.

EFFECTS ON TRANSCRIPTION

The occupation of TRs by T_3 leads to a change in the transcription rate of the target genes, although the precise way in which this occurs is not well understood. A depiction of the current model is shown in Figure 38-8. Studies in vitro have indicated that the TRs are bound to the TREs in both the presence and the absence of hormone. Therefore the hormone does not cause binding of the receptor to the target gene. Rather, T_3 binding to TR alters the interaction between this ligand-activated transcription factor and the proteins that constitute the basal transcriptional apparatus. Additional coregulatory proteins, called coactivators and corepressors, appear to mediate this linkage between the receptors and the transcriptional process (Cheng et al., 2010). The activation of transcription by T_3 is illustrated in Figure 38-8. In the absence of ligand, the TR–RXR heterodimer, bound to the response element, is associated with corepressor proteins, which mediate an inhibitory interaction with the proteins of the basal transcriptional apparatus. Addition of hormone leads to dissociation of corepressors and recruitment of coactivators, which then switches on transcription. In this model, absence of hormone is not just a lack of stimulation of transcription but actually an inhibition. In addition to direct interaction of coregulatory molecules with the basal transcriptional apparatus, evidence has accumulated that acetylation of histones may play an important role. Corepressor proteins associate not only with unliganded TR but also with proteins that are able to deacetylate histones. DNA can be wound more tightly around deacetylated histones and tends to be transcriptionally inactive. Therefore at least a part of the transcriptional inhibition in the absence of thyroid hormone may be explained by this mechanism. Coactivators, in contrast, are associated with histone acetylation, thereby opening up DNA structures and allowing transcription to occur.

Although the majority of the actions described are stimulatory, transcription can be either stimulated or inhibited by T_3, depending on the target gene. The autoregulation of thyroid hormone status itself is an example of negative transcriptional

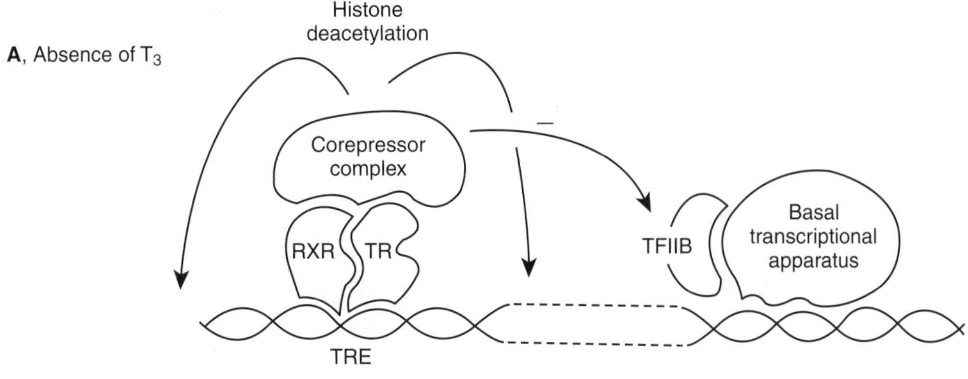

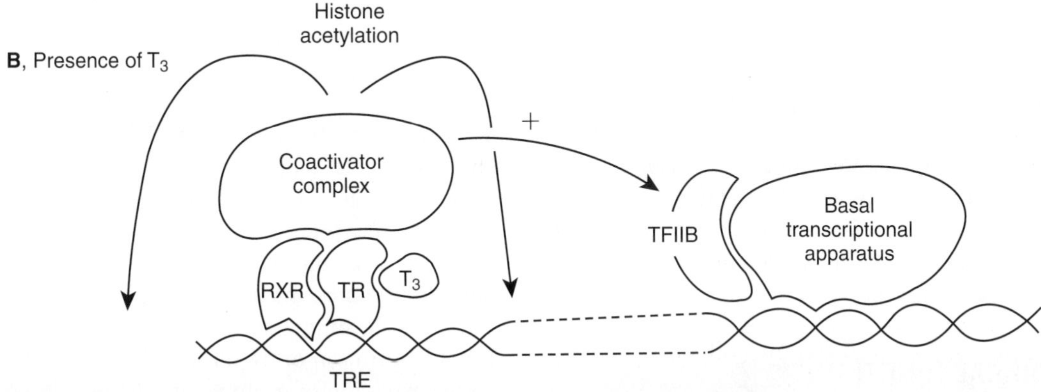

FIGURE 38-8 Thyroid hormone action in the nucleus. A heterodimer between a thyroid hormone receptor (*TR*) and a retinoid X receptor (*RXR*) binds to the thyroid hormone response element (*TRE*) of target genes. **A,** In the absence of T_3, this dimer is associated with a corepressor protein, which is part of a complex that has histone deacetylase activity. This complex also interacts with the basal transcriptional apparatus through one of its associated proteins, transcription factor IIB (*TFIIB*), and inhibits transcription. **B,** In the presence of T_3, a coactivating complex replaces the corepressor. This results in histone acetylation and initiation of transcription. The dotted lines between the two portions of the DNA indicate that TREs are often far upstream of the transcriptional start site, requiring folding of the DNA to bring the two regions together.

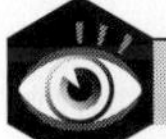

NUTRITION INSIGHT

Spot 14: A Model Thyroid Hormone-Responsive Gene

A key metabolic target for T_3 is the liver. In 1981 Oppenheimer, Towle, and co-workers sought to identify hepatic gene products that changed in abundance in response to thyroid hormone status (Seelig et al., 1981). Attention was particularly focused on one product, called spot 14 or S14, and a cDNA encoding this product was isolated. The identity of the S14 protein was and still is unknown, but T_3 treatment results in a rapid and large induction in the expression of the S14 mRNA. This stimulation occurs at the level of transcription and can be detected as soon as 10 minutes after intravenous T_3 injection into a hypothyroid rat.

It appears that S14 acts within the nucleus to coordinate the regulation of a subset of genes involved in lipid metabolism. Supporting this idea is the demonstration that specifically blocking the production of S14 protein within cultured hepatocytes also removed the ability of the cells to increase lipogenesis in response to T_3 and glucose (Brown et al., 1997). Most studies regarding the regulation of S14 have been limited to liver. The gene is expressed in several other tissues, in particular adipose tissue, and this distribution has supported a role for the protein in lipid metabolism. However, the responsiveness of *S14* gene expression to T_3 is quite tissue-specific. In contrast to liver, lung and brain do not alter either *S14* expression or lipogenesis in response to T_3 (Blennemann et al., 1995). Identifying the elements of the *S14* promoter and the nuclear proteins that interact with them to dictate this cell-specific regulation of expression is an important area of research for both *S14* and other T_3-regulated genes.

control. T_3 acts at the transcriptional level in the anterior pituitary gland to limit the production of TSH, which results in decreased production of thyroid hormones. Clearly negative regulation of gene transcription in response to T_3 must require a different relationship between TRs and coregulatory proteins from that described in the preceding text.

NONNUCLEAR PATHWAYS

The nuclear pathway for thyroid hormone action is now well established. Nonnuclear mechanisms have also been suggested, but evidence in their favor is much less complete and sometimes contradictory. The stimulatory effects of T_3 on oxygen consumption are well known, and this knowledge led to the suggestion that it might act directly on mitochondria. T_3 clearly affects mitochondrial structure and function, but it appears likely that such actions are mediated by the nuclear transcriptional pathway described previously. Binding proteins that recognize thyroid hormones have also been identified in the plasma membrane and the cytoplasm. These may serve transport functions governing the delivery of T_3 to the nucleus, rather than initiating biological functions independent of nuclear receptors. The means whereby T_3, which is not very soluble and binds easily to proteins, enters the cell and reaches the nucleus are not clear.

PHYSIOLOGICAL FUNCTIONS OF THYROID HORMONES

The physiological actions of T_3 can be divided into metabolic and developmental spheres, represented by the regulation of basal energy expenditure on the one hand and the thyroid hormone requirement for normal brain development on the other. It is interesting to note that, although these actions of thyroid hormone have been known for decades and although the molecular mechanism of T_3 action within the nucleus has been increasingly well delineated, large gaps remain in our physiological understanding of how thyroid hormone regulates these processes.

REGULATION OF BASAL METABOLIC RATE

Thyroid hormone increases oxygen consumption in all warm-blooded animals. The effect is seen in the basal portion of metabolic rate (i.e., that measured in the postabsorptive, resting state). Basal or resting oxygen consumption is reduced about 30% in hypothyroid individuals and is increased 50% in hyperthyroidism (Freake and Oppenheimer, 1995). Thus overall, basal metabolism can be doubled by alterations in thyroid state. It is generally assumed that most tissues, with the exception of brain, spleen, and testis, respond to thyroid hormone by increasing oxygen consumption. However, this is based on measuring oxygen consumption in vitro in preparations of tissue taken from animals of different thyroid states. The extent to which such measurements correspond to metabolic activity of tissues of intact animals is clearly open to question.

There is a considerable lag time following administration of thyroid hormone before an increase in oxygen consumption can be detected. This delay is approximately 1 day and is consistent with the nuclear pathway for thyroid hormone action. Appearance of the physiological effects requires the transcription of mRNAs and the translation and accumulation of the relevant proteins, a process that is likely to take hours. An early and attractive explanation for the stimulation of metabolic rate observed with thyroid hormone treatment was that the hormone acted directly on mitochondria to uncouple electron transport from ATP synthesis. Indeed, such effects could be demonstrated in vitro. However, this required very high concentrations of thyroid hormone and could not be reproduced at physiological levels. Thus this concept was discarded. More recently, it has been revived, although in different forms. Treatment with thyroid hormone produces numerous effects on mitochondria (Freake and Oppenheimer, 1995). These include induction of several components of the electron transport chain; increased activity of the ADP translocator protein, which is responsible for the import of ADP into mitochondria and therefore necessary for oxidative phosphorylation; increases in mitochondrial inner membrane surface area; and changes in inner membrane lipid composition. Some investigators believe that a considerable portion of resting oxygen consumption can be attributed to the passive leak of protons back into the mitochondrial matrix (Harper et al., 1993).

The operation of the electron transport chain is coupled to the extrusion of protons into the inter-membrane space. The inner mitochondrial membrane contains proton channels, which permit the return of these protons coupled to the synthesis of ATP. However, in addition to these channels, it has been shown that the inner mitochondrial membrane itself is not completely impermeable to protons. Moreover, such thyroid-induced effects as increased membrane surface area or changed membrane lipid composition may enhance this permeability; this could result in increased oxygen consumption without altering ATP production and thus enhance heat production uncoupled to ATP synthesis.

In addition, a role for uncoupling proteins (UCPs) in thyroid thermogenesis has been suggested (Lanni et al., 2003). UCP allows the return of protons across the inner mitochondrial membrane without the synthesis of ATP. UCP was originally thought to be confined to brown adipose tissue, explaining the heat production of that specialized tissue. It is now appreciated that there are several UCPs encoded by separate genes and expressed in various tissues. Some of these UCPs are induced by thyroid hormone and therefore could contribute to its thermogenic effects.

Although efficiency of energy production may be decreased, these effects likely account for only a part of the thyroid hormone–dependent increase in metabolic rate. Treatment with T_3 results not only in increased amounts of respiratory chain components but also in a greater state of reduction of these components. This implies an enhanced delivery of reducing equivalents to the electron transport chain and an increased production of ATP. An increased production of ATP is necessarily coupled with an increased expenditure of ATP. Otherwise respiration would be limited by a lack of

ADP. Numerous ATP-consuming processes are enhanced by thyroid hormone and collectively account for the increased load on mitochondria.

Effects on Energy-Consuming Processes

A well-known effect of hyperthyroidism is increased heart rate (Klein and Danzi, 2009). Cardiac size, stroke volume, and output are all increased. These changes may be partially attributed to direct transcriptional effects on cardiac genes, but the increased demand for oxygen delivery also plays an important role. Increased oxygen consumption overall results in an enhanced requirement for oxygen supply and therefore blood flow.

The cell membrane Na^+,K^+-ATPase is also a target of thyroid hormone action. This protein uses ATP to pump sodium out and potassium into cells, both against considerable concentration gradients (see Chapter 34). The expression of the gene encoding Na^+,K^+-ATPase is stimulated by thyroid hormone treatment, and earlier experiments suggested this could account for the major portion of increased oxygen consumption in some tissues. However, these experiments, which involved measurement of oxygen consumption in tissue preparations in vitro, have been criticized as nonphysiological. Subsequent studies in more intact systems have suggested a much more limited role for this protein, perhaps accounting for 5% to 10% of the enhanced oxygen consumption (Clausen et al., 1991).

Changes in heart rate and ion pumping provide only a partial explanation for the thyroid hormone–dependent increase in ATP consumption. Stimulation of fat, carbohydrate, and protein metabolism by T_3 also increases requirements for ATP, and these effects are discussed in the next section.

REGULATION OF MACRONUTRIENT METABOLISM

The nutritional significance of iodine and thyroid hormones is magnified by the fact that T_3 regulates the metabolism of all the macronutrients. An unusual characteristic of this regulation is that it operates on both the anabolic and the catabolic arms of these pathways to increase substrate cycling. Although construction and destruction of macromolecules may appear to be wasteful, it is completely consistent with the central role of thyroid hormones to generate heat for the maintenance of body temperature.

Lipids

Thyroid hormone stimulates fatty acid synthesis by enhancing expression of the genes involved in this process. The principal target is liver, but smaller inductions also occur in other tissues. The target genes, which respond in a coordinated fashion, include acetyl-CoA carboxylase and fatty acid synthase, which are directly responsible for assembling the carbon skeleton of palmitate. Target genes are also enzymes of the hexose monophosphate shunt and malic enzyme, which generate the required reducing equivalents as NADPH that are needed for lipid synthesis. The esterification of fatty acids into triacylglycerols and phospholipids is also increased by T_3 (see Chapter 16 for details of lipid metabolism).

Thyroid hormone also enhances lipolysis, probably by increasing the sensitivity of adipose cells to circulating catecholamines. The fatty acids released are also oxidized at an enhanced rate. This is because thyroid hormone also stimulates the expression of carnitine palmitoyltransferase, the protein that governs the entry of fatty acids into the mitochondria for β-oxidation. Many of these pathways of lipid metabolism are counter-regulated. For example, the activity of carnitine palmitoyltransferase is inhibited by malonyl-CoA, the product of acetyl-CoA carboxylase, which catalyzes the first step of fatty acid synthesis. Similarly, long-chain fatty acids, which are elevated in catabolic states, inhibit the activity of acetyl-CoA carboxylase and therefore limit fatty acid synthesis. This counter-regulation is overcome by effects of thyroid hormone to increase the expression of the genes encoding these enzymes. The increased enzyme mass then allows greater flux through both pathways, despite their normal reciprocal regulation.

An inverse relationship between thyroid hormone status and serum cholesterol levels is a feature of thyroid disease well known to clinicians. Regulation of cholesterol metabolism is also an example of the double action of thyroid hormone. T_3 treatment increases the levels of mRNA encoding the hydroxymethylglutaryl-CoA reductase enzyme, thereby increasing cholesterol synthesis. However, T_3 also increases the expression of cell surface low-density lipoprotein (LDL) receptors expressed in fibroblasts, liver, and other tissues. LDL receptor levels are regulated by negative feedback in the presence of high intracellular cholesterol levels. This is mediated through the sterol regulatory element-binding protein-2 (SREBP-2), which is directly regulated by T_3. Thus, thyroid hormone promotes a decrease in plasma cholesterol levels, despite its positive effect on hepatic cholesterol synthesis. Beneficial effects of thyroid hormone on reverse cholesterol transport, as illustrated in Figure 38-9, and also on weight loss have led to an active search for TRβ selective analogs that might activate these pathways while leaving heart rate unaffected (Baxter and Webb, 2009).

Carbohydrates

Hyperthyroidism increases and hypothyroidism decreases substrate cycling through multiple pathways of glucose metabolism. Both glycolysis and gluconeogenesis are stimulated by thyroid hormone. Glycogen stores are depleted in the hyperthyroid state, which further emphasizes the importance of lipid stores to meet the energy demands under this condition. It seems reasonable to suppose that these effects are mediated by transcriptional regulation of the enzymes involved. Perhaps the most investigated step in this context is phosphoenolpyruvate carboxykinase, which plays a key regulatory role in gluconeogenesis. Treatment with thyroid hormone stimulates transcription of this gene, at least in the rat, and a TRE has been identified in its promoter.

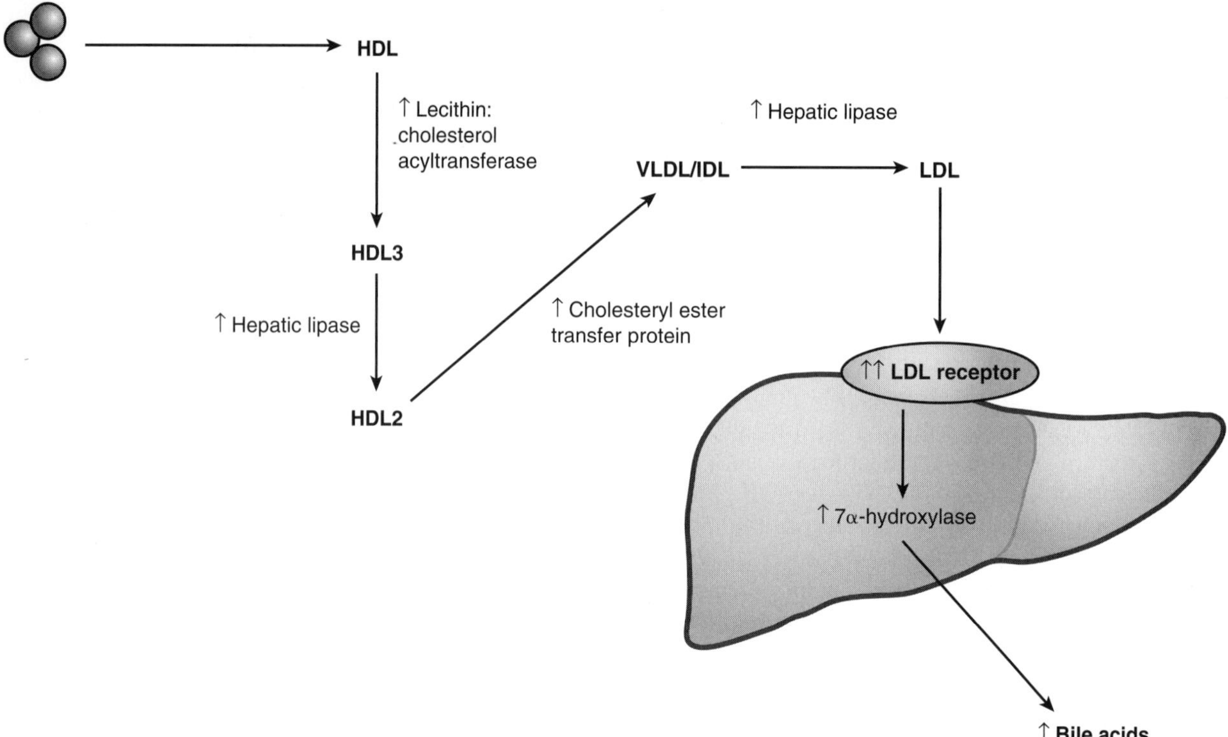

FIGURE 38-9 Thyroid hormone affects multiple steps in the reverse transport of cholesterol, or cholesterol efflux and excretion. Thyroid hormone increases expression of cholesteryl ester transfer protein, hepatic lipase, lecithin:cholesterol acyltransferase, and 7α-hydroxylase. Because thyroid hormone increases low-density lipoprotein (LDL) receptor expression in liver and increases loss of cholesterol in bile as bile acids, the net effect of thyroid hormone is to decrease plasma cholesterol levels.

Proteins

Protein turnover is also sensitive to thyroid state. Less is known about T_3 regulation of these pathways in comparison with those involving the other macronutrients. Hyperthyroidism leads to a generalized increase in RNA synthesis in both cardiac and skeletal muscle, which in turn accelerates protein synthesis. However, muscle mass has been shown to be decreased in the thyrotoxic state, so that, as with lipid and carbohydrate metabolism, the overall effect of elevated T_3 is catabolic.

The pathways underlying the thermogenic effects of thyroid hormone are summarized in Figure 38-10. Many specifics, including the relative contributions of these various components and of different organ systems to the overall effect, remain to be determined.

REGULATION OF GROWTH AND DEVELOPMENT

It is quite clear that T_3 stimulates transcription of the growth hormone gene in the rat, and indeed this system has been widely used as a model for the regulation of gene expression by thyroid hormone. The situation is less clear in humans, and attempts to demonstrate responsiveness of the human growth hormone gene to T_3 have yielded mixed results. However, it appears that growth hormone secretion is impaired in hypothyroid individuals, as is signaling through the insulin-like growth factor-1 pathway. Therefore T_3 does appear to be necessary for normal growth hormone activity in humans. The effects of thyroid hormone on growth and development, at the level of a particular tissue or organ system, are the aggregate of direct T_3 effects and of those produced by growth hormone as well as by other secondary signals influenced by thyroid state.

Brain Development

The brain has traditionally represented a fascinating conundrum to investigators of thyroid hormone action. On the one hand, the devastating effects of a lack of thyroid hormones are all too apparent in the syndrome of cretinism (discussed in the next section). On the other hand, the brain is one of the few organs that do not appear to respond to thyroid hormone in terms of alterations in metabolic rate. This illustrates the separation between the metabolic and developmental aspects of T_3 action.

Much of the work looking at thyroid hormones and brain development has been done in rodents. This is appropriate as long as it is appreciated that the chronology of brain development in these animals differs from that in humans. Although, of course, the human time line is much longer than that of the rat, brain development in the rat occurs relatively late so that more neurogenesis occurs postnatally. In humans, most neuronal cell division is complete at birth. However, the development of these neurons, including axonal outgrowth and synaptogenesis, continues into the first 2 years of life, as does the production of glial cells and the process

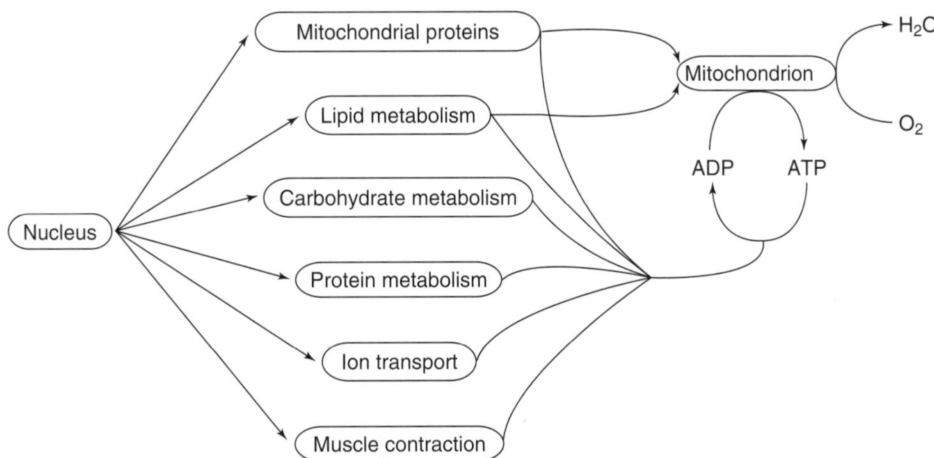

FIGURE 38-10 Mechanisms underlying the stimulation of oxygen consumption by thyroid hormone. T_3, acting via its nuclear receptors, regulates the levels of proteins required for the synthesis and breakdown of macronutrients, for ion transport, and for muscle contraction. Both the synthesis and the operation of these proteins consume ATP and therefore stimulate respiration. Thyroid hormone also affects mitochondrial function by changing the membrane lipid composition and by altering the level of mitochondrial proteins encoded by both the mitochondrial and the nuclear genomes. (Modified from Freake, H. C., & Oppenheimer, J. H. [1995]. Thermogenesis and thyroid function. *Annual Review of Nutrition, 15*, 263–291. Copyright 1995 by Annual Reviews Inc.)

of myelinogenesis. These processes (i.e., the development of appropriate brain architecture and organization) are thyroid hormone–dependent. The effects are likely mediated by the nuclear pathway at the transcriptional level. A growing list of gene targets has been identified, including those encoding myelin basic protein, cytoskeletal components, and various growth factors (Bernal et al., 2003).

In humans, the fetal thyroid begins to function by about 20 weeks gestation. Before that time, requirements for thyroid hormone are met by placental transport of maternally synthesized T_4 (de Escobar et al., 2007). During the second and third trimesters, fetal requirements are met by a combination of fetal and maternal sources. Iodine deficiency compromises both maternal and fetal thyroid hormone synthesis. The significance of the maternal supply is indicated by comparing the consequences of iodine deficiency with those of congenital hypothyroidism. In the latter condition, the maternal iodine supply is intact and the neurological symptoms in the newborn infant are distinctly milder.

Receptors for thyroid hormone are present in fetal brain by the 10th week of gestation. It appears likely that thyroid hormone plays a role in brain development from this early point through the first 2 years of life. The consequences of deficiency at any particular time may not be reversible by later supplementation. The extent of the reversibility will depend on the timing and the severity of the deficiency. Although in some cases brain damage may not be prevented by supplementation as early as the second trimester, the effects of congenital hypothyroidism are at least partially alleviated by treatment postnatally. The routine screening of the thyroid hormone status of neonates in the United States is useful because postnatal treatment with thyroid hormones can improve the status of these infants, even though as a group they still may have learning difficulties, depending on the severity of the hypothyroidism and the time of onset of thyroid hormone therapy postnatally. Although it is clear that thyroid hormone is required for normal brain development, it is less certain whether it plays a role in the functioning of the mature brain. However, experiments with mice lacking the various TRs have suggested a role for the receptor in modulating behavior (Bernal et al., 2003).

Developmental Effects on Other Tissues

Hypothyroidism leads to reduced muscle mass and delayed skeletal maturation (Brown et al., 1981). Lung maturation in the fetus has also been reported to be dependent on thyroid hormone. The effects of thyroid state on the heart have already been mentioned, in terms of their contribution to energy expenditure. Effects on skeletal and heart muscle are mediated in part by differential effects of T_3 on the expression of the myosin heavy chain genes (Izumo et al., 1986). There are two myosin heavy chain genes, α and β, and T_3 stimulates transcription of the α form. Growth hormone also has important influences, and thus at least some of the consequences of hypothyroidism on peripheral tissues are likely to be mediated by lack of this trophic hormone.

IODINE DEFICIENCY

SCOPE OF THE PROBLEM

Iodine deficiency is classically recognized by the enlargement of the thyroid gland, known as goiter. An insufficient supply of iodine results in reduced accumulation of the mineral and diminished production of thyroid hormones. Lower plasma levels of thyroid hormones lead to an increased production of TSH by the pituitary gland. This stimulates many aspects of thyroid gland function, including the hyperplasia that leads to goiter. This chronic stimulation of the thyroid gland also causes more efficient iodine uptake. This accelerated uptake may have led to increased thyroid cancer risk in iodine-deficient

TABLE 38-1 Populations at Risk of Iodine Deficiency and Their Access to Iodized Salt

WHO REGION	% GENERAL POPULATION WITH URINE IODINE CONCENTRATION <100 μg/L*	% HOUSEHOLDS WITH ACCESS TO IODIZED SALT
Africa	41.5	66.6
Americas	11.0	86.8
Eastern Mediterranean	47.2	47.3
Europe	52.0	49.2
Southeast Asia	30.0	61.0
Western Pacific	21.2	89.5
Total	30.6	70.0

Data from Zimmermann, M. (2009). Iodine deficiency. *Endocrine Reviews, 30*, 376–408.
*2006 estimates.

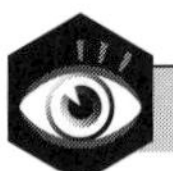

NUTRITION INSIGHT

Reemergence of Iodine Deficiency in Australia

Although Australia was historically iodine deficient, population surveys between 1985 and 1992 indicated that the country had become iodine sufficient, despite the fact that less than 10% of the population was using iodized salt. In 2003–2004, however, a national study demonstrated a reemergence of iodine deficiency. Although the reemergence of iodine deficiency was at first puzzling to public health investigators, it became clear that the replacement of iodophor cleansers by other sanitizers in the dairy industry was the primary reason for the decrease in the iodine content of Australian diet (Li et al., 2006).

Australian regulators considered mandating salt iodization, but concern was voiced over the possibility that this might encourage an increase in salt intake. Instead, regulations were established mandating the use of iodized salt instead of non-iodized salt in most bread. These regulations have been in effect since late 2009. Follow-up national surveys will be required to determine whether this measure has been successful.

individuals following exposure to radioactive iodine from the Chernobyl nuclear accident. Goiter is only one of many symptoms resulting from lack of iodide, and the broader term *iodine deficiency disorders* (IDDs) is now preferred. The WHO now assesses iodine deficiency using median urinary iodine concentrations as well as goiter rate to define population iodine status. A median urinary iodine concentration of 100 to 199 μg/L is consistent with optimal nutrition in nonpregnant populations, whereas among pregnant women a median concentration of 150 to 249 μg/L is optimal (WHO, 2007). Based on data for 2002, 35% of the world's population, or 2 billion people, were at risk for iodine deficiency (Table 38-1). Those afflicted were found in all regions of the world. IDD is widespread in areas of Southeast Asia and sub-Saharan Africa. In addition, of the 54 countries in which WHO data suggest that iodine deficiency is a significant problem, 23 are in Europe.

CRETINISM

Although goiter may be the most obvious form of IDD, the effects on neurological development are the most important. Iodine deficiency is generally considered to be the most significant preventable cause of brain damage and mental retardation in the world today. The extent of the neurological impairment depends on the timing and severity of the iodine deficiency. One critical period is the first trimester of pregnancy, when a lack of maternally supplied thyroid hormones at a time of very active fetal brain development has irreversible consequences. Severe effects of iodine lack are called cretinism and have classically been divided into two types: neurological and myxedematous. In the former, the neurological symptoms are severe and include mental retardation, deaf mutism, and motor spasticity. Myxedematous or hypothyroid cretinism has less severe neurological symptoms, but those affected are more clinically hypothyroid and growth retarded.

OTHER CONSEQUENCES

In addition to the long-term consequence of cretinism, an insufficient supply of iodine during pregnancy is also associated with an increased occurrence of spontaneous abortions, stillbirths, congenital abnormalities, and perinatal and infant mortality (Zimmermann, 2009). It is clear that profound iodine lack results in cretinism and that this damage is irreversible by later treatment with thyroid hormones. In areas of severe iodine deficiency, iodine supplementation of mothers before conception results in children with improved cognitive performance relative to those given a placebo (Pharoah et al., 1971). What is less apparent is the extent to which mild iodine deficiency causes much smaller decrements in neurological function and whether these may be reversible. A recent observational study suggested that mild to moderate maternal iodine deficiency may also be associated with attention deficit and hyperactivity disorders in offspring (Vermiglio et al., 2004).

Iodine deficiency after birth can result in hypothyroidism and goiter. Whether it also leads to impaired neurological function and, if so, whether these effects can be reversed by iodine supplementation is an open question. It used to be said that the adult brain was refractory to thyroid hormone treatment because animal studies had shown that brain was one of the few tissues in the body that did not increase oxygen consumption in response to administration of thyroid hormone. In addition, a number of morphological and biochemical parameters were identified that were sensitive to thyroid hormone in the neonatal period, but not at later times. However, with the rat as a model, some biochemical responses to thyroid hormone in adult brain have been identified and behavioral effects suggested (Bernal et al., 2003). If the adult brain is responsive, the possibility exists that milder consequences of thyroid insufficiency can be remedied at later ages.

OTHER THYROID ABNORMALITIES

Deficiencies of iodine are entirely manifested through abnormalities in thyroid hormone metabolism and function. Situations are often seen clinically, in which the latter are disordered in the face of normal iodine supply. Hypothyroidism can result from a primary defect in the thyroid gland itself (usually of autoimmune origin). Or, rarely, it may be caused by a pituitary or hypothalamic dysfunction, leading to insufficient stimulation of the gland by TSH or peripheral resistance to thyroid hormone. The latter has usually been attributed to a defect in the receptor-signaling pathway. The symptoms of hypothyroidism are fairly generalized, and most organ systems are affected. The signs and symptoms include fatigue, cold intolerance, constipation, mental slowness, reduced cardiac function, and increased serum cholesterol. Increased serum TSH is a biochemical characteristic of primary thyroid hormone deficiency, and patients are treated with sufficient T_4 to return TSH levels to the normal range.

Hyperthyroidism is most often caused by Graves disease, in which antibodies directed against the TSH receptor result in a continuous stimulation of the thyroid gland and overproduction of thyroid hormones. Like all autoimmune diseases, this is more often seen in women. Hyperthyroidism can also commonly result from hyperfunctioning thyroid adenomas or thyroiditis. The signs and symptoms include weight loss, heat intolerance, tachycardia, muscular tremor, irritability, and nervousness. Enlargement of the thyroid may be present. Treatment of Graves disease or hyperfunctioning adenomas is by antithyroid drugs, radioactive iodine to cause necrosis of the thyroid cells, or surgical thyroidectomy. The latter two treatments can result in hypothyroidism, which requires that the patient be treated with thyroid hormone replacement.

PREVENTION

Iodine deficiencies can be combated by programs directed at the whole population or targeted at those particularly at risk. Iodization of salt represents a simple, inexpensive, and effective measure to supply iodine to a population, and there are numerous examples of it being used to eliminate IDD. Either potassium iodide or potassium iodate (which is more stable) can be used. However, the high prevalence of IDD in the face of the decades-old knowledge of how to prevent the condition shows that reality is more complex. The amount of iodized salt required is enormous, and its distribution to many of the communities at risk is very difficult. Most if not all populations in the world use salt and so have developed their own local means to produce it. The introduction of iodized salt therefore either means replacing the local product with potentially unacceptable, centrally produced iodized salt or putting the technology in place to allow fortification locally. Ensuring a stable and reliable supply of iodized salt may be very difficult or impossible using the latter approach. Despite these difficulties, the WHO now estimates that 70% of the world's population consumes iodized salt (Table 38-2). Fortification of other foods (e.g., bread) has been attempted, often with success, but it is unlikely that this would have as widespread applicability as salt supplementation programs.

TABLE 38-2 World Health Organization Guidelines for Population Urinary Iodine Concentrations

IODINE INTAKE CATEGORY	Median Urinary Iodine Concentration (µg/L) NONPREGNANT ADULTS	PREGNANT WOMEN
Insufficient	<100	<150
Adequate	100–199	150–249
More than adequate	200–299	250–499
Excessive	>299	≥500

Data from WHO. (2007). *Assessment of the iodine deficiency disorders and monitoring their elimination: A guide for programme managers* (3rd ed.). Geneva, Switzerland: WHO.

In areas where universal salt iodization cannot be achieved, the most common vehicle used for delivery of iodine is iodized oil (WHO, 2007). The fatty acids of the oil are chemically modified by iodination and, once inside the body, the iodine is slowly released over a period of months to years. Injection of the oil is the usual route of administration; oral preparations, which are cheaper but less effective, are also available. These treatments are most often used in remote areas, where interactions with health services are rare and introduction of iodized salt is problematic. They permit the supply of iodine to those segments of the population who are particularly at risk (i.e., women of child-bearing age, infants, and children).

EFFECTS OF IODINE EXCESS

In the 1940s Wolff and Chaikoff reported that high iodide exposure in rats resulted in a transient inhibition of thyroid hormone synthesis lasting approximately 24 hours (acute

Wolff–Chaikoff effect) but that normal thyroid hormone synthesis resumed with continued administration of iodide. This phenomenon is sometimes described as an escape from or adaptation to the acute Wolff–Chaikoff effect—hypothyroidism following administration of iodine or iodide (Wolff and Chaikoff, 1948). The mechanism responsible for the acute Wolff–Chaikoff effect may be the generation of intrathyroidal iodolactones or iodolipids, which inhibit thyroid peroxidase activity. Escape from the acute Wolff–Chaikoff effect occurs through an inhibition of NIS synthesis, which then causes a reduction in intrathyroidal iodine and a consequent decrease in levels of the iodine-induced inhibitors of hormone synthesis (Eng et al., 1999). Failure to escape from the Wolff–Chaikoff effect results in iodine-induced hypothyroidism upon exposure to large amounts of iodine. Risk factors for iodine-induced hypothyroidism include underlying thyroid autoimmunity such as Hashimoto's thyroiditis or a history of partial thyroidectomy.

Another phenomenon that occurs in response to administration of iodine or iodide is called the Jöd–Basedow phenomenon. The Jöd–Basedow phenomenon refers to the iodine-induced hyperthyroidism that occurs when a person with a chronically iodide-deficient thyroid gland is suddenly exposed to iodine, resulting in overproduction of thyroid hormones. The Jöd–Basedow phenomenon typically occurs when an individual who lives in an iodine-deficient area with endemic goiter relocates to an iodine-abundant geographical area, is given a dietary supplement of iodide, is given iodine as contrast medium for radiographic procedures, or is given amiodarone, an antiarrhythmic medication that is 37% iodine by weight. Transient increases in rates of hyperthyroidism have been reported in historically iodine-deficient regions with the initiation of salt iodization.

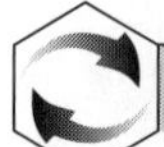

DRIs Across the Life Cycle: Iodine

	μg Iodine per Day	
Infants	RDA	UL
0 through 6 mo	110 (AI)	ND
7 through 12 mo	130 (AI)	ND
Children		
1 through 3 yr	90	200
4 through 8 yr	90	300
9 through 13 yr	120	600
14 through 18 yr	150	900
Adults		
≥19 yr	150	1,100
Pregnant	220	1,100
Lactating	290	1,100

Data from IOM. (2006). In J. J. Otten, J. P. Hellwig, & L. D. Meyers (Eds.), *Dietary Reference Intakes: The essential guide to nutrient requirements.* Washington, DC: The National Academies Press.
AI, Adequate Intake; *DRI*, Dietary Reference Intake; *ND*, not determinable; *RDA*, Recommended Dietary Allowance; *UL*, Tolerable Upper Intake Level.

DIETARY RECOMMENDATIONS, DIETARY INTAKE, AND TOXICITY

DIETARY REQUIREMENTS AND RECOMMENDATIONS

The Institute of Medicine (IOM, 2001) set the Estimated Average Requirement (EAR) for iodine at 95 μg for both male and female adults; the Recommended Dietary Allowance (RDA) for iodine was set as the EAR × 40%, rounded to the nearest 50 μg, and is 150 μg for both male and female adults. These values for adults are based on measurements of radioiodine turnover in a range of studies. The EAR for pregnant women was increased by 65 μg/day based on thyroid iodine content of the newborn and iodine balance studies; therefore the EAR and RDA for pregnant women are 160 and 220 μg/day of iodine, respectively. The EAR for lactating women is increased to allow for the average daily loss of iodine in human milk, approximately 114 μg/day; the EAR and RDA for lactating women are 209 and 290 μg/day of iodine, respectively. EARs and RDAs for children from 9 through 18 years of age were extrapolated down from adult data on the basis of metabolic body weight ($kg^{0.75}$); the EAR and RDA for children ages 9 through 13 years is 73 μg/day and 120 μg/day, respectively. For children ages 14 through 18 years, the EAR is 95 μg/day and the RDA is 150 μg/day. EARs and RDAs for children aged 1 through 8 years were based on balance study data; the EAR for this age-group is 65 μg/day and the RDA is 90 μg/day.

Adequate Intakes (AIs) were estimated for infants; the AI for infants from 0 through 6 months of age was based on the average iodine intake from human milk (146 μg/L × 0.78 L/day), and the AI for 7- through 12-month-old infants was extrapolated from the value for younger infants. Interestingly, the AIs for infants are greater than the RDAs for 1- through 3-year-olds (90 μg/day). This reflects the different methodologies used to calculate these values, rather than a true difference in requirements.

DIETARY INTAKE

Surveillance of urinary iodine values of the U.S. population has been carried out at intervals since 1971. Following a precipitous drop in urinary iodine values between NHANES I (1971–1974) and NHANES III (1988–1994), U.S. dietary iodine intake appears to have stabilized. Major contributors to U.S. iodine intake are iodized salt, which contains 76 μg of iodine per gram, and also the use of iodates in bread production (as dough improvers) and in dairy production (iodine-based antiseptics) (Pearce, 2008). The Total Diet Study (2003–2006) estimated average intakes from 138 to 353 μg/day in the United States.

TOXICITY

The IOM (2001) established a Tolerable Upper Intake Level (UL) for iodine. This was based on the amount of iodine that causes an elevated TSH concentration, which is an indicator for increased risk of developing hypothyroidism. The UL for adults is 1,100 μg/day of iodine. Those for children range from 200 μg/day of iodine for 1- to 3-year-old children up to 900 μg/day for adolescents.

THINKING CRITICALLY

1. Although rare, families have been described in which members have a hereditary resistance to thyroid hormone (decreased responsiveness of target tissue to thyroid hormone). What would you expect to be the clinical consequences of this disorder?
2. Assuming that infants are screened and treated for hypothyroidism at birth, which scenario might be expected to have the most severe consequences for fetal neurodevelopment: fetal thyroid agenesis (absence of the fetal thyroid), maternal iodine deficiency during pregnancy, or maternal hypothyroidism in an iodine sufficient mother?
3. In general, a single hormone is either anabolic or catabolic. Anabolic and catabolic pathways tend to be counter-regulated, so that activation of one is associated with inhibition of the other. Thyroid hormone breaks both of these rules. How and why?

REFERENCES

Aranda, A., & Pascual, A. (2001). Nuclear hormone receptors and gene expression. *Physiological Reviews, 81*, 1269–1304.

Baxter, J. D., & Webb, P. (2009). Thyroid hormone mimetics: Potential applications in atherosclerosis, obesity and type 2 diabetes. *Nature Reviews. Drug Discovery, 8*, 308–320.

Bernal, J., Guadano-Ferraz, A., & Morte, B. (2003). Perspectives in the study of thyroid hormone action on brain development and function. *Thyroid, 13*, 1005–1012.

Bianco, A. C., Salvatore, D., Gereben, B., Berry, M. J., & Larsen, P. R. (2002). Biochemistry, cellular and molecular biology, and physiological roles of the iodothyronine deiodinases. *Endocrine Reviews, 23*, 38–89.

Blennemann, B., Leahy, P., Kim, T.-S., & Freake, H. C. (1995). Tissue-specific regulation of lipogenic mRNAs by thyroid hormone. *Molecular and Cellular Endocrinology, 110*, 1–8.

Blount, B. C., Valentin-Blasini, L., Osterloh, J. D., Mauldin, J. P., & Pirkle, J. L. (2007). Perchlorate exposure of the US population, 2001–2002. *Journal of Exposure Science and Environmental Epidemiology, 17*, 400–407.

Brown, J. G., Bates, P. C., Holliday, M. A., & Millward, D. J. (1981). Thyroid hormones and muscle protein turnover. *The Biochemical Journal, 194*, 771–782.

Brown, S. B., Maloney, M., & Kinlaw, W. B. (1997). "Spot 14" protein functions at the pretranslation level in the regulation of hepatic metabolism by thyroid hormone and glucose. *The Journal of Biological Chemistry, 272*, 2163–2166.

Cheng, S. Y., Leonard, J. L., & Davis, P. J. (2010). Molecular aspects of thyroid hormone action. *Endocrine Reviews, 31*, 139–170.

Clausen, T., Van Hardeveld, C., & Everts, M. E. (1991). Significance of cation transport in control of energy metabolism and thermogenesis. *Physiological Reviews, 71*, 733–774.

de Escobar, G. M., Obregón, M. J., & del Rey, F. E. (2007). Iodine deficiency and brain development in the first half of pregnancy. *Public Health Nutrition, 10*, 1554–1570.

Eng, P. H., Cardona, G. R., Fang, S. L., Previti, M., Alex, S., Carrasco, N., ... Braverman, L. E. (1999). Escape from the acute Wolff-Chaikoff effect is associated with a decrease in thyroid sodium/iodide symporter messenger ribonucleic acid and protein. *Endocrinology, 140*, 3404–3410.

Environmental Protection Agency. (2011). Drinking water: Regulatory determination on perchlorate. *Federal Register, 76*, 7762–7767.

Freake, H. C., & Oppenheimer, J. H. (1995). Thermogenesis and thyroid function. *Annual Review of Nutrition, 15*, 263–291.

Harper, M. E., Ballantyne, J. S., Leach, M., & Brand, M. D. (1993). Effects of thyroid hormone on oxidative phosphorylation. *Biochemical Society Transactions, 21*, 785–792.

Heuer, H., & Visser, T. J. (2009). Minireview: Pathophysiological importance of thyroid hormone transporters. *Endocrinology, 150*, 1078–1083.

Institute of Medicine. (2001). *Dietary Reference Intakes for vitamin A, vitamin K, arsenic, boron, chromium, copper, iodine, iron, manganese, molybdenum, nickel, silicon, vanadium, and zinc.* (pp. 258–289). Washington, DC: National Academy Press.

Izumo, S., Nadal-Ginard, B., & Mahdavi, V. (1986). All members of the MHC multigene family respond to thyroid hormone in a highly tissue-specific manner. *Nature, 231*, 557–560.

Klein, I., & Danzi, S. (2009). Thyroid disease and the heart. *Circulation, 116*, 1725–1735.

Kopp, P., Pesce, L., & Solis, S. J. (2008). Pendred syndrome and iodide transport in the thyroid. *Trends in Endocrinology and Metabolism, 19*, 260–268.

Lanni, A., Moreno, M., Lombardi, A., & Goglia, F. (2003). Thyroid hormone and uncoupling proteins. *FEBS Letters, 543*, 5–10.

Lazar, M. A. (1993). Thyroid hormone receptors: Multiple forms, multiple possibilities. *Endocrine Reviews, 14*, 184–193.

Li, M., Waite, K. V., Ma, G., & Eastman, C. J. (2006). Declining iodine content of milk and re-emergence of iodine deficiency in Australia. *The Medical Journal of Australia, 184*, 307.

Marine, D., & Kimball, O. P. (1917). The prevention of simple goiter in man. *The Journal of Laboratory and Clinical Medicine, 3*, 40–48.

Markel, H. (1987). "When it rains it pours": Endemic goiter, iodized salt, and David Murray Cowie, MD. *American Journal of Public Health, 77*, 219–229.

Pearce, E. N. (2008). U.S. iodine nutrition: Where do we stand? *Thyroid, 18*, 1143–1145.

Pearce, E. N., Lazarus, J. H., Smyth, P. P., He, X., Dall'amico, D., Parkes, A. B., ... Braverman, L. E. (2010). Perchlorate and thiocyanate exposure and thyroid function in first-trimester pregnant women. *The Journal of Clinical Endocrinology and Metabolism, 5*, 3207–3215.

Pearce, E. N., Pino, S., He, X., Bazrafshan, H. R., Lee, S. L., & Braverman, L. E. (2004). Sources of dietary iodine: Bread, cows' milk, and infant formula in the Boston area. *The Journal of Clinical Endocrinology and Metabolism, 89*, 3421–3424.

Pharoah, P. O. D., Buttfield, I. H., & Hetzel, B. S. (1971). Neurological damage to the fetus resulting from severe iodine deficiency during pregnancy. *Lancet, 1*, 398–410.

Royaux, I. E., Suzuki, K., Mori, A., Katoh, R., Everett, L. A., Kohn, L. D., & Green, E. D. (2000). Pendrin, the protein encoded by the Pendred syndrome gene (PDS), is an apical porter of iodide in the thyroid and is regulated by thyroglobulin in FRTL-5 cells. *Endocrinology, 141*, 839–845.

Sap, J., Munoz, A., Damm, K., Goldberg, Y., Ghsydael, J., Leutz, A., ... Vennstrom, B. (1986). The c-erb-A protein is a high affinity receptor for thyroid hormone. *Nature, 324*, 635–640.

Seelig, S., Liaw, C., Towle, H. C., & Oppenheimer, J. H. (1981). Thyroid hormone attenuates and augments hepatic gene expression at a pretranslational level. *Proceedings of the National Academy of Sciences of the United States of America, 78*, 4733–4737.

Vermiglio, Z. F., Lo Presti, V. P., Moleti, M., Sidoti, M., Tortorella, G., Scaffidi, G., ... Trimarchi, F. (2004). Attention deficit and hyperactivity disorders in the offspring of mothers exposed to mild-moderate iodine deficiency: A possible novel iodine deficiency disorder in developed countries. *The Journal of Clinical Endocrinology and Metabolism, 89*, 60454–60460.

Weinberger, C., Thompson, C. C., Ong, E. S., Lebo, R., Gruol, D. J., & Evans, R. M. (1986). The c-erb-A gene encodes a thyroid hormone receptor. *Nature, 324*, 641–646.

Wolff, J., & Chaikoff, I. L. (1948). Plasma inorganic iodide as a homeostatic regulator of thyroid function. *The Journal of Biological Chemistry, 174*, 555–564.

World Health Organization. (2007). *Assessment of the iodine deficiency disorders and monitoring their elimination: A guide for programme managers* (3rd ed.). Geneva: WHO.

Zimmermann, M. (2009). Iodine deficiency. *Endocrine Reviews, 30*, 376–408.

RECOMMENDED READINGS

Cheng, S. Y., Leonard, J. L., & Davis, P. J. (2010). Molecular aspects of thyroid hormone action. *Endocrine Reviews, 31*, 139–170.

Freake, H. C., & Oppenheimer, J. H. (1995). Thermogenesis and thyroid function. *Annual Review of Nutrition, 15*, 263–291.

Zimmermann, M. (2009). Iodine deficiency. *Endocrine Reviews, 30*, 376–408.

RECOMMENDED WEBSITES

International Council for the Control of Iodine Deficiency Disorders. Links to website of ICCIDD, formed in 1985, the only international organization specifically constituted to promote optimal iodine nutrition and the elimination of iodine deficiency disorders (IDD). *http://www.iccidd.org*

National Institutes of Health Office of Dietary Supplements. Iodine fact sheet is available at *http://ods.od.nih.gov/factsheets/Iodine-HealthProfessional*

World Health Organization. Links to WHO publications and data on iodine deficiency disease throughout the world. *http://www.who.int/vmnis/iodine/en*

CHAPTER 39

Selenium

Gerald F. Combs, Jr., PhD*

COMMON ABBREVIATIONS

DI	iodothyronine-5′-deiodinase
eEFSeCys	selenocysteine-specific eukaryotic elongation factor
GPX	glutathione peroxidase
Se	selenium
SECIS	selenocysteine insertion sequence
SeCys	selenocysteine
SeMet	selenomethionine
SepP	selenoprotein P
$tRNA^{[Ser]SeCys}$	tRNA for selenocysteine
TRR	thioredoxin reductase

Selenium (Se) was discovered in 1817 by the Swedish chemist Jöns Jakob Berzelius, who found the element associated with tellurium. He named the new element selenium (from the Greek word *selene,* meaning moon) because it tends to be found in the earth along with tellurium (which had been named after the Latin word *tellus,* meaning earth). Not until the late 1950s, however, was selenium thought to play a role in normal metabolism. Until that time, the biomedical significance of selenium had been recognized only for its toxic properties. In 1957 it was discovered that trace amounts of Se could alleviate necrotic liver disease and capillary leakage in vitamin E–deficient animals, suggesting that Se spared the need for that fat-soluble vitamin (Schwarz and Foltz, 1957; Schwarz et al., 1957). Research in the 1970s revealed the basis of this interaction: Se is an essential constituent of the antioxidant enzyme glutathione peroxidase 1 (GPX1) (Rotruck et al., 1973). Since that time, an increasing understanding has emerged of the metabolic functions and health implications of this trace element, now known to be an essential constituent of some 25 selenoproteins, including the GPXs, each of which contains covalently linked selenium in the form of selenocysteine (SeCys). This previously unrecognized selenoamino acid, SeCys, was found to be incorporated into the selenoproteins cotranslationally by a process signaled by the TGA codon in DNA (UGA in mRNA), which normally functions as a stop codon. Because many, if not all, selenoproteins appear to have redox functions, selenium is now regarded as being important in the metabolic protection from cellular oxidative stress. In addition, selenium has been shown to have a role in anticarcinogenesis.

*This chapter is a revision of the chapter contributed by Roger A Sunde, PhD, for the second edition.

CHEMISTRY OF SELENIUM

Selenium is in group 16 (chalcogens) of the periodic table of elements. This group includes the nonmetallic elements sulfur and oxygen in the periods above Se, and the metallic elements tellurium and polonium in the periods below. Within period 3 of the periodic table, Se lies between the metal arsenic and the nonmetal bromine. Thus Se is often considered a metalloid, having both metallic and nonmetallic properties.

Inorganic selenium biochemistry involves mainly that of its nonmetallic anionic forms Se^{2-} (selenide, -2 oxidation state, H_2Se, hydrogen selenide), SeO_3^{2-} (selenite, +4 oxidation state, H_2SeO_3, selenous acid) and SeO_4^{2-} (selenate; +6 oxidation state, H_2SeO_4, selenic acid). Selenide (mainly in the anionic form of HSe^- at pH 7) plays a pivotal role in metabolism, being the obligate precursor for cotranslational synthesis of SeCys.

The major forms of selenium in cells are the selenoamino acids, in which selenium forms covalent bonds with carbon atoms. Selenium also forms covalent bonds with sulfur atoms. The selenoamino acids include SeCys, which is encoded in a special manner by DNA/mRNA and is cotranslationally synthesized, and the selenide-containing amino acid selenomethionine (SeMet, a selenoether), which originates in plants and microorganisms that use elemental selenium in place of sulfur for synthesis of sulfur (seleno) amino acids. SeMet can be incorporated into proteins in the body nonspecifically in place of methionine (Met). The selenium compounds of greatest relevance in biology are listed in Table 39-1.

Although selenium has many similarities to sulfur, selenium compounds are more nucleophilic and more acidic than the corresponding sulfur compounds. For example the pK_{a1} of H_2Se is 3.9 compared to 7.0 for H_2S, and the pK_a of the selenol group of selenocysteine (R-SeH) is 5.5 compared to 8.5 for the thiol group of cysteine (R-SH).

Thus, whereas thiols such as cysteine (Cys) tend to be protonated at physiological pH, selenols such as SeCys tend to be dissociated under the same conditions. This may have important implications for reaction chemistry catalyzed by selenoproteins.

In addition, the higher redox potentials of selenium compounds, compared with their sulfur analogs, cause selenium metabolism to be inclined toward reduction, whereas sulfur metabolism is generally oxidative. Thus sulfide is oxidized to sulfate but selenate is reduced to selenide.

Selenite (SeO_3^{2-}) readily accepts electrons and is therefore easily reduced. At low pH, it is readily reduced by such agents as ascorbic acid and SO_2. Selenite can readily react with nonprotein thiols (e.g., reduced glutathione, GSH) or with protein-sulfhydryl groups to be reduced to selenide via sequential formation of RSSeSR products called selenotrisulfides (e.g., GSSeSG) and RSSeH products called selenodisulfides (GSSeH).

Selenate (SeO_4^{2-}) is much more resistant to reduction, and activation of selenate to adenosine-5′-phosphoselenate appears to be required as a first step in its physiological reduction.

Selenium has five naturally occurring stable isotopes: ^{80}Se, the most abundant form, along with ^{74}Se, ^{76}Se, ^{77}Se, and ^{78}Se. Some of these stable isotopes of selenium have been employed in metabolic studies in humans. These can be detected by mass spectrometry. Thirteen radioisotopes of selenium can be produced by neutron activation or radionuclear decay, and some of these have found applications as well. Because of its emission of γ-radiation and its relatively long half-life (120 days), ^{75}Se has been widely employed in biological experimentation and in medical diagnostic work. The short-lived ^{77m}Se ($t_{1/2}$ = 17.5 sec) has been used in the neutron activation analysis of Se in biological materials.

SELENIUM IN FOODS

The selenium contents of foods vary widely, primarily because of variability in the soluble selenium content of the soil for plant species and in the biologically available selenium content of livestock diets. Because of the intimate relationship between plants and animals in the food chain, the selenium contents of foods from both plant and animal origins tend to be greatly influenced by the local soil selenium environment. The major forms of selenium in soil are selenite and selenate.

Foods of all types tend to show geographic patterns of variation in selenium content reflecting, in general, local soil selenium conditions. Variation in the selenium content of foods is readily seen by comparing the selenium contents of like foods from different countries (Combs and Combs, 1986). For example, whole wheat grain may contain more than 2 to 5 mg Se/kg (air-dried) if produced in the western parts of North and South Dakota in the United States or in Saskatchewan and Alberta in Canada. However, whole wheat grain may contain as little as 0.1 mg Se/kg if produced in Kansas or New Zealand, and only 0.005 mg Se/kg if produced in Shaanxi Province, China. On a global basis, foods with the lowest selenium contents are found in the provinces of Heilongjiang, northern Shaanxi, and Sichuan in China. Ironically, foods containing the greatest concentrations of selenium have also been found in China, though in different locales.

Most of the selenium taken up by plants is incorporated into organoselenium compounds such as SeMet, Se-methylselenocysteine, SeCys, and other related metabolites (Rayman et al., 2008). The selenoamino acids are synthesized

TABLE 39-1 Biologically Important Se Compounds

OXIDATION STATE	COMPOUND	BIOLOGICAL RELEVANCE
Se^{2-}	Hydrogen selenide, H_2Se	Obligate metabolic precursor to selenoproteins
	Methylselenol, CH_3SeH	Excretory form (lung); putative anticarcinogenic metabolite
	Dimethyl selenide, $(CH_3)_2Se$	Excretory form (lung)
	Trimethyl selenonium, $(CH_3)_3Se^+$	Excretory form (kidney)
	1β-Methylseleno-*N*-acetyl-D-galactosamine	Excretory form (kidney)
	Selenomethionine, SeMet	Common food form, non-specific Se-containing proteins (e.g., albumin); metabolized to selenocysteine (SeCys)
	Selenocysteine, SeCys	Common food form; form in selenoproteins; metabolized to hydrogen selenide
	Se-Methylselenomethionine	Form in some foods; metabolized to methylselenol
	Se-Methylselenocysteine	Form in some foods; metabolized to methylselenol
	Selenobetaine	Metabolic precursor of methylselenol
	Selenotaurine	Form in some foods
Se^0	Selenodiglutathione	Reductive metabolite of selenite/selenate with anticarcinogenic activity
Se^{4+}	Sodium selenite, Na_2SeO_3	Commonly used supplement for livestock feeds and ingredient in multivitamin/mineral supplements
Se^{6+}	Sodium selenate, Na_2SeO_4	Potential food/feed supplement form

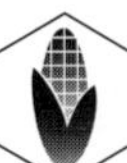

FOOD SOURCES OF SELENIUM

Nuts and Seeds
540 μg per 1 oz Brazil nuts
25 μg per ¼ cup (~1 oz) sunflower seeds

Fish, Meat, and Poultry
65 μg per 3 oz canned tuna
30 to 65 μg per 3 oz fish (swordfish, flounder, sole, halibut, or cod)
20 to 40 μg per 3 oz mollusks (oysters, scallops, or clams)
35 μg per 3 oz crustaceans (crab or shrimp)
20 to 40 μg per 3 oz pork
20 to 35 μg per 3 oz beef
20 to 30 μg per 3 oz lamb
25 to 35 μg per 3 oz turkey
15 to 25 μg per 3 oz chicken

Grains and Cereals
20 μg per ½ cup couscous, cooked
15 μg per ½ cup spaghetti or macaroni, cooked
18 μg per 1 waffle
10 μg per 1 pancake
31 μg per 1 cup cream of wheat, cooked with water
19 μg per 1 cup oatmeal, cooked in water
22 μg per 1 hard roll
11 to 14 μg per 1 English muffin
10 μg per ½ cup brown rice, cooked
6 to 7 μg per ½ cup white rice, cooked

Milk and Milk Products
18 μg per ½ cup ricotta cheese
8 to 12 μg per ½ cup cottage cheese

Miscellaneous
9 μg per ½ cup cooked mushrooms
6 μg per 1 large egg
5 to 7 μg per ½ cup beans, mature seeds (soybean, pinto, or lima, cooked)
12 μg per 1 cup soy milk

Data from U.S. Department of Agriculture, Agricultural Research Service. (2011). *USDA National Nutrient Database for Standard Reference, Release 24*. Retrieved from http://www.ars.usda.gov/ba/bhnrc/ndl

by plants and microorganisms when Se^{2-} replaces S^{2-} in the biosynthetic pathways for sulfur-amino acid synthesis. The selenoamino acids, particularly SeMet, then are incorporated into proteins. SeMet is the most abundant form of selenium in cereal grains and legumes, due mainly to the nonspecificity of the methionyl-tRNA synthetase which will use SeMet in place of Met for aminoacylation of the $tRNA^{Met}$.

Certain plant species called selenium accumulator plants, if grown on high-Se soils, can accumulate very large amounts of Se as non-protein selenoamino acids such as Se-methylselenocysteine, γ-glutamyl-Se-methylselenocysteine, and selenocystathionine. It is thought that these forms are less toxic because their formation prevents excess selenoamino acid incorporation into proteins. Se-methylselenocysteine is a major selenocompound in Se-enriched garlic, onions, broccoli florets, and broccoli sprouts, but γ-glutamyl-Se-methylselenocysteine becomes the major form when these vegetables are grown in soil with high selenium levels.

Animals ingest various forms of selenium, especially SeMet, in their diets. However, they do not have pathways for synthesis of cysteine or methionine from inorganic sulfur and hence do not incorporate large amounts of inorganic selenium into selenoamino acids. Of course, SeCys is synthesized cotranslationally in animals and is incorporated into selenoproteins at specific sites. However, animals can non-specifically incorporate SeMet from the diet into proteins in place of Met. SeMet is the dominant selenoamino acid in tissues of animals that are given high levels of SeMet in their feed, due to the nonspecific incorporation of SeMet in addition to selenoprotein synthesis. On the other hand, animals given selenite or selenate instead of SeMet incorporate selenium mostly as SeCys residues in selenoproteins because this is the only route for de novo selenoamino acid synthesis in animals. Thus, the total concentration of selenium in tissues of animals given selenite or selenate as the source of selenium is lower than that in tissues of animals given SeMet as the source of selenium. Because SeCys and SeMet are found mainly as part of proteins, the selenium content of foods tends to be correlated with protein content.

Small amounts of inorganic selenium compounds, especially selenate, are present in foods. Minor quantities of inorganic selenium are found in the drinking water, although the level depends on characteristics and the selenium concentration of the soil through which the water passes. Larger intakes of inorganic selenium occur only when selenium supplements in the form of selenate or selenite salts are taken.

The selenium content of foods of animal origin depends largely on the amount and form of selenium consumed by livestock. Food animals raised in regions with feeds of low selenium content deposit relatively low concentrations of selenium in their edible tissues and products (e.g., milk, eggs), whereas animals raised with relatively high selenium nutriture yield food products with much greater selenium concentrations, particularly if the feed contains SeMet. Because livestock need selenium to prevent debilitating deficiency syndromes, it is used as a feed supplement, usually as sodium selenite or sodium selenate, in animal agriculture in many parts of the world. This practice has reduced what would otherwise be a stronger geographic variation in the selenium content of animal food products. Within the normal ranges of selenium in livestock diets, muscle meats from most species tend to contain 0.3 to 0.5 mg Se/kg (fresh weight). Organ meats usually contain higher (4 to 15 times) concentrations of Se.

SELENIUM IN HUMAN DIETS

The average daily selenium intake of adults is estimated to vary widely among different regions. In most human diets, the dominant food sources of selenium are cereals, meats, and fish. The dominance of cereal-based foods as core

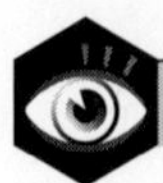

NUTRITION INSIGHT

Selenium-Accumulator Plants

Though the selenium contents of most plants generally reflect the selenium contents of the soil in which they are grown, certain species can accumulate appreciable amounts of the element. Cruciferous vegetables, for example, which are naturally rich in sulfur, can accumulate nutritionally significant amounts of selenium (up to 1 to 10 mg/kg, air-dried) if grown on high-Se soils or if fertilized with selenite or selenate salts. Others can accumulate much more selenium under such conditions. Species in the genera *Aster, Astriplex, Castilleja, Comandra, Grindelia, Gutierrezia, Machaeranthera,* and *Mentzelia* can accumulate as much as 25 to 100 mg Se/kg. Other plants in the genera *Astragalus, Machaeranthera, Haplopappus,* and *Stanleya* can accumulate hundreds to thousands of milligrams Se per kilogram. One species, *Astragalus bisulcatus,* has been found to accumulate as much as 10 g Se/kg (see Rosenfeld and Beath, 1964). Species in this latter group, referred to as Se-accumulator plants, were identified as causing "blind staggers" (a neuropathy apparently involving selenosis and, perhaps, plant alkaloids) among livestock grazing on seleniferous soils in northwestern Nebraska and western regions of North and South Dakota. Selenium-accumulator plants have been proposed for use in bioremediation of seleniferous soils.

More than a dozen selenium metabolites have been reported in the tissues of Se-accumulator plants, the dominant one being Se-methylselenocysteine (Shrift, 1969). The non-specific integration of the selenoamino acids into proteins is believed to be the major contributor of selenium toxicity in plants. The ability of Se-accumulator plants to convert these selenoamino acids into non-protein amino acids such as Se-methylselenocysteine (MeSeCys), γ-glutamyl-Se-methylselenocysteine (GGMeSeCys), and selenocystathionine reduces the incorporation of selenoamino acids into proteins and thus minimizes selenium toxicity. Non-accumulator plants, which are incapable of this metabolism, are sensitive to high soil Se levels. For this reason, the presence of Se-accumulator plants has been used to identify seleniferous rangeland.

sources of selenium means that, in many countries, selenium intakes can be affected by factors that influence the importation of grain from the world market, most of which is grown in areas of the United States, Canada, and Australia where the soil is rich in selenium.

Milk and milk products contribute small amounts of selenium to the total intake in most countries, although these foods may contribute a large proportion of total selenium intake in countries where their consumption is relatively high or where the rest of the diet provides little selenium, or both (e.g., New Zealand). Vegetables and fruits are uniformly low in selenium (fresh weight) and provide only small amounts (<8% of total Se intake) of the mineral in most human diets.

An analysis of American diets based on the U.S. Department of Agriculture 1977–1978 Nationwide Food Consumption Survey and published selenium contents of American foods revealed that a core of only 22 foods provided 80% of the total dietary selenium intake (Schubert et al., 1987). Five foods contributed half of total selenium in the "typical" American diet; these foods were beef, white bread, pork, chicken, and eggs.

The major forms of selenium in plant and animal tissues are analogs of the sulfur-containing amino acids, SeMet and SeCys. Plants tissues contain mostly SeMet, which plants synthesize. Animal and human tissues contain both SeMet obtained from dietary sources and SeCys in specific selenproteins which animals synthesize in conjunction with a specific tRNA. SeCys is the dominant form of selenium in livestock supplemented with inorganic forms of selenium.

UTILIZATION OF DIETARY SELENIUM

BIOAVAILABILITY OF DIETARY SELENIUM

The utilization of dietary selenium by the human body involves the metabolic conversion of a portion of ingested selenium to forms that can be incorporated into selenoproteins (as SeCys residues). Because most food selenium occurs as selenoamino acids in food proteins, the bioavailability of such selenium is determined in part by the digestibility of those proteins; poorly digested selenium-containing proteins, as well as dietary selenium compounds that are insoluble in the luminal environment of the small intestine, will pass through to be eliminated in the feces. Under normal circumstances, there appears to be only a small enterohepatic circulation of absorbed selenium; therefore fecal selenium constitutes mostly unabsorbed dietary selenium.

SELENIUM ABSORPTION

In general, the apparent absorption of selenium from food is efficient. Inorganic Se salts appear to be absorbed across the gut by diffusion, whereas SeMet is actively transported by the same system that transports methionine (Met). Accordingly, the enteric absorption of relatively large single doses (200 μg Se) was estimated to be 84% for selenite and 98% for SeMet (Patterson et al., 1989). The majority of selenium appears to be taken up by liver to reenter the circulation as selenoprotein P (SepP), which is essential for the normal distribution of selenium to extrahepatic tissues (Burk and Hill, 2009).

SELENIUM METABOLISM

Recognition that the metabolic function of selenium is related to that of vitamin E (α-tocopherol) emerged with the demonstration that selenium could prevent pathological conditions in vitamin E–deficient rats (Schwarz and Foltz, 1957) and chicks (Schwarz et al., 1957). From this origin came the view of selenium as an antioxidant nutrient. Indeed, combined deprivation of selenium and vitamin E yields elevated levels of products of free radical attack on polyunsaturated fatty acids that are detectable in tissues (malonyldialdehyde, F_2-isoprostanes) and exhaled breath (ethane, pentane). Thus it is clear that selenium and vitamin E function in concert in cellular antioxidant protection. In this system, α-tocopherol functions as a lipid-soluble, chain-breaking antioxidant, whereas selenium is involved as one or more SeCys residues in one or more redox-active selenoproteins. Because the physiological role of selenium is as SeCys residues in selenoproteins, an important aspect of selenium metabolism is the incorporation of dietary selenium into these selenoproteins.

Reduction of Selenate and Selenite to Selenide

The various forms of selenium that are taken up from the gastrointestinal tract are metabolized ultimately to selenide (Ganther, 1999) (Figure 39-1). For the oxidized inorganic forms, this involves reduction. Selenate is converted to selenite via activation to adenosine phosphoselenate and reduction by reactions with reduced glutathione (GSH). Selenite, whether from the diet or formed from selenate, is converted to selenide by reactions that require GSH and NADPH as reductants and involve formation of a glutathione selenopersulfide (GSSeH) intermediate.

Metabolism of Selenomethionine from the Diet

Ingested SeMet can be used in protein synthesis in place of Met, or it can be catabolized ultimately to selenide. It can charge $tRNA^{Met}$ at rates similar to that of Met (K_m values: 11 μmol/L for SeMet versus 7 μmol/L for Met) and is thus readily incorporated into proteins according to their Met contents. This nonspecific, protein-bound selenium accounts for most of the selenium in tissues (e.g., 20% to 60% of the selenium in plasma) of individuals fed normal diets containing SeMet. Metabolism of SeMet to selenide occurs by the same pathway used for the transmethylation and transsulfuration of Met to form Cys. This involves activation of SeMet to Se-adenosylselenomethionine, which in turn serves as a methyl donor and is converted to Se-adenosylselenohomocysteine. Se-adenosylselenohomocysteine is further metabolized to selenohomocysteine. Selenohomocysteine is further metabolized by the transsulfuration enzymes (see Figure 14-22 for Met metabolism Chapter 14), cystathionine β-synthase and cystathionine γ-lyase. These reactions yield SeCys, from which selenide is released by a specific γ-lyase. The SeCys produced from metabolism of ingested SeMet is not incorporated directly (i.e., nonspecifically) into proteins in animals. A third prospect for SeMet is metabolism to methylated forms and methylseleno-*N*-acetyl-galactosamine, which are excretable forms.

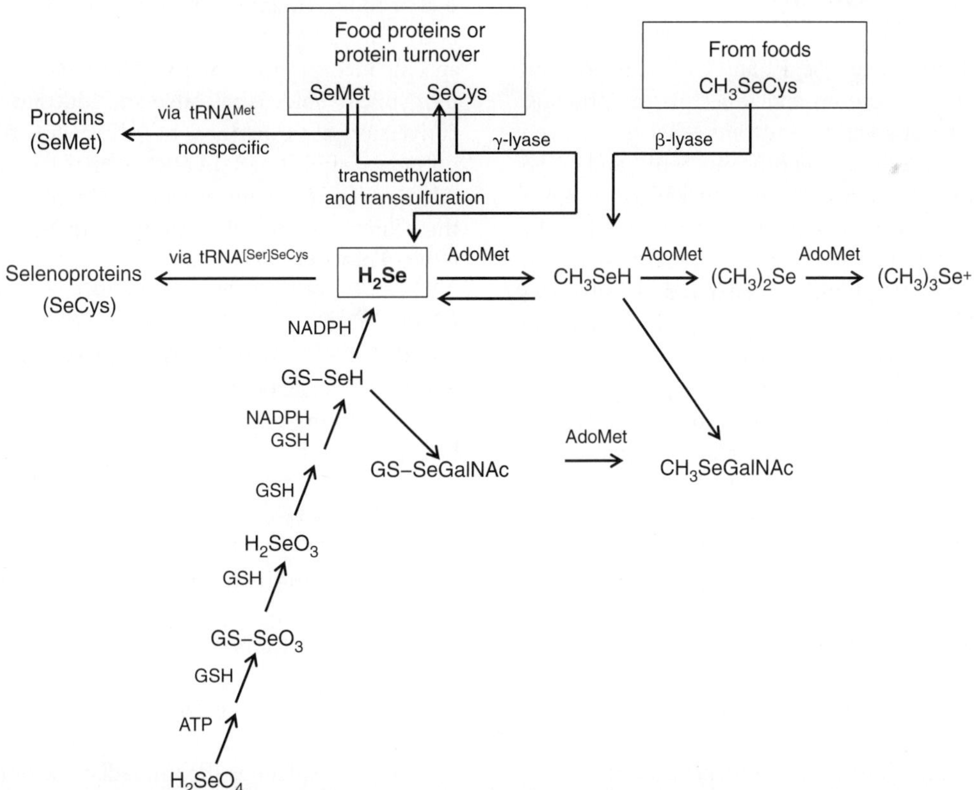

FIGURE 39-1 Selenium metabolism in humans, showing the central role of selenide as an intermediate in SeCys synthesis, selenoamino acid degradation, and Se excretion. The major forms of selenium ingested in the diet are shown in boxes. *AdoMet, S*-adenosylmethionine; *GalNAc, N*-acetylgalactosamine; *GSH*, reduced glutathione; *SeCys*, selenocysteine; *SeMet*, selenomethionine.

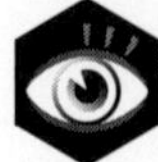

NUTRITION INSIGHT

Selenium Metabolism at a Glance

Ingested forms of Se have two fundamental metabolic fates (see Figure 39-1):

1. Nonspecific incorporation into proteins: SeMet is the major selenoamino acid non-specifically incorporated into animal proteins.
2. Conversion to selenide: This route can involve *any form of Se,* producing the obligate immediate precursor for:
   i. Biosynthesis of SeCys in the specific selenoproteins; a process that requires
      a. Five unique gene products:
         (1) Selenophosphate synthetase (SPS)
         (2) SeCys insertion sequence (SECIS)
         (3) SECIS-binding protein 2 (SBP2)
         (4) Selenocysteine-specific eukaryotic elongation factor (eEFSeCys)
         (5) SeCys synthase (SeCysS) a unique tRNA, Se-specific tRNA (tRNA$^{[Ser]SeCys}$)
      b. A specific mRNA with two unique features: a UGA codon and a SECIS element
   ii. Conversion to excretable metabolites

Use of Selenide for Selenoprotein Synthesis or Its Conversion to Excretory Forms

Selenide occupies a central position in selenium metabolism. It can be methylated to readily excretable forms by a sequential process yielding methylselenol (CH_3SeH), dimethylselenide ($[CH_3]_2Se$) and trimethylselenonium ($[CH_3]_3Se^+$). A substantial portion of selenide is converted to a selenosugar, 1β-methylseleno-*N*-acetyl-galactosamine. Selenide is also the obligate precursor for the specific incorporation of Se into the selenoproteins. This process involves the cotranslational modification of a serine (Ser) to SeCys while bound to a specific tRNA (see "Selenium Incorporation into Selenoproteins" below).

PLASMA FORMS OF SELENIUM

The circulating plasma pool of selenium comprises two functional, specific selenoproteins (SepP1 and GPX3); the general non-specific SeMet in albumin and other plasma proteins; and a small amount of selenium in forms other than amino acid residues in proteins (e.g., selenosugars). SepP1 and GXP3 accounted for about 34% and 20%, respectively, (or a total of 54%) of the total plasma selenium pool in a group of healthy adult subjects in North Dakota in the United States, a region with relatively high selenium intakes and a mean plasma selenium level of 142 ng/mL (Combs et al., 2011). The proportion of plasma selenium contributed by the two plasma selenoproteins was estimated to be slightly larger (64%) in a group of subjects with plasma total selenium concentrations of 125 ng/mL, which are closer to mean values for the U.S. population (Burk et al., 2006). Maximal expression of the plasma selenoproteins occurs at intakes yielding plasma levels above 70 ng/mL, which is close to the plasma selenium levels estimated to be contributed by maximal expression of SepP1 and GPX3. Higher intakes of foods containing SeMet result in increases in the nonspecific incorporation of SeMet into plasma proteins and thus higher plasma selenium levels. Intake of inorganic forms of selenium does not result in an increase in this component of plasma selenium because animals do not incorporate inorganic selenium into SeMet (Burke et al., 2001).

SELENIUM EXCRETION

Metabolic tracer studies have shown that over a 12-day period, Se-adequate adults excrete a total of 17% of selenium from an oral selenite dose, but only 11% of selenium from an oral SeMet dose (Patterson et al., 1989). The primary route of selenium excretion is across the kidney; the dominant urinary metabolite in individuals with low-to-moderate Se intakes is the selenosugar 1β-methylseleno-*N*-acetyl-galactosamine (Kobayashi et al., 2002). Individuals with relatively high selenium intakes may excrete other compounds such as trimethylselenonium or other selenosugars in the urine and methylselenol in the breath.

SELENIUM INCORPORATION INTO SELENOPROTEINS

Selenium is incorporated as SeCys in some 25 selenoproteins in animals (Kryukov et al., 2003). Neither SeCys from the diet or endogenous protein turnover nor SeCys formed in the body during SeMet catabolism can be used directly for the specific incorporation of SeCys into selenoproteins. Instead, inorganic selenide is activated and added in a cotranslational conversion of serine (Ser) to SeCys while the amino acid is bound to a specific tRNA (tRNA$^{[Ser]SeCys}$) (Figure 39-2). The selenium in selenoamino acids is used for selenoprotein synthesis only after the selenoamino acids have been catabolized to yield inorganic selenium.

tRNA$^{[Ser]SeCys}$

The tRNA$^{[Ser]SeCys}$ in mammals differs from other tRNAs by having 90 nucleotides (compared to the usual 76), a UCA (uracil–cytosine–adenine) anticodon sequence, 2 additional base pairs in the acceptor stem (9 compared to 7), and 11 additional bases (16 compared to 5, including 5 base pairs compared to none) in the D-loop (Carlson et al., 2006). Mammalian tRNA$^{[Ser]SeCys}$ has two isoforms arising from the same gene and differing in the modification of uridine at the 5′ position of the UCA anticodon (i.e., 5-methylcarboxymethyl uridine or 5-methylcarboxymethyl uridine-2′-*O*-methylribose). The tRNA$^{[Ser]SeCys}$ is charged with Ser at its 3′-terminal adenosine in a reaction catalyzed by seryl-tRNA synthetases, which do not distinguish between tRNA^{Ser} and tRNA$^{[Ser]SeCys}$.

Selenophosphate is the immediate Se donor for the conversion of Ser-tRNA$^{[Ser]SeCys}$ to SeCys-tRNA$^{[Ser]SeCys}$. The formation of selenophosphate is catalyzed by selenophosphate synthetase (SPS) (Salinas et al., 2006). Humans have two *SPS* genes; one encodes a selenoprotein (SPS2) and the

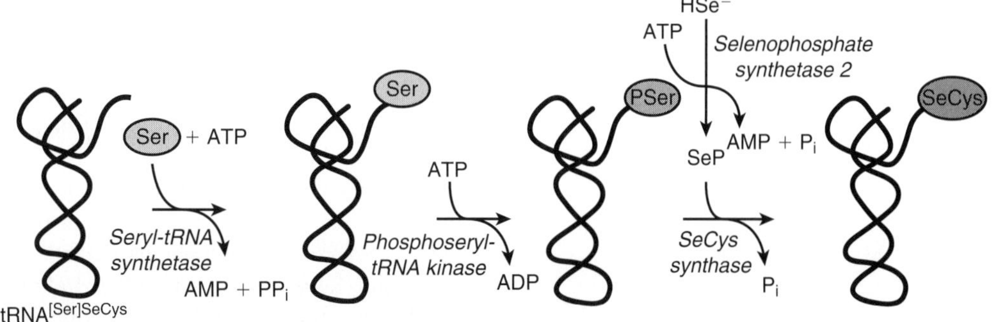

FIGURE 39-2 Cotranslational synthesis of selenocysteine (SeCys). The tRNA$^{[Ser]SeCys}$ is aminoacylated by seryl-tRNA synthetase, and then the attached serine residue is phosphorylated by action of *O*-phosphoseryl-tRNA$^{[Ser]SeCys}$ kinase. The next step involves the addition of selenide in the form of selenophosphate to the phosphoserine moiety in a reaction catalyzed by selenocysteine synthase. Selenophosphate for this reaction is formed by selenophosphate synthetase 2. *PSer,* Phosphoserine; *Sec,* selenocysteine; *Ser,* serine. Modified from Allmang, C., Wurth, L., & Krol, A. (2009). The selenium to selenoprotein pathway in eukaryotes: more molecular partners than anticipated. *Biochimica et Biophysica Acta,1790*, 1415–1423.

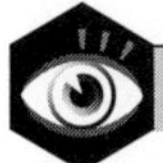

NUTRITION INSIGHT

Why Selenocysteine?

Selenoproteins are relatively rare in nature. Redox-active proteins containing Cys are far more common than those containing SeCys; indeed, Cys-analogues of most if not all selenoproteins occur. Yet, SeCys and Cys have similar chemical properties. How then does SeCys, with its energetically costly biosynthetic process, offer an evolutionary advantage over Cys in selenoproteins? Arner (2010) addressed this question. He pointed out that the common answer of its lower pK_a (~5.2 for the selenol of SeCys versus ~8.5 for the thiol of Cys), meaning that free SeCys is mainly deprotonated at physiological pH and thus more chemically reactive, may not apply to these residues in the microenvironment of the protein structure. He suggested two other features instead:

- The inherently high nucleophilicity of SeCys as compared to Cys, which gives SeCys greater initial reaction rates with nucleophiles and potentially more facile catalysis of single-electron transfers than Cys
- The lower reduction potentials of SeCys redox couples, which may facilitate the catalysis of both one- and two-electron reactions much more efficiently by SeCys than by Cys.

other encodes a non-selenoprotein (SPS1). SPS2 and SPS1 differ only in the amino acid residue at position 60 (threonine in SPS1, SeCys in SPS2). It is hypothesized that SPS1 may ensure continued synthesis of SeCys, albeit at low levels, under conditions of limited Se supply and diminished activity of SPS2. The reaction uses ATP as a cosubstrate for addition of phosphate to selenide (HSe^{2-}) to form selenophosphate ($HSePO_3^{2-}$).

The addition of selenide to the serine attached to Ser-tRNA$^{[Ser]SeCys}$ to form SeCys-tRNA$^{[Ser]SeCys}$ involves the action of two additional enzymes, a specific *O*-phosphoseryl-tRNA$^{[Ser]SeCys}$ kinase and selenocysteine synthase. *O*-phosphoseryl-tRNA$^{[Ser]SeCys}$ kinase catalyzes the phosphorylation of the serine residue of Ser-tRNA$^{[Ser]SeCys}$, and the pyridoxal phosphate-dependent selenocysteine synthase catalyzes the addition of selenium from selenophosphate to complete the conversion of the Ser attached to the tRNA$^{[Ser]SeCys}$ to a SeCys that is still esterified to the tRNA.

The UGA Codon in Selenoprotein mRNA

Each SeCys center of a selenoprotein is encoded by a TGA in the respective gene, which is transcribed as UGA in the mRNA. This phenomenon, first recognized with the sequencing of the cDNA for GPX1, was unexpected because a UGA in mRNAs typically serves as a stop codon in mammalian protein synthesis. Studies on translation of selenoprotein mRNAs revealed that the 3′-untranslated region (3′-UTR) of the mRNA was necessary for UGA-encoded SeCys incorporation. Berry and colleagues (1991) identified a consensus 87-base stem–loop element necessary for the insertion of Se in two selenoproteins of the rat (iodothyronine 5′-deiodinase-1 and GPX1). This SeCys insertion sequence (SECIS) element has been found in the 3′-UTRs of the mRNAs of all selenoproteins. Most selenoprotein mRNAs contain a single UGA codon encoding a single SeCys residue per polypeptide chain and a single SECIS element. Selenoprotein P is unique in that its mRNA encodes multiple SeCys residues and contains two SECIS elements in its 3′-UTR.

As shown in Figure 39-3, the mammalian SECIS element consists of a stem–loop structure with an apical loop and an internal loop between two helical regions (stems). The apical loop consists of 7 to 10 unpaired bases, including a consensus AA (adenine–adenine) sequence. The helix between the apical and the internal loops contains an AUGA (adenine–uracil–guanine–adenine) sequence 5′ to the apical

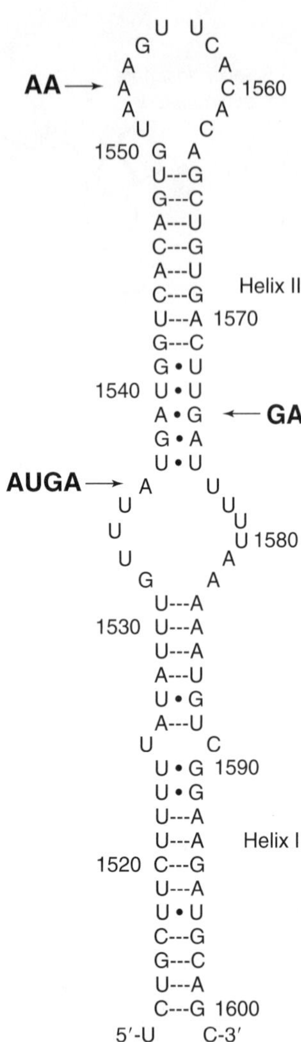

FIGURE 39-3 Selenocysteine insertion sequence (SECIS) element. Eukaryotic SECIS element that resides in the 3′-UTR of rat DI1. The AUGA...AA...GA motif is indicated. Modified from Walczak, R., Westhof, E., Carbon, P., & Krol, A. (1996). A novel RNA structural motif in the Sec insertion element of eukaryotic selenoprotein mRNAs. *RNA, 2*, 367–379, with permission from Cambridge University Press.

loop, and a GA (guanine–adenine) sequence 3′ to the apical loop. This AUGA … AA … GA motif is key to functionality, although a few mammalian SECIS elements have been found with a variant motif, AUGA … CC … GA. The conserved UGA and GA sequences form the core of a quartet motif of non–Watson and Crick base pairs (i.e., U-U and G-A), resulting in a greater than 90-degree kink in the stem–loop. Half of mammalian SECIS elements have an additional stem extending from the apical loop; it is thought that these specific secondary structures may affect the rate of SeCys insertion into various selenoproteins.

Archaea have the same SECIS element as eukaryotes. However, the prokaryotic SECIS consists of a 38-nucleotide stem–loop element located in the open reading frame of the selenoprotein mRNA immediately following the UGA codon (Bock et al., 2006). It is thought that constraints of maintaining this secondary structure may limit the capacity of bacterial genes to place SeCys at the active site of enzymes. In bacteria, a single elongation factor is required to bind the SECIS element and the SeCys-tRNA, whereas in eukaryotes and archaea, those roles are filled by different proteins: SECIS-binding protein (SBP2), which appears to bind to the AUGA/GA stem nucleotides, and a SeCys-specific elongation factor (eEF-SeCys) that partners with SBP2 for incorporation of UGA-encoded SeCys. That eEFSeCys binds to SeCys-$\text{tRNA}^{[Ser]SeCys}$ but not to Ser-tRNA^{Ser} prevents misincorporation of Ser in place of SeCys. Like other elongation factors, eEFSeCys binds GTP and is dependent upon GTP hydrolysis for activity.

This process of SeCys incorporation into selenoproteins is accomplished by a complex of these proteins on the ribosome: selenoprotein mRNA, SBP2, eEFSeCys–GTP, and SeCys-$\text{tRNA}^{[Ser]SeCys}$. The bases between the UGA and the SECIS element of the selenoprotein mRNA serve as a flexible tether, enabling the complex to orient the anticodon on the tRNA to interact with the approaching acceptor site on the ribosome. Peptide bond formation between SeCys and the nascent polypeptide is catalyzed by peptidyltransferase, as is the case for addition of other amino acids to the growing peptide chain.

THE SELENOPROTEINS

Genomic screening for selenoproteins has been accomplished by searching for conserved SECIS elements, conserved appropriate secondary structures, open reading frames containing in-frame TGA codons, and homologs in other species containing Cys (Kryukov et al., 2003). Most selenoproteins appear to be enzymes, or to have been derived from enzyme families, with their SeCys residues located in variants of the CxxC (where C = Cys and x = any amino acid) motif found in many redox proteins (Gladyshev, 2006). The selenoproteins appear to have a scattered phylogenetic distribution; most have homologs containing Cys instead of SeCys. For example, GPX6 is a selenoprotein (contains SeCys) in humans and swine but not in rodents. Other cross-species examples include methionine-*R*-sulfoxide reductase, which is a selenoprotein in green algae but not in vertebrates; and protein U, which contains SeCys in fish but exists as Cys-containing homologs in humans and worms. In general, the substitution of SeCys for Cys in the enzyme active site enhances its catalytic efficiency.

Selenoproteins are present in bacteria, archaea, and eukaryota, but not in all members of these domains. In addition, the size of the selenoproteome varies among domain members. For example, in eukaryotes, the highest number of selenoproteins is observed in aquatic organisms (e.g., more than 30 selenoproteins in many fishes and algae) whereas no selenoproteins have been identified in fungi and higher plants (Lobanov et al., 2009). In addition to use of selenium for synthesis of proteins that are translated with SeCys residues, some bacterial and archaeal cells use selenium for synthesis of selenouridine-modified tRNAs and/or post-translational maturation of selenium-molybdenum-cofactor containing enzymes such as xanthine dehydrogenase and purine hydroxylase (Haft and Self, 2008). The incorporation

TABLE 39-2 The Major Selenoproteins

SELENOPROTEIN	GENERAL FUNCTION	ISOFORMS	LOCALIZATION	SPECIAL FEATURES
Glutathione peroxidases	Antioxidant enzymes catalyzing the reduction of hydroperoxides using reducing equivalents from reduced glutathione (GSH)	GPX1	Cytosol, mitochondrial matrix space	Sensitive to dietary Se deprivation
		GPX2	Cytosol; mostly gastrointestinal cells	Relatively resistant to dietary Se deprivation
		GPX3	Plasma, milk	Sensitive to dietary Se deprivation
		GPX4	Cell membranes; mammalian sperm mid-piece	Relatively resistant to dietary Se deprivation
Thioredoxin reductases	Antioxidant flavoenzymes catalyzing the reduction of thioredoxin using reducing equivalents from NADPH	TRR1	Cytosol	
		TRR2	Mitochondria	Relatively resistant to dietary Se deprivation
		TRR3	Cytosol; mostly testes	
Deiodinases	Enzymes essential for thyroid hormone function; catalyze activation of T_4 to T_3	DI1	Cytosol; mostly liver, muscle	Catalyzes 5′-deiodination of T_4 outer ring; also can catalyze 5-deiodination of inner ring
		DI2	Cytosol; brain, pituitary, brown adipose, skin, placenta	Catalyzes 5′-deiodination of T_4 outer ring
		DI3	Cytosol; brain, skin, placenta	Catalyzes 5-deiodination of inner ring for conversion of T_3 to T_2 and T_4 to reverseT_3
Selenoprotein P	Major transporter for Se to peripheral tissues	SepP	Plasma; cytosol of most cells	Has 5–6 Se atoms per molecule
Selenoprotein W	Presumed to function in protecting muscle from oxidative damage	SepW	Cytosol; muscle, brain	Upregulated by supranutritional Se levels
Selenoprotein 15	Thought to be involved in protein folding	Sep15	Endoplasmic reticulum; most cells	A thiol-disulfide oxidase
Selenoprotein R	Reduces methionine *R*-sulfoxide (oxidized methionine)	SepR	Cytosol and nucleus; most cells	Also called methionine-*R*-sulfoxide reductase
Selenophosphate synthetase 2	Catalyzes ATP-dependent activation of selenide in the cotranslational synthesis of tRNA-bound SeCys	SPS2	Cytosol; most cells	Functions in the synthesis of all selenoproteins

of selenium into these latter compounds also appears to require the conversion of selenide to selenophosphate by selenophosphate synthetase.

The human selenoproteome consists of 25 selenoproteins broadly classified as antioxidant enzymes (Reeves and Hoffman, 2009) (Table 39-2). Of these, the first to be recognized, and thus the best studied, are the GPXs. Other well-studied selenoproteins include the iodothyronine 5′-deiodinases (DIs), the thioredoxin reductases (TRRs), and selenoproteins P (SepP) and W (SepW). Many selenoenzymes exist as multiple isoforms.

GLUTATHIONE PEROXIDASES

Most cells as well as blood plasma contain GPX (Flohé and Brigelius-Flohé, 2006). In most cases, GPX activities are reduced by selenium deprivation and restored by selenium refeeding. For this reason, GPX in accessible tissues (plasma, whole blood, buccal cells) has been used to diagnose nutritional selenium deficiency. GPXs catalyze the reduction of hydroperoxides using reducing equivalents from reduced glutathione (GSH): $2\ GSH + ROOH \rightarrow GSSG + ROH + H_2O$. There are at least six isoforms of GPX in higher animals:

- GPX1 is highly specific for GSH as the donor of reducing equivalents but can use many organic hydroperoxides (ROOH) as the acceptor substrate at rates very similar to those for hydrogen peroxide (H_2O_2). The enzyme is a homotetramer of 23 kDa subunits. Each subunit contains a SeCys residue in a UxxT amino acid sequence motif. This structure is thought to stabilize the Se atom as the attacking group through hydrogen bonding with the threonine hydroxyl group. Specificity for GSH as the donor substrate is conferred by other charged amino acids within the active site. The Se atom is essential for catalytic activity, and activity is lost if SeCys is replaced by either Ser or Cys. Knockout mice that do not express GXP1 show the normal phenotype unless they are exposed to oxidant drug stress to which their tolerance is markedly compromised (Zhu et al., 2006). Expression of GPX1 is regulated by selenium supply at the mRNA level (Sunde, 2006). Rats deprived of selenium show coordinated decreases in GPX1 mRNA, activity, and protein, but deficient rats refed with selenium show increases in mRNA prior to changes in enzyme activity. It has been proposed that selenium has a role in maintaining GPX1 mRNA stability.

- GPX2 is found primarily in gastrointestinal cells, where in the rat it constitutes more than 70% of total GPX activity. Its mRNA can also be detected in liver. The GPX2 knockout mouse is without phenotype, but the double-knockout of both GPX1 and GPX2 caused animals to develop ileocolitis by the time of weaning (Esworthy et al., 2005).
- GPX3 occurs in plasma and extracellular fluids, constituting 10% to 25% of total plasma selenium. Plasma GPX3 appears to be mostly of renal origin; dialysis patients with renal failure show very low levels.
- GPX4 is also called phospholipid hydroperoxide glutathione peroxidase. It is a monomeric, intracellular enzyme that reduces phospholipid hydroperoxides and cholesterol hydroperoxides (Maiorino et al., 1990). It is associated with cell membranes, where it is thought to detoxify hydroperoxides that would otherwise impair membrane function. It is found in mammalian sperm, where it undergoes oxidative cross-linking during maturation to comprise half of the structural material in the midpiece (Ursini et al., 1999). Knocking out GPX4 in mice is embryonically lethal (Yant et al., 2003).
- Other GPXs include a homolog of GPX3 (called GPX6), which has been identified in humans and swine where it appears to be expressed only in the Bowman gland (Kryukov et al., 2003). Cys homologs of seleno-GPXs have been identified in mammals; these include GPX5, an androgen-regulated protein secreted from the epididymis, and GPX7, a protein whose function has not been elucidated. The non–seleno glutathione *S*-transferases can also show GPX-like catalytic activity.

THIOREDOXIN REDUCTASES

The thioredoxin reductases (TRRs) are NADPH-dependent flavoenzymes that function as homodimers. Each monomer contains a flavin adenine dinucleotide (FAD) prosthetic group, an NADPH-binding domain, and a redox-active disulfide. The TRRs function in the regulation of intracellular redox state by transferring reducing equivalents from NADPH through the tightly bound FAD of the enzyme to reduce the enzyme's redox-active disulfide. The reduced TRR then transfers these reducing equivalents to the protein thioredoxin, reducing the redox-active disulfide of thioredoxin (Trx). The overall reaction catalyzed by TRR is: $NADPH + H^+ + Trx\text{-}S_2 \rightarrow NADP^+ + Trx\text{-}(SH)_2$. As the disulfide bond between the two Cys residues in Trx is reduced, the disulfide bond in TRR is reformed. The reduced Trx then serves as an electron donor for reduction of disulfides in a number of other proteins, including peroxidases and ribonucleotide reductase. The TRRs are selenoenzymes in mammals (Tamura and Stadtman, 1996), with three isoforms, each containing SeCys (U) as the penultimate amino acid adjacent to Cys (C) in a CU amino acid motif at the C-terminus. These isoforms are preferentially expressed in the cytosol (TRR1), mitochondria (TRR2), and testis (TRR3). Splicing variants also exist. Deletion of the gene is lethal in the fetal stage.

IODOTHYRONINE 5′-DEIODINASES

Selenium deprivation results in elevated circulating levels of thyroxine (T_4) with concomitant decreases in circulating levels of the metabolically active triiodothyronine (T_3). (See Chapter 38, Figure 38-1 for the chemical structures of thyroid hormones.) The observed effects of selenium deprivation on the conversion of T_4 to the active T_3 hormone led to the discovery that the enzyme responsible for this conversion is a SeCys-containing selenoprotein (Bianco and Larson, 2006). Three isoforms of iodothyronine deiodinases (DIs) are now recognized as arising from distinct genes:

- DI1 in liver, muscle, and kidney is responsible for producing more than 90% of circulating T_3. It appears to function as a 55-kDa homodimer localized in the endoplasmic reticulum (ER) of hepatic cells and in the basolateral membrane of cells of renal proximal convoluted tubules. The protein contains a single, N-terminal transmembrane segment that positions its catalytic portion in the cytosol where it catalyzes the deiodination of the T_4 outer and inner rings. It preferentially removes the outer ring 5′-iodine (I) from either T_4 or reverse T_3 (rT_3), yielding T_3 or T_2, respectively. The enzyme contains a SxxU (S = Ser, x = any amino acid, U = SeCys) amino acid motif involved in catalysis: $T_4 + 2\ GSH \rightarrow T_3 + GSSG + I^- + H^+$. This appears to proceed by a mechanism similar to that for GPX1, with the formation of an enzyme–Se-I intermediate. The enzyme also converts rT_3 to T_2 for the elimination of excess hormone from the circulation.
- DI2 catalyzes the 5′-deiodination of the T_4 outer ring. It is found in brain, pituitary, brown adipose tissue, placenta, and skin where it appears to be important for the local production of T_3.
- DI3 catalyzes the 5-deiodination of the T_4 inner ring, resulting in inactivation. It is found in brain, skin, and placenta. That it also occurs in fetal tissues (liver, muscle, brain, and central nervous system) suggests a role in protecting the fetus from the adverse effects of high levels of T_3 and T_4 by facilitating their conversion to the inactive forms, T_2 and rT_3, respectively.

This array of deiodinases facilitates the regulation of iodine metabolism (Kohrle and Gartner, 2009) and specifically the conservation of iodine during periods of deficiency. This is accomplished through the downregulation of DI1, which limits the conversion of T_4 to T_3, while still making T_4 available for activation by DI2 in key target organs. That both selenium and iodine play key roles in this system means that deficiencies of either nutrient have the potential to compromise thyroid hormone status. The combined deficiencies of selenium and iodine have been proposed as contributing to the etiology of endemic myxedematous cretinism in Central Africa (Vanderpas et al., 1990). This condition is exacerbated by supplementation with selenium alone: restoration of DI1 activity leads to increases in plasma T_3, which further reduces the concentration of T_4, the substrate for DI2 in critical endocrine tissues.

SELENOPROTEIN P

Selenoprotein P (SepP) is an extracellular selenoprotein. It is secreted within a few hours of selenium ingestion (Burk and Hill, 2009). SepP comprises 40% to 60% of total plasma selenium in individuals who are not Se-deficient. The major source of plasma SepP appears to be the liver, which contains the greatest amounts of SepP mRNA. Smaller amounts of SepP mRNA are found in kidney, heart, testis, and lung.

The mRNA for SepP differs from those of all other selenoproteins in that it contains 10 UGA codons and two SECIS elements in its 3′-UTR. Other selenoprotein mRNAs contain only a single UGA. The 10 UGAs in SepP are distributed with 1 early in the coding region for the N-terminus and 9 in the coding region for the C-terminal portion of the protein. The translated SepP has 360 amino acid residues and contains up to 10 SeCys moieties and at least 4 glycosylation sites per molecule. Purified plasma SepP has been found to contain only 5 to 6 Se atoms per molecule. This may reflect early termination at one of the later UGAs in the mRNA, resulting in smaller circulating forms. In rats, a full-length isoform of SepP along with three other isoforms that terminate at the positions of the second, third, and seventh selenocysteine residues are found, indicating that some of the in-frame UGAs code alternatively for insertion of SeCys or for termination of translation (Ma et al., 2002).

That SepP is necessary for the transport of selenium from the liver to the kidney was demonstrated by the conditional knockout of hepatic SepP in the mouse. This dramatically reduced plasma SepP and thereby plasma selenium levels and resulted in reduced selenium levels and GPX activity in the kidney (Schweizer et al., 2005). Surprisingly, brain selenium and GPX activity were not affected. Whereas the complete knockout of SepP from all tissues resulted in loss of coordination leading to paralysis and death, knockout of SepP only in liver did not result in any neurological symptoms (Schweizer et al., 2005; Burk et al., 2006). These results suggest that locally expressed SepP may be important in the retention of selenium in the brain. Tissue uptake of selenium is likely to involve the degradation of SepP to release its SeCys residues intracellularly. Immunohistochemical localization studies have shown that SepP associates with the luminal and interstitial surfaces of the vascular system; the brain is a notable exception, suggesting that SepP may not cross the blood–brain barrier.

SepP may also have a role in redox regulation. A redox role is supported by the presence of the N-terminal SeCys as a UxxC motif, which is common in redox-active selenoproteins, although this could simply indicate that this plasma protein evolved from redox-active selenoproteins. It has also been suggested that SepP may function in disulfide exchange and in metal binding, functions that could be associated with the histidine-rich regions of SepP.

SELENOPROTEIN W

Selenoprotein W (SepW) was recognized as a small selenoprotein absent from the skeletal muscles of Se-deficient lambs and calves, leading to a myopathy commonly called white muscle disease (Vendeland et al., 1995). Human SepW is an 85– to 88–amino acid polypeptide with a single UGA-encoded SeCys at residue 13 as part of a CxxU amino acid sequence motif. The purified protein is typically associated with a tightly bound GSH. Its mRNA is abundant in skeletal muscle and brain in both sheep and primates. Though SepW is presumed to function in the protection against muscle degeneration, the nature of this role has not been elucidated, although there is evidence that it responds to stress and may be involved in cellular immunity (Whanger, 2009). Hawkes and associates (2009) found that SepW mRNA is upregulated by supranutritional amounts of selenium, making it the only selenoprotein known to show a response to surplus selenium. This finding suggests a possible role of SepW in selenium anticarcinogenesis, which also involves supranutritonal selenium intakes (see section, "Selenium Anticarcinogenesis").

SELENOPROTEIN 15

Selenoprotein 15 is a 15-kDa protein, apparently expressed in all mammalian cells, with a single SeCys present in a CxU amino acid motif (Labunsky et al., 2006). The protein has an N-terminal signal peptide that directs it to the ER, where it associates with UDP-glucose:glycoprotein glucosyltransferase. Sep15 may be involved in protein folding or quality control of glycoprotein folding. Polymorphisms in the gene have been associated with differential cancer risk.

SELENOPROTEIN R

Selenoprotein R, also known as methionine-*R*-sulfoxide reductase (MsrB1), is present in the cytosol and nucleus (Kim and Gladyshev, 2004). It is a small (12-kDa) zinc-containing, thiol-dependent protein that reduces methionine-*R*-sulfoxide residues in proteins. It contains a SeCys present in a UxxS motif. Mammals have two other MsrB isoforms which contain Cys instead of SeCys; these isoforms have lower catalytic activities than the selenoprotein form. Because methionine sulfoxide is produced by oxidative attack on proteins, these reductases are essential in protecting against oxidative stress (Lee et al., 2009).

SELENOPHOSPHATE SYNTHETASE 2

As discussed previously (see "Selenium Incorporation into Selenoproteins"), one of the mammalian selenophosphate synthetases, SPS2, contains SeCys as a CxU motif. Studies in

SPS2 knockdown cells showed that reintroduction of SPS2 restored selenoprotein biosynthesis but expression of SPS1 did not (Xu et al., 2007). This study suggests that SPS2 may be essential for generating the selenium donor for selenocysteine biosynthesis in mammals, whereas SPS1 could have a different role.

OTHER SELENOPROTEINS

A number of other selenoproteins have been identified by genomic searching (Kryukov et al., 2003; Shchedrina et al., 2010):

- SepH: a nuclear-located protein with a CxxU motif. Its function is unknown.
- SepI: a protein homologous to human choline/ethanolamine phosphotransferase with seven putative transmembrane domains. In humans and mice, the SeCys is present in a SxU motif.
- SepK: a protein localized to ER and plasma membranes of mammalian cells. SepK contains a SeCys near the C-terminus with no adjacent cysteine, serine, or threonine residues.
- SepM: a protein with an in-frame TGA and SeCys is present in a CxxU motif in the N-terminal portion. This selenoprotein contains a variant SECIS in the 3′-UTR with an AUGA … CC … GA motif. It is homologous to Sep15 except that its SeCys sequence motif resembles that of SepW or SepT. SepM is localized to the ER lumen.
- SepN: a protein without homology to any other known protein. Its SeCys, present in the C-terminal half, is flanked by Cys in a CU motif similar to that in the TRRs. SepN is an integral ER membrane protein. Mutations in the *SepN* gene have been linked to various muscular disorders.
- SepO: the largest human selenoprotein (669 residues) with a single SeCys located three residues from the C terminus in a CxxU motif. Its SeCIS also has the AUGA … CC … GA motif. SepO is localized to the ER membrane.
- SepS: a protein localized to ER and plasma membranes of most cells. Its SeCys is the penultimate amino acid residue at the C-terminus in an SxxU motif. SepS is part of the ER associated protein degradation machinery that facilitates degradation of misfolded or aberrant proteins in the ER. Its expression is increased by disturbances in the ER that cause accumulation of misfolded proteins. Overexpression has been shown to increase cell tolerance to oxidative stress (Gao et al., 2004).
- SepT: a protein composed of 182 amino acid residues with SeCys in a CxxU motif. SepT is localized to the ER membrane, but its function is unknown.
- SepV: a paralog of SepW with SeCys in a CxxU motif; it appears to be expressed only in the seminiferous tubules of the testes.

SELENIUM-BINDING PROTEINS

Non-SeCys proteins capable of binding selenium have been found in cells incubated with radiolabeled selenite. These include a 56-kDa protein, referred to as SECIS-binding protein 1 (SBP1). SBP1 is regulated reciprocally to GPX1 levels. Increased expression of either SBP1 or GPX1 results in diminished levels of the other. GPX1 levels were increased and SBP1 levels were decreased by selenium supplementation of cell culture medium, and the effect of selenium on SBP1 was GPX1 dependent (Fang et al., 2010). That SBP1 and GPX1 physically interact raises the question of whether SBP1 may have a role in regulating GPX1 catalytic activity and/or turnover.

TISSUE DISTRIBUTION OF SELENIUM

The body content of selenium in adequately nourished humans was estimated to be 13 to 20 mg from analysis of cadavers (Schroeder et al., 1979) and 30 mg from metabolic studies using stable isotopic tracers (Patterson et al., 1989). Based on these reports, some 60% of total body selenium is contained in the muscles, liver, blood, and kidneys, with the skeleton accounting for 30%. Tissue selenium levels reflect selenium intakes over medium to long time frames. Differences in patterns of food consumption, which affect selenium intake, will necessarily affect tissue selenium concentrations. This is particularly true for selenium in foods, most of which is in the form of SeMet. Because of the nonspecific incorporation of SeMet into proteins during their biosynthesis, foods providing SeMet will support the nonspecific accumulation of that form in tissue proteins in humans. In contrast, the tissues of animals fed inorganic selenium salts or SeCys reflect only the contents of selenoproteins. Inorganic forms of selenium and the selenium in SeCys must to converted to selenide and then specifically incorporated into selenoproteins for these sources of selenium to appear in the proteins of humans.

Nève (1995) noted that the minimum concentration of selenium that might be expected in plasma under conditions of maximal expression of plasma GPX3 is 70 to 80 ng Se/mL. Accordingly, this level may be taken as a criterion of nutritional adequacy because it corresponds to the amount of selenium contained in maximally expressed plasma selenoproteins (Hill et al., 1996).

NUTRITIONAL ESSENTIALITY OF SELENIUM

SELENIUM DEFICIENCY IN ANIMALS

Selenium was not recognized as an essential nutrient until the 1950s, when it was found to be the active component of yeast that prevented necrotic liver degeneration in vitamin E–deficient rats and exudative diathesis in vitamin E–deficient chicks (Schwarz and Foltz, 1957; Schwarz et al., 1957). Thompson and Scott (1970) later showed that inorganic selenium per se was required for the prevention of pancreatic exocrine failure in the vitamin E–adequate chick. Selenium deficiency is now known to play roles, along with vitamin E, in several other nutritional diseases of livestock (see review by Combs and Combs, 1986).

SELENIUM DEFICIENCY IN HUMANS

The first evidence for the essentiality of selenium in humans came with the report of a selenium-deficient woman undergoing total parenteral nutrition (van Rij et al., 1979). The patient, a New Zealander from a low-selenium area, developed dermatologic lesions (dry, flaky skin) over a 30-day period, followed by severe muscular pain. During this time, plasma selenium dropped to only 9 ng/mL from a level at admission of 25 ng/mL, which is a third of the level associated with maximal GPX3 expression. The patient responded to treatment with selenium (100 μg/day given intravenously as selenite), proving this case to be one of inorganic selenium deficiency.

Two diseases have been associated with severe endemic Se deficiency in humans: a juvenile cardiomyopathy (Keshan disease) and an osteoarthropathy (Kashin-Beck disease). Each occurs in rural, mountainous areas of central and northeastern China and Russia (eastern Siberia) where the food systems are exceedingly low in selenium. Soil selenium levels are very low in these areas (less than 125 μg Se/kg soil), and grains generally contain less than 40 μg Se/kg grain (compared to 100 μg Se/kg for wheat grown in Kansas in the United States). In these areas, humans have been shown to have blood selenium levels below 25 ng/mL (compared to 85 to 200 ng/mL in the United States).

Dramatic reductions in Keshan disease incidence were achieved by the use of oral sodium selenite (0.5 to 1 mg Se/week) or selenite-fortified table salt (10 to 15 mg Se/kg body weight) (Keshan Disease Research Group, 1979; Chen et al., 1980). It appears likely that Keshan disease may actually be caused by cardiophilic RNA viruses, the virulence of which can be potentiated by severe selenium deficiency through increased viral mutation (Beck and Levander, 1998; Beck, 2007). This suggests that selenium deficiency may also increase risks for other diseases caused by RNA viruses (e.g., measles, influenza, hepatitis, and HIV/AIDS).

Kashin-Beck disease is an osteoarthropathy affecting the epiphyseal and articular cartilage and epiphyseal growth plates of growing bones. The disease is manifested as enlarged joints (especially of the fingers, toes, and knees); shortened fingers, toes, and extremities; and in severe cases, dwarfism. A recent meta-analysis of 15 clinical trials (Zou et al., 2009) suggested that selenium supplementation had some value in preventing the disease. However, additional factors, including iodine deficiency and exposure to fungal toxins, have been suggested as factors in the etiology of Kashin-Beck disease, and it is possible that the disease may be related to impaired thyroid hormone metabolism. Studies conducted in central Africa found that the prevalences of the iodine deficiency diseases, goiter and myxedematous cretinism, were greatest among populations of relatively low selenium status (Vanderpas et al., 1990). Because selenium-dependent DIs are essential in thyroid hormone metabolism, the efficacy of iodine supplementation alone may be limited in selenium-deficient populations.

Low blood selenium levels have been measured in patients with several other diseases (Combs and Combs, 1986). Children with protein-deficiency diseases, kwashiorkor or marasmus, tend to show low plasma levels of selenium, but

CLINICAL CORRELATION

Keshan Disease

Although prevalent in China for at least a century, the disease now known as Keshan disease was formally described in the mid 1930s based on cases observed in Keshan County, Heilongjiang Province. Since then, Keshan disease has been diagnosed among people living in mountainous parts of more than a dozen provinces and autonomous regions within a broad belt of endemic selenium deficiency. Affected areas have soil selenium levels less than 125 ng/kg, and less than 3% of this is available for uptake by plants. Foods and feed grains produced in these area generally contain less than 40 ng Se/kg; unless supplemented with selenium, residents typically have plasma selenium levels of 10 to 25 ng/mL—the lowest levels observed anywhere in the world.

Keshan disease is a multifocal myocarditis primarily affecting children between 2 and 10 years old and, to a lesser extent, women of child-bearing age. Diagnosis is based on signs of acute or chronic cardiac insufficiency, cardiac enlargement, arrhythmia, and electrocardiographic abnormalities. Affected individuals may show cardiogenic shock or congestive heart failure. Four clinical subtypes have been described: acute, chronic, subacute, and latent (Ge et al., 1983).

In the 1970s, Chinese scientists conducted a seminal selenium intervention study demonstrating that selenium was effective in preventing Keshan disease (Keshan Disease Research Group, 1979). In an area of Sichuan Province where Keshan disease is endemic, they randomized almost 21,000 children to treatment groups that received either sodium selenite (single weekly doses of 0.5 or 1.0 mg, depending on age) or a placebo. During 2 years of intervention, they found selenium treatment to reduce Keshan disease incidence by 86% (1.5 cases/1,000 in the selenium group versus 11 cases/1,000 in the control group) and case-fatality by 88% (5.9% in the selenium group versus 50% in the control group). In light of these results, the control group was abolished, and in the subsequent 2 years more than 25,000 children received selenium supplements. Only four new cases were identified (two of which were fatal), and all of these were attributed to noncompliance. This study and several other very successful intervention projects led to the widespread use of selenium supplements, which has virtually eliminated Keshan disease from previously affected areas.

Although it became clear that Keshan disease is endemic to selenium-deficient areas and can be prevented by selenium supplements, one question remained: Why should its incidence show distinct seasonal fluctuations? This question is informed by the findings of Beck and colleagues, (see "Clinical Correlation, Selenium and Viral Resistance") who demonstrated the importance of adequate selenium status in protecting hosts from cardiophilic viruses. These findings suggest that severe selenium deficiency may predispose people to Keshan disease, given its endemic distribution.

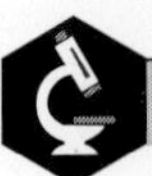

CLINICAL CORRELATION

Selenium and Viral Resistance

Efforts to understand the basis for seasonal fluctuations in the incidence of Keshan disease led to the recognition that selenium status can be an important determinant of resistance to viral infection. Chinese investigators, seeing those seasonal fluctuations as suggestive of an infectious component, isolated several viruses from the hearts of patients with fatal outcomes. Bai and colleagues (1980) found that one such RNA virus, coxsackievirus B4 (CVB4), caused more severe heart damage to selenium-deficient mice than it did to selenium-adequate mice.

This work was extended by Beck and colleagues (Beck and Levander, 1998; Beck, 2007), who demonstrated similar effects of selenium deficiency on the cardiac pathology of a virulent strain of coxsackievirus B3 (CVB3/20). They later found that selenium deprivation increased the virulence of a normally amyocarditic strain of the virus, CVB3/0; after being passed through a selenium-deficient host, CVB3/0 caused heart damage in selenium-adequate mice. This increased virulence was associated with changes in bases at seven sites in the consensus viral genome, which are profiles corresponding to previously sequenced strains associated with myocarditis. The dietary effect proved to be one of oxidative stress rather than selenium deficiency per se, because similar increases in CVB3/0 virulence were found when the virus was passed through mice deprived of vitamin E, particularly in the presence of high dietary iron, or through GXP1-deficient mice. Coxsackieviruses are a collection of RNA viruses that have related mutations and are often referred to as "quasispecies." Therefore it is not clear whether these effects involve oxidative damage to viral RNA or changes in the host that facilitate enhanced viral replication with attendant increases in mutation rate.

This finding raises the question of whether oxidative stress caused by poor nutritional status, infection, or inflammation may potentiate the virulence of other segmented RNA viruses, such as those responsible for important diseases that include influenza, measles, hepatitis, and HIV/AIDS.

this could reflect diminished levels of plasma proteins (e.g., albumin) as well as diminished selenium intake as part of dietary proteins. Malnourished children also appear to have increased needs for selenium and other antioxidant nutrients, due to the pro-oxidative effects of malnutrition and inflammation. Neonates typically have lower blood selenium levels than their mothers, and low plasma selenium levels have been associated with increased risk of respiratory morbidity among low-birth-weight newborns. Low blood selenium levels have been observed in infants with phenylketonuria, but these effects have been due to the use of parenteral feeding solutions containing negligible amounts of selenium.

SELENIUM TOXICITY

SELENOSIS IN ANIMALS

The first reports that selenium was biologically active came in the 1930s when it was identified as a toxic principle in neuropathies of grazing in horses and cattle in northwestern Nebraska and the western Dakotas. The immediate cause of these cases of "loco disease" was the ingestion of certain forage plants that were found to accumulate very high levels of selenium (hundreds of milligrams of Se per kilogram) when growing on the seleniferous soils of that region. Subsequent research has raised questions about possible contributions of intoxicating alkaloids that are also present in those plants.

The safe range of dietary selenium intake is relatively narrow. For example, the rat, which has a minimum dietary requirement of 0.1 mg Se/kg, shows impaired growth with dietary levels greater than 2 to 5 mg Se/kg (depending on the strain). Chronic dietary levels of 4 to 16 mg/kg have been shown to cause edema and poor hair quality and to reduce survival. Though the biochemical mechanisms underlying selenium toxicity have not been elucidated, they are likely to involve the inactivation of regulatory proteins through the formation of Se adducts of protein thiols.

SELENOSIS IN HUMANS

Acute Se toxicity in humans has been described in several cases of accidental overexposure involving ingestion of solutions containing a high concentration of selenium (e.g., gun bluing, sheep drench, antidandruff shampoo). These cases involved exposures to gram quantities of selenium; each involved the rapid development of severe gastrointestinal and neurological symptoms, followed by acute respiratory failure, myocardial infarction, and renal failure (Institute of Medicine [IOM], 2000).

Chronic selenosis of dietary origin was described in a county in southern China where residents were exposed, during drought years, to foods containing several hundreds of milligrams of selenium per kilogram as a result of the use of ash from high-selenium coal for amending local soils (Yang et al., 1983). Dietary selenium intakes were estimated to average 5 mg/day; individuals with intakes greater than 1.5 mg/day showed hair loss, pathological nails, and some elevated skin sensitivity. These symptoms resolved upon reduction of selenium intakes. This experience was used by the U.S. Food and Drug Administration to set a "no observed adverse effect level" (NOAEL) for selenium at 0.8 mg/day, which was associated with whole blood selenium levels of approximately 1000 ng/mL (Abernathy et al., 1993). The IOM (2000) set the Tolerable Upper Intake Level (UL) for selenium at half of the NOAEL, 0.4 mg/day for adults. Evidence that this level is safe comes from residents of high-selenium areas of South Dakota and Wyoming who have been observed to consume as much as 0.7 mg Se/day but show no signs of selenosis (Longnecker et al., 1991).

Some studies have suggested that high-Se status may be linked to diabetes risk. Type 2 diabetes was overrepresented among subjects in the National Health and Nutrition

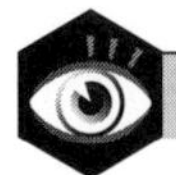

NUTRITION INSIGHT

Selenium Intoxication

Endemic selenosis occurred in the early 1960s in Enshi County, Hubei Province, China, although it was not reported in the English language literature until two decades later (Yang et al., 1983). During the years of peak prevalence (1961–1964), the five most heavily affected villages experienced morbidity rates approaching 50%. The most common signs were hair and nail loss, although lesions of the skin, nervous system, and teeth were also reported. Dietary selenium intakes of individuals in this population were not determined until some years later when they averaged almost 5 mg/day, with people having blood selenium levels as high as 3,200 ng/mL. The source of selenium was found to be local foods, which were produced in soils amended with ash from a source of coal that contained enormous amounts of Se (300 to 80,000 μg Se/g coal).

An episode of selenium intoxication occurred in the United States (Helzlsouer et al., 1985). It involved a formulation error in an over-the-counter dietary supplement: instead of providing the 150 μg Se as specified on the label, each tablet contained more than 27 mg Se. Symptoms were reported by 13 users of the supplement. They experienced nausea, abdominal pain, diarrhea, nail and hair changes, fatigue, and irritability; some reported symptoms of peripheral neuropathy.

Examination Survey 2003–2004 who had plasma levels of selenium that were at least 147 ng/mL (Bleys et al., 2007). In the Nutritional Prevention of Cancer Trial, supplementation of nondeficient subjects with SeMet appeared to increase type 2 diabetes risk (Stranges et al., 2005). Questions remain about the interpretation of these findings, both of which relied primarily on subject self-reports.

SELENIUM AND ANTICARCINOGENESIS

There has been much interest in a possible role of selenium in preventing carcinogenesis. Anti-tumorigenic effects of selenium supplementation have been noted in animal studies, and epidemiologic studies have shown lower incidence of cancer in regions with higher soil and crop selenium levels. However, there is much controversy about the association between selenium exposure and cancer risk and about whether selenium supplements are effective in decreasing the incidence or mortality of cancer. In the Nutritional Prevention of Cancer (NPC) study of dermatology patients with a history of basal cell or squamous cell carcinomas of the skin who were given a daily dose of 0.20 mg Se or a placebo for an average of 6.3 years, there was no effect of Se supplementation on the incidence of basal cell or squamous cell skin cancer (Clark et al., 1996). However, analysis of secondary end points indicated that the treatment group had a significant reduction in total cancer mortality, total cancer incidence, and incidences of lung, colorectal, and prostate cancers. The preventative effect was greatest in patients with the lowest baseline selenium levels, none of whom were of deficient selenium status. This study was followed by the SELECT prostate cancer prevention trial with a much larger sample size comprised of men of relatively high baseline selenium status. The SELECT study found no evidence for a preventative effect of selenium supplementation on incidence of prostate cancer over a 5-year intervention period (Lippman et al., 2009). Analysis of data from these two studies suggests that the anticarcinogenic effects of selenium may be observed only for populations who have relatively low, but nutritionally adequate, selenium status.

A 2011 Cochran review summarized evidence from prospective studies and intervention trials for the relationship between selenium exposure and cancer risk and for the efficacy of selenium supplementation for cancer prevention. The authors concluded that the literature indicated that people with higher selenium levels or intakes had a lower frequency of certain cancers (such as bladder or prostate cancer) but no difference in occurrence of other cancers such as breast cancer, although it is uncertain whether selenium itself was the reason for the differential risks. The Cochran review group also concluded that the trials with the most reliable results found that organic selenium did not prevent prostate cancer in men who had high baseline selenium status and may actually increase the risk of total non-melanoma skin cancer.

In contrast, a more recent meta-analysis (Lee et al, 2011) concluded that selenium supplementation in 9 randomized clinical trials had a preventive effect on cancer incidence in populations with low baseline serum selenium levels (<126 ng/ml) and in high-risk populations for cancer. Although there is not yet a consensus of the role of selenium in human cancer, it seems likely that selenium supplementation can reduce cancer risk in many people with nutritionally adequate but not high selenium status.

Selenium has been shown to be involved in several processes related to anticarcinogenesis. These include alteration of gene expression, stimulation of DNA damage, inhibition of metastatic tumor cell invasion, and inhibition of microvascular development of tumors. These effects are thought to involve the redox cycling and thiol attacks of methylated selenium metabolites, as well as the labilization of proteins critical for tumor cell growth due to replacement of methionine by selenomethionine (Jackson and Combs, 2008). Because most, if not all, of the selenoproteins have antioxidant functions, it is also possible that they participate in anticarcinogenesis.

HUMAN SELENIUM REQUIREMENTS

The Recommended Dietary Allowance (RDA) for Se, 55 μg/day for both men and women (IOM, 2000), is based on the maximal expression of GPX3. This was based on data from two studies. One study involved Chinese adults with a basal intake of 11 μg Se/day supplemented with graded levels of selenite (Yang et al., 1987). This study indicated that GPX3

CLINICAL CORRELATION

Selenium and Cancer

The findings of the SELECT trial (Lippmann et al., 2009) surprised the research community. That study, which was the largest selenium intervention study ever conducted, with more than 32,000 male subjects, found no reduction in prostate cancer risk due to supplemental selenium (200 μg Se/day as SeMet). Though the study was not a long one (only 5 years), its results nevertheless seemed at odds with the large body of evidence and particularly the dramatic results of the 7-year Nutritional Prevention of Cancer (NPC) trial (Clark et al., 1996). This study showed anticarcinogenic activities of selenium (see "Selenium Anticarcinogenesis") in its pool of 1,300 participants.

Rayman and associates (2009) interpreted the SELECT results in the context of the totality of clinical evidence, and pointed out that, in fact, the SELECT results confirm the outcomes in the NPC trial for participants with the highest baseline plasma selenium levels (>121 ng/mL) before supplementation. The conclusion from both NPC and SELECT trials is that daily selenium supplements will not benefit all persons. The NPC trial results indicate that cancer risk reduction with selenium should be expected only in men with low (<106 ng/mL) or suboptimal (<121 ng/mL) levels before supplementation—subgroups for which cancer risk was not evaluated by SELECT. After selenium supplementation, plasma selenium levels in SELECT subjects far exceeded the postsupplementation values of men in the highest baseline plasma selenium tertile of the NPC study, who experienced no prostate cancer risk reduction. Therefore Rayman and colleagues (2009) considered the results of SELECT and NPC to be consistent, not contradictory. They emphasized the need to individualize approaches to cancer prevention by identifying subsets of individuals most likely to benefit from selenium supplementation, for example, those with low selenium status or high-risk genotypes, or both.

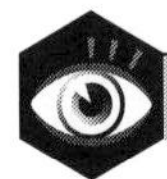

NUTRITION INSIGHT

Health Effects of Selenoprotein SNPs

Margaret P. Rayman, DPhil

The two most common types of human genetic variation are: (a) single nucleotide polymorphism and (b) insertion or deletion of one or more nucleotide(s). A variation at a single nucleotide in a gene that occurs in at least 1% of the population is known as a single nucleotide polymorphism, or SNP. SNPs may affect the structure and therefore the functionality of the encoded protein; the rate at which the gene is transcribed; or the processing, stability, or translation of the mRNA. SNPs may also serve as markers to identify and map other genes that cause disease when mutated. If these non-disease-causing variations are found to be inherited with a particular trait, but do not cause the trait, they not only serve as markers for the trait but may provide evidence for the location of the gene in the genome. SNPs deposited in the National Center for Biotechnology Information (NCBI) database are given a reference SNP (rs) number that identifies the particular SNP.

SNPs can alter selenoprotein expression, enzyme activity, and the plasma concentration of selenium with subsequent effects on the dietary requirement for selenium. Given such actions, it is not surprising that several SNPs in selenoprotein genes have been found to influence disease risk, progression, or mortality. SNPs in selenoprotein genes that have been shown to have functional consequences include: rs1050450, which causes a Pro-Leu amino acid change in GPX1 that affects its enzyme activity; rs713041, which causes a C-U nucleotide substitution in the 3′ untranslated region (3′UTR) of the *GPX4* mRNA; rs5859 in the 3′UTR of the *Sep15*; rs34713741 in the promoter region of the selenoprotein S (*SepS*) gene; and two SNPs in *SepP1*, rs7579 and rs3877899, which both affect blood selenoprotein levels.

An example of the possible link between SNPs in selenoproteins and disease risk is a study of a population from the Czech Republic, a region of Europe where residents are known to have low selenium status and where low selenium status had been associated with increased incidence of colorectal cancer (Meplan et al., 2010). Participants included 832 cases of colorectal cancer and 705 controls who were genotyped for twelve SNPs in selenoprotein genes. Results indicated that three of the twelve SNPs measured were associated with increased risk of colorectal cancer: rs7579 in *SepP1,* rs713041 in *GPX4,* and rs34713741 in *SepS*. In contrast, the rs1050450 allele in *GPX4* was associated with decreased risk of colorectal cancer. The rs2972994 allele of *SepP1* was associated with increased risk of colorectal cancer in women but with a decreased risk of colorectal cancer in men.

Thus variants in selenoprotein genes appear to play a role in cancer development and represent potential biomarkers of colorectal cancer risk. Functional effects of SNPs in these genes could lead to altered ability of cells to prevent oxidative damage, to prevent endoplasmic reticulum stress associated with misfolded proteins, or regulate apoptotic and inflammatory signaling. Effects of these variants on colorectal cancer risk are relatively small, as are those of many other individual variants underlying cancer and other complex, multigenic disease traits.

activity increased until it reached a plateau level with a total selenium intake of 41 μg/day. After adjusting for differences in the body weights of the subjects and most Americans, the Estimated Average Requirement (EAR) was set at 52 μg Se/day. The other study involved adult New Zealanders with a basal intake of 28 μg Se/day who were supplemented with graded levels of SeMet (Duffield-Lillico et al., 1999). Significant increases in GPX3 activity were seen with 10 μg supplemental Se/day, yielding an EAR of 38 μg Se/day. The average of these two estimates, 45 μg/day, was chosen as the EAR;

using an assumed 10% coefficient of variation, the RDA for Se was set at 55 μg/day (45 μg + 20%) for both men and women. The selenium RDAs for children were extrapolated from this value based on body weight. The RDAs for infants, however, were based on projected intakes of selenium from human milk (birth through 6 months: 15 μg/day), and from human milk plus complementary foods (6 months through 1 year: 20 μg/day). Additional selenium was recommended for pregnant (60 μg/day) and lactating (70 μg/day) women.

Dietary selenium requirements were estimated by the World Health Organization (1996) using a different approach. They were based on a study done in a Keshan disease area of China where normal intakes are relatively low (i.e., the same study used by the IOM in setting the DRIs). In this study, adult men were given graded doses of SeMet for 5 to 8 months, and the relationship between total selenium intake and plasma GPX3 activity was determined (Yang et al., 1987). From these values, normative requirements (to maintain desirable reserves) were estimated based on the selenium intake needed to support two thirds of maximal GPX3 activity: 26 μg Se/day. Adjustment for assumed interindividual variation yielded recommended intakes of 40 and 30 μg Se/day for men and women, respectively. The selenium intakes recommended by WHO are thus lower than those recommended by IOM largely due to the lower criterion used by WHO (GPX3 at two thirds of the plateau level) compared to that used by IOM (at the plateau level).

The results of a more recent study (Xia et al., 2005) are relevant to the estimation of the quantitative selenium needs of people. It involved individuals in China with an average basal selenium intake of 9 μg/day (women) and 11 μg/day (men). This low dietary intake was associated with plasma selenium levels (22 μg/L) of 18%, plasma GPX3 activities of 40%, and plasma SepP levels of 23%, respectively, of average levels found in Americans. The 4-month supplementation of this cohort with graded levels of selenium showed SeMet to be more effective than selenite in supporting GPX3 expression. Although SepP levels also increased, they did not reach plateau levels within the 4-month period of supplementation. These results indicate clear differences in the bioavailabilities of selenite and SeMet. These various

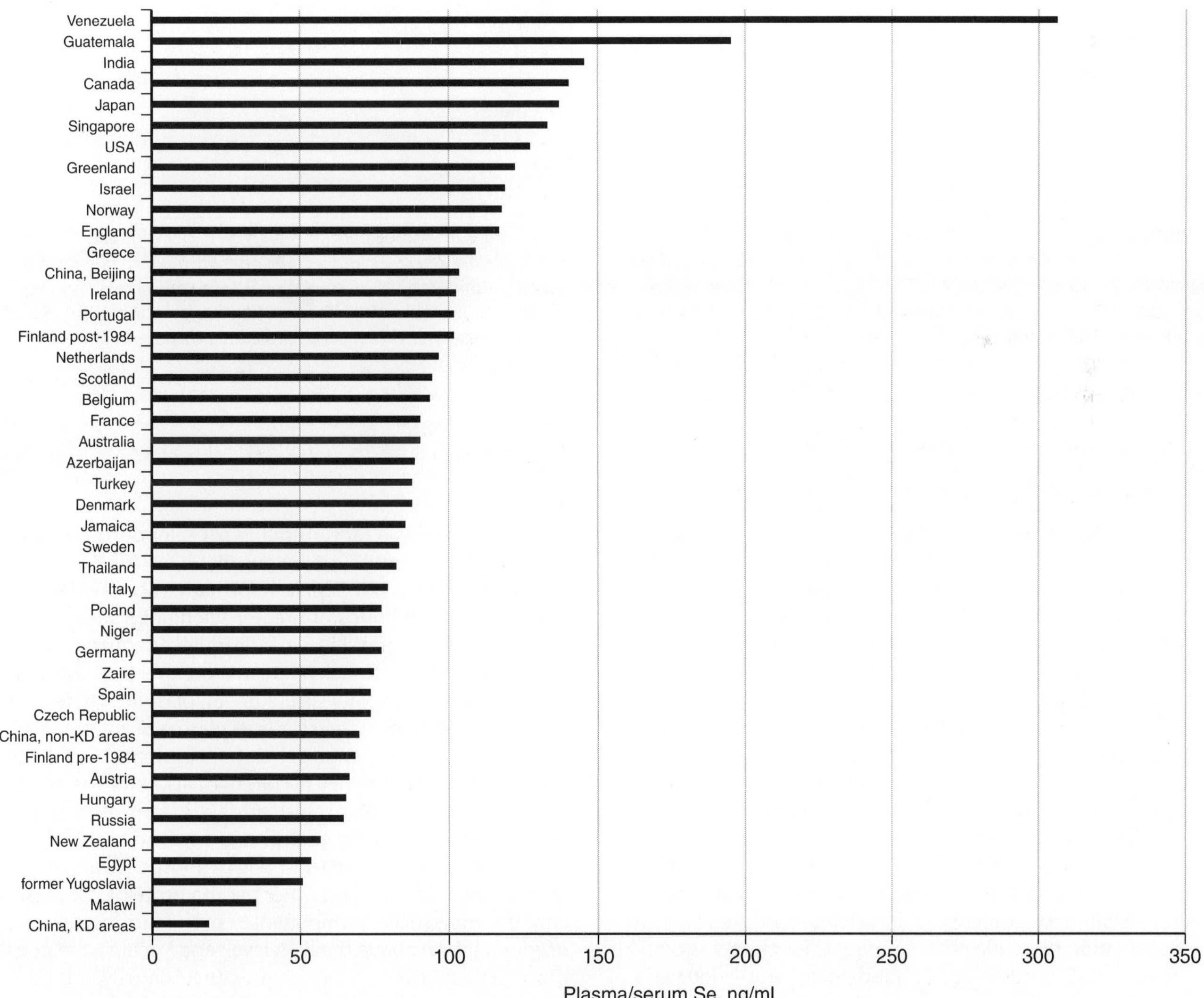

FIGURE 39-4 Global Se status, plasma/serum selenium levels of healthy adults (Combs, 2001). Note: selenium status increased as the result of adding selenate to agricultural fertilizers starting in 1984. *KD*, Keshan disease.

approaches highlight issues relevant to setting requirements such as which form of a nutrient should be used to establish requirements, which assessment parameter is most appropriate, and how long supplementation studies should continue.

SELENIUM INTAKES

Estimates of the average selenium intakes in 18 countries varied from as low as 3 μg/person/day in a Keshan disease–endemic part of China to as high as 224 μg/person/day in Canada and Venezuela. The estimated intakes of several countries (Greece, Libya, New Guinea, Sweden, Turkey, and the United Kingdom) fall below the U.S./Canadian RDA (see Navarro-Alarcon and Cabrera-Vique, 2008). These differences are reflected in the average plasma/serum selenium levels of residents of various countries, which span an order of magnitude (Combs, 2001) (Figure 39-4).

Americans consume 80 to 180 μg Se/day (Figure 39-5), with estimated average selenium intakes of 146 and 98 μg/day for men and women, respectively (IOM, 2000); these intake levels are two to five times those of residents of Finland, the United Kingdom, and New Zealand. Although these

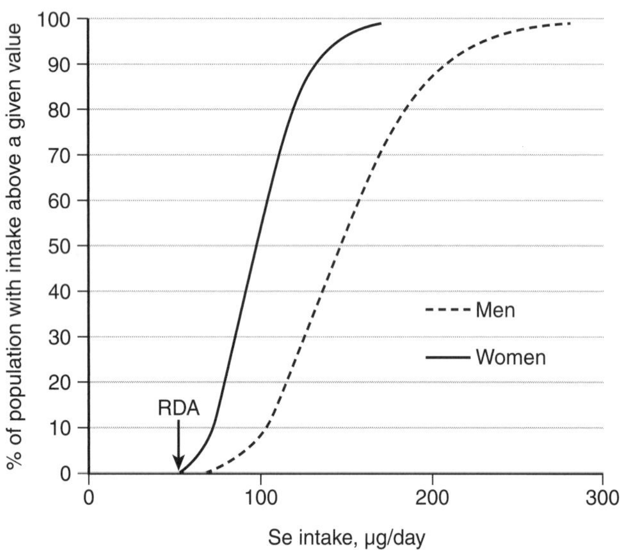

FIGURE 39-5 Distribution of dietary Se intakes of Americans. (Data from the third National Health and Nutrition Examination Survey [NHANES III, 1988–1994]. IOM. [2000]. *Dietary Reference Intakes for vitamin C, vitamin E, selenium and carotenoids* [pp. 446–447]. Washington, DC: National Academy Press.)

DRIs Across the Life Cycle: Selenium

	μg Selenium per Day	
Infant	RDA	UL
0 through 6 mo	15 (AI)	45
7 through 12 mo	20 (AI)	60
Children		
1 through 3 yr	20	90
4 through 8 yr	30	150
9 through 13 yr	40	280
Males		
≥14 yr	55	400
Females		
≥14 yr	55	400
Pregnant	60	400
Lactating	70	400

Data from IOM. (2006). In J. J. Otten, J. P. Hellwig, & L. D. Meyers (Eds.), *Dietary Reference Intakes: The essential guide to nutrient requirements.* Washington, DC: The National Academies Press.
AI, Adequate Intake; *DRI*, Dietary Reference Intake; *RDA*, Recommended Dietary Allowances; *UL*, Tolerable Upper Intake Level.

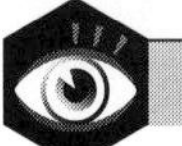

NUTRITION INSIGHT

Assessment of Selenium Status

The assessment of nutritional status in humans depends on the availability of variables that are responsive to the level of intake, are correlated with that nutrient's metabolic function, and most importantly can also be measured in accessible tissues and body fluids.

Several biomarkers of selenium status have been investigated. These include:

- In plasma or serum: total selenium, GPX3, SepP
- In urine: total selenium, selenosugars
- In buccal cells: total selenium, GPX1

The plasma biomarkers have been used most successfully. The plasma biomarkers have been validated in populations suboptimally nourished in selenium, in which they were correlated with differences in selenium intake and responded to increases in selenium intake. Two of the plasma biomarkers have direct functional significance. GPX3 participates in antioxidant protection, and SepP is involved in selenium transport. However, because expression of these (and perhaps all) selenoproteins plateau at intakes somewhat below the RDAs for Se intake, neither the GPX3s nor SepP is informative about selenium status under conditions of greater selenium intake.

Assessing selenium status in individuals adequately nourished with respect to selenium is therefore best assessed using measures of total selenium in plasma. There is a substantial body of research using plasma selenium level. It is important to recognize that measurement of total plasma selenium provides no direct measure of metabolic functionality of selenium. Instead it is a sum of selenium incorporated specifically as SeCys in SepP and GPX3 (i.e., functional selenoproteins) and SeMet nonspecifically incorporated into albumin and other plasma proteins. Of these, only the nonspecific component responds to increases in selenium intake above the RDA level; and because the nonspecific component cannot be measured directly, it is best assessed by measurement of total plasma selenium.

estimates indicate that the selenium intakes of most Americans exceed the RDA, a review of data from 68 countries (Combs, 2001) indicated that millions of people do not consume enough selenium to support maximal selenoenzyme expression, which is at least 40 μg Se/day (Yang et al., 1987). Suboptimal selenium status appeared to be prevalent in almost half of the countries that were surveyed (Combs, 2001).

Differences in selenium consumption by women in different parts of the world are reflected as differences in the selenium contents of human milk and therefore in the selenium intakes of breast-fed infants; estimates of selenium intakes have ranged from 7.5 to 212 μg per day for individual infants. Limited analyses of the selenium contents of human milk in the low-selenium areas of China indicate that the selenium intakes of nursing infants, particularly in areas of endemic Keshan disease, may be as little as 33% to 40% of those of breast-fed infants in Finland and New Zealand.

REFERENCES

Abernathy, C. O., Cantilli, R., Du, J. T., & Levander, O. A. (1993). Essentiality versus toxicity: Some considerations in the risk assessment of essential trace elements. In J. Saxena (Ed.), *Hazard assessment of chemicals*. Washington, DC: Taylor and Francis.

Arner, E. S. J. (2010). Selenoproteins—What unique properties can arise with selenocysteine in place of cysteine? *Experimental Cell Research, 316*, 1296–1303.

Arsova-Sarafinovska, Z., Matevska, N., Eken, A., Petrovski, D., Banev, S., Dzikova, S., Georgiev, V., Sikole, A., Erdem, O., Sayal, A., Aydin, A., & Dimovski, A. J. (2008). Glutathione peroxidase 1 (GPX1) genetic polymorphism, erythrocyte GPX activity, and prostate cancer risk. *International Urology and Nephrology, 41*, 63–70.

Bai, J., Wu, S., Ge, K., Den, X., & Su, C. (1980). The combined effect of selenium deficiency and viral infection of the myocardium in mice. *Acta Acadica Medica Sinica, 2*, 29–31.

Beck, M. A. (2007). Selenium and vitamin E status: Impact on viral pathology. *The Journal of Nutrition, 137*, 1338–1340.

Beck, M. A., & Levander, O. A. (1998). Dietary oxidative stress and the potential of viral infection. *Annual Review of Nutrition, 18*, 93–116.

Berry, M. J., Banu, L., Chen, Y., Mandel, S. J., Kieffer, J. D., Harney, J. W., & Larsen, P. R. (1991). Recognition of a UGA as a selenocysteine codon in Type I deiodinase requires sequences in the 3′ untranslated region. *Nature (London), 353*, 273–276.

Bianco, A. C., & Larsen, P. R. (2006). Selenium, deiodinases and endocrine function. In D. L. Hatfield, M. J. Berry, & V. N. Gladyshev (Eds.), *Selenium: Its molecular biology and role in human health* (pp. 207–220). New York: Springer.

Bleys, J., Navas-Ancien, A., & Guallar, E. (2007). Serum selenium and diabetes in U.S. adults. *Diabetes Care, 30*, 829–834.

Bock, A., Rother, M., Leibundgut, M., & Ban, N. (2006). Selenium metabolism in prokaryotes. In D. L. Hatfield, M. J. Berry, & V. N. Gladyshev (Eds.), *Selenium: Its molecular biology and role in human health* (pp. 9–28). New York: Springer.

Burk, R. F., & Hill, K. E. (2009). Selenoprotein P—Expression, functions and roles in mammals. *Biochimica et Biophysica Acta, 1790*, 1441–1447.

Burk, R. F., Hill, K. E., & Motley, A. K. (2001). Plasma selenium in specific and non-specific forms. *Biofactors, 14*, 107–114.

Burk, R. F., Hill, K. E., Motley, A. K., Austin, L. M., & Norsworthy, B. K. (2006). Deletion of selenoprotein P upregulates urinary selenium excretion and depresses whole-body selenium content. *Biochimica et Biophysica Acta, 1760*, 1789–1793.

Burk, R. F., Norsworthy, B. K., Hill, K. E., Motley, A. K., & Byrne, D. W. (2006). Effects of chemical form of selenium on plasma biomarkers in a high-dose human supplementation trial. *Cancer Epidemiology Biomarkers and Prevention, 15*, 804–810.

Carlson, B. A., Xu, X. M., Shrimali, R., Sengupta, A., Yoo, M. H., Irons, R., ... Gladyshev, V. N. (2006). Mammallian and other eukaryotic selenocysteine tRNAs. In D. L. Hatfield, M. J. Berry, & V. N. Gladyshev (Eds.), *Selenium: Its molecular biology and role in human health* (pp. 29–38). New York: Springer Science+Business Media.

Chen, X., Yang, G., Chen, J., Wen, Z., & Ge, K. (1980). Studies on the relations of selenium and Keshan disease. *Biological Trace Element Research, 2*, 91–107.

Clark, L. C., Combs, G. F., Jr., Turnbull, B. W., Slate, E. H., Chalker, D. K., Chow, J., ... Taylor, J. R. (1996). Effects of selenium supplementation for cancer prevention in patients with carcinoma of the skin. A randomized controlled trial. Nutritional Prevention of Cancer Study Group. *The Journal of the American Medical Association, 276*, 1957–1963.

Combs, G. F., Jr. (2001). Selenium in global food systems. *The British Journal of Nutrition, 85*, 517–547.

Combs, G. F., Jr., & Combs, S. (1986). *The role of selenium in nutrition*. New York: Academic Press.

Combs, G. F., Jr., Watts, J. C., Jackson, M. I., Johnson, L. K., Zeng, H., Scheett, A. J., Uthus, E. O., Schomburg, L., Hoeg, A., Hoefig, C. S., Davis, C. D., & Milner, J. A. (2011). Determinants of selenium status in healthy adults. *Nutrition Journal, 10*, 75.

Dennert, G., Zwahlen, M., Brinkman, M., Vinceti, M., Zeegers, M. P. A., & Horneber, M. (2011). Selenium for preventing cancer. *Cochrane Database of Systematic Reviews 2011, Issue, 5*. Art. No.: CD005195. DOI: 10.1002/14651858.CD005195.pub2.

Duffield-Lillico, A. J., Reid, M. E., Turnbull, B. W., Combs, G. F., Jr., Slate, E. H., Fischbach, L. A., ... Clark, L. C. (2002). Baseline characteristics and the effect of selenium supplementation on cancer incidence in a randomized clinical trial: A summary report of the Nutritional Prevention of Cancer Trial. *Cancer Epidemiology, Biomarkers & Prevention, 11*, 630–639.

Duffield-Lillico, A. J., Thomson, C. D., Hill, K. E., & Williams, S. (1999). An estimation of selenium requirements for New Zealanders. *The American Journal of Clinical Nutrition, 70*, 896–903.

Esworthy, R. S., Yang, L., Frankel, P. H., & Chu, F. F. (2005). Epithelium-specific glutathione peroxidase, GPX2, is involved in the prevention of intestinal inflammation in selenium-deficient mice. *The Journal of Nutrition, 135*, 740–745.

Fang, W., Goldberg, M. L., Pohl, N. M., Tong, C., Xiong, B., Koh, T. J., ... Yang, W. (2010). Functional and physical interaction between the selenium-binding protein 1 (SBP1) and the glutathione peroxidase 1 selenoprotein. *Carcinogenesis, 31*, 1360–1366.

Flohé, L., & Brigelius-Flohé, R. (2006). Selenoproteins of the glutathione system. In D. L. Hatfield, M. J. Berry, & V. N. Gladyshev (Eds.), *Selenium: Its molecular biology and role in human health* (pp. 161–172). New York: Springer.

Ganther, H. E. (1999). Selenium metabolism, selenoproteins and mechanisms of cancer prevention: Complexities with thioredoxin reductase. *Carcinogenesis, 20*, 1657–1666.

Gao, Y., Feng, H., Walder, K., Bolton, K., Sunderland, T., Bishara, N., ... Collier, G. (2004). Regulation of the selenoprotein SelS by glucose deprivation and ER stress: SelS is a novel glucose-regulated protein. *FEBS Letters, 563*, 185–190.

Ge, K., Xue, A., Bai, J., & Wang, S. (1983). Keshan disease—An endemic cardiomyopathy in China. *Virchows Archiv für Pathologische Anatomie und Physiologie und für Klinische Medizin, 410*, 1–12.

Gladyshev, V. N. (2006). Selenoproteins and selenoproteomes. In D. L. Hatfield, M. J. Berry, & V. N. Gladyshev (Eds.), *Selenium: Its molecular biology and role in human health* (pp. 99–110). New York: Springer.

Haft, D. H., & Self, W. T. (2008). Orphan SelD proteins and selenium-dependent molybdenum hydroxylases. *Biology Direct, 3*, 4.

Hatfield, D. L., Yoo, M. H., Carlson, B. A., & Gladyshev, V. N. (2009). Selenoproteins that function in cancer prevention and promotion. *Biochimica et Biophysica Acta, 1790*, 1541–1454.

Hawkes, W. C., Wang, T. T. Y., Alkan, Z. A., Rishter, B. D., & Dawson, K. (2009). Selenoprotein W modulates control of cell cycle entry. *Biological Trace Element Research, 131*, 229–244.

Helzlsouer, K., Jacobs, R., & Morris, S. (1985). Acute selenium intoxication in the United States. *Federation Proceedings, 44*, 1670.

Hill, K. E., Xia, Y., Akesson, B., Boeglin, M. E., & Burk, R. F. (1996). Selenoprotein P concentration in plasma is an index of selenium status in selenium-deficient and selenium-supplemented Chinese subjects. *The Journal of Nutrition, 126*, 138–145.

Institute of Medicine. (2000). *Dietary Reference Intakes for vitamin C, vitamin E, selenium and carotenoids*. Washington, DC: National Academy Press.

Jackson, M. I., & Combs, G. F., Jr. (2008). Selenium and anticarcinogenesis: Underlying mechanisms. *Current Opinion in Clinical Nutrition and Metabolic Care, 11*, 718–726.

Keshan Disease Research Group. (1979). Observations of the effect of sodium selenite in prevention of Keshan disease. *Chinese Medical Journal, 1*, 75–82.

Kim, H. Y., & Gladyshev, V. N. (2004). Methionine sulfoxide reduction in mammals: Characterization of methionine-R-sulfoxide reductase. *Molecular Biology of the Cell, 15*, 1055–1064.

Kobayashi, Y., Ogra, Y., Ishiwata, K., Takayama, H., Aimi, N., & Suzuki, K. T. (2002). Selenosugars are key and urinary metabolites for selenium excretion within the required to low-toxic range. *Proceedings of the National Academy of Sciences of the United States of America, 99*, 15932–15936.

Kohrle, J., & Gartner, R. (2009). Selenium and thyroid. *Best Practice & Research. Clinical Endocrinology & Metabolism, 23*, 815–827.

Kryukov, G. V., Castellano, S., Novoselov, S. V., Lobanov, A. V., Zehtab, O., Guigo, R., & Gladyshev, V. N. (2003). Characterization of mammalian selenoproteins. *Science, 300*, 1439–1443.

Labunsky, V. M., Gladyshev, V. N., & Hatfield, D. L. (2006). The 15-lDA selenoprotein (Sep15): Functional analysis and role. In D. L. Hatfield, M. J. Berry, & V. N. Gladyshev (Eds.), *Selenium: Its molecular biology and role in human health* (pp. 141–148). New York: Springer.

Lee, B. C., Dikiy, A., Kim, H. Y., & Gladyshev, V. N. (2009). Functions and evolution of selenoprotein methionine sulfoxide reductases. *Biochimica et Biophysica Acta, 1790*, 1471–1477.

Lee, E. H., Myung, S. K., Jeon, Y. J., Kim, Y., Chang, Y. J., Ju, W., Seo, H. G., & Huh, B. Y. (2011). Effects of selenium supplements on cancer prevention: meta-analysis of randomized controlled trials. *Nutrition and Cancer, 63*, 1–11.

Lippman, S. M., Klein, E. A., Goodman, P. J., Lucia, M. S., Thompson, I. M., Ford, L. G., ... Coltman, C. A., Jr. (2009). Effect of selenium and vitamin E on risk of prostate cancer and other cancers: The Selenium and Vitamin E Cancer Prevention Trial (SELECT). *The Journal of the American Medical Association, 301*, 39–51.

Lobanov, A. V., Hatfield, D. L., & Gladyshev, V. N. (2009). Eukaryotic selenoproteins and selenoproteomes. *Biochimica et Biophysica Acta, 1790*, 1424–1428.

Longnecker, M. P., Taylor, P. R., Levander, O. A., Howe, M., Veillon, C., McAdam, P. A., ... Willett, W. C. (1991). Selenium in diet, blood, and toenails in relation to human health in a seleniferous area. *The American Journal of Clinical Nutrition, 53*, 1288–1294.

Ma, S. G., Hill, K. E., Caprioli, R. M., & Burk, R. F. (2002). Mass spectrometric characterization of full-length rat selenoprotein P and three isoforms shortened at the C terminus. Evidence that three UGA codons in the mRNA open reading frame have alternative functions of specifying selenocysteine insertion or translation termination. *Journal of Biological Chemistry, 277*, 12749–12754.

Maiorino, M., Gregolin, C., & Ursini, F. (1990). Phospholipid hydroperoxide glutathione peroxidase. *Methods in Enzymology, 186*, 448–457.

Méplan, C., Hughes, D. J., Pardini, B., Naccarati, A., Soucek, P., Vodickova, L., Hlavatá, I., Vrána, D., Vodicka, P., & Hesketh, J. E. (2010). Genetic variants in selenoprotein genes increase risk of colorectal cancer. *Carcinogenesis, 31*, 1074–1079.

Navarro-Alarcon, M., & Cabrera-Vique, C. (2008). Selenium in food and the human body: A review. *The Science of the Total Environment, 400*, 115–141.

Nève, J. (1995). Human selenium supplementation as assessed by changes in blood selenium concentration and glutathione peroxidase activity. *The Journal of Trace Elements in Experimental Medicine, 9*, 65–73.

Patterson, B. H., Levander, O. A., Helzlsouer, K., McAdam, P. A., Lewis, S. A., Taylor, P. R., ... Zech, L. A. (1989). Human selenite metabolism: a kinetic model. *The American Journal of Physiology, 257*, R556–R567.

Rayman, M. P., Combs, G. F., Jr., & Waters, D. J. (2009). Selenium and vitamin E supplementation for cancer prevention. *The Journal of the American Medical Association, 301*, 1876.

Rayman, M. P., Infante, H. G., & Sargent, M. (2008). Food-chain selenium and human health: Spotlight on speciation. *The British Journal of Nutrition, 100*, 238–253.

Reeves, M. A., & Hoffman, P. R. (2009). The human selenoproteome: Recent insights into functions and regulation. *Cellular and Molecular Life Sciences, 66*, 2457–2478.

Rosenfeld, I., & Beath, O. A. (1964). *Selenium: Geobotany, biochemistry, toxicity and nutrition*. New York: Academic Press.

Rotruck, J. T., Pope, A. L., Ganther, H. E., Swanson, A. B., Hafeman, D. G., & Hoekstra, W. G. (1973). Selenium: Biochemical role as a component of glutathione peroxidase. *Science, 179*, 588–590.

Salinas, G., Romero, H., Xu, X. M., Carlson, B. A., Hatfield, D. L., & Gladyshev, V. N. (2006). Evolution of selenocysteine decoding and the key role of selenophosphate synthetase in the pathway of selenium utilization. In D. L. Hatfield, M. J. Berry, & V. N. Gladyshev (Eds.), *Selenium: Its molecular biology and role in human health* (pp. 39–50). New York: Springer.

Schroeder, H. A., Frost, D. V., & Balassa, J. J. (1979). Essential trace elements in man: Selenium. *Journal of Chronic Diseases, 23*, 277–285.

Schubert, A., Holden, J., & Wolf, W. R. (1987). Selenium content of a core group of foods based on a critical evaluation of published analytical data. *Journal of the American Dietetic Association, 87*, 285–299.

Schwarz, K., Bieri, J. G., Briggs, G. M., & Scott, M. L. (1957). Prevention of exudative diathesis in chicks by factor 3 and selenium. *Proceedings of the Society for Experimental Biology and Medicine, 95*, 621–629.

Schwarz, K., & Foltz, C. M. (1957). Selenium as an integral part of factor 3 against dietary necrotic liver degeneration. *Journal of the American Chemical Society, 79*, 3292–3293.

Schweizer, U., Streckfuss, F., Pelt, P., Carlson, B. A., Hatfield, D., Korhle, J., & Stombur, L. (2005). Hepatically derived selenoprotein P is a key factor for kidney but not brain selenium supply. *The Biochemical Journal, 386*, 221–226.

Shchedrina, V. A., Zhang, Y., Labunskyy, V. M., Hatfield, D. L., & Gladyshev, V. N. (2010). Structure-function relations, physiological roles, and evolution of mammalian ER-resident selenoproteins. *Antioxidants and Redox Signaling, 12*, 839–849.

Shrift, A. (1969). Aspects of selenium metabolism in higher plants. *Annual Review of Plant Physiology, 20*, 475–495.

Stranges, S., Marshall, J. R., Trevisan, M., Natarajan, R., Donahue, R. P., Combs, G. F., Jr., ... Reid, M. E. (2005). Effects of selenium supplementation on cardiovascular disease incidence and mortality: Secondary analyses in a randomized clinical trial. *American Journal of Epidemiology, 163*, 694–699.

Sunde, R. A. (2006). Regulation of glutathione peroxidase-1 expression. In D. L. Hatfield, M. J. Berry, & V. N. Gladyshev (Eds.), *Selenium: Its molecular biology and role in human health* (pp. 149–160). New York: Springer.

Tamura, T., & Stadtman, T. C. (1996). A new selenoprotein from human lung adenocarcinoma cells: Purification, properties, and thioredoxin reductase activity. *Proceedings of the National Academy of Sciences of the United States of America, 93*, 1006–1011.

Thompson, J. N., & Scott, M. L. (1970). Impaired lipid and vitamin E absorption related to atrophy of the pancreas in selenium-deficient chicks. *The Journal of Nutrition, 100*, 797–805.

Ursini, F., Heim, S., Kiess, M., Majorino, M., Roveri, A., Wissing, J., & Flohé, L. (1999). Dual function of the selenoprotein PHGPx during sperm maturation. *Science, 285*, 1393–1396.

Vanderpas, J., Contempre, B., Duale, M., Gosossens, W., Beebe, N., Ntambue, K., ... Diplock, A. T. (1990). Iodine and selenium deficiency associated with cretinism in northern Zaire. *The American Journal of Clinical Nutrition, 52*, 1087–1090.

van Rij, A. M., McKenzie, J. M., & Robinson, M. F. (1979). Selenium and total parenteral nutrition. *JPEN. Journal of Parenteral and Enteral Nutrition, 3*, 235–239.

Vendeland, S. C., Beilstein, M. A., Yeh, J. Y., Ream, W., & Whanger, P. D. (1995). Rat skeletal muscle selenoprotein W: cDNA clone and mRNA modulation by dietary selenium. *Proceedings of the National Academy of Sciences of the United States of America, 92*, 8749–8753.

Whanger, P. D. (2009). Selenoprotein expression and function—Selenoprotein W. *Biochimica et Biophysica Acta, 1790*, 1448–1452.

World Health Organization (1996). Selenium. In *Trace elements in human nutrition and health* (pp. 105–122). Geneva: WHO.

Xia, Y., Hill, K. E., Byrne, D. W., Xu, J., & Burk, R. F. (2005). Effectiveness of selenium supplements in a low-selenium area of China. *The American Journal of Clinical Nutrition, 81*, 829–834.

Xu, X. M., Carlson, B. A., Irons, R., Mix, H., Zhong, N., Gladyshev, V. N., & Hatfield, D. L. (2007). Selenophosphate synthetase 2 is essential for selenoprotein biosynthesis. *Biochemical Journal, 404*, 115–120.

Yang, G. Q., Wang, W., Zhou, R., & Sun, S. (1983). Endemic selenium intoxication of humans in China. *The American Journal of Clinical Nutrition, 37*, 872–881.

Yang, G. Q., Zhu, L. Z., Liu, S. J., Gu, L. Z., Qian, P. C., Huang, J. H., & Lu, M. D. (1987). Human selenium requirements in China. In G. F. Combs Jr., O. A. Levander, J. E. Spallholz, & J. E. Oldfield (Eds.), *Selenium in biology and medicine* (pp. 589–607). New York: AVI.

Yant, L. J., Ran, Q., Rao, L., Van Remmen, H., Shibatani, T., Belter, J. G., ... Prolla, T. A. (2003). The selenoprotein GPX4 is essential for mouse development and protects from radiation and oxidative damage insults. *Free Radical Biology & Medicine, 34*, 496–502.

Zeng, H. (2009). Selenium as an essential micronutrient: Roles in cell cycle and apoptosis. *Molecules, 14*, 1263–1278.

Zhu, J. H., Zhang, X., McClung, J. P., & Lei, X. G. (2006). Impact of Cu, Zn-superoxide dismutase and Se-dependent gluathione peroxidase-1 knockouts on acetaminophen-induced cell death and related signaling in murine liver. *Experimental Biology and Medicine (Maywood, N.J.), 231*, 1726–1732.

Zhuo, P., & Diamond, A. M. (2009). Molecular mechanisms by which selenoproteins affect cancer risk and progression. *Biochimica et Biophysica Acta, 1790*, 1546–1554.

Zou, K., Liu, G., Wu, T., & Du, L. (2009). Selenium for preventing Kashin-Beck osteoarthropathy in children: A meta-analysis. *Osteoarthritis Cartilage, 17*, 144–151.

RECOMMENDED READINGS

Bellinger, F. P., Raman, A. V., Reeves, M. A., & Berry, M. J. (2009). Regulation and function of selenoproteins in human disease. *The Biochemical Journal, 42*, 11–22.

Burk, R. F., & Hill, K. E. (2009). Selenoprotein P—Expression, functions and roles in mammals. *Biochimica et Biophysica Acta, 1790*, 1441–1447.

Hatfield, D. L., Berry, M. J., & Gladeshev, V. N. (Eds.). (2006). *Selenium: Its molecular biology and role in human health* (2nd ed., pp. 419). New York: Springer.

Institute of Medicine, Food and Nutrition Board. (2000). *Dietary Reference Intakes for vitamin C, vitamin E, selenium and carotenoids* (pp. 284–324). Washington, DC: National Academy Press.

Kryukov, G. V., Castellano, S., Novoselov, S. V., Lobanov, A. V., Zehtab, O., Guigo, R., & Gladyshev, V. N. (2003). Characterization of mammalian selenoproteins. *Science, 300*, 1439–1443.

Rayman, M. P. (2008). Food-chain selenium and health: Emphasis on intake. *The British Journal of Nutrition, 100*, 254–268.

Rayman, M. P., Infante, H. G., & Sargent, M. (2008). Food-chain selenium and health: Spotlight on speciation. *The British Journal of Nutrition, 100*, 238–253.

CHAPTER 40

Fluoride

Gary M. Whitford, PhD, DMD

COMMON ABBREVIATION

HF hydrofluoric acid

Fluoride (F^-), the ionic form of the element fluorine, is the thirteenth most abundant element in the crust of the earth and has been found in all naturally occurring animate and inanimate materials. Because of its high affinity for divalent and trivalent cations, fluoride exists in the earth mainly in combination with calcium, magnesium, aluminum, and other metals. Similarly, the bulk of fluoride in the human body (about 99%) is associated with the skeleton and teeth. Results from early studies with rodents suggested adverse effects on growth, reproduction, and hematopoiesis when the diet contained only traces of fluoride. Based on such findings, fluoride was classified as an essential element by the National Research Council in 1974. Subsequent studies were unable to confirm these effects. Although no longer considered essential, fluoride is regarded as beneficial, owing to its ability to prevent dental decay.

In high concentrations, fluoride has the ability to inhibit the activity of a wide variety of enzymes, and its potential to cause acute toxicity is relatively high. The ability of fluoride to stimulate new bone formation is unique among osteoactive agents. Its ability to inhibit the initiation and even reverse the progression of dental caries is also unique.

DENTAL FLUOROSIS AND DENTAL CARIES

Early in the twentieth century Frederick McKay and other investigators drew attention to several regions in the southwestern United States where opacities and discoloration of the teeth were endemic. The identification of fluoride as the etiological factor involved the efforts of chemists, biologists, and epidemiologists during the following three decades. The condition, previously known by several descriptive names such as "Colorado brown stain," is now called dental fluorosis.

CHARACTERISTICS OF DENTAL FLUOROSIS

Dental fluorosis is a developmental disorder of the enamel that occurs only preeruptively (Fejerskov et al., 1977). After enamel mineralization is complete, no amount of fluoride intake (or of topically applied fluoride) can cause dental fluorosis; it is classified as mild, moderate, or severe, with the degree of involvement depending on fluoride intake during tooth development. In the milder forms, the enamel has whitish, horizontal striations that may be localized to certain regions of the teeth, frequently the incisal thirds (biting edges) of the anterior teeth and cusps of the posterior teeth ("snow-capping"). Mild fluorosis is not easily noticed by the casual observer and requires some experience to recognize. The moderate and severe forms are characterized by graded degrees of brownish discoloration, sometimes with pitting of the enamel. Histologically, the enamel is more porous (i.e., less dense than normal enamel). The discoloration, which is due to diffusion of sulfur, iron, and other dietary pigments into the porous enamel, occurs slowly after the teeth have erupted. Chemically, the enamel has an abnormally high protein content, which accounts for the porosity. Dental fluorosis is generally regarded as an aesthetic problem, not an adverse health effect. The enamel of the incisors, which are the teeth most noticeable, appears to be most susceptible during the second and third years of life—the period when the teeth are in the late secretory and early maturation stages of development (Evans and Darvell, 1995).

FLUORIDE INTAKE AND THE PREVALENCE OF DENTAL FLUOROSIS

An average daily fluoride intake of 0.05 mg/kg body weight (range 0.03 to 0.07 mg/kg) by children with developing teeth is associated with the milder forms of fluorosis in approximately 10% of the population. These levels of fluoride intake (average and range) are those found when the water fluoride concentration is optimal (about 1.0 ppm or 1.0 mg/L) and the water is the main source of fluoride intake. An average daily intake of 0.10 mg/kg is associated with a prevalence of mild fluorosis of about 50% in a population, with about 5% of the population exhibiting moderate fluorosis.

WATER FLUORIDATION AND DENTAL CARIES

The investigators who documented the relationship between fluoride concentrations in drinking water and dental fluorosis in the 1930s unexpectedly recorded a striking effect on dental caries (Figure 40-1). It was concluded that the consumption of water containing 1.0 ppm fluoride was associated with the

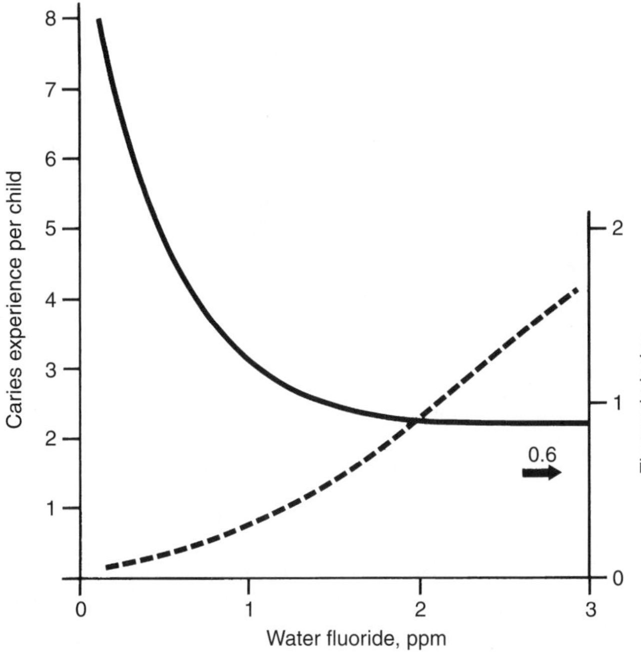

FIGURE 40-1 The relationships between caries experience (*solid line*) and the community dental fluorosis index (*dotted line*) and the fluoride concentration in drinking water as reported by Dean (1942). A total of 7,257 12- to 14-year-old children were examined. A fluorosis index value of 0.6, which occurred where the water fluoride concentration approached 2.0 ppm, was judged to represent the threshold for a problem of public health significance. (From Dean, H. T. [1942]. The investigation of physiologic effects by the epidemiologic method. In F. R. Moulton [Ed.], *Fluorine and dental health* [pp. 23–31]. Washington, DC: American Association for the Advancement of Science; Whitford, G. M. [1983]. Fluorides: Metabolism, mechanisms of action, and safety. *Dental Hygiene, 57*, 16–29. Copyright [1983] American Dental Hygienists' Association.)

near-maximum protection against dental caries in a community and an acceptably low prevalence of the milder forms of dental fluorosis. That is how 1.0 ppm was established as the "optimum" concentration in drinking water. The optimum range is from 0.7 to 1.2 ppm, depending on the average regional temperature. The lower concentrations are recommended for warmer climates, where water intake tends to be higher.

The first study of controlled water fluoridation began on January 25, 1945, in Grand Rapids, Michigan. After 6.5 years, the caries experience among 4- to 6-year-old children in Grand Rapids was approximately 50% lower than in the control city of Muskegon, Michigan. Many subsequent studies confirmed this effect with caries reductions ranging from 20% to 80% and averaging approximately 50%. At present, community water supply systems with controlled fluoride concentrations serve more than 60% of the American population. Another 4% of the population lives in some 3,340 communities with natural water fluoridation. Some of these water systems are equipped with defluoridating units because the natural concentrations are too high.

The difference in the prevalence of dental decay between American communities with and without water fluoridation is lower today than it was before 1970. A national survey conducted in 1979 to 1980 found a 33% lower prevalence among 5- to 17-year-old children who had always been exposed to fluoridated water compared with those who had never been exposed; a 1986–1987 survey found a 25% lower prevalence (Brunelle and Carlos, 1990). The widespread use of topical fluoride products and the "halo" effect, which is discussed in subsequent text, appear to largely account for the smaller difference.

TOPICAL FLUORIDE PRODUCTS

Several kinds of products designed for the topical application of fluoride to the teeth became available in the 1960s. These include gels and solutions with high fluoride concentrations, which are applied in the dental office, and toothpastes and mouth rinses used at home. The fluoride concentrations in these products range from 230 ppm in the over-the-counter mouth rinses to 12,300 ppm in the professionally applied gels. Fluoride toothpastes sold in the United States have a fluoride concentration in the 900 to 1,100 ppm (mg/kg) range as required by the U.S. Food and Drug Administration. Clinical studies with toothpastes found caries reductions that ranged from 18% to 28%, with an average reduction close to 25%. When water fluoridation and fluoridated toothpastes are used together, the reductions in dental caries are roughly additive.

Three national epidemiological surveys conducted in 1971 to 1973 (National Center for Health Statistics), 1979 to 1980, and 1986 to 1987 (National Institute of Dental Research) revealed a progressive decline in tooth decay. Compared with the 1971 to 1973 data, there were 53% fewer affected tooth surfaces in the 1986–1987 survey. In 1979 through 1980, 36.6% of the 5- to 17-year-old children surveyed had no dental decay; in 1986 to 1987 the percentage had increased to 49.9%. Data summarized by the National Center on Health Statistics (Dye et al., 2007) show that the prevalence of caries has declined further from 1988 to 2004. It is generally agreed that the combination of water fluoridation and increased uses of topical fluoride products and pit and fissure sealants have been responsible for these findings.

HOW FLUORIDE PREVENTS DENTAL CARIES

The main minerals of tooth enamel and dentin are various calcium phosphate salts, principally hydroxyapatite and hydroxyfluorapatite [$Ca_{10}(PO_4)_6(OH)_{2-n}F_n$; n = 0, 1, or 2]. Fluoride-containing apatite is less soluble in acid than is hydroxyapatite that contains no fluoride. Dental caries are caused by the action of acid produced several times each day during the metabolism of carbohydrates by bacteria in dental plaque. The mechanisms by which fluoride prevents dental caries include the following:

- Increased resistance of enamel to acid attack
- Promotion of remineralization of incipient enamel lesions, which are initiated at the ultrastructural level several times daily according to the frequency of eating or drinking foods containing carbohydrates (Ten Cate, 1990)
- Increasing the availability of minerals in plaque, which, especially under acidic conditions, provides mineral ions (ionized calcium, phosphate, and fluoride) that retard demineralization and promote remineralization (Tatevossian, 1990)
- A reduction in the amount of acid produced through inhibition of bacterial enzymes (especially enolase) and glucose uptake (Hamilton, 1990)

These various mechanisms require frequent exposure to fluoride throughout life to maintain adequate concentrations of the ion in the dental plaque and enamel. The plaque and enamel receive fluoride from the blood via the saliva (saliva is a continuous source of fluoride except during sleep) and from water, food, and dental products (Whitford, 1996).

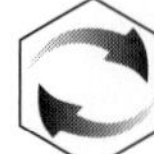

DRIs Across the Life Cycle: Fluoride

	mg Fluoride per Day	
Infants	AI	UL
0 through 6 mo	0.01	0.7
7 through 12 mo	0.5	0.9
Children		
1 through 3 yr	0.7	1.3
4 through 8 yr	1	2.2
9 through 13 yr	2	10
Males		
14 through 18 yr	3	10
≥19 yr	4	10
Females*		
14 through 18 yr	3	10
≥19 yr	3	10

Data from IOM. (2006). In J. J. Otten, J. P. Hellwig, & L. D. Meyers (Eds.), *Dietary Reference Intakes: The essential guide to nutrient requirements.* Washington, DC: The National Academies Press.

*No additional intake recommended for pregnant or lactating women.

AI, Adequate Intake; *DRI,* Dietary Reference Intake; *UL,* Tolerable Upper Intake Level.

FLUORIDE INTAKE

The major sources of ingested fluoride are the diet, especially water and beverages made with fluoride-containing water, and dental products. The ingestion of fluoride from dental products may be intentional, as with dietary supplements, or unintentional, which occurs to varying degrees when toothpastes or mouth rinses are used.

RECOMMENDED FLUORIDE INTAKE

In developing the Dietary Reference Intakes (DRIs), the Institute of Medicine (IOM, 2006) set Adequate Intakes (AIs) for fluoride across the life cycle. The AI is based on estimated intakes that have been shown to significantly reduce the occurrence of dental caries in a population without causing unwanted side effects, including moderate dental fluorosis. Except for infants through the age of 6 months, for whom intake from breast milk is regarded as adequate, the AI values are based on an average daily intake of 0.05 mg/kg body weight.

The IOM (2006) also established a Tolerable Upper Intake Level (UL) of 0.10 mg/kg/day (equating to 0.7 to 2.2 mg/day) for infants and children through 8 years of age to minimize the risk of moderate dental fluorosis. The UL was set at 10 mg/day for children older than 9 years and adults. That intake value was based on studies of fluoride exposure from dietary sources or work environments (Hodge and Smith, 1977) that indicated 10 mg/day for 10 or more years carries only a small risk for an individual to develop preclinical or stage 1 skeletal fluorosis.

FLUORIDE CONCENTRATIONS IN FOODS

The fluoride concentration of most unprepared foods is less than 0.5 ppm (0.5 mg/kg). The concentrations occurring naturally in drinking water supplies in the United States range from 0.05 to 6 ppm; the great majority are considerably less than 1.0 ppm. The higher concentrations are mainly found in the southwestern United States. The concentrations in foods may increase or decrease depending on the fluoride concentration of the water used for cooking. Tea and marine fish (without bones) have higher concentrations that typically range from 1 to 6 ppm (1 to 6 mg/L or mg/kg). The range for average dietary fluoride intakes as reported in seven studies conducted from 1958 to 1985 was 1.2 to 2.4 mg/day (Burt, 1992).

FLUORIDE INTAKE BY INFANTS AND YOUNG CHILDREN

Human milk, like cow and goat milk, has a low fluoride concentration (about 0.01 ppm). Therefore a liter of milk provides not more than 0.01 mg of fluoride, an intake level that has been shown to result in a negative fluoride balance (total excretion > total intake) in infants, which indicates a net loss from calcifying tissues of fluoride that was acquired in utero (Ekstrand et al., 1984).

Before 1980 many American manufacturers of ready-to-feed infant formulas prepared their products using fluoridated water, which resulted in concentrations ranging from 0.6 to 1.2 ppm and intakes in excess of 0.10 mg/kg by some infants. However, a number of reports in the 1980s began to show an increase in the prevalence of dental fluorosis and raised concern about this practice. At a meeting sponsored by the American Dental Association, investigators discussed the possible relationship between fluoride intake from infant formulas and an increased risk of dental fluorosis with the manufacturers, who then agreed to prepare their products with low-fluoride water (Pendrys and Stamm, 1990). Today ready-to-feed formulas manufactured in the United States have fluoride concentrations that range from 0.09 to 0.20 ppm (McKnight-Hanes et al., 1988; Siew et al., 2009).

These provide 0.20 mg or less of fluoride with each liter consumed. The fluoride concentrations of liquid concentrates and powdered formulas prepared in the home span a wide range (0.1 to 1.2 ppm), depending mainly on the water used in the home to reconstitute these products.

Of particular interest is fluoride intake by young children at risk of dental fluorosis. When drinking water containing 1.0 ppm fluoride is the major source of the ion, the average daily intake by young children is approximately 0.05 mg/kg. Table 40-1 shows the results of five studies of dietary fluoride intake by children up to 2 years of age (Burt, 1992). Data were obtained for diets prepared with or without fluoridated water. In 1979, daily fluoride intake by 2- to 6-month-old infants living in areas with fluoridated water ranged from 0.09 to 0.13 mg/kg. These levels of intake were well above the optimum range and due partly to high-fluoride formulas. The more recent studies found lower daily intakes that were remarkably similar and close to 0.05 mg/kg. Table 40-1 also shows lower intakes in areas with low water fluoride concentrations. Average daily dietary fluoride intakes by older children and adults are somewhat less than 0.05 mg/kg because intake does not keep up with body weight.

The diet, however, is not the only source of fluoride intake. In a more recent study, Levy and colleagues (2003) periodically monitored fluoride intake from water, other beverages, selected foods, toothpastes, and dietary supplements by 785 children from birth up to 72 months of age. The drinking water fluoride concentrations of nearly all of the children were either less than 0.3 ppm or between 0.6 and 1.1 ppm. Table 40-2 shows the history of intake (mean, 10th and 90th percentiles) by these children over the course of the study. The overall averages for the intakes of children at 6 months and at 2 years are close to the AI levels recommended by the IOM (0.05 mg/kg) and only slightly higher than those shown in Table 40-1 for children whose drinking water was fluoridated. The 90th percentile intake values, however, are substantially higher. These higher levels of intake occurred mainly for children whose drinking water contained 0.6 ppm or more of fluoride. During the second and third years of life when, as noted in the preceding text,

TABLE 40-1 Average Dietary Fluoride Intake by U.S. Children as Reported in Five Studies Conducted From 1979 to 1988

		mg Fluoride/Day		mg Fluoride/kg Body Weight/Day	
YEAR	AGE	F	No F	F	No F
1979	2 mo	0.63	0.05	0.13	0.01
	4 mo	0.68	0.10	0.10	0.02
	6 mo	0.76	0.15	0.09	0.02
1980	6 mo	0.21	0.35	0.03	0.04
	2 yr	0.61	0.32	0.05	0.03
1985	6 mo	0.42	0.23	0.05	0.03
	2 yr	0.62	0.21	0.05	0.02
1988	6 mo	0.4	0.2	0.05	0.03

Data from Burt, B. A. (1992). The changing patterns of systemic fluoride intake. *Journal of Dental Research, 71*(Spec. Issue), 1228–1237.
F, Foods processed and mixed with fluoridated water (>0.7 ppm); *No F,* foods not processed and mixed with fluoridated water (<0.4 ppm).

TABLE 40-2 Estimated Total Daily Fluoride Intake by Children From Water, Other Beverages, Selected Foods, Toothpaste, and Dietary Supplements

	10th Percentile		Mean (± SD)		90th Percentile	
AGE (mo)	mg	mg/kg	mg	mg/kg	mg	mg/kg
6	0.05	0.007	0.47 ± 0.39	0.060 ± 0.050	1.01	0.127
12	0.10	0.011	0.42 ± 0.33	0.042 ± 0.034	0.84	0.086
24	0.28	0.022	0.70 ± 0.43	0.055 ± 0.035	1.23	0.098
36	0.32	0.022	0.79 ± 0.45	0.054 ± 0.032	1.33	0.090
48	0.31	0.018	0.80 ± 0.49	0.047 ± 0.030	1.36	0.080
60	0.28	0.015	0.76 ± 0.46	0.040 ± 0.025	1.34	0.070
72	0.28	0.012	0.74 ± 0.47	0.034 ± 0.021	1.34	0.060

Data from Levy, S. M., Warren, J. J., & Broffitt, B. (2003). Patterns of fluoride intake from 36 to 72 months of age. *Journal of Public Health Dentistry, 63*, 211–220.

the incisors appear to be at greatest risk of dental fluorosis, the 90th percentile values are consistent with the occurrence of scattered cases of moderate dental fluorosis. In the cohort studied by Levy and colleagues (2003), the most important sources of fluoride intake (in descending order) were toothpaste, beverages, and drinking water.

FLUORIDE INTAKE FROM DENTAL PRODUCTS

Unlike the situation that existed 35 or more years ago when the diet was the only important source of fluoride intake, fluoridated dental products (toothpastes, rinses, dietary supplements) now contribute significantly to intake by both children and adults. An important observation that drew attention to this fact was the increase in the prevalence of dental fluorosis in the United States (Leverett, 1982). The products that are used most frequently and contribute most to fluoride intake are the toothpastes.

When the toothbrush bristles are covered with toothpaste, a weight of approximately 1.0 g is used, which, in the case of a standard 1,000-ppm product, contains 1.0 mg of fluoride. Studies have shown that from 10% to nearly 100% of the amount used by individual children is swallowed. Among children younger than 6 years of age, the amount ingested is inversely related to age because of inadequate control of the swallowing reflex. The overall average is close to 30%, so that about 0.3 mg of fluoride is ingested with each brushing. This is equal to or more than the average total daily intake from the diet in nonfluoridated areas and about 50% of the dietary intake where the water is optimally fluoridated (see Table 40-1).

Several studies have shown that the use of fluoridated toothpaste starting at an early age increases the risk of dental fluorosis (mostly the milder forms) by twofold to tenfold (Burt, 1992). As a result of such findings, several workshops conducted since 1985 have produced several precautionary recommendations for children with developing teeth, including (1) parental supervision of brushing, (2) the use of pea-sized portions of toothpaste, (3) teaching how to rinse and empty the mouth at an early age, and (4) the production of products with lower concentrations of fluoride. Some U.S. manufacturers of toothpastes that contain fluoride now market their products specifically for children, but so far the changes have been limited to flavors, appearance (e.g., sparkles), and colorful packaging because, unfortunately, the U.S. Food and Drug Administration requires the fluoride concentration to be between 900 and 1,100 ppm. Several European countries, however, market 250-ppm and 500-ppm toothpastes for use by children. The effectiveness of these products in controlling dental caries is virtually the same as that of the 1,000-ppm products.

ESTIMATING TOTAL FLUORIDE INTAKE: COMPLICATING FACTORS

As shown in Table 40-1, the average dietary fluoride intake by young children since 1980 has remained relatively constant, regardless of water fluoridation level. The literature indicates that intake with the diet has also been relatively constant among adults. Before the mid-1960s the diet accounted for nearly all fluoride intake so that total intake could be estimated rather easily. Today, however, the situation is considerably different. The variable intake associated with the use of dental products was discussed earlier. Other factors of current importance include (1) increased sales of bottled water, (2) the use of home water purification systems, and (3) the halo or "diffusion" effect.

The most popular bottled waters contain small amounts of fluoride (less than 0.2 ppm) but some, such as Vichy water from France, contain 5 ppm or more. However, nearly two dozen brands bottled in the United States contain added fluoride in concentrations ranging from 0.5 to 1.0 ppm. If the fluoride is added by the manufacturer, the law requires that the label show the concentration, but this is not required if the fluoride occurs naturally. The popular countertop water purification systems used in many homes today remove little or no fluoride from water, but fluoride is effectively removed by distillation or reverse osmosis systems. The halo effect refers to the distribution of foods and beverages prepared with fluoridated water to other communities where the water is not fluoridated. Dietary fluoride supplements are prescribed for children in communities where the water supplies are low in fluoride but, because of the halo effect, some children in these communities may already have sufficient fluoride intake. The ingestion of dietary supplements by such children increases their risk of dental fluorosis. Considering all of these variables, it is clear that some persons living in communities without water fluoridation can ingest as much or more fluoride as some persons in fluoridated communities.

FLUORIDE PHYSIOLOGY

Figure 40-2 shows the main features of fluoride metabolism, a subject covered in detail by Whitford (1996). The overall process is relatively uncomplicated because fluoride is not known to undergo biotransformation to form complex chemical compounds, each of which would have its own special metabolic characteristics.

FLUORIDE ABSORPTION

In the absence of high concentrations of calcium and certain other cations with which fluoride forms insoluble compounds that are poorly absorbed, 80% to 90% of ingested fluoride is absorbed. The average half-time for absorption is 30 minutes. When taken with milk or other foods high in calcium, absorption is reduced to 50% to 70%. Although the stomach is not structurally or functionally designed for absorption, as much as 40% of ingested fluoride can cross the gastric mucosa. The rate and extent of gastric absorption are directly related to the acidity of the stomach contents. This is due to the formation of hydrofluoric acid (HF, $pK_a = 3.4$) whose permeability coefficient across lipid membranes is only slightly less than that of water itself. Most of the fluoride not absorbed from the stomach will be absorbed from the upper intestine, where the pH of the contents appears to have little effect on fluoride absorption. Regardless of the site, there is no evidence for any absorptive mechanism other than diffusion.

FLUORIDE IN CALCIFIED TISSUES

Fluoride concentrations in plasma and most soft tissues are low and typically between 0.01 and 0.05 ppm. Approximately 99% of the fluoride in the body is contained in the skeleton and teeth, where it exists mainly as hydroxyfluorapatite. Fluoride concentrations in bone usually range from 600 to 1,500 ppm and depend on past intake and the age of the individual. Higher soft and hard tissue concentrations may occur in people who work in certain industries, such as phosphate fertilizer or aluminum processing factories, or who live in areas with unusually high fluoride concentrations in drinking water.

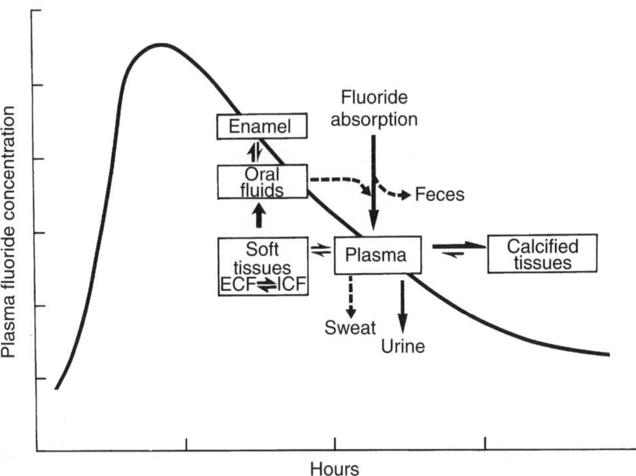

FIGURE 40-2 The major characteristics of fluoride metabolism and a curve showing typical plasma concentrations after ingestion of a small amount of fluoride. (From Whitford, G. M. [1990]. The physiological and toxicological characteristics of fluoride. *Journal of Dental Research, 69*[Spec. Issue], 539–549.)

As indicated by the double arrows in Figure 40-2, fluoride is strongly but not irreversibly bound in calcified tissues. The skeleton has both rapidly exchangeable and slowly exchangeable fluoride pools. Fluoride in the latter pool is found firmly bound within the mineral latticework of mature calcified tissues. Fluoride is mobilized from this pool during the slow but continuous process of bone resorption by osteoclasts.

The rapidly exchangeable pool is located in the hydration shells on the surface of bone crystallites to which fluoride is attracted electrostatically. There appears to be a fixed ratio for the fluoride concentration in the hydration shell and the surrounding extracellular fluid. Therefore when the plasma concentration increases, as after a meal, there is net uptake into the rapidly exchangeable pool. After approximately 30 minutes when the plasma concentration is falling, net migration of most of the fluoride back into the extracellular fluid occurs. A fraction of the fluoride, however, becomes associated with newly forming crystallites so that the skeletal concentration usually increases gradually throughout life. In the postabsorptive state when plasma concentrations are steady, there is little or no net fluoride uptake.

EXCRETION OF FLUORIDE

The excretion of fluoride occurs mainly via the kidneys. The fecal excretion of fluoride usually accounts for only 10% to 20% of daily intake. Even under extreme conditions of heat or exercise, only minor amounts of fluoride are excreted in sweat, which has a low fluoride concentration close to that in plasma (about 0.02 ppm). Therefore a liter of sweat contains only approximately 0.02 mg of fluoride.

NUTRITION INSIGHT

Prenatal Fluoride Supplementation Followed by Breast Feeding

Research on the benefits of prenatal fluoride supplementation for the deciduous teeth of the offspring has yielded conflicting results. A large and well-designed study (randomized and double blind; Leverett et al., 1997) was unable to detect a statistically significant difference in dental caries between two groups of 5-year-old children whose mothers did or did not take fluoride supplements during pregnancy. Although no longer recommended by professional pediatric or dental organizations, some physicians and dentists still recommend that women take additional fluoride during pregnancy, in the belief that it will make the deciduous teeth more resistant to dental caries. Much of the fluoride acquired by the fetal calcified tissues, however, could be lost if the infant is breast-fed.

Strong evidence for the mobilization of fluoride from the rapidly exchangeable pool in calcified tissues came from a Swedish study (Ekstrand et al., 1984). Two groups of infants born to mothers residing in the same community were studied for several weeks. One group was fed human milk, which has a low fluoride concentration (~0.01 ppm). The other group was fed a formula reconstituted using the local drinking water that contained 1.0 ppm. The average daily fluoride intakes by the two groups were 10.6 and 861 μg, respectively. The average daily excretions (urinary plus fecal) were 32 and 383 μg. Therefore the breast-fed infants were in a negative balance, whereas the formula-fed infants were in a strongly positive balance. These findings indicated that the higher fluoride intake was sufficient to maintain or increase the plasma concentrations established in utero and promote accumulation in calcifying tissues. The lower intake by the breast-fed infants, which would have resulted in gradually declining plasma concentrations, caused mobilization from the rapidly exchangeable pool.

Therefore if it is assumed that prenatal fluoride supplementation of the mother has some beneficial effect on the deciduous teeth, it appears that the practice is rational only if the infant's postnatal fluoride intake is substantially greater than that provided by breast-feeding.

The renal handling of fluoride is characterized by free filtration through the glomerular capillaries into the tubules, followed by a variable degree of tubular reabsorption. The renal clearance of fluoride, that is, the volume of plasma from which it is completely removed per unit time, is approximately 35 mL/min in healthy adults. Various studies found averages in adults ranging from 27 to 42 mL/min but a much wider range among individuals (12 to 71 mL/min). The clearances in children are lower, but when factored for body weight they are practically the same as for adults (Whitford, 1999). The efficiency with which the kidneys clear fluoride from the body is due to the relatively large hydrated radius of the ion that restricts its reabsorption from the renal tubular fluid back into the blood.

URINARY pH AND THE BALANCE OF FLUORIDE

Like absorption from the stomach, the reabsorption of fluoride from the renal tubular fluid is strongly dependent on pH and the diffusion of HF (Figure 40-3). The fraction of fluoride that exists in the form of HF is directly related to the acidity of the renal tubular fluid. When the pH is high, say 7.4, only 0.01% of the fluoride is in the form of HF and available for reabsorption. This results in a high clearance rate. When the pH is close to the physiologically possible lower limit (~4.0), nearly 20% exists as HF. Under this condition, reabsorption is more rapid and the clearance rate is low.

The dependence of the renal clearance on urinary pH is a major factor in determining the metabolic balance (intake minus excretion) of fluoride. Urinary pH may be affected significantly by several conditions or factors, including certain diseases such as diabetes mellitus, renal tubular acidosis, the chronic obstructive pulmonary diseases, and some hormonal disorders; acidifying or alkalinizing drugs; altitude of residence; and composition of the diet. The latter factor is probably the most important in that it affects the urinary pH of all people.

SKELETAL DEVELOPMENT AND THE BALANCE OF FLUORIDE

At the beginning of this chapter, it was stated that about 50% of the fluoride absorbed by adults each day is deposited in calcified tissues and the rest is excreted in the urine. This is only a rough generalization, however, as is indicated by the variability among individuals in the renal excretion of fluoride. Another factor important in determining fluoride balance is the stage of skeletal development. The uptake of fluoride by calcified tissues is directly related to the total surface area of the crystallites. During bone development they are small in size, large in number, loosely organized, and heavily hydrated, and they have a large surface-to-volume ratio. Therefore the fraction of absorbed fluoride that is retained in the body is inversely related to age during growth.

A longitudinal study with growing dogs determined the retention (percentage of dose not excreted in the urine) of intravenously administered fluoride for nearly 20 months (Whitford, 1990). The results are shown in Figure 40-4. Shortly after the pups were weaned, only about 10% of the dose was excreted so that retention was close to 90%. Retention declined throughout the study and reached a final value close to 50%, which is the average for adult dogs several years of age. These findings are similar to those from studies with human infants and adults (Ekstrand et al., 1994). Although there are no data with which to judge, it is likely that in the later years of life, when bone resorption begins to exceed accretion, retention of fluoride falls to even lower levels.

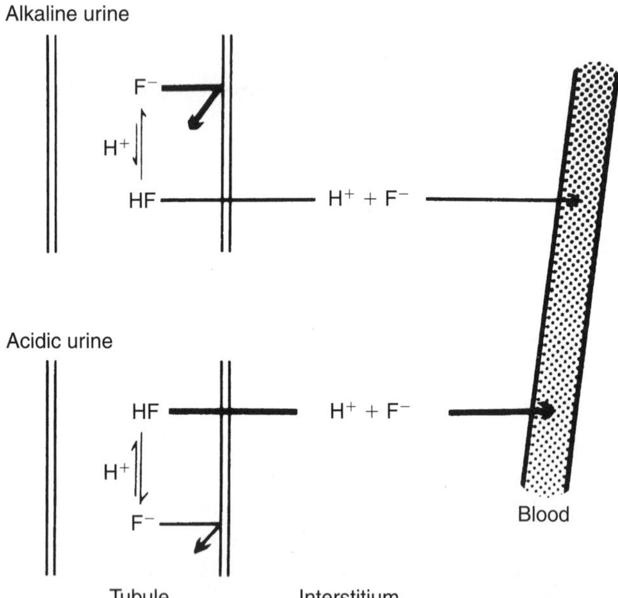

FIGURE 40-3 The mechanism for the reabsorption of fluoride from the kidney tubule. The tubular epithelium is virtually impermeable to ionic fluoride (F^-); it is easily permeated by the undissociated acid, hydrofluoric acid (HF), which lacks a charge. (From Whitford, G. M. [1990]. The physiological and toxicological characteristics of fluoride. *Journal of Dental Research, 69*[Spec. Issue], 539–549.)

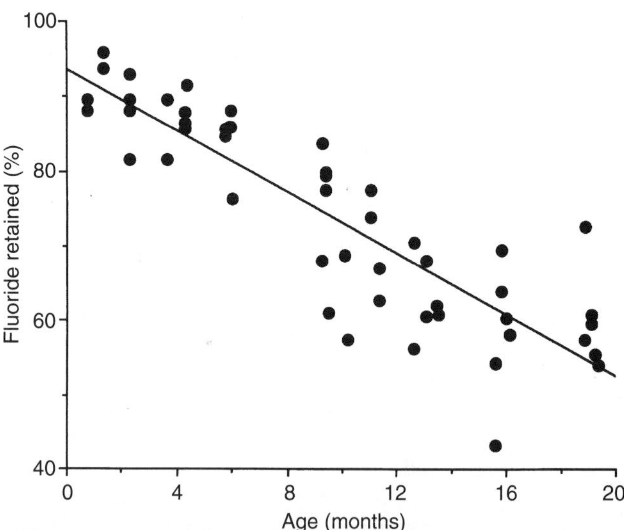

FIGURE 40-4 The inverse relationship between age and fluoride retention in growing dogs. (From Whitford, G. M. [1990]. The physiological and toxicological characteristics of fluoride. *Journal of Dental Research, 69*[Spec. Issue], 539–549.)

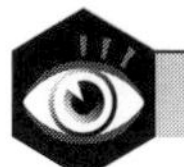

NUTRITION INSIGHT

Urinary pH and the Balance of Fluoride

Many infants are fed either breast milk, which has a low acid load, or a cow's milk–based formula, which has a much higher acid load. The urinary pH of breast-fed infants ranges from the middle 6s to the lower 7s, whereas that of infants fed a cow's milk formula ranges from the lower 5s to the lower 6s (Moore et al., 1977). A diet consisting largely of vegetables and fruits (excluding cranberries, plums, and prunes) produces urinary pH values in the upper 6s and middle 7s, whereas a diet of meats and dairy products causes distinctly acidic pH values ranging from the upper 4s to the upper 5s.

Although data showing the effects of feeding infants human milk or cow's milk formulas are not available, it is likely that fluoride excretion is higher and balance is lower in breast-fed infants because of their higher urinary pH. Research with young adults eating a vegetarian diet showed that the renal clearance of fluoride was significantly higher than when they were restricted to a meat and dairy product diet (Whitford and Weatherred, 1996). Compared with laboratory rats kept at sea level, rats residing at a simulated high altitude (hypobaric hypoxia) have a more acidic urine and significantly higher fluoride concentrations in plasma and calcified tissues. Therefore several environmental and physiological variables can influence urinary pH and the renal handling of fluoride sufficiently to alter fluoride retention and its actions in the body.

ACUTE FLUORIDE TOXICITY

Life-threatening or fatal cases of acute fluoride toxicity are now extremely rare. Substantial amounts of fluoride in toothpastes, mouth rinses, or dietary supplements, however, are found in most American homes. Because of the suspected or actual overingestion of these products, especially by young children, several thousand calls to poison control centers are made each year.

SIGNS, SYMPTOMS, AND TREATMENT OF ACUTE FLUORIDE TOXICITY

Acute fluoride toxicity can develop with alarming rapidity. Nausea and vomiting almost always occur immediately after swallowing a large amount of fluoride and should be treated as initial signs of a potentially serious sequence of events. A variety of nonspecific signs and symptoms, including excessive salivation and tearing, sweating, headache, diarrhea, and generalized weakness, may follow within minutes. Spasm of the extremities, tetany, and/or convulsions may develop if a potentially fatal dose has been swallowed. These effects will be accompanied by hypotension and possibly cardiac dysrhythmias, all of which are consequences of hyperkalemia and severe hypocalcemia. As renal function and respiration become depressed, a mixed metabolic and respiratory acidosis develops progressively and may end in coma.

Treatment on site and in the hospital is aimed at reducing absorption, promoting excretion, and supporting the vital signs. It should begin immediately. The oral administration of 1% calcium gluconate or calcium chloride reduces absorption. If calcium solutions are not available, milk may slow absorption. While these actions are being taken, the hospital should be advised that a case of acute fluoride poisoning is in progress so that preparations for appropriate treatment can be made before arrival.

DOSES PRODUCING ACUTE TOXICITY

The "probably toxic dose" (PTD) is defined as the "minimum dose that could cause serious or life-threatening systemic signs and symptoms and that should trigger immediate therapeutic intervention and hospitalization" (Whitford, 1996). Based on reasonably well-documented case reports, the PTD has been estimated at 5 mg fluoride per kg. One 3-year-old child died in an emergency room 3 hours after swallowing a fluoride solution in a dental office. The estimated dose was between 24 and 35 mg/kg. Another 3-year-old died in a hospital after swallowing about 200 1.0-mg fluoride tablets. In this case the dose was approximately 16 mg/kg. A third 27-month-old child died 5 days after swallowing an unknown number, but less than 100, of 0.5-mg fluoride tablets. The dose in this case was estimated to be slightly less than 5 mg/kg. In each of these cases, the child vomited almost immediately so that the absorbed dose was less than the ingested dose. Note that the survival times after the doses were inversely related to the size of the doses. Based on these reports, it has been concluded that a fluoride dose of 15 mg/kg will probably cause death and that a dose of 5 mg/kg may be fatal. It should be noted that acute toxicity stemming from the ingestion of optimally fluoridated water (1 mg/L) is not possible because 5 L/kg of body weight would be required to reach the PTD.

DENTAL PRODUCTS AS SOURCES OF HIGH FLUORIDE DOSES

During the first half of this century, sodium fluoride was a popular pesticide. Large amounts of it were stored in the kitchens of some homes and institutions. Being a finely divided white powder easily mistaken for powdered milk, flour, sodium bicarbonate, and similar products, there were numerous individual and several mass poisonings (Hodge and Smith, 1965). In 1941, for example, approximately 17 pounds of sodium fluoride was mistaken for powdered milk and used to prepare scrambled eggs at the Oregon State Hospital. There were 263 cases of poisoning, 47 of which were fatal. More than 600 deaths were due to fluoride ingestion in the United States between 1933 and 1965, which accounted for nearly 1% of all fatal poisonings during that period.

Other compounds have replaced sodium fluoride as a pesticide, and fluoride-related fatalities are now rare. Owing to the presence of vitamins, dietary supplement tablets, and dental products containing fluoride in most American homes, however, the number of nonfatal cases has increased sharply. The American Association of Poison Control Centers reported that about 30,000 fluoride-related reports were made to U.S. Poison Control Centers annually from 1998 to 2002. Among these, approximately 2.5% of the cases were treated in a health facility each year. Toothpastes and mouth washes were involved in approximately 79% of the total number of reports each year. More than 90% of the cases involved young children. The "medical outcome" classification of the great majority of cases was "none" (transient and minor signs and symptoms), but 32 to 56 cases each year were classified in the more serious "moderate" and "major" categories, including eight "major" cases (long-term sequelae) and one death. The fatality was listed as a suicide due to acute ingestion of toothpaste by a 51-year-old person (Watson et al., 2003).

The PTD for a 1-year-old child of average weight (10 kg) is 50 mg. Each gram of conventional, 1,000-ppm toothpaste contains 1.0 mg of fluoride, so ingestion of 50 g (1.6 oz.) could cause serious toxicity. For an average 5- to 6-year-old (20 kg), the PTD is contained in 100 g of toothpaste. Most of the over-the-counter mouth rinses have a fluoride concentration of 230 ppm or 0.23 mg/mL. Therefore the PTD for a 10-kg child is contained in 217 mL (7.3 oz.) of mouth rinse. These products should be stored out of the reach of small children, and their use should be supervised by an adult.

CHRONIC FLUORIDE TOXICITY

EFFECTS ON BONE

Perhaps because of its early use as a pesticide, fears and claims of harm surrounding the fluoridation of water, including a variety of allergic reactions, cancer, birth defects, and genetic disorders, were heard from the beginning. None of these claims has stood the test of controlled scientific research, as indicated in reviews by Kaminsky and colleagues (1990), the U.S. Public Health Service (1991), the National Research Council (1993), the U.K. National Health Service (NHS) Centre for Reviews and Dissemination (2000), and the Irish Forum on Fluoridation (2002).

The 1993 report by the National Research Council concluded that the database on the possible relationship between fluoride exposure and the risk of bone fracture was limited and inconsistent. Some studies found no relationship, others found an increased risk, and still others found a decreased risk. Most of the studies were "ecological" in design: they compared fracture rates in areas with or without significant concentrations of fluoride in the drinking water, but did not gather information concerning previous fluoride intake or bone fluoride concentrations for individuals with or without fractures. Furthermore, most of the studies failed to control for variables known to increase the risk of bone fractures. The report recommended that "additional studies of hip and other fractures be conducted in geographic areas with high and low concentrations in the drinking water, and that studies should use information from individuals rather than population groups." The recommendation for specific risk factors for individuals that should be evaluated in such studies included "fluoride intake from drinking water and from all other sources, reproductive history, past and current hormonal status, intake of dietary and supplemental calcium and other cations, bone density, and other factors that might influence risk of fracture" (National Research Council, 1993).

The report by the NHS Centre for Reviews and Dissemination (2000) critically evaluated 23 published studies dealing with the relationship between water fluoridation and the risk of bone fracture. Figure 8.1 of the NHS report shows that most of the 95% confidence intervals in the 23 studies included a relative risk of 1.0, which means that the difference between fluoridated and nonfluoridated populations was not statistically significant. Among those that did not include a relative risk of 1.0, five suggested an increased risk

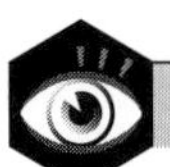

NUTRITION INSIGHT

Too Much of a Good Thing: "Tea Fluorosis"

Tea is one of the world's most popular beverages. The tea plant, *Camellia sinensis,* has the remarkable ability to accumulate large concentrations of fluoride (and aluminum) in its leaves, hundreds of milligrams per kilogram, depending on the age of the leaves before harvesting and the fluoride concentration in the soil. Green teas, the leaves of which are harvested at a young age, generally have lower concentrations than the more popular black teas. The fluoride concentration in brewed black tea typically range from 2 to 6 mg/L depending on the brand, brewing time, and fluoride concentration in the water used for brewing. Accordingly, an 8-oz cup of black tea contains 0.47 to 1.42 mg of fluoride. As noted in the text, a daily fluoride intake of approximately 20 mg for 10 or more years may lead to crippling skeletal fluorosis; intakes between 10 and 20 mg/day would be expected to cause less severe but clinically or radiographically recognizable skeletal changes. Recent reports have described cases of markedly elevated plasma fluoride concentrations and skeletal fluorosis in patients who consumed 1 to 2 gallons of tea daily for many years (Hallanger and Johnson, 2007; Whyte et al., 2008). The author is currently collaborating on three similar manuscripts. One of the three cases, a patient in England, had a plasma fluoride concentration of 44 μmol/L (normal ~1.0 μmol/L) and an iliac crest concentration of 15,144 mg/kg (normal <1,500 mg/kg). The long-term fluoride intake by the patients ranged from approximately 25 to nearly 50 mg/day. It is likely that more cases of tea fluorosis will be identified as the medical profession becomes more aware of tea as a potential source of excessive fluoride intake.

of fracture in the fluoridated population and four suggested a decreased risk of fracture. The report also noted that few of the studies controlled for all of the major variables known to influence the risk of fracture. It was concluded that "the best available evidence on the association of water fluoridation and bone fractures show no association."

Skeletal fluorosis is a condition characterized by several stages of severity. The changes progress according to the amount and duration of fluoride intake, from the asymptomatic preclinical stage in which there is a slight increase in cortical bone density (osteosclerosis) detectable on X-ray films; through stage I in which bone density is further increased; through stage II in which there is further osteosclerosis, some stiffness and pain in the joints, and slight calcification of ligaments; and ultimately to crippling skeletal fluorosis in which irregular, bony outgrowths (exostoses) on previously smooth bone surfaces are present and marked calcification of ligaments limits joint mobility. Among adults with lifelong exposure to optimally fluoridated water (about 1.0 mg/L), bone ash fluoride concentrations are usually less than 1,500 ppm, which are well below those associated with skeletal changes. Bone ash concentrations range from 3,500 to 5,500 ppm in the preclinical stage of skeletal fluorosis to over 9,000 ppm in the crippling stage. It may take 10 years or more of daily ingestion of approximately 20 mg of fluoride to reach the skeletal fluoride concentrations associated with crippling fluorosis. Only five cases of crippling fluorosis have been documented in the United States in the last 40 years. The U.S. Environmental Protection Agency (EPA) has set the MCL (maximum contaminant level) for fluoride in drinking water at 4 ppm to protect against the earliest signs of skeletal fluorosis.

REFERENCES

Brunelle, J. A., & Carlos, J. P. (1990). Recent trends in dental caries in U.S. children and the effect of water fluoridation. *Journal of Dental Research, 69*(Spec. Issue), 723–727.

Burt, B. A. (1992). The changing patterns of systemic fluoride intake. *Journal of Dental Research, 71*(Spec. Issue), 1228–1237.

Dean, H. T., Arnold, F. A., & Elvove, E. (1942). Domestic water and dental caries. *Public Health Rep, 57*, 1155–1179.

Dye, B. A., Tan, S., Smith, V., Lewis, B. G., Barker, L. K., Thornton-Evans, G. ... Li, C. H. (2007). Trends in oral health status: United States, 1988–1994 and 1999–2004. *Vital and Health Statistics, 11*(248), 1–92.

Ekstrand, J., Hardell, L. I., & Spak, C. J. (1984). Fluoride balance studies on infants in a 1-ppm-water-fluoride area. *Caries Research, 18*, 87–92.

Ekstrand, J., Ziegler, E. E., Nelson, S. E., & Fomon, S. J. (1994). Absorption and retention of dietary and supplemental fluoride by infants. *Advances in Dental Research, 8*, 175–180.

Evans, R. W., & Darvell, B. W. (1995). Refining the estimate of the critical period for susceptibility to enamel fluorosis in human maxillary central incisors. *Journal of Public Health Dentistry, 55*, 238–249.

Fejerskov, O., Thylstrup, A., & Larsen, M. J. (1977). Clinical and structural features and possible pathogenic mechanisms of dental fluorosis. *Scandinavian Journal of Dental Research, 85*, 510–534.

Hallanger Johnson, J. E., Kearns, A. E., Droan, P. M., Khoo, T. K., & Wermers, R. A. (2007). Fluoride-related bone disease associated with habitual tea consumption. *Mayo Clinic Proceedings, 82*, 719–724.

Hamilton, I. R. (1990). Biochemical effects of fluoride on oral bacteria. *Journal of Dental Research, 69*(Spec. Issue), 660–667.

Hodge, H. C., & Smith, F. A. (1965). Biological properties of inorganic fluorides. In J. H. Simons (Ed.), *Fluorine chemistry* (Vol. 4, pp. 1–42). New York: Academic Press.

Hodge, H. C., & Smith, F. A. (1977). Occupational fluoride exposure. *Journal of Occupational Medicine, 19*, 12–39.

Institute of Medicine. (2006). In J. J. Otten, J. P. Hellwig, & L. D. Meyers (Eds.), *Dietary Reference Intakes: The essential guide to nutrient requirements* (p. 313). Washington, DC: The National Academies Press.

Irish Forum on Fluoridation (2002). Dublin: Stationery Office.

Kaminsky, L. S., Mahoney, M. C., Leach, J., Melius, J., & Miller, M. J. (1990). Fluoride: Benefits and risks of exposure. *Critical Reviews in Oral Biology and Medicine, 1*, 261–281.

Leverett, D. H. (1982). Fluoride and the changing prevalence of dental caries. *Science, 217*, 26–30.

Leverett, D. H., Adair, S. M., Vaughan, B. W., Proskin, H. M., & Moss, M. E. (1997). Randomized clinical trial of the effect of prenatal fluoride supplements in preventing dental caries. *Caries Research, 31*, 174–179.

Levy, S. M., Warren, J. J., & Broffitt, B. (2003). Patterns of fluoride intake from 36 to 72 months of age. *Journal of Public Health Dentistry, 63*, 211–220.

McKnight-Hanes, M. C., Leverett, D. H., & Adair, S. M. (1988). Fluoride content of infant formulas: Soy-based formulas as a potential factor in dental fluorosis. *Pediatric Dentistry, 10*, 189–194.

Moore, A., Ansell, C., & Barrie, H. (1977). Metabolic acidosis and infant feeding. *British Medical Journal, 1*, 129–131.

National Health Service (NHS) Centre for Reviews and Dissemination. (2000). *A systematic review of water fluoridation. Report 18*. Heslington, United Kingdom: University of York.

National Research Council. (1993). *Health effects of ingested fluoride*. Washington, DC: National Academy Press.

Pendrys, D. G., & Stamm, J. W. (1990). Relationship of total fluoride intake to beneficial effects and enamel fluorosis. *Journal of Dental Research, 69*(Spec. Issue), 529–538.

Siew, C., Strock, S., Ristic, H., Kang, P., Chou, H. N., Chen, J. W., Frantsve-Hawley, J., & Meyer, D. M. (2009). Assessing a potential risk factor for enamel fluorosis: A preliminary evaluation of fluoride content in infant formulas. *Journal of the American Dental Association, 140*, 1228–1236.

Tatevossian, A. (1990). Fluoride in dental plaque and its effects. *Journal of Dental Research, 69*(Spec. Issue), 645–652.

Ten Cate, J. M. (1990). In vitro studies on the effects of fluoride on de- and remineralization. *Journal of Dental Research, 69*(Spec. Issue), 614–619.

U.S. Public Health Service. (1991). *Review of fluoride: Benefits and risks*. Bethesda, MD: U.S. Public Health Service, Department of Health and Human Services.

Watson, W. A., Litovitz, T. L., Rodgers, G. C., Jr., Klein-Schwartz, W., Youniss, J., Rose, S. R., ... May, M. E. (2003). 2002 annual report of the American Association of Poison Control Centers Toxic Exposure Surveillance System. *The American Journal of Emergency Medicine, 21*, 353–421.

Whitford, G. M. (1990). The physiological and toxicological characteristics of fluoride. *Journal of Dental Research, 69*(Spec. Issue), 539–549.

Whitford, G. M. (1996). The metabolism and toxicity of fluoride. In H. M. Myers (Ed.), *Monographs in oral science* (2nd ed.). Basel, Switzerland: S. Karger, No. 16.

Whitford, G. M. (1999). Fluoride metabolism and excretion in children. *Journal of Public Health Dentistry*, *59*, 2224–2228.
Whitford, G. M., & Weatherred, T. W. (1996). Fluoride pharmacokinetics: Effects of urinary pH changes induced by the diet. *Journal of Dental Research*, *75*(Spec. Issue), 354.
Whyte, M. P., Totty, W. G., Lim, V. T., & Whitford, G. M. (2008). Skeletal fluorosis from instant tea. *Journal of Bone and Mineral Research*, *23*, 759–769.

RECOMMENDED READINGS

Burt, B. A. (1992). The changing pattern of systemic fluoride intake. *Journal of Dental Research*, *71*, 1228–1237.
Proceedings, Joint IADR/ORCA International Symposium on Fluorides. (1990). Mechanisms of action and recommendations for use. *Journal of Dental Research*, *69*(Spec. Issue), 505–835.
Whitford, G. M. (1996). The metabolism and toxicity of fluoride. In H. M. Myers (Ed.), *Monographs in oral science 16* (2nd ed.). Basel: S. Karger.

CHAPTER 41

Molybdenum and Beneficial Bioactive Trace Elements

Forrest H. Nielsen, PhD

DEFINITION OF ULTRATRACE ELEMENTS

In 1980 the term *ultratrace element* began to appear in the nutritional literature; the definition for this term was an element required in amounts of 50 ng or less/g diet by animals, or in μg/day by humans. The term also has been applied to elements found to have beneficial bioactivity in animals or humans (including boron and silicon, whose dietary intakes are enumerated in mg/day) but not generally accepted as essential because they lacked a defined biochemical function.

The evidence for the essentiality of four ultratrace elements—cobalt, iodine, molybdenum, and selenium—is substantial and noncontroversial; specific biochemical functions have been defined for these elements. Iodine and selenium are recognized as elements of major nutritional importance and are the topics of Chapters 38 and 39. Although cobalt is required in ultratrace amounts, it has to be in the form of vitamin B_{12}; therefore cobalt as part of vitamin B_{12} is covered in Chapter 25. Very little nutritional attention is given to molybdenum because a deficiency has not been unequivocally identified in humans other than in an individual nourished by total parenteral nutrition or in individuals with rare genetic defects that cause metabolic disturbances involving the functional roles of this element. Therefore molybdenum is discussed in this chapter.

Boron and chromium have not been firmly established as nutritionally essential because they lack clearly defined essential biochemical functions. However, numerous human studies have shown that boron in nutritional amounts and chromium in supranutritional amounts may influence health and disease by directly or indirectly producing beneficial functional outcomes. Recent epidemiological studies have indicated that nutritional amounts of silicon also may have beneficial bioactivity in humans. Thus these three elements receive some attention here. Animal studies indicate that several other elements, some essential for lower forms of life (e.g., nickel and vanadium), may be bioactive beneficial food components. Because of the lack of findings from controlled human studies, they are only briefly summarized at the end of this chapter.

MOLYBDENUM

Molybdenum is an established essential element on the basis that it is used in the synthesis of a molybdenum cofactor required for the activity of sulfite oxidase, xanthine dehydrogenase, and aldehyde oxidase in mammals. The identification of inborn errors of metabolism that affected molybdenum cofactor synthesis provided the bulk of the evidence for its classification as essential.

BIOCHEMICAL FORMS AND PHYSIOLOGICAL ACTIONS

Molybdenum is a transition element that readily changes its oxidation state and can thus act as an electron transfer agent in oxidation–reduction reactions in which it cycles from Mo^{6+} to reduced states. This explains why molybdenum functions as an enzyme cofactor in all forms of life. Molybdenum is present at the active site in a small nonprotein cofactor containing a pterin nucleus in all known molybdoenzymes except nitrogenase (Johnson, 1997). More than 40% of the molybdenum not attached to an enzyme in the liver exists as this cofactor bound to the mitochondrial outer membrane. This form is transferred to an apomolybdoenzyme to make the holomolybdoenzyme (Rajagopalan, 1988). The molybdoenzymes in mammalian systems also contain Fe–S centers and flavin cofactors. Molybdoenzymes catalyze the hydroxylation of various substrates by using oxygen atoms from water. Aldehyde oxidase oxidizes and detoxifies various pyrimidines, purines, pteridines, and related compounds. Xanthine oxidase/dehydrogenase catalyzes the transformation of hypoxanthine to xanthine and of xanthine to uric acid. Hypoxanthine and xanthine are intermediates in the degradation of purines. Sulfite oxidase catalyzes the transformation of sulfite, formed mainly from cysteine catabolism, to sulfate.

ABSORPTION, TRANSPORT, AND EXCRETION

Documented cases of molybdenum deficiency and toxicity may be rare because the body is able to adapt to a wide range of intakes. Molybedenum is readily absorbed, with food-bound molybdenum about 16% less bioavailable than soluble complexes (e.g., ammonium molybdate), over a

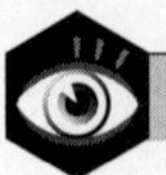

NUTRITION INSIGHT

Essential Elements

The concept of essential nutrients was well established by 1940 with a definition of food substances necessary for life, tissue growth, and repair that the body cannot synthesize. Essential nutrients were identified when dietary deficiency led to disease or failure to grow. In the 1960s and 1970s, new criteria appeared for establishing essentiality of mineral elements that could not be fed at dietary concentrations low enough to cause death or interrupt the life cycle (growth, development, or maturation such that procreation is prevented). The major criterion was that a dietary deficiency had to consistently and adversely change a biological function from optimal, and this change was preventable or reversible by physiological amounts of the element. In the 1980s and 1990s, establishing essentiality on the basis of this criterion began to receive resistance when many elements were suggested to be essential based on some small change in a physiological or biochemical variable after experimental animals were supposedly fed a diet deficient in an element. These elements included those in Table 41-1. Doubts arose about whether many of the changes were really the result of suboptimal functions. It was suggested that many of the changes were the result of pharmacological or supranutritional amounts of an element fed to supplemented controls having a beneficial effect through overcoming the lack of some other nutrient, preventing a detrimental effect caused by an inappropriate intake of another dietary substance, or affecting intestinal organisms. As a result, if the lack of an element cannot be shown to cause death or interrupt the life cycle, most nutritionists today do not consider an element essential unless it has a defined biochemical function. However, several mineral elements were often described as essential, including chromium and fluoride, before current criteria came into vogue. Therefore these are still often stated as essential in the literature when they probably should be reported as possibly essential or bioactive beneficial mineral elements.

broad range of intakes (Novotny and Turnland, 2006, 2007). Men absorbed 90% to 94% of daily intakes of molybdenum ranging from 22 to 1,490 μg. Molybdenum absorption was most efficient at the highest levels of dietary molybdenum. The amount and percentage of molybdenum excreted in the urine increased as dietary molybdenum increased, which suggests that urinary excretion rather than regulated absorption is the major homeostatic mechanism for molybdenum. The absorption of molybdenum can be reduced by diets high in sulfur, because the sulfate anion is a competitive inhibitor of molybdenum absorption (Mills and Davis, 1987).

Molybdate is transported loosely attached to erythrocytes in blood (Johnson, 1997). Concentrations of molybdenum in tissues, blood, and milk vary with molybdenum intake. For example, mean plasma concentration for men with an intake of 22 μg/day was 0.51 μg/L, with an intake of 121 μg/day it was 1.17 μg/L, and with an intake of 1,490 μg/day it was 6.22 μg/L (Novotny and Turnland, 2007). Highest concentrations of molybdenum are found in liver, kidney, and bone (normally >1 mg/kg dry weight) (Johnson, 1997). The concentration of molybdenum in other tissues usually is between 0.14 and 0.20 mg/kg dry weight.

MOLYBDENUM COFACTOR SYNTHESIS

The molybdenum cofactor is an unstable reduced pterin with a unique four-carbon side chain, which is synthesized by a complex pathway that requires the protein products encoded by at least four different genes (*MOCS1, MOCS2, MOCS3,* and *GEPH*) (Reiss and Johnson, 2003). Both *MOCS1* (molybdenum cofactor synthesis-step 1) and *MOCS2* (molybdenum cofactor synthesis-step 2) are bicistronic genes, encoding two proteins in different open reading frames. The protein products are designated MOCS1A, MOCS1B, MOCS2A, and MOCS2B and are required for synthesis of molybdopterin. Molybdopterin synthase (MOCS2A and MOCS2B) must be activated by a sulfotransferase that is the product of MOCS3. *GEPH* encodes gephyrin, which is required during cofactor assembly for insertion of molybdenum. Gephyrin is a bifunctional protein that is essential for synaptic clustering of inhibitory neurotransmitter receptors in the central nervous system as well as the biosynthesis of molybdopterin in peripheral tissues. The steps in molybdenum cofactor formation are illustrated in Figure 41-1.

INBORN ERRORS IN MOLYBDENUM COFACTOR SYNTHESIS

Molybdenum cofactor deficiency is a rare inborn error of metabolism. Mutations that affect molybdenum cofactor synthesis result in the simultaneous loss of activity of all human molybdenum cofactor–dependent enzymes. The combined deficiency of sulfite oxidase, xanthine dehydrogenase, and aldehyde oxidase results in a severe phenotype clinically similar to that in patients with the rarer isolated sulfite oxidase deficiency. The two conditions can easily be distinguished by diminished uric acid levels and elevated xanthine concentrations in plasma and urine that result from the decreased xanthine dehydrogenase activity in the combined cofactor deficiency but not in isolated sulfite oxidase deficiency. Diagnosis of molybdenum cofactor deficiency is usually made shortly after birth because of a failure to thrive and neonatal seizures that are unresponsive to therapy. The disease is associated with a pronounced and progressive loss of white matter in the brain. Biochemical diagnostic changes include elevated urinary sulfite and *S*-sulfocysteine, hypouricemia, elevated plasma *S*-sulfonated transthyretin, and deficient molybdoenzyme activity in fibroblasts. Mild cases of the disease have been reported, probably the result of a low level residual activity of the mutant protein. However, most recognized cases have been severe; most patients die in early childhood and some

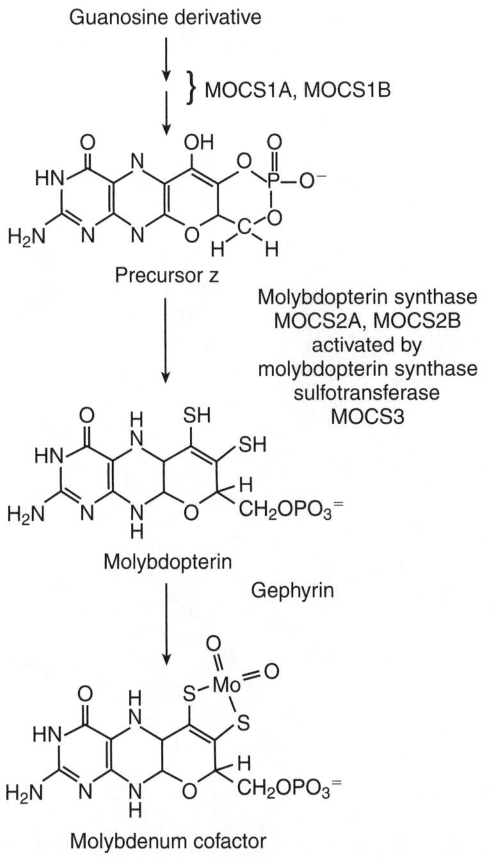

FIGURE 41-1 Pathway of molybdenum cofactor biosynthesis. The genes/proteins that are responsible for molybdenum cofactor synthesis are named MOCS for molybdenum cofactor synthesis and are numbered 1, 2, and 3. The gephyrin protein (encoded by *GEPH*) is necessary for insertion of molybdenum during cofactor assembly. (From Reiss, J., & Johnson, J. L. [2003]. Mutations in the molybdenum cofactor biosynthetic genes MOCS1, MOCS2, and GEPH. *Human Mutation, 21*, 570. Reprinted with permission of Wiley-Liss, Inc., a subsidiary of John Wiley & Sons, Inc.)

survive for only a few days. There currently is no effective dietary or oral therapy for molybdenum cofactor deficiency. However, a single case was successfully treated by daily intravenous administration of cyclic pyranopterin monophosphate (Veldman et al., 2010).

Most disease-producing mutations have been identified in *MOCS1* and *MOCS2* (Reiss and Johnson, 2003). Mutations of *MOCS3* are very rare (Yamamoto et al., 2003; Ichida et al., 2001). A mutation in *GEPH* was identified in fibroblasts of a patient from a family with three deceased children who had all been diagnosed as molybdenum cofactor–deficient (Reiss et al., 2001).

NUTRITIONAL REQUIREMENT

Although molybdenum is an established essential element, it is not of much practical concern in human nutrition. Reports describing signs of nutritional molybdenum deficiency in humans are rare. A convincing case of molybdenum deprivation was observed in a patient with Crohn's disease who was receiving prolonged parenteral nutrition therapy (Abumrad et al., 1981). Signs and symptoms exhibited by this patient, which were exacerbated by methionine administration, included high methionine and low uric acid levels in blood, high oxypurines and low uric acid in urine, and very low urinary sulfate excretion. This patient had mental disturbances that progressed to coma. Intravenous supplementation with ammonium molybdate improved the clinical condition, reversed the sulfur-handling defect, and normalized uric acid production. Men fed only 22 μg molybdenum/day for 102 days maintained molybdenum balance and exhibited no biochemical signs of deficiency (Turnlund et al., 1995). In a separate study, four men adapted to consuming diets that provided 22 μg daily exhibited decreased uric acid and increased xanthine excretion in urine in response to a load dose of adenosine monophosphate; these changes suggest that xanthine oxidase activity was decreased by the low-molybdenum regimen (Turnlund et al., 1995).

Molybdenum deficiency signs also are difficult to induce in animals (Mills and Davis, 1987). In rats and chicks, excessive dietary tungsten was used to restrict molybdenum absorption, and thus induce molybdenum deficiency signs, which included depressed activities of molybdoenzymes, disturbed uric acid metabolism, and increased susceptibility to sulfite toxicity.

Beneficial effects have been reported for supranutritional amounts of molybdenum in the form of tetrathiomolybdate, which inhibits metal transfer functions between copper trafficking proteins (Alvarez et al., 2010). Copper-lowering therapy by tetrathiomolybdate has been found to inhibit cancer growth in five rodent models, and in advanced and metastatic cancer in dogs and humans (Brewer, 2003). In animal studies, tetrathiomolybdate inhibited pulmonary fibrosis induced by bleomycin, hepatitis induced by concanavalin A, cirrhosis induced by carbon tetrachloride (Brewer, 2003), and hyperglycemia induced by streptozotocin (Zeng et al., 2008). Supranutritional amounts of sodium molybdate were found to prevent hyperinsulinemia and hypertension induced by fructose in rats (Güner et al., 2001).

DIETARY REFERENCE INTAKES

Although molybdenum deficiency has not been observed in healthy people, Dietary Reference Intakes (DRIs) have been set for molybdenum (Institute of Medicine [IOM], 2001). Based on the balance studies done by Turnlund and colleagues (1995), which indicated adults could achieve molybdenum balance on an intake of 22 μg/day, the requirement was estimated to be 25 μg/day (22 μg/day plus 3 μg/day to allow for miscellaneous losses not measured in the study). Because some foods, such as soy, have lower bioavailability than the foods provided in the balance studies done by Turnlund and co-workers (1995), an average bioavailability of 75% was used to set an Estimated Average Requirement (EAR) of 34 μg/day for adults. The Recommended Dietary Allowance (RDA) was set as the EAR + 30% and is 45 μg/day for adults. DRIs for children were extrapolated from the adult value, using metabolic weight ($kg^{0.75}$) as the base for extrapolation. Molybdenum has relatively low toxicity. Based largely on

DRIs Across the Life Cycle: Boron, Chromium, Molybdenum, Nickel, and Vanadium

	Boron UL mg/day	Chromium AI μg/day	Molybdenum RDA μg/day	Molybdenum UL mg/day	Nickel UL mg/day	Vanadium UL mg/day
Infants						
0 through 6 mo	ND	0.2	2 (AI)	ND	ND	ND
7 through 12 mo	ND	5.5	3 (AI)	ND	ND	ND
Children						
1 through 3 yr	3	11	17	0.3	0.2	ND
4 through 8 yr	6	15	22	0.6	0.3	ND
Males						
9 through 13 yr	11	25	34	1.1	0.6	ND
14 through 18 yr	17	35	43	1.7	1.0	ND
19 through 50 yr	20	35	45	2.0	1.0	1.8
≥51 yr	20	30	45	2.0	1.0	1.8
Females						
9 through 13 yr	11	21	34	1.1	0.6	ND
14 through 18 yr	17	24	43	1.7	1.0	ND
19 through 50 yr	20	25	45	2.0	1.0	1.8
≥51 yr	20	20	45	2.0	1.0	1.8
Pregnant						
<19 yr	17	29	50	1.7	1.0	ND
≥19 yr	20	30	50	2.0	1.0	ND
Lactating						
<19 yr	17	44	50	1.7	1.0	ND
≥19 yr	20	45	50	2.0	1.0	ND

Institute of Medicine. (2001). *Dietary Reference Intakes for vitamin A, vitamin K, arsenic, boron, chromium, copper, iodine, iron, manganese, molybdenum, nickel, silicon, vanadium, and zinc.* Washington, DC: National Academy Press.

AI, Adequate Intake; *DRI*, Dietary Reference Intake; *ND*, not determinable; *RDA*, Recommended Dietary Allowance; *UL*, Tolerable Upper Intake Level.

animal studies, the IOM (2001) set the UL for molybdenum at 2,000 μg/day (or 2.0 mg/day) for adults.

For most of the population, the diet is the most important source of molybdenum. Plant foods are the major sources of molybdenum in the diet, and their molybdenum content depends upon the content of the soil in which they are grown. Good food sources of molybdenum include legumes, grain products, and nuts. Two studies of molybdenum intake in the United States yielded average intakes ranging from 76 to 240 μg/day for adults (Pennington and Jones, 1987; Tsongas et al., 1980). Therefore almost all diets should meet the RDA for molybdenum.

BORON

NUTRITIONAL AND PHYSIOLOGICAL SIGNIFICANCE

Boron has been shown to be essential for the completion of the life cycle (i.e., deficiency causes impaired growth, development, or maturation such that procreation is prevented) for organisms in all phylogenetic kingdoms (Nielsen, 2008a). In the animal kingdom, the lack of boron was shown to adversely affect reproduction and embryo development in both the African clawed frog *(Xenopus laevis)* and zebra fish.

Experiments with mammals have not shown that the life cycle can be interrupted by boron deprivation, nor has a biochemical function been defined for it. However, substantial evidence exists for boron being a bioactive food component that is beneficial, if not required, for health (Nielsen, 2008a). Nutritional amounts of boron fed to animals consuming a low-boron diet induce biochemical and functional changes considered beneficial for bone growth and maintenance, brain function, and inflammatory response regulation. For humans, boron intakes of 1 to 3 mg/day compared to intakes of 0.25 to 0.50 mg/day apparently have beneficial effects on bone and brain health (Nielsen, 2008a). In addition, some recent epidemiological and cell culture studies suggest that boron may have a protective effect against prostate, cervical, breast, and lung cancers (Nielsen, 2008a).

Findings showing that nutritional intakes of boron influence central nervous system function are among the most supportive in demonstrating that boron is a beneficial bioactive element for humans. Boron deprivation of older men and women altered electroencephalograms (EEGs) such that they suggested states of reduced behavioral activation (i.e., drowsiness) and mental alertness. The EEG changes may have been responsible for boron deprivation impairing cognitive processes of attention, encoding skills and memory, and psychomotor measures of manual dexterity and fatigue.

Findings that boron deprivation decreased alveolar bone osteoblast surface in rats and mice, prevented maturation of bone growth plate in chicks, and induced limb teratogenesis in frogs suggest that boron is beneficial to bone growth and maintenance through affecting osteoblast and/or osteoclast presence or activity and not through affecting bone calcium concentrations. Boron, however, can be beneficial to calcium metabolism that ultimately affects bone composition through influencing the activity of hormones. Several studies have shown that when fed marginal amounts of vitamin D, classical signs of vitamin D deficiency were exhibited by boron-deprived animals but not by boron-supplemented animals. These signs included rachitic long bones with distortion of marrow sprouts and delayed initiation of cartilage calcification, decreased calcium and phosphorus apparent absorption and balance, and decreased femur calcium concentration. In addition, boron has been shown to work with estrogen to be beneficial for bone structure and calcium and magnesium metabolism in ovariectomized rats, and serum 17β-estradiol and 25-hydroxyvitamin D concentrations in humans.

POSSIBLE BIOCHEMICAL FORMS AND PHYSIOLOGICAL ACTIONS

The diverse responses reported for low intakes of boron have made it difficult to identify a primary mechanism responsible for the bioactivity of boron. The wide range of responses probably is secondary to boron influencing a cell signaling system, or the formation and/or activity of an entity that is involved in many biochemical processes. The biochemistry of boron and some recent animal, bacteria, and plant findings have given some insights as to the possible basis for the bioactivity of boron and have resulted in several hypothesized mechanisms of action.

Boron biochemistry is essentially that of boric acid. Boron has three L-shell electrons available for bonding as in boric acid, but there is a tendency for boron to acquire an additional electron pair to fill the fourth orbital. Therefore boric acid acts as a Lewis acid and accepts an electron pair from a base (H_2O) to form tetracovalent boron compounds, such as $B(OH)_4^-$. Thus the reaction:

$$B(OH)_3 + H_2O \rightleftharpoons B(OH)_4^- + H^+$$

At the pH of blood (7.4), this process results in dilute aqueous boric acid solutions composed of $B(OH)_3$ and $B(OH)_4^-$. Because the pK_a of boric acid is 9.25, the abundance of these two species in blood should be 98.4% and 1.6%, respectively. Boric acid forms ester complexes with hydroxyl groups of organic compounds, which preferably occurs when the hydroxyl groups are adjacent and *cis*. This property results in boron as boric acid forming complexes with several biologically important sugars, including ribose.

Ribose is a component of adenosine. The diverse actions of boron might occur through its reaction with biomolecules containing adenosine or formed from adenosine-containing precursors. *S*-Adenosylmethionine and diadenosine phosphates have higher affinities for boron than any other currently recognized boron ligands in animal tissues (Hunt, 2008). Diadenosine phosphates are present in all animal cells and function as signal nucleotides associated with neuronal response. *S*-Adenosylmethionine, which is synthesized from adenosine triphosphate and methionine, is one of the most frequently used enzyme substrates in the body (see Chapter 25). About 95% of *S*-adenosylmethionine is used in methylation reactions, which influences the activity of DNA, RNA, proteins, phospholipids, hormones, and neurotransmitters. The methylation reactions result in the formation of *S*-adenosylhomocysteine, which can be hydrolyzed into homocysteine. High circulating homocysteine and depleted *S*-adenosylmethionine have been implicated in many of the disorders suggested to be affected by nutritional intakes of boron, including osteoporosis, arthritis, cancer, diabetes, and impaired brain function. The suggestion that boron bioactivity may be associated with *S*-adenosylmethionine is supported by the finding that the bacterial quorum-sensing signal molecule, auto-inducer AI-2, is a furanosyl borate ester synthesized from *S*-adenosylmethionine (Chen et al., 2002). Quorum sensing is the cell-to-cell communication between bacteria accomplished through the exchange of extracellular signaling molecules (auto-inducers). Deprivation studies with rats also indicate that boron is bioactive through affecting *S*-adenosylmethionine. Boron deprivation increased plasma homocysteine and decreased liver *S*-adenosylmethionine and *S*-adenosylhomocysteine (Nielsen, 2009a).

Boron also strongly binds oxidized nicotinamide adenine dinucleotide (NAD^+) and thus may influence reactions in which NAD^+ is involved. For example, extracellular NAD^+ binds to the plasma membrane receptor, CD38, an adenosine diphosphate (ADP)-ribosyl cyclase that converts NAD^+ to cyclic ADP ribose (ADPR) (also see Chapter 24). ADPR is released intracellularly (Eckhert, 2006) where it binds to the ryanodine receptor and releases Ca^{2+} from the endoplasmic reticulum. Thus boron may be bioactive through binding NAD^+ and/or ADPR and inhibiting Ca^{2+} release. Ca^{2+} is a signal ion for many processes in which boron has been shown to have an effect, including insulin release, bone formation, immune response, and brain function.

Boron also may become bioactive through forming diester borate complexes with phosphoinositides, glycoproteins, and glycolipids, which contain *cis*-hydroxyl groups, in membranes. The finding that the borate transporter NaBC1, which apparently is essential for boron homeostasis in animal cells, conducts Na^+ and OH^- across cell membranes in the absence of boron (Park et al., 2004) supports the suggestion that boron affects the transduction of regulatory ions across cell membranes. It is speculated that the primary essential role of boron in plants, perhaps involving interplay between boron and calcium, is at the cell membrane level that affects signaling events (Bolaños et al., 2004).

Naturally occurring organoboron compounds identified to date contain boron bound to four oxygen groups or as stable boron diesters. Among these compounds are several antibiotics, including boromycin, an antibiotic synthesized by *Streptomyces antibioticus* that has the ability to encapsulate alkali metal cations and increase the permeability of the cytoplasmic membrane to potassium ions.

DIETARY CONSIDERATIONS

About 85% of ingested boron is absorbed and then efficiently excreted via the urine, mainly as boric acid. As a result, urinary boron mirrors boron intake. Boron is distributed throughout soft tissues at concentrations mostly between 1.39 and 1.85 μmol/kg fresh tissue (0.015 to 2.0 μg/g) (World Health Organization, 1998). Based on studies with postmenopausal women, fasting plasma boron concentrations range from 3.14 to 8.79 mmol/L (34 to 95 ng/mL) (Nielsen, 2006). The concentration of boron in human milk was found to be relatively stable, with mean concentrations ranging from 2.50 to 3.88 μmol/kg (27 to 42 μg/kg) (Hunt, 2008). As with other mineral elements, overcoming homeostatic mechanisms by high boron intakes will elevate tissue and blood boron concentrations.

The IOM (2001) did not set Recommended Dietary Allowances (RDAs) or Adequate Intakes (AIs) for boron, but did set Tolerable Upper Intake Levels (ULs) for different age groups. The UL for adults is 20 mg/day.

In human depletion–repletion experiments, participants responded to a boron supplement after consuming a diet supplying only 0.2 to 0.4 mg/day for 63 days (Nielsen, 2008a), which suggests that this intake of boron is inadequate. Thus a dietary boron intake higher than 0.4 mg/day may be needed to promote bone and brain health and immune function. Extrapolation of data from animal experiments suggests that 1.0 mg boron/day may provide optimal nutritional benefits. Both animal and human data were used by the World Health Organization (1996) to suggest that an acceptable safe range of population mean intakes of boron for adults could be 1 to 13 mg/day. Many people apparently have boron intakes of less than 1.0 mg/day. The Continuing Survey of Food Intakes by Individuals (CSFII), 1994–1996, indicated that boron intakes ranged from a low of about 0.35 to a high of about 3.0 mg/day for adults (IOM, 2001). The median boron intakes for various age groups of adults ranged from 0.81 to 1.22 mg/day. Rich food sources of boron are fruits, leafy vegetables, nuts, legumes, and pulses (e.g., dry beans).

CHROMIUM

NUTRITIONAL AND PHYSIOLOGICAL SIGNIFICANCE

Approximately 50 years ago, trivalent chromium was reported to be the active component of the "glucose tolerance factor" that alleviated impaired glucose tolerance in rats fed torula yeast–sucrose diets (Schwarz and Mertz, 1959). This change was accepted as proof for chromium essentiality for higher animals. Essentiality for humans gained acceptance when it was found between 1977 and 1986 that chromium supplementation alleviated glucose intolerance and neuropathy exhibited by three patients on long-term total parenteral nutrition (Moukarzel, 2009). Since then no reports of chromium supplementation helping patients on long-term parenteral nutrition have appeared. However, subsequent to these three cases, a number of reports from numerous research groups described beneficial effects provided by chromium supplementation in study participants with varying degrees of glucose intolerance, ranging from hypoglycemia (low blood sugar) to insulin-dependent diabetes (Anderson, 1998). Also, beneficial effects of chromium supplementation on blood lipid profiles were reported. These findings promoted the concept of chromium essentiality although most studies found that supranutritional amounts of chromium were required to be effective.

As the decades passed without a defined biochemical function for chromium, doubts arose about it being classified as essential. The development of the controversy about chromium essentiality has been reviewed by Vincent and Stallings (2007). Doubts about chromium essentiality were heightened by difficulties in inducing consistent signs of chromium deficiency in experimental animals. Nutritional, metabolic, physiological, or hormonal stressors generally had to be employed to induce experimental animals to respond to chromium deprivation; in most cases, the responses were not remarkable. In addition, a systematic review of randomized controlled trials (Balk et al., 2007) found no significant effects of chromium on lipid or glucose metabolism in people without diabetes. However, chromium supplementation slightly but significantly improved glycemia in patients with diabetes. Patient selection may be the basis for not finding a consistent beneficial effect of chromium on carbohydrate metabolism in individuals with metabolic syndrome, impaired glucose tolerance, or type 2 diabetes (Wang and Cefalu, 2010). A clinical response to chromium (i.e., decreased glucose level and improved insulin sensitivity) apparently is most likely in insulin-resistant individuals with type 2 diabetes and highly elevated fasting plasma glucose and hemoglobin A_{1c} concentrations; these individuals may be lacking chromium in an essential function. However, supranutritional amounts were usually needed to be therapeutically effective, which could mean that chromium was acting pharmacologically to alleviate another cause of pathology in these subjects. Thus whether chromium is an essential nutrient remains uncertain and still a controversial issue. However, substantial evidence exists to indicate that chromium has beneficial bioactivity under certain circumstances.

Among the circumstances hypothesized that would benefit from chromium supplementation were endeavors to decrease body fat (weight loss) and to increase muscle or lean body mass. These hypotheses were based on the assumption that chromium would amplify the action of insulin under all circumstances, and this amplification would result in less glucose being converted into fat and in an upregulation of protein synthesis for muscle gain. The lack of chromium supplementation affecting glucose metabolism or insulin action in people without insulin resistance and diabetes explains why well-conducted randomized controlled trials showed no effect of supplemental chromium on weight and body composition (Lukaski and Scrimgeour, 2009).

Low chromium concentration in toenails has been associated with cardiovascular disease (Guallar et al., 2005;

Rajpathak et al., 2004). However, these epidemiological findings do not reveal whether the low concentrations indicate a cause or effect of cardiovascular disease. Long-term supplementation trials are needed to ascertain whether chromium supplementation would be beneficial to cardiovascular health.

POSSIBLE BIOCHEMICAL FORMS AND PHYSIOLOGICAL ACTIONS

Cr^{3+} is the most stable oxidation state of chromium and most likely the valence state of importance in biological systems. Cr^{6+}, which is a byproduct of manufacturing stainless steel, pigments, chromate chemicals, and other products, also is stable. However, Cr^{6+} would presumably be readily reduced to Cr^{3+} by reducing agents in foods or within the upper gastrointestinal tract.

In aqueous solutions, Cr^{3+} complexes are relatively inert kinetically, such that ligand-displacement reactions have half-times in the range of several hours. Therefore chromium is unlikely to be involved as a metal catalyst at the active site of enzymes where the rate of exchange needs to be rapid. However, chromium may have a structural role such as in the tertiary structure of a protein or nucleic acid. In addition, chromium may bind ligands in the proper orientation to facilitate enzymatic catalysis; this may be the role for chromodulin, which was previously called low-molecular-weight Cr-binding substance. Chromodulin has been described as a naturally occurring mammalian oligopeptide with a mass of about 1.5 kDa; it is composed of glycine, cysteine, aspartate, and glutamate and binds four chromic ions tightly and cooperatively ($K_a \sim 10^{21}$ M^{-4}) (Vincent and Bennett, 2007). Apochromodulin (apparently the predominant form in vivo) can accept chromic ions from other biological molecules such as transferrin, which may serve as a transporter of chromium (Vincent and Bennett, 2007).

Two potential functions for chromodulin have been described. Chromodulin carries chromium into the urine after a large dose is given. Thus Stearns (2007) has suggested that chromodulin is nothing more than a molecule for the detoxification and excretion of chromium. However, Vincent and Bennett (2007) have described substantial evidence indicating that chromodulin potentiates insulin effects by amplifying insulin-dependent protein tyrosine kinase activity of the insulin receptor; this stimulation apparently is dependent upon the chrominum content of chromodulin. It is hypothesized (Vincent and Bennett, 2007) that the binding of insulin to its receptor on an insulin-sensitive cell causes a conformational change resulting in the autophosphorylation of tyrosine residues on the internal side of the receptor. The receptor becomes an active tyrosine kinase that transmits the insulin signal into the cell. In response to insulin, chromium also moves into insulin-sensitive cells, which contain apochromodulin, to form holochromodulin. The holochromodulin then binds to the receptor to assist in maintaining it in an active form, thus amplifying the receptor's kinase activity. When blood insulin decreases, a change in the conformation of the insulin receptor causes a release of the holochromodulin from the cell to blood and excretion in the urine. Chromium is specifically needed by the oligopeptide for activity. Apochromodulin is inactive in stimulating insulin receptor kinase activity. Titration with chromic ions completely restores activity, whereas other transition metals known to be essential fail to restore activity.

In cultured skeletal muscle cells, chromium upregulates mRNA levels of insulin receptor, GLUT 4 (glucose transporter), glycogen synthase, and uncoupling protein 3 (Qiao et al., 2009). This upregulation, however, may be occurring through the amplification of insulin, which also increases mRNA for glucose uptake and these metabolism substances. Nonetheless, chromium, or a biologically active form of chromium, might have a role in regulating gene expression of a critical substance in glucose metabolism. Ribonucleic acid (RNA) synthesis directed by free DNA in vitro has been shown to be enhanced by the binding of chromium to the template. Furthermore, chromium is concentrated in hepatic nuclei 48 hours after intraperitoneal injection of $CrCl_3$. The chromium is preferentially bound to DNA in chromatin and increases the number of initiation sites, which enhances RNA synthesis.

Another possible role suggested for chromium is the activation of GLUT4 trafficking via a cholesterol-dependent mechanism (Chen et al., 2006). Chromium altered plasma membrane cholesterol and mobilized GLUT4 to the plasma membrane in cultured cells. It was suggested that chromium may have reduced membrane cholesterol through an effect on AMP-activated protein kinase.

DIETARY CONSIDERATIONS

Estimates of Cr^{3+} absorption, based on metabolic balance studies or on urinary excretion during physiological intakes, range from 0.4% to 2.5%. Most ingested chromium is excreted unabsorbed in the feces. Most absorbed chromium is excreted rapidly in the urine. The highest levels of chromium in human tissues are found in liver, spleen, and bone. Cr^{3+} competes for one of the binding sites on transferrin, and most of the chromium in blood apparently is found bound to transferrin.

In the absence of a functional criterion for assessing chromium status, the IOM (2001) set AIs for chromium rather than EARs and RDAs. On the basis of a limited number of chromium balance studies and determinations of dietary intakes of chromium by adults, the mean chromium content of well-balanced daily diets was determined to be 13.4 μg/1,000 kcal (IOM, 2001). The AIs are based on this value and estimated energy intakes. No UL was set for dietary chromium (soluble Cr^{3+} salts) because of insufficient data and little evidence for adverse effects. Cr^{3+} is unlikely to be toxic because it forms complexes with oxygen-based ligands that are usually electrochemically inactive and thus have poor ability to cross cell membranes. However, Cr^{6+} has a much higher level of toxicity and is classified as a human carcinogen, mutagen, and clastogen.

No national survey data are available on chromium intakes. Chromium is widely distributed throughout the food supply, but the chromium content is highly variable among different lots of the same food and is subject to increases and decreases during food processing. Whole grains, pulses, some vegetables (e.g., broccoli and mushrooms), liver, processed meats, ready-to-eat cereals, spices, and beer are generally good sources. Dietary chromium content based on paired food or duplicate meal analyses for self-selected diets yielded mean chromium intakes of 22 to 48 μg/day for 10 adult men and 13 to 36 μg/day for 23 adult women (Anderson and Kozlovsky, 1985); these estimates are probably lower than normal intakes because of evidence that participants decrease their energy intake when involved in a dietary collection or study.

SILICON

NUTRITIONAL AND PHYSIOLOGICAL SIGNIFICANCE

Silicon is essential for lower forms of life (Carlisle, 1997; Řezanka and Sigler, 2007). Silicon plays a structural role in diatoms, radiolarians, and some sponges. It may be needed by some higher plants, including rice. Silicon is not generally accepted as a confirmed essential nutrient for animals and humans because it lacks a defined specific biochemical function. However, nutritional (10 to 35 mg/kg diet) and supranutritional (e.g., 100 to 500 mg/kg diet as a soluble salt) intakes prevent several physiological and biochemical abnormalities observed in animals fed diets low in silicon (<5 mg/kg). Older studies used supranutritional amounts but subsequent studies used nutritional amounts to show that silicon alleviated abnormal bone (including reduced growth plate and increased chondrocyte density), decreased hexosamine, and increased collagen exhibited by animals fed diets low in silicon (Carlisle, 1997; Nielsen, 2006; Jugdaohsingh et al., 2008). Nutritional amounts of silicon also may modulate the immune or inflammatory response (Nielsen, 2010). Silicon deprivation apparently causes mild chronic inflammation, and influences the chronic-phase inflammatory response as evidenced by a reduction in this response in an animal model of rheumatoid arthritis (Nielsen, 2008b).

Epidemiological, supplementation, and cell culture studies have suggested that nutritional intakes of silicon are beneficially bioactive in humans. Silicon intake was positively associated with bone mineral density in men and premenopausal women, and at the spine and femur in pre- and postmenopausal women on hormone replacement therapy (Jugdaohsingh, 2007). The beneficial effect of moderate beer consumption on hip and spine bone mineral density was associated with the silicon in beer (Tucker et al., 2009). Limited findings from supplementation trials suggest that silicon supplementation may increase bone mineral density in women with low bone mass (Jugdaohsingh, 2007). Increased silicon in drinking water has been associated with decreased incidence of Alzheimer disease and associated disorders (Gillette-Guyonnet et al., 2007).

POSSIBLE BIOLOGICAL FORMS AND PHYSIOLOGICAL ACTION

The mechanism of action for the beneficial bioactivity of silicon has not been identified. Silicon easily forms stable complexes with polyols that have at least four hydroxyl groups (Kinrade et al., 1999). The need for polyol compounds, such as hexosamines and ascorbate, to form glycosaminoglycans, mucopolysaccharides, and collagen involved in connective tissue stabilization or formation is affected by silicon status (Carlisle, 1997).

In plants, silicon apparently binds hydroxyl groups of proteins involved in signal transduction (Řezanka and Sigler, 2007). A similar action might be the basis for the finding that silicon in mice stimulated gene expression of factors involved in osteoblastogenesis and suppressed expression of factors involved in osteoclastogenesis (Maehira et al., 2009). The silicon in silica-based bioactive glass and ceramics has been implicated in the in vivo efficiency of bone implants through involvement in gene upregulation, osteoblast proliferation and differentation, type 1 collagen synthesis, and apatite formation (Jugdaohsingh, 2007). Silicon also might be affecting the inflammatory or immune response and cognitive function through an effect on cell components involved in signal transduction.

Another mechanism through which silicon may be beneficial is by altering the absorption or utilization of other mineral elements involved in bone metabolism, immune or inflammatory response, or cognitive function. Epidemiological findings indicate that silicon can alleviate the toxic actions of aluminum (Gillette-Guyonnet et al., 2007) and facilitate the absorption, retention, or utilization of copper, iron, and magnesium (Nielsen, 2006).

DIETARY CONSIDERATIONS

The IOM (2001) judged that animal and human data were too limited to allow setting any DRIs for silicon. On the basis of extrapolations from animal data, weak balance data from humans, and the usual amount of silicon excreted daily by urine, it has been suggested that a daily intake of 10 to 25 mg/day would be beneficial to humans (Nielsen, 2006, 2009b). High-fiber diets, aging, and high dietary molybdenum, calcium, and magnesium might necessitate an increase in this intake. The dietary intake of silicon is between 15 and 50 mg/day for most Western populations (Nielsen, 2006; Jugdaohsingh, 2007). Foods rich in silicon include unrefined grains, some vegetables, and seafood (Jugdaohsingh, 2007).

BIOACTIVE ULTRATRACE ELEMENTS: NICKEL, VANADIUM, AND ARSENIC

Nickel, vanadium, and arsenic are bioactive in higher animals and are components of naturally occurring and biologically important molecules. Biological roles for these elements have been established in lower forms of life, which indicate that they may be essential or have beneficial bioactive actions in humans.

NICKEL

Nickel is generally acknowledged as being essential for plants and some bacteria. In these lower forms of life, nickel has been identified as an essential component of eight different enzymes. Seven of the enzymes are involved in the use or production of gases: (1) urease produces NH_3, (2) Ni-Fe hydrogenase generates and utilizes H_2, (3) carbon monoxide (CO) dehydrogenase interconverts CO and CO_2, (4) methyl-coenzyme M reductase generates CH_4, (5) Ni superoxide dismutase generates O_2, (6) acireductone dioxygenase produces CO, and (7) acetyl-CoA synthase catalyzes acetyl-CoA synthesis from CO_2 (Ragsdale, 2009). These gases are essential components of the global carbon, nitrogen, and oxygen cycles. Nickel apparently is utilized in these enzymes because of its coordination and redox chemistry (Ragsdale, 2009). Nickel is able to cycle through three redox states (+1, +2, and +3) and to catalyze reactions spanning approximately 1.5 V. The other nickel enzyme, glyoxylase I converts methylglyoxal to lactate. A mammalian nickel-dependent enzyme has not been identified.

Although an essential biochemical function in higher animals has not been identified for nickel, deprivation studies show that it has beneficial if not essential functions in several experimental animal models. Among the detrimental changes described for nickel deprivation are impaired reproduction (decreased conception rate and sperm production and motility), impaired bone health (decreased strength and altered composition), undesirable changes in carbohydrate and lipid metabolism (e.g., increased plasma lipids), decreased iron status or utilization, impaired vitamin B_{12} action, and enhanced renal damage and high blood pressure induced by a high-salt diet (Nielsen, 2006).

One possible mechanism for nickel bioactivity in such a variety of processes is through affecting gaseous molecules that have signaling roles, such as O_2, nitric oxide (NO), and CO. Oxygen, a regulator of cellular energetics and maturation, is carefully regulated in higher animals. In most tissues, the molecular and cellular responses to a low O_2 tension is the activation of the transcription factor hypoxia-inducible factor 1 (HIF-1). Nickel has the ability to stabilize the HIF-1α protein and to activate hypoxia-inducible gene expression (Kang et al., 2006). These genes are involved in angiogenesis, glucose transport, glycolysis, erythropoiesis, and catecholamine metabolism. Activation of the HIF-1α pathway also increases osteogenesis (Wang et al., 2007) and preosteocyte maturation and mineralization (Zahm et al., 2008).

Nickel also potently induces the activity of heme oxygenase that produces CO. Carbon monoxide inhibits NO synthases activity and activates guanylate cyclase to produce cGMP. The cGMP signal transduction system has a crucial role in vision, taste, smell, blood pressure control, kidney function, and sperm motility, all of which are affected by nutritional amounts of nickel (Nielsen et al., 2002; Gordon and Zagotta, 1995).

Nickel also may be bioactive through altering methyl metabolism, which would have far-reaching effects through influencing the utilization of *S*-adenosylmethionine. The lack of vitamin B_{12}, which is involved in methyl metabolism, inhibits the response of rats to nickel supplementation when dietary nickel is low (Nielsen et al., 1989), and nickel can alleviate vitamin B_{12} deficiency in pigs, including an increase in serum homocysteine (Stangl et al., 2000).

Absorption of dietary nickel is typically less than 10% of intake and is increased by iron deficiency, pregnancy, and lactation. In the plasma, most nickel is bound to albumin. The transport of nickel into tissues may involve magnesium and/or iron transport mechanisms. Nickel is widely distributed in tissues in concentrations between 0.01 and 0.2 mg/kg wet weight.

The IOM (2001) did not set an RDA or AI for nickel because of lack of evidence for an essential function in humans. Based on animal studies, a beneficial intake of nickel for humans might be near 50 μg/day. Typical daily dietary intakes for nickel are 70 to 260 μg/day for adults in the United States and Canada. Rich sources of nickel include chocolate, nuts, legumes, and grains. The UL is 1.0 mg/day for adults, based on levels that caused general systemic toxicity in rats (IOM, 2001).

VANADIUM

Vanadium is essential for some lower forms of life (algae, seaweeds, a lichen, and a fungus) where it is a component of the haloperoxidases bromoperoxidase, iodoperoxidase, and chloroperoxidase. Haloperoxidases catalyze the oxidation of halide ions by hydrogen peroxide (H_2O_2), thereby facilitating the formation of a carbon–halogen bond (Crans et al., 2004). The mechanism of action of vanadium in the haloperoxidases is H_2O_2 reacting with vanadium as V^{5+} to form a dioxygen species that reacts with the halide to yield an oxidized halide species, which is the intermediate that forms the carbon–halogen bond.

Vanadium is generally not accepted as an essential nutrient for higher animals and humans, but there is no question that it is a bioactive element. Beneficial activity at nutritional intakes is indicated by findings from vanadium deprivation studies. Vanadium deprivation resulted in swollen joints, skeletal deformations, and decreased life span in goats (Anke et al., 2005). Also, an increased death rate, sometimes preceded by convulsions, occurred in kids of vanadium-deprived goats. Vanadium deprivation altered thyroid hormone metabolism, impaired reproduction, and altered bone morphology in rats (Nielsen, 1998).

Vanadium in pharmacological or supranutritional amounts has been repeatedly found to have beneficial bioactivity. Its ability to selectively inhibit protein tyrosine phosphatases probably explains the broad range of effects vanadium has on cellular regulatory cascades. The mechanism by which vanadium inhibits protein tyrosine phosphatases has been suggested to involve the generation of H_2O_2 upon the conversion of the pentavalent V^{5+} anion, vanadate (VO_3^-), to the intracellular tetravalent V^{4+} anion, vanadyl (VO_2^+), which is catalyzed by NADPH oxidase. The vanadyl may then react with H_2O_2 to form peroxovanadate (Hulley and Davison, 2003). Peroxovanadate quickly and irreversibly oxidizes the active site cysteine to cysteic acid in protein tyrosine phosphatase. Protein tyrosine phosphatase inhibition apparently is the basis for vanadium having insulin-like actions at the cellular level and stimulating cellular proliferation and differentiation. The insulin-mimetic action of vanadium has resulted in an effort to develop vanadium compounds that could be therapeutic agents for diabetes (Marzban and McNeill, 2003; Sakurai, 2007).

Because urine vanadium is usually less than 0.8 μg/L and the estimated daily intake of vanadium is 12 to 30 μg, apparently less than 5% of vanadium ingested normally is absorbed with the remainder being excreted in the feces (Nielsen, 1998). Vanadate is absorbed three to five times more effectively than vanadyl. When vanadate appears in the blood, it is quickly converted into the vanadyl cation. Vanadyl is bound and transported by transferrin and albumin. Vanadium is rapidly removed from plasma and is generally retained in tissues under normal conditions at concentrations less than 10 ng/g fresh weight. Urine is the major excretory route for absorbed vanadium.

No RDA or AI was set by the IOM (2001) for vanadium. Based on animal experiments, any requirement for vanadium would be small; a daily dietary intake of 10 μg probably would meet any postulated requirement. Good sources of vanadium include grains and grain products, mushrooms, parsley, and shellfish. Based on evidence for renal toxicity in animals, the UL for adults was set at 1,800 μg of vanadium per day (or 1.8 mg per day) (IOM, 2001).

ARSENIC

Arsenic is unquestionably a bioactive element in higher animals and humans. However, the concept that arsenic has beneficial activity at physiological intakes is not well accepted, although animal deprivation studies (<35 ng/g diet) indicate that arsenic is beneficial to chickens, hamsters, goats, pigs, and rats (Uthus, 1992; Anke, 2005). The most consistent signs of apparent arsenic deprivation were depressed growth and abnormal reproduction characterized by impaired fertility and increased perinatal mortality. Death with myocardial damage occurred in lactating goats. Limited in vitro and epidemiological studies also have suggested that arsenic can have beneficial effects at low exposures in humans. For example, one study found that humans exhibited a "J shaped response" to arsenic exposure via drinking water (Kayajanian, 2003). Compared to exposure to drinking water containing about 50 μg/L, both low exposure (<50 μg/L) and high exposure (>100 μg/L) resulted in a higher incidence of cancers. A similar response was seen in an animal study that determined the effects of arsenic on dimethylhydrazine-induced aberrant crypts (Uthus and Davis, 2005). The mechanism through which arsenic is bioactive most likely involves the utilization of labile methyl groups arising from methionine. By altering labile methyl group metabolism, arsenic affects the function of metabolically or genetically important molecules dependent on or regulated by methyl incorporation (Davis et al., 2000). In higher amounts (pharmacological) arsenic in the trioxide form is an effective treatment for some forms of cancer, especially promyelocytic leukemia. Arsenic promotes the degradation of an oncogenic protein (PML-RARα) that drives the growth of acute promyelocytic leukemia cells (Zhang et al., 2010).

Humans have enzymes that are used specifically to methylate inorganic arsenic (Thomas et al., 2007). Methylation of arsenic takes place in the liver, following glutathione-dependent reduction of arsenate (As^{5+}) to arsenite (As^{3+}), and is catalyzed by an arsenite methyltransferase that utilizes *S*-adenosylmethionine as the methyl donor. The monomethylarsonic acid formed is reduced to monomethylarsonous acid, which is rapidly methylated by a methyltransferase to form dimethylarsinic acid. Methylated arsenic compounds occur normally in all organisms (Le, 2002). Arsenolipids (arsenobeteine and arsenocholine) and arsenosugars are found in a variety of marine life. Arsenolipids are highly absorbed by humans and unchanged before excretion in the urine.

Absorption of arsenic from food is about 65% and absorption of inorganic arsenite or arsenate from water is about 90% of that ingested. With nontoxic or nutritional intakes of arsenic, dimethylarsinic acid is the final step in the metabolism of arsenic by the liver in humans and most animals, and is the major form in urine except when high amounts of seafood are eaten. Urine is the major excretory route for all forms of arsenic. Because mechanisms exist for riding the body of arsenic, no tissue significantly accumulates this element if low, or physiological amounts are ingested. Body arsenic is widely distributed in low concentrations (<1.0 μg/g fresh weight) under normal conditions, with the highest amounts usually found in skin, hair, and nails.

The Total Diet Study of 1991–1997, according to the IOM (2001), found that the median intake of arsenic from foods was 2.0 and 2.6 μg/day for women and men aged 19 to 70 years, respectively. Another report, however, estimated that the individual mean total intake from all food, excluding shellfish, in the United States was 30 μg/day (Adams et al., 1994). This intake is similar to intakes of arsenic that were found to be beneficial in animals and epidemiological studies. Sources of arsenic include fish, meat and poultry, grains and cereal products, grape juice, and spinach. The IOM (2001) did not set any DRIs for arsenic because of the lack of data supporting a biological role for arsenic in humans. Although no UL was set, high intakes of inorganic arsenic are clearly toxic. Organic forms of arsenic that occur naturally in foods have much lower toxicity than does inorganic arsenic.

ABSTRUSE ULTRATRACE ELEMENTS

The nutritional importance of the other ultratrace elements not specifically described in this chapter is quite limited and effectively summarized in Table 41-1. The evidence that these elements have beneficial effects or essential roles

TABLE 41-1 Reported Beneficial Bioactivity of Aluminum, Bromine, Cadmium, Germanium, Lead, Lithium, Rubidium, and Tin

ELEMENT	REPORTED DEPRIVATION SIGNS	REPORTED BENEFICIAL BIOACTIVITY	TYPICAL DAILY INTAKE AND FOOD SOURCES
Aluminum	*Goat:* ↑ spontaneous abortions, ↓ growth, ↓ life span, leg weakness and incoordination *Chick:* ↓ growth	Stimulated osteoblasts to form bone in vitro by activating a putative G protein–coupled system	2–25 mg Processed cheese, foods containing baking powder, grains, vegetables, herbs, tea
Bromine	*Goat:* ↑ spontaneous abortions, ↓ growth, ↓ fertility, ↓ life span ↓ hematocrit, ↓ hemoglobin *Human:* insomnia	Alleviated impaired growth caused by hyperthyroidism in mice and chicks; substitute for chloride requirement of chicks	2–5 mg Grains, nuts, fish
Cadmium	*Rat:* ↓ growth *Goat:* ↓ growth	Stimulated growth of cells in soft agar; mostly a toxicological concern	10–20 μg Shellfish, grains grown in high-cadmium soils
Germanium	*Rat:* Altered bone and liver mineral content, ↓ tibia DNA, ↓ growth *Chick:* ↓ growth	Antitumor and immune-enhancing action in animals; improved bone strength and mineral density in osteoporotic rats	0.4–1.5 mg Wheat bran, vegetables, pulses
Lead	*Rat:* ↓ growth, anemia, altered iron and lipid metabolism *Pig:* ↓ growth, ↑ serum cholesterol and phospholipids	Alleviated iron deficiency in young rats and depressed growth in rats fed unbalanced diet; mostly a toxicological concern	5–50 μg Seafood, foods grown on high-lead soils
Lithium	*Goat:* ↓ fertility, ↓ birth weight, ↓ life span *Rat:* ↓ fertility, ↓ birth weight, ↓ litter size, ↓ weaning weight	Enhanced growth of some cultured cells; insulin mimetic and immune modulating actions; antimanic action; low lithium status associated with violent crime, learning disability, and heart disease	0.2–0.6 mg Eggs, meat, fish, milk, potatoes, vegetables (content varies with geographic origin)
Rubidium	*Goat:* ↓ food intake, ↓ growth, ↓ life span, ↑ spontaneous abortions *Rat:* Altered tissue mineral concentrations	None found	1–5 mg Fruits and vegetables, especially asparagus; fish; poultry; black tea; coffee
Tin	*Rat:* ↓ growth, ↓ response to sound, ↓ feed efficiency, altered tissue mineral composition, alopecia	Associated with thymus immune function	1–40 mg Canned foods

Data from Nielsen, F. H. (2001). Boron, manganese, molybdenum, and other trace elements. In B. A. Bowman & R. M. Russell (Eds.), *Present knowledge in nutrition* (8th ed., pp. 384–400). Washington, DC: ILSI Press.

at physiological intakes is generally limited to a few gross observations in one or two species by one or two research groups. Moreover, some of the changes in deprivation studies were not very marked, not necessarily indicative of a suboptimal biological function, or obtained under less than satisfactory experimental conditions. Therefore discussion of their nutritional or biochemical significance is judged to be premature at this time.

THINKING CRITICALLY

1. Should dietary recommendations be made for mineral elements shown to have beneficial effects in amounts achievable from a mixed diet?
2. Should an element such as arsenic be considered toxic at low intakes (<50 μg/day) when enzymes exist that facilitate its excretion and thus prevent its accumulation in the body?

REFERENCES

Abumrad, N. N., Schneider, A. J., Steel, D., & Rogers, L. S. (1981). Amino acid intolerance during prolonged total parenteral nutrition reversed by molybdate therapy. *The American Journal of Clinical Nutrition, 34*, 2551–2559.

Adams, M. A., Bolger, P. M., & Gunderson, E. L. (1994). Dietary intake and hazards of arsenic. In W. R. Chappell, C. O. Abernathy, & C. R. Cothern (Eds.), *Arsenic: Exposure and health* (pp. 41–49). Northwood, United Kingdom: Science and Technology Letters.

Alvarez, H. M., Xue, Y., Robinson, C. D., Canalizo-Hernández, M. A., Marvin, R. G., Kelly, R. A., ... O'Halloran, T. O. (2010). Tetrathiomolybdate inhibits copper trafficking proteins through metal cluster formation. *Science, 327*, 331–334.

Anderson, R. A. (1998). Chromium, glucose intolerance and diabetes. *Journal of the American College of Nutrition, 17*, 548–555.

Anderson, R. A., & Kozlovsky, A. S. (1985). Chromium intake, absorption and excretion of subjects consuming self-selected diets. *The American Journal of Clinical Nutrition, 41*, 1177–1183.

Anke, M. (2005). Recent progress in exploring the essentiality of the non-metallic ultratrace elment arsenic to the nutrition of animals and man. *Biomedical Research on Trace Elements, 16*, 188–197.

Anke, M., Illing-Günther, H., & Schäfer, U. (2005). Recent progress on essentiality of the ultratrace element vanadium in the nutrition of animal and man. *Biomedical Research on Trace Elements, 16*, 208–214.

Balk, E., Tatsioni, A., Lichtenstein, A., Lau, J., & Pittas, A. G. (2007). Effect of chromium supplementation on glucose metabolism and lipids: A systematic review of randomized controlled trials. *Diabetes Care, 8*, 2154–2163.

Bolaños, L., Lukaszewski, K., Bonilla, I., & Blevins, D. (2004). Why boron? *Plant Physiology and Biochemistry, 42*, 907–912.

Brewer, G. J. (2003). Copper-lowering therapy with tetrathiomolybdate for cancer and diseases of fibrosis and inflammation. *The Journal of Trace Elements in Experimental Medicine, 16*, 191–199.

Carlisle, E. M. (1997). Silicon. In B. L. O'Dell & R. A. Sunde (Eds.), *Handbook of nutritionally essential minerals* (pp. 603–618). New York: Marcel Dekker.

Chen, G., Liu, P., Pattar, G. R., Tackett, L., Bhonagiri, P., Strawbridge, A. B., & Elmendorf, J. S. (2006). Chromium activates glucose transporter 4 trafficking and enhances insulin-stimulated glucose transport in 3T3-L1 adipocytes via a cholesterol-dependent mechanism. *Molecular Endocrinology, 20*, 857–870.

Chen, X., Schauder, S., Potier, N., Van Dorsselaer, A., Pelczer, I., Bassier, B. L., & Hughson, F. M. (2002). Structural identification of a bacterial quorum-sensing signal containing boron. *Nature, 415*, 545–549.

Crans, D. C., Smee, J. J., Gaidamauskas, E., & Yang, L. (2004). The chemistry and biochemistry of vanadium and the biological activities exerted by vanadium compounds. *Chemical Reviews, 104*, 849–902.

Davis, C. D., Uthus, E. O., & Finley, J. W. (2000). Dietary selenium and arsenic affect DNA methylation in vitro in Caco-2 cells and in vivo in rat liver and colon. *The Journal of Nutrition, 130*, 2903–2909.

Eckhert, C. D. (2006). Other trace elements. In M. E. Shils, M. Shike, B. Caballero, & R. J. Cousins (Eds.), *Modern nutrition in health and disease* (10th ed., pp. 338–350). Philadelphia: Lippincott Williams & Wilkins.

Gillette-Guyonnet, S., Andrieu, S., & Vellas, B. (2007). The potential influence of silica present in drinking water on Alzheimer's disease and associated disorders. *The Journal of Nutrition, Health & Aging, 11*, 119–124.

Gordon, S. E., & Zagotta, W. N. (1995). Subunit interactions in coordination of Ni2+ in cyclic nucleotide-gated channels. *Proceedings of the National Academy of Sciences of the United States of America, 92*, 10222–10226.

Guallar, E., Jiménez, F. J., van't Veer, P., Bode, P., Brimersma, R. A., Gómez-Aracena, J., ... Martin-Moreno, J. M., for the EURAMIC-Heavy Metals and Myocardial Infarction Study Group. (2005). Low toenail chromium concentration and increased risk of nonfatal myocardial infarction. *American Journal of Epidemiology, 162*, 157–164.

Güner, S., Tay, A., Altan, V. M., & Ölçelikay, A. T. (2001). Effect of sodium molybdate on fructose-induced hyperinsulinemia and hypertension in rats. *Trace Elements and Electrolytes, 18*, 39–46.

Hulley, P., & Davison, A. (2003). Regulation of tyrosine phosphorylation cascades by phosphatases: What the actions of vanadium teach us. *The Journal of Trace Elements in Experimental Medicine, 16*, 281–290.

Hunt, C. (2008). Dietary boron: Possible roles in human and animal physiology. *Biomedical Research on Trace Elements, 19*, 243–253.

Ichida, K., Matsumura, T., Sakuma, R., Hosoya, T., & Nishino, T. (2001). Mutation of human molybdenum cofactor sulfurase gene is responsible for classical xanthinuria type II. *Biochemical and Biophysical Research Communications, 282*, 1194–1200.

Institute of Medicine. (2001). *Dietary Reference Intakes for vitamin A, vitamin K, arsenic, boron, chromium, copper, iodine, iron, manganese, molybdenum, nickel, silicon, vanadium, and zinc.* Washington, DC: National Academy Press.

Johnson, J. L. (1997). Molybdenum. In B. L. O'Dell & R. A. Sunde (Eds.), *Handbook of nutritionally essential mineral elements* (pp. 413–438). New York: Marcel Dekker.

Jugdaohsingh, R. (2007). Silicon and bone health. *The Journal of Nutrition, Health & Aging, 11*, 99–110.

Jugdaohsingh, R., Calomme, M. R., Robinson, K., Robinson, K., Nielsen, F., Anderson, S. H. C., ... Powell, J. J. (2008). Increased longitudinal growth in rats on a silicon-depleted diet. *Bone, 43*, 596–606.

Kang, G. S., Li, Q., Chen, H., & Costa, M. (2006). Effect of metal ions on HIF-1α and Fe homeostasis in human A549 cells. *Mutation Research, 610*, 48–55.

Kayajanian, G. (2003). Arsenic, cancer, and thoughtless policy. *Ecotoxicology and Environmental Safety, 55*, 139–142.

Kinrade, S., Del Nin, J. W., Schach, A. S., Sloan, T. A., Wilson, K. L., & Knight, C. T. G. (1999). Stable five- and six-coordinated silicate anions in aqueous solution. *Science, 285*, 1542–1545.

Le, X. C. (2002). Arsenic speciation in the environment and humans. In W. T. Frankenberger, Jr. (Ed.), *Environmental chemistry of arsenic* (pp. 95–116). New York: Marcel Dekker.

Lukaski, H. C., & Scrimgeour, A. G. (2009). Trace elements excluding iron—Chromium and zinc. In J. A. Driskell (Ed.), *Nutrition and exercise concerns of middle age* (pp. 233–250). Boca Raton, FL: CRC Press, Taylor & Francis Group.

Maehira, F., Miyagi, I., & Eguchi, Y. (2009). Effects of calcium sources and soluble silicate on bone metabolism and the related gene expression in mice. *Nutrition, 25*, 581–589.

Marzban, L., & McNeill, J. H. (2003). Insulin-like actions of vanadium: Potential as a therapeutic agent. *The Journal of Trace Elements in Experimental Medicine, 16*, 253–267.

Mills, C. F., & Davis, G. K. (1987). Molybdenum. In W. Mertz (Ed.), *Trace elements in human and animal nutrition* (Vol. 1, pp. 429–463). San Diego: Academic Press.

Moukarzel, A. (2009). Chromium in parenteral nutrition: Too little or too much? *Gastroenterology, 137*, S18–S28.

Nielsen, F. H. (1998). The nutritional essentiality and physiological metabolism of vanadium in higher animals. In A. S. Tracey & D. C. Crans (Eds.), *Vanadium compounds: Chemistry, biochemistry, and therapeutic applications* (pp. 297–307). Washington, DC: American Chemical Society.

Nielsen, F. H. (2006). Boron manganese, molybdenum, and other trace elements. In B. A. Bowman & R. M. Russell (Eds.), *Present knowledge in nutrition, Vol 1* (9th ed., pp. 506–526). Washington, DC: ILSI Press.

Nielsen, F. H. (2008a). Is boron nutritionally relevant? *Nutrition Reviews, 66,* 183–191.

Nielsen, F. H. (2008b). A novel silicon complex is as effective as sodium metasilicate in enhancing the collagen-induced inflammatory response of silicon-deprived rats. *The Journal of Trace Elements in Experimental Medicine, 22,* 39–49.

Nielsen, F. H. (2009a). Boron deprivation decreases liver *S*-adenosylmethionine and spermidine and increases plasma homocysteine and cysteine in rats. *The Journal of Trace Elements in Experimental Medicine, 23,* 204–213.

Nielsen, F. H. (2009b). Micronutrients in parenteral nutrition: Boron, silicon, and fluoride. *Gastroenterology, 137,* S55–S60.

Nielsen, F. H. (2010). Silicon deprivation does not significantly modify the acute white blood cell response but does modify tissue mineral distribution response to an endotoxin challenge. *Biological Trace Element Research, 135,* 45–55.

Nielsen, F. H., Yokoi, K., & Uthus, E. O. (2002). The essential role of nickel affects physiological functions regulated by the cyclic-GMP signal transduction system. In L. Khassanova, P. H. Collery, I. Maymard, Z. Khassanova, & J.-C. Etienne (Eds.), *Metal ions in biology and medicine* (Vol. 7, pp. 29–33). Paris: John Libbey Eurotext.

Nielsen, F. H., Zimmerman, T. J., Shuler, T. R., Brossart, B., & Uthus, E. O. (1989). Evidence for a cooperative relationship between nickel and vitamin B_{12} in rats. *The Journal of Trace Elements in Experimental Medicine, 2,* 21–29.

Novotny, J. A., & Turnland, J. R. (2006). Molybdenum kinetics in men differ during molybdenum depletion and repletion. *The Journal of Nutrition, 136,* 953–957.

Novotny, J. A., & Turnland, J. R. (2007). Molybdenum intake influences molybdenum kinetics in men. *The Journal of Nutrition, 137,* 37–42.

Park, M., Li, Q., Shcheynikov, N., Zeng, W., & Muallem, S. (2004). NaBC1 is ubiquitous electrogenic Na+-coupled borate transporter essential for cellular boron homeostasis and cell growth and proliferation. *Molecular Cell, 16,* 331–341.

Pennington, J. A. T., & Jones, J. W. (1987). Molybdenum, nickel, cobalt, vanadium, and strontium in total diets. *Journal of the American Dietetic Association, 87,* 1644–1650.

Qiao, W., Peng, Z., Wang, Z., Wei, J., & Zhou, A. (2009). Chromium improves glucose uptake and metabolism through upregulating the mRNA levels of IR, Glut4, GS, and UCP3 in skeletal muscle cells. *Biological Trace Element Research, 131,* 133–142.

Ragsdale, S. W. (2009). Nickel-based enzyme systems. *The Journal of Biological Chemistry, 284,* 18571–18575.

Rajagopalan, K. V. (1988). Molybdenum: An essential trace element in human nutrition. *Annual Review of Nutrition, 8,* 401–427.

Rajpathak, S., Rimm, E. B., Li, T., Morris, J. S., Stamper, M. J., Willett, W. C., & Hu, F. B. (2004). Lower toenail chromium in men with diabetes and cardiovascular disease compared with healthy men. *Diabetes Care, 27,* 2211–2216.

Reiss, J., Gross-Hardt, S., Christensen, E., Schmidt, P., Mendel, R. R., & Schwarz, G. (2001). A mutation in the gene for the neurotransmitter receptor-clustering protein gephyrin causes a novel form of molybdenum cofactor deficiency. *American Journal of Human Genetics, 68,* 208–213.

Reiss, J., & Johnson, J. L. (2003). Mutations in the molybdenum cofactor biosynthetic genes MOCS1, MOCS2, and GEPH. *Human Mutation, 21,* 569–576.

Řezanka, T., & Sigler, K. (2007). Biologicially active compounds of semi-metals. *Phytochemistry, 69,* 585–606.

Sakurai, H. (2007). Medicinal aspects of vanadium complexes: Treatment of diabetes mellitus in model animals. *Biomedical Research on Trace Elements, 18,* 241–248.

Schwarz, K., & Mertz, W. (1959). Chromium (III) and the glucose tolerance factor. *Archives of Biochemistry and Biophysics, 85,* 292–295.

Stangl, G. I., Roth-Maier, D. A., & Kirchgessner, M. (2000). Vitamin B12 deficiency and hyperhomocytsteinemia are partly ameliorated by cobalt and nickel supplementation in pigs. *The Journal of Nutrition, 130,* 3038–3044.

Stearns, D. M. (2007). Multiple hypotheses for chromium (III) biochemistry: Why the essentiality of chromium (III) is still questioned. In J. B. Vincent (Ed.), *The nutritional biochemistry of chromium (III)* (pp. 57–70). Amsterdam: Elsevier.

Thomas, D. J., Li, J., Waters, S. B., Xing, W., Adair, B. M., Drobna, Z., ... Styblo, M. (2007). Arsenic (+3 oxidation state) methyltransferase and the methylation of arsenicals. *Experimental Biology and Medicine (Maywood, N.J.), 232,* 3–13.

Tsongas, T. A., Meglen, R. R., Walravens, P. A., & Chappell, W. R. (1980). Molybdenum in the diet: An estimate of average daily intake in the United States. *The American Journal of Clinical Nutrition, 33,* 1103–1107.

Tucker, K. L., Jugdaohsingh, R., Powell, J. J., Qiao, N., Hannan, M. T., Sripanyakorn, S., ... Kiel, D. (2009). Effects of beer, wine and liquor intakes on bone mineral density in older men and women. *The American Journal of Clinical Nutrition, 89,* 1188–1196.

Turnlund, J. R., Keyes, W. R., Peiffer, G. L., & Chiang, G. (1995). Molybdenum absorption, excretion, and retention studied with stable isotopes in young men during depletion and repletion. *The American Journal of Clinical Nutrition, 61,* 1102–1109.

Uthus, E. O. (1992). Evidence for arsenic essentiality. *Environmental Geochemistry and Health, 14,* 55–58.

Uthus, E. O., & Davis, C. D. (2005). Dietary arsenic affects dimethylhydrazine-induced aberrant crypt formation and hepatic global DNA methylation and DNA methyltransferase activity in rats. *Biological Trace Element Research, 103,* 133–146.

Veldman, A., Santamaria-Araujo, J. A., Sollazzo, S., Pitt, J., Gianello, R., Yaplito-Lee, J., ... Schwarz, G. (2010). Successful treatment of molybdenum cofactor deficiency type a with cPMP. *Pediatrics, 125,* e1249–e1254.

Vincent, J. B., & Bennett, R. (2007). Potential and purported roles for chomium in insulin signaling: The search for the holy grail. In *The nutritional biochemistry of chromium (III)* (pp. 139–160). Amsterdam: Elsevier.

Vincent, J. B., & Stallings, D. (2007). Introduction: A history of chromium studies (1955–1995). In *The nutritional biochemistry of chromium (III)* (pp. 1–40). Amsterdam: Elsevier.

Wang, Y., Wan, C., Deng, L., Liu, X., Cao, X., Gilbert, S. R., ... Clemens, T. L. (2007). The hypoxia-inducible factor α pathway couples angiogenesis to osteogenesis during skeletal development. *The Journal of Clinical Investigation, 117,* 1616–1626.

Wang, Z. Q., & Cefalu, W. T. (2010). Current concepts about chromium supplementation in type 2 diabetes and insulin resistance. *Current Diabetes Reports, 10,* 145–151.

World Health Organization. (1996). *Trace elements in human nutrition and health.* Geneva: WHO.

World Health Organization, International Programme on Chemical Safety. (1998). *Boron environmental health criteria 204.* Geneva: WHO.

Yamamoto, T., Moriwaki, Y., Takahashi, S., Tsutsumi, Z., Tuneyoshi, K., Matsui, K., ... Hada, T. (2003). Identification of a new point mutation in the human molybdenum cofactor sulferase gene that is responsible for xanthinuria type II. *Metabolism, 52,* 1501–1504.

Zahm, A. M., Bucaro, M. A., Srinivas, V., Shapiro, I. M., & Adams, C. S. (2008). Oxygen tension regulates preosteocyte maturation and mineralization. *Bone*, *43*, 25–31.

Zeng, C., Hou, G., Dick, R., & Brewer, G. J. (2008). Tetrathiomolybdate is partially protective against hyperglycemia in rodent models of diabetes. *Experimental Biology and Medicine (Maywood, N.J.)*, *233*, 1021–1025.

Zhang, X.-W., Yan, S.-J., Zhou, Z.-R., Yang, F.-F., Wu, Z.-Y., Sun, H.-B., ... Chen, Z. (2010). Arsenic trioxide controls the fate of the PML-RARα oncoprotein by directly binding PML. *Science*, *328*, 240–243.

RECOMMENDED READINGS

Nielsen, F. H. (2006). Boron, manganese, molybdenum, and other trace elements. In B. A. Bowman & R. M. Russell (Eds.), *Present knowledge in nutrition* (9th ed., Vol. 1, pp. 506–526). Washington, DC: ILSI Press.

Nielsen, F. H. (2008). Trace mineral deficiencies. In C. D. Berdanier, J. Dwyer, & E. B. Feldman (Eds.), *Handbook of nutrition and food* (2nd ed., pp. 159–176). Boca Raton, FL: CRC Press.

Index

Page numbers followed by *f*, *t*, and *b* indicate figures, tables, and boxes, respectively.

D

Q

R

S

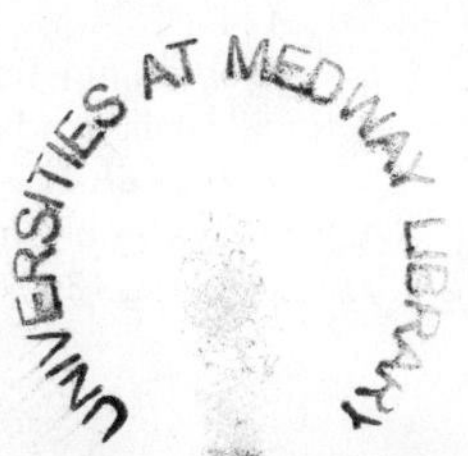

W

X